LNMP	last normal menstrual period
LP	lumbar puncture
LUL	left upper lobe
LUQ	left upper quadrant
LVH	left ventricular hypertrophy
m	meter
m, min, ♍	minum
MAP	mean arterial pressure
mcg	microgram
MCH	mean corpuscular hemoglobin
MCHC	mean corpuscular hemoglobin concentration
MCV	mean cell volume, mean corpuscular volume
mg	milligram
Mg	magnesium
MG	myasthenia gravis
MI	myocardial infarction
MICU	medical intensive care unit
ml	milliliter
mm	millimeter
mm^3	cubic millimeter
mm Hg	millimeters of mercury
MRI	magnetic resonance imaging
MS	multiple sclerosis
MW	molecular weight
N	nitrogen
Na	sodium
NICU	neonatal intensive care unit
NIH	National Institutes of Health
nm	nanometer
NMR	nuclear magnetic resonance
NPO	nothing by mouth
NS	normal saline
O_2	oxygen
OD	right eye; optical density; overdose
OL	left eye
OOB	out of bed
ORIF	open reduction and internal fixation
OS	left eye
OT	occupational therapy
OTC	over-the-counter
oz, ℥	ounce
P&A	percussion and auscultation
$Paco_2$	partial pressure of carbon dioxide (arterial blood)
Pao_2	partial pressure of oxygen (arterial blood)
para I, II, etc	unipara, bipara, etc
PAT	paroxysmal atrial tachycardia
pc	after meals
PCG	phonocardiogram
Pco_2	partial pressure of carbon dioxide
PCP	pulmonary capillary pressure, phencyclidine
PCV	packed cell volume
PCWP	pulmonary capillary wedge pressure
PD	interpupillary distance; postural drainage
PE	pulmonary embolism, physical examination
PEEP	positive end expiratory pressure
PEG	pneumoencephalography
per	through, by way of
PERRLA	pupils equal, round, and reactive to light and accommodation
PET	positron emission tomography
PG	prostaglandin
pH	hydrogen ion concentration (acidity and alkalinity)
PID	pelvic inflammatory disease
PKU	phenylketonuria
PM	postmortem
PM	evening
PMS	premenstrual syndrome
PND	paroxysmal nocturnal dyspnea, postnasal drip
Po_2	partial pressure of oxygen
PO, po	orally
PPD	purified protein derivative
ppm	parts per million
p.r.n.	when required, as often as necessary
PT	physical therapy; prothrombin time
PTT	partial thromboplastin time
PUO	pyrexia of unknown origin
PVC	premature ventricular contraction

q	every
q2h	every 2 hours
q3h	every 3 hours
q4h	every 4 hours
qd	every day
qh	every hour
qid	four times a day
qn	every night
qod	every other day
qns	quantity not sufficient
R/O	rule out
RA	rheumatoid arthritis
RBBB	right bundle branch block
RDA	recommended daily (dietary) allowance
RDS	respiratory distress syndrome
Rh+	positive Rh factor
Rh−	negative Rh factor
RHD	rheumatic heart disease
RLL	right lower lobe
RLQ	right lower quadrant
RML	right middle lobe
ROM	range of motion
ROS	review of systems
RS	Reiter's syndrome
RSV	Rous sarcoma virus
RUL	right upper lobe
RUQ	right upper quadrant
Rx	take; treatment
s̄	without
SB	sternal border
SC	subcutaneous
sib.	sibling
SICU	surgical intensive care unit
SIDS	sudden infant death syndrome
Sig	write on label
SLE	systemic lupus erythematosus
sol	solution, dissolved
sos	if necessary
sp. gr., SG, s.g.,	specific gravity
SQ, subq	subcutaneous
SR	sedimentation rate
ss	half
SSS	sick sinus syndrome, specific soluble substance, short-stay surgery
stat	immediately
STD	sexually transmitted disease
STS	serologic test for syphilis
susp	suspension
T_3	triiodothyronine
T_4	tetraiodothyronine
T&A	tonsillectomy and adenoidectomy
TAB	typhoid and paratyphoid A and B
TAH	total abdominal hysterectomy
TAT	tetanus antitoxin; thematic apperception test
TB, TBC	tuberculosis
TBG	thyroxin-binding globulin
TG	triglyceride
TIA	transient ischemic attack
TIBC	total iron-binding capacity
tid	three times a day
TKO	to keep open
TLC	total lung capacity; thin layer chromatography
TPN	total parenteral nutrition
TPR	temperature, pulse, and respirations
tr, tinct	tincture
TST	triple sugar iron test
UIBC	unsaturated iron-binding capacity
URI	upper respiratory infection
UTI	urinary tract infection
V&T	volume and tension
VC	vital capacity
VD	venereal disease
VDA	visual discriminatory acuity
VDH	valvular disease of the heart
VDRL	Venereal Disease Research Laboratory (test for syphilis)
VS	vital signs
VSD	ventricular septal defect
V_T	tidal volume
W/V	weight/volume
WBC	white blood cell, white blood count
WNL	within normal limits
WR	Wasserman reaction

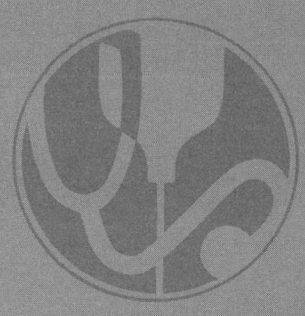

Fundamentals of Nursing

CONCEPTS, PROCESS, AND PRACTICE

Fundamentals of Nursing

CONCEPTS, PROCESS, AND PRACTICE

PATRICIA A. POTTER, RN, MSN

Director of Nursing Practice,
Barnes Hospital,
St. Louis, Missouri

ANNE G. PERRY, RN, MSN, ANP

Associate Professor,
St. Louis University School of Nursing,
St. Louis, Missouri;
Doctoral Candidate,
Southern Illinois University at Edwardsville,
Edwardsville, Illinois

SECOND EDITION

with over 700 illustrations,
including 29 in color

The C. V. Mosby Company

ST. LOUIS • BALTIMORE • TORONTO 1989

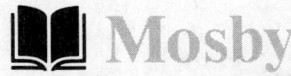

Editor: Thomas Lochhaas
Assistant editor: Laurie Sparks
Editorial assistant: Linda Stagg
Developmental editor: Susan Epstein
Project manager: Carol Sullivan Wiseman
Production editor: Pat Joiner
Book and cover design: Gail Morey Hudson

SECOND EDITION

Printed in the United States of America

The C.V. Mosby Company
11830 Westline Industrial Drive, St. Louis, Missouri 63146

Library of Congress Cataloging in Publication Data

Potter, Patricia Ann.
    Fundamentals of nursing.

    Includes bibliographies and index.
    1. Nursing.   2. Nursing—Examinations, questions,
etc.   3. Nursing—Study and teaching—Audio-visual
aids.   I. Perry, Anne Griffin.   II. Title.
[DNLM: 1. Nurse-Patient Relations.   2. Nursing Care.
3. Nursing Process.   WY 100 P868f]
RT42.P68   1989   610.73   88-23130
ISBN 0-8016-4257-4

C/VH/VH   9 8 7 6 5 4

Contributors

NANCY DICKENSON-HAZARD, RN, CPNP, MSN

Executive Director, National Board of PNP/As, Rockville, Maryland

CATHERINE FOGERTEY DOERRER, RN, MSN

Director of Surgical Nursing, Barnes Hospital, St. Louis, Missouri

CHERYL HALL HARRIS, RN, BSN

Staff Nurse, Children's Mercy Hospital, Kansas City, Missouri

GAIL KIECKHEFER, RN, PhD

Research Assistant Professor, Department of Parent-Child Nursing, University of Washington, Seattle, Washington

Sr. KATHLEEN KREKELER, RN, PhD

Professor of Nursing, St. Louis University, School of Nursing, St. Louis, Missouri

PAMELA A. LESSER, RN, MS

OB Patient Education Coordinator, Barnes Hospital, St. Louis, Missouri

ANNETTE GIESLER LUECKENOTTE, RN, GNP, MS

Gerontology Nurse Specialist, Barnes Hospital, St. Louis, Missouri

JILL FELDMAN MALEN, RN, MS, NS

Nurse Specialist, Barnes Hospital, St. Louis, Missouri

SHARON L. MERRITT, RN, EdD

Associate Professor, College of Nursing, University of Illinois, Chicago, Illinois

RUTH BECKMANN MURRAY, RN, MSN, EdD

Professor, Coordinator of Psychiatric/Mental Health Nursing Graduate Major, St. Louis University, School of Nursing, St. Louis, Missouri

ELIZABETH NICKSON, RN, MSN

Clinical Nurse Specialist, St. Anthony's Medical Center, St. Louis, Missouri

RACHEL E. SPECTOR, RN, PhD

Associate Professor, Boston College School of Nursing, Chestnut Hill, Massachusetts

ELEANOR J. SULLIVAN, RN, PhD

Dean, School of Nursing, University of Kansas, Kansas City, Kansas

FRANCES THOMAS, RN, MSN

Clinical Nurse Specialist, St. Anthony's Psychiatric Center— Stress Unit, St. Anthony's Medical Center, St. Louis, Missouri

JOETTA A. VERNON, RN, MS

Doctoral Student, University of Nebraska, Omaha, Nebraska

STEPHANIE A. WEISENBORN, RN, BSN

Physician's Assistant, Barnes Hospital, St. Louis, Missouri

LAUREL A. WIERSEMA, RN, MSN

Surgical Nurse Specialist, Barnes Hospital, St. Louis, Missouri

Consultants

FRANCES BRITTON ARONOVITZ, RN, PhD

Chairperson, Transitional Nursing, Miami-Dade Community College, Medical Center Campus, Miami, Florida

BARBARA BRILLHART, RN, PhD

Associate Professor, School of Nursing, University of Texas at Arlington, Arlington, Texas

MARGIE E. BROWN, RNC, MS, ANP

Professor of Nursing, Long Beach City College, Long Beach, California

ROBERTA BURRIS, RN, MS

Instructor, Division of Nursing, University of Texas at Tyler, Tyler, Texas

DAWN COX, RN, MSN

Assistant Professor, Troy State University, School of Nursing, Montgomery, Alabama

JUANITA Z. FLINT, RN, MS

Faculty/Coordinator, El Centro/Brookhaven College, Farmers Branch, Texas

MARY J. KEEGAN, RN, MSN

Trauma Nurse Specialist, St. Louis University Medical Center, St. Louis, Missouri

BARBARA R. KOLLATH, RN, MSN

Assistant Professor and Coordinator of Learning Resources, Marquette University, Milwaukee, Wisconsin

JOAN LEACH, RN, MS, CAGS

Doctoral Candidate, University of Connecticut; Associate Professor of Nursing, Greater Hartford Community College, Hartford, Connecticut

MARY KELLY MEMMER, RN, BS, MN

Professor of Nursing, California State University, Chico, California

CHARLOTTE NIKSCH, RN, MSN

Assistant Professor, University of Evansville, Evansville, Indiana

CYNTHIA E. NORTHROP, RN, MS, JD

Nurse Attorney; Adjunct Associate Professor, Teachers College, Columbia University, New York

OLGA CAROL PONCE PETROZELLA, RN, MSEd

Assistant Professor, Miami-Dade Community College, Miami, Florida

LEMBI SAARMANN, RN, EdD

Assistant Professor, School of Nursing, San Diego State University, San Diego, California

KAREN KELLY SCHUTZENHOFER, RN, EdD

Assistant Dean, Assistant Professor, School of Nursing, University of Missouri at St. Louis, St. Louis, Missouri

MARTHA A. SPIES, RN, MSN

Assistant Professor, Deaconess College of Nursing, St. Louis, Missouri

MARTHA A. THOMPSON, MAEd, MSN, RN

Professor, Department of Nursing, San Jose State University, San Jose, California

SARAH JANE TOBIASON, RN, MA

Assistant Professor, College of Nursing, Arizona State University, Tempe, Arizona

P. SUSAN WAGNER, RN, MSc

Assistant Professor, College of Nursing, University of Saskatchewan, Saskatoon, Saskatchewan, Canada

To the Nursing Profession

for the innumerable rewards
and opportunities it has provided us

A Special Tribute to Tom Lochhaas

His knowledge, talent, creativity,
and gentle forcefulness have been
a gift to both of us.
We will miss his leadership and support
but wish him well in life's pursuits.

PATRICIA A. POTTER

ANNE G. PERRY

Preface

As society changes, so too do the art and science of professional nursing practice. In response to new consumer needs and demands, health care services are increasingly moving into the home and community and alternative care settings. As a consequence of this and of changes within the profession, the nurse's roles and responsibilities are expanding to meet new challenges and expectations. More than ever, the nurse today must be able to apply a broad knowledge base in providing proficient and skillful care to clients, families, and communities. The development of nursing theories, the growing body of nursing research, and the continued expansion of knowledge in the physical, social, and behavioral sciences provide nurses with the fundamental tools to promote, maintain, and restore a client's well-being. Knowledge alone, however, is insufficient. If nurses are to provide quality care, they must also be sensitive to clients' needs as unique individuals and committed to achieving standards of excellence in nursing practice. This awareness leads to a truly holistic nursing perspective.

Fundamentals of Nursing: Concepts, Process, and Practice (second edition) is a basic textbook designed for beginning students in professional nursing programs. Comprehensive in scope and complete in its coverage, this text will not only introduce students to the basic concepts, process, skills, and techniques of nursing practice but also provide them with a firm foundation for more advanced areas of nursing study. Emphasizing cognitive, interpersonal, and psychomotor skills, the text presents the theoretical and practical knowledge needed to make sound clinical judgments and carry our fundamental nursing activities.

APPROACH

All units and chapters of the text have been designed to meet the specific needs of the learner. A chapter outline and learning objectives at the beginning of each chapter help students focus on the relevant issues in subject matter. Key terms are introduced in each chapter to familiarize students with the terms and basic concepts they will encounter in the detailed text discussion. Special attention has been paid to the reading level and clear presentation of material. In all chapters the subject is approached in a logical, building-block fashion. Realistic clinical examples are offered throughout to clearly illustrate the application of theoretical concepts in clinical practice. In addition, all clinical chapters use the nursing process format. New in this edition are detailed boxes that graphically help students to understand the steps of the nursing process.

To help students recognize and understand key issues and principles, tables, boxes and step-by-step procedural guides present information graphically, logically, and succinctly. Over 700 illustrations and photographs highlight the major concepts and procedures to supplement discussion with accurate and meaningful visual aids. Each chapter closes with a brief summary followed by a list of key concepts emphasizing the most important nursing principles presented in the chapter. The references, research articles, and additional readings for each chapter can be used as guides for students who desire to further explore the information in the nursing and applied sciences literature.

Although the emphasis of the text is on the clinical aspects of nursing care, we fully recognize that technical expertise alone will not prepare today's nurses to deliver care creatively and effectively. Fundamental concepts such as the health-illness continuum, basic human needs, self-awareness, nurse-client relationship, client teaching, research, leadership, and home care are therefore discussed in depth in individual chapters and referred to throughout the text. This approach helps students begin to incorporate nursing theory in clinical practice situations. For example, an entire unit is devoted to the principles of growth and development and the appropriate health care concerns of each developmental stage, but other chapters discuss developmental health care needs throughout the life span, along with appropriate nursing interventions.

The five-step nursing process serves as a framework in chapters discussing the physiological, psychosocial, and special needs of clients. Students learn to assess a broad range of factors related to the nature and extent of clients' health status and to cluster assessment data to identify actual or potential health problems. Nursing diagnoses are explored in these chapters, and their value for planning the direction and scope of nursing care is considered. Within the planning phase, students learn to establish goals of care, to set priorities for different aspects of care, and to integrate nursing activities within a care plan. In the implementation step, nursing interventions are discussed with scientific rationales and practical considerations for making nursing therapies more effective. Current nursing research findings help broaden the student's understanding of independent nursing functions. The ongoing evaluation of nursing care is discussed in terms of specific outcome criteria reflecting the long- and short-term goals of care.

The approach used throughout the text reflects the major premise that students must understand and master the performance of basic clinical skills. Skills and procedures are discussed in depth in the relevant chapters and presented in tabular form. The step-by-step, two-column format for each procedure provides the appropriate nursing action and the rationale for it. The procedures incorporate current scientific principles and research results to help students understand the reason for specific nursing interventions. Text discussions elaborate on the objectives and purposes of the procedures and relate the nursing actions to meaningful client assessments. In addition, the procedures include opportunities for heightened nurse-client interactions and integrate client-teaching activities with the performance of skills.

ORGANIZATION

The text comprises 10 units organized to enhance teaching strategies. Unit 1 introduces the student to the profession of nursing by presenting a historical overview of nursing practice. Current nursing theories are then discussed to help the student understand the health care consumer, the range of health care needs, the health-illness continuum, and different approaches to health care. In addition, areas of cultural and ethnic diversity and advances in home care have been added to Unit 1.

Unit 2 discusses the use of the nursing process as a whole and considers each component in detail. The unit introduces the skills needed to assess the client's health status through nursing history and physical assessment, to cluster and analyze data to formulate nursing diagnoses, to organize and write the nursing care plan, to select and implement appropriate nursing interventions, and to evaluate the care plan on an ongoing basis. The unit also includes a nursing research chapter as an introduction to the process of research and as an aid to help the student learn to form basic research questions, locate current nursing research findings, and apply them in nursing practice, and participate in data collection.

Unit 3 provides information about the fundamental skills essential for all areas of nursing practice. The unit progresses from the simple skills of measuring vital signs to the more complicated techniques of physical assessment and medication administration. Throughout this unit, illustrations and photographs and step-by-step descriptions clearly show how each skill should be performed. Each chapter also describes ways to implement skills with minimum stress to clients and to combine client teaching with skills performance. The unit also includes a chapter on recording and reporting techniques and the methods for complete and accurate documentation of nursing care.

The nurse learns to apply certain basic concepts of professional nursing practice in all encounters with clients. Unit 4 offers a comprehensive review of values, ethics, legal issues, and principles of communication and teaching. In the chapter dealing with values, students learn the importance of clarifying personal and professional values, as well as assisting clients in defining and understanding values related to health care beliefs and practices. Because of new ethical issues related to technology and a greater societal emphasis on clients' rights, the nurse must be aware of the importance of ethical decision making in health care. The chapter on ethics discusses the significance of an ethical code for nursing and provides guidelines for the resolution of ethical dilemmas in health care. The chapter discussing communication provides a solid introduction to communication principles, particularly as used in therapeutic nurse-client relationships. Client teaching is increasingly important in nursing, and the chapter on teaching and learning focuses on factors that promote or hinder learning and draws parallels between the teaching-learning process and the nursing process for establishing effective teaching plans for clients. The legal issues chapter helps students become acquainted with clients' legal rights and the increasingly complex legal issues that confront nurses in practice.

Because the student nurse cares for clients of all ages and because normal developmental tasks influence how the nurse promotes health and prevents illness, the student can gain from a developmental perspective in all areas of practice. In Unit 5, individual chapters are devoted to the family; the fetus, neonate, infant, and toddler; the school-age child and adolescent; the young and middle adult; and the older adult. In addition to describing theoretical views of growth and development for each stage, the unit explores the primary and developmental health care needs of all age groups. Last, the unit includes nursing measures for death, loss, and grieving.

Unit 6 explores the psychosocial needs of individuals in the community and institutional settings. The student learns how a client's basic needs, adaptation to stress, self-concept, sexuality, and spiritual health influence health beliefs and practices. The chapters in this unit explain how to assess needs in these areas and incorporate interventions in the nursing care plan.

Unit 7 details nursing care for clients with basic physiological needs in the areas of hygiene; nutrition; sleep; comfort; oxygenation; fluid, electrolyte, and acid-base balances; and urinary and bowel elimination. Each chapter discusses normal physiology and alterations that result in or result from a client's health problems. The emphasis on the physiological nature of health alterations and a comprehensive look at assessment criteria in each area help to prepare the student to develop individualized therapies in a clinical setting.

The need for safety is one of the client's most important needs, and the client is often unable to meet this need because of health problems. In Unit 8, the student learns about the importance of maintaining a safe environment, body mechanics, reducing the hazards of immobility, and infection control. The unit also includes chapters dealing with sensory alterations and substance abuse.

Unit 9 focuses on the care of clients with perioperative needs—those who have inpatient or outpatient surgery. Because the student nurse often works with such clients in early clinical experiences, a conceptual foundation and a familiarity with nursing interventions for wound healing are important. Each chapter provides the student with a broad understanding of the nature of clients' problems and gives specific guidelines for innovative nursing therapies.

Unit 10, unique in this fundamentals text, introduces the student to the principles of nursing leadership and management and the process of change. The leadership and management chapter discusses theories of effective leadership and the student's participation in the health care team. The student also gains valuable knowledge on ways to assume a leadership role in client care.

In organizing the text, every attempt was made to ensure a logical progression of concepts and skills and a meaningful grouping of related subjects. Only rarely, however, is a textbook read in sequence. Recognizing that instructors may assign chapters in different sequences, we make extensive use of cross-references throughout the text and include a thorough index. We hope this approach will provide easy access to information of particular interest.

TEACHING AND LEARNING PACKAGE

To help students and instructors use the text to its fullest potential, five ancillary materials have been developed: an instructor's manual, a student study guide, a computerized testbank, a computer-assisted instruction (CAI) tutorial, and a set of overhead transparencies. The *Instructor's Manual* comprises 49 chapters, each coordinated to one chapter of the text. The chapters include learning objectives, topical lecture outlines, a list of key terms introduced in the chapter, lecture notes, audiovisual resources, speaker suggestions, discussion/ essay questions, and suggestions for student learning activities/experiential exercises. In addition, performance checklists for the basic skills presented throughout the text are included in a format that allows convenient duplication for class use. Instructors or students may use these checklists as guides to evaluate skills performance in laboratory or clinical settings.

A Study Guide to Fundamentals of Nursing, by Kathleen Hoover, RN, MSN, and the authors, has been developed to furnish a meaningful self-instructional tool focusing on the essential concepts, principles, and skills presented in the text. Each chapter parallels a text chapter and includes chapter objectives, prerequisite readings, a review of key concepts, application exercises for each key concept, additional readings, and answers for all exercises.

Microtest, a computerized testbank of over 500 multiple choice questions carefully developed in direct relationship to the distribution of content in the text, aids instructors using the IBM PC and Apple IIe and IIc microcomputers in test construction. All questions on the floppy disks are also printed in the *Instructor's Manual.*

A CAI tutorial emphasizing the principles and practices of infection control is available on floppy disk for IBM or Apple computers, allowing instructors to provide another learning resource to students. This highly interactive program reinforces the student's learning of this material from the text by applying it in given situations.

The overhead transparency set includes nearly 100 illustrations and photographs, about a quarter of which are in full color, selected for their value as instructional tools. Many of the remaining transparencies are in two colors.

■ ■ ■

Throughout the text the clinical examples depict men and women who practice nursing in a variety of health care settings. We have attempted to delete sexist language and cumbersome terms such as "he/she" and "his/her" as much as possible when referring to clients and nurses in the text.

We acknowledge the differences in opinion related to use of the terms "client" and "patient." We have chosen to use the term "client" because it suggests a more active, participatory role for the person who has entered the health care delivery system. In its broadest sense "client" refers to the client-family unit and the client–significant other unit, as well as the individual.

Writing this book has been challenging and exciting for us, as has been the process of working with a team of expert reviewers and editors to produce a text of the highest quality. Of the many goals we set for ourselves during the development of the book, the first and foremost was to prepare a comprehensive resource to meet the varied needs of students and instructors. At the same time, however, we have attempted to remain responsive to the needs of the profession, and for this reason we welcome the comments and suggestions of readers. As practicing clinicians and instructors, we have, during the writing of the book, felt particularly close to our own clients, students, and colleagues, as if communicating directly with them rather than writing on a page. In this spirit, we hope that the reader may also participate in this larger communication that we believe essential for nursing education.

ACKNOWLEDGMENTS

The creation of this textbook has been a true labor of love. We wish to extend our thanks and gratitude for the many contributions made by the following individuals:

Our editor, Tom Lochhaas, a talented man who has taught us many lessons as authors. The long hours Tom contributed to this project have resulted in a textbook we believe is unique.

Our developmental editor, Susan Epstein, and editorial assistant, Linda Stagg, for their energy, commitment, and motivation.

The professional nursing staffs of Barnes Hospital and The St. Louis University Hospital. Their commitment to excellence in nursing care has instilled many ideas for this text. A special thanks to members of the administrative staffs for their support and belief in this project.

St. Louis University School of Nursing for providing an environment in which faculty and students can achieve their highest potential. Thanks to faculty members and students who lent their time and expertise for many of the photographic sessions.

Sherry Wiebe and Alice Baumgart for providing the Canadian chapters on the "Health Care Delivery System" and "Legal Issues in Nursing," which are printed in the *Instructor's Manual.*

Patrick Watson, a highly creative individual whose photographs are visually realistic. Through Pat's patience and a determination to achieve visual perfection, his photographs make each chapter very special.

Our illustrators, Vicki M. Freidman and Marcy H. Hartstein, for their meticulous line and full-color drawings.

Bess Arends for her limitless energy, commitment, and love for this project. She is a special person who always has the ability to instill confidence and support when it is most needed.

Our family and friends for their patience, understanding, and support during times that were often difficult at best. They provided an emotional strength that made all our efforts worthwhile.

Our reviewers and nursing advisory panel, whose knowledge, recommendations, and support helped develop this text to meet the needs of beginning nursing students.

The book editing, design, and production staff at The C.V. Mosby Company, whose talents and commitment to quality resulted in a visually appealing and much more readable textbook.

We also wish to acknowledge a friendship that has weathered many difficult decisions, crises, and revisions and will continue to be the basis for future creative efforts.

Patricia A. Potter
Anne G. Perry

Contents

Detailed Contents

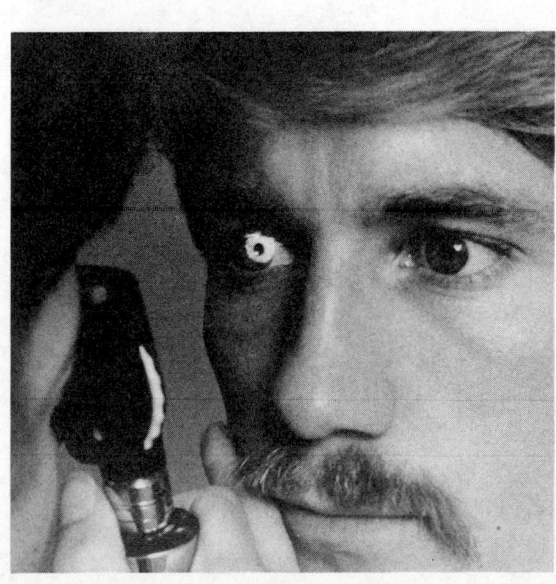

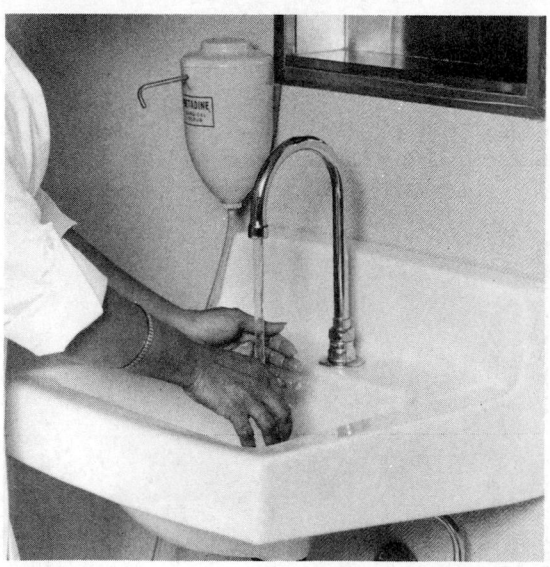

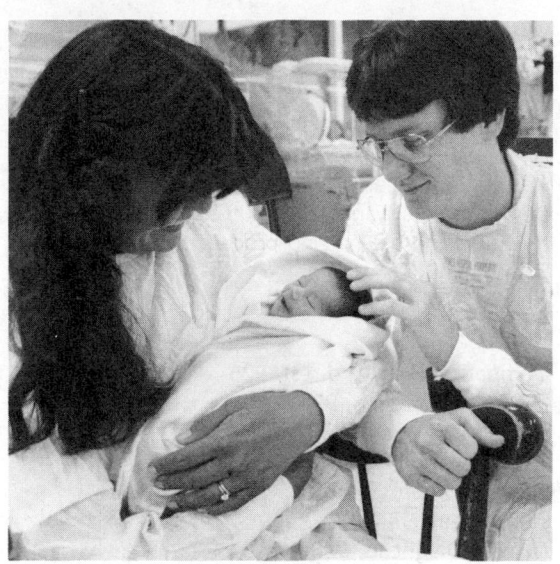

UNIT 6

Human Needs in Health and Illness

UNIT 7

Basic Physiological Needs

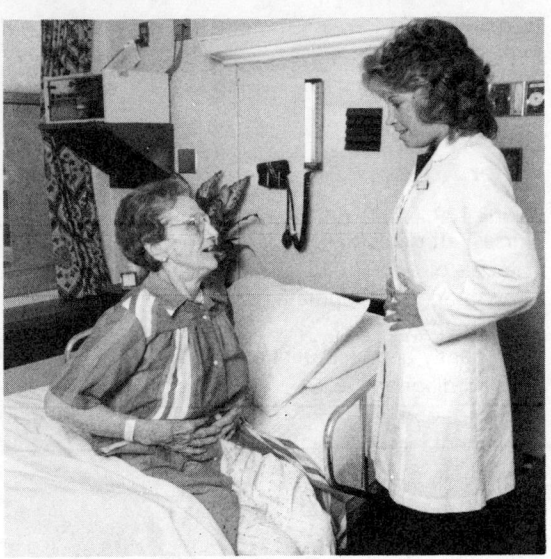

UNIT 9
Caring for the Perioperative Client

UNIT 10
Contemporary Issues

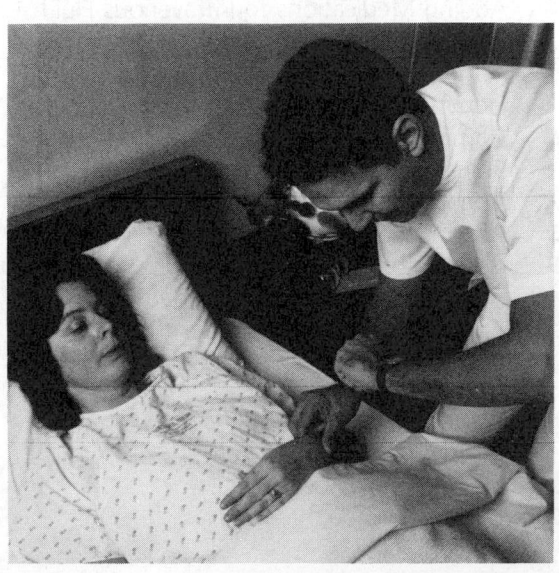

Clinical Procedures

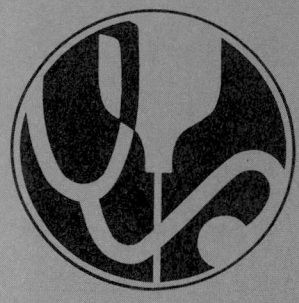

UNIT **1**

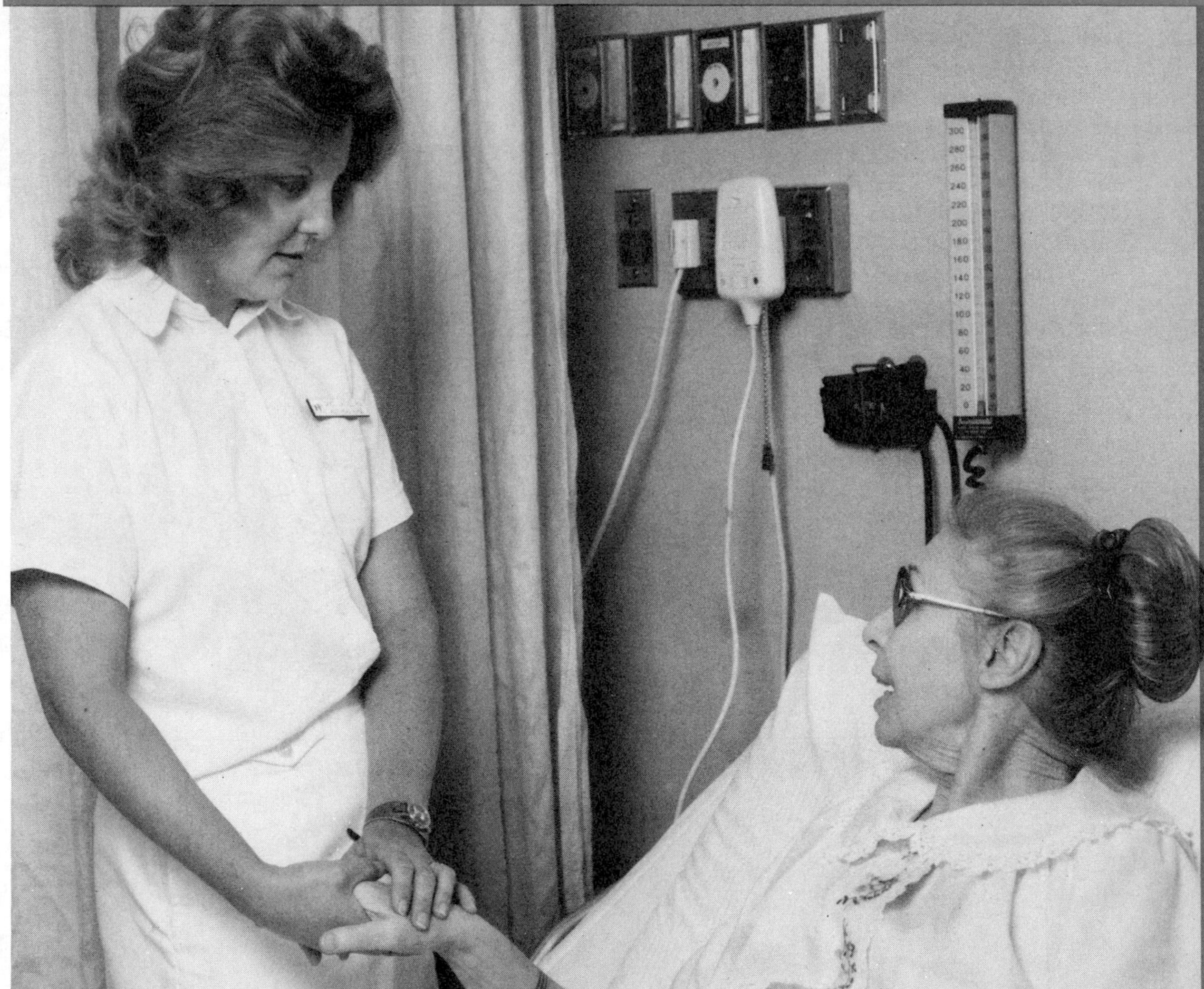

The Nurse, Client, and Health Care Environment

The five chapters in Unit 1 introduce many of the fundamental aspects of nursing by examining the profession itself, basic concepts of health and illness, and the world of health care services. Because nursing is a dynamic, growing profession and the roles of nurses have expanded to address the needs of the whole person in both illness and health, these chapters focus on the larger context of nursing as it is practiced today.

Nurses practice in a variety of settings and assume many roles as they provide care to culturally diverse clients. The first chapter explores these roles, prominent philosophies of nursing, the meaning of nursing as a profession, and current trends in nursing. The second chapter considers the relationship of health and illness, with emphasis on health promotion and illness prevention for the family and community, as well as the individual client. The subsequent chapters discuss complexities of the present health care system and the client's rights within it, the cultural diversity of clients and the impact of culture on health care, and the role of nursing in home health care.

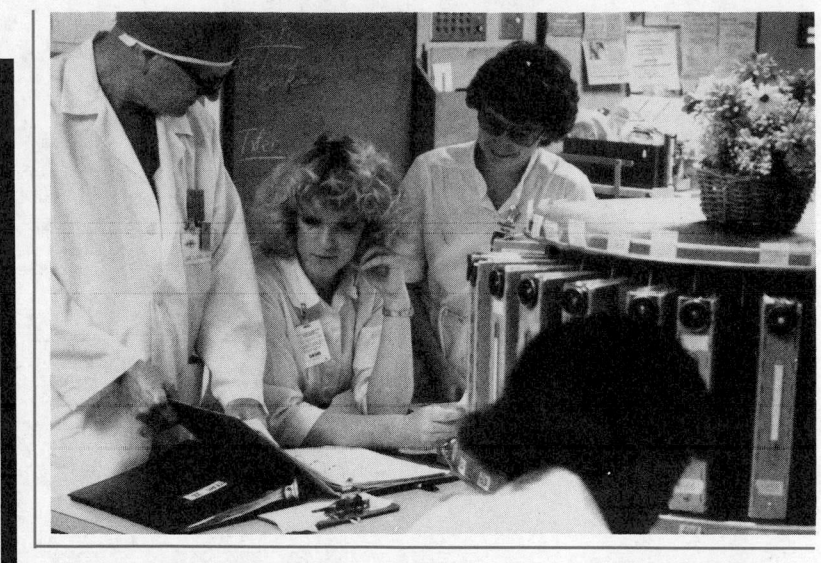

OBJECTIVES

Mastery of content in this chapter will enable the student to:

- Define the key terms listed.
- Discuss the historical development of professional nursing.
- Discuss the modern definitions and philosophies of nursing.
- Describe educational programs for becoming a registered nurse.
- Describe practice settings and roles for nurses.
- Describe at least three career roles for nurses.
- List the five characteristics of a profession and discuss how nursing demonstrates these characteristics.
- Discuss the influence of social and economic changes on nursing practice.
- Discuss the influence of nursing on political issues and health care policy.

KEY TERMS

American Nurses' Association (ANA)
Canadian Nurses Association (CNA)
Certified Nurse-midwife (CNM)
Clinical Nurse Specialist
Congress for Nursing Practice
Continuing Education
DRGs
In-Service Education
International Council of Nurses (ICN)
Licensed Practical or Vocational Nurse
National League for Nursing (NLN)
Nurse Administrator
Nurse Anesthetist
Nurse Educator
Nurse Practitioner
Nurse Researcher
Nursing Theory
Occupational Therapist
Pharmacist
Physical Therapist
Physician
Physician Assistant
Professional Organization
Registered Nurse
Respiratory Therapist
Social Worker

The Profession of Nursing

Modern nursing involves many different activities, concepts, and skills related to health sciences, social sciences, and other areas. Nursing as a profession is unique in that it addresses in a humanistic and holistic manner the responses of individual clients and their families to actual and potential health problems. The nurse has many roles, such as care giver, decision maker, client advocate, and teacher, and often acts in several roles at the same time. Because of this complex interrelationship of roles, practicing nurses need a philosophy of nursing to guide their delivery of care. Over the years, nurses have developed many philosophies and definitions of nursing. The following definition by the International Council of Nurses (1973) is a concise statement with which most nursing theorists would agree:

The unique function of the nurse is to assist the individual, sick or well, in the performance of those activities contributing to his health, its recovery, or to a peaceful death that he would perform unaided if he had the necessary strength, will, or knowledge.

The profession of nursing is complex and multifaceted in other ways as well. Nurses practice in many settings that emphasize different aspects of nursing care and nursing roles. In addition, there is a variety of educational programs by which one becomes a registered nurse and a variety of career opportunities open to nurses as they gain experience and continue their education.

Expertise in nursing is the result of theoretical knowledge and clinical experience. The expertise required to interpret clinical situations and make complex decisions plus the theoretical knowledge needed for this clinical

3

expertise is the basis for the advancement of nursing practice and the development of nursing science (Benner, 1984). Knowledge and expertise are gained over time through a continual process.

The profession of nursing evolves as society and health care continue to change. Nursing responds and adapts to such changes and meets new challenges as they arise. Nursing also influences political decisions related to health care and health care policy.

HISTORICAL PERSPECTIVE

Nursing is an essential, evolving part of society that has always been directed to serving health care needs. Nursing was distinguished in its early history as a form of community service and was originally related to a strong instinct to preserve and protect the family (Donahue, 1985). Nursing began as the desire to keep people healthy, as well as to provide comfort, care, and assurance to the sick. Although the general goals of nursing have remained relatively the same over the centuries, the practice of nursing has been influenced by characteristics of society that have changed with time, and thus nursing has gradually evolved into a modern profession.

Nursing did not begin with Florence Nightingale, since nursing is as old as medicine. Throughout history, nursing and medicine have had an interdependent relationship. During the Hippocrates era, medicine practiced without nursing, and during the middle ages, nursing practiced without rational medicine (Donahue, 1985).

In ancient cultures, religious beliefs and myths were the basis for health care and medical practice. Religious leaders assumed the responsibility for diagnosis and treatment, and many cultures believed that illness was caused by the gods' displeasure. In these cultures, nurses usually had a role subservient to religious leaders.

Many ancient societies did not value human life in the same way we do today, so the caretakers of life were less respected. Nurses delivered custodial care and depended on physicians or priests for direction (Kelly, 1981). Under the direct supervision of a physician the nurse tended to the hygiene of clients in the home. Nurses did not participate in any activities to promote health, nor did they teach families how to care for the ill.

One consistent role of the nurse from early civilization is the role of midwife. Throughout medical-nursing history the midwife has been accepted in her role to assist women during childbirth.

Under the influence of Christianity, nurses gained respect, and the practice of nursing expanded. Nursing records of early Christian workers to the present are continuous (Donahue, 1985). One of the earliest records of Christian nursing was the formation of the Order of the Deaconesses, a group somewhat like today's public health or visiting nurses.

Their goals included meeting the following basic needs of the society (Dolan, et al., 1983; Donahue, 1985):
1. To feed the hungry
2. To give water to the thirsty
3. To clothe the naked
4. To visit the imprisoned
5. To shelter the homeless
6. To care for the sick
7. To bury the dead

Historically, both men and women have held the role of nurse. The entry of women into nursing can be traced to approximately AD 300 (Shryock, 1959; Donahue, 1985). Women entered nursing because (1) the social position of Roman women improved (Shryock, 1959), (2) Christians taught that men and women are equal before God (Shryock, 1959; Dolan, et al., 1983), and (3) Christians appealed to women "to carry on His work in behalf of all who were in distress" (Shryock, 1959).

The Benedictine order, founded in the sixth century, increased the number of men entering nursing. Although the Benedictines were scholars, librarians, teachers, and agriculturalists, nursing the sick eventually became the chief function and duty of their community life (Donahue, 1985).

In the Middle Ages the Crusades were a stimulus for expanded nursing and health care. Military nursing orders for men were formed, and hospitals were established. After the Crusades, large cities began to develop with the decline of feudalism. The extensive population growth in cities led to certain health problems (see box) and increased need for health care. Some of these health problems still exist in urban areas today, although the mortality rate associated with them has greatly declined. During the Middle Ages, secular groups were formed to meet specific health care needs. The Hospital Brothers of St. Anthony was formed to care for victims of the

---

Health Problems Associated with the Growth of Cities

- Overcrowding and related stresses
- Poor ventilation
- Poor heating and cooling
- Poor sanitation, garbage collection, and plumbing
- Poor water supply
- Inadequate methods of preserving foods
- Ignorance of elementary hygiene

disease called St. Anthony's fire, the Misericordia in Italy provided transportation services for the ill (Fig. 1-1), and the Alexian Brothers (a group still active today) cared for victims of bubonic plague.

The lack of hygiene and sanitation and the increasing poverty in urban centers resulted in serious problems in health care in the fifteenth to seventeenth centuries. Societal factors, such as laws punishing the poor and the Window Tax (which led to decreased ventilation because landlords bricked in windows to avoid paying the tax), created conditions and health needs to which nursing responded.

The Sisters of Charity (1633) was founded by St. Vincent de Paul. The sisters cared for people in hospitals, asylums, and poor houses. In addition, the sisters became widely known as visiting nurses because they care for sick people in their homes. The first supervisor of the Sisters of Charity was Louise de Gras, a widow of high social standing. de Gras, who entered the order and was later known as St. Louise de Marillac, established perhaps the first educational program to be associated with a nursing order. The program included experience in the hospital, home visits, and the care of the sick. She recruited intelligent, refined, and compassionate women (Donahue, 1985). The Sisters of Charity were introduced in America by Mother Elizabeth Seton in 1809 and later changed their name to the Daughters of Charity (Donahue, 1985).

In the eighteenth century the growth of cities brought an increase in the number of hospitals and a larger role for nurses. The smallpox epidemics in the French colonies and during the Revolutionary War in the English colonies increased the need for nursing services. Nursing skills and knowledge were generally passed on by experienced nurses, since there was still little formal education for nurses.

During the nineteenth century, the Deaconess order was revived by Protestant churches. The Deaconess Institute at Kaiserswerth, Germany, was established in 1836 by Pastor Theodor Fliedner (Woodham-Smith, 1983; Donahue, 1985). The regeneration of this nursing order was stimulated by the recognition of the need for the services of women as nurses. Florence Nightingale received the *Yearbook of the Institution of Deaconesses at Kaiserswerth* in October 1846 (Woodham-Smith, 1983). In 1847, she went to Kaiserswerth to work with the Deaconesses (Woodham-Smith, 1983; Donahue, 1985).

In 1853, Nightingale went to Paris to study with the Sisters of Charity and was later appointed superintendent of the English General Hospitals in Turkey. During this period, she brought about major reforms in hygiene, sanitation, and nursing practice and reduced the mortality rate at the Barracks Hospital in Scutari, Turkey, from 42.7% to 2.2% in 6 months (Cohen, 1984; Woodham-Smith, 1983; Donahue, 1985).

In 1860, Nightingale wrote *Notes on Nursing: What it is and What it is not* for the lay person. Her philosophy of nursing practice reflected the changing needs of society. She saw the role of nursing as having "charge of somebody's health" based on the knowledge of "how to put the body in such a state to be free of disease or to recover from disease" (Nightingale, 1860). During the same year, she developed the first organized program of training for nurses, the Nightingale Training School for Nurses at St. Thomas' Hospital in London (Fig. 1-2).

The Civil War stimulated the growth of nursing in the United States. Clara Barton, founder of the American Red Cross, tended soldiers on the battlefields, cleansing their wounds, meeting their basic needs, and comforting them in death. The American Red Cross was ratified by the United States Congress in 1882 after 10 years of lobbying by Barton. Dorothea Lynde Dix, Mary Ann Ball (Mother Bickerdyke), and Harriet Tubman also influenced nursing during the Civil War (Donahue, 1985).

Fig. 1-1 The Brothers of Misericordia taking a patient to the hospital in Florence.

From Dolan, JA, et al.: Nursing in society, ed. 15, Philadelphia, 1983, W.B. Saunders Co.

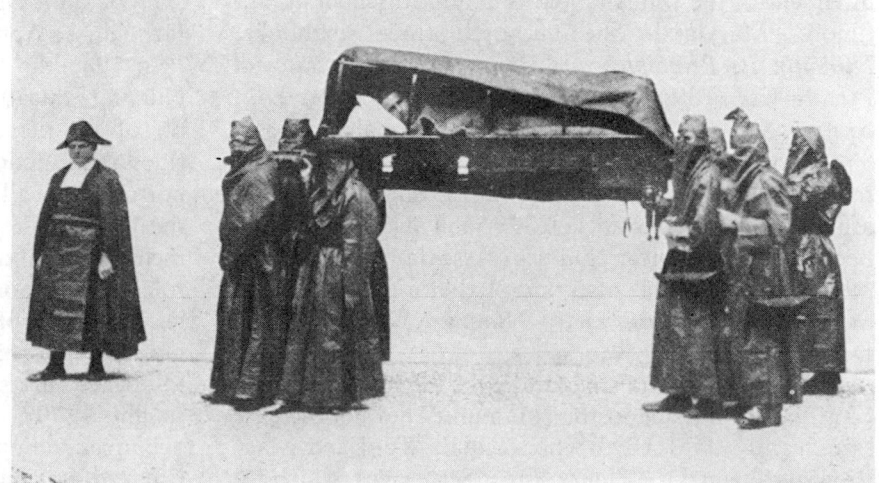

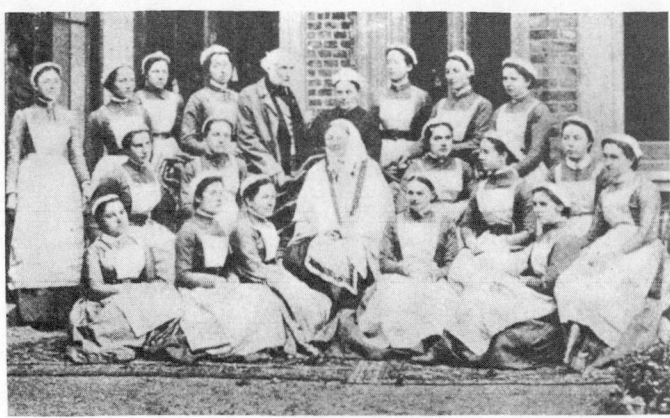

Fig. 1-2 Florence Nightingale *(center)* and students at St. Thomas' Hospital, London, 1887.

From Dolan, JA, et al.: Nursing in society, ed. 15, Philadelphia, 1983, W.B. Saunders Co.

As superintendent of the female nurses of the Union Army, Dix organized hospitals, appointed nurses, oversaw and regulated supplies to the troops. Mother Bickerdyke organized ambulance services, supervised nurses, and walked abandoned battlefields at night looking for wounded soldiers. Harriet Tubman was active in the Underground Railroad movement and assisted in leading over 300 slaves to freedom (Donahue, 1985).

After the Civil War, nursing schools in the United States and Canada began to follow Nightingale's plan. In Canada the first training school, St. Catherine's in Ontario, was founded in 1874 (Donahue, 1985; Raab, 1985). In 1884, Mary Agnes Snively took over the directorship of the Toronto General Hospital. She helped form the Canadian National Association of Trained Nurses in 1908 (Donahue, 1985; Raab, 1985). The name was later changed to the Canadian Nurses Association (CNA) in 1924 (Donahue, 1985).

Isabel Hampton (later Isabel Hampton Robb), a graduate of St. Catherine's in Ontario, was the first superintendent of the Johns Hopkins Training School in Baltimore, Maryland. She authored three textbooks: *Nursing: Its Principles and Practice for Hospital and Private Use* (1894), *Nursing Ethics* (1900), and *Educational Standards for Nurses* (1907) (Donahue, 1985). She helped found the Nurses' Associated Alumnae of the United States and Canada in 1896. The Canadian affiliation was removed in 1899, and the organization became the American Nurses' Association (ANA) in 1911. Hampton was also one of the original founders of the *American Journal of Nursing* (Wheeler, 1985; Donahue, 1985).

Nursing in hospitals expanded in the late nineteenth century, but nursing in the community did not increase significantly until 1893 when Lillian Wald and Mary Brewster opened the Henry Street Settlement, which fo-cused on the health needs of New York's poor people living in tenements (Silverstein, 1985; Donahue, 1985). Nurses working in this settlement had more responsibility for their clients than nurses working in hospitals because they frequently encountered situations requiring action independent of a physician's orders. In addition to the treatment of illness, poor people needed nursing therapies aimed at restoring nutrition status, providing shelter, and maintaining hygiene. Wald also authored the following books describing her activities: *The House on Henry Street* (1915) and *Windows on Henry Street* (1934).

Advances were made in hospital care, public health, and nursing education in the early twentieth century. Mary Adelaide Nutting, a member of the first graduating class at Johns Hopkins Hospital and successor to Isabel Hampton Robb as superintendent of the Johns Hopkins Training School, was instrumental in the affiliation of nursing education with universities. She became the first professor of nursing at Columbia University Teachers College in 1907 (Donahue, 1985).

In 1923 the Rockefeller Foundation funded a survey of nursing education, the Goldmark Report. The report concluded that nursing education needed financial support and suggested that such support be given to university schools of nursing. As a result the Rockefeller Foundation funded the expansion of nursing programs at Yale University, Vanderbilt University, and the University of Toronto. Frances Payne Bolton provided financial support for the nursing school at Western Reserve University.

As nursing education developed, nursing practice also expanded. In 1901 the Army Nurse Corps was established, followed in 1908 by the Navy Nurse Corps. Nursing specialization was also occurring. In the 1920s, graduate nurse-midwifery programs were initiated, and beginning in the 1950s, specialty nursing organizations such as the Association of Operating Room Nurses (1949), American Association of Critical Care Nurses (1969), and Oncology Nursing Society (1975) were formed (see Appendix A for a comprehensive list).

In 1965 the National Commission on Nursing and Nursing Education took up issues that included the supply of and demand for nurses, clarification of nursing roles and functions, education of nurses, and career opportunities available to nurses. Their report, often called the Lysaught report after Jerome P. Lysaught, the director of the study, called for clarification of nursing roles and responsibilities in relation to those of other health care professionals. It also advocated greater financial support for nurses and more career opportunities to attract nurses and retain them in the profession (Lysaught, 1970).

Nurses and nurse educators are revising nursing practice and curricula to meet the ever-changing needs of society. Advances in high technology, rising acuity of clients, and early discharge of clients from health care institutions require present and future nurses to have a strong knowledge base from which to practice.

CONCEPTUAL AND THEORETICAL MODELS OF NURSING PRACTICE

As nursing continues to evolve, nurses theorize about the nature of nursing practice, principles on which practice is based, and the proper goals and functions of nursing in society. Conceptual and theoretical nursing models provide knowledge to improve practice, guide research and nursing curricula, and identify the domain and goals of nursing practice. Theory provides the nurse with goals for assessment, diagnosis, and intervention; common ground for communication; and professional autonomy and accountability (Marriner, 1986; Chinn and Jacobs, 1987; Meleis, 1985; Torres, 1986; Parse, 1987) (see box).

Historical review demonstrates that nursing developed a growing body of knowledge for the last 120 years. The overall goal of this knowledge has been to explain the practice of nursing as different and distinct from the practice of medicine, psychology, and social work (Torres, 1986; Chinn and Jacobs, 1987).

Nursing concepts and theory have evolved since the era of Nightingale, who, in establishing the discipline of nursing, spoke with firm conviction about the "nature of nursing as a profession that required knowledge dis-

tinct from medical knowledge" (Nightingale, 1860). Nightingale wanted to provide a way for young women to make a meaningful contribution to society, a trait that gained importance as nursing developed (Torres, 1986).

Before 1955, the only significant milestone influencing the development of nursing concepts and theory was the establishment of the journal, *Nursing Research*, in 1952. This journal reported on the scientific investigations in nursing by nurses and other professionals. Ultimately the journal encouraged scientific productivity and provided the framework for a questioning attitude that may have set the stage for inquiries into theoretical nursing (Meleis, 1985).

In the mid-1950s, nurses began to formulate theoretical views of nursing and concerns about what to include or exclude from nursing curricula. Columbia University Teachers' College offered masters and doctoral programs focusing on education and administration (Meleis, 1985). Although the focus of these programs was not nursing science, prominent nurse theorists, such as Peplau, Henderson, Hall, Abdellah, King, Wiedenbach, and Rogers, graduated from this institution.

During the 1960s, Yale University School of Nursing defined nursing even further. "Nursing was considered a process rather than an end, an interaction rather than content, and a relationship between two human beings rather than an interaction between unrelated nurse and patient" (Meleis, 1985). In addition, the ANA's 1965 position paper defined nursing and concluded that one of the most significant goals for nursing was theory development. This supported the need for continuing efforts to develop the body of nursing knowledge (ANA, 1965; Meleis, 1985). During the 1960s, federal support was also provided to nurses pursuing masters and doctoral degrees.

Theory development was emphasized from the mid-1960s to 1970. A series of symposia, sponsored by Case Western Reserve University, was held to assist in the development of nursing theory. During the mid-1970s the National League for Nursing (NLN) made theory-based curriculum a requirement for accreditation. Thus schools of nursing were expected to select, develop, and implement a conceptual framework for their curricula (Meleis, 1985).

Definitions of nursing can help the nursing student understand how the roles and actions of nurses fit together in the unified profession of nursing. The following sections describe, in chronological order, the general focus of selected nursing theories (Table 1-1).

Nightingale's Theory

Contemporary authors are beginning to explore Nightingale's work as a potential theoretical and con-

---

Goals of Theoretical Nursing Models

- Formulate legislation governing nursing practice and education
- Formulate regulations interpreting nurse practice acts so nurses and others better understand the laws
- Develop curriculum plans for nursing education
- Establish criteria for measuring the quality of nursing care, education, and research
- Prepare job descriptions used by employers of nurses
- Guide the development of nursing care delivery systems
- Provide knowledge to improve nursing administration, practice, education, and research
- Guide research to establish an empirical knowledge base for nursing
- Identify the domain and goals of nursing

TABLE 1-1 Summary of Nursing Theories

Theorist	Goal of Nursing	Framework for Practice
Nightingale (1860)	To facilitate "the body's reparative processes" by manipulating the client's environment (Torres, 1986).	Manipulate the client's environment to include appropriate noise, nutrition, hygiene, light, comfort, socialization, and hope.
Peplau (1952)	To develop an interaction between the nurse and client (Peplau, 1952).	Nursing is a significant, therapeutic, interpersonal process (Peplau, 1952). Nurses participate in structuring the health care system to facilitate the natural ongoing tendency of humans to develop interpersonal relationships (Marriner, 1986).
Henderson (1955)	To work interdependently with other health care workers (Marriner, 1986), assisting the client to gain independence as quickly as possible (Henderson, 1955). To assist the client in gaining the strength he lacks (Torres, 1986).	Henderson's 14 basic needs (Henderson, 1966) (see p. 10).
Abdellah (1960)	To provide service to individuals, families, and society. To be kind and caring but also intelligent, competent, and technically well prepared to provide this service (Marriner, 1986).	Typology of 21 nursing problems (Abdellah, 1960) (see p. 10).
Orlando (1961)	To respond to the client's behavior in terms of his immediate need. To interact with the client to meet the immediate need for help by identifying the behavior of the client, the reaction of the nurse, and the nursing action to be taken (Torres, 1986; Chinn and Jacobs, 1987).	Three elements, including client behavior, nurse reaction, and nurse action, which compose a nursing situation (Orlando, 1961).
Hall (1962)	To provide care and comfort to the client during the disease process (Torres, 1986).	Client is composed of three overlapping parts: (1) a person (the core), (2) a pathology and treatment (the cure), and (3) a body (the care). The nurse is the care giver (Chinn and Jacobs, 1987; Marriner 1986).
Wiedenbach (1964)	To assist individuals in overcoming obstacles that interfere with their ability to meet the demands/needs brought about by a condition, environment, situation, or time (Torres, 1986).	Nursing as a practice is related to individuals who need help because of a behavioral stimulus. Clinical nursing has four components: philosophy, purpose, practice, and art (Chinn and Jacobs, 1987).
Levine (1966)	To use conservation activities aimed at optimal use of client's resources.	Adaptation model of human as an integral whole based on "four conservation principles of nursing" (Levine, 1973).
Johnson (1968)	To reduce stress so the client can move more easily through the recovery process.	Basic needs framework focusing on seven categories of behavior (see p. 11). The individual's goal is to achieve a behavioral

Theorist	Goal of Nursing	Framework for Practice
		balance and steady state by adjustment and adaptation to certain forces (Johnson, 1980; Torres, 1986).
Rogers (1970)	To maintain and promote health, prevent illness, and care for and rehabilitate the sick and disabled through the "humanistic science of nursing."	"Unitary man" evolving along a life process. Client continually changes and coexists with his environment.
Orem (1971)	To care for the client and help the client attain total self-care.	Self-care deficit theory. Nursing care becomes necessary when the client is unable to fulfill biological, psychological, developmental, or social needs.
King (1971)	To use communication to help the client reestablish a positive adaptation to his environment.	Nursing process defined as dynamic interpersonal process between the nurse, client, and health care system.
Travelbee (1971)	To assist an individual or family to prevent or cope with illness, regain health, find meaning in illness, or to maintain the highest maximal degree of health (Marriner, 1986).	Interpersonal process is viewed as a human-to-human relationship formed during illness and the "experience of suffering."
Neuman (1972)	To assist individuals, families, and groups to attain and maintain a maximal level of total wellness by purposeful interventions.	Systems model of nursing practice has stress reduction as its goal (Torres, 1986). Nursing actions are in one of three levels of prevention: primary, secondary, or tertiary.
Roy (1976)	To identify the types of demands placed on a client, assess the client's adaptation to the demands, and help the client adapt.	Adaptation model based on four adaptive modes: physiological, psychological, sociological, and dependence-independence (Roy, 1980).
Patterson and Zderad (1976)	To respond to human needs and to build humanistic nursing science (Patterson and Zderad, 1976; Chinn and Jacobs, 1987).	Humanistic nursing requires the participants to be aware of their "uniqueness," as well as their "commonality" with others (Chinn and Jacobs, 1987).
Leininger (1978)	To provide care consistent with nursing's emerging science and knowledge with caring as a central focus (Chinn and Jacobs, 1987).	Transcultural care theory: caring is the central and unifying domain for nursing knowledge and practice (Leininger, 1980).
Watson (1979)	To promote health, restore clients to health, and prevent illness (Marriner, 1986).	Philosophy and science of caring: caring is an interpersonal process comprised of interventions that result in meeting human needs (Torres, 1986).
Parse (1981)	To focus on man as a living unity and man's qualitative participation with health experience (Parse, 1981). Nursing is viewed as a science and an art (Marriner, 1986).	Man continually interacts with environment and participates in maintenance of health (Marriner, 1986). Health is a continual, open process, rather than a state of well-being or the absence of disease (Parse, 1981; Marriner, 1986; Chinn and Jacobs, 1987).

ceptual model for nursing (Chinn and Jacobs, 1986; Marriner, 1986; Meleis, 1985; Torres, 1986). Meleis (1985) notes that Nightingale's concept of environment as the focus of nursing care and her admonition that nurses need not know all about the disease process are early attempts to differentiate between nursing and medicine.

Nightingale did not view nursing as limited merely to the administration of medications and treatments but rather as oriented toward providing adequate fresh air, light, warmth, cleanliness, quiet, and adequate nutrition (Nightingale, 1860; Torres, 1986). Through observation and data collection, she linked the client's health status with environmental factors and, as a result, initiated improved hygiene and sanitary conditions during the Crimean war.

According to Chinn and Jacobs (1987), Nightingale presented many important theoretical ideas that potentially stimulated development. However, a community of scholars to collaborate and inspire one another was missing.

Torres (1986) notes that Nightingale provided basic concepts and propositions that could be validated and used for practice in nursing. Nightingale's "descriptive theory" provided nurses with a way to think about nursing or a frame of reference that focuses on patients and their environment (Torres, 1986). Nightingale's letters and writings direct the nurse to act on the behalf of the client. Her principles encompass the areas of practice, research, and education. Most important, her concepts and principles shape and delineate nursing practice (Marriner, 1986). Nightingale taught and used the nursing process, noting that "vital observation [assessment] . . . is not for the sake of piling up miscellaneous information or curious facts, but for the sake of saving life and increasing health and comfort."

Peplau's Theory

Hildegard Peplau's theory (1952) focuses on the individual, the nurse, and the interactive process, with the result being the nurse-client relationship (Torres, 1986; Marriner, 1986). Nursing's overall goal is to educate the client and family and to help the client reach mature personality development (Chinn and Jacobs, 1987). Therefore the nurse strives to develop a nurse-client relationship in which the nurse serves as a resource person, counselor, and surrogate.

When the client seeks help, the nurse first discusses the nature of the problem and explains the services available. As the nurse-client relationship develops, the nurse helps the client identify the problem and potential solutions. The client gains from this relationship by using available services to meet needs. When the original needs have been resolved, new needs may emerge.

The nurse-client interpersonal relationship is characterized by the following overlapping phases: orientation, identification, explanation, and resolution. The nurse and client have specific tasks and roles for each phase (Torres, 1986).

Peplau's theory and ideas provided a design for the practice of psychiatric nursing. Nursing research on anxiety, empathy, behavioral tools, and tools to evaluate verbal responses resulted from Peplau's conceptual model (Marriner, 1986).

Henderson's Theory

Virginia Henderson's nursing theory (1955) involves basic needs of the whole person. Henderson (1964) defines nursing as

assisting the individual sick or well in the performance of those activities contributing to health or its recovery . . . that he would perform unaided if he had the necessary strength, will, or knowledge. And to do this in such a way as to help him gain independence as rapidly as possible.

The following needs, often called "Henderson's 14 basic needs," provide a framework for nursing care (Henderson, 1966):
1. Breathe normally
2. Eat and drink adequately
3. Eliminate by all avenues of elimination
4. Move and maintain a desirable position
5. Sleep and rest
6. Select suitable clothing; dress and undress
7. Maintain body temperature within normal range
8. Keep the body clean and well groomed
9. Avoid dangers in the environment
10. Communicate with others
11. Worship according to faith
12. Work at something that provides a sense of accomplishment
13. Play or participate in various forms of recreation
14. Learn, discover, or satisfy the curiosity that leads to normal development and health

Abdellah's Theory

The nursing theory developed by Faye Abdellah et al. (1960) emphasizes delivering nursing care for the whole person to meet the physical, emotional, intellectual, social, and spiritual needs of clients and their families. In this approach the nurse needs knowledge and skills in interpersonal relations, psychology, growth and development, communication, and sociology, as well as the basic sciences and specific nursing skills. The nurse is seen as a problem solver and decision maker. The nurse formulates an individualized view of the client's needs, which may occur in the following four areas:

1. Comfort, hygiene, and safety
2. Physiological balance
3. Psychological and social factors
4. Sociological and community factors

In these four areas, Abdellah and colleagues identified the following specific client needs, which are often referred to as "Abdellah's 21 nursing problems":

1. To maintain good hygiene and physical comfort
2. To achieve optimal activity, exercise, rest, and sleep
3. To prevent accident, injury, or other trauma and prevent the spread of infection
4. To maintain good body mechanics and prevent and correct deformities
5. To facilitate the supply of oxygen to all body cells
6. To facilitate the maintenance of nutrition to all body cells
7. To facilitate the maintenance of elimination
8. To facilitate the maintenance of fluid and electrolyte balance
9. To recognize the physiological responses of the body to disease conditions—pathological, physiological, and compensatory
10. To facilitate the maintenance of regulatory mechanisms and functions
11. To facilitate the maintenance of sensory function
12. To identify and accept positive and negative expressions, feelings, and reactions
13. To identify and accept the interrelatedness of emotions and organic illness
14. To facilitate the maintenance of effective verbal and nonverbal communication
15. To facilitate the development of productive interpersonal relationships
16. To facilitate progress toward achievement of personal spiritual goals
17. To create and/or maintain a therapeutic environment
18. To facilitate awareness of self as an individual with varying physical, emotional, and developmental needs
19. To accept the optimum possible goals in light of limitations—physical and emotional
20. To use community resources as an aid in resolving problems arising from illness
21. To understand the role of social problems as influencing factors in the cause of illness

Orlando's Theory

Ida Orlando (1961) emphasized that the client is an individual with a need that, when met, diminishes distress, increases adequacy, or enhances well-being. Orlando's theory focuses on the nurse's reaction to the client's behavior in terms of his immediate need (Torres, 1986). Orlando's theory is a conceptual framework for the process of professional nursing (Marriner, 1986). Three elements—client behavior, nurse reaction, and nurse actions—compose the nursing situation. Once the nurse thoroughly assesses the client's needs, she recognizes the impact of that need on the client's level of health and then acts automatically or deliberately to meet the need, ultimately reducing the client's distress (Chinn and Jacobs, 1987).

Levine's Theory

Myra Levine's nursing theory, begun in 1966 and published in 1973, views the client as an integrated being who interacts with and adapts to his environment, with conservation of energy as a primary concern. Health is viewed in terms of the conservation of energy in the following areas, which Levine calls the "four conservation principles of nursing":

1. Conservation of client energy
2. Conservation of structural integrity
3. Conservation of personal integrity
4. Conservation of social integrity

With this approach, nursing care involves conservation activities aimed at optimal use of the client's resources.

Johnson's Theory

Dorothy Johnson's theory of nursing (1968) focuses on how the client adapts to his illness and how actual or potential stress can affect the client's ability to adapt. For Johnson the goal of nursing is to reduce stress so the client can move more easily through the recovery process. Her theory focuses on basic needs in terms of the following seven categories of behavior:

1. Security-seeking behavior
2. Nurturance-seeking behavior
3. Master of oneself and one's environment according to internalized standards of excellence
4. Taking in nourishment in socially and culturally acceptable ways
4. Ridding the body of waste in socially and culturally acceptable ways
6. Sexual and role identity behavior
7. Self-protective behavior

According to Johnson, the nurse assesses the client's needs in these categories of behavior, called behavioral subsystems. Under normal conditions the client functions fairly effectively in the environment. When stress disrupts normal adaptation, however, the client's behavior becomes erratic and less purposeful. The nurse identifies the client's inability to adapt and provides nursing care to resolve problems in meeting the client's needs.

Rogers' Theory

In her theory, Martha Rogers (1970) considers man (unitary human being) as an energy field coexisting within the universe. Man is in continuous interaction with his environment. In addition, man is a unified whole, possessing his own integrity and manifesting characteristics that are more than the sum of his parts (Rogers, 1970). Unitary man is a "four dimensional energy field identified by pattern and manifesting characteristics that are specific to the whole and which cannot be predicted from the knowledge of parts" (Marriner, 1986). The four dimensions used in Rogers' theory, energy fields, openness, pattern and organization, and four dimensionality, are used to derive principles about how human beings develop.

Rogers views nursing primarily as a science and is committed to nursing research. Nursing therefore incorporates knowledge of the basic sciences and physiology, as well as nursing knowledge:

The science of nursing aims to provide a body of abstract knowledge growing out of scientific research and logical analysis and capable of being translated into nursing practice. Nursing's body of scientific knowledge is a new product specific to nursing . . . . Nursing is a humanistic science.

Orem's Theory

Dorothea Orem (1971) developed a definition of nursing that emphasizes self-care needs of the client. Orem describes her philosophy of nursing in this way:

Nursing has as a special concern man's needs for self-care action and the provision and management of it on a continuous basis in order to sustain life and health, recover from disease or injury, and cope with their effects. Self-care is a requirement of every person—man, woman, and child. When self-care is not maintained, illness, disease, or death will occur. Nurses sometimes manage and maintain required self-care continually for persons who are totally incapacitated. In other instances, nurses help persons to maintain required self-care by performing some but not all care measures, by supervising others who assist patients, and by instructing and guiding individuals as they gradually move toward self-care.

The goal of Orem's self-care deficit theory of nursing is helping the client care for himself. According to Orem, nursing care is necessary when the client is unable to fulfill biological, psychological, developmental, or social needs. The nurse determines why a client is unable to meet these needs, what must be done to enable the client to meet them, and how much the client is able to do for himself.

King's Theory

Imogene King's theory (1971) focuses on the interpersonal relationship between client and nurse. The nurse-client relationship is the vehicle for the nursing process, which is defined as a dynamic interpersonal process in which the nurse and the client are affected by each other's behavior, as well as by the health care system. The nurse's goal is to use communication to assist the client in reestablishing or maintaining a positive adaptation to his environment.

Travelbee's Theory

Joyce Travelbee's theory, begun in 1966 and published in 1971, emphasizes nursing as an interpersonal process involving the nurse and client. Travelbee defines nursing as

an interpersonal process whereby the . . . nurse practitioner assists an individual or family to prevent, or cope with, the experience of illness and suffering, and, if necessary, assists the individual or family to find meaning in these experiences.

Because the client's whole self may be involved in coping with the experience of illness, this definition also addresses the individual in all dimensions.

Neuman's Theory

Betty Neuman (1972) defines a total person model incorporating the holistic concept and an open-systems approach (Marriner, 1987). Neuman views the person as a dynamic composite of physiological, sociocultural, and developmental variables functioning as an open system. As an open system the person interacts with, adjusts to, and is adjusted by the environment (Chinn and Jacobs, 1987), which is viewed as a stressor. Stressors disrupt the system. Neuman's model has three categories, including intrapersonal, interpersonal, and extrapersonal. Intrapersonal stressors are forces occurring within the person; interpersonal stressors such as role expectations occur between persons, and extrapersonal stressor such as financial circumstances occur outside the person (Neuman, 1982; Marriner, 1986).

Neuman's goal of nursing is to assist individuals, families, and groups to attain and maintain a maximal level of total wellness. The nurse assesses, manages, and evaluates client systems. Nursing focuses on the variables affecting the client's response to the stressor (Chinn and Jacobs, 1987). Nursing actions are in one of the following levels of prevention: primary, secondary, and tertiary. Primary prevention focuses on strengthening a line of defense through the identification of actual or potential risk factors associated with stressors. Secondary prevention strengthens internal defenses and resources by establishing priorities and treatment plans for identified symptoms, and tertiary prevention focuses on readaptation. The principal goal in tertiary prevention is to strengthen resistance to stressors through client education and to assist in preventing recurrence of the response to the stressor (Chinn and Jacobs, 1987; Marriner, 1986; Torres, 1986; Neuman, 1982).

Roy's Theory

Sister Callista Roy's adaptation theory (1976) views the client as an adaptive system. Roy believes that the need for nursing care arises when the client cannot adapt to internal and external environmental demands. All individuals must adapt to the following demands:
1. Meeting basic physiological needs
2. Developing a positive self-concept
3. Performing social roles
4. Achieving a balance between dependence and independence

The nurse determines what demands are causing problems for a client and assesses how well the client is adapting to these demands. Nursing care then helps the client adapt.

AMERICAN NURSES' ASSOCIATION DEFINITION

In 1955 the ANA published the following official definition of nursing practice*:

The practice of professional nursing means the performance for compensation of any act in the observation, care, and counsel of the ill, injured, or infirm or in the maintenance of health or prevention of illness of others, or in the supervision and teaching of other personnel, or the administration of medications and treatments as prescribed by licensed physician or dentist, requiring substantial specialized judgment and skill and based on knowledge and application of the principles of biological, physical, and social sciences. The foregoing shall not be deemed to include acts of diagnosis or prescription of therapeutic or corrective measures.

This early definition by the ANA is significant in its attempt to define nursing practice in a fairly specific manner. Nonetheless, it tends to stress nursing's dependent role, an emphasis that is no longer accepted. In 1965 the ANA Committee on Education issued a position paper that presents a fuller definition of nursing and emphasizes nursing as an independent profession[†]:

Nursing is a helping profession and, as such, provides services which contribute to the health and well-being of people.

Nursing is a vital consequence to the individual receiving services; it fills needs which cannot be met by the person, by the family, or by other persons in the community.

The essential components of professional nursing are care,

*From American Nurses' Association: Am J Nurs 55:1474, 1955.
[†]From American Nurses' Association: Am J Nurs 65:106, 1965.

cure, and coordination. The care aspect is more than "to take care of," it is "caring for" and "caring about" as well. It is dealing with human beings under stress, frequently over long periods of time. It is providing comfort and support in times of anxiety, loneliness, and helplessness. It is listening, evaluating, and intervening appropriately.

The promotion of health and healing is the cure aspect of professional nursing. It is assisting patients to understand their health problems and helping them to cope. It is the administration of medications and treatments. And it is the use of clinical nursing judgment in determining, on the basis of patients' reactions, whether the plan for care needs to be maintained or changed. It is knowing when and how to use existing and potential resources to help patients toward recovery and adjustment by mobilizing their own resources.

Professional nursing practice is this and more. It is sharing responsibility for the health and welfare of all those in the community, and participating in programs designed to prevent illness and maintain health. It is coordinating and synchronizing medical and other professional and technical services as these affect patients. It is supervising, teaching, and directing all those who give nursing care.

In 1979 the Committee of Chairpersons of the ANA determined that the Congress for Nursing Practice should define the nature and scope of nursing practice. The Congress for Nursing Practice is the part of the ANA concerned with legal aspects of nursing practice, public recognition of the significance of nursing practice to health care, and implications for nursing practice of trends in health care.

In 1980 the Congress for Nursing Practice defined nursing as the diagnosis and treatment of human responses to actual or potential health problems (ANA, 1980). This definition involves the following characteristics of nursing: phenomena, theory application, nursing action, and evaluation of the effects of action (Fig. 1-3). *Phenomena* are the human responses to actual or potential health problems. The nurse identifies the client's responses by assessing the client's health status and obtaining data about the client. The nurse uses nursing *theory* to understand the client's responses. The nurse takes *actions* to resolve actual or potential health care problems. The nurse then evaluates the *effects* of the actions on the client's responses. These four characteristics are related to the nursing process, which is described in Unit 2.

EDUCATIONAL PREPARATION

Licensed Practical Nurse Education

A licensed practical or vocational nurse is trained in basic nursing techniques and direct client care. The licensed practical nurse (LPN) practices under the supervision of a registered nurse in a hospital or community

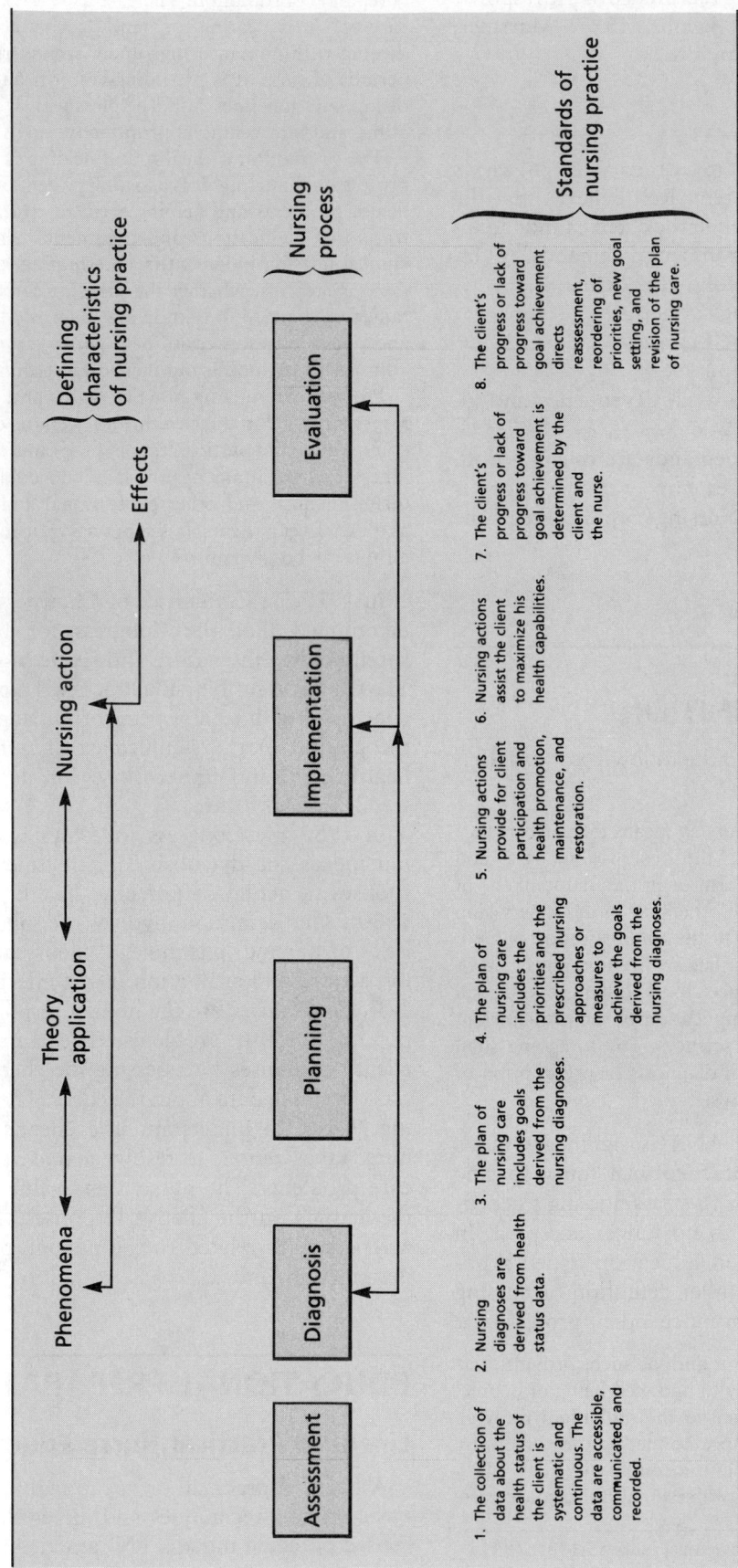

Fig. 1-3 Defining characteristics of nursing practice: relationship to the nursing process and the standards of nursing practice.

Modified from the American Nurses' Association: Nursing and social policy statement, Kansas City, Mo., 1980, The Association.

health practice setting. Licensed practical nurses, licensed vocational nurses (LVNs), and in Canada registered nurse's assistants (RNAs) generally receive 1 year of education and training in a hospital, community college, or other agency. The LPN is licensed by the state board of nursing after completing the educational program and passing the licensure examination.

Registered Nurse Education

The growth of nursing stimulated various educational routes for becoming a registered nurse (RN). Initially, training schools were usually associated with a specific hospital. The primary purpose of such a school was to train nurses who would work within that institution.

As nursing increasingly defined its own body of knowledge, formalized educational processes developed to ensure a consistent level of nursing education in institutions. Such consistency was also necessary for registered nurse licensure.

In the United States, there are three common types of programs through which an individual can become a registered nurse: the associate degree program, the diploma program, and the baccalaureate degree program. In Canada, there are diploma programs and baccalaureate degree programs.

ASSOCIATE DEGREE EDUCATION

The associate degree program in the United States is a 2-year program usually offered by a college or junior college. The major focus of this program is on theoretical and practical courses related to the practice of nursing. Graduates of this program take the state board examination for registered nurse licensure.

DIPLOMA EDUCATION

The diploma program in the United States is a 2- or 3-year program usually associated with a hospital. Some diploma programs are affiliated with a college or university, which grants college credit for nonnursing courses. Graduates of a diploma program receive a diploma from the hospital and take the state board examination for registered nurse licensure. In Canada, diploma programs are offered in community colleges or hospitals and are 2-year programs (or 3 years in some hospital-based programs) comparable to associate degree programs in the United States.

BACCALAUREATE EDUCATION

The baccalaureate degree program within a college or university usually encompasses 4 years of study. The program focuses on theoretical and practical courses but also includes courses in the social sciences, basic sciences, and humanities to support nursing theory. In Canada, a Bachelor of Science in Nursing (BScN) or a Bachelor in Nursing (BN) is the equivalent to the Bachelor of Science in Nursing (BSN) in the United States.

The American Association of Colleges of Nursing (AACN) published the *Essentials of College and University Education for Professional Nursing* (1986). This document delineated essential knowledge, practice and values, attitudes, personal qualities, and professional behaviors for the baccalaureate-prepared nurse. The goal of this document was to provide a standard by which "faculty can measure the content of the curriculum and the performance of the graduate" (AACN, 1986). In addition, the employer "can use them as a base for new graduate orientation programs." (AACN, 1986).

Two other types of degree programs offer eligibility to take the state board examinations. First, some programs offer a master's degree in nursing as the first professional degree. At present, these programs exist at Yale University and Massachusetts General Hospital. The second type of program, the nursing doctorate (ND) at Case Western Reserve University, offers the doctorate as the first professional degree.

Accreditation and Licensure

Associate degree, diploma, and baccalaureate degree programs must meet certain criteria established by the NLN in order to be accredited. This voluntary accreditation is available for basic nursing education programs and master's degree programs in nursing (National Commission on Nursing, 1983).

Registered nurse licensure for practice in most states and provinces requires that the student complete a prescribed course for study from an approved program. In the United States the program must be approved by the State Board of Nursing in the state in which the student is seeking licensure. In Canada the program must be approved by a Provincial Board of Nursing in the province in which the student is seeking licensure.

In the United States, registered nurse candidates must pass the National Council Licensure Examination for Registered Nurses (NCLEX-RN), which is administered by each state's board of nursing. In Canada the Canadian Nurses' Association Testing Service (CNATS) administers the test to qualified candidates in each province. Whether nurses can practice in a state or province other than their own depends on the reciprocal agreement between the states or provinces involved. In some instances reciprocity is considered on an individual basis.

Graduate Nursing Education

As expressed by the ANA (1969) the purpose of a graduate program in nursing is to prepare nurse clinicians capable of improving nursing care through the advancement of nursing theory and sciences. Those com-

---

Characteristics of Graduate Education in Nursing Leading to the Master's Degree

The master's program in nursing is offered by an educational institution of higher learning and is built on a baccalaureate curriculum including an upper division major in nursing. It provides students with an opportunity to: (1) acquire advanced knowledge from the sciences and the humanities to support advanced nursing practice and role development; (2) expand knowledge of nursing theory as a basis for advanced nursing practice; (3) develop expertise in a specialized area of clinical nursing practice; (4) acquire the knowledge and skills related to a specific functional role in nursing; (5) acquire initial competence in conducting research; (6) plan and initiate change in the health care system and in the practice and delivery of health care; (7) further develop and implement leadership strategies for the betterment of health care; (8) actively engage in collaborative relationships with others for the purpose of improving health care; and (9) acquire a foundation for doctoral study.

Modified from National League for Nursing: Characteristics of graduate education in nursing leading to the master's degree, New York, 1978, The League.

---

pleting a graduate program can receive the degree of Master of Arts in Nursing (MA), Master in Nursing (MN), or Master of Science in Nursing (MSN). The National League for Nursing has described the characteristics of and standards for accredited master's degree nursing programs (see box).

A master's degree in nursing can be valuable for nurses seeking expanded roles such as that of nurse educator, clinical nurse specialist, nurse administrator, or practitioner. These roles are described in a later section of this chapter.

The first nursing doctorate program opened in 1953 at the University of Pittsburgh. The need for nurses with doctorate degrees is rising (Institute of Medicine, 1983). By 1990, it is estimated that over 13,000 doctorally prepared nurses will be needed (Holzemer, 1987). Professional doctoral programs in nursing (DSN or DNSc) emphasize the application of research findings to clinical nursing. Other programs emphasize more basic research and theory and award the Doctor of Philosophy (PhD) in nursing (Holzemer, 1987).

Continuing Education

Changes occur continually in the sciences, in technology, and in nursing procedures. Continuing educa-

tion programs help nurses remain current in skills, knowledge, and theory.

Continuing education involves formal, organized, educational programs offered by educational and health care institutions. As expressed by the ANA (1975), the goals of continuing education in nursing are (1) to improve and maintain nursing practice, (2) to promote and exercise leadership in effecting change in health care delivery systems, and (3) to fulfill professional learning needs. Other goals include helping nurses become specialized in a particular area of practice and teaching nurses new skills and techniques.

In general, continuing education programs are short term and are designed for all professional nurses. The ANA or the state board of nursing is the accrediting agency for continuing education programs. The ANA awards continuing education units on completion of specific courses. Some states require nurses to take continuing education courses for license renewal (Table 1-2).

In-Service Education

An in-service education program is instruction or training provided by a health care agency or institution. An in-service program is held in the institution and is designed to increase the knowledge, skills, and competencies of nurses and other health care professionals employed by the institution. For example, a hospital might offer an in-service program to inform nurses about primary nursing before it is implemented at the hospital.

All nurses have access to continuing education and in-service programs organized and conducted by a university, private hospital, private continuing education service, or the employing institution or agency. Such programs assist the practicing nurse in acquiring new knowledge and skills necessary for today's highly technical and fast-changing health care delivery system.

Career Mobility and Clinical Ladder

Education continues to be important after the nurse begins to practice, whether the practice setting focuses on the adult or child, the chronically or acutely ill, or in the home or hospital. Nursing encompasses an ever-widening range of roles. Multiple career paths and goals are open to new and experienced practitioners (Hefferin and Kleinknecht, 1986).

In the past, career mobility for nurses was somewhat limited. However, with expanding roles in nursing practice, this situation has changed. The clinical ladder approach to advancement has been discussed in many nursing journals and put into practice in various settings (Anderson and Denyes, 1975; Colavecchio, Tescher, and Scalgi, 1975; Zimmer, 1975). The clinical ladder unifies clinical practice and nursing administration, fosters col-

TABLE 1-2 Mandatory Continuing Education

State	CE Contact Hours Required
FOR REGISTERED NURSES	
California	30 hours every 2-year relicensure period (all 30 may be in home study)
Colorado	20 hours every 2-year relicensure period (5 may be in home study)
Florida	24 hours every 2-year relicensure period (all 24 may be in home study)
Iowa	45 hours every 3-year relicensure period (15 may be in home study)
Kansas	30 hours every 2-year relicensure period: '82-'84 (6 may be in home study in '82-'84)
Kentucky	15 hours every 1-year relicensure period (home study permitted only for licensees living or working outside of United States)
Massachusetts	10 hours every 2-year relicensure period: '82-'84 15 hours every 2-year period: '84-'86 (all 10, 15 may be in home study)
Minnesota	30 hours every 2-year relicensure period (all 30 may be in home study)
Nebraska	75 hours every 5 years *or* 20 hours + 200 hours of practice every 5 years (licenses must be renewed every year; no provision for home study)
Nevada	30 hours every 2-year relicensure period (10 may be in home study)
New Mexico	30 hours every 2-year relicensure period (all 30 may be in home study)
FOR NURSE PRACTITIONERS	
Alaska	30 hours every 2-year relicensure period (home study provision is pending)
Idaho	60 hours every 2-year relicensure period (30 may be in home study)
Mississippi	40 hours every 2-year relicensure period (no home study permitted)
New Hampshire	20 hours every 2-year relicensure period (no home study permitted)
Oregon	100 hours every 2-year relicensure period + 25 hours pharmacological CE if NP prescribes (50 hours may be in home study)

laboration between nursing education and service, and is a professional advancement system.

The clinical ladder contains structure, criteria for clinical competencies, promotional procedures, and incentives for advancement (Huey, 1982). The structure is individualized for a specific institution and may include multiple levels on the following pathways: clinical, administration, research, and education (ANA, 1984). There are specific objective-measurable criteria for each level within the structure. Within a clinical ladder system, nurses are no longer promoted strictly on the basis of education and seniority within the institution. The promotional procedures within the clinical ladder are clearly delineated, thereby promoting self-appraisal and peer appraisal for career mobility within the system. The incentive for advancement may include increased autonomy of practice, raise in salary or promotion within the organizational structure itself, increased expertise, and personal self-fulfillment.

The clinical ladder is a method for career mobility by which one program can encourage and motivate nurses to remain in the health care setting. Career counseling is another method for retention and promoting within the various settings.

Hefferin and Kleinknecht (1986) developed the Nursing Career Preference Inventory to assist nurses in de-

termining which of the four primary nursing practice areas—clinical, administration, research, or education—reflects their personal work activity interests or preferences (see research highlight). Career inventories are

---

⚔ *Research Highlight* ⚔

Hefferin and Kleinknecht developed the Nursing Career Preference Inventory (NCPI) that would (1) assist individual nurses in identifying their personal patterns of nursing work interests or preferences and (2) determine the primary nursing practice areas and the customary hospital based nursing role positions that most often reflect the identified work interest patterns. The NCPI was developed from the response of 2735 nurses. The internal consistency of the four NCPI categories was high. The researchers noted that the NCPI filled a void in career counseling for nurses and assisted nurses in identifying and achieving career goals.

Hefferin, EA, and Kleinknecht, MK: Development of the nursing career preference inventory, Nurs Res 35(1):44, 1986.

valuable in retaining bright, talented nurses within an institution, as well as decreasing the risk of experienced nurses leaving the profession altogether.

Research has demonstrated that the first year of clinical practice is critical for the new graduate. During the first year job satisfaction, commitment to the employing institution, and professionalism decrease. New graduates and experienced nurses entering a new work environment are at risk. As the nurse gained graduate education, the decline in satisfaction was significantly reduced (McCloskey and McCain, 1987).

NURSING PRACTICE

Nurses practice in a variety of settings, in many roles within those settings, and with other care givers in the allied health professions. The practice of nursing is guided only in part by administrators in hospitals and other health care agencies and institutions. State and provincial nurse practice acts establish specific legal regulations for nursing practice, and professional organizations establish standards of nursing practice as criteria for nursing care.

Standards of Nursing Practice

As nursing has become more independent as a profession, it has increasingly set its own standards for practice. Such standards are important as guidelines for providing care and as criteria for evaluating care. When standards are clearly defined, clients can be assured they are receiving high-quality care, nurses know exactly what is necessary to give nursing care, and administrators can determine that care meets acceptable standards. Moreover, standards of practice are important if a legal dispute arises over whether adequate care was provided in a particular case (see Chapter 18). The ANA and the CNA have published standards of nursing practice (Tables 1-3 and 1-4).

Nurse Practice Acts

In all states in the United States and all provinces in Canada, nurse practice acts regulate the licensure and practice of nursing. Each state or province defines for

---

TABLE 1-3 American Nurses' Association Standards of Nursing Practice

Standard	Rationale
1. The collection of data about the health status of the client/patient is systematic and continuous. The data are accessible, communicated, and recorded.	Comprehensive care requires complete and ongoing collection of data about the client/patient to determine the nursing care and needs of the client/patient. All health status data about the client/patient must be available for all members of the health care team.
2. Nursing diagnoses are derived from health status data.	The health status of the client/patient is the basis for determining the nursing care needs. The data are analyzed and compared to norms when possible.
3. The plan of nursing care includes goals derived from the nursing diagnoses.	The determination of the results to be achieved is an essential part of planning care.
4. The plan of nursing care includes priorities and the prescribed nursing approaches or measures to achieve the goals derived from the nursing diagnoses.	Nursing actions are planned to promote, maintain, and restore the client/patient's well-being.
5. Nursing actions provide for client/patient participation in health promotion, maintenance, and restoration.	The client/patient and family are continually involved in nursing care.
6. The nursing actions assist the client/patient to maximize his health capabilities.	Nursing actions are designed to promote, maintain, and restore health.
7. The client/patient's progress or lack of progress toward goal achievements is determined by the client/patient and the nurse.	The quality of nursing care depends upon comprehensive and intelligent determination of nursing's impact upon the health status of the client/patient. The client/patient is an essential part of this determination.
8. The client/patient's progress or lack of progress toward goal achievement directs reassessment, reordering of priorities, new goal setting, and revision of the plan of nursing care.	The nursing process remains the same, but the input of new information may dictate new or revised approaches.

From American Nurses' Association: Standards of nursing practice, Kansas City, Mo., 1973, The Association.

itself the scope of nursing practice, but most have similar practice acts. The definition of nursing practice published by the ANA in 1955 (see p. 13) is in some ways representative of the scope of nursing practice as defined in most states and provinces. In the last decade, however, many states have revised their nurse practice acts to reflect nursing's growing autonomy and the expanded roles of nurses in practice. The 1955 ANA prohibition against diagnosis and treatment, for example, has been removed from nurse practice acts in many states or re-phrased to differentiate between nursing diagnosis and treatment and medical diagnosis and treatment. Nurse practice acts are discussed in more detail in Chapter 18.

Practice Settings

As nursing's role in the health care system has expanded, the settings in which nurses practice have also increased. Table 1-5 gives statistics on the numbers of nurses in practice settings.

TABLE 1-4   Summary of Canadian Nurses Association Standards for Nursing Practice

Standard	Elements
I. Nursing practice requires that a conceptual model for nursing be the basis for the independent part of that practice.	1. Nurses are required to have a clear idea or conception of the distinct goal of nursing. 2. Nurses are required to have a clear idea or conception of the client. 3. Nurses are required to have a clear idea or conception of their role in response to the health needs of society. 4. Nurses are required to have a clear idea or conception of the source of client difficulty. 5. Nurses are required to have a clear idea or conception of the focus and modes of nursing intervention. 6. Nurses are required to have a clear idea or conception of the expected consequences of nursing activities.
II. Nursing practice requires the effective use of the nursing process.	1. Nurses are required to collect data in accordance with their conception of the client. 2. Nurses are required to analyze data collected in accordance with their conception of the goal of nursing, their role, and the source of client difficulty. 3. Nurses are required to plan their nursing actions based on the identified actual and potential client problems and in accordance with their conception of the focus and modes of intervention. 4. Nurses are required to perform nursing actions that implement the plan. 5. Nurses are required to evaluate all steps of the nursing process in accordance with their conceptual models for nursing.
III. Nursing practice requires that the helping relationship be the nature of the client-nurse interaction.	1. Nurses are required to increase the likelihood that the client will perceive the health service experience as understandable, manageable, and meaningful at the outset. 2. Nurses are required to set mutually agreed upon expectations as a means of increasing the likelihood that the client will perceive the health service experience as understandable, manageable, and meaningful. 3. Nurses are required to ensure a successful termination of the helping relationship.
IV. Nursing practice requires nurses to fulfill professional responsibilities.	1. Nurses are required to respect statutes and policies relevant to the profession and the practice setting. 2. Nurses are required to comply with the Code of Ethics of their profession. 3. Nurses are required to function as members of a health team.

Modified from Canadian Nurses Association: A definition of nursing practice standards for nursing practice, Ottawa, 1980, (revised, 1987) The Canadian Nurses Association.

TABLE 1-5 Employment Settings of Registered Nurses

Setting	United States* (%)	Canada† (%)
Hospital	66	73
Nursing homes	8	6.5
Community health	7	9
Physician/dentist offices	6	2.5
Schools	4	—
Nursing education	4	3
Occupational health	4	—
Other	4	3
Unknown	—	3

*Data from American Nurses' Association: Facts about nursing 84-85, Kansas City, Mo., 1985, The Association.
†Data from Statistics Canada and Canadian Nurses' Association, Nursing in Canada: 1985, Ottawa, 1986, Canadian Nurses' Association.

HOSPITALS AND OTHER INSTITUTIONS

More nurses are employed in hospitals than in any other practice setting. The Diagnostic Related Groups (DRGs) have resulted in shorter hospital stays. Thus clients are being discharged from hospitals sooner, frequently requiring continued nursing care in the home. Today's hospital-based professional nurse is not only adept in providing nursing care but is also able, through early discharge planning, to meet the home care needs of her clients.

Hospital acuity rates have also risen in the 1980s. This rising acuity has resulted in part from new disease entities and new forms of supportive therapy. Opportunistic infections associated with acquired immunodeficiency syndrome (AIDS), organ transplantation, and technological equipment used in the critical care setting are a few factors contributing to a higher percentage of critically ill clients in hospitals. Today's professional nurses are meeting these health care needs. In hospitals, nursing services operate 24 hours a day. Hospitals use different staffing patterns to meet the need for nursing care. Some hospitals have three 8-hour shifts, whereas other hospitals use two 12-hour shifts or three 10-hour shifts that overlap during the early morning, late afternoon, and nighttime.

The roles and responsibilities of nurses employed in hospitals vary because hospitals differ widely in size and organizational structure. Hospitals usually have many policies and regulations governing nursing activities, as well as other health care activities, and responsibilities tend to be clearly divided among nurses and other health care professionals.

Clients in hospitals generally require 24-hour nursing care. Hospitals provide acute, long-term, and rehabili-

tational care. The nurse in an acute care setting cares for clients with severe illnesses and more complex problems. These clients are usually more dependent and more seriously ill than in the past because of shorter periods of hospitalization (Department of Health and Human Services, 1982). As a result, nursing practice in acute care settings has become more specialized and complex. The skills and knowledge needed to practice in an acute care setting depend on the clinical area.

The rapid rise in the number of the elderly, clients with chronic illnesses, and clients with functional impairments has resulted in the growth of long-term care facilities. Most long-term care is provided in institutions such as chronic disease hospitals, psychiatric hospitals, and nursing homes. Nursing homes are the most common agencies providing in-house long-term care.

Rehabilitation institutions generally employ many types of health professionals. The goal of these institutions is to teach the disabled client how to achieve a maximal level of function and to teach the family how to help him reach that level.

In chronic care and rehabilitation institutions, as in hospitals, nurses generally have multiple roles and responsibilities. The extent of specialization and nurses' independence from other health care professionals varies from institution to institution.

COMMUNITY SETTINGS

Since 1974 the number of nurses employed in community-based practice settings has increased substantially. Rising costs of institutional care have created the need for community-based nursing services aimed at health promotion and disease prevention.

Nursing in community-based settings is concerned primarily with health promotion, maintenance, education and management, and coordination and continuity of care within the community. Community-based nurses try to determine the health needs of individuals, families, and communities and help clients cope with threats to health and with problems of illness. Whereas institutional health care focuses on the individual and his family, community-based nursing is directed toward the health of the community and the interaction of individuals within that community. A community can be a particular location, as in an urban or rural area, or a group of people related by occupation, school, or some other common interest or characteristic. Thus community-based nurses are employed in a variety of practice settings, including community and occupational health centers, schools, home health care agencies, and private practices.

COMMUNITY HEALTH CENTERS. A community health center offers comprehensive programs for health maintenance, promotion, education and management, and coordination of care within the community. Community health centers provide ambulatory care (care sought by clients who are able to come to the centers), as well as care within the home. Persons seeking health care at a community health center usually live near the center.

Nurses employed in these centers often work more independently than nurses working in institutional settings. Community health centers also employ other health professionals, but nurses generally provide most of the care. In some settings physicians are called in only when specific needs arise. Examples of community health centers are planned parenthood clinics and family care and mental health centers.

SCHOOLS. Community-based health services are common in schools and on college campuses. Nursing services include health education in disease prevention, health promotion, and sex education. In addition, nurses working in schools may provide care for students with nonemergency acute illnesses such as upper respiratory tract infections, influenza, and viruses. School nurses also make referrals for students and their families when additional, more specialized health care is needed.

OCCUPATIONAL HEALTH. Health services are provided by many companies in large office buildings and factories. Nursing care in these settings involves five areas. The nurse may develop programs aimed at increasing health and safety in the workplace by reducing occupational accidents, the risk of occupational disease, or the transmission of a contagious disease among the work force. The nurse may provide programs for health promotion, disease prevention, and health education to employees. The nurse also treats nonemergency acute illnesses and provides first aid. In emergency situations, such as heart attacks or trauma, the nurse gives emergency care and arranges transportation to a hospital. The nurse also refers employees to additional health resources.

HOME HEALTH CARE AGENCIES. A client often needs specific nursing care that can be given efficiently in the home. Some hospital-based nursing services have initiated their own institutional-based home health care services. Nurses in these agencies provide home-based nursing care to clients discharged from that particular institution. Other agencies providing home health care include visiting nurse associations, public health nursing agencies, and private home care agencies.

The nurse who functions in the home setting must also be skilled at teaching. Rising health care costs have limited the duration and frequency of visits. As a result the home health care nurse often teaches the client, family, or significant other to competently perform nursing

activities and self-care. In addition, caring for the client in the home environment requires the nurse to be flexible, resourceful, creative, and self-confident, as well as clinically competent (see Chapter 5).

OTHER SETTINGS

The settings previously described are the most common areas in which nurses are employed, but there are a number of other settings in which nurses' roles and responsibilities vary widely. A nurse employed in a physician's office, for example, may have little independent responsibility, but a nurse in sole practice or joint practice with other nurses or other health care professionals may provide care with much independence. Nurses are also employed in educational and research positions.

ROLES AND FUNCTIONS OF THE NURSE

Contemporary nursing requires that the nurse possess knowledge and skills in a variety of areas. In the past the principal role of nurses was to provide care and comfort as they carried out specific nursing functions, but changes in nursing have expanded the role to include increased emphasis on health promotion and illness prevention, as well as concern for the client as a whole. The contemporary nurse functions in the interrelated roles of care giver, decision maker, client advocate, manager, rehabilitator, comforter, communicator, and teacher.

Care Giver

As care giver, the nurse helps the client regain health through the healing process. Healing is more than just curing a specific disease, although treatment skills that promote physical healing are important to care givers. The nurse addresses the holistic health care needs of the client, including measures to restore the client's emotional and social well-being. The care giver helps clients and their families set goals and meet those goals with a minimal cost of time and energy.

Decision Maker

To provide effective care, nurses use decision-making skills throughout the nursing process. Before undertaking any nursing action, whether it is assessing the client's condition, giving care, or evaluating the results of care, the nurse plans the action by deciding the best approach for each client. In some situations the nurse makes these decisions alone or with the client and family and in other cases works with other nurses or health care professionals.

Protector and Client Advocate

As protector the nurse helps maintain a safe environment for the client and takes steps to prevent injury and to protect the client from possible adverse effects of diagnostic or treatment measures. Confirming that a client does not have an allergy to a medication to be administered in a hospital and providing immunization against disease in a community-based practice are examples of the nurse's protective role. In the role of client advocate, the nurse protects the client's human and legal rights and provides assistance in asserting those rights if the need arises. For example, the nurse may provide additional information for a client who is trying to decide whether to accept treatment. The nurse may also defend clients' rights in a general way by speaking out against policies or actions that might endanger clients' well-being or conflict with their rights.

Manager

The nurse acts as manager and coordinator by delegating some responsibility to and supervising other health care workers. Nurses must also manage their own time and the resources of the practice setting when providing care to several clients concurrently. The nurse coordinates the activities of others in the health care team such as nutritionists and physical therapists in managing the client's total care.

Rehabilitator

Rehabilitation is the process by which a person returns to maximal functioning after an illness, accident, or other disabling event. Many of these clients experience alterations that change their lives, and the nurse helps them adapt as fully as possible. Rehabilitative activities range from teaching a client how to walk with crutches to helping a client cope with severe exacerbations of chronic illness.

Comforter

The role of comforter, caring for the client as a person, is a traditional and historical one in nursing and has continued to be important as nurses have assumed new roles. Because nursing care must be directed to the whole person rather than simply the body, comfort and emotional support often help give the client strength to recover. While carrying out nursing activities, the nurse can provide comfort by demonstrating care for the client as an individual human being with unique feelings and needs. As comforter, the nurse should help the client reach therapeutic goals rather than encouraging emotional or physical dependence.

Communicator

The role of communicator is central to all other nursing roles. Without clear communication, it is impossible to give care effectively, make decisions with the client and family, protect the client from threats to well-being, coordinate and manage client care, assist the client in rehabilitation, offer comfort, or teach the client. Nursing involves almost constant communication with clients and families, other nurses and health care professionals, resource persons, and the community. The quality of communication is a critical factor in meeting the health needs of individuals, families, and communities.

Teacher

As teacher, the nurse explains to clients concepts and facts about health, demonstrates procedures such as self-care activities, determines that the client fully understands, reinforces learning or client behavior, and evaluates the client's progress in learning. Some kinds of teaching are unplanned and informal, as when a nurse responds to a client's question about a health issue in casual conversation. Other teaching activities may be planned and more formal, as when the nurse teaches a diabetic client how to administer self-injections. Teaching is involved in the full range of nursing activities directed toward helping the client achieve a high level of health. The nurse uses teaching methods that match the client's capabilities and needs and incorporates other resources, such as the family, in teaching plans. An additional form of teaching is through staff development. In staff development the nurse educator provides new knowledge to nurses employed in a particular agency.

Career Roles

The preceding roles and functions of the nurse are true of most nurses in most practice settings. Career roles, on the other hand, are specific employment positions. With increasing educational opportunities for nurses and the growth of nursing as a profession, along with a greater concern for job enrichment, nursing offers expanded roles and different kinds of career opportunities. These include the nurse as educator, clinical nurse specialist, nurse practitioner, certified nurse-midwife, anesthetist, administrator, and researcher. Additional nonclinical roles include risk managers, quality assurance nurses, and product consultants. Many physicians and other health care professionals, in addition to nurses themselves, support these expanded nursing roles (White, 1977).

NURSE EDUCATOR

Nurse educators work primarily in three areas, including schools of nursing, staff development departments of health care agencies, and client education departments. Nursing educators generally have a background in clinical nursing, which provides them with practical skills as well as theoretical knowledge. A faculty member in a school of nursing prepares students to perform as nurses. Nursing faculty members are responsible for teaching current nursing practice, as well as necessary skills in laboratory or clinical settings.

Nurse educators in staff development departments of health care institutions provide educational programs for nurses within their institution. These programs include orientation of new personnel, critical care nursing courses, and instruction about new equipment or procedures.

The primary focus of the nurse educator in an agency's department of client education is to teach ill or disabled clients and families how to provide care in the home. In most health care agencies, however, the budget does not permit a separate client education department. Therefore staff nurses usually incorporate education into a client's plan of care.

Nurse educators in nursing schools are usually required to have graduate nursing education. In addition, they generally have a specific clinical specialty and advanced clinical experience.

CLINICAL NURSE SPECIALIST

The clinical nurse specialist has a master's degree in nursing and expertise in a specialized area of practice. Clinical nurse specialists work in critical care, acute care, long-term care, and community health care agencies. In addition, a clinical nurse specialist may specialize in the management of a disease such as cancer, diabetes, or cardiovascular or pulmonary disease or in a specific field such as pediatrics or gerontology. The clinical nurse specialist functions as a clinician, educator, manager, consultant, and researcher within the area of practice to plan, or improve the quality of, nursing care for the client and the family.

NURSE PRACTITIONER

The nurse practitioner provides health care to clients, usually in an outpatient, ambulatory care, or community-based setting (Roy and Obloy, 1978; Molde and Diers, 1986). A 1986 study by Diers and Molde noted that nurse practitioners care for clients with complex problems and attend more to symptoms of nonpathological conditions, comfort, and comprehensiveness of care.

A significant percentage of primary care encounters extend beyond the boundaries of medicine and demand the expertise of the nurse. The nurse practitioner is able to establish a collaborative provider-client relationship (Kasch, 1986).

A nurse practitioner may work with clients in a specific group or with clients of all ages. Five major practitioner categories are adult, family, pediatric, obstetrics-gynecology, and geriatric nurse practitioner. A nurse practitioner should have the knowledge and skills necessary to detect and manage acute self-limited and chronic stable conditions. The nurse practitioner's educational preparation includes either a practitioner program or a master's degree in nursing.

An *adult nurse practitioner* (ANP) provides primary, ambulatory care to adults with a nonemergency acute or chronic illness. ANPs are usually employed in ambulatory care centers or outpatient clinics and work in collaboration with a primary physician.

A *family nurse practitioner* (FNP) provides primary, ambulatory care for families, usually in collaboration with a family care physician. The FNP meets the family's general health care needs, manages some illnesses by providing direct care, and guides or counsels the family as needed.

A *pediatric nurse practitioner* (PNP) provides health care to infants and children.

An *obstetrics-gynecology nurse practitioner* provides primary ambulatory care to women seeking obstetrical or gynecological health care. The nurse practitioner who is also a certified nurse-midwife may independently deliver infants.

A *geriatric nurse practitioner* (GNP) provides ambulatory or inpatient care to older adults. The GNP's activities include interventions for health maintenance, illness prevention, or health restoration.

CERTIFIED NURSE-MIDWIFE

A certified nurse-midwife (CNM) is educated in nursing and midwifery and is certified by the American College of Nurse-Midwives. The practice of nurse-midwifery involves providing independent care for women during normal pregnancy, labor, and delivery and for the newborn. It may include some gynecological services such as routine Pap smears, family planning, and treatment for minor vaginal infections. Nurse-midwives practice in conjunction with a health care agency that provides medical consultation, collaborative management, and referral.

NURSE ANESTHETIST

A nurse anesthetist is an RN who has received advanced training in an accredited program in anesthesiology. Nurse anesthetists provide surgical anesthesia under the guidance and supervision of an anesthesiologist, who is a physician with advanced knowledge of surgical anesthesia. Nurse anesthetists frequently administer anesthetics to clients undergoing minor surgery.

NURSE ADMINISTRATOR

A nurse administrator manages client care and the delivery of specific nursing services within a health care agency. This administrator may hold a middle management position, such as head nurse or supervisor, or an upper-level management position, such as assistant or associate director or director of nursing services. Middle management positions usually require at least a baccalaureate degree in nursing, and upper-level positions generally require a master's degree in nursing.

NURSE RESEARCHER

The nurse researcher investigates problems to improve nursing care and to further define and expand the scope of nursing practice. The nurse researcher may be employed in an academic setting or in an independent professional or community service agency. The minimum educational requirement is a graduate degree in nursing.

Health Care Team

In most practice settings the nurse works with other health care professionals to provide total care for clients. The health care team is comprised of four general types of professionals, including nurses, physicians, allied health professionals such as therapists and technicians, and other specialists such as social workers and chaplains. The involvement of many different persons in the client's health care, however, holds the risk of fragmenting care. Because nurses have the greatest opportunity to interact with all the other professionals in the health care team, they often have the role of coordinating and integrating services within the plan of care.

PHYSICIAN

A physician is a professional who has earned a degree of Doctor of Medicine (MD) or Doctor of Osteopathy (DO). The physician has completed a required curriculum, has had a specific period of postgraduate training, and has passed a licensing examination. A physician is licensed for the medical diagnosis and treatment of clients.

Most physicians specialize in diseases involving one body system (for example, a cardiologist specializes in heart diseases) or in one specific disease (for example, an oncologist specializes in cancer). Physicians may also specialize in surgery or in treating a certain age group.

Nurses work with physicians in many capacities. One nurse may work in a setting in which most nursing care depends on the physician's orders. An intensive care nurse may follow written guidelines that permit more independent nursing actions. A clinical nurse specialist or nurse practitioner may function in a collaborative capacity with a physician; for example, in preparing a client with newly diagnosed diabetes for discharge, the nurse and physician work together to teach the client and family about home care.

PHYSICIAN ASSISTANT

A physician assistant (PA) is trained in certain aspects of the practice of medicine to provide support to physicians. PAs practice in the United States but not in Canada and must work under the direction and supervision of a physician. PAs practice in hospitals, clinics, or private physicians' offices.

Nurses usually work with PAs in the same way they work with physicians. In some rural areas the PA is always present in the hospital or clinic and may assume some of the tasks of the physician.

ALLIED HEALTH PROFESSIONALS

THERAPIST. A physical therapist (PT) is licensed to assist in the examination, testing, and treatment of physically disabled or handicapped people through the use of special exercises, the application of heat and cold, the use of sonar waves, and other techniques. PTs usually receive their training in a 4-year college course leading to a bachelor of science degree in physical therapy. They practice in hospitals, clinics, rehabilitation centers, and community-based agencies.

An *occupational therapist* (OT) is licensed or certified to develop and use adaptive devices that help chronically ill or handicapped clients carry out activities of daily living. OTs usually receive education and training in a 4-year college program. Like PTs, they work in a variety of settings.

A respiratory therapist (RT) is licensed to deliver treatment that is designed to improve clients' ventilatory function or oxygenation. Educational and training programs for RTs vary. They may participate in 6-month training programs or educational programs in 4-year colleges. RTs are usually employed in institutional health care settings.

Nurses work with therapists in a collaborative capacity. Care initiated by therapists is frequently continued and evaluated by a nurse. Nurses and therapists together consider the client's progress and develop goals and discharge plans that include the client and family. In addition, nurses refer clients to therapists for further care. For example, a nurse caring for a person with severe pulmonary disease may refer the client to a PT to learn exercises for strengthening the upper arm muscles, to an OT to learn energy-saving techniques for activities of daily living, and to an RT for techniques to promote airway clearance.

PHARMACIST. A pharmacist is a licensed professional who formulates and dispenses medications. The pharmacist may practice only within a pharmacy or may be involved in client care conferences or in the development of medication administration systems (see Chapter 15). The pharmacist's education ranges from a bachelor of science degree to a doctorate in pharmacology.

Pharmacists practice in institutional and outpatient settings.

The pharmacist is a valuable resource for nurses. For example, the nurse can request information about new drugs from the pharmacist. The nurse must know the action, desired effect, correct dosage, and side effects of all drugs administered. If this information is not available in standard reference books such as textbooks or hospital formularies, the nurse should consult the pharmacist.

Pharmacists also provide information about which drugs are compatible and which can be mixed or administered together. In addition, pharmacists can tell the nurse which over-the-counter drugs may interact adversely with prescribed drugs so that this information can be incorporated into the discharge teaching plan.

SOCIAL WORKER. A social worker is trained to counsel clients and their families. Counseling services may include providing emotional support for a client and family during a severe or terminal illness, arranging placement in an extended care facility, and locating financial resources for clients. The social worker generally has a baccalaureate or master's degree in social work and are employed in every type of agency in the health care system.

Nurses frequently refer clients to social workers, and they work together to identify resources for meeting the client's present and future health care needs.

CHAPLAIN. Chaplains offer spiritual support and guidance to clients and their families and may be employed by an agency or institution or be provided by a church within the community. A client may request to see a chaplain, or the nurse may initiate a referral.

NURSING AS A PROFESSION

Professionalism

Nursing is not simply a collection of specific skills, and the nurse is not simply a person trained to perform specific tasks. Nursing has evolved into a profession.

There is no one factor that absolutely differentiates a job from a profession, but the difference is important in terms of how nurses practice. When we say a person acts "professionally," for example, we imply that the person is conscientious in actions, knowledgeable in the subject, and responsible to self and others.

Etzioni (1961) describes professions in terms of the following primary characteristics:

1. A profession requires an extended education of its members, in addition to a basic liberal foundation.

2. A profession has a theoretical body of knowledge leading to defined skills, abilities, and norms.
3. A profession provides a specific service.
4. Members of a profession have autonomy in decision making and practice.
5. The profession as a whole has a code of ethics for practice.

Nursing clearly shares, to some extent, each of these characteristics of a profession. Nursing is still evolving as a profession, however, and faces controversial issues as nurses strive for greater professionalism.

EDUCATION

As a profession, nursing requires that its members possess a significant education. The issue of standard-

---

Eight Premises for ANA's First Position Paper on Education for Nursing

- Nursing is a helping profession and, as such, provides services which contribute to the health and well-being of people.
- Nursing is of vital consequence to the individual receiving services; it fills needs which cannot be met by the person, by the family, or by other persons in the community.
- The demand for services of nurses will continue to increase.
- The professional practitioner is responsible for the nature and quality of all nursing care patients receive.
- The services of professional practitioners of nursing will continue to be supplemented and complemented by the services of nurse practitioners who will be licensed.
- Education for those in the health professions must increase in depth and breadth as scientific knowledge expands.
- In addition to those licensed as nurses, the health care of the public, in the amount and to the extent needed and demanded, requires the services of large numbers of health occupation workers to function as assistants to nurses. These workers are presently designated: nurses' aids, orderlies, assistants, attendants, etc.
- The professional association must concern itself with the nature of nursing practice, the means for improving nursing practice, the education necessary for such practice, and the standards for membership in the professional association.

From American Nurses' Association: A position paper: educational preparation for nurse practitioners and assistants to nurses, Kansas City, Mo., 1965, The Association.

ization of nursing education is a major controversy today. Most nurses agree that nursing education is important to practice and that it must respond to changes in health care created by scientific and technological advances. The ANA's 1965 position paper on nursing education emphasizes the role of education in the profession (see box on p. 25).

In 1984 the ANA described two levels of practice, the associate nurse and the professional nurse. The NLN also supports a proposal that associate and diploma graduates take one licensing examination. North Dakota was the first state to implement such a policy. In January 1987, North Dakota's Supreme Court ruled that the state board "has the authority . . . to direct that only associate and baccalaureate degree graduates may sit for practical and registered nursing license examinations respectively" (News, 1987).

THEORY

As nursing has emerged as a profession, nursing knowledge has been developed through nursing theories. Theoretical models serve as a framework for both nursing curricula and clinical practice. Nursing theories also lead to research that increases the scientific basis of nursing practice.

A theory is a way of understanding a reality, and in this general sense, all practicing nurses use the theories they have learned. Several of the approaches described previously in the section on definitions and philosophies are parts of fully developed nursing theories.

SERVICE

Nursing has always been a service profession, although in the past the service was usually viewed as a charitable one. Today, nursing is a vital and indispensable component of the health care delivery system.

AUTONOMY

Autonomy means that one is reasonably independent and self-governing in decision making and practice. It has been difficult for nurses to attain the degree of autonomy enjoyed by some other professionals. In the past, physicians, hospital administrators, and others in the health care delivery system have found nursing autonomy difficult to understand and support. Through clinical competence and greater educational preparation, however, nurses are increasingly taking on independent roles in nurse-run clinics, collaborative practice, and advanced nursing careers.

With increased autonomy come greater responsibility and accountability. Accountability means that the nurse is held responsible, professionally and legally, for the type and quality of nursing care provided. The nurse is accountable for keeping abreast of technical skills and knowledge needed to perform nursing care. The nursing profession itself regulates accountability through nursing audits and standards of practice.

CODE OF ETHICS

Nursing has a code of ethics, which defines the principles by which nurses function. In addition, nurses incorporate their own values and ethics into practice. Chapter 17 gives several examples of specific statements of nursing's code of ethics.

Professional Organizations

A professional organization is created to deal with issues of concern to those practicing in the profession. In North America the major professional nursing organizations are the American Nurses' Association (ANA), the Canadian Nurses' Association (CNA), and the National League for Nursing (NLN). The CNA and the ANA were formed in the late nineteenth century to improve standards of health and availability of health care, to foster high standards for nursing, and to promote the professional development and general and economic welfare of nurses. The ANA and CNA are part of the International Council of Nurses (ICN). The objectives of the ICN parallel those of the CNA and ANA in that the ICN promotoes national associations of nurses, improves standards of nursing practice, seeks a higher status for nurses, and provides an international power base for nurses.

The NLN is concerned with the improvement of nursing education, nursing service, and health care delivery in the United States. In Canada the Canadian Association of University Schools of Nursing and the Canadian Association of Practical and Nursing Assistants perform similar functions.

Nursing students also take part in organizations such as the National Student Nurses' Association (NSNA) in the United States and the Canadian Student Nurses' Association (CSNA) in Canada. These organizations consider issues of importance to nursing students and often cooperate in activities and programs with the professional organizations.

Some professional organizations are special interest groups focusing on specific areas such as critical care, nursing administration or research, or nurse-midwifery. The goal of these organizations is to improve the standards of practice, expand nursing roles, and foster the welfare of nurses within the specialty areas. In addition, professional organizations present education programs and publish journals. Some representative specialty organizations are discussed in the following paragraphs. Appendix A gives a comprehensive list of these organizations in the United States and Canada.

The Association of Operating Room Nurses (AORN) in the United States and the National Conference of

Operating Room Nurses in Canada are concerned with continuing education for operating room nurses, higher standards for operating room care, and increased research activities.

The Nurses' Association of the American College of Obstetricians and Gynecologists (NAACOG) includes Canadian and American nurses and promotes standards of practice in obstetrical and gynecological nursing, encourages professional growth for its members, and is an accrediting body for advanced programs in obstetrical and gynecological nursing.

The National Association of Pediatric Nurse Associates/Practitioners (NAPNAP) is a national organization for nurses prepared by training or experience to give primary care to children. NAPNAP works in conjunction with the American Academy of Pediatrics.

The American Association of Critical Care Nurses (AACN) is a national organization of nurses working in critical care areas. The AACN is concerned with nursing education, practice, and research as they involve critical care nursing.

SOCIETY'S INFLUENCE ON NURSING

Throughout history, nursing has responded to changes in other areas of society. The contemporary nursing profession continues to respond to the needs and influences of society as a whole. Nursing is currently responding to technological advances, demographic changes, the consumer movement, the increased emphasis on health promotion, and the women's and human rights movements.

Technological Advances

In recent years, scientific and technological advances have affected almost every aspect of life. Health care has changed in many ways, including the use of new equipment, new diagnostic tests and treatment measures, and new drugs. Nursing had adapted and will continue to respond to these changes with continuing education, inservice programs, and other educational approaches. Nursing is also uniquely concerned with the *human* side of technological advances. Society as a whole seems to accept technological advances in health care, but clients often experience problems related to technology. For example, dialysis machines have been used for many years to treat clients with kidney problems, but that fact does not lessen the emotional conflict a client may experience on learning dialysis is needed. As health care technology becomes increasingly complex and sophisticated, nurses have the growing role of helping clients adjust to the use of technology in their care.

Demographic Changes

Demographic changes affect the population as a whole. Changes that have influenced health care in recent decades include the population shift from rural areas to urban centers, the increasing life span, the higher incidence of chronic, long-term illness, and the increased incidence of diseases such as alcoholism and lung cancer. Nursing as a profession responds to such changes by exploring new methods for providing care, by changing educational emphases, by establishing practice standards in new areas, and so on. The individual nurse also responds to demographic changes in the population served by the practice setting to better meet the changing health care needs of clients.

Consumer Movement

The consumer movement is a heightened awareness of the value and costs of products and services; in short, consumers want their money's worth. Health care in general has been influenced by the consumer movement in ways as diverse as new kinds of health care agencies such as health maintenance organizations, new forms of health insurance, and concern about the rising costs of health care. Also, consumers are more knowledgeable about health and illness and are becoming more vocal in their desire for high-quality care. Because nurses generally interact more with clients than other health care professionals, they must often answer questions about the quality and costs of health care. Health care consumers are also more aware of their rights as clients, and the nurse supports these rights in the role of client advocate.

Health Promotion

Related to the consumer movement is a greater emphasis in society on health promotion and illness prevention. Exercise and nutrition are subjects that interest an increasing number of people. Nursing has responded to this greater concern for health promotion in many ways, from programs in the community to specific health promotion and teaching activities for clients in hospitals and other health care settings. Health promotion activities are a part of many of the roles of nurses, including those of care giver, client advocate, rehabilitator, communicator, and teacher.

Women's Movement

The women's movement has brought about many changes in society as women have increasingly sought economic, political, occupational, and educational equality. Nursing is responding in two ways. Because most nurses are women, they are increasingly asserting their equal rights as human beings, as employees, and as health care professionals. The women's movement has encouraged nurses to seek greater autonomy and responsibility in providing care. The women's movement has caused women clients to seek more responsibility for and control over their bodies, their health, and their lives in general. As women become more aware of their own needs and unique qualities, they seek health care that can help them meet those needs.

Human Rights Movement

Like the women's movement, the human rights movement is changing the way society views the rights of *all* its members, including minorities, clients with terminal illness, pregnant women, and the elderly. Many groups have special health care needs, and nursing has responded by respecting all clients as individuals with a right to good care and with basic human rights. Nurses advocate the rights of all clients, but they have also recognized the special needs of some groups and thus have created bills of rights for dying, hospitalized, and pregnant clients, as well as other groups, to ensure that quality care is provided without sacrificing the client's rights.

TRENDS IN NURSING

This chapter has emphasized that nursing is not a static, unchanging profession but is continually growing and evolving as society changes, as health care emphases and methods change, as the life-styles of clients change— and as nurses themselves change. To speak of nursing at all is to speak of nursing as it is at a given time, and in this sense, this chapter is about trends in nursing.

The current philosophies and definitions of nursing demonstrate the holistic trend in nursing—to address the whole person in all dimensions, in health and illness, as an individual but also in interaction with the family and community. Nursing continues to draw on the social sciences and other fields as the focus of nursing care expands.

One trend in nursing education is the growing number of students receiving basic nursing education in community colleges and universities. Professional nursing organizations continue to stress the importance of education for nurses seeking new and expanded roles.

Nursing practice trends include a growing variety of settings in which nurses practice greater independence. Nurses continue to gain autonomy and respect as members of the health care team. Nursing roles continue to expand with the broadening focus of nursing care. The clinical ladder and new career roles also represent current trends in nursing practice.

Trends in nursing as a profession include the growing emphasis on those aspects of nursing characterizing it as a profession, including education, theory, service, autonomy, and ethical codes. The activities of nursing's professional organizations reflect all the trends in nursing education and practice. Finally, all the influences of society on nursing also reflect trends in contemporary nursing.

Two other trends remain to be discussed: the increasing political influence of nursing and nursing's influence on health care policy and practice.

Political Influence of Professional Nursing

Historically, nurses' involvement in politics has been limited. Although individual nurses such as Florence Nightingale and Margaret Sanger have influenced decision making in such areas as sanitation, nutrition, and birth control, nurses have accomplished less as a group. The recent women's movement, however, has inspired nurses to address health care issues. In addition, as more college-educated people enter the profession, they bring to nursing the activism and involvement of the university campuses (Deloughery and Gebbie, 1975).

Political power is the ability to influence or persuade an individual holding a government office to exert the power of that office to affect a desired outcome (Rogge, 1987). Traditionally, nurses have been uncomfortable with politics because the majority of nurses are women, and politics has been male dominated. They are also unaware of historical precedents established by nurses in the political arena and because they are not politically astute, lack the political education to successfully compete in politics (Mason and Talbott, 1985).

Nurses' involvement in politics is receiving greater emphasis in nursing curricula, in the professional organizations, and in health care settings (Stanhope and Belcher, 1982). Professional nursing organizations have employed lobbyists to urge state legislatures and the U.S. Congress to improve the quality of health care. Kalisch and Kalisch (1982) note that the ANA

works for the improvement of health standards and the availability of health care services for all people; fosters high standards of nursing, stimulates and promotes the professional development of nurses, and advances their economic and general welfare. The purposes are unrestricted by considerations of nationality, race, creed, lifestyle, color, sex, or age.

The ANA employs registered nurses as lobbyists at the federal level, and state nursing organizations also hire lobbyists and legislative specialists to work on state nursing issues and assist with federal efforts. Finally, lobbyists working on behalf of nursing are employed in

Washington by professional interest groups such as the American Federation of Teachers, NLN, American College of Nurse Midwives, American Public Health Association, and American Association of Colleges of Nursing. The overall political purposes of these groups are to remove financial barriers to health care, to increase the quality of nursing care available, to increase economic rewards to nurses, and to expand professional nursing roles (Aiken, 1982).

In addition, individual nurses work to effect change in the health care system. According to Mullane (1975), if nurses become serious students of social needs, activists in influencing policy to meet those needs, and generous contributors of time and money to nursing and their organizations and to candidates working for universal good health care, then the future is bright indeed.

Nursing's Influence on Health Care Policy and Practice

Nurses are still on the outer edge of the health care power system, perhaps partly because the public has assumed that nurses, most of whom are women and thus traditionally viewed as followers, do not need representation on advisory committees or boards. In addition, many nurses seem to be content with "over-the-fence" methods, offering assistance individually on specific issues but avoiding political involvement (Deloughery and Gebbie, 1975).

Political activism and commitment are a part of professionalism, however, and politics are an important aspect of the delivery of health care. Therefore nurses should not view politics as "dirty business" but as a reality that includes the arts of influence, compromise, and social interaction. Nurses have been involved in a different sort of politics in schools of nursing and in health care settings when seeking additional resources,

more self-direction, and accountability with authority. The skills gained in such experiences can be transferred to the politics of health care policymaking.

As long as nurses avoid involvement in health care policy and practice, misinformed outsiders can attempt to impose their will on nursing and nursing practice. Nonnursing groups, often led by other health care providers, have made attempts to impose institutional licensure, mandatory continuing education, curtailment of advanced nursing practice, and other constraints on a profession that should have its own voice in decisions made in these and numerous other areas affecting the quality of nursing care. Although nurses have often successfully prevented infringement on the profession's self-governance, the future of nursing requires that nurses individually and collectively seek a greater influence on health care policies affecting nursing practice.

SUMMARY

Nursing as a profession is complex and multifaceted. The nurse's role includes that of care giver, teacher, counselor, advocate, and researcher. This diverse education prepares the nurse to function in a multidimensional role. The nurse needs a theoretical or conceptual model from which to practice in a variety of settings. The professional growth and development of today's nurse requires information on research and on how to carry out a research study, as well as on the utilization of findings in a clinical practice setting. The standards of practice set forth by professional nursing associations provide guidelines for competent, safe, and professional practice. Historical origins of nursing have assisted today's professionals in their development and future needs.

KEY CONCEPTS

✓ Nursing is an essential part of society, out of which it has grown and with which it evolves.

✓ Nursing has responded to the health needs of society, which were influenced by economic, social, and cultural variables of a specific era.

✓ Formalized education programs for professional nursing were established in the nineteenth century by Florence Nightingale.

✓ The growth of nursing and nursing education in the United States was stimulated by the Civil War.

✓ The Canadian Nurses' Association and the American Nurses' Association were established in the late nineteenth century.

✓ The opening of the Henry Street Settlement by Lillian Wald and Mary Brewster marked the expansion of nursing into the community setting.

✓ Nursing education became affiliated with universities early in the twentieth century.

✓ Expansion of nursing into the military occurred in the early twentieth century, and the development of specialty nursing organizations began in the 1950s and has continued to the present.

✓ The Lysaught Report (1970) emphasized the need for clarification of nursing roles and responsibilities, greater financial support for nurses, and more career opportunities.

✓ Nursing definitions reflect changes in the practice of nursing and help bring about changes by identifying the domain of nursing practice and guiding research, practice, and education.

✓ Conceptual and theoretical nursing models provide knowledge to improve practice, guide research and nursing curricula, and identify the domain and goals of nursing practice.

✓ Peplau's nursing theory focuses on interpersonal relationships that people establish as they pass through various developmental stages.

✓ Henderson's theory involves 14 basic needs of the whole person through which the nurse assists "the individual sick or well in the performance of those activities contributing to health or its recovery . . . that he would perform unaided if he had the necessary strength, will, or knowledge."

✓ Abdellah's theory emphasizes the delivery of nursing care for the whole person as an individual.

✓ Levine's theory views the client as an integrated whole interacting with and adapting to his environment with the conservation of energy as a primary concern.

✓ Johnson's theory focuses on the client's ability to adapt to his illness and the impact of actual or potential stressors on his adaptation. The client's adaptation is based on basic needs in terms of seven categories of behavior.

✓ Rogers' theory approaches the client as a whole person ("unitary man") who is continually evolving and changing.

✓ Orem's theory emphasizes the self-care needs of the client, in which the goals of nursing care are to help the client care for himself.

✓ King's theory focuses on the relationship between the client and the nurse. This relationship is the vehicle for the nursing process in which the nurse uses communication to help the client adapt to his illness.

✓ Travelbee emphasizes nursing as an interpersonal process involving the nurse-client relationship and the client's ability to cope with the experience of illness.

✓ Neuman's theory assists clients to attain and maintain a maximal level of total wellness.

✓ Roy's theory views the client as an adaptive system, in which the need for nursing care developed when the client was unable to adapt to internal and external environmental demands.

✓ Educational preparation of the registered nurse can be through one of three programs in the United States or one of two programs in Canada.

✓ A license for a registered nurse in each state or province is granted after a candidate has completed a prescribed course of study in an accredited program and passed a licensing examination.

✓ Graduate nursing programs prepare nurse clinicians to improve nursing care through the advancement of nursing theory and sciences.

✓ Continuing education programs can be accredited by the American Nurses' Association or the state board of nursing.

✓ The clinical ladder is a mechanism for career mobility that incorporates opportunities for advancement in nursing through either an administrative or a clinical track.

✓ Nursing standards provide the guidelines for implementing and evaluating nursing care.

✓ Rapid rise in the elderly population, chronic illnesses, and functional impairments has resulted in an increased number of long-term care facilities.

✓ Community-based agencies focus primarily on health promotion, maintenance, education and management, as well as coordination and continuity of care within the community.

✓ The multiple roles and functions of the nurse include care giver, decision maker, client advocate, manager, rehabilitator, comforter, communicator, and teacher.

✓ Specific employment positions include educator, clinical nurse specialist, nurse practitioner, certified nurse-midwife, nurse anesthetist, administrator, and researcher.

✓ The health care team is multidisciplinary and may include a physician, physician assistant, physical therapist, ocupational therapist, respiratory therapist, pharmacist, social worker, and chaplain.

✓ Nursing is a profession in which there are established educational preparation for the nurse, nursing theory, a service provided, autonomy, and a code of ethics.

✓ Professional nursing organizations deal with issues of concern to specialist groups within the nursing profession.

✓ Changes in society, such as increased technology, new demographic patterns, consumerism, health promotion, and the women's and human rights movements, have led to changes in nursing.

✓ Nurses are becoming more politically sophisticated and, as a result, are able to increase nursing's influence on health care policy and practice.

REFERENCES

Abdellah, FG, et al.: Patient-centered approaches to nursing, New York, 1960, Macmillan Publishing Co.

Aiken, LH: The impact of federal health policy on nursing. In Aiken, LH, editor: Nursing in the 80's: crises, opportunities, challenges, Philadelphia, 1982, J.B. Lippincott Co.

American Association of Colleges of Nursing: Essentials of college and university education for professional nursing: a final report, Washington, D.C., 1986, American Association of College of Nursing.

American Nurses' Association: Educational preparation for nurse practitioners, Am J Nurs 65(12):106, 1965.

American Nurses' Association: Statement on graduate education in nursing, New York, 1969, The Association.

American Nurses' Association: Standards for continuing education in nursing, Kansas City, Mo., 1975, The Association.

American Nurses' Association: Nursing and social policy statement, Kansas City, Mo., 1980, The Association.

American Nurses' Association: Career ladders: an approach to professional productivity and job satisfaction, American Nurses' Association, Kansas City, Mo., Pub. No. N5-27, 1984, The Association.

American Nurses' Association Committee on Education: A position paper, New York, 1965, The Association.

Anderson, MI, and Denyes, MJ: A ladder for clinical advancement in nursing practice, J Nurs Adm 5(2):16, 1975.

Benner, P: From novice to expert: excellence and power in clinical nursing practice, Menlo Park, Calif., 1984, Addison-Wesley Publishing Co., Inc.

Chinn, PL, and Jacobs, MK: Theory and nursing: a systematic approach, ed. 2, St. Louis, 1987, The C.V. Mosby Co.

Cohen, IB: Florence Nightingale, Sci Am 250(128):137, 1984.

Colavecchio, R, Tescher, B, Scalgi, C: A clinical ladder for nursing practice, J Nurs Admin 5:54, 1974.

Deloughery, GL, and Gebbie, KM: Political dynamics: impact on nurses and nursing, St. Louis, 1975, The C.V. Mosby Co.

Department of Health and Human Services: The registered nurse population: an overview, DHHS Pub. No. HRS-P-00-83-1, 1982, Washington, D.C., U.S. Government Printing Office.

Dolan, JA, et al.: Nursing in society: a historical perspective, ed. 15, Philadelphia, 1983, W.B. Saunders Co.

Donahue, MP: Nursing: the finest art, an illustrated history, St. Louis, 1985, The C.V. Mosby Co.

Etzioni, A: The semiprofessionals and their organizations, New York, 1961, The Free Press.

Henderson, V: The nature of nursing, Am J Nurs 64:62, 1964.

Henderson, V: The nature of nursing, New York, 1966, Macmillan Publishing Co.

Huey, FL: Looking at ladders, Am J Nurs 82:1520, 1982.

Institute of Medicine, Division of Health Care Services: Nursing and nursing education: public policies and private actions, Washington, D.C., 1983, National Academy Press.

International Council of Nurses: Code for nurses, Geneva, 1973, The Council.

Johnson, DE: Theory in nursing: borrowed and unique, Nurs Res 11:206, 1968.

Kalish, BJ, and Kalish, PA: Politics of nursing, Philadelphia, 1982, J.B. Lippincott Co.

Kasch, CR: Establishing a collaborative nurse-patient relationship: a distince focus of nursing action of primary care, Image: J Nurs Sch 18:44, 1986.

Kelly, LY: Dimensions of professional nursing, New York, 1981, Macmillan Publishing Co.

King, IM: Toward a theory for nursing, New York, 1971, John Wiley & Sons, Inc.

Levine, MC: An introduction to clinical nursing, ed. 2, Philadelphia, 1973, F.A. Davis Co.

Lysaught, JP: An abstract for action, New York, 1970, McGraw-Hill Book Co.

Marriner, A: Nursing theorists and their work, St. Louis, 1986, The C.V. Mosby Co.

Mason, DJ, and Talbott, SW: Political action handbook for nurses, Menlo Park, Calif., 1985, Addison-Wesley Publishing Co., Inc.

Meleis, AI: Theoretical nursing: development and progress, Philadelphia, 1985, J.B. Lippincott Co.

Molde, S, and Diers, D: Nurse practitioner research: selected literature review and research agenda, Nurs Res 34(6):362, 1986.

Mullane, MK: Nursing care and the political arena, Nurs Outlook 23:699, 1975.

National Commission on Nursing: Source book, National Commission on Nursing, Chicago, 1983, American Hospital Association.

Neuman, B: The Neuman systems model: application to nursing education and practice, New York, 1982, Appleton-Century-Crofts.

Neuman, BM, and Young, RJ: A model for teaching total person approach to patient problems, Nurs Res 21:264, 1972.

News: North Dakota's High Court frees nursing board to enforce its BSN requirement for RN licensure, Am J Nurs 87(3):372, 1987.

Nightingale, F: Notes on nursing: what it is and what it is not, London, 1860, Harrison & Sons.

Orlando, IJ: The dynamic nurse-patient relationship: function, process, and principles, New York, 1961, G.P. Putnam's Sons.

Orem, DE: Nursing: concepts of practice, New York, 1971, McGraw-Hill Book Co.

Parse, RR: Man-living-health: theory of nursing, New York, 1981, John Wiley & Sons, Inc.

Parse, RR: Nursing Science: major paradigms, theories, and critiques, Philadelphia, 1987, W.B. Saunders Co.

Peplau, HE: Interpersonal relations in nursing, New York, 1952, G.P. Putnam's Sons.

Raab, DM: Nursing in Canada: perserverance in practice, Health Care, p. 27, September 1985.

Rogers, ME: An introduction to the theoretical basis of nursing, Philadelphia, 1979, F.A. Davis Co.

Rogge, MM: Nursing and politics: a forgotten legacy, Nurs Res 36(1):26, 1987.

Roy, C: The Roy adaptation model. In Riehl, JP, and Roy, C, editors: Conceptual models for nursing practice, New York, 1980, Appleton-Century-Crofts.

Roy, C, and Obloy, SM: The practitioner movement: toward a science of nursing, Am J Nurs 79:1698, 1978.

Shryock, RH: The history of nursing: an interpretation of the social and medical factors involved, Philadelphia, 1959, W.B. Saunders Co.

Silverstein, NG: Lillian Wald at Henry Street 1893-1895, ANS 7(2):1, 1985.

Stanhope, M, and Belcher, AE: Political imperatives for nursing practice. In Lancaster, J, and Lancaster, W, editors: Concepts for advanced nursing practice, St. Louis, 1982, The C.V. Mosby Co.

Stevens, BJ: Nursing theory: analysis, application, evaluation, ed. 2, Boston, 1984, Little, Brown & Co., Inc.

Torres, G: Theoretical foundations of nursing, Norwalk, Conn., 1986, Appleton-Century-Crofts.

Travelbee, J: Interpersonal agents of nursing, ed. 2, Philadelphia, 1971, F.A. Davis Co.

Wheeler, CE: The American Journal of Nursing and the socialization of a profession, 1900-1920, ANS 7(2):20, 1985.

White, S: The expanded role for nurses, Nurs '77 7:90, 1977.

Wiedenbach, E: Clinical nursing: a helping art, New York, 1964, Springer Publishing Co., Inc.

Woodham-Smith, C: Florence Nightingale, New York, 1983, McGraw-Hill Book Co.

Zimmer, MJ: Rationale for a ladder for clinical advancement, J Nurs Adm 5:18, 1975.

Research Articles

Hefferin, EA, and Kleinknecht, MK: Development of the nursing career preference inventory, Nurs Res 35(1):44, 1986.

Holzemer, W: Doctoral education in nursing: an assessment of quality, 1979-1984, Nurs Res 36(2):110, 1987.

McCloskey, JC, and McCain, BE: Satisfaction, commitment, and professionalism of newly employed nurses, Image: J Nurs Sch 19(1):20, 1987.

ADDITIONAL READINGS

Canadian Nurses Association: Nursing in Canada: 1985, Ontario, Canada, 1986, Canadian Nurses' Association.

Crosby, LJ, Facteau, LM, and Donley, R: Priorities for nurse training act legislation: a national survey of nursing deans, Image: J Nurs Sch 15(4):107, 1983.

Curran, CR, Minnick, G, and Moss, J: Who needs nurses? Am J Nurs 87:444, 1987.

Dennis, KE, and Prescott, PA: Florence Nightingale: yesterday, today, and tomorrow, ANS 7(2):66, 1985.

Dickoff, J, and James, P: A theory of theories: a position paper, Nurs Res 17(3):197, 1968.

Diers, D, Hamman, A, and Molde, S: Complexity of ambulatory care: nurse practitioner and physician caseloads, Nurs Res 35(5):310, 1986.

Fairman, JA: Sources and references for research in nursing history, Nurs Res 36(1):56, 1987.

Fawcett, J: Analysis and evaluation of conceptual models of nursing, Philadelphia, 1984, F.A. Davis Co.

Johnson, DE: The behavioral system for nursing. In Riehl, JP, and Roy, C, editors: Conceptual models for nursing practice, ed. 2, New York, 1980, Appleton-Century-Crofts.

King, IM: A theory for nursing: system, concepts, process, New York, 1971, John Wiley & Sons, Inc.

Knox, SL: A clinical advancement program, J Nurs 10(7):29, 1980.

Leininger, M: Conference on the nature of science and nursing, Nurs Res 17(6):484, 1968.

Leininger, MM: Transcultural nursing: concepts, theories and practices, New York, 1978, John Wiley & Sons, Inc.

Leininger, MM: Caring: a central focus of nursing and health care services, Nurs Health Care 1(3):135, 1980.

Leininger, MM: Transcultural care, diversity and universality: a theory of nursing, Thorofore, N.J., 1985, Slack, Inc.

Newman, MA: Nursing's theoretical evolution, Nurs Outlook 20(7):449, 1972.

Parse, RR, Cogne, AB, and Smith, MJ: Nursing research: qualitative methods, Bowie, Md., 1985, Brady.

Patterson, JG, and Zderad, LT: Humanistic nursing, New York, 1976, John Wiley & Sons, Inc.

Roy, C: Adaptation: a conceptual framework for nursing, Nurs Outlook 18(3):42, 1970.

Roy, C: Introduction to nursing: an adaptation model, ed. 2, Englewood Cliffs, N.J., 1984, Prentice Hall, Inc.

Roy, C, and Roberts, S: Theory construction in nursing: an adaptation model, Englewood Cliffs, N.J., 1981, Prentice Hall, Inc.

Shamansky, SL, Schilling, LS, and Holbrook, TL: Determining the market for nurse practitioner services: the New Haven experience. Nurs Res 34(4):242, 1985.

Silva, MC, and Rothbart, D: An analysis of changing trends in philosophies of science on nursing theory development and testing, ANS 6(2):1, 1984.

Stevens, BJ: Nursing theory: analysis, application, evaluation, ed. 2, Boston, 1984, Little, Brown & Co., Inc.

Taylor, MS, and Covaleski, MA: Predicting nurse's turnover and internal transfer behavior, Nurs Res 34(4):237, 1985.

Walker, LO: Toward a clearer understanding of the concept of nursing theory, Nurs Res 20(5):428, 1971.

Watson, J: Nursing: human science and human care, New York, 1985, Appleton-Century-Crofts.

Watson, J, et al.: A model of caring: an alternative health care model for nursing practice and research, Pub. NP-59-3M 8179 190, Kansas City, Mo., 1979, American Nurses' Association.

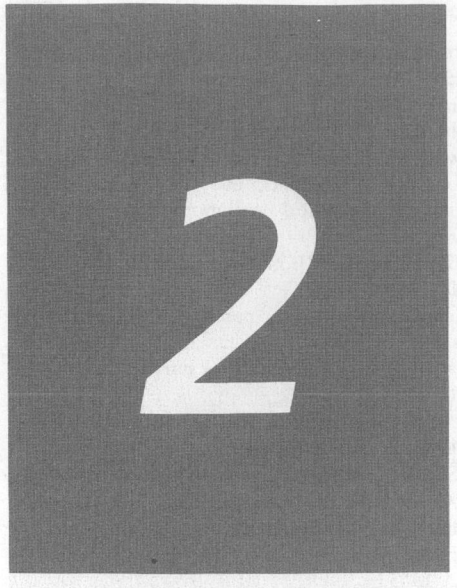

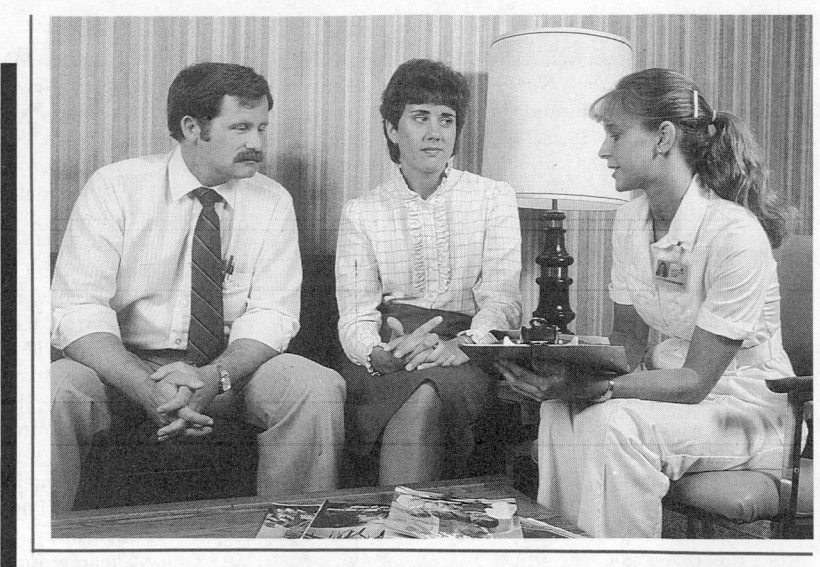

OBJECTIVES

Mastery of concept in this chapter will enable the student to:

- Define the key terms listed.
- Discuss health definition and concepts.
- Discuss the health-illness continuum model, the high-level wellness model, the agent-host-environment model, the health belief model, the evolutionary-based model, and the health promotion model.
- Describe health promotion and illness prevention activities.
- List and discuss the three levels of preventive care.
- List and explain four kinds of risk factors.
- Describe variables influencing a person's health beliefs and practices.
- Describe variables influencing illness behavior.
- State and discuss the stages of illness behavior.
- Describe the impact of illness on the client and family.
- Discuss the nurse's role for clients in health and illness.

KEY TERMS

Active Strategies of Health Promotion
Acute Illness
Agent
Anxiety
Body Image
Chronic Illness
Denial
External Environment
Health
Health Behavior
Health Belief Model
Health Promotion
Health-Illness Continuum
Host
Illness
Illness Behavior
Illness Prevention
Internal Environment
Passive Strategies of Health Promotion
Primary Nursing
Primary Prevention
Secondary Prevention
Tertiary Prevention

Health and Illness

In the past, most individuals and societies have viewed good health or wellness as the opposite or absence of disease. This attitude toward health remains popular with many health professionals. It assumes that people are normally healthy and that people with disease are unhealthy and in an abnormal state. This simple, either-or attitude can be easily applied: a person is considered either healthy or ill, with no range in between. Of course, this attitude ignores states of health between disease and good health, and it emphasizes the physiological dimension of a person, considering only the body as either ill or healthy and overlooking the complex interrelationships between a person's physiological, emotional, intellectual, sociocultural, developmental, and spiritual dimensions.

Today's health and medical care services are shaped largely by the way health professionals define health and illness (Balog, 1982). Health professional's definitions of health and illness serve as a basis for determinations about the types and quality of health care services that should be provided. Not all health care professionals, however, agree about how these concepts should be defined.

The definition of good health or wellness adhered to by health care workers may not always correspond with a client's concept, which is unique to each person. An individual's life-style, cultural background, and economic and psychosocial status influence personal beliefs about health and practices related to health care. Nurses therefore need to be aware of variables influencing a client's health beliefs and practices in order to provide individualized care for the client.

People also have different attitudes toward illness and

react to it in different ways. Medical sociologists call the reaction to illness *illness behavior.* The nurse needs to understand how clients react to illness and how illness affects clients and their families. Illness can have an enormous impact on a client and the family, and the nurse who recognizes this impact and the factors involved can take steps to minimize the effects and assist the client and family in maintaining or returning to the highest level of functioning.

The nurse also identifies actual and potential risk factors predisposing a person or group to illness. Nursing actions involving health promotion and illness prevention assist the client not only in regaining optimal health but also in maintaining and enhancing the existing level of health.

The nurse assesses the whole person, including the physical, intellectual, emotional, developmental, and spiritual dimensions, as well as interactions with family and community. To best assist clients in health maintenance and promotion, illness prevention, and adaptation to changes illness produces in every dimension of functioning, the nurse must understand clients' psychosocial, cultural, and economic backgrounds, as well as physical conditions.

DEFINITION OF HEALTH

Good health or wellness is not merely the absence of illness. Defining good health is difficult because every person has his own concept. Health is not an acquired piece of scientific knowledge, nor is it a thing, a part of the body, or a function of the body, like hearing, seeing, or breathing. Health is a state of being that people define in relation to their own values.

No universal definition of health is acceptable to all health care workers and to consumers. The World Health Organization (WHO) defines health as a "state of complete physical, mental and social well-being, not merely the absence of disease or infirmity" (1974). Yet this definition of health has not been totally accepted. Those opposed to it believe that, for underdeveloped countries and for persons of low economic status, the WHO definition is unrealistic because many people would not be considered healthy (Fuchs, 1974). In addition, with the WHO definition, it is difficult to determine scientifically who is or is not healthy or to determine the point at which a person becomes ill rather than healthy (Breslow, 1972).

Thus it is difficult for health care professionals to agree on a clear, workable definition. A related issue is the unique attitude of each client toward health, which involves much more than the absence of illness or disability. Each client's concept is very important to the

nurse in helping the client identify and reach health goals, which may be different for all clients.

Nurses also have an attitude toward health. They plan care for clients in order to help meet their health care needs and achieve maximal independence. Nurses plan care based on a definition of health and accepted standards of health care. Health in its broadest sense is a dynamic state in which the individual adapts to changes in internal and external environments to maintain a state of well-being in all dimensions. The internal environment includes many factors influencing a person's health, including genetic and psychological variables, intellectual and spiritual dimensions, and the physiological and physical disease processes. The external environment includes factors outside the person that may influence health, including the physical environment, social relationships and economic variables. Because both environments may continually change, the person must adapt in order to maintain a state of well-being.

"Health" and "illness" therefore must be defined in terms of the individual. Health can include conditions that the client or nurse may have previously considered to be illness. Health is also closely related to an individual's life-style, and some illnesses can be considered to be the result of that life-style. A client who reacts continually to stress may have frequent gastrointestinal upsets. In such a case, treating the condition may have no effect on the pattern of the person's behavior, and he may not even consider a gastrointestinal upset an illness at all if it seems a "normal" or usual aspect of his life. A rigid attitude toward health and illness by a health professional may have little meaning for such a person's future health, since the whole person is not considered.

Therefore, because the attitudes of client and nurse toward health may not coincide exactly, the nurse works with the client and family throughout the nursing process to mutually establish the client's goals of care and to plan individualized care.

MODELS OF HEALTH AND ILLNESS

A model is a theoretical way of understanding a complex phenomenon. Because health and illness are complex concepts, it helps to use models of health to understand the relationships between them and attitudes toward health and health practices.

Health beliefs are a person's ideas, convictions, and attitudes about health and illness. Health beliefs may be based on factual information or misinformation, common sense or common myths, or reality or false expectations. Health behaviors usually result from health beliefs, and can therefore positively or negatively affect health. Positive health behaviors are activities related to maintaining, attaining, or regaining good health, and preventing illness. Common positive health behaviors include immunizations, proper sleep patterns, and adequate exercise, diet, and nutrition. Negative health behaviors include practices actually or potentially detrimental to health, such as smoking, drug or alcohol abuse, poor diet, and refusal to take necessary medications.

To understand a client's health behaviors and beliefs so effective health care can be provided, nurses have developed health models. These models allow them to understand and predict a client's health behavior, including the use of health services and compliance with recommended therapies.

A client's health beliefs depend on many factors, including perception of the level of health, modifying factors such as demographics, personality, and perception of benefits resulting from positive health behaviors. Health models usually consider these components. The following health models are described in this chapter: the health-illness continuum, the high-level wellness model, the agent-host-environment model, and health belief model, the evolutionary-based model, and the health promotion model. The first three models describe the relationships between health and illness, and the fourth explains and predicts a client's health behavior. The last two models were developed by nurses and focus on health promotion.

Health-Illness Continuum

According to the health-illness continuum model, health is a dynamic state that continually alters as a person adapts to changes in the internal and external environments to maintain a state of physical, emotional, intellectual, social, developmental, and spiritual well-being. Illness is an abnormal process in which the functioning of a person is diminished or impaired in one or more dimensions, compared with the person's previous condition. Because both health and illness are relative qualities, existing in varying degrees or levels, it is more accurate to consider health and illness in terms of a scale or continuum rather than an either-or, absolute state (Fig. 2-1).

A nurse can locate a client's level of health at any point on the health-illness continuum. High-level wellness and severe illness are the opposite ends of the continuum, with a full range of states in between. A client's risk factors (variables in any dimension making illness more likely) are important in identifying the level of health. Risk factors include variables related to genetic and physiological factors, age, life-style, and environment (see later sections in this chapter). As a person progresses through the developmental stages of life, certain risk factors are more common than others. An adolescent, for example, is more likely than an adult to experience stresses related to body image and self-concept, and an older adult is more likely than a child to

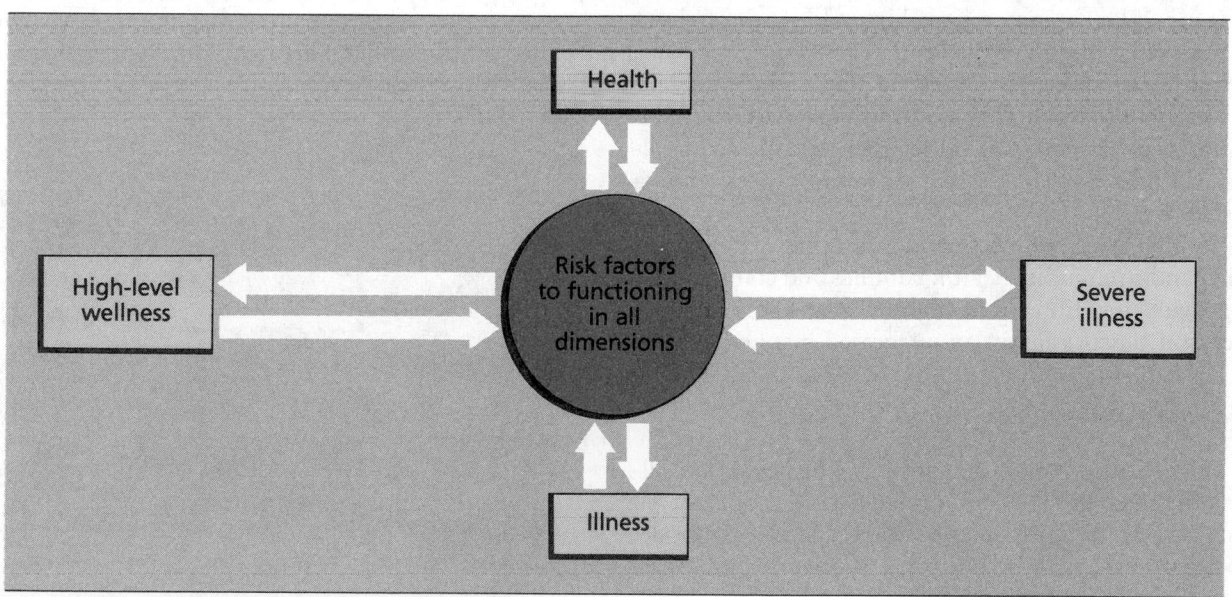

Fig. 2-1 The health-illness continuum, ranging from high-level wellness to severe illness, provides a method of identifying a client's level of health. A person's level of health is a reflection of his level of functioning in all dimensions.

develop cardiac illness. In addition, within any one developmental stage, a person may experience many health-illness states.

The way clients view their level of health depends on their attitudes toward health and their values, beliefs, and perceptions of their physical, emotional, intellectual, social, developmental, and spiritual well-being. The nurse's role is to help clients identify their position on the health-illness continuum in order to help them reach an optimal level of health.

The drawback of the health-illness continuum is that it is not always easy to describe a client's level of health in terms of one point between two extremes. For example, is a man who has his broken leg in a cast but who has adapted to limited mobility more or less healthy than a man experiencing severe depression after the death of his spouse but who is physiologically healthy? The model is effective, nonetheless, when it is used for comparing a client's present level of health with previous levels and for setting goals for nursing care to attain a future level of health.

High-Level Wellness Model

In the model developed by Dunn (1977), high-level wellness is a method of functioning oriented toward maximizing the potential of which an individual is capable. It requires the individual to maintain a continuum of balance and purposeful direction within his environment and involves the following components: (1) progress toward a higher level of functioning, (2) an open-ended and ever-expanding challenge to live at the fullest potential, and (3) progressive integration or maturation of the individual at increasingly higher levels throughout the life cycle (Dunn, 1959; Pender, 1987).

Health care directed toward helping a client achieve high-level wellness emphasizes health promotion and illness prevention activities rather than treatment for illness. High-level wellness is a dynamic process, not a passive, static state.

The high-level wellness model is applicable also to family and community health. Families and communities have many functions, and high-level wellness involves successful functioning in an integrated manner.

Agent-Host-Environment Model

The agent-host-environment model of health and illness originated in the community health work of Leavell et al. (1965) and has since been expanded as a model for describing the cause of illness in other health areas. According to this approach, the level of health or illness of an individual or group depends on the dynamic relationship among three variables: agent, host, and environment.

The *agent* is any factor, internal or external, that by its presence or absence can lead to disease or illness. Agents can be biological, chemical, physical, mechanical, or psychosocial. The presence of these agents does not mean a person will become ill, but an agent must be present (or absent, as in a lack of adequate nutrition) for a particular illness to occur.

The *host* is the individual person or group who may or many not be susceptible to a particular illness or disease. Host factors are those physical or psychosocial situations or conditions putting an individual or group at risk for becoming ill. Such factors may be related to the host's family history, age, or life-style. The presence of host factors does not mean a person will become ill. However, illness is more likely if these factors are present.

The *environment* consists of all factors outside the host. Physical environment includes economic level, climate, living conditions, and elements such as light and sound levels. Social environment consists of factors involving a person or group's interaction with others, including stress, conflicts with others, economic hardships, and life crises such as the death of a spouse. Environmental factors do not usually cause illness in themselves but can increase or decrease susceptibility to disease.

The agent-host-environment model emphasizes that both health and illness depend on the dynamic interaction of all three variables (Fig. 2-2). For example, a person does not contract a respiratory infection simply because a microorganism has entered his respiratory system. The microorganism alone does not *cause* the illness, which depends on host and environmental factors as well. It has been shown that the presence of an infectious organism may affect one individual in one environment but not affect another person in a different environment.

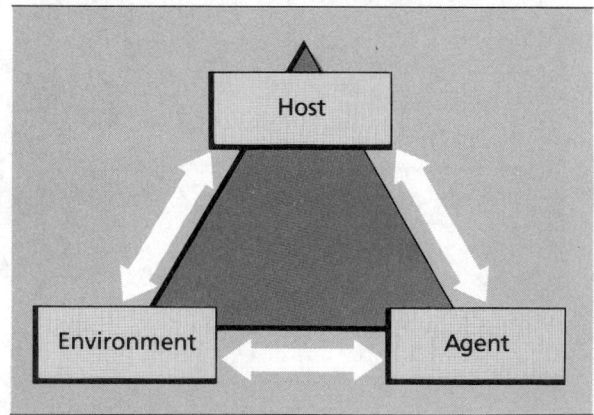

***Fig.* 2-2** Interaction of agent, host, and environment as causes of disease and illness. The double arrows indicate that each factor can be affected by the other two.

These factors continually interact. No one can be totally free of all agents of illness. For example, people are frequently exposed to microorganisms in food and water, to toxic fumes such as automobile emissions, and to psychosocial stresses. But in health the defense mechanisms of the body and mind allow them to resist or minimize the threats of such agents, depending on host and environmental factors. Health, then, can be considered a state in which these three areas interact positively and maintain a dynamic state of adaptation to changes in any of the areas. Illness occurs when the interaction of two or more factors leads to failure of the person to adapt.

The agent-host-environment model has been expanded into a general theory of the multiple cause of disease. Until recent decades, it was commonly believed that single causes of diseases could be identified. Infectious diseases in particular were thought to have single causes: the bacterium or virus that is the agent was considered solely responsible. It is now recognized that most diseases have multiple causes, as the agent-host-environment model demonstrates. The theory of the multiple cause of disease is important to nurses because nursing emphasizes holistic care of the client, which is based on knowledge of environmental, psychosocial, and life-style factors.

Health Belief Model

Rosenstock's (1974) health belief model (Fig. 2-3) addresses the relationship between what a person believes and how he acts. It provides a way of understanding and predicting how clients behave in relation to their health and how they will comply with health care therapies.

The first component in this model involves the individual's perception of susceptibility to an illness. The second component is the individual's perception of the seriousness of the illness. This perception is influenced and modified by demographic and sociopsychological

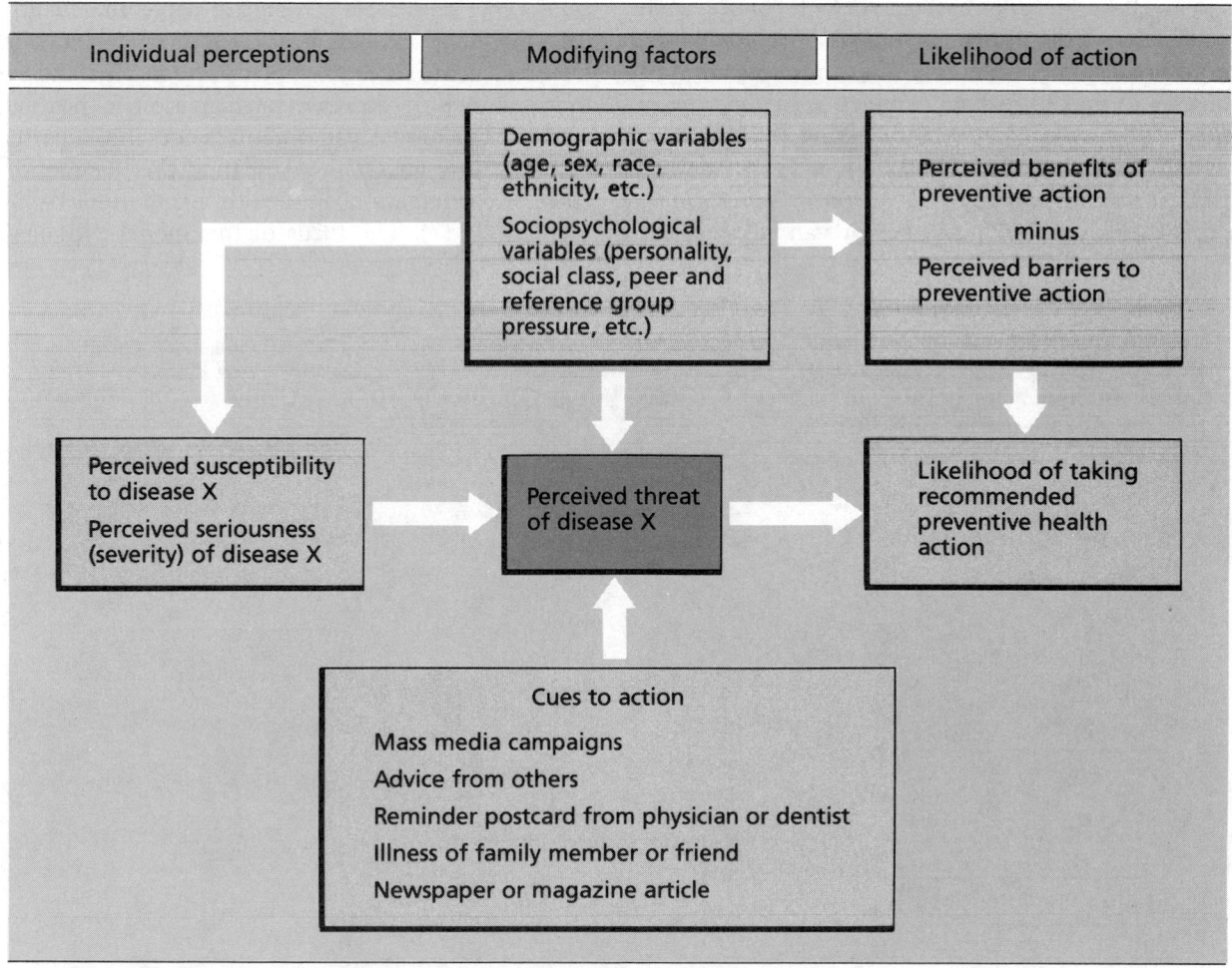

Fig. 2-3 Health belief model.
From Becker, MH, and Maiman, LA: Med Care 13:12, 1975.

variables, perceived threats of the illness, and cues to action (for example, mass media campaigns and advice from family, friends, and medical professionals).

The third component—the likelihood that a person will take preventive action—is the person's perception of the benefits of taking action. Preventive action may include life-style changes, increased adherence to medical therapies, or a search for medical advice or treatment.

The health belief model can help nurses understand factors influencing client's perceptions, beliefs, and behavior and plan care that will most effectively assist a client in maintaining or regaining health and preventing illness.

Evolutionary-Based Model

The evolutionary-based model of health and viability is supported by the principle that illness and death sometime serve an evolutionary function (Dixon and Dixon, 1984). The model (Fig. 2-4) interrelates the following elements: (1) *life events,* reflecting developmental variables, as well as variables associated with chance, such as accidents or relocation, (2) *life-style determinants,* those personal and learned adaptive strategies an individual uses to make life-style changes, (3) *evolutionary viability within social context,* reflecting the extent to which individuals function to promote survival and well-being (Dixon and Dixon, 1984), (4) *control perceptions,* reflecting the extent to which a person can influence the

circumstances of life, (5) *viability emotions,* "affective reactions" developed from life events or life-style determinants, and (6) *health outcomes,* the physiological, behavioral, and psychological states resulting from viability emotions in combination with the other factors within the model.

With this model, nursing interventions can be developed for all six client dimensions. The full scope of clinical experience may require assisting clients to regain a sense of viability. This is particularly important in nursing because of the opportunity for long-term contact with the client and family (Dixon and Dixon, 1984).

Health Promotion Model

The health promotion model proposed by Pender (1982) was designed to be a "complimentary counterpart to models of health protection." Health promotion is directed toward increasing a client's level of well-being and self-actualization (Pender, 1987). The model focuses on three functions (Fig. 2-5), setting an order on why clients engage in certain cognitive-perceptual health factors that may explain health-promoting behaviors. It identifies factors (for example, demographic and social) that enhance or decrease participation in health promotion. The model also organizes cues into a pattern to explain, through nursing research, the likelihood of a client's participation in health promotion behaviors (Pender, 1987). The focus of this model explains why

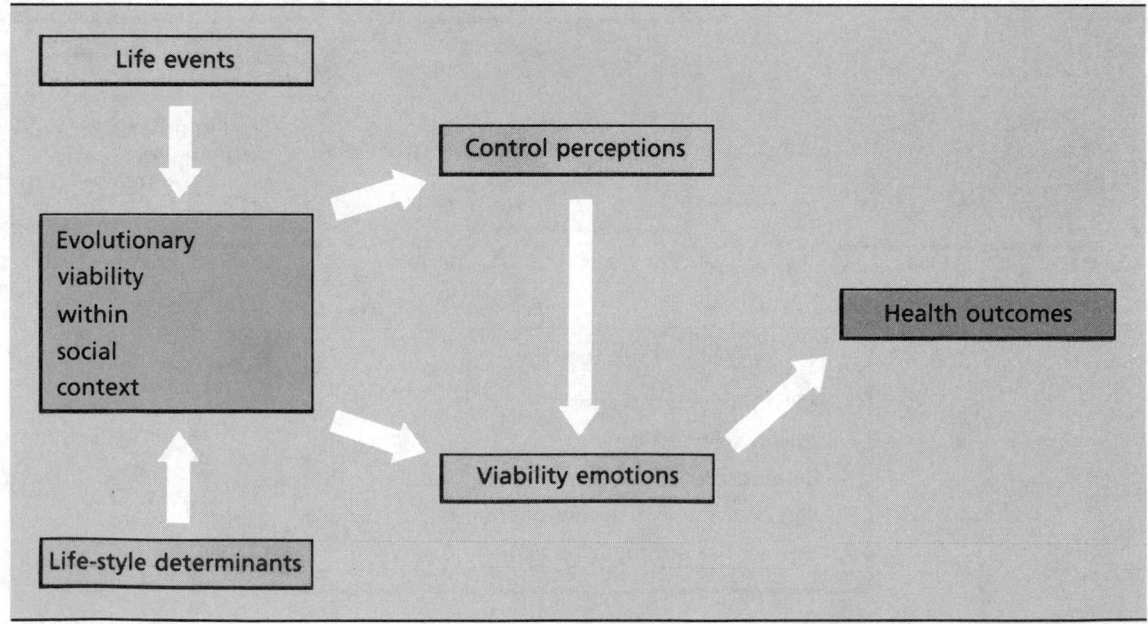

Fig. 2-4 Evolutionary-based model of viability and health.
Redrawn from Dixon, JK, and Dixon, JP: ANS 6(3):5, 1984.

individuals engage in health activities. It is not designed for use with families or communities.

■ ■ ■

The six models of health and illness presented here are not conflicting theories but represent ways of approaching complex issues and of understanding how clients' attitudes toward health and illness differ and thus lead to different kinds of health behaviors. The following section continues this discussion by examining in more detail the primary variables of health beliefs and practices.

VARIABLES INFLUENCING HEALTH BELIEFS AND PRACTICES

Nurses need to understand the variables that influence clients' health beliefs and practices. Both internal and external variables can influence how a person thinks and

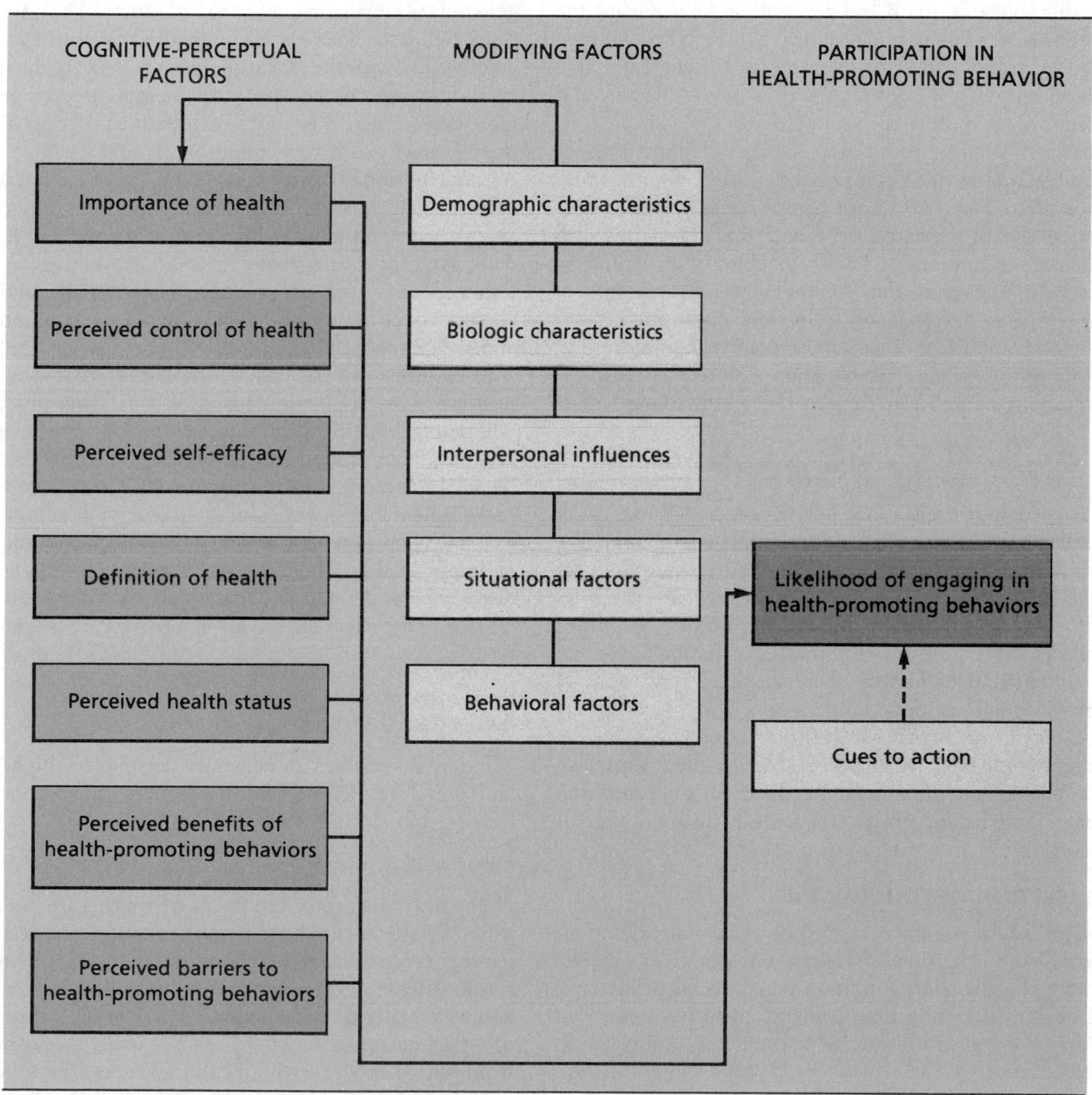

Fig. 2-5   Health promotion model.
From Pender, NJ: Health promotion in nursing practice, ed. 2, Norwalk, Conn., 1987, Appleton Lange.

acts. Understanding the way in which these variables affect a client allows the nurse to plan and deliver individualized care for that client.

Internal Variables

Internal variables include a person's developmental stage, intellectual background, perception of personal functioning, and emotional and spiritual factors.

DEVELOPMENTAL STAGE

A person's thought and behavior patterns change through the stages of life. The nurse must consider a client's level of growth and development when using the client's health beliefs and practices as a basis for planning care. A young child, for example is not generally able to conceptualize the potential seriousness of illnesses and needs to be motivated to act in ways beneficial to a treatment plan or to develop habits for illness prevention. An adolescent's emotional development may influence personal beliefs about health-related matters such as the use of contraception, and the nurse thus uses different techniques of health teaching than would be used for a young adult. Knowledge of the stages of growth and development helps the nurse predict the client's response to illness or the threat of illness. The planning of nursing care is then adapted to these expectations, as well as to the client's abilities to participate in self-care.

INTELLECTUAL BACKGROUND

A person's beliefs about health are shaped in part by intellectual variables, including knowledge (or misinformation) about body functions and illnesses, educational background, and past experiences. These variables influence what a person thinks. In addition, cognitive abilities shape *how* a person thinks, including the ability to understand factors involved in illness and to apply knowledge of health and illness to personal health practices. A person's cognitive abilities also relate to his developmental stage. A nurse considers a client's intellectual background to understand the client's beliefs about health and health practices so these variables can be incorporated into nursing care.

PERCEPTION OF FUNCTIONING

The way a person perceives physical functioning affects health beliefs and practices. For example, a person with a chronic heart condition perceives his or her level of health differently than someone who has never had a major health problem. As a result, the health beliefs and practices of these two persons tend to be different. In addition, a person who has successfully recovered from a severe acute illness may change health beliefs and practices as a result of the illness.

When nurses assess a client's level of health, they gather subjective data about the way the client perceives physical functioning, as well as objective data about actual functioning. This information allows nurses to plan and implement individualized care more successfully.

EMOTIONAL AND SPIRITUAL FACTORS

Emotional and spiritual factors also influence health beliefs and practices. A person experiencing a stress response with each change in life tends to respond stressfully to any sign of illness (see Chapter 28), such as worrying that illness is life threatening. A person who generally is very calm may have little emotional response during illness, whereas an individual unable to cope emotionally with the threat of illness may deny the presence of symptoms and not take therapeutic actions. A man who finds he is short of breath and coughs frequently may blame this condition on cold weather if he cannot emotionally accept the possibility of a respiratory illness. Many people have strong emotional reactions against even thinking about the risk of cancer and will deny symptoms and refuse to take preventive action. Other illnesses are more emotionally acceptable, and the person will be more likely to acknowledge the symptoms and seek appropriate care.

If religious beliefs include the belief that physical health is necessary for spiritual health, a clients' practices will reflect that belief. On the other hand, if the person's religious beliefs require abstention from certain kinds of medical treatment, health care may be avoided. In some cases a client may believe illness is a deserved punishment that must be accepted and does nothing to regain or maintain health. Thus, as with emotional variables, a nurse must understand a client's spiritual values in order to involve the client effectively in nursing care (see Chapter 31).

External Variables

External variables influencing a person's health beliefs and practices include family practices, socioeconomic factors, and cultural variables.

FAMILY PRACTICES

The way a client's family uses health care services generally affects the client's health practices. If a person's parents treated every virus and illness as a potentially severe disease and immediately sought health care, the adult generally does the same. A person with this type of family background would be more likely to stay home from school or work with a cold, whereas others would attempt to carry on as usual. In addition, the adult clients are also more likely to practice prevention if their families did so. For example, people whose parents took them for annual checkups as children are more likely to take their own children for regular checkups.

SOCIOECONOMIC FACTORS

Social and psychosocial factors can increase a person's risk for illness, as well as influence how that person defines and reacts to illness. Psychosocial variables include the stability of the person's marital or intimate relationship, life-style habits, and occupational environment.

A person's social network has also been shown to be related to health behavior (Steele, 1982; Parsons, 1958). Neighbors, peers, and co-workers are usually aware of a person's level of health, and if the person is unexpectedly absent from work or a planned activity or is experiencing a symptom of illness, a member of his social network may encourage medical attention. People generally seek approval and support from their social groups, and this desire for approval and support affects their health beliefs and practices. For example, if it is socially acceptable in a particular peer group for teenage girls to smoke, the pressure to conform may be stronger in that group than the concern about smoking being potentially harmful to health.

Social variables partly determine how the health care delivery system provides medical care. Because the health care system is organized in certain ways, it determines how clients can obtain the care they seek. The system provides care for clients with health problems society considers "legitimate" and "acceptable." In addition, the system defines the treatment method, the economic cost to the client, and potential reimbursement to the health care agency or client. The health care system is a complex structure on which clients depend for care. Chapter 3 describes this system in detail.

Economic factors, like social factors, can affect a client's level of health by increasing the risk for disease, by influencing how or at what point the client enters the health care system, or by limiting compliance with a prescribed treatment plan. Epidemiological studies have shown that persons at low economic levels have a greater risk for pulmonary disease, cancer, and diabetes mellitus than persons at higher levels (Goldsmith, 1975; Davidson, 1971). In addition, a large proportion of people at low economic levels live in urban areas and therefore have a greater risk for disease because of their environment.

Economic factors also influence the way a client enters the health care system. A worker who has health insurance benefits is more likely to seek care and treatment for a chronic cough than an individual who is out of work and no longer has insurance.

A person's compliance with treatment designed to maintain or improve health is also affected by economic status. A person with high utility bills, a large family, and low income tends to give higher priority to food and shelter than to costly drugs or treatment or to expensive foods for special diets.

CULTURAL BACKGROUND

Cultural background influences individual beliefs, values, and customs. It influences how a client enters the health care system, as well as personal health practices. For example, a study of the illness referral practices of Spanish-speaking cultural groups showed that most individuals in such a group generally did not use health care services but practiced self-medication (Allinger, 1977).

Sociocultural differences between clients and nurses can affect the nurse-client relationship and the quality of nursing care delivered. If nurses are not aware of their own and other cultural patterns of behavior, language, and action, they may not be able to recognize and understand a client's behavior and beliefs and may have difficulty interacting with the client. For example, a client from a culture that strongly values and expects close, warm, and supportive family relationships may experience cultural conflict with a nurse who does not value or has not experienced close kinship ties (Leininger, 1977).

Cultural factors must be identified and incorporated into a client's care plan to avoid conflict between goals and methods of care and the client's cultural background (see Chapter 4).

HEALTH PROMOTION AND ILLNESS PREVENTION

Nurses emphasize health promotion and illness prevention activities as important forms of health care, since nurses assist clients in maintaining good health and improving their levels of health instead of merely providing care after illness occurs. Health promotion and illness prevention are closely related concepts and, in practice, overlap to some extent. Health promotion activities help clients maintain their present level of health or enhance it in the future. Illness prevention activities protect a client from actual or potential threats to health. Both types of activities are oriented to the future. The difference between them involves motivations and goals. Health promotion activities motivate a person to act positively to reach the goal of a higher level of health and well-being. Illness prevention activities motivate a person to avoid a negative condition rather than to take a positive action, with the goal of maintaining, rather than attempting to improve, a level of health.

Health promotion activities can be passive or active. With passive strategies, an individual gains from the

---

Categories of the Life-Style and Health Habits Assessment*

- General competencies of self-care
- Nutritional practices
- Physical or recreational activities
- Sleep patterns
- Stress management
- Self-actualization
- Sense of purpose
- Relationships with others
- Environmental control
- Use of health care system

*The complete LHHA is described in detail, along with the rating scale, in Pender, NJ: Health promotion in nursing practice, ed. 2, Norwalk, Conn., 1987, Appleton & Lange.

✂ Research Highlight ✂

Walker et al. developed an instrument focusing on health-promoting behaviors. The 48-item, Health-promoting Life-Style Profile (HPLP) was administered to 952 adults and was evaluated and statistically analyzed. As a result, six dimensions were isolated, meaning that, as a result of factor analysis, each of the 48 items on the HPLP inventory was placed into one of the following categories: self-actualization, health responsibility, exercise, nutrition, interpersonal support, and stress management. The researchers noted that their results were similar to other findings on health practice and high-level wellness dimensions.

Walker SN, Sechrist KR, and Pender, NJ: The Health-Promoting Life-Style Profile: development and psychometric characteristics, Nursing Research, 36:76, 1987.

---

activities of others without acting himself. The fluoridation of municipal drinking water and the fortification of homogenized milk with vitamin D are two examples of passive health promotion strategies.

With active strategies, an individual is motivated to adopt a specific health program. Weight reduction and smoking cessation programs require clients to be actively involved in measures to improve their present and future levels of wellness while at the same time decreasing the risk of disease.

Health promotion and illness prevention activities have become an important focus of health care. Although scientific and medical advances since the 1940s have resulted in cures for many infectious diseases, there are still no cures for many chronic diseases. Thus there is greater motivation for preventing the occurrence of these diseases. In addition, the rapid escalation of health care costs has motivated consumers to seek ways of decreasing the incidence and minimizing the results of illness or disability. Also, society as a whole has become increasingly conscious of health and the value of maintaining or increasing the level of health.

Pender (1987) has developed the Life-Style and Health Habits Assessment (LHHA), which is divided into 10 sections (see box). The assessment tool uses yes and no responses. The rating in each section, as well as the total score, provides the nurse with the information necessary to design an individualized health protection-promotion program for the client. It is hoped that use of the LHHA will increase the client's self-awareness of living patterns and assist in motivating behavior changes (Pender, 1987).

The LHHA provided a starting point for the Health-Promoting Life-Style Profile (HPLP) (Walker, Sechrist, and Pender, 1987). The instrument focuses on health-promoting behaviors and is currently being validated (see research highlight).

The HPLP focuses on health-promoting behaviors. Health-damaging behaviors (e.g., smoking and alcohol) did not conceptually fit with health-promotion activities and were deleted from the profile, further supporting the idea that health promotion and illness prevention are different activities (Pender, 1987).

Other tools for health promotion and illness prevention have been developed. The goal of a total health program is to improve a client's level of well-being in all dimensions, not just physical health. Total programs are based on the belief that many factors can affect a person's level of health (Fig. 2-6). Health can be influenced by an individual's practices, such as poor eating habits and little or no exercise. Health can also be affected by physical stressors, a poor living environment, exposure to air pollutants, and an unsafe environment. Psychological stressors can influence an individual's level of health, as can hereditary factors. Total health promotion programs are directed toward changing a person's life-style to develop habits that can improve the level of health. The following habits have been shown to promote total health, help prevent illness, and improve life expectancy (Belloc and Breslow, 1972):

1. Three meals a day with no snacking
2. Breakfast every day
3. Moderate exercise two or three times a week
4. Seven to 8 hours uninterrupted sleep a day

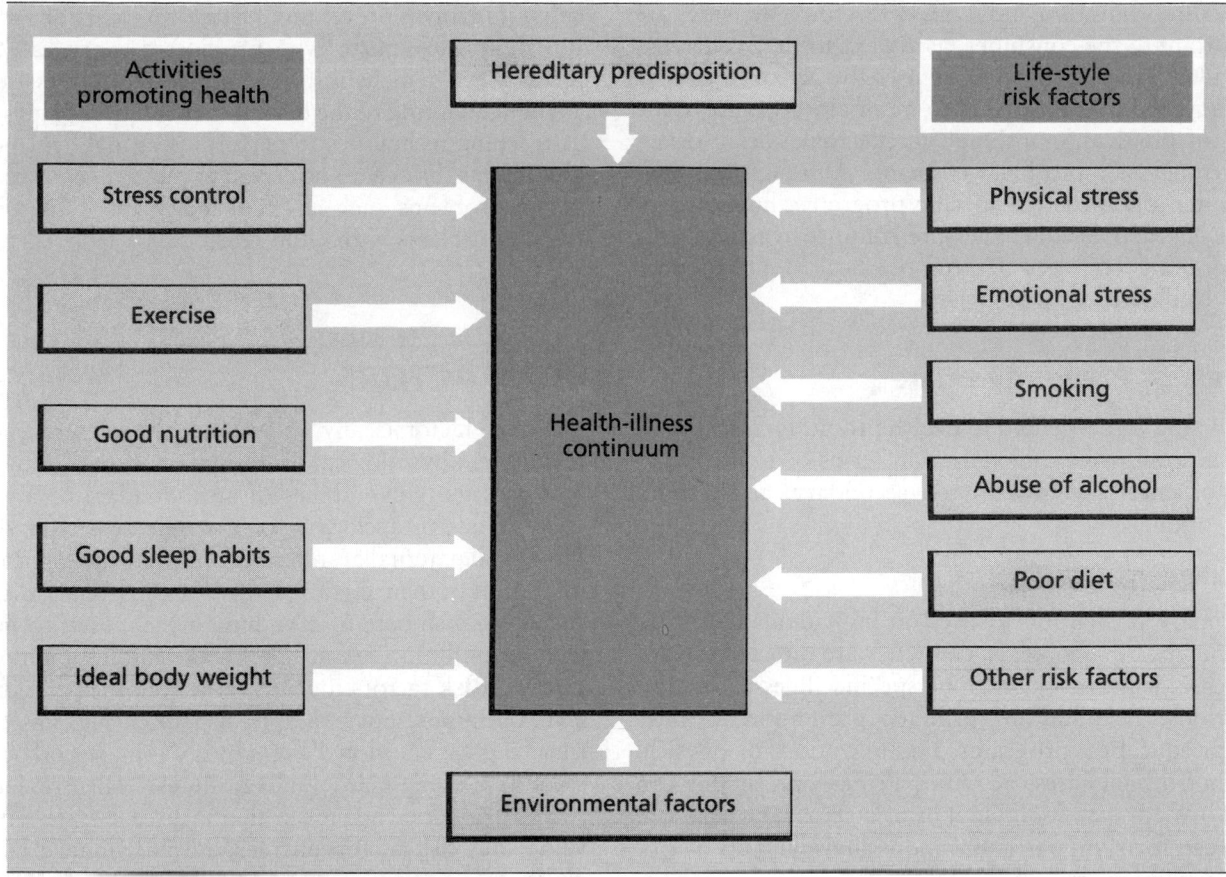

Fig. 2-6   Multifactorial health-illness dynamics.
From Milsum, JH: Fam Community Health 3:1, 1980. Reprinted with permission of Aspen Publishers, Inc.

5. No smoking
6. Ideal body weight for sex, age, height, and body build
7. Alcohol only in moderation

Other programs are aimed at specific health care problems. For example, the American Lung Association has developed smoking cessation clinics that include group support (Fig. 2-7). Exercise programs encourage participants to regularly schedule exercise. Stress reduction programs teach participants to cope with stressors in their personal lives.

Some health promotion and illness prevention programs are operated by health care agencies. Others are independently operated. Many corporations have developed health promotion activities for employees. Likewise, colleges and community centers offer health promotion and illness prevention programs. Nurses may be actively involved in these programs or may serve as consultants or give referrals. The goal of these activities is to improve the client's level of health through preventive health services, environmental protection, and health education.

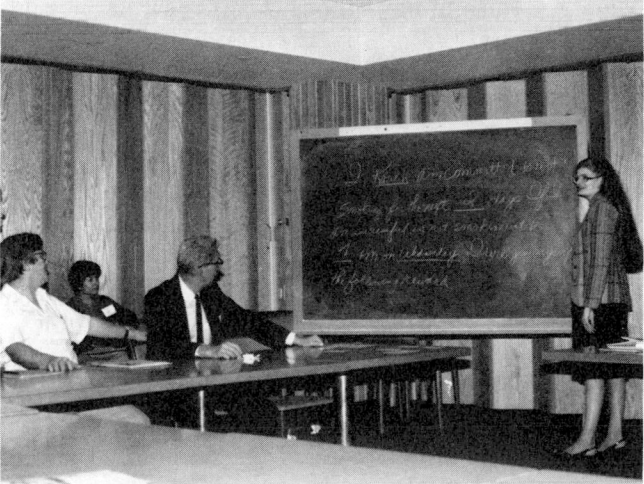

Fig. 2-7   The American Lung Association has developed client-centered smoking cessation clinics that include group support.
Courtesy American Lung Association of Eastern Missouri.

Health promotion and illness prevention activities are important to the consumer, as well as to the health care provider. Whether an activity uses the active or passive strategy, the overall goal is to maintain or improve the level of physical, emotional, intellectual, social, developmental, and spiritual well-being. Although activities are often organized in specific programs, nurses in all areas of practice often have opportunities to assist clients in adopting activities to promote health and decrease risks of illness.

Levels of Preventive Care

Nursing care oriented to health promotion and illness prevention can be understood in terms of health activities on three levels, primary, secondary, and tertiary prevention.

PRIMARY PREVENTION

Primary prevention focuses on individuals not experiencing health problems. Activities are directed toward decreasing the probability of specific illnesses or dysfunctions. In addition, primary prevention includes health education programs, immunization, or physical and nutritional fitness activities. Primary prevention can be provided to an individual or to a general population, or it can focus on particular individuals who are at risk for developing specific diseases.

SECONDARY PREVENTION

Secondary prevention focuses on individuals experiencing health problems or illnesses and who are at risk for developing complications or worsening conditions. Activities are directed toward diagnosis and prompt intervention, thereby reducing severity and enabling the client to return to normal health at the earliest possible point (Pender, 1987). A large portion of nursing care is delivered in the home, the hospital, or skilled nursing facilities at a secondary level designed to prevent complications. Secondary prevention includes preventing wound infections, administering medications and intravenous fluids, assisting with personal hygiene, and promoting physical activities. In addition, other secondary prevention nursing activities include educating clients about self-care and providing emotional support to help them adapt to illnesses.

TERTIARY PREVENTION

Tertiary prevention focuses on individuals with short- or long-term disabilities. Activities are directed toward rehabilitation rather than diagnosis and treatment (Pender, 1987). The goal of care at this level is to help clients achieve as high a level of functioning as possible compared to limitations caused by illness or impaired functioning. This level of care is called *preventive care* because it involves preventing further disability or reduced functioning. A nurse who provides tertiary care to a recently blinded client, for example, not only assists the client in adapting to the disability through activities such as teaching techniques to perform personal hygiene but also directs the client's attention to the goal of preventing future problems such as accidents in the home or potential problems with child rearing.

RISK FACTORS

A risk factor is any situation, habit, environmental condition, physiological condition, or other variable that increases the vulnerability of an individual or a group to an illness or accident. For example, a person whose father and paternal grandfather died of acute myocardial infarction in their forties is at risk for coronary disease. Likewise, members of a community exposed to industrial air pollution are at risk for developing pulmonary disease. Risk factors include variables other than physical conditions. For example, a person who has experienced great emotional stress over a long period of time risks developing many kinds of illness. The presence of risk factors does not mean that a disease state will develop, but risk factors increase an individual's vulnerability to a particular disease. Risk factors can occur in different aspects of a person's internal or external environment. Nurses and other health care professionals are concerned with them for several reasons. Risk factors play a major role in how a nurse identifies a client's health status. They can also influence a person's health beliefs and practices, if the person is aware of their presence. Identifying risk factors is also important for health promotion and illness prevention activities, which are often based on reducing or eliminating risk factors.

Risk factors can be placed in the following interrelated categories: genetic and physiological factors, age, physical environment, and life-style.

Genetic and Physiological Factors

Physiological risk factors involve the physical functioning of the body. Certain physical conditions, such as pregnancy or being overweight, place increased stress on a person's physiological systems (e.g., the circulatory system) increasing the person's susceptibility to illness in these areas. Heredity, or an individual's genetic predisposition to specific illness, is a major physical risk factor. For example, a person with a family history of diabetes mellitus is at risk for developing the disease later in life. Other documented genetic risk factors include family histories of cancer, coronary disease, and renal disease.

Age

Age increases an individual's susceptibility to certain illnesses. For example, the risk of cardiovascular disease increases with age for both sexes. The risks of birth defects and complications of pregnancy increase after age 35. Many kinds of cancer pose a greater risk for persons over age 45 than for younger persons. Age risk factors are often closely associated with other risk factors such as family history and personal habits. For example, a man at age 60 who has smoked 40 years is at a greater risk for developing lung cancer than a man at age 30 who has smoked 10 years.

Environment

The physical environment in which a person works or lives can increase the likelihood that certain illnesses will occur. Studies have shown, for example, that some kinds of cancer and other diseases are more likely to develop in industrial workers exposed to certain chemicals or residents living near toxic waste disposal sites.

Air, water, and noise pollution increase the risk of illness. High crime rates or overcrowding can also lead to stresses that make individuals more susceptible to disease.

In the home the physical environment may include conditions that pose risks to an individual or to a whole family. Unclean, poorly heated or cooled, or overcrowded dwellings increase the likelihood that infections and other diseases will be contracted and spread. Within the family, conflicts or other problems may create stresses that put individual members, or the family as a whole, at increased risk of illness.

Life-Style

Many activities, habits, and practices involve risk factors, as do the stresses of life crises and frequent lifestyle changes. A person's health practices and behaviors can have a positive or negative effect on health. Practices with potential negative effects, including overeating or poor nutrition, insufficient rest and sleep, and poor personal hygiene, are risk factors. Other habits that put a person at risk for illness include smoking, alcohol or drug abuse, and activities involving a threat or injury, such as skydiving or mountain climbing. Some habits are risk factors for specific diseases. For example, ex-

TABLE 2-1   Social Readjustment Rating Scale

Rank	Life Event	Mean Value	Rank	Life Event	Mean Value
1	Death of spouse	100	23	Son or daughter leaving home	29
2	Divorce	73	24	Trouble with in-laws	29
3	Marital separation	65	25	Outstanding personal achievement	28
4	Jail term	63	26	Wife begins or stops work	26
5	Death of close family member	63	27	Begin or end school	26
6	Personal injury or illness	53	28	Change in living conditions	25
7	Marriage	50	29	Revision of personal habits	24
8	Fired at work	47	30	Trouble with boss	23
9	Marital reconciliation	45	31	Change in work hours or conditions	20
10	Retirement	45	32	Change in residence	20
11	Change in health of family member	44	33	Change in schools	20
12	Pregnancy	40	34	Change in recreation	19
13	Sex difficulties	39	35	Change in church activities	19
14	Gain of new family member	39	36	Change in social activities	18
15	Business readjustment	39	37	Mortgage or loan less than $10,000	17
16	Change in financial state	38	38	Change in sleeping habits	16
17	Death of close friend	37	39	Change in number of family get-togethers	15
18	Change to different line of work	36	40	Change in eating habits	15
19	Change in number of arguments with spouse	35	41	Vacation	13
20	Mortgage over $10,000	31	42	Christmas	12
21	Foreclosure of mortgage or loan	30	43	Minor violations of the law	11
22	Change in responsibilities at work	29			

Reprinted with permission from J Psychosom Res 11:213. Holmes, TH, and Rahe, RH: Social readjustment rating scale. Copyright 1967, Pergamon Press Ltd.

cessive sunbathing increases the risk of skin cancer, and being overweight increases the risk of cardiovascular disease.

Any emotional stress can be a risk factor if it is severe or prolonged or the person is unable to cope adequately with it. In such a case, emotional stress may increase the chance of illness. Emotional stresses may occur with events such as divorce, pregnancy, and arguments. Any area of life that leads to long-term emotional stress can be a risk factor. Job-related stresses, for example, may

TABLE 2-2 Hospital Stress Rating Scale

Rank	Event	Mean
1	Possibility of loss of function of senses (e.g., eyesight, hearing)	116.8
2	Admission for life-threatening illness	107.1
3	Possibility of loss of an organ	92.1
4	Anticipated bad experience with medications	80.3
5	Inadequate insurance to cover hospitalization	78.5
6	Possibility of disfigurement	75.8
7	Anticipated future loss of income as a result of illness	75.5
8	Admission for surgery	73.7
9	Inadequate explanation of diagnosis	71.8
10	Undiagnosed ailment at time of admission	71.1
11	Inadequate finances for family during hospital stay	71.0
12	Being away from home	60.4
13	Inadequate explanation of treatment	58.0
14	Presence of severely ill roommate	57.8
15	Isolation for contagious condition	57.5
16	Anticipated improvement in functioning	56.8
17	Unconcerned attitude of hospital staff	56.4
18	Spouse at home	55.7
19	Anticipated pain or discomfort as a result of treatment	54.6
20	Dependent children at home	53.9
21	Hospitalization at considerable distance from home	53.2
22	Hospitalization as the result of an accident	50.7
23	Anticipated relief of pain or discomfort	50.2
24	Emergency admission	50.0
25	Experience of esthetically unpleasant surroundings	47.7
26	Admission for diagnostic tests only	46.2
27	Not having visitors	44.5
28	Prior hospitalization experience	43.3
29	Anticipated improved appearance	43.0
30	Change in amount of physical activity	41.6
31	Holiday or special family occasion during hospitalization	41.3
32	Change in amount of independent behavior	41.0
33	Major change in eating habits	40.1
34	Cared for by unfamiliar physician	39.6
35	Major change in sleeping habits	38.8
36	Being away from job	38.0
37	Language problem in communication with staff	36.2
38	Presence of unfamiliar machines or mechanical devices	35.1
39	Isolation from friends	34.5
40	Acquaintance with someone else with the same medical problem	34.3
41	Change in amount of personal privacy	33.6
42	Change in amount of interaction with other people	32.2
43	Extensive medical knowledge	30.7
44	Change in awareness of world or local events	27.2
45	Being away from school	26.3

From Volicer, BJ: Copyright © 1974, American Journal of Nursing Company. Reproduced with permission from Nursing Research, May/June, vol. 23, no. 3.

overtax a person's cognitive skills and decision-making ability, leading to what is sometimes called "mental overload" or "burnout."

Holmes and Rahe (1967) have developed a social readjustment rating scale (Table 2-1, p. 47) that correlates life-style changes with the risk of illness. Research has shown that there is a greater risk for illness when a person has a change in life-style.

Adjustments that clients must make in hospitals and other health care settings also involve a risk for further illness. Volicer (1974) developed a hospital stress rating scale (Table 2-2) that closely parallels the Holmes and Rahe scale. The objective of the scale is to predict the risk of a long hospital stay, complications, and pain, all of which may be linked to further disability or prolonged illness. The hospital stress rating scale assigns a numerical value to actual or potential stressors experienced during hospitalization. The higher the client's total score, the greater the risk that complications will develop, that pain medications will be necessary, and that the hospital stay will be prolonged. A high score on the scale does not mean a client will experience complications or a long hospital stay. However, it does predict general risks and therefore helps a nurse identify risks in order to develop nursing interventions to reduce hospital stress and the incidence of complications (Volicer, 1974).

ILLNESS AND ILLNESS BEHAVIOR

Illness is not merely the presence of a disease process. Illness is an abnormal state in which a person's physical, emotional, intellectual, social, developmental, or spiritual functioning is diminished or impaired compared with that person's previous experience. Cancer is a disease process, but one client with leukemia who is responding to treatment may not perceive himself as ill and may continue to function as usual, whereas another client with breast cancer who is preparing for surgery may perceive herself as ill and be affected in dimensions other than the physical.

Illness therefore is not synonymous with disease, although nurses must be familiar with different kinds of diseases and their treatments. Nurses are concerned more with illness, which includes disease but also the effects on functioning and well-being in all dimensions.

People who are ill generally act in a way that medical sociologists call *illness behavior*. Illness behavior involves the ways persons monitor their bodies, define and interpret their symptoms, take remedial actions, and use the health care system (Mechanic, 1982). If an individual perceives himself to be ill, illness behavior can serve as a coping mechanism. For example, illness behavior may

serve as a means of obtaining reassurance. A person who has been off work for a week because of illness may need to be reassured that his employer missed his contribution and that others care about him. The health team can also be a source of support and reassurance for the client. This support is particularly important for a client with a chronic disease. Clients with severe cardiac impairments who are unable to care for themselves look to the health team for support. Clients may need reassurance that the inability to care for themselves is due to the physical disease and not to a lack of motivation or desire. In addition, illness behavior can result in the client being released from a role, social expectation, or responsibility. For a housewife, for example, the "flu" may be a temporary release from child care and household responsibilities.

Variables Influencing Illness Behavior

Just as health behavior is affected by internal and external variables, so is illness behavior. The nurse needs to understand the influences of these variables in order to understand the client's behavior and plan individualized care. These variables are complex in their origins and effects.

INTERNAL VARIABLES

Important internal variables influencing the way clients behave when they are ill are their perceptions of symptoms and the nature of the illness itself.

If a client believes the symptoms of his illness disrupt his normal routine, he is more likely to seek health care assistance than if he did not perceive the symptoms to be disruptive. If a client perceives his symptoms as serious or perhaps life threatening, he is also more likely to seek assistance. A person awakened in the middle of the night with crushing chest pain generally views this as a symptom of a potentially serious and life-threatening illness and will probably be motivated to seek assistance. However, such a perception can also have the opposite effect. A person may fear a serious illness, react by denying it, and not seek medical assistance.

Rotter's (1966) social learning theory describes people's motivation for health behavior on the basis of a trait predisposing them to an internal or external orientation of control. People more internally controlled are likely to take the initiative in their own health care practices. Externally controlled individuals perceive their illness as a matter attributed to luck, fate, or a supreme being and thus beyond their control. Cox (1985) investigated the reliability of the Health Self-Determination Index (HSDI) and noted that, while further testing is needed, the tool could assist nurses in determining and predicting client's responses to health problems and needs. Therefore knowing how clients react to health problems enables the nurse to anticipate their needs, questions, and concerns and ultimately, to assist them in adopting positive health practices.

A client's illness behavior can also be affected by the nature of the illness. Acute illnesses involve symptoms of relatively short duration that are usually severe and that may affect the client's functioning in any dimension. Chronic illnesses persist over a long period of time, usually longer than 6 months and can affect functioning in any dimension. Several variables influence the illness behavior of a client with a chronic illness. The client may fluctuate between a state of maximal functioning and serious exacerbations that may be life threatening.

If a chronic illness cannot be cured and the symptoms are only partially relieved by therapy, the client may not be highly motivated to comply with the therapy plan. In addition, in the present system, health care professionals are sometimes not highly motivated to remain involved in a client's care, and the client's own motivation may lessen correspondingly. The present system is geared to short, intensive client interactions. Continuity is often lacking in the provision of health care, and health care services and community support systems vital for management of chronic illness do not always maintain adequate communication with one another (Aiken, 1976).

Clients with acute illness are more likely to seek health care and to comply readily with therapy. Chronically ill clients may become less actively involved in their care, may experience greater frustration, and may comply less readily with care. Because nurses generally spend more time with chronically ill clients than other health care professionals do, they are in the unique position of being able to assist these clients in overcoming problems related to illness behavior.

EXTERNAL VARIABLES

External variables influencing a client's illness behavior include the visibility of symptoms, social group, cultural background, economic variables, accessibility of the health care system, and social support.

The visibility of the symptoms of an illness can affect a client's body image and illness behavior. For example, a person who has a draining sore on the lip may seek assistance sooner than a person with a sore throat because people may comment on the sore, the sore changes the person's appearance, and the drainage requires continual care.

A client's social group may assist the client in recognizing the threat of an illness or support the denial of a potential illness. Assume, for example, that two 35-year-old women in two different social groups have identified a breast mass while performing breast self-examination. Both women discuss the finding with their friends. The first woman's friends might encourage her to seek medical attention to determine if a biopsy is necessary, whereas the second woman's friends might tell her that the lump probably represents only fibrocystic disease and that she does not need to rush to a doctor. In a third situation, the social group might forbid the discussion of such subjects altogether, with the result that a woman would neither seek medical attention nor feel reassured that there is no risk. These examples illustrate the influence that friends may have on a client. The client's interaction with family members, peers, and others may have similar results.

Illness behavior can be interpreted and explained in terms of personal experiences and expectations. An individual's cultural and ethnic background teaches him how to be healthy, how to recognize illness, and how to be ill. Meanings attached to health and illness are related to the basic culture-bound values by which people define a given experience and perception (Spector, 1985).

Western culture has emphasized a specific, systematic, causal explanation for trying to understand diseases. In addition the effects of diseases and their interpretation also vary according to cultural circumstances. For example, there is a higher mortality rate from measles in underdeveloped countries, than in Western cultures (Moore et al., 1980). Therefore a nurse needs to understand a client's cultural background in order to develop individualized therapy. For example, two studies of how cultural groups respond to pain (Leininger, 1977; Zborowski, 1952) demonstrated several cultural variations. Older New Englanders, for instance, were found to avoid responding to pain and tended to suffer in silence and not seek relief. Members of the Irish cultural group tended to deny pain. Members of the Italian and Jewish cultural groups sought relief for pain, but Italians were more concerned about the implications of pain for their future levels of wellness and functioning.

The concepts of health and illness can continually change. They vary because of society's interpretation of health and illness, changes in the biological and cultural factors causing illness, and biological and cultural adaptations to health.

Economic variables also influence how a client reacts to an illness. Because of economic constraints an individual may delay treatment, and in many cases continue to work, rear children, or go to school despite an illness. People of higher economic status tend to practice preventive health care more frequently than people of lower economic status, perhaps because middle- and upper-class persons have more resources to devote to preventive health care. Frequently the resources of lower-class and lower-middle-class persons are devoted to the basic needs of food and shelter.

The effect of the client's accessibility to the health care system is closely related to the influence of economic factors. The health care system is a socioeconomic system that a client must enter, interact in, and exit. To many clients, entry into the system itself is complex or confusing, and some clients may seek nonemergency medical care in an emergency room because they do not know how to obtain health services otherwise. The physical proximity of clients to a hospital, clinic, or health care agency often influences how soon they enter the system after deciding to seek care. In addition, some clients are reluctant to seek care from a large, complex medical center and will more readily visit a community agency. Clients frequently feel that a large medical center is impersonal, that care is provided in a mechanized, assembly-line approach, and that health care personnel are always looking for the worst. Some clients, however, may seek care only from a large medical center because they believe diagnosis and treatment procedures are more modern.

Social support has been linked to health practices such as seat belt use, exercise, nutrition, smoking cessation,

---

Ten Determinants of Illness Behavior

- The visibility and recognizability of the illness's symptoms
- The extent to which the person perceives the symptoms as serious (the person's estimate of the present and future risks)
- The person's information, knowledge, and cultural assumptions and understanding related to the perceived symptoms
- The extent to which symptoms disrupt family, work, and social activities
- The frequency of the appearance of the symptoms and their persistence
- The extent to which others exposed to the person tolerate the symptoms
- The extent to which basic needs are denied because of the illness
- The extent to which meeting other needs competes with illness responses
- The extent to which the person gives other possible interpretations to the symptoms
- The availability and physical proximity of treatment resources and the psychological and monetary costs of taking action (including costs in time and effort, as well as costs such as stigma, social distance, and feelings of humiliation)

Modified from Mechanic, D: The epidemiology of illness behavior and its relationship to physical and psychological distress. In Mechanic, D: Symptoms, illness behavior, and help seeking, New York, 1982, Prodist.

---

and health screening practices (Muhlenkamp and Sayles, 1986). In addition, research has noted that clients reacted positively to social support during participation in positive health practices (Hubbard, Muhlenkamp, and Brown, 1984). Thus persons who view themselves as being part of a social group and having emotional and personal resources on which they can rely are more likely to practice positive health behaviors.

These internal and external factors can interact in various ways to influence how persons behave when ill and how and when they seek health care. Mechanic (1982) summarized the influences on illness behavior in a list of 10 primary determinants (see box). A nurse who knows the variables affecting illness behavior can better understand a client's illness behavior. Nursing care can then be planned and delivered in a way that involves the client's resources so he is restored to a maximal level of health.

Stages of Illness Behavior

Although the behavior of ill individuals is influenced by internal and external variables, people generally pass through five stages of illness behavior (Fig. 2-8). This behavior pattern involves how a person seeks, finds, and completes health care.

Nurses encounter clients in various stages of illness behavior. Knowledge of these stages enables a nurse to assess a client's behavior, determine the stage of illness behavior, and develop nursing interventions to promote optimal physical, emotional, intellectual, social, and spiritual functioning throughout the client's illness.

STAGE 1: SYMPTOM EXPERIENCE

During this initial stage a person is aware that "something is wrong." A person usually recognizes a physical sensation or a limitation in functioning but does not suspect a specific diagnosis.

The person's perception of a symptom includes three components: awareness of a physical change such as pain, a rash, or a lump; evaluation of this change and a decision that it is a symptom of an illness; and then an emotional response.

For example, a 38-year-old woman detects a lump during monthly breast self-examination. She knows the lump is not related to hormonal changes because she recently completed her menstrual period. She decides that the lump means "something is wrong" and that it may be a symptom of cancer. She becomes anxious and fearful about this potential diagnosis.

Once a person acknowledges the presence of a symptom or symptoms he may behave in many ways. A man decides the symptoms are mild or are not life threatening, as in the case of a cold, so he attempts self-medication strategies rather than seek health care. Frequently, he

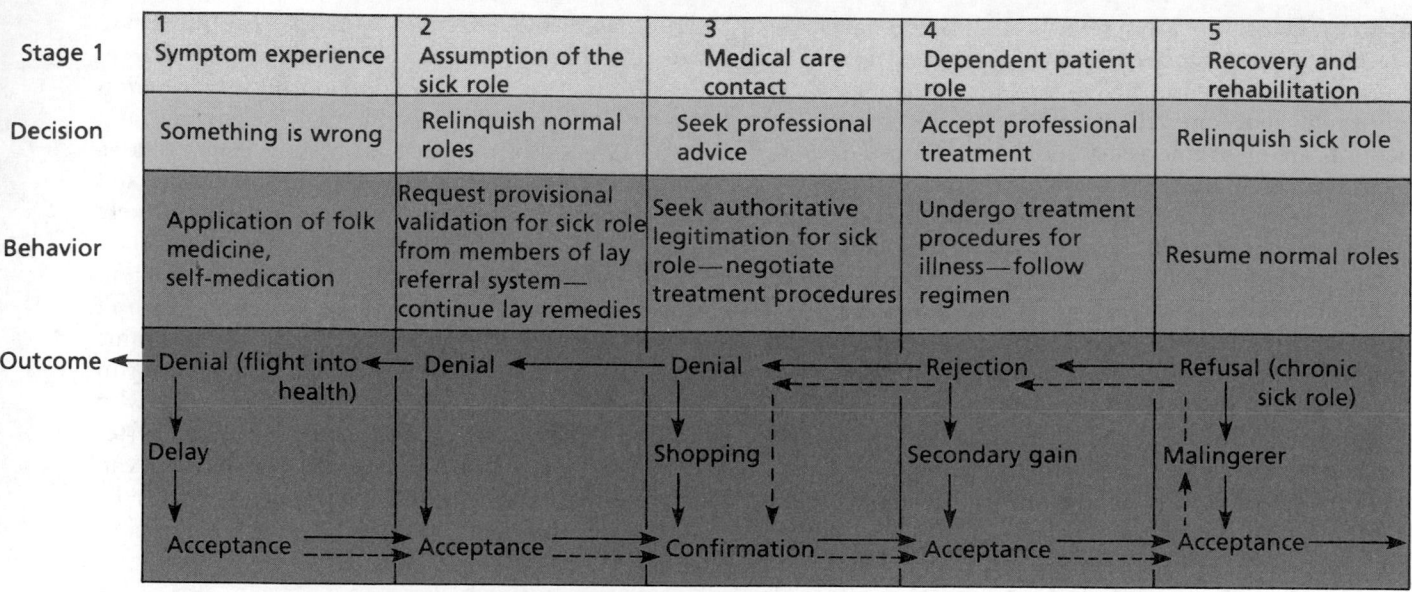

Stage 1	1 Symptom experience	2 Assumption of the sick role	3 Medical care contact	4 Dependent patient role	5 Recovery and rehabilitation
Decision	Something is wrong	Relinquish normal roles	Seek professional advice	Accept professional treatment	Relinquish sick role
Behavior	Application of folk medicine, self-medication	Request provisional validation for sick role from members of lay referral system—continue lay remedies	Seek authoritative legitimation for sick role—negotiate treatment procedures	Undergo treatment procedures for illness—follow regimen	Resume normal roles
Outcome	←Denial (flight into health) ↓ Delay ↓ Acceptance	←Denial ↓ ↓ Acceptance	←Denial ↓ Shopping ↓ Confirmation	←Rejection ↓ Secondary gain ↓ Acceptance	←Refusal (chronic sick role) ↓ Malingerer ↓ Acceptance→

Fig. 2-8 Stages of illness behavior.
From Suchman, EA: Health Hum Behav 6:114, 1965.

treats himself with over-the-counter drugs and home remedies.

If the person regards the symptoms as severe or life threatening, immediate care may be sought or the symptoms' presence or implications may be denied. If a person denies the symptoms or their meaning for future wellness, advice or treatment may be delayed. Before progressing to the next stage of illness behavior, the person must first acknowledge the presence of a health problem.

STAGE 2: ASSUMPTION OF THE SICK ROLE

If symptoms persist and become severe, clients assume the sick role. At this point the illness becomes a social phenomenon, and the sick person seeks confirmation from family and social group that he is indeed ill and that he should be excused from normal duties and role expectations (Coe, 1978). The social group validates the person's illness and may also support continued self-medication.

The assumption of the sick role results in emotional changes such as withdrawal or depression, as well as physical changes. Emotional changes may be simple or complex, depending on the severity of the illness, the degree of disability, and the anticipated length of the illness.

In the case of an illness requiring intervention from health professionals, the person may deny that such intervention is necessary and thus delay contact with the health care system.

Once the person accepts the persistent nature of the symptoms or the potential threat to present and future

levels of wellness, he seeks contact with the health care system and becomes a client.

STAGE 3: MEDICAL CARE CONTACT

If symptoms persist despite home remedies, become severe, or require emergency care, the person is motivated to seek professional health services. In this stage the client seeks expert validation of illness, as well as treatment. In addition, the client seeks an explanation of the symptoms, the cause of the symptoms, the course of the illness, and the implications of the illness for future health.

The severity of the illness influences how long the person waits before making contact with health care professionals. A person with a life-threatening illness or trauma may seek immediate contact, whereas a person with a persistent skin rash may delay contact for several weeks or months. In addition, the psychosocial and cultural variables affecting illness behavior may influence the length of the delay.

The client's illness can be validated at any point on the health-illness continuum. A health professional may determine that the client does not have an illness or that an illness is present and may be life threatening. The client then accepts or denies this diagnosis, depending on several factors. The variables affecting illness behavior in general influence how the client reacts to illness. If the client accepts the diagnosis, the client usually follows through with the prescribed treatment plan. If the client denies the diagnosis, he may begin "shopping" within the health care system. In such a case the client consults several health care providers until one who makes the desired diagnosis is found or until the client changes his mind and accepts the initial diagnosis. A client who considers himself ill, even if health professionals regard him as healthy, may explore nontraditional health settings to obtain the desired diagnosis of illness. Conversely, a client initially diagnosed as ill, particularly with a life-threatening illness, may seek another expert to tell him that his health or life is not threatened. Clients with diagnosed cancer may seek opinions from several physicians in an attempt to avoid facing the diagnosis.

STAGE 4: DEPENDENT CLIENT ROLE

Once the client accepts the illness and seeks treatment, the fourth stage of illness behavior is entered, in which health professionals are depended on for the relief of symptoms. In the dependent role the client accepts care, sympathy, and protection from the demands and stresses of life. A client can adopt the dependent role in a health care institution, at home, or in a community setting.

In the dependent role, it is socially permissible for the client to be relieved of normal obligations and tasks. The more ill the client, the more he is exempted from responsibilities.

Once the client enters the dependent stage, he must also adjust to the disruption of his daily schedule. This disruption affects the client's role in occupation, family, and community and may lead to stress in the emotional, intellectual, social, developmental, and spiritual dimensions.

STAGE 5: RECOVERY AND REHABILITATION

The final stage of illness behavior—recovery and rehabilitation—can arrive abruptly, such as with the subsiding of a fever. If recovery is not abrupt, long-term care may be required, before the client is able to resume an optimal level of functioning as in the case of a fractured leg. In the case of chronic illness, the final stage may involve adjustment to a prolonged reduction in the level of health and functioning.

■　■　■

Not all clients go through each of these five stages, nor do they all move through them at the same rate or in the same manner. A person who has been in good health but suddenly suffers a heart attack and is taken to an emergency room, for example, is put immediately into the dependent client role, even though he has not progressed emotionally through the earlier stages. Nonetheless, this pattern of illness behavior occurs in many cases, and an understanding of these stages helps a nurse identify a client's changing illness behavior to provide effective nursing care.

IMPACT OF ILLNESS ON CLIENT AND FAMILY

Illness is never an isolated event. The client and family must deal with changes resulting from illness and treatment. Each client responds uniquely to illness, and therefore nursing interventions must be individualized. The client and family commonly experience behavioral and emotional changes, as well as changes in roles, body image, self-concept, and family dynamics.

Environment, personal behaviors, and psychosocial factors play an interactive role in illness and health. The health care professional can no longer focus only on the client's physical functioning. Diagnostic assessment from a biopsychosocial perspective is more comprehensive and results in more specific diagnoses and interventions (Shaver, 1985).

Behavioral and Emotional Changes

People react differently to illness or the threat of illness. Individual behavioral and emotional reactions depend on the nature of the illness, the client's attitude toward it, the reaction of others to it, and the variables of illness behavior.

Short-term, non-life-threatening illnesses evoke few behavioral changes in the functioning of the client or family. A husband and father who has a cold, for example, may lack the energy and patience to spend time in family activities and may be irritable and prefer not to interact with his family. This is a behavioral change, but the change is subtle and does not last long. Some may even consider such a change to be a normal response to illness.

Severe illnesses, particularly those that are life threatening, can lead to more extensive emotional and behavioral changes, such as anxiety, shock, denial, anger, and withdrawal. These are common responses to the stress of illness. The nurse develops interventions to assist the client and family to cope with this stress because the stressor itself cannot usually be changed (see Chapter 28).

ANXIETY

Anxiety is a feeling of apprehension, uneasiness, agitation, uncertainty, and fear occurring when a person anticipates threat. The symptoms of an illness do not necessarily create as much anxiety for clients and their families as the anticipation of the way the illness may affect their future health. For some, the anxiety is a fear of a possible diagnosis, particularly a diagnosis of cancer. Others may become more anxious over impending surgery and anticipated pain. Anxiety responses vary from client to client, from family to family, and from stage to stage in illness behavior, but the nurse who knows the signs of anxiety develops appropriate nursing interventions (see Chapter 28).

SHOCK

When a client or his family is informed of the presence of a severe or life-threatening illness, a shock response may occur. The shock response is a powerful emotional state. For some, the state of emotional shock may be an adaptive mechanism allowing them time to absorb what they have been told. Some people describe themselves as "numb" or "immobilized." People hearing that they have cancer or a severely debilitating disease such as parkinsonism may react with shock. They hear what has been said to them but fail to respond or respond in a totally inappropriate manner.

DENIAL

Denial is a mechanism by which the client or family avoids emotional conflict and anxiety by refusing to acknowledge intolerable facts. A family learning that a loved one has cancer may deny the diagnosis and attempt to continue as though nothing were wrong. Denial, however, can be an effective way for a client or family to cope with an illness. The nurse must determine when denial is no longer productive and may be a hindrance to therapy.

ANGER

The client or family may experience anger because of the illness. The anger of family members might be directed toward the client because the illness has disrupted their routine, their plans, and, in some cases, their economic and emotional support. The family members' anger might also be directed toward themselves. Assume, for example, that a 50-year-old man has a heart attack while cleaning the garage and that throughout hospitalization and the recovery phase his teenage son is very angry and makes no attempt to hide his anger. The nurse might discover that the son has been angry at himself for not cleaning the garage because he thinks that if he had, his father would not have suffered the heart attack. In addition, the client or family might become angry with the health care team for making the diagnosis.

Anger, like other emotions, may take irrational forms. The client who suffered the heart attack may be angry at the disease process itself, as if it had singled him out. Anger also may have effects on a client's social or spiritual dimensions. For example, a client may become unsociable or blame a supreme being for his illness (see Chapter 31). Regardless of the kind of anger, the nurse helps the client and family work through his emotion and cope with the associated stresses.

WITHDRAWAL

Illness, particularly long-term or severe illness, may cause a client to withdraw. Regardless of whether the client is in a hospital or at home, she may avoid interaction, remain in her room, or resort to solitary activities such as continuously watching television. Withdrawal is a symptom of depression and may be an effect of the illness or the diagnosis. Family members may also withdraw from contact with the ill person because of anger or depression, in which case the nurse needs to plan care activities promoting the continuation of family functioning and support for the client.

Impact on Family Roles

People have many roles in life such as wage earner, decision maker, professional, and parent. When an illness occurs, the roles of both client and family may change. Such a change may be subtle and short-term or drastic and long-term. Clients and families generally adjust more easily to subtle, short-term changes. In most cases the client and family know that the role change is only temporary. Assume, for example, that the mother of two preschool children acquires a viral infection and that her illness continues for a week, during which time she relinquishes her roles of housewife and child care provider. Initially she may welcome giving up these roles to be able to care for herself. As she gets better, however, she begins to look forward to resuming her roles.

With short-term role changes a client does not go through prolonged adjustment phases. Long-term changes, however, require an adjustment process similar to the grief process (see Chapter 26). The client and family members often require specific counseling and guidance to assist them in coping with the role changes. The following example illustrates how such changes can occur:

Mr. Lampe is a married 40-year-old construction worker with three sons. The family is very active in outdoor activities and goes hiking and camping every 2 weeks during the summer and fall. Mr. Lampe is injured while hiking, and his injury necessitates the amputation of one leg. Because of the injury Mr. Lampe has to change jobs, with the result that he receives a lower salary. The family activities change from active outdoor ones to passive indoor ones. Mrs. Lampe becomes angry because the reduction in income makes it difficult for the family to maintain its previous standard of living. The three sons become angry because their dad no longer takes them camping and hiking. Mr. Lampe becomes angry because he feels that his wife and children should be grateful that he is alive and should not worry about material things. The anger in the family gradually increases to the point that Mr. Lampe becomes unable to function at his highest level. The visiting nurse notices these changes in the family and observes the family members' angry outbursts. She refers the family for counseling sessions with a family therapist to help the family members cope with the anger resulting from the changes in Mr. Lampe's roles.

In some cases the family takes over all the roles of the client, including those of wage earner and decision maker, because family members mistakenly assume the ill person needs to be free of decisions and responsibilities in order to recover. Although Mr. Lampe does need to recover physically from his illness, he does not have to relinquish all his roles in the family. If the family attempts to relieve him of all responsibility, he may feel isolated and withdraw from it. Because changes in a client's role affect his family, nurses must incorporate the family into the plan of care.

Impact on Body Image

Body image is the subjective concept of physical appearance. Some illnesses result in changes in the client's physical appearance, which can affect the client and family. Clients and families react differently to these changes.

The reactions of a client and family to a change in body image depend on (1) the type of change (for example, loss of a limb, loss of a special sense, or loss of an organ); (2) the adaptive capacity of the client and family; (3) the rate at which the change takes place; and (4) supportive services available to the client and family (see Chapter 29).

When such a change occurs, the client generally adjusts in the following phases: shock, withdrawal, acknowledgment, acceptance, and rehabilitation. Initially the client may be shocked by the change or impending change in body image. The client may depersonalize it and talk about it as though it were happening to someone else. As the client and family recognize the reality of the change, they become anxious and may withdraw, refusing to discuss it. Withdrawal is an adaptive coping mechanism and can assist the client in making the adjustment. As the client and family acknowledge the change, they move through a period of grieving. At the end of the acknowledgment phase, they accept the loss. During rehabilitation the client is ready to learn how to adapt to the body image change through use of a prosthesis or changes in life-style and goals.

Impact on Self-Concept

A person's self-concept is his mental image of himself, including how he views his strengths and weaknesses in all aspects of his personality. A person's self-concept depends in part on his body image and roles but also includes other aspects of his psychological and spiritual self. The impact of illness on the self-concept of the client and the members of his family may be more complex and less readily observed than role changes.

A person's self-concept is important in his relationships with other family members. For example, a client whose self-concept changes because of illness may no longer meet the expectations of family members, leading to tension or conflict. As a result, family members may

change their interactions with the client. For example, the client may no longer be part of the family's decision-making process or may not be perceived as being able to provide emotional support to other family members or friends. Finally, the client may be left out of social functions.

In the course of providing care, a nurse is able to observe such changes in the client's self-concept—or in the self-concepts of family members—and to develop a care plan to help them adjust to the impact of illness.

Impact on Family Dynamics

Because of the effects of illness on the client and his family, family dynamics is often changed. Family dynamics is the process by which the family functions, makes decisions, gives support to individual members, and copes with everyday changes and challenges. If a parent in a family becomes ill, family activities and decision making often come to a halt as the other family members wait for the illness to pass, or they delay action because they are reluctant to assume the ill person's roles or responsibilities. In some cases of prolonged illness, the family often has to shift to a new pattern of functioning, a change that can lead to emotional stresses. Young children, for example, may experience a strong sense of loss if either parent is hospitalized or unable to provide affection and a sense of security. Such emotional difficulty may persist even when the other parent or family members are successful in assuming the roles and responsibilities of the hospitalized parent. If a parent of an adult becomes ill and cannot carry out usual activities, the adult child often assumes many of the parent's responsibilities and in essence becomes a parent to his own parent. Such a reversal of the usual situation can lead to emotional stresses, conflicting responsibilities for the adult child, or even direct conflict over who is to make decisions.

Chapter 21 discusses in more detail family dynamics and the impact of illness on family functioning. Illness can disrupt a family's patterns of living, just as it can disrupt the functioning of the client himself in all dimensions. A nurse must view the whole family as a client and plan care to meet the same goal that must be met for the ill person—to regain the maximal level of functioning and well-being.

SUMMARY

Health is not merely the absence of illness or disability. It is a dynamic state in which individuals adapt to internal and external environments to maintain the condition of physiological, emotional, intellectual, sociocultural, developmental, and spiritual well-being.

To provide effective nursing care and assist clients in regaining and maintaining high levels of wellness, nurses must understand each client's concept of health and his or her health beliefs and practices. Successful nursing care requires nurses to work with clients and their families, so the success of this relationship depends on nurses' awareness of the unique feelings, beliefs, and practices of clients and family members.

Most nurses practice in hospitals, and most clients entering the health care system to receive care perceive themselves as ill. Nurses practicing within home health care or community agencies also care for clients whose health beliefs and practices also vary.

Health professionals are emphasizing health promotion and illness prevention activities, which are designed to help clients reduce the risks of illness and maintain maximal levels of health. Consumers of health care are also making health promotion activities a higher priority.

When persons become ill, they progress through stages of illness behavior, which are influenced by psychosocial and cultural factors, the accessibility of the health care system, and the nature of the illness itself. If the illness is serious enough for a person to enter the health care system and receive nursing care, a nurse should be able to identify the factors influencing behavior and the impact of the illness on the client and family. In this way the nurse establishes a nursing care plan that helps the client achieve a high level of wellness in all dimensions. Nursing care is thus directed toward preventing illness and promoting health, helping the client adjust to an illness and its impact, and helping regain maximal functioning.

KEY CONCEPTS

✓ Health is a dynamic state in which the individual adapts to changes in the internal and external environment and thus maintains a state of well-being in all dimensions.

✓ An illness may be a disease but also includes reduced functioning in any of the human dimensions.

✓ A person's state of health or illness should be considered in relation to individual values, personality, and life-style rather than measured by any absolute standard.

✓ According to the health-illness continuum model, health and illness are in a dynamic, relative relationship. This model allows a nurse to compare a client's state of health with past states.

✓ The high-level wellness model describes health as an integrated method of functioning oriented toward maximizing an individual's potential.

✓ The agent-host-environment model describes disease or illness as the result of the dynamic interaction of factors related to the agent, host, and environment. No one factor is the cause of disease or illness.

✓ The health belief model considers factors influencing a person's health beliefs. This model helps nurses understand and predict the behaviors of clients in seeking or complying with health care.

✓ The evolutionary-based model of health and viability is based on the principle that illness and death sometimes serve as evolutionary functions.

✓ The health promotion model is directed toward increasing an individual's level of well-being and self-actualization.

✓ A person's health beliefs and practices are influenced by internal variables, including developmental stage, intellectual background, perception of functioning, and emotional and spiritual factors, and by external variables, including family practices and socioeconomic and cultural factors.

✓ To individualize care for a client and ensure his maximal participation in that care, the nurse considers his health beliefs and practices when planning care.

✓ Health promotion activities seek to maintain or enhance a person's health.

✓ Illness prevention activities seek to protect a person against risk factors and thus maintain his level of health.

✓ Nursing incorporates health promotion and illness prevention activities rather than simply treating illness once it occurs.

✓ Primary preventive care helps healthy people maintain and increase their levels of health.

✓ Secondary preventive care seeks to help already ill persons avoid complications or further health problems.

✓ Tertiary preventive care helps clients to adapt to or overcome disability or reduced functioning caused by illness.

✓ Risk factors threaten a person's health, influence health practices, and are important considerations in illness prevention activities.

✓ Risk factors are commonly associated with genetic or physiological variables, age, environment, and life-style.

✓ A person's illness behavior, like his health practices, is influenced by a number of variables and must be considered by the nurse when planning care.

✓ Although no two ill individuals behave in exactly the same way, most pass through the following stages of illness behavior: symptom experience, assumption of the sick role, medical care contact, the dependent role, and recovery and rehabilitation.

✓ Illness can have a number of effects on the client and family, including behavioral and emotional changes and changes in roles, body image, self-concept, and family dynamics.

✓ A nurse must consider all the effects of an illness on a client and family to plan and implement holistic nursing care that assists both in attaining a state of maximal functioning and well-being.

REFERENCES

Aiken, LH: Chronic illness and responsive ambulatory care. In Mechanic, D: The growth of bureaucratic medicine, New York, 1976, John Wiley & Sons, Inc.

Balog, JE: The concepts of health and disease: a relativistic perspective, Health Values 6:7, 1982.

Becker, MH: The health belief model and personal health behavior, Thorofare, N.J., 1974, Slack, Inc.

Belloc, NB, and Breslow, L: Relationship of physical health status and health practices, Prev Med 1:409, 1972.

Breslow, L: A quantitative approach to the World Health Organization definition of health: physical, mental and social well-being, Int J Epidemiol 1:347, 1972.

Coe, R: Sociology of medicine, ed. 2, New York, 1978, McGraw-Hill Book Co.

Davidson, JK: Diabetes in socioeconomically deprived neighborhoods. In Diabetes mellitus: diagnosis and treatment, New York, 1971, American Diabetes Association.

Dixon, JK, and Dixon, JP: An evolutionary-based model of health and viability, ANS 6(3):1, 1984.

Dunn H: What high level wellness means, Health Values 1:9, 1977.

Dunn, HL: High-level wellness for man and society, Am J Public Health 49:789, 1959.

Fuchs, VR: Who shall live? Health, economics, and social choice, New York, 1974, Basic Books, Inc., Publishers.

Goldsmith, JR: Health effects of air pollution, Basics RD 4(2):4, 1975.

Holmes, TH, and Rahe, RH: Social readjustment rating scale, J Psychosom Res 11:213, 1967.

Leavell, HR, et al.: Preventive medicine for the doctor in his community, ed. 3, New York, 1965, McGraw-Hill Book Co.

Leininger, M: Cultural diversities of health and nursing care, Nurs Clin North Am 12(1):5, 1977.

Mechanic, D: The epidemiology of illness behavior and its relationship to physical and psychological distress. In Mechanic, D: Symptoms, illness behavior, and help seeking, New York, 1982, Prodist.

Moore, LG, et al.: The biocultural basis of health: expanding views of medicine anthropology, Prospect Heights, Ill., 1980, Waveland Press, Inc.

Parsons, T: Definitions of health and illness in light of American values and social structures. In Joco, EG, editor: Patients, physicians, and illness, New York, 1958, The Free Press.

Pender, NJ: Health promotion in nursing practice, ed. 2, Norwalk, Conn., 1987, Appleton & Lange.

Rosenstock, I: Historical origin of the health belief model, Health Educ Monogr 2:334, 1974.

Shaver, JF: A biopsychosocial view of human health, Nurs Outlook 33:186, 1985.

Spector RE: Cultural diversity in health and illness, ed. 2, Norwalk, Conn., 1985, Appleton & Lange.

Steele, RL: Social networks as a means of health maintenance, Health Values 6(6):6, 1982.

Suchman, EA: Stages of illness and medical care, J Health Human Behav 6:114, 1965.

World Health Organization: Chronicle of WHO, Geneva, 1974, The Organization, Interim Commission.

Research Articles

Allinger, RL: Study of illness referral in a Spanish speaking community, Nurs Res 26:53, 1977.

Cox, CL: The health self-determination index, Nurs Res 34:177, 1985.

Hubbard, P, Muhlenkamp, AF, and Brown, N: The relationship between social support and self-care practices, Nurs Res 33:266, 1984.

Muhlenkamp, AF, and Sayles, JA: Self-esteem, social support and positive health practices, Nurs Res 35:334, 1986.

Rotter, J: Generalized expectancies for internal versus external control of reinforcement, Psychol Monogr, 80:1, 1966.

Suchman, EA: Health attitudes and behavior, Arch Environ Health 20:105, 1970.

Volicer, BJ: Patient's perceptions of stressful events associated with hospitalization, Nurs Res 23:235, 1974.

Walker, SN, Sechrist, KR, and Pender, NJ: The health-promoting lifestyle profile: development and psychometric characteristics, Nurs Res 36:76, 1987.

Zborowski, M: Cultural components in response to pain, J Soc Issues 8:16, 1952.

ADDITIONAL READINGS

Alexy, B: Goal setting and health risk reduction, Nurs Res 34(5):283, 1985.

Brown BJ: Reorganizing hospital-based nursing practice: an analysis of patient outcomes, provider satisfaction and costs. In Aiken, LH, editor: Health policy and nursing practice, New York, 1981, McGraw-Hill Book Co.

Dunn, H: High level wellness, Arlington, Va., 1961, R.W. Beatty, Ltd.

Dunn, HL: What high-level wellness means, Can J Public Health 50:447, 1959.

Edelman, C, and Mandle, CL: Health promotion throughout the life span, St. Louis, 1986, The C.V. Mosby Co.

Ferrans, CE, and Powers, MJ: Quality of life index: development and psychometric properties, ANS 8(1):15, 1985.

Fries, JF: The future of disease and treatment: changing health conditions, changing behaviors, and new medical technology, J Prof Nurs 2(1):10, 1986.

Holmes, TH, and Rahe, RH: Social readjustment rating scale, J Psychosom Res 11:213, 1967.

Hyman, RB, and Woog, P: Stressful life events and illness onset: a review of crucial variables, Res Nurs Health 5:155, 1982.

Jonas, S: Hospitals adopt new roles, Hospitals 53:84, 1979.

Lenz, ER: Information seeking: a component of client decisions and health behaviors, ANS 6:59, 1984.

Mechanic, D: Medical sociology, ed. 2, New York, 1978, The Free Press.

Milsum, JH: Health, risk factor reduction and life-style changes, Fam Community Health 3:1, 1980.

Parsons, T: The social system, New York, 1951, The Free Press.

Pender, NJ: A conceptual model for preventive health behavior, Nurs Outlook 23:385, 1975.

Pender, NJ, and Pender, AR: Attitudes, subjective norms, and intentions to engage in health behaviors, Nurs Res 35(1):15, 1986.

Pollock, SE: Human responses to chronic illness: physiologic and psychosocial adaptation, Nurs Res 35:90, 1986.

Steinfels, P: The concept of health: an introduction, The Hastings Cent Rep 1(3):3, 1973.

Tripp-Reimer, T: Reconceptualizing the construct of health: integrating emic and etic perspectives, Res Nurs Health 1:101, 1984.

Volicer, BJ: Perceived stress levels of events associated with the experience of hospitalization: development and testing of a measurement tool, Nurs Res 22:491, 1973.

Volicer, BJ, and Bahannon, MW: A hospital stress rating scale, Nurs Res 24:354, 1975.

Wolinsky, FD: The sociology of health: principles, professionals and issues, Boston, 1980, Little, Brown & Co., Inc.

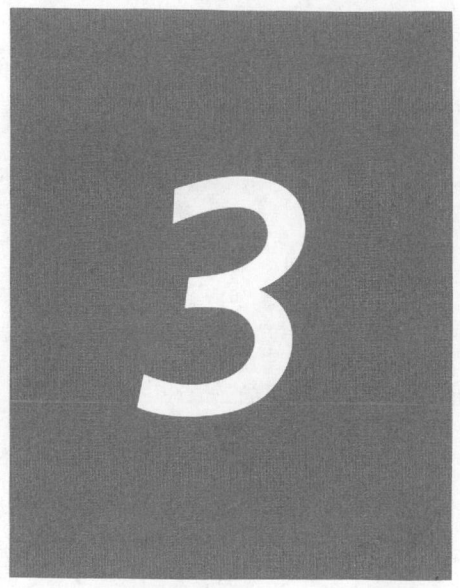

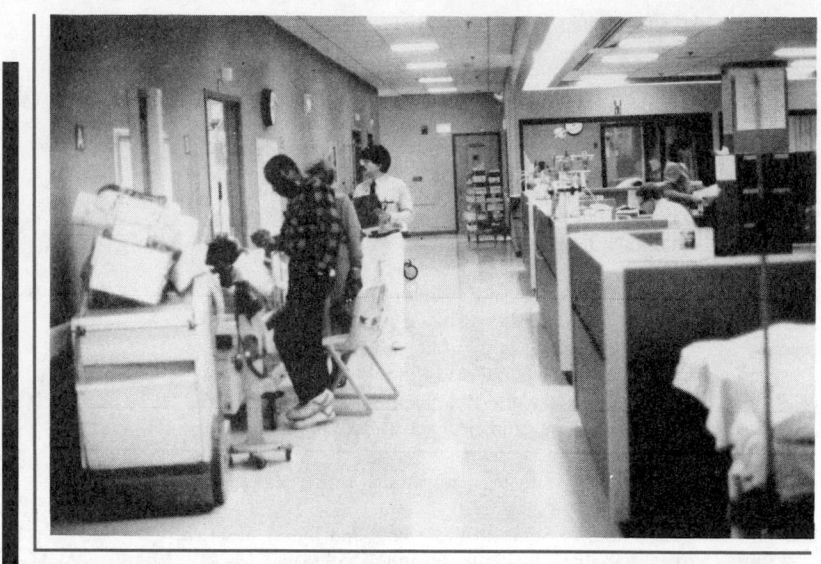

OBJECTIVES

Mastery of content in this chapter will enable the student to:

- Define the key terms listed.
- Describe society's influence on the health care delivery system.
- Discuss the client's entry into the system.
- Discuss how a client can use the system.
- Describe the six types of health care agencies.
- Discuss the client's right to health care and describe client rights within the health care delivery system.
- State various methods for financing health care.
- Describe the problems of the system.

KEY TERMS

Alcoholics Anonymous
Crisis Intervention Centers
Day-Care Centers
Diagnostic Related Groups
Drug Rehabilitation Centers
Extended Care Facilities
Governmental Agencies
Health Care Delivery System
Health Maintenance Organizations
Home Health Care Agencies
Hospice
Individual Practice Associations
Informed Consent
Medicaid
Medicare
Nursing Care Strategy
Outpatient Setting
Preferred Provider Organization
Prospective Payment
Psychiatric Hospital
Rehabilitation
Rehabilitation Center
Volunteer Agencies

The Health Care Delivery System

The health care system is being restructured with revolutionary changes. For example, it is predicted that the fee-for-service, solo-practice physician will be modified within the next 10 years (Griffith, 1985). The source of this change is the skyrocketing cost of medical services. Consumer demand, third-party reimbursement (payment by insurance), and federal legislation have attempted to slow the spiraling costs. However, health care costs continue to rise, and the financing for such services has become expensive for persons with private health insurance and for government agencies providing assistance to meet health care costs.

Rising costs of and restrictions placed on health care services by private and governmental third-party payers may further lower the frequency and quality of care of people from varying socioeconomic backgrounds, thus further promoting the two-tiered health care system in which clients with private insurance may receive a different quality of care than those with public insurance. Income, social class, and place of residence frequently dictate the client's accessibility to and type of health care received. Leah Curtin (1980) states that the interests of health care professionals lie in the individual first and society second, whereas the interests of health care administrators and representatives of the people lie in society first and the individual second.

Nursing is a major component of the health care delivery system, and nurses make up the largest single employment group within the system. Nursing services are necessary for virtually every client seeking care of any type, including health promotion, diagnosis and treatment, and rehabilitation. Because nursing is such an important part of the health care system and because the delivery of nursing services is tied to other components of the health care delivery system, the nurse needs to understand the system to most effectively deliver quality care within it. The changing health care delivery system includes a complex array of agencies providing specialized care. This complexity may at times confuse clients and threaten their entry into the system.

FACTORS INFLUENCING HEALTH CARE DELIVERY

The health care delivery system provides services related to health promotion, illness prevention, diagnosis and treatment of diseases, and rehabilitation. These services are provided by many kinds of agencies in different settings, including outpatient settings such as hospital clinics and physicians' offices, community settings such as day-care centers and home health care, and institutional settings such as hospitals or nursing homes.

Changes in the health care delivery system have increased rapidly within the last decade. The present system is the result of changes associated with social and consumer influences, new knowledge and technology, and economic and political factors.

Health Care Delivery System

The health care delivery system involves a combination of preventive, remedial, and therapeutic services provided by hospitals and other institutions, governmental and voluntary agencies, health care professionals, pharmaceutical and medical equipment manufacturers, and governmental and private insurance agencies. Changes within the system are related to Medicare and Medicaid, technological advances, and increased knowledge required of all health care workers.

In 1965, Title 18 of the Social Security Act and the introduction of Medicare changed the demographics of clients seeking access to the system. The older, retired population now had a government-supported insurance policy to partially pay for hospitalization and elective procedures.

Scientific and technological advances have increased the complexity of the industry. An explosion in knowledge created a need for specialization among health care professionals. Thus the consumer could seek care from professionals in the different specializations.

The health care industry became so complex that consumers were confused in all aspects of their involvement with the system. Money was needed to train technicians and buy equipment developed as a result of scientific advances. The system increasingly became a business, and business objectives sometimes seemed to threaten service goals. Therefore there was a risk that the system would lose touch with the needs of the consumer and

that the delivery of care would be impeded. Planners of health care services need to remain aware of consumer needs rather than requiring the consumer to fit into the services of the system (Brown, 1979).

Societal and Consumer Influences

Consumers of health care delivery services have increased their knowledge and awareness of health promotion, illness prevention, and treatment practices. As a result, these consumers are exerting influence on health care and its delivery.

As consumers have become more knowledgeable about health in general, they have gained a greater awareness of the impact of life-style on health. As a result, consumers have expressed a greater need for knowledge and services related to illness prevention and health promotion (see Chapter 2). Consumers seek diagnosis and treatment of illness, but this is no longer the exclusive or even primary focus of health care.

In addition, clients with chronic disease or disability seek more information about self-care, wishing to remain as independent as possible. Thus clients demand more health maintenance services, which allow those with chronic disease to achieve the highest level of wellness and functioning.

The health care beliefs and practices of society are as complex as those of an individual, depending on continually evolving values, ethics, concepts of health, and other factors. In general, however, consumers' desire for health promotion, health maintenance, and new cures and treatments has led to changes in the health care delivery system. Many institutions and community-based agencies provide a wide range of health promotion and health maintenance programs on a regular basis. Volunteer agencies have arisen to meet specific needs in health maintenance and promotion, and consumers have become more active in fund raising to support research in these areas.

Influence of New Knowledge and Technology

Scientific knowledge continues to grow rapidly. Research has led to new treatments and cures for life-threatening diseases such as cancer, cardiovascular diseases, and diabetes mellitus. Clients have the opportunity to receive the most advanced treatment for specific illnesses.

The disadvantages of this knowledge explosion are related to four factors. It is increasingly difficult for health care professionals to remain well informed about advances in their field. Increasing technology causes increasing cost, and care is more fragmented because of increased specialization.

Equipment is becoming more specialized and costly. A very expensive and sophisticated piece of equipment such as a gallium scanner may be needed for only a few clients. The health care delivery system must investigate the best uses for new knowledge and technology. The ultimate factors in the use of this technology may be the economic resources available and the wants and needs of society as a whole.

Economic Influences

Ultimately, someone must pay for all health care services. Clients with private resources or insurance policies are generally able to seek health promotion and maintenance services, but, too often, those with lower economic status must defer seeking health services until they are very ill because their income goes to meet other needs. As the total economy of a community or a country declines, its overall use of health care services also declines.

During inflationary times and periods of high unemployment, more people defer seeking diagnosis and treatment, and the use of health care services declines because of the high personal cost of services. In some situations the health care delivery system responds to declining use of inhospital services by expanding less costly services such as health promotion activities.

Political Influences

The health care delivery system is also influenced by political decisions and factors. Through health care legislation, government at all levels affects how health care is provided and who pays for it. A federal administration making health care a high priority, for example, can benefit the health care delivery system by introducing legislation that increases funding for health education and research.

Although politics influences the health care delivery system, it is the client who must adjust to changes caused by health care legislation. The poor frequently must delay seeking preventive or tertiary care because of economic restraints resulting from government policies such as increasing Medicare copayments.

EVOLUTION OF THE HEALTH CARE DELIVERY SYSTEM

Before 1945 the U.S. government was not involved in the health care industry. In 1945 the Hill-Burton Act was passed, providing money for hospital construction, expansion, or improvement (Beck, 1985). As a result, new hospitals were built in suburban and rural settings.

Large urban medical centers were expanded for scientific research and technological advances.

With the passage of the Medicare and Medicaid amendments to the Social Security Act in 1965, the U.S. government established a national and state health insurance program for certain segments of the population. The Medicare program provides medical and hospital insurance for persons who are over 65 years of age or disabled. The Medicaid program provides a joint federal and state health insurance program for low-income persons in specific groups, including families with dependent children, the aged, the blind, the disabled, and those who cannot afford medical care. In Canada, similar but more inclusive medical services are provided by provincial medical care plans.

The National Health Planning and Resources Development Act of 1974 (PL 93-641) introduced a comprehensive system of health planning. This law brought together into one system the previously existing but fragmented federal programs involved in health planning and resource development, including the Hill-Burton program for health facility construction, Regional Medical Programs for categorical health delivery programs, and the Comprehensive Health Planning Act of 1966.

Although legislation was designed to provide for the expansion of hospitals and the payment of services and to develop a system of health planning, some legislation did affect certain professionals. The Rural Health Clinics Act of 1978 represents the U.S. government's willingness to allow nurse practitioners to deliver primary health care. This act provides for the development of rural health clinics in medically undeserved areas, for the use of nurse practitioners as clinic staff, and for direct reimbursement to clinics for services provided by nurse practitioners to Medicare and Medicaid recipients. This law demonstrates the trend toward involving nurses in primary health care delivery.

In 1982, Congress passed the Tax Equity and Fiscal Responsibility Act (TEFRA) to set limits in cost-based reimbursement (Beck, 1985). This program lasted only about 6 months and was replaced by a newer, prospective-payment legislation. In 1983 the U.S. Congress approved a Medicare prospective pricing plan for most inpatient services as part of the Social Security Amendments of 1983, thus initiating prospective reimbursement as the basis for payment for hospital services. The amount of reimbursement is based on diagnostic related groups (DRGs), the type of hospital, and the geographical region. DRGs were developed at Yale University's Center for Health Studies and were based on the following variables: primary and secondary diagnoses, primary and secondary procedures, the client's age, and the length of stay. The 467 DRGs were formulated through research into usual procedures and treatments for different illnesses.

TYPES OF HEALTH CARE SERVICES

Health Promotion

Health promotion services have developed rapidly within the health care delivery system. Health promotion activities, including specific health education programs, are designed to help clients reduce the risk of illness, maintain maximal function, and promote habits related to good health. Health promotion activities take place in many settings. Hospitals, for example, offer programs such as prenatal nutrition classes in which pregnant women are taught the essentials of good nutrition during pregnancy, after childbirth, and for the infant. These classes thus promote the general health of the woman, the fetus, and the infant. Many kinds of health promotion activities exist within the community. For example, exercise classes such as those in aerobic dance encourage participants to exercise the body and cardiovascular system.

Illness Prevention

Illness prevention is another type of service provided by the health care delivery system. The nurse helps prevent illness by assisting the client and family in reducing risk factors and avoiding the need for primary, secondary, or tertiary health care. Prevention activities usually directly involve the client and include things such as periodical physical examinations and identification of familial risk factors for illnesses such as cardiovascular disease. Once a client's risk factors are identified, the client can engage in positive health practices such as giving up smoking to prevent illness. Community and family mental health programs have been created to provide support and counseling to individuals and families in crises.

Illness prevention activities also include environmental programs to reduce the threat of illness or disability. For example, controlling the breeding of mosquitoes with insecticides during hot, humid weather can reduce the risk of an encephalitis outbreak.

Occupational safety measures and educational programs also are illness prevention activities. In the painting and construction industry, for example, the use of respirators by employees exposed to dust and paint fumes reduces the risk of lung disease.

Public education programs and legislation are also involved in illness and injury prevention. Laws requiring the use of an approved infant or toddler restraint seat in automobiles, for example, are directed toward preventing severe injury or death.

Preventive health education and health practices are generally very effective in reducing the risk of disease and disability, and prevention activities help to improve the client's and community's level of health. Furthermore, it is becoming evident that preventive measures, such as smoking cessation, stress management, or weight control, reduce the costs of health care.

Diagnosis and Treatment

The diagnosis and treatment of illness have traditionally been the most commonly used services of the health care delivery system. Advances in scientific knowledge of space-age technology and computers have resulted in more sophisticated diagnostic procedures and greater chances for early diagnosis. Many new diagnostic tests are noninvasive and painless.

Nurses' activities in the community can be directed toward early diagnosis. For example, nurses teach female clients about breast self-examination (see Chapter 13), enabling them to discover a breast mass at an early stage and thus seek early treatment. In other community settings, such as schools, special programs have been organized to detect certain conditions, such as hypertension, elevated cholesterol, or visual or hearing impairments, in early stages.

Nurses are also involved in diagnosis when they take the client's history in the assessment phase of the nursing process (Chapter 6).

The nurse is responsible for client education during the diagnosing process. When the client understands the procedure, anxiety about it and the equipment used is reduced. The client is better informed and can participate more fully and efficiently in the tests.

Treatment methods have also expanded because of advances in technology and knowledge. Clients are receiving newer, more innovative health care treatments based on the most recent research. The treatment of illnesses has also expanded outside hospitals and other institutions. Even when treatment is initiated within an institution, nurses teach the client and family how to complete the treatment plan at home and in outpatient settings.

Rehabilitation

Rehabilitation is the restoration of a person to normal or near-normal function after a physical or mental illness, injury, or chemical addiction. Rehabilitation was once available primarily for clients with illnesses or injury to the nervous system, but the health care delivery system has expanded its rehabilitative services. Today, cardiovascular rehabilitation programs help clients and their families adjust to necessary changes in life-style after a heart attack. Pulmonary rehabilitation programs aim to increase the exercise tolerance of clients with chronic pulmonary diseases. In addition, specific rehabilitation programs have been designed for those with physical impairments such as stroke, spinal cord trauma, or head or orthopedic injuries; those with chemically induced impairments such as alcohol or drug dependencies; and those with mental illnesses such as depression.

Rehabilitation services begin the moment a client with an illness or injury enters the health care system. Initially, rehabilitation may focus on the prevention of complications related to the illness or injury. As the client's condition stabilizes, rehabilitation is directed toward maximizing the client's functioning and increasing his level of independence.

These programs take place in many health care settings, including specific rehabilitation institutions. Frequently, clients needing long-term rehabilitation have severe disabilities affecting their ability to carry out the activities of daily living. Rehabilitation services are also provided by outpatient settings, in which the client receives treatment at specified times during the week but remains at home the rest of the time.

Many rehabilitation services are provided in outpatient settings or in the home, particularly when rehabilitation strategies will be applied to the client's home environment so a maximal level of function and independence can be achieved. Nurses and other members of the health care team visit the client's home and help the client and family learn to adapt to the illness or injury.

TYPES OF AGENCIES

As a result of the expansion of the health care system and increasing specialization, the variety and numbers of health care agencies have increased. Services once delivered primarily by hospitals are now provided in many other types of settings. The range of health care agencies includes outpatient, community-based, volunteer, institutional, hospice, and governmental.

Outpatient Agencies

Clients who do not require hospitalization can receive treatment in a physician's office, clinic, or another ambulatory care facility. Most receive health care through these outpatient services. Outpatient services are generally directed toward the diagnosis and treatment of both acute and chronic illnesses.

Physicians' offices provide primary care for a large segment of the population. Physicians in office practice tend to focus on the diagnosis and treatment of specific illnesses rather than on health promotion and other health services. Some physicians' offices have complete laboratory facilities for analyzing blood specimens and urine samples and obtaining electrocardiograms and ra-

diographs (x-ray films). Nurses employed in physicians' offices can assume many roles. Some nurses have the traditional role of registering clients, taking vital signs, preparing the client for examination or laboratory studies, and providing basic information. Other nurses working with physicians have the expanded role of nurse practitioner with responsibility for the primary care of clients in stable health states.

Clinics traditionally involve the following kinds of settings: (1) a department in a hospital where clients not requiring hospitalization receive medical care and (2) a group practice of physicians, or (3) a community agency that delivers a particular type of health service such as immunizations. The roles of nurses in a clinic closely parallel those of nurses in a physician's office.

Ambulatory care centers, like clinics, provide health services on an outpatient basis. Nurses providing primary care in an ambulatory setting work in a more expanded role as a nurse practitioner or clinical nurse specialist. These nurses have a specific caseload of clients and provide follow-up care for these clients when the clients visit the care center.

Community-Based Agencies

Community-based health care agencies focus on providing health care to clients within their neighborhoods. Examples of community-based agencies are day-care centers, home health care agencies, crisis intervention centers, drug rehabilitation centers, and specialized organizations such as Alcoholics Anonymous. Nurses may have a variety of roles within community-based agencies.

Day-care centers provide health care to specific client populations during the day. They may be associated with a hospital or other institution or may function independently. Frequently the clients of such centers do not require hospitalization but need continuous health care services while their family or support persons work. These clients include elderly individuals needing daily physical rehabilitation, individuals with emotional illnesses needing daily counseling, and individuals with chemical dependence problems who are involved in a rehabilitation program. Day-care centers reduce the cost of health care and allow the client to retain more independence by living at home.

Nurses working in day-care centers provide continuity between the care delivered in the home and the care delivered in the center. For instance, nurses can ensure that the client continues to take prescribed medication, administer specific treatments, and assist the client through counseling sessions.

Home health care agencies are organizations providing professional and nonprofessional health care services in the home. Community health nursing is one such type of service. Community health nurses employed by agencies deliver continuing and comprehensive care that can be preventive, curative, and rehabilitative. Home health care agencies, like community health care agencies in general, provide care based on the belief that care directed to the individual, the family, and the group contributes to the health of the population as a whole.

Crisis intervention centers provide emergency psychiatric care and counseling to clients experiencing extreme stress or conflict, often involving suicide attempts or drug or alcohol abuse. These centers, which are usually self-contained units within a hospital or community health care center, provide services 24 hours a day. The services may be delivered directly on the premises, or counseling may be provided over the telephone. The primary objectives of crisis intervention centers are to help the person cope with the immediate problem and to offer guidance and support for long-term therapy (see Chapter 28).

Drug rehabilitation centers provide to a client with chemical drug dependency long-term care and a gradual return to the community. These rehabilitation centers may operate in association with a hospital or other institution or may function independently. Nurses employed in these centers must be knowledgeable about chemical dependencies and community resources, as well as counseling and communication techniques.

Specialized organizations provide services for clients with select health problems. For example, Alcoholics Anonymous is an international nonprofit organization of recovering alcoholics whose purpose is to help alcoholics stop drinking and remain sober through group support, shared experiences, and faith in a higher power. Meetings are held in a central community location such as a church, school, or hospital. A group called Al-Anon assists families in helping alcoholic family members, and Alateen helps teenagers cope with alcoholism in their families.

Volunteer Agencies

Volunteer agencies are not-for-profit health care agencies established nationally or within a community to meet a specific need. Examples are the American Lung Association and the American Cancer Society and, in Canada, the Canadian Lung Association and the Canadian Heart Foundation. Most volunteer agencies do not provide treatment but have programs focused on the prevention and detection of specific illnesses. In addition, some volunteer agencies provide financial support for training of physicians and nurses, as well as for biomedical research directed toward the prevention, detection, or treatment of certain diseases.

Volunteer agencies depend heavily on professional and lay volunteers to carry out many of the activities of the agency. Financial support is generally derived from fund-raising activities, federal grants, and donations from individuals supporting the agency. Many health professionals donate time and resources to agencies within their specialty.

Institutional Settings

Institutional settings include hospitals, nursing homes, extended care facilities, and some rehabilitation centers offering health care services to inpatients (clients admitted to a stay within the institution for the purpose of diagnosis, treatment, or rehabilitation).

Hospitals traditionally have been the major agency of the health care system. They vary in size from small rural hospitals of perhaps only 20 beds to large urban medical centers with hundreds of beds. Public and private hospitals exist throughout Canada and the United States. A public hospital is financed and operated by a government agency at the local, state, provincial, or national level. Many clients in public hospitals cannot afford to pay for care. Private hospitals are owned and operated by groups such as churches, corporations, businesses, and charitable organizations. Clients of private hospitals generally have some type of insurance or medical assistance to pay for hospital care.

Hospitals generally provide inpatient, outpatient, and support group services to answer the needs of the community. Because of the number of services, nurses working in hospitals have a variety of roles, including opportunities for specialization.

An *extended care facility* is an institution providing long-term medical, nursing, or custodial care for clients with chronic illnesses or disabilities. Extended care facilities include intermediate care and skilled nursing facilities, convalescent and nursing homes, and some residential institutions.

Extended care facilities offer the client many levels of skilled nursing care. One client may require only minimal nursing care, such as ensuring that medications are taken each day and the presence of health care professionals in case other problems develop. Another client may need some assistance with the activities of daily living such as dressing. Still another client may need considerable assistance with bathing, dressing, and feeding. Extended care facilities provide round-the-clock nursing coverage. Nurses employed in such a setting have expertise in the nursing skills required for the clients to whom the facility provides care.

A *rehabilitation center* is a residential institution providing therapy and training to restore a client to optimal level of functioning and independence. Rehabilitation centers actively involve the client and family in providing health care. The goal of rehabilitation is to decrease the client's dependence on the care provided so that the client assumes responsibility for personal care.

Rehabilitation centers employ persons from nursing, medicine, and the allied health fields. Many rehabilitation centers focus on physical rehabilitation programs to teach the client and family how to achieve maximal physical function after a stroke, head, or spinal cord injury or physical impairment. Drug rehabilitation centers help the client become free from drug dependence and return to the community. Mental health rehabilitation centers help the mentally ill to cope with their problems and return to independent functioning. Nurses employed in rehabilitation centers are committed to long-term continuity of nursing services and must be knowledgeable in their specialized area.

Psychiatric hospitals or mental health hospitals provide inpatient and outpatient counseling services to clients with behavioral or emotional illnesses. Treatment in psychiatric hospitals is directed toward helping clients control their behavior. Psychiatric hospitals may be operated within large medical centers or hospitals or may be independent, government-supported, or private hospitals.

Nurses working in psychiatric hospitals use communication skills as a major basis for care (see Chapter 19). Effective care depends on use of communication and other skills to develop a nurse-client relationship.

Hospices

The trend of seeking care outside of institutions has led to the development of hospices to meet the needs of the terminally ill. A hospice is a system of family-centered care designed to make the terminally ill person comfortable and to ensure a satisfactory life-style through the terminal phase of the illness. Hospice care can benefit a client in the terminal phases of any disease, such as a cardiomyopathy, multiple sclerosis, AIDS, cancer, emphysema, or renal disease.

A client entering a hospice has reached the terminal phase of illness, and the client, family, and physician have agreed that no further treatment could reverse the disease process. The client and family must accept the fact that the hospice will not use emergency measures such as cardiopulmonary resuscitation to prolong life. Instead, the hospice provides pain control and comfort measures to maintain the quality of life. Hospices do not have rigid visiting policies or other prescribed limits, and the environment for the clients and health care workers is very relaxed.

Hospices are operated in many settings. Independent hospices provide only hospice care and are not affiliated with a hospital or medical center. Other hospices operate within a hospital setting, and many hospitals are now developing hospice units in a separate area of the institution. Many home care agencies also offer these services and involve neighborhood and community resources in providing care and emotional support for terminally ill clients and their family.

Nurses who work in hospices are employed in both institutional and community settings. A hospice nurse is committed to the philosophy and objectives of the facility for which he or she works. The nurse provides care and support for the client and family during the terminal phase and continues to give the family emotional support throughout the grieving period.

Governmental Agencies

Governmental agencies are clinics, hospitals, and other health services supported by local, state, provincial, or national taxes. Local governmental agencies include city hospitals and public health clinics. Agencies at the state or provincial level include state psychiatric hospitals and hospitals for clients with pulmonary disease. National agencies include primary research institutions such as the National Institutes of Health (NIH) and agencies administering health and welfare programs for a country such as the Canadian Department of Health and Welfare.

The types of local and state or provincial agencies and the allocation of resources for these agencies vary from one city, state, or province to another. Usually, agency funds originate in the tax base and are controlled by elected or appointed officials.

Health departments at the city or county level are generally concerned with specific health needs of the community and may receive additional support from the state or provincial health organization. Federal agencies provide specific kinds of health services on a national level. Of the many health-related national agencies in the United States and Canada, two are described in the following paragraphs: the Veterans Administration hospitals and the Canadian health care system.

The *Veterans Administration (VA) hospitals* were established after World War II to provide care for injured veterans. They are generally near major medical centers with teaching and training functions and a medical school. Many of the medical staff members in a VA hospital are supplied by the medical school.

Nursing services in VA hospitals are provided around the clock. Nursing services and nursing roles in these hospitals are similar to those in nongovernmental hospitals.

The *Canadian health care system* includes a Department of National Health and Welfare, which is responsible for (1) enforcing federal laws about harmful foods and drugs, (2) providing health care services for certain categories of people, (3) promoting fitness and amateur sports, (4) administering social welfare programs, and (5) overseeing financial and technical programs (Stewart, 1985).

Most general and specialized hospital costs are financed by provincial hospital insurance plans. Each province organizes and administers its own plan, but plans have many common features, and each plan must meet certain federal standards (Soderstrom, 1981). In all provincial plans, insured services must be available to all residents. Members of the military and the Royal Canadian Mounted Police and inmates of federal prisons are excluded because their insurance is financed through other federal agencies.

THE CLIENT AND THE HEALTH CARE DELIVERY SYSTEM

A person may have little or no interaction with the health care delivery system while experiencing good health. However, if the person becomes ill, feels illness threatening, or is motivated for other reasons to seek health care, the health care delivery system must be entered. Some clients enter the system easily by walking into a clinic or hospital emergency room or by making an appointment with a physician in private practice. Other clients experience difficulties in entering the system because of confusion or unfamiliarity with the agencies or because of low economic status.

Clients entering the system have rights. Society generally believes that all people have a right to health care, but once a person enters the health care delivery system, he becomes a client and thus has certain rights *within* the system. People as health care consumers have a general right to determine *what* kind of health care should be available for present and future needs. Each of these rights affects how health care is delivered, but practices ensured by these rights are also influenced by society's attitudes and the delivery system itself.

Right to Health Care

Society has generally come to believe that all people have a right to health care, regardless of cultural, economic, or other factors. In the 1960s, this belief led to the development of the federal Medicare and Medicaid programs, directed toward providing health care for those otherwise unable to afford care. These two programs seek to meet the health care needs of the elderly and the poor, the groups generally least able to afford health care on their own. However, the Medicare and Medicaid programs do not cover all health care costs. Rising costs require the client to assume more and more of the cost of health care needs.

To control rising costs, Medicare and Medicaid were changed in 1983 so payment for services would become prospective, meaning the amount of payment is known in advance (Beck, 1985). This payment plan is deter-mined from the DRGs and has many implications for the future. Since the program began, the length of hospital stay has decreased, and many clients needing acute care services are sent home. One result is an increase in home health care agencies, which are equipped to provide competent, complex nursing care that may also require the use of sophisticated equipment (Smith, 1985).

Nursing services have also been affected. Discharge planning has a high priority and must be implemented the first day of hospital admission. In some institutions, a high ratio of RN staff is viewed as too expensive, so there has been a reanalysis of the appropriate methods for delivering care with fewer RNs. In addition, in an attempt to further reduce nursing costs, lower-salaried, nonprofessional health care workers may be hired (Smith, 1985).

Rising costs, nursing shortages, and changing demographics have forced smaller, rural hospitals to close or consolidate with larger medical centers. In addition, smaller, rural hospitals are unable to diversify services (for example, 1-day surgery centers, home health care, fitness programs) to compete with larger centers.

Health care costs continue to rise for three reasons. Rising poverty levels reduce the percentage of low-income mothers receiving prenatal care. Hence, premature births, low-birth-weight infants, and infant mortality and morbidity rates increase in the indigent population. The increase in the numbers of clients with AIDS or AIDS-related illness is costly to the health care system, as well as to the public and private insurance carriers. Modern technology also provides physicians and nurses with skills and treatments to care for trauma and disease victims who would have died 10 years ago.

Rights Within the System

In 1973 the American Hospital Association developed a Patient's Bill of Rights (see Chapter 18), which lists 12 specific rights of hospitalized clients. The bill offers some guidance and protection to clients by stating the responsibilities of the hospital and staff toward clients and their families. However, it is not a legally binding document. The Patient's Bill of Rights supports consumer activities for clients in the health care system. The client has the right to information pertaining to diagnosis and treatment, fees for services, and continuity of care. The client has the right to refuse diagnostic or treatment procedures. Above all, the Patient's Bill of Rights reaffirms the client's right to both information and privacy while receiving health care.

One of the client's specific legal rights in any health care facility is informed consent, which is obtaining permission from the client to perform certain kinds of actions. Informed consent must be obtained before beginning any invasive procedure, administering an experimental drug, or placing a client in a research study. Informed consent must meet the following criteria:

1. The consent document must be written in language that the client or guardian can understand.
2. The consent document must delineate all possible risks and actions of the physician or researcher to minimize the risks.
3. The consent document must list the benefit of the procedure to the client; if there is no known benefit at present, the consent document must state that fact.
4. Any alternatives to the procedure must be specified, even if the only alternative is nonparticipation.
5. The document must state that participation is voluntary and that clients can refuse to participate or withdraw from participation without having further health care withheld.
6. Clients who give informed consent must be rational and competent or represented by a competent guardian and must be told how they can reach the physician or researcher performing the procedure.

Clients' rights and informed consent affect the way the health care system delivers care. Most agencies now have committees to evaluate clients' suggestions and complaints about the delivery of health care. In many institutions, this committee is called a *patient care committee*. Another committee, an institutional review board, ensures that elements of informed consent are consistent with federal guidelines. Although the need to protect clients' rights sometimes results in increased work and paperwork, this protection is necessary to ensure that all clients maintain their rights within the health care delivery system.

Entry of the Client into the System

The three most common ways clients enter the health care system are (1) entry by referral from a health team member, (2) entry when the client has a specific health need, and (3) entry related to financial resources. Other methods of entry are (1) self-referral (2) employer referral, and (3) social referral.

A client may enter the system by referral from a health team member in the case of an acute, potentially life-threatening problem, such as the presence of an angina-like chest pain, or in the case of a less threatening problem such as a rash of unknown cause. The nurse is frequently the professional in a position to refer clients to the system. Such referrals may be given to neighbors seeking advice, children and their families at a school where the nurse practices or does volunteer work, and families of clients to whom the nurse has previously provided care.

Clients also enter the system on their own because of a specific need. For example, a college student may seek health care for treatment of a complaint such as a sore throat or gastrointestinal upset and so may enter the health care system at the primary care level through the student health center. Another student may be involved in a severe automobile accident and enter the health care system through a hospital emergency room.

Finally, entry into the health care system may be influenced by financial situations. An employed person with insurance may readily enter a hospital for elective surgical or diagnostic procedures because he has the financial resources to seek and pay for primary health care. An unemployed person with limited resources may seek care only if an illness becomes acute and may then go to a hospital emergency room. Frequently the only type of care some clients can obtain is that supported by local, state, provincial, or federal programs.

Regardless of the manner of entry into the system, all clients encounter nurses and nursing services. The first impression the client has of nursing services may stay with him and become a significant and lasting impression of nursing. Nurses therefore have the opportunity to increase clients' awareness of such services and the types of quality care they can and should expect.

FINANCING HEALTH CARE SERVICES

The rapid rise in health care costs has been the subject of discussion by governmental officials, the media, health care professionals, and consumers. It has become increasingly difficult, if not impossible, for people to meet these costs with their own resources. Therefore government agencies and private companies have developed a variety of prepaid health care programs, insurance programs, and social services to subsidize the cost of health care.

Private and Group Health Insurance Plans

The traditional insurance policy can be obtained by the individual or through a group plan offered by employers. This plan is a retrospective fee-for-service option. Health insurance programs pay for some, most, or all of the expenses of health care for the client. Such payments are called third-party reimbursements because the costs of health care services are met, not by the health care agency or the client, but by the third party, the insurer. Ultimately, of course, consumers bear the costs through insurance premiums.

Group health plans are another method of financing health care services. Health maintenance organizations (HMO) deliver care based on a prepaid fee. HMOs provide all types of health care services and emphasize health promotion and illness prevention more than other agencies.

A second type of group health plan is a preferred provider organization (PPO). A PPO is a group of physicians or a hospital agreeing to provide comprehensive health services at a discount to companies under contract. These plans are also called industry-based health plans. The PPO benefits the client and the hospital. The client receives care at a reduced rate, and the hospital gains because it can provide services at lower cost when its services are used by more clients.

Individual practice associations (IPAs) are also prospective payment plans. The client pays a fixed annual payment to the IPA, and the IPA pays the care provider (Griffith, 1985). The client must select from member providers.

HMOs, PPOs, and IPAs are directed toward cost reduction. Each requires utilization review services to avoid exceeding cost limits. HMOs and IPAs are regulated by federal legislation (HMO Act of 1973) (Griffith, 1985).

Governmental Insurance Plans

The U.S. government's commitment to financing medical care for the elderly and poor has been reduced by federal budget cuts. The 1983 changes in federal health policy have led to reductions in Medicare and Medicaid payments, with the prospective-pricing plan using DRGs being phased in over a 4-year period.

Prospective pricing affects all hospitals except children's, psychiatric, rehabilitation, and long-term care facilities. Separate psychiatric and rehabilitation units of general hospitals are also exempt.

In theory the objective of the prospective payment system is to provide incentives for hospitals to lower costs. For example, the DRG fee for gallbladder removal requiring an 8-day hospital stay might be set at $2500, a figure set on the basis of what the services should total. In hospital X, however, these services have typically been billed at $3000. Because Medicare reimburses the hospital only $2500, regardless of actual costs, the hospital has the incentive to investigate other methods of providing quality care. The hospital is also motivated not to keep the client hospitalized longer than necessary, since the reimbursement is the same regardless of length of stay. In theory, then, prospective payments should help contain costs. On the other hand, some people are concerned that this policy might reduce the quality of care in certain cases. The hospital might, in the example here, be tempted to discharge the client before 8 days even though, by its past standards, the client would have remained in the hospital another day or two.

Although DRGs provide incentives for hospitals to lower costs, they also protect clients from premature discharge and reduced standards of care. Protection of clients is ensured by audits of records by federal authorities. If these audits identify a hospital's trend to premature discharge resulting in clients' readmission to the hospital within 7 days, the hospital risks losing reimbursement funds.

At present, prospective payments are intended only for federally supported health insurance programs. In 1988 the prospective payment system applied only for the hospital stay, not for physician services.

PROBLEMS WITH THE PRESENT SYSTEM

Although the health care delivery system is increasingly responsive to the needs of the community by offering more services for health promotion and maintenance, it still has a number of problems, including the high costs of care, fragmentation of care, inability to meet the special needs of the chronically ill and elderly, and uneven distribution of services. These problems are not particularly new in the health care delivery system but have been aggravated by modern conditions in many cases.

Because nurses make up the largest segment of health professionals and because they are able to provide 24-hour-a-day care for clients, they have an opportunity to work toward solutions to the problems of the health care system.

Affordability of Care

In recent decades the costs of overall health care in the United States and Canada have tripled (Soderstrom, 1983). Some of the causes of the high costs of care follow:

1. Increased population and demand for services
2. Larger number of people with chronic illnesses
3. Growing cost of new technology and equipment
4. Inflation
5. Increased specialization of care
6. Increased number of people over 65 years of age
7. Increased number of clients surviving traumatic, disabling injuries or life-threatening illnesses
8. Increased survival rates of infants with low birth weight and ill neonates

Nursing must address the need for cost containment. If the prospective hospitalization payment system proves to be an effective method of reducing costs, nursing should also determine the costs of nursing service based on DRGs. One method for determining price rates for nursing services based on DRGs is to use detailed nursing care plans that include direct and indirect client care and that should allow for variances in both the independent and interdependent functions of nurses. According to Curtin (1983), nursing care strategies should reflect the nursing time needed to deliver care to clients, thus quantifying nursing care. To establish nursing care strategies, the nurse must correctly assess the client's needs and develop an individualized and accurate nursing care plan (see Unit 2).

Fragmentation of Care

Advanced scientific knowledge and technology have resulted in increasing specialization of health care in areas such as cardiac disease, kidney disease, and cancer. Although specialization allows each professional on the health care team to provide clients with highly advanced care, the delivery of the total care for the client is often fragmented. The number of primary physicians and care givers has gradually declined, and many families find themselves in the position of having a different physician for each family member or illness. As a result, care is not provided for the family as a unit or for the whole person. The care giver is therefore not able to assess family or personal dynamics and their impact on the person's level of health. With so many specialists involved in the care of clients, the client can be lost to health care follow-up simply because it is too difficult for him to cope with so many specialists. Furthermore, as the client goes from one specialist to another the cost of care increases, the client can be overmedicated or undermedicated, and the client's quality of life is changed because of the time involved in obtaining health care.

Nurses employed in community health, outpatient, psychiatric, and institutional settings have the opportunity to reduce the fragmentation of care. Primary care nursing is a delivery of care system that reduces fragmentation because one nurse manages the total care of the client. The primary nurse coordinates care given by other nurses, physicians, and other personnel and assists with scheduling of tests, procedures, and daily activities for the client. In addition, the primary nurse may personally care for the client when on duty. The primary nurse can thus continually monitor and assess the client's condition, relate information to him, and maintain continuity between specialists who may make recommendations for his care. Also, the nurse can give support to the client and help him cope with what otherwise might be a confusing situation.

Special Needs of the Chronically Ill and Elderly

The health care delivery system, and particularly the hospital, were developed primarily to meet the needs of the acutely ill. As a result, the needs of the chronically ill are frequently not met, or met only partially, in this system. The chronically ill commonly receive care in health care settings, such as outpatient clinics, where there is little continuity of care. In such cases clients and their families receive very little support to help them adapt to changes in life-style resulting from chronic illness.

Chronic illnesses affect the elderly more frequently than children or young or middle-aged adults, and, because people are living longer in North America, the number of clients with chronic diseases is growing. Thus there is an increasing need for the health care system to address the special care requirements of the chronically ill, including adaptation to changing roles, changes in family structure and cognitive and functional abilities, as well as physical and other needs related to disease processes.

Nursing is increasing its knowledge and expertise in caring for the chronically ill in all age groups. Nurses coordinate efforts to provide care designed to return chronically ill clients to their homes and to achieve and maintain the highest possible level of functioning.

The nursing profession is also giving more attention to the special needs of geriatric clients. The rapidly growing specialty of gerontological nursing prepares nurses to design strategies aimed at helping these clients maintain functioning and independence. Geriatrics involves the collaboration of all the health care disciplines. Nurses are able to coordinate the health care team and in many cases direct this care.

Availability of Health Care Services

The number of health care workers in North America has increased, but for several reasons, low-income and rural areas still lack adequate health care professionals and services. Low-income communities do not often have the fiscal resources necessary to establish or maintain major health care services. Increased specialization by health care professionals has led to fewer family and general practitioners meeting the need in some rural areas, and these areas often do not need or cannot support the services of specialists. Some rural areas even have seasonal population fluctuations, resulting in varying needs for health care services.

Nursing is able to meet some of these special health care needs. Nurse practitioners specializing in family, pediatric, adult, and obstetrical-gynecological services can provide services. Many community health agencies have expanded their nursing staff in rural areas to provide better care. School health nurses can provide health education and referral to members of the community.

■ ■ ■

Nursing alone certainly cannot solve all the problems of the present health care delivery system. However, nursing can influence the system by

1. Implementing cost containment measures
2. Providing total care to coordinate the client's care and to decrease fragmentation
3. Designing nursing strategies to meet the special needs of the elderly and chronically ill
4. Providing low-income and rural regions with more nursing services

SUMMARY

The health care industry is the most rapidly growing and changing industry in North America. Because of its rapid expansion, patterns of use by clients have changed, and new emphases are emerging. Consumers of health care have demanded health promotion and maintenance services, and the health care delivery system is changing to meet these needs.

The costs of health care are growing as rapidly as the health care system itself. This trend has led to the development of new and different kinds of outpatient and community-based health agencies, as consumers increasingly desire to receive health care outside the traditional hospital setting.

Today's health care delivery system is much better than in the past, but it is not without problems. Financing health care puts a burden on private and governmental resources. Technological advances have resulted in high-quality specialized care, but specialization has led to fragmentation of care. Finally, health care services are still unevenly distributed.

KEY CONCEPTS

✓ Health care services are provided in a large number of settings, across all age groups, and for the chronically, as well as the acutely ill.

✓ The explosion of the health care industry has resulted in specialization of health care professionals.

✓ Consumers are requesting more information, especially on services related to illness prevention and health promotion.

✓ Chronically ill and disabled clients are seeking knowledge and skills to maximize their levels of wellness and independence.

✓ Increased technology and new biomedical equipment increase the risk of health care professionals giving greater attention to the machine than to the client.

✓ A nation's economy directly affects the fiscal resources of the health care delivery system.

✓ Health promotion activities are designed to help clients reduce the risk of illness, maintain maximal function, and promote life-style habits related to good health.

✓ Illness prevention activities are directed toward helping the client and family reduce risk factors.

✓ Diagnosis and treatment activities are usually disease specific, with the goal of curing the client.

✓ Rehabilitation is the restoration of an individual to normal or near-normal function after a physical or mental illness, injury, or chemical dependency.

✓ Community-based agencies focus on providing health care to clients within their neighborhoods.

✓ Crisis intervention centers provide emergency psychiatric treatment and counseling to clients experiencing extreme stress or conflict.

✓ Extended care is the provision of medical, nursing, or custodial care for clients needing long-term care because of chronic illness or disability.

✓ Rehabilitation centers use a multidisciplinary health care team to restore the client to the maximal level of physical, emotional, or mental wellness.

✓ Psychiatric mental health agencies provide inpatient and outpatient counseling services to clients with behavioral or emotional illnesses.

✓ A hospice provides family-centered care to help clients maintain a satisfactory level of comfort and life-style through the terminal phase of illness.

✓ Governmental agencies can be local, regional, or national and are supported by revenues obtained through taxes.

✓ Prepaid health care can be obtained through health maintenance organizations, preferred provider organizations, or individual practice associations.

✓ Clients may enter the health care system through referral and specific health need.

✓ Financing of health care services is primarily through private and group health plans or governmental support.

✓ The high cost of health care is the result of increased population and demand for services, increased number of people with chronic illness, cost of technology, inflation, specialization, increased number of clients over 65 years of age and surviving illness and injury, and increased survival rates of ill infants.

✓ Nursing is able to reduce health care costs by implementing cost containment measures, implementing primary care, meeting special needs of the elderly and chronically ill, and expanding nursing activities into low-income and rural regions.

REFERENCES

Beck, DF: The hospital's financial future: DRGs and beyond, Health Care Superv 3:1, 1985.

Brown, RE: Consumerism in health care delivery: the harbinger of opportunity. In Cooper, PD, editor: Health care marketing, Rockville, Md., 1979, Aspen Publishers, Inc.

Curtin, L: Is there a right to health care, Am J Nurs 80:462, 1980.

Curtin, L: Determining costs of nursing services per DRG, Nurs Manage 14(4):16, 1983.

Griffith, H: Who will become the preferred providers? Am J Nurs 85:538, 1985.

Smith, CE: DRGs: making them work for you, Nurs 85, 15:1, 1985.

Soderstrom, L: The Canadian health system, London, 1981, Croom Helm, Ltd.

Soderstrom, L: Soaring hospital costs: the brewing revolt, U.S. News and World Report, Aug. 22, 1983.

Stewart, M, et al.: Community health nursing in Canada, Toronto, 1985, Gage Educational Publishing, Ltd.

Research Article

Shukla, RK, and Tuner, WE: Patient's perception of care under primary nursing and team nursing, Res Nurs Health 7:93, 1984.

ADDITIONAL READINGS

American Hospital Association: AHA Medicare payment: special report 3, Chicago, 1983, The Association.

Canadian Hospital Association: Introduction to nursing management: a Canadian perspective to nursing management, Ottawa, 1985, Canadian Hospital Association.

Department of Health and Human Services: Health United States, Pub. No. (PHS) 83-1232, Washington, D.C., 1982, U.S. Government Printing Office.

Fagin, CM: Nursing as an alternative to high-cost care, Am J Nurs 82:56, 1982.

Flomann, MP, and Shaffer, FA: DRG's as one of nine approaches to case mix in transition, Nurs Health Care 4(8):438, 1983.

Fox, RT: DRGs: a management control tool in hospitals and multi-institutional systems, Hosp Prog 62:52, 1981.

Fromer, MJ: What's fair? Forum, Health Care Financing Administration, Washington, D.C., April 16 to 21, 1985.

Halloran, E, and Halloran, DC: Exploring the DRG/Nursing equation, Am J Nurs 85:1093, 1985.

Hunt, K: DRG: what it is, how it works, and why it will hurt, Med Econ 60:262, 1983.

Inglehart, JK: Federal health policies and the poor, N Engl J Med 307:836, 1982.

Johnson, WL: Supply and demand for registered nurses. I. Nurs Health Care 1:16, 1980.

Johnson, WL: Supply and demand for registered nurses. II. Nurs Health Care 1:73, 1980.

Maraldo, PJ and Solomon, SB: Nursing's window of opportunity, Image: J Nurs Sch 19:83, 1987.

Moccin, P, and Pfordresner, K: If nurses had their way, Ms 146:104, 1983.

Waters, S: What happens if your hospital bills separately for nursing? RN 48(7):18, 1985.

White, CH: Redefining professional nursing: solution to the chronic shortage? Hosp Prog 62:40, 1981.

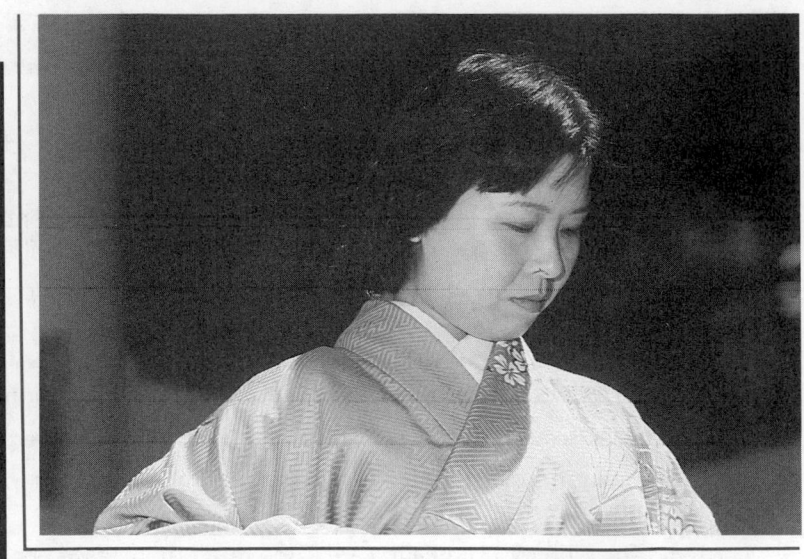

OBJECTIVES

Mastery of content in this chapter will enable the student to:

- Define the key terms listed.
- Describe the relationship of sociocultural background to health and illness beliefs and practices.
- Explain the need for a nurse's self-evaluation when providing care to clients from other sociocultural backgrounds.
- Compare concepts of traditional and modern health and illness beliefs and practices.
- Describe *heritage consistent* and *heritage inconsistent* attributes.
- Perform a cultural assessment using heritage consistency.
- List traditional health and illness beliefs and practices of Asian Americans, black Americans, Native Americans, and Americans of Spanish origin, and Americans of European origin.
- Describe sociocultural barriers—communication and economic—to health care.
- List potential nursing diagnoses related to a client's ethnicity.
- Discuss several ways planning and implementation of nursing interventions can be adapted to a client's ethnicity.

KEY TERMS

Acculturation

Assimilation

Culture

Culture shock

Curing

Ethnicity

Ethnocentrism

Healing

Health

Illness

Modern

Religion

Socialization

Traditional

.Xenophobia

Culture, Ethnicity, and Nursing

Nurses often come from different ethnic, cultural, and religious backgrounds than their clients and must understand that clients have differing world views and interpretations about health and illness based on sociocultural and religious beliefs. When the nurse conveys awareness of and sensitivity to a client's unique health and illness beliefs and practices, good rapport is established. This rapport facilitates the delivery of safe and effective nursing care.

A broad range of health and illness beliefs exist in the United States. Many of these beliefs have roots in the cultural, ethnic, religious, or social background of a person, family, or community. When people anticipate fear or experience an illness or crisis, they may use a *modern* or *traditional* approach toward prevention and healing. These approaches may originate in culture, ethnicity, or religion. These beliefs and practices may be internal or personal, and the person may be able to define and describe them. However, they may be due to external social forces not within the person's control. Examples of external forces include communication barriers, such as language differences, or economic barriers causing limited access or lack of access to modern, health care facilities.

For a nurse to successfully provide care for a client of a different cultural or ethnic background, effective intercultural communication must take place. Intercultural communication occurs when each person attempts to understand the other's point of view from his or her own cultural frame of reference. Effective intercultural communication is facilitated by the nurse's identification of areas of commonalities. After reaching a cultural understanding, the nurse must consider cultural factors throughout the nursing process. Major nursing organizations have emphasized in the last decade the importance of considering cultural factors when delivering nursing care. According to the American Nurses' Association (1976), "Consideration of individual value systems and lifestyles should be included in the planning and health care for each client." Nursing curricula recognize the contribution of nursing to the health care needs of a diverse and multicultural society.

IMMIGRATION

The population of the United States consists largely of the descendants of immigrants. The only truly native Americans are the American Indians, Aleuts, and Eskimos because they settled here thousands of years before the Europeans, Asians, and Africans. People have come to this land from every nation of the world and continue to immigrate, both legally and illegally. The passage of Public Law 99-603, The Immigration Reform and Control Act of 1986, made it possible for several million people to become legal aliens in this country if they have lived here continuously since 1982 and have proof of employment.

The social explosion in the United States in the mid-1960s resulted in a surge of group consciousness. Blacks, Americans of Spanish origin, Asian Americans, Native Americans, and white ethnic groups have asserted their cultural group identities. The rejuvenation of ethnic identity eroded both the "melting pot" myth and the belief that an American culture would decrease group awareness (Giordano and Giordano, 1977).

Every immigrant group has its own cultural attitudes toward health and illness. Each group also has widely ranging beliefs and practices regarding these areas. Health and illness can be interpreted in terms of personal experience and expectations. There are countless ways to explain health and illness, and people base their responses on cultural, religious, and ethnic backgrounds. The responses are culture specific, based on a client's experience and perception.

HERITAGE CONSISTENCY

One way of analyzing belief systems is through the *melting pot* theory in which people are acculturated into the dominant culture via schools, televisions, radio, and motion pictures. Another theory is *heritage consistency*, which looks at acculturation on a continuum. Using this theory, the degree to which a person identifies with the dominant culture is analyzed, as well as how the person identifies with his traditional culture. It is possible to assess health beliefs by determining a person's ties to traditional beliefs, as well as by their stage of acculturation. A relationship exists between strong personal identities and heritage or level of acculturation and health beliefs.

Heritage consistency was originally developed in 1980 by Estes and Zitzow to assess and counsel Native American alcoholics within a cultural context. It describes the degree to which a client's life-style reflects tribal culture. The theory has now expanded in an attempt to study the degree to which any person's life-style reflects the traditional culture, whether it is European, Asian, African, or Spanish. For the same person, some aspects of life-style may reflect cultural heritage, whereas other aspects are inconsistent with that heritage because the person has undergone acculturation.

Culture

Culture is nonphysical traits, such as values, beliefs attitudes, and customs, shared by a group of people and passed from one generation to the next. Culture is also the sum of beliefs, practices, habits, likes, dislikes, norms, customs, and rituals learned from the family during the years of socialization. Many people's beliefs, thoughts, and actions, both conscious and unconscious, are determined by their cultural background (Spector, 1985).

Ethnicity

Ethnicity is a cultural group's sense of identification associated with the group's common social and cultural heritage. The phenomenon of ethnicity is "complex, ambivalent, paradoxical, and elusive" (Senior, 1965). A person is born into an ethnic group but may also adopt characteristics of an ethnic group. The characteristics of an ethnic group include common language and dialect, migratory status, race, and religious faith and practices, extending to kinship, neighborhood, and community boundaries; shared traditions, values, and symbols; literature, folklore, and music; food preferences and settlement and employment patterns; special political interests; and an internal and external sense of distinctiveness. There are at least 106 different ethnic groups in North America and more than 170 Native American tribes (Thernstrom, 1980).

Religion

Religion is a belief in a divine or superhuman power (or powers) to be obeyed and worshipped as the creator and ruler of the universe. Ethical values and religion, a system of beliefs and practices, further clarify ethnicity

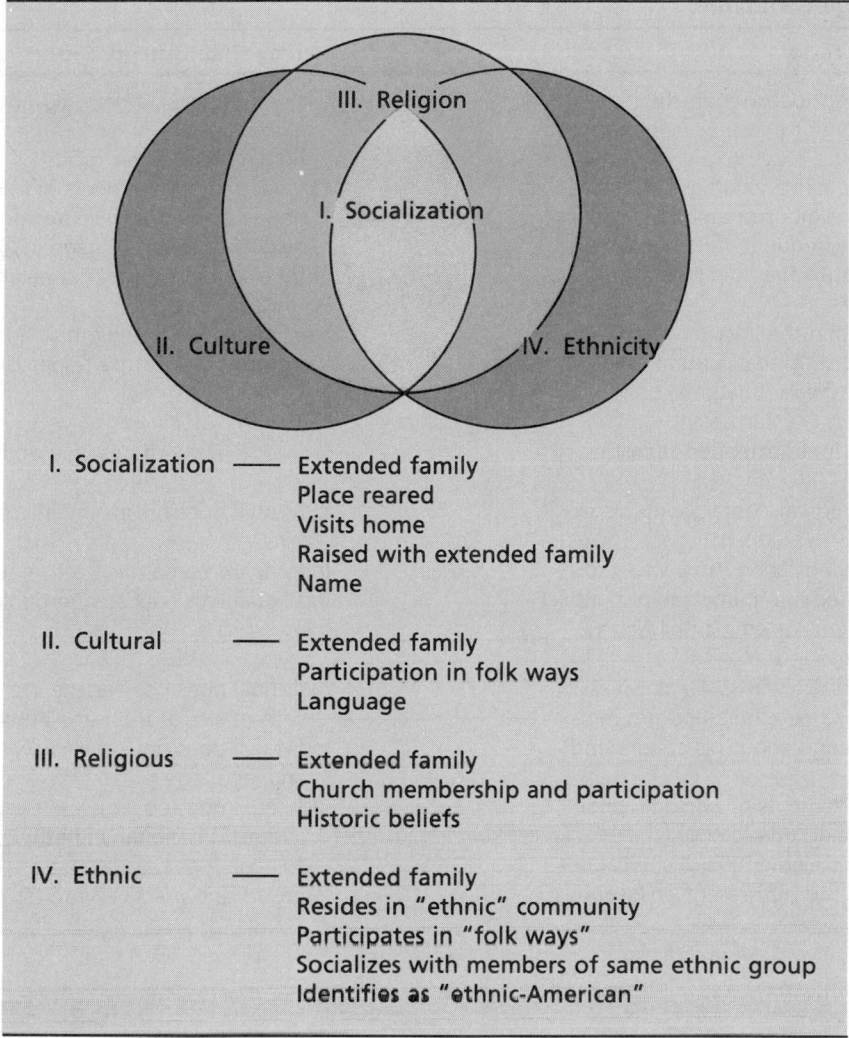

Fig. 4-1   Model of heritage consistency.
From Spector, R: Cultural diversity in health and illness, ed. 2, Norwalk, Conn., 1985, Appleton-Century-Crofts.

(Abramson, 1980) by providing a frame of reference and a perspective within which to organize information. Religious teachings help formulate a meaningful philosophy and system of practices through a system of beliefs, practices, and social controls having specific values, norms, and ethics that vary between religious groups. Some religious practices are related to health. For example, some religions teach that adherence to a code or mandate is conducive to holistic harmony and health and that breaking this code may cause disharmony or illness (Thernstrom, 1980).

The degree of heritage consistency is evaluated by determining the importance of culture, ethnicity, and religion to a person, although it is difficult to isolate the specific aspects of culture, ethnicity, and religion that shape a person's world view. Figure 4-1 illustrates the way these three variables intertwine in the socialization

of the person. When religion is discussed culture and ethnicity must also be included. However, within the diverse U.S. society, descriptions and comparisons of ethnic, religious, and cultural behavior in health and illness may be made.

ETHNIC AND CULTURAL ASSESSMENT OF FAMILIES

Heritage consistency is evaluated on an ever-changing continuum. It is not designed to stereotype or diagnose. Rather, it is a method of understanding whether a person interprets an event through a modern viewpoint or through a more traditional viewpoint, depending on the way persons with the same heritage would define it. The

TABLE 4-1 Heritage Continuum

Heritage Consistency Factors	Heritage Inconsistency Factors
Childhood development occurred in the individual's country of origin or in a U.S. neighborhood of like ethnic group.	Childhood development did not occur in the individual's country of origin or in an immigrant neighborhood of like ethnic group.
Extended family members encouraged participation in traditional religious or cultural activities.	Extended family members did not encourage participation in traditional religious or cultural activities.
Individual engaged in frequent visits home to his country of origin or to the "old neighborhood" in the United States.	Individual does not engage in visits home to his country of origin or the "old neighborhood" in the United States.
Family homes are within the ethnic community.	Family was not in the ethnic community.
Individual participates in ethnic cultural events such as religious festivals, "national holidays," singing, dancing, and costumes.	Individual does not participate in ethnic cultural events.
Individual was raised in an extended family setting.	Individual was not raised in an extended family setting.
Individual maintains regular contact with his extended family	Individual does not maintain contact with his extended family.
Individual's name has not been Americanized.	Individual's name has been Americanized.
Individual was educated in a parochial (nonpublic) school with a religious or ethnic philosophy similar to his background.	Individual was educated in public schools.
Individual engages primarily in social activities with others of the same ethnic background.	Individual does not engage primarily in social activities with others of the same ethnic background.
Individual has knowledge about his culture and language.	Individual does not have knowledge about his culture and language.
Individual possesses elements of personal pride about his national and ethnic origin.	Individual does not possess elements of personal pride about his national and ethnic origin.
Individual incorporates elements of historical beliefs and practices into his present philosophy.	Individual does not incorporate elements of historical beliefs and practices into his present philosophy.

Modified from Spector, RE: Cultural diversity in health and illness, ed. 2, Norwalk, Conn., 1985, Appleton-Century-Crofts.

factors constituting heritage consistency and inconsistency are presented in Table 4-1.

TRADITIONAL HEALTH AND ILLNESS BELIEFS

In discussing health beliefs and practices as they stem from a cultural, ethnic, and religious framework, the word *may* should be used to prevent any stereotyping. The range of health and illness definitions, beliefs, and practices is infinite, and there are differences within and between groups. However, some discernible commonalities do exist. The nurse must remember that it is imperative to constantly assess and communicate with clients to clarify their beliefs about health and illness.

Traditional Beliefs

Culturally based folk beliefs often determine the definitions of health and illness of people who have tra-

ditional belief systems. The prevention and treatment of illness depend on understanding its cause, and traditional health beliefs about the cause of illness may differ vastly from the Western model of epidemiology. It is therefore important to understand traditional epidemiology, or what may be considered the cause of illness within a belief system. Cultural, ethnic, and religious backgrounds quite often reflect the beliefs held about this phenomena. In the modern epidemiological model, the causes of an illness may be stress and maladaption, viruses, bacteria, or carcinogens (agents causing cancer). In the traditional epidemiological model, there are vastly different causative agents, including "soul loss," "spirit possession," "spells," "evil eyes," and "hexes." Illness may be attributed to people who have the ability to make others ill (e.g., witches). People who believe in these forces must exercise great care to protect themselves. Envy, hate, and jealousy are also forces to be avoided. A person may practice prevention by avoiding situations that could provoke the envy, hate, or jealousy of another. If health is viewed as the reward for good behavior, every effort is made to avoid situations in which a person's behavior, social or religious, is compromised (Spector, 1985).

Traditional Practices

Many traditional practices are used to prevent and treat illness, including objects and substances and religious practices.

USE OF PROTECTIVE OBJECTS

Protective objects can be worn or carried or hung in the home. Amulets are objects with magical powers, for example, charms worn on a string or chain around the neck, wrist, or waist to protect the wearer from the evil eye or evil spirts. Amulets exist in societies all over the world and are associated with protection from trouble (Budge, 1978). People may also use a talismans or "consecrated religious objects" (Budge, 1978). Talismans are believed to possess extraordinary powers and may be worn on a rope around the waist or carried in a pocket or purse. *It is recommended that people who wear amulets or carry a talisman be allowed to do so in a health care institution.*

USE OF SUBSTANCES

Substances are ingested in certain ways or amounts or are worn or hung in the home. This practice uses diet and consists of many different observances. It is believed that the body is kept in balance or harmony by the type of food eaten so many food taboos and combinations exist in traditional belief systems. For example, it is believed that some food substances can be ingested to prevent illness. People from many ethnic backgrounds eat raw garlic or onion in an effort to prevent illness or may wear them on the body or hang them in the home. The rules of kosher practiced among Jewish people mandate the elimination of pork and shellfish from the diet. They are allowed fish with scales and fins and only certain cuts of beef from animals with cleft hooves that chew cud (cattle and lambs). Moslems also adhere to many of these dietary practices. Jews also believe that milk and meat must never be mixed or eaten at the same meal (Steinberg, 1947).

RELIGIOUS PRACTICES

Another traditional approach to illness prevention centers around religion and includes practices such as the burning of candles, rituals of redemption, and prayer. Religion strongly affects the way people attempt to prevent illness, and it plays a strong role in rituals associated with health protection. Religion dictates social, moral, and dietary practices designed to keep a person healthy and in balance and plays a vital role in that person's perception of illness prevention. Many people believe illness can be prevented by strict adherence

to religious codes, morals, and practices and view illness as punishment for violating a religious code. Religious practices such as the Catholic custom of "blessing of the throats" on St. Blaise Day are performed to prevent sore throats and choking. Baptism is a ritual of cleansing and prevents evil from harming the person. Circumcision is a redemptive practice used to prevent illness and harm. (Morgenstern, 1966).

Traditional Remedies

The admitted use of folk or traditional medicine is increasing, and the practice is seen among people from all walks of life and cultural and ethnic backgrounds. Use of folk medicine is not a new practice among heritage consistent people, so many of the remedies have been used and passed on for generations. The pharmaceutical properties of vegetation—plants, roots, stems, flowers, seeds, and herbs—have been studied, tested, cataloged, and used for countless centuries. Many of these plants are used by specific communities. Others cross ethnic and community lines and are used in certain geographic areas. These remedies are purchased in special stores or market places and may also be purchased in the person's country of origin.

When patients do not adhere to a pharmacological regimen, an effort must be made to determine if they are taking traditional remedies. Frequently, the active ingredients of traditional remedies are unknown. If a client is believed to be taking them, an effort must be made to determine the remedy, as well as its active ingredients. Often, these ingredients can be antagonistic or synergistic to prescribed medications. If this is the situation, the medication may have no effect or a severe overdose may occur.

The richness of this *pharmacopoeia* far exceeds the limits of this chapter, thus only a limited sample of the remedies of each population will be highlighted.

Healers

In the traditional context, healing is the restoration of the person to a state of harmony between the body, mind, and spirit, or the restoration of holistic health. Within a given community, specific people are known to have the power to heal. The healer may be male or female and is thought to have received the gift of healing from a divine source.

In many instances a heritage consistent person may consult a traditional healer before, instead of, or in conjunction with a modern health care provider. Many differences exist between the Western physician and the traditional healer (Kaptchuk and Croucher, 1987) (Table 4-2). The relationship between the person and the healer, for example, is often much closer than that between the person and the health care professional. The

TABLE 4-2 Comparisons: Traditional Healer Versus Physician

Healer	Physician
Maintains an informal, friendly, affective relationship with the entire family.	Business-like and formal, dealing primarily with the client.
Comes to the house day or night.	Client must go to the physician's office or clinic. Home visits are rarely, if ever, made.
For diagnosis, consults with head of house, creates a mood of awe, talks to all family memers, is not authoritarian, has social rapport, builds expectation of cure.	Deals primarily with the ill person, may address only person's illness. Authoritarian manner can create fear.
Generally less expensive than the physician.	Generally more expensive than the healer.
Has ties to the "world of the sacred," has rapport with the symbolic, spiritual, creative, or holy force.	Primarily secular, pays little attention to the religious beliefs of a client or meanings of an illness.
Shares the world view of the client, that is, speaks the same language, lives in the same neighborhood or in the same similar socioeconomic conditions, may know the same people, understands the life-style of the client.	Generally does not share the world view of the client, that is, may not speak the same language, live in the same neighborhood or in the same socioeconomic conditions, may not understand the life-style of the client.

Modified from Spector, RE: Cultural diversity in health and illness, ed. 2, Norwalk, Conn., 1985, Appleton-Century-Crofts.

person sees the healer as one who understands the problem within his cultural context, speaks the same language, and shares a similar world view. Examples of traditional healers follow:

1. Medicine man: the traditional healer of the Native Americans.
2. *Senora:* a Puerto Rican woman knowledgeable in the treatment of illness.
3. *Espiritista:* a person possessing more sophisticated skills than the *Senora*.
4. *Curandero:* a person with God-given ability to heal using a religious-psychiatric approach.
5. *Partera:* a Mexican-American midwife.
6. Root-worker: a black person able to determine the cause of an illness and the treatment.

Traditional healers have always been a part of cultures. The methods used by these healers were developed over generations by trial and error, with religious beliefs and social circumstances contributing to them. Effective methods have been preserved and adapted to meet the needs of the present time. The traditional healer is aware of the cultural and personal needs of the client and is able to understand him within the context of his problem in today's world.

CULTURAL ASPECTS OF HEALTH AND ILLNESS

Many cultures exist in the United States today (Fig. 4-2). Nurses must be aware of these groups and be familiar with the basic characteristics of each. The follow-ing "culture capsules" provide a general overview of Asian, black, Native American, Spanish or hispanic-origin, and white cultures. Each capsule includes a synopsis of the background, traditional definitions of health and illness, and traditional beliefs about the causes of illness, methods of prevention, and remedies.

These culture capsules illustrate the dynamic similarities and differences existing between groups of people. Nurses should remember that clients must be assessed as individuals. Characteristic beliefs of a cultural group are not necessarily shared by each individual in that group.

Asian Americans

Asian Americans originated in China, Hawaii, the Philippines, Korea, Japan, Laos, Cambodia, and Viet Nam. Many Asian Americans have lived in the United States for several generations. Others arrived more recently, and still others enter the country now, especially in California.

HEALTH AND ILLNESS

Within the Asian community, Chinese medicine provides an overall framework for Asian cultures and teaches that health is a state of spiritual and physical harmony between a body, mind, and spirit in harmony with nature. In addition, the forces of *yin* (female, negative energy) and *yang* (male, positive energy) must be in balance. Illness is the result of imbalance between yin and yang. The body is viewed as a gift given by parents and forebears. It is not the person's personal property and must be cared for and maintained. The primary role

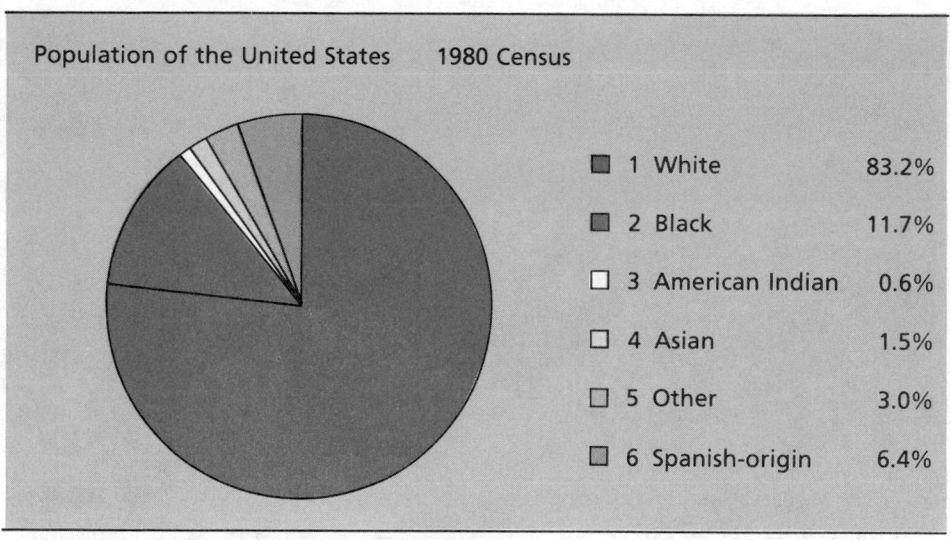

Fig. 4-2 Population of the United States.

From U.S. Bureau of the Census: Current population reports: population characteristics, Series P-20, No. 374, Population profile of the central states: 1981, Washington, D.C., 1982, U.S. Government Printing Office.

of the physician in ancient China was to help safeguard the body and to prevent illness. If a person became ill despite preventive measures, it was not necessary to pay the physician for treatment.

ILLNESS CAUSE AND PREVENTION. Illness may be caused by an upset in the balance of yin and yang. The weather, overexertion, and prolonged sitting may also cause illness, which may be prevented by adhering to a proper diet to maintain the body's balance, exercising, avoiding temperature changes, and taking certain remedies.

REMEDIES. The following examples are a few of the traditional remedies used to prevent and treat ailments among Asian Americans (Fig. 4-3):

Jen Shen Lu Jung Wan is a brown-colored, thick liquid used as a general tonic to brace up the whole system and as an aid to improve digestion. It may be taken before elective surgery.

Thousand Year Eggs are uncooked eggs covered with carbon or straw and stored in large vases for a long time. They are eaten daily with rice for good health.

Huo Li Jian Mei Su are small, brown, coated pills taken twice a day as a counteraction against senility, for the relief of fatigue, and for the maintenance of youth, health, and beauty.

Tiger Balm is a salve used for temporary relief of minor aches and pains.

Ginseng root is the most famous of the Chinese medicines. It has universal medicinal usage in "building the blood," especially after childbirth. Chinese legend states

that the more the root looks like a man, the more effective it is. Ginseng is native to the United States and is used in this country as a restorative tonic.

White Flower is a liquid used to treat colds, influenza, headaches, and coughs.

Other methods of treatment include the use of *acupuncture*, a method of treating disease by puncturing the skin at certain points of the body with metal needles, and *moxibustion*, the application of heat to these same points. (Spector, 1985).

Blacks

Most members of the black community originated in Africa. The majority were brought here as slaves between 1619 and 1860 from the west coast of Africa. Today, a number of blacks have immigrated to the United States from African countries, the West Indies, the Dominican Republic, Haiti, and Jamaica.

HEALTH AND ILLNESS

The traditional definition of health stems from the African belief about life and the nature of being. Life is a process rather than a state, and the nature of a person is viewed in terms of energy force rather than matter. When healthy, a person is in harmony with nature. Illness is seen as disharmony of the mind, body, and spirit or as disharmony between man and nature. Researchers and epidemiologists have noted chronic illnesses and illness patterns associated with cultural and ethnic groups. The research highlight describes the correlation between psychological stress and hypertension.

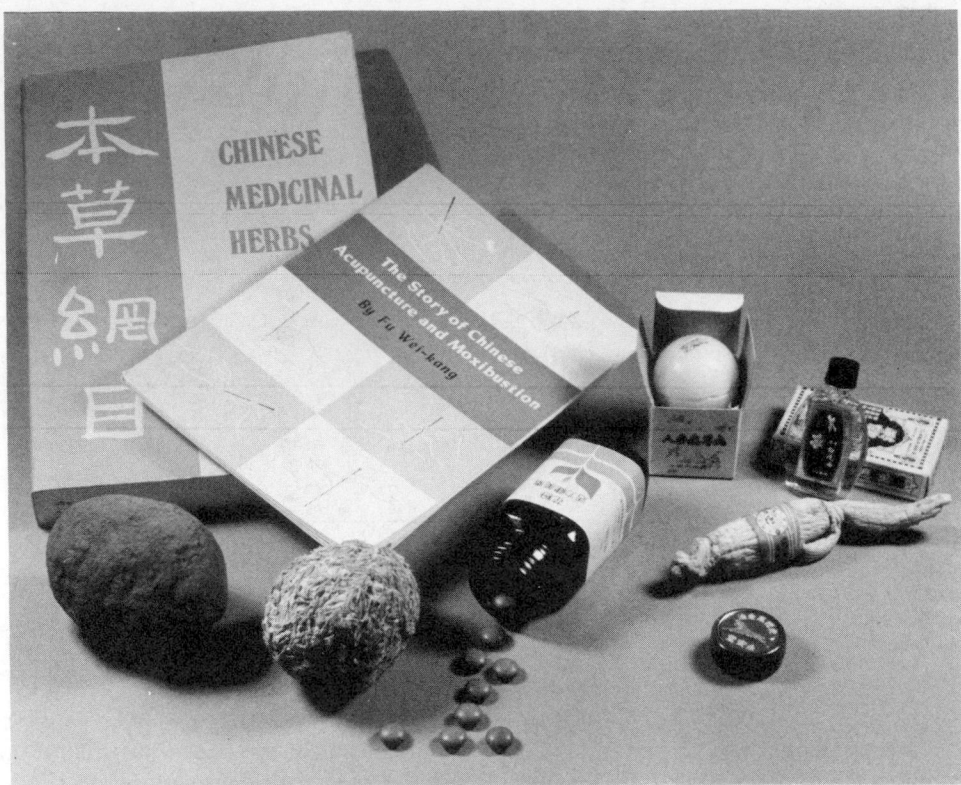

Fig. 4-3   Asian American remedies include *Jen Shen Lu Jung Wan,* Thousand Year Eggs, *Huo Li Jian Mei Su,* Tiger Balm, Ginseng root, White Flower.

Photograph by Lucy Rozier, Boston College Audio Visual Services, Boston College, Chestnut Hill, Mass., from the author's private collection.

❧ Research Highlight ❧

Johnson et al. studied associative patterns and relationships between psychological variables—Type A/B behavior, life satisfaction, and interpersonal trust—and blood pressure levels. The sample, consisting of 179 black adult women in three age groups, was tested with a 53-item risk factor questionnaire that measured the three variables. Blood pressures were then taken. The findings indicated significant relationships between Type A/B behavior, life satisfaction, trust, and blood pressure; between trust and life satisfaction; and between diastolic blood pressure and Type A behaviors. The researchers also reported a significant increase in diastolic blood pressure in younger persons and a significant increase in systolic blood pressure in older persons as a result of stress.

Johnson, M, et al.: Psychological stress and blood pressure levels in black women, J Natl Black Nurses Assoc 12:41, 1987.

ILLNESS CAUSE AND PREVENTION. Illness (disharmony) is often attributed to demons and evil spirits. Several methods are used as protection from these forces, including the ancient belief and practice of voodoo. Voodoo is believed to cause, as well as prevent, the action of malevolent forces. "White" magic protects against these forces, and "black" magic directs their energy to a specific person or body area. Belief in both exists today, but the extent of this belief is unknown. Traditional beliefs about prevention of illness focus on avoiding people believed to carry evil spirits or becoming evil spirits themselves. Prayer and a well-balanced diet are also considered helpful.

REMEDIES. The following examples are a few of the traditional remedies used to prevent or treat ailments among Black Americans (Fig. 4-4).

Bangles are silver bracelets worn by people originating from the West Indies. They overlap and are open to "let out evil" yet closed to prevent evil from entering the body. They are worn from infancy and are replaced as the person grows. These bracelets tend to tarnish and leave a black ring on the skin when a person is becoming ill. The black ring serves as a signal to rest, improve diet, and take any other needed precautions. Some people wear many bangles, believing that their sound frightens away evil spirits. Many people believe that they are extremely vulnerable to evil, even to death, when these bracelets are removed, so removal of these bracelets can cause a great deal of anxiety.

Talismans protect the wearer from all sickness and are worn on a string around the waist or carried in a pocket or in a purse. *Asafoetida* is a foul-smelling, gummy substance worn to ward off colds and evil. It is known as the "incense of the devil." A dehydrated garden *snake* is ground into a powder and dissolved in water. The liquid is applied to skin lesions such as poison ivy. *Voodoo candles* have a peculiar spiritualistic character and are used for sacred rituals and rites. Colors also have significance. For example, pink means love; white, peace; blue, success and protection from harm (Spector, 1985).

Native Americans

There are approximately 170 Native American tribes in the United States, predominantly in the Western states. Although many Native Americans remain on reservations, many also live off the reservation.

HEALTH AND ILLNESS

Health reflects the ability to live in total harmony with nature and the ability to survive under extremely difficult circumstances. People are believed to have an intimate spiritual relationship with nature. The earth is considered a living organism, the body of a higher individual, with a will and a desire to be well and experiences health and illness like a person. The body and the earth must be treated with respect. Since the earth provides food, shelter, and medicine to man, it must be protected. According to Basque (1975), "The land belongs to life, life belongs to the land, and the land belongs to itself." Thus to stay healthy a person must maintain a positive, balanced relationship with nature.

Another explanation of the Native American view of health is that the body is divided into two halves, plus and minus. There are also, in every whole, two energy poles, positive and negative. Every individual has the power to control himself and, with this potency, spiritual power (control of the body's energy) is derived. Health is described as the harmony or balance between the two halves or the two energy poles. Illness is the disharmony of the body, mind, and spirit (Boyd, 1974).

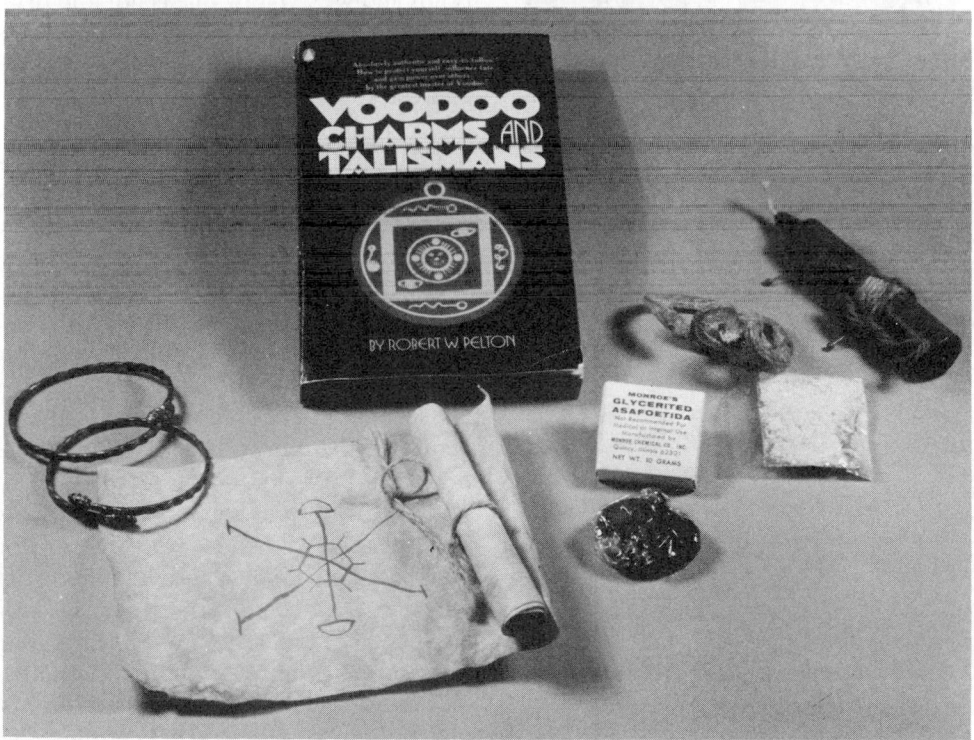

Fig. 4-4 Black American remedies include bangles, talisman, Asafoetida, snake, Voo Doo candle.
Photograph by Lucy Rozier, Boston College Audio Visual Services, Boston College, Chestnut Hill, Mass., from the author's private collection.

ILLNESS CAUSE AND PREVENTION. Sources causing illness vary from nation to nation or tribe to tribe. Hopi Indians associate illness with evil spirits and therefore strive to avoid or ward off these spirits. Navahos see illness as the result of displeasing the holy people, annoying the elements, disturbing animal and plant life, neglecting the celestial bodies, misusing a sacred Indian ceremony, or tampering with witches or witchcraft. Hawk Littlejohn, an Eastern Band Cherokee medicine man, describes illness as the imbalance of the body, mind, or spirit caused by an excess in one domain and the neglect of the other two. For example, a student who spends too much time studying—developing the mind— may neglect his body and spirit and will therefore be vulnerable to disharmony and illness. The main principle for the prevention of illness is the maintenance of harmony with the body, mind, and spirit and the avoidance of factors that cause disharmony.

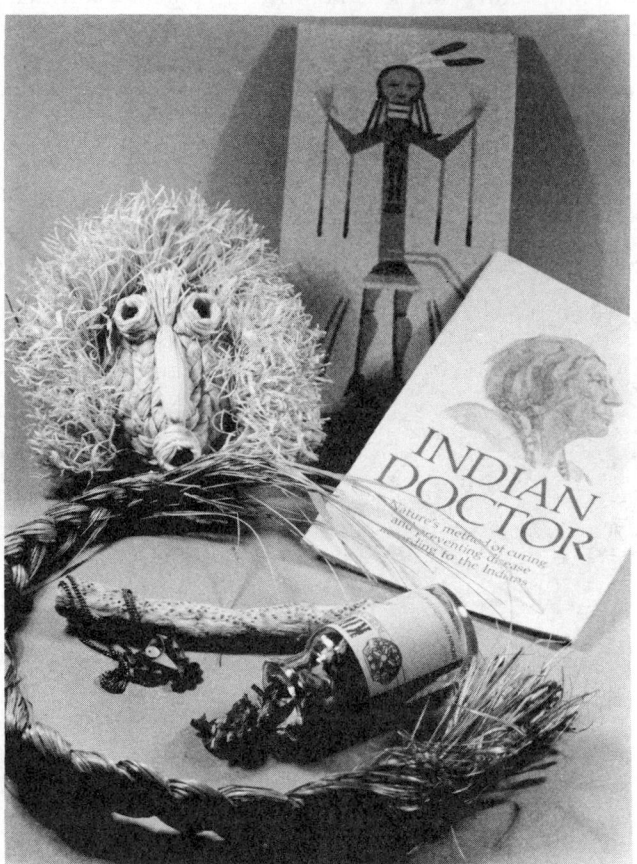

Fig. 4-5 Native American remedies include sand painting, mask, sweet grass, Thunderbird, Estafiate.

Photography by Lucy Rozier, Boston College Audio Visual Services, Boston College, Chestnut Hill, Mass., from the author's private collection.

REMEDIES. The following examples are remedies used by Native Americans to prevent or treat illness (Fig. 4-5):

Sand painting is the creation of a sand painting by the Navaho medicine man while diagnosing an ailment. The painting is created by the medicine man in an elaborate diagnostic ceremony of motion of the hand. When the hand moves in a certain way, the medicine man knows that it is indicative of a specific illness and he is able to prescribe the correct treatment.

A *mask* is worn to hide the self from the devil or evil spirits. *Sweet grass* is burned as a rite of purification by the medicine man. A *Thunderbird* is an amulet worn for good luck and protection. *Estafiate* are dried leaves used in a tea to treat stomach problems (Spector, 1985).

Spanish-Origin Americans

Members of the Spanish-origin community originate in Spain, Cuba, Mexico, Puerto Rico, and other Spanish-speaking countries.

HEALTH AND ILLNESS

Health is often believed to be the result of good luck or a reward from God for good behavior. Health represents a state of equilibrium within the universe where the forces of hot, cold, wet, and dry are balanced. Blood is hot and wet, yellow bile is hot and dry, phlegm is cold and wet, and black bile is cold and dry. The concept originated with the early Hippocratic theory of health and the four humors. Health exists when the four humors are in a balanced state. Health is maintained by the diet and other practices that keep the humors balanced. Illness is viewed as misfortune or bad luck, punishment from God for evil thoughts or actions, or the imbalance of hot and cold.

ILLNESS CAUSE AND PREVENTION. Several factors cause illness. A hot-cold imbalance, for example, is primarily-caused by improper diet. Food substances are classified as hot or cold with and without regard to their actual temperature. This classification can vary from person to person, but essentially, certain foods are known to be hot, and others are known to be cold. Examples of cold food are chicken, honey, avocados, bananas, and lima beans. Examples of hot foods are chocolate, coffee, corn meal, garlic, kidney beans, onions, and peas. Illness can occur if these foods are eaten in improper combinations or amounts. For example, *Friadad del estomago,* "cold stomach," is caused by eating too many cold foods. There are several "healthy" conditions in which a person maintains health by adhering to the "hot-cold" system. A pregnant woman avoids "hot" foods. During menstruation and after childbirth, she avoids "cold" foods. An infant who requires formula that contains a "hot" food such as evaporated milk may be fed a "cold" food such as whole milk.

Other factors believed to cause illness are the "dislocation of body parts" and magic or supernatural causes outside the body such as *Mal ojo* or "bad eye." *Envidia* (envy) is also a cause of illness and bad luck, and many means are used to prevent it. Many people of Spanish origin believe that to succeed is to fail, that is, when a person's success provokes the envy of friends and neighbors, misfortune or illness may follow.

Illness may be prevented by proper diet, avoidance of "harmful" people, the wearing of amulets for protection, the use of candles, and prayer.

REMEDIES. The following remedies are used among people of Spanish origin (Fig. 4-6) for the prevention or treatment of illness:

All kinds of novena *candles* may be burned to ward off evil. *Jabon de la Mano Milagrosa* (soap of the miraculous hand) is used to cleanse and protect a person. *Amulets* such as Milagros (Mexican) are worn as pro-

tection from evil. The *Mano Negro* (Blackhand) amulet of Puerto Rico may be placed on a baby at birth and is believed to protect it from the "evil eye."

Manzanilla is a herb made into tea and used to treat stomach and intestinal pain, uterine cramps, anxiety, and insomnia. *Anis* are star-shaped seeds used to treat painful gases, upset stomach, colic, and anorexia and to increase breast milk (Spector, 1985).

Whites

Members of most white ethnic communities originated in Europe and have been migrating to this country since 1620. The white population is a diverse mixture of people from many countries, speaking numerous languages and observing a wide variety of health beliefs and practices. The 1980 census was the first to attempt to break down the population by country of origin. The largest groups were found to be from England, Germany, Ireland, and France.

HEALTH AND ILLNESS

Health and illness are defined in many ways, including the ability to do activities of daily living, a state of physical and emotional well-being, and a state free of illness. Illness is described as the inability to do activities of daily living, the presence of disease symptoms and pain, and the malformation of body organs.

ILLNESS CAUSE AND PREVENTION. Traditional beliefs about the cause of illness are many and varied. Examples of these causes include breaking of religious rules, exposure to causative agents, punishment from God, drafts, climatic changes, and the abuse of the body. An wide variety of methods for preventing illness may be found among the Europeans, including diet, exercise, religious rituals, and the wearing of amulets.

REMEDIES. The following are a few examples of remedies reported among whites (Fig 4-7):

Sloan's Liniment aids in the temporary relief of minor pains resulting from arthritis and other ailments. *Malocchio* is an Italian horn worn to prevent the "evil eye." The hunchbacked man *Gobo* on this horn offers extra protection. He is holding a horseshoe for luck in his left hand and is pointing the index and baby finger of his right hand to ward off the evil spirit.

Olbas and *Magentropfen* are medicines sold in Germany to treat sore throats and lack of appetite. *Swamp root* is an over-the-counter liquid used as a diuretic and sold in the United States. *Syrup of Black Draught* is used as an over-the-counter laxative. *Father John's Medicine* is a wholesome, family medicine that has been used for colds and coughs since 1855 (Spector, 1985).

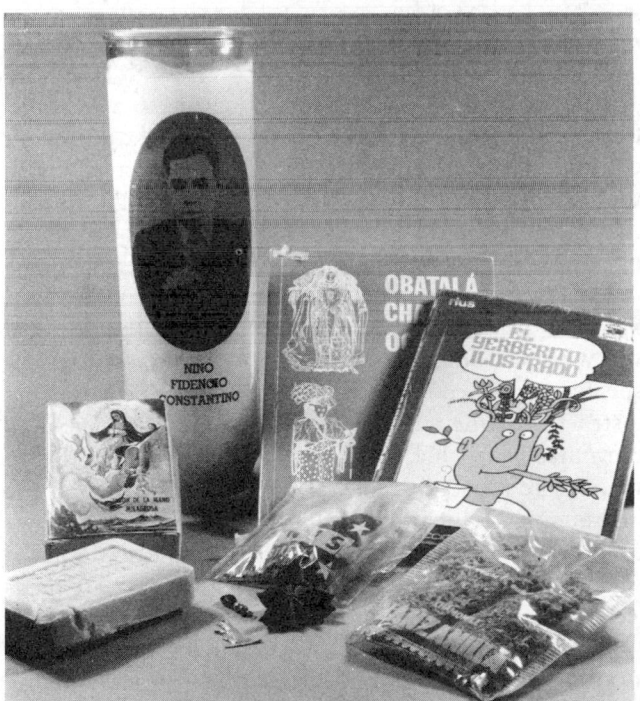

Fig. 4-6 Spanish-origin remedies include candles, *Jabon de la Mano Milagrosa*, amulets—*Milagros* (Mexican), *Mano Negro* (Puerto Rican), *Manzanilla*, *Anis*.

Photograph by Lucy Rozier, Boston College Audio Visual Services, Boston College, Chestnut Hill, Mass., from the author's private collection.

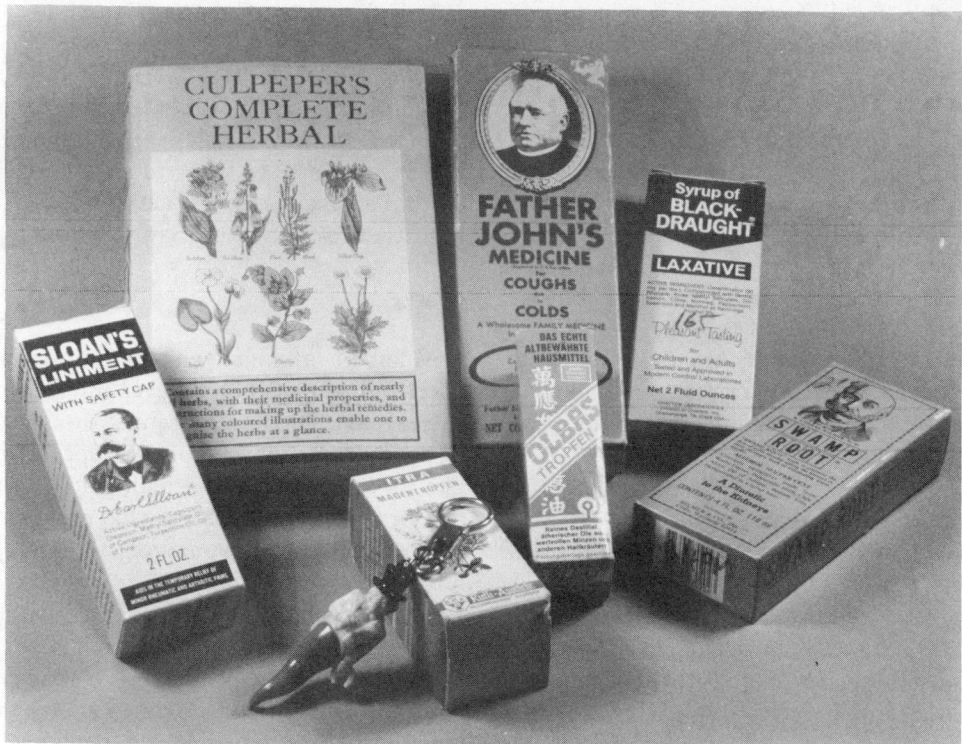

Fig. 4-7 Remedies used by whites. Sloan's Liniment, *Malocchio, Olbas* and *Magentropfen*, swamp root, Syrup of Black Draught, Father John's Medicine.

Photograph by Lucy Rozier, Boston College Audio Visual Services, Boston College, Chestnut Hill, Mass., from the author's private collection.

ETHNIC AND CULTURAL FACTORS AFFECTING HEALTH CARE

Communication

Communication barriers are manifested in many ways, including language differences, time orientation, and personal space and territoriality.

LANGUAGE

Language differences are possibly the most important factor in providing nursing care to ethnic group clients because they can affect all stages of the nursing process. Clear and effective communication is important when dealing with any client and is crucial if language differences create a cultural barrier between the nurse and the client. If the client does not speak the nurse's language, a translator is necessary. More often, however, the client speaks the nurse's language with limited ability or uses language with denotative or connotative meanings different from the nurse's meanings. For example, a client with limited language ability might know customary greetings such as "How are you?" or "Hello" but not understand health terms such as "pain" or "tempera-

ture" usually understood by lay persons in the dominant cultural group. Failure to communicate effectively with the client not only may cause delays in diagnosis and treatment but may also lead to tragic consequences. In one incident, for example, an English-Speaking nurse failed to ascertain that the client truly understood preoperative instructions about washing the surgical site with povidone-iodine (Betadine). The non-English-speaking Asian client, throughout the time she was being instructed by the nurse, kept nodding and smiling when the nurse asked her, "Do you understand what I told you?" The nurse judged that the client understood the instructions. Much to the nurse's dismay, the client drank the whole bottle of povidone-iodine solution instead of washing with it. Fortunately appropriate medical measures were instituted to save the client's life.

The nurse should not assume that the client understood her communication. A more appropriate nursing intervention is for the nurse to demonstrate using the providone-iodine and showing the client *how* to wash the area and to have the client return the demonstration. No words have to be spoken, yet by actually doing this procedure or any other procedure in pantomime, the client grasps what the nurse is teaching and is then able to follow directions.

Nurses need the ability to communicate with clients limited in the use of the nurse's language, because when deprived of the most common medium of interaction with clients—the spoken word—nurses often become frustrated and ineffective. Some nurses tend to avoid clients with whom they cannot communicate. This creates a vicious circle of cultural misunderstandings. According to Muecke (1970) the nurse might behave toward the client in ways that could be misconstrued:

1. The nurse shouts the same words louder. Raising the voice will not make the words more understandable, and such actions could also suggest hostility to the client.
2. The nurse focuses on the task rather than on the client, possibly suggesting that the nurse is more interested in doing the task than in concentrating on the client.
3. The nurse stops talking with the client altogether and starts doing things for him instead of with him, possibly implying the client's inferiority.

The consequence of the nurse's actions is the painful isolation of the non-English-speaking client in an unfamiliar environment. Consequently, the client experiences cultural shock and may react by withdrawing, becoming hostile or belligerent, or being uncooperative.

Language differences can be bridged, however. The nurse can ask family members fluent in English to interpret. In this way the family can also provide information about the client's background that could be valuable in holistic care. The health institution can also facilitate the search for an interpreter. For example, a list of bilingual or multilingual staff members and volunteers in a hospital might be kept in a central place such as the information desk.

Medical terms must be clearly explained to all clients, especially those with limited skills in the dominant language. Hospital jargon presents problems even for alert, oriented, adult clients who speak the dominant language. For example, there may be many clients who think that "force fluids" means "force urination" or "force elimination of fluids."

Differences in denotative meanings may exist between members of two cultures, causing miscommunications. For instance, when a black youth says "That's bad" and means "That's good," a white adult might be confused. The black youth is speaking in an argot, or a special linguistic code of his cultural group. Another linguistic block to communication between ethnic groups comes from differences in connotative meanings for certain words, even when the denotative meanings are the same. For example, to a white person, "hospital" may mean a facility where modern health care is provided. Navajos, however, associate hospitals with death, since they believe the ground and the building where any person dies become contaminated for an indeterminate period with evil spirits that will infect anyone who steps on this ground (Hall, 1963). Thus they avoid hospitals.

By giving special attention to the communication process, nurses can work to overcome language barriers with non-English-speaking clients. Observing nonverbal behaviors, for example, can help clarify a client's communication, although nonverbal communication is also influenced by culture. Nurses can also learn how to phrase questions and statements to elicit information from clients whose ethnic background shapes their response. For example, when a Mexican American man is asked if he feels pain, he may simply say no if he believes that admitting pain is a sign he is not manly. The nurse might ask instead when he feels pain.

Finally, the nurse who practices in an area where many members of an ethnic minority live should attempt to learn the clients' language. No nurse can learn all the languages that may be encountered in practice, but it is possible for a nurse to learn one other language, such as Spanish. With more difficult languages, such as Vietnamese, the nurse can learn some basic terms. Many community health nurses have learned the languages of their clients, and nurses in other settings also should be aware of the problems that may arise because of language differences.

TIME ORIENTATION

Certain cultures in the United States and Canada tend to be future oriented. The members of these cultures are concerned with long-range goals and with health care measures in the present to prevent the occurrence of illness in the future. They prefer to plan ahead in making schedules, setting appointments, and organizing activities. Time orientation varies among different cultural groups, however, and a nurse who has an ethnocentric attitude toward time may find it difficult to understand and plan care for clients with a different time orientation. Some blacks, some persons of Spanish origin, and some persons of Southern European origin are oriented more to the present than the future. These clients may not share the nurse's attitude toward matters related to time. A client may be late for an appointment not because of reluctance or lack of respect for the nurse but because he is less concerned about planning ahead to be on time than with the activity in which he is currently engaged. This time orientation difference may become important in health care measures such as long-term planning and explaining when medications should be taken. For example, if a client has not been regularly taking the medication prescribed to lower his blood pressure, teaching about the potential effects of hypertension should emphasize short-term problems rather than only long-term problems, which may be less important to the client.

PERSONAL SPACE AND TERRITORIALITY

Personal space involves a person's set of behaviors and attitudes toward the space around himself. Territoriality is an attitude toward an area a person has claimed and defends or reacts emotionally about when another encroaches on it. Both are influenced by culture, and thus different ethnic groups have varying norms related to the use of space.

Staff members and other clients frequently encroach on a client's territory in the hospital, which includes his room, bed, closet, and belongings. The nurse should try to respect the client's territory as much as possible, especially when performing nursing procedures. The nurse should also welcome visiting members of the family and extended family. This can remind the client of home, lessening the effects of isolation and shock from hospitalization.

Personal space is involved in many nursing activities, and the nurse should be sensitive about the client's attitudes toward personal space. For example, providing nursing care often involves touching the client, an action that has different meanings in different cultures and for different individuals. What is comforting to one client may be threatening to another. Standards of behavior vary also in terms of who, male or female, can touch the client, and where. The meaning of personal space also varies among cultures. Hall (1963) has studied the meaning of space and has identified behaviors common in the following zones:

1. *Intimate zone* extends up to 1½ feet. Since this distance allows adults to have the most bodily contacts for perception of breath and odor, they do not find this acceptable in public places. Visual distortions are also present.
2. *Personal distance* extends from 1½ to 4 feet. This is an extension of the self that is like having a "bubble" of space surrounding the body. At this distance the voice may be moderate, the body odor may not be apparent, and visual distortion may have disappeared.
3. *Social distance* extends from 4 to 12 feet. This is reserved for impersonal business transactions. Perceptual information in much less detailed.
4. *Public distance* extends 12 feet or more. Individuals interact only impersonally. Communicators' voices must be projected, and subtle facial expressions may be lost.

These generalizations about the use of personal space are based on studies of the behavior of white North Americans. Use of personal space varies between individuals and ethnic groups. The extreme modesty practiced by members of some cultural groups and lower socioeconomic groups may prevent members from seeking preventive health care.

Economic Barriers

Several economic barriers, such as unemployment, underemployment, homelessness, lack of health insurance, and poverty prevent people from entering the health care system. Poverty is by far the most critical factor. *Poverty* is a relative term and changes from time and place. In the United States, poverty is pervasive and found extensively among people in certain geographical areas, such as Appalachia, other rural areas, and urban areas, and certain groups, such as blacks, Spanish-origin Americans, Native Americans, rural populations, the elderly, migrant workers, and illegal aliens. Poor health, crippling diseases, drug and alcohol abuse, poor education, and inferior education are contributing social causes of poverty.

Several programs, both governmental and private, aid people with short- and long-term problems. It is important for the nurse to be aware of a client's needs and financial resources available in the local community. An in-depth analysis of poverty and poverty programs is presented in Chapter 3.

SOCIOCULTURAL FACTORS AND THE NURSING PROCESS

When nurses provide care to clients from a background other than their own, they must be aware of and sensitive to the clients' sociocultural background, assess and listen carefully to health and illness beliefs and practices, and respect and not challenge cultural, ethnic, or religious values and health care beliefs. The nursing process enables the nurse to provide individualized care (see Unit 2).

The nurse should begin the *assessment* by attempting to determine the client's cultural heritage (see Table 4-1) and English language skills. The client should be asked if any of his health beliefs relate to the cause of the illness or to the problem. The nurse should then determine what, if any, home remedies the person is taking to treat the symptoms.

Assessment enables the nurse to cluster relevant data and develop actual or potential *nursing diagnoses* related to the cultural or ethnic need of the client. In addition, the nursing diagnosis should state the probable cause. The identification of the cause of the problem further individualizes the nursing care plan and encourages selection of appropriate interventions.

When establishing the goals of care and *planning* specific interventions, the nurse again considers cultural variables as they relate to the client. The extended family should be involved in care, for example, if the family is the client's strongest support group. Cultural beliefs and practices can be incorporated into therapy. The client's educational level and language skills should be considered when planning teaching activities. Explanations of aspects of care usually not questioned by acculturated clients may be required for non-English-speaking or non-acculturated clients to avoid confusion, misunderstanding, or cultural conflict. The nurse may have to alter her usual ways of interacting with clients to avoid offending or alienating a client with different attitudes toward social interaction and etiquette. A client who is modest and self-conscious about the body may need psychological preparation before some procedures and tests.

The nurse can find out what care the client considers appropriate by involving him and his family in planning care and asking about their expectations. This should be done in every case, even if the nursing care cannot be modified. Because both the nurse and the client are likely to take many aspects of their cultures for granted, questions should be clear and explanations should be explicit.

Discussing cultural questions related to care with the client and family during the planning stage helps the nurse understand how cultural variables are related to the client's health beliefs and practices, so that interventions can be individualized for the client.

The nurse *evaluates* the results of nursing care for ethnic clients as for all clients, determining the extent to which the goals of care have been met. Evaluation continues throughout the nursing process and should include feedback from the client and family. With an ethnic minority client, however, self-evaluation by the nurse is crucial as he or she increases skills for interaction. The nurse should consider questions such as the following:

1. Am I open to understanding ways in which the client's values differ from mine?
2. Have I given sufficient attention to communicating with the client with limited language skills?
3. Have I successfully involved the client's family in the nursing process?
4. Am I incorporating the client's traditional beliefs and practices into nursing therapies?
5. Is my therapeutic relationship with the client grounded on respect for the client regardless of cultural differences?

Nurses should evaluate their attitudes toward ethnic nursing care. Some nurses may believe they should treat all clients the same and simply act naturally, but this attitude fails to acknowledge that cultural differences do exist and that there is no one "natural" human behavior. The nurse cannot act the same with all clients and still hope to deliver effective, individualized, holistic care. Sometimes, inexperienced nurses are so self-conscious about cultural differences and so afraid of making a mistake that they impede the nursing process by not asking questions about areas of difference or by asking so many questions that they seem to pry into the client's personal life. The process of self-evaluation can help the nurse become more comfortable when providing care to clients from diverse backgrounds.

SUMMARY

Nurses need to be aware of and sensitive to the cultural needs of clients. The body of knowledge relevant to this sensitive area is growing, and it is imperative that nurses from all cultural backgrounds be aware of nursing implications in this area. The practice of nursing today demands that the nurse identify and meet the cultural needs of diverse groups, understand the social and cultural reality of the client, family, and community, develop expertise to implement culturally acceptable strategies to provide nursing care, and identify and use resources acceptable to the client (Boyle, 1987).

KEY CONCEPTS

✓ Cultural background affects a person's health in all dimensions, so the nurse should consider the client's cultural background when planning care.

✓ Many ethnic and cultural groups in North America retain the cultural heritage of their original culture.

✓ How culture influences behaviors, attitudes, and values depends on many factors and thus is not the same for different members of a cultural group.

✓ Although basic human needs are the same for all people, the way a person seeks to meet those needs is influenced by culture.

✓ Ethnocentrism can impede the delivery of care to ethnic minority clients and, when pervasive, can become cultural racism.

✓ Stereotyping ethnic group members can lead to mistaken assumptions about a client.

✓ The nurse should have an understanding of the general characteristics of the five major groups in North America—Asian, American, black, Native American, Spanish-origin, and white—but should always individualize care rather than generalize about all clients in these groups.

✓ Before assessing the cultural background of a client, nurses should assess how they are influenced by their own culture.

✓ The nursing diagnosis for clients should include potential problems in their interaction with the health care system and problems involving the effects of culture.

✓ The planning and implementation of nursing interventions should be adapted as much as possible to the client's cultural background.

✓ Evaluation should include the nurse's self-evaluation of attitudes and emotions toward providing nursing care to clients from diverse sociocultural backgrounds.

REFERENCES

Abramson, HJ: Religion. In Thermstrom, S, editor: Harvard encyclopedia of American ethnic groups, Cambridge, Mass., 1980, Harvard University Press.

Basque, W: Lecture notes, Boston, 1975.

Boyd, D: Rolling thunder, New York, 1974, Random House, Inc.

Boyle, JS: The practice of transcultural nursing, Transcultural Nursing Society Newsletter, 7:2, 1987.

Budge, EAW: Amulets and superstitions, New York, 1978, Dover Publications, Inc. (Originally published in London, 1930, by Oxford University Press).

Estes, G, and Zitzow, D: Heritage consistency as a consideration in counseling Native Americans, Paper presented at the convention of the National Indian Education Association, Dallas, 1980.

Giordano, J, and Giordano, GP: The ethno-cultural factor in mental health, New York, 1977, Institute of Pluralism and Group Identity.

Hall, ET: Proxemics: the study of man's spatial relations. In Goldstein, I., editor: Man's image in medicine and anthropology, New York, 1963, International Universities Press, Inc.

Kaptchuk, T, and Croucher, M: The healing arts, New York, 1987, Summit Books.

Kleinman, A: Patients and healers in the context of culture, Berkeley, 1980, University of California Press.

Littlejohn, H.: Interview, Boston, 1979.

Morgenstern, J: Rites of birth, marriage, death, and kindred occasions among the Semites, Chicago, 1966, Quadrangle.

Muecke, MA: Overcoming the language barrier, Nurs Outlook 18:53, 1970.

Senior, C: The Puerto Ricans: strangers then neighbors, Chicago, 1965, Quadrangle.

Spector, RE: Cultural diversity in health and illness, ed. 2, Norwalk, Conn., 1985, Appleton-Century-Crofts.

Steinberg, M: Basic Judaism, New York, 1947, Harcourt, Brace, & World.

Thernstrom, S, editor: The Harvard encyclopedia of American ethnic groups, Cambridge, Mass., 1980, Harvard University Press.

ADDITIONAL READINGS

Alvarez, RR: Familia, Berkeley, 1987, University of California Press.

American Nurses' Association: Code for nurses with interpretive statements, Kansas City, Mo., 1976, The Association.

Angelou, M: I know why the caged bird sings, New York, 1970, Random House, Inc.

Bauwens, EE: The anthropology of health, St. Louis, 1983, The C.V. Mosby Co.

Branch, MR, and Paxton, PP: Providing safe nursing care for ethnic people of color, New York, 1976, Appleton-Century-Crofts,

Brink, PJ, and Saunders, JM: Cultural shock: theoretical and applied. In Brink, PJ, editor: Transcultural nursing: a book of readings, Englewood Cliffs, N.J., 1976, Prentice-Hall, Inc.

Culpeper, N: Complete herbal, London, 1640, W. Foulsham & Co., Ltd.

Dalmau, F: Obatala, chango, y ochun, Barcelona, Italy, 1971, I.G. Manuel. El Yerberito Ilustrado, Mexico, 1975.

Densmore, F: How Indians use wild plants for food, medicine, and crafts, New York, 1974, Dover Publications, Inc.

Doane, NL: Indian doctor book, Charlotte, N.C., 1985, Aerial Photography Services, Inc.

Evaneshko, V, and Kay, M: The ethnoscience research technique, West J Nurs Res 4:49, 1982.

Fabrega, H: Medical anthropology. In Siegel, BJ, editor: Biennial review of anthropology, Stanford, Calif., 1971, Stanford University Press.

Fejos, P: Man, magic, and medicine. In Goldstone, I, editor: Medicine and anthropology, New York, 1959, International Universities Press, Inc.

Greeley, A: Why can't they be like us? America's white ethnic groups, New York, 1975, E.P. Dutton.

Gutman, HG: The black family in slavery and freedom, 1750-1925, New York, 1976, Pantheon Books, Inc.

Johnson, MN, et al.: Psychological stress and blood pressure levels in black women, J Natl Black Nurses Assoc 12:41, 1987.

Kleinman, A: Patients and healers in the context of culture, Berkeley, 1980, University of California Press.

Leininger, M: Transcultural nursing: concepts, theories and practices, New York, 1978, John Wiley & Sons, Inc.

Leininger, MM, editor: Transcultural nursing care: teaching, practice, research, Salt Lake City, 1980, University of Utah Press.

Maloney, C, editor: The evil eye, New York, 1976, Columbia University Press.

McLemore, SD: Racial and ethnic relations in America, Newton, Mass., 1980, Allyn & Bacon, Inc.

National League for Nursing: Criteria for the appraisal of baccalaureate and high degree programs in nursing, ed. 4, Pub. No. 15-1251, New York, 1977, The League.

O'Brien, ME: Transcultural nursing research: alien in an alien land, Image: J Nurs Sch 13:37, June 1981.

Orque, MS, Bloch B, and Monrroy, LS: Ethnic nursing care, St. Louis, 1983, The C.V. Mosby Co.

Painter, MT: With good heart: Yaqui beliefs and ceremonies in Pascua village, Tucson, 1986, University of Arizona press.

Parsons, T: The social system, Glencoe, N.Y., 1951, The Free Press.

Pelton, RW: Voodoo charms and talismans, New York, 1973, Popular Library.

Saunders, L: Cultural difference and medical care: the case of the Spanish-speaking people of the Southwest, New York, 1954, Russell Sage Foundation.

Shih-Chen, Li: Chinese medicinal herbs, San Francisco, 1973, Georgetown Press.

Torres, E: Green medicine, Kingsville, Tex, 1983, Nieves Press.

U.S. Department of Commerce, Bureau of Census: Current population reports: population characteristics, Series P-20, No. 374, Population profile of the United States, 1981, Washington, D.C., 1982, U.S. Government Printing Office.

Unschuld, PU: Medicine in China: a history of pharmaceuticsm, Berkeley, 1986, University of California Press.

Wei-kang, F: The story of Chinese acupuncture and moxibustion, Peking, 1975, Foreign Languages Press.

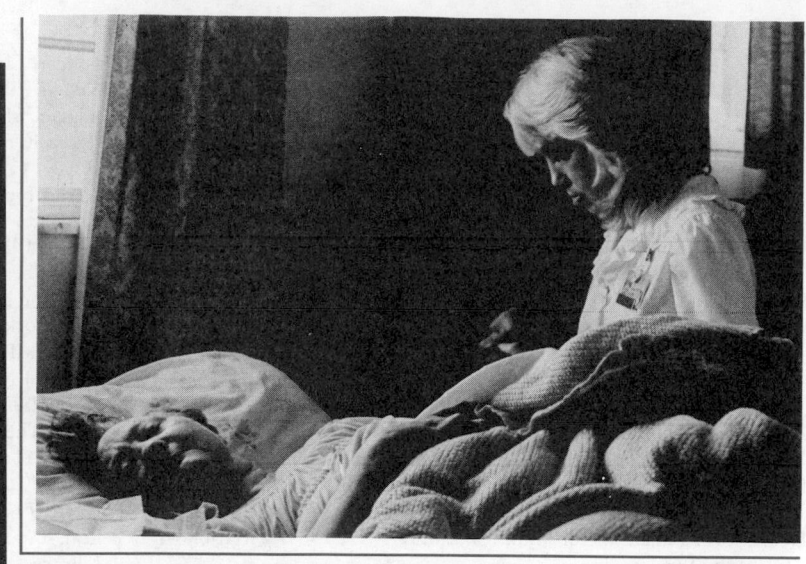

OBJECTIVES

Mastery of content in this chapter will enable the student to:

- Define the key terms listed.
- Identify the types of home health care agencies and reimbursement mechanisms.
- Identify recent social, economic, technological, and governmental forces that have influenced the development of home health nursing.
- Describe roles and responsibilities of nurses in home health care.
- Describe how regulatory standards and quality assurance guidelines affect the clinical practice of home health nursing.
- Identify at least two areas of specialized nursing care in the home setting.
- Identify future trends in home health care and the way they affect clinical practice.

KEY TERMS

Acuity
Case Management
Chemotherapy
Discharge Planning
Home Health Agency
Home Health Care
Hospice
Intravenous (IV) Therapy
Medicaid
Medicare
Private Duty Agencies
Private Insurance
Quality Assurance
Ventilators

Home Health Care

Home health care is the provision of medically related professional and paraprofessional services and equipment to clients and families in their places of residence for health maintenance, client and family education, illness prevention, diagnosis and treatment of disease, palliation, and rehabilitation. The most common professional services provided in the home include nursing; physical, occupational, speech, and respiratory therapy; medical social work; nutrition; and physician care. Of these services, nursing is predominant.

Paraprofessional services include home health aides, choreworkers, sitters, and companions. Many of these care givers provide personal care and household support services that prevent the need for costly hospitalization or nursing home placement.

Home health care equipment is any medically related product adapted for home use, including highly technical items such as mechanical ventilators and intravenous (IV) infusion pumps and nontechnical items such as hospital beds and walkers.

Home health care agencies have extended almost every type of health care service into the client's residence. Health promotion and education are traditionally the primary objectives of home care. The focus is encouragement of client and family independence through teaching of self-care. Recovery and stabilization of illness must be addressed in the home setting, where problems related to life-style, safety, environment, family dynamics, and health care practices can be readily identified.

Clients needing home health care have a variety of medical, socioeconomic, and psychological problems.

Most of these clients are medically unstable and have an acute problem such as wound infection or exacerbation of a chronic condition such as lung disease. They usually require home treatment, professional assessment, education, and frequent changes in therapy. Some clients may be medically stable but require long-term care to prevent exacerbations and the need for institutionalization. Insurance reimbursement for medically unstable clients has improved, but most policies and governmental funds do not reimburse clients for long-term care.

TYPES OF HOME HEALTH SERVICES AND REIMBURSEMENT

To meet client needs for home health care services and equipment and to ensure adequate reimbursement, nurses must understand the services available and the way clients are reimbursed. Home health care services are reimbursed by three mechanisms, including governmental funds, private insurance, and private pay.

Home Health Agencies

Home health agencies provide intermittent professional and home health aide services, usually once a day or two to three times a week. Visits usually last 45 minutes to 1 hour. Professional services are provided for implementing skilled assessment, treatment plan, and teaching programs. Home health aides provide personal care such as bathing, feeding, and bed making. Use of these services allows clients to live independently, usually with the help of family members.

Approved agencies providing these services usually receive reimbursement from the government (such as Medicare and Medicaid in the United States), private insurance, and private pay. The Medicare and Medicaid programs have strict and elaborate regulations governing reimbursement for home health care services. The Canadian national health insurance program administers and coordinates home health care services.

Private Duty Agencies

Private duty agencies provide professional and paraprofessional home health care services on a more continuous basis, usually by registered nurses, licensed practical nurses, choreworkers, homemakers, sitters, or home health aides. These agencies provide nursing coverage for 4 to 24 hours a day.

The cost of 24-hour, private-duty nursing care ranges from $7000 to $12,000 (U.S.) a month, depending on the level of the professional providing the care. Governmental funds will not pay for private duty nursing, so

reimbursement is provided primarily by private insurance and private pay. Some governmental programs are available for homemaker services.

Durable Medical Equipment Companies

Most durable medical equipment (DME) companies provide medical equipment, such as hospital beds, wheelchairs, commodes, and ventilators, and disposable supplies. Home oxygen is also available from most DME companies. Reimbursement is through government and private insurance. Fairly stringent guidelines exist for determining reimbursement for equipment.

The DME industry is one of the most rapidly growing areas in the health care field. Nurses and therapists are frequently employed by these companies to provide client education and assist with sales and marketing activities. Referral to these companies should be made after scrutiny of quality control measures and ability to provide good service and client education.

INCREASED DEMAND FOR HOME HEALTH CARE

Home health care has evolved into a challenging, and rapidly growing field. Because of recent economic, social, governmental, and technological developments, home health professionals are caring for clients who are more ill, who go home from the hospital sooner, and who have more needs for highly technical care and complex equipment than ever before.

The U.S. government's health care payment system has resulted in major cutbacks that have made an impact on the home health care industry. Funding for hospital care has been drastically cut, especially for the elderly, resulting in a tremendous increase in the need for home health care services by clients who would have previously been hospitalized. As a result, many of these clients require more highly skilled and technical services.

Other forces causing more demand for home health care services include increases in the number of elderly and chronically ill, advances in home care technology, and a breakdown in the extended family. Most households require two incomes, which leaves fewer family members at home to care for the elderly and disabled. Clients are more acutely ill when discharged from the hospital and require more intensive services.

NURSING ROLES AND RESPONSIBILITIES

Nurses assume many roles in home health care, from nurse to agency owner and director. Home health care provides a great deal of autonomy and flexibility and offers opportunities for independent clinical practice, management, marketing, teaching, clinical specialization, and research.

Clinical Practice

Home health nurses provide creative and adaptive care to clients in the home setting. A holistic, nonjudgmental, and family-centered philosophy is essential for the nurse in the home. The nurse must understand another's value systems and beliefs. The nurse helps clients grow and develop independence and usually has an interest in health promotion and maintenance. Most of all, home health nurses must take initiative to identify, solve, and follow up on client problems.

Home health nurses provide individualized care and have one-on-one contact with clients and families. They are independent and have their own caseloads, and they help clients to adapt to treatment plans and disease processes. They also help clients to adjust to the influences of cultural and environmental factors and have the opportunity to develop the nurse-client relationship more fully than nurses in short-term hospital care.

Home health nursing requires clinical assessment and teaching skills, as well as the ability to coordinate and document care provided. A home care nurse needs a broad knowledge of community resources, cultural and socioeconomic factors, family dynamics, and psychology, as well as writing skills and knowledge and application of regulatory and reimbursement guidelines.

Home Health Management

Most home health agency directors and field supervisors are nurses possessing advanced training in administration and experience in home health care practice. They provide a vital link among care givers, clients, physicians, community resources, advisory board members, and regulatory and reimbursement agencies. In addition to clinical and personnel management, they are responsible for financial management, quality assurance, and program development.

Home health nursing management requires a strong ability to promote staff excellence while containing costs and complying with reimbursement and regulatory guidelines.

Teaching and Research Activities

Most nurses in home health agencies are involved in many educational activities. In fact, the primary focus of home health care nursing is client and family education to establish self-care and independence, so nurses need to establish teaching objectives and develop and implement teaching plans for clients and family members. Nurses must determine the client's learning abilities and develop individualized teaching plans, which should be evaluated in terms of the client's objectives.

Most home health care agencies coordinate staff educational activities, including orientation, case conferences, monthly in-service workshops, and physical assessment courses. Workshops about specialty services are also important as home care becomes more technical and intensive.

The home health care nurse must know how to solve problems. Managers and field staff must refine problem-solving skills and further develop them into more formalized research activities. Many agencies are engaged in formalized studies to document the following:

1. Cost effectiveness of clinical problems
2. Staffing needs
3. Consumer satisfaction
4. Quality assurance activities

These research activities will become important as competition and regulations increase and funding sources decrease.

Legal and Ethical Responsibilities

Nurses are legally able to perform in the home independent nursing activities based on educational preparation and experience. Nurses can evaluate clients for the need for home health care services without a medical order but must provide care under the direction of a written plan of treatment signed by a physician. Home health nurses often establish the plan of care and then collaborate with the physician for medical treatment plans.

The most controversial legal issues in home health clinical practice are

1. Risks associated with providing highly technical procedures, such as administration of IV medication and blood products, in the home
2. Legal aspects of client teaching such as liability for errors made by family care givers based on misuse of information provided by the nurse
3. Compliance with Medicare or other governmental home health regulations

When nurses care for clients, they frequently find it difficult to close cases once financial reimbursement is no longer possible. Many nurses face ethical dilemmas when torn between complying with regulations and caring for the needs of elderly, indigent, and chronically ill clients. The nurse must be very knowledgeable about home health care policies to provide clinical documentation that will result in optimal reimbursement for the client. Nursing managers must also be very knowledgeable about regulations and follow the legal steps necessary to overturn coverage denials when appropriate.

Discharge Planning

Discharge planning is a major function of most home health agencies, especially those affiliated with hospitals. Agencies hire experienced nurses to function as home health coordinators or discharge planners. Nurses attend discharge planning rounds and consult with medical, nursing, and social work staffs in hospitals and clinics. They facilitate access to all home health equipment and services during a client's discharge from the hospital or clinic. The coordinator screens all referrals to see if the client is eligible for home health services in terms of insurance coverage, health care needs, and family and home situation.

Once a client is determined to be eligible for home health services, the coordinator completes a referral form based on information obtained from the following:

1. Client and family interviews
2. Consultation with physicians, other nurses, and staff members
3. The client's medical records

Thorough assessment and data collection by the coordinator before hospital discharge facilitates continuity of care and, in many cases, can speed the discharge process. A complete discharge assessment allows home health nurses to better understand the client's medical problems. It provides more information for making decisions about home health care planning.

Another aspect of discharge planning occurs when the client is discharged from home health care. The home health nurse (case manager) usually collaborates with the client and family and other home health care staff (such as nurses, therapists, and social workers) to plan the discharge. All necessary referrals are made to community resources for follow-up care. For example, a patient with chronic lung disease may be referred to breathing clubs, support groups, or outpatient rehabilitation programs. Home health staff follow up on these referrals to assess client satisfaction and to evaluate effectiveness.

DELIVERY OF HOME HEALTH NURSING CARE

ASSESSMENT

Client and family assessment begins at referral. The coordinator submits written referral forms to the home health nurses. These forms usually include (1) demographic data, (2) physician's orders, (3) medications, (4) treatments, (5) nursing and medical diagnoses, (6) goals and prognoses, and (7) functional limitations and activities.

Special problems and concerns at discharge should be communicated to the home health staff. In complicated specialty cases (for example, IV therapy, mechanical ventilation, and hospice care), home health nurses may also visit the client in the hospital before discharge to identify needs, initiate discharge teaching, and prepare the client and family for care.

Before the nurse can thoroughly assess the client and family, a "preassessment phase" must take place. This phase involves incorporating information about the client's environment and gradually establishing a nurse-client relationship. The preassessment phase is based on acceptance of individuals and families (Stuart-Siddall, 1986). The nurse combines information from the referral with an assessment of the client and family in the home setting, including interviews, physical assessments, and history. For this reason, the assessment is complex and time consuming. An assessment usually includes data about the following areas:

1. Physical assessment and history of all body systems, with emphasis on present illness
2. Psychosocial assessment (education, ethnicity, and social relations)
3. Family dynamics (decision making and rituals)
4. Community resources (need for financial assistance and follow-up health care)
5. Environmental factors (housing, transportation, and neighborhood)
6. Functional limitations (problems resulting in inabilities related to activities of daily living).
7. Client and family knowledge and attitudes toward illness and health behaviors and the impact on their life-style

NURSING DIAGNOSIS AND PLANNING

The plan of care identifies nursing diagnoses and establishes long- and short-term goals. The goals and nursing diagnoses should be related to the primary disease processes, treatment plan, functional limitations, and psychosocial, financial, and environmental problems.

The planning process in home health care requires involvement of the client and the family. All care is given in the home. It is the family's environment, where they are accustomed to having control, and the nurse must not lose sight of this fact. Home care professionals have minimal control over the environment, unlike hospital nurses who work in a very controlled environment. Client involvement in care planning and teaching leads to better compliance with care. The client is urged to take an active role.

The following factors must be considered when planning home care:

1. Socioeconomic, cultural, and environmental factors
2. Family and community resources
3. Client teaching
4. Interdisciplinary collaboration between home health and hospital professionals involved in care
5. The client's physician, who must be consulted and informed on a regular basis

Short- and long-term goals must be realistic and measurable. They are planned with involvement of the client and family, who are also involved in discharge planning. Home health staff must foster the client's independence to prepare him for discharge.

IMPLEMENTATION

Implementation of the plan of care requires close collaboration among clients, family members, home health personnel, and physicians. Skilled interventions include assessments, teaching, consultation with physicians about changes in therapy, and initiation of complex procedures such as Foley catheter changes, IV therapy, intramuscular injections, and mechanical ventilation. Most procedures can be taught to the client and family. Governmental and private insurers pay for visits only until the client and family have had time to learn procedures.

Planned interventions are not always easily achieved in many home settings. Nurses in home care must adapt interventions to all types of environmental, social, financial, and cultural constraints. Family and community resources must be used to assist with implementation.

EVALUATION

Evaluation of outcomes of care is an ongoing process, which is the key to the success of home health care. Outcomes of care must be documented for continuity of care, reimbursement, and research. Evaluation of client response to teaching, treatments, and medications usually result in identification of changes needed in therapy. It also helps to identify obstacles that may interfere with the effectiveness of the care plan. Effective, ongoing evaluation of outcomes and thorough follow-up for necessary changes are the most important functions of home health care personnel.

CLINICAL ASPECTS OF QUALITY ASSURANCE

Many governmental and private regulatory agencies have established standards and guidelines for the operation and reimbursement of home health agencies. All regulations directly or indirectly have impact on the clinical and administrative practice of home health nurses.

The U.S. and Canadian governments have established specific reimbursement guidelines for coverage of home health care services. Governmental agencies distribute funds for all claims and monitor for compliance with guidelines.

In the United States the Joint Commission for Accreditation of Healthcare Organizations (JCAHO) has established comprehensive home health care standards. All hospital-based home health care agencies must meet these standards to receive JCAHO accreditation. Documentation and case management most frequently affect the day-to-day clinical practice of home health nurses.

The client's clinical record must contain comprehensive, updated care plans and detailed notes from each visit. Visit reports must contain evidence that a visit was necessary and that skilled care was given (for example, assessments, which reflect medical instability, and client teaching and consultation with physicians). Homebound status, safety measures, and functional limitations must also be well documented.

Each client must be assigned a case manager who coordinates all aspects of care, including planning and collaboration with all home health care disciplines, community resources, and physicians. The case manager is a home health nurse who plans the client's discharge from a home health care program and implements postdischarge follow-up as needed. A monthly case conference must be held on each client and followed up by written documentation. The goal of case management is to ensure the quality of interdisciplinary planning and coordination of care.

The purpose of quality assurance is to ensure delivery and documentation of quality care and agency compliance with regulatory and reimbursement guidelines. Even though direct client care must be the primary consideration of the home health nurse, these regulatory procedures must also be performed. Failure to comply with these guidelines can result in considerable damage to clients and possibly the lifetime loss of their home health care benefits.

SPECIALTY NURSING AREAS

Home health care clients increasingly need more specialized and technically advanced services. Most agencies have come to realize that general home health nurses are not trained to provide this level of care. As a result, agencies have developed specialty nursing teams in areas such as hospice care, IV and pulmonary therapy, obstetrics, psychiatry, pediatrics, oncology, and diabetes care. Many larger agencies employ clinical nurse specialists to develop and manage specialty nursing programs.

Hospice

Hospice is a philosophy of care. It exists to provide support and care for persons in the last months of an incurable illness so life can be lived as fully and comfortably as possible.

Hospice care has evolved into a specialization. Nurses working in this area require highly technical skills related to pain control and other palliative therapies. They also need to know the psychology of dealing with dying patients and their families (see Chapter 26).

This specialized philosophy of care is applied to clients and families in the comfort of their own home. In the United States, about 80% of certified hospice care is provided in the home. Most programs are managed by home health care agencies. Home hospice care is preferred over inpatient hospice care for clients whose family members provide home care.

Home IV Therapy

Clients are now undergoing home IV therapies, including fluids, antibiotic medications, parenteral nutrition, blood products, and narcotic and chemotherapeutic agents.

In the United States, many agencies require national IV therapy certification for nurses administering home IV therapy. These nurses are usually certified in chemotherapy as well. IV therapy nurses must have good teaching and assessment skills. Comprehensive discharge planning is needed to ensure safe and effective home care.

Home Respiratory Care

Clients with chronic lung diseases are discharged sooner, are more ill, and need more complicated and technical care and equipment. They may require not only oxygen, but also mechanical ventilation and tracheostomy (see Chapter 36).

Respiratory care technology has responded to the needs of these clients. Small, portable ventilators are now as efficient and effective as most hospital ventilators.

Nurses caring for these clients not only need to know how to operate this equipment but must also have advanced knowledge and skills in respiratory nursing care and client and family teaching.

FUTURE TRENDS

Home health care will continue to grow. Many persons in the field project a 30% growth in client referrals, programs, and revenues in the next 15 years. Today's trends will continue to grow and will create many new challenges. The following list projects developments in the home health care field (Stuart-Siddall, 1986):

1. New roles and responsibilities in home care will develop for nursing, which will become the most essential element in home health care. Nursing educational programs will put more emphasis on home care management, documentation, teaching, and adaptation of acute care skills to the home. Graduate programs in home health nursing will expand and be more prevalent.

2. Home health research must be developed so practitioners and managers can make more informed decisions. The industry must prove its cost effectiveness for reimbursement to keep pace with growth.

3. Efforts to improve reimbursement will escalate, and the government will be pressured to respond to the expanding needs of home health care consumers. It is hoped that reimbursement for prevention and long-term care will occur.

4. The physician's role in home care will also expand. More physicians will provide care in the home and will become a direct part of the home health care team rather than just being involved only by referral.

5. Cost containment will be a primary focus of most home health care agencies. Research and innovative measures in this area are needed. Management and staffing needs must be studied more closely. Standards regarding the interrelationships of staffing needs, client acuity, and quality of care issues must be studied.

6. Computerization and high technology will revolutionize the home health care industry. Computer systems will help the efficiency of the clinical, management, and financial aspects of home health.

Home health care agencies will focus on high technology, cost containment, reimbursement reform, and rapid growth for many years to come. Nursing will be one of the primary forces in making these changes occur.

SUMMARY

Because of economic and other factors, increasing numbers of clients are receiving health care in their own homes. Nurses assume many roles in home health care through different types of agencies. Although some aspects of nursing care in the home are the same as practiced in other health care settings, home health nurses pay particular attention to collaboration among family members, the client, and other members of the health care team. Quality assurance of safe and effective care in the home is also particularly important.

KEY CONCEPTS

✓ Home health care is a rapidly changing field affected by many forces and trends in society.

✓ Nursing is the essential and predominant component of home health care. Nurses hold many roles from top management to bedside clinician.

✓ Delivery of home health nursing care involves assessment, nursing diagnosis and planning, implementation, evaluation, as well as accurate documentation.

✓ Home health care is closely regulated by governmental and accreditation agencies, which have a tremendous impact on the clinical practice of home health nurses.

✓ Home health care nursing is becoming highly specialized and technical.

✓ The future of home health care nursing will be marked by rapid growth, high technology, reimbursement reform, and specialization.

REFERENCE

Stuart-Siddall, S: Home health care nursing: administrative and clinical perspectives, Rockville, Md., 1986, Aspen Publishers, Inc.

ADDITIONAL READINGS

American Nurses' Association: Standards of nursing care for home health care practice, Kansas City, Mo., 1986, The Association.

Fortinshy, RH, Granger, CV, and Seltzer, GB: The use of functional assessment in understanding home care needs, Med Care 19(5):489, 1981.

Home health and hospice manual regulations and guidelines, National Health Publishing, Owings Mills, Md., 1985, Rynd Communications.

Stewart, JE: Home health care, St. Louis, 1979, The C.V. Mosby Co.

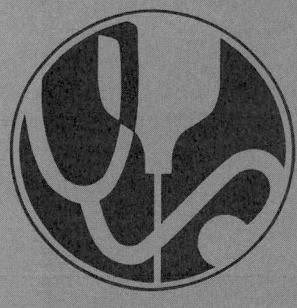

UNIT 2

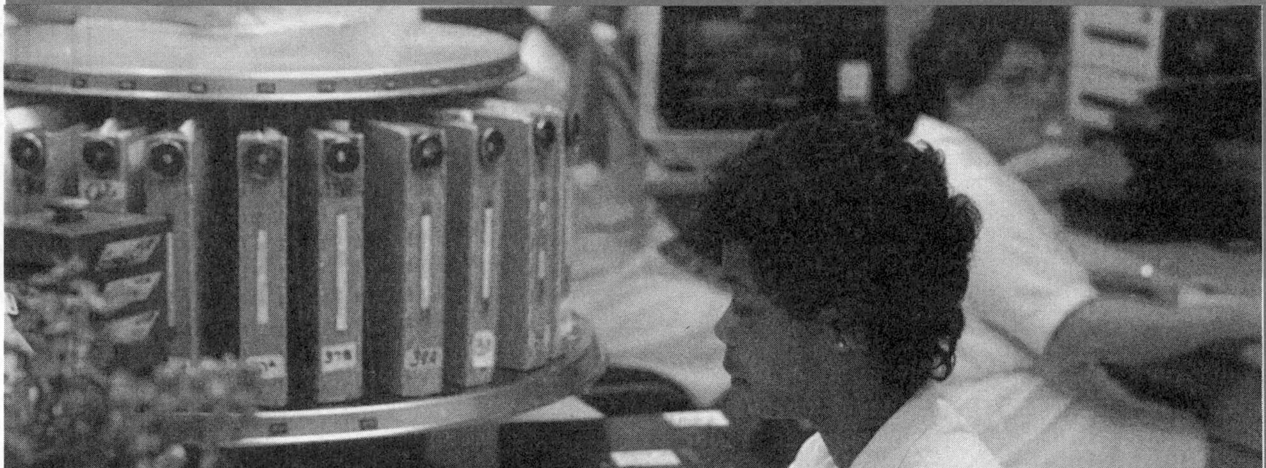

The Nursing Process

The six chapters in Unit 2 discuss the nursing process, which is an organized method of providing individualized care for clients in all states of health and illness, and the role of nursing research throughout the nursing process. A five-step approach is used: assessment, nursing diagnosis, planning, implementation, and evaluation.

The process is a systematic, purposeful method of helping clients regain, maintain, or promote health. The concept of nursing as a process is relatively new, having been introduced in the 1950s, and the steps in the nursing process are defined in many ways. Although some educational and health care institutions use a process that divides the steps in a different way, in most cases these different models correspond to the same essential principles. The five-step model, however, is most easily applied in all nursing situations.

Nursing research is discussed in Unit 2 to define the role of nursing research through the nursing process and to set the stage for the role of research in later chapters.

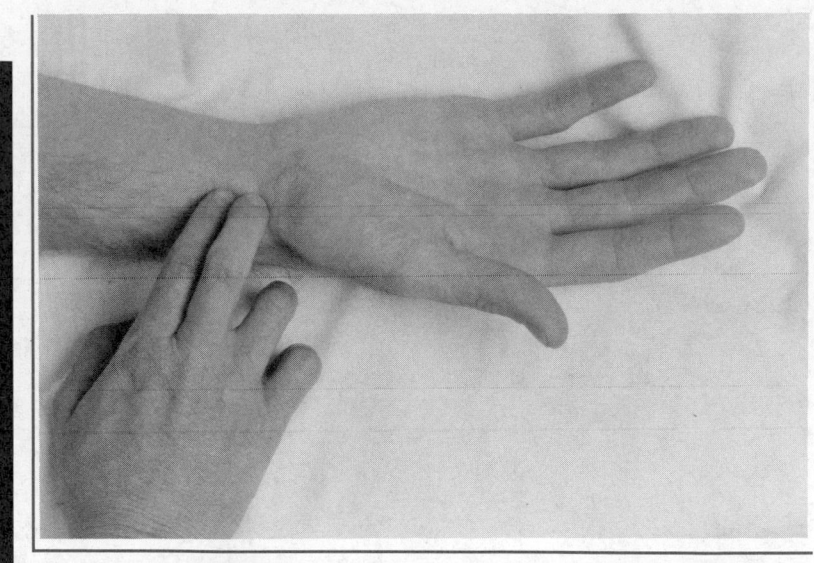

OBJECTIVES

Mastery of content in this chapter will enable the student to:

- Define the key terms listed.
- State the five components of the nursing process.
- Describe the three components of the nursing assessment.
- Discuss the purposes of nursing assessment.
- Differentiate between objective and subjective data.
- State the sources of data for a nursing assessment.
- Describe the interviewing techniques.
- State the purpose of a nursing history.
- State the purpose of a physical examination.
- Demonstrate the four skills of physical examination.
- Conduct and record a nursing assessment.

KEY TERMS

Auscultation

Data Source

Direct-Question Interview

Inspection

Interview

Norm

Nurse-Client Relationship

Nursing Health History

Objective Data

Observation

Open-Ended Question Interview

Palpation

Percussion

Physical Examination

Problem-Seeking Interview

Problem-Solving Interview

Standard

Subjective Data

Assessment

The nursing process is a method for organizing and delivering nursing care. To understand its functions, components, and interactions, it helps to have a working knowledge of the nature of a process, which is a series of steps or components leading to achievement of a goal. The three characteristics of a process are purpose, organization, and creativity (Bevis, 1978). Purpose is the goal or specific aim of the process. Organization is the series of steps or components needed to achieve the goal. Creativity is the continual development of the process itself. A process is a continuous progression from one point to another to achieve a specific goal.

The nursing process provides the creative and organizational structure and framework for nursing care, yet is flexible enough to be used in all nursing settings. The purposes of the nursing process are to identify the client's health care needs, to establish a nursing care plan to meet those needs, to complete the nursing interventions designed to meet the needs, and to evaluate the effectiveness of interventions.

The components of the nursing process—assessment, nursing diagnosis, planning, implementation, and evaluation—provide the organizational structure for achieving the purpose of the process (Fig. 6-1) (Table 6-1). Throughout the process the nurse collects and analyzes data to identify clients' actual or potential health care needs. The nurse then develops and implements an individualized care plan and evaluates the client's response to the plan, determining whether health care needs have changed or remain the same. If they have changed, the nurse may modify the original plan of care.

TABLE 6-1 Summary of Nursing Process

Component	Purpose	Steps
Assessment	To gather, verify, and communicate data about client so data base is established	1. Collecting nursing health history 2. Performing physical examination 3. Collecting laboratory data

Nursing diagnosis	To identify health care needs of client, to formulate nursing diagnoses	1. Interpreting data
		  a. Validating
		  b. Clustering
		2. Formulating nursing diagnoses

Planning	To identify client's goals; to determine priorities of care, to design nursing strategies to achieve goals of care, to determine outcome criteria	1. Identifying client goals 2. Establishing evaluation criteria 3. Selecting nursing actions 4. Delegating actions 5. Consulting 6. Writing nursing care plan
Implementation	To complete nursing actions necessary for accomplishing plan	1. Reassessing client 2. Reviewing and modifying existing care plan 3. Performing nursing actions
Evaluation	To determine extent to which goals of care have been achieved	1. Comparing client response to criteria 2. Analyzing reasons for results and conclusions 3. Modifying care plan

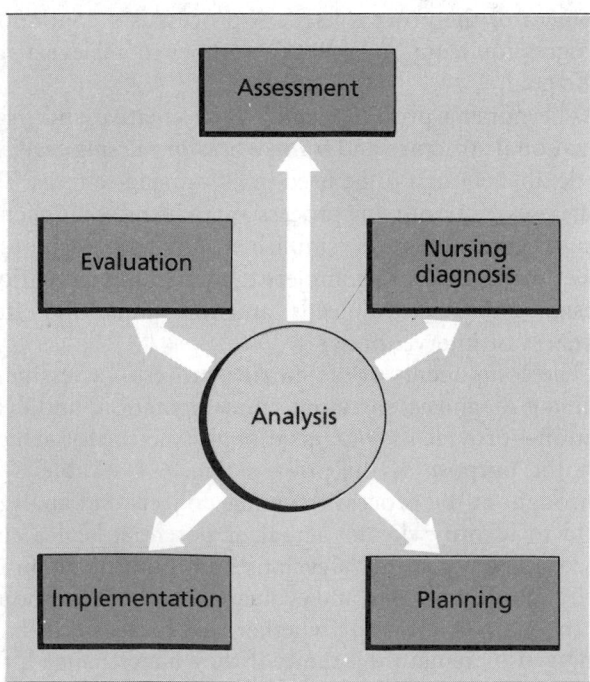

Fig. 6-1 Five-step nursing process model.

Evaluation and modification bring creativity to the nursing process. In addition the evaluation and modification of the existing care plan provide for the continual growth of the nursing process. With this process the nurse is able to meet the client's health care needs as they arise or change. The creativity of the nursing process is also demonstrated by its application in a wide variety of health care settings. For example, the nursing process is readily applicable for the neonate or the geriatric client and for clients in critical care or general medical-surgical units and inpatient or community-based settings.

HISTORICAL PERSPECTIVE

The nursing process has traditionally been defined as a systematic method for assessing health status, diagnosing health care needs, formulating a plan of care, initiating the plan, and evaluating the effectiveness of the plan. The use of the nursing process in providing individualized care requires the nurse to rely on scientific knowledge to make clinical nursing judgments and to set priorities.

The term "nursing process" was first introduced by Lydia Hall in 1955. Although this term has been used in education and practice for 30 years, the definition of the process has evolved and been modified (Table 6-2). Hall described the following types of relationships between nursing and the client: nursing at the client, to the client, for the client, and with the client (Hall, 1955 and 1963).

Dorothy Johnson (1959), Ida Orlando (1961), and Ernestine Wiedenbach (1963) introduced a three-step nursing process model into nursing education and practice. In all of these models the nurse must first identify or assess client needs. However, steps two and three differ. Only Wiedenbach includes an evaluation component within her model.

In 1967, Lois Knowles presented a process model she called the "five D's": discover, delve, decide, do, and discriminate. During the first two phases (discover and delve) the nurse collects data on the health status of the client, then selects a plan of action (decide) and carries it out (do). During the last phase (discriminate), the nurse establishes health care priorities and assesses the client's reaction to the nursing actions (Knowles, 1967).

In 1967 the Western Interstate Commission of Higher Education (WICHE) defined the nursing process as "the interrelationship between a patient and a nurse in a given setting; it incorporates the behaviors of patient and nurse and the resulting interaction." They listed the steps in the process as perception, communication, interpretation, intervention, and evaluation. The faculty at the Catholic University of America (1967) divided the nursing process into the following phases: assessment, planning, intervention, and evaluation (Yura and Walsh, 1983).

In 1969 Dolores Little and Doris Carnevali used a four-step process in the development of written nursing care plans, combining health assessment and designation of the problem into the first step.

In 1981, Ruth Freeman and Janet Heinrich introduced a six-step nursing process for community health nursing. The first step of their process is the establishment of a working relationship. Second is the assessment of the situation as it relates to health and nursing care, as well as to the balance between health conditions and the reinforcing or counteracting forces that mediate them. The third and fourth steps are the development and negotiation of action goals with the client and the collaboration between nurse and client to decide possible courses of action. The fifth step is the implementation phase in which the step-by-step course of action is taken. The sixth and final step is validation of the effectiveness of the action taken. In this model the decisions and actions of multiple health care professionals are continually coordinated.

Typology of 11 Functional Health Patterns

- Health perception–health management pattern
- Nutritional-metabolic pattern
- Elimination pattern
- Activity-exercise pattern
- Cognitive-perceptual pattern
- Sleep-rest pattern
- Self-perception–self-concept pattern
- Role-relationship pattern
- Sexuality-reproductive pattern
- Coping-stress-tolerance pattern
- Value-belief pattern

From Gordon, M: Nursing diagnosis process and application, ed. 2, New York, 1987, McGraw-Hill Book Co.

In 1973 Kristine Gebbie and Mary Ann Lavin at St. Louis University School of Nursing initiated national conferences on the classification of nursing diagnoses. In addition, nursing educators and practicing nurses began to use the five-step nursing process model on a regular basis. Since 1973, conferences on the classification of nursing diagnoses have been held every 2 years.

In 1982, Marjory Gordon introduced a typology of functional health patterns (see box). This framework is not conceptually linked to one nursing theoretical model. Thus it is adaptable to all models. The 11 categories are short and lend themselves to nursing diagnoses as opposed to medical diagnoses. The typology also focuses on wellness, as well as illness, patterns. The nurse assesses clients by organizing patterns of behavior as the behaviors pertain to a functional category.

ASSESSMENT

Nursing assessment is the process of gathering, verifying, and communicating data about a client. The purpose of the assessment is to establish a data base about the client's level of wellness, health practices, past illnesses and related experiences, and health care goals. The information contained in the data base is the basis for an individualized plan of nursing care developed throughout the nursing process.

The collection of data includes the nursing health history, physical examination, and results of laboratory and diagnostic tests. The data gathered during the health history are obtained when the nurse interviews the client. To collect data from an interview, the nurse initiates the

TABLE 6-2 Evolution of the Five-Step Nursing Process Model

Hall (1955)	Johnson (1959)	Orlando (1961)	Wiedenbach (1963)	Knowles (1967)	WICHE (1967)
"Nursing is a process"	1. Assessment	1. Behavior of the client	1. Identify	1. Discover	1. Perception and communication
				2. Delve	
	2. Decision	2. Reaction to the nurse		3. Decide	2. Interpretation
	3. Action	3. Nursing action	2. Act	4. Do	3. Intervention
			3. Evaluate	5. Discriminate	4. Discrimination

nurse-client relationship (see Chapter 19), uses various interview techniques, and progresses through the following phases of an interview: orientation, working, and termination. The skills of inspection, palpation, percussion, and auscultation permit the nurse to collect data from the physical examination. Laboratory and diagnostic tests validate the findings of the history and examination and can lead to identification of other problems not previously noted.

DATA COLLECTION

Data collected during assessment should be descriptive, concise, and complete and should not include interpretative statements. Descriptive data originate in the client's perception of any symptom, the perceptions and observations of family or significant others, the nurse's observations, or reports from other members of the health team. For example, a client may describe pain as a "sharp, throbbing pain in the abdomen." The nurse's observation may be, "The client lies on his side holding his abdomen. Facial grimacing present throughout assessment." The nurse records only what is observed and does not interpret the client's behavior such as by writing, "The client tolerates pain poorly." Concise data briefly describe the information obtained. The information is summarized in a short format using correct medical terms (for example, "Patient describes a constant sharp throbbing pain in the upper right quadrant of the abdomen. Pain began 48 hours before hospitalization, 2 hours after a high-fat meal. Pain was not relieved by antacids."). Complete data collection results when the nurse obtains all the information relevant to the actual or potential health problem. To confirm that complete data have been collected, the nurse might ask, "Do I have the information to answer the questions:

when, where, and what are the duration and influencing factors?" For example, a nurse in an outpatient clinic might write the following information on the assessment form of a client seeking treatment for recurrent headaches:

Mrs. Cooper is seeking treatment for recurrent headaches. She describes the headaches as occurring every morning after she rises from bed. The pain is localized over the left front maxillary sinus and is described by Mrs. Cooper as "pulsating." The headaches last anywhere from 1 hour to "all day." In the past the pain has been relieved with 10 grains of aspirin, but the client states that the aspirin has not been effective during the past 10 days. Mrs. Cooper notices an increase in the intensity of the headache during cold, damp weather.

The collection of inaccurate, incomplete, or inappropriate data leads to incorrect identification of the client's health care needs and subsequent inaccurate, incomplete, or inappropriate nursing diagnoses. Inaccurate data result if the nurse fails to collect information relevant to a specific area or if the nurse is disorganized or unskilled in assessment techniques. Data are incomplete if the nurse neglects to obtain all information about a specific area, jumps to conclusions about a potential problem, or makes assumptions without validation. Inappropriate data are those unrelated to the area being assessed.

TYPES OF DATA

During the assessment the nurse obtains two types of data, objective and subjective. Objective data are observations or measurements made by the data collector. Identifying the presence of a total body rash is an example of observed objective data. The measurement of objective data is based on an accepted standard, such as a thermometer or unit of measure. An elevated body

Catholic University (1967) (Yura and Walsh [1983])	**Little and Carnevali (1969)**	**Freeman (1970)**	**Gebbie and Lavin (1973)**
1. Assessment	1. Health assessment and designation of the problem	1. Establishment of working relationship	1. Assessment
		2. Assessment	2. Nursing diagnosis
2. Planning	2. Goals	3. Development and negotiation of action goals	3. Planning
3. Intervention	3. Nursing action	4. Implementation of step-by-step actions	4. Intervention
4. Evaluation	4. Evaluation	5. Validation of action taken	5. Evaluation

temperature and measurement of a child's head circumference are examples of measured objective data.

Subjective data are clients' perceptions about their health problems. Only clients can provide this kind of information. For example, the presence of pain is a subjective finding. Only the client can provide information about the frequency, duration, location, and intensity of it. Subjective data usually include feelings of anxiety, physical discomfort, or mental stress. Although only the client can provide subjective data relevant to these feelings, the nurse must be aware that these problems can result in physiological changes, which are identified through objective data collection.

Ms. Johnson is taking care of Mr. Woods 1 day after an appendectomy. Ms. Johnson asks Mr. Woods about any pain or discomfort. He replies, "I have an occasional twinge in my right side, but I'm fine." Ms. Johnson observes that he is diaphoretic and has tachycardia and that his blood pressure is elevated.

Mr. Woods' description of his pain is subjective, but the physiological changes of elevated blood pressure, tachycardia, and diaphoresis are the bases for additional objective data.

SOURCES OF DATA

Data are obtained from the client, the family or significant others, health team members, the health record, other records, and pertinent nursing and medical literature. Each source provides information about the client's level of wellness, risk factors, health practices and goals, and patterns of illness, as well as information relevant to the client's health care needs. The physical examination and diagnostic and laboratory tests are also sources of data.

Client

In most situations the client is the best source of information. The client who is oriented and answers questions appropriately can provide the most accurate information about his health care needs, life-style patterns, and present and past illnesses.

Family or Significant Others

The family or significant others can be interviewed as primary sources of information about infants or children and critically ill, mentally handicapped, disoriented, or unconscious clients. In cases of severe illness or emergency situations the family or significant others may be the only available source of data about the client's health-illness patterns, current medications, allergies, onset of illness, and other information needed by nurses and physicians.

In addition to serving as a primary source of information, the family or significant others can supply additional data about the client's health status and may be able to indicate how the client reacts to changes in level of wellness and functioning. Finally, the family or significant others can make pertinent observations about the client's needs that can affect the delivery of care.

Health Team Members

The health team consists of physicians, nurses, allied health professionals, and nonprofessional employees working in a health care setting (see Chapter 3). Because assessment is an ongoing process, the nurse must communicate with other health team members, including physical therapists, clergy, social workers, and community health workers. Health team members can provide data about the way the client interacts within the health care environment, reacts to information about diagnostic tests, and responds to visitors. Every member of the health team interacting with a client is a potential source of information, and the health team can identify and communicate data, as well as verify information from other sources.

Medical Records

The present and past medical records of the client can verify information about past health patterns or can provide new information. By reviewing medical records the nurse can identify patterns of illness and a client's past methods of coping.

Other Records

Other records such as educational, military, and employment records may contain pertinent health care information. If the client received services at a community health center or day-care clinic, the nurse should obtain data from these records but must first obtain written permission from the client or guardian to see them. Any information obtained is confidential and is treated as part of the client's legal medical record (see Chapter 18).

Literature Review

Reviewing nursing and medical literature about the client's illness helps to complete the data base. The review increases the nurse's knowledge about the symptoms, treatment, and prognosis of specific illnesses. The knowledgeable nurse is able to obtain pertinent information for the assessment and for planning care.

METHODS OF DATA COLLECTION

The nurse uses the following methods of data collection to establish the data base: the interview, the nursing health history, the physical examination, and results of laboratory and diagnostic tests. Each method allows the nurse to collect complete information about a client's past and present level of wellness.

Interview

The interview is a pattern of communication initiated for a specific purpose and focused on a specific content area. In nursing, the major purposes of the interview are to obtain a nursing health history, identify health needs and risk factors, and determine specific changes in level of wellness and pattern of living. The interviewer obtains information about the client's health state, life-style, support systems, patterns of illness, patterns of adaptation, strengths and limitations, and resources.

Objectives of the Nursing Interview

- Initiates nurse-client relationship
- Obtains information from the client in all dimensions
- Provides the nurse with an opportunity to observe the client
- Provides the client with an opportunity to obtain information
- Provides the first step toward establishing a therapeutic relationship between the nurse and client

---

In conducting the interview the nurse uses specific communication skills to focus attention on the client's level of wellness. The nurse also helps clients understand the changes that are occurring or will occur in their pattern of living. This chapter describes communication skills and the interview, whereas Chapter 19 discusses the total communication process and details the various communication techniques necessary for nursing practice.

The nursing interview achieves several objectives (see box). First, the nurse-client relationship is initiated. A nurse-client relationship is the association between the nurse and the client that has a mutual concern, the client's well-being. The nurse-client relationship encourages the sharing of information, ideas, and emotions.

During the interview, the nurse obtains information about a client's physical, developmental, emotional, intellectual, social, and spiritual dimensions. Physical and developmental information reflects normal functioning and the pathological changes induced by illness, trauma, or developmental stage as they affect the client's pattern of living. Emotional information includes the behavioral responses to changes in health and pattern of living. Relevant emotional information includes mood, perceptions, body image, self-concept, and attitudes about sexuality. Intellectual information includes intellectual performance, problem-solving ability, educational level, communication patterns, and attention span. Social information involves environmental, cultural, ethnic, or social patterns that can affect the present or future level of wellness. The nurse also collects information about values, beliefs, and religious practices, which are part of the spiritual dimension.

The interview also provides the nurse with the opportunity to observe the client. The nurse observes interactions between the client and family and between the client and the health care environment, as well as the use of eye contact, nonverbal communication, and other body language. While observing this behavior, appearance, and interaction with the environment, the nurse determines whether the data obtained by observation are consistent with those obtained by verbal communication. For example, if the client states no concern about an upcoming diagnostic test but appears anxious and irritable, the data conflict. The observation provides additional data for the health history.

The interview is a mechanism by which the client can obtain information as well. If a positive nurse-client relationship has been established, the client will feel comfortable enough to ask the nurse questions about the health care environment, treatments, diagnostic testing, and available resources. The client needs this information to participate in establishing goals and planning care.

In addition, the interview is a first step toward establishing a therapeutic relationship between the nurse and client so health interventions such as education or counseling can occur.

To interview a client successfully and to achieve the purpose and objectives of the interview, the nurse needs skills in initiating the nurse-client relationship, using the various types of interviews, and moving from one phase of the interview to the next.

INITIATING THE NURSE-CLIENT RELATIONSHIP

Perhaps the most difficult client interview for a nurse to conduct is the first. For some clients, being interviewed by a nurse is a new experience. Therefore it is important that the nurse establish an effective nurse-client relationship before proceeding to the nursing health history.

The first step in initiating the relationship is for the nurse to introduce himself or herself as the interviewer, stating name, position, and the purpose of the interview.

Good afternoon, Mr. Carney. I am Miss West, the student nurse who will be taking care of you tomorrow. I would like to talk to you for 30 to 40 minutes about your health and answer any questions you may have about your care. The reason for the interview is so I can plan your nursing care. Do you have any questions at this time? May I talk to you now?

In this example the nurse introduced herself as the interviewer, gave an estimate of the time needed for the interview, and told Mr. Carney the reason for the interview. Indicating the interview length in advance is important because it helps ensure the client's cooperation. Clients, even those in a hospital, should not be considered captive audiences, and the nurse should take steps to ensure that a client's time is not used inappropriately. Stating the length of the inteview demonstrates to clients that their time will not be abused. In the example, the nurse also gave Mr. Carney an opportunity to ask questions. It is important to determine if the client has any pressing questions before beginning the interview. By answering these questions the nurse can meet some of the client's immediate needs, and the client may feel more comfortable about completely answering the nurse's questions. For example, a client who is unsure about how the hospital bed operates may be thinking about the bed instead of the interviewer's questions and therefore may not provide complete information for the data base. Finally, the nurse asked if it was all right to conduct the interview at that time, thereby giving the client a choice.

The next step in initiating the nurse-client relationship is to communicate trust and confidentiality to the client. Illnesses that cause people to seek help are often accompanied by anxiety, helplessness, disruption of family relationships, and changes in self-image. Frequently, clients are asked to provide very personal information about themselves and their families. Generally, people share such information only with close friends, and there is a certain amount of trust that this information will not be shared with others. The nurse assures the client that the interview is confidential before asking the client to share personal information concerning past or present levels of wellness or family relationships.

Finally, the nurse-client relationship is enhanced by the professionalism and competence conveyed by the nurse. The nurse's attitude of professionalism and professional manner and appearance encourages a supportive therapeutic relationship with the client so the nurse and client can communicate freely, thereby allowing the nurse to identify health care needs and objectives. The nurse is involved with the client and family or significant others and becomes an advocate for the client. The nurse as a client advocate intercedes for the client and encourages others to put the client's needs high on their list of priorities.

TYPES OF INTERVIEW TECHNIQUES

The client's personality and health care needs and the health care setting affect the interview process. An emergency situation may require one type of interview technique, whereas a chronic illness requires another. The interview in an emergency room usually centers on the present illness or trauma, precipitating factors, medications the client is taking, and allergies. By contrast, an interview with a client undergoing extensive rehabilitation may focus on past and present illnesses and coping strategies, family and community resources, and the client's present limitations and goals for rehabilitation. The nurse can use many interview techniques to elicit the necessary information from the client or other data sources.

PROBLEM-SEEKING TECHNIQUE. The problem-seeking technique identifies the client's potential problems, and subsequent data collection focuses on those problems. For example, the nurse may ask the client if there are changes in digestion such as lack of appetite, nausea, vomiting, or diarrhea. If the client says that some of these symptoms have occurred, the nurse may proceed with problem-solving questions.

PROBLEM-SOLVING TECHNIQUE. The problem-solving interview technique focuses on gathering in-depth data on specific problems identified by the client or nurse (Yarnall and Atwood, 1974). If, for example, the client has experienced nausea, the interviewer gathers information about the onset, aggravating factors, associated symptoms, and relief measures the client has tried.

DIRECT-QUESTION TECHNIQUE. The direct-question technique is a structured format requiring one- or two-word answers and is frequently used to clarify previous information or provide additional information (Enelow and Swisher, 1979). With this technique the questions do not encourage the client to volunteer more information than is directly requested. This type of questioning is useful in obtaining biographical data, as well as specific information about health problems such as symptoms, precipitating factors, and relief measures.

OPEN-ENDED QUESTION TECHNIQUE. The open-ended question is aimed at obtaining a response of more than one or two words. This technique leads to a discussion between the client and the nurse in which the client actively describes his or her health status. This method strengthens the nurse-client relationship because it demonstrates that the nurse wants to invest time in hearing the client's thoughts. Examples of open-ended questions are, "What are your health care needs? How have you been feeling? What can you tell me about your problem?"

PHASES OF THE INTERVIEW

The interview involves three phases, orientation, working, and termination. Before interviewing the client, the nurse prepares by reading the past medical record, obtaining information about the client's present illness, reviewing literature on the health problem, and creating an environment conducive to an interview. An interview with a hospitalized client should be scheduled for a time when interruptions by other health care professionals or families will be minimal and the client will not be receiving visitors. An environment in which the client is comfortable and relaxed is also conducive to a good interview. Clients interviewed at home may prefer the interview to take place in a bedroom away from other family members. Finally, the nurse selects a place private enough to allow the client to be comfortable when providing personal information.

ORIENTATION PHASE. Before beginning the nurse reviews the purposes for the interview, the types of data to be obtained, and the methods most appropriate for conducting the interview. The review encourages the nurse to consider why the interview is being done, what specific data are needed from the client, and which interview techniques will be used to obtain those data. The interview helps establish the nurse-client relationship. While conducting the interview the nurse remains aware that the client is forming an impression about nursing.

The nurse opens the interview by explaining the purposes of the interview. The nurse also tells the client about the types of questions that will be asked and about the client's role in the interview process. Then the nurse spends 5 to 10 minutes becoming acquainted with the client.

Mr. Coffey is preparing an admission history on Mr. Rose, a 21-year-old man hospitalized for the first time.

Mr. Coffey: Good afternoon, Mr. Rose. I'm Bill Coffey and I'm your primary nurse for your hospital stay.

Mr. Rose: Hi, Bill. Please call me Jim. What's a primary nurse?

Mr. Coffey: Jim, "primary nurse" means I'm totally responsible for all your nursing care while you're hospitalized. Although other nurses will sometimes take care of you when I'm off, I'm the nurse who plans your care.

Mr. Rose: I guess that's a lot like being a coach. You may not play the game, but you're responsible for winning or losing.

Mr. Coffey: I suppose that's one way of looking at it. Sometime this afternoon I'd like to ask you some questions about your health. We call this a health interview. The interview is done so I can best plan your care, and any information you give me is confidential. The total interview should take about 20 to 30 minutes. When could I interview you?

Mr. Rose: Could I do it now? My girl friend is coming to visit later this afternoon. We coach a Little League team in the evenings, so she'll have to be at the game tonight.

Mr. Coffey: That's fine. Since you're in a private room, is it OK if we stay here? (Mr. Rose nods yes.) Good, let me close the door. Before we start, do you have any questions about anything in your room?

Mr. Rose: Yes. Why is there an outlet for oxygen on the wall above my bed? Does that mean that I'm really sick—did they put me in a special room?

Mr. Coffey: No, that's not it. Every bed in this hospital has an oxygen outlet located on the wall above the head of the bed. The reason is that this hospital has a central oxygen delivery system, and when a patient needs oxygen, we're able to supply it quickly, easily, and safely.

Mr. Rose: OK. I wasn't actually worried. I was basically just curious. That was the only piece of equipment I couldn't explain.

Mr. Coffey: (pause) Jim, you mentioned that you and your girl friend are coaches for a Little League team. What's that like?

In this example Mr. Coffey introduced his role to the client. He reviewed the interview process, and its objectives, confidentiality, and length. The nurse and client agreed mutually on an interview time. Before beginning the interview, Mr. Coffey asked his client if he had any questions. Mr. Coffey's answer about the oxygen allowed Mr. Rose to clarify his concern so he would not be distracted during the interview. Mr. Coffey used the client's experience with coaching as a means of becoming acquainted before proceeding to the health interview. He chose coaching because Mr. Rose had made reference to his coaching experience. Mr. Coffey asked an open-ended question about coaching to encourage Mr. Rose to talk.

WORKING PHASE. As the interview progresses, the nurse asks questions to form a data base from which the nursing care plan will be developed. The four techniques of interviewing are implemented as needed. In addition, the nurse uses 10 strategies (see box) to facilitate communication and ensure that nurse and client clearly understand what the other is saying (see Chapter 19).

TERMINATION PHASE. As in the other phases of the interview, termination requires skill on the part of the interviewer. Ideally the client should be given a clue that the interview is coming to an end. For example, the nurse may say, "There are just two more questions," or "We'll be finished in 5 to 6 minutes." With this method the client can maintain attention without being distracted by wondering how much longer the interview will last. Also, the client may ask any final questions before the interview ends.

The nurse should be as organized during this phase as during the opening. The interview is terminated in a friendly manner, with the nurse indicating specifically when there will be additional contact. For example, an appropriate way to end an interview would be, "Thank you for answering these questions. They'll be helpful in planning your nursing care. Another nurse will be caring for you this evening, but I'll be back on duty tomorrow morning. Do you have any other questions? Is there anything I can do for you now?"

The nurse's interviewing skills and techniques are essential in developing a data base. The skillful interviewer is able to adapt interview strategies to different clients and health care environments. Pertinent health data are obtained when the nurse is prepared for the interview and is able to carry out each of the three interview phases.

Nursing Health History

The nursing health history is the data collected about the client's level of wellness, changes in life patterns, sociocultural role, and mental and emotional reactions to illness. The nursing history is obtained during the interview and is the first step in carrying out the nursing assessment. The objectives of the nursing health history

---

Ten Strategies for Effective Communication

- *Silence* is helpful for making observations about the client and provides the client with time to organize thoughts and to present complete information to the interviewer.
- *Attentive listening* demonstrates interest in the client's needs, concerns, and problems. Listening can be facilitated by maintaining eye contact, remaining relaxed, and using appropriate touch techniques.
- *Conveying acceptance* demonstrates the interviewer's willingness to listen to the client's beliefs, values, and practices without being judgmental.
- *Related questions* are planned in which the nurse uses words and word patterns in the client's normal sociocultural context.
- *Paraphrasing* provides an opportunity for the interviewer to validate information from the client without changing the meaning of the client's statement. Paraphrasing is the interviewer's formulation of what the client has said in more specific words.
- *Clarifying* facilitates correct communication of information. It is achieved by asking the client to restate the information or by providing an example.
- *Focusing* eliminates vagueness in communication, limits the area of discussion for the client, and helps the interviewer direct attention to the pertinent aspects of a client's message.
- *Stating observations* provides the client with feedback about how the interviewer observes the client's behavior, action, facial expression or activities.
- *Offering information* allows the interviewer to clarify treatments, initiate health teaching, and identify and correct misconceptions.
- *Summarizing* condenses the data into an organized review. It validates data because the client has the opportunity to confirm that the data are correct. Summarizing indicates the end to a particular part of the interview.

---

are to identify patterns of health and illness, the presence of risk factors for physical and behavioral health problems, any deviations from normal, and available resources for adaptation (Perry, 1982).

Patterns of health and illness are identified by collecting data about the physical, developmental, intellectual, emotional, social, and spiritual dimensions (Fig. 6-2). Incorporating data from all these dimensions into the nursing health history ultimately enables the nurse to develop a complete plan of care.

Although many formats for the nursing health history have been given in the literature, all contain similar basic components (see box on p. 113).

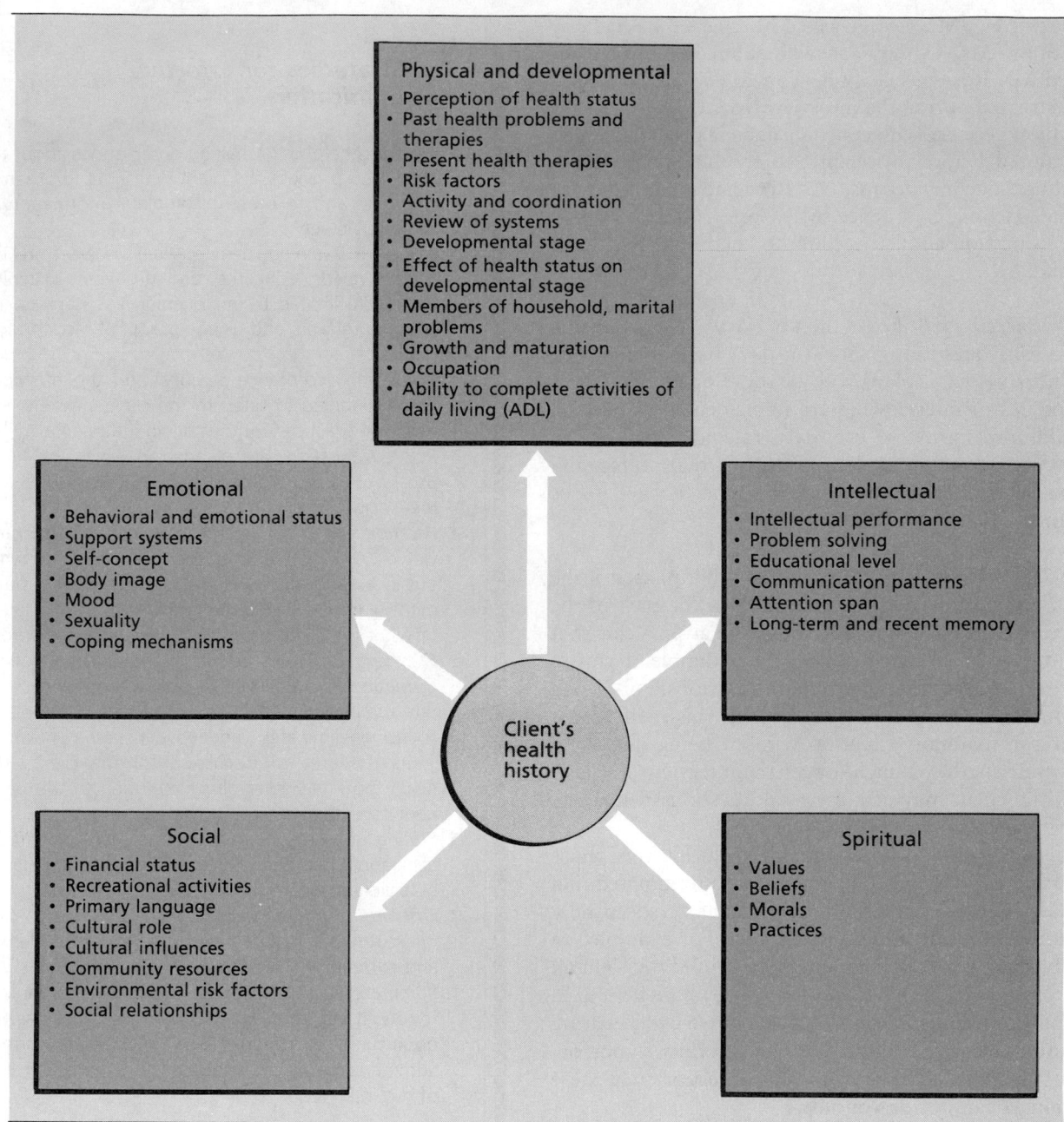

Physical and developmental
• Perception of health status
• Past health problems and therapies
• Present health therapies
• Risk factors
• Activity and coordination
• Review of systems
• Developmental stage
• Effect of health status on developmental stage
• Members of household, marital problems
• Growth and maturation
• Occupation
• Ability to complete activities of daily living (ADL)

Emotional
• Behavioral and emotional status
• Support systems
• Self-concept
• Body image
• Mood
• Sexuality
• Coping mechanisms

Intellectual
• Intellectual performance
• Problem solving
• Educational level
• Communication patterns
• Attention span
• Long-term and recent memory

Client's health history

Social
• Financial status
• Recreational activities
• Primary language
• Cultural role
• Cultural influences
• Community resources
• Environmental risk factors
• Social relationships

Spiritual
• Values
• Beliefs
• Morals
• Practices

Fig. 6-2   Dimensions for gathering data for a health history.

BIOGRAPHICAL INFORMATION

Biographical information is factual demographic data about the client. The client's age, address, working status, marital status, and types of insurance coverage should be included.

REASON FOR SEEKING HEALTH CARE

The nurse asks why the client sought health care because the information contained on the client's admission form may differ greatly from the client's subjective reason for seeking health care, as in the following example:

Mr. Jones has been seen in the outpatient clinic for chronic diarrhea and is scheduled for a series of gastrointestinal diagnostic tests.

During the nursing health history the nurse asks Mr. Jones his reason for seeking health care. "To find out why I have this pain in my stomach," the client replies. The information can make the nurse aware of any discomfort that Mr. Jones has that may or may not be related to chronic diarrhea.

Basic Components for a Nursing Health History

- *Biographical information:* date of birth, sex, address, family members or significant others' names and addresses, marital status, religious preference and practices, occupation, source of health care, and insurance.
- *Reasons for seeking health care:* goals of care, expectation of the services and care delivered, and what the client expects the health care system to provide.
- *Present illness or health concern:* onset, symptoms, nature of symptoms (for example, sudden or gradual), duration, precipitating factors, relief measure(s), and presence of weight loss or gain.
- *Past health history:* prior illnesses throughout client's development, injuries and hospitalizations, surgeries, blood transfusions, allergies, immunizations, habits (smoking, caffeine, alcohol or drug abuse), prescribed and self-prescribed medications, work habits, relaxation activities, and sleep, exercise, and eating or nutritional patterns.
- *Family history:* health status of the immediate family and living blood relatives, the cause of death of blood relatives, and risk factor analyses for cancer, heart disease, diabetes mellitus, kidney disease, hypertension, or mental disorders.
- *Environmental history:* hazards, pollutants, and physical safety.
- *Psychosocial and cultural history:* primary language, cultural group, community resources, mood, attention span, and developmental stage.
- *Review of systems (ROS):* head-to-toe review of all major body systems, as well as the client's knowledge of and compliance with health care (for example, frequency of breast or testicular self-examination or last visual acuity examination).

The statement made by the client is not a diagnostic statement but is the client's perception of reasons for seeking health care. Clarification of the client's perception identifies potential areas for education, counseling, or community resources the client may require throughout all phases of diagnoses and recovery. When recorded, the statement is enclosed in quotation marks to indicate the client's own words.

PRESENT ILLNESS

If an illness is present, the nurse gathers essential and relevant data about the onset of symptoms. Did the symptoms begin suddenly or gradually? What is their duration? Are they always present or do they come and go? In the section of the history on present illness the nurse records specific information such as location, intensity, and quality of a symptom. The nurse needs to know if any action precipitates the symptoms, makes them worse, or provides relief.

While the nurse is discovering why the client is seeking health care, it is appropriate to learn the client's expectations of the health care providers. Does the client expect to be "cured," "free of pain," or "able to care for myself?" This information assists in establishing the goals of nursing care, as well as in determining whether the client's expectations of self and the health care providers are realistic. In addition, the client's expectations provide the nurse with information on the client's perceptions about any patterns of illness or changes in lifestyle.

PAST HEALTH HISTORY

The information collected about the client's past history provides data on the client's health care experiences. The nurse determines if the client has ever been hospitalized or undergone surgery. Also essential in planning nursing care are descriptions of any allergies, including if the allergic reaction is caused by food, drugs, or pollutants. If an allergy is present, the specific reaction and treatment are noted on the assessment form.

While collecting information on the client's history, the nurse identifies habits and life-style patterns. Use of alcohol, tobacco, caffeine, or drugs or routinely taken medications can place the client at risk for diseases involving the liver, lungs, heart, nervous system, or thought processes. Noting the type of habit, as well as the frequency and duration of use, provides essential data.

Assessing patterns of sleep, exercise, and nutrition is important in planning nursing care. Whenever possible the nursing care plan within a health care setting should be correlated with a client's life-style patterns. Frequently, variations in sleep, activity, and nutritional patterns can be accommodated.

FAMILY HISTORY

The purpose of the family history is to obtain data about immediate and blood relatives. The objectives are to determine whether the client is at risk for illnesses of a genetic or familial nature and to identify areas of health promotion and illness prevention. The family history also provides information about family structure, interaction, and function that may be useful in planning care. For example, a cohesive, supportive family can be a resource in helping a client adjust to an illness or disability and should be incorporated into the plan of care. On the other hand, if the client's family is nonsupportive, it may be better not to involve them in the client's care, particularly if the family history reveals that the client is experiencing stress related to familial relationships.

Date *April 10, 19--*

Biographical information

Name *William Brown*   Date of birth *06/20/19*   Sex *M*

Address *4511 Front Street*

Family member or significant other name *Hannah — 40 years*

Address *same*

Marital status   S Ⓜ D W   Religious preference *Methodist*

Religious practices *Attends church weekly*

Occupation (present) *carpenter*

Length of occupation *32 years   client has owned his own remodeling firm for the past 20 years*

Source of health care *private doctor, Dr. Kelly*

Insurance *Blue Cross - Blue Shield*

Client's reason for seeking health care *"To find out why I've had diarrhea for 3 weeks"*

Present illness

Onset *3 weeks ago*   , Sudden or gradual *sudden*

Duration *continued to present*

Symptoms *watery diarrhea, no cramping or GI pain noted*

Precipitating factors *occurs following a meal, diarrhea is sudden*

Relief measures *some relief noted when client eats small meals*

Expectations of health care providers *"to stop diarrhea" and "to tell me I don't have stomach cancer"*

Past history

Illnesses: Childhood *measles, mumps, and chickenpox*

Injuries & hospitalizations *(1) age 12 - tonsillectomy, (2) age 46 - broken leg*

Operations *see above*

Major illnesses *none*

Allergies: Type *roses, no drugs or food allergies stated*

Reaction *sneezing, runny nose*

Treatment *Allerest tablets*

Immunizations: *current*

Habits: ETHANOL *6-pack/day* SMOKING *2 packs/day for 20 years*   DRUGS *none*

Duration of each

Medications: Prescribed *none*

Self-medicated *Allerest*

Sleep patterns *usually retires at 11pm and rises at 6 AM*

Exercise patterns *plays tennis or racquetball 3 times a week*

Nutritional patterns *large breakfast-lunch, salad for evening meal*

Work patterns *works 50-60 hours a week*

Fig. 6-3   Nursing health history.

Family history

Health of parents, siblings, spouse, children _____

Risk factor analysis: cancer, heart disease, diabetes mellitus, kidney disease, hypertension, mental disorders

mother died at 58 from stomach cancer; father died at 75 from heart attack; brother died at 42 from stomach cancer; 2 sisters, 50 and 48, alive and well; 1 son, 35, alive and well

Environmental history

Cleanliness *lives in rehabilitated city home*

Hazards *some street crime*

Pollutants *auto fumes*

Psychosocial/cultural history

Primary language *English*

Cultural group *neighbors* _____ Community resources *his church*

Mood *sociable, talkative, asked if symptoms were cancer related.*

Developmental stage *an adult male who appears to assume the responsibilities of an adult role.*

Review of systems (ROS) _____

Head, eyes, ears, nose, and throat (HEENT)

Head: Headaches *occasional* Dizziness *no*

Vision: Last eye exam *2 months ago*

Glasses *yes, bifocals* Contacts _____ (Hard _____ Soft _____ Long wearing _____)

Blurring *no*

Diplopia *no* Pain *no* Inflammation *yes, during allergy season*

Surgery *no*

Hearing: Impaired *no* Type of hearing aid _____

Date of new batteries _____

Pain *no* Drainage *no* Tinnitus *occasionally*

Nose: Allergic rhinitis *yes* Type allergen *roses*

Relief measures *Allerest tablets*

Frequency of colds per year *1*

History of polyps *no*

Sinuses *no problems*

Nose bleeds *none*

Throat & mouth: Last dental exam *6 months ago*

Dentures *no*

Speech disorders _____

Swallowing problem *no*

Respiratory: Cough *yes* Sputum *yes on rising in the morning*

Dyspnea *no* Dyspnea on exertion *no*

Activity tolerance *plays racquetball 3 times per week*

Last chest x-ray *this hospitalization*

Pain *no* Hemoptysis *no*

Fig. 6-3 cont'd Nursing health history.

Continued.

Circulatory: Pain _no_____ Palpitations _no_____

Edema _no_____ Numbness _no_____ Tingling _no_____

Changes in color _no_____ Changes in hair _no_____

Distribution on extremities _no_____

Syncope _no_____ Dizziness _no_____

PND _no_____

Nutritional: Appetite _good until 3 weeks ago_____

Nausea_____ Vomiting _____

Elimination (bowel):

Routine pattern _every other day_ Use of laxatives _none_____

Colostomy _____ Ileostomy _____

Constipation _____ Diarrhea _began 3 weeks ago_____

Melena _____

(Urine) incontinence _no_____ Infections _once — 10 years ago_____

Hematuria _no_____ Catheter _no_____

Reproductive:

Pregnancies _N/A_____ Children _____

Last Pap test _____ Results_____ LMP_____

Excessive bleeding _____ Vaginal discharge _____

Self breast exam

Prostate problems

Neurological:

Confusion _no_____ Convulsions _no_____

Paralysis _no_____ Paresthesia _no_____ Weakness _no_____

Incoordination _no____ Headaches _relieved with ASA 10 gr_____

Musculoskeletal:

Pain _no_____ Stiffness _no_____

Exercise patterns _racquetball 3 times a week_____

Adaptive responses _no_____

Skin: Rashes _no____ Lesions _no_____ Color _white_____

Texture _smooth_ Turgor _good_____

Fig. 6-3 cont'd   Nursing health history.

ENVIRONMENTAL HISTORY

The environmental and psychosocial histories provide data about clients' home environments and any support systems that clients or family members may need to use in the future. The environmental history, for example, identifies exposure to pollutants that can affect clients' health, high crime that prevents clients from walking around their neighborhoods, and resources that can assist clients in the return to the community.

PSYCHOSOCIAL HISTORY

The psychosocial history includes information about how the client and family cope with stressors. Questions about resolved stressors indicate to the nurse the types of stressors encountered by the client and the resources available to deal with any impending stressors (see Chapter 28).

REVIEW OF SYSTEMS

The review of systems (ROS) is a systematic method for collecting data on all body systems. During the ROS the nurse asks the client about the normal functioning of each system, as well as any changes noted by the client. Changes noted by the client are usually subjective data because they are described as perceived by the client.

As the nurse proceeds through the nursing health history, the data obtained are recorded in a clear, concise manner using appropriate terminology. A clear, concise record is necessary because other health care professionals may use the nursing health history in delivering health care. The sample in Fig. 6-3 shows the correct way to record information on a nursing health history. Chapters in this unit present sections of a care plan devised for Mr. Brown, who has entered the hospital after having diarrhea for 3 weeks.

Physical Examination

The physical examination is the taking of vital signs and other measurements and the examination of all body parts using the techniques of inspection, palpation, percussion, and auscultation. The examiner looks for abnormalities that may yield information about past, present, and future health problems. The physical examination is conducted after the nursing health history so data gathered during the history can be verified. In addition, new data are obtained during the examination.

Throughout the examination, data are measured against a standard, which is an established rule or basis of comparison in measuring or judging capacity, quantity, content, and value of objects in the same category. The term "norm" is frequently used synonymously with "standard" in the literature. Selected standards are reliable and relevant for the category being compared. For example, established standards for ideal height and weight are used to determine if an individual is taller or shorter than the standard or is overweight or underweight. The nurse conducting the physical examination uses inspection, palpation, percussion, and auscultation to verify information and to collect further data, which are compared with the standards to determine whether the findings are normal or abnormal. Chapter 13 discusses these skills in more detail, but they are presented here as an overview of the physical examination.

Before conducting the physical examination, the nurse prepares the client, the environment, and the necessary equipment. The nurse informs the client about the process of the physical examination, specifically its purposes, the nurse's role, the client's role, and the approximate duration.

INSPECTION

The nurse inspects the client's body and observes his or her mood, including all responses and nonverbal behavior. The inspection begins with the nurse's first contact with the client and continues throughout the nursing history. Inspection is used by the nurse to systematically collect data about significant behaviors or physical features. It is important to be accurate and thorough, using a systematic method such as head to toe.

PALPATION

With palpation the examiner uses the hands and sense of touch to gather data. Palpation is used to detect tenderness, temperature, texture, vibration, pulsations, masses, and other changes in structural integrity. Each body part is palpated, usually after a systematic assessment pattern. Palpation rules out or confirms suspicions raised during interview and inspection. Because touching may elicit fear, embarrassment, pain, or other strong emotions, it is important to explain the actions and reasons for them. In addition, the client should be instructed to let the nurse know if the palpation procedures produce tenderness, pressure, or pain. The two palpation techniques, light and deep, are described in detail in Chapter 13.

PERCUSSION

Percussion is the tapping of the body's surface to produce vibration and sound. The sounds indicate the density of the underlying tissue and thus detect the location of body organs and structures. For example, percussion over a hollow organ such as the stomach produces a high-pitched, drumlike sound called *tympany*, whereas percussion over a dense organ such as the liver produces a low-pitched, thudlike sound called *dullness*. The technique of percussion requires the examiner to place the palmar surface of one hand against the client's body while tapping with the other.

AUSCULTATION.

Auscultation is the process of listening to sounds produced by the body. Three systems produce sounds for the examiner to auscultate, including the cardiovascular system, the respiratory system, and the gastrointestinal system. For auscultation of these systems the nurse uses a stethoscope, an instrument that amplifies sounds produced by internal organs.

Order of Examination

The physical examination is carried out in a systematic manner similar to the review of systems (see Chapter 13). This component of the assessment usually begins with data on the client's height, weight, and vital signs.

Next the examiner writes a general statement about perceptions of the client and the client's level of health. This statement, usually called the *general survey*, includes information about mental status, body development, nutritional status, sex and race, chronological versus apparent age, appearance, and speech.

Last is a head-to-toe examination of the body systems. The examiner records objective data obtained during the examination, using clear, concise, and appropriate language in describing each system examined.

Laboratory Data

The final source of assessment data is the results of laboratory tests. Laboratory data verify alterations identified in the nursing health history and physical examination. The data are baseline information about the client's response to illness and information about the effects of later treatment measures.

Laboratory data are compared with the established norms for a particular test, age group, and sex. The nurse identifies variations from the normal and interprets the findings according to the disease process and treatments. In addition, laboratory data can be used to evaluate the success or failure of nursing, as well as medical, interventions.

Laboratory tests are selected according to the symptoms or disease. However, common laboratory tests may be used for a large number of clients (see box). Specific laboratory tests and the nursing responsibilities associated with them are detailed in Unit 7.

Laboratory data are one more source of information the nurse uses in completing a data base. In addition to verifying abnormal findings noted in the history and examination, laboratory data can identify actual or potential health care problems not previously noted by the client or examiner.

Common Laboratory and Diagnostic Tests

BLOOD

- Complete blood count (CBC)
- Electrolytes—SMA_6, SMA_{12}
- Arterial blood gases (ABGs)
- Fasting blood sugar (FBS)
- Glucose tolerance test (GTT)

URINE

- Urinalysis (UA)
- Urine culture and sensitivity

RADIOLOGICAL EXAMINATIONS

- Chest roentgenogram (CXR)
- Upper gastrointestinal (UGI)
- Lower gastrointestinal (LGI)
- Scans: body, head, chest, bone

STOOL

- Guaiac
- Ova and parasites

SPUTUM

- Culture and sensitivity
- Acid-fast bacilli (AFB)
- Cytology

SUMMARY

Nursing assessment is the gathering and verifying of data about a client to establish a data base. The nursing health history, physical examination, and collection of laboratory data are all components of the nursing assessment. To complete the assessment phase, the nurse implements proper interview techniques, is systematic, and correctly inspects, palpates, percusses, and auscultates the client's body systems.

The professionalism, competency, and organization of the nurse promote an environment in which the client is able to share appropriate, pertinent data about previous levels of wellness, health practices, past illness, and health care goals. The data gathered enable the nurse to draw conclusions about the client's needs and to plan individualized care.

KEY CONCEPTS

✓ Assessment is the gathering, verification, and communication of data about a client by means of interview, nursing health history, physical examination, and laboratory and diagnostic tests.

✓ Written data statements should be descriptive, concise, and complete and should not include interpretative statements.

✓ Collection of inaccurate, incomplete, or inappropriate data may result in incorrect identification of the client's health care needs.

✓ Objective data are observations or measurements by the data collector.

✓ Subjective data are the client's or family's perceptions.

✓ The client is the principal source of data.

✓ Families or significant others can be a primary source of information about the client's health status.

✓ Every member of the health care team is a potential source of information.

✓ Other data sources include the health record, other records, and pertinent literature.

✓ Review of the pertinent literature increases the nurse's knowledge about the symptoms, treatment, and prognosis of specific illnesses.

✓ The interview is the mechanism for obtaining the nursing health history.

✓ The interviewer identifies the client's needs and risk factors, as well as specific changes in the client's level of wellness and pattern of living.

✓ Use of effective communication skills enables the nurse to initiate the nurse-client relationship and complete the interview.

✓ The interview comprises three phases: orientation, working, and termination.

✓ During the interview process, the following information is obtained about the dimensions of the client: physical, developmental, intellectual, emotional, social, and spiritual.

✓ The nursing process is a method for organizing and delivering nursing care.

✓ The purpose of the nursing process if to identify the client's health care needs, establish a nursing care plan, and complete nursing interventions designed to meet the needs of the client.

✓ Organization of the nursing process is based on five components, including assessment, nursing diagnosis, planning, implementation, and evaluation.

✓ The interview allows the nurse to observe the client and any interaction between the client and family.

✓ The four primary interview techniques include problem solving, problem seeking, direct question, and open-ended question.

✓ The nursing health history obtains data from the client and family about the level of wellness, past medical history, family history, environmental history, psychosocial and cultural history, and a review of the body systems.

✓ Physical examination requires the skills of inspection, palpation, auscultation, and percussion.

✓ Laboratory and diagnostic tests add to the data base and verify data gathered through the nursing health history and physical examination.

REFERENCES

Bevis, EM: Curriculum building in nursing: a process, St. Louis, 1978, The C.V. Mosby Co.

Enelow, AJ, and Swisher, SN: Interviewing and patient care, ed. 2, New York, 1979, Oxford University Press, Inc.

Gordon, M: Nursing diagnosis process and application, ed. 2, New York, 1987, McGraw-Hill Book Co.

Hall, LE: Quality of nuring care. Address given at the Department of Baccalaureate and Higher Degree programs of the New Jersey League for Nursing, Public Health News, New Jersey Department of Health, 1955.

Hall, LE: A center for nursing, Nurs Outlook 11:805, 1963.

Knowles, L: Decision making in nursing: a necessity for doing, 1966 ANA clinical sessions, New York, 1967, Appleton-Century-Crofts.

Perry, AG: Analysis of the components of the nursing process. In Carlson, JH, Craft, CA, and McGuire, AD, editors: Nursing diagnosis, Philadelphia, 1982, W.B. Saunders Co.

Yarnall, S, and Atwood, J: Problem-oriented practice for nurses and physicians, Nurs Clin North Am 9:215, 1974.

Yura, H, and Walsh, M: The nursing process: assessing, planning, implementing, and evaluation, ed. 4, New York, 1983, Appleton-Century-Crofts.

ADDITIONAL READINGS

Alexander, MM, and Brown, MS: The why and how of examination. I. Physical examination, Nurs 73 3:25, 1973.

Alexander, MM, and Brown, MS: The why and how of examination. II. History taking, Nurs 73 3:35, 1973.

Bellack, JP, and Bamford, DA: Nursing assessment: a multidimensional approach, 1984, Belmont, Calif., Wadsworth, Inc.

Bermost, LS: Interviewing: a key to therapeutic communication in nursing practice, Nurs Clin North Am 1:205, 1966.

Bowers, AC, and Thompson, JM: Clinical manual of health assessment, ed. 2, St. Louis, 1984, The C.V. Mosby Co.

Edelman, C, and Mandle, CC: Health promotion throughout the lifespan, St. Louis, 1986, The C.V. Mosby Co.

Eggland, ET: How to take a meaningful nursing history, Nurs 77 7:22, 1977.

Fields, WL, and McGinn-Campbell, KM: Introduction to health assessment, Reston, Va. 1983, Reston Publishing Co., Inc.

Jones, DA: Health assessment manual, New York, 1984, McGraw-Hill Book Co.

Jones, DA, Lepley, MK, and Baker, BA: Health assessment across the life span, New York, 1984, McGraw-Hill Book Co.

Kesler, AR: Pitfalls to avoid in interviewing outpatients, Nurs 77 7:70, 1977.

Malasanos, L, et al.: Health assessment, ed. 3, St. Louis, 1986, The C.V. Mosby Co.

Marriner, A: The nursing process: a scientific approach to nursing care, ed. 4, St. Louis, 1987, The C.V. Mosby Co.

McCain, RF: Nursing by assessment, not intuition, Am J Nurs 65:82, 1965.

Mengel, A: Getting the most from patient interviews, Nurs 82, 12(11):46, 1982.

Norris, L: Coaching the question, Nurs 86, 16(5):100, 1986.

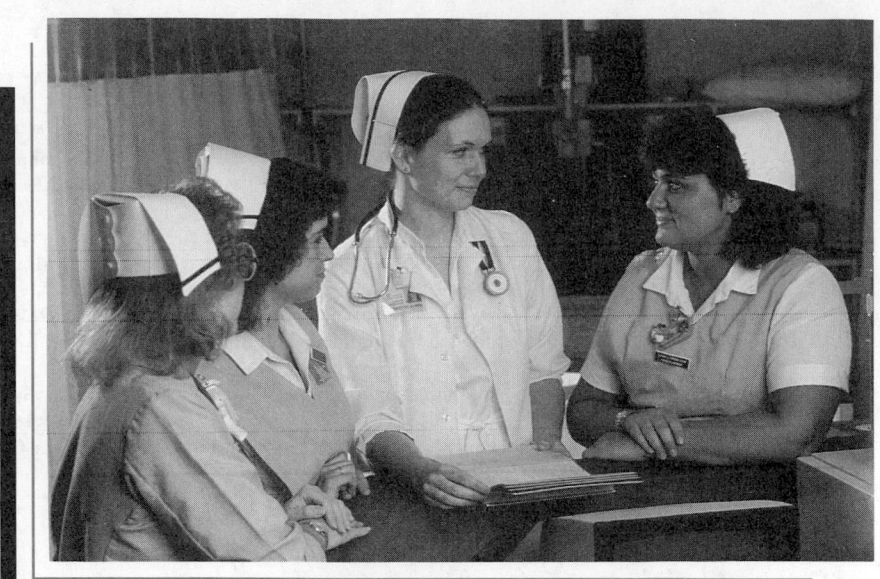

OBJECTIVES

Mastery of content in this chapter will enable the student to:

- Define the key terms listed.
- Describe the way defining characteristics and the etiological process individualizes a nursing diagnosis.
- List and discuss the steps of the nursing diagnostic process.
- Demonstrate the nursing diagnostic process.
- Differentiate between a nursing diagnosis and a medical diagnosis.
- Explain what makes a nursing diagnosis correct.
- Discuss the advantages of nursing diagnoses for the client.
- Discuss the advantages of nursing diagnoses for the profession of nursing.
- Discuss the limitations of nursing diagnoses.
- Formulate nursing diagnoses from a nursing assessment.

KEY TERMS

Actual Health Care Problem
Clinical Reasoning
Data Clustering
Data Validation
Diagnosis
Diagnostic Process
Discharge Planning
Error of Commission
Error of Omission
Etiological Factor
Health Care Need
Medical Diagnosis
Nursing Diagnosis
Peer Review
Potential Health Care Problem
Quality Assurance

Nursing Diagnosis

After completing the nursing assessment the nurse proceeds to the nursing diagnosis, a statement of the potential or actual problem in the client's health status that the nurse is licensed and competent to treat. The overall purpose of the nursing diagnosis is to analyze assessment data and identify health problems involving the client, family, and significant others.

The statement of a nursing diagnosis is the culmination of a diagnostic process during which the nurse analyzes assessment data to determine the client's health problems. The problems are then stated as a nursing diagnosis.

Nursing diagnoses are developed for a client, family, or community, taking into account the physical, developmental, intellectual, emotional, social, and spiritual dimensions of the person or persons being assessed.

NURSING DIAGNOSTIC PROCESS

The diagnostic process includes the following elements: analysis and interpretation of data, identification of problems, and formulation of nursing diagnoses (Fig. 7-1). Analysis and interpretation of data require data validation and clustering. Through data validation the nurse determines whether the information gathered during assessment is complete and accurate. It is important for the nurse to do this early in the diagnostic process, since the formulation of correct, appropriate nursing diagnoses depends on accurate data collection. The nurse uses data clustering to group related data or defining characteristics from the nursing health history,

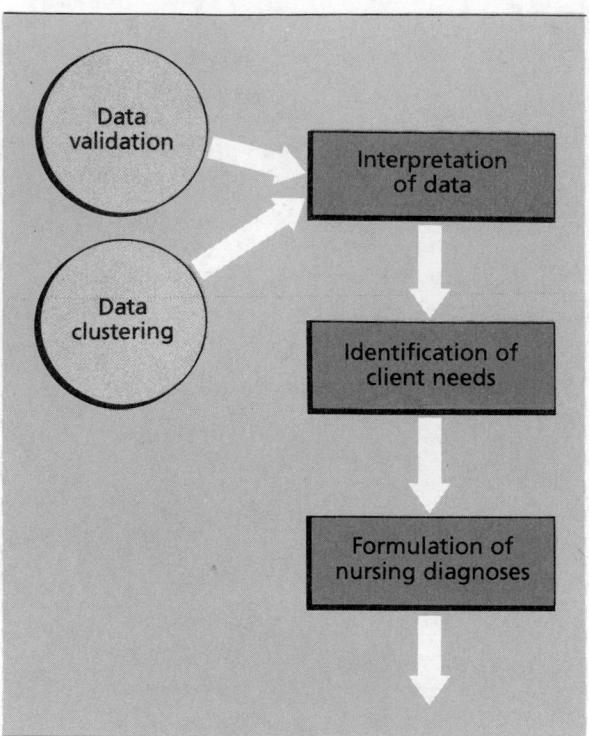

Fig. 7-1 Nursing diagnostic process.

physical examination, and laboratory findings, forming a picture of the client health needs. The statement of the client's needs then describes the general health care problem, after which the nurse formulates a statement of the client's actual or potential specific health problems, written as nursing diagnoses.

Analysis and Interpretation of Data

As the nurse examines assessment data, information about the client's health status is validated. Validation involves determining the relationship between data and health needs and confirming their accuracy. Data obtained during assessment are valid if they relate to the area being examined. For example, data collected about eating habits, nausea, vomiting, diarrhea, weight, height, muscle mass, adipose tissue, serum albumin, and hemoglobin are valid for assessment of nutritional status. However, these data would not be valid for assessment of the ability to complete activities of daily living.

The nurse continually revises the data base to include changes in the client's physical and emotional status, as well as the results of laboratory and diagnostic tests. Many sources are used to support data, including the client, family, health care team members, and the medical record. The nurse supports data through several methods. The nurse can verify data obtained from another source of information. For example, if a family member of a client who is an outpatient says the client is unable to leave home due to increased fatigue, the nurse can support this information by asking the client about activity patterns. The nurse also verifies data obtained during the nursing history by physical examination. For example, if a client says she has a lump in her left breast, the nurse can verify the presence of the lump by physical examination. The nurse can validate physical examination findings by reexamining the client later or requesting a colleague to verify the data by physical examination. For example, a client with pulmonary disease may have a slight inspiratory wheeze auscultated during the physical examination. The nurse later reevaluates the lung to determine if the wheeze is still present. In addition, the nurse validates data obtained with the history or physical examination by the results of laboratory or diagnostic tests. For example, during the history the client complains about increased fatigue and during physical examination the nurse notes that the client's pulse is 108 and the blood pressure is 110/60. The nurse knows that fatigue, a rapid pulse, and a lowered blood pressure are signs of anemia. Laboratory results reveal the client's hemoglobin level is 9.6 g, consistent with anemia. While validating existing data, the nurse also verifies that findings in the physical examination are based on fact rather than intuition.

Data clustering is the process used to group related information. These data are usually signs and symptoms indicating a general problem. The nurse clusters data as they relate to mental or emotional status, to individual body systems, to risk factors, to family data, or to community factors. This clustering identifies related changes in the client's needs and ultimately leads to the formulation of a nursing diagnosis.

During assessment the nurse gathers a large amount of data that at first may appear irrelevant and unrelated. However, as data are clustered, a pattern begins to emerge. The nurse begins clustering once the information is obtained and continues throughout the nursing diagnostic process.

When the nurse clusters data, the result is a grouping of signs and symptoms, or defining characteristics (Carpenito, 1983). The presence of one sign or symptom does not support the nursing diagnostic label. Instead, the clustering of multiple defining characteristics supports the diagnosis. Absence of these characteristics suggests that the diagnosis should be rejected. Diagnostic categories and their defining characteristics provide structure for the cognitive process in the identification of client need and actual formulation of the nursing diagnoses (Hurley, 1986).

The clustering process is perhaps best demonstrated through an example showing the way certain characteristics relate to a concept. For example, gray hair does not necessarily indicate that a person is an older adult.

TABLE 7-1 Comparison of Interventions for Nursing Diagnoses with Different Etiologies

Nursing Diagnoses	Interventions
CLIENT A	
Ineffective airway clearance related to obesity	Place in high fowler's position.
	Cough and deep breathe every 2 hours while awake.
	Start weight reduction diet (1200 calories) to decrease obesity.
Self-care deficit in feeding related to bilateral arm casts	Encourage family to visit during meals.
	Be certain staff or family members are available to feed client.
	Provide high-calorie milkshakes with straw at 3 PM and 8 PM.
Social isolation related to protective isolation for wound infection	Plan staffing patterns to include visits to client's room four times a day.
	Relax visiting hours for client's family.
CLIENT B	
Ineffective airway clearance related to poor coughing	Teach client deep breathing and coughing.
	Splint client's abdominal incision during coughing.
Self-care deficit in feeding related to inability to grasp feeding utensils	Provide large-handled eating utensils.
	Offer finger foods cut in large pieces for between-meal snacks: 10-2-8.
Social isolation related to recent move into neighborhood	Provide client with phone numbers and location of local senior citizens' center.
	Draw client a map of neighborhood stores, restaurants, libraries.

However, if gray hair is clustered with wrinkled skin, age spots, and slowed gait, then these characteristics probably indicate that the person is an older adult.

Identification of Client Problems

Before formulating the nursing diagnosis the nurse identifies the client's general health care needs. It may help the beginning nurse to think of the identification of client needs as the general health care problem and the formulation of the nursing diagnosis as the specific health care problem. Thus the nurse, in describing health care problems, moves from general to specific. After the general health care problem has been identified, the assessment data are refined to support a nursing diagnosis.

To identify the client's need, the nurse first determines what the client's health problems are and whether they are actual or potential problems. An actual health problem is one that is perceived or experienced by the client, such as a sleep pattern disturbance caused by a noisy environment. A potential health problem is one for which the client is at risk, such as an overweight smoker at risk for ineffective airway clearance related to incisional pain.

When identifying client needs, the nurse considers all assessment data and focuses on pertinent and abnormal findings. The nurse groups, or clusters, related findings to identify actual or potential health problems.

The problem-identification step brings the nurse closer to forming a nursing diagnosis and making general analyses of the clustered data, thus assisting her in making a nursing diagnosis.

Formulation of Nursing Diagnoses

Formulation of the nursing diagnosis is based on identification of client needs. The diagnostic statement should include the problem (for example, knowledge deficit) and its etiology (for example, related to unfamiliarity with diagnostic procedure). The problem is the actual or potential client, and the etiology is that which will be affected by nursing interventions.

The etiology identifies the cause of the problem. It may be a direct or contributing factor in the development of the client need and subsequent nursing diagnosis. The etiology is represented in the nursing diagnostic statement by the phrase *related to*. In some cases the etiological label is used as an explanatory concept to explain the reason the nursing diagnosis exists (for example, ineffective airway clearance related to obesity). Inclusion of the etiology individualizes the nursing diagnosis and subsequent interventions (Table 7-1).

Etiological factors are difficult to validate. In some settings, medical diagnoses are recorded as the etiology of the nursing diagnosis. This is incorrect. Nursing interventions cannot change the medical diagnosis. However, nursing interventions can be directed toward etiological factors, as well as toward the diagnostic label.

For example, the nursing diagnosis, "alteration in comfort related to mastectomy," is incorrect. Nursing actions cannot affect the medical diagnosis of mastectomy. Rewording the diagnosis to read, "alteration in comfort related to incisional pain" results in nursing interventions directed toward improving comfort and pain control.

As the client's needs change, nursing diagnoses are modified. For example, a client's pertinent assessment data included decreased dietary fiber and limited fluid intake, no bowel movement for 3 days, presence of bowel sounds, distention of the lower abdomen, hard fecal material extracted during digital rectal examination, and guaiac-negative stool specimen. The nursing diagnosis was "impairment of bowel elimination: constipation related to limited fiber intake." After appropriate nursing interventions, the constipation was resolved, and the nursing diagnosis was modified to read "potential impairment of bowel elimination: constipation related to limited fiber intake." Once the health problem has been resolved, the nursing diagnosis for that problem is no longer relevant. In addition, as the client's physiological and emotional status changes, the health problem may remain relevant, but the cause may change. Therefore the nursing diagnosis must be restated. New nursing diagnoses are developed as the client's needs and status change.

The modification of nursing diagnoses is ongoing. As the level of nursing care and level of wellness change, these changes are reflected in the statement of nursing diagnoses. Outdated nursing diagnoses do not accurately reflect the client's current needs and result in a lower quality of nursing care.

The box contains a summary of the pertinent assessment data that may lead to the identification of an actual or potential health care problem. Table 7-2 demonstrates data clustering, identification of client need, and formulation of nursing diagnoses in the analysis process for select nursing diagnoses.

Table 7-3 uses the three nursing diagnoses, "potential ineffective airway clearance, potential disturbance in self-concept, and potential ineffective coping," to demonstrate the way the defining characteristics and probable etiologies assist in the development of the total diagnostic label. The defining characteristics and relevant etiologies are from the North American Nursing Diagnosis Association (NANDA) classification (Hurley, 1986). A complete list of the current NANDA classification of nursing diagnostic labels is on p. 130.

Summary of Relevant Assessment Data

PHYSICAL AND DEVELOPMENTAL

- Diarrhea for 3 weeks
- Productive cough on rising each morning
- 15-pound weight loss 2 weeks before hospitalization
- Hemoglobin 10 g
- Slight change of emphysema shown on chest roentgenogram
- Crackles in bilateral lung bases
- Distended abdomen
- Squamous cell cancer
- Smoked for 20 years, 2 packs a day (40 pack-years)
- Family history of stomach cancer
- Family history of heart attack
- Married for 40 years
- Self-employed for 20 years
- One adult son, 35 years old
- Two sisters, 50 and 48, with no major health problems
- Temporary colostomy
- Abdominal incision

INTELLECTUAL

- Talkative
- Frequently asks nurses if he has cancer
- Good attention span

EMOTIONAL

- Anxious
- Withdrawn after biopsy report of squamous cell cancer
- Avoids viewing abdomen

SOCIAL

- Plays tennis three times a week
- Active in his neighborhood

SPIRITUAL

- Methodist
- Attends church weekly
- Reads Bible daily

NURSING DIAGNOSIS

Nursing Diagnosis and Medical Diagnosis

Until recent years the term *diagnosis* was almost exclusive to the medical profession. A medical diagnosis is the identification of a disease condition based on a specific evaluation of physical signs, symptoms, history, laboratory tests, and procedures. Physicians are licensed to treat these diseases or pathological processes by performing surgery, prescribing medication, and ordering specific invasive and noninvasive therapies. During the

TABLE 7-2 Formulation of Nursing Diagnoses

Clustering Data	Identification of Client Need	Nursing Diagnosis Formulation
Diarrhea for 3 weeks Distended abdomen Family history of stomach cancer	Alteration in elimination patterns	Diarrhea related to unknown cause
Weight loss: 15 pounds total Diarrhea Anemia, hemogloin level 10 g	Excessive weight loss	Altered nutrition: potential for less than body requirements related to chronic diarrhea for 3 weeks
40 pack/year history of smoking Slight change of emphysema shown on chest roentgenogram Crackles auscultated in lung fields	At risk for postoperative respiratory complications	Potential ineffective airway clearance post-operatively related to incisional pain
Temporary colostomy Abdominal incision Avoids viewing abdomen	Change in body image	Potential disturbance in self-concept related to change in body image
Verbalizes fear of stomach cancer Becomes withdrawn after biopsy report	Changes in interpersonal interactions	Potential ineffective coping related to unknown prognosis

TABLE 7-3 Defining Characteristics and Etiologies to Support Nursing Diagnoses

Defining Characteristics	Nursing Diagnoses	Etiologies "Related to"
Abnormal breath sounds Changes in rate or depth of respiration Cough Cyanosis Dyspnea Smoking history	Actual or potential ineffective airway clearance	• Decreased energy/fatigue • Tracheobronchial infection, obstruction, secretion • Pain
Verbal or nonverbal response to actual or perceived change in structure of function Missing or impaired body part, not looking or touching body or body part Trauma to body Refusal to acknowledge change	Actual or potential disturbance in self-concept	• Biophysical (e.g., amputation or loss of function of extremity) • Cognitive/perceptual (e.g., expressions of worthlessness, sorrow) • Psychosocial (e.g., withdrawal behavior, excessive crying)
Verbalization of inability to cope Inability to meet role expectations Inability to problem solve Inability to meet basic needs Alteration in societal participation Destructive behavior Inappropriate use of defense mechanisms Verbal manipulation Change in usual communication patterns High rate of illness High rate of accidents	Actual or potential ineffective coping	• Situational crises (e.g., unexpected illness, financial difficulties) • Maturational crises (e.g., marriage, parenthood)

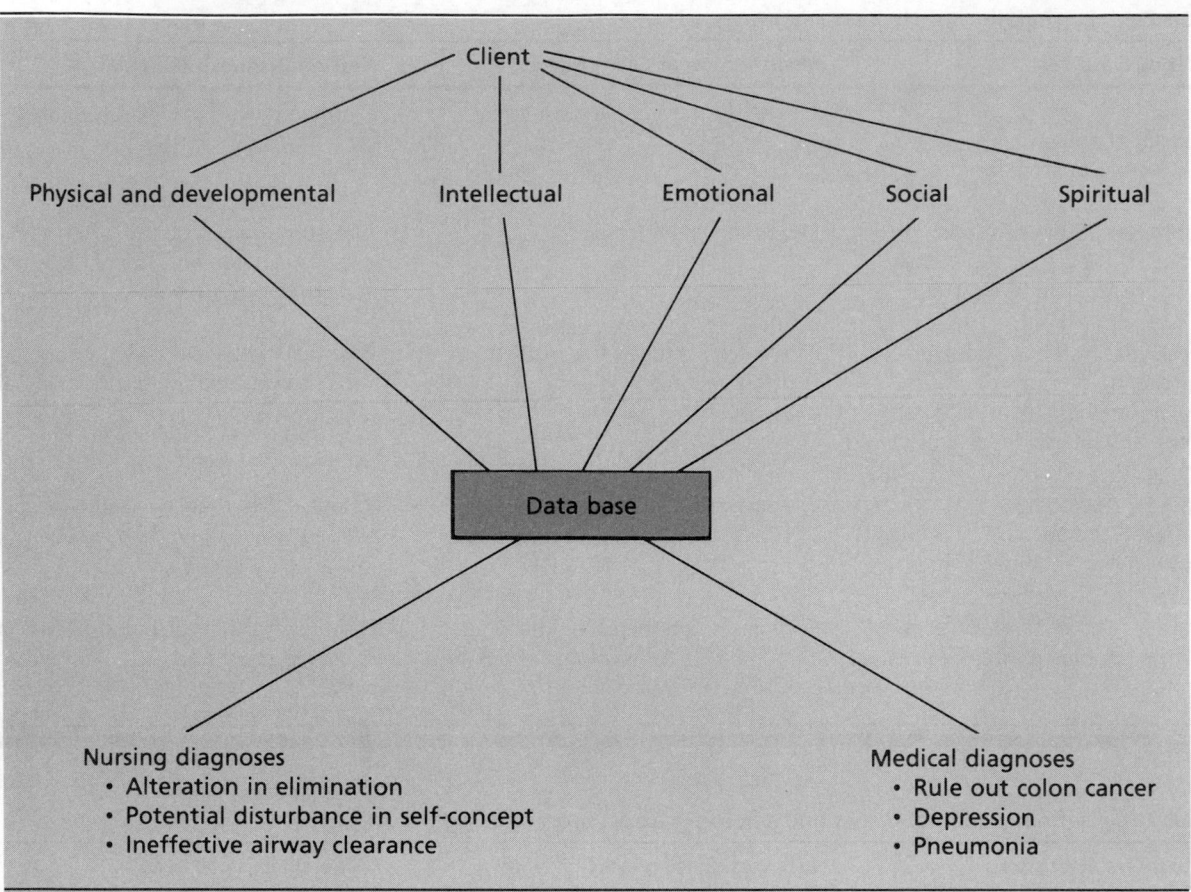

Fig. 7-2 Comparison of nursing and medical diagnoses using the same data base.

last two decades, however, the term *nursing diagnosis* has appeared more frequently in the literature. A nursing diagnosis is a statement of a potential or actual health problem that the nurse is licensed and competent to treat. It reflects the client's level of health or response to a disease or pathological process. Both medical and nursing diagnoses are derived from the physiological, psychological, sociocultural, developmental, and spiritual dimensions of the client (Fig. 7-2). In some institutions physicians and nurses use the same data base to formulate diagnoses.

The goals and objectives of a nursing diagnosis differ from those of a medical diagnosis. The goal of a nursing diagnosis is to identify actual and potential health problems of the client; the goals of a medical diagnosis are to identify and, in some cases, cure the disease or the pathological process. The objective of a nursing diagnosis is to develop a plan of care so the client and family are able to adapt to changes resulting from health problems. The objectives of the medical diagnosis are to prescribe treatment. Thus the focus of a medical diagnosis is to identify and treat a disease or pathological process, whereas the nursing diagnosis focuses on helping the

client reach a maximal level of wellness. A medical diagnosis of appendicitis, for example, requires the physician to remove the infected appendix. After the appendectomy the client may have a nursing diagnosis of impaired mobility related to surgical incision. The nursing care would be directed toward gradually increasing the client's mobility to preoperative levels.

Advantages of Nursing Diagnoses

The nursing diagnosis is advantageous for both nurses and clients. It facilitates communication among nurses about a client's level of wellness and discharge planning. The health care delivery system today requires greater numbers of health care professionals. As more people become responsible for the care of a single client, it is essential that these professionals be able to clearly communicate with one another about clients' problems. Nursing diagnoses facilitate communication in several ways. The initial list of nursing diagnoses is an easily obtainable reference to the client's current health care needs. Nursing diagnoses also encourage the nurse to develop organizational skills, since they help to prioritize the client's needs. As the nurse communicates with other professionals, the use of the nursing diagnoses encourages organized communication relevant to the client's goals and priorities. Nursing diagnoses are also used for charting in the nurse's notes, writing referrals, and providing effective transition of care from one unit to another, from one clinic to another, or from the hospital to the community setting. Discharge planning is the set of decisions and activities involved in giving continuity and coordination to nursing care (McKeehan, 1979). Discharge planning is necessary when a client is discharged from one hospital to another or from the hospital to the community. In discharge planning, nursing diagnoses are the mechanism for communicating and delineating care the client still requires.

Nursing diagnoses can also serve as focuses for quality assurance and peer review. Quality assurance is the monitoring and evaluation of the quality and appropriateness of patient care compared to accepted standards. In nursing, peer review is an appraisal by professional co-workers of equal status of the way a nurse conducts practice, education, or research. Both quality assurance and peer review use accepted standards as measures against which performance is weighed. The nursing diagnosis is a method of identifying the focus of nursing activity. In focusing on the nursing diagnosis, the reviewer can determine whether nursing care was correct and delivered according to standards of practice.

The benefits of nursing diagnosis for the profession are also important for the client and the family. Better communication among health care professionals helps eliminate potential problems in giving care and maintains a focus on meeting the client's health care goals. Similarly, the ultimate reason for quality assurance and peer review is to ensure that high-quality care is given to clients and families. Furthermore, the client benefits from the individualization of nursing care resulting from appropriate goal setting, correct selection of priorities, selection of appropriate interventions, and establishment of outcome criteria.

Limitations of Nursing Diagnoses

Nursing diagnoses have limitations, and the beginning practitioner should be aware of their existence. Because of the continuous evolution of the term and use of nursing diagnoses, the language can occasionally be verbose and contain jargon. This may limit use of nursing diagnoses to only nursing professionals and result in confusion among other members of the health care team (Shamansky and Yanni, 1985).

Imprecise language of the diagnostic statement may incorrectly "label" a client. One such diagnostic label is "noncompliance." The term is value ladened and incomplete (Edel, 1985; Stantis and Ryan, 1982). In addition, the evolving process of standardized terminology in the form of a taxonomy has resulted in confusion about the language of the diagnostic statement (Lunney, 1986; Porter, 1986). The 1986 National Conference for the Classification of Nursing Diagnosis proposed a taxonomic structure for an organizational framework of current and future diagnostic labels (McLane, 1987).

Nursing diagnoses are problem oriented and have limited focus on health promotion and health maintenance activities and needs (Martens, 1986; Gleit and Tatro 1981; Popkess, 1981). Because a client's state of health is viewed along a continuum, the strengths or positives related to health care should also be assessed and diagnosed. A positive nursing diagnosis exists when it has been established that the client has resources from which he can draw emotional or physical energy or an established life-style that fosters wellness (Martens, 1986).

Controversy exists in nursing literature and practice about whether physiological diagnoses are within the domain of nursing practice (Jacoby, 1985). Some believe the nurse does not possess the skills or the license to diagnose and intervene with certain diagnostic labels. Gordon (1982) proposes that physiological dysfunctions are medical diagnoses. Physicians focus on the functioning of the physical systems and diagnose organic pathological conditions. Nurses, however, focus on health patterns.

Kim (1984) proposes that pathophysiological nursing diagnoses are a legitimate part of the classification system. She argues that when a truly interdependent role of the nurse exists, diagnoses require collaborative and interdependent nursing interventions (see Chapter 9). Shoemaker (1984) notes that diagnosis is clinical judgment derived through a deliberate, systematic process of data collection and analysis and provides the basis for prescribing definitive therapy for which the nurse is accountable. A nurse must function interdependently in many settings, inside and outside the hospital, to diagnose and treat physiological conditions.

The incomplete taxonomy limits nursing practice. Nursing diagnoses, developed by the Task Force of the National Group for the Classification of Nursing Diagnoses, are only the beginning of a total classification system (see box). Through formulation and use of other nursing diagnoses, the taxonomy will grow and expand the focus of professional nursing.

SOURCES OF ERROR

The diagnostic process has potential for errors. An error is identifying a client need incorrectly or not at all, or identifying a need important to the nurse and not the client. Errors in the diagnostic process result in the de-

NANDA-Approved Nursing Diagnoses

Activity intolerance
Altered family processes
Altered growth and development
Altered health maintenance
Altered nutrition: less than body requirements
Altered nutrition: more than body requirements
Altered nutrition: potential for more than body requirements
Altered oral mucous membrane
Altered parenting
Altered patterns of urinary elimination
Altered role performance
Altered sexuality patterns
Altered thought processes
Altered (specify type) tissue perfusion, (cerebral, cardiopulmonary, renal, gastrointestinal, peripheral)
Anticipatory grieving
Anxiety
Bathing/hygiene self-care deficit
Body-image disturbance
Bowel incontinence
Chronic low self-esteem*
Chronic pain
Colonic constipation*
Constipation
Decisional conflict (specify)*
Decreased cardiac output
Defensive coping*
Diarrhea
Dressing/grooming self-care deficit
Dysfunctional grieving
Dysreflexia*
Family coping: potential for growth
Fatigue*
Fear
Feeding self-care deficit
Fluid volume deficit (1)
Fluid volume deficit (2)
Fluid volume excess
Functional incontinence
Health seeking behaviors (specify) or desire for high-level wellness (specify)*
Hopelessness
Hyperthermia
Hypothermia
Impaired adjustment
Impaired gas exchange
Impaired home maintenance management
Impaired physical mobility
Impaired skin integrity

Impaired social interaction
Impaired swallowing
Impaired tissue integrity
Impaired verbal communication
Ineffective airway clearance
Ineffective breastfeeding*
Ineffective breathing pattern
Ineffective denial*
Ineffective family coping: compromised
Ineffective family coping: disabled
Ineffective individual coping
Ineffective thermoregulation
Knowledge deficit (specify)
Noncompliance (specify)
Pain
Parental role conflict*
Perceived constipation*
Personal identity disturbance
Post-trauma response
Potential activity intolerance
Potential altered body temperature
Potential fluid volume deficit
Potential for aspiration*
Potential for disuse syndrome*
Potential for infection
Potential for injury
Potential for poisoning
Potential for suffocating
Potential for trauma
Potential for violence: self-directed or directed at others
Potential impaired skin integrity
Powerlessness
Rape-trauma syndrome
Rape-trauma syndrome: compound reaction
Rape-trauma syndrome: silent reaction
Reflex incontinence
Self-esteem disturbance*
Sensory/perceptual alterations (specify) (auditory, gustatory, kinesthetic, olfactory, tactile, visual)
Sexual dysfunction
Situational low self-esteem*
Sleep pattern disturbance
Social isolation
Spiritual distress (distress of the human spirit)
Stress incontinence
Toileting self-care deficit
Total incontinence
Unilateral neglect
Urge incontinence
Urinary retention

*Diagnosis accepted in 1988.

velopment of an incomplete or inappropriate nursing care plan.

Gordon (1982) groups errors into the following categories: errors of omission and errors of commission. An error of omission occurs when the nurse fails to identify a health care problem, which can occur when incomplete data are collected from the client, when data are clustered incorrectly in the analysis process, or when data are interpreted improperly. Errors of commission occur from overdiagnosis or diagnosing nonexistent health care problems. For example, a client who enters a hospital for a diagnostic test may be prematurely diagnosed as having "knowledge deficit related to unfamiliarity with procedure." However, on further assessment the nurse may learn that the client has undergone the test before and has no questions about its implications.

Although these errors occur during any step of the diagnostic process, they often originate in the nursing assessment. When collecting data, the interviewer can fail to use the problem-solving interview technique. As Chapter 6 explains, the interviewer asks specific questions focused on a particular problem in the problem-solving technique. For example, when a client reports abdominal pain, the nurse uses the problem-solving technique to determine its location, intensity, duration, precipitating causes, and relief factors. It may be possible to identify a problem without this method, but important information and potential solutions remain unde-

tected because incomplete, inaccurate, or irrelevant data have been collected. While analyzing the client's response to actual or potential health care problems, the nurse relies on verbal and nonverbal communication patterns. The alert nurse changes interview techniques to obtain the most complete, accurate, and relevant data base.

Errors in data clustering can lead to errors of commission because data are clustered prematurely, incorrectly, or not at all (Gordon, 1982). Premature closure of clustering occurs when the nurse makes the nursing diagnosis before all data have been grouped. For example, when a client with a cast on the right arm is assessed, data concerning the immobilized arm are clustered, but relevant information on the client's perception of being able to carry out activities of daily living are not included. Because the similar data are not grouped, the nurse develops an incorrect nursing diagnosis. Incorrect clustering occurs when the nurse tries to make the nursing diagnosis fit the signs and symptoms obtained in data collection. For example, a nurse has assessed a client with a medical diagnosis of an acute myocardial infarction. The nurse knows that chest pain occurs with a myocardial infarction, and thus concludes "pain related to myocardial ischemia" is a relevant nursing diagnosis. However, the nurse did not validate the presence of pain with the client, who actually has none. The nurse implemented pain-reducing activities based on the incorrect diagnosis. The nursing diagnosis should

TABLE 7-4   Examples of Errors in Formulating the Nursing Diagnostic Statement

Correct Statement	Stated as a Medical Diagnosis	Stated in Medical Terminolgy	Stated as a Nursing Intervention
Diarrhea related to unknown cause	Diarrhea	Alteration in bowel elimination related to lesion in descending colon	Offer bedpan frequently because of alteration in elimination.
Altered nutrition: potential for less than body requirements related to chronic diarrhea for 3 weeks	Potential malnutrition	Potential alteration in nutrition: less than body requirements owing to malnutrition	Client needs high-protein diet owing to potential alteration in nutrition.
Potential ineffective airway clearance postoperatively related to abdominal incisional pain	Potential pneumonia	Potential ineffective airway clearance owing to emphysema	Cough frequently because of ineffective airway clearance.
Potential disturbance in self-concept related to change in body image	Avoidance reaction to colostomy	Potential disturbance in self-concept owing to colostomy	Client needs to be encouraged to interact with others.
Potential ineffective coping related to terminal prognosis	Fear of cancer	Potential ineffective coping owing to squamous cell cancer	Client needs to verbalize fear.

be derived from the data, not the other way around. An incorrect nursing diagnosis affects quality of care.

Another type of error can occur in the manner in which the nursing diagnosis is stated. Although the nursing diagnosis should be stated in the format designated by a particular school or agency, some common guidelines will reduce errors in the diagnostic statement itself. The statement should be worded in appropriate, concise, and precise language, which involves using correct terminology reflecting the *nursing* needs of the client. Concise wording ensures that the nursing need can be easily communicated intraprofessionally and interprofessionally. The diagnostic statement should also be precise, identifying unique nursing needs, and should be stated in the problem-cause format. A diagnostic statement such as "unhappy and worried about health" can lead to errors. The language needs to be more precise and appropriate, such as "potential ineffective coping related to fear of medical diagnosis of cancer."

There are three other potential sources of error in writing the diagnostic statement, including nursing diagnoses stated as medical diagnoses, use of medical terminology to describe the cause, and statement of the nursing diagnosis as an intervention. These are errors because they shift the focus of the statement from nursing to medicine or shift the focus from the cause to the intervention. Table 7-4 states the correct nursing diagnoses formulated from Mr. Brown's assessment data from the previous chapter and compares them with the three errors of medical diagnosis, medical terminology, and nursing intervention.

As expertise with the diagnostic process is gained, the likelihood of errors is reduced, and the nurse is able to develop the nursing diagnoses based on the actual or potential nursing needs of the client.

SUMMARY

The analysis of data obtained during nursing assessment results in the formulation of nursing diagnoses. Nursing diagnoses are developed through a process in which data are validated and clustered, the client's needs are identified, and the specific nursing diagnoses are formulated. The stated nursing diagnoses reflect the client's individual needs and response to a disease or pathological process.

Formulation of the nursing diagnosis is a cognitive activity focusing on the client's health care needs and expectations. The formulation of nursing diagnoses enables the nurse and client to determine client goals, priorities, and projected outcomes of nursing care in the planning component of the nursing process.

KEY CONCEPTS

✓ The statement of nursing diagnoses is the result of the diagnostic process.

✓ The diagnostic process includes analysis and interpretation of data, identification of client problems, and formulation of nursing diagnoses.

✓ The interpretation of data requires the nurse to validate and cluster data.

✓ Nursing diagnoses state the actual or potential problems in the client's health status.

✓ Nursing diagnoses are written for the physical, developmental, intellectual, emotional, social, and spiritual dimensions of the client.

✓ Nursing diagnoses are necessary to develop a plan of care that will help the client and family adapt to changes resulting from an illness or change in life-style.

✓ Nursing diagnoses improve communication between nurses and other health professionals.

✓ Nursing diagnoses can serve as a focus for quality assurance and peer review.

✓ Nursing diagnostic errors can occur by omission or commission.

✓ Errors of omission occur when the nurse has failed to identify a health problem.

✓ Causes of errors of omission are incomplete data collection, incorrect data clustering, or improper interpretation of data.

✓ Errors of commission occur when the nurse overdiagnoses or diagnoses nonexistent health problems.

✓ Causes of errors of commission are incomplete data collection and incorrect data clustering.

✓ Diagnostic statement errors include using inappropriate or imprecise language, stating a nursing diagnosis as a medical diagnosis, using medical terminology to describe the cause, and stating the nursing diagnosis as an intervention.

REFERENCES

Carpenito, LJ: Nursing diagnoses: application to clinical practice, Philadelphia, 1983, J.B. Lippincott Co.

Edel, MK: Noncompliance: an appropriate nursing diagnosis? Nurs Outlook 33:183, 1985.

Gleit, CJ, and Tatro, S: Nursing diagnoses for healthy individuals, Nurs Health Care 8:456, 1981.

Gordon, M: Nursing diagnosis: process and application, New York, 1982, McGraw-Hill Book Co.

Hurley, ME: Classification of nursing diagnoses, St. Louis, 1986, The C.V. Mosby Co.

Jacoby, MK: The dilemma of physiological problems: eliminating the double standard, Am J Nurs 85:281, 1985.

Kim, MJ, McFarland, GR, and McLane, AM, editors: Classification of nursing diagnoses: proceedings of the Fifth Conference (NANDA), St. Louis, 1984, The C.V. Mosby Co.

Lunney, M: Nursing diagnoses: refining the system, Am J Nurs 82:456, 1986.

Martens, K: Let's diagnose strengths, not just problems, Am J Nurs 86:192, 1986.

McKeehan, KM: Nursing diagnosis in a discharge planning program, Nurs Clin North Am 14:517, 1979.

McLane, AM, editor: Classification of nursing diagnoses: proceedings from the Seventh Conference (NANDA), St. Louis, 1987, The C.V. Mosby Co.

Popkess, SA: Diagnosing your patient's strengths, Nurs 81 11:34, 1981.

Porter, EJ: Critical analysis of NANDA nursing diagnoses taxonomy. I. Image: Nurs Sch 18:137, 1986.

Shamansky, SL, and Yanni, CR: In opposition to nursing diagnosis: a minority opinion, Image: J Nurs Sch 17:47, 1985.

Shoemaker, JK: Essential features of a nursing diagnosis. In Kim, MJ, et al., editors: Classification of nursing diagnoses: proceedings of the Fifth Conference (NANDA), St. Louis, 1984, The C.V. Mosby Co.

Stantis, MA, and Ryan, J: Noncompliance, an unacceptable diagnosis, Am J Nurs 82:941, 1982.

Research Article

Kim, MJ: Nursing diagnoses in critical care, Dimens Crit Care Nurs 2:5, 1983.

ADDITIONAL READINGS

Aspinall, MJ: Nursing diagnosis: the weak link, Nurs Outlook 24: 433, 1976.

Aspinall, MJ: Use of a decision tree to improve diagnostic accuracy, Nurs Res 28:182, 1979.

Benner, P, and Tanner, C: How expert nurses use intuition, Am J Nurs 87: 23, 1987.

Campbell, C: Nursing diagnosis and intervention in nursing practice, New York, 1978, John Wiley & Sons, Inc.

Carnevali, DL, et al., Diagnostic reasoning in nursing, Philadephia, 1984, J.B. Lippincott Co.

Dalton, J: A descriptive study: defining characteristics of the nursing diagnosis: cardiac output, alterations in, decreased. Image: J Nurs Sch 17:113, 1985.

Fehring, RJ: Validating diagnositic labels: standardized methodology. In Hurley, M, editor: Classification of nursing diagnoses: proceedings of the Sixth Conference (NANDA), St. Louis, 1986, The C.V. Mosby Co.

Gebbie, KM, and Lavin, MA: Classifying nursing diagnoses, Am J Nurs 74:250, 1974.

Gordon, M: Nursing diagnoses and the diagnostic process, Am J Nurs 76:1298, 1976.

Gordon, M: Classification of nursing diagnoses, J NY Nurses Assoc 9:5, 1978.

Gordon, M: The concept of nursing diagnoses, Nurs Clin North Am 14:487, 1979.

Hagey, RS, and McDonough, P: The problem of professional labeling, Nurs Outlook 32:151, 1984.

Halloran, EJ: Nursing workload, medical diagnosis related groups and nursing diagnoses, Res Nurs Health 8:421, 1985.

Iyer, PW, Taptich, BJ, and Bernocchi-Losey, D: Nursing process and nursing diagnoses, Philadelphia, 1986, W.B. Saunders Co.

Lee, HA, and Strong, KA: Using nursing diagnoses to describe the clinical competence of baccalaureate and associate degree graduating students: a comparative study, Image: J Nurs Sch 17:82, 1985.

Kim, MJ: Without collaboration, what's left? Am J Nurs 85:281, 1985.

Kim, MJ, et al., editors: Pocket guide for nursing diagnoses, ed. 2, St. Louis, 1987, The C.V. Mosby Co.

Levin, RF, and Crosley, JM: Focused data collection for the generation of nursing diagnoses, Nurs Staff 2(2):56, 1986.

Price, BR: Nursing diagnoses: making a concept come alive, Am J Nurs 80:668, 1980.

Shoemaker, J: How nursing diagnoses helps focus your care, RN 8:56, 1979.

Walker, L: Nursing diagnoses and interventions: new tools to define nursing's unique role, Nurs Health Care 7(6):323, 1986.

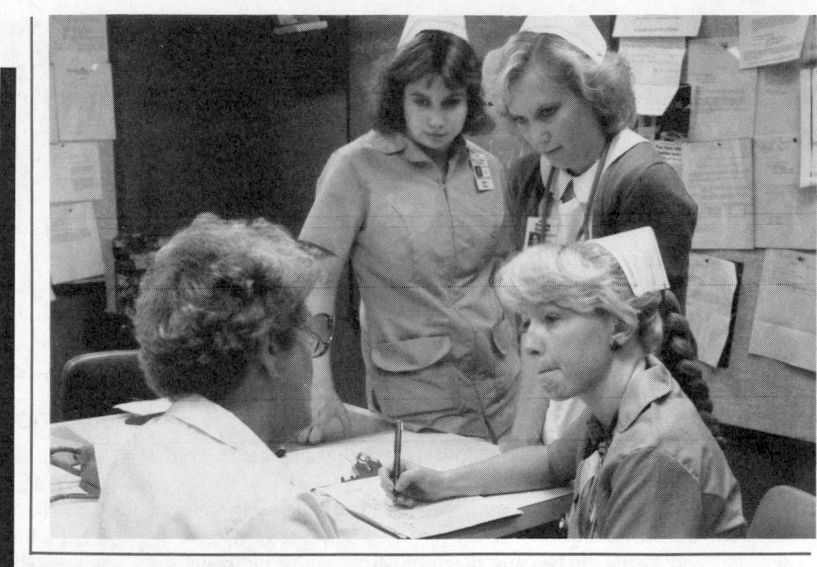

OBJECTIVES

Mastery of content in this chapter will enable the student to:

- Define the key terms listed.
- List the purposes of the nursing care plan.
- Discuss differences between institutional, standardized, and student care plans.
- Describe the differences between care plans used in hospital and community health settings.
- Identify incorrect nursing interventions developed during the planning component.
- Develop a nursing care plan from a nursing assessment.
- List the six steps involved in obtaining consultation.
- Discuss the consultant process.

KEY TERMS

Anticipatory Guidance
Client-Centered Goal
Consultation
Kardex
Nursing Care Plan
Expected Outcome
Scientific Rationale

Planning

Nursing assessment and the formulation of nursing diagnoses initiate the planning step of the nursing process. Planning is a category of nursing behaviors in which client-centered goals are established and strategies are designed to achieve the goals. During planning, goals are determined, priorities are set, expected outcomes are developed, and a nursing care plan is formulated. Planning includes consulting with other members of the health care team, modifying care, and recording relevant information about the client's health care needs and clinical management.

ESTABLISHING PRIORITIES

After specific nursing diagnoses have been formulated, the nurse establishes the priorities of each diagnosis by ranking the nursing diagnoses in order of importance. Developing client goals may occur simultaneously with or even before the establishment of priorities. However, for clarity and explanation purposes, determining goals is presented in the next section.

Maslow's hierarchy of needs can be useful in designating priorities. Basic physiological needs are given priority over safety needs. The needs for love, esteem, and self-actualization have a lower priority. The nurse may encounter situations in which there are no emergency physical needs but in which high priority must be given to psychological, sociocultural, developmental, or spiritual needs of the client. Chapter 27 discusses in detail Maslow's hierarchy of needs and its implications for nursing practice.

TABLE 8-1 Priority Setting

Nursing Diagnoses	Rationale
HIGH PRIORITY	
Alteration in bowel elimination: diarrhea related to unknown cause	Prompt resolution of diarrhea and cause prevents further decline in physiological and emotional status.
Potential ineffective coping, related to unknown medical diagnosis	Dealing early with ineffective coping will help client prepare for a diagnostic test, treatment, or diagnosis.
Potential ineffective airway clearance, postoperatively related to abdominal incisional pain	Because of the risk of postoperative complications, the nurse will institute preventive client education early in nursing care.
INTERMEDIATE PRIORITY	
Potential alteration in nutrition: less than body requirements related to chronic diarrhea for 3 weeks	This nursing diagnosis does not affect the client's immediate physiological or emotional status. Possible surgery will also assist the nurse in resolving the diagnosis.
LOW PRIORITY	
Potential for chronic infections related to history of smoking for 20 years	This nursing diagnosis reflects the long-term needs of the client.

Priorities are classified as high, intermediate, or low. High-priority nursing diagnoses are the urgent or immediate needs of the client. High priorities occur in the psychological and physiological dimensions, and the nurse should avoid classifying only physiological nursing diagnoses as high priority. Intermediate-priority nursing diagnoses involve the nonemergency, non-life-threatening needs of the client. Low-priority nursing diagnoses are client needs that may not be directly related to a specific illness or prognosis.

Whenever possible, the client should be involved in priority setting. In some situations the client and nurse will assign different priority rankings to the nursing diagnoses. If both place a different value on health care needs and treatments, these differences can be resolved through open communication. However, when the client's physiological and emotional needs are at stake, the nurse may need to assume primary responsibility for setting priorities.

When the nurse assigns priorities to nursing diagnoses, the needs of the client, the resources of the health care

system, and the limitations of time are considered. Table 8-1 displays priority settings and rationales. These priorities involve client needs and resources and limitations of the health care system.

DETERMINING GOALS OF CARE

Nursing care planned according to nursing diagnoses and priority setting will reflect the goals of care established by the client and nurse. The nursing diagnoses formulated are based on the client's response and perception of changes in level of wellness, activities of daily living, life-style patterns, and role performance. Because each person responds uniquely to a situation, the nursing diagnoses and client goals of health care are also unique.

Individual nursing diagnoses and priority setting helps determine the goals of care. Setting goals is an activity that includes the family and significant others, as well as the client.

A *client-centered goal* is a specific and measurable objective designed to reflect the client's highest level of wellness and independence in function. Client-centered goals require active involvement on the part of the client in goal setting and the development of projected outcomes and plan of care. Because clients participate during client-centered goal setting, they should be alert and have some degree of independence in completing activities of daily living, problem solving, and decision making. When developing goals, the nurse can act as an advocate for the client to prevent further deterioration in the level of wellness or cognitive and physical functioning.

When clients' cognitive and physical impairments are so severe that they are unable to actively participate in goal setting, the nursing team acts in the client's behalf to develop client-centered goals. These clients may include comatose individuals who have no family, totally disoriented individuals, individuals unable to participate in decision making, and abandoned infants or infants removed by the courts from parental custody and decision making.

Goals should not only meet the immediate needs of the client, but should also include prevention and rehabilitation. Two types of goals are developed for the client, short-term and long-term goals.

Short-Term Goals

A short-term goal can be achieved quickly, during a clinic visit, hospitalization, or a home visit, for example. A short-term goal for a client with ineffective airway clearance, for example, may be "maintain a patent airway."

TABLE 8-2   Goal Setting

Nursing Diagnoses	Short-Term Goals	Long-Term Goals
Potential ineffective airway clearance postoperatively related to abdominal incisional pain	Lungs remain clear postoperatively.	Absence of postoperative pulmonary complication.
Potential disturbance in self-concept related to change in body image	Client views the incision and colostomy by fifth postoperative day.	Client cares for colostomy independently 2 weeks after surger.
Potential ineffective coping related to unknown medical diagnoses.	Client asks pertinent questions about cancer.	Client will attend "I can cope" classes at the Cancer Society.
Potential for infection related to retained secretions resulting from inability to cough	Lungs remain clear on auscultation. Sputum becomes white and frothy.	Client does not exhibit signs and symptoms of pulmonary infiltrate. Sputum does not show signs of infection.
Impaired skin integrity related to immobility resulting from coma	Prevent future skin breakdown.	Skin returns to healed and intact status.

Long-Term Goals

A long-term goal is a goal that will be achieved in the future. A long-term goal for a client with an ineffective airway clearance may be to "remain free of upper respiratory infection for 6 months." These goals often focus on prevention, rehabilitation, discharge, and health education. Failure to set long-term goals may prevent the client from achieving a maximal level of wellness.

Goal setting establishes the framework for the nursing care plan. Table 8-2 shows short- and long-term goals, which are individualized to meet client needs. Through goals the nurse is able to provide continuity of care. In addition, goal setting promotes optimal use of time and resources. Ultimately the goal results in development of expected outcome of the nursing interventions.

EXPECTED OUTCOMES

The expected outcome is the specific, desired change in the client's condition in the physiological, social, emotional, developmental, or spiritual dimensions. Change in condition is documented through observable or measurable client responses. The expected outcomes define when a specific, client-centered goal has been met and later assist in evaluating the extent to which the nursing diagnosis has been resolved.

Expected outcomes can provide five functions. They are projected before nursing actions are formulated, providing a direction for nursing activities (Gordon, 1982). They include client observable behaviors and measurable outcomes for each goal. They provide a projected time span for goal attainment and provide an opportunity to state any additional resources that may be required to achieve the goal, including additional equipment, personnel, or knowledge. The nurse also uses the outcomes as criteria to evaluate the effectiveness of nursing activities.

Expected outcomes are derived from client-centered goals, both short- and long-term goals, and are based on nursing diagnoses developed during the second component of the nursing process (Table 8-3). In addition, expected outcomes are important in evaluation.

NURSING CARE PLAN

The final product of planning is the nursing care plan, which is based on data obtained and the nursing diagnoses, priorities, and goals developed. Generally, nursing care plans involve the following areas: nursing diagnoses, goals, specific action by the nurse, and expected outcomes of the client's responses to nursing actions. Specific care plans may include the additional area of assessment and may not include evaluation.

Purpose of Care Plans

The nursing care plan is a written guideline for client care. Written care plans document the client's health care needs, which are determined by assessment and the nursing diagnosis, priorities, and goals formulated during planning. Care plans also coordinate nursing care, promote continuity of care, and list outcome criteria to be used in the evaluation of nursing care (Little and Carnevali, 1983). In addition, the written care plan communicates to other nurses and health care professionals pertinent assessment data, a list of problems, and therapies. A written care plan decreases the risk of incomplete, incorrect, or inaccurate care.

TABLE 8-3 Expected Outcomes

Nursing Diagnoses	Goals	Expected Outcomes
Potential ineffective airway clearance postoperatively related to abdominal incisional pain	Lungs remain clear immediately after surgery.	Client able to clear airway with deep breathing and coughing. Sputum remains white. Client remains afebrile. Lungs clear to auscultation. Chest x-rays film free of pneumonia, atelectasis, or infiltrate.
Impaired skin integrity related to immobility resulting from coma	**Short-Term Goal** Prevent future skin breakdown	Absence of prolonged erythema or skin breakdown in unaffected areas. Skin remains dry. Absence of prolonged pressure over bony prominences.
	Long-Term Goal Skin returns to healed, intact status	Affected area shows signs of wound granulation: decreased drainage decreased wound size decreased erythemia Absence of erythemia and skin breakdown in unaffected areas. Absence of prolonged pressure over bony prominences.

The nursing care plan is organized in such a way that any nurse can quickly identify the nursing actions to be delivered. In hospitals and outpatient and community-based settings the client often receives care from more than one nurse, more than one physician, several allied health professionals, and many health technicians. The written nursing care plan makes possible the coordination of nursing care, subspecialty consultations, and scheduling of diagnostic tests.

The care plan can also identify and coordinate resources used to deliver nursing care. The listing of specific equipment and supplies necessary for nursing actions is an economically efficient mechanism for selecting equipment. If all equipment and supplies are included in the care plan, the nurse's time is more effectively used in providing care as opposed to locating supplies.

The nursing care plan enhances the continuity of nursing care by listing the specific nursing actions necessary to achieve the goals of care. These nursing activities can be carried out throughout the day and from day to day. A correctly formulated nursing care plan facilitates the continuity of care from one nurse to another. As a result, all nurses have the opportunity to deliver the same quality of care.

The written nursing care plan organizes the information exchanged by nurses in the change-of-shift report. Nurses focus their report on the nursing care and treatments delineated in the care plan. At the end of a scheduled shift, the nurse discusses the care plan with the next care giver. Thus all nurses are able to discuss current and pertinent information about the client's plan of care.

The written care plan can also be adapted to the discharge needs of the client. Incorporating the goals of the care plan into discharge is particularly important for a client who will be undergoing long-term rehabilitation in the community. The adaptation of the care plan enhances the continuity of nursing care between nurses in the hospital and nurses in the community.

Same-day surgeries and earlier discharges from hospitals require the nurse to plan discharge needs on the client's care plan the moment the health care agency is entered. Mortensen and McMullin (1986) noted that incomplete assessments and the absence of measurable outcome criteria extended client stays in short-term, one-day surgical centers. Client stays were lengthened because there were no documented, measurable criteria for discharge readiness on the postoperative nursing care plan, resulting in confusion among all the health care professionals as to when the client could safely be discharged from the setting.

In developing an individualized care plan the nurse

involves the family, significant others, and the client. The family is a resource that can be used to help the client meet health goals. In addition, meeting some of the family's needs can improve the client's level of wellness.

The last item documented on the nursing care plan is the outcome criteria used in evaluation of care. Proper listing of the outcome criteria provides the nurse with objective statements that help determine whether the goals of care have been achieved.

The development of the nursing care plan is the end point of the planning phase. The complete care plan is the blueprint for nursing action, providing direction for implementation of the plan and a framework for evaluation of the client's response to nursing actions.

Medical Diagnosis and other pertinent medical information:
10/25 LBP c̄ RLE SCIATICA
10/26 LAMINECTOMY L4-L5 c̄ BONE GRAFT

Condition SATIS — PMH: DM
Allergies (Drugs, food, other) PCN, ASA, CODEINE

1083 13160 23-4
SMITH, PHIL
Stamp Addressograph Plate Here

Adm. Date 10/23	Age 64	Religion CATH	Mode of Travel
Service ORTHO	Doctor FORD	Resident KOWALSKI	Intern

FREQUENTLY ORDERED ITEMS

Temp.
Pulse & Resp. q 4°
BP
I & O q 8°
Weights
Spot Checks
Chest P.T.
Incentive Spirometer
P.T.

ACTIVITIES	NUTRITION
Ad lib	Diet REGULAR
Ambulate x 2	
Chair	
BRP	
Bedrest	
Bath	Feedings
Self	
Tub	Assist c̄ meals
Shower	FLUID BALANCE
Bed ✓	Force
Assist.	D E N
	Restrict
	D E N
Orderlies Needed	

Family:

Date	Specimens/Daily Lab
10/25	ADM. BLOOD WORK
10/25	UA c̄ MICRO
10/25	BS

Date	Diagnostic Procedures
10/25	MYELOGRAM
	CT SCAN
10/25	CXR
10/25	EKG

Date	Treatments
10/24	BR AND LOGROLL q 2°

NURSING CARE PLAN

Date	Nursing Diagnosis	Expected Outcomes	Nursing Plan/Orders
10/26	ALTERED COMFORT, PAIN	1. PT. REQUESTS FOR PAIN MED. DECREASES 2. PT. RESPIRATORY EXPANSION ↑	1. ENCOURAGE PATIENT TO SPLINT INCISION WHEN TURNING 2. INSTRUCT PATIENT IN RELAXATION EXERCISES
10/27	IMPAIRED PHYSICAL MOBILITY RELATED TO PAIN	1. PT. INCREASES AMBULATION FROM BID TO QID OR GREATER	1. AMBULATE IN HALL c̄ PT 20 MINUTES AFTER ADMINISTRATION OF ANALGESIC 2. ENCOURAGE FAMILY TO WALK PATIENT
		2. PT. ASSUMES ADL	1. ALLOW PT. EXTRA TIME TO DO SELF CARE FOR HYGIENE NEEDS

Discharge Planning: Destination: Transportation: Probable Date: Referral Agencies: Appointment:
Supplies:

Patient Name

Fig. 8-1 Nursing care plan on a nursing Kardex.

Care Plans in Various Settings

The structure of the nursing care plan varies from one health care setting to another. For example, the nursing care plan used in a hospital is different from one used in a community health setting. The nursing care plan developed for the client returning home is usually based solely on long-term health needs. In addition, the client and family or significant others are more involved and assume more responsibility for care because the client is receiving nursing care in the home. Although the structure of the care plan varies depending on the setting, its overall purpose remains the same: to provide a written guideline for client care so the health care needs of the client and subsequent therapies are communicated among the health care team.

INSTITUTIONAL (STAFF) CARE PLANS

Staff care plans are concise documents that become part of the client's medical record. Many hospitals use the Kardex nursing care plan. Kardex is a trade name for a card-filing system allowing quick reference to the particular needs of the client for certain aspects of nursing care. Each card is folded once. Information about medications, activity levels, level of self-care, diet, treatments, and procedures is usually included on the outside of the card. The nursing care plan is commonly placed on the inside (Fig. 8-1). Each institution has its own format for the Kardex, but the basic information con-tained on it is universal. The nursing care plan section of the Kardex also has institutional variations. One institution might use a three-column nursing care plan, which includes the problem, goal, and nursing action. Another institution may incorporate a four-column nursing care plan on the Kardex, which includes the nursing diagnosis, goal, nursing action, and evaluation. As the five-step nursing process has gained popularity, the nursing care plan on the Kardex in many hospitals has been revised to include the following components of the nursing process: assessment, nursing diagnosis, goal, implementation, and evaluation (Fig. 8-2).

STANDARDIZED CARE PLANS. The use of computers and the need to efficiently organize the nurse's time have resulted in standardized nursing care plans, which are forms created for a specific clinical area (for example, coronary care, abdominal surgery, postpartum, and same-day surgery units). Each care plan lists generalized nursing diagnoses, goals, outcome criteria, and nursing interventions for a specific group of clients (Fig. 8-3).

After a complete nursing assessment, the nurse, using a standardized format, determines if it should be used for that particular client. Even if the care plan is generally appropriate on a client, the nurse must add or delete information on the standardized form to individualize it for the client's needs. Failure to do so can result in incomplete and inaccurate care.

Standardized nursing care plans are a method to

Assessment	Nursing diagnosis	Goal	Implementation	Evaluation
Weight loss: 15 lbs in 10 days. Eats only portion of meal due to full feeling immediately after beginning a meal	Potential alteration in nutrition: less than body requirements related to sensation of fullness c̄ meals	Weight remains 185 lbs	1. Weigh daily 2. Small frequent high calorie feedings 8-10-12-2-4-6	Weight remains 185 lbs Consumes all food delivered on meal tray

Fig. 8-2 Five-column nursing care plan.

NURSING STANDARD CARE PLAN

Nursing Diagnosis: ALTERATION IN COMFORT

Related to _____

(inadequate pain relief, fear of drug dependence, vomiting, nausea, other)

Addressograph

Expected Outcomes:

☐ Patient will demonstrate increased comfort as evidenced by:
  ☐ ability to sleep within patient's normal limits.
  ☐ fewer signs and symptoms of discomfort.
  ☐ verbalization of comfort level.
  ☐ participation in self-care activities, i.e., eating, bathing, etc.
☐ Patient/support person will demonstrate effective use of medication and/or pain control devices.
☐ Patient will verbalize and demonstrate understanding of specific teaching plan.
☐ Other: _____
☐ Other: _____

Date Initiated /Initials	Nursing Interventions	Date Inactivated /Initials
_____	1. Evaluate pain/effectiveness of relief measures every _____	_____
_____	2. Establish a trusting relationship with patient, communicate that you know the pain is real by: _____	_____
_____	3. Measure for pain/relief: ☐ position _____ ☐ administer analgesics prior to/during _____ ☐ minimize negative environmental stimuli by _____ ☐ administer cutaneous stimulation (TENS, aquakpad, ice bags) of _____ during _____ ☐ assist patient with relaxation techniques including _____ every _____ ☐ promote distraction measures including _____ ☐ possible meditation techniques including _____ ☐ other _____	_____
_____	4. Assess bowel function and skin integrity every _____	_____
_____	5. Assess potential for injury while receiving therapy by: _____	_____
_____	6. Provide teaching specific to patient/support person needs (e.g. use of medications, other relief measures). Initiate individual plan. _____	_____
_____	7. Initiate consults/referrals. _____	_____
_____	8. Other interventions specific to patient: _____	_____
	Signature/Initials: _____	

Fig. 8-3 Standardized nursing care plan.

streamline and augment care planning. They are not intended to replace the nursing care plan process but to avoid a situation in which the nurse must write the same generalized plan again.

STUDENT CARE PLANS

Nursing students learn to write and use a nursing care plan as part of their education. The student care plan is essential for learning the problem-solving technique, the nursing process, skills of written and verbal communication, and organizational skills needed for nursing care. Most important, by using the nursing care plan, students can apply the knowledge gained from nursing and medical literature and the classroom in a practice situation.

The student care plan is more elaborate than care plans in hospital or community health agencies because its purpose is to teach the process of planning care. To learn the care-planning process, the student must progress in a step-by-step manner, beginning with assessment and ending with evaluation. Student care plans vary from one educational program to another and between beginning and more advanced students. Some educational institutions model the student care plan on the care plan used in the affiliated health agency. The only modification may be that the instructor requires the beginning student to include the scientific rationale for the nursing actions selected (Table 8-4). A scientific rationale is the reason, based on supporting literature, a specific nursing action was chosen.

WRITING THE NURSING CARE PLAN

As an initial step in planning, the nurse assigns a priority to each nursing diagnosis, such as those based on Maslow's hierarchy of needs, urgent client physiological and safety needs, and important needs perceived by the client. The nursing diagnosis with the highest priority is the beginning point for the nursing care plan and is followed by other nursing diagnoses in order of assigned priority.

When using the five-column plan, in the assessment column (column 1), the nurse includes all data relevant to the corresponding nursing diagnosis (column 2). The nurse includes the previously developed goals in the next column (column 3). At this point the nurse begins to translate the short- and long-term goals into action plans that anticipate the needs of the client, coordinate nursing care, and select the appropriate nursing measures.

The nurse writes the action plan in the implementation column (column 4) of the nursing care plan. Each nursing action is written to include information necessary to implement nursing care. It may help the beginning nurse to ask if the stated interventions answer the following questions: *What* is the intervention? *When* should each intervention be implemented? *How* should the intervention be performed? *Who* should be involved in each aspect of intervention? In addition, the nurse should understand the reason for a specific intervention. Nonspecific nursing interventions result in incomplete or in-

TABLE 8-4　Scientific Rationale for the Student Care Plan

Assessment	Nursing Diagnosis	Goals	Implementation	Rationale	Evaluation (Expected Outcomes)
Fever: higher than 102° F for 72 hours Diaphoresis Incontinence of urine	Potential impairment of skin integrity related to immobility resulting from coma	Reduce pressure on bony prominences.	Primary nurse will turn client every 2 hours in the following sequence: 8 AM—supine 10 AM—left side 12 noon—prone Repeat, begin with supine position.	Critical time for skin tissue breakdown is between 1 and 2 hours of constant pressure.*	No skin breakdown noted. Skin color is normal, temperature normal, capillary return normal. Client is afebrile.
Decreased skin turgor No skin breakdown noted		Avoid future skin breakdown.	All nursing personnel will keep client's skin dry at all times.	Moisture increases maceration of the skin and promotes bacterial growth.†	Skin remains dry and intact. Skin turgor is improved.

*Data from Bereck, KH: Etiology of decubitus ulcers, Nurs Clin North Am 10(1):160, 1975.
†Data from Kavchack-Keys, MA: Four proven steps for preventing decubitus ulcers, Nurs 77 7:60, 1977.

accurate nursing care, lack of continuity among care givers, and poor use of resources.

Common omissions in writing nursing interventions include action, frequency, quantity, method, or person to perform them. These errors can occur if the nurse is unfamiliar with the planning process. Table 8-5 illustrates these types of errors by showing incorrect and correct statements of nursing interventions.

The column (column 5) in the nursing care plan contains the projected outcome criteria previously identified. Listing the criteria on the nursing care plan gives a written estimation of when the goal of care has been achieved, thus indicating when a particular nursing diagnosis is no longer relevant to the plan of care.

CONSULTATION WITH OTHER HEALTH CARE PROFESSIONALS

Planning nursing care involves consultation with other members of the health care team. Consultation may occur at any step in the nursing process but is needed most often in the planning and intervention steps, because at these points the nurse is more likely to identify a problem requiring additional knowledge or skills or a need to

obtain community or agency resources. Consultation is a process in which the help of a specialist is sought to identify ways to handle problems in client management or the planning and implementation of programs. Consultation is based on the problem-solving approach, and the consultant is the stimulus for change.

In clinical nursing, consultation is used to solve problems in the delivery of nursing care or use of resources. Nurse consultants are most frequently approached for advice about difficult clinical problems. Nurses are consulted for their clinical expertise, patient education skills, or staff education skills.

Nurses also obtain consultations from other members of the health care team, such as physical therapists, nutritionists, and social workers. Again the consultant focuses on problems in nursing.

When to Consult

The need for consultation in nursing occurs when the nurse has identified a problem that cannot solved using the nurse's knowledge, skills, and resources. The consultation process increases the nurse's knowledge about the problem and helps in learning skills and obtaining the resources needed to solve the problem. After the consultation, the nurse may be able to resolve similar

---

TABLE 8-5 Frequent Errors in Writing Nursing Interventions

Type of Error	Incorrectly Stated Nursing Intervention	Correctly Stated Nursing Intervention
Failure to precisely or completely indicate nursing actions	Primary nurse will turn client every 2 hours.	Primary nurse will turn client every 2 hours, using the following schedule: 8 AM—supine, 10 AM—left side, 12 noon—prone, 2 PM—right side } Repeat sequence at 4 PM and 2 AM
Failure to indicate frequency	Primary nurse will observe client cough and deep breathe.	Primary nurse will observe client cough and deep breathe at 10 AM—2 PM—6 PM—10 PM.
Failure to indicate quantity	Primary nurse will provide hydrogen peroxide (H_2O_2) mouthwash to client every 2 hours while awake: 8-10-12-2-4-6-8-10.	Primary nurse will provide 50 ml of H_2O_2 mouthwash to client every 2 hours while awake: 8-10-12-2-4-6-8-10.
Failure to indicate method	Primary nurse will change client's dressing once a shift: 6 AM—2 PM—10 PM.	Primary nurse will replace client's dressing, with Neosporin ointment to wound and two dry 4 × 4's secured with hypoallergenic tape, once a shift: 2 PM—10 PM—6 AM.
Failure to indicate person to perform the action	Irrigate nasogastric (NG) tube every 2 hours (even) round the clock with 30 ml of normal saline (NS).	Primary nurse will irrigate NG tube every 2 hours (even) round the clock with 30 ml NS.

problems in the future. For example, a nurse encountering a patient with a recent colostomy might request a consultation from an enterostomal therapist to determine the materials needed to clean the colostomy site and the specific techniques to use during the procedure.

Consultation is also used when the exact problem remains unclear. A consultant objectively entering a situation is able to more clearly assess and identify the exact nature of the problem, whether it be client oriented, personnel oriented, or equipment oriented. A consultant entering the environment unbiased can often objectively identify the problem and outline a method for resolving it.

How to Consult

The first step in the consultation process is identification of the general problem area, which will give the consultant a starting point for identifying the specific problem.

Second, the consultation should be directed to the appropriate professional, who may be another nurse or another member of the health care team. Consultations requested of the wrong individual delay problem solving and diminish the quality of care delivered to the client.

Third, the nurse provides the consultant with pertinent information and resources about the problem area. Pertinent information includes a brief summary of the problem, methods used to resolve the problem, and outcome of those methods. Other resources can include the patient's medical record, nurses and other members of the health team, and the client's family.

Fourth, it is important that the nurse not bias consultants. Consultants are in the clinical setting to identify and resolve a nursing problem, and biasing them can hinder problem resolution. Bias can be avoided by not overloading consultants with subjective and emotional conclusions about the client and the problem.

Fifth, the nurse requesting consultation should be available to discuss the findings and recommendations. When a consultation is requested, the nurse provides a private, comfortable atmosphere in which the consultant and the client can meet. However, this does not mean that the nurse leaves the environment. A common mistake is turning the whole problem over to the consultant. The consultant is not there to take over the problem but rather to assist the nurse in resolving it. The nurse requesting assistance should request the consultation for a day when she is scheduled to work and at a time when distractions are minimal. Thus the consultant is available to the nurse, and the nurse is also available to the consultant.

Finally, the nurse incorporates the consultant's recommendations into the nursing care plan. The success of the consultant's advice depends on the nurse's implementation of the problem-solving techniques suggested.

The use of consultants is a valuable adjunct to nursing care. In clinical nursing practice, a competent and experienced nurse even encounters problems beyond his or her knowledge or experience. Professional and competent nurses recognize their limitations, seek appropriate consultation, and learn from the findings and recommendations.

SUMMARY

The planning component of the nursing process results in the development of the nursing care plan, which details the selected nursing interventions and the apropriate evaluation criteria for each client. The nursing student learns the process of planning care in the educational and the clinical settings. Although the format of the nursing care plan varies from one educational institution to another and from one health care setting to another, the student nurse will encounter the student care plan and the institutional care plan throughout the educational process.

Planning nursing care involves a cognitive and written process. The student learns to solve a client's health care problems by selecting appropriate nursing interventions. In addition, the student learns to communicate the client's health care needs through the written nursing care plan. Individual nursing care plans are the result of the nurse's knowledge and expertise, as well as the knowledge and expertise gained through use of consultants.

Complete and accurate planning of nursing care results in individualization, coordination, and continuity of nursing care. Planning establishes the framework of nursing care to be delivered during implementation.

KEY CONCEPTS

✓ During the planning component, client goals are determined, priorities are established, expected outcomes of nursing care are developed, and a nursing care plan is written.

✓ Nursing care is planned and organized around specific nursing diagnoses, resulting in an individualized nursing care plan.

✓ Establishing priorities means the nursing diagnoses and goals are ranked in order of importance.

✓ The nurse begins the nursing care plan with the nursing diagnoses that have the highest priority.

✓ The goal is the intended outcome of the nursing intervention.

✓ Goals include prevention and rehabilitation, as well as the crisis or urgent needs of the client.

✓ Goal setting establishes a framework for the nursing care plan.

✓ Expected outcomes serve as a basis for the criteria that the nurse uses to evaluate the effectiveness of the nursing care plan.

✓ In general, nursing care plans include the nursing diagnosis, goals, specific actions by the nurse, and projected client response to the nursing action.

✓ The nursing care plan is a written guideline for client care so such care can be quickly understood.

✓ The nursing care plan increases communication among nurses and facilitates the continuity of care from one nurse to another and from one health care setting to another.

✓ The development of an individualized care plan requires involvement of the family or significant others during the planning phase.

✓ Staff care plans may become part of a client's medical record.

✓ The nursing care plan is a method for teaching students to transfer knowledge gained from nursing and medical literature and the classroom into practical experience.

✓ A scientific rationale is the reason, based on supporting literature, a specific nursing action was chosen.

✓ Poorly written nursing care plans result in incomplete or inaccurate nursing care, lack of continuity among care givers, and poor use of resources.

✓ Correctly written nursing interventions include actions, frequency, quantity, method, and the person to perform them.

✓ Planning nursing care often involves consultation with other members of the health care team.

✓ The need for consultation in nursing occurs when the nurse identifies a problem that cannot be solved using his or her knowledge, skills, and resources.

REFERENCES

Gordon, M: Nursing diagnosis: process and application, New York, 1982, McGraw-Hill Book Co.

Little, DE, and Carnevali, DC: Nursing care planning, ed. 3, Philadelphia, 1983, J.B. Lippincott Co.

Mortensen, M, and McMullin, C: Discharge score for surgical outpatients, Am J Nurs 86:1347, 1986.

ADDITIONAL READINGS

Bower, FL: The process of planning nursing care, St. Louis, 1983, The C.V. Mosby Co.

Caplan, G: The theory and practice of mental health consultation, New York, 1970, Basic books, Inc. Publishers.

Hendrix, MJ, and LaGodna, GE: Consultation: a political process aimed at change. In Lancaster, J, and Lancaster, W, editors: Concepts for advanced clinical nursing practice, St. Louis, 1982, The C.V. Mosby Co.

Iyer, PW, Taptich, BJ, and Bernocchi-Losey, D: Nursing process and nursing diagnosis, Philadelphia, 1986, W.B. Saunders Co.

Kissinger, JF, and Munjas, BA: Nursing process: student attributes and teaching methodologies, Nurs Res 30:242, 1981.

Mayers, MG: A systematic approach to the nursing care plan, ed. 2, New York, 1978, Appleton-Century-Crofts.

McHugh, M: Nursing process: musings on the method, Holistic Nurs Prac 1:21, 1986.

Pilcher, MW: Post-discharge care: how to follow-up, Nurs 86, 16:50, 1986.

Sanborn, CW, and Blount, M: Standard plans for care and discharge, Am J Nurs 84:1394, 1984.

Westfall, UE: Outcome criteria genisation: a process and product. In Harley, MA, editor: Classification of nursing diagnoses: proceedings of the sixth National Conference, St. Louis, 1986, The C.V. Mosby Co.

Yura, H, and Walsh, MB: The nursing process: assessment, planning, implementing, evaluation, ed. 4, New York, 1983, Appleton-Century-Crofts.

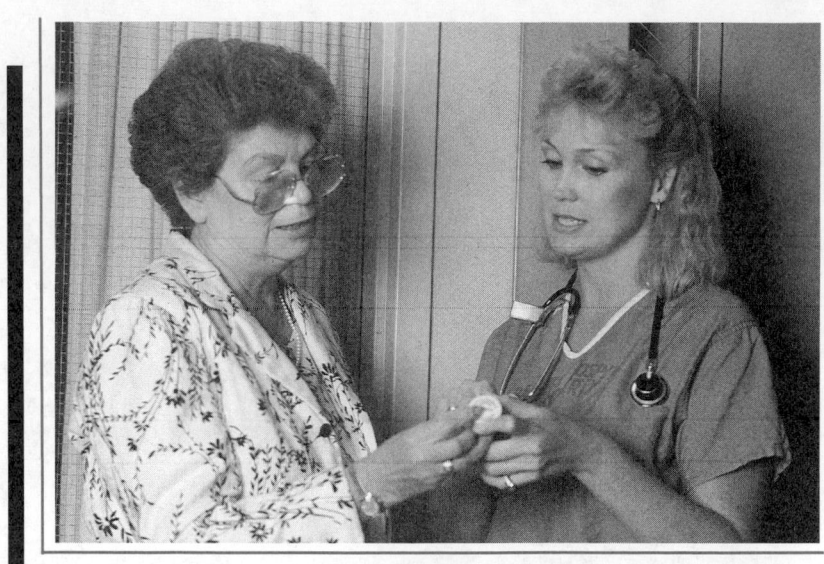

OBJECTIVES

Mastery of content in this chapter will enable the student to:

- Define the key terms listed.
- Discuss the differences between dependent, independent, and interdependent interventions.
- List and discuss the five steps of the implementation process.
- Describe the five different implementation methods.
- Select appropriate implementation methods for an assigned client.

KEY TERMS

Activities of Daily Living

Adherence

Adverse Reaction

Counseling

Dependent Intervention

Implementation

Independent Intervention

Interdependent Intervention

Lifesaving Measure

Nurse Practice Act

Nursing Intervention

Preventive Nursing Action

Protocol

Standing Order

Teaching

Teaching-Learning Process

Technique

Implementation

In theory, implementation of the nursing care plan follows the planning component of the nursing process. However, in practice settings, implementation may begin directly after nursing assessment. Immediate implementation is necessary when the nurse identifies urgent needs of the client, such as a threat to the client's physiological status (for example, a cardiac arrest), psychological status (for example, a sudden death of a loved one), socioeconomic status (for example, sudden loss of a home in a fire), or spiritual status (for example, illness viewed as God's punishment).

Implementation is a category of nursing behavior in which the actions necessary for achieving the expected outcomes of the nursing care plan are initiated and completed. Implementing includes the nurse's performing or assisting in the performance of the client's activities of daily living, counseling and teaching the client or client's family, giving care to achieve client-centered goals, supervising and evaluating the work of staff members, and recording and exchanging information relevant to the client's continued health care.

Implementation begins after the care plan has been developed and focuses on the initiation of nursing interventions to achieve the goals of the care plan. A nursing intervention is any act by a nurse that implements the nursing care plan or any specific objective of the plan. The client may require intervention in the form of support, medication, treatment for the current condition, client-family education or treatment to prevent future health problems.

Implementation is continuous and interacts with the other components of the nursing process. During implementation the nurse reassesses the client, modifies the plan of care, and rewrites expected outcomes as necessary. To complete implementation effectively, the nurse is knowledgeable about types of interventions, and the implementation process, and specific implementation methods.

TYPES OF NURSING INTERVENTIONS

Implementation puts the plan of care into action. Once the plan has been developed according to the client's needs and priorities, the nurse carries out specific nursing interventions, which can be dependent, independent, or interdependent.

Dependent Interventions

A dependent nursing intervention is a nursing action that is completed with a physician's order and that requires nursing judgment or decision making. Examples of dependent nursing interventions include following physician's orders about the type, dosage, and frequency of medication; completing an invasive procedure such as inserting a Foley catheter; and requesting specific diagnostic and laboratory tests. Each dependent nursing intervention involves specific nursing responsibilities.

When administering medications, the nurse is responsible for knowing the classification of the drug, its physiological action, normal dosage, side effects, and nursing interventions related to the drug's action or side effects (see Chapter 15). The nursing interventions associated with administering medication depend on the physician's written order.

Ms. Kline is caring for a preoperative client, Mrs. Wells, who has the following medication order: "Atropine sulfate 0.4 mg IM at 8:00 AM today." Ms. Kline recalls that atropine is an anticholinergic drug and that the desired preoperative effect is to control salivation, bronchial secretions, and rhinorrhea during surgical anesthesia. She consults a resource to determine that 0.4 mg is a normal preoperative dose. Ms. Kline prepares Mrs. Wells for the injection and tells Mrs. Wells to expect an increase in thirst caused by medication. After administration of the drug she observes the client for any side effects such as flushing, tachycardia, restlessness, or disorientation, and she records in the client's medical record that the drug has been administered.

With an invasive procedure the nurse is responsible for knowing when the procedure is necessary, the clinical skills necessary to complete it, and its expected outcome and possible side effects, as well as adequate preparation of the client and proper communication of the results.

When a specific diagnostic or laboratory test is ordered by a physician, the nurse is responsible for scheduling the test, preparing the client, and knowing the normal findings and nursing implications associated with the test.

Although it is not within the legal practice of nursing for the nurse to prescribe and order medications, invasive procedures, and diagnostic tests, it is within the practice of nursing to complete such orders. Administering medications, implementing an invasive procedure, and preparing a client for diagnostic tests are dependent nursing interventions. The student nurse becomes familiar with dependent nursing interventions throughout the educational process.

When encountering an order for a dependent intervention, the nurse does not automatically implement the order but stops to determine whether the requested order is appropriate for the client. Every nurse encounters an inappropriate or incorrect order at some time. The nurse with a strong knowledge base will recognize the error and seek clarification of it. The ability to recognize incorrect orders is particularly important when administering medications or implementing procedures. An error can occur in writing the order or transcribing it to the Kardex or medication card. Clarifying an order is competent nursing practice, and it protects the client and members of the health care delivery system. The nurse carrying out an incorrect or inappropriate order is as much in error as the person who wrote or transcribed the original order and is liable for any complications resulting from the error. Chapter 18 explains legal issues affecting nursing practice.

Independent Interventions

An independent nursing intervention can solve the client's problems without consultation or collaboration with physicians or other nonnursing health professionals (Kim, 1986). Examples of independent nursing interventions include progressive relaxation and guided imagery techniques and therapeutic touch and massage (Snyder, 1985).

In delineating the scope of nursing practice, the ANA (1980) listed ten areas among those in nursing's domain (see box). This list, along with the continuing work of NANDA and nurse researchers, clarifies and elaborates the realm of independent nursing practice.

Independent nursing interventions do not require a physician's order or an order from another professional. Physicians frequently include in their written orders the specifics of independent nursing interventions. However, according to the nurse practice acts in a majority of states, nursing actions pertaining to activities of daily living, health education, health promotion, and counseling are in the domain of nursing practice. These acts

---

Delineation of Nursing Practice

1. Self-care limitations
2. Impaired functioning in areas such as rest, sleep, ventilation, circulation, activity, nutrition, elimination, skin, or sexuality
3. Pain and discomfort
4. Emotional problems related to illness and treatment, life-threatening events, or daily experiences such as anxiety, loss, loneliness, or grief
5. Distortion of symbolic function, reflected in interpersonal and intellectual processes such as hallucinations
6. Deficiencies in decision making and the ability to make personal choices
7. Self-image changes required by health status
8. Dysfunctional perceptual orientations to health
9. Strains related to life processes such as birth, growth and development, and death
10. Problematic affiliative relationships

Used with permission: American Nurses' Association: Nursing: a social policy statement, Kansas City, Mo., 1980, p. 10, The Association.

---

delineate the legal scope of the practice of nursing within the geographical boundaries of the jurisdiction (see Chapter 18).

Interdependent Interventions

An interdependent nursing intervention is completed with or without a physician's order or is written at a nurse's suggestion. It can also provide a solution to a client's problem in a collaborative manner through judgment and recommendations of the interdisciplinary health team. The ANA (1980) defines *collaboration* as a "partnership in which the power on both sides is valued by both, with recognition and acceptance of separate and combined spheres of activity and responsibility, mutual safeguarding of legitimate interests of each party, and a commonality of goals that is recognized by both parties."

Protocols and Standing Orders

A protocol is a written plan specifying the procedures to be followed during an assessment or in providing treatment. For example, nurses providing primary care for a caseload of clients in an outpatient setting follow a protocol. In such a setting the nurse assesses the client and identifies abnormalities. The established protocol delineates the conditions the nurse is permitted to treat and the types of treatment the nurse is permitted to administer.

A protocol can also be strictly within the framework of nursing such as a protocol for admission and discharge, relaxation training, or pain management. Protocols are also used in interdisciplinary settings for diagnostic testing and physical, occupational, and speech therapies.

A standing order is a written document containing rules, policies, procedures, regulations, and orders for the conduct of client care in various stipulated clinical settings. Standing orders are commonly found in critical care settings, in which the nurse continually assesses the client's urgent needs and intervenes appropriately. An example of such a standing order is one that specifies a certain drug for an irregular heart rhythm. When the critical care nurse assesses the client and identifies the irregular rhythm, he or she gives the appropriate medication without first notifying the physician. Standing orders are also common in the community health setting, in which the nurse encounters situations that do not permit contacting a physician immediately. Thus standing orders and protocols give the nurse the legal protection to intervene appropriately in the client's best interest.

■ ■ ■

Nursing interventions implemented during the nursing process include dependent, independent, and interdependent interventions. The nurse implementing any intervention has the responsibility to obtain correct theoretical knowledge and to develop the clinical competency necessary to carry out the intervention. Nursing responsibility is equally great for all types of interventions.

DECISION-MAKING STRATEGIES FOR CHOOSING NURSING INTERVENTIONS

Nurses using the nursing process make two major types of decisions. The diagnostic process defines the client's strengths and problems at the conclusion of the assessment and throughout the diagnostic stage. Specific nursing interventions are also selected during the planning stage. (Grier, 1981).

The student must carefully select the interventions designed to achieve expected outcomes and know the difference between dependent, independent, and interdependent interventions. Several factors make the process of decision making more difficult when choosing among independent nursing interventions (Snyder,

TABLE 9-1 Information-Processing Model. Sample Nursing Diagnosis: Alteration in Comfort Related to Abdominal Incisional Pain

Possible Actions	Possible Consequences Associated with the Action	Probability of Consequence Occurring	Value of Consequence to Client
Teach relaxation exercises.	Client able to control perception of pain.	Moderate	Ability to control perception and response to pain
	Pain is unrelieved.	Moderate	
	Pain increases.	Low	
Client uses controlled analgesia.	Client able to control administration of analgesia within preset limits.	High	Ability to use analgesia to continuously relieve pain
	Pain is relieved.	High	
	Pain is unrelieved.	Moderate	
	Pain increases.	Low	
Nurse administers narcotic analgesia every 4 hours.	Client is unable to control administration of analgesia.	High	Inability to control administration of analgesia
	Pain increases in intensity before nurse administers narcotic analgesia.	Moderate to high	Pain perception increases or decreases based on blood levels of narcotic analgesia
	Pain is relieved.	Moderate to high	
	Client is confused after administration of narcotic analgesia.	Low to moderate	

1985). One factor is the absence of objective data concerning the probable consequences of the interventions. Another is that independent nursing interventions are often not mutually exclusive from medical therapies. For example, the nurse may need to augment relaxation, massage, and guided imagery techniques with prescribed analgesics for pain management (see Chapter 35).

Snyder (1985) proposes an information-processing model of decision making (Table 9-1). The objective of this model is to characterize the sequence of the thought process used by problem solvers. In addition, Snyder incorporates a behavioral decision model of decision making, focusing on what decisions are to be made rather than how they are made. Therefore the information-processing model identifies how decisions are made, and the behavioral decision model denotes what decisions are made. Because of the information-processing model, a student uses the following components of decision making when determining nursing interventions (Snyder, 1985): (1) the set of all possible nursing actions, (2) a listing of all possible consequences associated with each possible nursing action, (3) the determination of the probability that each of the consequences will occur, and (4) a judgment based on the value of that consequence to the client. This model is effective in assisting the student with clinical decision making. However, the beginning student or practitioner

still needs supervision from an instructor or experienced nurse.

IMPLEMENTATION PROCESS

The implementation component of the nursing process has five steps: reassessing the client, reviewing and modifying the existing nursing care plan, identifying areas of assistance, implementing nursing strategies, and communicating nursing strategies.

Reassessing the Client

Assessment is a continuous process. Each time a nurse interacts with a client, additional data is gathered to reflect physical, developmental, intellectual, emotional, social, and spiritual needs. The student nurse begins to reassess the client's needs each time the client and student interact. Whenever new data are assessed and a new need is identified, the nurse modifies nursing care.

During the initial phase of implementation the nurse reassesses the client. This is a partial assessment and may focus on one dimension of the client or on one system. The purpose of the reassessment is to gather new data that can affect the implementation or outcome of care.

TABLE 9-2 Nursing Care Plan for Mrs. Coyle

Assessment	Nursing Diagnosis	Goal	Implementation	Evaluation
Has not voided in 8 hours Fluid intake for last 8 hours 2400 ml Patient status: she "feels the urge to void," bladder discomfort Bladder palpable to 2 cm below umbilicus	Impaired urinary elimination related to perineal swelling following vaginal delivery of 8-pound, 15-ounce, baby girl	Facilitate emptying of bladder	Insert straight catheter, using sterile technique, if patient has not voided in 8 hours and bladder is palpable	1000 ml of clear yellow urine returned via straight catheter Bladder not palpable Client no longer has sensation to void Client no longer complains of bladder discomfort

A nursing care plan has been developed for Mrs. Coyle (Table 9-2). The nursing diagnosis, "Impaired urinary elimination related to perineal swelling following vaginal delivery of 8-pound, 15-ounce baby girl," provided the focus for the plan. Before inserting the straight catheter, the nurse conducts reassessment to determine that Mrs. Coyle has not voided spontaneously, for if she has, the catheterization procedure would no longer be appropriate.

The reassessment phase of the implementation component thus provides a mechanism for the nurse to determine that the proposed nursing action is appropriate for the client's level of wellness.

Reviewing and Modifying the Existing Nursing Care Plan

Although the nursing care plan was developed according to the nursing diagnoses identified during assessment, changes in the client's status can necessitate modification of planned nursing care. Before beginning care, the nurse reviews the plan of care and compares the established plan with the assessment to validate the stated nursing diagnoses and to determine if the nursing interventions are the most appropriate for the clinical situation. If it is discovered that the client's status has changed and the nursing diagnosis and related nursing interventions are no longer appropriate, the nursing care plan needs to be modified.

Modification of the existing nursing care plan includes several steps. First, data in the assessment column are revised to reflect the client's current status. New data entered in the nursing care plan should be dated to inform other members of the health care team when the

change occurred. Whenever possible, new data should be recorded in a different color to alert other care givers to changes.

Second, nursing diagnoses are revised. Nursing diagnoses that are no longer relevant are deleted, and new nursing diagnoses are added. Because the client's status and health care needs have changed, the priorities, goals, and expected outcomes need revision. The revisions are also dated and noted in a different color on the nursing care plan.

Third, specific implementation methods are revised to correspond to the new nursing diagnoses and client goals. This revision reflects the client's present status. The new implementation methods indicate the client's greater independence from or dependence on nursing. In addition, the revised implementation can include the client's specific needs for health care resources.

Finally, the evaluation section of the nursing care plan is changed to correspond to the other modifications in the plan. Changes in the expected outcomes and evaluation criteria further indicate the desired level of wellness for the client and indicate when the need has been resolved and the nursing diagnosis is no longer relevant.

For example, a preoperative nursing care plan was developed for Mr. Brown. As he progressed through the postoperative period, his nursing needs changed. New data were noted in blue ink and dated. The nurse made modifications in the nursing care plan for one nursing diagnosis: potential effective airway clearance postoperatively related to abdominal incisional pain (Table 9-3).

On the second postoperative day the nurse assessed Mr. Brown and noted decreased chest wall movements,

TABLE 9-3 Modified Nursing Care Plan for Mr. Brown

Assessment	Nursing Diagnoses	Goals	Implementation	Evaluation
Has smoked two packs/day for 20 years; chest roentgenogram shows slight change of emphysema; crackles auscultated in lung field; scheduled for abdominal surgery	Potential ineffective airway clearance postoperatively related to abdominal incision	Maintain a patent airway.	Mr. Brown demonstrates turn, cough, and deep breathing.	Productive cough produced. Airways clear to auscultation.
Decreased chest wall movements; crackles in bases, do not clear with coughing	Ineffective airway clearance postoperatively related to abdominal incisional pain		Nurse administers chest physiotherapy to all lobes of the lung: 8-12-4-8-12-4.	Lung fields are clear on auscultation. Patient becomes afebrile.
		Promote airway clearance.	Mr. Brown coughs and deep breathes every 2 hours around the clock.	Chest roentgenogram demonstrates atelectasis resolving.
Chest roentgenogram shows right lower lobe atelectasis: 101°R		Promote lung expansion. Resolve atelectasis.	Nurse to suction nasotracheally every 2 hours if patient is unable to cough productively.	
		Control abdominal incisional pain.	Teach client to splint incision with pillow before and during coughing procedure.	Client does not report increased pain during coughing.

basilar rales, and elevated temperature (39° C). Mr. Brown had a standing order for a chest x-ray examination, which was taken immediately and revealed collapse of alveoli in the right lower lobe. The nursing diagnosis was revised to read "Ineffective airway clearance related to abdominal incision." The goal of "maintaining a patent airway" was still appropriate. Specific nursing interventions were developed to assist in achieving a patent airway. Finally, the projected evaluation criteria were rewritten to reflect the desired level of wellness and to indicate when the need had been resolved.

The astute nurse is sensitive to changes in the client's status and readily incorporates these changes into the nursing care plan. The health status of clients is dynamic and continuously changing. Therefore the plan of care needs to be flexible to incorporate necessary changes.

An out-of-date or incorrect nursing care plan compromises the quality of nursing care, whereas review and modification of the plan enable the nurse to provide nursing care that meets the client's needs.

Identifying Areas of Assistance

Some nursing situations require the nurse to seek assistance. The assistance can fall in the following categories: additional personnel, additional knowledge, and additional nursing skills. Before implementing care, the nurse evaluates the plan to determine the need for assistance and the type required.

Situations requiring additional personnel vary. For example, a nurse assigned to care for an overweight, immobilized client may need additional personnel to help turn, transfer, and position the client because of the physical work involved. The nurse also needs to determine when the personnel are needed. If the client is to be turned and repositioned every 2 hours, additional personnel will be needed every 2 hours. The nurse then must determine how many persons are needed and must discuss the need for assistance with potential resources. Finally, the nurse needs to take time to plan care so the additional personnel do not become overburdened.

Additional personnel are also required when a client's health status declines or when the number of clients in a unit increases. In both situations the required level of nursing care is too much for one nurse to deliver safely.

Mr. Douglas is assigned to care for two postoperative clients, Mr. West and Mrs. Jade. Two hours into the shift, Mr. West begins to hemorrhage and goes into shock. Mr. Douglas spends the next hour stabilizing Mr. West's condition. At this point he reviews the care plan for Mrs. Jade and the new care plan for Mr. West. The nurse's assessment of the situation is that for next 2 hours he will need to spend all of his time with Mr. West. He approaches his supervisor with this assessment and requests additional help for the next 2 hours.

Some nursing situations require additional knowledge and skills, as well as additional personnel. A nurse needs additional knowledge when administering a new medication or implementing a new procedure. Such information can be obtained from a hospital's formulary or procedure book. If the nurse still is uncertain about the new medication or procedure, other members of the health care team can be consulted.

Because of the continual growth of health care professions and related technology, a nurse may lack the skills needed to carry out a procedure. When this occurs, information about the procedure is obtained from the literature and the agency's procedure book. Next all the equipment necessary for the procedure is collected. Finally, another nurse who has completed the procedure correctly and safely provides assistance. The assistance can come from another staff nurse, a supervisor, an educator, or a nurse specialist.

Requesting assistance occurs frequently in all types of nursing practice and is a learning process that continues throughout educational experiences and into professional development.

Implementing Nursing Strategies

The nurse implements nursing strategies to achieve the goals of care, selecting from several methods to achieve the goals of nursing care:

1. Assisting in the performance of the activities of daily living
2. Counseling and educating the client and family
3. Giving care to achieve therapeutic goals

4. Giving care to facilitate attainment of therapeutic goals by the client
5. Supervising and evaluating the work of other staff members

The nurse is responsible for knowing when one of these methods is preferred over another and for having the necessary theoretical knowledge and psychomotor skills to implement each method. A later section introduces the general theoretical information for each method and refers to subsequent chapters that detail the necessary theoretical and psychomotor skills.

Communicating Nursing Strategies

Nursing strategies are written or communicated orally. When written, nursing strategies are incorporated into the nursing care plan and client's medical record. The nursing care plan usually reflects proposed nursing strategies. After the strategies are implemented, pertinent information is written in the client's record. This information usually includes a brief description of the nursing assessment, the specific procedure, and the client's response to nursing care.

A brief description of pertinent assessment findings in the client's medical record validates the need for a specific nursing intervention. Writing the time and the details of the intervention document that the procedure was completed. A summary of the client's response to the procedure evaluates its effectiveness.

Nursing strategies are also communicated orally from one nurse to another or to other health professionals. Nurses commonly communicate orally when changing shifts, transferring a client to another unit, or discharging a client to another health agency. Whether the nursing strategy is written or communicated orally, the language should be clear, concise, and to the point. Chapter 19 discusses communication skills necessary in nursing practice, and Chapter 14 describes skills needed to record pertinent information in the client's medical record.

IMPLEMENTATION METHODS

The nurse carries out the nursing care plan by using several implementation methods. For example, the client with a nursing diagnosis of "impaired mobility related to bilateral arm casts" may require assistance in performing activities of daily living. The client coping inadequately because of fear of a medical diagnosis requires counseling as a method of nursing action. The client with a diagnosed knowledge deficit needs interventions through health education. The totally immobilized or disoriented client requires nursing interventions providing total client care. Yet another method of implementation of the nursing care plan involves the supervision and evaluation of other members of the health care team.

For each nursing diagnosis the nurse is able to identify the need for one specific implementation method rather than another. Each method of implementation includes specific theoretical knowledge and clinical skills.

Assisting with Activities of Daily Living

Activities of daily living (ADLs) are activities usually performed in the course of a normal day, such as eating, dressing, bathing, brushing the teeth, or grooming. Conditions resulting in the need for assistance with ADLs can be acute, chronic, temporary, permanent, or rehabilitative. An acute disease is characterized by symptoms that are usually severe and that are present for a relatively short period of time, usually less than 6 months. An episode of acute disease results in (1) recovery to a state of health and activity comparable to the client's state before the disease, (2) passage into a chronic phase of the disease, or (3) death. For example, the postoperative client is unable to complete ADLs independently because of the acute health problem, surgery. As the client progresses through the postoperative period, he gradually depends less on nurses for completing ADLs.

A chronic disease persists longer. Although the symptoms of chronic disease are usually less severe than those of the acute phase of the same disease, chronic disease may result in complete or partial disability. A client with partial paralysis after a cerebrovascular accident has a chronic impairment requiring long-term assistance with ADLs.

The client's need for assistance with ADLs may be temporary, permanent, or rehabilitative. In the case of temporary assistance with ADLs, the client needs assistance during a specific time period. A client with impaired mobility because of bilateral arm casts has a temporary need for assistance. After removal of the casts the client will gradually assume responsibility for ADLs. A client with a total self-care deficit related to an injury high in the cervical spinal cord has a permanent need for assistance. It is unrealistic for the nurse to plan a rehabilitation program with the goal that the client will be able to independently complete all ADLs. This client may have a rehabilitative need for assistance with ADLs. Through rehabilitation the client will learn new ways to perform ADLs, thus becoming more independent and better able to perform self-care.

Through the assessment the nurse collects data that verify the need for assistance with ADLs. As the nurse analyzes this data, nursing diagnoses are formed in relation to such assistance.

Counseling

Counseling is an implementation method that helps the client use a problem-solving process to recognize and manage stress and that facilitates interpersonal relationships between the client and family, significant others, or health care team. Nurses provide counseling to help the client accept actual or impending changes resulting from stress. Counseling is emotional, intellectual, spiritual, and psychological support. Clients and their families in need of nursing counseling are those who have "normal" adjustment difficulties and are upset or frustrated but who are not psychologically disabled (McGowan and Schmidt, 1962). Psychologically disabled clients require counseling by nurses specializing in psychiatric nursing, social workers, psychiatrists, or psychologists.

Many counseling techniques are used to foster cognitive, behavioral, developmental, experiential, and emotional growth in clients (see box). Counseling encourages individuals to examine available alternatives and to decide which choices are useful and appropriate. When clients are able to examine alternatives, they can develop a sense of control and are able to better manage stress. To assist clients in need of counseling techniques, the nurse must be able to identify the need for counseling and possess communication skills to develop a therapeutic relationship with clients (Sundeen et al., 1988).

Clients, families, or significant others needing counseling include persons who must adjust their life-style patterns, such as stopping smoking, reducing weight, or decreasing their activity levels. Clients coping with chronic or disabling diseases require counseling to help them accept changes in life-style or body image as the disease progresses. During life-threatening illnesses, clients and families or significant others need counseling to cope with the possibility of death.

Teaching

Counseling is closely aligned to teaching. Both involve using communication skills to effect a change in the

---

Examples of Counseling Strategies Used by Nurses

- Behavior modification
- Bereavement counseling
- Biofeedback
- Relaxation training
- Reality orientation
- Crisis intervention
- Guided imagery
- Play therapy

client. However, with counseling the change results in the development of new attitudes and feelings, whereas in teaching the focus of change is intellectual growth or the acquisition of new knowledge or psychomotor skills (Redman, 1988).

Teaching is an implementation method used to present correct principles, procedures, and techniques of health care to clients and to inform clients about their health status. As a nursing responsibility, teaching is implemented in all health care settings. The nurse is responsible for assessing the learning needs of clients and is accountable for the quality of education delivered.

The teaching-learning process is an interaction between the teacher and learner in which specific learning objectives are presented (Redman, 1988). The teaching-learning process provides the organizational structure and framework for client education. The teaching-learning process is much like the basic nursing process and has the following components: assessment, diagnosis, planning, implementation, and evaluation.

During assessment the nurse determines the client's learning needs and readiness to learn. The nurse then intreprets the data to formulate nursing diagnoses reflecting these learning needs. In planning, the nurse and client establish learning goals. Implementation is the initiation of the teaching strategies that are designed to achieve the learning goal. Finally, evaluation measures the learning that has occurred. The purpose of the teaching-learning process is to develop and implement a teaching plan individualized for the client's needs, level of knowledge, and learning resources.

Giving Care to Achieve the Client's Goals

To achieve the therapeutic goals for the client, the nurse initiates interventions to compensate for adverse reactions, uses precautionary and preventive measures in providing care, applies correct techniques in administering care and preparing the client for special procedures, and initiates lifesaving measures in emergency situations. The following sections briefly discuss the nursing interventions in these areas. The specific knowledge and skills needed to carry out these nursing procedures are detailed in subsequent chapters to which the student is referred.

COMPENSATION FOR ADVERSE REACTIONS

An adverse reaction is a harmful or unintended effect of a medication, diagnostic test, or therapeutic intervention. Adverse reactions can follow independent, dependent, or interdependent nursing interventions. Nursing actions that compensate for adverse reactions reduce or counteract the reaction. To intervene, the nurse must have knowledge about the potential undesired effects. For example, when administering a medication, the

nurse understands the known and potential side effects of the drug. After administration of the medication the nurse assesses the client for any side effects. The nurse should be aware of drugs that can counteract the side effects. For example, a client may have an unknown hypersensitivity to penicillin, and hives develop after three doses. The nurse records the reaction and stops administration of the drug. The nurse also consults the physician's standing orders and administers an antipruritic medication to relieve the itching and an antihistamine to reduce the allergic response.

In caring for a client who is undergoing or who has undergone a particular diagnostic test, the nurse uses an understanding of the test and its potential adverse effects. For example, a client has not had a bowel movement in 24 hours after a barium enema. Because a bowel impaction is a potential side effect of a barium enema, the nurse administers increased fluids, gives a stool-softening medication, and instructs the client to let the nursing personnel know when a bowel movement occurs.

Therapeutic interventions may also have potential harmful side effects.

Ms. Rice, the nurse, assesses that Mr. Allen has a small area of skin breakdown. Ms. Rice develops interventions designed to prevent further skin breakdown and to promote wound healing. She plans a heat lamp treatment to the skin for 20 minutes twice a day, selects the wattage for the bulb of the lamp, places the lamp 24 inches from the client's skin, and checks the client after 10 minutes. When reassessing the client's skin, Ms. Rice finds that there are no adverse effects of the treatment and resumes the treatment for another 10 minutes. After the second 10 minutes of treatment the nurse notices that the skin is reddened and the area of breakdown has increased. To counteract the increased skin breakdown, the nurse discontinues the treatment and institutes another skin care measure to reduce skin breakdown and promote wound healing.

Although adverse effects are not common, they do occur. The nurse learns potential side effects, is able to recognize the presence of an adverse reaction, and is able to intervene accordingly.

PREVENTIVE MEASURES

Preventive nursing actions are directed toward preventing illness and promoting health to avoid the need for secondary or tertiary health care. Prevention includes assessment and promotion of the client's health potential, application of prescribed measures such as immunizations, health teaching, early diagnosis and treatment, and development of rehabilitation potential.

In the case of a client who has a hypersensitivity to penicillin, the nurse can implement several preventive measures. The nurse indicates the penicillin allergy in the client's medical record, informs the client and family of the need for a Medic-Alert bracelet, and teaches them actions they should take if the client is given penicillin again. The nurse also teaches the client and family about the allergy and specific drugs to avoid.

Preventive nursing actions are used to meet the therapeutic goals of the client. Through preventive actions the nurse is able to help the client attain the highest level of wellness.

CORRECT TECHNIQUES IN ADMINISTERING CARE AND PREPARING A CLIENT FOR PROCEDURES

The administration of nursing care requires the nurse to be experienced in many techniques, methods followed in performing specific procedures such as administering medications, changing clients' dressings, or inserting Foley catheters. Client care, particularly in the hospital setting, involves many techniques. Every procedure the nurse does for the client is carried out by a specific method.

To carry out a procedure, the nurse must be knowledgeable about the procedure itself, when it is needed, how to do it, and its expected outcome. In a hospital the nurse is required to complete many procedures each day. Some of these procedures might be new, so before entering into a new procedure the nurse assesses personal competencies and determines the need for assistance, new knowledge, or new skills.

LIFESAVING MEASURES

A lifesaving measure is an independent, dependent, or interdependent nursing intervention implemented when a client's physiological or psychological state is threatened. The purpose of the lifesaving measure is to restore physiological or psychological equilibrium. Such measures include administering emergency medications, instituting cardiopulmonary resuscitation (CPR), restraining a confused or violent client, and obtaining immediate counseling from a crisis center for a severely anxious client.

The initiation of lifesaving measures is an essential component of nursing practice. As with any procedure the nurse must be knowledgeable about the lifesaving procedure itself, when it is necessary, how to do it, and its expected outcome. If an inexperienced nurse happens on a situation requiring emergency measures, the proper nursing action is to get an experienced professional.

Giving Care to Facilitate the Client's Attainment of Health Goals

The nurse facilitates the attainment of health goals by providing an environment conducive to meeting health care goals, adjusting care in accordance with clients' expressed or implied needs, stimulating and motivating clients thereby enabling them to achieve self-care and independence, and encouraging them to accept care or adhere to the treatment regimen. In each of the nursing interventions the nurse and client work together to meet the goals they developed during the analysis component. With some interventions nurses assume a more active role, and with others they assume a more passive role.

Nurses have the capacity to create a health care environment conducive to achieving the client's goals. Ideally the nurse develops an environment that provides the client with adequate privacy for meeting basic needs and that allows him to feel safe and free to interact with the health care team. An early step in creating an appropriate environment is to orient the client and family to the health care agency. If it is a hospital, the client needs to be acquainted with the room, the health care team, and other clients. A client in a clinic should be made acquainted with clinic policies and procedures, location of restrooms and cafeterias, and the health care team. When the client receives care in the home, the nurse should take time to acquaint the client and family with the purposes of and expectations about the home visit.

Whether the client is in the hospital, an outpatient clinic, or a community setting, the nurse takes measures to provide for privacy. Obviously, clients need privacy to carry out activities of hygiene, grooming, and elimination. In addition, they need privacy to talk with their families, friends, or members of the health care team. In an environment of privacy the client feels free to share concerns, ask questions about diagnosis and treatment, and resolve personal problems.

Nursing care and other therapeutic measures are designed to meet the client's needs. As a further aid in the attainment of health care goals, the nursing care plan includes some flexibility so the client is not placed into a fixed routine. Obviously the degree of flexibility depends on the nature of the need, the severity of the client's disability or illness, and the client's dependence on nursing care. However, even the smallest degree of flexibility, giving the client an opportunity to have some choice about the type or timing of nursing care, is valuable.

Clients with severe and chronic diseases need to be encouraged to increase their level of self-care and independence, a difficult task often disheartening for the client and nurse. To avoid discouraging the client, it is best to attempt to achieve this nursing goal gradually. The nursing care plan is implemented so the client successfully achieves one level of independence before attempting the next.

Mr. Porter is a 50-year-old executive, husband, and father of three teenagers. He is recovering from a severe myocardial infarction and cardiac arrest. For the past 10 days all of Mr.

Porter's hygiene and grooming needs have been met by the nursing staff. One day Mr. Porter expresses doubts of ever getting his energy back and being able to care for himself. That evening Mr. Martin, a student nurse, assesses Mr. Porter and develops a nursing care plan. One of the goals is complete self-care by Mr. Porter within 1 week. With the help of his instructor, Mr. Martin implements the following nursing care plan, which is designed to achieve the overall goal of independence in various phases:

Day 1	Wash face and comb hair
Day 2	Wash face, shave, and comb hair
Day 3	Feed himself breakfast, wash face, shave, and comb hair
Day 4	Feed himself meals, wash face, shave, and comb hair
Day 5	Perform grooming activities and feed himself
Day 6	Perform grooming activities and feed himself
Day 7	Shower

Each day included achievable tasks for Mr. Porter. Placing the tasks in sequential order served the following purposes: (1) each task was developed with the knowledge that Mr. Porter could indeed successfully complete the activity, (2) a sequence of successes motivated Mr. Porter to continue with the plan, and (3) the sequence was designed to gradually increase Mr. Porter's activity tolerance.

Clients with chronic diseases are frequently on a regimen that requires strict adherence to the treatment modalities. Client adherence means the client and family must invest time in carrying out the required home treatments. For example, a client with chronic obstructive pulmonary disease must spend several hours a day performing respiratory therapies designed to keep the airway open and to maintain an acceptable level of wellness.

Some treatment plans include the need for the client and the family to adjust to functional changes as a result of medications. For example, a client with high blood pressure treated with methyldopa (Aldomet) occasionally feels increasingly fatigued during the early stages of treatment, or a client with cancer who is undergoing chemotherapy has changes in energy level and body image as a result of the medication.

Finally, adherence to treatment plans can require an increased financial investment by the client and family. For example, a cardiac client's two-story house may no longer be suitable, since the client is unable to climb stairs without feeling short of breath. Thus the client and family must invest in a new house.

Investments of time, money, and personal resources for a long period of time can discourage the client and his family. The discouraged client may neglect the treatment regimen. Once the client begins to reduce his adherence to treatment, his level of wellness declines.

Nurses are able to intervene and assist clients in adhering to a treatment plan. Adequate discharge planning and education of the client and family help promote a smooth transition from one health care setting to another or to the home and help to increase the client's level of knowledge about the treatment plan. Counseling the client and family helps them adapt to change resulting from the disease process or treatment. Continuity of care also provides a supportive professional familiar with the client's pattern of living, pattern of wellness, and treatment. In addition, reinforcing successes with the treatment plan encourages the client to adhere to the regimen.

Supervising and Evaluating the Work of Other Staff Members

The nurse who develops the nursing care plan frequently does not perform all the nursing interventions. Some of these interventions may be delegated to another member of the health care team. Noninvasive interventions such as skin care, range of joint motion exercises, ambulating, grooming, and performing hygiene measures can be assigned to another staff nurse, a nursing assistant, or a licensed practical nurse. The nurse assigning tasks is responsible for ensuring that each task is assigned to an individual skilled in it. The nurse is also responsible for ensuring that the delegated task was completed according to the standard of care.

SUMMARY

In the fourth component of the nursing process, implementation, the nurse initiates and carries out the objectives of the nursing care plan. During implementation the nurse completes dependent, independent, and interdependent nursing interventions.

As with the other components of the nursing process, implementation itself is a process. It is comprised of the following steps: reassessing the client, reviewing and modifying the existing nursing care plan, identifying areas of assistance, implementing nursing strategies, and communicating nursing strategies. During reassessment the nurse focuses on one part of the total nursing assessment to determine the presence of changes affecting nursing interventions. The nurse gathers and analyzes data from the reassessment and reviews or modifies the nursing care plan as needed. The review and modification of the plan reflect the client's current health care needs and appropriate nursing actions. Before implementing nursing strategies the nurse identifies areas of assistance requiring additional personnel, knowledge, or nursing skills. After the implementation of nursing strategies the nurse writes or communicates orally the specific nursing intervention and client responses.

Nursing strategies are selected from five methods, including assisting with activities of daily living, counseling and teaching, giving care to achieve the therapeutic goals for the client, giving care to facilitate the attainment of health care goals by the client, and supervising and evaluating the work of other staff members. Each implementation method requires the nurse to use theoretical knowledge and clinical skills.

Knowledge of the implementation process and the selection of appropriate nursing strategies enable the nurse to provide individualized and competent care. Through implementation, strategies are designed to accomplish the goals delineated in the nursing care plan.

KEY CONCEPTS

✓ The purpose of implementation is to carry out the nursing care plan developed in the planning component.

✓ Three types of interventions exist, including dependent, independent, and interdependent.

✓ Dependent nursing interventions are completed with a physician's order but require nursing judgment or decision making.

✓ Independent nursing interventions can solve the client's problems without consultation or collaboration with physicians or other nonnursing professionals.

✓ Interdependent nursing interventions are completed with or without a physician's order or are written at a nurse's suggestion and can provide the solution to the client's problem in a collaborative manner with judgment and recommendations of the interdisciplinary health team.

✓ A protocol is a written plan specifying a procedure or a series of procedures to be followed for selected situations.

✓ A standing order is a written document containing rules, policies, procedures, regulations, and orders for the conduct of client care in various stipulated settings.

✓ Implementation requires the nurse to reassess the client, review and modify the existing nursing care plan, identify areas in which assistance is needed, implement nursing strategies, and communicate nursing strategies.

✓ The nursing care plan is modified as a client's level of wellness and health care needs change.

✓ The implementation of nursing care may require additional knowledge, nursing skills, and personnel.

✓ After implementation the nurse writes in the client's record a brief description of the nursing assessment, specific procedures, and client's response to nursing care.

✓ Implementation methods fall into the following categories: assisting with activities of daily living, counseling and teaching, giving care to achieve therapeutic goals, giving care to facilitate attainment of health goals, and supervising other personnel.

✓ Counseling helps the client use problem solving to recognize and manage stress and facilitates interpersonal relationships between the client and the family, significant others, or health care team.

✓ Teaching is used to present correct principles, procedures, and techniques of health care to the client, to inform clients about their health status, and to refer the client and family to appropriate resources.

✓ Nursing actions to achieve therapeutic goals include compensation for adverse reactions, preventive measures, correct techniques for administering care and preparing the client for procedures, and lifesaving measures.

✓ Nursing actions facilitating attainment of health goals include providing a conducive environment, adjusting care to fit the client's needs, and stimulating and motivating the client.

✓ Delegating care to other personnel involves ensuring that the individuals assigned are skilled in the tasks and evaluating that each task was completed according to the standard of care.

✓ To complete any nursing procedure the nurse must be knowledgeable about the procedure, when it is needed, how to do it, and its expected outcome.

REFERENCES

American Nurses' Association: Nursing: A social policy statement, Kansas City, Mo, 1980, The Association.

Grier, M: The need for data in making nursing decisions. In Werley, H, and Grier, M, editors: Nursing information systems, New York, 1981, Springer Publishing Co., Inc.

Kim, MJ: Degree of independence of nursing interventions for nursing diagnoses. In Hurley, MA, editor: Classification of nursing diagnoses: Proceedings of the Sixth Conference, (NANDA), St. Louis, 1986, The C.V. Mosby Co.

McGowan, JF, and Schmidt, JF: Counseling: readings in theory and practice, New York, 1962, Holt, Rinehart, & Winston, Inc.

Redman, BK: The process of patient teaching in nursing, ed. 6, St. Louis, 1988, The C.V. Mosby Co.

Snyder, M: Independent nursing interventions, New York, 1985, John Wiley & Sons, Inc.

Sundeen, SJ, et al.: Nurse-client interaction: implementing the nursing process, St. Louis, ed. 4, 1988, The C.V. Mosby Co.

Research Article

Kim, MJ: Nursing diagnoses: a Janus view. In Hurley, ME, editor: Classification of nursing diagnoses: Proceedings of the Sixth Conference (NANDA), St. Louis, 1986, The C.V. Mosby Co.

ADDITIONAL READINGS

Brown, JJ, Fanner, CA, and Padrick, KP: Nursing's search for scientific knowledge, Nurs Res 33:26, 1984.

Carpenito, LJ: Nursing diagnosis application to clinical practice, Philadelphia, 1983, J.B. Lippincott Co.

Chesney, MA: Behavior modification and health enhancement. In Matarazzo, JD, et al.: Behavioral health: a handbook of health enhancement and disease prevention, New York, 1984, John Wiley & Sons, Inc.

Duff, RS, and Hollingshead, AB: Sickness and society, New York, 1968, Harper & Row, Publishers, Inc.

Halloran, E, and Kiley, M: Case mix management for nurses, Nurs Manage 15(2):39, 1984.

Iyer, PW, Taptich, BJ, and Bernocchi-Losey, D: Nursing process and nursing diagnosis, Philadelphia, 1986, W.B. Saunders Co.

LeBou, MD: Behavior modification: a significant method in nursing practice, Englewood Cliffs, N.J., 1973, Prentice-Hall, Inc.

Marriner, A: The nursing process: a scientific approach to nursing care, ed. 4, St. Louis, 1987, The C.V. Mosby Co.

McMurrey, PH: Toward a unique knowledge base in nursing, Image: J Nurs Sch 14:12, 1982.

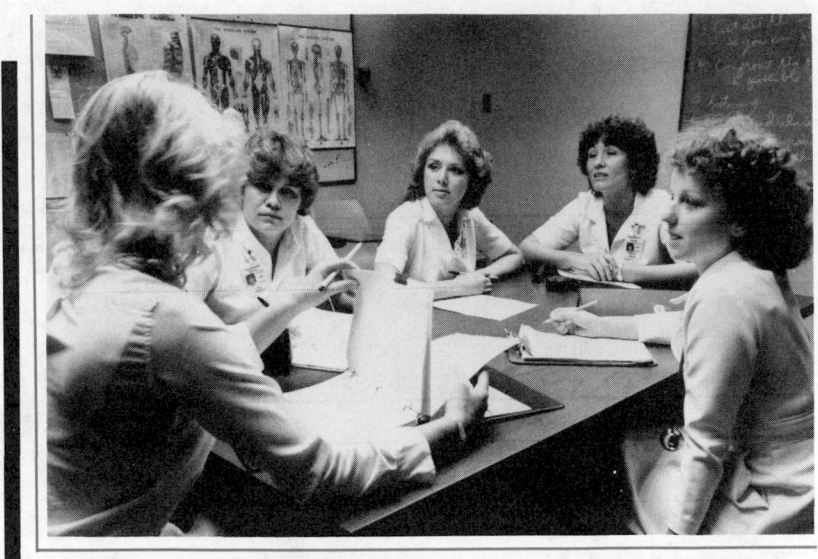

OBJECTIVES

Mastery of content in this chapter will enable the student to:

- Define the key terms listed.
- State and discuss the four steps of the evaluation process.
- Describe interaction between the components of the nursing process.
- Evaluate the nursing actions selected for an assigned client.

KEY TERMS

Concurrent Nursing Audit

Evaluation

Nursing Audit

Nursing Research

Outcome

Quality Assurance

Evaluation

The evaluation component of the nursing process measures the client's response to nursing actions, progress toward achieving goals, the quality of nursing care provided in an institution or agency, and the level of nursing care for a client. Evaluation is a category of nursing behavior in which the nurse makes and records a determination about the extent to which the client's goals have been met.

The consequences of nursing intervention can be positive or negative or expected or unexpected. The effects of intervention must be evaluated periodically and the nursing implementation changed accordingly. The frequency of evaluation and reevaluation depends on the situation (Marriner, 1983). A client whose health status is continually changing requires more frequent evaluations or reassessments.

Nursing care is evaluated through a continuous process determining:

1. The client's response to nursing actions as measured against the expected outcomes established during planning
2. The client's progress toward achieving short- and long-term goals
3. The presence of new health care needs
4. The need to modify the existing nursing care plan

Evaluation includes comparison of observed results, such as reversal of symptoms, improved energy level, and proper use of equipment by the client, with outcome criteria. Positive evaluations can lead the nurse to conclude that the plan was effective in meeting the client's goals. Negative evaluations indicate that the problem was not solved and that modifications in the plan are necessary. In addition, the evaluation process can identify specific factors resulting in the success or failure of the plan.

The evaluation component of the nursing process is oriented toward the client receiving nursing care, as well as toward the institution providing the care. Individual evaluation focuses on the client's response to nursing therapies, the progress of the client toward achieving goals of nursing care, and the development of new health care needs. Institutional evaluation uses legal criteria and professional standards to judge quality of care.

EVALUATION PROCESS

Establishment of Outcome Criteria

The criteria for the effectiveness of nursing actions are based on the expected outcomes developed during planning (see Chapter 8). Expected outcomes are stated in behavioral terms to describe the desired effect of nursing actions. Inclusion of expected outcomes in the care plan gives the nurse an objective determinant as to when and how goals have been achieved.

Scientific principles, supported by nursing research findings, increase the theoretical base from which the expected outcomes are derived. Nursing research is a detailed process in which a systematic study of a problem in the field of nursing is performed (see Chapter 11). The problem may be identified in areas of clinical practice, and the scientific method is implemented to solve the problem. Nursing research is essential for the continued development of the scientific aspects of professional nursing.

The evaluation process determines the quality of nursing care in relation to accepted standards of care. A standard is an established basis of comparison in measuring or judging capacity, quantity, content, and value of objects in the same category. The ANA (1974) has developed eight standards of nursing practice used to promote high-quality care (Table 10-1). These standards encourage the nurse to assess the total client, to analyze his health care needs, to develop goals and nursing actions, and to evaluate the client's response to the nursing actions (Barba, Bennett, and Shaw, 1978). Furthermore, the ANA standards are based on the nursing process (Table 10-1). The evaluation of the quality of nursing care is also based on the correct use of the components of the nursing process.

Each hospital uses evaluation to establish its own system for nursing audits. These audits resulted from the 1972 and 1973 revisions of the standards of the Joint Commission on Accreditation of Health Care Organizations. Basically the revisions required medical and nursing audits in hospitals seeking accreditation (Barba, Bennett, and Shaw, 1987).

More detail on nursing audits is presented in the "Quality Assurance" section of this chapter.

Comparison of Client Response to Outcome Criteria

After the expected outcomes have been established and recorded, the nurse compares the client response with expected outcomes. After completing the nursing action, the nurse collects additional data, for example, through the use of one of the following assessment techniques: observation, palpation, percussion, and auscultation. The new data are compared with the outcome

TABLE 10-1 Correlation of the ANA Standards of Practice and the Components of the Nursing Process

Standard	Nursing Process
The collection of data about the health status of the client is systematic and continuous. The data are accessible, communicated, and recorded.	Assessment
Nursing diagnoses are derived from health status data.	Nursing diagnosis
The plan of nursing care includes goals derived from the nursing diagnoses.	Planning
The plan of nursing care includes priorities and prescribed nursing approaches or measures to achieve the goals derived from the nursing diagnoses.	
Nursing actions provide for client participation in health promotion, maintenance, and restoration.	Implementation
Nursing actions assist the client to maximize his health capabilities.	
The client's progress or lack of progress toward goal achievement is determined by the client and the nurse.	Evaluation
The client's progress or lack of progress toward goal achievement directs reassessment, recording of priorities, new goal setting, and revision of the plan of care.	

From ANA standards of nursing practice, Am Nurs 6:11, 1974.

TABLE 10-2   Use of Evaluation Measures to Determine the Success of Client Goals and Expected Outcomes

Goals	Evaluation Measures	Expected Outcomes
Client maintains patent airway	Auscultate client's lungs.	All lung fields clear to auscultation.
	Observe client's ability to cough.	Client able to cough productively.
Improved activity tolerance	Palpate client's radial pulse.	Pulse remains below 110 BPM.
	Palpate client's radial pulse 10 minutes after exercise.	Return to baseline pulse rate within 10 minutes after exercise.
	Observe and ask client about perception of dyspnea or breathlessness.	Decreased reports of dyspnea. Respiratory rate remains within 2 breaths of client's baseline rate.

criteria to determine what changes have occurred and if the changes were predicted (Table 10-2).

A decision is then made about the success or failure of the nursing therapies (Iyer, Taptich, and Bernocchi-Losey, 1986). Use of selected evaluation methods results in reassessment of client, which starts the nursing process over. Once again, the nurse collects and validates data, clusters and interprets the data, formulates new or modified nursing diagnoses, establishes priorities, develops client goals, selects outcome criteria, and plans and implements nursing therapies (Marriner, 1983).

Analysis of Variables Affecting Outcomes and Conclusions

The data and comparisons obtained during the second step of the evaluation process enable the nurse to determine the degree to which the plan of care was effective. In addition, the nurse is able to draw conclusions about possible factors that led to the success or failure of the plan of care.

The new data collected about Mr. Brown indicate the plan (Table 10-3) was not effective for "maintaining a patent airway postoperatively." The nurse must reassess, reanalyze client data, and evaluate the nursing plan to determine the reason the plan was ineffective.

To determine the reason the plan failed, the nurse first reassesses the client for new data. During the reassessment of Mr. Brown, the nurse notes that he is well hydrated, has symmetrical chest wall movements, has crackles in the right middle lobe, has a rectal temperature of 102°F, does not splint the abdominal incision, has requested an analgesic five times since surgery, and has clear chest x-rays. During reanalysis the significant new assessment findings of not splinting the abdominal incision and frequent need for analgesia lead the nurse to revise the nursing diagnosis to read "ineffective airway clearance related to abdominal incisional pain."

Perhaps one reason for the failure of the initial plan for Mr. Brown was that an incorrect nursing diagnosis was initially developed. The first nursing diagnosis of "potential ineffective airway clearance postoperatively related to abdominal incision" did not include incisional pain as a probable cause. Therefore the plan and subsequent implementation did not provide any nursing actions for the control of incisional pain.

TABLE 10-3   Nursing Care Plan for Mr. Brown

Assessment	Nursing Diagnosis	Goal	Implementation	Evaluation (Expected Outcomes)
40 pack-year history of smoking	Potential ineffective airway clearance postoperatively related to abdominal incision	Maintain a patent airway postoperatively.	Demonstrate turn, cough, and deep breathing.	Mr. Brown correctly demonstrates procedures.
Chest roentgenogram shows flattened diaphragms and hyperinflated lungs			Turn, cough, and deep breathe every 2 hours around the clock on first and second postoperative days.	Lung fields clear on auscultation.
Crackles auscultated in lung fields				Patient remains afebrile.
Scheduled for abdominal surgery				Chest roentgenogram does not show infiltrate on auscultation.

TABLE 10-4   Modification of Nursing Care Plan for Mr. Brown

Assessment	Nursing Diagnosis	Goal	Implementation	Evaluation (Expected Outcomes)
40 pack-year history of smoking	Ineffective airway clearance related to abdominal incisional pain	Client reports less abdominal pain while maintaining a patent airway.	Administer analgesics every 4 hours during first 48 hours.	Pain controlled by analgesics and splinting of incision
Chest x-ray examination shows no evidence of consolidation			Splint abdominal incision with two pillows during coughing.	Lung fields clear on auscultation
Crackles present in right middle lobe			Turn, cough, and deep breathe every 2 hours around the clock for 48 hours.	Afebrile Chest x-ray film clear
Rectal temperature of 102°F				
Does not splint abdominal incision				
Used analgesics five times since surgery				

A second factor in the failure of the plan can be found in implementation. Nursing actions should be safe, effective, and efficient and should provide comfort. The nursing action of turn, cough, and deep breathe every 2 hours is a safe intervention. Nursing research has documented that this is an effective, efficient, and comfortable method for mobilizing pulmonary secretions postoperatively. However, because the initial nursing diagnosis for Mr. Brown was incorrect, he was uncomfortable during the procedure and was unable to cough as productively as he might have if the nursing actions implemented had included measures for minimizing his abdominal incisional pain, such as timed analgesic medication and splinting the abdominal incision.

Therefore the plan for Mr. Brown was ineffective because of an inaccurate nursing diagnosis and subsequent nursing strategies. With these conclusions the nurse knows why the plan failed and what modifications are necessary.

Modifications in the Nursing Care Plan

Modifications in the plan of care are based on conclusions developed during the third step of the evaluation process. Two conclusions were made for Mr. Brown. First, the nursing diagnosis should have read "potential ineffective airway clearance related to abdominal incisional pain." Second, the nursing actions developed for the implementation component should have included nursing strategies to control his incisional pain. Once these conclusions were reached, the nursing care plan for Mr. Brown was modified (Table 10-4)

Modifications alone are not enough. The nurse must implement the new plan and reevaluate the client's response to the nursing actions. Therefore evaluation of care is a continuous process. Reevaluation showed that Mr. Brown was afebrile, coughing productively, and properly splinting his incision, and that his lung fields were clear on auscultation.

BENEFITS OF EVALUATION

Evaluation of nursing care, the nursing audit, is time consuming and in some situations can be perceived by the nurse as threatening. However, changes in nursing procedures and health care delivery cannot be achieved without changes in the knowledge, abilities, awareness, and perceptions of the nurses providing care.

Clients benefit from well-developed quality assurance programs because they receive better care. Nurses benefit from such a program because it stresses the need to know, to do, to evaluate, and to document (Moore, 1979). Therefore nurses expand their knowledge and skills and become more proficient professionals.

Quality Monitoring Incident

SECTION A

Information to be Obtained from Recorded Patient Information

1.302   ARE RESPIRATORY RATE AND QUALITY RECORDED?

     Applies to patients with respiratory conditions, conditions in which respiratory involvement is anticipated, or when otherwise necessary, e.g., stroke patient, patient on respirator, hyperglycemic patient, etc.

     Quality refers to descriptions, such as shallow, labored Cheyne-Stokes, retracting, etc. Must be recorded within past 48 hours. Both rate and quality necessary for yes answer.

        No   1
        Yes   2
        Not Applicable   3

1.408   IS THE PLAN FOR TURNING AND POSITIONING THE PATIENT STATED IN WRITING, E.G., IN THE NURSING CARE PLAN, KARDEX, ETC.?

     If not stated in writing to see if applicable, may ask nurse: "IS MR.   ABLE TO TURN AND POSITION HIMSELF?"

        Code NA only if patient does not need to be turned or positioned. Accept only written plan.

        No   1
        Yes   2
        Not Applicable   3

2.603   IF ATTENTION TO THE PATIENT'S ORAL FLUID INTAKE IS INDICATED, E.G., ENCOURAGE, FORCE OR RESTRICT FLUIDS, ARE THE FOLLOWING STATED?

   A.   TIME FLUIDS ARE TO BE GIVEN.

        No   1
        Yes   2
        Not Applicable   3

   B.   KINDS OF FLUIDS TO BE GIVEN

        No   1
        Yes   2
        Not Applicable   3

   C.   AMOUNT OF FLUIDS TO BE GIVEN.

        No   1
        Yes   2
        Not Applicable   3

4001, 01

Fig. 10-1 Nursing audit form.

Quality Assurance

Quality assurance is an ongoing, systematic, comprehensive evaluation of health care services and the impact of those services on the health care consumer. The overall goal of a quality assurance program is to ensure excellent health care. These programs contain two components, including the documentation that standards of care are met and the introduction of changes in health care delivery based on objective measurements (Maciorowski, Larson, and Keane, 1985).

The Joint Commission on Accreditation of Healthcare Organizations (JCAHO) requirement for quality assurance includes seven components (see box). These components result in problem resolution based on explicit, knowledgeable use of a logical approach to problem solving (Meisenheimer, 1983).

A nursing audit is a thorough investigation designed to identify, examine, or verify the performance of certain specified aspects of nursing care using established professional standards. Only a concurrent nursing audit—an evaluation of nursing care while the client receives care—is required of health care agencies. The concurrent nursing audit occurs frequently while the client is in the hospital.

The purpose of the audit is to evaluate the overall nursing care the client receives. Frequently the person who performs the audit is a nurse working in a different nursing unit from the one for which the audit is taking place. To ensure consistency in audits from one nurse to another, each agency develops its own form. The audit form is a checklist including specific criteria for each category of care (Fig. 10-1). Although different in structure and style, audit forms are consistent in evaluating all levels of nursing care activities as included within the nursing process and the ANA standards of nursing practice.

The establishment and use of evaluation criteria provide a standard for determining the client's response to a specific nursing action, as well as the quality of nursing care being delivered. The criteria are a mechanism for improving delivery of health care to clients.

Nursing Process

Because health care delivery agencies provide nursing care, it is imperative that these agencies measure the quality of that care. One such method of measuring the quality of health care is through quality assurance programs. However, the evaluation component of the nursing process can assure assessment of care delivered to all clients, whose nursing care plan was based on a nursing process model.

Lillisand and Korff (1983) have documented the following benefits of nursing process evaluation: (1) improved quality of nursing care, (2) improved attitude and motivation on the part of staff nurses to improve knowledge and skills, and (3) staff growth and development. The last benefit assists nurses in self-appraisal of assessment competencies, knowledge, and delivery of care. As a result, nurses independently seek informal and formal education and continuing education to resolve any perceived deficiencies.

SUMMARY

The evaluation process determines the effectiveness of the nursing care plan, is continuous, and interacts with other components of the nursing process. During evaluation the nurse compares client response with expected outcomes, which serve as evaluation criteria. As the nurse assesses the client's response, he or she determines whether the plan was a success or failure and why.

If the goals were achieved, the nursing plan was successful. A successful plan can be individualized for use with other clients with similar health care needs and goals.

If the plan failed, the nurse uses problem solving to determine why. The nurse must determine why it failed before the problem can be resolved.

If a plan has failed to meet the client's health care needs and the goals of nursing care, the needs must be reassessed and rediagnosed, and the plan must be modified, reimplemented, and reevaluated. This shows the continuous nature of the nursing process.

Quality assurance programs in agencies assist in evaluating the quality of total care provided for all clients. These programs enable nurses to define where strengths, as well as errors or omissions, occur in nursing care.

> ### *Seven Components of a Quality Assurance Program*
>
> - Identification of problems
> - Setting of priorities for problem assessment and problem resolution
> - Establishment of clinically valid criteria
> - Selection of assessment methodology
> - Identification of problem causes
> - Implementation of corrective action
> - Evaluation of problem resolution

KEY CONCEPTS

✓ Evaluation determines the extent to which goals of care have been met.

✓ The nurse evaluates the client response to nursing actions against expected outcomes established during the planning component.

✓ The nurse evaluates the client's progress toward achieving goals.

✓ Evaluation may uncover new health care needs.

✓ The nursing care plan is modified based on data obtained during evaluation.

✓ Projected outcomes are stated in behavioral terms to describe the desired effect of nursing actions.

✓ Projected outcomes provide an objective determinant as to when and how nursing goals have been achieved.

✓ Evaluation of client response determines the degree of success of the nursing care plan.

✓ Assessment data gathered during evaluation determine the need to revise and modify the plan of care.

✓ The evaluation process enables the nurse to determine the reason the nursing plan was successful or unsuccessful.

REFERENCES

ANA standards of nursing practice, Am Nurse 6:11, 1974.

Barba, M, Bennett, B, and Shaw, WJ: The evaluation of patient care through use of ANA's standards of nursing practice, Superv Nurse 9:42, 1978.

Iyer, PW, Taptich, BJ, and Bernocchi-Losey, D: Nursing process and nursing diagnosis, Philadelphia, 1986, W.B. Saunders Co.

Maciorowski, LF, Larson, E, and Keane, A: Quality assurance evaluate thyself, J Nurs Adm 15(6):38, 1985.

Marriner, A: The nursing process; a scientific approach to nursing care, St. Louis, 1983, The C.V. Mosby Co.

Meisenheimer, CG: Incorporating JCAH standards into a quality assurance program, Nurs Adm Q 7(3):1, 1983.

Moore, KR: What nurses learn from nursing audit, Nurs Outlook 27(4):254, 1979.

Research Article

Lillesand, KM, and Korff, S: Nursing process evaluation: a quality assurance tool, Nurs Adm Q 7(3):9, 1983.

ADDITIONAL READINGS

Anderson, PA, and Davis, SE: Nursing peer review: a developmental process, Nurs Manage 18(1):46, 1987.

Cobb, MD: Evaluating medication errors, J Nurs Adm 16(4):41, 1986.

Crockett, D, and Sutcliffe, S: Staff participation in nursing quality assurance, Nurs Manage 17(10):41, 1986.

Davis-Martin, S: Outcome and accountability: getting into the consumer dimension, Nurs Manage 17(10):25, 1986.

Decker, F, et al.: Using patient outcomes to evaluate community health nursing, Nurs Outlook 27(4):278, 1979.

Foglesong, D: Standards promote effective production, Nurs Manage 18(1):24, 1987.

Greaves, PE, and Loquist, RS: Impact evaluation: a competency-based approach, Nurs Adm Q 7(3):81, 1983.

Grohar, ME, Myers, J, and McSweeney, M: A comparison of patient acuity and nursing resource use, J Nurs Adm 16(6):19, 1986.

Joint Commission on Accreditation of Hospitals: The QA Guide: a resource for hospital quality assurance, Chicago, 1980, JCAH.

Kunkle, V: Accountability standards balance quality and efficiency, Nurs Manage 18(1):34, 1987.

Lunde, KF, and Durbin-Lafferty, E: Evaluating clinical competency in nursing, Nurs Manage 17(8):47, 1986.

Standards of nursing practice, Am Nurse 6:11, 1974.

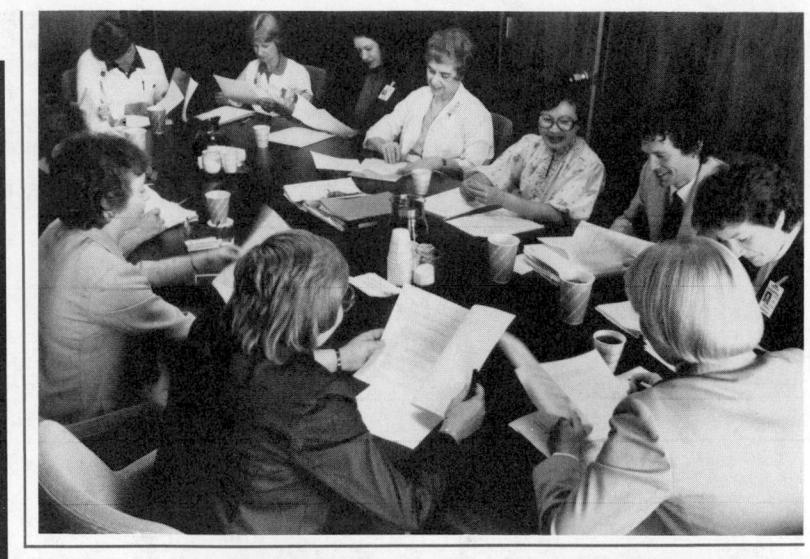

OBJECTIVES

Mastery of content in this chapter will enable the student to:

- Define the key terms listed.
- Compare the various ways to acquire knowledge.
- List the characteristics of scientific investigation.
- Compare methods for developing new knowledge in nursing.
- Define scientific and nursing research.
- Compare the research process with the nursing process.
- List the ANA priorities for nursing research.
- Explain the rights of human research subjects.
- Explain the rights of others who assist in the conduct of human research studies.
- Describe a typical research report.
- Discuss methods of locating research reports in nursing and related areas.
- Explain how to organize information from a research report.
- List the characteristics of a clinical nursing problem that can be researched.
- List the criteria for using research findings in nursing practice.

KEY TERMS

Anonymity
Bias
Citation
Comparison Group
Concept
Confidentiality
Control
Empirical Data
Experiment
Generalization
Phenomena
Primary Source
Proposition
Random Selection
Research Process
Research Utilization
Sample
Secondary Source
Statistics
Subjects
Theory

Research in Nursing Care

For over 20 years, many nursing leaders and organizations have made considerable efforts to increase nurses' awareness of the importance of conducting nursing studies and using research as a foundation for practice. In 1974 the ANA House of Delegates passed a resolution calling for more nursing research to focus on clinical problems nurses face in professional practice. Until the 1970s, nursing studies tended to focus on the roles and characteristics of nurses rather than on problems in delivering professional care to clients (Gortner, 1980). In 1976 the ANA published specific recommendations for studying research at the different nursing education levels. The Institute of Medicine's (IOM) study of nursing (1983) recommended that the federal government increase funds for scientific research in nursing and that steps be taken to establish a national organization to place nursing research "in the mainstream of scientific investigation." Acting on this recommendation in 1985, the U.S. Congress overrode two presidential vetoes to establish the National Center for Nursing Research under the National Institutes of Health. This center was established "for the pupose of conducting a program of grants and awards supporting nursing research and research training related to patient care, the promotion of health, and the prevention of disease and the mitigation of the effects of acute and chronic illnesses and disabilities" (Merritt, 1986).

Nursing research is important, even for nursing students studying the fundamentals of the profession. This chapter should help the student gain an appreciation of the importance of research in furthering the status of nursing as a science and develop basic skills for understanding and using nursing research to gain knowledge and practice skills.

SCIENTIFIC RESEARCH IN NURSING

Acquiring Knowledge

Human beings acquire knowledge in many ways. A person continuously takes in and processes numerous pieces of information to understand experiences. The scientific researcher also seeks to explain or understand reality, but the scientist's process of acquiring knowledge is systematic and logical. This process, or *scientific method*, is the foundation of research. Scientific research is the most reliable and objective of all methods of gaining knowledge.

One way of learning is by tradition. One generation passes knowledge to the next. For example, children often learn about traditional holidays such as Christmas and Passover through traditional or customary family practices. In nursing, certain traditional methods of practice such as the change-of-shift report and other daily hospital work practices are passed from one practitioner to the next. Tradition is an efficient way of learning, although it can also limit the ability to seek new ways of doing things. If tradition becomes so ingrained that a person does not question the custom, other more appropriate or efficient ways may be overlooked.

Knowledge is also acquired by seeking information from experts in a particular field. Experts are often asked to solve problems or to answer questions. For example, at income tax time an accountant's help is sought to fill out tax forms. Similarly, nursing students often seek the advice of instructors and practicing nurses in assessing and caring for clients. Authority, like tradition, is not infallible, although it is commonly treated as absolute truth.

A person also learns through experience. Without this process, a person would have to relearn a procedure every time it was performed. Practice leads to the development of routines that help build skills. For example, a student nurse taking blood pressure for the first time may feel awkward and unsure of hearing the sounds, but with pratice the student's technique and confidence improve. Although experience is an important way of learning, it has limitations. A person may continue to do something simply because it was learned that way and may overlook improved or other ways of doing the same thing. If experience causes a person to learn something incorrectly, it is used inappropriately.

Learning by trial and error is yet another way of gaining knowledge. Making mistakes or repeatedly trying various ways of accomplishing something will result in

a better way of solving the problem. This method of learning is practical, but it is unsystematic and often a haphazard way of acquiring knowledge. In nursing, trial and error is not an appropriate way of acquiring new knowledge because a client's health status depends on nursing actions.

The scientific method is the most advanced, objective means of acquiring knowledge. It is characterized by systematic, orderly procedures that, although not infallible, seek to limit the possibility for error and minimize the likelihood that any bias or opinion by the researcher might influence the results of research and thus the knowledge gained. Polit and Hungler (1987) describe the characteristics of scientific investigation as follows:

1. The steps of planning and conducting an investigation are undertaken in a *systematic*, orderly fashion.
2. Scientists attempt to *control* external factors that are not under direct investigation but which can influence a relationship between phenomena they are studying. For example, if a scientist were studying the relationship between diet and heart disease, other characteristics such as stress would have to be eliminated as contributing factors to this disease.
3. Evidence that is part of reality (empirical data) is gathered directly or indirectly through use of the human senses and is the basis for discovering new knowledge.
4. The goal is to understand phenomena in such a way that the knowledge gained can be applied *generally*, not just to isolated cases or circumstances.
5. Scientists strive to conduct investigations that contribute to testing or developing *theories*, thereby advancing the knowledge that can be applied toward increasing understanding of people, places, or life events.

Nursing and the Scientific Method

Compared with other ways of acquiring knowledge, the scientific method is more orderly and objective in its approach. Nurses are now using this approach to develop knowledge. In the past, much of the information used in nursing practice was borrowed from biology, physiology, psychology, and sociology. Often, this information was applied to nursing without testing or comparing ways for caring for clients. For example, nurses use several methods to help clients sleep. Interventions such as giving a client a backrub, making sure the bed is clean and comfortable, preparing the environment by dimming the lights, and talking to a worried or anxious client are frequently used nursing measures and, in general, are logical, common sense approaches. However, when these measures are considered in greater depth, questions may arise about their applications for clients in different situations. Will all these approaches work with all clients at all times? If not, why? Which are more effective and why? In what order should a nurse try them? How can the nurse know which interventions are appropriate for certain clients? What are the sleep problems clients with a particular health care problem tend to experience? Through research these questions can be studied in greater depth. At present, nurses generally rely on personal experience or what nursing experts say should work to help clients sleep. If an intervention works for most clients, the nurse may be satisfied with this success without questioning whether there might be a better way. If the intervention is not successful, the nurse might resort to trial and error by trying different approaches or a different sequence of accepted measures to promote sleep. Even if an intervention discovered with this approach is effective for one or more clients, however, the questions raised above about applications for other clients in other settings remain.

Definitions of Scientific and Nursing Research

According to Kerlinger (1986), "scientific research is systematic, controlled, empirical, and critical investigation of natural phenomena guided by theory and hypotheses about the presumed relations among such phenomena." When scientists use systematic, controlled methods for studying events or problems, they have more confidence that the results are accurate and are not influenced by opinion or belief. For a study to be empirical, the evidence collected must come from objective findings. Other researchers should be able to examine the evidence and see the same phenomena. To guide the design of a research study, scientists create a hypothetical proposition (hypothesis) about what they expect to see before conducting the study. Finally, scientists generally study the way characteristics or events are related. A relationship may mean that one attribute changes as another changes, but this does not necessarily mean that a change in one causes a change in the other. For example, as people get older, they tend to lose their hair and their skin becomes wrinkled. Hair loss and skin wrinkles are related to each other as part of the aging process, but this does not mean that either factor causes the other to occur. The cause of aging is not known. Scientists can only study how attributes or events cause other things to happen, as well as other kinds of relationships. When reading research studies, it is important to avoid interpreting results in terms of cause and effect because there is a difference between cause-and-effect relationships and other kinds of relationships. Researchers often study how changes in attributes are related to

each other without being able to determine why or how these changes take place.

The Commission on Nursing Research of the ANA (1981a) has defined nursing research as follows:

Nursing research develops knowledge about health and the promotion of health over the full life span, care of persons with health problems and disabilities, and nursing actions to enhance the ability of individuals to respond effectively to actual or potential health problems.

Biomedical research is concerned mainly with discovering the causes and treatments of disease. In contrast, nursing research is directed toward helping well people improve their health status and stay healthy, as well as assisting clients who are sick or disabled by an illness. Nursing also focuses on the full range of human responses rather than the biological or physical ones. For example, the effects of preoperative teaching on postoperative recovery is an area that has been studied extensively. Some studies (Schmidt and Woolridge, 1973; Wolfer and Davis, 1970) have examined the emotional reaction of clients to a surgical experience, such as postoperative anxiety and fear, as well as physiological responses such as the return to usual oral intake and urinary retention. Teaching clients what they can expect on the day of surgery and in the immediate postoperative period is now a widely implemented and accepted nursing measure. Such teaching often includes, for example, information about when vital signs will be monitored after surgery and the deep breathing and coughing techniques they will be asked to perform. This information is provided to relieve clients' fear and anxiety and to help them recover from surgery.

Because nurses are interested in acquiring knowledge about a wide range of human needs and responses to health problems, nursing research uses many methods to study clinical problems. The hallmark of scientific research is the experiment. In a true experimental study, the conditions under which a measure is investigated are tightly controlled. The study usually includes a comparison or control group that does not receive the nursing measure being investigated. The results for this group are compared with those of a study or *experimental group* that receives some form of treatment or intervention. The subjects selected for the comparison and experimental groups are chosen at random from among those eligible for the study. Designing an experiment to study physical causes of disease is less difficult than designing an investigation that also includes psychological or social aspects of health. For example, to study the relationship between postoperative anxiety and preoperative teaching, the researcher can control one psychological factor by using only subjects having surgery for the first time. However, the researcher cannot control other experiences the clients may have had, such as hearing a friend's "horror" stories about surgery or reading about surgical experiences in the newspapers. These psychological factors that cannot be controlled may influence the subject client's level of anxiety.

Nursing studies use many methods for investigating clinical problems, some of which may be similar to the experimental approach. Other methods may be similar to those used in the social sciences such as anthropology and sociology. The problem being investigated is one of the factors that determines the appropriate method. To the extent the particular research problem allows, a study strives to follow the criteria of scientific investigation.

Nursing Research and the Nursing Process

The research process (Seaman and Verhonick, 1982; Abdellah and Levine, 1986) consists of phases or steps that can be compared and contrasted with those of the nursing process. Both are problem-solving processes used by nurses in practice (Table 11-1) but are very different. The nursing process is used to determine health

TABLE 11-1 Comparison of Phases of the Nursing Process and the Research Process

Nursing Process	Research Process
Assessment	Select the topic and identify the research problem
	Formulate a summary of the proposed research
Nursing Diagnosis	Review the literature for theory and other related studies
	Define concepts and variables to be studied
	State hypotheses about expected observation or questions to be studied
Planning	Determine ethical implications of the proposed study
	Identify assumptions and limitations
	Describe the research design and methods for data collection
	Define the study population and sample
	Determine how to process, analyze, and summarize data
	Plan for communicating findings
Implementation	Collect data from subjects
Evaluation	Analyze and interpret data
	Communicate findings in written and other forms

Data from Seaman, CH, and Verhonick, PJ: Research methods for undergraduate students in nursing, ed. 2, Norwalk, Conn., 1982, Appleton-Century-Crofts and Abdellah, FG, and Levine, E: Better patient care through nursing research, ed. 3, New York, 1986, Macmillan Publishing Co.

needs and plan nursing care for clients. It is used as a basis for gaining and using information about clients to help them restore, maintain, or promote health. Depending on the nursing diagnosis, knowledge from a number of disciplines may be used in the nursing process to help clients solve particular health problems.

In contrast, the *research process* is used to gain knowledge that can be used in other similar situations. Nurses may want to gain knowledge about the reason a particular event happens or the best way to provide care for clients with a certain health problem. The research process is used to gain knowledge that can be applied to a whole group or class of clients.

During assessment, the nurse caring for a client with sleeping difficulties determines the factors that might interfere with the client's ability to sleep. Is the client concerned about his health status? Is the client experiencing pain? Is the environment noisy? Is the bed messy or uncomfortable? After assessing these aspects, the nurse formulates a nursing diagnosis, plans interventions, implements these interventions, and evaluates the subjective and objective evidence indicating whether the client is able to sleep.

In contrast, a researcher studying sleeping difficulties seeks new information that can be applied to more than one client. For example, a nurse notices that many clients seem to have a difficult time sleeping the night before a particular diagnostic procedure. Based on work with these clients, the nurse determines that most of them express concerns about what may be discovered by the test. In this situation the nurse might design a research study in which some of the clients receive the usual nursing care and others receive an approach based on relieving their anxiety. After collecting information about the effects of the usual care for one group and the new approach for the other, the nurse researcher compares the results to determine if clients who received the new care had less difficulty sleeping than those who received the normal nursing care. If the clients receiving the new care slept better, the nurse has acquired new knowledge about how to help clients undergoing the diagnostic procedure to sleep better.

Nurse Researchers

In 1981 the ANA published the following list of priorities for nursing research*:

1. Promoting health, well-being, and competency for personal care among all age groups.
2. Preventing health problems throughout the life span that have the potential to reduce productivity and satisfaction.

---
*Commission on Nursing Research, American Nurses' Association: Research priorities for the 1980's: generating a scientific basis for nursing practice, Kansas City, Mo., 1981b, The Association.

3. Decreasing the negative impact of health problems on coping abilities, productivity, and life satisfaction of individuals and families.
4. Ensuring that the care needs of particularly vulnerable groups are met through appropriate strategies.
5. Designing and developing health care systems that are cost effective in meeting the nursing needs of the population.

In 1985 the Cabinet on Nursing Research of the ANA outlined predictions about (1) consumers of nursing ser-

---

ANA Nursing Research Priorities

**GENERATION OF KNOWLEDGE
ENABLING NURSES TO**

- Promote health, well-being, and ability to care for oneself among all age, social, and cultural groups.
- Minimize and prevent behaviorally and environmentally induced health problems that compromise the quality of life and reduce productivity.
- Minimize the negative effects of new health technologies on the adaptive abilities of individuals and families experiencing acute or chronic health problems.
- Ensure that the care needs of particularly vulnerable groups, such as the elderly, children with congenital health problems, individuals from diverse cultures, the mentally ill, and the poor, are met in effective and acceptable ways.
- Classify nursing practice pheonomena.
- Ensure that principles of ethics guide nursing research.
- Develop instruments to measure nursing outcomes.
- Develop integrative methodologies for the holistic study of human beings as they relate to their families and life-styles.
- Design and evaluate alternative models for delivering health care and for administering health care systems so that nurses will be able to balance high quality and cost-effectiveness in meeting the nursing needs of identified populations.
- Evaluate the effectiveness of alternative approaches to nursing education for the kind of practice that requires broad knowledge and a wide repertoire of skills, and for the kind of practice that requires specialized knowledge and a focused set of skills.
- Identify and analyze historical and contemporary factors that influence the shaping of nursing professionals' involvement in national health policy development.

From ANA; Directions for nursing research: toward the twenty-first century, Kansas City, Mo. 1985a, The Association.

---

vices, (2) health care systems, and (3) nursing for the year 2000 (ANA, 1985a). On the basis of these predictions, priorities for nursing research were further specified (see box).

These priorities demonstrate to nurses, other health care professionals, and the general public what the profession sees as important areas in which nurses need further knowledge to improve services they provide. Researchers can use these priorities to develop research projects by funding agencies to set priorities for funding research. Student nurses can use these priorities to determine whether to participate in a research project.

Nurses conduct research in a variety of settings. Student nurses and practitioners may be asked to participate in research that investigates client outcomes and the effectiveness of nursing care. These types of research are commonly called *quality assurance studies*. Data are collected to determine the impact nurses have on achievement of client care objectives in a particular clinical setting. Because the results of such research are usually applicable only in one institution, this is not scientific research as discussed earlier. However, such research is important to the institution because the nursing department can use it to demonstrate the contributions made by nurses to client care. For example, a recent editorial in the *American Journal of Nursing* (Mallison, 1987) urged nurses to participate in client outcome studies to determine how staffing levels affect the quality of care. The editor sees these types of studies as important in light of a growing nursing shortage and the understaffing experienced in many clinical agencies.

Clinical nursing research should be undertaken by nurses trained to conduct scientific investigations. Generally, nurse researchers hold master's and doctoral degrees. A student nurse asked to participate in a nursing study as a subject or by collecting data is entitled to receive information about the qualifications of the person conducting the study. The researcher's educational background and biographical sketch give some information about the person's qualifications for conducting research. An experienced researcher is usually more qualified to undertake a complex, long-term project than a beginning researcher. Nurses new to research may, however, make an important contribution by conducting less complex studies investigating important nursing problems (Seaman and Verhonick, 1982.)

ETHICAL ISSUES IN RESEARCH

Rights of Human Subjects

To refine existing knowledge and develop new knowledge, clinical research is sometimes directed toward trying new procedures whose outcome is doubtful or unknown (ANA, 1975). This kind of research may conflict with the purpose of nursing practice, which is to meet specific clients' needs. In such cases the researcher is responsible for structuring the investigation to avoid or minimize harm to the subjects. Although it is not always possible to anticipate all potential undesirable effects, researchers are obligated to inform everyone involved about the known potential risks. Other basic human rights must also be observed. These principles,

---

Ethical Guidelines for Conducting Nursing Research with Human Subjects

I. Scientific merit of the research
   A. Study of the problem or question(s) under study must be ethical.
   B. The problem or question(s) must be worthwhile, e.g., significant ones for nursing.
   C. The design and methods of the study must meet established scientific criteria, e.g., meet reliability and validity criteria, make optimal use of time and resources.
   D. The study must be designed with accepted ethical boundaries.
II. Consent and human subject protection and confidentiality
   A. Informed consent
      1. Information must be provided so that subjects can make an informed and educated decision about participation, including the following:
         a. Nature/purpose of study
         b. Purpose, extent and duration of participation
         c. Type of information that is requested
         d. Use of records
         e. Use of information during and after study
         f. Inconvenience, potential risks and potential benefits
         g. Standard treatment that may be withheld
         h. Freedom to withdraw at any time without recrimination
         i. How anonymity and confidentiality will be maintained
      2. Persons who are competent to consent must be free to do so without threat that they must participate to maintain benefits, e.g., high quality care. If not competent to give consent, it must be sought from an individual who can act as an advocate for the non-competent person.
      3. Verbal or written consent may be obtained, provided ethical considerations are observed. Who consented, under what circumstances, the information provided to subjects, and assurance of the right to withdraw and that no coercion was used must be documented by the investigator.
      4. Other persons affected by the subject's participation must be informed of the study and consent obtained if necessary, e.g., staff nurse, spouse.
   B. Confidentiality
      1. Information must be handled so that confidentiality and anonymity are maintained.
      2. Information may not be used or released outside the terms of the agreement.
   C. Protection of subjects
      1. Subjects must be protected from all types of harm.
      2. Potential benefits must outweigh potential risks.
      3. When the well-being of the subject conflicts with the integrity of the research, a decision must be made that favors the subject.
III. The research setting
   A. The investigator must make a specific request to the agency where the research is to be conducted and provide the agency with the knowledge needed to make an informed consent about approval.
   B. The agency has an obligation to provide a valid system for review.
   C. All nurses have an obligation to collaborate in the research process with the investigator.
   D. Investigators have a responsibility to provide adequate information to the staff members involved in or affected by the study.
   E. Staff members have the right to participate or not, and should be informed if this is a condition of employment in a particular agency.

From Canadian Nurses Association: Ethical guidelines for nursing research involving human subjects, Ottawa, 1983, The Association.

as set forth by the CNA (1983), are outlined in the box.

Informed consent means that research subjects are (1) given full and complete information about the purpose of the study, procedures, data collection, potential harm and benefits, and alternative methods of treatment; (2) capable of fully understanding the research and the implications of participation; and (3) assured of free choice in giving consent, including the right to withdraw from the study at any time. Procedures for obtaining informed consent must be outlined in the study protocol.

Confidentiality means that the privacy of subjects will be respected. Anonymity is often used to ensure privacy and, if promised, must be respected.

In addition the researcher planning to conduct a study must possess the knowledge and skills necessary to undertake the research. For example, a nurse planning to conduct a study involving psychiatric clients should be familiar with psychiatric nursing principles and theory. Current ANA (1985b) and CNA (1983) guidelines state that qualified nurse researchers have a right to engage in research and have a right of access to resources needed to conduct studies.

In the United States, any agency receiving federal funds must have an institutional review board (Armiger, 1977). This group reviews all studies conducted in the institution to ensure ethical principles (see Chapter 17) are observed. Not all research undertaken in clinical areas involves experimentation with human subjects. Research not using a new treatment with subjects may involve minimal or no risk to clients. For example, a survey designed to measure clients' perceptions of stress in intensive care units holds little risk for participants. Nonetheless, a major responsibility of the institutional board is to determine the risk status of all research projects.

Rights of Other Research Participants

Student and practicing nurses may be asked to participate in research as data collectors or may be involved in the care of clients participating in a study. All participants, including health care professionals caring for clients, have the right to be fully informed about the study, its procedures (including informed consent and risk factors), and any physical or emotional injury that clients could experience as a result of participation. Often the physical risks are more obvious than emotional risks. Depending on the problem being studied, clients may be asked to give highly personal and intrusive information. Because this type of research can lead to anxiety or stress for some clients, the researcher should prepare all participants, including nurses delivering care, for this possibility and assist them in coping with the effects. Participants also have the right to see review forms from the institutional review board certifying approval of the study. Any student, nurse, or other participant has the right to refuse to carry out any research procedures if concerned about its ethical aspects.

Besides dealing with the harmful effects of a research project, nurses may be faced with other ethical dilemmas (Brink and Wood, 1983). For example, some clients may feel they have to participate in an investigation to please the health care professionals on whom they depend for care. They may feel that they will receive inferior care if they refuse to participate. Research ethics require that clients not be made to feel that they are obliged to participate in a study. The ultimate decision rests with the client. Withholding proper care or in any way implying that care will be withheld from clients who refuse to participate is unethical.

Another ethical dilemma in research involves withholding a new intervention from clients who might benefit from its use. In an experiment investigating a new intervention, for example, the experimental group may receive the new intervention while the comparison group receives the usual care. In such cases, comparison group clients are deprived of a new treatment that could be beneficial to them. One way of managing this dilemma is to offer the new nursing care to the comparison group after data necessary to the experimental study have been collected.

NURSING RESEARCH IN NURSING PRACTICE

Identifying Research Studies

When reading nursing literature, the practicing or student nurse must be able to differentiate a research report or article from other types of writing. This may not be as simple as it seems. Even if the title has the word *research* in it, the article does not necessarily report the results of a research study. The nurse can determine whether an article reports a research study only by examining its contents.

Sometimes, however, an article's title can give a clue to its contents. Phrases such as "a study of" or "comparison of" suggest a research report. The abstract and the introductory paragraphs of an article can also indicate whether the article is based on research. The *abstract* is a short summary of the purpose of a study, the subjects included in the research, the way the study was conducted, and the results obtained in the investigation. An abstract is often very brief and does not contain all the essential information from the article. The first few paragraphs of the article should provide further clues about whether it describes a research study. Phrases such as "the purpose of this study was" and "this research was carried out to determine" are indications that the article is a research report. If the article describes only the author's experience with a particular aspect of nursing care, it probably is not a research article.

In addition to the abstract, a typical research report (1) includes an introductory section presenting the purpose, a summary of literature used to formulate the study, and the hypotheses tested (the *introduction* section); (2) describes the methods used to conduct the study, including the sample (what or who was studied), and to collect data, including the device or instrument used to measure empirical information (the *methods* section); (3) describes the results obtained in the study, including statistical tests used to analyze data (the *results* section); (4) presents the author's interpretation of the results, including conclusions and implications that can be drawn from the study (the *discussion* section); and (5) a *reference* list.

If the report is written by one of the researchers in the study, it is a primary source. Any other article about the study is considered a secondary source (for example, an article in which the author was not directly involved in conducting the study but collected the information from a primary or another secondary source). Most nursing textbooks are secondary sources of information. Authors of these texts incorporate knowledge and information gathered from nursing and related literature, including research written by original investigators.

The fact that a report is a primary source does not guarantee its accuracy, which depends on the ability of researchers to be scientific, impersonal, and impartial in conducting studies. However, a primary source does report firsthand knowledge, whereas secondary sources may include another person's interpretation of the original work.

Finding Research Studies

Students and practicing nurses often need to find research articles on subjects that interest them. In the health care field a number of resources are useful when searching the literature for research articles.

To find primary research sources related to a particular subject, the first source is the journals where original research reports are usually published. The most efficient way to locate research articles is to consult an index of journal articles. The *Cumulative Index to Nursing and Allied Health Literature* (CINAHL), published bimonthly, contains listings from over 300 English-language nursing and allied health journals, as well as ANA and NLN publications. The *International Nursing Index*, published four times a year, contains listings from over 200 nursing journals from around the world. *Index Medicus*, an international index published monthly, includes listings from approximately 2200 biomedical

journals, including about 60 nursing journals. The *Hospital Literature Index*, published quarterly, contains listings from journals dealing with planning and providing health care programs and services. These indexes are generally found in reference sections of medical and nursing libraries.

These indexes can save time in finding articles. Each index uses a list of key words that form subject headings and subheadings, under which article listings are grouped or organized. An author listing is also available, making it possible to find articles published during a certain time period by a particular person. Articles on a particular subject are found by first checking the subject headings to see if the key term listed in the index matches the subject. The key term listing may also lead to other subject groupings that contain articles similar in content. Using an index may at first seem time consuming, but it saves time, since the alternative is looking through many journals trying to find articles pertinent to the subject.

Many nursing and medical libraries provide computerized searches for articles. MEDLINE, a data base available through the Medical Literature Analysis and Retrieval System (MEDLARS), is a system available in many libraries for locating research materials. Information in this system is retrieved from *Index Medicus* and the *International Nursing Index*. In addition the CINAHL is available as a computerized data base. A list of articles and abstracts is transmitted over telephone lines within hours of being requested. Computer searches generally involve a user's fee. Reference librarians have information about this type of resource.

Nurses having access to a microcomputer and a modem may subscribe individually to bibliographic services available through a data base vendor. Some of the more popular services include *Knowledge Index* available through *DIALOG Information Services, GRATEFUL MED* available through the National Library of Medice and *BRS Colleague* available through W.B. Saunders Co. Most of these vendors charge an initial subscription fee and an hourly fee for time connected to the central computer. There are also charges for telephone time. These services often provide access to data bases in other disciplines (for example, psychology and sociology).

Major nursing journals publishing research studies include *Nursing Research, Research in Nursing and Health, Western Journal of Nursing Research,* and the *International Journal of Nursing Studies.* Although not all articles published in these journals are research reports, most issues are devoted to primary reports of nursing studies. Other nursing journals also publish original reports of research studies. For example, *Heart and Lung,* a specialty journal published under the auspices of the American Association of Critical Care Nurses, often includes research reports. Recently, more speciality practice journals appear to be publishing research articles.

Secondary literature sources such as books can be helpful in finding primary research sources. Nursing students seeking research articles should use reference lists or bibliographies at the end of textbook chapters. To document the scientific basis for their writing, authors frequently cite primary sources as references, and these references are a valuable resource for nursing students who want more information.

Other secondary resources helpful in finding primary nursing research articles are research reviews such as the *Annual Review of Nursing Research* and the *Review of Research in Nursing Education*. Each volume is devoted to certain topics. For example, the 1986 edition of the *Annual Review of Nursing Research* (Werley and Fitzpatrick, 1986) contains a chapter on historical research in nursing written by Irene Palmer, who is a prominent nurse researcher in this area. A review can help determine the status of research on a topic and can direct the reader toward other primary research sources. Research reviews are relatively new in nursing.

Organizing Information from a Research Study

Articles listed in a bibliography or reference section are called *citations*. A citation provides the author's name and information about where "ideas" or "quotations" were originally published. Writers are ethically obligated to give credit to others whose thoughts are used, even if the original author's exact words are not quoted.

There are many ways to list a citation. The style recommended by the American Psychological Association (1983) is widely used. This format avoids footnotes. All citations are arranged alphabetically at the end of the report. Schools of nursing use many formats, however, and nursing students should determine which citation format is used at their own school. Listing citations according to the recommended guidelines prevents incomplete citations.

A book citation includes author names, date of publication, title, edition if appropriate, place of publication, and publisher. Journal citations include author names, date of publication, title of article, name of the journal in which the article appeared, volume and issue numbers, and the exact page numbers of the article. The page numbers of direct quotations should be noted. The order of information in citations, the punctuation used, and the use of underlining and quotation marks depend on the particular format.

The use of index cards for recording information helps to maintain consistency and accuracy in record keeping. One card is used for notations about each article. Other categories of information should be noted for future use of the research study as a foundation for nursing practice. These categories include (1) *when* the study was conducted; (2) *what* problem area was studied; (3) *how* information and data were collected and compared; (4) the subjects *who* were included in the study; (5) *where* the study was conducted (including type of setting and geographical region); (6) a brief summary of the *results* (including major findings and conclusions of the study); and (7) the number of *citations* or references used in the report. Any direct quotation from the report should be noted on the index card with quotation marks and the exact page number on which the quotation appears (see box).

The date of publication gives the approximate time when the study was conducted. Sometimes, researchers define the exact time period in the article because a considerable time (as long as 2 years) may pass between the time a study was completed and the time the article was published. Noting when a study was conducted allows tracking the development of knowledge in a particular area.

In nursing, many kinds of clinical problems can be studied. Knowing exactly what was studied provides information about the topics that have been investigated by nurse researchers. Studies undertaken in a particular problem area can then be collected and evaluated.

There are often many ways to investigate a particular research problem. Knowing how researchers studied a question helps evaluate how thoroughly aspects of the problem have been investigated.

A major purpose of scientific research is to increase knowledge about general classes of people or events. Knowing who the subjects were in a research study gives information about to whom the conclusions may be applied. When similar results are obtained with different groups of clients, nurses can be more confident when using the new methods with other clients.

Since nursing care is provided for clients in varying circumstances, knowing where the research was done can influence whether the results might apply in a different setting or region. This information is particularly relevant for research involving psychological aspects of nursing care. Different regions of the country have unique traditions and customs. Nursing interventions appropriate for people with certain attitudes and beliefs may not be relevant in regions or settings where attitudes and beliefs differ substantially.

A summary of the results concerns what has or has not been demonstrated in a particular problem area. When the findings and conclusions are similar in a number of research studies, the conclusions are considered more significant than in the case of an isolated research project. The effects of preoperative teaching on the postoperative recovery of clients is an example of a problem

Sample Bibliography Card

WHEN

Walike, B.C. & Walike, J.W. (1977). Relative lactose intolerance: A clinical study of tube-fed patients. *Journal of American Medical Association, 238,* 948-951.

WHAT	Lactose intolerance of tube-fed patients.
HOW	Consistency, frequency and composition of stools; body weight; selected blood studies including electrolyte levels, protein, glucose, cholesterol, total bilirubin, and BUN; 24-hour urine studies; glucose tolerance test; lactose tolerance test; symptoms of gastrointestinal distress.
WHO	20 white patients between the ages of 46 and 74 receiving both lactose and lactose-free nasogastric tube feedings after head or neck surgery for cancer; 4 patients were dropped from the study due to complications unrelated to tube feeding.
WHERE	Inpatient hospital clinical research unit (14 patients) in Seattle, WA; location of 6 patients not stated.
RESULTS	Significant differences in stool frequency and consistency were found for patients on tube feeding diets that contained lactose (milk sugar) when compared to how these same patients tolerated lactose-free diets. Nine patients also experienced at least one other symptom of gastrointestinal distress. Lactose intolerance is relative and should be viewed in relation to both increased amount and ability of the intestines to break down milk sugar.

"The results indicate that lactose should be reduced or eliminated from tube-feeding diets to improve patient tolerance and comfort and to reduce diarrhea." (p. 948)

CITATIONS   18 references

area in which collective evidence provides a reasonable scientific foundation for nursing practice.

■ ■ ■

Many books and journal articles in nursing and related disciplines provide more detailed information about reading and evaluating research studies. Learning to find and read nursing research studies is not a simple task, but nursing research is based on principles of logic, and with a thoughtful approach, the nursing student can learn to understand and evaluate nursing research studies.

Identifying Clinical Nursing Problems

Diers (1979) defined a clinical nursing problem as "a difference between two state of affairs, a discrepancy between the way things are and the way they ought to be, or between what one knows and what one needs to know to eliminate the problem." The questions raised in this definition are: Given the nursing interventions recommended for clients with a particular health care problem, how might the suggested care be improved so the results or outcomes of care are better? Given the knowledge about how to provide nursing care, what additional information would be needed to plan new interventions for clients with a particular health care problem? Unanswered questions and the desire to improve nursing practice can provide the stimulus for conducting a research study.

Experience can make it possible to identify a researchable clinical nursing problem, but a nurse does not need to have years of clinical practice to identify a nursing problem. Sometimes a person who is relatively new in a situation can more easily see how things could be improved than those who have more experience and who take present conditions for granted. The nurse also needs to consider whether the problem frequently occurs in a particular client goup, whether it can be consistently and accurately measured, and whether a possible nursing solution might change how care is delivered (Fuller, 1982).

Sometimes nursing students or practicing nurses think their ideas about nursing problems for study are not worthwhile unless they are certain in advance that the proposed clinical study would make a radical change in client care. However, research efforts also may have to refine ideas about a clinical problem before the investigator can test alternative nursing interventions. In fact, some nurse researchers think that more investigative work needs to be done to describe the client phenomena before research to test an alternative intervention is undertaken. In addition the researcher may have to devise correct ways for measuring results before the study can proceed. All these factors may discourage a nurse from undertaking a nursing research project. On the other hand, they can be viewed as stimulating challenges because much information has yet to be scientifically tested for its relevance to nursing practice.

Studies by Barbara Walike Hansen et al. (Walike et al., 1974) illustrates how research can progress from the phase of clinical problem refinement to the testing of new nursing measures. This early study documented the need for further research into tube feeding procedures and the way clients are affected by this method of meeting nutritional needs. Flynn, et al. (1987) found that tube-fed patients experience problems similar to those identified by Walike. A number of factors associated with clients' responses to tube feedings have been studied, including (1) tube location for proper formula administration, (2) temperature, volume, and rate of formula administration, (3) the attitudes and adjustments of clients toward tube feeding procedures, and (4) responses to the formula contents and other complications experienced by clients receiving tube feedings. Some of the studies dealing with these aspects of caring for people receiving tube feedings are outlined in Table 11-2.

Determining the proper insertion length for a nasogastric tube so it is located properly in the stomach is a topic frequently covered in nursing texts. Hanson (1979, 1980) described an improved method for determining the proper insertion length that increased from 72% to 91% the likelihood that the tube would be properly located in the body or fundus of the stomach. Metheny, Spies, and Eisenberg investigated risk factors associated with tube displacement (1986) and the accuracy of methods used to monitor tube location (1988).

The temperature, volume, and rate of administration of tube-feeding formula are regulated and monitored by nurses. The effects of cold, room-temperature, and warm (body-temperature) feedings on gastrointestinal function have been reported by Kugawa-Busby et al. (1980), who found that healthy volunteers tolerated room-temperature feedings as well as they did warm formula. Some subjects experienced cramping and diarrhea 6 to 9 hours after receiving cold feedings. The volume and rate of administering feedings to normal volunteer subjects have been found to be related to subjective symptoms of gastrointestinal distress (Heitkemper et al., 1981). The recommended rate for tube feeding in this study was less than 60 ml/min for the usual volume feeding of 250 ml. When larger volumes (up to 750 ml per feeding) were needed to meet nutritional needs, subjects were able to tolerate them when administered at a rate of 30 ml/min. Six of the fourteen subjects experienced nausea or abdominal discomfort with the first feeding. Tolerance improved with subsequent formula administrations.

Other studies investigated the distressful objective and subjective symptoms experienced by tube-fed clients. The first study (Padilla et al., 1979) described the psychosensory irritations and deprivations commonly experienced by 30 clients. Sensory irritations included dry mouth, sore throat, and thirst. Deprivation of taste when chewing and swallowing food were reported by these clients. A follow-up study (Padilla et al., 1981) explored the effects on reducing client distress of four different ways of providing information about tube feeding procedures. The teaching intervention most effective for subjects in this study provided sensory information about the procedure and coping behaviors to increase comfort during and after feeding tube insertion. In addition, clients perceiving they had control over their environment and behavior did not express less distress than clients perceiving they had no control.

Results of the Walike and Walike study (1977) dealing with the effects of lactose (milk sugar) on stool frequency and consistency are shown in the box on p. 180. As a result of this research, commercially prepared tube-feeding formulas that do not contain lactose are now available. One problem in this study was the difficulty experienced by the researcher in finding a reliable and uniform way to measure stool consistency (Hansen, 1984). The investigators found that the nurses used "very creative and imaginative descriptions" to describe the characteristics of stool, and these descriptions differed among nurses participating in data collection. A stool consistency diagram (Fig. 11-1) was developed to group descriptions into nine categories. The actual water content of stools in each category was analyzed to confirm these categories objectively. At the time of the study, only one rating form for stool consistency of meconium existed in the research literature. The experience of these investigators in having to develop a reliable, valid way of measuring a human phenomenon is common among nursing researchers. Much of nursing practice deals with identifying and describing human responses to health care problems insufficiently defined and classified to permit general agreement about observations among nurses. Other studies dealing with complications associated with tube feedings are outlined in Table 11-2.

These articles represent a sample of tube feeding research conducted. Through collaborative efforts, the Tube Feeding Consortium Group (Bergstrom et al., 1984) was able to study a large number of subjects in many locations to make the findings more generalized. The clinical nursing problems addressed in the tube feeding studies outlined in Table 11-2 involve aspects of care with which nurses must deal in everyday practice. Client safety might be improved, for example, if the new method for determining length of inserting a feeding tube

TABLE 11-2   Summaries of Selected Tube Feeding Studies

Topic	Author and Purpose(s)	Subjects and Procedure(s)	Major Findings
General exploratory/descriptive	*Walike et al. (1974): Assess and describe problems associated with tube feeding, develop hypotheses about methods for reducing eliminating problems.	121 adults: 48 female, 73 male (age range, 14-90). Survey (145 variables) record review of factors influencing incidence and causes of tube feeding problems: demographic and health status data; tube feeding method, diet, intake and output, vital signs; physical/emotional status, drug therapy, attitudes/reactions to diet; blood chemistry; hematology and urine data. Data collection tools were investigator developed.	Various types and tube sizes were used with patients. Variations in procedure were found for client position during feeding, use of gastric aspiration, rate, temperature and volume of administration, number of feedings per day and contents of solutions. Adverse client responses to feedings included diarrhea, gastrointestinal complications, weight loss, and elevated BUN. Scant information about attitudes and adjustments to feedings was found.
Tube location and placement	*Hanson (1979): Identification of noninvasive techniques and criteria for predicting proper length of stomach tube placement and clinical means for determining appropriate tube length.	104 adults: 99 cadavers, 5 normal volunteers. Comparison of external body measurements to actual distance from the tip of the nose to the lower esophageal sphincter.	New formula for predicting length was found to accurately predict length needed 91% of the time, compared to a 72% accuracy rate using traditional nose-to-ear-to-ziphoid measurement.
	Metheny, Spies, and Eisenberg (1986): Describe frequency with which nurses reported being able to aspirate fluid and measure gastric retention, predict accurate tube placement by client's ability to speak and predict accurate placement by auscultation of air.	Staff nurses supplied data for 20 nasogastric tube-fed patients (128 tube days) and 55 nasointestinal tube-fed patients (247 tube days). Data included results of withdrawing 5 ml of fluid, air auscultation, speaking ability and gastric retention.	Ability to aspirate fluid varied from 79% (large bore tubes) to 33% (small bore tubes) and check for gastric retention (90% large and 45% small). All clients were able to speak. 47% of time, nurses reported hearing epigastric air when the tube was located somewhere else besides the stomach. New methods for checking placement need to be developed and tubes that will allow proper monitoring need to be identified.
Rate, volume, and temperature of administration	*Heitkemper et al. (1981): Determine effects of volume and rate of administration of enteral tube feedings on subject tolerance and gastric pressure changes.	14 healthy volunteers: 9 females, 5 males (age range, 21-35). Studied for 10-12 trials on separate days. Feedings were administered at various volumes and rates after 10 hr of fasting.	First time feedings are more likely to be associated with feelings of discomfort, which subside with subsequent feedings. Rate of infusion should be no greater than 60 ml/min. Volume of feeding does not affect subjective tolerance as long as the rate per minute is within the suggested guideline.
	*Kagawa-Busby et al. (1980): Determine the effects of nasogastric tube feedings at various temperatures on gastric motility, total GI transit time and diarrhea, and subjective distress symptoms.	6 healthy volunteers: 4 female, 2 male. Nine trials per subject, for a total of 54 at 3 different temperatures for infusion. Rate was 50 ml/min for all administrations.	All three temperatures resulted in similiar gastric motility pattern after feeding. All showed a similiar decrease in gastric contraction and return of gastric activity during and after feeding. Two subjects reported diarrhea after cold feedings; no GI disturbances were found after warm feeding.

TABLE 11-2, cont'd

Topic	Author and Purpose(s)	Subjects and Procedure(s)	Major Findings
Attitudes and adjustments	*Padilla et al. (1979): Determine the type, incidence and subjective level of distress experienced by patients with tube feedings.	30 alert adult tube feeding patients. Interviewed via 47-item tube feeding and hospital experience checklist, a tool developed by the investigators to measure distress associated with tube feedings and hospitalization.	Clients identified a sore nose or throat, being NPO, limited mobility, dry mouth and runny nose as some of the more uncomfortable aspects of having a feeding tube. Interventions to reduce the unpleasant experiences were identified by health care professionals familiar with the problems of tube-fed patients.
Formula contents and/or complications	Cataldi-Betcher et al. (1983): Evaluate the incidence of complications for patients receiving enteral nutrition support.	253 subjects: 53% male (mean age 62.8), 47% female (mean age, 63.8). Standardized protocols for enteral feedings were followed by majority of physicians ordering enteral feedings. Most clients had weighted nasogastric tubes. 30 (11.7%) experienced GI (6.2%) mechanical (3.5%), or metabolic (2%) complications.	For clients with functioning GI tract, enteral feedings are preferred method of support. Diarrhea is the most frequent GI complication; cause is multifactorial. Correct tube selection is important to prevent mechanical complications; both small and large bore tubes have strengths and limitations. Metabolic complications are often less severe than those associated with parenteral nutrition. Recommendations for preventing all complications were discussed.
	Taylor (1982): Compare the incidence of diarrhea and/or aspiration pneumonia in neurosurgical clients receiving continuous versus intermittent infusion tube feeding.	13 clients (5 on intermittent, 7 on continuous, and 1 on both) (age range, 19 to 64). Investigator developed instruments to measure vital signs, relevant laboratory data, medications, incidence of diarrhea and/or aspiration.	Descriptive study documented that diarrhea and aspiration occur with both continuous and intermittent feedings. Procedure used in both protocols may reduce the incidence of aspiration. Further research needs to be done on the use of tube feedings with clients with neurological problems.
	*Walike and Walike (1973): Determine what proportion of diarrhea could be accounted for in tube-fed clients by lactose content of the diet and other factors that contribute to the remaining GI symptoms.	11 clients studied for a mean of 9.4 days on both lactose and lactose free N/G diets (9 males, 2 females). Data collected included relevant lab data, frequency and consistency of stools and lactose tolerance tests.	Lactose content of diets commonly used for N/G tube fed patients is major cause of diarrhea. Intolerance to lactose cannot be determined by traditional test with N/G patients. Relative lactose intolerance may be present in a great majority of adults; this becomes important when size of lactose load is beyond the client's ability to hydrolyze it. Elimination of lactose from tube feeding diets will reduce GI side effects.
	*Walike and Walike (1977)	(see box on p. 180 for summary of results.)	

*Tube Feeding Consortium Group Study.

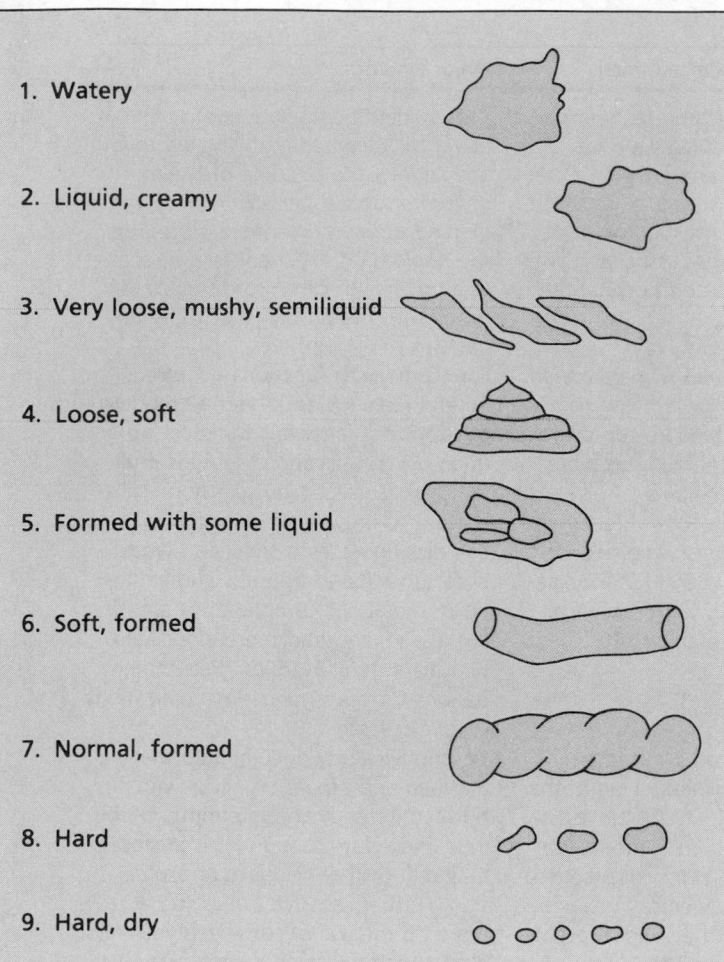

1. Watery

2. Liquid, creamy

3. Very loose, mushy, semiliquid

4. Loose, soft

5. Formed with some liquid

6. Soft, formed

7. Normal, formed

8. Hard

9. Hard, dry

Fig. 11-1 Stool consistency diagram.

Modified from Horsley, JA, Crane, J, and Haller, KB: Reducing diarrhea in tube-fed patients, CURN project, San Diego, 1981, Grune & Stratton, Inc.

were widely used in professional nursing practice. The problem of diarrhea in clients receiving tube feedings can be minimized by changing the contents of the tube-feeding formula. This has been a significant nursing problem, especially with clients who are bedridden or who have a decreased level of consciousness. The scientific foundation on which decisions about the nursing care of tube-fed patients can be based has been strengthened by the work of researchers investigating tube feeding. These studies originated in questions about procedures and clients' responses to a common nursing measure. The results of these studies did not lead to the invention of a completely new nursing intervention, but a substantial scientific basis has been established for improving nursing care for tube-fed patients.

Using Findings in Nursing Practice

To use findings in clinical practice, the nurse must be aware of the problems already studied. Therefore nurses should read journals that contain research reports, as well as textbooks and other sources, in nursing and related fields.

Not all research related to clinical nursing problems can or should be applied in practice. The nurse must judge the scientific worth of a study before considering its use in practice. This chapter can provide only a foundation for judging the worth of a research study. Other aspects that should be considered follow (Stetler and Marram, 1976; Setler, 1985):

1. How much substantiating evidence is provided by other scientific studies that have obtained similar results,
2. Whether the subjects and environment in the study are similar to the patients for whom the nurse provides care in the particular practice setting,
3. The theoretical basis for present nursing care and the effectiveness of current theory in solving clinical nursing problems,
4. The feasibility of applying findings, including ethical and legal limitations, institutional policy, changes in the organization of nursing services that might be required, and potential costs in time, money, and equipment.

The nurse must make judgements that involve validating the scientific soundness of a study, comparatively evaluating whether or not any use can be made of the findings, and deciding what type of application would be appropriate (Stetler, 1985).

Haller, Reynolds and Horsley (1979) note the research utilization process begins with the identification of a nursing problem area that has been investigated through conceptually related studies having the potential for use in clinical practice. The problem area chosen must have an established research base, be relevant to practice, and be capable of being reliably evaluated by nurses in clinical settings. In selecting the problem area the nurse is concerned with whether a solid research base exists for changing practice, the scientific merit of the studies constituting the research base, and the potential risk to the client in implementing the practice change. The final phases include developing a clinical protocol to be used to implement the change and clinically evaluating the outcomes of the new nursing care to determine its effectiveness.

Nurses should not change from accepted to unproven ways of providing client care without careful deliberation and consultation with colleagues. Experimenting with new nursing measures is inappropriate, especially if an increased risk to clients' health is possible.

Some people estimate that the half-life of knowledge in the health care field is 5 years. This means that half of what a nurse learns today may be out of date in 5 years. By developing skills necessary to read and understand nursing research studies, nurses can remain current throughout their careers.

SUMMARY

Research is an essential part of the nursing profession because it is an advanced, objective method of gaining new knowledge about human needs and people's responses to illness, treatments and therapies, and other health-related factors. The research process, a problem-solving method, involves a number of phases from the identification of the problem to the development and testing of hypotheses to the analysis, interpretation, and communication of findings. To gain new knowledge in a variety of nursing areas, nurses conduct clinical research in many settings, involving many kinds of research subjects whose rights must carefully be protected.

Nurses indirectly involved in conducting research also gain from research findings. Nurses therefore must develop skills for finding and identifying research studies and for organizing research information for clinical application. Successful use of research findings in nursing practice depends on the skills of the nurse to judge the scientific worth of a study, determine whether findings can be applied to a particular clinical setting and group of clients, and consider other practical issues such as ethical implications, institutional policies, and implementation costs. These skills are important for all nurses because of continuously evolving nursing knowledge about skills needed to practice professional nursing in all settings.

KEY CONCEPTS

✓ People acquire knowledge through tradition, from authorities in a field, through experience, by trial and error, and through application of the scientific method.

✓ The scientific method is the most objective method of gaining new knowledge.

✓ A scientific investigation is an orderly, planned, and controlled way of studying reality that can be applied to general situations and contributes to the testing of theories about people, places, or life events.

✓ Nursing research is conducted to study the physical or psychosocial responses of people of all ages in both health and illness.

✓ An experimental research study controls factors that could influence the results , includes comparison and experimental treatment groups of subjects, and uses random means for selecting study subjects.

✓ The research process is a systematic means of gaining knowledge about how to provide care for a group of people with a particular health care problem.

✓ Participation of human subjects in research studies requires the researcher to obtain informed consent of study subjects, to maintain the confidentiality of subjects, and to protect subjects from undue risk or injury.

✓ The researcher conducting a study is required to inform everyone assisting in the study about the purposes of the research and to prepare them for any adverse effects the subjects could experience.

✓ Research reports are most commonly found in specialized journals.

✓ A number of indexes for health care field are available for finding research articles.

✓ When summarizing data reported in a research study, the nurse should note when, how, where, and by whom the investigation was conducted and who and what was studied.

✓ A researchable clinical nursing problem is one that is not satisfactorily resolved by present nursing interventions, that occurs frequently in a particular group, that can be consistently and accurately measured, and that has a possible solution within the realm of nursing practice.

✓ To determine whether research findings can be used as a basis for nursing practice, the nurse should consider the scientific worth of the study, the substantiating evidence provided in other studies, the similarity of the research setting to the nurse's own clinical practice setting, the status of current nursing theory, and factors affecting the feasibility of application.

REFERENCES

Abdellah, FG, and Levine, E: Better patient care through nursing research, ed. 3, New York, 1986, Macmillan Publishing Co.

American Nurses' Association: Human rights guidelines for nurses in clinical and other research, Kansas City, Mo., 1975, The Association.

American Nurses' Association: Directions for nursing research: toward the twenty-first century, Kansas City, Mo., 1985a, The Association.

American Nurses' Association: Human rights guidelines for nurses in clinical and other research, Kansas City, Mo., 1985b, The Association.

American Psychological Association: Publication manual of the American Psychological Association, ed. 3, Washington, D.C., 1983, The Association.

Armiger, B: Ethics of nursing research: profile, principles, perspective, Nurs Res 26:330, 1977.

Bergstrom, N, et al.: Collaborative nursing research: anatomy of a successful consortium, Nurs Res 33:20, 1984.

Brink, PJ, and Wood, MJ: Basic steps in planning nursing research: from question to proposal, ed. 2, North Scituate, Mass., 1983, Duxbury Press.

Canadian Nurses Association, Ethical guidelines for nursing research involving human subjects, Ottawa, 1983, The Association.

Commission on Nursing Research, American Nurses' Association: Guidelines for the investigative function of nurses, Kansas City, Mo., 1981a, The Association.

Commission on Nursing Research, American Nurses' Association: Research priorities for the 1980's: generating a scientific basis for nursing practice, Kansas City, Mo., 1981b, The Association.

Diers, D: Research in nursing practice, Philadelphia, 1979, J.B. Lippincott Co.

Fuller, ED: Selecting a clinical nursing problem, Image: J Nurs Sch 14:60, 1982.

Gortner, SR: Nursing research: out of the past and into the future, Nurs Res 29:204, 1980.

Haller, KB, Reynolds, MA, and Horsley, JA: Developing research-based innovation protocols: process, criteria, and issues, Res Nurs Health 2:45, 1979.

Hansen, BW: Personal communication, Feb. 14, 1984.

Hanson, RL: New approach to measuring adult nasogastric tubes for insertion, Am J Nurs 80:1334, 1980.

Heitkemper, ME, et al.: Rate and volume of intermittent enteral feeding, J Parenter Enter Nutr 5:125, 1981.

Institute of Medicine, Division of Health Care Services: Nursing and nursing education: public policies and private actions, Washington, D.C., 1983, National Academy Press.

Kerlinger, FN: Foundations of behavioral research, ed. 3, New York, 1986, Holt, Rinehart & Winston, Inc.

Mallison, MB: The shortage that destroys, Am J Nurs 87:899, 1987.

Merritt, DH: The National Center for Nursing Research, Image: J Nurs Sch 18:84, 1986.

Polit, DV, and Hungler, BP: Nursing research: principles and practice, ed. 3, Philadelphia, 1987, J.B. Lippincott Co.

Seaman, CH, and Verhonick, PJ: Research methods for undergraduate students in nursing, ed. 2, Norwalk, Conn., 1982, Appleton-Century-Crofts.

Stetler, CB: Research utilization: defining the concept, Image: J Nurs Sch 17:40, 1985.

Stetler, CB, and Marram, G: Evaluating research findings for applicability in practice, Nurs Outlook 24:559, 1976.

Werley, HH, and Fitzpatrick, J: Annual review of nursing research, vol. 4, New York, 1986, Springer Publishing Co., Inc.

Research Articles

Flynn, KT, et al.: Enteral tube feedings: indications, practices and outcomes, Image: J Nurs Sch 19:16, 1987.

Hanson, RL: Predictive criteria for length of nasogastric tube insertion for tube feedings, JPEN 3:160, 1979.

Kagawa-Busby, KS, et al.: Effects of diet temperature on tolerance of enteral feedings, Nurs Res 29:276, 1980.

Metheny, NA, Spies, MA, and Eisenberg, P: Frequency of nasoenteral tube displacement and associated risk factors, Res Nurs Health 9:241, 1986.

Metheny NA, Spies, MA, and Eisenberg, P: Measures to test placement of nasoenteral feeding tubes, West J Nurs Res Aug. 1988.

Padilla, GV, et al.: Subjective distresses of nasogastric tube feeding, JPEN 3:53, 1979.

Padilla, GV, et al.: Distress reduction and the effects of preparatory teaching films and patient control, Res Nurs Health 4:375, 1981.

Schmidt, FE, and Woolridge, PJ: Psychological preparation of surgical patients, Nurs Res 22:108, 1973.

Walike, BC, and Walike JW: Relative lactose intolerance: a clinical study of tube-fed patients, JAMA 238:948, 1977.

Walike, BC, et al.: Patient problems related to tube feeding. In Batey, MV, editor: Communicating nursing research, vol. 7, Boulder, Colo., 1974, Western Interstate Commission for Higher Education.

Wolfer, JA, and Davis, CE: Assessment of surgical patients' preoperative emotional condition and postoperative welfare, Nurs Res 19:402, 1970.

ADDITIONAL READINGS

Binger, JL, and Jensen, LM: Lippincott's guide to nursing literature: a handbook for students, writers, and researchers, Philadelphia, 1980, J.B. Lippincott Co.

Cabinet on Nursing Research, American Nurses' Association: Establishment of a National Institute of Nursing: a statement of rationale (mimeograph), Kansas City, Mo., 1983, The Association.

Cataldi-Betcher, EL, et al.: Complications occurring during enteral nutrition support: a prospective study, JPEN 7:546, 1983.

Eisenberg, P, et al.: Characteristics of patients who remove their nasal feeding tube, Clinical Nurse Specialist 1(3):94, 1987.

Fox, DA: Fundamentals of research in nursing, Norwalk, Conn., 1983, Appleton-Century-Crofts.

Horsley, JA, Crane, J, and Haller, KB: Reducing diarrhea in tube-fed patients, conduct and utilization of Research in Nursing (CURN) project, New York, 1981, Grune & Stratton, Inc.

Keohane, PP, et al.: Relation between osmolality of diet and gastrointestinal side effects in enteral nutrition, Br Med J [Clin Res] 288:678, 1984.

Metheny, NA, Eisenberg, P, and Spies, MA: Aspiration pneumonia in patients fed through nasoenteral tubes, Heart Lung 15:256, 1986.

Taylor, TT: A comparison of two methods of nasogastric tube feedings, J Neurosurg Nurs 14:49, 1982.

Trussell, P, Brandt, A, and Knapp, S: Using nursing research: discovery, analysis and interpretation, Wakefield, Mass., 1981, Nursing Resources.

Williams, KR: Effect of the temperature of tube feeding on gastric motility in monkeys, Nurs Res 24:4, 1975.

Woods, NF, and Catanzaro, M: Nursing research: theory and practice, St. Louis, 1987, The C.V. Mosby Co.

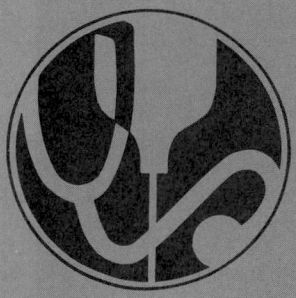

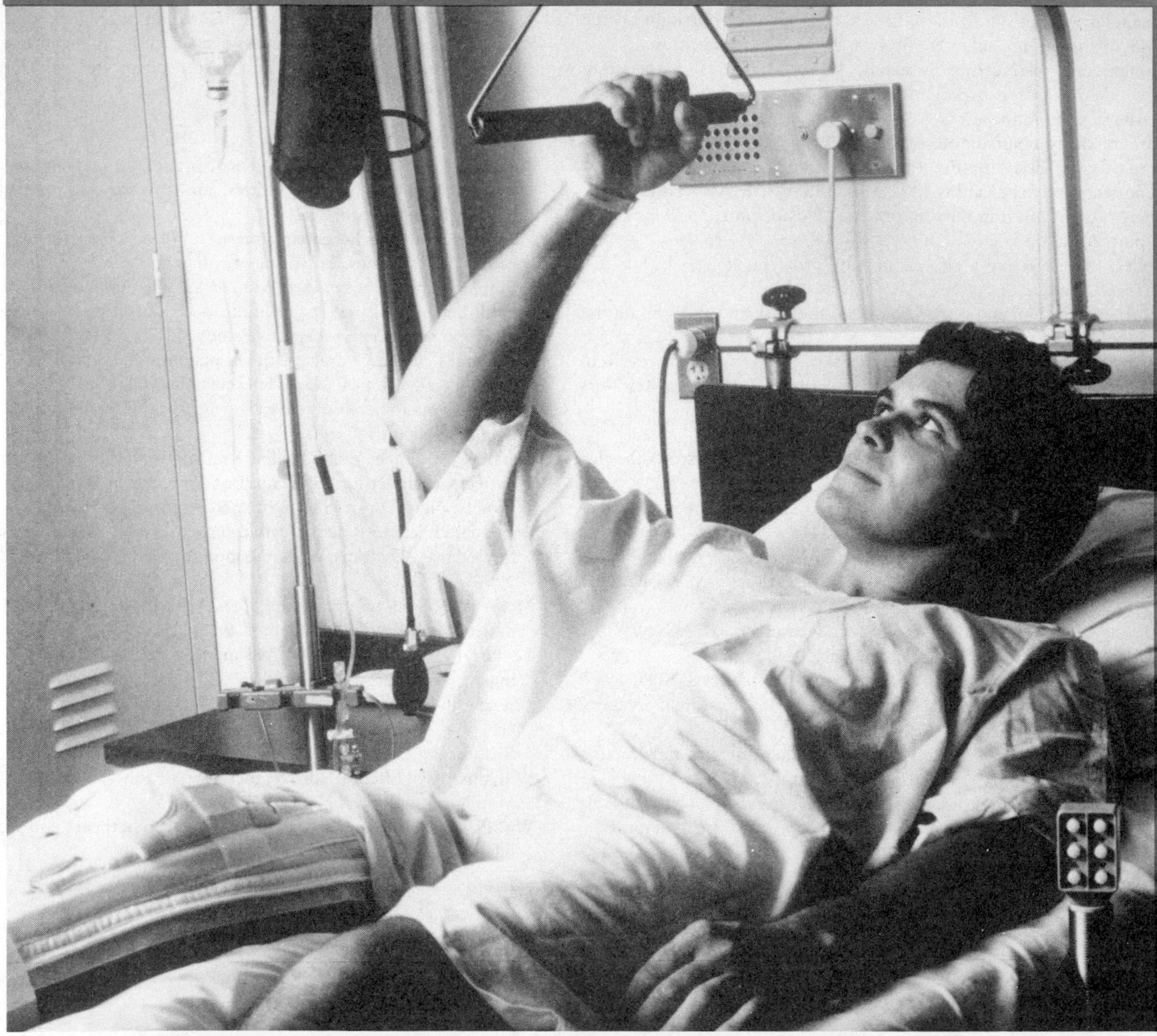

Professional Nursing Skills

Nursing practice in all settings involves a wide range of professional skills used in the care of clients. The four chapters in Unit 3 discuss these commonly used nursing skills. The skills for vital sign measurement and physical assessment are basic to nursing practice and are used frequently. Nursing care throughout the nursing process depends on effective recording and reporting skills, which are the bases of communication among health care professionals. Finally, the nurse's skills in administering medications are essential when providing care for clients with different health needs.

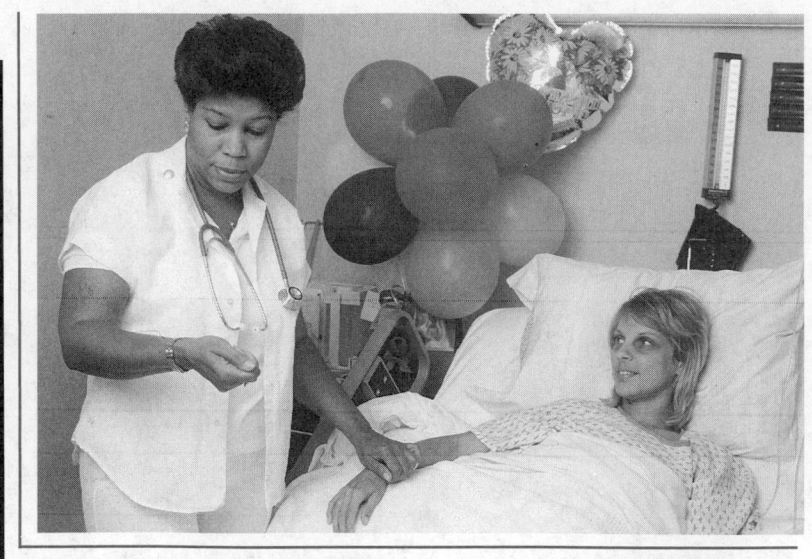

OBJECTIVES

Mastery of content in this chapter will enable the student to:

- Define the key terms listed.
- Explain the principles and mechanisms of thermoregulation.
- Discuss the rationale for a nursing care plan for a client with a fever.
- Identify steps used to assess a client's oral, rectal, and axillary temperature.
- Explain the physiology for the normal regulation of blood pressure, pulse, and respirations.
- Describe the types of factors that normally cause variations in body temperature, pulse, respirations, and blood pressure.
- Identify steps used to assess a client's pulse, respirations, and blood pressure.
- Identify normal vital sign values for an adult and an infant.
- Explain variations in technique used to assess an infant's and child's vital signs.
- Describe the benefits and precautions involving self-measurement of blood pressure.
- Accurately record and report vital sign measurements.

KEY TERMS

Auscultation
Bradycardia
Calorie
Cardiac Telemetry
Centigrade
Costal
Cyanosis
Diaphoresis
Diurnal
Dysrhythmia
Eupnea
Fever
Febrile
Hematocrit
Hemodynamics
Hemorrhage
Holter Monitor
Hypercarbia

Hypertension
Hyperthermia
Hypotension
Hypothermia
Hypoventilation
Insensible Water Loss
Meniscus
Myalgia
Neurotransmitter
Orthostatic Hypotension
Pyrogen
Spirometer
Tachycardia
Thermoregulation
Tidal Volume
Viscera
Vital Signs

Vital Signs

Vital signs—temperature, pulse, respirations, and blood pressure—are indicators of health status. Many factors such as the temperature of the environment, physical activity, and the effects of illness cause vital signs to change, sometimes beyond a normal range. Measurement of vital signs provides data that can be used to determine a client's usual state of health (baseline data), as well as his or her response to physical and psychological stress and medical and nursing therapy. An alteration in normal vital signs may signal the need for medical or nursing intervention.

When a client comes to a health care agency or is seen by a nurse at home, measurement of vital signs is a routine part of the complete physical assessment (see Chapter 13). They may also be measured separately as part of a review of the client's condition. Vital signs are a quick and efficient way of monitoring a condition or identifying the presence of problems. The basic skills required to measure vital signs are simple but should not be taken for granted. Vital signs and other physiological measurements can be the basis for clinical problem solving. Careful measurement techniques ensure accurate findings.

GUIDELINES FOR TAKING VITAL SIGNS

Vital signs are a part of the data base a nurse collects during assessment. The process of taking vital signs is not routine but is individualized to the client's needs and condition. The nurse must be able to measure vital signs correctly, understand and interpret the values, communicate findings appropriately, and begin interventions as needed. The nurse's judgment helps determine the need for and frequency of vital sign measurement.

The following guidelines help the nurse incorporate vital sign measurement into nursing practice:

1. *The nurse caring for the client measures vital signs*—Throughout the course of a shift, the nurse makes observations of the client's condition. Vital signs give important information about the client's state of health. The nurse caring for a client is the best one to take vital signs, interpret their significance, and make decisions about care.

2. *Equipment should be functional and appropriate*—Equipment used to measure vital signs (for example, a thermometer or stethoscope) must work properly to ensure accurate findings.

3. *Know the normal range for all vital signs*—This knowledge helps the nurse detect abnormalities.

4. *Know the client's normal range of vital signs*—A client's normal values may differ from the standard range for that age or physical state. Normal values for a client serve as a baseline for comparison with findings taken later. Thus a nurse can detect a change in condition over time.

5. *Know the client's medical history and any therapies or medications prescribed*—Some illnesses or treatments cause predictable vital sign changes.

6. *Control or minimize any environmental factors that may affect vital signs*—Measuring a pulse after the client exercises or experiences an emotional upset or checking temperature in a warm, humid room may yield values that are not true indicators of the client's condition.

7. *Use an organized, systematic approach when taking vital signs*—The nurse uses a systematic method to assess vital signs. For example, many nurses measure temperature first. By using a glass thermometer, the nurse can measure the temperature while checking pulse, respirations, and blood pressure. Each procedure requires a step-by-step approach.

8. *Decide the frequency of vital sign assessment on the basis of the client's condition*—In the hospital the physician orders a minimum frequency of vital sign measurements for each client, but the nurse is responsible for judging if more frequent assessments are needed. If a client's physical condition begins to worsen, the nurse takes vital signs more often, perhaps as often as every 5 to 10 minutes. After a client returns from surgery or a major diagnostic examination such as cardiac catheterization, frequent measurements are taken until the vital signs stabilize to the before-pro-

cedure range. Taking vital signs as a basis for determining changes and trends is useful in making therapeutic decisions.

9. *Analyze the results of vital sign measurement*—The nurse is often in the best position to assess all the clinical findings about a client. Vital signs are not assessed in isolation. The nurse must also know other physical signs or symptoms and be aware of the client's ongoing health status. Vital signs can be just part of the puzzle the nurse solves when assessing the client's physical and psychological condition.

10. *Verify and communicate significant changes in vital signs*—Baseline measurements allow a nurse to identify changes in vital signs. When vital signs reach an abnormal range, it may help to have another nurse or a physician repeat a measurement to verify it. The nurse tells a physician when vital signs become abnormal. It is also important for the nurse to record and report any changes to the nurses working the next shift.

Vital signs are physiological data that assist the nurse in performing routine care measures and critical interventions. For example, to determine if a client tolerates exercise, the nurse may assess pulse rate. When a client experiences excessive blood loss after injury or surgery, blood pressure measurement can reveal the seriousness of the hemorrhage. Continued blood pressure checks help determine when to administer fluids or medications to restore blood pressure to normal. The box provides information about when nurses should assess vital signs.

When to Take Vital Signs

- On the client's admission to a health care facility
- In a hospital on a routine schedule according to a physician's order or hospital policy
- Before and after any surgical procedure
- Before and after any invasive diagnostic procedure
- Before and after the administration of certain medications that affect cardiovascular, respiratory, and temperature control function
- When the client's general physical condition changes (as with loss of consciousness or increased intensity of pain)
- Before and after nursing interventions influencing any one of the vital signs (such as before a client previously on bed rest ambulates or before a client performs range of motion exercises)
- Whenever the client reports any nonspecific symptoms of physical distress (such as feeling "funny" or "different")

BODY TEMPERATURE

The body's tissues and cells normally function best within a relatively narrow temperature range. Humans are warm-blooded animals. A person's body temperature remains relatively stable despite internal extremes (for example, metabolic changes) or external conditions (for example, climatic temperature). Temperature-control mechanisms keep the body's *core temperature*, or temperature of deep tissues, in a relatively constant range, 37° C (98.6° F) ± 1° F. The body's surface temperature rises and falls with the temperature of the environment. The layers of skin, subcutaneous tissues, and fat may fluctuate between 20° and 40° C (68° and 104° F) without damage.

When a nurse measures a client's body temperature, the thermometer registers the body's core temperature. In clinical practice, nurses learn the normal temperature range of individuals. No single temperature is normal for all people. The temperature range for a normal active adult is larger than might be expected (Fig. 12-1), depending in part on a person's range of activity.

Body Temperature Regulation

The balance of body temperature is precisely regulated by physiological and behavioral mechanisms. For the body temperature to stay constant, heat produced in the body must equal heat lost to the environment. A nurse applies knowledge of temperature control mechanisms to promote temperature regulation.

NEURAL CONTROL

The hypothalamus, located between the cerebral hemispheres, controls body temperature the same way a thermostat works in the home. A comfortable temperature is the "set point" at which a heating system operates. In the home a fall in environmental temperature activates the furnace, whereas a rise in temperature shuts the system down. The hypothalamus senses minor changes in body temperature. When body temperature deviates from the set point, the thermoregulatory center of the hypothalamus activates heat loss or production so the core temperature stays in a safe physiological range.

When nerve cells in the hypothalamus become heated, impulses are sent out to reduce body temperature (Fig. 12-2). Mechanisms of heat loss include sweating, dilation of blood vessels, and inhibition of heat production. If the hypothalamus senses that the body's temperature is too low, signals are sent out to increase heat production and conservation through vasoconstriction, muscle shivering, and piloerection. Lesions or trauma to the hypothalamus or spinal cord, which carries hypothalamic messages, can cause serious alterations in temperature control.

HEAT PRODUCTION. Heat is produced in the body by metabolism, which is the sum of the chemical reactions in all body cells. Food is the primary fuel source for metabolism. Although heat production increases when a person is active, it is a constant process. Most heat comes from the body's core during quiet times and rest. During work the main site of heat production is the muscles. Table 12-1 reviews the sources and mechanisms of heat production.

SKIN IN TEMPERATURE REGULATION

The skin has the following roles in temperature regulation: (1) insulation of the body, (2) vasoconstriction,

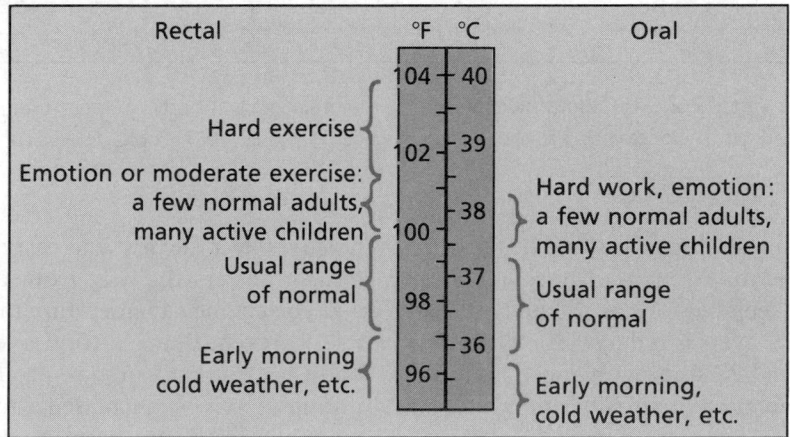

Fig. 12-1 Ranges of rectal and oral temperatures found in normal persons.
Redrawn from Mountcastle, VB: Medical physiology, vol. 2, ed. 14, St. Louis, 1980, The C.V. Mosby Co.; based on Dubois, EF: Fever and the regulation of body temperature, Springfield, Ill., 1948, Charles C Thomas, Publisher.

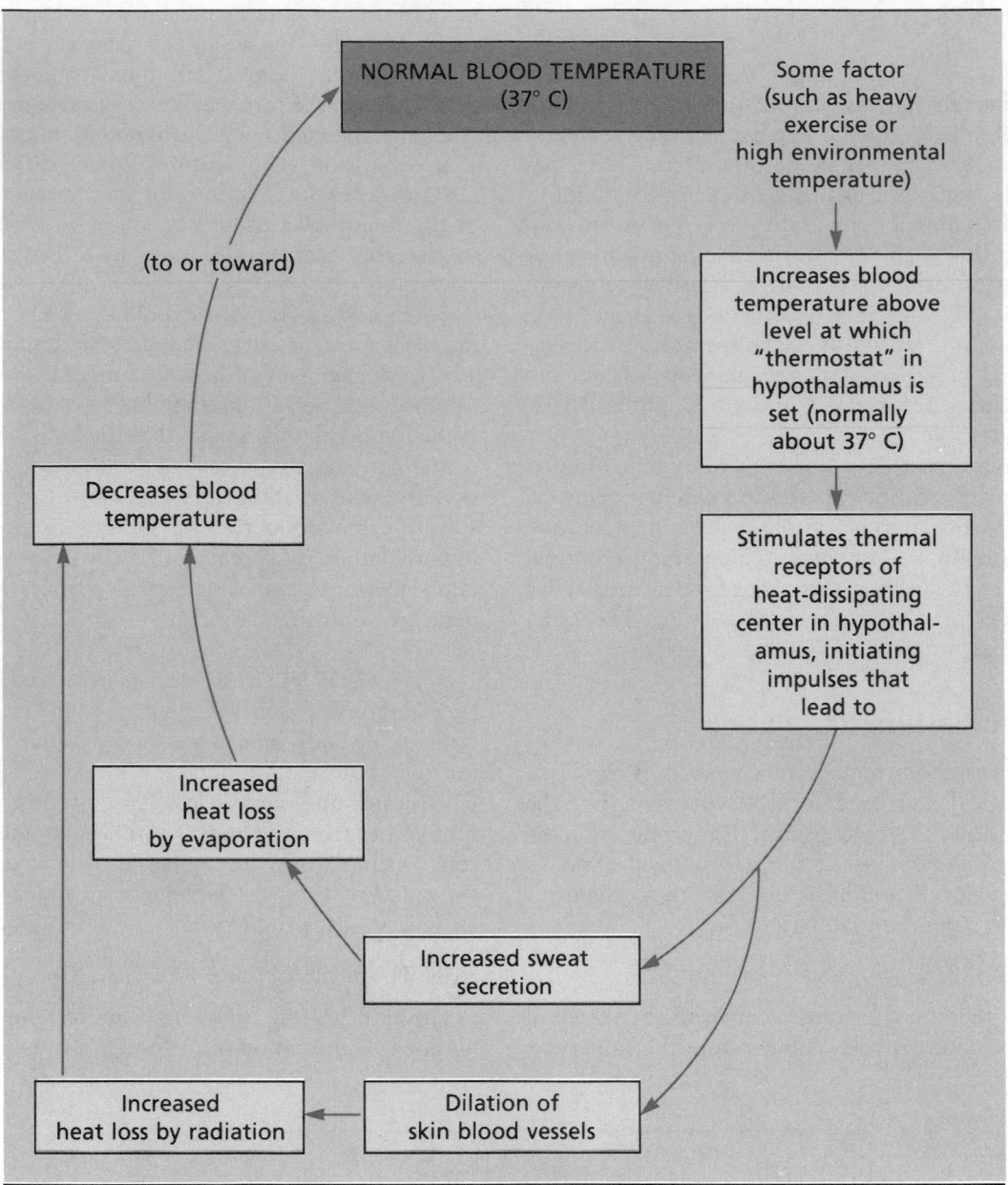

Fig. 12-2 Heat loss mechanisms to maintain normal body temperature.
From Thibodeau, GA: Anatomy and physiology, St. Louis, 1987, The C.V. Mosby Co.

which affects the amount of blood flow and heat loss to the skin, and (3) temperature sensor. The skin, subcutaneous tissue, and fat keep heat inside the body. When blood flow between skin layers is reduced, the skin alone is an excellent insulator. Persons with more body fat have better natural insulation than slim and muscular people.

The way the skin controls body temperature is similar to the way an automobile radiator controls engine temperature. The engine of an automobile generates a great deal of heat. Water is pumped through the engine's sys-

tem to collect the heat and carry it to the radiator, where a fan transfers the heat from the water to the outside air. The engine's temperature thus stays within safe limits to prevent damage from overheating. In the human body the internal organs produce heat, and at times during exercise or increased sympathetic stimulation the amount of heat produced is greater than normal body core temperature. Blood flows from the internal organs, carrying heat to the body surface. The skin is well supplied with blood vessels. In the most exposed areas of the body—the hands, feet, and ears—blood can flow

TABLE 12-1   Sources and Mechanisms of Heat Production

Source	Mechanism	Nursing Implications
Metabolism	Basal metabolic rate (BMR) is the smallest amount of energy expenditure needed to sustain life and maintain a normal body temperature in a comfortable, warm environment. BMR is a measure of the kilocalories of energy expended per hour per square meter of surface area. The BMR constitutes 55% to 60% of a person's total metabolic rate or the amount of energy used or expended by the body at any time.	Food intake and exercise influence metabolic rate. Seriously ill clients benefit from increased calorie intake and reduced activity so that energy is available for healing and vital functions.
Muscle activity	As exercise levels increase, the amount of energy or muscular work increases. The energy of muscular work comes from oxidation of carbohydrates and fats. Even minor activity such as bathing can raise the metabolic rate and therefore heat production.	Clients whose energy reserves are minimal and whose body temperatures are already elevated can suffer increased temperature from any physical exertion.
	Shivering of skeletal muscles also increases body heat production. When body temperature becomes too low, the tone of all skeletal muscles increase. Maximal shivering can increase heat production four to five times greater than normal (Guyton, 1986).	Nurses may give medications that reduce shivering to prevent a rise in a fever. Apply extra clothing or bed coverings to prevent or reduce shivering.
Thyroid hormone	Thyroxine and triiodothyronine increase basal metabolism by breaking down glucose and fat. The anterior pituitary gland releases thyroid-stimulating hormone (TSH) according to metabolic demands. Both thyroid hormones must be present for maintenance of a normal BMR. Deficient thyroid secretion slows metabolism. In cold temperatures, neither hormone assists in temperature regulation.	Clients with thyroid disorders may have intolerances to heat or cold.
Sympathetic stimulation	Norepinephrine and epinephrine stimulate the sympathetic nervous system to increase metabolism when a drop in blood glucose levels occurs. This results in glycogen metabolism, which makes glucose available to cells for energy.	For ill clients, nutritional maintenance prevents depletion of energy stores and supports normal temperature.

directly from arteries to veins, bypassing capillaries. Blood flow through the more vascular areas of the skin may vary from minimal flow to as much as 30% of the cardiac output (Guyton, 1986). Heat transfers from the blood, through vessel walls, to the skin's surface and is lost to the environment through heat loss mechanisms. The body's core temperature remains within safe limits.

The degree of vasoconstriction determines the amount of blood flow and heat loss to the skin. If the core temperature must be lowered, the hypothalamus inhibits sympathetic impulses, blood vessels dilate, and more

blood reaches the skin's surface. On a hot, humid day the blood vessels in the hands are dilated and easily visible. In contrast, if the core temperature becomes too low, the hypothalamus initiates vasoconstriction and blood flow to the skin lessens. Thus body heat is conserved.

The skin is well supplied with heat and cold receptors. Since the cold receptors are more plentiful, however, the skin functions primarily to detect cold surface temperatures. When the skin becomes chilled, its sensors send information to the hypothalamus, which initiates the following reflexes: shivering to increase body heat production, inhibition of sweating, and vasoconstriction of blood vessels.

HEAT LOSS

As the body produces heat, it also loses heat. The skin's structure and exposure to the environment result in constant, normal heat loss through the following processes: radiation, conduction, convection, and evaporation.

RADIATION. Radiation is the transfer of heat from the surface of one object to the surface of another without actual contact between the two (Thibodeau, 1987). Heat radiates from the skin to nearby objects that are cooler and radiates to the skin from those that are warmer. The amount of heat lost by radiation from the skin varies according to dilation of surface blood vessels when heat must be lost and by vasoconstriction when heat loss must be reduced.

Heat loss through radiation can be reduced by covering the body with clothing, especially dark, closely woven clothes. Body positioning also affects heat loss through radiation. A person standing with arms and legs extended radiates more heat than a person lying down in a fetal position.

CONDUCTION. Conduction is the transfer of heat to any object or surface actually in contact with the body. The process of conduction accounts for a small amount of heat loss. Heat conducts through solids, gases, and liquids.

When a person sits on a chair, there is heat conduction until the chair's surface temperature begins to rise. When the skin surface and chair temperature are the same, conductive heat loss stops. If the air next to the skin is cooler than the skin's surface, the body's heat warms the air. Wearing several layers of clothing creates layers of warmed air surrounding the body, which keeps the person warm and reduces conductive heat loss.

CONVECTION. Convection is the transfer of heat away from a surface, such as the skin, by movement of heated air or fluid particles (Thibodeau, 1987). Normally a warm layer of air exists close to the skin's surface. Heated air rises from the skin and passes to cooler air by convection currents, causing little heat loss from the skin.

However, considerable heat loss can occur when moistened skin comes into contact with slightly moving air. The body cannot create a warm layer of water next to the skin as it does in the air. The rate of heat loss from the skin can be high. Thus water used to bathe clients should be above body temperature. However, if a client's temperature is abnormally high, the nurse can lower the client's fever by bathing the person in tepid water that is below body temperature. The water will absorb heat. Cold water is not used because of the danger of causing chills, which will actually raise body temperature through muscle shivering.

EVAPORATION. Heat energy is needed to change water from a liquid to a gas. For each gram of water that evaporates from the body surface, approximately 0.6 kilocalorie (kcal) of heat is lost (Mountcastle, 1980). The body always loses some heat by evaporation. Normally, this insensible water loss occurs from the skin and lungs. The drying effect from evaporation can cause skin scaling and itching, as well as drying of the nares and pharynx. An average adult may lose 280 to 380 kcal per day by insensible loss. However, insensible loss occurs regardless of body temperature and thus plays no major role in temperature regulation.

Sweating controls body temperature through evaporative heat loss. Millions of sweat glands lie deep below the dermal layer of the skin. The glands secrete sweat, a watery solution containing sodium and chloride, which passes through tiny ducts on the skin's surface. The glands are controlled by sympathetic nerve fibers. Acetylcholine is the main neurotransmitter stimulating sweat glands. When the body's temperature rises, sweat glands release sweat, which evaporates from the skin's surface to promote heat loss. Exercise causes a significant rise in body temperature to stimulate sweating. Emotional or mental stress causes sweating through sympathetic stimulation. When temperatures are cold, sweat gland secretion is inhibited. Sweating is less efficient when air currents are reduced or when the humidity of the air is high. People who have a congenital absence of sweat glands or who have a serious skin disease that impairs sweating are not able to tolerate warm temperatures.

BEHAVIORAL CONTROL

Behavioral regulation involves the voluntary acts persons take to maintain a comfortable body temperature. Humans alter their behavior when exposed to temperature extremes. The ability of a person to control body temperature depends on the degree of temperature extreme, the person's ability to sense feeling comfortable or uncomfortable, and the person's thought processes or emotions. When the temperature in the environment falls, a person can add clothing, move to a warmer place, raise the temperature setting on a furnace thermostat, increase muscular activity by running in place, or sit with arms and legs tightly wrapped together. In contrast, when the temperature becomes hot, a person can remove clothing, stop activity, lower the thermostat on an air conditioner, turn on a fan, seek a cooler place, or take a cool shower or bath.

Persons with altered temperature control mechanisms, such as an infant or elderly person, have difficulty maintaining body temperature. These persons may need assistance in changing their environment so that exposure to temperature extremes is limited. An individual suffering from an illness or injury that lowers consciousness or causes an impairment in thought processes may also be unable to recognize the need to change behavior for temperature control. When temperatures become extremely hot or cold, behavioral modifications have a limited effect on controlling temperature loss or gain.

Factors Affecting Body Temperature

The nurse must be aware of factors affecting body temperature to assess temperature variations and evaluate the significance of changes from normal.

AGE

At birth the newborn leaves a warm, relatively constant environment and enters one in which temperatures fluctuate widely. Thermoregulatory mechanisms are not fully developed. An infant's temperature may change drastically with changes in the environment. Extra care is therefore needed to protect the newborn. Clothing must be adequate, and exposure to temperature extremes must be avoided. When protected from environmental extremes, the newborn's body temperature is maintained within the range of 35.5° to 37.5° C (96° to 99.5° F). Heat production steadily declines as the infant grows into childhood. Individual differences of 0.5° to 1° F are normal (Whaley and Wong, 1987).

Temperature regulation is unstable until a child reaches puberty. The normal temperature range gradually drops as an individual approaches old age. A temperature of 35° C (95° F) orally is not unusual for an elderly person in cold weather. However, the average body temperature of an older adult is approximately 36° C (96.8° F). Older adults are particularly sensitive to temperature extremes because of a deterioration in thermoregulation, including poor vasomotor control, reduced subcutaneous tissue, reduced sweat gland activity, and reduced metabolism. Some elderly clients are especially at risk when temperatures fall if they are not physically active or have limited incomes that prevent them from heating their homes adequately.

EXERCISE

Muscle activity increases heat production, so any form of exercise can increase body temperature. After prolonged exercise, such as long-distance running, body temperatures may temporarily reach levels as high as 39° to 41° C (103.2° to 105.8° F) (Petersdorf, 1980).

HORMONES

Women generally experience greater fluctuations in body temperature than men. Hormonal variations during the menstrual cycle cause body temperature fluctuations. Progesterone levels rise and fall cyclically during the menstrual cycle. Before the menstrual cycle, progesterone levels are low and the body temperature falls a few tenths of a degree Fahrenheit below the baseline level. The lower temperature persists until ovulation occurs. At ovulation, greater amounts of progesterone enter the circulatory system and raise the body temperature to previous baseline levels or higher. Plotting out temperature variations during the menstrual cycle to determine when ovulation occurs and avoiding sexual intercourse during ovulation is a form of birth control.

CIRCADIAN RHYTHMS

Body temperatures normally change 0.5° to 1° C (0.9° to 1.8° F) during 24 hours. However, temperature is one of the most stable rhythms in humans. The temperature is usually lowest between 1 and 4 AM (Fig. 12-3). During the day, body temperature rises steadily, peaking between 4 and 7 PM, and then declining to early morning levels. At one time, daily temperature variations were believed to be a result of greater daytime activity. However, temperature patterns are not automatically reversed in people who work during the night and sleep during the day. It takes 1 to 3 weeks for the cycle to reverse. Each client has a different temperature pattern, which the nurse must assess to identify a change in health. Studies (Angerami, 1980; Samples et al., 1985) show that the optimal time to screen for fever is 6 PM.

STRESS

Physical and emotional stress increase body temperature through hormonal and neural stimulation. The client who is anxious about entering a hospital or a physician's office may register a higher-than-normal temperature. The nurse can obtain a more accurate tem-

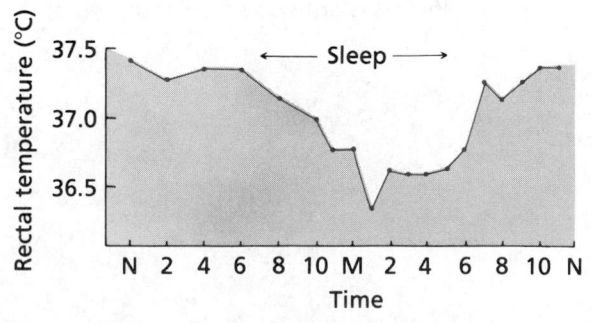

Fig. 12-3   24-hour temperature cycle.
From Mountcastle, VB: Medical physiology, vol. 2, ed. 14, St. Louis, 1980, The C.V. Mosby Co.

perature reading by waiting until the client's emotional stress subsides.

ENVIRONMENT

Environment influences body temperature. If a client's temperature is assessed in a very warm room or if he or she has just been outside on a cold blustery day, the nurse can expect to see a temperature variation. The very young and old are most likely to be affected by environmental temperatures.

Temperature Alterations

Body temperature becomes altered as a result of a change in temperature-regulating mechanisms or a change in environmental temperature. The nature of the change affects the type of clinical problems a client experiences.

FEVER

The simplest definition of a fever is a body temperature above 38° C (100.4° F) rectally measured under resting conditions. However, since each person's temperature range varies, a fever may exist in a person whose temperature is within the normal accepted range. A true fever results from an alteration in the hypothalamic set point (Fig. 12-4). Bacteria, viruses, fungi, and certain antigens are pyrogens, substances that cause a rise in body temperature. Once pyrogens enter the body, the white blood cells, called *macrophages,* produce the hormonelike substance, interleukin-1 (Atkins, 1983). Interleukin-1 helps promote the body's immunity and defense against infection but also acts on cells in the hypothalamus to cause synthesis of prostaglandin E, which raises the set point. Once the set point is increased, physiological and behavioral mechanisms go to work. During the chill phase of a fever, the body acts to produce and conserve heat. It may take several hours before the body temperature reaches the new set point. During this time, neural mechanisms cause vasoconstriction. A person experiences chills, shivers, and feels cold even though the body temperature is rising. Once the body temperature reaches the new set point, the chills subside, and the person then feels warm.

During the course of a fever, the body's metabolism increases and oxygen consumption rises. Heart and respiratory rates also increase. If the client has a cardiac or respiratory problem, the stress of fever can be great. A prolonged fever can seriously weaken a client because of exhaustion of the body's energy stores and the increased work of breathing. Confusion can result because of reduced oxygen to the brain (although this condition is completely reversible in some cases). The increased metabolism places a client at risk for dehydration. De-

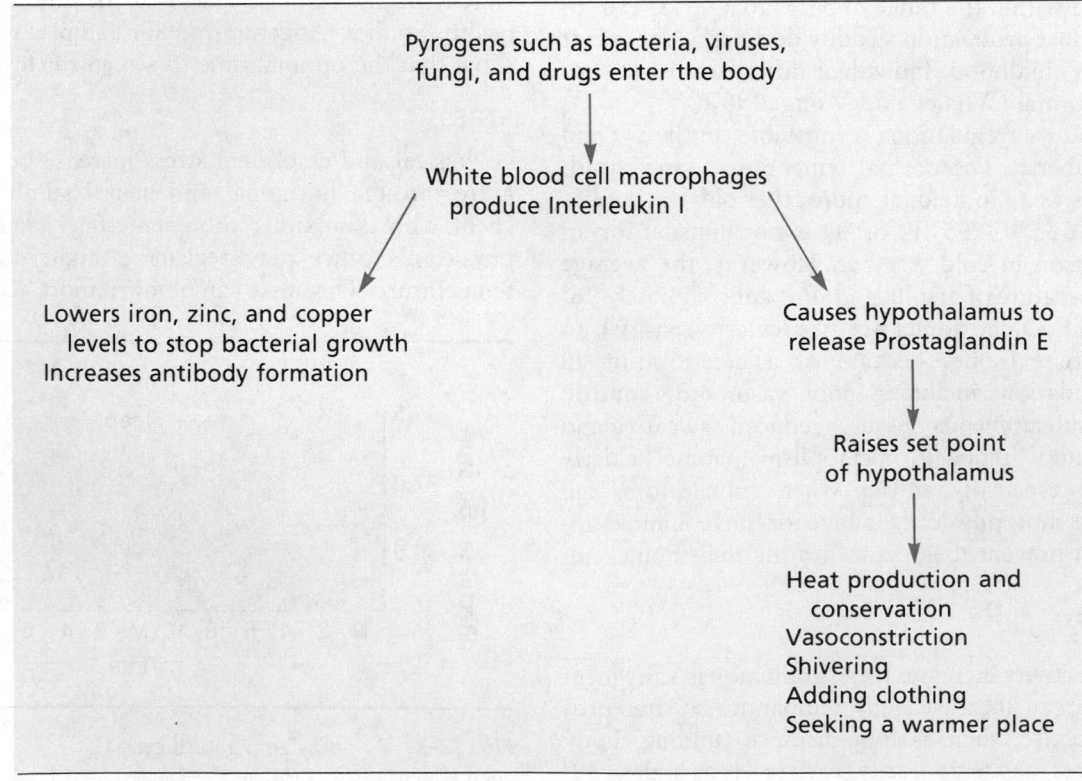

Fig. 12-4 Mechanism of a fever.

hydration is a problem especially for children because they can quickly lose large amounts of fluids in proportion to their body weight.

Once the cause of the fever is removed (for example, by destruction of bacteria by antibiotic medication), the hypothalamic set point drops. The body begins to initiate heat loss mechanisms. The skin becomes warm and flushed because of vasodilation. Diaphoresis, or excess sweating, helps lower the body's temperature. The client feels more alert with renewed energy.

Fevers may also be caused by central nervous system problems. Increased intracranial pressure caused by inflammation or bleeding may result in a very high fever, 41° C (106° F) or above. Clients with this type of fever do not sweat and fail to respond to antipyretic medication (for example, aspirin).

TREATMENT ISSUES. Physicians often disagree about when to treat a fever. A fever is usually not harmful if it stays below 39° C (102° F). Recent research (Dinarello, 1984) suggests that fever is an important defense mechanism. Moderate fevers, those between 37° and 38° C (98.6° and 100.4° F), may help activate the body's immune system. Interleukin-1 stimulates antibody production. These disease-fighting agents work best at higher temperatures. Fever also fights viral infections by stimulating interferon, the body's natural virus-fighting substance. Fevers also serve a diagnostic purpose. The natural pattern of a fever may reveal its cause (Table 12-2).

Physicians sometimes hesitate to treat fevers. Most fevers in children are of a viral origin, brief duration, and have limited effects (Lovejoy, 1978). However, controversy exists over when to treat fevers aggressively in children. Because of unstable temperature control mechanisms, children may become easily dehydrated or suffer convulsions.

ASSESSMENT OF FEVER. The nurse caring for clients with fever performs the following assessments through all stages of the febrile episode:
1. Measure vital signs when a fever is suspected and on an ongoing basis as ordered (for example, every 2 to 4 hours) until body temperature returns to normal. An increase in temperature is usually paired with tachycardia (increased heart rate) and tachypnea (increased respiratory rate).
2. Inspect and palpate the client's skin and check for turgor (see Chapter 13). As a fever develops, the skin may feel cool and dry and looks pale. At the height of the fever the skin becomes warm. Once a fever begins to break, the skin is flushed, warm, and moist from sweating. Reduced skin turgor is a sign of dehydration.
3. Ask how the client feels. Common symptoms of fever include headache, myalgia (muscle aches), chills, nausea, photophobia (sensitivity of the eyes to light), weakness, fatigue, and loss of appetite. A client will often complain of thirst.
4. Note the presence of vomiting or diarrhea, which can increase fluid and electrolyte loss (see Chapter 37).
5. Observe the client for behavioral changes such as confusion, restlessness, or disorientation.
6. Monitor test results for electrolyte levels. An excessive loss of fluids will cause electrolyte imbalance (sodium, potassium, and chloride are most likely to be altered).
7. Inspect the condition of the oral mucosa (see Chapter 13) for dryness resulting from dehydration. Small herpetic lesions characteristic of a fever may also be found on the mucosa.

NURSING DIAGNOSIS. The nurse reviews assessment findings to identify the nursing diagnoses related to prob-

TABLE 12-2   Common Fever Patterns

Type of Fever	Nature of Pattern	Possible Cause
Sustained	Shows little fluctuation	Scarlet fever Pneumococcal pneumonia Rickettsial fever Central nervous system problems
Intermittent	Wide temperature variations with return to normal at least once daily	Bacterial or viral infection Acute pyelonephritis Malaria
Remittent	Fluctuate less than intermittent; does not return to normal	Endocarditis Lung infection
Recurrent	Lasts a few days; temperature returns to normal a day or so, then fever returns	Hodgkin's disease Rat-bite fever Yellow fever
Night	Occurs late in evening or night	Tuberculosis

Examples of Nursing Diagnoses Related to Fever

NANDA-APPROVED NURSING DIAGNOSES

Pain related to:
- Fever

Activity intolerance related to:
- Reduced energy stores

Impaired gas exchange, related to
- Increased oxygen consumption

Potential or actual fluid volume deficit: related to:
- Increased metabolism

Hyperthermia related to:
- Infectious process
- Central nervous system injury

Altered nutrition: less than body requirements related to:
- Increased metabolism

lems caused by fever (see nursing diagnoses box). The diagnosis of hyperthermia directs the nurse to a comprehensive approach of care. However, the nurse may choose to separately diagnose the specific problems the client experiences as a result of fever (see sample nursing diagnoses box).

PLANNING. A client who has a fever often has other medical problems. The nurse must be able to consider how the problems interact. An example of a care plan for a client with a fever is listed in the care plan box. Goals of care for clients with fever include the following:

1. Attaining a sense of comfort and rest
2. Returning to a normal range of body temperature
3. Maintaining adequate nutrition
4. Maintaining fluid and electrolyte balance

IMPLEMENTATION. Once a client becomes febrile, the physician tries to determine the cause of the fever. The nurse obtains necessary culture specimens (such as urine, blood, and sputum) for diagnostic testing. When an infection is suspected, the physician will order antibiotic medications for the nurse to administer. The physician will also order the temperature value for giving antipyretic medications. For example, "Give 10 grains of aspirin for temperature of 39° C or over." Antipyretic medications (aspirin and acetaminophen) act to prevent the hypothalamus from synthesizing prostaglandin E, thus preventing the set point from rising further.

The nurse can also provide a number of independent measures (see box on p. 202) for clients with fever.

EVALUATION. After any intervention, the nurse measures the client's temperature to evaluate for change. If therapies are effective, body temperature will decrease.

The nurse also evaluates success at meeting the goals of care. The evaluation box lists evaluative criteria used by the nurse.

HEAT EXHAUSTION

Heat exhaustion occurs when a person loses excessive amounts of water and sodium from profuse sweating.

Sample Nursing Diagnoses for Fever

Defining Characteristics	Nursing Diagnoses	Related Factors
High body temperature Tachycardia Tachypnea Warm skin Restlessness	Hyperthermia	- Infectious process - Exposure to hot environment - Vigorous exercise - Central nervous system injury
Malaise Myalgia Diaphoresis Nausea	Pain	- Fever
Tachycardia Reduced skin turgor Dry skin and mucous membranes Vomiting Reduced intake of fluids Altered electrolyte values	Fluid volume deficit	- Diaphoresis because of fever - Increased metabolism because of fever

Sample Nursing Care Plan for Hyperthermia

Nursing Diagnosis	Goals	Expected Outcomes	Nursing Interventions
Hyperthermia related to infectious process	Client will regain a normal range of body temperature.	Temperature level will fall.	Administer tepid sponge bath for 15 minutes. Keep room temperature at 70° F unless shivering develops (then raise thermostat). Administer acetaminophen (Tylenol) or aspirin grains 10 as ordered for a temperature higher than 39° C (102° F). Provide dry clothes and bed linens. Maintain light covering of bed clothes.
	Fluid and electrolyte levels remain normal.	Skin turgor is normal. Skin is moist and supple. Serum, sodium, potassium, and chloride levels stay in normal range.	Provide at least 3000 ml of oral liquids daily (must exceed urine output). Measure intake and output every shift.

The reduction in fluid volume and electrolytes causes extreme thirst, nausea and vomiting, weakness, headache, confusion, normal or slightly elevated body temperature, tachycardia, and a drop in blood pressure when the person stands or sits (postural hypotension). Exposure to high environmental temperature causes this common heat-related illness. Placing a person immediately in a cool environment to rest and stop sweating is the first treatment. Fluid and electrolyte replacement (see Chapter 37) will restore any imbalances.

HEAT STROKE

Heat stroke is a dangerous heat emergency because the fatality rate from it is very high. Persons most at risk

Sample Evaluation of Interventions for Fever

Goals	Evaluative Measures	Expected Outcomes
Client attains sense of comfort and rest.	Question client as to how he or she feels. Observe for restlessness.	Client will describe sense of relaxation with renewed energy. Client will be able to rest or sleep quietly.
Client regains a normal body temperature range.	Measure temperature after interventions (for example, sponging) designed to lower fever.	Temperature level will decline after therapy.
Adequate nutrition is maintained.	Monitor client's weight daily during febrile episode.	Body weight will remain stable.
Fluid and electrolyte balance is maintained.	Assess skin turgor and texture.	Skin remains supple with normal texture.
	Monitor serum electrolyte values. Measure intake and output.	Electrolytes remain in normal range. Output does not exceed intake.

Nursing Measures for a Fever

CHILL STAGE

- Reduce frequency of activities that increase oxygen demand such as excessive turning and ambulation. Allow for rest periods.
- Provide supplemental oxygen therapy as ordered to improve oxygen delivery to body cells.
- Provide measures to stimulate client's appetite and offer well-balanced meals to meet increased metabolic needs.
- Offer extra blankets and raise the room temperature to keep the client warm during chills. Remove blankets when the client feels warm.
- Provide extra fluids to replace fluids lost through increased metabolism.
- Assess onset and duration of chill. Take temperature immediately after episode.

COURSE OF FEVER

- Provide fluids (at least 3 liters per day for a client with normal cardiac and renal function) to replace fluids lost through insensible water loss and sweating.
- Bathe the client with tepid water to reduce the body's surface temperature.
- Encourage oral hygiene because oral mucous membranes dry easily as a result of dehydration.
- Reduce external covering on the client's body to promote heat loss through radiation and conduction. Do not induce chills.
- Keep clothing and bed linen dry to increase heat loss through conduction and convection.
- Control temperature of the environment without causing chills. Provide cool, circulating air.
- Limit physical activity to minimize heat production.

include the very young and old; obese people; clients with cardiovascular disease, hyperthyroidism, diabetes, and alcoholism; clients taking medications (phenothiazines, anticholinergics, diuretics, amphetamines, and beta-adrenergic receptor antagonists) that decrease the body's ability to lose heat; and persons who exercise or work strenuously in the heat (athletes, construction workers, and farmers).

A person with heat stroke suddenly becomes giddy, confused, or delirious. Extreme thirst, nausea, muscle cramps, and visual disturbances are common. The most important sign of heat stroke is hot, dry skin. The victim does not sweat because of severe electrolyte loss and impaired hypothalamic function. Vital signs reveal an elevated temperature, sometimes as high as 45° C (113° F), tachycardia, and hypotension. Clients are often un-

conscious by the time they reach an emergency room and have fixed, unreactive pupils, incontinence, and blotchy redness of the skin.

Moving the person to a cool environment is not enough to affect heat stroke. Immersion in tubs of ice water is no longer recommended because it causes severe peripheral vasoconstriction and shivering, which raises the body's core temperature. Because most victims are discovered outdoors, Marine Corps physicians recommend placing the client in a mesh hammock and directing an electric fan at the body while spraying the skin with mists of warm water (Barner et al., 1984). If a hammock is unavailable, the number of coverings in contact with the client must be reduced. Undressing the heat stroke victim allows air to circulate around the skin. Placement of wet towels over the skin and ice packs at vascular areas such as the neck, axilla, or groin can promote heat loss.

The best treatment for heat stroke is prevention. The nurse can teach people to (1) avoid strenuous exercise in hot, humid weather; (2) drink fluids such as clear fruit juices before, during, and after exercise; (3) wear light, loose-fitting, light-colored clothing; (4) avoid exercising in areas with poor ventilation; (5) wear protective covering over the head when outdoors; and (6) expose themselves to hot climates gradually.

HYPOTHERMIA

When a person is found ill or injured in cold weather or immersed in cold water, hypothermia should be suspected. This condition usually develops gradually and may not be noticed for several hours. Skin temperature drops to around 35° C (95° F), and uncontrolled shivering begins. A loss of memory, depression, and signs of poor judgment may be early indications of hypothermia. If body temperature falls to below 34.4° C (94° F), heart and respiratory rates and blood pressure begin to fall and the skin becomes cyanotic. If hypothermia progresses, the client may experience cardiac dysrhythmia, lose consciousness, and become unresponsive to painful stimuli. In cases of severe hypothermia a person may demonstrate clinical signs similar to death (for example, unresponsiveness to stimuli and slow respirations and pulse).

The priority treatment for hypothermia is prevention of further decrease in body temperature. The nurse should remove any wet clothes, replace them with dry ones, and wrap the client in blankets. In emergencies away from a hospital or health care setting, it helps to have the client lie under blankets next to a warm person. A conscious client will benefit from drinking hot liquids such as soup. Placing the client near a fire, in a warm room, or placing heating pads next to areas of the body (head and neck) that lose heat the quickest also helps. Once the person reaches an emergency department, the form of treatment depends on the severity of the condition. Infusion of warmed intravenous fluids (see Chapter 37), application of heating blankets, and instillation of warm fluids into the stomach may be used. Clients with hypothermia must be watched closely for cardiac irregularities and electrolyte imbalances.

Prevention is the key for clients at risk for hypothermia. Prevention involves education of clients or family members and friends. Clients most at risk include the very young and the elderly and persons debilitated by trauma, stroke, diabetes, drug or alcohol intoxication, sepsis, and Raynaud's Disease (LaVoy, 1985). The mentally ill or retarded may fall victim to hypothermia because they are unaware of the potential dangers of cold conditions. Persons who have inadequate home heating, poor diet, and lack of warm clothing are also at risk.

Assessment of Body Temperature

SITES

The mouth, rectum, and axilla are common sites for measuring body temperature. Special chemically prepared thermometer strips or patches can also be applied to the forehead. Each site has advantages and disadvantages (Table 12-3). Oral temperatures can be affected by a number of variables. The nurse waits 20 to 30 minutes to measure oral temperature after a client ingests hot or cold liquids or food, has been smoking, or has been involved in strenuous exercise. An oral thermometer should not be used if the client is receiving continuous oxygen therapy. Cooled oxygen will lower the reading, and temporary removal of the oxygen mask for an oral temperature measurement seriously reduces arterial oxygen levels (Felton, 1978). If a client is receiving oxygen, rectal or axillary temperature measurement is best.

The rectal site is believed to provide the most reliable measurement because few factors can alter the results. A rectal thermometer is used for infants and young children, except in the case of newborns, who may experience rectal trauma. A person's rectal temperature is usually a few tenths of a degree higher than the oral temperature. Even within the rectum, variations of 0.1° to 0.9° C exist, depending on the position of the thermometer (Mountcastle, 1980).

The axilla is the safest site for temperature measurement, especially with newborns. However, the time required for measurement with a thermometer and the difficulty with thermometer placement makes the axillary area less convenient and less accurate. When chemical thermometer strips are used, an axillary temperature can be obtained within a minute.

THERMOMETERS

Three types of thermometers are available for determining body temperature: mercury in glass, electronic, and disposable.

The mercury-in-glass thermometer is the most familiar. It consists of a glass tube sealed at one end and a mercury-filled bulb at the other. Exposure of the bulb to heat causes the mercury to expand and rise in the enclosed tube. The length of the thermometer is marked with either Fahrenheit or centigrade calibrations (Fig. 12-5). The mercury will not fluctuate or fall unless the thermometer is shaken vigorously.

A mercury thermometer is read by holding it with the fingertips horizontally at eye level, with the bulb pointed to the left (Fig. 12-6). *The bulb should not be touched.* Touching it might bring the fingers into contact with the client's body secretions and may cause a change in the thermometer reading. The thermometer is rotated slowly until the column of silver mercury appears. The cali-

TABLE 12-3 Selection of Sites for Temperature Measurement

Common Sites	Advantages	Disadvantages
Mouth	Most accessible site; more comfortable for client	Should not be used for clients who could be injured by thermometer, who are unable to hold thermometer properly, or who might bite down on thermometer: infants or small children, confused or unconscious clients, clients who have had oral surgery, clients with trauma to face or mouth, clients experiencing oral pain, clients who breathe only with mouth open, clients with history of convulsions, clients experiencing a shaking chill
Rectum	Thought to provide most reliable measurement	Should not be used for clients after rectal surgery, clients who have a rectal disorder such as tumor or severe hemorrhoids, clients who cannot be positioned for proper thermometer placement such as those in traction, or newborns
Axilla	Safest method because noninvasive	Requires nurse to hold thermometer in position; less accurate

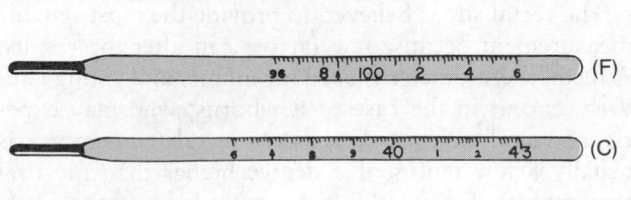

Fig. 12-5 Comparison of Fahrenheit and centigrade calibrations.

brated line at the end of the mercury column is the temperature reading.

Glass thermometers, the oral or slim tipped, the stubby, and the pear-shaped rectal, are all available in centigrade or Fahrenheit. The oral thermometer is slender, allowing for greater exposure of the bulb against the blood vessels in the mouth. It usually has a blue tip. The stubby thermometer is shorter and thicker than the oral type. It can be used to measure temperature at any site. The pear-shaped rectal thermometer has a blunt end designed to prevent trauma during rectal insertion. It usually has a red tip.

Time delay for recordings and easy breakability are disadvantages of mercury-in-glass thermometers. Advantages are low price, wide availability, and reliable accuracy.

The electronic thermometer consists of a battery-powered display unit, a thin wire cord, and a temperature-sensitive probe covered by a disposable plastic sheath to prevent the transmission of infection. (Fig. 12-7) Separate probes are available for oral and rectal use. Within only a few seconds of insertion a reading appears on the display unit. Temperature readings appear in Fahrenheit,

centigrade, or both. An electronic thermometer is not necessarily more accurate than a glass thermometer (Baker et al., 1984). For example, variables that alter oral temperature measurements affect all types of thermometers. An electronic thermometer may be less accurate because the sensor probe is inserted for a shorter time. However, a study by Baker et al. (1984) showed that although length of insertion may result in different temperature values, the difference is not likely to be clinically significant. The study found mercury-in-glass thermometers with insertion times of 2 minutes to be essentially no different than readings on the quicker electronic thermometers.

Electronic thermometers have many advantages. They can be inserted immediately. Their readings appear within seconds, and they are easy to read. The duration of the client's discomfort is also minimized.

Disposable, single-use thermometers are thin strips of plastic with chemically impregnated paper. They are used for oral or axillary temperatures, particularly with children. They can be inserted in the same way as an oral thermometer or can be applied to the skin. The chemical dots on the thermometer change color to reflect the temperature reading. Only 45 seconds are needed to record a temperature.

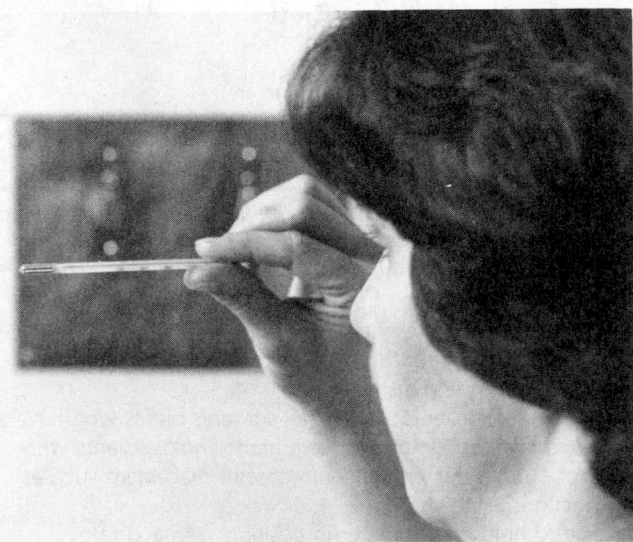

Fig. 12-6 Reading a thermometer.

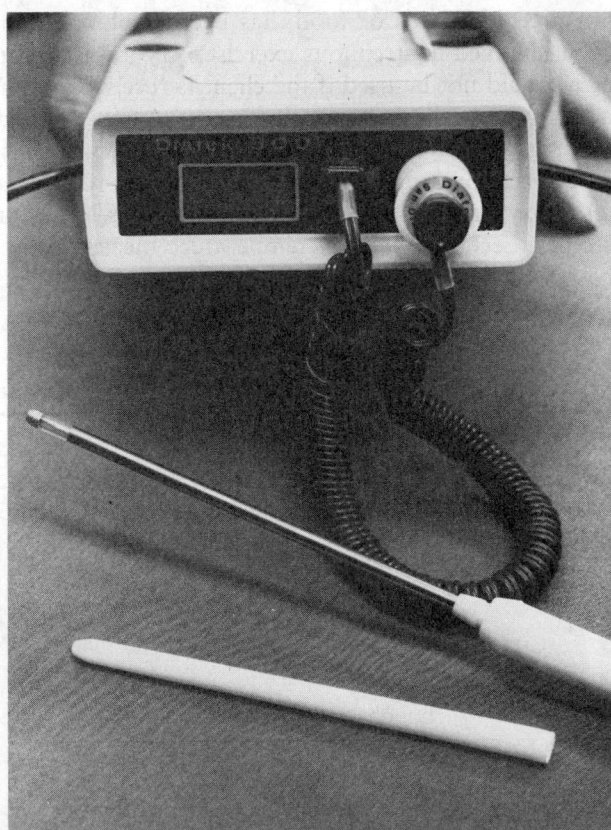

Fig. 12-7 Electronic thermometer.

PROCEDURE 12-1

Measuring Body Temperature

STEPS	RATIONALE
1. Assess for signs and symptoms of temperature alterations and for factors that normally influence body temperature.	Physical signs and symptoms may indicate abnormal body temperature. Nurse can accurately assess nature of temperature variations.
2. Explain to client how temperature is to be taken and importance of maintaining proper position until reading is complete.	Clients are often curious as to what their temperatures are and should be cautioned against prematurely removing thermometer to read results.
3. When taking oral temperature, wait 20 to 30 minutes before measuring temperature if client has smoked or ingested hot or cold liquids or foods.	Smoking and hot or cold substances can cause false temperature readings in oral cavity (Erickson, 1980).
4. Prepare needed equipment and supplies: a. Appropriate thermometer b. Soft tissues c. Lubricant (for rectal only) d. Pen, pencil, flowsheet or record form e. Disposable gloves	Chosen on basis of preferred site for temperature measurement.
5. Oral temperature—glass thermometer a. Wash hands. b. Assist client in assuming comfortable position that provides easy access to mouth. c. Apply disposable gloves.	Reduces transmission of microorganisms. Ensures client's comfort and accuracy of temperature reading. Gloves should be worn for handling items soiled with body fluids (for example, saliva) (CDC, 1987).
d. Hold color-coded end of glass thermometer with fingertips.	Reduces contamination of thermometer bulb.
e. If thermometer is stored in disinfectant solution, rinse in cold water before using.	Removes solution irritating to oral mucosa. Hot water can cause mercury to expand and break bulb.
f. Take soft tissue and wipe thermometer bulb end toward fingers in rotating fashion. Dispose of tissue.	Reduces contamination of bulb end.
g. Read mercury level while holding thermometer at eye level and gently rotating it.	Mercury is to be below 35.5° C (96° F). Thermometer reading must be below client's actual temperature before use.
h. If mercury is above desired level, shake thermometer down. Grasp tip of thermometer securely and stand away from any solid objects. Sharply flick wrist downward as though cracking a whip. Continue shaking until reading is below 35.5° C (96° F).	Brisk shaking lowers mercury level in glass tube. Standing in open spot avoids breakage of thermometer.
i. Ask client to open the mouth and gently place thermometer under tongue in posterior sublingual pocket lateral to center of lower jaw.	Heat from superficial blood vessels in sublingual pocket produces temperature reading.
j. Ask client to hold thermometer with lips closed. Caution against biting down on thermometer.	Maintains proper position of thermometer during recording. Breakage of thermometer may injure mucosa and cause mercury poisoning.
k. Leave thermometer in place for 2 min or according to agency policy.	Studies vary as to proper length of time for recording. Graves and Markarian (1980) found that glass thermometers kept in place for 8 min recorded values averaging only 0.7° F higher than those kept in place for 3 min. Baker et al. (1984) found that 2-min insertions did not cause clinically significant variations.
l. Carefully remove the thermometer and read at eye level.	Ensures accurate reading.
m. Inform client of temperature reading.	Promotes participation in care and understanding of health status.
n. Wipe secretions from thermometer with soft tissue. Wipe in rotating fashion from fingers toward bulb. Dispose of tissue.	Wipe from area of least contamination to area of most contamination.

Continued.

PROCEDURE 12-1, cont'd

Measuring Body Temperature

STEPS	RATIONALE
o. Wash thermometer in lukewarm soapy water, rinse in cool water, dry, and replace in storage container.	Mechanically removes organic material that can harbor microorangisms and hinder action of disinfectant. Storage container prevents breakage.
p. Remove and dispose of gloves. Wash hands.	Reduces transmission of microorganisms.
6. Oral temperature—electronic thermometer	
a. Wash hands.	Reduces transmission of microorganisms.
b. Assist client in assuming position of comfort that provides easy access to mouth.	Ensures client's comfort and accuracy of temperature reading.
c. Apply disposable gloves.	Gloves should be worn for handling items soiled with body fluids (for example, saliva) (CDC, 1987).
d. Attach oral probe (blue tip) to thermometer unit. Grasp top of stem, being careful not to apply pressure to ejection button.	Ejection button releases plastic cover from probe.
e. Slide disposable plastic probe cover over thermometer probe until it locks in place.	Soft plastic cover will not break in client's mouth, and prevents transmission of microorganisms between clients.
f. Ask client to open the mouth and gently place probe under tongue in posterior sublingual pocket lateral to center of lower jaw.	Heat from superficial blood vessels in sublingual pocket produces temperature reading. With electronic thermometer, temperatures in right and left posterior sublingual pocket are significantly higher than in area under front of tongue (Erickson, 1980).
g. Ask client to hold thermometer with lips closed.	Maintains proper position of thermometer during recording.
h. Leave probe in place until audible signal occurs. Client's temperature appears on digital display.	Probe must stay in place until signal occurs to ensure an accurate reading.
i. Remove probe from under client's tongue and inform client of temperature reading.	Promotes participation in care and understanding of health status.
j. Push ejection button on thermometer probe to discard plastic probe cover into proper receptacle.	Reduces transmission of microorganisms.
k. Return probe to storage well.	Protects probe from damage. Automatically causes digital reading to disappear.
l. Remove and dispose of gloves. Wash hands.	Reduces transmission of microorganisms.
m. Return thermometer to charger after temperature reading.	Maintains battery charge.
7. Rectal temperature—glass thermometer	
a. Wash hands.	Reduces transmission of microorganisms.
b. Draw curtain around client's bed and/or close room door. Keep client's upper body and lower extremities covered with sheet or blanket.	Maintains client's privacy, minimizes embarrassment, and promotes comfort.
c. Assist client in assuming Sim's position with upper leg flexed. Move aside bed linen to expose only anal area.	Exposes anal area for correct thermometer placement.
d. Prepare thermometer following Steps 5d to 5h for oral temperature measurement with glass thermometer.	Mercury must be below client's temperature level before insertion.
e. Squeeze liberal portion of lubricant onto tissue. Dip thermometer's blunt end into lubricant, covering 2.5 to 3.5 cm (1 to 1½ in) for adult or 1.2 to 2.5 cm (½ to 1 in) for infant.	Lubrication minimizes trauma to rectal mucosa during insertion. Tissue avoids contamination of all lubricant in container.
f. Apply disposable gloves.	Gloves should be worn for handling items soiled by body fluids (for example, feces) (CDC, 1987).
g. With nondominant hand, separate client's buttocks to expose anus.	Fully expose anus for thermometer insertion.
h. Ask client to breathe slowly and relax.	Relaxes anal sphincter for easier thermometer insertion.
i. Gently insert thermometer into anus in direction of umbilicus. Insert 1.2 cm (½ in) for infant and 3.5 cm (1½ in) for adult. Do not force thermometer.	Ensures adequate exposure against blood vessels in rectal wall.
j. If resistance is felt during insertion, withdraw thermometer immediately. Never force thermometer.	Prevents trauma to mucosa. Glass thermometers can break.

STEPS	RATIONALE
k. Hold thermometer in place for 2 min or according to agency policy.	Prevents injury to client. Recommended times vary among institutions. Nichols and Kucha (1972) identified optimal placement time as 2 min.
l. Carefully remove thermometer and wipe off secretions with tissue. Wipe in rotating fashion from fingers toward bulb. Dispose of tissue.	Avoids nurse's contact with microorganisms. Wipe from area of least contamination to area of most contamination.
m. Read thermometer at eye level.	Ensures accurate reading.
n. Inform client of temperature reading.	Promotes participation in care and understanding of status.
o. Wipe client's anal area to remove lubricant or feces.	Provides for client's comfort.
p. Help client return to comfortable position.	Restores client's comfort.
q. Wash thermometer in lukewarm soapy water, rinse in cool water, dry, and replace in storage container.	Mechanically removes organic material that can harbor microorganisms and hinder action of disinfectant. Storage container prevents breakage.
r. Dispose of gloves. Wash hands.	Reduces transmission of microorganisms.
8. Rectal temperature—electronic thermometer	
a. Wash hands.	Reduces transmission of microorganisms.
b. Draw curtain around client's bed and/or close room door. Keep client's upper body and lower extremities covered with sheet or blanket.	Maintains client's privacy, minimizes embarrassment, and promotes comfort.
c. Assist client in assuming Sim's position with upper leg flexed. Move aside bed linen to expose only anal area.	Exposes anal area for correct thermometer placement.
d. Attach rectal probe (red tip) to thermometer unit. Grasp top of stem, being careful not to apply pressure to ejection button.	Ejection button releases plastic cover from probe.
e. Slide disposable plastic cover over thermometer probe until it locks in place.	Probe cover prevents transmission of microorganisms between clients.
f. Squeeze liberal portion of lubricant onto tissue. Dip probe cover into lubricant, covering 2.5 to 3.5 cm (1 to 1½ in) for adult or 1.2 to 2.5 cm (½ to 1 in) for infant.	Lubrication minimizes trauma to rectal mucosa during insertion.
g. Apply disposable gloves.	Gloves should be worn for handling items soiled with body fluids (for example, feces) (CDC, 1987).
h. With nondominant hand, separate client's buttocks to expose anus.	Fully exposes anus for thermometer insertion.
i. Ask client to breathe slowly and relax.	Relaxes anal sphincter for easier thermometer insertion.
j. Gently insert probe into anus in direction of umbilicus. Insert 1.2 cm (½ in) for infant and 3.5 cm (1½ in) for adult.	Ensures adequate exposure against blood vessels in rectal wall.
k. If resistance is felt during insertion, withdraw thermometer immediately. Never force thermometer.	Prevents trauma to mucosa.
l. Hold electronic probe until audible signal occurs. Read temperature on digital display.	Reading occurs within seconds after insertion.
m. Carefully remove probe from rectum and inform client of temperature reading.	Promotes participation in care and understanding of health status.
n. Push ejection button to discard plastic probe cover into receptacle.	Reduces transmission of microorganisms.
o. Return probe to storage well.	Protects probe from damage. Automatically causes digital reading to disappear.
p. Wipe client's anal area to remove lubricant or feces. Remove and dispose of gloves.	Provides for client's comfort. Reduces transmission of microorganisms.
q. Help client return to comfortable position.	Restores client's comfort.
r. Wash hands.	Reduces transmission of microorganisms.
9. Axillary temperature—glass thermometer	
a. Wash hands.	Reduces transmission of microorganisms.
b. Draw curtain around client's bed or close door.	Provides privacy and minimizes client's embarrassment.

Continued.

PROCEDURE 12-1, cont'd

Measuring Body Temperature

STEPS	RATIONALE
c. Position client lying supine or sitting.	Provides easy access to axilla.
d. Move clothing or gown away from client's shoulder and arm.	Provides optimal exposure of axilla.
e. Prepare glass thermometer following Steps 5d to 5h of oral measurement.	Mercury must be below client's temperature level before insertion.
f. Insert thermometer into center of axilla, lower client's arm over thermometer, and place arm across client's chest.	Maintains proper position of thermometer against blood vessels in axilla.
g. Hold thermometer in place for 5 to 10 min or according to agency policy.	Recommended time varies among institutions. Eoff and Joyce (1981) recommend 5 min for children.
h. Remove thermometer and wipe off any secretions with tissue. Wipe in rotating fashion from fingers toward bulb. Dispose of tissue.	Avoids nurse's contact with microorganisms. Wipe from area of least contamination to area of most contamination.
i. Read thermometer at eye level.	Ensures accurate reading.
j. Inform client of temperature reading.	Promotes participation in care and understanding of health status.
k. Wash thermometer in lukewarm soapy water, rinse in cool water, dry, and replace in storage container.	Mechanically removes organic material that can harbor microorganisms and hinder action of disinfectant. Storage container prevents breakage.
l. Assist client in replacing clothing or gown.	Restores client's sense of well-being.
m. Wash hands.	Reduces transmission of microorganisms.
10. Axillary temperature—electronic thermometer	
a. Wash hands.	Reduces transmission of microorganisms.
b. Draw curtain around client's bed and/or close room door.	Provides privacy and minimizes client's embarrassment.
c. Position client lying supine or sitting.	Provides easy access to axilla.
d. Move clothing or gown away from client's shoulder and arm.	Provides optimal exposure of axilla.
e. Attach rectal probe (red) to thermometer unit. Prepare electronic thermometer following Steps 8d and 8e for rectal temperature measurement.	Probe cover prevents transmission of microorganisms between clients.
f. Insert probe into center of axilla, lower client's arm over thermometer, and place arm across client's chest.	Maintains proper position of thermometer against blood vessels in axilla.
g. Hold electronic probe in place until audible signal occurs. Read temperature on digital display.	Reading occurs within seconds after insertion.
h. Remove probe from axilla and inform client of temperature reading.	Promotes participation in care and understanding of health status.
i. Push ejection button to discard plastic probe into proper receptacle.	Reduces transmission of microorganisms.
j. Return electronic probe to storage well.	Protects probe from damage. Automatically causes digital reading to disappear.
k. Assist client in replacing clothing or gown.	Restores client's comfort.
l. Wash hands.	Reduces transmission of infection.
11. Compare temperature reading with client's baseline and normal temperature range for client's age group.	Normal body temperature fluctuates within narrow range. Comparison reveals presence of abnormality.
12. If temperature is abnormal, measure it again.	Improper placement or movement of thermometer can cause inaccuracies. Second reading confirms initial finding of abnormal body temperature.
13. Record temperature on vital sign flowsheet or nurses' notes and report any abnormal findings to nurse in charge or physician.	Vital sign measurements should be recorded promptly on flowsheets to avoid omissions from client's record. Abnormalities may require immediate therapy.

GUIDELINES FOR TAKING TEMPERATURE

When measuring body temperature at any site, the following basic principles should be carefully followed to maintain the client's safety and ensure accuracy in measurement (Procedure 12-1):

1. The most appropriate site for measuring the client's temperature is assessed.
2. All necessary equipment is assembled to ensure an uninterrupted procedure.
3. The hands are washed using medically aseptic technique (see Chapter 43) to prevent spread of infection.
4. The client is positioned properly and the purpose and method for the procedure are explained.

When it is necessary to convert temperature readings, the following formulas can be used:

- To convert Fahrenheit to centigrade, subtract 32° from the Fahrenheit reading and multiply the result by $5/9$.

$$C = (F - 32°) \times 5/9$$

- To convert centigrade to Fahrenheit, multiply the centigrade reading by $9/5$ and add 32° to the product.

$$F = (9/5 \times C) + 32°$$

PULSE

The pulse is an indicator of circulatory status. Circulation is the means by which cells receive nutrients and remove waste products of metabolism. For cells to function normally, there must be a continuous blood flow and an appropriate volume and distribution of blood to cells that most need nutrients.

Physiology of Pulse Regulation

Blood flows through the body in a continuous circuit. The heart is a pulsatile pump, ejecting blood intermittently into the arterial system. Cardiac centers located in the medulla of the brainstem receive impulses from sensory receptors. These sensory impulses then cause the cardiac centers in the medulla to accelerate or inhibit the heart rate through sympathetic or parasympathetic innervation. For example, if baroreceptors located in the wall of the aortic arch are stretched by increased blood volume, sensory impulses travel to the medulla. The cardioinhibitory center becomes stimulated and causes a reflex slowing of the heart rate to compensate for the increase in blood volume.

A person's heart rate varies throughout the day. Nevertheless, the heart functions to maintain a relatively constant circulatory blood flow. Approximately 60 to 70 ml of blood enters the aorta with each ventricular contraction (stroke volume). With each stroke volume

ejection the walls of the aorta distend, creating a pulse wave that travels rapidly toward the distal ends of the arteries. The pulse wave moves 15 times faster through the aorta and 100 times faster through the small arteries than the ejected volume of blood (Guyton, 1986). When a pulse wave reaches a peripheral artery, it can be palpated by pressing the artery lightly against underlying bone or muscle. The pulse rate is an indirect measurement of cardiac output. The volume of blood pumped by the heart during 1 minute is the cardiac output, the product of heart rate and the ventricle's stroke volume. In an adult the heart normally pumps 5000 to 6000 ml of blood per minute throughout the circulation.

A change in heart rate or stroke volume does not always change the heart's output or the amount of blood in the arteries (Thibodeau, 1987). For example, if a person's heart rate is 70 beats per minute and the stroke volume is 70 ml, the cardiac output is 4900 ml per min. What happens if the heart rate drops to 60 beats per minute and the stroke volume rises to 100 ml? The resultant cardiac output would be 6000 ml per min. A change in heart rate alone does not alter cardiac output. Mechanical, neural, and chemical factors regulate the strength of heart contractions and its stroke volume.

If a client develops an abnormally slow, rapid, or irregular pulse, it may indicate a problem in circulatory regulation. The pathological process causing a change from the normal heart beat may ultimately alter cardiac output. The nurse assesses the heart's function by palpating a peripheral pulse or by using a stethoscope to listen to heart sounds (apical pulse).

Pulse Assessment

The radial and carotid arteries are the most accessible peripheral pulse sites for assessment. When a client's condition suddenly deteriorates, the carotid site is the best for finding a pulse quickly. The heart will continue delivering blood through the carotid artery to the brain as long as possible, whereas peripheral pulses will weaken. The radial and apical pulses are the most common sites for assessment of vital signs. The radial and carotid sites are used by persons learning to monitor their own heart rates (for example, athletes).

Assessment of other peripheral pulse sites (Table 12-4) such as the brachial or femoral (see Chapter 13) is unnecessary unless a complete physical assessment is conducted, unless surgery or treatment have impaired blood flow to a body part, or unless there are clinical indications of impaired peripheral blood flow. If the radial pulse is thought to be abnormal or if it is inaccessible because of a dressing, cast, or other encumbrance, the apical pulse is assessed. The apical pulse is the best site for assessing an infant's or young child's pulse. When a client takes medication that affects heart

TABLE 12-4 Pulse Sites

Site	Location	Assessment Criteria
Temporal	Over temporal bone of the head, above and lateral to the eye	Easily accessible site to assess pulse in children.
Carotid	Along medial edge of sternoclei-domastoid muscle in the neck	Easily accessible site to assess character of pulse peripherally. Used during physiological shock or cardiac arrest when other sites are not palpable.
Apical	Fourth to fifth intercostal space at midclavicular line	Site for auscultation of heart sounds.
Brachial	Groove between biceps and triceps muscles at the antecubital fossa	Assess status of circulation to lower arm. Site used to auscultate blood pressure.
Radial	Radial or thumb side of forearm at the wrist	Common site to assess character of pulse peripherally. Assess status of circulation to hand.
Ulnar	Ulnar side of forearm at the wrist	Assess status of circulation to ulnar side of hand. Used to assess an Allen test.
Femoral	Below the inguinal ligament, midway between symphysis pubis and anterior superior iliac spine	Assess character of pulse during physiological shock or cardiac arrest when other pulses are not palpable. Assess status of circulation to the leg.
Popliteal	Behind the knee in popliteal fossa	Assess status of circulation to the lower leg.
Posterior tibial	Inner side of each ankle, below medial malleolus	Assess status of circulation to the foot.
Dorsalis pedis	Along top of foot between extension tendons of great and first toe	Assess status of circulation to the foot.

rate, the apical pulse may provide a more accurate assessment of heart function.

The first two fingers of the hand are used to palpate a peripheral pulse. The tips are the most sensitive parts of the fingers for detecting the pulsation of the arterial wall. Beginning students sometimes apply excessive pressure over the artery and totally obliterate the pulse. It helps to imagine the anatomical position of the artery when attempting to locate it. If the pulse is not easily located on one side, the other can be tried. The client's extremity should be kept in a relaxed position to permit full exposure of an artery. For assessment of the radial artery, the client's wrist should be extended and relaxed (Fig. 12-8). This position ensures that the artery lies superficially above the radius. Procedure 12-2 outlines pulse assessment. If the nurse is unable to palpate a pulse, a doppler electronic stethoscope can be used (see Chapter 13). This instrument magnifies sounds produced by the heart and blood vessels.

STETHOSCOPE

When assessing the apical pulse the nurse uses an acoustical stethoscope (Fig. 12-9). Sound waves originating from an internal organ usually reach the body's surface and are dissipated into the air. Unless the sounds are of a high amplitude, the unassisted ear cannot hear them clearly. The stethoscope is a closed cylinder that prevents the dissipation of sound waves as they reach the body's surface and amplifies them for the examiner. The four major parts of the stethoscope are the earpieces, binaurals, plastic or rubber tubing, and chestpiece.

The earpieces should fit snugly and comfortably in the nurse's ears. The binaurals should be angled and strong enough so the earpieces stay firmly in the ears without causing discomfort. To ensure the best reception of sound, the earpieces follow the contour of the ear canal. For most persons therefore the earpieces should point toward the face as the stethoscope is put on.

The rubber or plastic tubing should be flexible and 30 to 40 cm (12 to 18 inches) in length. Longer tubing decreases the transmission of sound waves. The tubing should be thick walled to help eliminate transmission of noises when the tubing rubs against other surfaces.

The chestpiece consists of a bell and a diaphragm. The diaphragm is the circular, flatsurfaced portion of the chestpiece and has a thin plastic disk on the end. It transmits high-pitched sounds, such as bowel and lung sounds, best. The examiner holds the diaphragm firmly

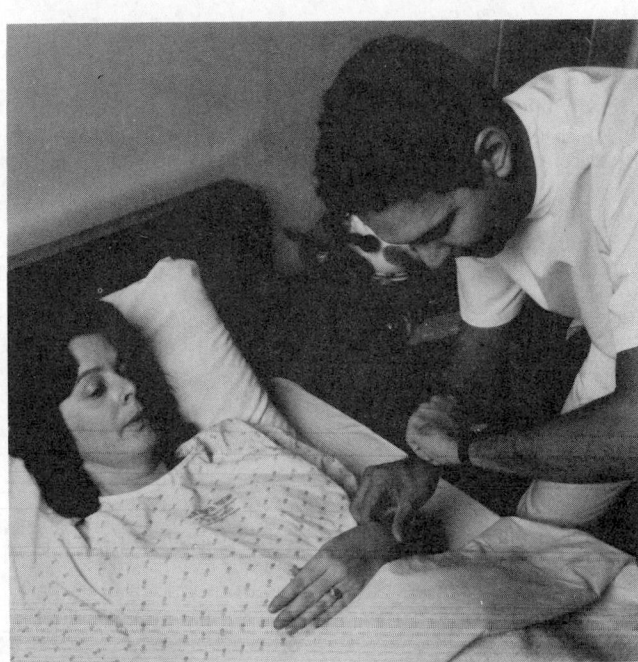

Fig. 12-8   Palpation of radial pulse.

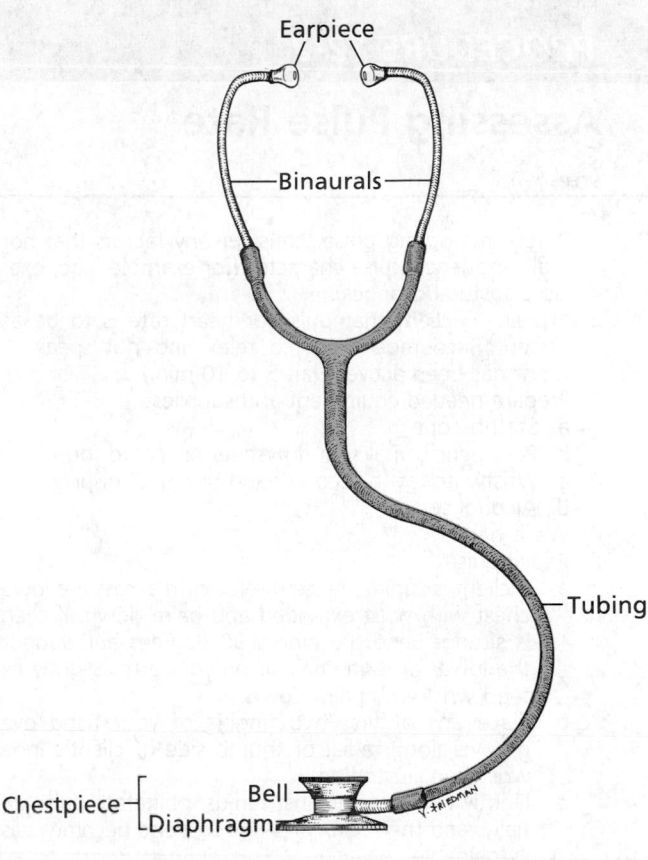

Fig. 12-9   Acoustical stethoscope.

against the skin for full sound amplification. The bell transmits low-pitched sounds such as heart and vascular sounds. It is held lightly against the skin. Compressing the bell against the skin reduces sound amplification. The bell and diaphragm are rotated into position on the chestpiece, depending on which part the nurse chooses to use. The diaphragm or bell must be in proper position during use for the nurse to hear sounds through the stethoscope.

Character of the Pulse

Assessment of the radial pulse includes measurement of the pulse rate, rhythm, strength, elasticity, and equality. When auscultating an apical pulse, the nurse assesses the heart rate and rhythm only.

RATE

Before measuring a pulse, the nurse should know the baseline heart rate for comparison (Table 12-5). Pulse rates vary, depending on age, level of activity, and a variety of other factors (see box on p. 214). The client shoud be at rest during measurement of the pulse because

physical activity increases the heart rate. It may be necessary to wait 5 to 10 minutes after activity before measuring the pulse.

Some practitioners prefer to make baseline measurements of the pulse rate as the client assumes sitting, standing, and lying positions. Postural changes cause changes in pulse rate due to alterations in blood volume

TABLE 12-5   Normal Heart Rates

Age	Heart Rate (Beats/Min)		
	Resting (Awake)	Resting (Sleeping)	Exercise or Fever
Newborn	100-180	80-160	Up to 220
1 week to 3 months	100-220	80-200	Up to 220
3 months to 2 years	80-150	70-120	Up to 200
2 years to 10 years	70-110	60-90	Up to 200
10 years to adult	55-90	50-90	Up to 200

From Gillette, PC: Dysrhythmias. In Adams, FH, and Emmanouilides, GC, editors: Moss' heart disease in infants, children, and adolescents, ed. 3, © 1983, the Williams & Wilkins Co., Baltimore.

PROCEDURE 12-2

Assessing Pulse Rate

STEPS	RATIONALE
1. Before measuring pulse, consider any factors that normally influence pulse character (for example, age, exercise, postural changes).	Allows nurse to accurately assess presence and significance of pulse alterations.
2. Explain to client that pulse or heart rate is to be assessed. Encourage client to relax and not speak. (If client has been active, wait 5 to 10 min.)	Activity and anxiety can cause elevated heart rate. Client's voice interferes with nurse's ability to hear sound when apical pulse is measured.
3. Prepare needed equipment and supplies:	
a. Stethoscope	Used for apical pulse assessment.
b. Pen, pencil, vital sign flowsheet or record form	
c. Wristwatch with second hand or digital display	
d. Alcohol swab	
4. Wash hands	Reduces transmission of microorganisms.
5. Radial pulse	
a. If client is supine, place the forearm across the lower chest with wrist extended and palm down. If client is sitting, bend the elbow 90 degrees and support the lower arm on chair or on your arm. Slightly extend wrist with palm down.	Relaxed position of lower arm and extension of wrist permits full exposure of artery to palpation.
b. Place tips of first two fingers of your hand over groove along radial or thumb side of client's inner wrist (see illustration).	Fingertips are most sensitive parts of hand to palpate arterial pulsation. Nurse's thumb has pulsation that may interfere with accuracy.
c. Lightly compress against radius, obliterate pulse initially, and then relax pressure so pulse becomes easily palpable.	Pulse is more accurately assessed with moderate pressure. Too much pressure occludes pulse and impairs blood flow.
d. Once pulse can be felt regularly, look at watch's second hand and begin to count rate: when sweep hand hits number on dial, start counting with zero, then one, and so on.	Rate is determined accurately only after assessor is assured pulse can be palpated. Timing begins with zero. Count of one is first beat palpated after timing begins.
e. If pulse is regular, count rate for 15 sec and multiply total by 4.	Regular heart rate can be accurately assessed in 15 sec.
f. If pulse is irregular, count for full minute.	Longer time period ensures accurate count.
g. Assess regularity and frequency of any existing dysrhythmia.	Inefficient contraction of heart fails to transmit pulse wave and can interfere with cardiac output. Determines need to assess for pulse deficit.
h. Determine strength of pulse. Note thrust of vessel against fingertips.	Strength reflects volume of blood ejected against arterial wall with each heart contraction.
i. Palpate with two fingers along course of artery toward wrist to determine elasticity of arterial wall.	Degree of elasticity reflects quality of arterial wall and reveals general condition of peripheral vascular system.

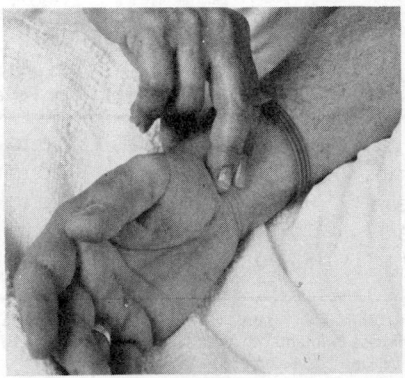

Step 5b

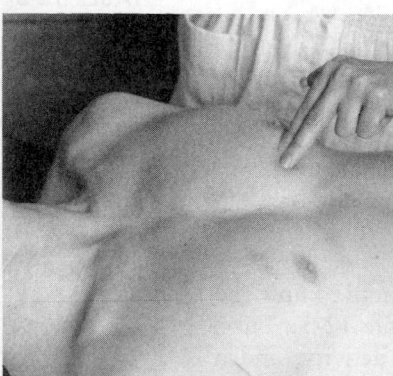

Step 6c

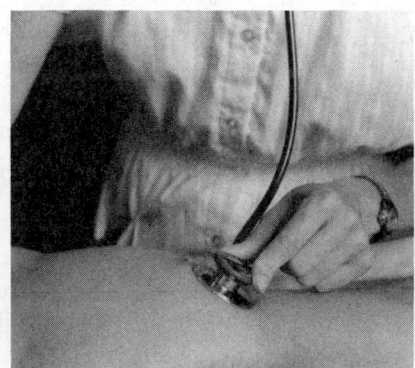

Step 6e

STEPS	RATIONALE
j. Assist client in returning to comfortable position.	Promotes sense of well-being.
k. Discuss findings with client.	Promotes client's participation in care and understanding of health status.
l. Wash hands.	Reduces transmission of microorganisms.
6. Apical pulse	
a. Clean earpieces and diaphragm of stethoscope with alcohol swab as needed (optional).	Controls transmission of microorganisms when nurses share stethoscope.
b. With client in supine or sitting position, turn down bed linen and raise gown to expose sternum and left side of chest.	Exposes portion of chest wall for selection of auscultatory site.
c. Palpate angle of Louis, located just below suprasternal notch at point where horizontal ridge is felt along body of sternum. Place index finger just to the left of client's sternum and palpate second intercostal space. Place next finger in intercostal space below and proceed downward until fifth intercostal space is located. Move index finger horizontally along fifth intercostal space to left midclavicular line (see illustration). Palpate point of maximal impulse (PMI), also called Erb's point.	Use of anatomical landmarks allows nurse to place stethoscope over apex of heart, which lies just under fifth intercostal space along left midclavicular line. This position enhances ability to hear heart sounds clearly. PMI is over apex of heart.
d. Place diaphragm of stethoscope in palm of your hand for 5 to 10 sec.	Warming of metal or plastic diaphragm prevents client from being startled and promotes comfort.
e. Place diaphragm over PMI and auscultate for normal S_1 and S_2 heart sounds (heard as "lub dub") (see illustration).	Heart sounds are caused by movement of blood through heart valves.
f. Once occurrence of S_1 and S_2 can be heard with regularity, use watch's second hand and begin to count rate: when sweep hand hits number on dial, start counting with zero, then one, and so on.	Rate is determined accurately only after nurse is able to auscultate sounds clearly.
g. If heart rate is regular, count for 30 sec and multiply by 2.	Regular apical rate can be assessed within 30 sec.
h. If heart rate is irregular, count for 1 min.	Rate determined is more accurate when measured over longer interval.
i. Note regularity of any existing dysrhythmia (S_1 and S_2 occurs early or later after previous sequence of sounds; S_1 or S_2 is absent for a beat).	Regular occurrence of dysrhythmia within 1 min may indicate inadequate cardiac function.
j. Replace client's gown and bed linen. Assist client in returning to comfortable position.	Maintains client's comfort.
k. Discuss findings with client.	Promotes client's participation in care and understanding of health status.
l. Wash hands.	Reduces transmission of microorganisms.
7. Compare client's pulse rate and character with previous baseline and/or normal pulse range for age group.	Allows nurse to assess for change in client's condition and for presence of cardiac alteration.
8. Record pulse characteristics on vital signs flowsheet or nurses' notes and report any abnormal findings.	Immediate documentation ensures accuracy in medical record. Abnormalities may require therapy.

Factors Influencing Pulse Rates

- **Exercise.** Short-term exercise increases pulse rate. Long-term exercise strengthens heart muscle, resulting in a lower-than-normal rate at rest and a quicker return to the resting rate after exercise.
- **Fever, Heat.** Both increase the pulse rate because of increased metabolic rate.
- **Acute Pain, Anxiety.** Both increase the pulse rate because of sympathetic stimulation.
- **Unrelieved Severe and Chronic Pain.** These decrease the pulse rate because of parasympathetic stimulation.
- **Medications.** Some medications alter pulse rate. For example, digitalis decreases the pulse rate, whereas atropine increases it.
- **Hemorrhage.** Loss of blood increases the pulse rate because of sympathetic stimulation.
- **Postural Changes.** Lying down decreases the pulse rate. Standing or sitting increases it.

and distribution and sympathetic activity. The heart rate typically increases when a person moves from a lying to a sitting or standing position. To assess peripheral pulse rate, the nurse counts the number of arterial pulsations for a select number of seconds. Then the nurse calculates the number of pulsations that would occur in 60 seconds. If a pulse is irregular, an accurate measurement is made by counting pulsations a full minute.

The nurse assesses an apical pulse by listening for heart sounds (see Chapter 13). The nurse tries to identify the first and second heart sounds (S_1 and S_2). At normal slow rates, S_1 is low pitched and dull in quality, sounding like a "lub." S_2 is a higher pitched and shorter sound and creates the sound, "dub." Using the diaphragm or bell of the stethoscope the nurse counts the number of "lub-dubs" occurring in a minute. For the beginning student a bell may be more difficult to use. However, it is best for detecting vascular sounds.

The nurse may assess common variations in heart rate. Tachycardia is an abnormally elevated heart rate, above 100 beats per minute. Bradycardia is a rate below 60 beats per minute. The nurse assesses an apical pulse when tachycardia or bradycardia are detected at peripheral pulse sites.

RHYTHM

Successive heart beats normally occur at regular intervals. If an interval is interrupted by an early beat or if a beat is late or missed, the individual has an abnormal rhythm or dysrhythmia (see Chapter 13). A dysrhythmia alters the heart's ability to pump properly, particularly if it occurs repetitively. The nurse assesses dysrhythmia by palpating interruption in the successive pulse waves or auscultating an interruption between sounds. If dysrhythmia is present, the regularity of its occurrence is assessed. It may be intermittent (occasional missed beats) or irregularly irregular (variation in frequency). To confirm presence of a dysrhythmia, the physician may order an electrocardiogram or place the client on a Holter monitor or cardiac telemetry.

When palpating for an irregular peripheral pulse, the nurse should also assess for a pulse deficit, which occurs when the heart ejects a volume of blood so small that it goes to the brain and peripheral pulse waves cannot be felt. Therefore the nurse auscultates more apical contractions than number of pulse waves palpated. Chapter 13 describes the technique used to assess for a pulse deficit.

STRENGTH

The strength or amplitude of a pulse reflects the volume of blood ejected against the arterial wall with each heart contraction. Assessing the pulse strength is a subjective process and requires considerable practice. Normally the pulse strength remains the same with each heartbeat. A normal pulse is full, easily palpable, and not easily obliterated by the assessor's fingers. A bounding pulse is easily palpated and difficult to obliterate. A weak pulse is difficult to palpate and easy for the assessor to lose during palpation. The weak pulse is thready and often rapid. Some institutions use a classification system for pulse strength (see Chapter 13).

ELASTICITY

A normal artery feels straight, smooth, round, and elastic when palpated. Certain conditions change the quality of the arterial wall. For example, in arteriosclerosis the vessel walls harden and become cordlike, and the artery becomes torturous and twisted.

The elasticity or expansibility of an artery does not affect the pulse rate, rhythm, or strength. However, elasticity does reflect the general status of the peripheral vascular system.

EQUALITY

Pulses on both sides of the peripheral vascular system should be assessed. The nurse assesses both radial pulses to compare the characteristics of each. A pulse in one extremity may be unequal in strength or absent in many disease states (for example, thrombus [clot] formation, aberrant blood vessels, or cervical rib syndrome).

RESPIRATION

Human survival depends on the ability of oxygen (O_2) to reach body cells and for carbon dioxide (CO_2) to be removed from the cells. Respiration involves two distinctly different processes: *external respiration,* or the movement of air between the environment and lungs, and *internal respiration,* or the movement of oxygen between hemoglobin and single cells. External respiration further involves the following complex but interrelated processes: *ventilation,* the mechanical movement of air to and from the lungs and the exchange of respiratory gases; *conduction,* the movement of air through the airways of the lungs; *diffusion,* movement of O_2 and CO_2 between alveoli and red blood cells; and *perfusion,* distribution of blood through the pulmonary capillaries.

The nurse can directly assess only the process of external respiration, specifically by assessing ventilation. The rate, depth, and rhythm of ventilatory movements indicate the quality and efficiency of the respiratory process. Diagnostic tests that measure respiratory function and O_2 and CO_2 levels in arterial blood also provide useful data to assess ventilation.

Physiological Control of Respiration

Breathing is generally a passive process. Normally a person thinks little about it. The respiratory center in the brainstem regulates the involuntary control of respirations. Adults normally breathe smoothly and uninterrupted, 12 to 20 times a minute.

Ventilation is regulated by levels of CO_2, O_2, and hydrogen ion concentration (pH) in the arterial blood. The most important factor in the control of ventilation is the P_{CO_2} of arterial blood. An elevation in the P_{CO_2} causes the respiratory center to increase the rate and depth of breathing. The increased ventilatory effort removes excess CO_2 during exhalation. Hypercarbia, a chronic excess of CO_2 in arterial blood, can eventually depress ventilation.

Chemoreceptors (carotid and aortic bodies) located in the periphery are sensitive to CO_2, pH, and hypoxia, or low levels of arterial O_2. If arterial O_2 levels fall, the chemoreceptors signal the respiratory center to increase the rate and depth of ventilation. Normally, rising CO_2 levels stimulate the initiation of inhalation, and hypoxia has limited impact on the control of ventilation. However, in clients with chronic lung disease such as emphysema or bronchitis the hypoxic drive to increase ventilation is very important. These persons have chronic hypercarbia and thus have lost the normal stimulus for ventilation. A low level of arterial O_2 is the only stimulus that allows a client with chronic lung disease to breathe.

Mechanics of Breathing

Although breathing is normally passive, muscular work moves the lung and chest wall. Inspiration is relatively more active than expiration. During inspiration the respiratory center sends impulses along the phrenic

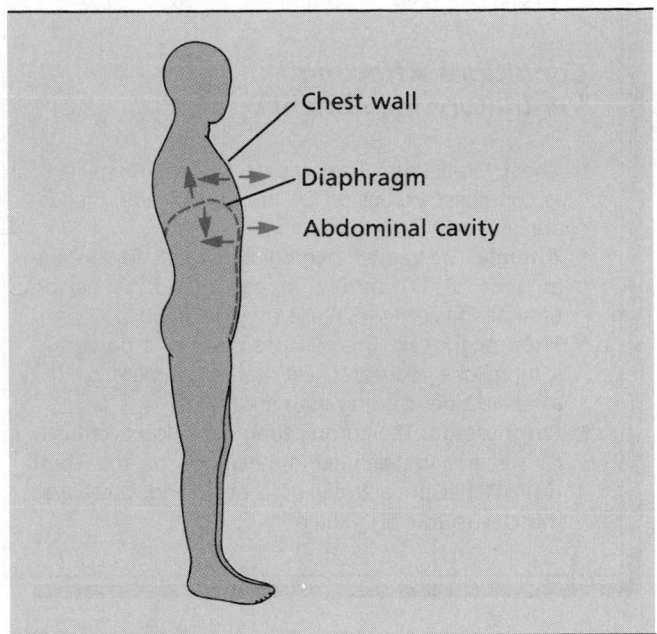

Fig. 12-10 Illustration of diaphragmatic movement during inspiration and expiration.

nerve, causing the diaphragm, a thin dome-shaped muscle connected to the lower ribs, to contract. As the diaphragm contracts, the abdominal organs move downward and forward, increasing the vertical dimension of the chest cavity. At the same time the ribs lift upward and outward, causing transverse expansion of the lungs. Fig. 12-10 shows the way diaphragmatic movement affects the size of the chest cavity. On expiration the diaphragm relaxes and the abdominal organs return to their original positions. The elastic lung and chest wall also return to a relaxed state. Little energy is required to move air out of the lungs. Expiration becomes an active process only during exercise, voluntary hyperventilation (increased ventilation), and certain disease states.

The nurse assesses respirations by observing for normal thoracic and abdominal movements and symmetry in chest wall movement. During quiet breathing the chest wall gently rises and falls. Contraction of the intercostal muscles between the ribs or of the accessory muscles in the neck and shoulders is not visible. Passive breathing is more diaphragmatic as the abdominal cavity slowly rises and falls.

When breathing requires more effort, rib (costal) movement increases. The intercostal and accessory muscles work actively to move air in and out. The shoulders may rise and fall, and the accessory muscles in the neck visibly contract. Diaphragmatic movement is less noticeable when rib movement increases. Certain clinical conditions (see box) affect ventilatory movement. With practice the nurse learns to recognize these conditions.

Conditions Affecting Ventilatory Movement

- **Chest Wall Pain.** Pain causes a client to splint or inhibit chest expansion on the painful side. Breaths are shallow.
- **Anemia.** Decreased hemoglobin levels lowers the amount of O_2 carried in the blood. A person breathes faster to increase oxygen delivery.
- **Pneumothorax.** The collapse of all or a portion of a lung lobe reduces chest wall movement on the affected side, causing asymmetry.
- **Emphysema.** The chronic lung condition eventually causes a barrel-shaped appearance of the chest wall. A person actively uses neck and chest wall muscles to forcibly exhale.

Assessment of Respirations

Respirations are the easiest of all vital signs to assess but are often the most haphazardly measured. Sometimes a nurse merely estimates the respiratory rate. However, recognition of a sudden change in the character of respirations is important. Consider the following clinical example:

After surgery, Mr. Troy's respirations are 16 per minute, regular, and shallow. Thirty minutes later, he complains of pain across his abdominal incision. The nurse assesses respirations at 28 per minute, regular, and labored. Mr. Troy's physical status has obviously changed, requiring assessment of all vital signs.

A nurse assesses respirations when a client is at rest. If a client is anxious, in pain, or fearful, the respirations will probably be increased in rate and depth. A skillful nurse does not let a client know that respirations are being assessed. A client who is aware of the nurse's intentions may consciously alter the rate and depth of breathing. Assessment is best done immediately after measuring pulse rate, with the nurse's hand still on the client's wrist. The nurse should always assess respirations carefully to avoid overlooking signs that may be relevant to a client's physiological needs. When assessing respirations, the nurse should keep in mind (1) the client's normal ventilatory pattern, (2) the influences any disease or illness has on respiratory function, (3) the relationship between respiratory and cardiovascular function, and (4) the influence of some therapies on respirations. Objective measurements composing an assessment of respiratory status include the rate and depth of breathing and the rhythm of ventilatory movements (Procedure 12-3).

TABLE 12-6 Normal Average Respiratory Rates by Age

Age Group	Rate	Age Group	Rate
Newborn	35	10 years	19
1-11 months	30	12 years	19
2 years	25	14 years	18
4 years	23	16 years	17
6 years	21	18 years	16-18
8 years	20	Adult	12-20

RATE

The nurse observes a full inspiration and expiration when counting a respiration. The respiratory rate varies with age (Table 12-6). An infant breathes quite rapidly. Throughout childhood, respiratory rate declines. Among adults, normal rates vary from 12 to 20 respirations per minute. The box lists factors affecting character of respirations.

DEPTH

The depth of respirations is assessed by observing the degree of excursion or movement in the chest wall. The nurse subjectively describes ventilatory movements as shallow, normal, or deep. Chapter 13 describes a more objective means of measuring chest excursions by palpation of chest wall movement. This technique can be

Factors Influencing Character of Respirations

- **Exercise.** Increases rate and depth to meet body's greater O_2 needs.
- **Acute Pain.** Increases rate and depth as a result of sympathetic stimulation. Client may inhibit or splint chest wall movement when pain is in area of chest or abdomen.
- **Anxiety.** Increases rate and depth as a result of sympathetic stimulation.
- **Smoking.** Chronic smoking changes lung's airways, resulting in an increased rate.
- **Body Position.** Straight, erect posture promotes full chest expansion. Stooped or slumped position impairs ventilatory movement.
- **Medications.** Narcotic analgesics and sedatives depress rate and depth. Amphetamines and cocaine may increase rate and depth.
- **Brainstem Injury.** Impairs respiratory center and inhibits respiratory rate and rhythm.

PROCEDURE 12-3

Assessing Respirations

STEPS	RATIONALE
1. Assess for factors that normally influence character of respirations.	Allows nurse to accurately assess for presence and significance of respiratory alterations.
2. If client has been active, wait 5 to 10 min before assessing respirations.	Exercise increases respiratory rate and depth.
3. Be sure client is in comfortable position, preferably sitting or lying with head of bed elevated 45 to 60 degrees.	Uncomfortable position may cause client to breathe more rapidly. An erect, sitting position promotes full ventilatory movement.

4. Prepare needed equipment and supplies:
  a. Watch with second hand or digital display.
  b. Pen, pencil, flow sheet or record form.	

5. Draw curtain around client's bed and/or close room door. Wash hands.	Maintains client's privacy. Prevents transmission of microorganisms.
6. Be sure client's chest is visible. If necessary, move bed linen or gown.	Ensures clear view of chest wall and abdominal movements.
7. Place client's arm in relaxed position across the abdomen or lower chest, or place your hand directly over client's upper abdomen.	This position is used during assessment of pulse and allows nurse to be inconspicuous. Client's or nurse's hand rises and falls during respiratory cycle.
8. Observe complete respiratory cycle (one inspiration and one expiration).	Rate is accurately determined only after nurse has viewed respiratory cycle.
9. Once cycle has been observed, look at watch's second hand and begin to count rate: when sweep hand hits number on dial, begin time frame, counting *one* with first full respiratory cycle.	Timing begins with count of one. Respirations occur more slowly than pulse; thus timing does not begin with zero.
10. If rhythm is regular in adult, count number of respirations in 30 sec and multiply by 2. In infant or young child count respirations for full minute.	Respiratory rate is equivalent to number of respirations per minute. Young infants and children normally breathe irregularly.
11. If adult's respirations have irregular rhythm or are abnormally slow or fast, count for full minute.	Accurate interpretation with irregularities requires assessment for at least 1 min.
12. Note depth of respirations. This can be assessed subjectively by observing degree of chest wall movement while counting rate. Nurse can also objectively assess depth by palpating chest wall excursion (see Chapter 13) after rate has been counted. Depth is shallow, normal, or deep.	Depth of respirations helps reveal volume of air moving to and from lungs. Character of ventilatory movements may reveal specific alterations or disease status.
13. Note rhythm of ventilatory cycle. (Normal breathing is regular and uninterrupted.)	Character of ventilations can reveal specific types of alterations.
14. Replace client's gown and cover with bed linen.	Restores client's comfort.
15. Wash hands.	Reduces transmission of microorganisms.
16. Discuss findings with client as needed.	Promote participation in care and understanding of health status.
17. Compare respirations with previous baseline and/or normal respiratory rate for age group.	Allows nurse to assess for change in condition and for presence of respiratory alterations.
18. Record respiratory rate and character on vital sign flow sheet or nurses' notes and report any abnormal findings.	Vital signs should be recorded immediately for accuracy and inclusion in medical record. Abnormalities may require therapy.

used if the nurse observes that chest excursion is unusually shallow.

During a normal relaxed breath (tidal breath) a person inhales 500 cc of air. The diaphragm moves approximately 1 cm (⁴/₁₀ inch), and the ribs retract upward from the body's midline approximately 1.2 to 2.5 cm (½ to 1 inch). A deep respiration involves a full expansion of the lungs with full exhalation. Respirations are shallow when only a small quantity of air passes through the lungs and ventilatory movement is difficult to see.

The capacity of the lungs to take in air depends on sex and age. Full capacity is determined by taking as deep a breath as possible and then blowing it all the way out into a spirometer, which measures air volume. The amount of air exhaled after a full inspiration is the lung's vital capacity. Men tend to have a larger vital capacity than women of the same age. Infants and young children have smaller vital capacities than adolescents and adults. With advancing age the lung loses its elasticity, and the capacity for forcible exhalation declines. Nursing care may focus on increasing the client's efforts to breathe deeply. The nurse's knowledge of the client's normal capacity to move air is helpful in planning realistic therapy.

RHYTHM

Normal breathing is regular and uninterrupted. A regular interval occurs after each respiratory cycle. Infants tend to breathe less regularly. The young child may breathe slowly for a few seconds and then suddenly breathe more rapidly.

While assessing respirations, the nurse estimates the time interval between respiratory cycles. Respiration is either regular or irregular in rhythm.

GENERAL RESPIRATORY CHARACTER

While assessing the three objective qualities of rate, depth, and rhythm, the nurse also observes factors related to the general character of respirations.

Depending on the level of oxygenation, respiratory alterations may cause changes in skin color and level of consciousness. The nail beds, lips, and skin may take on a bluish or cyanotic appearance when arterial O_2 levels are reduced (see Chapter 13). As oxygenation decreases, a person typically becomes more restless and anxious and tries harder to breathe.

Difficulty in breathing is defined as dyspnea. As breathing becomes labored a person uses accessory muscles in the chest and neck to breathe. A dyspneic client usually feels short of breath.

Sounds of breathing may indicate a respiratory disorder. Inflammation or stricture of the trachea or larynx causes obstruction to airflow. As a client inhales, air passing the obstruction creates a harsh crowing sound or respiratory stridor, which can easily be heard without a stethoscope. Chapter 13 describes in detail the normal and abnormal breath sounds that can be heard by auscultation with a stethoscope.

TABLE 12-7 Alterations in Respiration

Term	Description
Bradypnea	Rate of breathing is abnormally slow but regular.
Tachypnea	Rate of breathing is abnormally rapid but regular.
Hyperpnea	Respirations are increased in depth and rate. This occurs normally with exercise.
Apnea	Respirations cease for several seconds. Persistent cessation is called respiratory arrest.
Hyperventilation	The rate of ventilation exceeds normal metabolic requirements for exchange of respiratory gases. The rate and depth of respirations increase. There is an excessive intake of O_2 and blowing off of CO_2.
Hypoventilation	The volume of air entering the lungs is insufficient for the body's metabolic needs. The respiratory rate is below normal and the depth of ventilation is depressed. There is decreased O_2 intake and CO_2 exhalation.
Cheyne-Stokes respiration	Respiratory rhythm is irregular, characterized by alternating periods of apnea and hyperventilation. The respiratory cycle begins with slow, shallow breaths that gradually increase to abnormal depth and rapidity. Gradually breathing slows and becomes shallower, climaxing in a 10 to 20 second period of apnea before respiration resumes.
Kussmaul respiration	Respirations are abnormally deep but regular, similar to hyperventilation. This is characteristic of clients with diabetic ketoacidosis.
Dyspnea	Breathing is difficult and characterized by increased effort to inhale and exhale. The person actively uses intercostal and accessory muscles to breathe.
Sighing	Not to be confused with abnormal ventilatory rhythm, a sigh is a protective physiological mechanism for expanding small airways and alveoli not used during a normal tidal breath.
Orthopnea	Respiratory condition in which a person must sit or stand in order to breathe deeply or comfortably.

Respiratory alterations may cause changes in the features or characteristics of breathing. Table 12-7 describes several common respiratory alterations.

BLOOD PRESSURE

To cause blood to flow throughout the circulatory system, the heart pumps blood into the arteries under high pressure. Blood pressure is the force exerted by the blood against a vessel wall. The standard unit for measuring blood pressure is millimeters of mercury (mm Hg). The measurement indicates the height to which the blood pressure can raise a column of mercury. During a normal cardiac cycle (see Chapter 13), blood pressure reaches a peak that is followed by a trough. The peak or maximum pressure occurs during **systole** as the left ventricle pumps blood into the aorta. The trough occurs during **diastole** as the ventricles relax. Diastolic pressure is the minimal pressure exerted against the arterial walls at all times. The nurse records blood pressure with the systolic reading before the diastolic (for example, 120/80). The difference between systolic and diastolic pressure is the pulse pressure. Thus if the blood pressure is 120/80, the pulse pressure is 40 mm Hg.

Physiology of Arterial Blood Pressure

Blood pressure reflects the balance among hemodynamic factors, including cardiac output, peripheral vascular resistance, blood volume, blood viscosity, and elasticity of arteries. Each factor can affect another. For example, an increase in blood volume increases cardiac output. The box lists how hemodynamic factors can affect blood pressure.

Hemodynamic Effects on Blood Pressure

INCREASES BLOOD PRESSURE

- Increased cardiac output
- Increased peripheral vascular resistance
- Increased blood volume
- Increased blood viscosity
- Decreased arterial elasticity

DECREASES BLOOD PRESSURE

- Decreased cardiac output
- Decreased peripheral vascular resistance
- Decreased blood volume
- Decreased blood viscosity

The complex control of the cardiovascular system normally prevents any single factor from permanently changing blood pressure. For example, if blood volume falls, the body compensates with increased peripheral resistance to maintain the blood pressure at a normal level. Knowledge of the hemodynamic variables helps the nurse assess blood pressure alterations.

The blood pressure (BP) is a product of the cardiac output (CO) and peripheral vascular resistance (R), so $BP = CO \times R$. When volume increases in an enclosed space, the pressure in that space rises. Thus, as the cardiac output increases, more blood is pumped against the arterial walls, causing elevation in blood pressure. Exercise temporarily elevates blood pressure as the demand for cardiac output increases.

When vascular resistance increases, the blood pressure rises. The size of arteries and arterioles change to adjust blood flow to the needs of local tissues. The smaller the lumen of a vessel, the greater its peripheral vascular resistance to blood flow. When blood flow to a major organ falls sharply, peripheral arteries vasoconstrict to shunt blood to the major vessels supplying the organ. Arterial pressure rises to push blood through narrowed vessels. In contrast, as vessels dilate and vascular resistance falls, blood pressure drops.

The volume of blood circulating within the vascular system affects blood pressure. Most adults have a circulating blood volume of 5000 ml. Normally the blood volume remains constant. However, if volume increases, more pressure is exerted against arterial walls. The rapid, uncontrolled infusion of intravenous fluids is a typical cause of elevated blood pressure. When circulating blood volume falls, as in the case of hemorrhage or dehydration, blood pressure falls.

The thickness or viscosity of blood affects the ease with which blood flows through small vessels. The hematocrit, or percentage of red blood cells in the blood, determines blood viscosity. When the hematocrit rises and blood flow slows, arterial blood pressure increases. Normally the walls of an artery are elastic and easily distensible. As pressure within the arteries increases, the diameter of vessel walls also increases. Arterial distensibility prevents wide fluctuations in blood pressure. For example, if the volume pumped by the heart suddenly increases, arteries can distend and absorb much of the increase in pressure. However, in certain diseases such as arteriosclerosis the vessel walls lose their elasticity and are replaced by fibrous tissue that cannot stretch well. With reduced elasticity, there is greater resistance to blood flow. As a result, when the left ventricle ejects its stroke volume, the vessels no longer yield to the pressure. Instead, a given volume of blood is forced through the rigid arterial walls, and the pressure rises. Systolic pressure is more significantly elevated than diastolic because of reduced arterial elasticity.

Factors Influencing Blood Pressure

Blood pressure does not stay constant. Many factors influence it throughout the day. An understanding of these factors ensures a more accurate interpretation of blood pressure readings.

AGE

Normal blood pressure levels vary throughout life. It increases during the preadult years. The level of a child's or adolescent's blood pressure is assessed with respect to body size and age (Task Force on Blood Pressure Control in Children, 1987). Larger children (heavier and/or taller) have higher blood pressures than smaller children of the same age.

Once a child reaches adolescence, blood pressure continues to vary according to body size. However, the normal range for 13 to 18 year olds at the 90th percentile is 124-136/77-84 for boys and 124-127/63-74 for girls.

An adult's blood pressure tends to increase with advancing age. The standard norm for a healthy middle aged adult is 120/80. A systolic pressure below 140 mm and a diastolic pressure below 90 mm are still considered normal. The older adult's blood pressure range is 140-160/80-90.

STRESS

Anxiety, fear, pain, and emotional stress initiate sympathetic stimulation, causing blood pressure to rise. Sympathetic stimulation increases the heart rate, which in turn increases cardiac output and peripheral vascular resistance through vasoconstriction.

SEX

Through childhood, no clinically significant difference in blood pressure levels exists between boys and girls. After puberty, males have higher readings because of hormonal variations. When a woman reaches menopause, however, her blood pressure tends to be higher than that of a man of the same age.

RACE

The rate of hypertension (high blood pressure) is higher in urban black Americans than in white Americans (Joint National Committee on Detection, Evaluation, and Treatment of High Blood Pressure, 1984). Hypertension-related deaths are also higher among blacks. The tendency for blacks to have hypertension is believed to be genetically and environmentally related.

MEDICATIONS

Some medications can directly or indirectly affect blood pressure. During blood pressure assessment the nurse asks if the client is receiving drugs for hypertension. Antihypertensive medications lower blood pressure by different actions (Table 12-8). Another class of medications affecting blood pressure is narcotic analgesics, which can lower blood pressure.

DIURNAL VARIATION

Blood pressure levels vary over the course of a day. The blood pressure is typically lowest in the early morning. It gradually rises during the morning and afternoon, peaking in late afternoon or evening. No two persons have the same pattern or degree of variation. A student may find it interesting to have a friend check blood pressure at intervals during 24 hours.

Hypertension

High blood pressure is a major factor underlying death from strokes in the United States annually, and it also contributes to heart attacks. The Joint National Committee on Detection, Evaluation, and Treatment of High Blood Pressure (1984) has set criteria for determining categories of hypertension (Table 12-9). The diagnosis of hypertension in adults is made when an average of

TABLE 12-8   Antihypertensive Medications

Medication Type	Generic Names	Effects
Diuretic	Furosemide, spironolactone, metolazone, polythizide, benzthiazide	Lowers blood pressure by reducing reabsorption of sodium and water by the kidneys, thus lowering circulating fluid volume.
Beta-adrenergic blockers	Atenolol (Tenormin), nadolol (Corgard), timolol maleate (Blocadren)	Beta-adrenergic blocking agents combine with beta-adrenergic receptors in the heart, arteries, and arterioles to block response to sympathetic nerve impulses. Reduces heart rate and thus cardiac output.
Vasodilators	Hydralazine hydrochloride (Apresoline Hydrochloride), minoxidil (Loniten)	Act on arteriolar smooth muscle to cause relaxation and reduce peripheral vascular resistance.
Calcium channel blockers	Verapamil hydrochloride, nifedipine	Reduce peripheral vascular resistance by a systemic vasodilation.

two or more diastolic readings on at least two subsequent visits is 90 mm Hg or higher or when the average of multiple systolic blood pressures on two or more subsequent visits is consistently higher than 140 mm Hg. One blood pressure recording does not qualify as a diagnosis of hypertension. However, if the nurse assesses a high reading (for example, 150/90 mm Hg), the client should be encouraged to return for another check-up within two months (Table 12-10). When a nurse assesses a client's blood pressure for the first time, an average of two or more measurements should be taken with the client positioned comfortably (Joint National Committee on Detection, Evaluation, and Treatment of High Blood Pressure, 1984).

Hypertension causes thickening and loss of elasticity in the arterial walls. Peripheral vascular resistance increases within the affected vessels. As a result, blood flow to vital organs such as the heart, brain, and kidney decreases. The heart must continually pump against greater resistance.

The nurse can educate clients about their risks for hypertension. Persons with family members who have had hypertension are at significant risk. Obesity, cigarette smoking, heavy alcohol consumption, high blood cholesterol levels, and continued exposure to stress are all factors linked to hypertension. When clients are diagnosed with hypertension the nurse helps to educate them about (1) BP values, (2) long-term follow-up care and therapy, (3) the usual lack of symptoms (the fact that it may not be "felt"), (4) therapy's ability to control but not cure it, and (5) a consistently followed treatment plan that can ensure a relatively normal life-style (Joint National Committee on Detection, Evaluation, and Treatment of High Blood Pressure, 1984).

Blood Pressure Equipment

To assess blood pressure the nurse must have equipment that functions properly. The nurse also must be competent and feel comfortable when using a stethoscope and sphygmomanometer.

SPHYGMOMANOMETER

A sphygmomanometer consists of a pressure manometer, an occlusive cloth cuff enclosing an inflatable rubber bladder, and a pressure bulb with a release valve to inflate the cuff (Fig. 12-11).

There are two types of manometers, mercury and aneroid. The mercury manometer is the most accurate. It is an upright tube containing mercury. Pressure created by inflation of the compression cuff moves the column of mercury upward against the force of gravity. Millimeter calibrations mark the height of the mercury column. To ensure accurate readings, the mercury column should always be at 0 when the cuff is deflated and it should fall freely as pressure is released. Repeated calibrations are not needed as long as this is done. Deviations indicate that the manometer is malfunctioning. Mercury manometers are wall mounted or portable. Accurate readings are made by looking at the mercury meniscus at eye level. Looking up or down at the mercury results in measurement distortions.

TABLE 12-9 Classification of Blood Pressure

Range (mm Hg)	Category
DIASTOLIC	
<85	Normal blood pressure
85-89	High normal blood pressure
90-104	Mild hypertension
105-114	Moderate hypertension
≥115	Severe hypertension
SYSTOLIC, WHEN DIASTOLIC BP IS <90	
<140	Normal blood pressure
140-159	Borderline isolated systolic hypertension
≥160	Isolated systolic hypertension

From The Joint National Committee on Detection, Evaluation and Treatment of High Blood Pressure: The 1984 report of the Joint National Committee on Detection, Evaluation, and Treatment of High Blood Pressure, Arch Intern Med 144:1045, May 1984. Copyright 1984, American Medical Association.

TABLE 12-10 Follow-Up Criteria for First-Occasion Measurement

Range (mm Hg)	Recommended Follow-Up
DIASTOLIC	
<85	Recheck within 2 years.
85-89	Recheck within 1 year.
90-104	Confirm promptly (not to exceed 2 months).
105-114	Evaluate or refer to source of care (not to exceed 2 weeks).
≥115	Evaluate or refer immediately to a source of care.
SYSTOLIC, WHEN DIASTOLIC PRESSURE IS 90	
<140	Recheck within 2 years.
140-199	Confirm promptly (not to exceed 2 months).
≥200	Evaluate or refer promptly to source of care (not to exceed 2 weeks).

From The Joint National Committee on Detection, Evaluation, and Treatment of High Blood Pressure: The 1984 report of the Joint National Committee on Detection, Evaluation, and Treatment of High Blood Pressure, Arch Intern Med 144:1045, May 1984. Copyright 1984, American Medical Association.

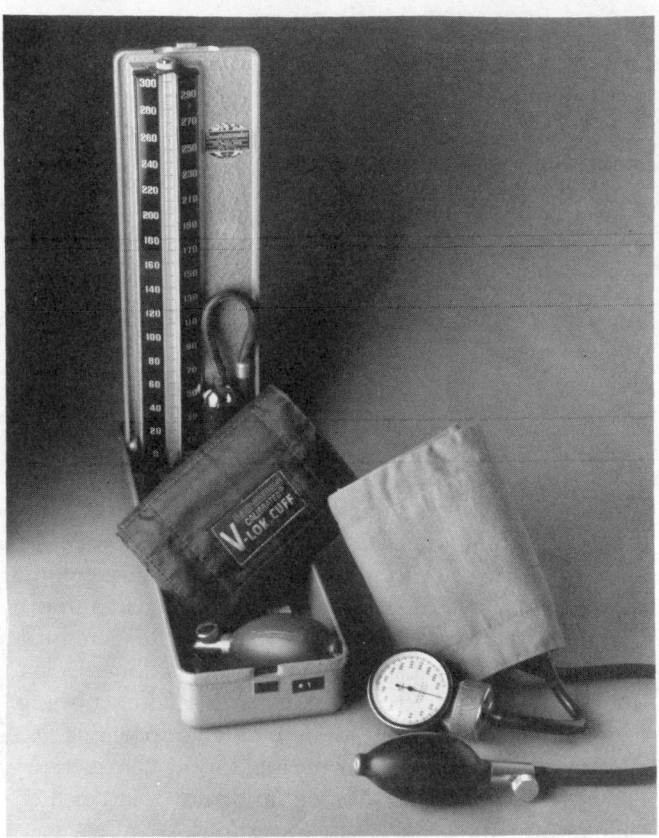

Fig. 12-11 Sphygmomanometer.

The aneroid manometer has a glass-enclosed circular gauge containing a needle that registers millimeter calibrations. A metal bellows within the gauge expands and collapses in response to pressure variations in the inflated cuff. Because metal parts in the aneroid model are subject to temperature expansion or contraction, the aneroid instrument is perhaps less reliable than the mercury type. Before using the aneroid model, the nurse must be sure that the needle points to 0 and that the manometer is correctly calibrated. An aneroid manometer should be recalibrated against a perfectly working mercury manometer at least once a year. Aneroid manometers have the advantages of being lightweight, portable, and compact.

Cloth cuffs used with the sphygmomanometer come in several sizes. Ideally the width of the cuff should be 40% of the circumference (or 20% wider than the diameter) of the midpoint of the limb on which the cuff is to be used (American Heart Association, 1980). The length of the enclosed bladder should be approximately twice the recommended width. A bladder of this length nearly encircles the arm and minimizes the risk of misapplication. In an adult the average bladder width is 12 to 13 cm and the length is 22 to 23 cm. In children the lower edge of the cuff should be above the antecubital

fossa, allowing room for placement of the stethoscope. An improperly fitting cuff causes inaccurate readings (Table 12-11).

Before using a sphygmomanometer the nurse should inspect the parts of the release valve and the pressure bulb. The valve should be clean and freely movable in either direction. If it sticks or becomes too tightly closed, the deflation of the pressure cuff will be hard to regulate. The pressure bulb is made of tough rubber and should be free of leaks.

Assessment of Blood Pressure

Blood pressure may be measured directly or indirectly. The direct method requires the insertion of a thin intravenous catheter into an artery. Tubing connects the catheter with an electronic sensor. Pressure within the artery transmits pressure along the fluid-filled tubing to the sensor that then displays a blood pressure reading on an electronic display. Direct monitoring is used only in an operating room or intensive care unit.

The indirect method requires use of the sphygmomanometer. The nurse may use either or both of two indirect techniques, auscultation and palpation. Assessing the blood pressure indirectly by auscultation is the most common technique (Procedure 12-4).

AUSCULTATION

The best environment for blood pressure measurement by auscultation is a quiet room at a comfortable temperature. The nurse attempts to control the client's pain, anxiety, or exertion and asks the client to refrain from eating or smoking before the assessment because these factors can cause false high readings.

Although the client may lie or stand, sitting is the preferred position. Some clients, especially the elderly, may experience orthostatic hypotension, the lowering of blood pressure when they move from a lying to sitting or a sitting to standing position. Orthostatic hypotension is a common side effect of antihypertensive medications. The nurse may compare blood pressure taken with clients sitting and standing to detect variations. Normally, blood pressures obtained with a client in different positions are similar. The nurse should initially measure blood pressure in both arms, especially if the client has heart disease or if the reading in the first arm is abnormal. Normally a difference of 5 to 10 mm Hg exists between the arms. In subsequent assessments the blood pressure should be measured in the arm with the higher pressure. Pressure differences higher than 10 mm Hg indicate conditions such as aortic stenosis or an arterial occlusion in the arm with the lower pressure.

The Joint National Commission on Detection, Evaluation, and Treatment of High Blood Pressure (1984) suggests assessing an average of two or more blood pres-

PROCEDURE 12-4

Assessment of Blood Pressure by Auscultation

STEPS	RATIONALE
1. Assess for factors that normally influence blood pressure.	Allows nurse to accurately assess blood pressure and significance of any pressure changes.
2. Determine best site for blood pressure assessment. Avoid applying cuff to arm: when IV catheter is in antecubital fossa and IV fluids are infusing; in the presence of arteriovenous shunt; when breast or axillary surgery has been performed on that side; if arm or hand has been traumatized or diseased; if lower arm is enclosed by cast or bulky bandage.	Inappropriate site selection may result in poor amplification of sounds, causing inaccurate readings. Application of pressure from inflated bladder can temporarily impair blood flow and compromise circulation in extremity that already has impaired circulation.
3. Prepare needed equipment and supplies and make sure they are in working order:	
a. Mercury sphygmomanometer: control valve should be clear and freely adjustable; when closed, valve should hold mercury constant; when released, valve allows controlled fall in mercury level; air vent at top of mercury manometer should be patent; rubber tubing connecting bladder to manometer should be at least 80 cm (32 in) long and with airtight connections	Used to measure arterial blood pressure indirectly. Accurate measurements depend on functional equipment.
b. Bladder and cuff: bladder should completely encircle arm without overlapping; tapering cuff should be long enough to encircle arm several times	Secure-fitting cuff and proper-sized bladder are needed to exert equal pressure around artery being auscultated. Too narrow bladder causes false high reading.
c. Stethoscope	Auscultates arterial pressure waves.
d. Pen, pencil, and flow sheet or record form	Provide for timely documentation of findings.
4. Encourage client to avoid exercise and smoking for 30 min before assessment.	These factors can cause false elevations in blood pressure.
5. Have client assume sitting or lying position. Be sure room is warm and quiet.	Maintains client's comfort during measurement.
6. Explain procedure to client and have client rest at least 5 min before measurement.	Reduces anxiety that can falsely elevate readings. Blood pressure readings taken at different times can be objectively compared when all are assessed with client at rest.
7. Wash hands.	Reduces transmission of microorganisms.
8. Support client's upper arm (while client is sitting or lying) at heart level with palm turned up (see illustration).	If arm is unsupported, client may perform isometric exercise that can increase diastolic pressure 10%. Placement of arm above heart level causes false low reading.

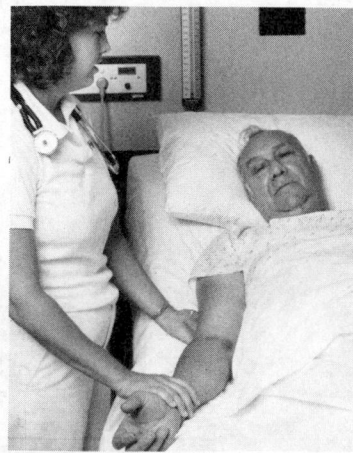

Step 8

Continued.

PROCEDURE 12-4, cont'd

Assessment of Blood Pressure by Auscultation

STEPS	RATIONALE
9. Expose upper arm fully by removing constricting clothing.	Ensures proper cuff application.
10. Palpate brachial artery (see illustration). Position cuff 2.5 cm (1 in) above site of brachial pulsation (antecubital space). Center bladder of cuff above artery (see illustration).	Inflating bladder directly over brachial artery ensures the proper pressure is applied during inflation.
11. With cuff fully deflated, wrap cuff evenly and snugly around upper arm (see illustration).	Loose-fitting cuff causes false high readings.
12. Be sure manometer is positioned vertically at eye level. Observer should be no further than 1 m (approximately 1 yd) away.	Eye level placement ensures accurate reading of mercury level.
13. Palpate brachial or radial artery with fingertips of one hand while inflating cuff rapidly to pressure 30 mm Hg above point at which pulse disappears. Slowly deflate cuff and note point when pulse reappears.	Identifies approximate systolic pressure and determines maximal inflation point for accurate reading. Prevents auscultatory gap.
14. Deflate cuff fully and wait 30 sec.	Prevents venous congestion and false high readings.
15. Place stethoscope earpieces in ears and be sure sounds are clear, not muffled.	Each earpiece should follow angle of ear canal to facilitate hearing.
16. Relocate brachial artery and place bell or diaphragm chestpiece over it. Do not allow chestpiece to touch cuff or clothing (see illustration).	Proper stethoscope placement ensures optimal sound reception. Stethoscope improperly positioned causes muffled sounds that often result in false low systolic and false high diastolic readings.
17. Close valve of pressure bulb clockwise until tight.	Tightening of valve prevents air leak during inflation.
18. Inflate cuff to 30 mm Hg above palpated systolic pressure.	Ensures accurate measurement of systolic pressure.
19. Slowly release valve and allow mercury to fall at rate of 2 to 3 mm Hg/sec.	Too rapid or slow a decline in mercury level can cause inaccurate readings.
20. Note point on manometer when first clear sound is heard.	First Korotkoff sound indicates systolic pressure.
21. Continue to deflate cuff gradually, noting point at which muffled or dampened sound appears.	Fourth Korotkoff sound involves distinct muffling of sounds and is recommended by American Heart Association as indication of diastolic pressure in children.
22. Continue cuff deflation, noting point on manometer at which sound disappears. (Note pressure to nearest 2 mm Hg.)	American Heart Association recommends recording fifth Korotkoff sound as diastolic pressure in adults.

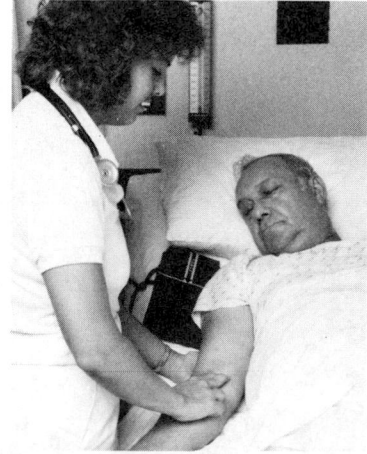

Step 10

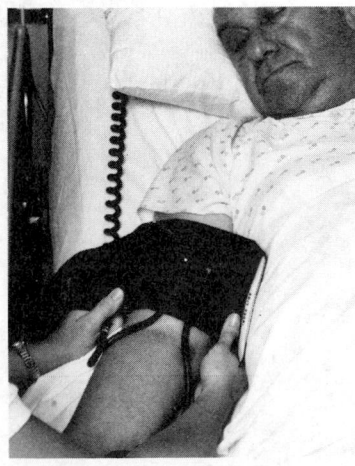

Step 10

STEPS	RATIONALE
23. Deflate cuff rapidly and completely. Remove from client's arm unless you plan to repeat measurement.	Continuous cuff inflation causes arterial occlusion, resulting in numbness and tingling of client's arm.
24. If this is first assessment of client, repeat procedure on other arm.	Comparison of pressure in both arms serves to detect any circulatory problems. (Normal difference of 5 to 10 mm Hg exists between arms.)
25. Assist client in returning to comfortable position and cover the upper arm if previously clothed.	Restores client's comfort.
26. Inform client of blood pressure reading.	Promotes participation in care and understanding of health status.
27. Wash hands.	Prevents transmission of microorganisms.
28. Compare blood pressure reading with previous baseline and/or normal average pressure for client's age.	Evaluates for change in condition and presence of blood pressure alterations.
29. Record blood pressure in nurses' notes or flowsheet and report any abnormal findings immediately.	Vital signs should be recorded immediately to ensure accuracy.

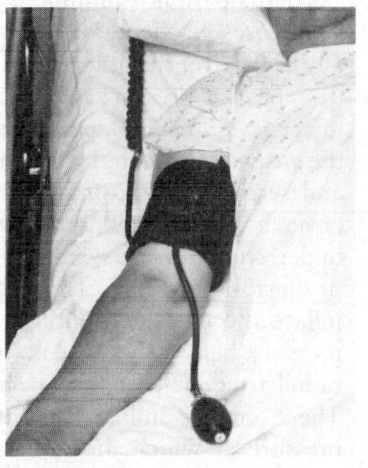

Step 11

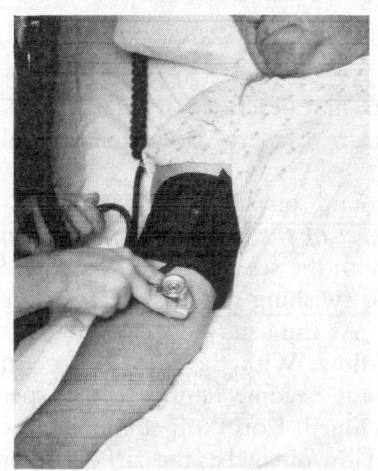

Step 16

sure values per visit to a health agency. This allows for more accurate detection of abnormalities. The nurse waits 2 minutes before repeating a measurement in the same arm. The nurse asks clients if they know their normal blood pressures. If so, comparisons can be made with the nurse's measurements. When assessing blood pressure, the nurse can discuss the following:

1. The numerical blood pressure value
2. The need for periodic remeasurement
3. Compliance with any present antihypertensive therapy

PRESSURE DYNAMICS.   Indirect measurement of arterial blood pressure works on a basic principle of pressure. The external application of pressure beyond that which keeps a vessel open causes the vessel to close. For example, in a client with a normal blood pressure of 120/80 mm Hg, blood flows freely through the brachial artery at a systolic pressure of 120 mm Hg. Inflation of the cuff gradually applies pressure to tissues surrounding the brachial artery. When the cuff pressure exceeds 120 mm Hg, the artery collapses, blood flow ceases, and auscultation reveals absence of sounds. When the cuff pressure is released, the point on the manometer at which sounds reappear through auscultation is the systolic pressure.

KOROTKOFF SOUNDS.   With the stethoscope placed over the artery the nurse listens for sounds created by blood flowing through it. In 1905, Nikdai S. Korot-

TABLE 12-11   Common Mistakes in Blood
                  Pressure Assessment

Error	Effect
Bladder or cuff too wide	False low reading
Bladder or cuff too narrow	False high reading
Cuff wrapped too loosely	False high reading
Deflating cuff too slowly	False high diastolic reading
Deflating cuff too quickly	False low systolic and false high diastolic reading
Stethoscope that fits poorly or impairment of the examiner's hearing, causing sounds to be muffled	False low systolic and false high diastolic reading
Inaccurate inflation level	False low systolic reading
Multiple examiners using different Korotkoff sounds for diastolic readings	Inaccurate interpretation of systolic and diastolic readings

koff, a Russian surgeon, first described arterial sounds. The Korotkoff sounds are used to assess the arterial blood pressure values.

The first Korotkoff sound (phase I) is a clear rhythmical tapping sound. *Onset of the sound corresponds to the systolic pressure.* With the second Korotkoff sound (phase II), a murmur or swishing sound appears as the cuff is further deflated. As the artery distends, there is a turbulence of blood flow. With the third Korotkoff sound (phase III), sounds become temporarily crisper and more intense. The fourth Korotkoff sounds (phase IV) become muffled and low pitched as the cuff is further deflated. Cuff pressure falls below the pressure within the vessel walls. *This sound is the diastolic pressure in infants and children.* The fifth Korotkoff Sound (Phase V) is actually a disappearance of all sounds. *In adolescents and adults, this sound corresponds with the diastolic pressure.*

RECORDING BLOOD PRESSURE READINGS. Several causes exist for error in blood pressure readings if the auscultation method is not performed correctly. Table 12-11 summarizes common mistakes in measurement.

The nurse records the position of the client and the arm in which the pressure was assessed. Most institutions record only the systolic and diastolic pressures (for example, 120/80). However, if both the fourth and fifth Korotkoff sounds are used for diastolic readings, the pressure may be recorded with three numbers (for example, 110/78/70). When a nurse is unsure of a reading, a colleague should reassess the blood pressure.

PALPATION

The indirect palpation technique is useful for clients whose arterial pulsations are too weak to create Korotkoff sounds. Severe blood loss and weakened myocardial contractility are examples of conditions that result in blood pressures too low to auscultate accurately.

The blood pressure cuff is applied in the same manner as in the auscultation method. The nurse palpates the radial artery throughout the procedure instead of using a stethoscope. When the cuff is inflated to the desired level, the valve is released and the mercury is allowed to fall 2 mm Hg per second. As soon as the radial pulse is again palpable, the manometer reading is noted. This reading is the systolic blood pressure. The diastolic pressure is difficult to determine by palpation. A subtle change in sensation, usually in the form of a thin snapping vibration, marks the diastolic level. When the palpation technique is used, the systolic value and the manner in which it was measured are recorded (for example, "120 systolic by palpation").

The palpation technique is used with auscultation in some cases. In clients with hypertension, the sounds usually heard over the brachial artery with high cuff pressure disappear as pressure is reduced and then reappear at a lower level. This temporary disappearance of sound is the *auscultatory gap.* It typically occurs between the first and second Korotkoff sounds. The gap in sound may cover a range of 40 mm Hg and thus may cause an underestimation of systolic pressure or overestimation of diastolic pressure. The examiner must be certain to inflate the cuff high enough to hear the true systolic pressure before the auscultatory gap. Palpation of the radial artery helps determine how high to inflate the cuff. The examiner inflates the cuff 30 mm Hg above the pressure at which the radial pulse was palpated. The range of pressures in which the auscultatory gap occurs is recorded (for example, "BP 180/94, with an auscultatory gap from 180 to 160").

ULTRASONIC STETHOSCOPE

If a nurse is unable to auscultate sounds because of a weakened arterial pulse, an ultrasonic stethoscope can be used (see Chapter 13). This stethoscope allows the nurse to hear low-frequency sounds and is commonly used with infants and children.

ASSESSMENT OF BLOOD PRESSURE IN CHILDREN

The nurse should include blood pressure measurement in the routine assessment of any child. The Task Force on Blood Pressure Control in Children (1987) recommends that all children age 3 through adolescence should have blood pressures checked at least yearly. The nurse can help parents understand the importance of this routine screening to detect children who may be at risk for hypertension.

The measurement and interpretation of blood pressure in infants and children is difficult for the following reasons:

1. Various arm sizes require careful and appropriate cuff size selection.
2. Readings are difficult to obtain in restless or anxious infants and children.
3. Placing stethoscope too firmly on the antecubital fossa can cause errors in auscultation of Korotkoff sounds.
4. Korotkoff sounds are difficult to hear in children because of low frequency and amplitude.
5. Blood pressure in children changes with growth and development.

The nurse can use the same auscultation method used with adults. An infant or child under 5 years of age should lie supine with the arms supported at heart level. Older children may sit. It is important to have the child relaxed and calm. A delay of at least 15 minutes before taking a reading is recommended to allow the child to recover from recent activity or apprehension. Those 15 minutes can be used for other quiet nursing activities. It may help to have a parent nearby.

ASSESSMENT OF BLOOD PRESSURE IN LOWER EXTREMITIES

Occasionally, dressings, casts, intravenous catheters, or other devices make the upper extremities inaccessible, and blood pressure must be measured in the lower extremities. Also, in clients with certain blood pressure abnormalities, it helps to compare upper extremity blood pressure with that in the legs. The popliteal artery, located behind the knee in the popliteal space, is the site for auscultation. The cuff must be wide and long enough to allow for the larger girth of the thigh and is positioned with the bladder over the posterior aspect of the midthigh. Placing the client in a prone position is best. If such a position is impossible, the client should be asked to flex the knee slightly for easier access to the artery. The procedure is the same as that for brachial artery auscultation. Systolic pressure in the legs is usually higher by 10 to 40 mm Hg than that in the brachial artery, but the diastolic pressure is essentially the same.

SELF-MEASUREMENT OF BLOOD PRESSURE

More people measure their own blood pressure because of improved technology in home monitoring devices and a greater interest in health promotion. Two of the more common devices used by the general public include portable home devices and stationary automated machines.

The portable home devices include the mercury and aneroid sphygmomanometers and electronic digital readout devices that do not require use of a stethoscope. The electronic devices inflate and deflate cuffs with the push of a button. The electronic devices may be easier to manipulate but can easily become inaccurate and require recalibration more than once a year. Because of their sensitivity, improper cuff placement or movement of the arm can cause electronic devices to give incorrect readings.

Stationary automated machines can be found in public places such as grocery stores, fitness clubs, banks, airports, or work sites. Users simply rest their arms within the machine's inflatable cuff, which contains a pressure sensor. The cuff fits over the clothing. A visual display tells users their blood pressure within 60 to 90 seconds. The reliability of the stationary machines is limited. Blood pressure values may vary by 5 to 10 mm Hg or more (for both systolic and diastolic values) compared with pressures taken with a manual sphygmomanometer. The stationary machines are often placed in public areas where environmental noise is high and capable of interfering with the machine's computer.

The National High Blood Pressure Education Program Coordinating Committee (Hunt et al., 1985) has identified the following benefits of blood pressure self-measurement:

1. Self-administered blood pressure measurement can detect an elevated blood pressure in persons previously unaware of a problem.
2. When persons have borderline hypertension, self-measurement can provide information about the pattern of blood pressure values.
3. Clients with hypertension can benefit from participating actively in their treatment through self-monitoring.
4. For some clients undergoing treatment for hypertension, visual evidence of blood pressure may help compliance with treatment.

The Coordinating Committee (Hunt et al., 1985) also cites the following concerns about self-measurement of blood pressure:

1. There is the possibility persons will be inadequately trained in using the devices. Printed instructions accompanying the equipment may be incomplete.
2. One elevated reading is not enough to diagnose hypertension and only indicates that further evaluation is needed by health care personnel. Thus a client may be needlessly alarmed.
3. Clients with hypertension may become overly conscious of their pressures and make inappropriate self-adjustment of medications.

Consumers can learn to use self-measurement devices if they have the information needed to perform the procedure correctly and if they know when to seek medical attention. The nurse can advise clients of possible inaccuracies in the machines, help clients understand the meaning and implications of reading, and teach them proper measurement techniques.

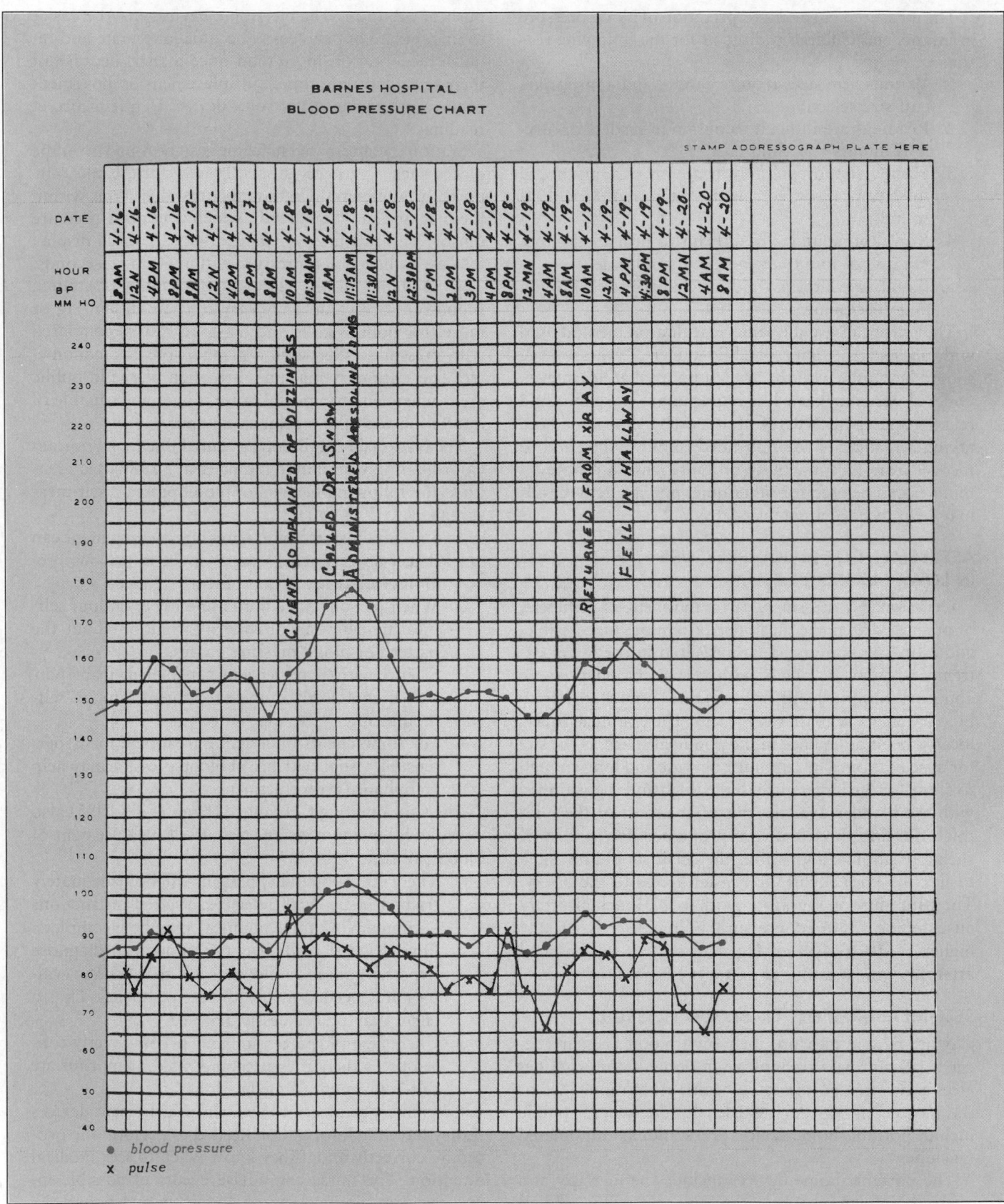

Fig. 12-12 Graphic flow sheet.
Courtesy Barnes Hospital, St. Louis.

REPORTING AND RECORDING VITAL SIGNS

The nurse is responsible for recording all vital signs accurately and in a timely manner. When a change or abnormality is assessed, the nurse reports the problem to the physician and the nurse on the next shift. The nurse decides when an abnormality has been assessed or reports a problem in response to a preexisting order such as "Call physician when systolic pressure $\geqq$180 mm Hg or diastolic $\geqq$100 mm Hg, or pulse >120 beats per minute."

Special graphic flow sheets exist for recording vital signs (Fig. 12-12). In addition to the actual vital sign values the nurse records in the nurses' notes any accompanying or precipitating symptoms such as chest pain and dizziness with abnormal blood pressure, shortness of breath with abnormal respirations, or flushing and diaphoresis with an elevated temperature. The nurse documents any interventions initiated as a result of vital sign measurement such as administration of tepid sponging or an antihypertensive medication.

SUMMARY

Vital signs measurements are a basic series of physiological assessments reflecting a client's health status. The nurse uses these data to make clinical decisions. Physical and psychological factors can create changes in vital signs. The nurse often decides the need for and frequency of vital sign assessment, which is not simply a routine chore but rather an integral part of a nurse's practice.

Before measuring any vital sign, the nurse should understand the physiological controls governing it. Each physiological control is influenced by certain variables such as age, physical exercise, or hormonal changes. The nurse who understands the effects of these variables is better prepared to anticipate normal variations. A nurse cannot recognize abnormalities without first knowing what is normal.

Basic principles apply in the procedures for assessing vital signs accurately. Medical aseptic technique should be used. The client should be placed in the most comfortable position for measurements. Procedures should be explained to the client to reduce anxiety. The nurse should not rush through an assessment and should not estimate values. All characteristics of a vital sign are assessed. Results are recorded promptly and accurately.

KEY CONCEPTS

✓ Vital signs include the physiological measurements of temperature, pulse, respirations, and blood pressure.

✓ Vital signs may be measured as part of a complete physical examination or more commonly in a review of the client's condition.

✓ The nurse assesses vital sign changes in conjunction with other physical assessment findings.

✓ The nurse uses judgment to determine the frequency of vital sign measurement.

✓ Knowledge of the factors influencing vital signs assists the nurse to interpret abnormal values.

✓ Vital signs are a basis for evaluating response to nursing interventions.

✓ Assessment of vital signs yields the most accurate values when the client is inactive and the environment is controlled for the client's comfort.

✓ Normally, heat production balances heat loss to maintain body temperature.

✓ The nurse assists the client in maintaining body temperature by initiating interventions promoting heat loss or production.

✓ A fever is one of the body's normal defense mechanisms and often does not require treatment.

✓ The oral route is the most accessible and acceptable site for temperature measurement.

✓ Rectal temperature measurements should not be performed on newborn infants or adults with rectal alterations.

✓ To assess cardiac function, pulse rate and rhythm are most easily measured using the radial or apical pulse.

✓ The nurse assesses the presence and character of peripheral pulses to determine the adequacy of local blood flow.

✓ Assessment of respirations involves observation of ventilatory movements.

✓ Blood pressure levels reflect the relationship among severel hemodynamic variables.

✓ Blood pressure can be measured by either auscultation or palpation.

✓ The diagnosis of hypertension can only be made after averaging pressure readings made on at least two occasions.

✓ Changes in any vital sign can influence characteristics of the other vital signs.

✓ Self-measurement of blood pressure can be useful in detecting an elevated blood pressure in persons previously unaware of a problem or in monitoring blood pressure in those persons already diagnosed with hypertension.

REFERENCES

American Heart Association: Recommendations for human blood pressure determination by sphygomomanometers, Dallas, 1980, The Association.

Atkins, E: Fever: a new perspective on an old phenomenon, New Engl J Med 308:958, 1983.

Barner, HB, et al.: Field evaluation of a new simplified method for cooling of heat casualties in the desert, Military Med 149:95, 1984.

Centers for Disease Control: Recommendations for prevention of HIV transmission in health-care settings, Morbidity and Mortality Weekly Report (suppl) 36:SS, Aug. 21, 1987.

Dinarello, C: Interleukin-1: Rev Infect Dis 6:51, 1984.

Eoff, M, and Joyce, B: Temperature measurements in children, Am J Nurs 81:1010, 1981.

Guerevich, I: Fever: when to worry about it, RN 48:14, Dec. 1985.

Guyton, AC: Textbook of medical physiology, ed. 6, Philadelphia, 1986, W.B. Saunders Co.

Joint National Committee on Detection, Evaluation, and Treatment of High Blood Pressure: The 1984 report of the Joint National Committee on Detection, Evaluation and Treatment of High Blood Pressure, Arch Intern Med 144:1045, May 1984.

LaVoy, K: Dealing with hypothermia and frostbite, RN 48:53, Jan. 1985.

Lovejoy, FH Jr.: Aspirin and acetaminophen: a comparative view of their anti-pyretic and analgesic activity, Pediatrics 62(suppl): 904, 1978.

Mountcastle, VB: Medical physiology, vol. 2, ed. 14, St. Louis, 1980, The C.V. Mosby Co.

Petersdorf, RC: Disturbances of heat regulation. In Isselbacher, KJ, et al., editors: Harrison's principles of internal medicine, ed. 9, New York, 1980, McGraw-Hill Book Co.

Task Force on Blood Pressure Control in Children: Report of Second Task Force on Blood Pressure Control in Children—1987, Pediatrics, 79:1-15, Jan. 1987.

Thibodeau, GA: Anatomy and physiology, St. Louis, 1987, The C.V. Mosby Co.

Whaley, LF, and Wong, DL: Nursing care of infants and children, ed. 3, St. Louis, 1987, The C.V. Mosby Co.

Research Articles

Angerami, ELS: Epidemiological study of a body temperature in patients in a teaching hospital, Int J Nurs Stud 17:91, 1980.

Baker, NC, et al.: The effect of type of thermometer and length of time inserted on oral temperature measurements of afebrile subjects, Nurs Res 33:109, March-April 1984.

Erickson, R: Oral temperature differences in relation to thermometer and technique, Nurs Res 29:157, 1980.

Graves, RP, and Markarian, MF: Three minute time intervals when using an oral mercury-in-glass thermometer with or without J-temp sheaths, Nurs Res 29:323, 1980.

Hunt, JC, et al.: Devices used for self-measurement of blood pressure: revised statement of the National High Blood Pressure Education Program, Arch Intern Med 145:2231, Dec. 1985.

Nichols, GA, and Kucha, DH: Oral measurements, Am J Nurs 72:1091, 1972.

Samples, JF, et al.: Circadian rhythms: basis for screening for fever, Nurs Res 34:377, Nov.-Dec. 1985.

ADDITIONAL READINGS

Adelman, EM: When patient's blood pressure falls, what does it mean? What should you do? Nurs 80 10:26, 1980.

Bernheim, HA, et al.: Fever: pathogenesis, pathophysiology, and purpose, Ann Intern Med 91:261, 1979.

Birdsall, C: How accurate are your blood pressures? Am J Nurs 84:1414, 1984.

Birdsall, C: How do you handle heat loss? Am J Nurs 85:367, 1985.

Birdsall, C: How do you interpret pulses? Am J Nurs 85:785, 1985.

Donaldson, JF: Therapy of acute fever: a comparative approach, Hosp Pract [Off] 9:125, 1981.

Dressler, DK, et al.: A comparison of oral and rectal temperature measurement on patients receiving oxygen by mask, Nurs Res 32:373, 1983.

Electronic thermometers: the better alternative? Health Devices 12:18, 1982.

Griffin, JP: Fever: when to leave it alone, Nurs 86 16:58, 1986.

Hayes, KB: Dealing with heat injuries, RN 47:41, 1984.

Lim-Levy, F: The effect of oxygen inhalation on oral temperature, Nur Res 31:150, 1982.

McCarron, K: Fever: the cardinal vital sign, CCQ, 15, July 1986.

Nichols, GA: Time analysis of afebrile and febrile temperature reading, Nurs Res 21:463, 1972.

Nichols, GA, et al.: Oral, axillary, and rectal temperature determinations and relationships, Nurs Res 15:307, 1966.

Nichols, GA, et al.: Taking oral temperature of febrile patients, Nurs Res 18:448, 1969.

Nichols, GA, et al.: Measuring oral and rectal temperatures of febrile children, Nurs Res 21:261, 1972.

Rayburn, W, et al.: Self-monitoring of blood pressure during pregnancy, Am J Obstet Gynecol 148:159, 1984.

Thomas, DO: Fever in children, RN 48:18, 1985.

Thomas, SP, and Groer, MW: Relationship of demographic lifestyle and stress variables to blood pressure in adolescents, Nurs Res 35:169, 1986.

Working Group on Hypertension in the Elderly: Statement on hypertension in the elderly, JAMA 256:70, 1986.

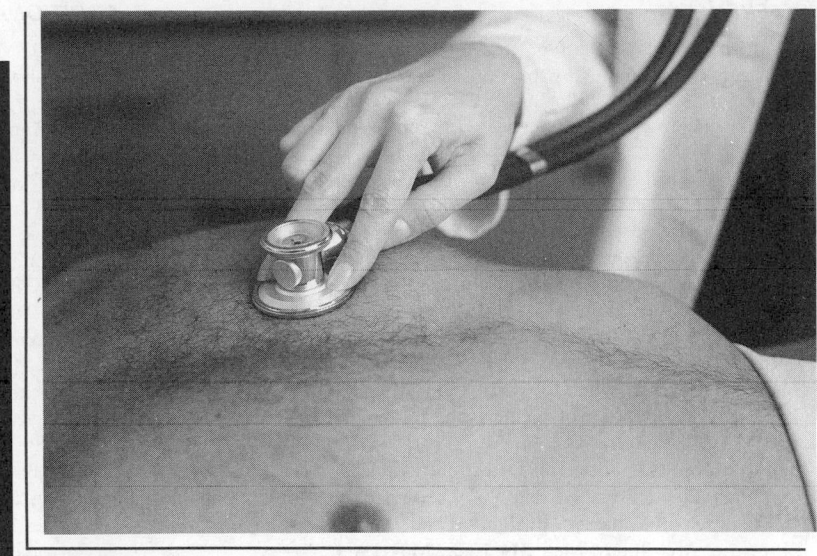

OBJECTIVES

Mastery of content in this chapter will enable the student to:

- Define the key terms listed.
- Discuss the purposes of physical assessment.
- Describe the techniques used with each of the physical assessment skills.
- Describe the proper position for the client during each phase of the examination.
- List techniques used to promote the client's physical and psychological comfort during an examination.
- Make environmental preparations before an examination.
- Use physical assessment skills during the performance of routine nursing care measures.
- Conduct physical assessments in an organized and proper fashion.
- Identify information to collect from the nursing history before an examination.
- Discuss normal physical findings in a young and middle adult compared with an elderly client.
- Discuss ways to incorporate health teaching into the examination process.
- Describe physical measurements made in assessment of each body system.
- Summarize assessment findings on a physical examination form.

KEY TERMS

Accommodation Reflex	Melanin
Alopecia	Melena
Aneurysm	Ophthalmic
Atrophy	Orthopnea
Bilirubin	Pallor
Borborygmus	Palpebra
Bruit	PERRLA
Buccal	Pigmentation
Carcinoma	Pleura
Cirrhosis	Pleural Cavity
Consensual Light Reflex	PMI
Crackle	Ptosis
Dorsal	Recumbent
Edema	Rigidity
Emphysematous	Sebaceous Gland
Exophthalmos	Serous Fluid
Friction Rub	Sign
Gait	Spasm
Gurgle	Stridor
Hematemesis	Systemic
Hirsutism	Tracheostomy
Hyperpigmentation	Turgor
Integument	Varicosity
Jaundice	Ventral
Malabsorption Syndrome	Vitiligo
Malignant Tumor	

Physical Examination and Health Assessment

The nurse works in a variety of settings, seeking information about clients' health status. The nurse conducts health assessments at health fairs, at screening clinics, in physician's offices, or in hospitals to identify the client's physical and psychosocial needs. Health screenings involve measurement of specific physical functions or diagnostic tests to detect persons with a high probability of having a characteristic (Larson, 1986). For example, blood pressure screenings detect high blood pressure. Tine tests identify persons who have been exposed to tuberculosis. Information from health screenings determine the need for more comprehensive examinations.

A complete health assessment involves a more detailed review of a condition. The nurse collects a nursing history (see Chapter 6) and performs a physical examination. The nurse uses the skills of physical assessment to make clinical judgements. The client's condition and response affects the extent of the examination. The accuracy of the physical assessment influences the choice of therapies a client receives. Continuity in health care improves when the nurse makes ongoing, objective, and comprehensive assessments.

PURPOSES OF PHYSICAL EXAMINATION

An examination should be designed for the client's needs. If a client is acutely ill, the nurse may assess only the involved body systems. A more comprehensive examination is conducted when the client feels more at ease, and the nurse then learns about the client's total health status. A complete physical examination is performed for

1. Routine screening to promote preventive health care.
2. Determination of eligibility for health insurance, military service, or a new job.
3. Admission to a hospital or long-term care facility.

The nurse uses physical assessment skills to

1. Gather baseline data about the client's health.
2. Supplement, confirm, or refute data obtained in the nursing history.
3. Confirm and identify nursing diagnoses.
4. Make clinical judgments about a client's changing health status and management.
5. Evaluate the physiological outcomes of care.

Gathering a Data Base

The nurse initially gathers thorough and detailed information about the client's health status with the nursing health history. However, a client may be unaware of a physical problem, so a thorough assessment of physical status is necessary. Even if a history is complete, a physical assessment reveals information that refutes, confirms, or supplements the existing data base. For example, a client may complain of back pain. The nurse asks several questions to clarify the nature of the pain. However, unless the nurse sees the bruise across the client's back, the symptom of pain could suggest several ailments.

One assessment finding cannot conclusively reveal the nature of an abnormality. A complete assessment is needed to form a definitive diagnosis. The nurse learns to group significant findings into patterns of data. In addition, each abnormal finding directs the nurse to gather additional information as needed. Information gathered during an initial physical assessment provides a baseline of functional abilities. The baseline is not the normal range of physical findings but rather the pattern of findings identified when the client was first assessed. This baseline serves as a comparison for future assessment findings. During a subsequent hospital or clinic visit the nurse can determine if changes in the client's condition have occurred.

Developing Diagnoses and a Plan of Care

The accuracy of the data base allows the nurse to develop individualized nursing diagnoses. Physical assessment findings help determine the etiology of diagnoses and thus the type of interventions required in the plan of care. Physical assessment is ongoing. The nurse

monitors the progress of the disease and response to therapies to review existing diagnoses and identify new problems.

Managing Client Problems

When caring for clients, nurses make many observations and perform a variety of therapies. Yet, the nurse's success in giving care depends on the ability to recognize change in status and to modify therapies so clients gain the most desirable outcome. Physical assessment skills allow nurses to judge the status of clients' health and direct the management of care. For example, the nurse inspects the skin during a routine bath and finds it excessively dry. The nurse does not use soap and applies body lotion to the skin. The nurse revises the written plan of care so other nurses know the type of skin care to provide. Instruction is also given to the client about skin care. Performing the mechanics of physical assessment is relatively simple. The more difficult challenge lies in using findings to make decisions.

Evaluating Nursing Care

Nurses are made accountable for their actions by evaluating the results of care, the final stage of the nursing process. Physical assessment skills enhance the evaluation of nursing measures through monitoring physiological outcomes of care. The same physical assessment skill used to assess a condition (for example, palpation of the client's pulse) can be used as an evaluative measure after care is administered (for example, an exercise plan) to determine tolerance and response to therapy.

Physical assessment skills allow a nurse to make detailed, objective measurements. The nurse does not depend on a guess when physical assessment can be used to evaluate effectiveness of nursing care.

INTEGRATION OF PHYSICAL ASSESSMENT WITH NURSING CARE

Whether a complete or partial physical assessment is performed, an examination should be integrated into routine care. For example, the nurse can assess the condition of body parts during a bed bath. When a client undergoes oral hygiene, the nurse can carefully assess oral cavity structures. This practice makes more efficient use of time. The nurse also learns that physical assessment should become an automatic behavior when nurse and client interact. The result is the nurse's ability to gather more comprehensive and relevant assessment findings.

SKILLS OF PHYSICAL ASSESSMENT

Chapter 6 briefly describes the skills of inspection, palpation, percussion, and auscultation. This chapter provides a more detailed description of those skills, and their application in the physical examination.

Inspection

The nurse inspects or looks at body parts to detect normal characteristics or significant physical signs. It helps to know normal physical characteristics before trying to distinguish abnormal findings. Experience is needed to recognize normal variations among clients, as well as ranges of normal in an individual. Inspection is a simple technique but is often underused. For example, when hurrying to complete a bath a nurse may fail to inspect all skin surfaces and overlook a rash under the client's arm. The quality of an inspection depends on the nurse's willingness to spend time doing a thorough job.

To inspect body parts accurately the nurse follows these principles:

1. Have good lighting available.
2. Position and expose body parts so all surfaces can be viewed.
3. Inspect each area for size, shape, color, symmetry, position, and abnormalities.
4. If possible, compare each area inspected with the same area on the opposite side of the body.
5. Use additional light (for example, a penlight) to inspect body cavities.

After a nurse completes inspection of a body part, findings may indicate further examination. Palpation is often used with or after visual inspection.

Palpation

Further assessment of body parts is made through the sense of touch. The hands can make delicate and sensitive measurements of specific physical signs, so palpation is used to examine all accessible parts of the body. The nurse uses different parts of the hand to detect characteristics such as texture, temperature, and the perception of movement.

The client should be relaxed and positioned comfortably because muscle tension during palpation impairs the ability to use palpation effectively. For example, tension of the abdominal muscles makes palpation of underlying organs impossible and mimics muscle rigidity. Asking the client to take slow deep breaths enhances muscle relaxation. Tender areas are palpated last. The nurse asks the client to point out the more sensitive areas and notes any nonverbal signs of discomfort.

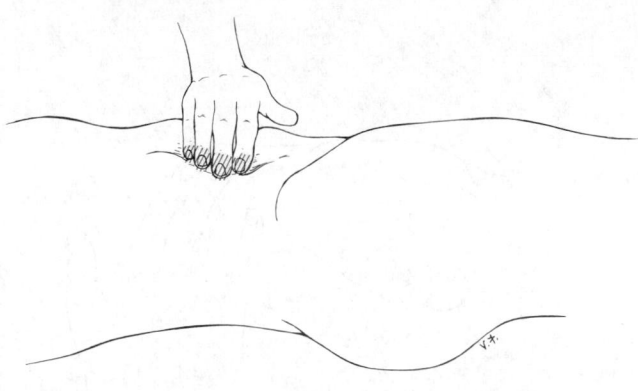

Fig. 13-1   During light palpation the nurse uses gentle pressure to depress the underlying body part. If areas of tenderness are detected, the area is examined further.

Clients appreciate warm hands, short fingernails, and a gentle approach. The nurse applies tactile pressure slowly and gently. Light palpation of structures such as the abdomen is performed to determine areas of tenderness. The nurse's hand is placed on the part to be examined and depressed about 1 cm (½ inch) (Fig. 13-1). Any tender areas found are examined further. The sensation of touch is best preserved with light, intermittent pressure. Heavy, prolonged pressure causes a loss of sensitivity in the nurse's hand.

The most sensitive parts of the hand, the pads of the fingertips, are used to assess texture, shape, size, consistency, and pulsation (Fig. 13-2, *A*). Temperature is best measured using the dorsum or back of the hand (Fig. 13-2, *B*) and fingers, where the skin is thinnest. The palm of the hand (Fig. 13-2, *C*) is more sensitive to vibration. The nurse measures position, consistency, and turgor by lightly grasping the body part with the fingertips (Fig. 13-2, *D*).

After light palpation has been applied, deeper palpation is used to examine the condition of organs, such as those in the abdomen. The nurse depresses the area being examined approximately 2 cm (1 inch). Caution is the rule. A student nurse should not attempt deep palpation without the assistance of a qualified instructor because prolonged pressure could cause internal injury. Deep palpation may be applied with one hand or both hands (bimanually) (Fig. 13-3). When the nurse uses bimanual palpation, one hand (called the sensing hand) is relaxed and placed lightly over the client's skin. The other hand (active hand) applies pressure to the sensing hand. The lower hand does not exert pressure directly and thus retains the sensitivity needed to detect organ characteristics.

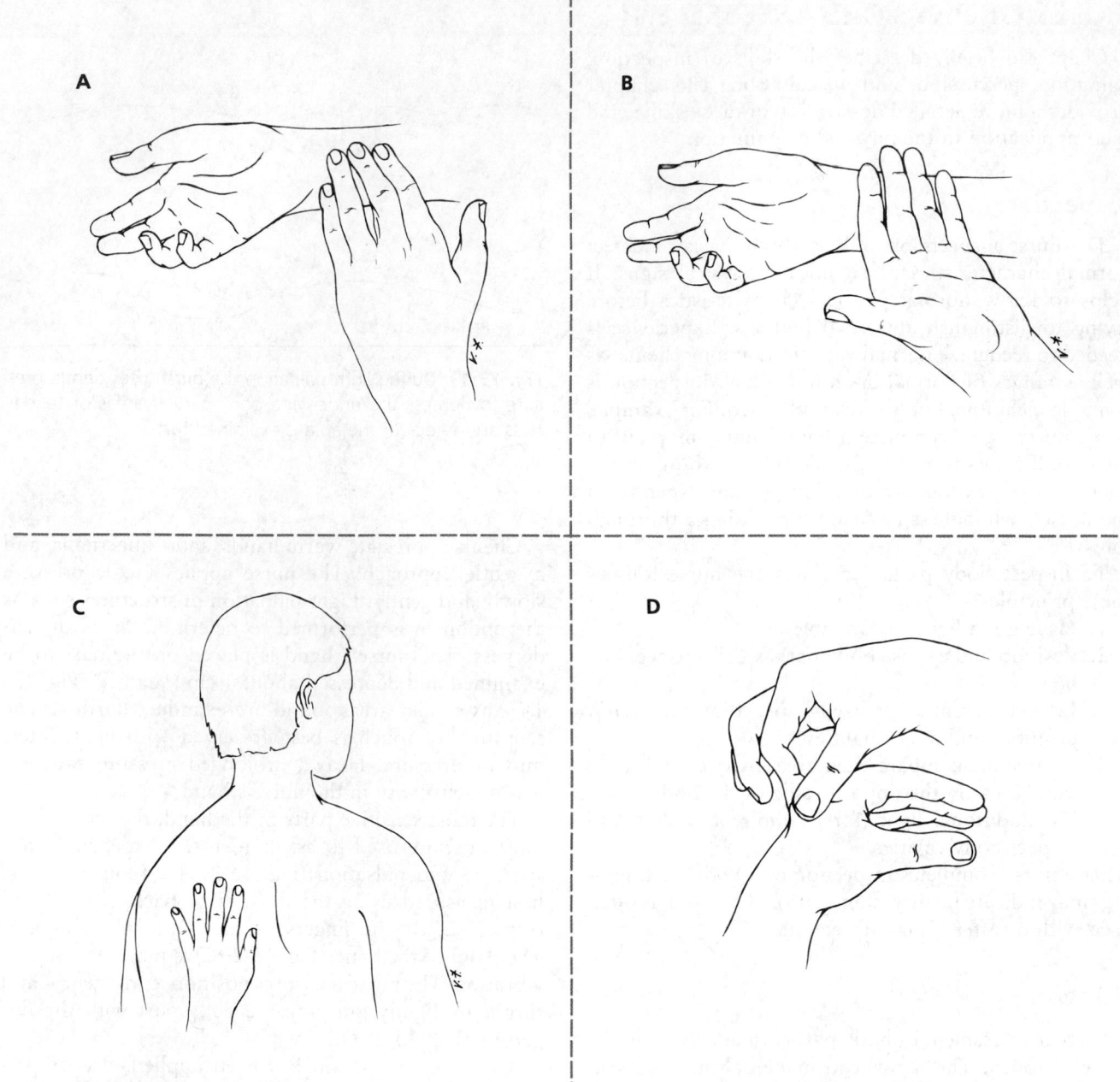

Fig. 13-2 **A,** The radial pulse is detected with the pads of the fingertips, the most sensitive part of the hand. **B,** The dorsum of the hand allows the nurse to detect temperature variations in the client's skin. **C,** The nurse uses the palm of the hand to detect vibration. **D,** The nurse grasps the skin with the fingertips to assess skin turgor.

The nurse must not palpate without considering the client's condition. For example, if the client has a fractured rib, extra care is used to locate the painful area. A vital artery is not palpated with pressure that obstructs blood flow. The nurse must also consider the body area being palpated and the reason for using palpation and must be able to discriminate and interpret the significance of what is sensed.

Percussion

Percussion requires dexterity. Through percussion the location, size, and density of an underlying structure are determined. Percussion helps to verify abnormalities assessed through palpation and auscultation. For example, if the nurse hears abnormal breath sounds when auscultating the lungs, percussion may rule out the presence of consolidated fluids.

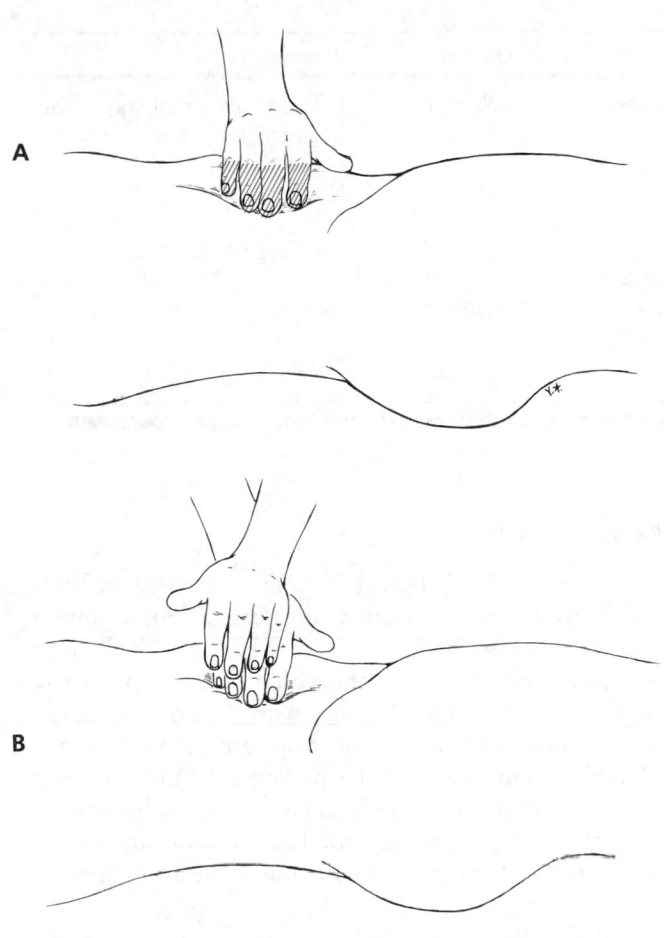

Fig. 13-3 **A,** During deep palpation the nurse depresses the underlying tissues approximately 2 cm (1 inch). Deep palpation allows the nurse to assess the condition of underlying organs. **B,** Position of hands for bimanual palpation. The underlying sensing hand detects the condition of underlying tissues and organs.

Fig. 13-4 To perform indirect percussion, the nurse places the middle finger of the nondominant hand against the body's surface. The tip of the middle finger of the dominant hand strikes the top of the middle finger of the nondominant hand.

When the examiner strikes the body's surface with a finger, vibration and sound are produced. This vibration is transmitted through the body tissues, and the character of the sound depends on the density of the underlying tissue. For example, the normal lung transmits sounds with high intensity and low pitch, whereas the more solid liver transmits a high-pitched sound of soft intensity. By knowing the way densities influence sound, the nurse is able to locate organs or masses, map their boundaries, and determine their size. An abnormal sound suggests the presence of a mass or substance such as fluid within an organ or body cavity.

The two methods of percussion are direct and indirect. The direct method involves striking the body surface directly with one or two fingers. The indirect technique is performed by placing the middle finger of the nondominant hand (called the pleximeter) firmly against the body surface, keeping the palm and remaining fingers off the skin. The tip of the middle finger of the dominant hand (called the plexor) strikes the base of the distal joint of the pleximeter (Fig. 13-4). The examiner uses a quick, sharp stroke with the plexor finger, keeping the forearm stationary. The wrist remains relaxed to deliver the proper blow. If the blow is not sharp, if the pleximeter is held loosely, or if the palm rests on the body surface, the sound is dampened or softened, preventing transmission of sound to underlying structures. The same force must be applied to each area so an accurate comparison of sounds can be made. A light, quick blow usually produces the clearest sound.

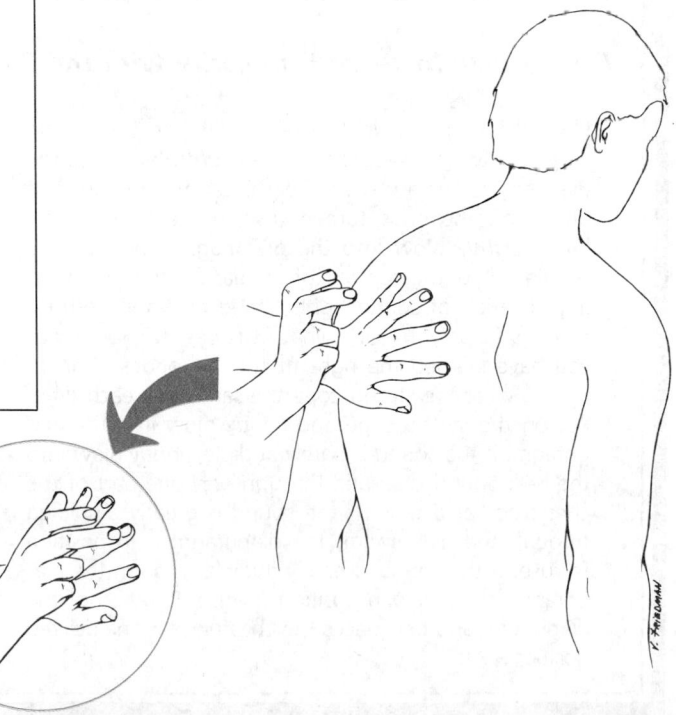

TABLE 13-1   Sounds Produced by Percussion

Sound	Intensity	Pitch	Duration	Quality	Percussion
Tympany	Loud	High	Moderate	Drumlike	Enclosed air-containing space: gastric air bubble, puffed-out cheek
Resonance	Moderate to loud	Low	Long	Hollow	Normal lung
Hyperresonance	Very loud	Very low	Longer than resonance	Booming	Emphysematous lung
Dullness	Soft to moderate	Moderate	Moderate	Thudlike	Liver
Flatness	Soft	High	Short	Flat	Muscle

Percussion produces five types of sounds: tympany, resonance, hyperresonance, dullness, and flatness. Each sound is created by certain types of underlying tissues and is judged by its intensity of pitch, duration, and quality (Table 13-1).

Percussion takes practice. The wrist is flexed by keeping the forearm stationary. For practice, the hand can be placed on the surface of a table and the middle finger struck with the middle finger of the opposite hand. The character of the sound changes when the blow is not light and quick.

Auscultation

Auscultation is listening to sounds created in body organs to detect variations from normal. Some sounds can be heard with the unassisted ear, although most sounds can be heard only through a stethoscope. A student must first become familiar with the normal sounds created by the cardiovascular, respiratory, and gastrointestinal systems, such as the passage of blood through an artery. Abnormal sounds can be recognized only after normal variations are learned. The nurse becomes more successful in auscultation by knowing the types of

Exercises to Increase Familiarity with the Stethoscope

- Place the earpieces in your ears with the tips of the earpieces turned toward the face. *Lightly* blow into the diaphragm. Again place the earpieces in your ears, this time with the ends turned toward the back of the head. *Lightly* blow into the diaphragm. The earpiece should follow the contour of the ear canal. Comparing amplification of sounds with the earpieces in both directions helps you learn what fit is best for you. Once you have learned the right fit for the loudest amplification, wear the stethoscope the same way each time.
- Put on the stethoscope and *lightly* blow into the diaphragm. If the sound is barely audible, *lightly* blow into the bell. Sound is carried through only one part of the chestpiece at a time. If the sound is greatly amplified through the diaphragm, the diaphragm is in position for use. If the sound is barely audible through the diaphragm, the bell is in position for use. Rotation of the diaphragm and bell places the chestpiece in the desired position.

- Put on the stethoscope and place the diaphragm over a friend's arm. Move the diaphragm lightly over the hair on the arm. The bristling sound created by the rubbing of hair against the diaphragm mimics a sound heard in the lungs. The diaphragm should be held firmly and stationary to eliminate extraneous sounds.
- Place the diphragm over the anterior part of your chest. Ask a friend to speak in a normal conversational tone. Environmental noise seriously detracts from hearing the noise created by body organs. When a stethoscope is used, the client and the examiner should remain quiet.
- Place the stethoscope on and gently tap the tubing. It is often difficult to avoid stretching or movement of the stethoscope's tubing. The examiner should be in a position so that the tubing hangs free. Moving or touching the tubing creates extraneous sounds.

sounds arising from each body structure and the location in which they can most easily be heard. Likewise, the nurse will become familiar with the areas that normally do not emit sounds.

To auscultate correctly the nurse needs good hearing acuity, a good stethoscope, and knowledge of how to use the stethoscope properly. Nurses with hearing disorders should purchase stethoscopes with greater sound amplification or ask colleagues to check findings through auscultation.

Chapter 12 describes the parts of the acoustical stethoscope and the general use of the bell and diaphragm. The bell is best for low-pitched sounds, such as heart and vascular sounds, and the diaphragm is best for high-pitched sounds, such as bowel and lung sounds.

A nurse must become familiar with the stethoscope before attempting to use it with a client. It helps to practice using it with a friend. A number of extraneous sounds created by movement of the tubing or chestpiece will interfere with auscultation of body organ sounds. By deliberately producing these sounds, the nurse learns to recognize and disregard them during the actual examination (see box).

Through auscultation the nurse notes the following characteristics of sound:

Frequency Number of sound wave cycles generated per second by a vibrating object. The higher the frequency, the higher the pitch of a sound and vice versa.

Loudness Amplitude of a sound wave. Auscultated sounds are described as *loud* or *soft*.

Quality The sounds of similar frequency and loudness from different sources. Terms such as *blowing* or *gurgling* describe the quality of sound.

Duration The length of time that sound vibrations last. The duration of sound is short, medium, or long. Layers of soft tissue dampen the duration of sounds from deep internal organs.

Auscultation requires concentration, practice, and application of knowledge. The nurse must consider the part of the body auscultated. What causes the sounds to be produced? For example, the first heart sound is caused by closure of the mitral valve. Where can the sound best be heard? The first heart sound is best auscultated at the fifth intercostal space along the midclavicular line. How is the sound heard normally? The first heart sound has the quality of a loud "lub," whereas the second sound is a "dub." Once the nature of auscultated sounds are understood, it becomes easier to recognize abnormal sounds and their origins.

Olfaction

Certain alterations in body function create characteristic body odors (Table 13-2). The sense of smell helps the nurse detect abnormalities that cannot be recognized by any other means. For example, a client with a cast is expected to experience discomfort after an injury. However, the nurse who notes a strong odor will suspect that the discomfort may also be related to wound infection. The discomfort alone does not reveal the presence of infection. Findings from olfaction and other as-

TABLE 13-2 Assessment of Characteristic Odors

Odor	Site or Source	Potential Causes
Alcohol	Oral cavity	Ingestion of alcohol
Ammonia	Urine	Urinary tract infection
Body	Skin, particularly in areas where body parts rub together (under arms, beneath breasts)	Poor hygiene, excess perspiration (hyperhidrosis), foul-smelling perspiration (bromhidrosis)
Fecal	Wound site	Wound abscess
	Vomitus	Bowel obstruction
	Rectal area	Fecal incontinence
Foul-smelling stools in infant	Stool	Malabsorption syndrome
Halitosis	Oral cavity	Poor dental and oral hygiene, gum disease
Sweet fruity, ketones	Oral cavity	Diabetic acidosis
Stale urine	Skin	Uremic acidosis
Sweet, heavy, thick	Draining wound	*Pseudomonas* (bacterial) infection
Musty	Casted body part	Infection inside cast
Fetid sweet	Tracheostomy or mucous secretions	Infection of bronchial tree (*Pseudomonas* bacteria)

sessment skills allow the nurse to detect serious abnormalities. If a nurse notices an unfamiliar odor, a colleague may be able to identify the problem.

PREPARATION FOR EXAMINATION

A haphazard approach when preparing for a physical examination can cause errors and incomplete findings. An efficient examination involves preparation of the environment, equipment, and client.

Preparation of Environment

A physical examination requires privacy. In a hospital, clients are often examined in their rooms. In a semiprivate room, room curtains or dividers around the bed can be closed. In physician's offices or clinics, special examination rooms provide privacy. In the home, the nurse may perform an examination in the bedroom.

Any examination room should be well equipped for all necessary procedures. Adequate lighting is needed for proper illumination of body parts. Ideally an examination room is soundproofed so clients feel comfortable discussing illnesses with nurses. The nurse eliminates any sources of noise such as a television or radio and takes steps to prevent interruptions from others.

Sometimes, it is difficult to perform a complete examination with a client in a bed or on a stretcher. Special examination tables make clients easily accessible and help them assume positions. The tables are high and narrow so the nurse must carefully assist clients so they do not fall when getting on and off them. A confused, combative, or uncooperative client should not be left on an examination table without supervision.

Examination tables are often hard and uncomfortable. When the client lies supine, the head of the table can be raised about 30 degrees. The client may also be given a small pillow. When examining a client in bed, the nurse can raise the bed to reach body parts more easily.

Before equipment preparation and the examination, handwashing must occur. Handwashing reduces the transmission of microorganisms.

Preparation of Equipment

The equipment needed for an examination should be readily available and arranged in order for easy use (Fig. 13-5). It should be kept warm. The diaphragm of the stethoscope may be briskly rubbed between the hands before it is applied to the skin. Warm water should be run over the vaginal speculum. The examiner's hands should also be warmed. All equipment must be checked to see that it functions properly. The ophthalmoscope and otoscope require good batteries and light bulbs. Equipment typically used is listed in the box.

Physical Preparation of Client

The client's physical comfort is vital to the success of the examination. Before starting, the nurse asks if the client needs to use the toilet. An empty bladder and

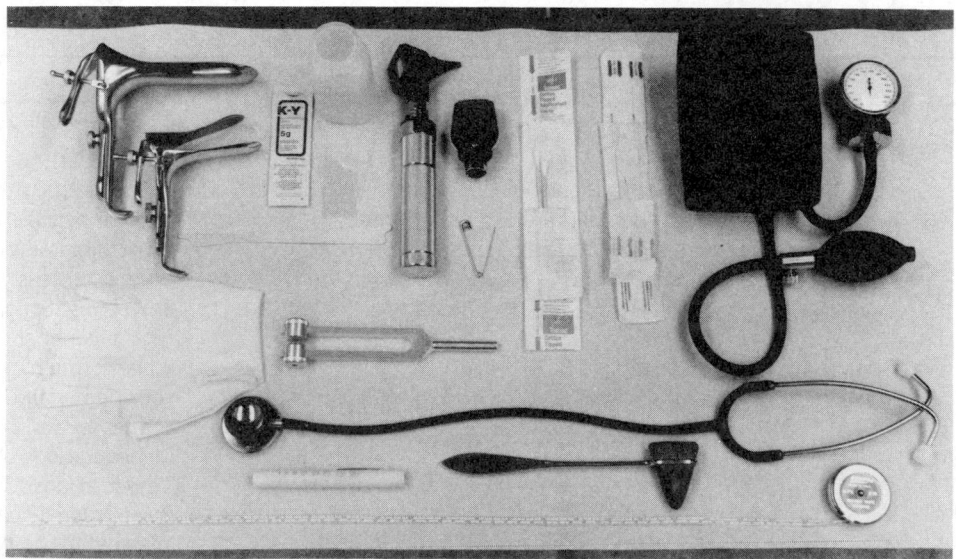

Fig. 13-5 Equipment used during a physical examination (clockwise from upper right): Sphygmomanometer, stethoscope, tape measure, reflex hammer, penlight, disposable gloves, vaginal speculums, cervical spatula, petrolatum jelly, specimen container and slides, otoscope, ophthalmoscope attachment, safety pins, cotton-tip swabs, and tongue blades.

Equipment and Supplies for Physical Assessment

- Cotton applicators
- Disposable pad
- Drapes
- Eye chart (for example, Snellen chart)
- Flashlight and spotlight
- Forms (for example, physical, laboratory)
- Gloves (sterile or clean)
- Gown for client
- Lubricant
- Ophthalmoscope
- Otoscope
- Papanicolaou smear slides
- Paper towels
- Percussion hammer
- Safety pin
- Scale with height measurement rod
- Specimen containers and microscope slides
- Sphygmomanometer and cuff
- Stethoscope
- Swabs or sponge forceps
- Tape measure
- Thermometer
- Tissues
- Tongue depressor
- Tuning fork
- Vaginal speculum
- Wristwatch with second hand

bowel facilitate examination of the abdomen, genitalia, and rectum and provides time to collect any needed urine or fecal specimens. The nurse explains the proper method for collecting specimens and ensures that each specimen is properly labeled.

Physical preparation involves being sure the client is dressed and draped properly. A client in the hospital will likely be wearing only a simple gown. An outpatient will have to undress. If the examination is limited to certain body systems, it may be unnecessary for the client to undress completely. The client should have privacy during undressing and plenty of time to finish. Walking into the room as the client undresses causes embarrassment.

Drapes and gowns are made of linen or disposable paper. Once clients have undressed and donned the gown, they should sit or lie down on the examination table with the drape over the lap or lower trunk. The examiner makes sure the client stays warm by eliminating drafts, controlling room temperature, and providing warm blankets. Seriously ill and elderly clients are more susceptible to chills. The nurse should ask if the client is comfortable. The client may become more relaxed if offered a pillow, sip of water, or tissue.

POSITIONING

During the examination the client is asked to assume certain positions to facilitate the assessment. Table 13-3 lists the preferred positions for each part of the examination and contains figures illustrating these positions. Clients' abilities to assume positions will depend on their physical strength and degree of wellness. Many of the positions, such as the lithotomy and knee-chest, are embarrassing and uncomfortable. Therefore the client should be kept in those positions no longer than necessary. The examiner should explain the position and assist the client in attaining it. The drapes should be adjusted to be sure that the area to be examined is accessible and that no body part is unnecessarily exposed. More than one position can be assumed for the same part of an examination (for example, supine and sitting for assessment of the anterior thorax), so the nurse first chooses the position that provides greater accessibility and accuracy in assessing body parts (sitting for anterior thorax). However, if the client is too weak or is physically unable to assume a position, the nurse may choose an alternative position.

Psychological Preparation of Client

The client is easily embarrassed when forced to answer sensitive questions about bodily functions or when body parts are exposed and examined. The possibility that the examiner will find something abnormal also creates anxiety, so reduction of the client's anxiety may be the nurse's highest priority before the examination. A thorough explanation lets clients know what to expect and gives them the knowledge they need to cooperate during the examination (Fig. 13-6, p. 243). The nurse first tells the client about the examination in general terms.

Ms. Bryce, I'm going to do a complete physical examination so I can have a good idea of whether you have any health problems. As we go along, I'll explain to you exactly what I'll be doing. Feel free to ask any questions. If you become uncomfortable, please tell me.

Then as the nurse examines each body system, a more detailed explanation is given.

As I examine your breasts, I want you to relax lying down. First I want to look at the color, size, and shape of your breasts. Then I'll gently use my hands to feel the breast tissue itself.

The nurse uses simple terms when describing actions. Complicated terminology confuses clients and adds to their fears. The nurse's manner should be professional. Yet, voice tone and facial expressions should be relaxed to put the client at ease. The nurse encourages clients to mention any discomfort they feel during the assessment.

TABLE 13-3 Positions for Examination

Position		Areas Assessed	Rationale	Limitations
Sitting		Head and neck, back, posterior thorax and lungs, anterior thorax and lungs, breasts, axilla, heart vital signs, and upper extremities	Sitting upright provides full expansion of lungs and provides better visualization of symmetry of upper body parts.	A physically weakened client may be unable to sit. Use supine position with head of bed elevated instead.
Supine		Head and neck, anterior thorax and lungs, breasts, axilla, heart, abdomen, extremities, pulses	This is the most normally relaxed position. It prevents contracture of abdominal muscles and provides easy access to pulse sites.	If client becomes short of breath easily, examiner may need to raise head of bed.
Dorsal recumbent		Head and neck, anterior thorax and lungs, breasts, axilla, heart	Some clients with painful disorders are more comfortable with knees flexed.	Position is not used for abdominal assessment because it promotes contracture of abdominal muscles.
Lithotomy		Female genitalia and genital tract	This position provides maximal exposure of genitalia and facilitates insertion of vaginal speculum.	This position is embarrassing and uncomfortable, so minimize time the client spends in it. Keep client well draped. A client with severe arthritis or other joint deformity may be unable to assume this position.
Sims'		Rectum	Flexion of hip and knee improves exposure of rectal area.	Joint deformities may hinder the client's ability to bend hip and knee.
Prone		Musculoskeletal	This position is used only to assess extension of the hip joint.	This position is not tolerated by a client with respiratory difficulties or the elderly.

When the client and examiner are of opposite sexes, it helps to have a third person of the client's sex in the room, especially when examination of the sexual organs is required. The presence of a third person assures the client that the examiner will behave ethically, and the third person acts as a witness to the examiner's proper conduct.

During the examination the nurse watches the client's emotional responses. Does the client's facial expression convey fear or concern? Does the client's body move-

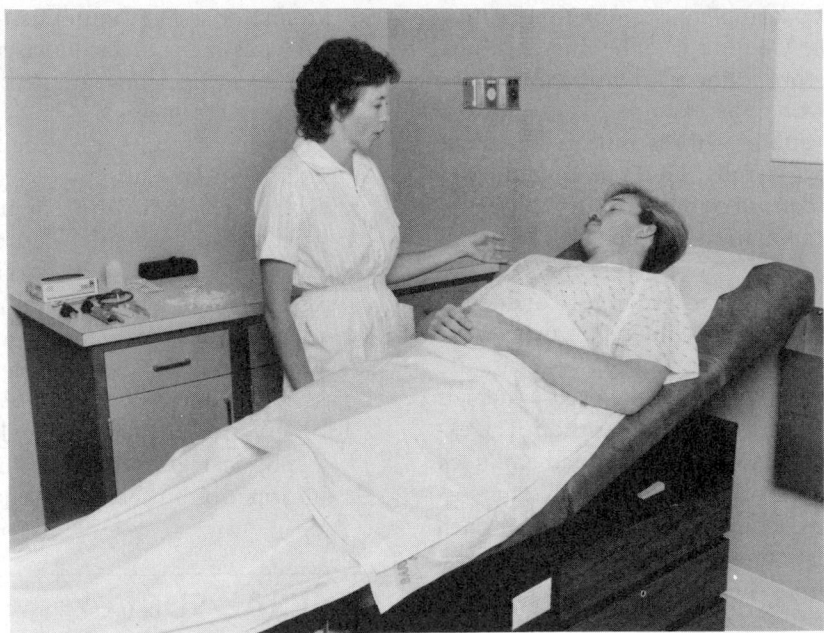

Fig. 13-6 The nurse explains the purpose and steps of the physical examination to the client.

ments reveal anxiety, such as frequently pulling the drape around the body or tensing up as the examiner touches the body? The nurse must remain calm and explain each step of the assessment clearly. It may be necessary to stop the examination and ask if the client feels anxious, afraid, or uncomfortable. The client should not be forced to continue. Postponing the examination until a later time may be advantageous because the findings may be more accurate when the client can cooperate and relax. If the fears are the result of misconceptions, the examiner attempts to clarify the purpose of the examination and how it is to be performed.

Assessment of Age Groups

The nurse uses different interview styles when talking with clients of different ages and with parents of clients. The following tips will assist in data collection during physical examination:

1. When obtaining histories on infants and children, gather all or part of the information from the parent or guardian.
2. Parents may think they are being tested by the examiner. Offer support during the examination and do not pass judgment.
3. Call children by their first name, and address the parents as "Mr. and Mrs. Brown" rather than by their first names.
4. Open-ended questions often allow parents to share more information and to describe more of the child's problems.

5. Interviewing older children allows the nurse to observe parent-child interactions.
6. Older children often can provide details about their health history and severity of symptoms.
7. Adolescents tend to respond best when treated as adults and individuals.
8. The adolescent has a right to confidentiality. After talking with parents about historical information the nurse speaks alone with the adolescent.
9. Do not stereotype aging clients. Most are able to adapt to change and to learn about their health.
10. Sensory or physical limitations can affect how quickly the nurse is able to interview older clients and conduct examinations. Plan for more than one examination session.

ORGANIZATION OF THE EXAMINATION

The extent of an examination depends on its purpose. A client who comes to the clinic with symptoms of a severe chest cold will not routinely require a neurological assessment. A client returning from surgery for repair of a fractured leg will require assessment of circulatory and musculoskeletal function rather than a breast examination. When a client is admitted to the hospital, a complete examination is usually performed. Clients with specific symptoms or needs often require only portions of an examination.

The performance of a complete examination follows the nursing history (see Chapter 6). The nurse uses information from the history to focus attention on specific parts of the examination. For example, if the history revealed symptoms of abdominal discomfort, the nurse examines the abdomen carefully. Findings from the history generally reveal a pattern of related signs and symptoms. The physical examination supplements information from the history to confirm or refute the data.

Each nurse develops a personal system for conducting a physical examination. The nurse must be sure that the system is well organized so important assessments are not forgotten or deleted. A commonly used system is one organized by the "head-to-toe" orientation. The examiner begins with an assessment of the head and neck area, progressing methodically down the body to incorporate all body systems. Using a head-to-toe approach helps the nurse anticipate the order of systems to assess.

The following tips may help the nurse keep an examination well organized:

1. Compare both sides of the body for symmetry. A degree of asymmetry is normal (for example, the bicep muscles in the dominant arm may be more developed than the same muscles in the nondominant arm).
2. If a client is seriously ill, assess first the systems of the body more at risk for being abnormal. For example, a client with chest pain should undergo an assessment of cardiovascular function first.
3. If a client becomes fatigued, offer rest periods between assessments.
4. Perform painful procedures near the end of the examination.
5. Record results of the examination in specific anatomical and scientific terms so any professional can interpret the findings (Fig. 13-7).
6. Use common and accepted medical abbreviations to keep notes brief and concise.
7. Record quick notes during the examination to avoid keeping the client waiting. Complete any observations at the end of the examination.
8. A physical assessment form allows recording of information in the same sequence it is gathered.

GENERAL SURVEY

The nurse begins an examination by observing a client's general appearance and behavior and by measuring vital signs and height and weight. At times the nurse may also make anthropometric measurements, including head circumference in infants.

General Appearance and Behavior

Assessment begins from the time the nurse first sees a client. During the nursing history the nurse makes mental notes of behavior and appearance. Any abnormalities or signs of problems revealed during the survey direct the nurse to examine body parts more carefully later. For example, if a client's appearance seems unkempt, the nurse will later carefully inspect the skin and nails to determine adequacy of hygiene. Information gained about general features may reveal characteristics of illness (for example, the facial appearance of a depressed client). The nurse's review of general appearance and behavior includes the following:

1. *Sex and Race*—a person's sex affects the type of examination performed and the manner in which assessments are made. Different physical features are related to sex and race.
2. *Signs of Distress*—There may be obvious signs or symptoms indicating a problem such as pain, difficulty in breathing, or anxiety.
3. *Body Type*—The nurse observes if a client appears trim and muscular, obese, or excessively thin. Body type can reflect level of health, age, and life-style.
4. *Posture*—Normal standing posture is an upright stance with parallel alignment of hips and shoulders. Normal sitting posture involves some degree of rounding of the shoulders. Observe if client has a slumped, erect, or bent posture. Posture may re-

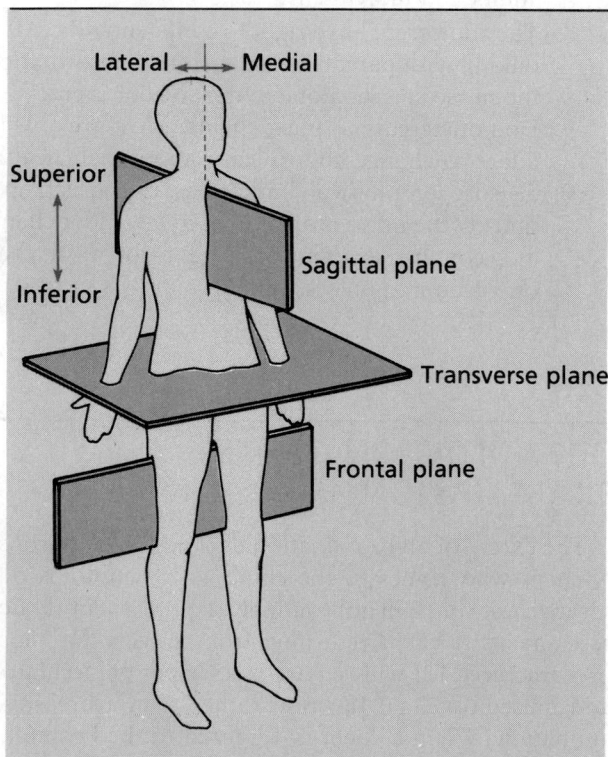

Fig. 13-7 The nurse describes assessment findings in terms of the anatomical position within body planes.

flect mood or presence of pain. Many elderly persons assume a stooped, forward-bent posture, with hips and knees somewhat flexed and arms bent at the elbows, raising the level of the arms.

5. *Gait*—Observe when client walks into examination room or at bedside (if client is ambulatory). Note if movements are coordinated or uncoordinated. A person normally walks with arms swinging freely at the sides, with the head and face leading the body.

6. *Body Movements*—Observe if movements are purposeful. Note if there are any tremors involving the extremities. Observe if any body parts are immobile.

7. *Age*—Age influences the normal features or physical characteristics a nurse observes. The ability to participate in some parts of the examination will also be influenced by age.

8. *Hygiene and Grooming*—Note the client's level of cleanliness by observing the appearance of the hair, skin, or fingernails. Note if the client's clothes are clean. A person's grooming may depend on the activities being performed just before the examination. Notice the amount and type of cosmetics used.

8. *Dress*—A person's culture, life-style, socioeconomic level, and personal preference will affect the type of clothes worn. Note if the type of clothing worn is appropriate for temperature and weather conditions. Depressed or mentally ill persons may be unable to choose proper clothing. The elderly tend to wear extra clothing because of their sensitivity to cold.

9. *Body Odor*—An unpleasant body odor may simply be the result of physical exercise. Poor hygiene may result in body odor, and poor oral hygiene may result in bad breath. A breath with alcohol on it does not always mean alcoholism.

10. *Mood and Affect*—*Affect* is the person's feelings as they appear to others. A person's mood or emotional state is expressed verbally and nonverbally. Note if verbal expressions match nonverbal behavior. Observe if the client's mood is appropriate for the situation. For example, after recently being diagnosed with cancer, does the client seem unusually happy? Observe facial expressions as questions are asked.

11. *Speech*—Normal speech is understandable and moderately paced and shows an association with the person's thoughts. Note if the client talks rapidly or slowly. An abnormal pace may be caused by emotions or neurological impairment. Observe if the client speaks in a normal tone with clear inflection of words.

Vital Signs

Most nurses prefer measuring vital signs before assessing individual body systems because positioning or

TABLE 13-4   1983 Metropolitan Height and Weight Tables

Men					Women				
Height		Small Frame	Medium Frame	Large Frame	Height		Small Frame	Medium Frame	Large Frame
Feet	Inches				Feet	Inches			
5	2	128-134	131-141	138-150	4	10	102-111	109-121	118-131
5	3	130-136	133-143	140-153	4	11	103-113	111-123	120-134
5	4	132-138	135-145	142-156	5	0	104-115	113-126	122-137
5	5	134-140	137-148	144-160	5	1	106-118	115-129	125-140
5	6	136-142	139-151	146-164	5	2	108-121	118-132	128-143
5	7	138-145	142-154	149-168	5	3	111-124	121-135	131-147
5	8	140-148	145-157	152-172	5	4	114-127	124-138	134-151
5	9	142-151	148-160	155-176	5	5	117-130	127-141	137-155
5	10	144-154	151-163	158-180	5	6	120-133	130-144	140-159
5	11	146-157	154-166	161-184	5	7	123-136	133-147	143-163
6	0	149-160	157-170	164-188	5	8	126-139	136-150	146-167
6	1	152-164	160-174	168-192	5	9	129-142	139-153	149-170
6	2	155-168	164-178	172-197	5	10	132-145	142-156	152-173
6	3	158-172	167-182	176-202	5	11	135-148	145-159	155-176
6	4	162-176	171-187	181-207	6	0	138-151	148-162	158-179

Copyright 1983 Metropolitan Life Insurance Company.
Source of basic data: 1979 Build Study, Society of Actuaries and Association of Life Insurance Medical Directors of America, 1980.
*Weights at ages 25-59 based on lowest mortality. Weight in pounds according to frame (in indoor clothing weighing 5 lb for men and 3 lb for women; shoes with 1-in heels).

moving the client during the examination could interfere with accurate recording of temperature, pulse, respirations, and blood pressure. However, it is also appropriate for the nurse to measure specific vital signs during assessment of individual body systems. For example, the pulse can be assessed during examination of the peripheral pulses or the heart and respirations during examination of the thorax. Body temperature is always measured during the general survey.

Height and Weight

A person's general level of health can be reflected in the ratio of height to weight. A nurse measures infants' and children's height and weight to assess growth and development and to calculate body surface area for medication administration (see Chapter 15). Before this measurement, the nurse asks clients their height and weight. It may help to know the client's satisfaction or perception of body image. The nurse also determines if the client has had a recent weight gain or loss. If a change exists, the nurse determines the amount and the period of time over which weight change occurred. A sudden loss in weight may indicate serious disease or a major

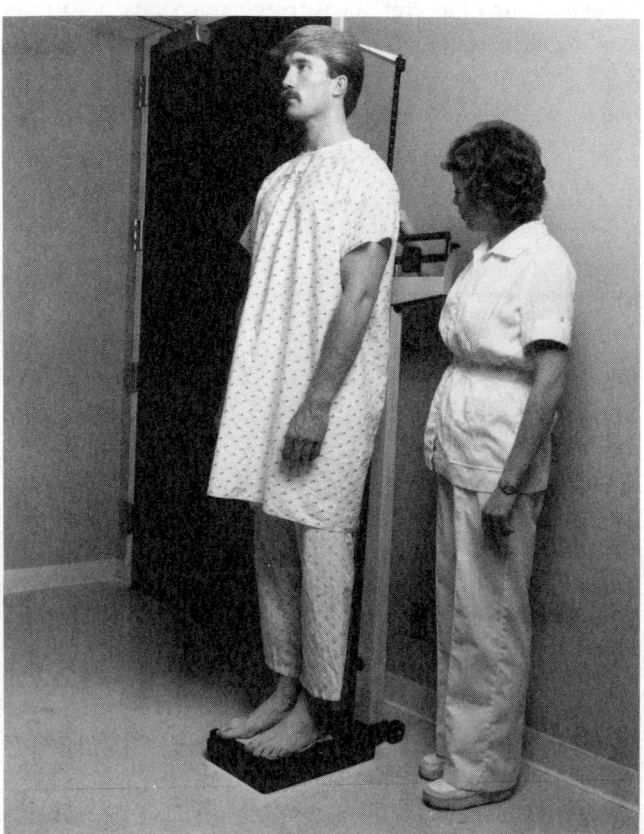

Fig. 13-8 The client stands erect to permit an accurate measurement of height.

change in dietary habits. This is a good time to question clients about current dietary habits. It is normal for weight to vary each day because of fluid loss or retention. Standardized charts list the average heights and weights of adults (Table 13-4) and children. The charts offer only general guidelines for assessing growth, development, and nutritional status.

HEIGHT

Different techniques exist for measuring the height of weight-bearing and non-weight-bearing clients. A client able to stand removes his or his shoes. A paper towel is placed on the scale platform or floor so the client's feet remain clean. A measuring stick or tape is attached vertically to the weight scales or wall. The nurse asks the client to stand erect, exercising good posture (Fig. 13-8). On a standing scale, a metal rod, which is attached to the back of the scale, swings out and over the top of the client's head. A measuring stick or flat book can also be placed on the client's head when a scale is unavailable. With the rod or stick placed level horizontally at a 90-degree angle to the measuring stick, the nurse measures height in inches or centimeters.

A non-weight-bearing client (such as an infant) is positioned supine on a firm surface. The legs are extended straight with the soles of the feet supported upright. The nurse places a tape measure from the soles of the feet to the vertex of the head to measure the recumbent length.

WEIGHT

Weight is a routine measure for any client visiting a physician's office or clinic, and many health screenings routinely include height and weight. When a client is admitted to a health care agency, weight may be recorded daily to assess nutritional pattern or fluid balance.

To ensure accuracy in a hospital setting a client is weighed at the same time, on the same scale, and wearing the same or equivalent clothing. In a clinic or office setting, weighing the client at the same time for each visit is difficult. Clients in hospitals usually wear the same type of gown or pajamas each day, but in a clinic or office the client should remove shoes and coat if a gown is not worn.

Clients capable of bearing their own weight use a standing scale. The nurse calibrates the scale by setting the weight at zero and noting if the balance beam registers in the middle of the mark. Scales with a digital display should read at zero before each use. The client stands on the scale platform and remains still (Fig. 13-9). The nurse slowly adjusts the scale weight on the balance beam until the tip of the beam registers in the middle of the mark. Digital scale readouts display weight in a matter of seconds.

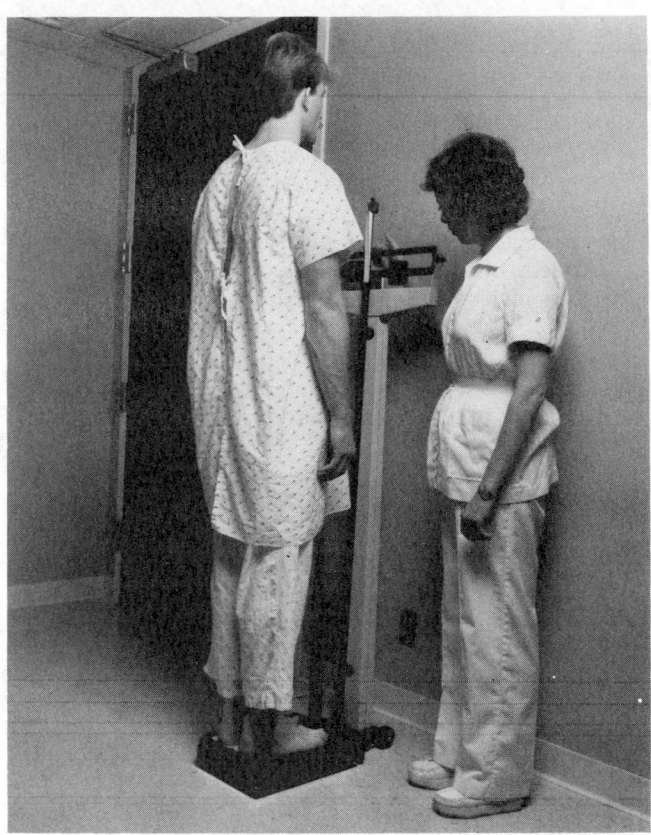

Fig. 13-9 The client stands on the scale as the nurse adjusts the balance.

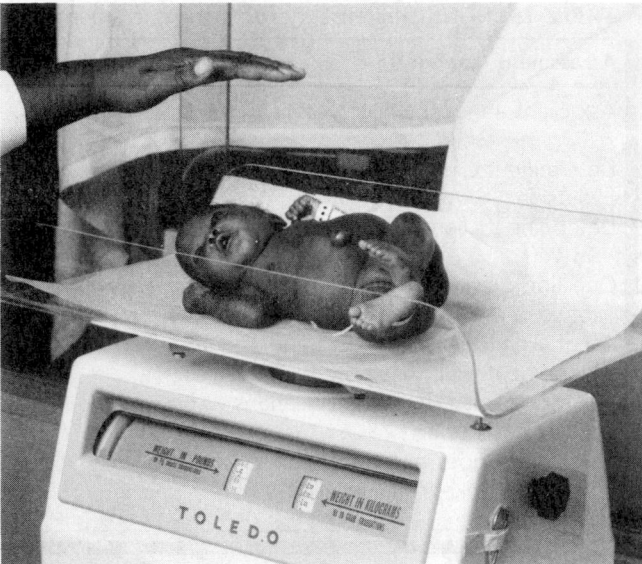

Fig. 13-10 When weighing an infant on the platform scale, the nurse keeps a hand just above the infant for safety.

Stretcher and chair scales are available for clients unable to bear weight. After being transferred to the scale the client is lifted above the bed by a hydraulic device, and the weight is measured on a balance beam or digital display. Caution must be used when transferring clients to and from the scales.

Infants can be weighed in baskets or on platform scales. The nurse removes the infant's clothing and diaper to ensure an accurate reading. The room should be warm to prevent chills. A light cloth or paper placed on the scale's surface will prevent cross-infection from urine or feces. The nurse places the infant in the basket or on the platform and holds a hand lightly above him to prevent accidental falls (Fig. 13-10). An infant's weight is measured in grams or pounds.

INTEGUMENT

The skin or integumentary system provides the body's external protection, regulates body temperature, and acts as a sensory organ for pain, temperature, and touch. Assessment of the integument includes the skin, hair, scalp, and nails. The nurse may initially take the time to observe all skin surfaces or may assess the skin gradually while other body systems are examined. The nurse uses assessment findings to determine the type of hygiene measures required to maintain integrity of the integument (see Chapter 32). Adequate nutrition and hydration become goals of therapy if the nurse identifies alterations in the integument's status (see Chapter 33). When assessing the integument, the nurse uses inspection, palpation, and olfaction.

Skin

Adequate illumination of the skin is required during assessment. If moist or draining skin lesions are palpated, disposable gloves are also needed. Because the nurse inspects all skin surfaces, the client must assume several positions. The nursing history for skin assessment is outlined in Table 13-5. The examination includes inspection of the skin's color, moisture, temperature, texture and thickness, and turgor. The presence of vascular changes, edema, and any lesions is also noted. If abnormalities are seen, the nurse palpates the involved areas. Skin odors are usually noted in the skin folds, such as the axilla or under the female client's breasts. Fig. 13-11 illustrates a normal cross section of the skin.

COLOR

Skin color varies from body part to body part and from person to person. Table 13-6 lists common variations. Normal skin pigmentation ranges in tone from ivory to deep brown, ruddy pink to light pink, or yellow to olive. Race affects skin color. The assessment of color first involves areas of the skin not exposed to the sun,

TABLE 13-5 Nursing History for Skin Assessment

Assessment Category	Rationale
Ask client about the history of changes in skin color.	Client is the best source to note change. Skin cancer may first be noticed as a localized change in skin color.
Determine if client works or spends excessive time outside.	Exposed areas such as face and arms will be more pigmented than rest of body.
Determine if client has noted any lesions or changes in skin.	Most skin changes do not develop suddenly. Change in character of a skin lesion might indicate cancer.
Question client about frequency of bathing and type of soap used.	Excessive bathing and use of harsh soaps can cause dry skin.
Ask if client has had recent trauma to skin.	Injury can cause bruising and changes in skin texture.
Determine if client has history of allergies.	Skin rashes commonly occur from allergies.
Ask if client uses topical medications or home remedies on the skin.	Incorrect use of topical agents may cause inflammation or irritation.
Ask if client goes to tanning parlors, uses sun lamps, or takes tanning pills?	Overexposure of skin to these irritants can cause skin cancer.

such as the palms of the hands. Exposed areas such as the face and arms will be darker. It is more difficult to note changes such as pallor or cyanosis in clients with dark skin.

The nurse focuses on sites where abnormalities are more easily identified. For example, pallor is most easily perceived in the buccal mucosa of the mouth, particularly in individuals with dark skin. Cyanosis is more readily seen in areas of least pigmentation such as lips, nail beds, palpebral conjunctiva, and palms. The best site to inspect for jaundice is the sclera. Localized skin changes, such as pallor or redness, may indicate circu-

latory changes. For example, an inflamed area of the skin is reddened due to an increased delivery of blood to an injured site. An area of an extremity that appears unusually pale may result from arterial occlusion or edema.

Although individual variations in skin color exist, skin color is usually uniform over the body. Clients with dark skin have lighter areas of pigmentation in the palms, soles of the feet, lips and nail beds. Areas of increased color (hyperpigmentation) and decreased color (hypopigmentation) are common.

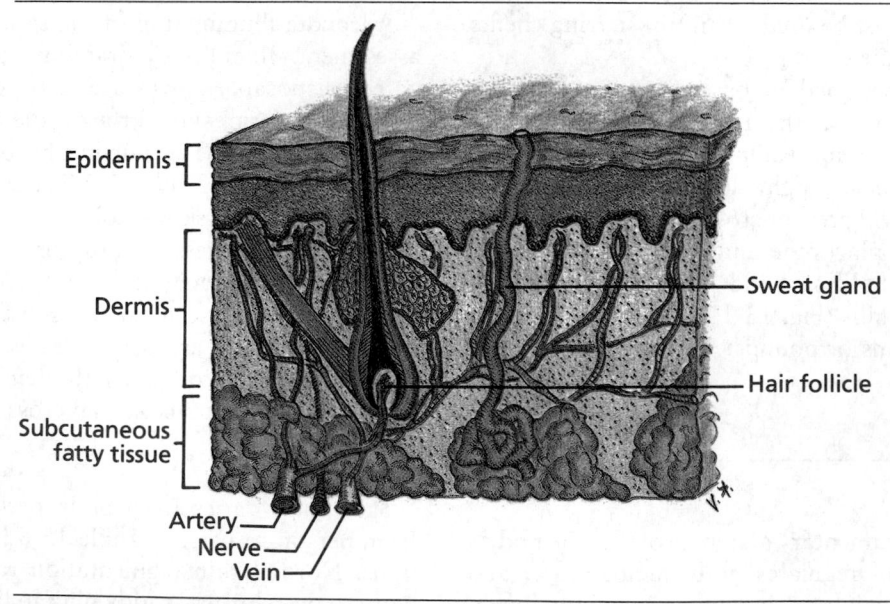

Fig. 13-11 A cross section of the skin reveals three layers, epidermis, dermis, and subcutaneous fatty tissues.

TABLE 13-6 Skin Color Variations

Color	Condition	Causes	Assessment Locations
Bluish (cyanosis)	Increased amount of deoxygenated hemoglobin; associated with hypoxia	Heart or lung disease, cold environment	Nail beds, lips, mouth, skin (severe cases)
Pallor (decrease in color)	Reduced amount of oxyhemoglobin	Anemia	Face, conjunctiva, nail beds
	Reduced visibility of oxyhemoglobin resulting from decreased blood flow	Shock	Skin, nail beds, conjunctiva, lips
	Congenital or autoimmune condition causing lack of pigment	Vitiligo	Patchy areas on skin
Yellow-orange (jaundice)	Increased deposit of bilirubin in tissues	Liver disease, destruction of red blood cells	Sclera, mucous membranes, skin
Red (erythema)	Increased visibility of oxyhemoglobin caused by dilation or increased blood flow	Fever, direct trauma, blushing, alcohol intake	Face; area of trauma
Tan-brown	Increased amount of melanin	Suntan, pregnancy	Areas exposed to sun; face, areola, nipples

MOISTURE

The hydration of skin and mucous membranes helps to reveal body fluid imbalances, changes in the integument's environment, and regulation of body temperature. Moisture refers to wetness and oiliness. It is normal for skin folds such as the axilla to be moist. After excessive exercise or exposure to warm temperatures, the skin may be moist from perspiration. Dry skin is common in the elderly and in persons who use excessive amounts of soap during bathing.

The nurse palpates to feel moisture on the skin. Skin that appears thin and watery may be thick and oily. If lesions ooze fluid, the color, odor, amount, and consistency are noted. The nurse may choose to wear gloves to avoid exposure to purulent discharge.

TEMPERATURE

The temperature of the skin depends on the amount of blood circulating through the dermis. Increased or decreased skin temperature indicates an increase or decrease in blood flow. Temperature is more accurately assessed by palpating the skin with the dorsum or back of the hand. Skin temperature may be the same throughout the body or may vary in one area, such as the localized warmth at an infected wound site or the coldness of fingers resulting from reduced blood flow. Assessment of skin temperature is a basic assessment whenever the client is at risk for having impaired circulation (for example, after application of a cast or tight bandage or after vascular surgery).

TEXTURE

The character of the skin's surface and the feel of deeper portions are its texture. The nurse determines if the client's skin is smooth or rough by stroking it lightly with the fingertips. The texture of the skin is normally smooth, soft, and flexible in children and adults. However, the texture is usually not uniform throughout. The palms of the hand and soles of the feet tend to be thicker. In the elderly the skin becomes wrinkled and leathery because of a decrease in collagen, subcutaneous fat, and sweat glands.

Localized changes may result from trauma or lesions. When irregularities in texture are found, the nurse asks if the client has experienced any recent injury to the skin. Deep palpation may reveal irregularities such as localized areas of hardness commonly caused by repeated intramuscular or subcutaneous injections. If the client has diabetes or receives vitamin B_{12} or iron injections, hardened areas are common.

TURGOR

Turgor is the skin's elasticity, which can be diminished by edema or dehydration. Normally the skin loses its elasticity with age.

To assess the skin turgor, a fold of skin on the back of the client's hand or forearm is grasped with the fingertips and released (Fig. 13-12). The nurse notes the ease with which the skin moves and the speed at which it returns to place. Normally the skin snaps back immediately to its resting position. The client with poor

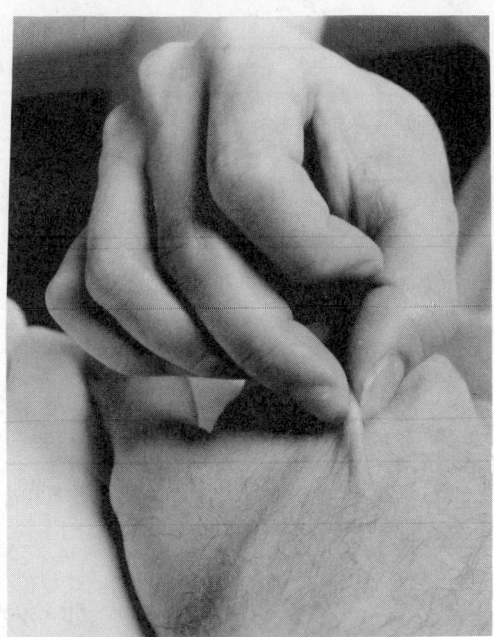

Fig. 13-12 Assessment for skin turgor.

skin turgor does not have a resilience to the normal wear and tear on the skin. The skin tends to stay pinched or tented when turgor is poor. A decrease in turgor predisposes the client to skin breakdown.

VASCULARITY

The circulation of the skin affects color in localized areas and the appearance of superficial blood vessels. With aging, capillaries become fragile. Localized pressure spots, found after a client has lain or sat in one position, appear reddened, pink, or pale. Petechiae are tiny, pinpoint-sized, red or purple spots on the skin caused by small hemorrhages in the skin layers. Presence of petechiae may indicate serious blood-clotting disorders.

EDEMA

Areas of the skin become swollen or edematous because of a build up of fluid in the tissues. Direct trauma and impairment of venous return are two common causes of edema. Edematous areas should be inspected for location, color, and shape. For the client with dependent edema caused by poor venous return, typical sites of edema are the feet, ankles, and sacrum. The formation of edema separates the skin's surface from the pigmented and vascular layers, masking skin color. The skin often becomes stretched and takes on a shiny appearance. The nurse palpates areas of edema to determine mobility, consistency, and tenderness. When pressure from the examiner's finger leaves an indentation in the edematous area, it is called *pitting edema*. To check the degree of pitting edema the nurse presses the edematous area firmly with the thumb for 5 seconds. The depth of pitting determines the degree of edema. For each centimeter in depth, the nurse records a plus sign (for example, 1 cm equals 1 + edema and 2 cm equal 2 + edema).

LESIONS

The skin is normally free of lesions, except common freckles or age-related changes such as skin tags. When a lesion is detected, it is inspected for color, location, size, type (see box), grouping (for example, clustered or linear), and distribution (localized or generalized). Palpation determines the lesion's mobility, contour (flat, raised, or depressed), and consistency (soft or hard). Certain types of lesions present a characteristic pattern. For example, a tumor is usually hard, localized, and immobile. Primary lesions such as macules and nodules arise from some stimulus to the skin. Secondary lesions such as ulcers occur as alterations in primary lesions.

Once identified, a lesion is closely inspected with good illumination. The lesion is palpated gently, covering its entire area. If the lesion is moist or draining fluid, gloves are worn during palpation because contact with drainage could spread infectious organisms.

It helps to ask clients if they notice any lesions of the skin and if a lesion has recently changed in character (see client-teaching box). Cancerous lesions frequently undergo changes in color and size. Any abnormal lesions are reported to the physician because further examination may be required.

Client Teaching After Skin Assessment

- Instruct client how to prevent skin cancer by avoiding overexposure to the sun: wear wide-brimmed hats and long sleeves, use sunscreens before going into the sun and after swimming or perspiring, avoid tanning under the direct sun at midday (11 AM to 2 PM).
- Teach client to conduct a monthly self-examination of the skin, noting any moles, blemishes, or birth marks.
- Tell client to report any changes in size, shape, or color of lesions. If a sore does not heal, report it to a physician.
- The elderly tend to have delayed wound healing. Instruct client to report any lesion that bleeds or fails to heal to a physician.
- Teach client to avoid applying drying agents such as rubbing alcohol or soap to the skin.
- Tell client to apply lotion and moisturizers to the skin regularly to reduce itching and drying.

Types of Skin Lesions

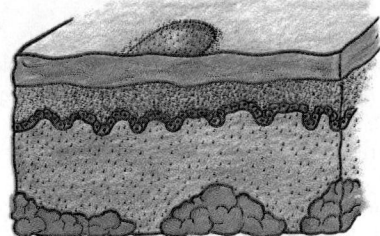

Macule flat, nonpalpable, change in skin color, smaller than 1 cm (for example, freckle, petechia).

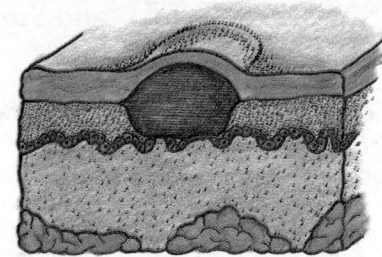

Papule: palpable, circumscribed, solid elevation in skin, smaller than 0.5 cm (for example, elevated nevus).

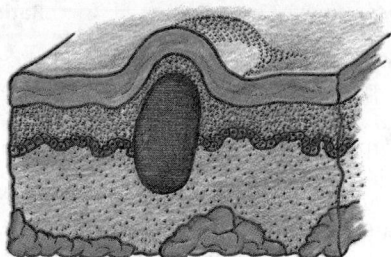

Nodule: elevated solid mass, deeper and firmer than papule, 0.5-0.2 cm (for example, wart).

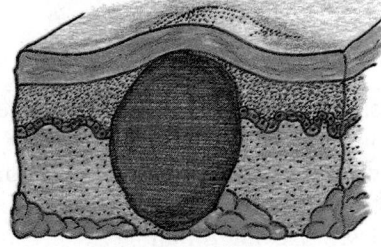

Tumor: solid mass that may extend deep through subcutaneous tissue, larger than 1-2 cm (for example, epithelioma).

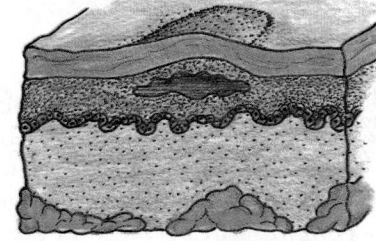

Wheal: irregularly shaped, elevated area or superficial localized edema, varies in size (for example, hive, mosquito bite).

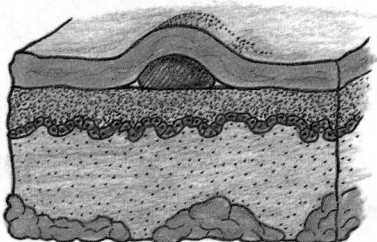

Vesicle: circumscribed elevation of skin filled with serous fluid, smaller than 0.5 cm (for example, herpes simplex, chickenpox).

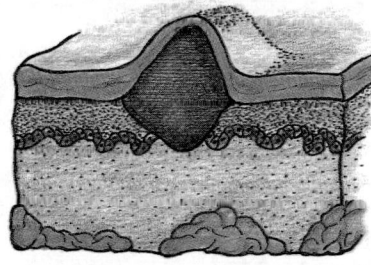

Pustule: circumscribed elevation of skin similar to vesicle but filled with pus, varies in size (for example, acne, staphylococcal infection).

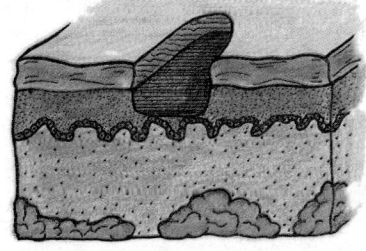

Ulcer: deep loss of skin surface that may extend to dermis and frequently bleeds and scars, varies in size (for example, venous stasis ulcer).

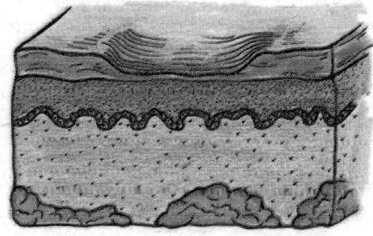

Atrophy: thinning of skin with loss of normal skin furrow with skin appearing shiny and translucent, varies in size (for example, arterial insufficiency).

Hair and Scalp

Good lighting allows the nurse to inspect the condition and distribution of hair and integrity of the scalp. Assessment of the hair occurs during all portions of the examination. Clients are sensitive about personal appearance. Thus the nurse explains the need to separate parts of the hair to detect any obvious problems. If lesions or lice are probable, the nurse applies disposable gloves to avoid spread of infection. Table 13-7 describes the nursing history for a hair and scalp assessment.

Two types of hair cover the body, terminal hair (long, coarse, thick hair easily visible on the scalp, axilla, and pubic areas) and vellus hair (small, soft, tiny hairs covering the whole body except for palms and soles). The nurse assesses the distribution, thickness, texture, and lubrication of the hair. In addition, the nurse inspects for infection or infestation of the scalp.

TABLE 13-7　Nursing History for Hair and Scalp Assessment

Assessment Category	Rationale
Ask client if a wig or hair-piece is being worn and request that it be removed.	Wigs or hairpieces interfere with inspection of hair and scalp. (Client may request to omit this part of the examination.)
Determine if client has noted change in growth or loss of hair.	Change may occur slowly over time.
Identify type of shampoo, other hair care products, or curling irons used for grooming.	Excessive use of chemical agents and burning of hair will cause drying and brittleness.
Determine if client has recently taken chemotherapy (if hair loss noted).	Chemotherapeutic agents kill cells that rapidly multiply such as tumor cells and normal hair cells.

Client Teaching after Hair and Scalp Assessment

- Clients may require instruction about basic hygiene measures, including shampooing and combing of the hair (see Chapter 32).
- Instruct clients who have lice about the frequency of using Kwell shampoo or soap.
- Instruct clients who have lice about the risks for transmitting the infestation.
- Instruct the client that his or her partner must be notified if lice were sexually transmitted.

Much of the information gathered about characteristics of hair growth comes from the client. In addition, the nurse needs to be aware of the normal distribution of hair growth in males and females.

Both sexes have the fine vellus hair covering the body and scalp hair, eyebrows, and eyelashes. At puberty, a change in the amount and distribution of hair growth occurs. Clients with hormone disorders may experience an unusual distribution and growth. Females with hirsutism have hair growth on the upper lip, chin, and cheeks, with vellus hair becoming coarser over the body. A change in hair growth can negatively affect body image and emotional well-being. Asian and black Americans have less hair than whites, and Native Americans have little or no hair on their bodies (Rossman, 1979).

Normal, terminal hair is black, brown, red, yellow, or variations in shades of these colors. The hair is coarse or fine. Normal variations exist in the shape of hair fibers. Clients' hair may be straight, curly, spiral, or wavy. The hair of black clients is usually thicker, curlier, and drier than the hair of white clients. The hair shaft is usually shiny and pliant.

In the elderly, the hair becomes dull gray, white, or yellow. It also thins over the scalp, axillar, and pubic areas. Elderly males lose facial hair, whereas elderly females may develop hair on the chin and upper lip.

Changes may occur in the thickness, texture, and lubrication of scalp hair. A number of disturbances in body function, such as a febrile illness can result in hair loss. Scalp disease can also cause loss of hair. Baldness (alopecia) or thinning of the hair is usually related to genetic tendencies. The hair is lubricated from the oil of sebaceous glands. Excessively oily hair is associated with androgen hormone stimulation. Dry, brittle hair occurs with aging and with excessive use of shampoo or other chemical agents. Poor nutrition often causes development of dry, coarse, discolored hair.

The amount of hair covering the extremities may be reduced as a result of aging and arterial insufficiency and is most commonly seen over the lower extremities. In females, loss of hair should not be confused with shaven legs.

The nurse inspects hair follicles on the scalp and pubic areas for lice or other parasites. The three types of lice are *Pediculus humanus* var. *capitis* or head lice, *Pediculus corporis* or body lice, and *Pediculus pubis* or crab lice. Head and crab lice attach their eggs to hair. The tiny eggs look like oval particles of dandruff. The lice themselves are difficult to see. Head and body lice are very small with grayish white bodies. Crab lice have red legs. The nurse looks for bites or pustular eruptions in the hair follicles and in areas where skin surfaces meet, such as behind the ears and in the groin. The discovery of lice requires immediate treatment (see client-teaching box).

When inspecting the scalp the nurse asks the client if he or she has noticed anything unusual. Lesions can easily go unnoticed in a thick growth of hair. By carefully separating strands of hair the nurse can thoroughly examine the scalp. The nurse assesses any lesion using the guidelines for skin lesions. If lumps or bruises are found, the nurse asks if the client has experienced recent trauma to the head. Moles on the scalp are not unusual. The nurse should warn the client that combing or brushing can cause a mole to bleed. Scaliness or dryness of the scalp is frequently caused by dandruff or psoriasis.

Nails

The most visible portion of the nails is the nail plate, the transparent layer of epithelial cells covering the nail

TABLE 13-8 Nursing History for Nail Assessment

Assessment Category	Rationale
Ask if client has experienced any recent trauma to the nails.	Trauma may change shape and growth of nail. All or a portion of the nail plate can be lost.
Question client's nail care practices.	Chemical agents can cause drying of the nails. Improper care may damage nails and cuticles.
Determine if client has noticed changes in nail appearance or growth.	Alterations may occur slowly over time.

bed. The vascularity of the nail bed creates the nail's underlying color. The semilunar, whitish area at the base of the nail bed is called the lunula, from which the nail plate develops. The nails can reflect general state of health. After gathering a brief history (Table 13-8), the nurse inspects the nail bed color, the thickness and shape of the nail plate, texture of the nail, the angle between the nail and the nail bed, and the condition of tissues around the nail. The nurse also palpates the nail base.

The nails are normally transparent, smooth, and convex, with a nail bed angle of about 160 degrees. In whites the nail beds are pink with translucent white tips. In blacks a brown or black pigmentation is normally present in longitudinal streaks. The nail bed is normally firm on palpation. Nails normally grow at a constant rate, but direct injury or generalized disease can impair

TABLE 13-9 Abnormalities of the Nail Bed

Type	Description	Causes
Normal nail 160°	Approximately a 160-degree angle between nail-plate and nail-base	
Clubbing 180° > 180°	Change in the angle between nail and nail base (the angle is eventually larger than 180 degrees); nail bed softens, with nail flattening; fingertips often enlarged	Chronic lack of oxygen: heart or pulmonary disease
Beau's lines	Transverse depressions in the nails indicating nail growth was temporarily disturbed; grows out over several months	Systemic illness such as severe infection; injury to the nail
Koilonychia (spoon nail)	Concave curves	Iron deficiency anemia; syphilis; use of strong detergents
Splinter hemorrhages	Red or brown linear streaks in the nail bed	Minor trauma; subacute bacterial endocarditis; trichinosis
Paronychia	Inflammation of skin at base of nail	Local infection; trauma

---

Client Teaching after Nail Assessment

- Instruct clients to cut nails only after soaking them about 10 minutes in warm water.
- Instruct client to avoid use of over-the-counter preparations to treat corns, calluses, or ingrown toenails.
- Tell client to cut nails straight across and even with the tops of the fingers.
- Instruct client to shape nails with a file or emery board.

TABLE 13-10 Nursing History for Head Assessment

Assessment Category	Rationale
Determine if client experienced recent trauma to the head.	Trauma is major cause for lumps, bumps, cuts, bruises, or deformities of the scalp or skull.
Ask if client has noticed any neurological symptoms such as headaches, dizziness, loss of consciousness, seizures, or blurred vision.	Head trauma may cause damage to brain tissues and change in neurological function.
Determine the length of time client has experienced neurological symptoms.	The duration of any signs or symptoms may reveal severity of the problem.

---

growth. The surrounding cuticles are normally smooth and intact without inflammation.

With aging, the nails of the fingers and toes develop longitudinal striations. The rate of nail growth also slows (Jacobs, 1981). The color of nails is an indicator of blood oxygenation. A bluish or purplish cast to the nail bed occurs with cyanosis. A white cast or pallor is the result of anemia. Thin nails can be a sign of poor circulation and nutritional deficiency. Extremely short nails with rough edges indicate nail biting, which is common in persons who frequently feel anxious. Changes in the shape and curvature of nails are indications of systemic disease (Table 13-9). Palpation of the nails also assesses adequacy of circulation or capillary refill. To palpate, the nurse gently grasps the client's finger and observes the color of the nail bed. Next, gentle, firm pressure is quickly applied with the thumb to the nail bed and released. As pressure is applied, the nail bed appears white or blanched. However, the pink color should return immediately after the release of pressure. Failure of the pinkness to promptly return indicates circulatory insufficiency.

Calluses and corns are commonly found on the toes or fingers. A callus is flat and painless. It results from a thickening of the epidermis. Corns are caused by friction and pressure from shoes and can usually be seen over a bony prominence. During the examination the nurse instructs clients on proper nail care (see client-teaching box).

HEAD AND NECK

An examination of the head and neck includes the head, eyes, ears, nose, mouth, pharynx, and neck (lymph nodes, carotid arteries, thyroid gland, and trachea). The carotid arteries can also be assessed during assessment of arteries. The nurse needs to understand each anatomical area and its normal physiological function. Assessment of the head and neck uses the skills of inspection, palpation, and auscultation, with inspection and palpation often used simultaneously.

Head

The nursing history (Table 13-10) will reveal risk for intracranial injury and local or congenital deformities. The nurse inspects the client's head, noting the size, shape, and contour. The skull is generally round with prominences in the frontal area anteriorly and the occipital area posteriorly. Local skull deformities are typically caused by trauma. In infants a large head may result from congenital anomalies or the build up of cerebrospinal fluid in the ventricles (hydrocephalus). Adults may have enlarged jaw and facial bones resulting from acromegaly, a disorder caused by excessive growth hormone secretion.

The nurse palpates the skull for nodules or masses. Gentle rotation of the fingertips down the midline of the scalp and then along the sides of the head will reveal any abnormalities.

Eyes

Examination of the eye includes assessment of visual acuity, visual fields, extraocular movements, and external and internal eye structures. Fig. 13-13 shows a cross section of the eye.

The assessment is very useful in determining the level of assistance clients require when ambulating or performing self-care activities. Clients with visual problems may also need special aids for reading teaching materials or instructions (for example, medication labels). Table 13-11 reviews the nursing history for an eye examination. The box describes common types of visual problems.

TABLE 13-11 Nursing History for Eye Assessment

Assessment Category	Rationale
Determine if client has history of eye disease, diabetes, or hypertension.	Some diseases can cause risk for partial or complete visual loss.
Ask client about presence of eye pain, photophobia (sensitivity to light), burning, itching, excess tearing or crusting, diplopia (double vision), blurred vision, floaters (small, black spots that seem to float across the field of vision), flashing lights, or halos around lights.	Common symptoms of eye disease indicate need for physician referral.
Assess client's occupational history.	Performance of close, intricate work can cause eye fatigue. Certain occupational tasks (for example, welding or working with chemicals) place persons at risk for eye injury unless precautions are taken.
Ask client if glasses or contacts are normally worn.	Glasses or contacts should be worn during certain portions of the examination for accurate assessment.
Determine when client last visited an eye doctor (ophthalmologist).	Date of last eye examination reveals level of preventive care taken by client.

Common Eye and Visual Problems

HYPEROPIA

- Farsightedness, a refractive error in which rays of light enter the eye and focus behind the retina. Persons are able to see distant objects but not close objects.

MYOPIA

- Nearsightedness, a refractive error in which rays of light enter the eye and focus in front of the retina. Persons are able to see close objects but not distant objects.

PRESBYOPIA

- Impaired near vision in middle-age and elderly adults.

STRABISMUS

- Congenital problem in which the eyes appear crossed. The muscles controlling movement of the eyes are not coordinated.

CATARACTS

- Loss of transparency of the lens, blocking light rays entering the eye. Cataracts may develop slowly and progressively after age 50 or suddenly after trauma.

GLAUCOMA

- Abnormal condition of elevated pressure within an eye caused by obstruction of the outflow of aqueous humor. Without treatment the disorder can cause blindness.

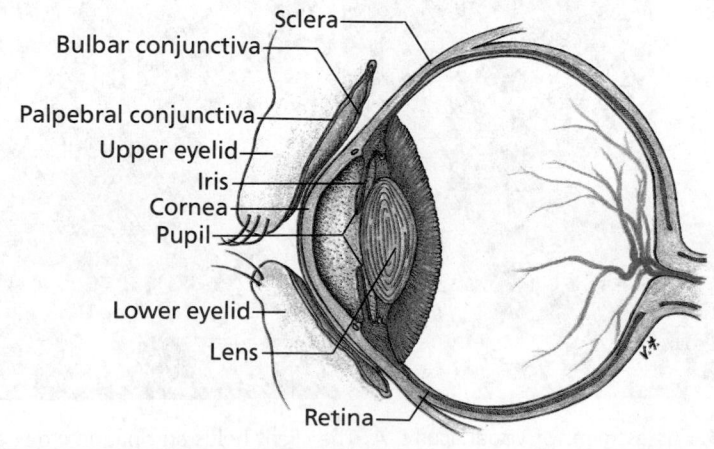

Fig. 13-13   Cross section of the eye.

VISUAL ACUITY

The easiest way to initially assess visual acuity is to ask the client to read printed material under adequate lighting. If a client wears glasses, he or she should wear them. The nurse should know the language a client speaks and whether the client is literate and able to read. Asking the client to read aloud can help determine literacy.

For a more accurate assessment of visual acuity, a Snellen chart is used. The client wears glasses but not if they are prescribed for reading. The client is positioned 20 feet from the chart and tries to read the smallest line of print possible three times, once with both eyes, then with each eye separately when the opposite eye is covered with an opaque card (Fig. 13-14). For clients unable to read, the E chart is used. Instead of reading letters the client tells the examiner which direction each E is pointing. The client is successful when he or she is able to read more than half the letters or figures in a line. The visual acuity score is recorded for each eye and both eyes. The Snellen chart has standardized numbers at the end of each line of the chart. The numerator is the number 20 or the standard distance the client stands from the chart. The denominator is the distance from which the normal eye can read the chart. Normal vision is 20/20. The larger the denominator, the poorer the client's

visual acuity. For example, a value of 20/40 means the client, standing 20 feet away, can read a line that a person with normal vision can read from 40 feet away. The nurse also records visual acuity as $\bar{s}c$ (without correction) or $\bar{c}c$ (with correction), depending on whether the client wears glasses or contact lenses.

If clients cannot read even the largest letters or figures of a Snellen chart, the nurse tests their ability to count upraised fingers or distinguish light. The nurse holds a hand 30 cm (1 foot) from the client's face and instructs the client to count the upraised fingers. To check light perception, the nurse shines a penlight into the eye and then turns the light off. If the client notes when the light is turned on or off, light perception is intact.

VISUAL FIELDS

As a person looks straight ahead, all objects in the periphery can normally be seen. To assess visual fields the nurse has the client stand or sit 60 cm (2 feet) away, facing the nurse at eye level. The client gently closes or covers one eye (such as the left) and looks across at the nurse's eye directly opposite. The nurse closes her other eye (in this case the right) so the field of vision is superimposed on that of the client. The nurse moves a finger outside the field of vision, then slowly brings it back. The object should be equidistant from the client

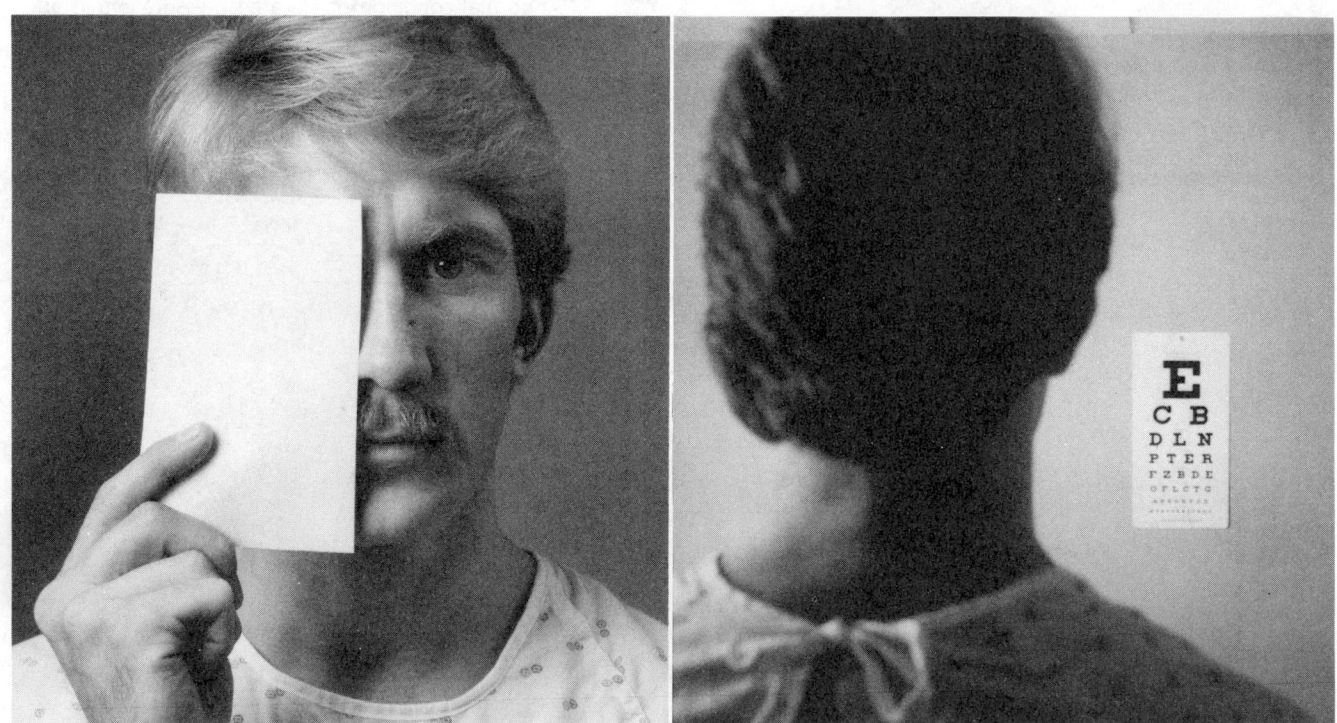

Fig. 13-14 Assessment of visual acuity. **A,** The client holds an opaque index card over one eye. The nurse assesses each eye separately for visual acuity. **B,** The client stands 20 feet away while reading the Snellen chart. The procedure is repeated for the other eye.

and nurse, except in the temporal field. To test temporal field vision, the object should be slightly behind the client (NOTE: The nurse will be able to see the finger.) The client is asked to tell the nurse when the finger is seen. If the nurse sees the finger before the client does, a portion of the client's visual field is reduced. The procedure is repeated for each field of vision for the other eye. Clients with visual field problems may be at risk for injury because they cannot see all objects in front of them. The elderly commonly have a loss of peripheral vision caused by changes in the lens.

EXTRAOCULAR MOVEMENTS

Six small muscles guide the movement of each eye. Both eyes move parallel to each other in each direction of gaze. When looking straight ahead toward the nurse, the client follows the movement of the nurse's finger through the eight cardinal gazes (Fig. 13-15). The finger is kept at a comfortable distance (6 to 12 inches or 15 to 30 cm) from the client. The client looks to the right, to the left, up, down, and diagonally up and down to the left and right. The examiner's finger stays within the normal field of vision. The client should not move or turn the head. As the client gazes in each direction, the nurse moves the finger slowly and smoothly.

The nurse observes for parallel eye movement, the position of the upper eyelid in relation to the iris, and the presence of abnormal movements such as nystagmus. With nystagmus a fine, rhythmical oscillation of the eyes is present. The nurse can often initiate nystagmus in a client with normal eye movement by having him or her gaze to the far left or right. As the eyes move through each direction of gaze, the upper eyelid only covers the iris slightly.

Disturbances in eye movement reflect local injury to eye muscles and supporting structures or a disorder of the cranial nerves innervating the muscles.

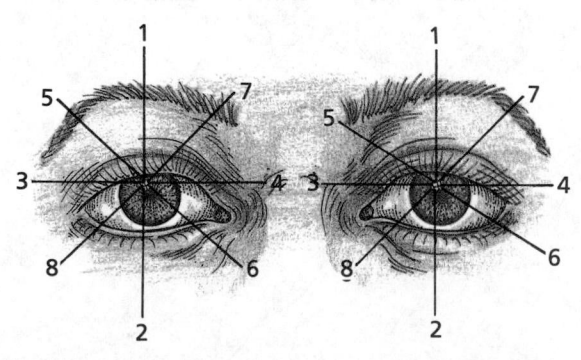

Fig. 13-15 The eight directions of gaze. The nurse directs the client to follow the movement of her finger through each of the gazes.

The nurse can also check for weakness or imbalance of the extraocular muscles by shining a light onto the client's eyes from 60 to 90 cm (2 to 3 feet) away in a darkened room. Normally the light reflects on the cornea in the same spot on both eyes. If an abnormality is present, the light shines on a different spot on each eye.

EXTERNAL EYE STRUCTURES

To inspect the external eye structures, the nurse stands directly in front of the client at eye level and asks the client to look at his or her face.

POSITION AND ALIGNMENT. The eyes are normally parallel to each other. Bulging (exophthalmos) is usually caused by hyperthyroidism when both eyes are involved. Abnormal protrusion of one eye may be caused by a tumor or inflammation of the eye's orbit.

EYEBROWS. The eyebrows are normally symmetrical. The eyebrows are inspected for quantity of hair and movement. A loss or absence of hair is indicative of hormonal disturbance. Aging causes loss of the lateral third of the eyebrows. Flaking of skin around the brows may be a form of dandruff, which can cause chronic eye irritation. The brows should raise and lower symmetrically. Paralysis of the facial nerve exists if a client cannot move the eyebrows.

EYELIDS. The nurse inspects the eyelids for position, color, condition of surface, condition and direction of eyelashes, and the client's ability to close and blink.

When the eyes are open in a normal position, the lids do not cover the pupil and sclera cannot be seen above the iris. The lids are also close to the eyeball. An abnormal drooping of the lid over the pupil is called ptosis (pronounced "toe-sis") and is caused by edema or impairment of the third cranial nerve. Defects in the position of the lid margins may be observed. Elderly clients frequently have lid margins that turn out or in. A disruption of the lid margin may lead to irritation of the conjunctiva. To inspect the surface of the upper lids, ask clients to close their eyes. The lids are normally the same color as the skin. Redness indicates inflammation or infection. Heart and kidney failure and allergies can cause edema of the eyelids, which prevents them from closing. Any lesions are inspected for typical characteristics and discomfort or drainage.

The eyelashes are normally distributed evenly and curved outward away from the eye. If the eyelid becomes inverted the lashes may turn inward and irritate the eye.

The nurse asks clients to close their eyes. Failure of the lids to close exposes the cornea to drying. This condition is common in unconscious clients or those with facial nerve paralysis. Normally a person blinks up to 20 times a minute, involuntarily, and bilaterally. The blink reflex helps to lubricate the cornea.

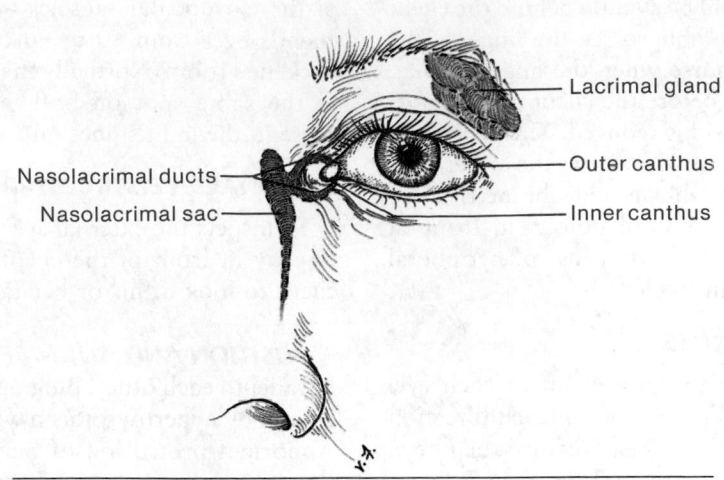

Fig. 13-16 The lacrimal apparatus secretes and drains tears, which moisten and lubricate eye structures.

LACRIMAL APPARATUS. The anterior surface of the eye, comprising the sensitive cornea and conjunctiva, is moistened or lubricated by tears secreted from the lacrimal gland (Fig. 13-16). The gland is located in the upper outer wall of the anterior part of the orbit. Tears flow from the gland across the eye's surface to the lacrimal duct, which is located in the nasal corner or inner canthus of the eye. The lacrimal gland can be the site of tumors or infections. The area of the gland is inspected for edema and redness and palpated gently to detect tenderness. Normally the gland cannot be felt.

The nasolacrimal duct may become obstructed, blocking the flow of tears. The client will complain of excess tearing. The nurse looks for evidence of edema in the inner canthus. Mild palpation of the duct at the lower eyelid just inside the orbital rim, not on the side of the nose, may cause a regurgitation of tears.

CONJUNCTIVAE AND SCLERAE. The bulbar conjunctiva covers the exposed surface of the eyeball up to the outer edge of the cornea, and the palpebral conjunctiva is the delicate membrane lining the eyelids. Normally the conjunctiva is transparent, enabling the examiner to view the tiny underlying blood vessels that give it a light pink color. The sclera is seen under the bulbar conjunctiva and normally has the color of white porcelain in white persons and light yellow in black persons.

Care must be taken when inspecting the conjunctiva. For adequate exposure the eyelids must be retracted without placing pressure directly on the eyeball. The lower lid is gently depressed with the thumb pressed against the bony orbit, and the client is asked to look up (Fig. 13-17). Many clients begin to blink, making the

examination difficult. Often the client can depress the eyelid to facilitate examination. The conjunctiva's color and the presence of edema or lesions are noted. A pale conjunctiva results from anemia, whereas a fiery red appearance is the result of inflammation (conjunctivitis). Conjunctivitis is a highly contagious infection. The nurse may choose to wear gloves during the examination. Thorough handwashing is necessary after the examination is completed.

A special technique is used to inspect the upper palpebral conjunctiva (Fig. 13-18) and should not be attempted the first time without qualified assistance. The technique is useful if the nurse suspects a foreign body under the lid. The client is asked to look down, relax the eyes, and avoid any sudden movement. The upper lid is gently grasped with a gloved hand and the lashes

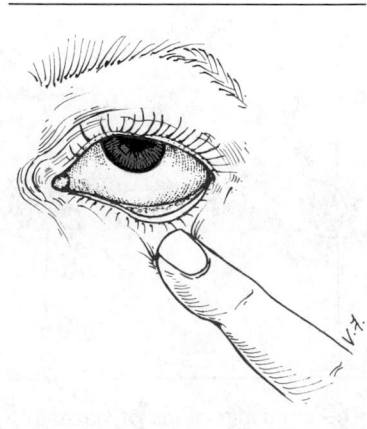

Fig. 13-17 Technique for retracting lower eyelid.

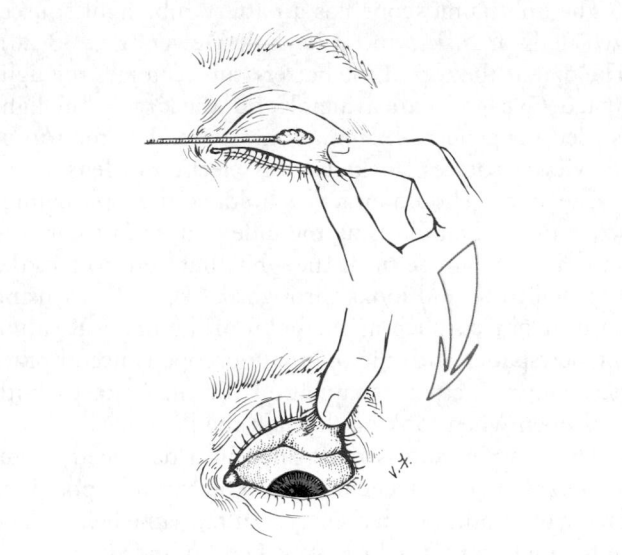

Fig. 13-18 Technique for inspecting upper palpebral conjunctiva.

are pulled down and forward. The end of a cotton applicator is placed 1 cm (½ inch) above the lid margin. The nurse pushes down on the upper eyelid, turning it inside out. A light grasp on the upper lashes keeps the lid inverted. After inspection the eyelashes are gently pulled forward and the client is instructed to look up. The eyelid will return to its normal position.

If a foreign body appears to be embedded in the eye, the nurse *should not attempt to remove it* and should notify a physician immediately.

CORNEAS. The cornea is the transparent, colorless portion of the eye covering the pupil and iris. From a side view, the cornea looks like the crystal of a wrist watch. The nurse inspects it for clarity and texture while shining a penlight on each cornea's surface. The cornea is normally shiny, transparent, and smooth. However, in the elderly, the cornea loses its luster. Any irregularity in the surface may indicate an abrasion or tear. The color and details of the underlying iris should be easy to see. In the elderly the iris becomes faded. A thin, white ring along the margin of the iris, called an *arcus senilis*, is common with aging.

PUPILS AND IRISES. When a beam of light is shined through the pupil and onto the retina, the third cranial nerve is stimulated and innervates the muscles of the iris to constrict. Any abnormality along the nerve pathways from the retina to the iris will alter the ability of the pupils to react to light. Changes in intracranial pressure, lesions along the nerve pathways, locally applied ophthalmic medications, and direct trauma to the eye may alter pupillary reaction.

The nurse observes the pupils for size, shape, equality, accommodation, and reaction to light. The pupils are normally round and equal in size. Dilated or constricted pupils can result from neurological disorders or the effect of eye drugs. The surrounding iris is inspected for defects

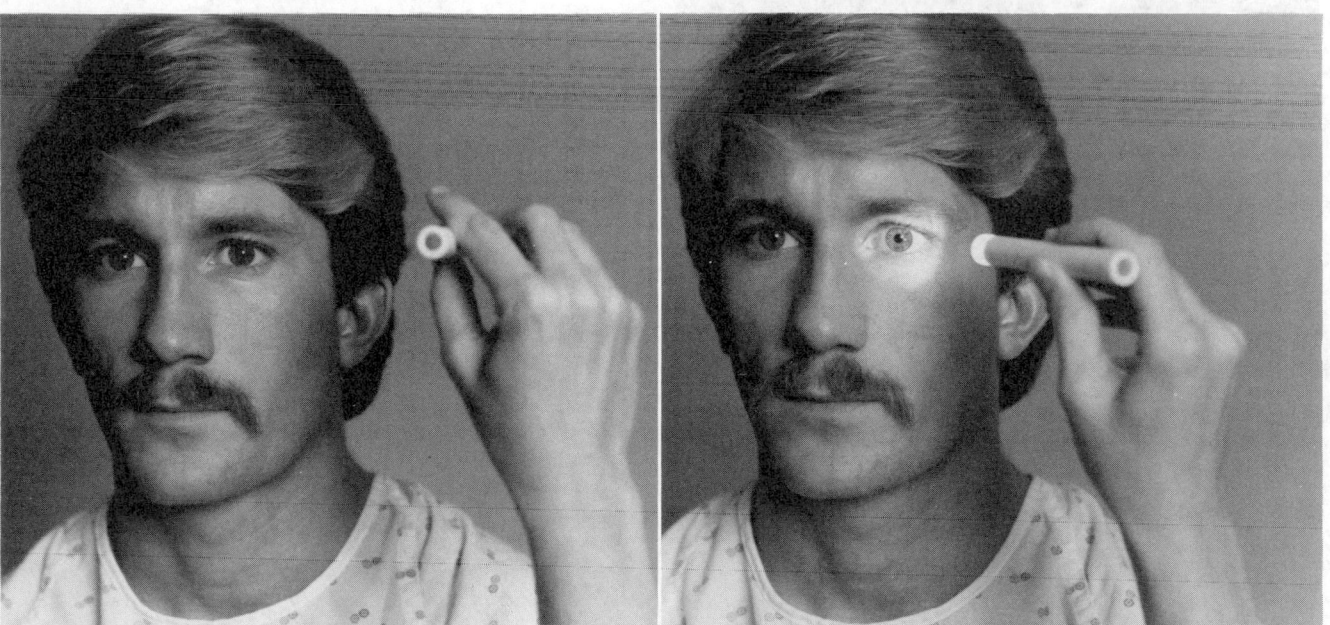

Fig. 13-19   **A,** To check pupil reflexes, the nurse first holds the penlight to the side of the client's face. **B,** Illumination of the pupil causes pupillary constriction.

along its margins. Pupillary reflexes (to light and accommodation) should be tested in a dimly lit room. As the client looks straight ahead, the nurse takes a penlight and brings it from the side of the client's face, directing the light onto the pupil (Fig. 13-19). If the client looks at the light there will be a false reaction to accommodation. A directly illuminated pupil constricts, and the opposite pupil constricts consensually. The nurse observes the quickness and equality of the reflex.

To test accommodation, the nurse holds a finger 10 to 15 cm (4 to 6 inches) from the client's nose. The client is asked to gaze at the finger and then at the wall in the distance. The pupils normally constrict when looking at the examiner's finger and dilate when looking at the wall, showing the pupil's ability to accommodate near and distant vision.

If assessment of pupillary reaction is normal in all tests the nurse records the abbreviation PERRLA (pupils equal, round, reactive to light, and accommodation).

INTERNAL EYE STRUCTURES

The internal eye cannot be observed without an instrument to illuminate its structures. The ophthalmoscope is used to inspect the fundus, which includes the retina, choroid, optic nerve disc, macula, fovea centralis, and retinal vessels. Clients in greatest need of an examination are those with diabetes, hypertension, and intracranial disorders.

The ophthalmoscope has a battery tube light source, two dials or disks, and a keyhole viewer (Fig. 13-20). The dial at the top of the battery tube changes the light image. Five lenses are available, but the large white light is used for general examination. The dial at the top of the viewer rotates clockwise for selection of lenses.

The nurse should practice holding the ophthalmoscope in each hand, using the index finger to rotate the lens dial. The nurse turns the white light on, rotates the lens dial to 0, and looks through the keyhole, focusing on near objects such as the palm of the hand. Reading the newspaper with the ophthalmoscope is useful practice. During actual examination the nurse keeps both eyes open when looking through the keyhole.

The examination is performed in a darkened room. The examiner and client sit in comfortable positions facing each other with their eyes at the same height. The ophthalmoscope's light is switched on and the lens rotated to 0. The index finger is kept on the lens dial to refocus the ophthalmoscope.

The examiner's right hand and eye are used to examine the client's right eye, and the left hand and eye are used for the client's left eye. The client is asked to gaze straight ahead over the examiner's shoulder throughout the examination.

The ophthalmoscope is held firmly against the nurse's face. At a distance of approximately 25 cm (10 inches) from the client and lateral to his line of vision, the examiner shines the light on the pupil. A bright orange glow in the pupil, called the red reflex, can then normally be seen. The light from the ophthalmoscope causes the

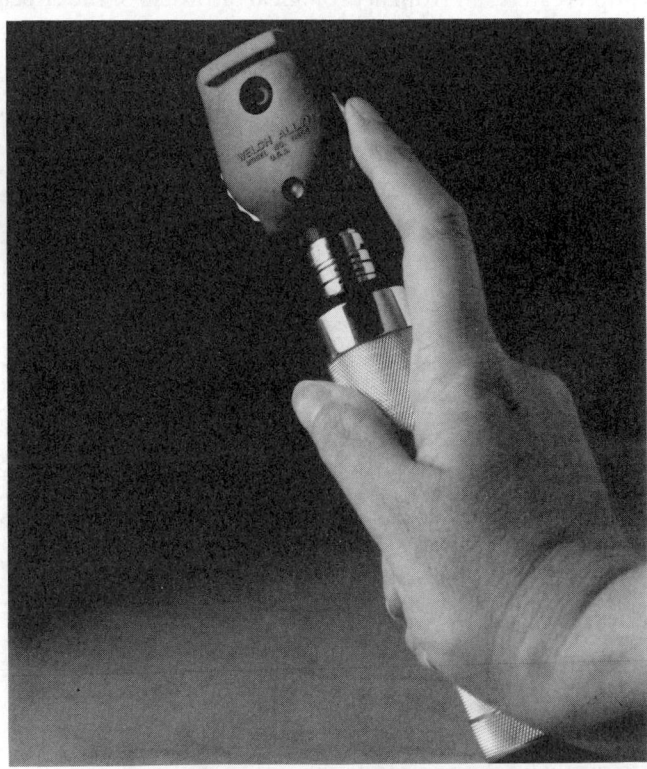

Fig. 13-20 An ophthalmoscope.

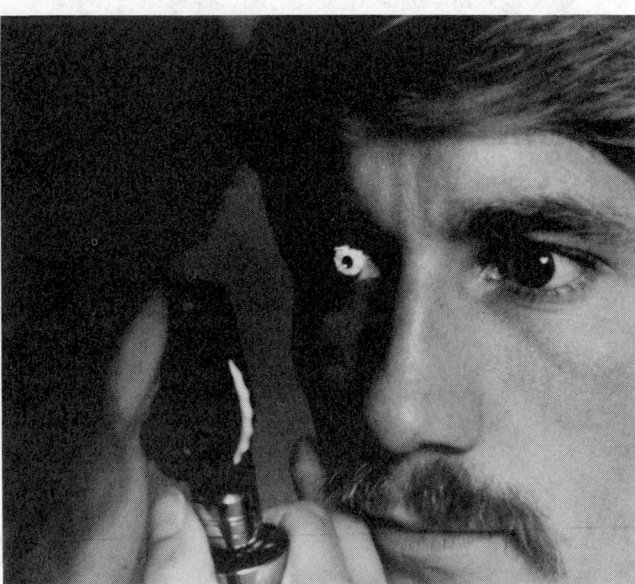

Fig. 13-21 To visualize internal eye structures, the nurse moves in toward the pupil with the light focused on the red reflex.

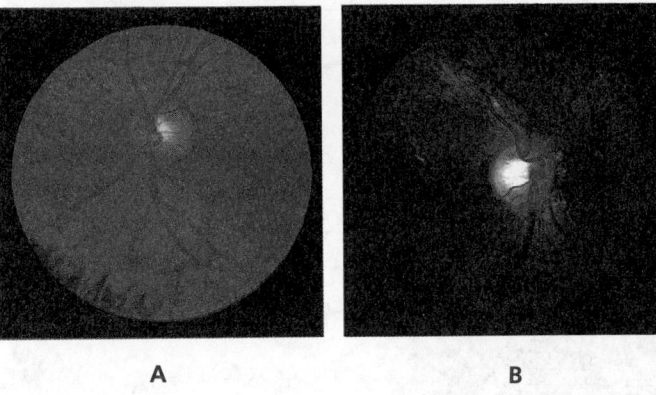

A   **B**

Fig. 13-22 Normal fundus. **A,** White adult. **B,** Black adult.

From Selected topics in ophthalmology, Medcom clinical lecture guides, Garden Grove, Calif., copyright 1973, Medcom, Inc.

pupil to constrict. The light is slowly moved in toward the pupil, while the examiner keeps it focused on the red reflex (Fig. 13-21). The nurse must relax and keep both eyes open. As the light approaches the pupil, the nurse begins to see structures of the fundus. Rotating the lens dial brings the internal structures into focus. The examiner inspects the size, color, and clarity of the disc, integrity of vessels, presence of retinal lesions, and appearance of the macula and fovea (Fig. 13-22). Normally the following structures are observed:

1. A clear, yellow optic nerve disc
2. Reddish-pink retina (white clients)
3. Darkened retina (black clients)
4. Light red arteries and dark red veins
5. A 3:2 vein to artery ratio in size proportion
6. The avascular macula

If any abnormalities are observed, the client should be examined by an ophthalmologist (see client-teaching box). The client's fundus should not be illuminated for extended periods. The bright light of the ophthalmoscope is very irritating and can cause discomfort and tearing. During the examination, assess the client for discomfort.

Ears

The ears are easy to examine because of their accessibility. The three parts of the ear are external, middle, and inner ear (Fig. 13-23). The nurse inspects and palpates external ear structures, which consist of the auricle, outer ear canal, and tympanic membrane. Inspection of middle ear structures, including the malleus, incus, and stapes, is performed with the use of an otoscope. To assess inner ear structures, the nurse tests hearing acuity.

The nurse assesses the ears to determine the integrity of ear structures and the condition of hearing. Nursing history data (Table 13-12) aids in identifying risks for hearing disorders.

Understanding the mechanisms for sound transmission helps the nurse to identify the nature of hearing disorders. Sound travels through the ear by air and bone conduction:

1. Sound waves in the air enter the external ear, passing through the outer ear canal.
2. The sound waves reach the tympanic membrane, causing it to vibrate.
3. Vibrations are transmitted through the middle ear by way of the bony ossicular chain to the oval window at the opening of the inner ear.
4. The cochlea receives the sound vibration.
5. Nerve impulses from the cochlea travel to the auditory nerve (eighth cranial) and to the cerebral cortex.

Disorders of the ear result from one of four types of problems, including mechanical dysfunction (blockage by ear wax or foreign body), trauma (foreign bodies or noise exposure), neurological disorders (auditory nerve damage), and acute illnesses (viral infection).

AURICLES

With the client sitting the nurse inspects the auricle's placement, color, size, and symmetry. The auricles are normally level with each other. The upper point of attachment to the head is in a straight line with the lateral canthus or corner of the eye. Low-set ears are a sign of congenital abnormality. The color of the auricle should be the same as that of the face. Any redness is a sign of inflammation or fever. Pallor can indicate frostbite.

The nurse palpates the auricles for texture and lumps or skin lesions. The auricle is normally smooth without lesions. If the client complains of pain, the nurse gently

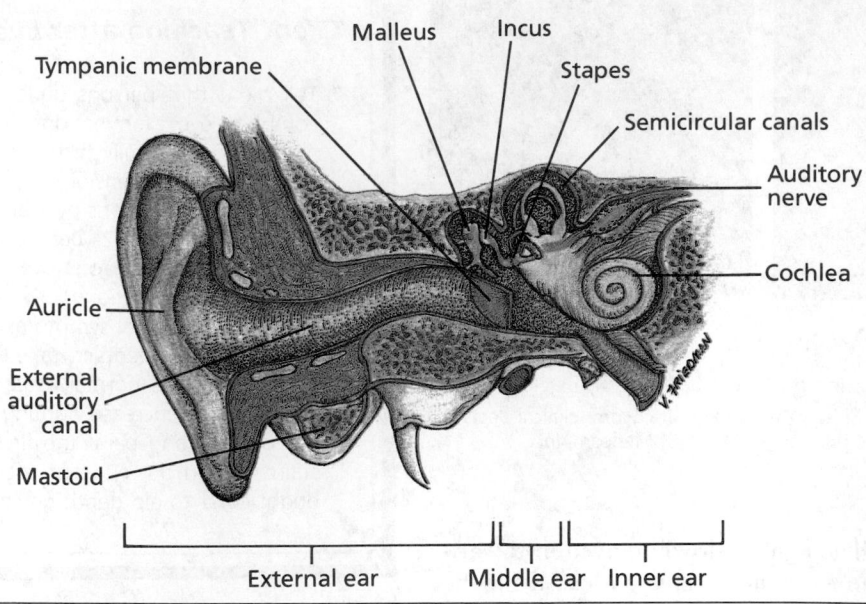

Fig. 13-23 The structures of the external, middle, and inner ear.

pulls the auricle and presses on the tragus and behind the ear. If palpating the external ear increases the pain, an external ear infection is likely. If palpation of the auricle and tragus cause no pain, the client may have a middle ear infection.

The nurse inspects the opening of the ear canal for size and presence of discharge. The meatus should not be swollen or occluded. A yellow, waxy substance called cerumen is common. Yellow or green discharge may indicate infection.

EAR CANALS AND EARDRUMS

The deeper structures of the external and middle ear can be observed only with an otoscope. A special ear

TABLE 13-12 Nursing History for Ear Assessment

Assessment Category	Rationale
Ask if client has experienced ear pain, itching, discharge, tinnitus (ringing in ears), or change in hearing.	These signs and symptoms indicate infection or hearing loss.
Assess risks for hearing problem: hypoxia at birth, meningitis, birth weight less than 1500 g, family history of hearing loss, congenital anomalies of skull or face, nonbacterial intrauterine infections (rubella, herpes), constant exposure to high levels of noise	Risk factors predispose child to permanent hearing loss. It may be difficult to assess an infant's hearing status with only an examination.
Determine client's exposure to loud noises at work and availability of protective devices.	Prolonged noise exposure can cause temporary or permanent hearing loss.
Note behaviors indicative of hearing loss such as failure to respond when spoken to; repetition of question, "what did you say?"; leaning forward to hear; and a child's inattentiveness or use of monotonous voice tone.	Persons with hearing loss cope with sensory deficit through a variety of behavioral cues.
Assess if client takes large doses of aspirin or antibiotics.	Medications have side effects of hearing disorders.
Determine whether client uses a hearing aid.	This determination allows nurse to assess client's ability to care for device and allows nurse to adjust voice tone to communicate with client.
If client has had a recent hearing problem, note onset, contributing factors, and effect on activities of daily living.	Nature and severity of hearing problem are determined.

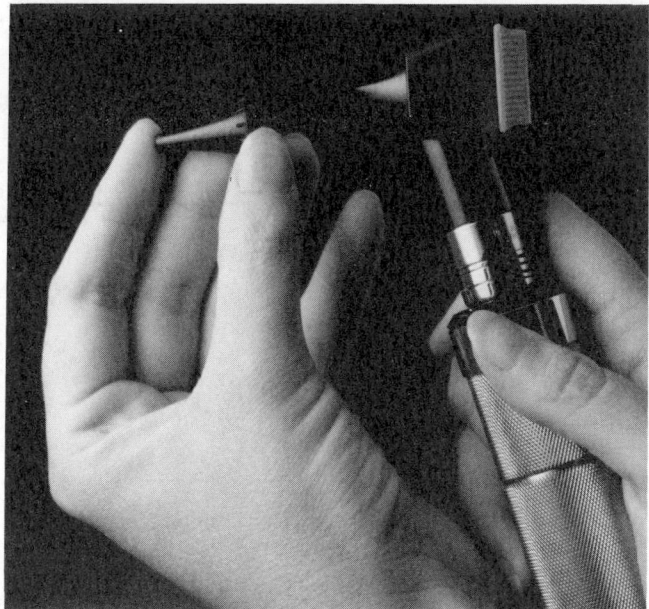

Fig. 13-24 The otoscope has speculums of many sizes to fit the ear canal.

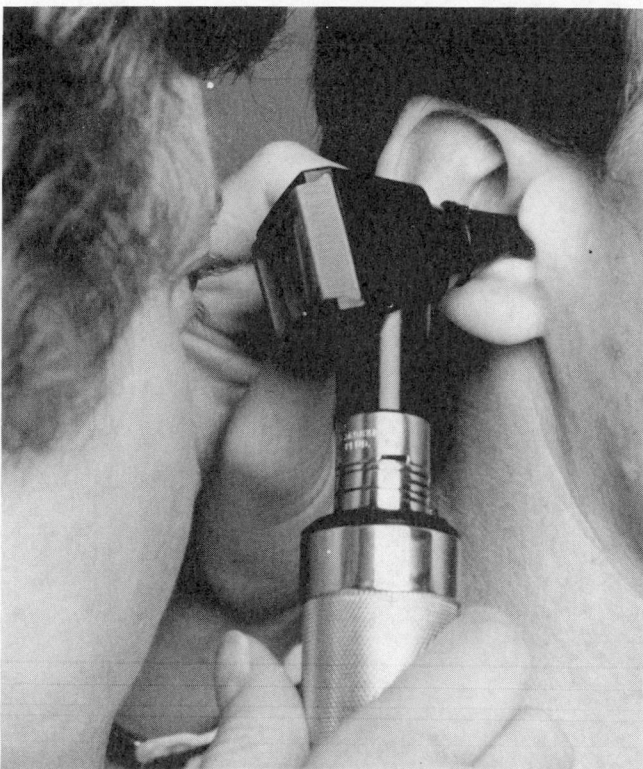

Fig. 13-25 In an adult, pulling the auricle upward and backward straightens the ear canal for easier otoscope placement.

speculum attaches to the battery tube of the ophthalmoscope. Speculums come in different sizes to conform to the size of clients' ear canals. For best visualization the largest speculum that fits comfortably into the ear canal should be used (Fig. 13-24).

Before inserting the speculum, the examiner checks for foreign bodies in the opening of the auditory canal. The client must avoid moving the head during the examination to avoid damage to the canal and tympanic membrane. Infants and young children often need to be restrained. Infants should lie supine with their heads turned to one side and their arms held securely at their sides. Young children can sit on their parent's lap with their legs held between the parent's knees.

The nurse turns on the otoscope by rotating the dial at the top of the battery tube. To insert the speculum properly the nurse asks the client to tip the head slightly toward the shoulder opposite the ear being examined. Pulling the auricle gently up, back, and slightly out in the adult or older child straightens the ear canal (Fig. 13-25). In infants the nurse pulls the auricle back and down. The nurse inserts the speculum into the ear canal slightly down and forward. Care should be taken to avoid abrading the sensitive lining of the ear canal. The nurse keeps the otoscope braced against the client's head to avoid sudden movement. Two grips on the otoscope may be used. In one, the examiner holds the battery tube along the client's neck with the fingers against the neck. In the other grip (Fig. 13-26), the inverted otoscope is lightly braced against the side of the client's head or cheek. This grip, used commonly with children, prevents

accidental movement of the otoscope deeper into the ear canal.

The nurse identifies the presence of cerumen and observes for lesions, foreign bodies, or discharge in the canal. A reddened canal is a sign of inflammation. During the examination the examiner asks the client how the ear canal is normally cleaned (see client-teaching box).

Client Teaching after Ear and Hearing Assessment

- Instruct client about the proper way to clean outer ear (see Chapter 32), avoiding use of cotton-tipped applicators and sharp objects such as hairpins.
- Tell client to avoid inserting pointed objects into the ear canal.
- Encourage clients over 65 to have regular hearing checks.
- Instruct family members of clients with hearing losses to avoid shouting and speak instead in low tones.

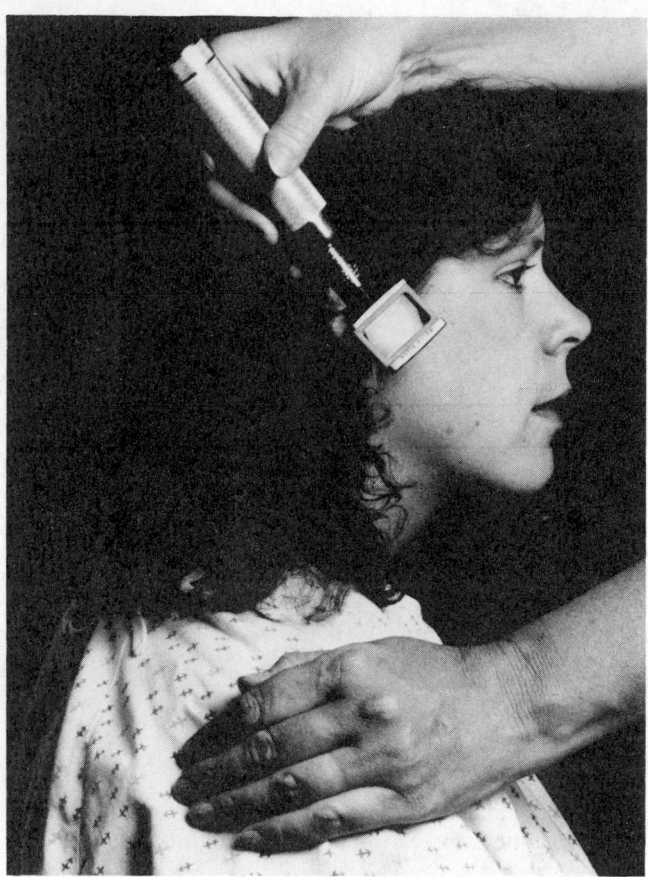

Fig. 13-26 Insertion of otoscope in inverted position.

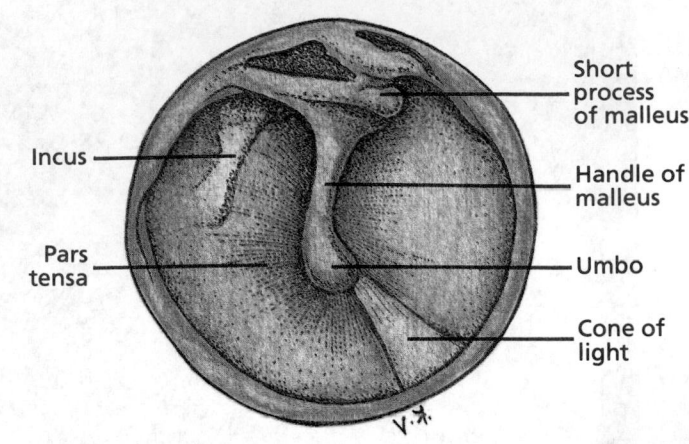

Fig. 13-27 Normal tympanic membrane.

The light from the otoscope allows visualization of the eardrum (tympanic membrane). The nurse must be familiar with the common anatomical landmarks and their appearances (Fig. 13-27). The otoscope is slowly moved to see the entire drum and its periphery. The normal eardrum is translucent or pearly gray. A pink or red eardrum indicates inflammation. A white color reveals pus behind the tympanic membrane. Because the eardrum is angled away from the ear canal, the light from the otoscope appears as a cone shape rather than a circle. The umbo is near the center of the drum, and the attachment of the malleus is behind it. A knoblike structure at the top of the drum is created by the underlying short process of the malleus. The examiner should check carefully to be sure there are no tears or breaks in the eardrum's membrane.

HEARING ACUITY

Often the nurse can tell if the client has a hearing loss from his or her response to conversation. The three types of hearing loss are conduction, sensorineural, and mixed. A conduction loss involves an interruption of sound waves as they travel from the outer ear to the cochlea of the inner ear, because they are not transmitted through the outer and middle ear structures. Examples of causes of a conduction loss are swelling of the auditory canal or tears in the eardrum. A sensorineural loss involves the inner ear, the auditory nerve, or the hearing center of the brain. Sound is conducted through the outer and middle ear structures, but the continued transmission of sound becomes interrupted at some point beyond the bony ossicles. A mixed loss involves a combination of conduction and sensorineural loss.

Clients working or living around loud noises are at risk for hearing loss. The elderly experience an inability to hear high-frequency sounds and consonants (for example, S, Z, T, G). Deterioration of the cochlea and a thickening of the tympanic membrane cause the elderly to gradually lose hearing acuity.

The simplest test for hearing acuity is identification of voice tones. One ear is tested at a time. The client occludes one ear with a finger, or the nurse occludes it for him. While standing 1 to 2 feet (30 to 60 cm) away the nurse covers the mouth so the client is unable to read lips. After exhaling fully, the nurse whispers softly toward the unoccluded ear, reciting numbers with two equally accented syllables such as "nine-four." If necessary the nurse gradually increases voice intensity until the client correctly repeats the numbers. A ticking watch may be used to test hearing acuity, but the spoken word allows for more accuracy and control.

If a hearing loss is present, the nurse can assess for conduction and sensorineural deafness through use of a tuning fork. A tuning fork of 512 or 1024 hertz (Hz) produces sound frequencies within the range of human speech. The fork should be lightly vibrated by tapping it on the heel of the palm or by stroking it between the thumb and index finger (Table 13-13).

TABLE 13-13   Tuning Fork Tests

Test and Steps	Rationale
WEBER'S TEST (LATERALIZATION OF SOUND)	
Hold the fork at its base and tap it lightly against the heel of the palm. Place the base of the vibrating fork on the top of the client's head or middle of forehead. Ask the client where sound is heard (on one or both sides).	A client with normal hearing hears sound equally in both ears or in midline of head. In conduction deafness, sound is heard in the impaired ear. In unilateral sensorineural hearing loss, sound is identified in the good ear.

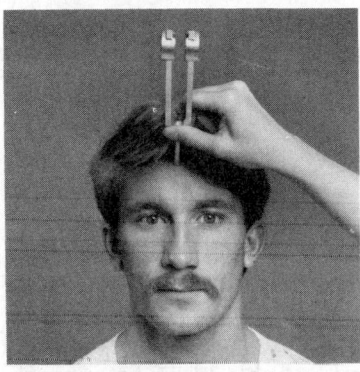

RINNE'S TEST (COMPARISON OF AIR AND BONE CONDUCTION)	
Strike the tuning fork against the knuckle. Place the vibrating fork on the mastoid process. Ask the client to inform you when sound is no longer heard. Immediately place the vibrating fork close to the external ear meatus. Ask the client to inform you if sound can be heard.	Normally, sound can be heard longer through air than through bone (positive Rinne). In conduction deafness, sounds through bone conduction can be heard after air conduction sounds become inaudible (negative Rinne). In sensorineural deafness, sound is heard longer through air.

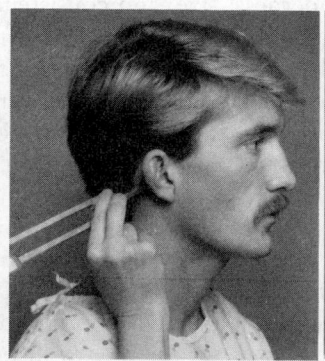 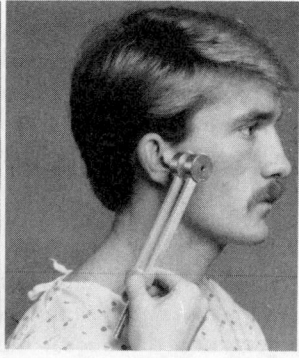

Nose and Sinuses

The nurse uses inspection and palpation to assess the nose and sinuses. A penlight allows the nurse to perform a gross examination of each naris. A more detailed examination requires use of a nasal speculum to inspect the deeper nasal turbinates. A student should not use a speculum unless a qualified practitioner is present. Table 13-14 lists components of the nursing history.

NOSE

When inspecting the nose the nurse observes for asymmetry, inflammation, or deformity. Recent trauma may have caused edema and discoloration. If swelling or deformities exist, the nose is palpated gently for tenderness, swelling and underlying deviations. Normally the nose is symmetrical and straight.

Air normally passes freely through the nose as a person breathes. As the nurse illuminates the anterior nares the mucosa is inspected for its color, presence of lesions, discharge, swelling, and evidence of bleeding. Normal mucosa is pink. Discharge resulting from sinus irritation is clear and watery. A sinus infection results in yellowish or greenish discharge. A pale mucosa with clear discharge is a sign of allergy. For the client with a nasogastric tube, the nurse routinely checks for local excoriation of the naris, characterized by redness and sloughing of the skin.

The client tips the head back slightly to give the nurse a clearer view of the septum and turbinates. The septum is inspected for deviation, lesions, and superficial blood vessels. Normally the septum is midline. A deviated septum can obstruct breathing and interfere with passage of a nasogastric tube.

TABLE 13-14   Nursing History for Nose and Sinus Assessment

Assessment Category	Rationale
Determine if client has experienced any trauma to the nose.	Trauma can cause deviation of septum and asymmetry of external nose.
Ask if client has history of allergies, nasal discharge, epistaxis (nose bleeds), or postnasal drip.	This history is useful in determining source or nature of nasal and sinus drainage.
Ask if client uses a nasal spray or drops.	Overuse of over-the-counter nasal preparations can cause physical change in mucosa.
Ask if client snores at night or has difficulty breathing.	Difficulty in breathing or snoring may indicate septal deviation or obstruction.

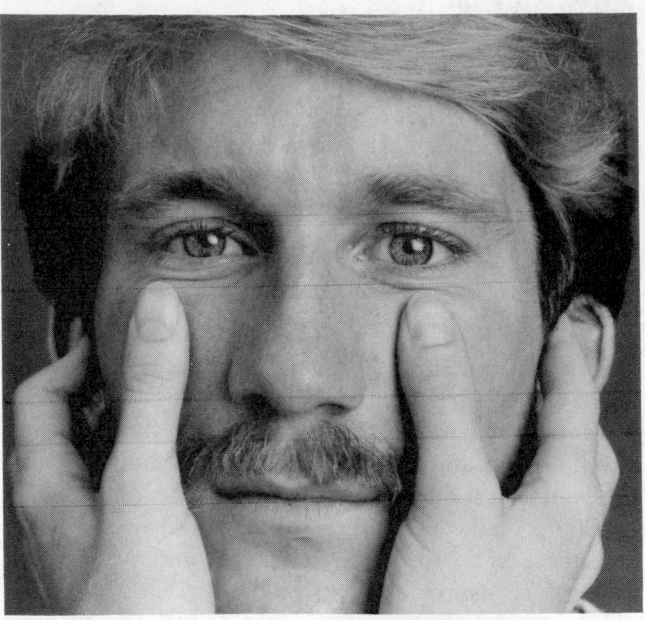

Fig. 13-28 Palpation of maxillary sinuses.

SINUSES

Examination of the sinuses is limited to palpation. In cases of allergies or infection, the interior of the sinuses becomes inflamed and swollen. The most effective way to assess for tenderness is by externally palpating the frontal and maxillary facial areas (Fig. 13-28). Gentle, upward pressure elicits tenderness easily and reveals the severity of sinus irritation. Pressure should not be applied to the eyes. Fig. 13-29 is a cross section of the nasal sinus cavities. The box describes client-teaching guidelines after nose and sinus assessment.

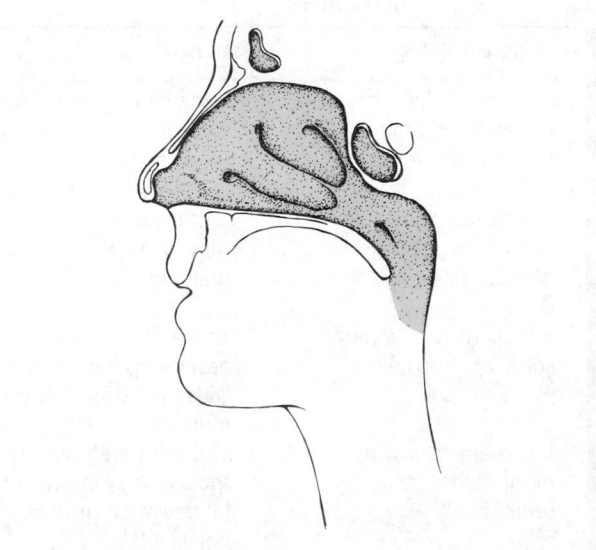

Fig. 13-29 Cross section of nasal sinus cavities.

> ### Client Teaching after Nose and Sinus Assessment
>
> - Caution clients against overuse of over-the-counter nasal sprays.
> - Instruct parents on care of children with nose bleeds: Have child sit up and lean forward to avoid aspiration of blood, apply pressure to anterior of nose with thumb and forefinger as child breathes through mouth, apply ice or a cold cloth to bridge of nose if pressure fails to stop bleeding.
> - The elderly lose the sense of smell and thus should have smoke detectors in their homes.

Mouth and Pharynx

To assess the oral cavity the nurse uses a penlight and tongue depressor or single gauze square. The CDC recommends wearing gloves when contacting mucous membranes (see Chapter 43). Assessment of the oral cavity can be made during administration of oral hygiene (see Chapter 32). Table 13-15 describes the nursing history.

LIPS

The lips are inspected for color, texture, hydration, contour, and lesions. As the client opens the mouth, the nurse views the lips from end to end. Normally they are pink, moist, symmetrical, and smooth (Fig. 13-30).

INNER AND BUCCAL MUCOSAS

To view the inner oral mucosa, the nurse has the client open the mouth slightly and then gently pulls the client's lower lip away from the teeth (Fig. 13-31, *A*). This process is repeated for the upper lip. The mucosa is inspected for color, hydration, texture, and lesions such as ulcers, abrasions, or cysts. If lesions are present, the nurse palpates them gently for tenderness, size, and consistency.

To visualize the buccal mucosa, the nurse asks the client to open the mouth and then gently retracts the cheeks with a tongue depressor or gloved finger covered with gauze (Fig. 13-31, *B*). The surface of the mucosa must be viewed from right to left and top to bottom. A penlight illuminates the most posterior portion of the mucosa. Normal mucosa is glistening, pink, soft, moist, and smooth. An increase in color or hyperpigmentation is normal in 10% of whites after age 50 and up to 90% of blacks by the same age. For clients with normal pigmentation the buccal mucosa is a good site to inspect for jaundice and pallor. In the elderly, the mucosa is normally dry because of reduced salivation. The ap-

TABLE 13-15 Nursing History for Mouth and Pharynx Assessment

Assessment Category	Rationale
Determine if client wears dentures and if they are comfortable	Dentures must be removed to visualize and palpate gums. Ill-fitting dentures irritate mucosa and gums and may be a risk for mouth cancer (U.S. Department of Health and Human Services, 1985).
Determine if client has had recent change in appetite or weight.	Symptoms may result from painful conditions of mouth. These findings may result from poor hygiene.
Assess dental hygiene practices and determine when client last visited dentist.	Reveals client's need for education or finances.
Determine if client smokes or chews tobacco.	Tobacco users have 4 to 15 times greater risk for mouth and throat cancers than nonusers (Mahboubi and Sayed, 1982)
Review history for alcohol consumption.	Heavy drinkers appear to have a greater risk for oral cancer.

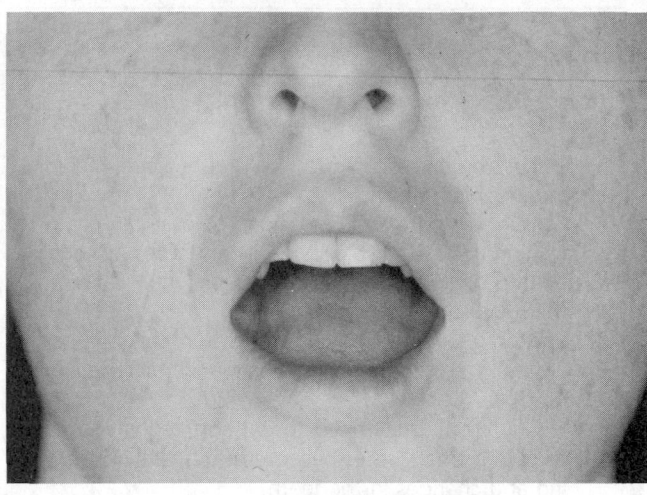

Fig. 13-30 The lips are normally pink, symmetrical, smooth, and moist.

pearance of thick, white patches (leukoplakia) can be seen in heavy smokers and alcoholics. Leukoplakia should be reported because it can also be a precancerous lesion. The nurse palpates the cheek between the thumb and index finger for deep-seated lumps.

GUMS AND TEETH

While the nurse retracts the cheeks, the gums or gingivae are inspected for color, edema, retraction, bleeding, and lesions. The gums around the back molars should be viewed because it is a difficult area to reach when cleaning teeth. Healthy gums are pink, smooth, and moist. Black clients may have patchy pigmentation. In the elderly the gums are usually pale. The nurse pal-

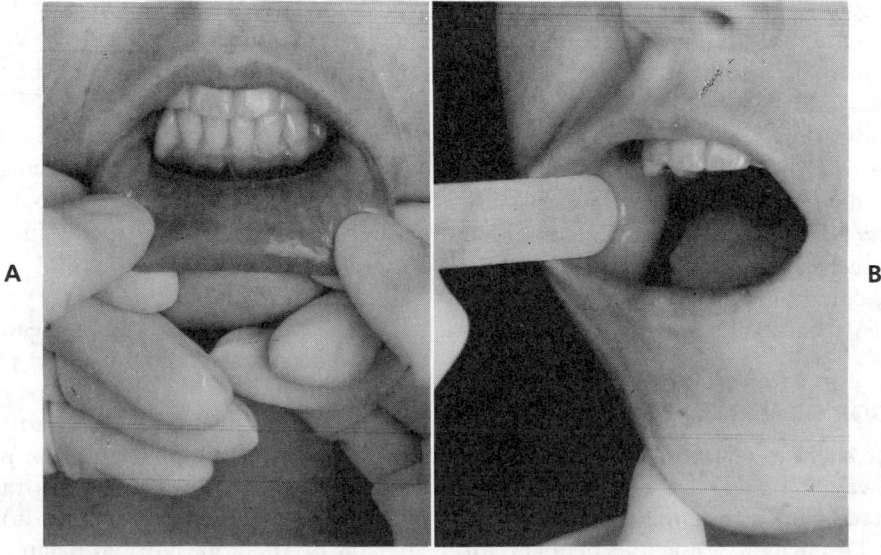

Fig. 13-31 A, Inspection of inner oral mucosa of lower lip. B, Retraction of the lips permits visualization of the buccal mucosa.

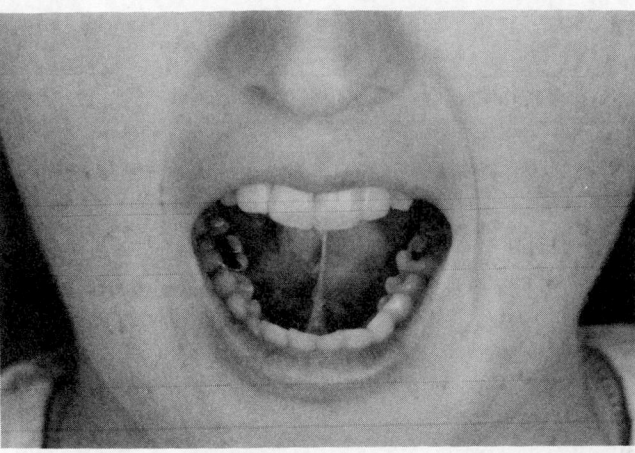

Fig. 13-32 The undersurface of the tongue is highly vascular.

pates the gums with a tongue depressor to determine if they are firm. Spongy gums that bleed easily indicate periodontal disease.

If a client wears dentures, any irregularity or lesions of the gums can cause discomfort and impair chewing. The nurse asks the client to remove dentures so a complete assessment can be performed. Any roughness on the denture surface can be smoothed out by a dentist.

The quality of dental hygiene is easily determined by inspecting the teeth. The client should open the lips and clench the teeth (see client-teaching box). The position and alignment of teeth are noted. To examine the posterior surface of the teeth the nurse has the client open the mouth with lips relaxed. A tongue depressor may be needed to retract the lips and cheeks, especially when one is viewing the molars. Tartar along the base of the teeth, dental caries, extraction sites, and the teeth's color should be noted. Normal, healthy teeth are smooth, white, and shiny. A chalky white discoloration of the enamel is an early indication of caries formation. Brown or black discolorations indicate formation of caries. In the elderly, loose or missing teeth are common because bone resorption increases. An older person's teeth often feel rough when tooth enamel calcifies. Yellow or darkened teeth are also common in the elderly because of general wear and tear that exposes the darker, underlying dentin.

TONGUE AND FLOOR OF MOUTH

The nurse asks the client to relax the mouth and stick the tongue out halfway.

If the client is forced to protrude the tongue too far, the gag reflex may be elicited. Using the penlight for illumination, the nurse examines the tongue for color, size, position, texture, and the presence of coating or lesions. The number of papillae (taste buds) varies throughout life. The tongue should be medium red or pink in color, moist, slightly rough on the top surface, and smooth along the lateral margins. When the tongue protrudes, it lies midline.

To test for tongue mobility the nurse asks the client to raise the tongue up and move it side to side. The tongue should move freely.

The tongue is highly vascular, particularly on the undersurface (Fig. 13-32). Extra care is taken to inspect the undersurface, a common site of origin for oral cancer lesions. The client lifts the tongue to permit adequate inspection. The nurse looks for white or red areas, nodules, or cysts. To palpate the tongue, the nurse explains the procedure and then asks the client to protrude the tongue. The nurse grasps the tip with a gauze square and gently pulls it to one side. With a gloved hand the nurse palpates the full length of the tongue and the base for any areas of hardening.

The floor of the mouth is also a site for oral cancer. Varicosities (swollen, tortuous veins) may be seen. Varicosities rarely cause problems but are common in the elderly. The nurse palpates any lumps or nodules.

PALATE

The client should extend the head backward, holding the mouth open so the nurse can inspect the hard and soft palates (Fig. 13-33). The hard palate or roof of the mouth is located anteriorly. The soft palate extends posteriorly toward the pharynx. The palates are observed for color, shape, texture, and extra bony prominences or defects. A bony growth or exostosis between the two palates is common. Normal palates are light pink. The soft palate appears smooth, whereas the hard palate is rough.

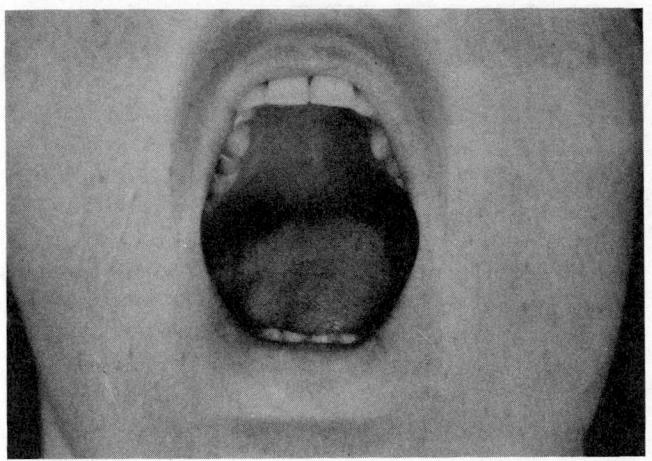

Fig. 13-33 The hard palate is located anteriorly in the roof of the mouth.

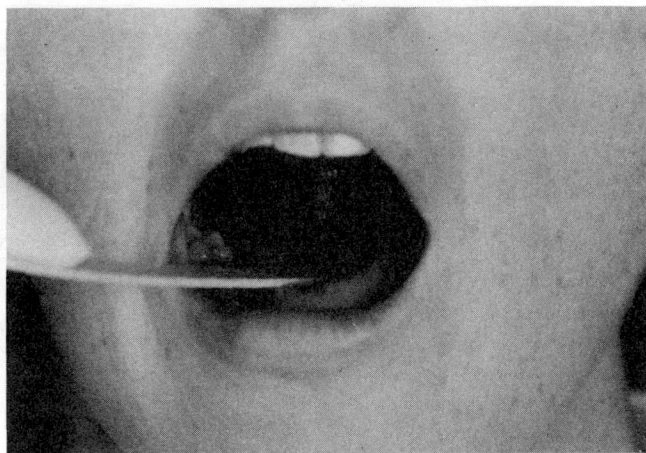

Fig. 13-34 A tongue depressor allows the nurse to visualize the uvula and posterior soft palate.

PHARYNX

Before examining the pharynx the nurse explains the procedure to the client. The client tips the head back slightly, opens the mouth wide, and says "ah." The nurse places the tip of a tongue depressor on the middle third of the tongue, taking care not to press the lower lip against the teeth. If the tongue depressor is placed too far anteriorly, the posterior part of the tongue mounds up, obstructing the view. The gag reflex is elicited when the tongue depressor touches the posterior tongue.

With a penlight, the nurse inspects the uvula and soft palate (Fig. 13-34). Both structures, which are innervated by the tenth cranial nerve (vagus), should rise centrally as the client says "ah." The nurse also inspects the arch formed by the anterior and posterior pillars, soft palate, and uvula. The tonsils can be viewed in the cavities between the anterior and posterior pillars and are oval with infoldings of tissue. The posterior pharynx is behind the pillars. The pharyngeal tissues are normally pink and smooth. Edema, ulcerations, or inflammation indicate infection or abnormal lesions. Clients with chronic sinus problems frequently exhibit a clear exudate that drains along the wall of the posterior pharynx. Yellow or green exudate indicates infection. A client with a typical sore throat has a reddened and edematous uvula and tonsillar pillars with the possible presence of yellow exudate.

Neck

The neck muscles, lymph nodes of the head, carotid arteries, jugular veins, thyroid gland, and trachea are located within the neck (Fig. 13-35). The nurse inspects and palpates these structures and auscultates the carotid arteries. Examination is best performed with the client

sitting. Areas of the neck are outlined by the sternocleidomastoid and trapezius muscles, which divide each side of the neck into two triangles (Fig. 13-36). The anterior triangle contains the trachea, thyroid gland, carotid artery, and anterior cervical lymph nodes. The posterior triangle contains the posterior lymph nodes. Table 13-16 reviews the nursing history for the neck examination.

NECK MUSCLES

To test the function of the sternocleidomastoid muscle, the nurse asks the client to flex the neck with the chin to the chest. The client hyperextends the neck back-

TABLE 13-16 Nursing History for Neck Assessment

Assessment Category	Rationale
Assess the client for a history of recent cold or infection.	Colds or infections can cause temporary or permanent lymph node enlargement.
Determine if client has history of thyroid problem or takes thyroid medication.	Disease or medications may influence tissue growth in thyroid gland.
Ask if client has had a history of neck pain.	Neck pain may be indicative of muscle strain, local nerve injury, or an enlarged or swollen lymph node.
Review history of pneumothorax (collapsed lung) or bronchial tumor.	These conditions place client at risk for tracheal displacement or lateral deviation.

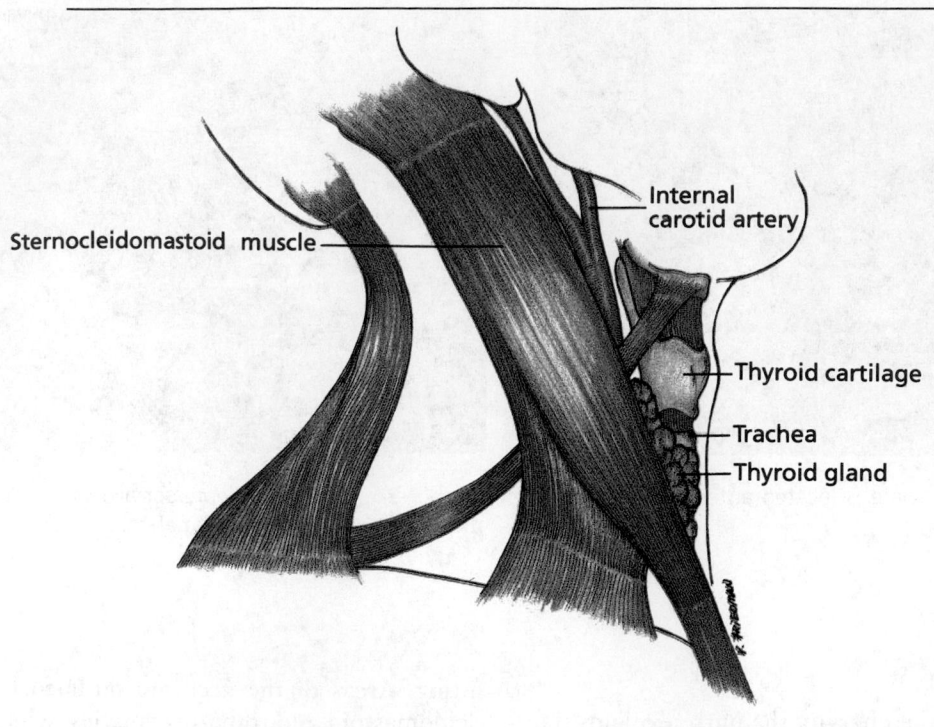

Fig. 13-35 Anatomical position of major neck structures. Note the triangles formed by the sternocleidomastoid muscle, lower jaw and anterior neck anteriorly and sternocleidomastoid muscle, trapezius muscle, and lower neck posteriorly.

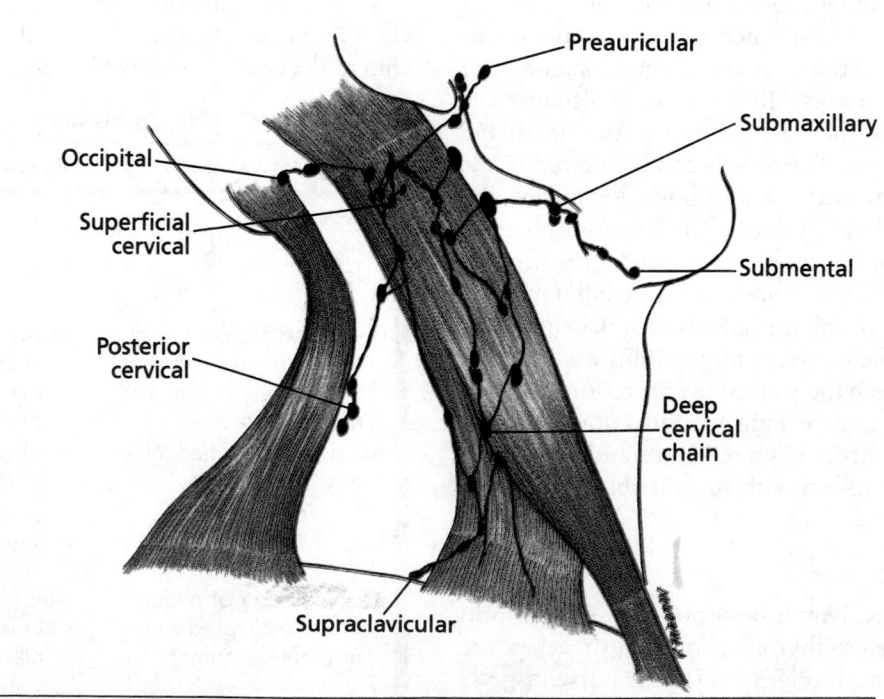

Fig. 13-36 Head and neck lymphatic system.

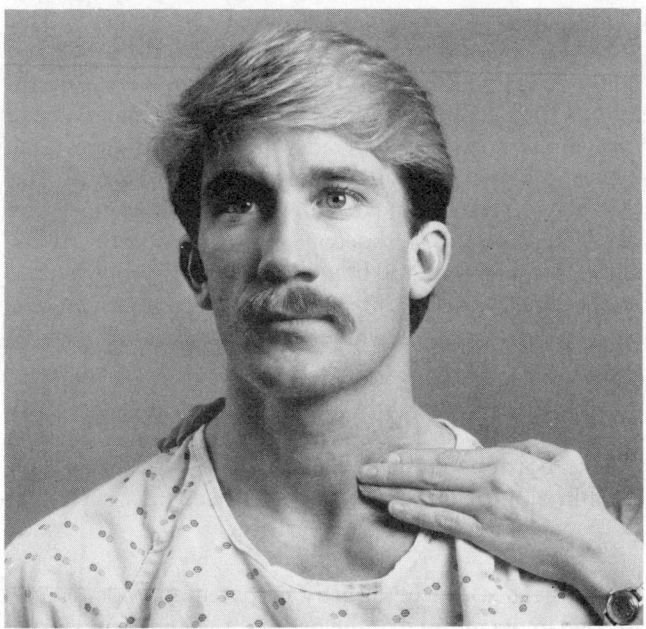

Fig. 13-37   Palpation of cervical lymph nodes.

ward to check for trapezius muscle function. Movement of the head sideways so the ear moves toward the shoulder further tests function of the sternocleidomastoid muscle. Other tests for muscle strength and function can be also performed (see "Musculoskeletal System").

LYMPH NODES

With the client's chin raised and head tilted backwards, the nurse inspects the neck for symmetry, masses, or scars. If masses are seen, they should be palpated to assess size, shape, tenderness, consistency, and mobility. An extensive system of lymph nodes collects lymph from the head, ears, nose, cheeks, and lips. Fig. 13-36 illustrates the location of each major lymphatic center in the head and neck.

A methodical approach is used to examine the lymph nodes to avoid overlooking any single node or chain. The client relaxes with the neck flexed slightly forward and, if needed, toward the side of the examiner. This maneuver relaxes tissues and muscles. Both sides of the neck are inspected and palpated for comparison. During palpation the nurse faces or stands to the side of the client for easy access to all nodes. Using the pads of the middle three fingers of each hand, the nurse palpates gently in a rotary motion over the nodes (Fig. 13-37). If excessive pressure is applied, small nodes are missed and palpable nodes are obliterated.

To palpate supraclavicular nodes the nurse asks the client to bend the head forward and relax the shoulders. The nurse may have to hook the index and third finger over the clavicle, lateral to the sternocleidomastoid muscle, to palpate nodes. The deep cervical nodes can only be palpated with the nurse's fingers hooked around the sternocleidomastoid muscle.

The lymph nodes serve as collecting sites for lymphatic fluid. Normally the nodes are not easily palpable. However, small, mobile, nontender nodes are not uncommon. The nodes become enlarged from localized and systemic infection.

The lymph nodes can also be the site of malignant tumors. A malignancy is usually hard, immobile, irregularly shaped, and often nontender (see client-teaching box).

THYROID GLAND

The thyroid gland lies in the anterior lower neck, in front of and to both sides of the trachea. The gland is fixed to the trachea with the isthmus overlying the trachea and connecting the two irregular, cone-shaped lobes (Fig. 13-38). The nurse assesses the gland by inspection, palpation, and auscultation.

The nurse stands in front of the client and inspects the area of the lower neck overlying the thyroid gland for visible masses and symmetry. The client should extend the neck and swallow, with the nurse noting whether these maneuvers cause a bulging of the gland. Normally the thyroid cannot be visualized.

To palpate the gland, the examiner stands either in front of or behind the client. For the posterior approach the client lowers the chin to relax the neck muscles. Both of the nurse's hands are placed around the neck with the fingertips overlying the lower trachea. The thyroid isthmus is palpated and the client swallows. Any enlargement of the isthmus as it rises should be noted. To examine each lobe, the nurse has the client turn the head slightly toward the side being examined (Fig. 13-39). For example, during examination of the left lobe the client lowers the chin and turns the head slightly to the left. The examiner's right hand gently displaces the thyroid to the left while the left hand palpates the lobe. This procedure is repeated for the right lobe. Normally the thyroid gland is not enlarged. However, in extremely thin individuals the thyroid is more easily palpable. Enlargement is a manifestation of thyroid dysfunction. Masses or nodules can be signs of malignant disease.

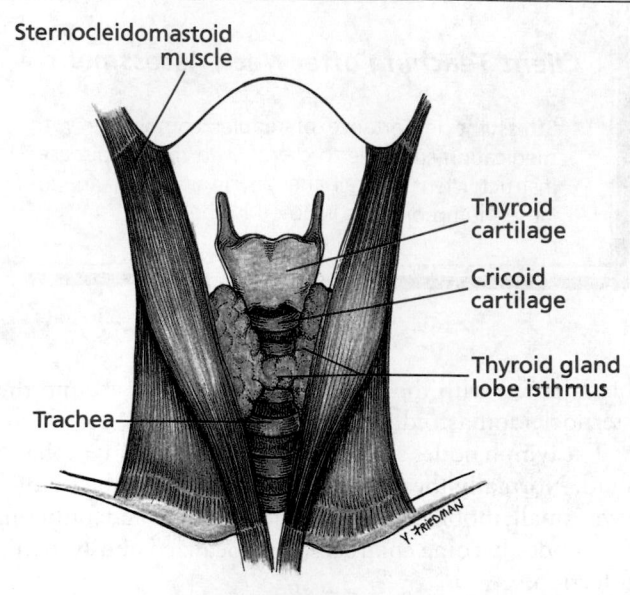

Fig. 13-38 The thyroid gland lies anteriorly in the neck. It is fixed to both sides of the trachea, with the isthmus overlying the trachea.

The anterior approach follows the same maneuvers as the posterior approach. The nurse uses the index and middle fingers of the dominant hand to palpate the isthmus as the client swallows. Then, with the client's head turned alternately to each side, the nurse displaces each lobe and palpates it with the other hand.

When the gland appears enlarged, the nurse places the diaphragm of the stethoscope over the thyroid. If the gland is enlarged, blood flow through the thyroid arteries increases and causes a fine vibration. The nurse can auscultate the vibration, which is heard as a soft, rushing sound or bruit.

CAROTID ARTERY AND JUGULAR VEIN

This portion of the examination is described under examination of the vascular system (see later section).

TRACHEA

The trachea can be directly palpated and is normally located in the midline of the neck, above the suprasternal notch. Masses in the neck or mediastinum and pulmonary abnormalities can cause displacement laterally. The client may sit or lie down during palpation. The position of the trachea is determined by palpating at the suprasternal notch, slipping the thumb and index fingers to each side (Fig. 13-40). Forceful pressure must not be applied because this action may elicit a cough.

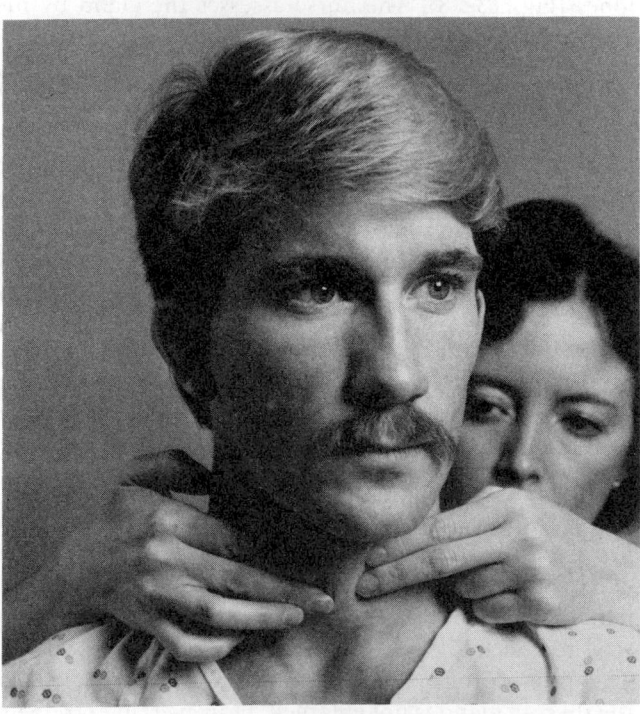

Fig. 13-39 The nurse palpates each thyroid lobe by having the client lower the chin and turn the head toward the side being examined.

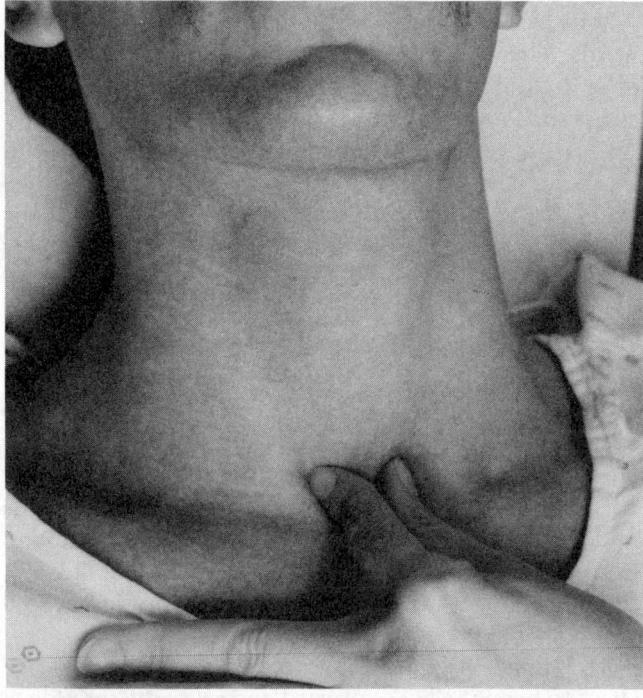

Fig. 13-40 The nurse palpates the trachea just above the suprasternal notch.

THORAX AND LUNGS

Physical assessment of the thorax and lungs takes into consideration the vital ventilatory and respiratory roles of the lungs. If the lungs are affected by disease, other body systems will reflect alterations. For example, reduced oxygenation can cause changes in a person's mental alertness because of the brain's sensitivity to lowered oxygen levels. The alert nurse uses the data from all body systems to determine the nature of pulmonary alterations.

Before assessing the thorax and lungs, the nurse must be familiar with the landmarks of the chest (Fig. 13-41). These landmarks help the nurse describe the location of findings and use assessment skills correctly. For example, by knowing the position of underlying organs in relation to the landmarks, the nurse can anticipate where to percuss or auscultate the chest wall. The landmarks are a series of imaginary lines and easily identifiable anatomical landmarks such as the ribs and spine. The lungs and thorax are assessed anteriorly, laterally (on both sides), and posteriorly, with the nurse using landmarks to record localized findings.

During the examination, the nurse keeps a mental image of the location of the lobes of the lung (Fig. 13-42). Locating the position of each rib is critical to visualizing the lobe of the lung being assessed. The angle of Louis, at the junction between the manubrium and the body of the sternum, is the starting point for locating the ribs anteriorly. Knowing that the second rib extends from the angle makes it easy to locate and palpate the intercostal spaces (between the ribs) in succession. The spinous process of the third thoracic vertebra and the fourth, fifth, and sixth ribs helps to locate the lung's lobes laterally. The lower lobes project laterally and anteriorly (Fig. 13-43). Posteriorly the tip or inferior margin of the scapula lies approximately at the level of the seventh rib (Fig. 13-44). Once the seventh rib is identified, the examiner can count upward to locate the third thoracic vertebra and align it with the inner borders of the scapula to locate the posterior lobes.

Examination of the lungs and thorax requires the client to be undressed to the waist. Good lighting is essential. The nurse uses each physical assessment skill in an orderly, systematic fashion. The nurse should assess clients at risk for pulmonary problems, such as the client confined to bed rest or the client with chest pain who cannot fully expand the lungs. The examination begins with the client sitting for assessment of the posterior and lateral chest. To assess the anterior chest, the

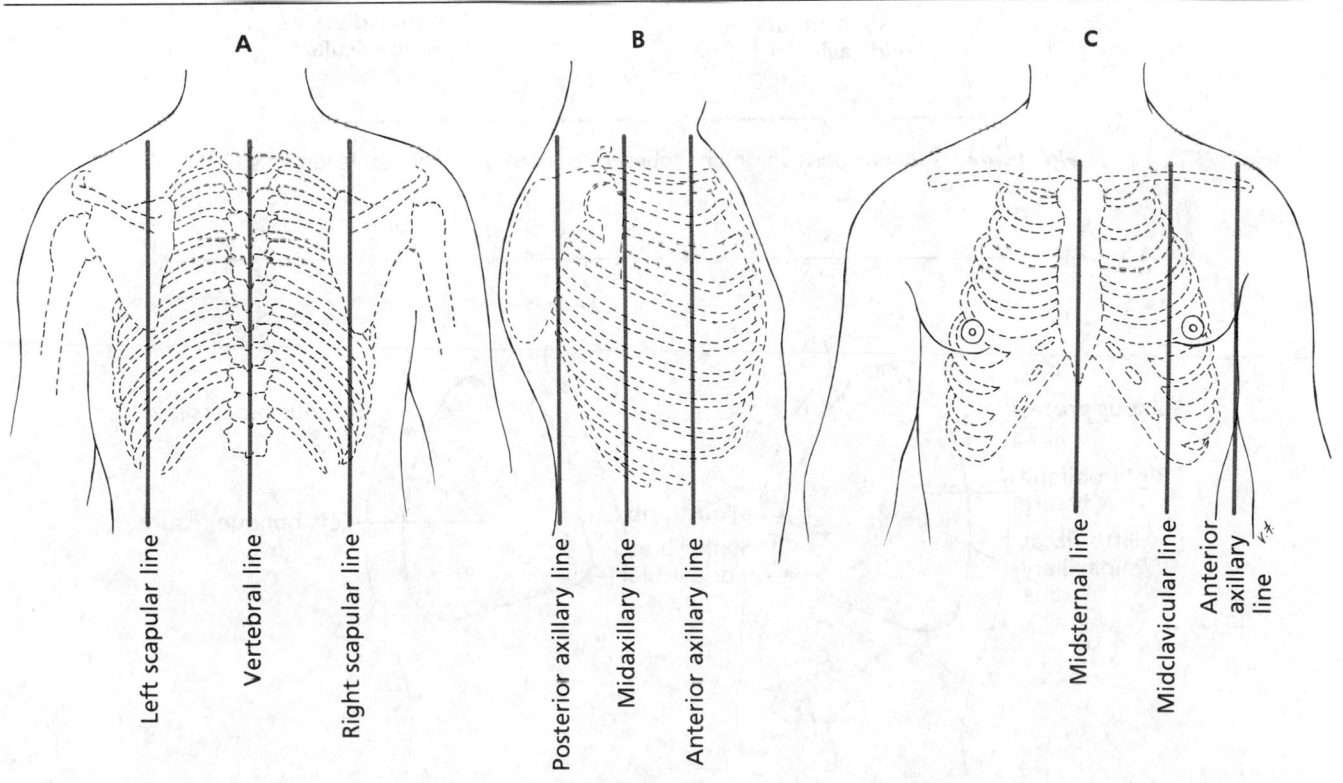

Fig. 13-41   Anatomical chest wall landmarks. **A,** Posterior chest landmarks. **B,** Anterior chest landmarks. **C,** Lateral chest landmarks.

nurse positions the client sitting or lying. Table 13-17 reviews the nursing history for lung examination.

Posterior Thorax

The nurse first inspects the shape of the client's chest. Shape or posture can significantly impair ventilatory movement. Normally the chest contour is symmetrical and the chest is twice as wide as deep (anteroposterior diameter in a 1:2 ratio) (Fig. 13-45). A small infant has a 1:1 ratio, with the chest having an almost round shape. Abnormal contours are caused by congenital and pos-

tural alterations. Aging and chronic lung disease are characterized by a barrel-shaped chest (anteroposterior to lateral diameter become 1:1).

Standing at a midline position behind the client, the nurse looks for deformities, position of the spine, slope of the ribs, retraction of the intercostal spaces on inspiration, and bulging of the intercostal spaces on expiration. The scapulae are normally symmetrical and closely attached to the thoracic wall. The normal spine is straight without lateral deviation. Posteriorly, the ribs tend to slope across and down. The ribs and intercostal spaces are easier to see in a thin person. Normally, no

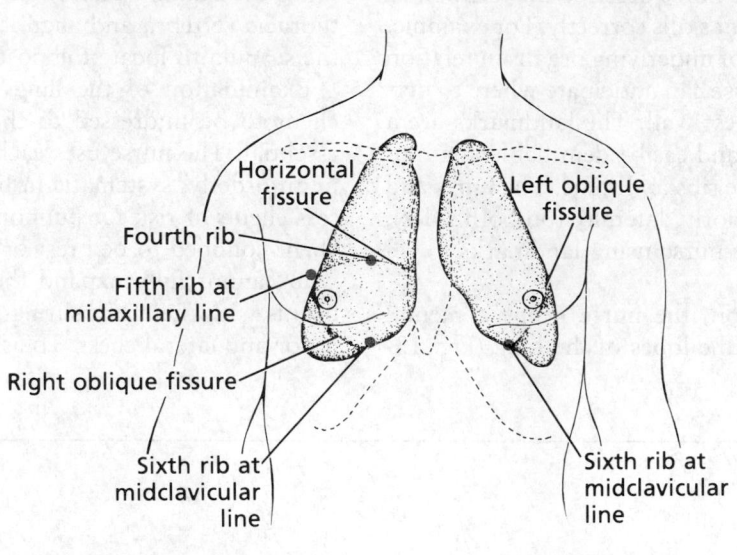

Fig. 13-42 Anterior position of lung lobes in relation to anatomical landmarks.

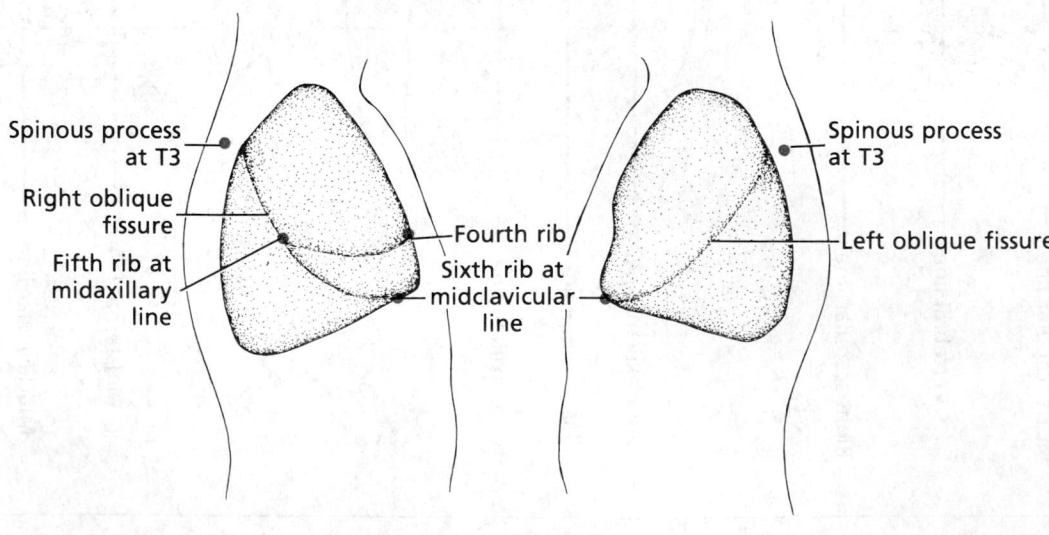

Fig. 13-43 Lateral position of lung lobes in relation to anatomical landmarks.

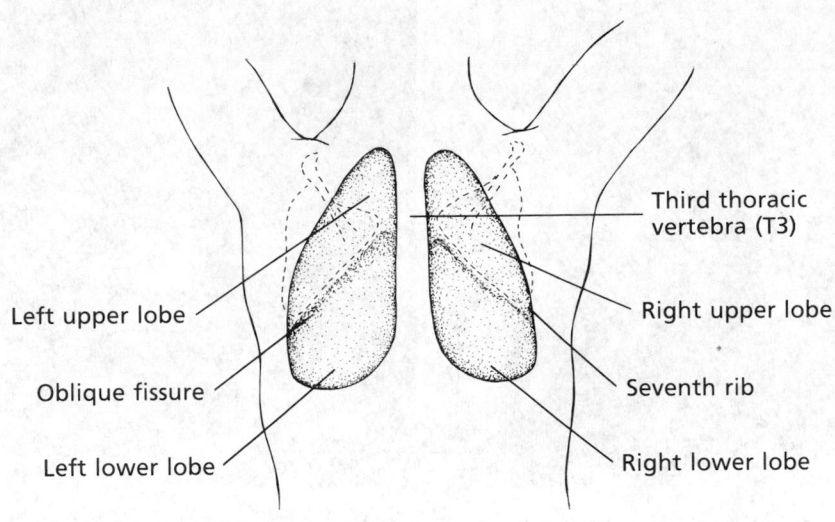

Fig. 13-44 Posterior position of lung lobes in relation to anatomical landmarks.

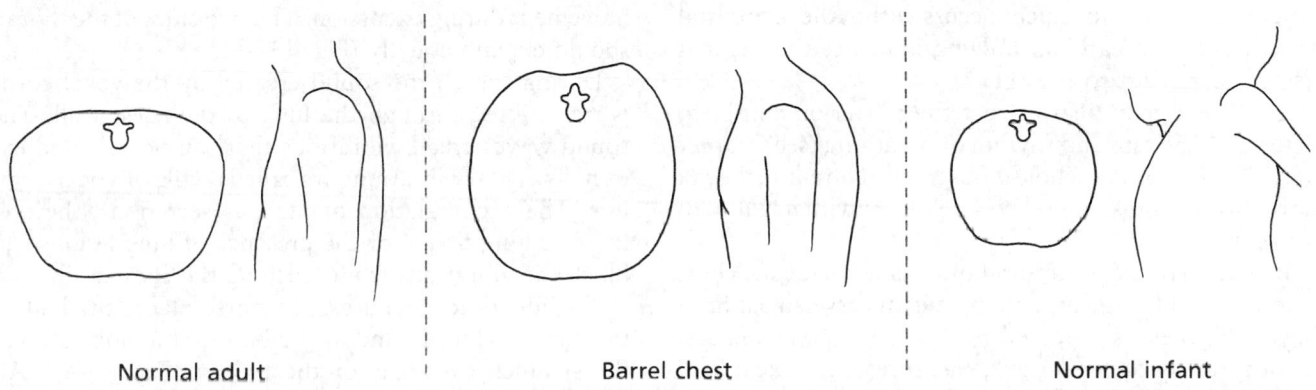

Fig. 13-45 Anteroposterior diameter of normal chest, barrel chest, and infant chest.

TABLE 13-17 Nursing History for Lung Assessment

Assessment Category	Rationale
Assess history of smoking, including number of years smoked, number of cigarettes per day, cigar or pipe-smoking, and length of time since stopping smoking.	Smoking is risk factor for lung cancer, heart disease, and emphysema or bronchitis. Smoking accounts for 30% of all cancer deaths (American Cancer Society, 1986).
Ask client if he has any of the following symptoms: cough (productive or nonproductive), amount of sputum production, shortness of breath, orthopnea, and poor activity tolerance.	Symptoms of respiratory alterations may help nurse localize any objective physical findings.
Determine if client works in environment containing pollutants, (for example, asbestos, coal dust, or chemical irritants).	These risk factors indicate various lung diseases.
Assess history of allergies to pollens, dust, or other airborne irritants, as well as to foods, drugs, or chemical substances.	Symptoms such as choking feeling, bronchospasm with respiratory stridor, wheezes on auscultation, and dyspnea may be caused by allergic response.
Review family history for cancer, tuberculosis, allergies, or chronic obstructive pulmonary disease (COPD).	These conditions may place client at risk for lung disease.

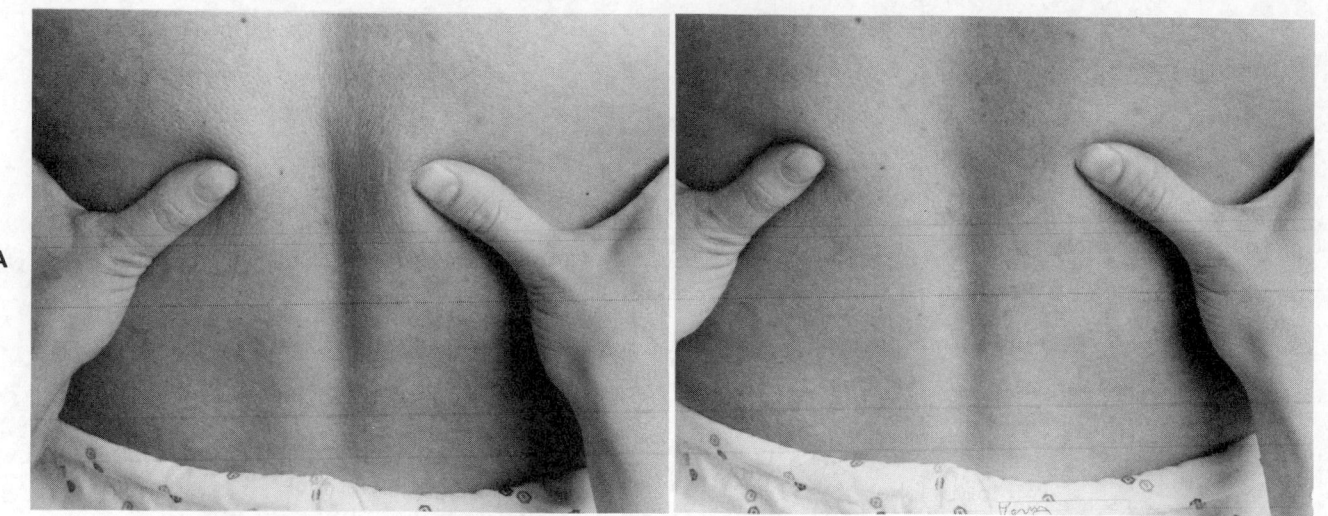

Fig. 13-46 A, Position of nurse's hands for palpation of posterior thorax excursion. B, As the client inhales the movement of chest excursion separates the nurse's thumbs.

bulging or active movement occurs within the intercostal spaces during breathing. Bulging indicates the client is using great effort to breathe.

The nurse may also inspect the posterior thorax to determine the rate and rhythm of breathing (see Chapter 36). The thorax as a whole is observed. The entire thorax normally expands and relaxes regularly with equality of movement.

Palpation of the posterior thorax assesses further characteristics and confirms or supplements assessment findings. The chest is palpated to detect lumps or masses, identify areas of tenderness, measure chest excursion, and elicit tactile fremitus.

If a suspicious mass or swollen area is detected, it is lightly palpated for size, shape, and the typical qualities of a lesion. When pain or tenderness is elicited, deep palpation is not used because deep palpation of a fractured rib segment could displace the bone fragment against vital organs.

Chest excursion is used to determine the depth of breathing. While standing behind the client the nurse places the hands on the lower portion of each rib cage. The hands are held parallel with the thumbs at the level of the tenth ribs, 2 inches apart and pointing toward the spine. The fingers point out laterally. The hands are pressed toward the spine so a small fold of skin appears between the thumbs. The nurse does not slide the hands over the skin. After exhalation, the client takes a deep breath and the movement of the examiner's thumbs is noted. Normally the thumbs are separated 1½ to 2 inches (3 to 5 cm) during excursion.

In the elderly, chest movement declines because of costal cartilage calcification and respiratory muscle atrophy. The nurse normally feels symmetry of respiratory movement during excursion. The two sides of the thorax should expand equally (Fig. 13-46).

During speech the sound created by the vocal cords is transmitted through the lung to the chest wall. The sound waves create vibrations that can be palpated externally. These vibrations are called tactile or vocal fremitus. The accumulation of mucous secretions, the collapse of lung tissue, or the presence of lung lesions can block the vibrations from reaching the chest wall.

To palpate for fremitus, the nurse places the ball of the hand (palm of hand at the base of the fingers) over the symmetrical areas of the thorax (Fig. 13-47, *A*), beginning at the lung apex. The nurse asks the client to repeat the words "ninety-nine" or "one-one-one." Normally there is a faint vibration as the client speaks. Both sides of the thorax are compared, moving from top to bottom. Only one hand is used to ensure accuracy. If fremitus is faint, it may be necessary to ask the client to speak in a louder or lower tone of voice. Symmetry of fremitus is normal. Vibrations are strongest at the top, near the level of the tracheal bifurcation. It is easy to assess for fremitus in a crying infant because strong vibrations can be felt through the chest wall.

Percussion of the chest wall determines whether underlying lung tissue is air filled, fluid filled, or solid. However, percussion only reaches 5 to 7 cm into the chest wall and thus cannot detect deep lesions. The client folds the arms forward across the chest. This position separates the scapulae further to expose more lung to assessment. Using the indirect technique, the nurse percusses in the intercostal spaces over symmetrical areas of the lungs. Resonance, the sound created by air-filled lungs, is heard over the posterior thorax. The chest is normally more resonant in the child than in the adult.

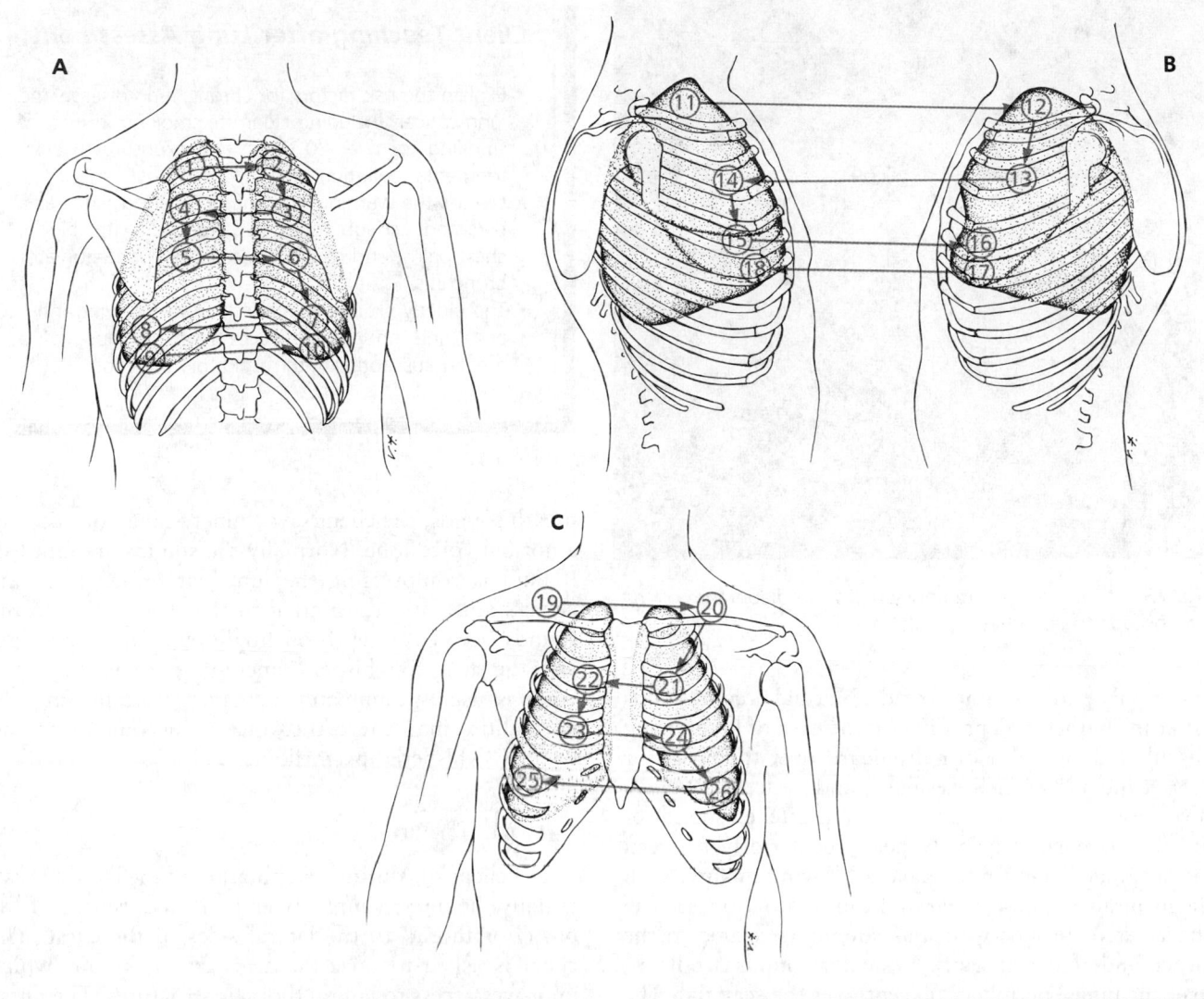

Fig. 13-47 A to C, The nurse follows a systematic pattern (posterior-lateral-anterior) when comparing fremitus, percussion notes, and auscultation.

If the nurse percusses over the scapulae, ribs, spine, or muscle, the percussion note will sound flat. A lung mass also causes a flat sound. An examiner may percuss over a bony area to compare sounds to be assured that flatness is the sound being identified.

Auscultation assesses the movement of air through the tracheobronchial tree. Air flows through the airways in an unobstructed pattern. Recognizing the sounds created by normal airflow allows the nurse to detect sounds caused by obstruction.

In an adult the diaphragm of the stethoscope is placed over the posterior chest wall between the ribs (Fig. 13-48). The bell works best in a child because of the small chest. The client should take slow, deep breaths with the mouth slightly open. The examiner listens to an entire inspiration and expiration at each position of the stethoscope. If sounds are faint, as in the case of the obese client, the client should be asked to breathe harder and faster. Breath sounds are much louder in children because of the thinness of the chest wall. The systematic pattern used in percussion should be used when comparing the right and left sides. An inexperienced student may attempt to auscultate all the left side and then return to the right side. This is incorrect. The assessor compares the sounds in one region on one side of the body with sounds in the same region on the opposite side. It is impossible to remember the quality of all sounds noted on one side of the body and then compare them with the other side.

The nurse auscultates for normal breath sounds and

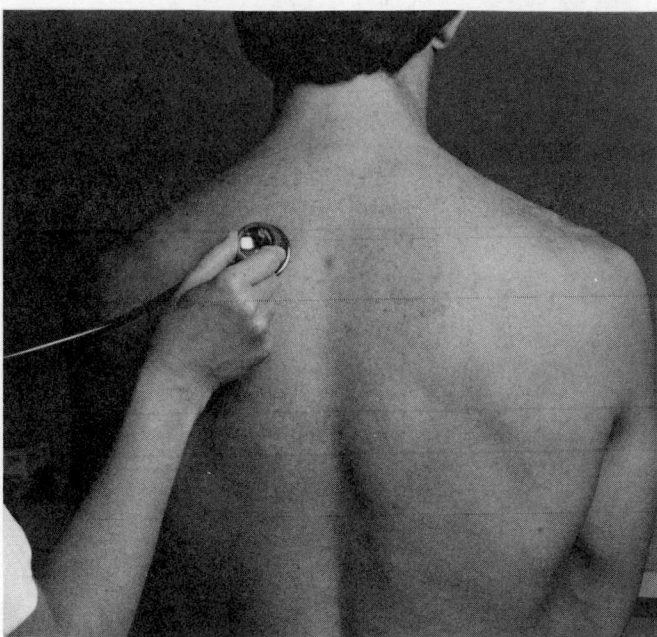

Fig. 13-48 In an adult the nurse uses the diaphragm of the stethoscope to auscultate breath sounds.

abnormal or adventitious sounds. Normal breath sounds differ in character, depending on the area of lungs being auscultated. Sounds normally heard over the posterior thorax include bronchovesicular and vesicular sounds. Bronchovesicular sounds are medium-pitched sounds of medium intensity normally heard posteriorly between the scapulae. The sounds have a blowing quality, with the inspiratory phase equal to the expiratory phase. The character of bronchovesicular sounds is related to the larger underlying airways. Vesicular sounds are heard over the lungs' periphery (except over the scapula). The sounds are created by air moving through the smaller airways. Vesicular sounds are soft, breezy, and low-pitched, and the inspiratory phase is about three times longer than the expiratory phase.

Abnormal sounds result from air passing through moisture, mucus, or narrowed airways, from alveoli suddenly reinflating, or from an inflammation between the lung's pleural linings. Adventitious sounds often occur superimposed over normal sounds. The four types of adventitious sounds include *crackles* (previously called *rales*), *rhonchi, wheezes,* and *pleural friction rub.* Each sound is caused by a specific entity and is characterized by typical auditory features (Table 13-18).

The location and characteristics of the sounds should be noted, as should the absence of breath sounds (found in clients with collapsed or surgically removed lobes).

If the nurse assesses abnormalities in tactile fremitus, percussion, or auscultation, another test is performed for spoken and whispered voice sounds. With the stethoscope placed over the same locations used to assess breath sounds, the client says "ninety-nine" or "eee" in a normal voice tone. Normally the sounds are muffled. If fluid is compressing the lung, vibrations from the client's voice are transmitted to the chest wall and the sounds become clear (bronchophony). The nurse then asks the client to whisper "ninety-nine." The whispered voice is usually faint and indistinct. Certain lung abnormalities may cause the voice to become clear and distinct (whispered pectoriloquy).

Lateral Thorax

The client sits during examination of the lateral chest. Usually the nurse simply extends the assessment of the posterior thorax to the lateral sides of the chest. The client is asked to raise the arms up in the air, which improves access to lateral thoracic structures. The nurse uses all four assessment skills (Fig. 13-47, *B*). Excursion cannot be assessed laterally. Normally, percussion notes are resonant and breath sounds are vesicular.

Anterior Thorax

The anterior thorax is inspected for the same features as the posterior thorax. The client sits or lies down. Anteriorly, the width of the costal angle is noted. It is usually larger than 90 degrees between the two costal margins. The nurse observes the breathing pattern. Normal breathing is quiet and barely audible near the open mouth. Clients with chronic obstructive pulmonary disease (COPD) (emphysema and chronic bronchitis) breathe noisily and may produce a grunting sound (see client-teaching box).

The accessory muscles of breathing—sternocleidomastoids and trapezius in the neck and abdominal muscles—are observed. Breathing is usually a passive activity with little effort required to ventilate. When the client

TABLE 13-18   Adventitious Sounds

Sound	Site Auscultated	Cause	Character
Crackles (previously called rales)	Most common in dependent lobes: right and left lung bases	Random, sudden reinflation of groups of alveoli (Forgacs, 1978)	Fine, short, interrupted crackling sounds heard during inspiration, expiration, or both; vary in pitch: high or low; may or may not change with coughing (Forgacs, 1978)
Rhonchi	Primarily over trachea and bronchi, if loud enough, can be heard over most lung fields	Fluid or mucus in larger airways, causing turbulence	Low-pitched, continuous musical sounds heard more during expiration; may be cleared by coughing
Wheezes	Can be heard over all lung fields	Severely narrowed bronchus	High-pitched, continuous musical sounds heard during inspiration or expiration; do not clear with coughing. (Wilkins, 1987)
Pleural friction rub	Anterior lateral lung field (if client sitting upright)	Pleura becomes inflamed; parietal pleura rubs against visceral pleura	Has grating quality; heard best on inspiration; does not clear with coughing

is forced to use effort to ventilate, the accessory muscles are used and can be seen contracting.

Respiratory rate and rhythm are more often assessed anteriorly. The male client's respirations are usually diaphragmatic, whereas the female's are more costal. The examiner palpates anteriorly for areas of abnormality, tenderness, chest excursion, and tactile fremitus. To measure chest excursion anteriorly, the nurse places the hands on the lateral rib cage, with the thumbs approximately 2 inches (5 cm) apart and angled along each costal margin (Fig. 13-49, *A*). The thumbs are pushed toward the midline to create a fold of skin between the thumbs. As the client inhales deeply, the thumbs should normally separate approximately 1½ to 2 inches (3 to 5 cm), with each side expanding equally (Fig. 13-49, *B*).

Tactile fremitus is assessed over the chest wall. Anterior findings differ from posterior findings because of the heart and female breast tissue. Fremitus is decreased over the precordium (area over the heart and lower thorax). The nurse will not be able to sense vibrations over breast tissue and thus must retract the breasts gently during palpation. If the breasts are large, this portion of the examination may be omitted.

Percussion of the anterior thorax follows a systematic

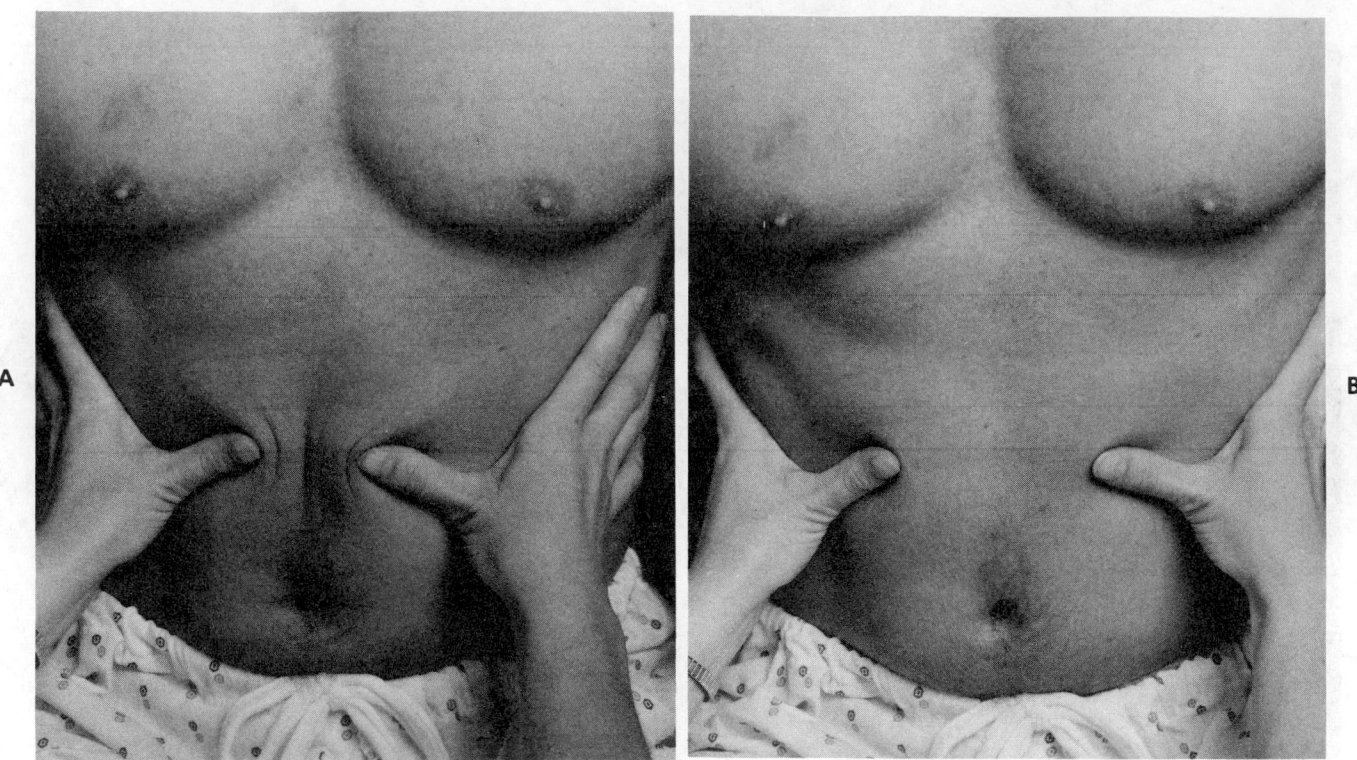

Fig. 13-49 **A**, Position of nurse's hands before excursion of the anterior chest wall. **B**, As the client inhales, the nurse's hands normally separate 3 to 5 cm (1½ to 2 inches).

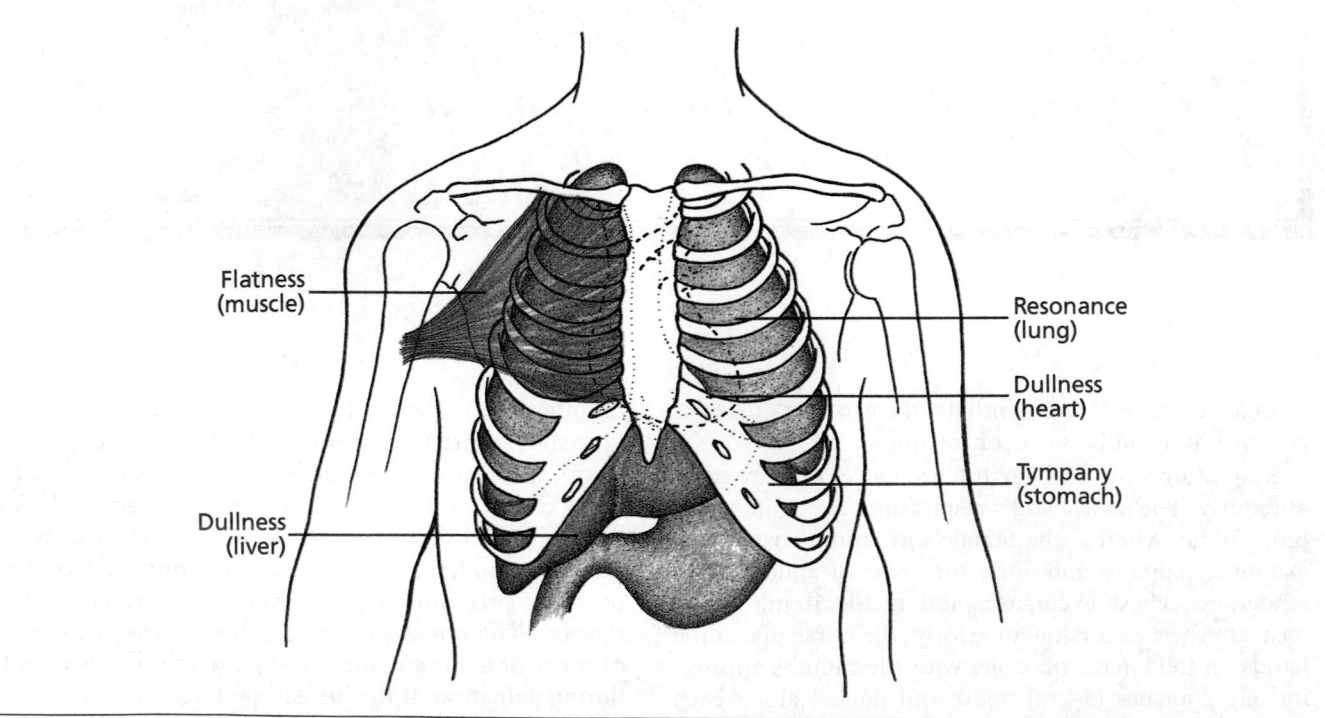

Fig. 13-50 Variations in percussion notes in normal thorax and upper abdomen.

pattern. The nurse must imagine the location of all internal organs accessible to examination anteriorly. The underlying liver, heart, and stomach create percussion notes characteristically different from those of the lung (Fig. 13-50). Percussion may be conducted with the client in a sitting or lying position. However, the procedure is easier for the examiner if the client lies down. The examiner starts above the clavicles and moves across and then down. The female breasts are displaced as needed. The normal lung is resonant. As the examiner proceeds downward, the areas of heart and liver dullness and the tympanic gastric air bubble will be detectable.

Auscultation of the anterior thorax follows the same pattern as percussion (Fig. 13-47, C, p. 277). The client should sit if possible to maximize chest expansion. In addition to bronchovesicular and vesicular sounds, a normal breath sound can be heard anteriorly. This bronchial sound is loud and high pitched. It has a hollow quality, with expiration lasting longer than inspiration (3:2 ratio). It is normally heard only over the trachea.

HEART

A client who has signs or symptoms of heart (cardiac) problems may be suffering a life-threatening condition requiring immediate attention. The nurse must sense which portions of an examination are absolutely necessary. When a client's condition is stable, assessment can reveal risks for heart disease or findings requiring a physician's attention. The nurse performing a cardiac assessment compares findings with those made in the vascular examination (see "Vascular System"). The nursing history (Table 13-19) provides data that helps to interpret physical findings.

Assessment of heart (cardiac) function is performed through the anterior thorax. The nurse forms a mental image of the heart's exact location. In the adult it is in the center of the chest (precordium) behind and to the left of the sternum, with a small section of the right atrium extending to the sternum's right. The base of the heart is the upper portion and the apex is the bottom tip. The surface of the right ventricle composes most of the heart's anterior surface. A section of the left ventricle shapes the left anterior side of the apex. The apex actually touches the anterior chest wall at approximately the fourth to fifth intercostal space along the midclavicular line, known as the *point of maximal impulse (PMI)*.

An infant's heart is positioned more horizontally and has a larger diameter compared with the total chest diameter than in an adult. The apex of the heart in an infant is at the third or fourth intercostal space, just to the left of the midclavicular line. By the age of 7 a child's PMI is in the same location as the adult's.

To understand the significance of assessment findings, the nurse must first understand timing in relation to the cardiac cycle (Fig. 13-51). The heart normally pumps blood through its four chambers in a methodical, even sequence. As the blood flows through each chamber, valves open and close, pressures within chambers rise and fall, and chambers contract. Each event creates a physiological sign that can be detected by an examiner.

TABLE 13-19 Nursing History for Heart Assessment

Assessment Category	Rationale
Determine history of smoking, exercise habits, and dietary patterns and intake.	Smoking, absent or reduced regular exercise, and intake of foods high in carbohydrates and cholesterol are risk factors for heart and vascular disease.
Determine if client is taking medications for cardiovascular function (for example, antidysrhythmics or antihypertensives) and if client knows their purpose, dosage, and side effects.	This knowledge allows nurse to assess compliance with drug therapies. Medications may affect vital sign values.
Assess for chest pain, palpitations, excess fatigue, dyspnea, edema of feet, cyanosis, fainting, or orthopnea. Ask if symptoms occur at rest or during exercise.	These are key symptoms of heart disease. Cardiovascular function may be adequate during rest but not during exercise.
Determine if client has a stressful life-style.	Repeated exposure to stress may increase the risk for heart disease.
Assess client's and family's history for heart problems (for example, heart attack, murmurs, or rheumatic heart disease).	Family history of heart problems increases the risk for heart disease.
Ask client about a history of heart trouble (for example, congestive heart failure, congenital heart disease, coronary artery disease, dysrhythmias).	This knowledge reveals client's level of understanding of condition. A condition will influence examination techniques used by nurse.

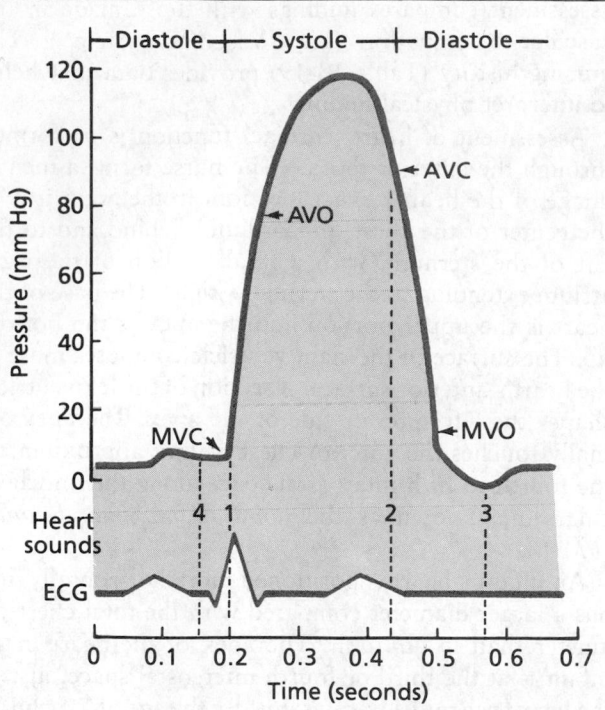

Fig. 13-51 Cardiac cycle.

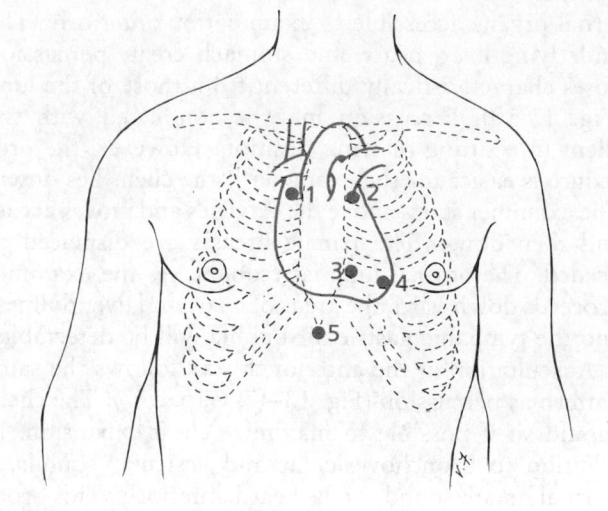

Fig. 13-52 Anatomical sites for assessment of cardiac function.

Both the right and left sides of the heart function in a coordinated fashion. Blood flows from the right atrium to the right ventricle and from the left atrium to the left ventricle through the atrioventricular valves. The tricuspid valve separates the right atrium and ventricle, and the mitral valve separates the left atrium and ventricle. Blood passes from the right ventricle through the pulmonic valve to the pulmonary artery. Similarly, blood leaves the left ventricle through the aortic valve into the aorta.

Events occurring on the left side of the heart have the most dramatic effect on assessment findings. Pressure is greatest on the left side, so longer and louder sounds are created. Events on the left side slightly precede those on the right. When the left ventricle is at rest (diastolic phase), the pressure in the left atrium exceeds that in the ventricle, creating a pressure gradient that moves blood through the opened mitral valve. During ventricular filling, pressure rises in the ventricle to exceed the pressure in the left atrium. Just before the ventricle contracts, the mitral valve closes to prevent regurgitation of blood back into the atrium, creating the first heart sound (S_1). Ventricular pressure builds, causing the aortic valve to open as the ventricle contracts (systolic phase). Blood flows into the aorta, elevating aortic pressure. When the ventricle empties, pressure within the chamber falls. To prevent regurgitation from the aorta back into the left ventricle, the aortic valve closes, creating the second heart sound (S_2). As ventricular pressure continues to fall, it drops below that of the left atrium. The mitral valve reopens to again allow ventricular filling. The rapid filling of the ventricle may create a third heart sound (S_3), heard more often in children and young adults. An S_3 can also be heard as an abnormality in older adults. When the atria contract to enhance ventricular filling, a fourth heart sound (S_4) is produced. The S_4 is not normally heard in adults.

Inspection and Palpation

The nurse uses inspection and palpation simultaneously. The examination begins with the client in the supine position or with the upper body elevated 45 degrees, since clients with heart disease frequently suffer shortness of breath while lying flat. The nurse stands on the client's right side. The client must refrain from talking, especially after the nurse begins auscultation of heart sounds. The nurse directs attention to the anatomical sites best suited for assessment of cardiac function. Louis' angle lies between the sternal body and manubrium and can be felt as a prominence on the sternum. The nurse can slip the fingers down each side of the angle, until he or she is able to feel the second intercostal spaces (Fig. 13-52, *dot 1*). The second intercostal space on the right is the aortic area, and the left second intercostal space is the pulmonic area. Deeper palpation is required to feel the spaces in obese clients or those with well-developed chest muscles.

The aortic and pulmonic areas are inspected for pulsations. Viewing these areas at an angle to the side im-

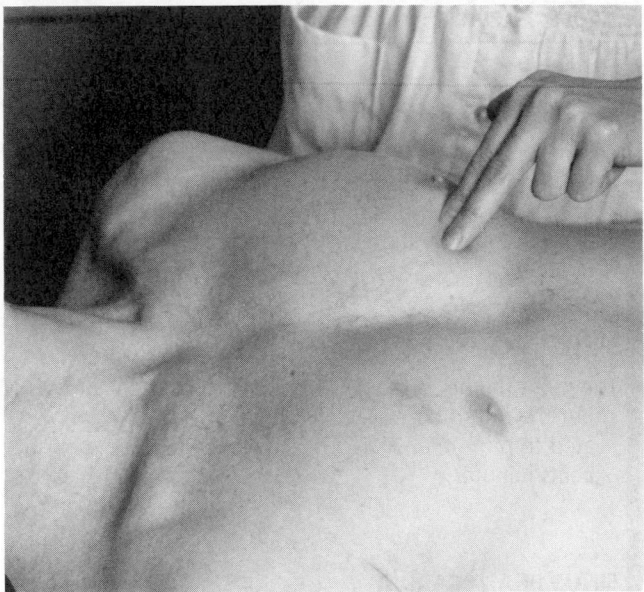

Fig. 13-53 Palpation of PMI at fourth to fifth intercostal space along midclavicular line.

proves the likelihood of detecting pulsation, which may arise from abnormalities in major vessels of the heart or improper valve closure. Pulsations are more easily felt with the fingertips. A vibration, felt best with the ball of the hand, is caused by loud murmurs. If pulsations or vibrations are palpated, the nurse times their occurrence in relation to systole or diastole by auscultating heart sounds simultaneously.

Inspection and palpation continue over the other anatomical sites. Once the pulmonic area is located (Fig. 13-52, *dot 2*), the nurse simply moves the fingers along the client's left sternal border to the fifth intercostal space to the tricuspid area (Fig. 13-52, *dot 3*). To find the apical area the nurse locates the fifth intercostal space just to the left of the sternum and moves the fingers laterally to the left midclavicular line (LMCL). Some examiners are able to locate the apical area with the palm of the hand but others use their fingertips (Fig. 13-52, *dot 4*). Normally, the apical impulse, or PMI, is a light tap felt in an area 1 to 2 cm (½ inch) in diameter (Fig. 13-53). If the apical pulse is more forceful, like a heave, it can be a sign of left ventricular failure. If the PMI cannot be found with the client in the supine position, the nurse asks the client to roll onto the left side, which moves the heart closer to the chest wall. The nurse estimates the heart's size by noting the diameter of the PMI and its position relative to the midclavicular line. In cases of serious heart disease, the cardiac muscle enlarges, with the PMI found to the left of the midclavicular line. The PMI may be difficult to find in the elderly because the chest deepens in its anteroposterior diameters. The PMI of an infant can usually be found near

the third or fourth intercostal space. It is easy to palpate the child's PMI because of the thin chest wall.

The final area to inspect and palpate is the epigastric area at the tip of the sternum (Fig. 13-52, *dot 5*). In clients with normal aortic structure and function, the pulsation of the abdominal aorta may be seen and felt.

Percussion

Percussion is rarely used during assessment of the adult heart. Chest x-ray studies are much more efficient in determining heart size. In infants, percussion can more easily detect the heart's borders because of the heart's proximity to the chest wall, a particularly important point for children with congenital defects whose hearts may be enlarged or malpositioned.

Auscultation

Auscultation of the heart detects normal heart sounds, extra heart sounds, and murmurs. The nursing student should first become skilled in detecting normal heart sounds. These low-intensity sounds, created by the closing of the valves, are often difficult to hear. Concentration is needed in detecting heart sounds. To begin auscultation the nurse eliminates all sources of room noise and explains the procedure to relieve the client's anxiety. The nurse must lift the female client's left breast to listen better to the chest wall.

The nurse first identifies the first (S_1) and second (S_2) heart sounds:

1. Auscultate using the diaphragm of the stethoscope because S_1 and S_2 are high-pitched sounds.
2. Begin auscultating at the apex or PMI (Fig. 13-54), then move systematically to the tricuspid, pulmonic, and aortic areas (Fig. 13-52, *dots 1 and 2*). A methodical approach ensures that all areas are assessed.
3. At normal slow rates, S_1 is high-pitched and dull in quality and sounds like a "lub." It is heard best at the apex and precedes the short systolic phase of heart contraction. If it is difficult to detect S_1, it should be timed in relation to the carotid pulse (see "Vascular System"). It occurs just before the carotid pulsation at systole.

Examiners learn first to hear the sound of S_2 at the aortic area. By slowly inching the stethoscope diagonally toward the apex and keeping the sound in focus, the nurse notes that S_2 begins to diminish in sound. S_1 gets louder, and soon, both sounds are heard as "lub dub." Once S_1 and S_2 are identified, the nurse assesses heart rate and rhythm:

1. Each combination of S_1 and S_2 counts as one heartbeat. The apical is assessed for one minute.
2. To assess heart rhythm, note the time between S_1 and S_2 (systole) and then the time between S_2 and the next

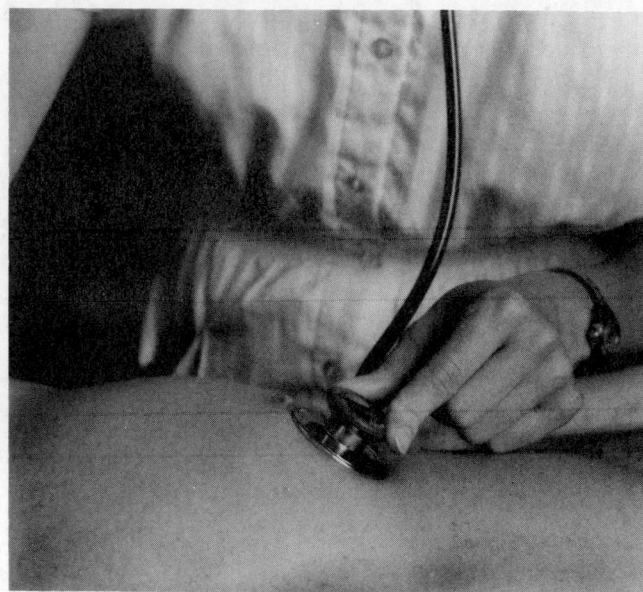

Fig. 13-54 Auscultation of heart sounds at the PMI using the diaphragm of the stethoscope.

S_1 (diastole). Listen to the full cycle at each auscultation area. A regular rhythm involves regular intervals of time between each sequence of beats.

3. Failure of the heart to beat at regular successive intervals is a dysrhythmia. Some dysrhythmias can be life threatening. Table 13-20 summarizes common dysrhythmias.

4. When the heart rhythm is irregular, apical and radial pulse rates are compared to determine if a pulse deficit exists. Auscultate the apical pulse first and then immediately palpate the radial pulse (see Chapter 12).

Compare the two rates. (Two nurses can work together, one assessing the apical and the other assessing the radial). With a deficit, the radial pulse is slower than the apical because ineffective contractions fail to send pulse waves to the periphery.

The next portion of the examination involves auscultation for extra heart sounds:

1. Apply the bell of the stethoscope, and listen for low-pitched extra heart sounds such as S_3 and S_4. Auscultate over each area.

2. S_3 occurs just after S_2 and S_4 occurs just before S_1. Both sounds occur during the diastolic phase of the cardiac cycle. S_3 and S_4 are common in children. Adults with extra sounds may suffer hypertension or enlargement of the left ventricle.

3. The nurse often hears S_3 and S_4 best with the client on his left side with the bell placed over the apex or PMI (Fig. 13-52, *dot 4*).

The final portion of the examination includes assessment for heart murmurs. Murmurs are sustained noises,

TABLE 13-20 Common Types of Dysrhythmias

Definition	Cause
SINUS DYSRHYTHMIA	
The pulse rate changes during respiration increasing at the peak of inspiration and declining during expiration.	Blood is momentarily trapped in the lungs during inspiration, causing a fall in the heart's stroke volume. This is a normal condition for children.
SINUS TACHYCARDIA	
The pulse rhythm is regular, but the rate is accelerated to more than 100 beats/minute.	Exercise, emotional stress, and caffeine or alcohol ingestion are common factors that cause increased firing of the sinoatrial node.
SINUS BRADYCARDIA	
Pulse rhythm is regular, but the rate is slower than normal at 40 to 60 beats/minute.	The sinoatrial node fires less frequently. This is common in well-conditioned athletes.
PREMATURE VENTRICULAR CONTRACTION	
Premature beat occurs before regularly expected heart contraction.	The ventricle contracts prematurely because of electrical impulse bypassing the normal conduction pathway. It may occur so early that it is difficult to detect as a second beat. It may be followed by a pause.
ATRIAL FIBRILLATION	
Rapid, random contractions of the atria cause irregular ventricular beats at 130 to 150 beats/minue.	Atria discharge very rapidly with some impulses not reaching ventricles. This condition occurs in rheumatic heart disease and mitral stenosis. It causes reduced cardiac output.

heard during systole, diastole, or both. They are caused by increased blood flow through a normal valve, forward flow through a stenotic valve or into a dilated vessel or heart chamber, or backward flow through a valve that fails to close. A murmur can thus be a sign of heart disease (see client-teaching box).

1. As the nurse auscultates each area over the heart, six factors are assessed when a murmur is detected: timing, location, radiation, intensity, pitch, and quality.

2. If a murmur occurs between S_1 and S_2, it is a systolic

Client Teaching after Heart Assessment

- Explain the risk factors for heart disease: high dietary intake of cholesterol, lack of regular aerobic exercise, smoking, stressful life-style, and family history of heart disease.
- Refer client (if appropriate) to resources available for controlling or reducing risks (for example, nutritional counseling, exercise class, and stress-reduction programs).
- For clients with heart disease, explain importance of compliance with complete treatment plan.

---

murmur. If it occurs between S_2 and the next S_1, it is a diastolic murmur.

3. The location of a murmur is not necessarily directly over the valves. With experience, a nurse can learn where each type of murmur is best heard. For example, mitral murmurs are heard best at the apex of the heart.

4. To assess for radiation the nurse listens for a murmur over areas besides where it is heard best. Murmurs can also sometimes be heard over the neck or back.

5. Intensity or loudness is related to the rate of blood flow through the heart or the amount of blood regurgitated. In serious murmurs the nurse may feel a thrust or intermittent palpable sensation at the auscultation site. A thrill is a continuous palpable sensation like the purring of a cat. Intensity is recorded in grades:

Grade I	Barely audible
Grade II	Audible immediately but faint
Grade III	Loud, without thrust or thrill
Grade IV	Loud, with thrust or thrill
Grade V	Very loud, with thrust or thrill; audible with stethoscope only partially applied.
Grade VI	Louder, may be heard without stethoscope

VASCULAR SYSTEM

Examination of the vascular system includes measurement of the blood pressure (see Chapter 12) and a thorough assessment of the integrity of the peripheral vascular system. Table 13-21 reviews the nursing history data collected before the examination. The nurse may perform portions of the vascular examination during assessment of other body systems. For example, the carotid pulse may be checked after palpation of cervical

TABLE 13-21 Nursing History for Vascular Assessment

Assessment Category	Rationale
Determine if the client experiences leg cramps, numbness, pain, or burning in the extremities or edema around the ankles.	These signs and symptoms indicate vascular disease.
If client experiences pain or cramping in the lower extremities ask if it is relieved or aggravated by walking.	Relationship of symptoms to exercise can clarify whether the problem is vascular or musculoskeletal. Pain caused by a vascular condition tends to increase with activity.
Ask female clients if they wear tight-fitting garters or knee-length nylons.	Tight clothing around lower extremities can impair venous return.
Assess medical history for heart disease, hypertension, phlebitis, diabetes, or varicose veins.	Circulatory and vascular disorders influence findings gathered during examination.

lymph nodes. As the nurse inspects the skin, signs and symptoms of arterial and venous insufficiency are noted. An experienced nurse integrates vascular assessment with other portions of the examination to minimize time spent in the total examination.

Blood Pressure

The nurse auscultates the blood pressure at the brachial artery site in both arms. Systolic readings that differ by 15 mm Hg or more suggest atherosclerosis or disease of the aorta. The nurse also compares the blood pressure in the lying position with the blood pressure in the sitting or standing position to assess for postural hypotension (see Chapter 42).

Arteries and Veins

Examination of the vascular system involves palpation, inspection, and auscultation. The nurse begins with an assessment of the integrity of accessible arteries and veins. In addition, the nurse notes the condition of the extremities perfused by the vascular system. Abnormalities interfering with arterial perfusion or venous return cause changes in the skin and tissues of affected extremities.

CAROTID ARTERIES

When the left ventricle pumps blood into the aorta, pressure waves are transmitted throughout the arterial

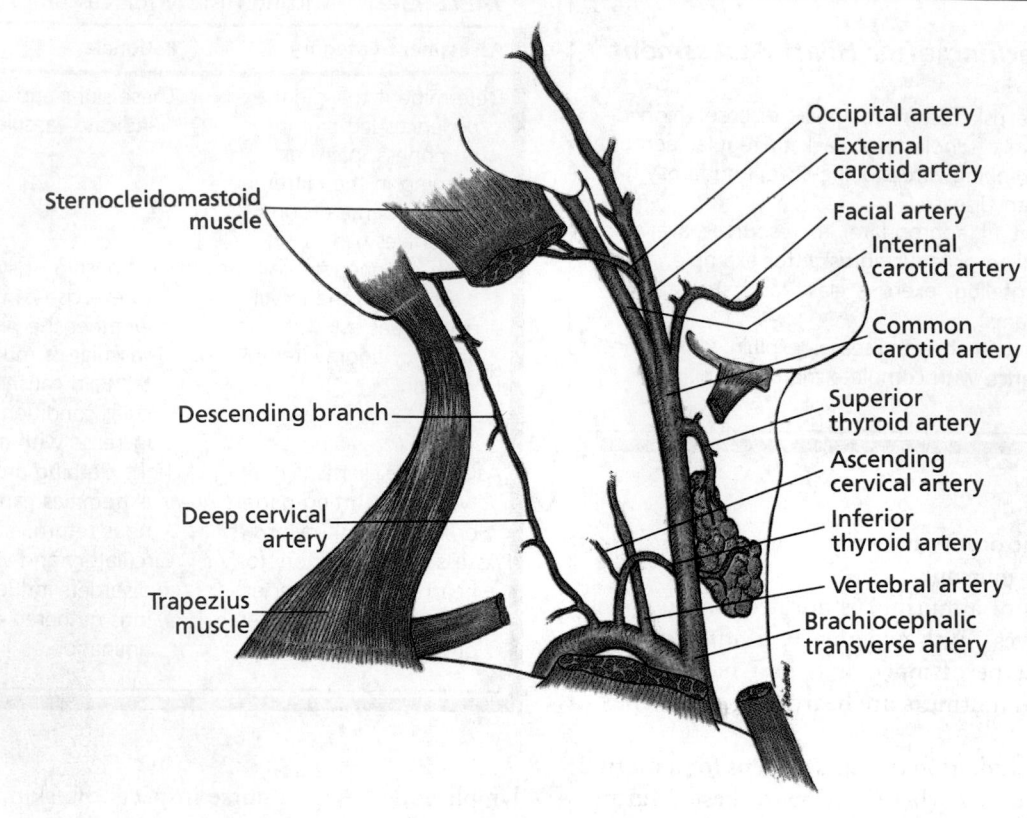

Fig. 13-55 Anatomical position of carotid artery.

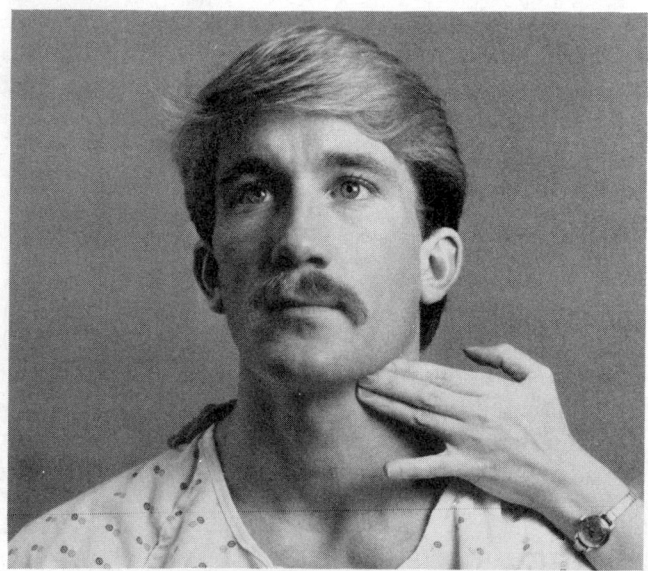

Fig. 13-56 Palpation of internal carotid artery along margin of the sternomastoid muscle.

system. Pressure waves are manifested as pulses that are palpable in arteries close to the skin or overlying bone. The carotid artery reflects heart function better than peripheral arteries because its pressure correlates with that of the aorta.

The carotid artery supplies oxygenated blood to the head and neck (Fig. 13-55) and is protected by the overlying sternocleidomastoid muscle.

To examine the carotid arteries, the nurse has the client sit. *One carotid artery is examined at a time.* If both arteries were to be occluded during palpation, the client could lose consciousness as a result of inadequate circulation to the brain. *The carotids must not be vigorously palpated or massaged.* The carotid sinus is in the upper third of the neck. Its stimulation can cause a reflex drop in heart rate and blood pressure.

The neck is inspected for obvious pulsation of the artery. Sometimes, the wave of the pulse can actually be seen. The carotid is the only site for assessing the quality of a pulse wave. Only an experienced assessor can evaluate the quality of the wave in relation to systole and diastole of the cardiac cycle.

To palpate the pulse, the nurse slides the index and middle fingers around the medial edge of the sterno-

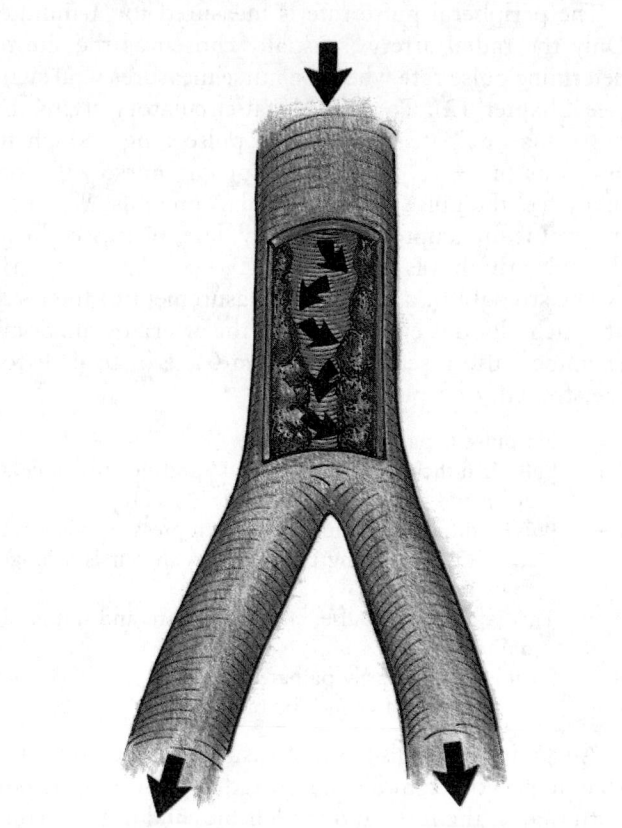

Fig. 13-57 Occlusion or narrowing of the carotid artery disrupts normal blood flow. The resultant turbulence creates a sound (bruit) the nurse can auscultate.

cleidomastoid muscle. The client turns the head slightly toward the side examined. This maneuver permits better access to the artery. The nurse palpates gently to avoid occlusion of circulation (Fig. 13-56).

The normal *carotid pulse* is localized rather than diffuse. A strong pulse, the carotid has a thrusting quality. As the client breathes, no change occurs during inspiration or expiration. Rotation of the neck or a shift from a sitting to a supine position does not change the carotid's quality. Both carotid arteries should be equal in pulse rate, rhythm, and strength and should be equally elastic.

The carotid is the only pulse that is auscultated. Auscultation is especially important for middle-age or elderly clients or clients suspected of having cerebrovascular disease. When the lumen of a blood vessel is narrowed, its blood flow is disturbed. As blood passes through the narrowed section, a turbulence is created, causing a blowing or swishing sound. The blowing sound is called a bruit (pronounced "brew-ee") (Fig. 13-57). The diaphragm of the stethoscope is placed over the carotid artery. The nurse asks the client to hold his

breath so breath sounds do not obscure a bruit. Normally, no sound is heard.

JUGULAR VEINS

The most accessible veins are the internal and external jugular veins in the neck. Both veins drain from the head and neck into the superior vena cava. The external jugular lies superficially and can be seen just above the clavicle. The internal jugular lies deeper, along the carotid artery. When a client lies in the supine position, the external jugular commonly distends and becomes easily visible. The jugular veins normally flatten when the client is in a sitting position. A client with heart disease may have distended jugular veins when sitting.

The jugular veins are inspected to measure venous pressures, which are influenced by blood volume, the capacity of the right atrium to receive blood and send it to the right ventricle, and the ability of the right ventricle to contract and force blood into the pulmonary artery. Any factor resulting in greater blood volume within the venous system results in elevated venous pressure. The nurse assesses venous pressure by following these steps:

1. Have the client lie supine with head elevated 30 to 45 degrees (semi-Fowler's position). Normal veins should be flat.
2. Be sure the neck and upper thorax is exposed. Use a small pillow to align the head straight. Avoid hyperextension or flexion of the neck to ensure that the vein is not stretched or kinked.
3. If the jugular vein is visible, measure venous pressure by first finding the highest visible point of the internal jugular vein.
4. Measure in centimeters the vertical height of this point from the sternal angle or suprasternal notch (Fig. 13-58).
5. Repeat the same measurement on the other side. Bilateral pressures higher than 3 cm are considered elevated and are a sign of heart failure. One-sided pressure elevation can be caused by obstruction.

PERIPHERAL ARTERIES AND VEINS

To examine the peripheral vascular system the nurse first assesses the adequacy of blood flow to the extremities by measuring arterial pulses and by inspecting the condition of the skin and nails. The integrity of the venous system is also assessed, with attention given to determining whether the client has abnormalities. A number of factors can impair circulation to the extremities (Table 13-22). Altered blood vessel integrity, mechanical obstruction to blood flow, and overlying constriction on vessel walls reduce perfusion of tissues. The nurse should anticipate a client's risk for circulatory impairment (see client-teaching box, p. 288). Some clients, such as elderly and diabetic persons, suffer phys-

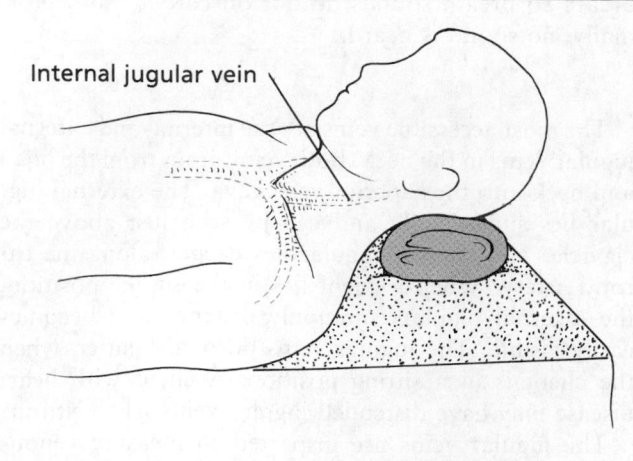

Fig. 13-58 Position of jugular vein distention.

ical changes in blood vessel walls that increase their risk for perfusion problems.

ARTERIAL PULSES. The nurse palpates peripheral arteries for elasticity of the vessel wall, rate and rhythm of pulse, strength of pulse, and equality of pulses. A systematic technique is useful, starting with the temporal arteries in the head and moving down to the arteries in the upper and lower extremities.

The wall of an artery is normally elastic, making it easily palpable. After the artery is depressed, it will spring back to shape when pressure is released. An abnormal artery may be described as hard, inelastic, or calcified.

The peripheral pulse rate is measured for 1 minute. Only the radial artery is usually chosen as the site to determine pulse rate when the nurse measures vital signs (see Chapter 12). To check local circulatory status the nurse may palpate a peripheral pulse long enough to assess its presence. With palpation the nurse will normally feel the pulse wave at regular intervals. When an interval is interrupted by an early, late, or missed beat, the pulse rhythm is irregular.

The strength of a pulse is a measurement of the force at which blood is ejected against the arterial wall. Some examiners use a scale rating from 0 (zero) to 4 + for the strength of a pulse:

0   No pulse is palpable.
1 +   Pulse is difficult to palpate, weak, and thready in character and is easy to obliterate.
2 +   Pulse is difficult to palpate, and light pressure will locate it. A discriminating touch senses that it is stronger than 1.
3 +   This is a normal pulse, easy to palpate and not easily obliterated.
4 +   Strong pulse is easily palpated, seems to bound against fingertips, and cannot be obliterated.

All peripheral pulses are measured for equality and symmetry. For example, the left radial pulse is compared with that of the right and the left brachial pulse is compared with the left radial. An inequality may indicate localized obstruction or an abnormally positioned artery.

In the upper extremities the primary artery is the brachial, which channels blood to the radial and ulnar arteries of the forearm and hand. If circulation in the brachial artery is blocked, the hands will not receive adequate blood flow. If circulation in the radial or ulnar arteries is impaired, the hand will still receive adequate

TABLE 13-22 Indicators for Assessing Local Blood Flow

Indicator	Rationale
Systemic diseases (arteriosclerosis, atherosclerosis, diabetes)	Disease results in changes in the integrity of the walls of arteries and smaller blood vessels.
Coagulation disorders (thrombosis, embolus)	Blood clot causes mechanical obstruction to blood flow.
Local trauma or surgery (contusion, fracture, vascular surgery)	Direct manipulation of vessels or localized edema impairs blood flow.
Application of constricting devices (casts, dressings, elastic bandages, restraints)	Constriction causes a tourniquet effect, impairing blood flow to areas below site of constriction.

Client Teaching after Vascular Assessment

- Tell clients their blood pressure reading. Explain the normal reading for the clients' ages. Discuss implications of abnormalities.
- Instruct clients with risk or evidence of vascular insufficiency in the lower extremities to avoid tight clothing over the lower body or legs, to avoid sitting or standing for long periods of time, to walk regularly, and to elevate feet when sitting.
- Elderly clients with hypertension may benefit from regular monitoring of blood pressure (daily, weekly, or monthly). Home monitoring kits are available (see chapter 12). Teach clients how to use them.

perfusion. An interconnection between the radial and ulnar arteries guards against arterial occlusion (Fig. 13-59).

The nurse should practice locating pulses on a friend. To locate pulses in the arm, the nurse has the client sit or lie down. The *radial pulse* is found along the radial side of the forearm, at the wrist. In a thin individual, a groove is formed lateral to the flexor tendon of the wrist. The radial pulse can be felt with light palpation in the groove (Fig. 13-60).

The *ulnar pulse* is on the opposite side of the wrist and tends to feel less prominent than the radial pulse (Fig. 13-61). An examiner palpates the ulnar pulse only when arterial insufficiency to the hand is expected.

To palpate the *brachial pulse,* the nurse finds the groove between the biceps and triceps muscles above the elbow at the antecubital fossa (Fig. 13-62). The artery runs along the medial side of the extended arm. The

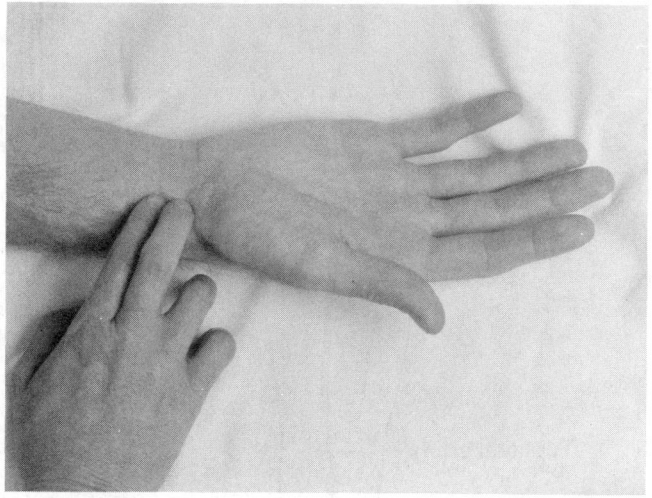

Fig. 13-60 Palpation of the radial pulse along the radial side of the forearm.

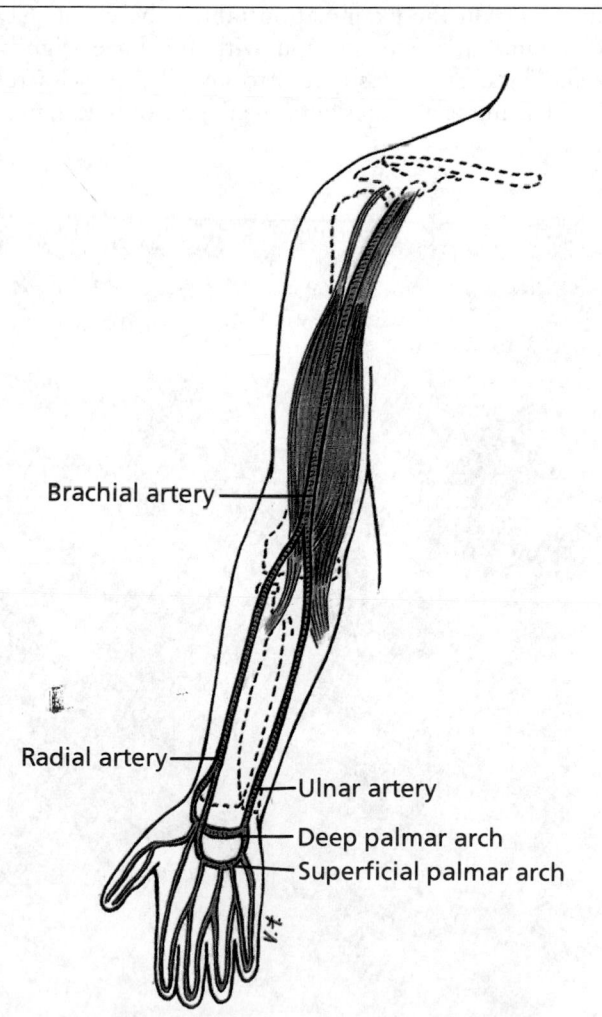

Fig. 13-59 Anatomical positions of brachial, radial, and ulnar arteries.

Brachial artery
Radial artery
Ulnar artery
Deep palmar arch
Superficial palmar arch

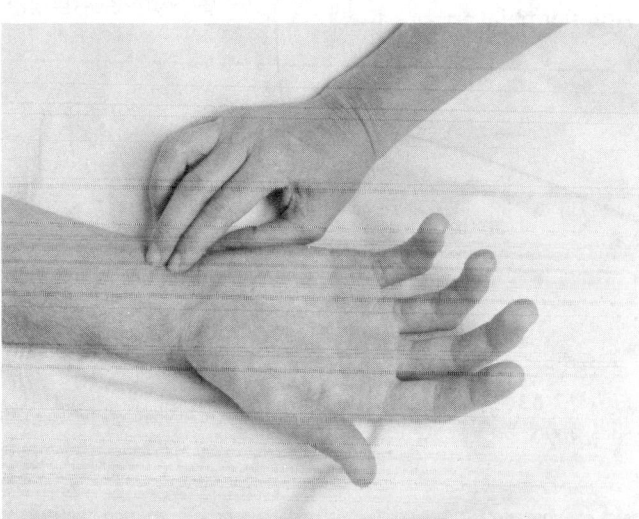

Fig. 13-61 Palpation of the ulnar pulse.

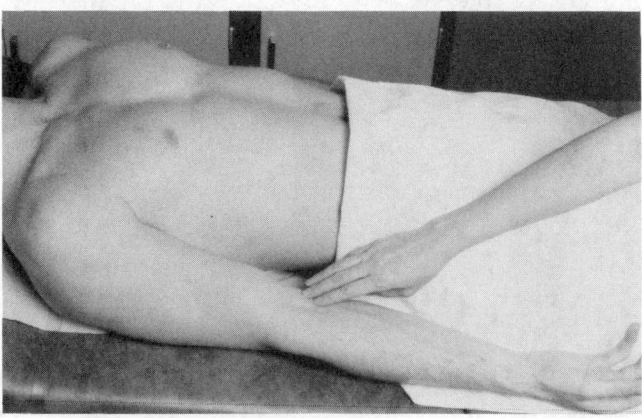

Fig. 13-62 The nurse palpates the brachial pulse by placing the fingertips in the groove between the biceps and triceps muscle.

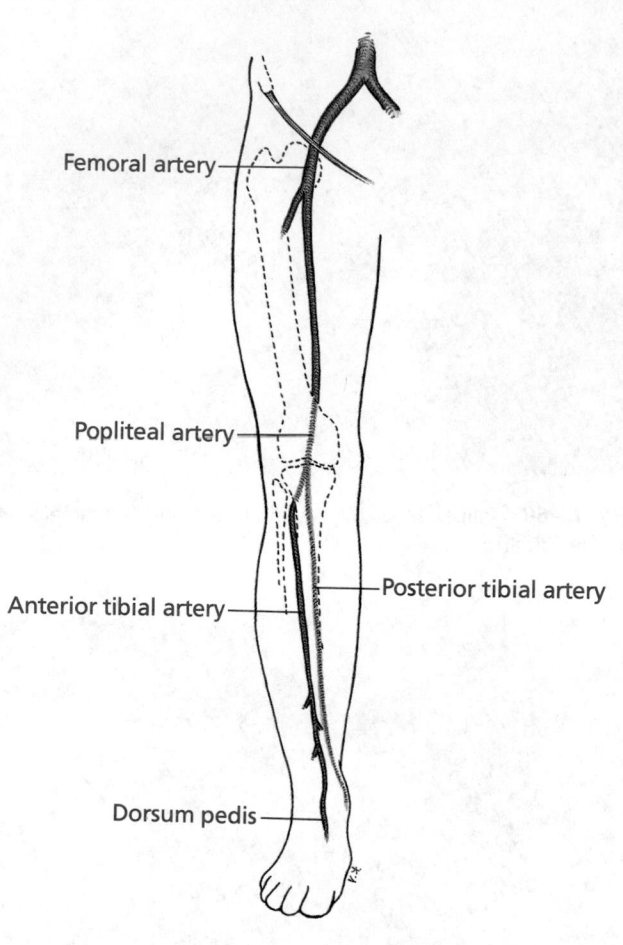

Fig. 13-63 Anatomical position of femoral, popliteal, dorsalis pedis, and posterior tibial arteries.

nurse palpates the artery with the fingertips of the first three fingers in the muscle groove.

The femoral artery is the primary artery in the leg, delivering blood to the popliteal, posterior tibial, and dorsalis pedis arteries (Fig. 13-63). An interconnection between the posterior tibial and dorsalis pedis arteries guards against local arterial occlusion.

The *femoral pulse* is found best with the client lying down with the inguinal area exposed (Fig. 13-64). The femoral artery runs below the inguinal ligament, midway between the symphysis pubis and the anterosuperior iliac spine. Deep palpation may be required to feel the pulse. Bimanual palpation is effective in obese clients. This technique differs from the previous description of bimanual palpation. The nurse places the fingertips of both hands on opposite sides of the pulse site. A pulsatile sensation can be felt as the fingertips are pushed apart by arterial pulsation.

The *popliteal pulse* is found behind the knee (Fig. 13-65). The client should slightly flex the knee, with the foot resting on the examination table. The client may also assume a prone position with the knee slightly flexed. The client is instructed to keep leg mescles relaxed. The nurse palpates with the fingers of both hands

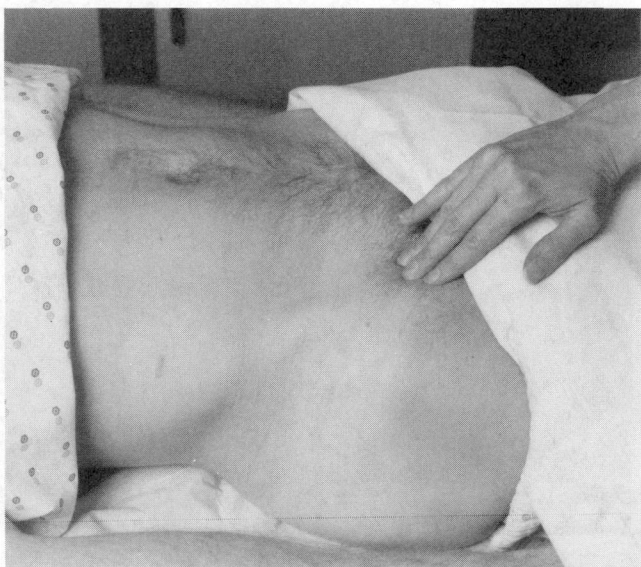

Fig. 13-64 The femoral pulse is usually palpated at the inguinal area midway between the symphysis pubis and anterosuperior iliac spine.

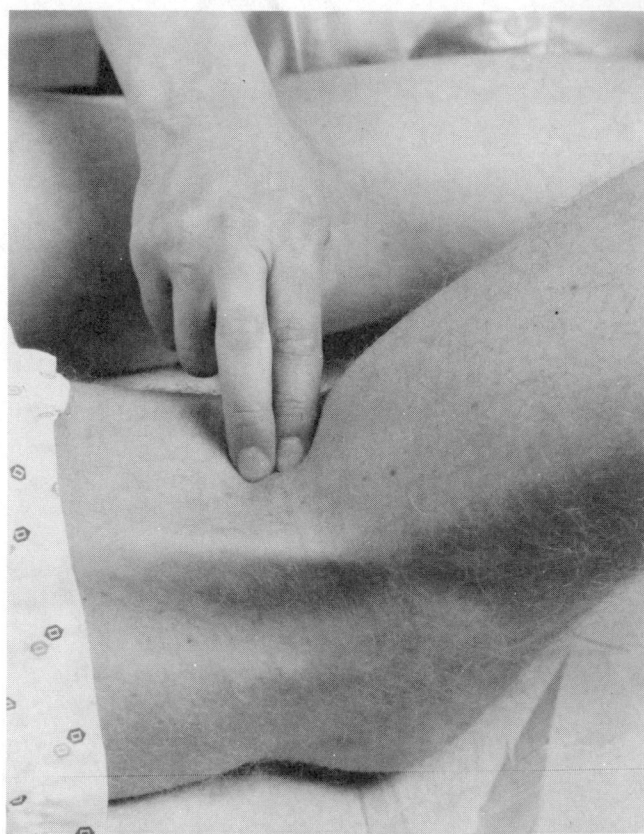

Fig. 13-65 The client lies with knee slightly flexed to give the nurse access to the popliteal pulse.

deeply into the popliteal fossa, just lateral to the midline. The popliteal is one of the more difficult pulses to locate.

With the client's foot relaxed the nurse locates the *dorsalis pedis pulse.* The artery runs along the top of the foot in a line with the groove between the extensor tendons of the great toe and first toe (Fig. 13-66). Often an examiner finds the pulse by placing the fingertips between the great and first toe and slowly inching up the foot. This pulse may be congenitally absent.

The *posterior tibial pulse* is found on the inner side of each ankle (Fig. 13-67). The nurse places the fingers behind and below the medial malleolus (ankle bone). The artery is easily located with the foot relaxed and slightly extended.

Ultrasound Stethoscopes. Occasionally a nurse has difficulty palpating a pulse. A pulse wave may not be

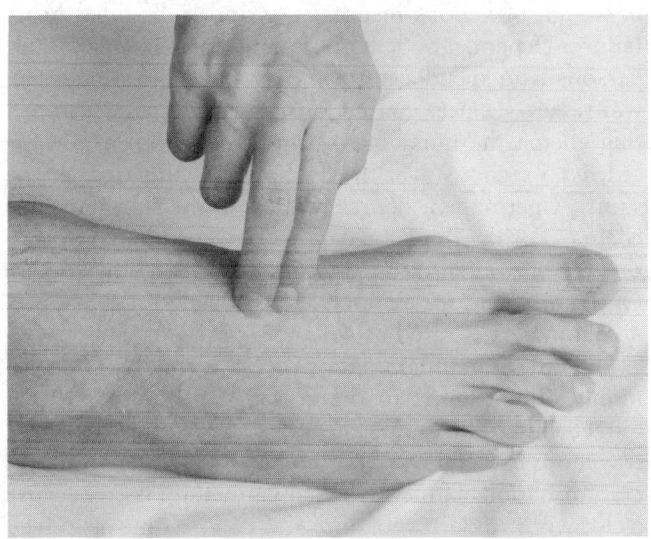

Fig. 13-66 The dorsalis pedis pulse is palpated at a point along a line with the groove between the extensor tendons of the great and first toes.

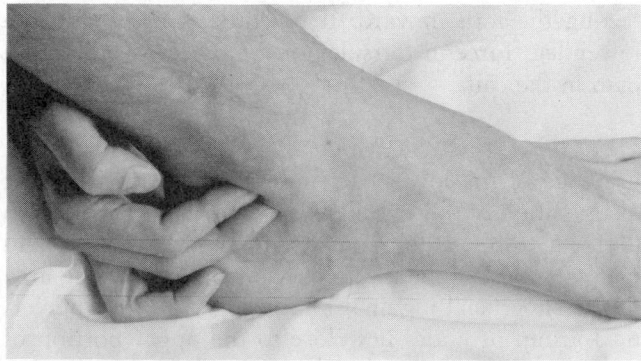

Fig. 13-67 Palpation of posterior tibial pulse below the medial malleolus.

manually palpable if the client is obese, if the heart's stroke volume is seriously reduced, if the blood volume is diminished, or if there is an obstruction of the artery. An ultrasound stethoscope will amplify sounds, allowing the nurse to hear low-velocity blood flow. Use of the stethoscope involves these steps:

1. Connect the stethoscope headset to the ultrasound probe.
2. Apply transmission gel to the client's skin at the pulse site or directly onto the transducer tip of the probe. (The gel creates an airtight seal for transmission of sound waves).
3. Turn the stethoscope's volume control to "on."
4. Gently apply the probe at a 45- to 90-degree angle on the skin at the pulse site (Fig. 13-68). Excess pressure might obliterate the pulse.
5. Move the probe over the pulse site until a pulsating "whooshing" sound, which indicates arterial blood flow, is heard. Do not be fooled by more intermittent and faint venous sounds.

TISSUE PERFUSION. The condition of the skin and nail beds offer useful data about the status of local tissue blood flow. The nurse first examines the upper extremities, looking at the color and texture of the skin and nail beds and for the presence of edema. If an arterial occlusion is present, the client has signs resulting from an absence in blood flow (Table 13-23). Venous conges-

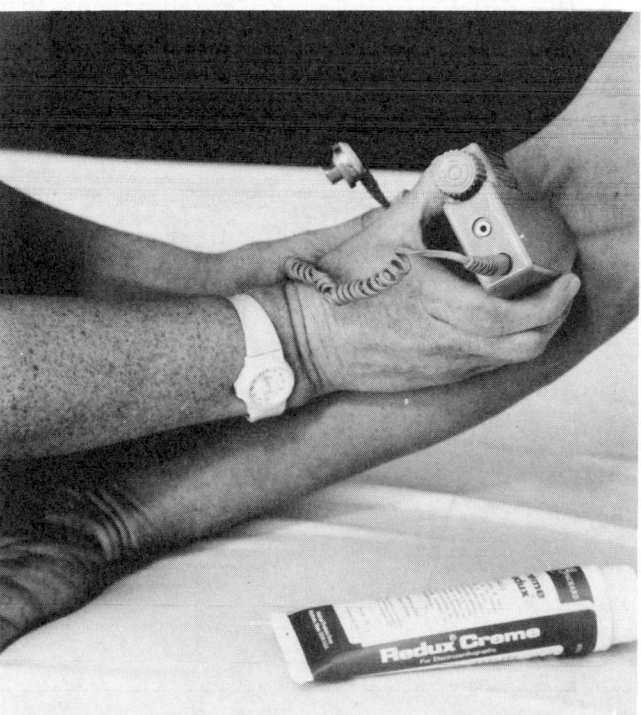

Fig. 13-68 Ultrasound stethoscope in position on brachial artery.

TABLE 13-23   Signs of Venous and Arterial Insufficiency

Assessment Criterion	Venous	Arterial
Color	Normal or cyanotic	Pale; worsened by elevation of extremity; dusky red when extremity lowered
Temperature	Normal	Cool (blood flow blocked to extremity)
Pulse	Normal	Decreased or absent
Edema	Often marked	Absent or mild
Skin changes	Brown pigmentation around ankles	Thin, shiny skin; decreased hair growth; thickened nails

tion causes tissue changes indicating an inadequate circulatory flow.

During examination of the lower extremities the nurse inspects skin and nail texture; hair distribution on the lower legs, feet, and toes; edema; venous pattern, and scars, pigmentation, or ulcers. The nurse should not be misled by women who shave their lower legs.

PERIPHERAL VEINS. The status of the peripheral venous system is examined when the nurse inspects for varicosities, peripheral edema, and phlebitis. Varicosities are superficial veins that become dilated, especially when the legs are in a dependent position. They are common in the elderly because the veins normally fibrose, dilate, and stretch. Varicosities in the anterior or medial part of the thigh and the posterolateral part of the calf are abnormal.

Dependent edema around the area of the ankle can be a sign of venous insufficiency and right-sided heart failure. Dependent edema is common in the elderly and persons who spend a lot of time standing (for example, waitresses, security guards, or nurses). To assess for pitting edema the nurse uses a thumb to press firmly for at least 5 seconds over the medial malleolus or over the shins. A permanent depression left in the skin indicates edema. The depth of the depression is estimated in centimeters (1 to 4 cm) to determine severity of the edema. One centimeter, for example, is rated as 1+ edema, and 4 centimeters is rated as 4+.

Phlebitis is an inflammation of a vein that occurs commonly after trauma to the vessel wall, infection, prolonged immobilization, and prolonged insertion of intravenous catheters (see Chapter 37). Phlebitis promotes clot formation, a potentially dangerous situation because a clot within a deep vein of the leg can become dislodged and travel through the heart, causing a pulmonary embolus. To assess for phlebitis the nurse inspects the calves for localized redness, tenderness, and swelling over vein sites. Gentle palpation of calf muscles will reveal tenderness and firmness of the muscle. The nurse may also check for a Homans' sign by supporting the leg while flexing the foot upward. If phlebitis is present in the lower leg, forceful dorsiflexion of the foot will cause pain in the calf.

LYMPHATIC SYSTEM. Assessment of the lymphatic drainage of the lower extremities is performed during examination of the vascular system. The nurse may also perform this examination just before the female and male genital examination. The nurse palpates the area of the superficial inguinal nodes (Fig. 13-69). The vertical group of nodes lies close to the upper portion of the great saphenous vein. The horizontal group lies below the inguinal ligament. The nurse uses a firm but gentle pressure when palpating over each lymphatic

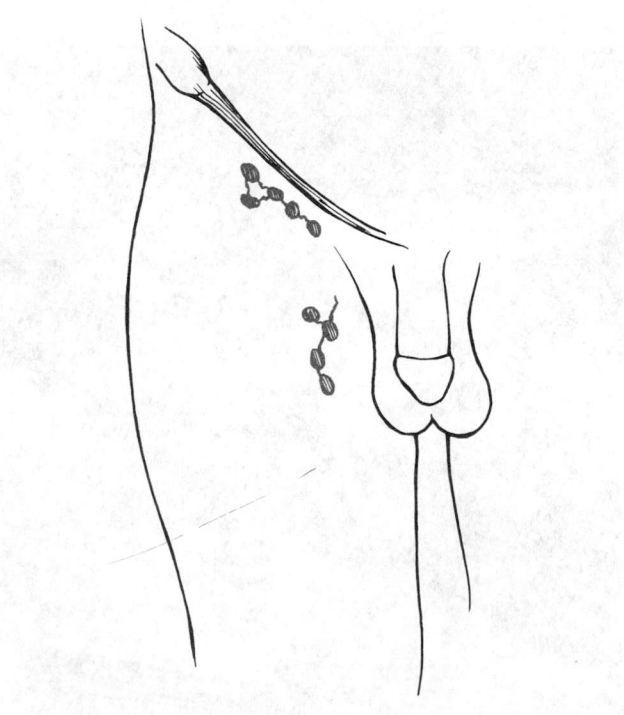

Fig. 13-69   Inguinal lymph nodes.

chain. The nodes are not normally palpable, although a single soft, nontender node is not unusual. Enlarged, hardened, tender nodes can reveal potential sites of infection or metastatic disease. An infection site can be identified by drainage collected by the nodes. For example, the horizontal group drains lymph from the skin of the lower abdominal wall, the external genitalia, anal canal, and lower vagina.

BREASTS

It is important to examine the breasts of both the female and the male client. A small amount of glandular tissue, a potential site for the growth of cancer cells, is located in the male breast. In contrast, the majority of the female breast is glandular tissue.

Female Breasts

Breast cancer will affect 1 out of every 11 women in the United States (American Cancer Society, 1986). The disease is the second leading cause of death in women with cancer (lung cancer is the first). Early detection is the key to cure. Women with benign fibrocystic breast conditions have been found to be at high risk for breast cancer (U.S. Department of Health and Human Services, 1985).

The American Cancer Society (1986) recommends the following guidelines for the detection of breast cancer:

1. Breast self-examination (BSE) should be performed monthly by women 20 years of age and older.
2. An examination by a physician should be performed every 3 years from ages 20 to 40, and after 40, the examination should be performed every year.
3. Women with a family history of breast cancer should have a physician's examination yearly.
4. A diagnostic mammogram (x-ray study of the breast) should be performed every year for women age 50 and over, for women age 40 or over with a family history of cancer of the breast, and for women age 35 or over with a history of breast cancer.

During an examination the nurse can explain how to perform a BSE. As the nurse assesses the client's breasts, he or she uses many of the same techniques the client will adapt for home use.

If the client already performs self-examinations, the nurse can ask what method she uses and when she does the examination in relation to her menstrual cycle. The best time for a self-examination is on the last day of the menstrual period, when the breast is no longer swollen or tender from hormone elevations. If the woman is postmenopausal, she should check her breasts the same time each month. The pregnant woman also must check her breasts on a routine monthly basis.

The client's history (Table 13-24) should alert the nurse to any signs of breast disease and normal developmental changes. Because of its glandular structure, the breast undergoes changes during a woman's life. Knowledge of these changes (see box on next page) helps the nurse complete an accurate assessment.

TABLE 13-24   Nursing History for Breast Assessment

Assessment Category	Rationale
Determine if the woman is over age 50, has a family history of breast cancer, had previous breast cancer, never had children, or had a first child after age 30, or did not breast-feed any children.	These risk factors indicate breast cancer.
Ask if client (both sexes) has noticed pain or tenderness of breast, discharge from nipple, change in size of breast, or presence of a lump or mass. Have the client point out any masses.	Potential signs and symptoms of breast cancer allow the nurse to focus on specific areas of the breast during assessment.
Ask if client performs monthly breast self-examinations. If so, determine the time of month she performs examination in relation to menstrual cycle. Have client describe the method she uses for examination.	The role of the nurse is to educate the client about breast cancer and techniques for self-examination.
Assess client's age at menarche, menopause, and first pregnancy.	The risk of cancer is greater in women who reach menarche early (before age 13), have menopause late (after age 50), and who had their first child after age 30.
Determine if client is taking oral contraceptives, digitalis, diuretics, steroids, or estrogen hormones.	Medications may cause nipple discharge. Hormones may cause fibrocystic changes in the breast.

Normal Changes in the Breast During a Woman's Life Span

PUBERTY (8 TO 13 YEARS)

Breasts mature in five stages. One breast may grow more rapidly than the other.

Stage 1 (Preadolescent)

▪ This stage involves elevation of the nipple only.

Stage 2

▪ In this stage, the breast and nipple elevate as a small mound, and the areolar diameters enlarge.

Stage 3

▪ This stage involves further enlargement and elevation of the breast and areola, with no separation of contour.

Stage 4

▪ The areola and nipple project into the secondary mound above the level of the breast.

Stage 5 (The Mature Breast)

▪ Only the nipple projects, and the areola recedes (may vary in some women).

YOUNG ADULTHOOD (20 TO 30 YEARS)

▪ Breasts reach full (nonpregnant) size. Shape is generally symmetrical. Breasts may be unequal in size.

PREGNANCY

▪ Breast size gradually enlarges to two to three times the previous size. Nipples enlarge and may become erect. Areola darkens. Superficial veins become prominent. A yellowish fluid (colostrum) may be expelled from the nipple.

MENOPAUSE

▪ Breasts shrink. Tissue becomes softer, sometimes flabby.

OLDER ADULTHOOD

▪ Breasts sag and nipples become smaller.

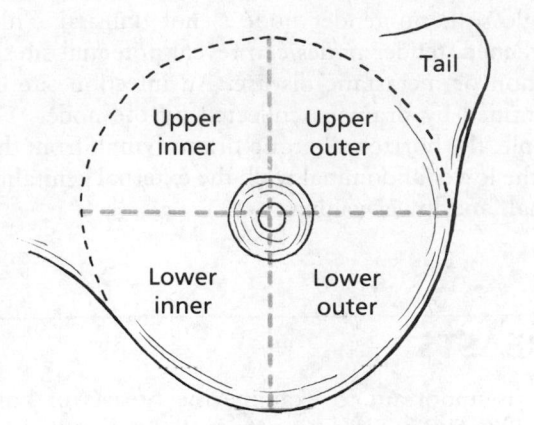

Fig. 13-70 The nurse localizes assessment findings by dividing each breast into four quadrants and an axillary tail.

INSPECTION

The client removes the top gown or drape to allow simultaneous visualization of both breasts. The client may stand or sit with arms at her side. If possible, the nurse places a mirror in front of the client during inspection so she can see what to look for when performing a self-examination. To recognize abnormalities, the client must be familiar with the normal appearance of her breasts.

The nurse describes observations or findings in relation to imaginary lines that divide the breast into four quadrants and a tail. The lines cross at the center of the nipple. Each tail extends outward from the upper outer quadrant (Fig. 13-70).

The breasts are inspected for size and symmetry. One breast is commonly larger than the other. However, a difference in size may be caused by inflammation or presence of a mass. The breasts usually extend in area from the third to the sixth ribs. The nipple is usually at the level of the fourth intercostal space. As the woman becomes older, the ligaments supporting the breast tissue weaken, causing the breasts to sag and the nipples to lower.

The nurse observes the contour or shape of the breasts and notes any masses, retraction, or flattening. Retraction or dimpling results from invasion of underlying ligaments by tumors. The ligaments become fibrotic and pull the overlying skin inward toward the tumor.

The client raises her arms high over her head, chest forward, to expose the extreme lateral portions and undersurface of the breast. This maneuver also causes contraction of the pectoral muscles, which will accentuate the presence of retraction or surface flattening.

The overlying skin is carefully inspected for color and venous pattern. Venous patterns are more easily seen in thin clients or pregnant women. The presence of edema or inflammation is noted. For women with large breasts the nurse should be sure to look carefully at the undersurface, a common site for redness and excoriation caused by rubbing of skin surfaces.

The normal areolae and nipples of a white female are pink, becoming brown with pregnancy. In dark-skinned

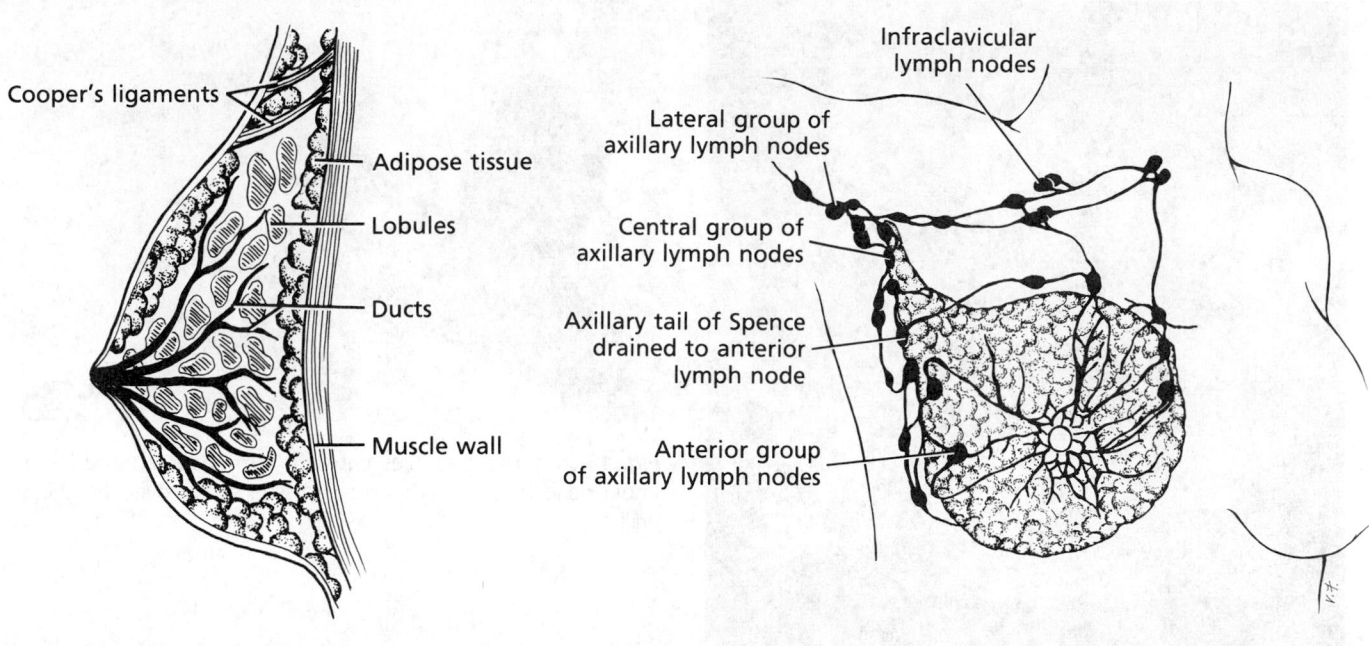

Fig. 13-71   Cross section of breast tissue.   **Fig. 13-72**   Anatomical position of axillary and clavicular lymph nodes.

clients the nipple is darker than other skin surfaces. Pregnancy causes an even darker color to develop. The nipple and areola are inspected for size and shape. A slight asymmetry is common. The nurse also observes the direction in which the nipples point. Normally they point in symmetrical directions. A recently inverted (turned inward) nipple may indicate an underlying growth. Rashes or ulcerations are not normal. Bleeding or discharge from the nipple is noted. The color of a discharge may range from clear yellow to green.

While inspecting the breasts, the nurse explains the characteristics observed. The client must be taught the significance of abnormal signs or symptoms.

PALPATION

Palpation allows the nurse to determine the condition of underlying breast tissue and lymph nodes. Breast tissue consists of glandular tissue, fibrous supportive ligaments, and fat (Fig. 13-71). Glandular tissue is organized into lobes that end in ducts that open onto the nipple's surface. The largest portion of glandular tissue is located in the upper outer quadrant and tail of each breast. Suspensory ligaments connect to skin and fascia underlying the breast to support the breast and maintain its upright position. Fatty tissue is located superficially and to the sides of the breast.

A large portion of lymph from the breasts drains into axillary lymph nodes. If cancerous lesions metastasize or spread, the nodes are commonly involved. The nurse must know the location of supraclavicular, infraclavi-

cular, and axillary nodes (Fig. 13-72). A tumor of one breast may also involve nodes on the opposite side.

The lymph nodes are palpated when the client sits. Easy access is gained to the axillary nodes with the client's arms at her sides and muscles relaxed. The nurse faces the client and supports her arm, while abducting that arm away from the chest wall. Then the nurse places her own hand against the client's chest wall and high in the axilla. The axillary nodes are palpated, with the fingertips of the nurse's hand pressing gently down over the surface of the ribs and muscles (Fig. 13-73).

The following areas of the axilla are palpated: (1) the edge of the pectoralis major muscle along the anterior axillary line, (2) the chest wall in the midaxillary area, (3) the upper part of the humerus, and (4) the anterior edge of the latissimus dorsi muscle along the posterior axillary line.

Each area must be assessed carefully because these nodes are easily missed. The nurse notes their number, consistency, movability, and size.

Normally lymph nodes are not palpable. However, one or two small, soft, nontender nodes may be normal. A palpable node feels like a small mass that may be hard, tender, and immobile. The supraclavicular and infraclavicular nodes are also palpated as the nurse stands at the client's right side. The procedure is reversed for the left side.

It may be difficult for the client to learn to palpate for lymph nodes. Lying down with the arm abducted makes the area more accessible. The client is instructed

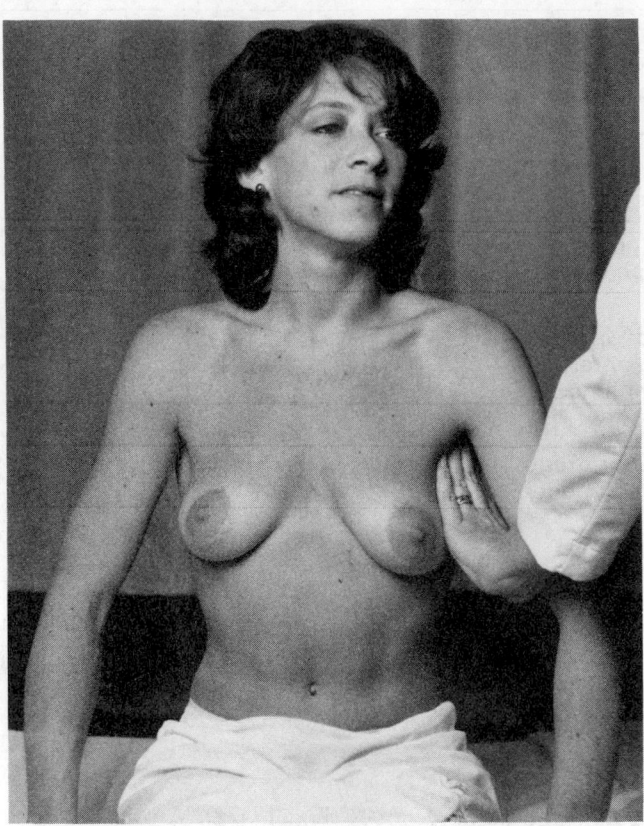

Fig. 13-73 The nurse supports the client's arm and palpates axillary lymph nodes.

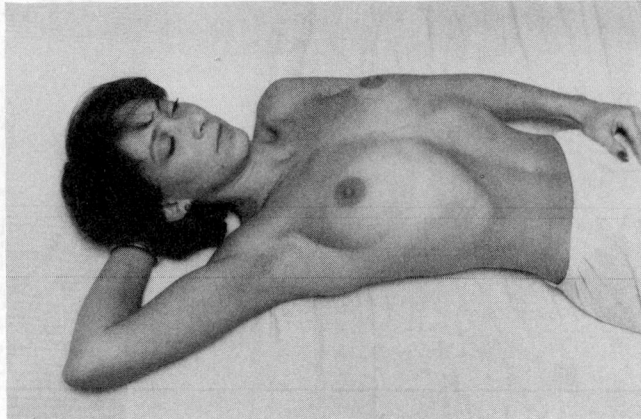

Fig. 13-74 The client lies flat with arm abducted and hand under head to help flatten breast tissue evenly over the chest wall.

to use her left hand for the right axillary and clavicular areas. The nurse can take the client's fingertips and move them in the proper circular fashion. The client then uses her right hand to palpate left-sided nodes.

Palpation of breast tissue is performed with the client lying supine or sitting. The supine position allows the breast tissue to flatten evenly against the chest wall. The client should raise her hand and place it behind the neck to further stretch and position breast tissue evenly (Fig. 13-74). The examiner often places a small pillow or towel under the shoulder blade to further position breast tissue.

The consistency of normal breast tissue varies widely. The breasts of a young client are firm and elastic. In an older client the tissue may feel stringy and nodular. The client's familiarity with the texture of her own breasts is very important. This familiarity is gained through monthly self-examination (see client-teaching box).

If the client complains of a mass, the nurse examines the opposite breast first to ensure an objective comparison of normal and abnormal tissue. The palmar surface of the first three fingers is used to compress breast tissue gently against the chest wall (Fig. 13-75). Palpation is performed in a rotary motion, using an organized ap-

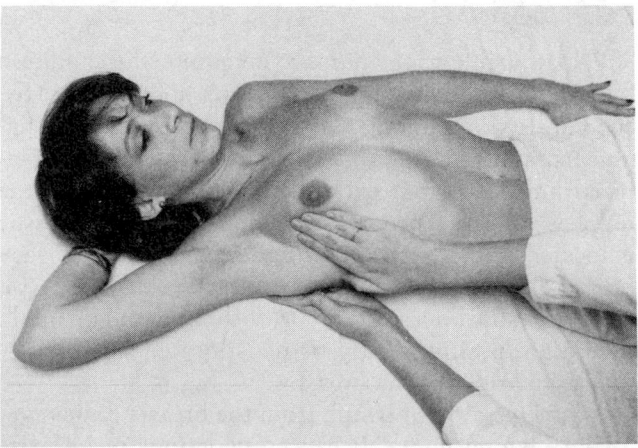

Fig. 13-75 The nurse palpates each breast quadrant using a rotary motion of the fingerpads.

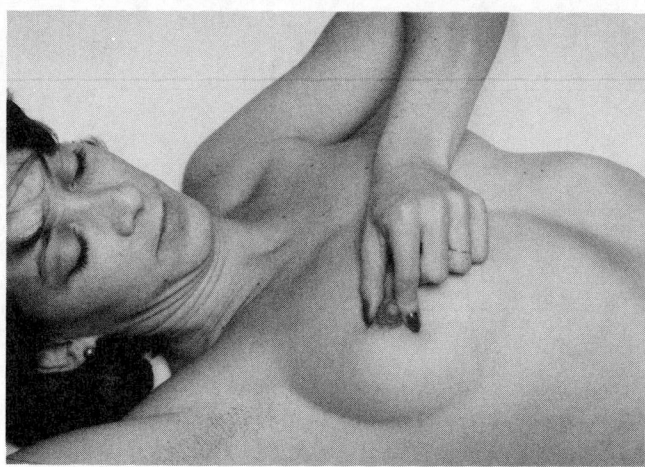

Fig. 13-76 The client palpates the nipple for presence of discharge.

proach. Some examiners start in the upper outer quadrant, where tumors develop most frequently. After the entire quadrant is palpated, the nurse moves systematically to the lower outer, lower inner, and upper inner quadrants. Another method is to proceed in and out, starting at the nipple. This pattern of palpation appears like the spokes of a wheel. The nurse must be sure to cover the entire breast and tail, directing attention to any areas of tenderness.

When palpating large, pendulous breasts, the nurse uses a bimanual technique. The inferior portion of the breast is supported in one hand while the nurse uses the other hand to palpate breast tissue against the supporting hand.

During palpation the nurse notes the consistency of breast tissue. The lobular feel of glandular tissue is normal. The lower edge of each breast may feel firm and hard. This is the normal inframammary ridge and not a tumor. It may be helpful to move the client's hand so she can feel normal tissue variations. Abnormal masses are palpated to determine the following:

1. Location in relation to quadrants
2. Size in centimeters
3. Shape (for example, round or discoid)
4. Consistency (soft, firm, or hard)
5. Tenderness
6. Mobility
7. Discreteness (whether boundaries of mass are easily detected)

Cancerous lesions are hard, fixed, nontender, and irregular in shape.

Special attention is given to gentle palpation of the nipple and areola. The thumb and index finger compress the nipple, and the nurse notes any discharge. As the nurse examines the nipple and areola, the nipple may become erect with wrinkling of the areola. These changes are normal.

After the nurse completes the examination, the client can demonstrate self-palpation (Fig. 13-76). Observing the client's technique helps the nurse emphasize the importance of a systematic approach. The client is urged to see her physician is she discovers any abnormal mass during routine monthly self-examination.

Male Breasts

Examination of the male breast is relatively easy. The nipple and areola are inspected for nodules, edema, and ulceration. An enlarged male breast may result from obesity or glandular enlargement. Fatty tissue feels soft, whereas glandular tissue is firm. Any masses are palpated for the same characteristics as the female breast. Because breast cancer in men is relatively rare, routine self-examinations are unnecessary.

ABDOMEN

The abdominal examination can be complex because of the organs located within and near the abdominal cavity. A thorough nursing history (Table 13-25, p. 299) helps the nurse interpret physical signs. A client with abdominal pain may suffer problems involving abdominal organs (for example, liver, stomach, and colon) or tissues and bones outside the abdominal cavity (for example, spine and muscles). Familiarity with common signs and symptoms, as well as the location of organs, helps the nurse make an accurate assessment. When assessing the abdomen the nurse may use two systems of landmarks to map out the abdominal region. In both systems the xiphoid process (tip of the sternum) marks the upper boundary of the abdominal region and the symphysis pubis delineates the lowermost boundary. One system divides the abdomen into quadrants by two imaginary lines crossing at the umbilicus (Fig 13-77, *A*). The second system divides the abdomen into nine sections (Fig. 13-77, *B*). Assessment findings are recorded in relation to the quadrants or sections. For example, the nurse may determine that the client is experiencing tenderness over the left lower quadrant (LLQ) with normal bowel sounds present.

The examiner also assesses abdominal organs that lie posteriorly. The kidneys are protected by the lower ribs and heavy back muscles. The costovertebral angle is used as a landmark during palpation of the kidney (Fig. 13-78). The client must be relaxed. A tightening of abdominal muscles hinders accuracy with palpation.

To help the client relax, the nurse asks if he or she needs to void. The room should be warm, and the client's upper chest and legs draped. The abdomen is exposed

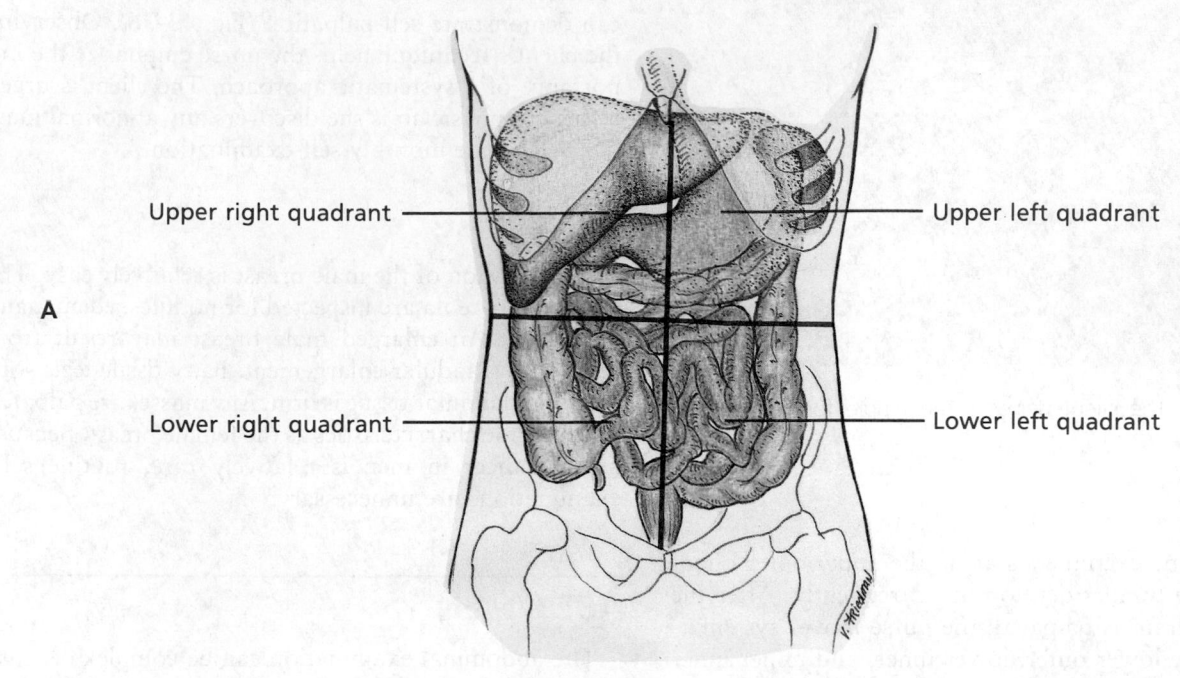

Upper right quadrant

Upper left quadrant

Lower right quadrant

Lower left quadrant

A

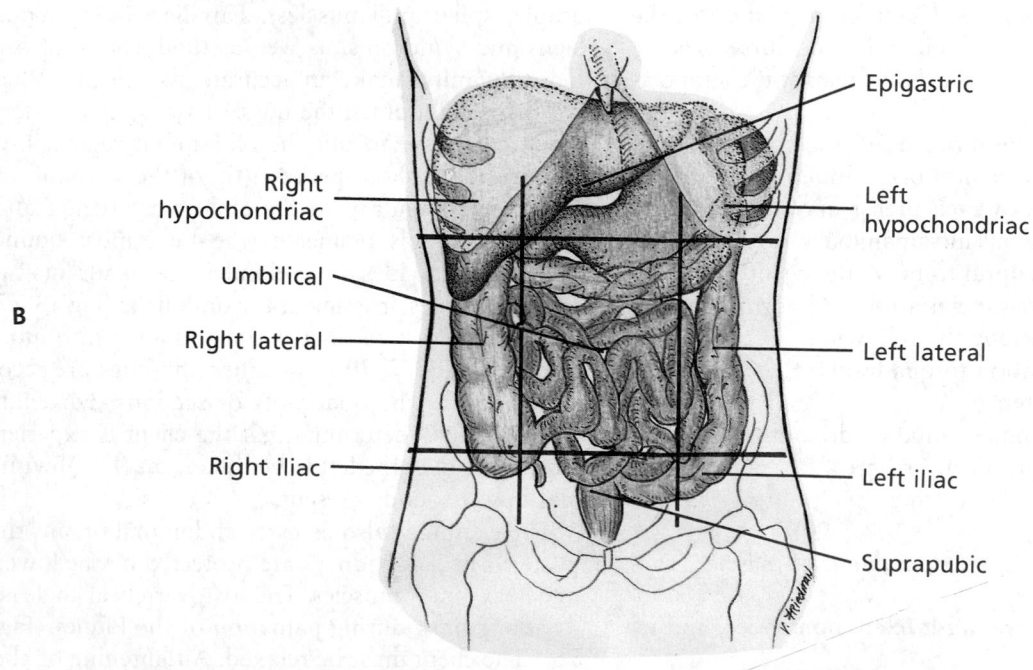

Epigastric

Right hypochondriac

Left hypochondriac

Umbilical

Right lateral

Left lateral

Right iliac

Left iliac

Suprapubic

B

Fig. 13-77   **A,** Division of abdomen into quadrants. **B,** Division of abdomen into nine anatomical sections.

TABLE 13-25 Nursing History for Abdomen Assessment

Assessment Category	Rationale
If client has abdominal or low back pain, assess the character of pain in detail (location, onset, frequency, precipitating factors, aggravating factors, type of pain, severity, etc.)	Pattern of characteristics of pain help determine its source.
Carefully observe the client's movement and position such as 1. Lying still with knees updrawn. 2. Moving restlessly to find a comfortable position. 3. Lying on one side or sitting with knees drawn up to chest	Positions assumed by client may reveal nature and source of pain: 1. Peritonitis 2. Renal stone 3. Pancreatitis
Assess normal bowel habits.	Data compared with physical findings can help to identify cause and nature of elimination problems.
Determine if client has had abdominal surgery or trauma.	Surgical or traumatic alterations of abdominal organs may cause changes in expected findings (for example, position of underlying organs).
Assess if client has had recent weight changes or intolerance to diet (for example, nausea, vomiting, or cramping, especially in last 24 hours).	Data may indicate alterations in upper gastrointestinal tract (stomach or gallbladder) or lower colon.
Assess for difficulty in swallowing, belching, or flatulence, bloody emesis (hematemesis), black or tarry stools (melena), or heartburn.	These characteristic signs and symptoms indicate abdominal alterations.
Ask client to locate any tender areas.	Nurse assesses painful areas last to minimize discomfort and anxiety.

from just above the xiphoid process down to the symphysis pubis. A good examination light is essential. The client lies in the supine position with arms down at the sides or folded across the chest. If the nurse allows the client to place the arms under the head, the abdominal muscles may tighten. A small pillow may be placed under the head or knees. Warm hands and stethoscope further promote relaxation. Maintaining conversation except during auscultation helps to distract the client. The nurse performs the examination slowly and calmly. The client should be asked to report pain and point out tender areas.

The order of an abdominal examination differs slightly from previous assessments. The nurse begins with inspection, then follows with auscultation. It is important to auscultate before palpation and percussion

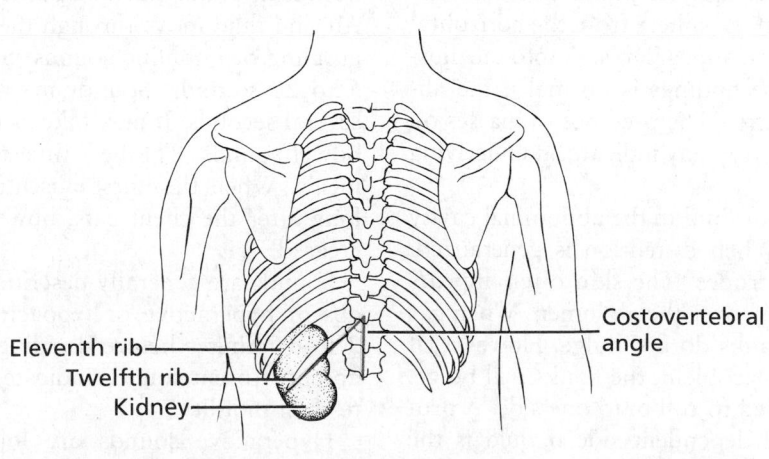

Fig. 13-78 The kidneys normally lie behind the lower ribs at a point even with the costovertebral angle.

because palpation and percussion may alter frequency and character of bowel sounds. The nurse will also need a tape measure.

Inspection

The nurse stands on the client's right side and inspects the abdomen, then sits to look across the abdomen's surface. Standing helps detect abnormal shadows and movement. The sitting position provides a horizontal view allowing for detection of abnormal protuberances. The examination light is directed over the abdomen.

SKIN

The location of scars, venous patterns, rashes, lesions, and striae, or stretch marks are noted. Artificial openings may indicate drainage sites resulting from surgery (see Chapter 47) or an ostomy. Scars indicate past trauma or surgery that may have created permanent changes in underlying organ anatomy. Venous patterns are usually faint, except in very thin clients. Striae result from stretching of tissue by obesity or pregnancy.

UMBILICUS

The position, shape, color, and signs of inflammation, discharge, or protruding masses are noted. Normally the umbilicus is a flat or concave hemisphere positioned midway between the xiphoid process and symphysis pubis. The color is the same as that of the surrounding skin. The presence of underlying masses can cause displacement of the umbilicus. Hernias, protrusions of abdominal organs through the muscle wall, cause upward protrusion of the umbilicus. Normally, no discharge is emitted from the umbilical area.

CONTOUR AND SYMMETRY

A flat abdomen forms a horizontal plane from the xiphoid process to the symphysis pubis. A round abdomen protrudes in a convex sphere from the horizontal plane. A concave abdomen appears to sink into the muscular wall. Each of these findings is normal if the abdomen's shape is symmetric. The presence of masses on only one side, or asymmetry, may indicate an underlying pathological condition.

Intestinal gas, tumor, or fluid in the abdominal cavity may cause distention. When distention is generalized, the entire abdomen protrudes. The skin often appears taut as if it were stretched over the abdomen. When gas causes distention, the flanks do not bulge. However, if fluid is the source of the problem, the flanks will bulge. The client should be asked to roll onto one side. A protuberance forms on the dependent side if fluid is the cause of the distention. The nurse asks the client if the abdomen feels unusually tight. The nurse must be careful not to confuse distention with obesity. In obesity the abdomen is large, rolls of adipose tissue are often present along the flanks, and the client does not complain of tightness in the abdomen. If abdominal distention is expected, the nurse may choose to measure the abdomen's girth by placing a tape measure around the abdomen at the level of the umbilicus. Consecutive measurements will show any increase or decrease in distention.

ENLARGED ORGANS

The nurse observes the abdominal contour while client takes a deep breath. Any enlarged organs in the upper abdominal cavity (for example, liver or spleen) may descend below the rib cage to cause a bulge. Closer examination can be performed with palpation.

MOVEMENT OR PULSATIONS

The nurse should remember that males breathe abdominally and females breathe more costally. If the client has severe pain, respiratory movement is diminished and the client tightens abdominal muscles to guard against the pain. On closer inspection the nurse may see peristaltic movement and aortic pulsation by looking across the abdomen from the side to detect movement. It may take several minutes to see a peristaltic wave. In contrast, aortic pulsations occur with each beat of systole and appear in the midline above the umbilicus (epigastric area).

Auscultation

The nurse asks the client to refrain from talking. If a client has a nasogastric or intestinal tube connected to intermittent suction, it should be momentarily turned off.

BOWEL MOTILITY

The warmed diaphragm of the stethoscope is placed over each of the four quadrants to detect bowel sounds. Air and fluid move through the intestines, creating soft gurgling or bubbling sounds that normally occur every 5 to 20 seconds. Sounds may last one-half second to several seconds. It may take as long as a minute to hear bowel sounds. The best time to auscultate is between meals. When the nurse auscultates just after meals or long after the client eats, bowel sounds tend to be increased.

Sounds are generally described as normal or audible, absent, hyperactive, or hypoactive. The nurse must listen 3 to 5 minutes before deciding that bowel sounds are absent. Absent sounds indicate a cessation of gastrointestinal motility.

Hyperactive sounds are loud, "growling" sounds called *borborygmi*, which indicate increased gastrointestinal motility. Inflammation of the bowel, anxiety, excess ingestion of laxatives, and reaction of the intes-

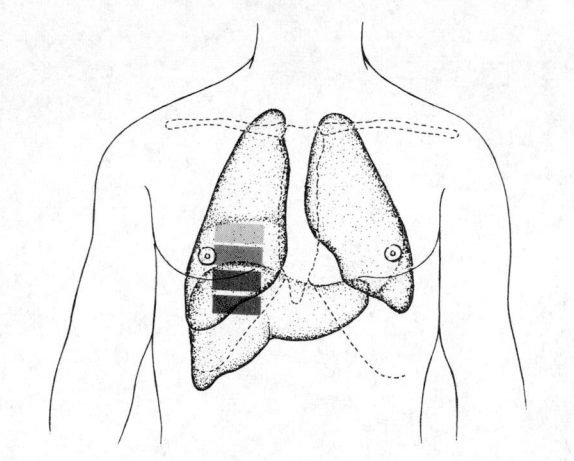

Fig. 13-79 To locate the liver's upper border, the nurse percusses downward, noting the change in sound from resonance (lung) to dullness (liver).

tines to certain foods cause increased motility (see client-teaching box).

VASCULAR SOUNDS

The nurse applies the bell of the stethoscope over the epigastrium for bruits. These blowing sounds often originate from a narrowing of the thoracic aorta. Renal artery bruits can be heard by placing the stethoscope over each upper quadrant anteriorly or the costovertebral angle posteriorly (which can be done when the client sits).

FRICTION RUBS

An inflamed liver or spleen may rub against the peritoneum during inspiration, creating a grating sound with respiratory variations. Friction rubs are heard best with the stethoscope's bell placed above the liver and spleen.

Percussion

Percussion of the abdomen maps out underlying organs and masses and helps to reveal the presence of air or fluid within the abdomen. The beginning student uses this skill in a limited fashion. Practice is needed to ensure accuracy.

ORGANS AND MASSES

The nurse systematically percusses each of the four quadrants to assess areas of tympany and dullness. Tympany usually predominates because of air in the stomach and intestines. A dull percussion note indicates solid masses such as an enlarged liver or spleen, tumors, a distended bladder, or ascites. When dullness is noted, it may be useful to also use palpation to complete a detailed assessment.

LIVER SIZE

Percussion allows the nurse to identify borders of the liver to detect enlargement. The nurse starts at the right midclavicular line, just below the umbilicus in an area of tympany. As the nurse slowly percusses upward, the percussion note changes from tympanic to dull at the liver's lower border. Usually the border is at the right costal margin. The upper border is found by percussing down from the clavicle. The nurse also percusses in the intercostal spaces, and the note changes from resonant to dull (Fig. 13-79). The liver's upper border is usually found in the fifth, sixth, or seventh intercostal space. The distance between the points where dullness is percussed along the midclavicular line should be 6 to 12 cm (2½ to 5 inches). Diseases such as cirrhosis and hepatitis cause liver enlargement.

STOMACH POSITION

With practice the nurse can locate the tympanic air bubble of the stomach by percussing over the left lower anterior rib cage. The bubble's size varies.

KIDNEY TENDERNESS

With the client sitting or standing erect, the nurse uses direct or indirect percussion to assess for kidney inflammation. With the ulnar surface of the partially closed fist, the nurse percusses the costovertebral angle at the scapular line (Fig. 13-80). If the kidneys are inflamed the client feels tenderness during percussion.

Palpation

With palpation, nursing students are primarily concerned with detecting areas of abdominal tenderness and noting the quality of abnormal distentions or masses. As students become more skilled, they learn to palpate

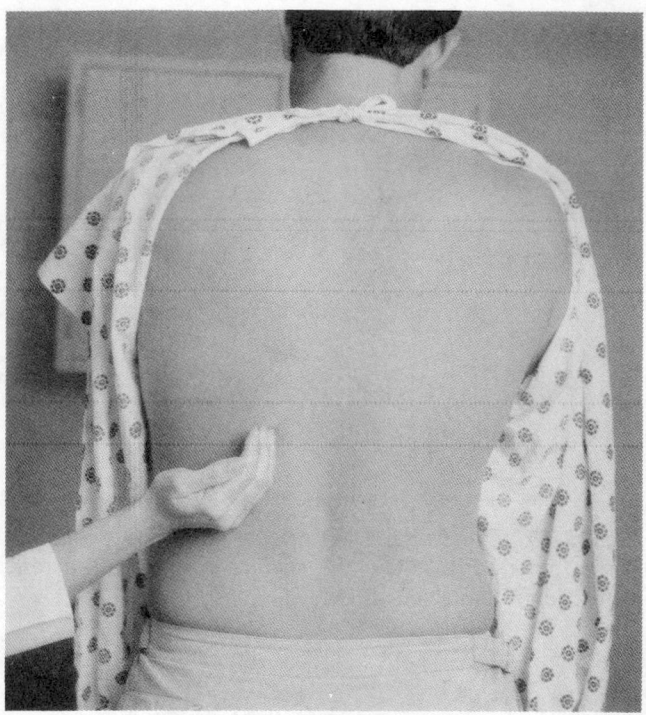

Fig. 13-80 Percussion for kidney tenderness along costo-vertebral angle.

for the presence of specific organs such as the liver, spleen, and kidney. Two types of palpation are used by the nurse, including light and deep.

After rubbing the hands together, the nurse, uses *light palpation* over each quadrant. The palm of the hand and forearm are kept horizontal as the nurse places the hand on the client's abdomen (Fig. 13-81). The skin is depressed approximately 1.3 cm (½ inch) with the fingertips in a gentle, dipping motion. The nurse avoids quick jabs. If the client is ticklish, the nurse places the hand under the client's until he tolerates the touch.

A systematic palpation of each quadrant assesses for muscular resistance, tenderness, and superficial organs or masses. If the nurse palpates a sensitive area, guarding, a voluntary tightening of underlying abdominal muscles, may occur. If tightening remains after the client is helped to relax, peritonitis may be the cause. A distended bladder is easy to detect with light palpation. Normally the bladder lies below the umbilicus and above the symphysis pubis. The nurse routinely checks for a distended bladder if a client has been unable to void.

A nurse must have experience to perform *deep palpation* successfully. Short fingernails are needed. One or two hands may be used (Fig. 13-82). The client must be relaxed as the nurse's hands are depressed approximately 2.5 to 7.5 cm (1 to 3 inches) into the abdomen. Deep palpation is never used over a surgical incision or over extremely tender organs. It is also unwise to use palpation on abnormal masses.

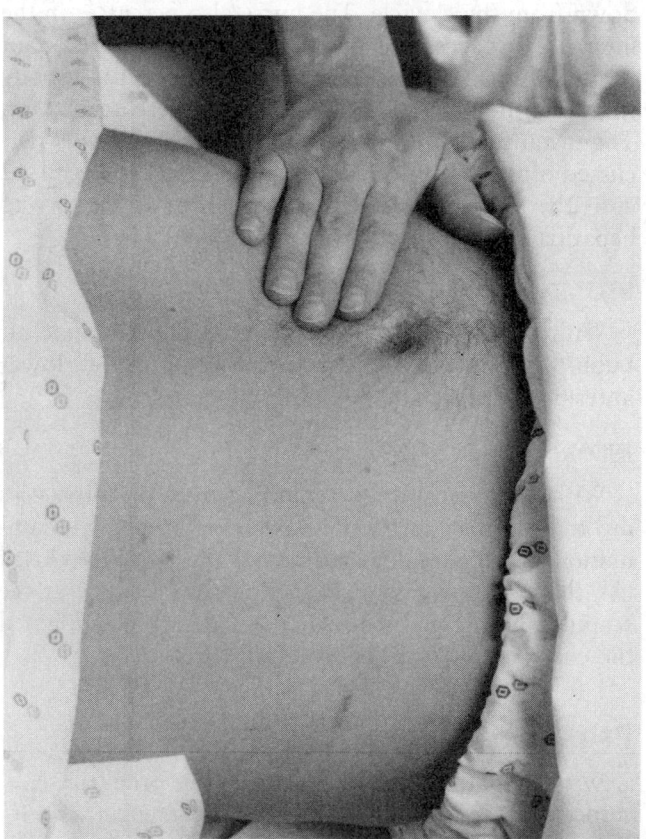

Fig. 13-81 Light palpation of the abdomen.

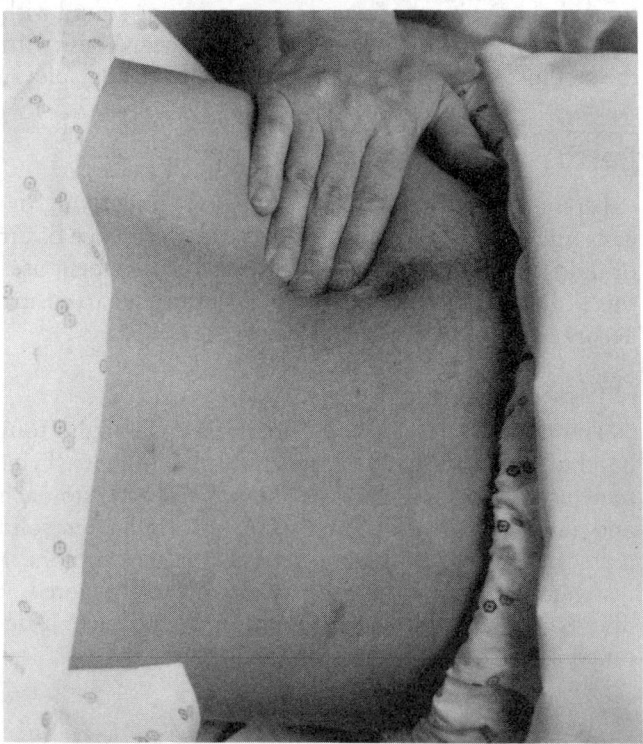

Fig. 13-82 Deep palpation of the abdomen.

Each quadrant is surveyed systematically. Masses palpated are assessed for size, location, shape, consistency, tenderness, mobility (for example, during respiration), and palpation. If tenderness is found, the examiner checks for rebound tenderness. With this test the examiner presses a hand slowly and deeply into the involved area and then lets go quickly. If pain is aggravated with the release of the hand, the test is positive. Rebound tenderness occurs in clients with inflammation of the abdominal cavity (peritonitis).

LIVER PALPATION

The liver normally lies in the right upper quadrant under the rib cage. The nurse uses deep palpation to locate the liver's lower edge. This technique detects liver enlargement.

To palpate the liver, the nurse places the left hand under the client's right posterior thorax at the eleventh and twelfth ribs and then applies upward pressure. This maneuver makes it easier to feel the liver anteriorly. With the fingers of the right hand pointing toward the right costal margin, the nurse places the hand on the right upper quadrant well below the liver's lower border, then presses gently in and up (Fig. 13-83). The client should take a deep breath, using the abdominal muscles. As the client inhales, the nurse tries to palpate the liver's edge

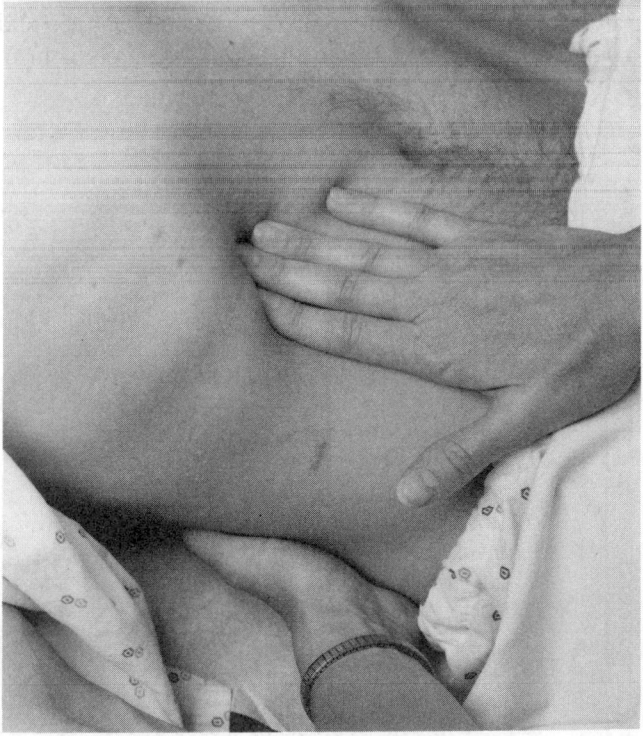

Fig. 13-83 The nurse's left hand is placed under the client's posterior thorax at the eleventh and twelfth ribs. The nurse's right hand palpates in and up to feel the liver's edge as the client inhales.

as it descends. The normal liver is nontender and has a firm, regular, and sharp edge. If the liver is palpable, the nurse traces its edge medially and laterally by repeating the maneuver.

AORTIC PALPATION

To assess aortic pulsation, the nurse palpates with the thumb and forefinger of one hand deeply into the upper abdomen, just left of the midline. Normally a pulsation is transmitted forward. If there is enlargement of the aorta from an aneurysm, the pulsation expands laterally. In obese clients, it may be necessary to palpate with both hands, one on each side of the aorta.

BLADDER PALPATION

It is usually unnecessary to palpate the bladder routinely. However, clients who are still under the effects of anesthesia postoperatively, who have received large doses of analgesic medications, who have spinal cord injuries, or who suffer incontinence should be examined for bladder retention. The nurse places one hand just above the symphysis pubis and palpates, feeling for the smooth bladder dome. An empty bladder is not palpable.

RECTUM AND ANUS

An examination of the rectum and anus can be conducted separately or as a continuation of the examination of the genitalia and reproductive organs. Usually the examination is not performed in young children or adolescents. The examination detects colorectal cancer in its early stages. In males the rectal examination can also detect prostatic tumors. The nurse collects a thorough history (Table 13-26) to detect risk for bowel or rectal disease.

The rectal examination can be uncomfortable and embarrassing, so the nurse uses a calm, gentle approach. Explanation of the procedure helps clients to relax and lessens discomfort during the digital examination. The left lateral sidelying (Sims) position is preferred. Clients are draped with only the anal area exposed. In females, the rectal examination may be done with clients in the lithotomy or dorsal recumbent position. The nurse uses disposable gloves and lubricant.

Inspection

Using the ungloved, nondominant hand the nurse gently retracts the buttocks as needed to visualize the perianal and saccrococcygeal areas. Anal tissues are normally moist and hairless compared with perianal skin. The anus is held closed by the voluntary external muscle sphincter. The nurse inspects for lumps, hemorrhoids

TABLE 13-26 Nursing History for Rectum and Anus Assessment

Assessment Category	Rationale
Determine if client has experienced bleeding from the rectum, black or tarry stools (melena), rectal pain, or change in bowel habits (constipation or diarrhea).	These are warning signs of colorectal cancer or other gastrointestinal alterations.
Determine if client has personal or family history of colorectal cancer, polyps, or inflammatory bowel disease.	These are risk factors for colorectal cancer.
Assess dietary habits for high-fat intake or deficient fiber content.	Bowel cancer may be linked to dietary intake of fat or insufficient fiber intake.
Determine if client has undergone screening for colorectal cancer (digital exam, stool blood slide test, proctoscopy).	Undergoing this screening reflects understanding and compliance with preventive health care measures.
Assess medication history for use of laxatives or cathartic medications.	Repeated use can cause diarrhea and eventual loss of intestinal muscle tone.
Assess use of codeine or iron preparations.	Codeine causes constipation. Iron turns the color of feces black and tarry.

(dilated veins that appear as reddened pretrusions of the skin), ulcers, inflammation, rashes, or excoriations. The perianal skin is normally intact, more pigmented, and coarser than the skin overlying the buttocks. The nurse then asks the client to bear down. This manuever helps to reveal presence of internal hemorrhoids or fissures in the anal lining. Normally the anal lining is intact.

Digital Palpation

Some institutions do not permit nurses to perform digital examinations. When policy permits, the nursing student should have a qualified examiner present during the first examination.

The nurse lubricates the index finger of the gloved dominant hand. The procedure is explained, then the client is asked to bear down gently as if having a bowel movement. As the anal sphincter relaxes, the nurse's fingertip is gently inserted into the anal canal, in a direction toward the umbilicus. Normally the client feels as though he must pass stool. The nurse should never force digital insertion.

The anal canal is the distal portion of the gastrointestinal tract. The canal extends in a line toward the umbilicus before turning into the mucus-lined rectum. The anus contains a rich supply of sensory nerve fibers. Thus digital manipulation can be painful. At the junction of the anal canal and rectum, the rectum balloons out and turns posteriorly into the hollow of the coccyx and sacrum. The nurse notes the tone of the anal sphincter as the muscle closes snugly around the finger. Careful palpation of each side of the rectal wall detects tenderness, irregularities, or nodules. Once the finger is advanced to its full extent, the client is asked to bear down

again. High lesions within the rectum will descend against the fingertip (see client-teaching box).

In male clients the nurse turns the hand so the finger palpates the anterior rectal wall. The prostate gland is palpable anteriorly as a rounded, heart-shaped structure about 2.5 to 4 cm (1 to 1½ inches) in length (Fig. 13-84). A small medial groove separates the gland into two lateral lobes. The nurse palpates the size, shape, and consistency of the prostate. The gland normally is firm, without bogginess, tenderness, or nodules.

Client Teaching after Rectum and Anus Assessment

- Discuss the American Cancer Society's guidelines for early detection of colorectal cancer:
  □ Digital rectal examination performed yearly after age 40.
  □ Stool blood slide test (guaiac test) performed yearly after age 50.
  □ Proctosigmoidoscopy, involving visual inspection of the rectum and lower colon with a hollow, lighted tube. The test, performed by a physician, should be performed every 3 to 5 years after age 50, after two annual examinations with negative results.
- Discuss dietary planning to reduce fat and increase fiber content.
- Warn clients against problems caused by overuse of laxatives, cathartic medications, codeine, or enemas.

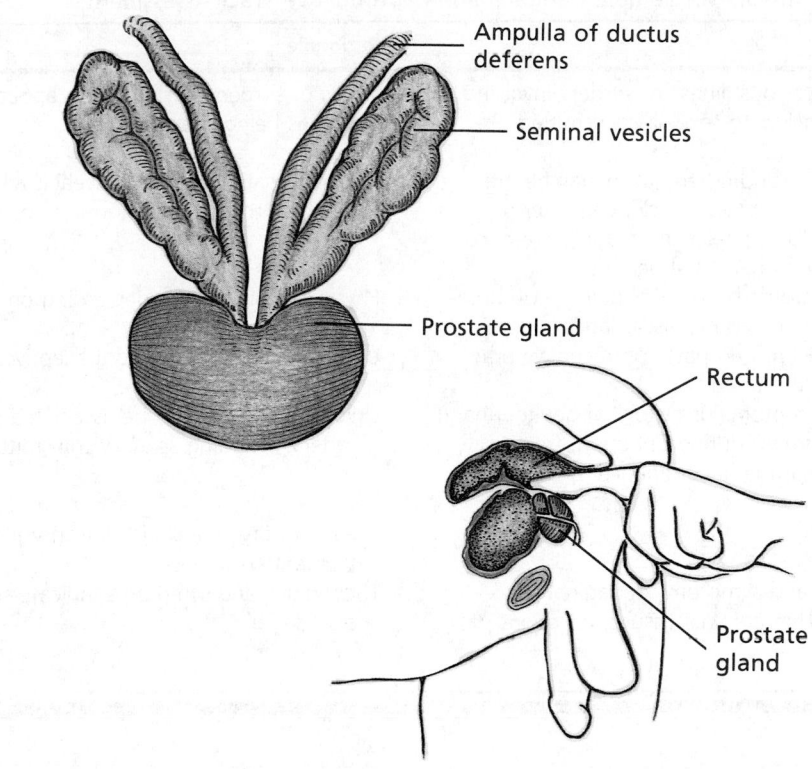

Ampulla of ductus deferens

Seminal vesicles

Prostate gland

Rectum

Prostate gland

Fig. 13-84   Palpation of the prostate gland during the rectal examination.

In females, it may be possible to palpate the cervix through the anterior rectal wall. It is common to mistake the cervix or an inserted tampon for a rectal tumor.

Once palpation is completed the nurse gently withdraws the finger and observes it for feces. Feces are normally brown. The presence of mucus, blood, or black, tarry stool should be reported. A sample of the feces is tested for occult blood (see Chapter 39). For women suspected of having sexually transmitted disease, a rectal culture is taken to rule out the presence of cross-infection from vaginal discharge. The nurse cleans the perianal area before continuing to the next part of the examination.

FEMALE GENITALIA AND REPRODUCTIVE TRACT

An examination of the genital area is viewed with uncertainty by many women. The adolescent will probably be fearful of the unknown. A woman's cultural background may add to her apprehension. The lithotomy position assumed during the examination is often a source of embarrassment so the nurse uses a calm, reassuring, and attentive approach. The client's comfort

is determined by the way she is positioned and draped. Each portion of the examination is explained in advance so the client can anticipate the nurse's actions. Delays that might aggravate embarrassment should be avoided.

The examination is relatively simple and should be a part of each women's preventive health care because uterine and vaginal cancer have a high incidence rate. Adolescents should be examined because of the growing incidence of sexually transmitted diseases. The nurse collects a complete history (Table 13-27) to assess the client's health status. The examination maybe part of a complete physical examination or an assessment conducted while the nurse performs routine hygiene measures or inserts a urinary catheter.

Preparing the Client

If the client is having a complete examination, the following special equipment will be needed:
1. Examination table with stirrups
2. Vaginal speculum
3. Adjustable light source
4. Sink
5. Lubricant
6. Clean, disposable gloves

TABLE 13-27 Nursing History for Female Genitalia and Reproductive Tract Assessment

Assessment Category	Rationale
Determine if client has previous illness or surgery involving reproductive organs, including sexually transmitted disease.	Illness or surgery can influence appearance and position of organs being examined.
Review menstrual history including age at menarche, frequency and duration of menstrual cycle, character of flow (for example, amount, presence of clots), presence of pain, dates of last two menstrual periods.	This information helps to reveal level of female's reproductive health, including normalcy of menstrual cycle.
Ask client to describe obstetric history, including each pregnancy and history of abortions or miscarriages.	Physical findings vary, depending on woman's history of pregnancy.
Ask client to describe current and past contraceptive practices and problems encountered.	Use of certain types of contraceptives may influence reproductive health.
Determine if client has symptoms or history of genitourinary problems, including burning during urination, frequency, urgency, nocturia, hematuria, incontinence, or stress incontinence.	Urinary problems may be associated with gynecological disorders, including sexually transmitted diseases.
Assess client's sexual history.	Sexual history reveals risk for and understanding of sexually transmitted disease.
Assess if client has signs and symptoms of vaginal discharge, painful or swollen perianal tissues, or lesions of the genitalia.	These signs and symptoms indicate sexually transmitted disease.

7. Glass microscopic slides
8. Sponge forceps or swabs
9. Wooden spatulas
10. Specimen bottles with fixative solution.

All equipment must be ready before the examination begins.

Often it will be necessary to collect a urine specimen. If this is the only examination, the client should empty her bladder before the examination begins. If a vaginal examination is to be performed, the client should be placed in a lithotomy position. This position is most practical because it allows full visualization of the genital area. The client lies on her back, the thighs are flexed and abducted, the knees are flexed, and the feet rest in stirrups. The client's arms should be at her sides or folded across the chest to prevent tightening of abdominal muscles.

A square drape or sheet is given to the client. She holds one corner over her sternum, the adjacent corners fall over each knee, and the fourth corner covers the perineum. Once the examination begins, the drape over the perineum is lifted.

If the nurse wishes to examine only the external genitalia, she helps the client assume the lithotomy position in bed or on the examination table. The client flexes her knees perpendicular to the bed and is then asked to relax her thighs, allowing each leg to abduct to the side. The client's head may be elevated for comfort. A woman suffering pain or deformity of the joints may be unable to assume a lithotomy position. In this situation it may

be necessary to have the client abduct only one leg or to have another nurse assist in separating the client's thighs.

The male examiner should always have a female in attendance during the examination. A female examiner may prefer to work alone but should have a female attendant if the client is particularly anxious or emotionally unstable.

External Genitalia

The perineal area must be well illuminated. The nurse gloves both hands to prevent the spread of infection.

The perineum is extremely sensitive and tender. The area is not touched without warning the client. It is best to touch the neighboring thigh first before advancing to the perineum.

To assess sexual maturity, quantity and distribution of hair growth is noted. A preadolescent has no pubic hair except for fine body hair like that on the abdomen. During adolescence, hair growth begins along the labia, becoming darker, coarser, and curlier as it spreads over the pubic symphysis. Hair growth eventually forms a triangle over the female perineum and along the medial surfaces of the thighs. Hair growth should not spread up over the abdomen. The nurse also inspects the skin of the pubic hair for lice, inflammation, irritation, or lesions.

The skin of the perineum is slightly darker than the skin of the rest of the body. The labia majora are usually

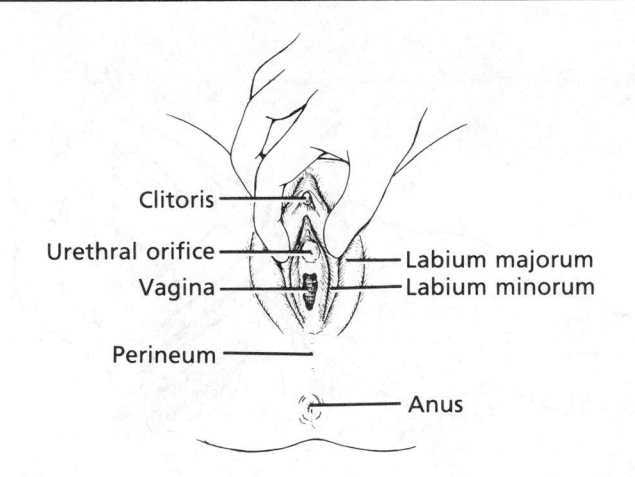

Fig. 13-85 Female external genitalia.

plump and well formed in a normal adult female. After childbirth the labia majora are separated, causing the labia minora to become more prominent. When a woman reaches menopause, the labia majora become thinned and with advancing age they become atrophied. The labia majora are normally without inflammation, edema, lesions, or lacerations.

To inspect the remaining external structures, the nurse gently places the thumb and index finger inside the labia minora and retracts the tissues outwardly with the non-dominant hand (Fig. 13-85). The nurse should have a firm hold to avoid repeated retraction against the sensitive tissues. The clitoris, labia minora, urethral orifice, hymen, and vaginal orifice are then examined, paying particular attention to discharge, inflammation, edema, ulceration, or lesions.

The size of the clitoris is variable. However, it normally is 0.5 cm (⅕ inch) in diameter. If inflamed, the clitoris will be a bright cherry red. In young women it is a common site for syphilitic lesions or chancres, which appear as small open ulcers that drain serous material. Elderly women may have malignant changes that result in dry, scaly, nodular lesions.

The labia minora are normally thinner than the labia majora. One side is usually larger than the other. In the female who is a virgin, the labia normally lie together. As a result of vaginal childbirth or intercourse they tend to gape more and fall to the sides.

When inspecting the vaginal orifice or introitus, the examiner notices the condition of the hymen, which is just inside the introitus. In the virgin the hymen may restrict the opening of the vagina. Only remnants of the hymen remain after sexual intercourse.

If inflammation and edema are found near the posterior end of the introitus, Bartholin's glands may be infected. The glands cannot normally be palpated. To

attempt palpation the nurse places a thumb and index finger between the labia majora and introitus and palpates one side at a time.

The urethral orifice is carefully observed for inflammation. The urethra is often difficult to locate. It is a small slit or pinhole opening just above the vaginal canal. In women who have had several vaginal childbirths, the opening to the vaginal canal often extends upward, interfering with the view of the urethra.

Minute openings of the Skene's gland are around the urethra. The nurse suspecting inflammation checks for urethral discharge. The nurse gently places an index finger 2.5 cm (1 inch) in the vaginal orifice and milks the urethra gently from inside outward. Drainage will be manually expressed if inflammation is present. If drainage is found, the nurse changes gloves for the remainder of the examination.

With the gloved index and middle fingers in the vaginal orifice, the nurse asks the client to strain downwards as if she was voiding. If the client lacks adequate muscular support, the vaginal walls will bulge, blocking the introitus opening. A portion of the vaginal wall and bladder (cystocele) may prolapse or fall into the orifice anteriorly. A bulging of the posterior wall may be caused by a prolapse of the rectum (rectocele). Normally when a client is asked to constrict or close the vaginal orifice, the nurse will palpate tension in the muscles. A female who has undergone vaginal childbirth has less muscle tone than one who has not.

After completing the external examination the nurse disposes of the examination gloves. The client is offered perineal hygiene for her comfort.

Internal Genitalia

To view the internal walls of the vagina and the cervix a speculum examination is needed. *Beginning students are unlikely to perform a speculum examination because the procedure requires considerable practice.* The procedure should *not* be attempted without supervision by an experienced examiner because incorrect use of the speculum can cause trauma to vaginal tissues. During the examination, specimens are collected for testing for cervical and vaginal cancer (Papanicolaou [Pap] smears). The speculum consists of two blades: the top, which is movable, and the bottom, which is fixed. The blades are attached by a thumbscrew that can be adjusted to open or close the blades. It helps to practice opening and closing the speculum before using it with a client. The nurse must select the proper size speculum to avoid causing discomfort. The smallest size will fit the virginal female. If the woman is sexually active, a medium-sized speculum is best. For women who have had children vaginally, the examiner uses a medium-to-large speculum.

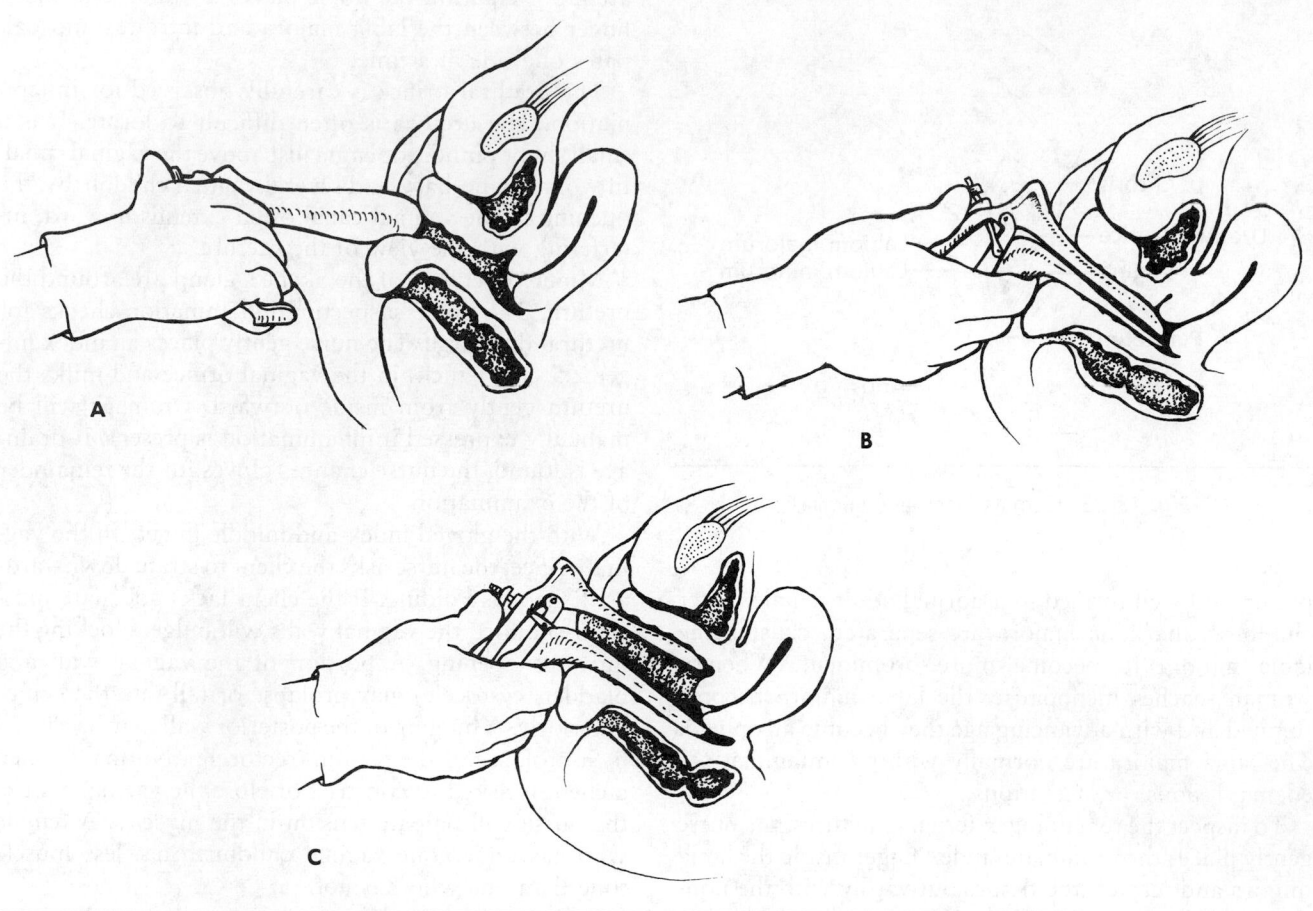

Fig. 13-86 Insertion of vaginal speculum. **A,** Speculum is introduced at oblique angle. **B,** Speculum is inserted downward at 45-degree angle to table. **C,** Blades are opened after full insertion.

Before the examination begins, the sterilized speculum blades are warmed in warm running water. Water is the ideal lubricant because commercially prepared lubricants interfere with Pap smear studies. The nurse sits on a stool facing the client's perineum. The adjustable light is placed over the examiner's shoulder, directed toward the examination site. The nurse applies a new pair of disposable gloves.

The nurse holds the speculum in the dominant hand and explains the procedure to the client. If the woman has never been examined, two fingers are gently inserted into the vagina to explore for abnormalities. Then with two fingers the nurse presses down on the perineal body just inside the introitus. After checking to be sure the speculum blades are closed, the nurse introduces the closed speculum obliquely (rotated 50 degrees counterclockwise from the vertical position) past the fingers (Fig. 13-86). The speculum is inserted downward at a 45-degree angle toward the examination table to avoid

trauma to the urethra (this maneuver corresponds with the normal downward slope of the vaginal canal). Care is taken to avoid pulling the pubic hair or pinching the labia.

After the wide portions of the blades have passed the introitus, the speculum is rotated so the blades are horizontal. The blades are opened slowly after full insertion and the speculum is moved to visualize the cervix. When the cervix is in full view, the blades are locked in the open position.

CERVIX

The nurse inspects the cervix and its opening or os. The normal cervix is a glistening pink color. The cervical diameter is approximately 2.5 to 3 cm (1 to 1$\frac{2}{10}$ inches) in a normal young female. In an elderly woman the cervix is smaller. The cervix of a nulliparous female (woman who has not delivered a viable fetus) is round whereas that of a multiparous female (woman who has

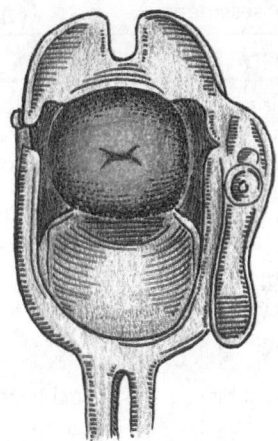

Fig. 13-87 Appearance of cervix through vaginal speculum.

delivered one or more viable newborns) is slitlike (Fig. 13-87). Discharge, lacerations, ulcerations, or lesions are abnormal.

Any discharge is examined carefully for color, odor, quantity, and consistency. Chronic infections yield thick, malodorous discharges.

PAP SMEAR

A Papanicolaou smear is a screening test for cervical cancer. Women who are sexually active and women over the age of 20 who do not have symptoms of disease are advised to have annual tests until two smears are negative. Thereafter, tests are to be done every 3 years until the age of 65. Women at risk for cervical cancer should have annual checkups (see client-teaching box).

Client Teaching after Female Genitalia and Reproductive Tract Assessment

- Instruct client about recommended frequency of Pap smears and gynecological examinations.
- Counsel clients with sexually transmitted disease about diagnosis and treatment. Teach preventive measures (for example, male partner's use of condoms, restricting number of sexual partners, avoiding sex with persons who have several other partners, and perineal hygiene measures).
- Tell clients with sexually transmitted diseases that they must inform sexual partners of the need for an examination.
- Reinforce the importance of perineal hygiene (as appropriate).

TABLE 13-28 Methods for Obtaining Pap Smears

Location	Technique
Endocervical	Use a cotton swab or applicator. Gently insert swab through the cervical os. Rotate the swab 360 degrees. Apply cells and secretions to glass slide. Apply fixative solution and label slide.
Outer cervix	Use the wooden Ayre spatula. Place tip of longer arm in cervical os. Rotate spatula, scraping the outer surface of the cervix. Apply cells to glass slide. Apply fixative solution and label slide.
Vaginal pool	Rotate spatula, inserting handle into vagina. Place handle on vaginal floor. Apply cells and secretions to glass slide. Apply fixative and label slide.

The examiner collects smear samples from three sites: the endocervical area, the outer cervix, and the vaginal pool (Table 13-28). After specimens are obtained, the nurse prepares slides with the fixative solution. The specimens are labeled with the client's name and source of the specimen.

VAGINA

The vaginal walls are viewed more easily as the speculum is withdrawn. As the speculum leaves the cervix, the thumbscrew is loosened but the blades are kept open with the thumb. During the withdrawal the nurse inspects the vaginal wall's texture, color, and support. Any discharge or lesions are noted. The color is normally pink throughout. Women commonly acquire yeast infections, which cause a thick, white, patchy, curdlike discharge that clings to the vaginal walls. The nurse closes the blades gradually as the speculum is removed to avoid excess stretching and pinching of the mucosa. The blades should be closed completely as the speculum emerges from the introitus. The nurse removes the disposable gloves and discards them in a proper receptacle. Perineal hygiene is provided for the client.

MALE GENITALIA

An examination of the male genitalia includes assessment of the external genitalia and the inguinal ring. Because the incidence of sexually transmitted disease in adolescents and young adults is high, an assessment of the genitalia should be a routine part of any health maintenance examination for this age group (see client-teaching box). If this is the only assessment to be performed on a client, the nurse must be sure to collect a thorough nursing history (Table 13-29).

The female nurse must learn to relax during the male client's genital examination, because her anxiety would make the procedure highly embarrassing for herself and the client. If the female nurse feels uncomfortable, she should ask a male nurse or male physician to perform the examination. The nurse should not discuss the client's sexual activity during the examination, because the client might perceive this discussion as evaluative or judgmental (see client-teaching box).

The client's modesty must be preserved. The genitalia are gently manipulated to avoid causing discomfort. The

---

TABLE 13-29 Nursing History for Male Genitalia Assessment

Assessment Category	Rationale
Review normal urinary elimination pattern: frequency of voiding; history of nocturia; character and volume of urine; fluid intake daily; symptoms of burning, urgency, frequency; difficulty starting stream; hematuria.	Urinary problems can be directly associated with gynecological problems because of the anatomy of males' reproductive and urinary systems.
Assess client's sexual history	Sexual history reveals risk for and understanding of sexually transmitted disease.
Determine if client has had previous surgery or illness involving urinary or reproductive organs.	Alterations resulting from disease or surgery may be responsible for symptoms or changes in organ structure or function.
Ask if client has noted penile pain or swelling, lesions of the genitalia, urethral discharge.	These signs and symptoms indicate sexually transmitted disease.

---

examination begins with the client lying supine with the chest, abdomen, and lower legs draped. Inspection and palpation are used. The nurse applies disposable gloves to prevent cross-infection from urethral discharge.

External Genitalia

The nurse begins by assessing the sexual maturity of the client, noting the size and shape of the penis and testes, the color and texture of the scrotal skin, and the character and distribution of pubic hair. The first sign of puberty, involving an increase in the size of the testes begins between 9.5 and 13.5 years of age. During the preadolescent stage, there is no pubic hair except for the fine body hair found on the abdomen. As a boy matures the pubic hair first begins to grow at the base of the penis and then begins to spread over the symphysis pubis. The hair changes from straight and soft to coarse and curly. By the end of puberty the testes and penis have enlarged to adult size and shape. The scrotal skin darkens and becomes wrinkled in texture. The pubic hair forms a triangle, covering the symphysis pubis and medial surfaces of the thighs.

The nurse inspects the skin covering the genitalia for lice, rashes, excoriations, or lesions.

> ### Client Teaching after Male Genitalia Assessment
>
> - Instruct client about testicular self-examination (see box, p. 312) and allow for return demonstration.
> - Counsel clients with sexually transmitted diseases about diagnosis and treatment. Teach preventive measures (for example, using condoms, restricting the number of sexual partners, avoiding sex with persons who have several other partners, and using perineal hygiene).
> - Tell clients with sexually transmitted disease that they must inform sexual partners of the need for an examination.

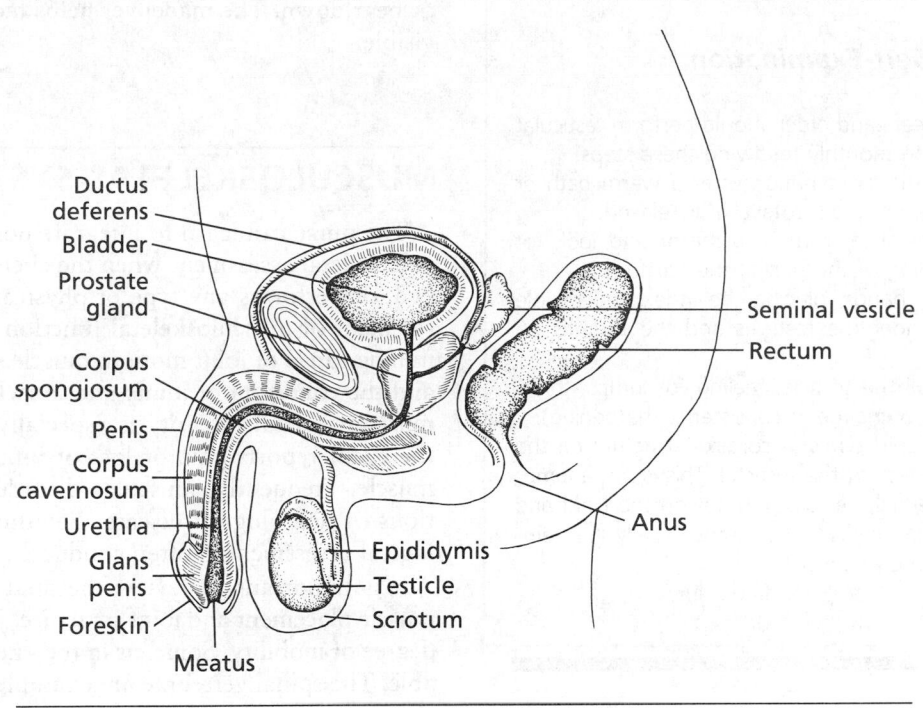

Fig. 13-88 External and internal male sex organs.

Labels: Ductus deferens, Bladder, Prostate gland, Corpus spongiosum, Penis, Corpus cavernosum, Urethra, Glans penis, Foreskin, Meatus, Seminal vesicle, Rectum, Anus, Epididymis, Testicle, Scrotum

PENIS

The nurse inspects the structures of the penis, including the shaft, corona, prepuce (foreskin), glans, and urethral meatus (Fig. 13-88). The penile structures should not be excessively manipulated because an erection may be caused.

If the foreskin is present, retract it or ask the client to do so. The foreskin should retract easily. A small amount of thick, white secretion between the glans and foreskin is normal. If there is evidence of abnormal discharge, a culture is usually obtained. The urethral meatus should be positioned at the tip of the glans. In some congenital conditions the meatus is displaced along the penile shaft. Gentle compression of the glans between the nurse's thumb and index finger opens the urethral meatus to allow inspection for discharge. The meatus is also inspected for lesions, edema, and inflammation.

The glans is carefully checked around its entire circumference for lesions. The area between the foreskin and glans is a common site for venereal lesions. Any lesion is palpated gently to note tenderness, size, consistency, and shape. When inspection of the glans is completed, the foreskin is pulled down to its original position.

The nurse continues to inspect the entire shaft of the penis, including the undersurface, looking for any lesions, scars, or areas of edema. The shaft is palpated between the thumb and first two fingers to detect any localized areas of hardness.

Scrotum

The nurse must be particularly cautious when inspecting and palpating the scrotum, because the structures lying within the scrotal sac are very sensitive.

The scrotum is a saclike structure divided internally into two halves. Each half contains a testicle, epididymis, and the vas deferens, which travels upward into the inguinal ring. It is normal to find the left testicle lower than the right. The nurse inspects size, shape, and symmetry while observing for lesions or edema. The scrotum is gently lifted to view the posterior surface. The scrotal skin is usually loose. A tightening of the skin may reveal edema. The scrotum's size normally changes with temperature variations as its dartos muscle contracts in cold and relaxes in warm temperature.

The underlying testicles are normally ovoid and approximately 2×4 cm ($\frac{4}{5} \times 1\frac{3}{5}$ inch) in size. The testicles and epididymis are gently palpated between the nurse's thumb and first two fingers. The nurse explains how to perform testicular self-examinations (see box on next page). The most common symptom of testicular cancer is a small, hard lump, about the size of a pea, on the front or side of the testicle. The size, shape, and consistency of the organs are noted. The testicles normally feel smooth and firm. The epididymis is resilient. In the elderly client, the testicles decrease in size and are less firm in palpation. The client should be asked about any unusual tenderness. The nurse continues palpating the vas deferens separately as it forms the spermatic cord

Testicular Self-Examination

All males 15 years and older should perform testicular self-examination monthly following these steps:

1. Perform the examination after a warm bath or shower when the scrotal skin is relaxed.
2. Stand naked in front of a mirror and look for any swelling of the skin of the scrotum.
3. Use both hands, placing the index and middle fingers under the testicles and the thumbs on top.
4. Gently roll the testicle, feeling for lumps, thickening, or a change in consistency (hardening).
5. Find the epididymis (a cordlike structure on the top and back of the testicle). This is *not* a lump.
6. Feel for small, pea-sized lumps on the front and side of the testicle. The lumps usually are painless and are abnormal.
7. Call your doctor if you find a lump.

toward the inguinal ring, noting the presence of nodules or swelling.

Inguinal Ring and Canal

The external inguinal ring provides the opening for the spermatic cord to pass into the inguinal canal. The canal forms a passage through the abdominal wall, a potential site for hernia formation. A hernia is a protrusion of a portion of intestine through the inguinal wall or canal. An intestinal loop may even enter the scrotum. The client stands during this portion of the examination.

Both inguinal areas are inspected for signs of obvious bulging. During inspection the client is asked to strain or bear down. The maneuver helps make a hernia more visible.

MUSCULOSKELETAL SYSTEM

The nurse can learn to integrate portions of the musculoskeletal assessment when the client walks, moves in bed, or performs any type of physical activity. The assessment of musculoskeletal function focuses on determining range of joint motion, muscle strength and tone, and the condition of joints and muscles. Assessment of musculoskeletal integrity is especially important when the client reports pain or loss of function in a joint or muscle. Frequently, muscular disorders are manifestations of neurological disease. For this reason a neurological assessment is often conducted simultaneously.

It is important to review the anatomy of bone and muscle placement and joint structure. Joints vary in their degree of mobility. Some, as in the knee, are freely movable. The spinal vertebrae are examples of slightly movable joints.

The examination uses inspection and palpation. The muscles and joints should be exposed and free to move. Depending on the muscle groups assessed, the client assumes a sitting, supine, prone, or standing position. Table 13-30 lists the information gathered in the nursing history.

General Inspection

The nurse observes gait and posture as the client walks into the examination room. When the client is unaware of the nature of the observations, his gait is more natural. Later a more formal test involves having the client walk in a straight line away from the nurse and then return. The nurse looks for foot dragging, limping, shuffling,

TABLE 13-30 Nursing History for Musculoskeletal System Assessment

Assessment Category	Rationale
Ask client to describe history of alteration in bone, muscle, or joint function (for example, recent fall, trauma, lifting heavy objects, history of bone or joint disease with sudden or gradual onset, and location of alteration).	History assists in assessing nature of musculoskeletal problem.
Assess nature and extent of pain, including location, duration, severity, predisposing and aggravating factors, relieving factors, and type of pain.	Alterations in bone, joints, or muscle are frequently accompanied by pain, which has implications for not only comfort but also the ability to perform ADL.
Determine how alteration influences ability to perform ADL (for example, bathing, feeding, dressing, toileting, and ambulating) and social functions (for example, household chores, work, recreation, sexual activities.	Level of nursing care will be determined by extent to which client is able to perform self-care. Type and degree of restriction in continuing social activities influences topics for client education and ability of nurse to identify alternative ways to maintain function.

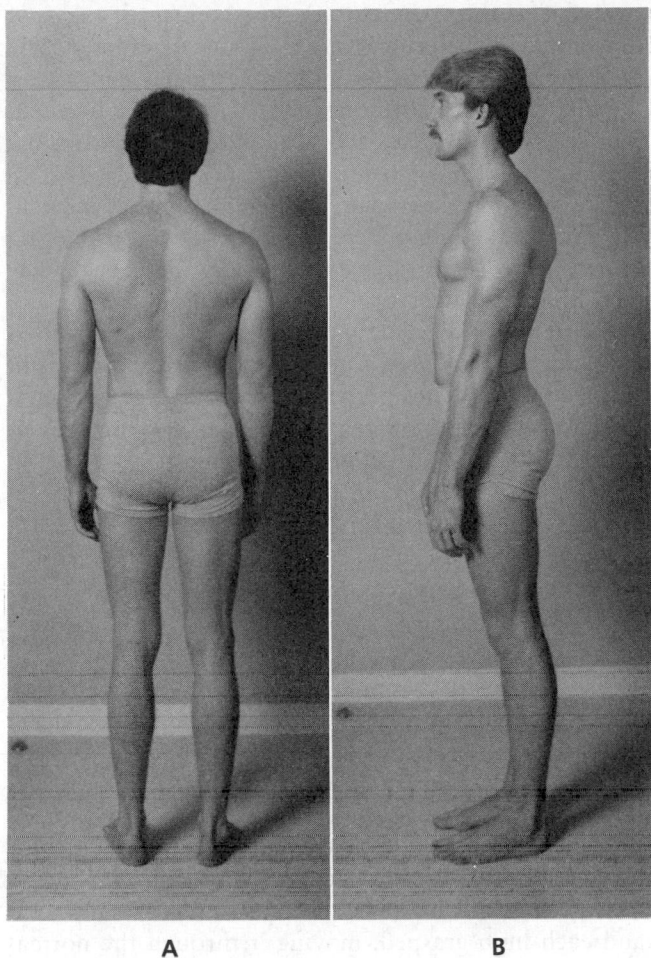

A   **B**

Fig. 13-89 **A,** Normal standing position. Client's hips and shoulders are aligned in parallel. **B,** Viewing the client sideways allows the nurse to observe the cervical, thoracic, and lumbar curves.

and the position of the trunk in relation to the legs. Normally the client walks with arms swinging freely at the sides and the head and face leading the body. An elderly client often walks with smaller steps and a wider base of support.

The normal standing posture is an upright stance with parallel alignment of the hips and shoulders (Fig. 13-89). Looking sideways at the client, the nurse notes the normal cervical, thoracic, and lumbar curves. The head is held erect. As the client sits, some degree of rounding of the shoulders is normal. Common postural abnormalities include lordosis, kyphosis, and scoliosis (Fig. 13-90). Kyphosis or hunchback is an exaggeration of the posterior curvature of the thoracic spine. This postural abnormality is common in the elderly. Lordosis or swayback is an increased lumbar curvature. A lateral spinal curvature is called scoliosis (see client-teaching box on next page).

During general inspection the nurse looks for symmetry of joints, muscles, and extremity length and obvious musculoskeletal deformities. A general review pinpoints areas requiring specialized assessment.

Range of Joint Motion

The nurse asks the client to put each joint through its full range of motion. If the client is weakened by illness, the nurse assesses range of motion passively by gently supporting and moving the extremities through their range of movement. The nurse must learn the correct terminology for the movements the joints are capable of making (Table 13-31). It also helps to practice range of motion of one's own joints to learn the limits of mobility. The same body parts are compared for equality in movement.

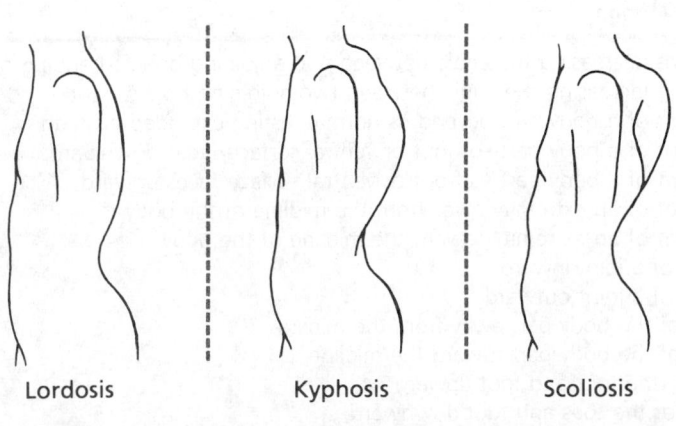

Lordosis   Kyphosis   Scoliosis

Fig. 13-90 Common postural abnormalities.

When assessing the client's range of motion, the nurse does not force a joint into a painful position. The nurse must know the joint's normal range and the extent to which it can be moved (see Chapter 41). Ideally, the normal range is assessed to determine a baseline for assessing later change.

A goniometer measures the precise degree of motion in a particular joint and is used mainly in clients who have a suspected reduction in joint movement. The instrument has two flexible arms with a 180-degree protractor in the center. The center of the protractor is positioned at the center of the joint being measured (Fig. 13-91, *A*). The arms extend along the body parts on each side of the protractor. A measurement is taken of the joint angle before moving the joint. After taking the joint through a full range of motion, the nurse measures the angle again to determine the degree of movement (Fig. 13-91, *B*). The reading is compared with the normal degree of joint movement.

When putting each joint through its range of motion, the nurse makes a number of basic observations, noting any swelling, stiffness, instability, deformity, or tenderness. Normal joints are nontender, without swelling, and move freely. In the elderly, joints often become swollen and stiff, with reduced range of motion resulting from cartilage erosion and fibrosis of synovial membranes.

The nurse also palpates for unusual joint movement and for nodules. Crepitus (a crackling sensation and noise caused by rubbing of bone fragments) may be noted. A normal joint has no nodules or crepitus. If a joint appears swollen and inflamed, the nurse may be able to detect warmth in the tissues.

Muscle Tone and Strength

The nurse may assess muscle strength and tone during measurement of range of motion. Tone is the slight muscular resistance felt by the examiner as the relaxed extremity is passively moved through its range of motion.

The client is asked to allow an extremity to relax or hang limp. This is often difficult, particularly if the client feels pain in the extremity. The extremity is supported and each limb grasped, moving it through the normal range of motion. Normal tone causes a mild, even resistance to movement through the entire range (Fig. 13-92).

If a muscle has increased tone or hypertonicity, any sudden passive movement of a joint is met with considerable resistance. Continued movement eventually causes the muscle to relax. A hypotonic muscle that has

TABLE 13-31 Terminology for Normal Range of Motion Positions

Term	Range of Motion	Examples of Joints
Flexion	Movement decreasing the angle between two adjoining bones; bending of a limb	Elbow, fingers, knee
Extension	Movement increasing the angle between two adjoining bones	Elbow, knee, fingers
Hyperextension	Movement of a body part beyond its normal resting extended position	Head
Pronation	Movement of a body part so front or ventral surface faces downward	Hand, forearm
Supination	Movement of a body part so front or ventral surface faces upward	Hand, forearm
Abduction	Movement of an extremity away from the midline of the body	Leg, arm, fingers
Adduction	Movement of an extremity toward the midline of the body	Leg, arm, fingers
Internal rotation	Rotation of a joint inward	Knee, hip
External rotation	Rotation of a joint outward	Knee, hip
Eversion	Turning of the body part away from the midline	Foot
Inversion	Turning of the body part toward the midline	Foot
Dorsiflexion	Flexion of the toes and foot upward	Foot
Plantar flexion	Bending of the toes and foot downward	Foot

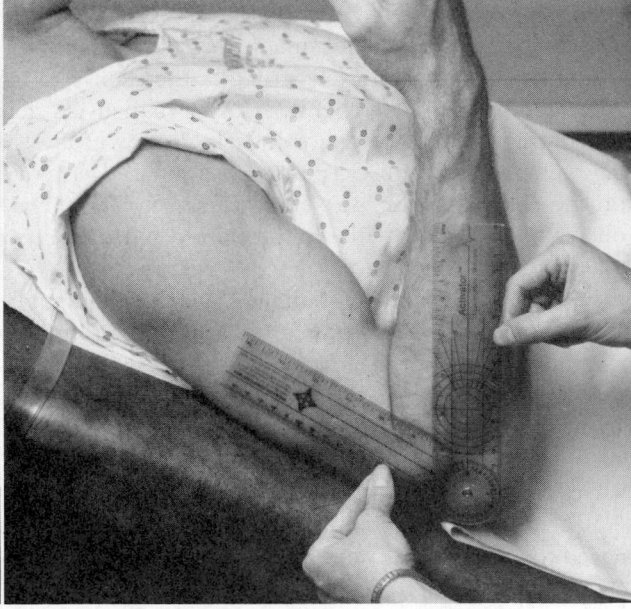

Fig. 13-91   A, The nurse positions the goniometer at the center of the elbow with the arms extending along the client's upper and lower arms. B, After the client flexes the arm the goniometer measures the degree of joint flexion.

TABLE 13-32   Maneuvers to Assess Muscle Strength

Muscle Group	Maneuver
Neck (sternocleido-mastoid)	Place hand firmly against client's upper jaw. Ask client to turn head laterally against resistance.
Shoulder (trapezius)	Place hand over midline of client's shoulder, exerting firm pressure. Have client raise shoulders against resistance.
Elbow	
Biceps	Pull down on forearm as client attempts to flex arm.
Triceps	As client's arm is flexed, apply pressure against the forearm. Ask the client to straighten his arm.
Hip	
Quadriceps	When the client is sitting, apply downward pressure to the thigh. Ask the client to raise the leg up from table.
Gastrocnemius	Client sits, holding the shin of his flexed leg. Ask the client to straighten the leg against resistance.

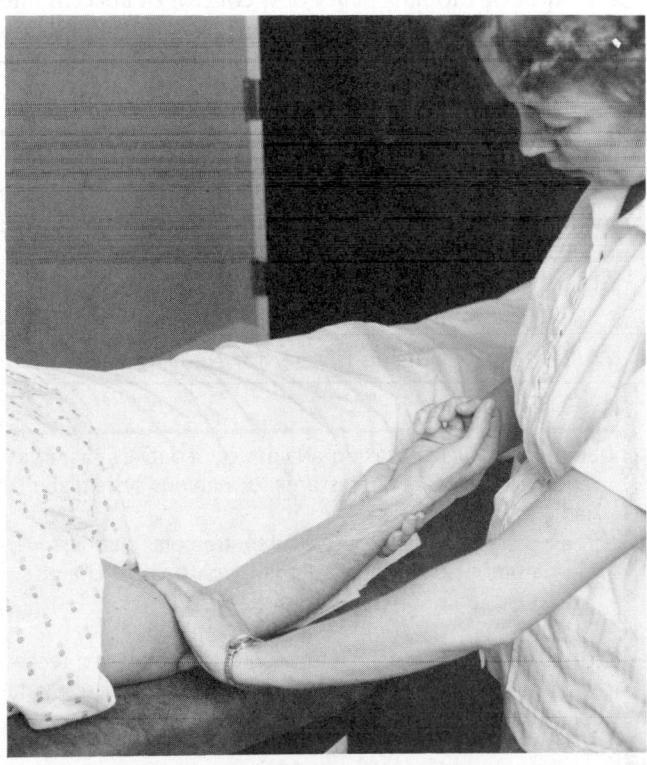

Fig. 13-92   The nurse palpates muscle tone when moving the extremity passively.

little tone feels flabby. The involved extremity hangs loosely in a position determined by gravity.

For assessment of muscle strength, the client assumes a stable position. The client performs maneuvers demonstrating strength of major muscle groups (Table 13-32). Symmetrical muscle pairs are compared. The arm on the dominant side is normally stronger than the arm on the nondominant side. In the elderly a loss of muscle mass causes bilateral weakness.

Each muscle group is examined. The examiner applies a gradual increase in pressure to a muscle group, (for example, elbow extension). The client resists the pressure applied by the examiner by attempting to move against resistance (for example, elbow flexion). The client resists until instructed to stop. As the examiner varies the amount of pressure applied, the joint moves.

If a weakness is identified, the muscle's size is compared to its opposite counterpart by measuring the muscle body's circumference with a tape measure. A muscle that has atrophied or become reduced in size may feel soft and boggy when palpated.

NEUROLOGICAL SYSTEM

The neurological system is responsible for many functions, including initiation and coordination of movement, reception and perception of sensory stimuli, organization of thought processes, control of speech, and storage of memory. A close integration exists between the neurological system and all other body systems. For example, urine production relies in part on the adequacy of blood flow to the kidneys, and the size of arterioles supplying the kidneys is under neural control.

An assessment of neurological function can be time consuming. An efficient nurse integrates neurological measurements with other parts of the physical examination. Cranial nerve function can be tested during the survey of the head and neck. Mental and emotional status is observed as the nursing history is collected. Reflexes are measured when the musculoskeletal system is assessed.

Many variables must be considered when deciding how extensive the examination should be. The client's level of consciousness influences his ability to follow directions. His physical status influences assessment. For example, an inability to walk makes a detailed assessment of coordination difficult. The client's chief complaint also helps determine the need for a thorough neurological assessment. If the client complains of headache or a recent loss of function in an extremity, a complete neurological review is needed. Table 13-33 reviews the data collected in the nursing history. If a complete examination will be given, the following special equipment will be needed:

1. Reading material
2. Vials containing aromatic substances (for example, vanilla and coffee)
3. Safety pins (sterile)
4. Snellen chart
5. Penlight
6. Vials containing sugar or salt
7. Tongue blade
8. Two test tubes, one filled with hot water, the other with cold water
9. Cotton balls or cotton-tipped applicators
10. Tuning fork
11. Reflex hammer

Mental and Emotional Status

A great deal can be learned about the client's mental capacities and emotional state by simply interacting with him. A nurse can pose questions throughout an examination to gather data and observe the appropriateness of emotions and ideas.

TABLE 13-33 Nursing History for Neurological System Assessment

Assessment Category	Rationale
Determine if client is taking analgesics, sedatives, hypnotics, antipsychotics, antidepressants, or nervous system stimulants as medications.	These drugs can alter level of consciousness or cause behavioral changes.
Screen client for headache, seizures, tremors, dizziness, vertigo, numbness or tingling of body part, visual changes, weakness, pain, or changes in speech.	These symptoms frequently originate from alterations in central nervous system or peripheral nervous system function. Identification of specific patterns of these symptoms may aid in diagnosis of pathological condition.
Discuss with spouse, family members, or friends any recent changes in client's behavior (for example, increased irritability, mood swings, or memory loss).	Behavioral changes may result from intracranial pathological states.
Assess client for history of change in vision, hearing, smell, taste, or touch.	Major sensory nerves originate from the brainstem. These symptoms may help to localize nature of the problem.

An alteration in mental or emotional status may reflect a disturbance in cerebral functioning. The cerebral cortex controls and integrates intellectual and emotional functioning. Primary brain disorders, drug effects, and metabolic changes are examples of alterations leading to changes in cerebral function.

To ensure an objective assessment the nurse must consider the client's cultural and educational background, values, beliefs, previous experiences, and current level of coping. It is easy to assume a client has an emotional problem if the nurse is too quick to judge how he responds to questions.

LEVEL OF CONSCIOUSNESS

The level of consciousness exists along a continuum, from full awakening, alertness, and cooperation to unresponsiveness to any form of external stimuli. A fully conscious client responds to questions spontaneously. As consciousness lowers, a client may show irritability, a shortened attention span, or an unwillingness to cooperate. To avoid ambiguity in the assessment of the level of consciousness, the Glasgow Coma Scale (GCS) measures consciousness by an objective numerical scale (Table 13-34). Caution is needed in using the scale with clients who have sensory losses. For example, a client may not respond to a nurse's presence if both sight and hearing are impaired.

As consciousness deteriorates, a client becomes disoriented to name, time, and place. The nurse asks questions regarding information that the client knows and that are short and to the point: "Tell me your name," "What's the name of this place?" "What day is this?" The client's ability to understand and answer questions has a direct effect on the nurse's ability to perform a complete examination. The client must be aroused to full alertness before the assessment can be conducted.

Eventually a client may be unable to follow simple commands such as "Squeeze my finger" or "Move your toes." At this lowered level of consciousness the client often is responsive only to painful stimuli. The nurse tests the client by applying firm pressure with the thumb over the root of the fingernail. The client should withdraw the hand from the painful stimulus. In cases of serious neurological impairment a client exhibits abnormal posturing in response to pain. A flaccid response indicates an absence of muscle tone in the extremities.

The GCS score allows nurses to evaluate neurological status over a period of time. The higher the score, the more improved or normal the level of functioning.

BEHAVIOR AND APPEARANCE

Behaviors, moods, hygiene, grooming, and choice of dress reveal pertinent information about a client's mental status. The nurse must be perceptive of mannerisms and actions during the entire physical assessment. The nurse notes whether the client responds appropriately to directions and observes his mood throughout the examination. The nurse notices the manner of the client's speech and his level of participation in the examination procedures (see client-teaching box).

Appearance reflects how a client feels about himself. Personal hygiene, such as unkempt hair, a dirty body, or broken, dirty fingernails, should be noted. The nurse observes the cleanliness, fit, and state of repair of clothes. Also the nurse can observe whether the client's choice of clothing is appropriate to the setting or type of weather. An unkempt appearance can be due to a poor self-image, an unexpected emergency, or an inability to perform grooming, rather than a mental problem.

Elderly clients frequently wear clothing that fits improperly. Many ready-to-wear garments are not de-

TABLE 13-34 Glasgow Coma Scale

Action	Response	Score
Eyes open	Spontaneously	④
	To speech	3
	To pain	2
	None	1
Best verbal response	Oriented	⑤
	Confused	4
	Inappropriate words	3
	Incomprehensible sounds	2
	None	1
Best motor response	Obeys commands	⑥
	Localized pain	5
	Flexion withdrawal	4
	Abnormal flexion	3
	Abnormal extension	2
	Flaccid	1
	Total Score	⑮

Client Teaching after Neurological System Assessment

- Explain to family or friends the implications of any mental impairment shown by the client.
- If the client has sensory or motor impairments, explain measures to ensure his safety (for example, use of ambulation aids or use of safety bars in bathrooms or stairways).
- Teach the elderly to plan enough time to complete tasks because reaction time is slowed.
- Teach elderly clients to observe skin surfaces for areas of trauma because their perception of pain is reduced.

signed to fit physical changes resulting from aging. Often the elderly ignore their appearance because of a lack of energy, finances, incentive, or reduced vision. The nurse considers these factors before assuming the elderly person has altered mental function.

LANGUAGE

The ability of an individual to understand spoken or written words and to express himself through writing, words, or gestures is a function of the cerebral cortex. An injury to the cortex may result in a disorder known as aphasia. There are two types of aphasia, sensory (or receptive) and motor (or expressive). With receptive aphasia a person cannot understand written or verbal speech. With expressive aphasia a person understands written and verbal speech but cannot write or speak appropriately when attempting to communicate. Often a client may suffer a combination of receptive and expressive aphasia.

The nurse assesses language capabilities when it is clear that communication with the client is ineffective. Some simple assessment techniques include:

1. Asking the client to name familiar object to which the nurse points.
2. Asking the client to respond to simple verbal and written commands such as "Stand up" or "Sit down."
3. Asking the client to read simple sentences out loud.

Intellectual Function

A person's intellectual function includes memory (recent, immediate, and past), knowledge, abstract thinking, association, and judgment. Each aspect of intellectual function is tested through a specific assessment technique. However, because cultural and educational background has a significant bearing on the ability to respond to the test questions, the nurse should not ask questions related to concepts or ideas with which the client is unfamiliar.

MEMORY

The nurse assesses immediate recall and recent and remote memory. Often a problem with memory becomes apparent when the nurse takes the nursing history. To assess immediate recall:

1. Have the client repeat a series of numbers (for example, 7, 4, 1) or repeat a series of number backwards.
2. Gradually increase the number of digits (for example, 7, 4, 1, 8, 6) until the client fails to repeat the digits correctly. Normally an individual is able to repeat a series of 5 to 8 digits forward and 4 to 6 digits backward.

To assess recent memory:

1. Ask the client to recall events occurring during the same day (for example, what he had for breakfast and how he came to the hospital). Accuracy of this information should be validated with a family member or witness.
2. Have the client recall information shared earlier during the interview (for example, name of nurse).

To assess remote memory:

1. Ask the client to recall previous medical history or family history.
2. Ask the client when his birthday or anniversary occurs.

It is common for the elderly to show symptoms of confusion and forgetfulness due to normal neurological changes. Sudden confusion, however, is usually not related to age. The elderly person is simply at greater risk to become confused by acute conditions such as dehydration, infection, drug toxicity, or hypoglycemia. In addition, hearing loss often leads to a decision that the person is confused.

KNOWLEDGE

The nurse can assess the client's knowledge by asking him what he knows about his illness or the reason for being hospitalized. By assessing knowledge, the nurse determines the client's ability to learn or understand. If an opportunity to teach exists, the nurse can test the client's mental status by asking for feedback during a follow-up visit.

ABSTRACT THINKING

Interpreting abstract ideas or concepts reflects the capacity for abstract thinking. A higher level of intellectual functioning is required for an individual to explain such phrases as "A stitch in time saves nine" or "Don't count your chickens before they're hatched." The nurse notes if the explanations are relevant and concrete. The client with altered mentation will likely interpret the phrase literally or merely rephrase the words.

ASSOCIATION

Another higher level of intellectual function involves finding similarities or associations between concepts: a dog is to a beagle as a cat is to a Siamese. The nurse names related concepts and asks the client to identify their associations. It is sufficient to use simple concepts.

JUDGMENT

Judgment requires a comparison and evaluation of facts and ideas to understand their relationships and to form appropriate conclusions. The nurse attempts to measure the client's ability to make logical decisions. By assessing judgment the nurse also measures the ability to organize thought processes. The nurse may choose to ask the client why he decided to seek health care or how he plans to adjust to his limitations when he returns home after his illness. A simpler test would involve asking the client what he would do if placed in a situation such as being locked out of his home or suddenly becoming ill when alone at home.

Cranial Nerve Function

Many measurements used to assess the integrity of organs within the head and neck also assess cranial nerve function. For example, the cochlear branch of the eighth cranial nerve is tested during a hearing assessment. The function of the ninth and tenth nerves can be assessed during examination of the pharynx. A dysfunction in any nerve reflects an alteration at some point along the cranial nerve's distribution. Cranial nerve assessment is easy once the nurse is familiar with the nerve's normal functions. To remember the order of the 12 nerves, the nurse can use this simple phrase: "On old Olympus' towering tops, a Finn and German viewed some hops." The first letter of each word in the phrase is the same as the first letter of the names of the cranial nerves (Table 13-35).

Sensory Function

The sensory pathways of the central nervous system conduct sensations of pain, temperature, position, vibration, and crude and finely localized touch. Different nerve pathways relay the sensations. For most clients a

TABLE 13-35   Cranial Nerve Function and Assessment

Number	Nerve Name	Type	Function	Method of Assessment
I	Olfactory	Sensory	Sense of smell	Ask client to identify different nonirritating aromas such as coffee and vanilla.
II	Optic	Sensory	Vision	Use Snellen chart; ask client to read printed material.
III	Oculomotor	Motor	Extraocular eye movement	Assess directions of gaze.
			Pupil constriction and dilation	Measure pupil reaction to light reflex.
IV	Trochlear	Motor	Upward and downward movement of eyeball	Assess directions of gaze.
V	Trigeminal	Sensory and motor	Sensory nerve to skin of face	Assess corneal reflex. Measure sensation of light, pain, and touch across skin of face.
			Motor nerve to muscles of jaw	Assess ability to clench teeth.
VI	Abducens	Motor	Lateral movement of eyeballs	Assess directions of gaze.
VII	Facial	Sensory and motor	Facial expression	Ask client to smile, frown, puff out cheeks, and raise and lower eyebrows.
			Taste	Have client identify salty or sweet tastes on front of tongue.
VIII	Auditory	Sensory	Hearing	Assess ability to hear spoken word.
IX	Glossopharyngeal	Sensory and motor	Taste	Ask client to identify sour, salty, or sweet taste on back of tongue.
			Ability to swallow	Use tongue blade to elicit gag reflex.
X	Vagus	Sensory and motor	Sensation of pharynx	Ask client to say "ah." Observe palate and pharynx movement.
			Ability to swallow	Use tongue blade to elicit gag reflex.
			Movement of vocal cords	Assess speech for hoarseness.
XI	Spinal accessory	Motor	Movement of head and shoulders	Ask client to shrug shoulders and turn head against passive resistance.
XII	Hypoglossal	Motor	Position of tongue	Ask client to stick out his tongue to the midline.

TABLE 13-36 Assessment of Sensory Nerve Function

Sensory Function	Equipment	Method*	Precautions
Pain	Sterile safety pin	Ask client to tell you when he feels a dull or sharp sensation. Alternately apply the pointed and blunt ends of the pin to the skin's surface. Note areas of numbness or increased sensitivity.	Areas where the skin is thickened, such as heel or sole of foot, may be less sensitive to pain. The elderly have reduced pain sensation bilaterally.
Temperature	Two test tubes, one filled with hot water, the other with cold	Touch the skin with the tube. Ask the client to identify hot versus cold sensation.	May omit test if pain sensation is normal.
Light touch	Cotton ball or cotton-tip applicator	Apply a light wisp of cotton to different points along the skin surface. After touching one specific spot touch the same spot on the opposite side of the body. Ask the client to tell you when he feels a sensation.	Apply along areas where the skin is thin or more sensitive (that is, face, neck, inner aspect of arms, or top of feet and hands). Be sure to test all major dermatomes (Fig. 12-91).
Vibration	Tuning fork	Apply vibrating fork to distal interphalangeal joint of fingers and interphalangeal joint of the great toe.	Be sure the client feels vibration and not merely pressure. Have him tell you when the vibration stops.
Position		Grasp the client's finger, holding it by its sides with your thumb and index finger. Alternate moving the finger up and down. Ask the client to tell you whether the finger is up or down. Repeat procedure with the toes.	Avoid rubbing adjacent appendages as the finger or toe is moved.
Two-point discrimination	Two safety pins	Lightly apply the points of two safety pins simultaneously to the skin's surface. Ask the client if he feels one or two pinpricks.	Apply pins to same anatomical site by fingertips, palm of hand, or upper arms. Minimal distance at which a client can discriminate two points varies (normally 2 or 3 mm on fingertips).

*All testing must be done with the client's eyes closed.

quick screening of sensory function is sufficient. However, the client who has symptoms of altered or decreased sensation, motor impairment, or paralysis requires a more extensive examination.

Normally a client has sensory responses to all stimuli tested. Sensations along the body's surface are felt equally on both sides of the face, trunk, and extremities. A nurse can assess the major sensory nerves by knowing the sensory dermatone zones. Some areas of the skin are innervated by specific dorsal root cutaneous nerves. For example, if the nurse notes reduced sensation when checking for light touch along an area of the skin (for example, the lower neck) the nurse can determine, in general, where a neurological lesion may exist (for example, fourth cervical spinal cord segment).

All sensory testing is performed with the client's eyes closed so he is unable to see when or where a stimulus strikes the skin (Table 13-36). Stimuli are applied in a random, unpredictable order to maintain attention. The client should say when he perceives the particular stimulus. The nurse compares symmetrical areas of the body as she applies stimuli to the arms, trunk, and legs.

Motor Function

An assessment of motor function includes the same measurements made during the musculoskeletal examination. In addition, cerebellar function is assessed. The cerebellum coordinates muscular activity by producing smooth, steady, and efficient movements of muscle groups. The maintenance of balance and equilibrium is also a function of the cerebellum. Sensory impulses from the vestibular portion of the inner ear travel to the cerebellum, where impulses are relayed to proper motor nerves to maintain body equilibrium. The cerebellum also controls posture.

COORDINATION

It is difficult for the nurse to explain the tests used to measure coordination. To avoid confusion the nurse simply demonstrates each assessment maneuver and then has the client repeat it after determining that he is physically able to make the necessary movements. The nurse observes the smoothness and balance of movements tested. In the elderly a normally slow reaction time may cause movements to be less rhythmical.

Performing rapid, rhythmical, alternating movements demonstrates coordination in the upper extremities. First, the client pats his hand against his thigh as fast as he can when sitting. The client should be able to strike the thigh rapidly and evenly without hesitation. Next the client alternately strikes the thigh with the hand supinated and then pronated. The speed and symmetry of movement are noted. An additional maneuver for upper extremity coordination involves touching each finger with the thumb of the same hand in rapid sequence. The client's dominant hand is slightly less awkward when performing this movement.

A final measurement of upper extremity coordination involves the point-to-point test. The nurse stands in front of the client holding her index finger 2 feet in front of the client's face. She asks the client to touch her finger with his index finger and then to touch his nose alternately. The client moves his finger back and forth repeatedly. The nurse looks for any tremor of the hand or awkwardness in movement. The test may be repeated with the client's eyes closed.

Lower extremity coordination is tested with the client in a supine position. The nurse places her hand at the ball of the client's foot. The client taps the nurse's hand with his foot as quickly as possible. Each foot is tested for speed and smoothness. The feet do not move as rapidly or evenly as the hands.

A final test involves having the client sit with his eyes closed and place the heel of his foot on the opposite knee. The client then slides his heel down the opposite leg to his foot. This maneuver normally is performed evenly without the heel sliding off the leg.

BALANCE

The nurse may use one or two of the following tests to assess balance and gross motor function:
1. Have the client perform a Romberg test by standing with feet together and eyes closed. Observe for presence of swaying while protecting the client's safety by standing at his side. Slight swaying is normal in an elderly client. The client normally does not have to break his stance.
2. Have the client close the eyes and stand on one foot and then the other.
3. Ask the client to walk a straight line by placing the heel of one foot directly in front of the toes of the other foot.

Reflexes

Eliciting reflex reactions allows the nurse to assess the integrity of sensory and motor pathways of the reflex arc and specific spinal cord segments. The assessment of reflexes does not determine higher neural center functioning. Fig. 13-93 traces the pathway of the reflex arc. When the muscle and tendon are stretched, nerve impulses travel along afferent nerve pathways to the dorsal horn of the spinal cord segment. Impulses synapse and travel to the efferent motor neuron in the spinal cord. A motor nerve then sends the impulses back to the muscle, causing the reflex response.

The two categories of normal reflexes are deep tendon reflexes, elicited by mildly stretching a muscle and tapping a tendon, and cutaneous reflexes, elicited by stim-

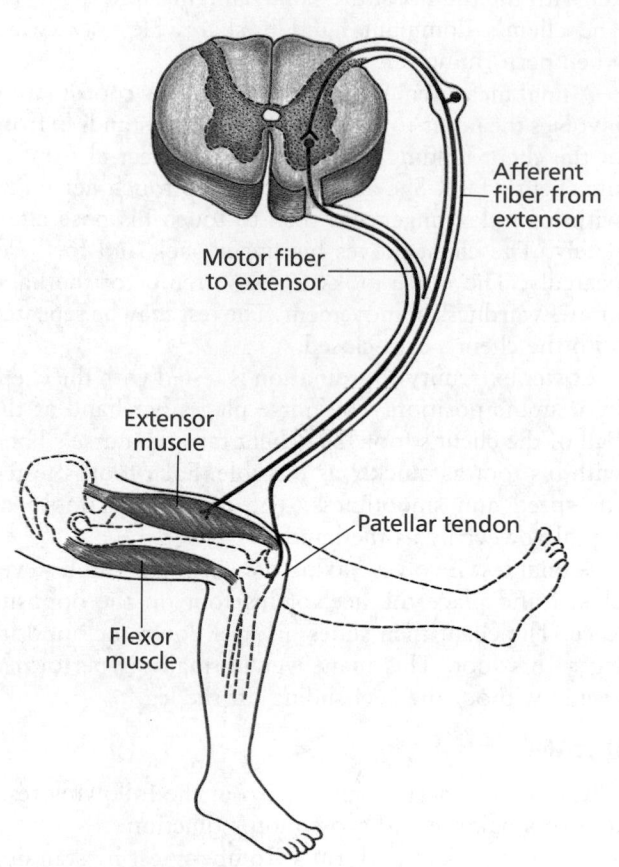

Fig. 13-93 Pathway of reflex arc.

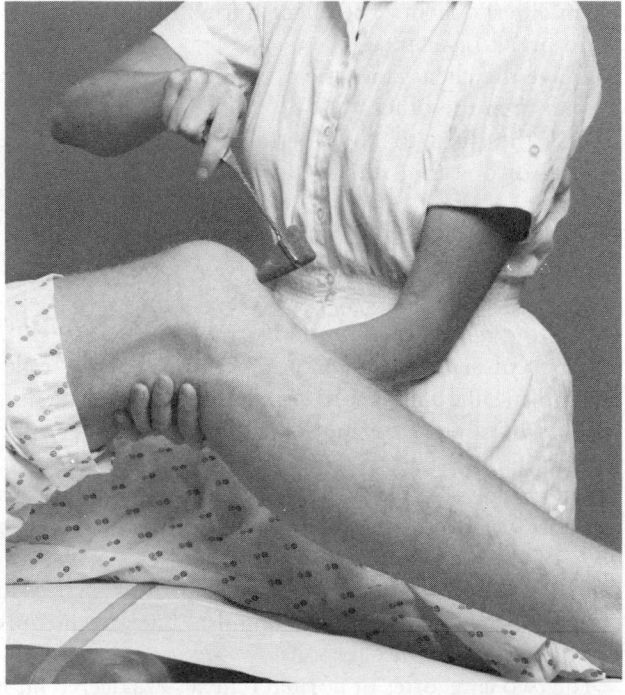

Fig. 13-94 Position for eliciting patellar tendon reflex. The lower leg normally extends.

ulating the skin superficially. Reflexes are graded as follows:

0	No response
1+	Low normal or diminished response
2+	Normal
3+	Brisker than normal; may not indicate disease
4+	Hyperactive and very brisk; often associated with spinal cord disorders

When reflexes are being assessed, the client should relax as much as possible to avoid voluntary movement or tensing of muscles. The nurse positions the limbs to slightly stretch the muscle being tested. The reflex hammer is held loosely between the nurse's thumb and fingers so it can swing freely and tap the tendon briskly (Fig. 13-94). The nurse compares the symmetry of the reflex from one side of the body to the other. In the elderly, reflexes are normally slowed. Practitioners often use stick figures to record reflexes. Table 13-37 summarizes common deep tendon and cutaneous reflexes.

AFTER THE EXAMINATION

After completing the assessment the nurse assists the client in dressing if necessary. The hospitalized client may need help in returning to bed and assuming a comfortable position. When the client is comfortable, it is helpful to share a summary of the assessment findings. If the findings have revealed serious abnormalities such as a tumor or highly irregular heart rate, the client's physician should be consulted before any findings are revealed. It is the physician's responsibility to make definitive medical diagnoses. The nurse can explain the type of abnormality found and the need for the physician to conduct an additional examination.

The nurse also cleans the examination area, storing all reusable equipment and disposing of materials that cannot be reused. Afterward, the nurse washes hands. If the client's bedside was the examination site, the nurse clears away soiled items from the table and makes sure the bed linen is dry and clean. The client may appreciate a clean gown and the opportunity to wash his face and hands.

The nurse checks to be sure the recording of the assessment is complete. If the nurse delayed making any entries in the assessment form, she records them at this time to avoid forgetting any important information. If entries were made periodically during the examination, they are reviewed for accuracy and thoroughness. Significant findings are communicated to appropriate medical and nursing personnel, either verbally or in the written care plan.

The client often needs a number of ancillary examinations such as x-ray examinations laboratory tests, or ultrasonography after a physical examination. These

TABLE 13-37 Assessment of Common Reflexes

Type	Procedure	Normal Reflex
DEEP TENDON REFLEXES		
Biceps	Flex the client's arm at the elbow with palms down. Place your thumb in the antecubital fossa at the base of the biceps tendon. Strike the thumb with the reflex hammer	Flexion of arm at elbow
Triceps	Flex the client's elbow, holding the arm across the chest, or hold the upper arm horizontally and allow the lower arm to go limp. Strike the triceps tendon just above the elbow.	Extension at elbow
Patellar	Have the client sit with his legs hanging freely over the side of the bed or chair or have the client lie supine and support his knee in a flexed position. Briskly tap the patellar tendon just below the patella.	Extension of lower leg at knee
Archilles	Have the client assume the same position as for the patellar reflex. Slightly dorsiflex the client's ankle by grasping the toes in the palm of your hand. Strike the Achilles tendon just above the heel.	Plantar flexion of the foot
Plantar (Babinski's)	Have the client lie supine with legs straight and feet relaxed. Take the handle end of the reflex hammer and stroke the lateral aspect of the sole from the heel to the ball of the foot, curving across the ball of the foot toward the big toe.	Bending of toes downward
CUTANEOUS REFLEXES		
Gluteal	Have the client assume a side-lying position. Spread apart the client's buttocks and lightly stimulate the perineal area with a cotton applicator.	Contraction of anal sphincter
Abdominal	Have the client stand or lie supine. Stroke the abdominal skin with the base of a cotton applicator over the lateral borders of the rectus abdominis muscle toward the midline. Repeat the test in each abdominal quadrant.	Contraction of rectus abdominis muscle with pulling of umbilicus toward the stimulated side

tests provide additional screening information to rule out the presence of abnormalities and help in the diagnosis of specific abnormalities found during the examination. Unit 7 describes ancillary tests in detail.

SUMMARY

Through physical assessment, the nurse makes insightful clinical decisions that contribute to the client's health management. Each body system is reviewed after a methodical sequence of observations and measurements. Information gathered during physical assessment supplements data obtained in the nursing history and from ongoing nurse-client interactions. As a result of more thorough data gathering, the nurse is able to make nursing diagnoses with greater precision. Therefore the plan of care becomes more individualized and comprehensive. Physical assessment findings also reveal whether specific nursing measures were successful in managing client problems.

Before an examination begins, the nurse takes the necessary steps to prepare the client and setting. Measures are taken to ensure privacy and psychological and physical comfort and to reduce the transmission of microorganisms. The client becomes an active participant as the nurse carefully explains each step of the examination. It is important to organize the examination. Each system review entails many observations. Basic principles for a thorough examination include comparing both sides of the body for symmetry, completing each system before moving to the next, using each skill as appropriate, and recognizing the observations that have priority for a client.

KEY CONCEPTS

✓ Baseline assessment findings reflect functional abilities when the nurse first assesses the client and serve as the basis for comparison with subsequent assessment findings.

✓ Assessment data can be used to evaluate the physiological outcomes of nursing care.

✓ Physical assessment of a child or infant requires the nurse to apply principles of physical growth and development.

✓ The nurse recognizes that the normal process of aging affects physical findings collected from an elderly client.

✓ Client teaching should be integrated throughout the examination to help clients understand the implications of all findings.

✓ The nurse can use time more efficiently by integrating physical assessment with routine nursing care.

✓ Inspection requires good lighting, full exposure of the body part, and a careful comparison of the part with its counterpart on the opposite side of the body.

✓ Palpation involves the use of different parts of the hand to detect different types of physical characteristics.

✓ Percussion is the detection of differences in density of underlying tissues by listening to sounds produced when striking the body's surface.

✓ Through auscultation the nurse assesses the character of sounds created in body organs.

✓ A good stethoscope should have earpieces that fit snugly, a flexible thick-walled tubing of the proper length, and a chestpiece with a bell and diaphragm.

✓ Correct use of a stethoscope involves holding the diaphragm firmly against the skin and applying the bell lightly against the skin's surface.

✓ A physical examination should be performed only after proper preparation of the environment and equipment and after preparing the client physically and psychologically.

✓ Throughout the examination the nurse should keep the client warm, comfortable, and informed of each step of the process.

✓ The client assumes various positions during the physical examination to provide greater accessibility of body parts and increase accuracy in assessment.

✓ The nurse should use a systematic approach whenever conducting a physical assessment.

✓ When assessing a seriously ill client the nurse concentrates on the body systems most likely to be affected.

✓ Information from the nursing history helps the nurse focus on specific parts of the examination.

✓ When assessing weight, the nurse should ask if the client has recently experienced a significant change in weight.

✓ Findings from the skin assessment may determine the need for better nutrition, hydration, and hygiene.

✓ Changes in the distribution of hair may be caused by hormonal and circulation alterations.

✓ A client should be warned against moving during examination of ear structures with an otoscope.

✓ Examination of the oral cavity is a basic part of assessment before administering oral hygiene.

✓ An enlarged lymph node may be the sign of localized or systemic infection or a malignant growth.

✓ Accuracy in assessing the thorax, heart, and abdomen is enhanced by creating a mental image of internal organs in relation to external anatomical landmarks.

✓ During assessment of the thorax the nurse compares both sides, moving from top to bottom.

✓ The nurse uses the diaphragm of the stethoscope to auscultate breath sounds in an adult, but the bell amplifies sounds best in a child.

✓ The apical pulse is more easily auscultated at the point of maximal impulse, along the fifth intercostal space at the midclavicular line.

✓ When assessing heart sounds, the nurse imagines events occurring during the cardiac cycle.

✓ The carotid arteries should never be palpated simultaneously.

✓ When it is difficult to palpate a peripheral pulse, the nurse assesses circulatory adequacy by noting color, temperature, skin changes, and the presence of edema in the extremities.

✓ When examining a woman's breasts the nurse explains the techniques for breast self-examinations.

✓ The abdominal assessment differs from other portions of the examination in that auscultation follows inspection.

✓ If the client and nurse are of opposite sexes, a nurse of the same sex as the client should be present during examination of the genitalia.

✓ During assessment of the male genitalia, the nurse explains the techniques for testicular self-examination.

✓ Assessment of musculoskeletal function can easily be conducted when observing the client ambulate or participate in other active movements.

✓ The nurse assesses mental and emotional status by interacting with the client throughout the examination.

✓ At the end of the examination the nurse provides for the client's comfort and completes a detailed review of physical assessment findings.

REFERENCES

American Cancer Society: 1986 Cancer facts and figures, New York, 1986, The Society.

Forgacs, P: The functional basis of pulmonary sounds, Chest 73:399, 1978.

Jacobs, R: Physical changes in the aged. In Devereaux, M, et al., editors: Elder care: a guide to clinical geriatrics, New York, 1981, Grune & Stratton, Inc.

Larson, E: Evaluating validity of screening tests, Nurs Res 35:186, 1986.

Mahboub, E, and Sayed, GM: oral cavity and pharynx. In Schottenfeld, D, and Fraumeni, JF Jr., editors: Cancer epidemiology and prevention, Philadelphia, 1982, W.B. Saunders Co.

Rossman, I: Anatomy of aging. In Rossman, I, editor: Clinical geriatrics, ed. 2, Philadelphia, 1979, J.B. Lippincott Co.

U.S. Department of Health and Human Services, Cancer Rates and Risks, ed. 3, 1985, National Institute of Health.

Wilkins, RL: Lung sounds, St. Louis, 1987, The C.V. Mosby Co.

Yacone, LA: Cardiac assessment: what to do, how to do it, RN 50:42, May 1987.

ADDITIONAL READINGS

American Cancer Society: Guidelines for the cancer-related checkup: recommendations and rationale, New York, 1980, The Society.

Berliner, H: Aging skin. I. Am J Nurs 86:1138, 1986.

Berliner, H: Aging skin. II. Am J Nurs 86:1259, 1986.

Blair, JD: A quick, high-yield mouth exam, Patient Care 19:33, Oct. 30, 1985.

Block, G, et al.: Health assessment for professional nursing, New York, 1981, Appleton-Century-Crofts.

Burger, D: Breast self-examination, Am J Nurs 79:1088, 1979.

Burggraf, V, and Donlon, B: Assessing the elderly, system by system, Am J Nurs 85:974, 1985.

Calvani, D: Assessing the elderly. II. Am J Nurs 85:1103, 1985.

Casey, MP: Testicular cancer: the worst disease at the worst time, RN 50:36, 1987.

Dennison, R: Cardiopulmonary assessment, Nurs 86, 16:34, April 1986.

Ebersole, P, and Hess, P: Toward healthy aging, ed. 3, St. Louis, 1989, The C.V. Mosby Co.

Erickson, BA: Detecting abnormal heart sounds, Nurs 86 16:58, 1986.

Fraser, MC, and McGuire, DB: Skin cancer's early warning system, Am J Nurs 84:1232, 1984.

Hays, AM, and Borger, F: Assessing the elderly: a test in-time, Am J Nurs 85:1107, 1985.

Henderson, ML: Assessing the elderly: altered perception, Am J Nurs 85:1104, 1985.

Hurst, JW, et al.: Noises in the neck, N Engl J Med 302:862, 1980.

Malkiewicz, J: A pragmatic approach to musculoskeletal assessment, RN 45:56, 1982.

Miracle, VA: Anatomy of a murmur, Nurs 86 16:26, 1986.

Norman, S: The pupil check, Am J Nurs 82:588, 1982.

Phipps, W, et al.: Medical-surgical nursing: concepts and clinical practice, ed. 3, St. Louis, 1987, The C.V. Mosby Co.

Reynolds, JI, and Logsdon, JB: Assessing your patients' mental status, Nurs 79 9:26, 1979.

Rutledge, DN: Factors related to women's practice of breast self-examination, Nurs Res 36:117, 1987.

Sana, JM, and Judge, RD: Physical assessment skills for nursing practice, ed. 2, Boston, 1982, Little, Brown, & Co.

Schweiger, JL, et al.: Oral assessment: how to do it, Am J Nurs 80:654, 1980.

Seidel, HM, et al.: Mosby's guide to physical examination, St. Louis, 1987, The C.V. Mosby Co.

Silverberg, E: Cancer statistics, 1984, New York, 1984, American Cancer Society.

Smith, C: Abdominal assessment: a blending of science and art, Nurs 81 11:42, 1981.

Tanner, JM: Growth of adolescence, ed. 2, Oxford, 1962, Blackwell Scientific Publications.

Tishknobf, MK: Breast cancer, the treatment evolution, Am J Nurs 84:1110, 1984.

Visich, MA: Breath and heart sounds, Nurs 81 11:64, 1981.

Whaley, LF, and Wong, DL: Nursing care of infants and children, ed. 3, St. Louis, 1987, The C.V. Mosby Co.

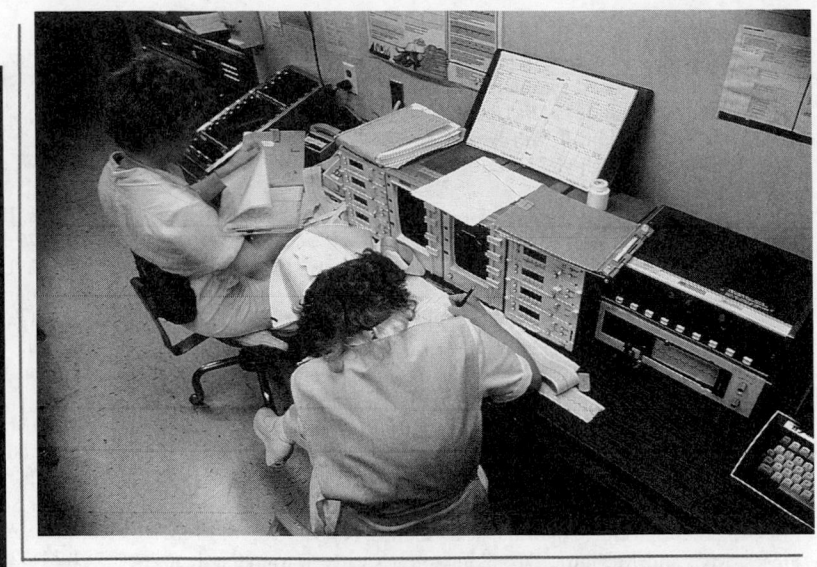

OBJECTIVES

Mastery of content in this chapter will enable the student to:

- Define the key terms listed.
- Describe guidelines for effectively communicating through reporting and recording.
- Discuss the relationship between documentation and health care financial reimbursement.
- Identify ways to maintain confidentiality of records and reports.
- Describe the purpose of a change-of-shift report.
- Explain how to verify telephone reports.
- Identify six purposes of a health care record.
- Discuss legal guidelines for recording.
- Differentiate between a source record and a problem-oriented record.
- Discuss the advantages and disadvantages of standardized documentation forms.
- Identify computerized applications for documentation.

KEY TERMS

Audit

Chart

Computer-Assisted Instruction (CAI)

Documentation

Incident Report

Inpatient

Litigation

Objective Data

Oral Report

Outpatient

PIE

Precipitating Factor

Problem-Oriented Medical Record (POMR)

Prospective Reimbursement

Quality Assurance

Record

Relieving Factor

SOAP

Standardized Care Plan

Sign

Subjective Data

Symptom

Recording and Reporting

All members of the health care team must have the same information about clients to ensure an organized and comprehensive plan of care. Unless the client's care plan is communicated to all members of the health team, care becomes fragmented, repetition of tasks occurs, and therapies often become delayed. Records and reports serve to communicate specific information about a client's health care so all interventions are directed toward the same goals.

A report involves an oral or written exchange of information. When nurses complete a shift or tour of duty, they provide an oral report to nurses on the next shift. Support services such as the laboratory or the radiology department issue written reports describing results of diagnostic tests. Information from written reports is incorporated into the client's permanent medical record or chart.

A client's record is a written communication that permanently documents information relevant to his or her health care management. An example is a clinic record or chart. After each clinic visit, information about the reasons a client sought medical care, the medical history, results of diagnostic tests, and the plan of therapy is recorded. With each successive visit the record is available to the physician and nurse. It is a continuing account of the client's health care needs.

Documentation and reporting are two of the most important functions a nurse performs. Unless information about a client's care is communicated with careful thought, serious errors can occur. Good documentation and reporting must reflect accurately the status of the client. All members of the health care team depend on this recorded and reported information. Accurate information ensures continuity and quality of care.

GUIDELINES FOR GOOD REPORTING AND RECORDING

When nurses fail to take reporting and recording seriously, many problems can arise. Consider the following situations:

Mrs. Blake has recently been diagnosed with diabetes. She must learn to give herself insulin injections before going home. A nurse on the day shift fails to document the teaching session about syringe parts and the method for preparing insulin dosage. During the evening shift, another nurse spends time assessing Mrs. Blake's learning needs because the teaching plan was not communicated. Valuable time is wasted, and Mrs. Blake becomes frustrated with the nurses' failure to know her needs.

Mr. Ryan returned from major abdominal surgery just before change of shift. The day nurse, Mr. Wells, measures the client's vital signs and gives a medication for pain. The evening nurse, Miss Tally, learns during report that Mr. Ryan received an analgesic medication but is not told his response to the drug. When Miss Tally enters Mr. Ryan's room, she measures his blood pressure at 90/60. She leaves the room to check the chart because she is concerned that the pain medication has lowered Mr. Ryan's blood pressure. If Mr. Wells had given a thorough report, Miss Tally would have known the client's blood pressure was normally low.

Both case examples demonstrate that quality recording and reporting are necessary to enhance efficient, individualized client care. Six important guidelines must be followed for quality documentation and reporting.

Accuracy

Information about clients and their care must be correct. Factual information is less likely to be misleading or to cause misinterpretation. A nurse should not try to make assumptions when data are not complete. It is important for the nurse to report objective data resulting from specific observations and measurements. An example of an objective description is, "Respirations 14 per minute, regular, with 2 cm chest excursion." If subjective data are communicated, they should be recognized as such, for example, "Client states pain 'feels like a burning sensation.' " Client's perceptions are important to know, but they cannot be evaluated by objective standards.

Documentation should clearly explain the nurse's observations of client's behaviors and not interpret those observations. An example of an accurate observation might include, "Mr. Lamb walked with a staggering gait

to the bathroom." The nurse never records what he or she thinks the problem might be. For example, the statement, "Mr. Lamb walked as though he was drunk," is an unacceptable, subjective interpretation of a client's behavior.

The use of precise measurements ensures accuracy. The nurse makes descriptions such as "intake 360 ml of water" rather than "client drank an adequate amount of fluid." Measurements are later used as a means to determine if a client's condition improves or worsens. Charting that an abdominal wound is "5 cm in length" is more accurate than "large and gaping." Use of an institution's accepted abbreviations, symbols, and system of measurement (for example, metric) ensures that all staff members will use the same language in reports and records (see Appendix).

Correct spelling is also important for accurate recording and reporting. Terms can easily be confused or misinterpreted (for example, dysphagia or dysphasia and dram or gram). Simple spelling mistakes can also cause serious treatment errors. Medications such as digitoxin or digoxin and morphine or Numorphan must be spelled carefully. If a mistake is made on a medication record, a client may receive the wrong medication.

Any descriptive entry in a client's record ends with the health team member's signature. An accurate signature includes first initial, complete surname, and status, such as "S. Day, RN." Nicknames are not used. The signature holds a nurse accountable for information recorded.

Conciseness

Concise data are easy to understand. Lengthy notes are difficult to read. Sketchy notes may leave an impression that nursing care was hurried or incomplete. A long report wastes time and is often boring. Clear, succinct recording and reporting gives only essential information and avoids the use of unnecessary words or irrelevant detail. A comparison of a concise and lengthy record entry follows.

CONCISE ENTRY	LENGTHY ENTRY
Ⓛ toes are warm, color pink, nail beds show good capillary return, dorsalis pedis pulse strong 4+, no inflammation or pain present.	The client's left toes appear to be warm with color pink. There is no inflammation. There is good capillary return present. Dorsalis pedis pulse in left foot is strong. The client denies pain.

Thoroughness

A good report or record is thorough, with complete information about a client. Criteria to provide for thorough communication exist for certain health problems

TABLE 14-1 Examples of Criteria for Reporting and Recording

Topic	What to Report or Record
Symptom (pain, nausea, headache, dizziness)	Description of episode, location of symptom, severity, onset, precipitating factor(s), frequency, duration, aggravating factor(s), relieving factor(s), associated symptom(s)
Sign (rash, tenderness on palpation of body part, diminished breath sounds)	Location of sign, description or quality of finding, aggravating or relieving factor(s)
Nursing care measures (enema, bath, dressing change)	Time administered, equipment used if appropriate, client's response (positive* or negative†), nurse's observations
Client behavior (anxiety, confusion, hostility)	Time of occurrence, behaviors exhibited, precipitating factor(s), nursing response or action, client response to nursing action
Medication administration (analgesic)	Time administered, any required preliminary observations (pulse, blood pressure), client response (positive‡) or nursing measures taken if negative response occurs§
Patient teaching	Information or topic presented, method of instruction (discussion, role-playing, demonstration), resources used (videotape, booklet), and evidence that client understands instruction

*For example, client denied pain during dressing change.
†For example, client experienced severe abdominal cramping during enema.
‡For example, client reports pain was reduced by analgesic.
§For example, rash noted on abdomen.

or nursing activities (Table 14-1). The nurse will make written entries in the client's medical record, describing nursing care administered and the client's response. An example of a thorough nurses' note is written below:

7:15 PM Client has sharp, throbbing localized pain along radial side of right wrist. Pain began approximately 5 minutes ago. Pain increased with movement of wrist and slightly relieved with elevation of hand on pillow. Radial pulse strong. Right wrist circumference 1 cm larger than left wrist. MD notified. Percocet 2 tabs given for pain.

L. Turno, RN

Currentness

Delays in recording or reporting can result in serious omissions and untimely delays for needed care. Decisions about a client's care are based on currently reported information. Activities that must be communicated at the time they occur include administration of medications or other treatments; preparation of clients for diagnostic tests or surgery; change in a client's status; admission, transfer, or discharge of a client; and treatment initiated for sudden changes in a client's condition. Routine activities such as bedmaking or giving a bath do not need to be charted immediately.

Each institution uses a system to report the time of day. Military time, a 24-hour system, avoids misinterpretation of AM and PM times that occur with the 12-hour system. A 4-digit number indicates the hours and minutes (Table 14-2).

Organization

The nurse communicates information in a logical format or order. Health team members will better understand information given in the order in which it occurred. The following example compares a well-organized note with a disorganized note.

ORGANIZED NOTE
Client reports sharp pain in left lower quadrant of abdomen, worsened by turning. Positioning on left side offers minimal relief. Abdomen is tender to touch, rigid, dull to percussion. Bowel sounds are absent. Dr. Phillips notified; ordered Demerol 75 mg IM for pain and a CT scan of abdomen.

DISORGANIZED NOTE
Client experiencing sharp pain in lower quadrant of abdomen. MD notified. Abdomen tender to touch, rigid with bowel sounds absent. Percussion note is dull. Demerol 75 mg IM ordered for pain. Positioning on left side offers minimal relief of pain. CT scan ordered of the abdomen.

TABLE 14-2 Comparison of Military and Civilian Times

Military	Civilian	Military	Civilian
0100	1:00 AM	1420	2:20 PM
0200	2:00 AM	1800	6:00 PM
0215	2:15 AM	2400	12:00 PM
1200	12:00 Noon	0001	12:01 AM
1300	1:00 PM		

The organized note describes the client's pain, nurse's assessment, and physician's order in a logical order of occurrence. The disorganized note is fragmented and does not clearly explain what happened first. Poorly organized notes can lead to confusion about whether proper care was given.

Confidentiality

A confidential communication is information given by one person to another with trust and confidence that such information will not be disclosed. The law protects information about a client that is gathered by examination, observation, conversation, or treatment. All health team members must keep confidential any information noted in the record and avoid repeating what is heard from other staff members who might reveal a diagnosis to others or discuss a client with other clients. The nurse is legally and ethically obligated to keep information about a client's illness and treatment confidential. A legal suit can be brought against any nurse who discloses information about clients without their consent. Only staff members directly involved in the client's care have legitimate access to the client's record. Nurses and other health care professionals may have reason to use records for data gathering, research, or continuing education. These are not breaches of confidentiality as long as the records are used as specified.

Written documentation of a client's health care is accessible to many personnel. Nurses are responsible for protecting records from unauthorized readers such as visitors. The nurse should know the location of the client's record at all times. If it is misplaced, every effort should be made to find it. The record is stored by the health care agency once treatment ends.

REPORTING

A large amount of information is exchanged between health care team members. Nurses must work professionally to ensure that quality reports are shared so all team members can make the best decisions about clients and their care. Three types of reports made by nurses include the change-of-shift report, telephone reports, and incident reports.

Change-of-Shift Reports

The change-of-shift report or intershift report occurs two or three times a day in every type of nursing unit in all types of health care settings. At the end of a shift, nurses share information about their assigned clients to the nurses working on the next shift. The report is a system of communication aimed at transferring essential information necessary for safe and holistic client care (Riegel, 1985). The process ensures better continuity of care. Nurses must exchange adequate knowledge about clients so all health care needs can be met.

For a report to be concise, clear, comprehensive, and give an accurate interpretation of a client's situation, Budziszewski (1960) suggests the following areas of reporting: selection, comparison, summary, and interpretation. A good report includes selection of significant facts about a client (for example, the condition of a wound or an episode of chest pain). Data have little

TABLE 14-3 Do's and Don't's of Intershift Report

Do's	Don't's
Provide only essential background information about client (name, sex, age, physician's diagnosis, medical history).	Don't review all routine care procedures or tasks (bathing or I & O).
Identify client's nursing diagnosis or health care problems and their related causes.	Don't review all biographical information already available on Kardex.
Describe objective measurements or observations about the client's condition and response to health problem. Stress any recent changes.	Don't use critical comments about the client's behavior.
Share significant information about family members as it relates to client's problems.	Don't make assumptions about relationships between family members.
Continuously review ongoing discharge plan (need for resources, client's level of preparation to go home).	Don't engage in idle gossip.
Relay to staff any significant changes in the way therapies are given (different gauze used in dressing change, new medication ordered).	Don't describe the basic steps of a procedure.
Describe instructions given in teaching plan and client's response.	Don't explain detailed content unless staff asks for clarification.
Evaluate results of nursing or medical care measures (effect of position change, backrub, analgesic administration).	Don't simply describe results as "good" or "poor." Be specific.
Be clear on priorities to which the oncoming staff must attend.	Don't force oncoming staff to guess what to do first.

meaning unless a comparison is made with previous information. Thus a nurse cannot make a conclusion about a client unless it is known if a change has occurred (for example, improvement in wound healing or the episode of chest pain as a first-time occurrence). A summary of important data helps if it is objective and concise. Interpretation, the result of selecting, comparing, and summarizing, is important because the nurse can report the clinical significance of the shift's events (Table 14-3).

A report should be given as quickly as possible. Even though it is the responsibility of a nurse to carefully review a client's Kardex before care begins, it is not necessary to report routine nursing orders or information available in the Kardex. A systematic approach to reporting using the nursing process can provide staff with critical information needed to continue the client's care. The basis for report is the client's health problems. At the time of the intershift report the nurse can be in any phase of the nursing process. Thus the actual report should reflect the ongoing, continuous nature of care.

The following is an example of an intershift report:

Background information	Cy Tolan, a 32-year-old client of Dr. Lang, in bed 4, is scheduled for a colon resection this morning. He has had ulcerative colitis for 2 years. This is his first experience with surgery.
Nursing diagnoses or problem(s)	He has anxiety related to inexperience with scheduled surgery.
Objective measurements	Mr. Tolan slept poorly last night. After receiving cleansing enemas until clear, he complained of some lower abdominal cramping. He received a Dalmane 15 mg at 11:30 PM, and I gave him a backrub.
Teaching plan	He asks good questions about the surgical procedure but admits to being anxious. Dr. Lang has explained to him that a colostomy may be needed. Staff on evenings explained postoperative routines. He fell asleep around midnight but woke at least twice during the night.
Family information	His wife remained with him last evening until the end of visiting hours. She has returned and is in the room this morning.
Discharge plan	Mr. Tolan is a very active person at home. He plays tennis and basketball and swims. Mrs.
	Tolan is concerned about how he might react to a colostomy. I believe we should call the enterostomal therapist in early if the colostomy is performed.
Priority needs	Right now, Mr. Tolan is relaxing in his room. He has his gown on. All preoperative procedures have been completed except for his p.r.n. medications.

In the previous example the nurse gives a clear picture of Mr. Tolan's anxiety about surgery. If anxiety is Mr. Tolan's only problem, the report would be complete. However, if the client had additional problems the nurse's report uses a similar format for each problem. An organized comprehensive approach lessens the chance of important information being deleted. It is important that members of the next shift know exactly what their responsibilities in caring for the client will be.

A report can be given orally in person or by audiotape. An in-person report permits nurses to obtain immediate feedback about unclear or incomplete information. The report may be conducted in a conference room (Fig. 14-1) or during nurses' "walking rounds." During walking rounds the client meets the staff who will care for him and learns of activities or treatment to expect during the shift, and the nurse meets and observes the client. Information that might alarm a client is reported out of hearing range, usually in the hallway just outside the room. The nurse also takes precautions to ensure that other clients do not hear confidential information.

When giving a report the nurse discusses the client or family in a professional and dignified manner. It is often necessary to describe the interactions between client, nurse, and family members in behavioral terms. The nurse avoids using labels such as "uncooperative," "difficult," or "bad" when describing client behaviors. Any derogatory statements overheard by the client could lead to a lawsuit against the nurse (see Chapter 18). A good report is objective and nonjudgmental. Value-laden terms are not conducive for establishing working relationships between staff members and clients. Staff members may unintentionally form a prejudicial opinion about clients before even meeting them. The content of reports should be pertinent to clients' health care.

Telephone Reports

Health care workers frequently communicate orders to one another by telephone. Reports may include a nurse informing a physician of changes in a client's condition, a nurse from one unit communicating information to a nurse in another unit about a client transfer, or the laboratory staff or radiologist reporting results of

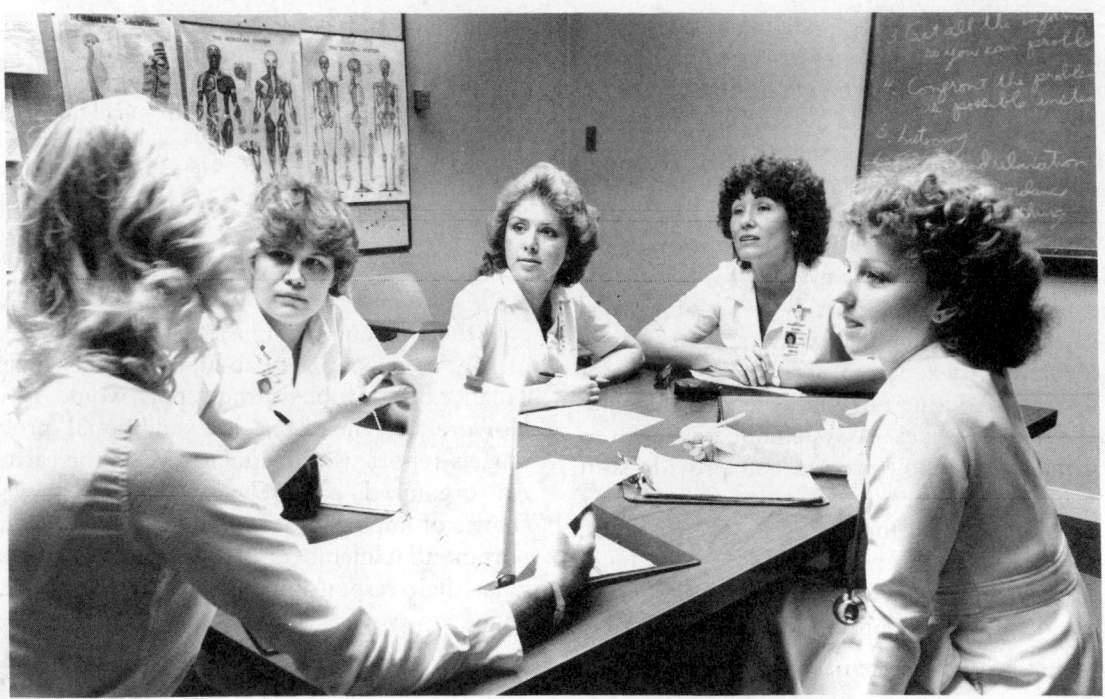

Fig. 14-1 Members of the nursing team meet at the change of shift for a report on each client's progress and specific health care needs.

Telephone Techniques

INCOMING CALLS

- Cue yourself to smile before picking up the phone.
- Identify the nursing division and yourself.
- Be natural. Use your real voice, tone, and volume.
- Treat each call as important.
- Give the caller your full attention.
- Listen carefully.
- Use words of courtesy and politeness.
- Take notes as pertinent information is communicated.
- If there are any questions, ask them after the caller has finished speaking.
- End the call graciously.
- Let the caller hang up first.

OUTGOING CALLS

- Place your call.
- When the other person answers, identify yourself.
- Use the person's name. State *why* you are calling.
- If the report is lengthy, have notes in front of you.
- Ask the other person if he has any other questions.
- End the call graciously.

diagnostic tests. Information in a telephone report may not be permanently documented in a written form. Thus the persons involved with a telephone report should be sure the information is clear, accurate, and concise. If any doubt exists about the information conveyed over the telephone, the receiver repeats the message back to the sender.

Nurse: This is Ms. Towns from 3200. Do you have the results of Mr. Tom Rush's potassium level?
Laboratory technician: Yes. Mr. Tom Rush's potassium is 3.2.
Nurse: Let me repeat that, 3.2?
Laboratory technician: Yes, that's correct.

Clarifying messages is important when nurses accept physician's orders over the telephone. The order must be verified by repeating it clearly and precisely. Then the nurse writes the order on the physician's order sheet in the client's permanent record and signs it. The physician later verifies the telephone order legally by signing it within a set time period.

It is important to be as courteous as possible when making or receiving phone calls (see box). Anyone calling a nursing unit should be treated as a consumer needing a service. Courtesy conveys a sense of professionalism and promotes cooperation of all health team members.

Incident Reports

An *incident* is any event not consistent with the routine operation of a health care unit or routine care of a client (Blake, 1984). Examples of incidents include client falls or accidental injuries, medication administration errors, loss of narcotic cabinet keys, accidental deletion of ordered therapies, or carelessness in performance of a procedure that led to actual or potential client injury. When an incident occurs, the nurse involved in the incident or the nurse who witnesses an injury completes a report. Most institutions have specific incident report forms (Fig. 14-2). The report documents an unusual situation that may possibly lead to a lawsuit or that indicates a failure to follow an institution's policy and procedures. The nurse describes details of the incident, and the physician examines the client to determine if any effects of the error occurred. The physician should also document the examination and findings in the client's medical record. The nurse does not duplicate all information from the incident report in the client's medical record. Only an objective description of what happened and any follow-up care is documented in the record.

Nurses usually become involved in client-related incidents at some point in their careers. They must understand the purpose of incident reports and the correct way to report information. The following list provides some guidelines for correctly completing an incident report:

1. The nurse who witnessed the incident or who found the client at the time of the incident should file the report.
2. Describe specifically what happened in concise, objective terms.
3. Do not interpret or attempt to explain the cause of the incident.
4. Describe objectively the client's condition when the incident was discovered.
5. Report any measures taken by you, other nurses, or physicians at the time of the incident.
6. Do not blame any nurse for guilt in an incident report.
7. Submit the report as soon as possible to the appropriate administrator.

Many nurses are reluctant to file incident reports because they believe such reports are detrimental to their employment record. Actually, incident reports are used by the institution's administration for quality assurance and risk management. By reviewing incident reports, administrators can identify areas of client risk. For example, if many incident reports reflect a growing increase in the number of client falls, the risk manager may recommend that nursing service provide inservice training about safety in transferring and ambulating clients. Incident reports can help to identify and eliminate significant problems in nursing practice or delivery of care methods.

RECORDING

Documentation is becoming very important in health care today. A medical record should be a comprehensive description of the client's health status and needs, as well as the services provided for the client's care. Good documentation reflects not only quality of care but evidence of each health care member's accountability in giving care. The record is also a document that shows to what extent hospitals should be reimbursed for services. The medical record is essentially the client's health care bill.

Several types of records are used to communicate information about clients. Although each agency uses a different record format, all records contain basically the following information:

1. Demographic data
2. Consent forms
3. Admission nursing history
4. Medical history
5. Reports of physical examinations
6. Reports of diagnostic studies
7. Medical diagnosis
8. Therapeutic orders
9. Progress notes
10. Nursing care plans
11. Record of care and treatment
12. Discharge plan and summary

Purpose of Records

A record is a valuable source of data used by all members of the health care team. Its purposes include communication, education, assessment, research, auditing, and legal documentation.

COMMUNICATION

The record is a means by which health team members communicate contributions to the client's care. A plan of care should be clear to anyone reading the chart. When a staff member is caring for a client, the record should explain the measures needed to maintain continuity and consistency of care.

EDUCATION

A client's record contains a variety of information, including medical and nursing diagnoses, signs and symptoms of disease, successful and unsuccessful therapies, diagnostic findings, and client behaviors. Students of nursing, medicine, and other health-related disciplines use these records as an educational resource. An effective

INCIDENT REPORT / Patient-Visitor

Barnes Hospital — St. Louis, Missouri

NOTICE: Consider whether Security should be called immediately, especially in cases of theft or disappearance of patient or employe valuables, hospital property - including narcotics, keys to offices or narcotics cabinets—automobiles and contents thereof, as well as vandalism, fights, or threats of physical harm.

"An incident is any happening which is not consistent with the routine operation of the hospital or the routine care of a particular patient. It may be an accident or a situation which might result in an accident".

INSTRUCTIONS FOR USE

TIMELY SUBMISSION

The last part of form (White Sheet - front and back) must be fully completed by the Department Head, Head Nurse, or Nurse-in-Charge or their representative and submitted within 72 hours to the appropriate administrator. Any delay in these reporting procedures must be accompanied by a written explanation for the lateness, and an endorsement by the appropriate administrator.

DEPT. HEAD/HEAD NURSE/NURSE-IN-CHARGE/EMPLOYE

1. COMPLETE LIGHT GREEN COPY of form and forward immediately to Safety Director.
2. PUMPKIN COLORED SHEET to the Head Nurse or Dept. Head. (EXCEPTION: SEE VISITOR NOT ON NURSING DIVISION)
3. COMPLETE THE FOLLOWING ON WHITE SHEET - FRONT AND BACK
   a. Description of Incident (what happened) by Patient, Visitor or Employe.
   b. What was accomplished prior to this incident to prevent its occurrence?
   c. Obtain Report and Signature of physician involved in treating patient.
   FORWARD FORM TO RESPONSIBLE ADMINISTRATOR.

ADMINISTRATOR

When the Administrator has completed his/her investigation, forward form to Safety Director.

VISITOR NOT ON NURSING DIVISION

Employe witnessing, involved in or informed of an incident should take visitor to the Emergency Room. IF VISITOR REFUSES TO GO TO EMERGENCY ROOM, employe should obtain PATIENT-VISITOR INCIDENT REPORT form from nearest department (DO NOT DETACH) obtain as much information as possible on LIGHT GREEN SHEET and forward ENTIRE FORM immediately to Safety Director.

EMERGENCY ROOM

With these incidents, the staff should complete the following portions of the PATIENT-VISITOR INCIDENT REPORT form:
1. LIGHT GREEN SHEET of Patient-Visitor Incident Report.
2. WHITE SHEET - Description of incident (what happened) by Visitor.
   Obtain physician's report and signature.

Contact Administrator on Duty for verification of charging or discount. Attach copy of Emergency Room note and forward completed form to Safety Director.

THIS DATA IS PROVIDED FOR THE LEGAL COUNSEL OF THE DIRECTORS OF BARNES HOSPITAL IN THE EVENT OF POSSIBLE LITIGATION AND IS TO BE CONSIDERED CONFIDENTIAL AND PRIVILEGED INFORMATION.

Fig. 14-2 Incident report form.
Courtesy Barnes Hospital, St. Louis.

INCIDENT REPORT / Patient-Visitor

Barnes Hospital — St. Louis, Missouri

THIS DATA IS PROVIDED FOR THE LEGAL COUNSEL OF THE
DIRECTORS OF BARNES HOSPITAL IN THE EVENT OF POSSIBLE
LITIGATION AND IS TO BE CONSIDERED CONFIDENTIAL AND
PRIVILEGED INFORMATION.

USE ADDRESSOGRAPH IF PATIENT

REPORT NO.	PERSON INVOLVED			Age 68	Date of Incident 1/8/--	Time (Military) 0915	Tele. No.
	PETERS (Last Name)	RON (First Name)	L (M.I.)	Sex M	Date Reported 1/8/--	Exact location of incident ROOM 6201A	

PATIENT ☒

Rm. No. 6201A   Reason for hospitalization (Diagnosis) ALZHEIMERS WORK UP   Attending Physician ROGERS

Mental condition of patient before incident:

Normal ☐ Senile ☐

Disoriented ☒ Sedated ☐ Other_____

Bedrails: Up ☒ Down ☐ Restraints: Yes ☐ No ☒

Activity Orders: Restraints ☐ Bed Rest ☐

Up privileges with assistance ☒ Without assistance ☐

Brief description of incident: PATIENT FOUND ON FLOOR AT SIDE OF BED. SMALL, 2CM ABRASION NOTED OVER Ⓛ FOREHEAD. CONSCIOUS AND RESPONDS TO VOICE.

VISTOR ☐   **OTHER** ☐

By whom employed_____   Occupation_____

Home Address_____   Home Phone_____

Nature of Incident   Reason in Hospital

ACCIDENT FACTS

Name, Address, Tele. No. of Witnesses, if any:

Was patient seen by physician: Yes ☒ No ☐ Not indicated ☐

Time called _1000_ a.m./p.m.   Time arrived _1030_ a.m./p.m.

Physician's Name.

Was treatment initiated by physician: Yes ☒ No ☐   X-Rays: Yes ☒ No ☐

I DO NOT WISH TO BE EXAMINED BY A PHYSICIAN: Signed:_____

DESCRIPTION OF INCIDENT

State what you saw and/or what you were told. Give names and addresses of all individuals who provided information concerning this incident.

ENTERED ROOM. FOUND PT. ON FLOOR AT SIDE OF BED. STATED "WHERE IS MARIE?" NOTED SMALL, 2CM ABRASION OVER Ⓛ FOREHEAD. AREA TENDER TO PALPATION. PT. ABLE TO MOVE ALL EXTREMITIES FULL ROM. ABLE TO RAISE FROM FLOOR INDEPENDENTLY. CALLED DR. ROGERS. SKULL-FILM ORDERED.

Date of Report 1/8/--   Signature of person preparing report _Rita Woods RN_

PROPERTY DAMAGE ☐

Owner of Property   If theft, what day   and hour   last seen.

Home Address   Tele. No.

MISSING ARTICLE ☐

Nature and Extent of Damage or Loss

Estimated replacement or repair cost: $

Fig. 14-2, cont'd Incident report form.

WHAT WAS ACCOMPLISHED PRIOR TO THIS INCIDENT TO PREVENT ITS OCCURRENCE? (Department Head/Head Nurse/Nurse-in-charge/Employe witnessing or involved in an incident)

_____

_____

_____

_____

_____

_____

Signature of Dept. Head/Head Nurse/Nurse-in-Charge/Employe

Medical Findings by M.D. Related to Incident

_____

_____

_____

Signature of Physician

ADMINISTRATIVE ACTION

_____

_____

Signature of Administrator

SAFETY DIRECTOR

_____

_____

_____

_____

_____

_____

_____

_____

_____

_____

_____

Signature of Safety Director

Fig. 14-2, cont'd   Incident report form.

way to learn the nature of an illness and the response to it is to read the medical record. Although no two clients have identical records, patterns of information can be identified in records of clients who have similar medical problems. With this information, students learn the patterns to look for in various health problems or diseases and become better able to anticipate the type of care required for a client.

ASSESSMENT

The record provides data for nurses to use to identify nursing diagnoses and plan proper interventions for care. Information from the record adds to the nurse's own observations and assessment findings. The medical history, for example, is in the record. Thus it is unnecessary for the nurse to collect information that is already available, unless there is reason to believe the information is inaccurate. Before caring for any client, the nurse refers to the medical record for new and relevant assessment findings.

The record provides a total picture of the client's health status. Assessment data entered by each health care member do not simply describe isolated happenings. Each observation is part of a larger puzzle, which when solved reveals the client's health status. The record contains data to explain and confirm observations or refute interpretations. After inspection of a wound, for example, the nurse may conclude that it is healing poorly. What clues to understanding the problem might be found in the record? What has the client's appetite been like? Have nurses on previous shifts also described the wound's poor appearance? Are there any laboratory results indicating onset of infection? Has the physician observed the wound in the last 24 hours? Any obser-

vations or interpretations made by the nurse are compared with data from the record. The record helps to explain the reasons for and implications of any findings the nurse gathers.

RESEARCH

Statistical data relating to the frequency of clinical disorders, complications, use of specific medical and nursing therapies, deaths, and recovery from illness can be gathered from client records. Records are a valuable resource for describing characteristics of the client populations using a specific health agency.

A nurse may use clients' records during a research study to collect information on certain factors. For example, if a nurse uses a new method of pain control on a group of clients, the records could provide data on the success of therapy. Record entries describing the number of analgesic medications used or the client's subjective report of pain relief could be used to evaluate the new pain-control measure. Nurses may also research records of previously discharged clients to identify nursing care problems. For example, a study to determine the incidence of infection in clients with specific types of intravenous catheters might be performed with a chart review.

AUDITING

A regular review of information in client records gives a basis to evaluate the level of health care provided in an institution. The JCAHO requires hospitals to establish quality assurance programs to conduct objective, ongoing reviews of client care. The JCAHO has standards for types of information to be found in the client's record, such as indications that care is individualized

---

Examples of JCAHO Nursing Service Standards

The nursing process (assessment, nursing diagnosis, planning, implementation, and evaluation) is documented for each hospitalized client from admission through discharge.

The plan of care is documented and reflects current standards of nursing practice.
- The plan includes nursing measures that will facilitate medical care prescribed and will restore, maintain, or promote the client's well being.
- As appropriate, such measures include physiological, psychosocial, and environmental factors; client and family education; and client discharge planning.

Documentation of nursing care is pertinent and concise and reflects client status.
- Nursing documentation addresses the client's needs, problems, capabilities, and limitations.
- Nursing intervention and client responses are noted.
- When a client is transfered within or discharged from the hospital, a nurse notes his status in his medical record.
- Evidence of instructions and the client's or family's understanding of these instructions is noted in the medical record.
- The nursing department or service is encouraged to standardize documentation of routine elements of care and repeated monitoring of, for example, personal hygiene and administration of medication.

and that discharge planning and client education have occurred. The JCAHO also asks institutions to establish standards for quality care (see box). Nurses conduct audits of records throughout the year to determine the degree to which quality assurance standards are met. Deficiencies identified during audits are shared with all members of the nursing staff so corrections in policy or practice can be made. Quality assurance programs keep nurses informed to maintain excellence in nursing care.

Medical records are also audited to establish a health care bill. Private insurance carriers and auditors from the federal government review records to determine the reimbursement a client or a health care agency receives. Hospitals now receive prospective payment for the DRG by which a client is discharged. Accurate charting allows for accurate DRG assessment and the fullest possible reimbursement (Hoke, 1985). Nurses must carefully record all therapies clients receive. Thorough documentation ensures that costs are recovered and that clients receive the care they require.

LEGAL DOCUMENTATION

A medical record must be accurate because it is a legal document. In the case of a lawsuit, the medical record, not the nursing care, is on trial. The record serves as a description of exactly what happened to a client. Nursing care may have been excellent. However, if a nurse failed to document care thoroughly, an incomplete record can become a lawyer's weapon in a lawsuit. Clients frequently request copies of their medical records, and they have the right to read those records. Each institution has policies for controlling the manner in which records are shared.

Recording should not become merely routine or superficial. Nor should nurses wait until the end of a tiring day to record the client's care. Good documentation should be done in a timely manner with careful thought. Table 14-4 provides guidelines to ensure that a client's record is legally sound.

TABLE 14-4 Legal Guidelines for Recording

Guideline	Rationale	Correct Action
Do not erase, apply correction fluid, or scratch out an error made while recording.	Charting becomes illegible. It may appear as though a nurse was attempting to hide information or deface the record.	Draw a single line through the error, write the word "error" above it and sign your name or initials. Then record the note correctly.
Do not write retaliatory or critical comments about the client or care of other health care professionals.	Statements can be used as evidence for nonprofessional behavior or poor quality of care.	Only enter objective descriptions of client's behavior and care administered by others.
Correct all errors promptly.	Errors in recording can lead to errors in treatment.	Avoid rushing to complete charting. Be sure information is accurate.
Record only facts.	Record must be accurate and reliable.	Be certain entry is factual. Do not speculate or guess.
Do not leave blank spaces in a nurse's notes.	Another person can add incorrect information to the space.	Draw a line horizontally through the space and sign your name at its end.
All record entries should be legible and written in ink.	Illegible entries can be misinterpreted, causing errors and lawsuits. Ink cannot be erased. Records are photocopied and stored on microfilm.	Never erase entries or use correction fluid, and never use a pencil.
If you question an order, record that a clarification was sought.	If a nurse performs an order known to be incorrect, he or she is just as liable for prosecution as the physician.	Do not record "physician made an error." Instead chart that "Dr. Smith was called to clarify order for . . . ."
Chart only for yourself.	A nurse is accountable for information he or she enters into the chart.	Never chart for someone else.
Avoid using generalized, empty phrases such as "status unchanged" or "had a good day."	Specific information about a client's condition or case can be accidentally deleted if information is too generalized.	Use complete, concise descriptions of care.
Begin each entry with the time and end with your signature and title.	Ensures that the correct sequence of events is recorded. Signature documents who is accountable for care delivered.	Do not wait until the end of the shift to record important changes that occurred several hours earlier. Be sure to sign.

TABLE 14-5 Components of Traditional Source Record

Section	Contents
Admission fact sheet	Specific demographic data about client (name, identification number, sex, age, marital status, occupation, employer, health insurance, nearest relative)
Physician's order sheet	Record of physician's orders, each order entered with date, time, and physician's signature. Orders prescribe specific therapies for client
Graphic/flow sheet	Record of repeated observations and tests and measurements (vital signs and weight)
Medical data base	All observations and interpretations of client's condition made by physicians (physical examination, history, progress notes)
Nursing notes	Narrative record of nursing process (assessment, nursing diagnosis, planning, implementation, and evaluation of care provided)
Medication records	Accurate documentation of all medications administered to client. Date, time, and signature of nurse are recorded.
Health care disciplines	Entries made into record by all health-related disciplines (physical therapy, dietary department, radiology, social work, and laboratories)
Discharge summary	Summary of client's condition, progress, prognosis, rehabilitation, and teaching needs at time of dismissal from hospital or agency

Methods of Recording

The nursing service department of each health care agency selects the method used for documentation of client's care. The method should consider the philosophy of the nursing service and the way nursing care is given to clients. For example, if a professional model is used to deliver care, a documentation system should be based on the nursing process.

Three common methods of record-keeping include traditional source records, problem-oriented records, and modified problem-oriented records. The primary difference between these types is the manner in which information is organized.

SOURCE RECORDS

In a source record the client's chart is organized so each discipline (for example, nursing, medicine, social work, or respiratory therapy) has a separate section in which to record data. The advantage of a source record is that care givers can easily locate the proper section of the record in which to make entries. Table 14-5 lists the components of a source record.

A disadvantage of the source record is that information is fragmented. Each care giver's notes may be well organized. However, it may become necessary to extract data from several different sections before identifying the client's problems and the plan of care. For example, the nurse describes the character of abdominal pain and use of relaxation therapy and analgesic medication in the nurse's notes. The physician's notes describe the progress of the client's bowel obstruction and the plan for surgery in a separate section of the record. The results of x-ray examinations showing the location of the bowel obstruction is in the test results section of the record.

The method by which source records are organized does not show how information from the various health care disciplines is related or how care is coordinated to meet all the client's needs.

The nurses' notes section is where nurses enter a narrative description of nursing care and the client's response (see box below). It is also a section for documenting care provided by the physician in the nurse's presence. The nurse may record key diagnostic test results from other sections of the record in the nurses' notes if they are of major importance in the care of the client. In a hospital an entry is usually made in the nurses'

Sample Nurses' Note

8/6/88 1100 Client states, "I'm having a hard time catching my breath." Respirations are labored at 28/min. P96, BP 112/70. Client using intercostal muscles during inhalation, breathing primarily costal. Breath sounds auscultated, crackles over both lower lobes. Chest excursion equal bilaterally. Elevated head of bed to Fowler's position. Obtained arterial blood gases at 1045 per order. Results are pH 7.31, $Pco_2$44, $Po_2$80. Dr. Stein called. Applied O_2 at 4 L/min per mask as ordered. Remained at bedside to calm client. P. Haske, RN.

notes for each shift or tour of duty. If a hospital uses several flow sheets for repetitive data it may only be necessary to record a note once every 24 hours or as a client's condition changes. If the client is seen in a clinic or at home, the nurse documents care provided during each visit.

PROBLEM-ORIENTED MEDICAL RECORDS

The problem-oriented medical record (POMR) is a structured method of documentation that places emphasis on the client's problems. The method corresponds to the nursing process and facilitates communication of client needs (Gawlinski and Rasmussen, 1984). Data are organized by problem rather than by the source of information. Each member of the health care team contributes to a single list of identified client problems. With the POMR the client's problems are easy to recognize and locate, data are well coordinated, and each discipline records progress notes on the same form. The client benefits from this charting method because all health care team members contribute to a common, coordinated plan of care. The box below describes advantages of the POMR method.

The POMR has the following major sections: data base, problem list, initial plan, and progress notes.

DATA BASE. This section contains all available assessment information pertaining to the client (for example, the physician's physical examination and medical history, the nurse's admission history and assessment, the dietitian's assessment, laboratory reports, and radiological test results). The data base provides a foundation for identifying client problems and planning an effective course of action. The data base should remain active and current with revisions made as new data become available. The data base will accompany clients through successive hospitalizations or clinic visits.

Advantages of POMR Charting Method

- Places emphasis on clients and their problems.
- Increases efficiency in gathering data about clients from all health care givers.
- Gives emphasis to clients' perceptions of their problems.
- Requires continuous evaluation and revision of plan of care.
- Provides greater continuity of care between health care team members.
- Enhances effective communication among health care team members.

PROBLEM LIST. Once data are analyzed, problems are identified and a single list is made (Fig. 14-3). The problems are listed in chronological order according to the date each was identified (not in order of priority). The list is an organizing guide by which all health care disciplines plan the client's care.

A problem may be well defined, such as a specific medical or nursing diagnosis. Signs, symptoms, or syndromes such as pain or diarrhea may be stated as problems when insufficient data have been recorded to diagnose a problem or when complications of a medical diagnosis arise. Problems include the client's physiological, psychological, social, cultural, spiritual, developmental, and environmental needs.

It is important to avoid listing problems that are vague or unsubstantiated by data. The nurse lists a diagnosis if one can be established, rather than a less specific term. For example, the nursing diagnosis of ineffective airway clearance is characterized by a cough, dyspnea, and abnormal breath sounds. Impaired breathing or coughing would be unacceptable nursing diagnoses. Manifestations or criteria for diagnoses or problems should not be listed separately. This can cause a fragmentation of care. Integration of data to form specific well-defined diagnoses or problems results in more goal-directed care.

The list of problems is filed in the front of the client's record to serve as an organizer or table of contents. New problems are added as they are identified. Once a problem has been resolved, the date of resolution is recorded and a line is drawn through the problem and its number on the problem sheet. The number for a resolved problem is not used again. This system keeps the problem list simple yet meaningful. Once a problem list is developed, succeeding record entries such as in the progress notes are coded by the problem number.

INITIAL PLAN. An initial plan is developed for each active problem identified. There are three parts to a plan:
1. *Diagnostic workup*—The physician indicates what diagnostic studies should be initiated first. Setting priorities prevents duplication of efforts and delay in dealing with the client's needs. During a time of cost containment in health care a coordination of diagnostic testing is very important.
2. *Proposed therapy*—The physician orders specific therapies by problem. The orders may include medications, activity restrictions, diet, special treatments, precautions to follow or observations to make. If the original problem is a nursing diagnosis, the nurse may outline the proposed interventions for care. The format of a POMR allows each health care worker to understand the rationale for all orders.
3. *Client education*—Identifying the client's educational needs addresses the long-term implications

Problem number	Date onset	Problem	Inactive or resolved	Date resolved
~~1~~	~~7/8/88~~	~~Ⓡ breast mass~~	~~Resolved~~	~~7/9/88~~
2	7/8/88	Anxiety over impending surgery		
3	7/9/88	Ⓡ sub-total mastectomy		
4	7/9/88	Alteration in comfort related to incisional pain	Controlled	7/12/88
5	7/10/88	Disturbance in self-concept		
6	7/11/88	Inadequate family support systems		

Fig. 14-3 POMR problem list.

of illness. Health team members identify the types of information or skills required by a client to adapt to any health-related problems.

PROGRESS NOTES. Health team members must monitor and record the progress of a client's problems. Progress notes follow a special format (for example, SOAP or PIE) so information is communicated clearly to all who read them (Fig. 14-4). SOAP is an acronym for subjective data, objective data, assessment, and plan. The logic for SOAP notes is similar to that of the nursing process. Data is collected about each of the client's problems, a conclusion is made, and a plan of care is developed. Each SOAP note is numbered and titled according to the problem on the list it addresses. The numbering system makes it easy to find notes about the same problem. The notes help communicate an on-going plan of care.

S—This section includes subjective data or information gathered from the client. For example, the client will describe a symptom such as pain or discuss an interest in learning about a medication. Whether the

1/19/88   Knowledge deficit related to inexperi-
4:30 PM   ence with surgery

S— "I'm worried about what it will be like after surgery." O—Client asking frequent questions about surgery. Has had no previous experience with surgery. Wife present, acts as a support person. A—Knowledge deficit related to inexperience with surgery. Client also expressing anxiety. P— Explain routine preoperative preparation. Demonstrate and explain rationale for TCDB exercises. Provide explanation and teaching booklet on postoperative nursing care.—S. Lazarus, RN	P—Knowledge deficit related to inexperience with surgery I— Explained to client normal preoperative preparations for surgery. Demonstrated TCDB exercises. Provided booklet to client on postoperative nursing care. E—Client able to demonstrate TCDB exercises correctly. Needs review of postoperative nursing care.—S. Lazarus, RN

Fig. 14-4 Examples of progress notes written in the SOAP and PIE formats.

Courtesy Barnes Hospital, St. Louis.

progress note includes subjective data depends on the acuteness of the client's illness or the nature of the problem.

O—Objective data consists of information that can be observed or measured. Physical findings, laboratory results, observations, or results of x-ray examinations are examples of objective data.

A—The individual who writes a SOAP note takes both the subjective and objective data and forms conclusions. The assessment is an interpretation of the client's condition or level of progress. It is a statement of the status of the diagnosis or problem. The assessment determines whether the problem has been resolved or if further care is required.

P—Depending on the assessment of the situation the health care member then develops a plan of care. Plans may include specific orders designed to manage the client's problem, collection of additional data about the problem, individual or family education,

and goals of care. The plan in each SOAP note is compared with the plan in previous notes. A decision is made to revise, modify, or continue previously proposed interventions.

PIE is an acronym for Problem-Intervention-Evaluation. This format simplifies documentation by unifying the care plan and progress notes into a complete record (Siegrist, 1985). The PIE format differs from SOAP because the narrative note does not include assessment information. Daily assessment data appears instead on special flow sheets (Fig 14-4) thus preventing duplication of information. The PIE notes can be numbered or labeled according to the client's problems. Resolved problems are dropped from daily documentation after the nurse's review. Continuing problems are documented daily.

P—Problem or nursing diagnosis applicable to client

I—Interventions or actions taken

E—Evaluation of the outcomes of nursing interventions and the client's response to nursing therapies

MODIFIED PROBLEM-ORIENTED MEDICAL RECORDS

In some institutions the POMR method of charting may only be used in the nursing records. POMR takes the place of narrative notes seen in the traditional source record.

At the time of a client's admission, an initial nursing assessment (Fig. 14-5, p. 346) identifies the nursing diagnoses or client problems. The diagnoses are dated and then numbered in order of occurrence or by priority on the basis of the initial assessment. The nurse then lists the number each time the problem is recorded in the SOAP or PIE notes. It is also acceptable to underline the number, diagnosis, or problem in the notes so it can easily be spotted. Once a diagnosis is resolved the nurse enters the date, notes that the problem is resolved, and initials it.

Nurses record SOAP or PIE notes on each pertinent problem daily or every shift, depending on agency policy. This continues until problems are resolved. The SOAP or PIE format helps nurses be aware of the care plan and the client response to interventions. New problems may be added to the problem list as they are identified.

Alternative Record-Keeping Forms

A client's medical record may use a variety of forms to make documentation easy and quick, yet comprehensive. Many of the forms eliminate the need to duplicate repeated data in the nursing notes. The forms present special types of information in a format more accessible than reviewing all progress notes.

NURSING HISTORY FORMS

A nursing history form is a special form completed at the time a client is admitted to a nursing care unit (Fig. 14-5). The form usually contains basic biographical data (age, method of admission, physician), a brief history (surgical history, allergies, medication history, previous illnesses), the client's perceptions about illness or hospitalization, and a physical assessment of all body systems. The form allows the admitting nurse to make a thorough client assessment to identify relevant nursing diagnoses or problems. Data on history forms provide baseline data that can be compared with changes that occur later in the client's condition. Each institution designs a nursing history form differently, depending on the philosophy of nursing care.

FLOW SHEETS

Flow sheets are forms that allow nurses to record specific measurements or observations that occur on a repeated basis. For example, it is unnecessary to chart a narrative progress note each time vital signs are checked, a bath is given, or a drug is administered. The flow sheet is a quicker and more efficient way to record information. Fig. 14-6 (p. 348) is an example of a vital sign flow sheet. Fig. 14-7 (p. 350) is an example of a nursing assessment flow sheet.

The only time the nurse may wish to duplicate information from a flow sheet into a narrative or progress note is when a significant change that results in specific therapies occurs. For example, if a client's blood pressure becomes dangerously high, the nurse may record the pressure in the narrative progress note, along with the medication administered to lower the pressure.

One value of a flow sheet is that it can show important clinical trends graphically without the nurse or physician having to locate the source information in several notes. Critical care units commonly use flow sheets for all types of physiological data.

NURSING KARDEX

Nursing information needed for the daily care of a client is readily accessible in the nursing Kardex (Fig. 14-8, p. 352). The Kardex is a flip-over card usually kept in a portable index file or notebook at the nurses' station. Nurses refer to the Kardex throughout the day. It organizes information in a useful manner as nurses give change-of-shift reports or make walking rounds. The Kardex contains pertinent information about clients and their ongoing plan of care. An updated Kardex eliminates the need for continual referral to the client's chart for routine information. Information commonly found in the Kardex includes the following:

1. Basic demographic data (for example, age, religion)
2. Primary medical diagnosis
3. Current physician's orders to be carried out by the nurse
4. A written nursing care plan (used when a formal plan is not found in the client's record)
5. Nursing orders
6. Scheduled tests and procedures
7. Safety precautions to be used in the client's care
8. Factors related to activities of daily living

In many institutions, nurses make Kardex entries in pencil since it is usually necessary to make frequent revisions as the client's needs change. However, entries should be made in ink if the Kardex is a permanent part of the client's record. The Kardex provides the nurse an opportunity to communicate useful information to the nursing team about the client's unique needs. Within the care plan or in the order entries sections the nurse can communicate information such as preferences in diet, specific methods to perform a treatment, methods to incorporate the client participation in care, or preferred times to perform a nursing order. Information within the Kardex should not simply be a reflection of routine nursing responsibilities or standardized care. The box below summarizes guidelines for Kardex care plans.

For example, for a client who has a urinary tract infection and is required to drink large amounts of fluids, a Kardex entry of "increase fluid intake" is relevant but not particularly individualized. If, however, the nurse's

---

Tips on Writing Kardex Care Plans

WHEN TO WRITE A CARE PLAN

- During a report as nurses discuss client problems and needs
- On rounds after client problems are identified and reviewed
- After discussions with other health team members responsible for client care
- After interactions with the client and family members

WHAT TO INCLUDE

- Pertinent nursing assessment data
- Nursing diagnoses
- Nursing orders
  - Observations to make and frequency required
  - Nursing measures aimed at restoring, maintaining, or promoting health
  - Specific methods used to implement nursing measures
  - Appropriate inclusion of family participation
  - Discharge planning
- Expected outcomes of nursing care

Barnes Hospital

NURSES ADMISSION NOTE   C-2

Date _10/13/--_ Time _1400_ Informant _PATIENT_   Age _71_

T _36⁸_ P _92_ R _22_ B/P _160/90_ Ht. _5'4"_ Wt. _165 LB_

Chief Complaint and History of Present Illness:

"_I'VE HAD THIS SORE ON MY FOOT FOR_
2 MONTHS AND IT WON'T HEAL."
ADMITTED FOR EVALUATION OF
VASCULAR DISEASE.

ADDRESSOGRAPH

Type of previous illness/surgery	Date	Type of previous illness/surgery	Date
DIABETES	1968		
HYSTERECTOMY	1958		

Has received blood products in the past: ☐ Yes ☒ No If yes, List dates _____   Reactions: ☐ Yes ☐ No

Allergies: _PENICILLIN_

Medication Name	Dose/Frequency	Time of Last Dose	Name	Dose/Frequency	Time of Last Dose
INSULIN (NPH)	30 UNITS qAM	0800			
INSULIN (REG)	8 UNITS qAM	0800			
METAMUCIL	↑ Tasp qAM	0900			

Patient Provided: ☒ Admission Kit ☒ I.D. Band ☒ Sensitivity/Allergy Band

Patient Instructed: ☒ Valuables Policy ☒ Waiver signed ☒ Smoking/Visitor policy ☒ Nurses Call/Emergency/TV/Phone
☒ Chaplain availability ☐ Patient rights (Psych. only) SIGNATURE: _L. Reed RN_

DIRECTIONS: Circle those that apply. Comment on those circled if needed.

Sensory

Sensory Alteration

• EYES: (Decreased acuity) (Blurred vision) Photophobia Discharge Prosthesis
EARS: Tinnitus Discharge Hard of hearing (R or L)
NOSE: Congestion Obstruction Discharge Epistaxis
THROAT: Sore throat Hoarseness   TOUCH: (Reduced)/absent tactile perception
ASSIST DEVICES/MEASURES: (Glasses) Contacts Hearing aid Tracheostomy
Comments: _ABLE TO READ ONLY LARGE PRINT WITH GLASSES._
HAS REDUCED SENSATION IN BOTH FEET UP TO ANKLE LEVEL.

Skin/Mucous Membrane

Impaired Skin Integrity
Alt. in mucous membranes

• Poor hygiene Poor turgor Diaphoretic Bruises Scars Erythema Petechiae Rash
Itching Jaundice (Wound (describe)) Pale/dry membranes Coated tongue Stomatitis
Carious teeth Halitosis
Comments: _3 CM OPEN AREA OVER (L) METATARSAL OF (L) FOOT,_
DRAINING MODERATE AMOUNT OF YELLOW DISCHARGE.

Respiratory

Ineffective airway clearance
Ineffective breathing patterns
Impaired gas exchange

• Cough Hemoptysis Dyspnea Orthopnea Cyanosis Restlessness Home 02 ____ L/min
Use of accessory muscles Pursed lip breathing Pain with breathing
Smoker (packs/day _____ years _____) (Lung sounds (describe))
Comments: _LUNGS CLEAR TO AUSCULTATION BILATERALLY_

Circulatory

Decreased cardiac output
Alt. periph. tissue perfusion
Alt. fluid volume

• Fatigue Chest pain Palpitations Syncope (Numbness) (Tingling) Edema
(Weak)/absent peripheral pulse Capillary refill (describe) (Extremities (describe color/temperature))
Comments: _BOTH LOWER FEET COOL TO PALPATION, MOTTLING NOTED_
AROUND (L) FOOT ULCER, DORSALIS PEDIS PULSES WEAK BILATERALLY.

Nutrition

Alt. in nutrition

• Diet: _1800 CAL ADA DIET AT HOME._
Dysphagia Heartburn Nausea Vomiting Appetite increase/decrease Decreased taste
Weight gain/loss _____ lbs. (Difficulty chewing) (Dentures - lower/upper)
Comments: _DENTURES LOOSE FITTING._

Fig. 14-5 Nursing history form.
Courtesy Barnes Hospital, St. Louis.

Elimination

Alt. in bowel elimination
Alt. in urinary elimination

- BOWEL: Constipation   Diarrhea   Incontinence   Melena   Tarry stools   Ostomy
  Abd. pain/cramps/gas   Hemorrhoids   (Last BM) *10/12*   Usual pattern *(describe)* **EVERY OTHER DAY**
  Medications/Enemas **METAMUCIL**   (Bowel Sounds) *(describe)*
  Comments: **NORMAL IN ALL 4 QUADRANTS**

  URINARY: (Frequency)   Urgency   Incontinence   Polyuria   Dysuria   Hematuria
  (Nocturia)   Anuria   Retention   Urinary appliance
  Comments: **URINE PALE YELLOW, CLEAR. PATIENT REPORTS THAT SHE VOIDS HOURLY. VOIDS AT LEAST TWICE NIGHTLY.**

Activity/Exercise Alteration

Impaired physical mobility
Self care deficit
Activity intolerance

- Self Care *(describe limitations to eat/bathe/dress/toilet/ambulate)*   Fatigue   Purposeful movement limited/absent
  Decreased strength   (Altered weight bearing)   Limited ROM   Abnormal gait   Impaired coordination
  Exercise routine **MILE A DAY, PRIOR TO ILLNESS** Assist devices used _____
  Comments: **DISCOMFORT WHILE BEARING WEIGHT ON Ⓛ FOOT. HAS BEEN UNABLE TO WALK REGULARLY IN LAST 3 WEEKS.**

Comfort

Alteration in comfort
Alteration in sleep pattern

- Pain *(describe character and patient behaviors)*   Restlessness   Sleep pattern *(Describe)* **7-8 HRS NIGHTLY**
  Pain control/sleeping aids used **ENJOYS HOT CHOCOLATE @ BEDTIME**
  Comments: _____

Immune Function

Potential for infection

- Fever in last 48°   Lymphadenopathy   Transplant history   Chemotherapy *(date)*_____
  Radiation therapy *(date)*_____   Venous access device _____
  Comments: **NO ABNORMAL FINDINGS**

Sexuality/ Reproductive

Alt. in sexual function/ response

- Vaginal/urethral discharge   Pap smear **UNSURE**   LMP **AGE 48**   Mammogram **1985**
  (Knowledge of self breast exam/testicular exam   Change in relationship with partner
  Limitation imposed by disease/therapy
  Comments: **DOES PERFORM A SELF-BREAST EXAM, BUT NOT REGULARLY**

Neuro/Cerebral Function

Alt. in thought process
Alt. in communication
Potential for violence

- (Alert)   Oriented x **3**   Memory impairment   Impaired attention span   H/A   Dizziness
  Inappropriate behavior   Inaccurate interpretation of environment   Difficulty expressing self verbally
  Numbness   Impaired judgement/perception
  Comments: _____

Cognitive Response

Lack of knowledge

- Foreign language   Poor understanding   Inexperience with therapy   (Requests information)
  Comments: **DESIRES TO HAVE MORE INFORMATION REGARDING SKIN CARE TO ULCER SITE AND ASSISTANCE WITH MENU PLANNING.**

Emotional Response

Alt. in coping mechanism
Alt. in self concept

- VERBALIZES: (Fear) of therapy or surgery   Loss of control   Inability to cope   Poor self-esteem
  Identifies stressors *(describe)* (Anxious)   Angry   Crying   Irritable   Inappropriate affect   Low mood
  Comments: **EXPRESSES CONCERN REGARDING IMPLICATIONS IF FOOT ULCER DOES NOT HEAL.**

Social System

Alt. in support system

- Employed/unemployed   Lives: **FOUR-ROOM APARTMENT**
  In nursing home/other _____   Support person **HUSBAND, JOHN OWENS**
  Ability to assist after discharge **HUSBAND IS ABLE TO ASSIST WITH ADL**
  Home environment affecting self-care _____
  Comments: **HUSBAND'S HOME PHONE   427-1060**

Values/Beliefs

Value/belief conflict

- Expresses attitudes/beliefs re: Hospitalization (Implications of care)
  Inappropriate perceptions of illness *(patient/family)* _____
  Patient preference for spiritual assistance **CATHOLIC, REQUESTS VISIT BY PRIEST**
  Comments: **DOES NOT WANT TO BECOME DEPENDENT PHYSICALLY.**

Health Management Pattern

Alt. in health maintenance
Potential for injury

- Last physical **1/88**   Alcohol use **DENIES**   Drug Use **DENIES**
  Noncompliance with therapies   Lack of knowledge *(describe)*   Needs equipment/finances/resources
  Comments: _____

Referrals

- (Dietitian)   Social service   (Nurse specialist)   AT/OT/PT   (Pastoral care)   Speech therapy
  Nurse Signature **L. Read RN**

Fig. 14-5, cont'd   Nursing history form.

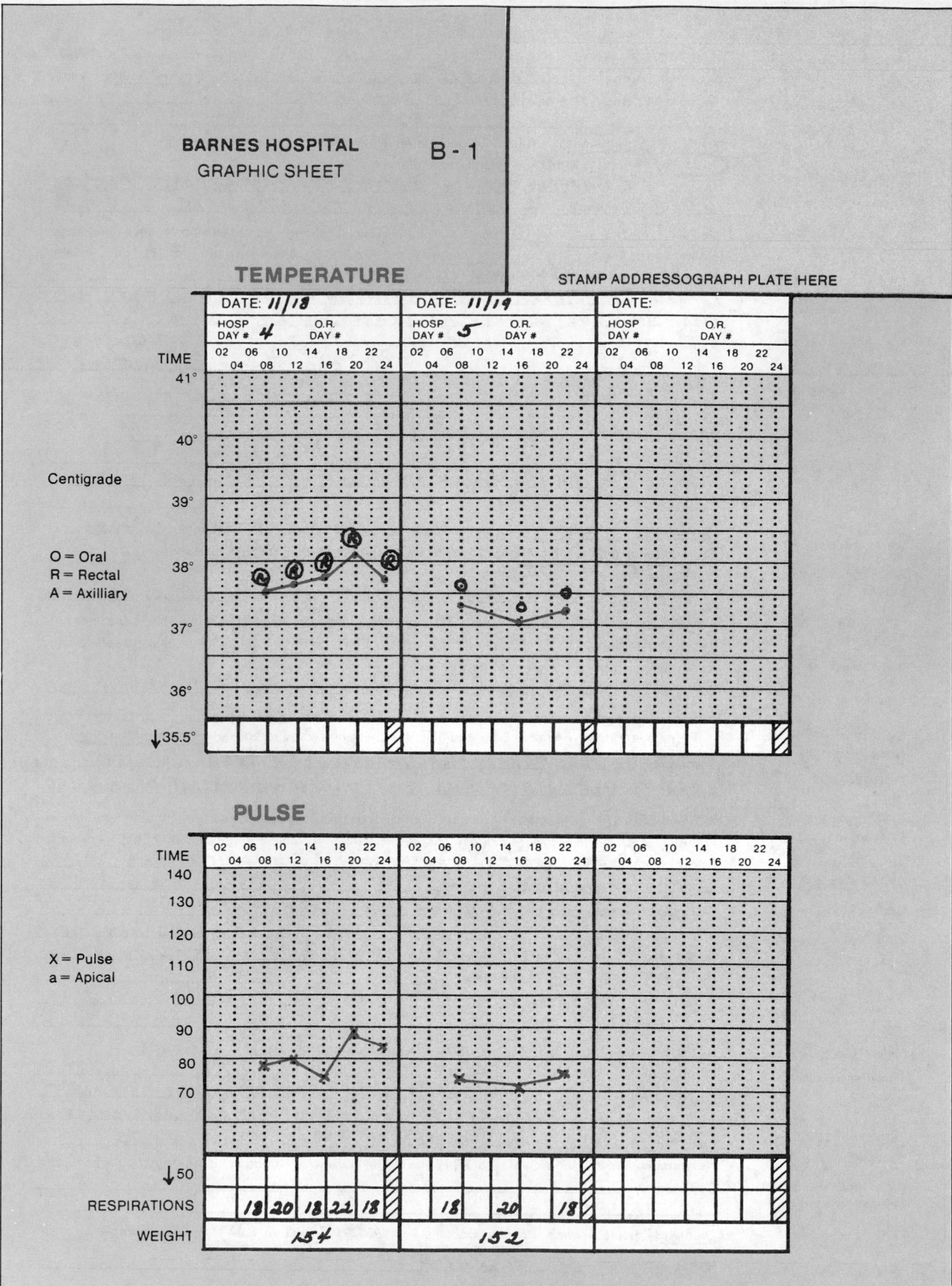

Fig. 14-6 Vital signs flowsheet.
Courtesy Barnes Hospital, St. Louis.

assessment has revealed that the client prefers iced tea and cranberry juice, a Kardex entry of "offer cranberry juice and iced tea, 1000 ml per shift" addresses the client's preferences and tailors the care plan to the client's needs.

The Kardex care plan has some disadvantages. Access is usually limited to nursing members of the health care team. Also, the Kardex does not offer space for writing an extensive plan for the client with multiple problems.

STANDARDIZED CARE PLANS

Although it is every professional nurse's responsibility to develop an individualized plan of care for a client, the process of writing the plan is time consuming. Nurses caring for several clients may need to write extensive plans of care. Many institutions have attempted to make documentation easier for nurses with standardized care plans. The plans, based on the institution's philosophy of nursing care, are preprinted, established guidelines used to care for clients with similar health problems. Once a nursing assessment is completed, the staff nurse identifies the standard care plans appropriate to the client. The care plans are placed in the client's record. Modifications can be made to the standardized plans in ink to individualize the nursing therapies. Most standardized plans also allow the nurse to write in specific goals or desired outcomes of care, as well as the dates when these outcomes should be achieved.

There are several advantages and disadvantages to standardized care plans. One advantage is the establishment of clinically sound standards of care for similar groups of clients. These standards can be useful when quality assurance audits are conducted. Standardized plans are easy to locate in a client's record, and thus all staff can quickly refer to the plan of care. Another advantage is the education. Nurses learn to recognize the accepted requirements of care for clients. The standardized plans can also improve continuity of care among professional nurses. Finally, even though the plans must be modified for each client, documentation takes less time.

Controversy exists over the use of standardized care plans. The major disadvantage is the risk that the standardized plans inhibit nurses' identification of unique, individualized therapies for clients. A second disadvantage is the need to formally update the plans on a routine basis to ensure that content is current and appropriate. Staff members often develop many standardized plans for clients seen in their institution. Large numbers of plans take up space for storage and are more costly to print than one common care plan form.

When standardized care plans are used in a health care facility, the nurse remains responsible for an individualized approach to care.

DISCHARGE SUMMARY FORMS. Much emphasis is placed on preparing clients for an efficient and timely discharge from a health care institution. A prospective payment system based on DRGs encourages health care institutions to be more efficient. The Health Care Financing Administration (HCFA) uses DRGs to establish expected time frames during which a client is expected to be hospitalized. Regardless of the client's actual length of stay, the hospital is reimbursed only for the established time period. The earlier a client is discharged, the more likely a hospital will be fully reimbursed. HCFA requires multidisciplinary involvement in discharge planning to ensure that clients leave hospitals in a timely manner with the resources necessary.

Ideally, discharge planning begins at the time of a client's admission. Nurses revise the plan as the client's condition changes. There should be evidence of the client's and family members' involvement in the discharge planning process. There should be no surprises by the time the client is discharged. The client should have the necessary information and resources to return home. The box below includes tips on completing discharge summary forms.

Tips on Writing Discharge Summary Forms

INFORMATION FOR HOME HEALTH CARE NURSES

- Describe nursing interventions (for example, dressing changes, step-by-step wound care).
- Describe information presented to client.
- Describe client's ability to perform health care skills (for example, administering medications, use of crutches).
- Explain family members' involvement in care.
- Describe resources needed in the home (for example, Meals On Wheels, self-help devices).

INFORMATION FOR CLIENTS

- Use clear, concise descriptions in client's own language.
- Explain step-by-step description of how to perform a procedure (for example, home drug administration). Reinforce explanation with printed instructions.
- Identify precautions to follow when performing self-care or administering medications.
- Review signs and symptoms of complications that should be reported to physician.
- List names and phone numbers of health care providers the client can contact.

BARNES HOSPITAL
Nursing Assessment Flowsheet

Date 10/14/88   C-10b

Instructions: Circle if Present.
Write in Assessment.
Indicate N/A if not applicable or not assessed.

Code: S - Self, A - Assist, T - Total
I - Instructed, C - Collected

Addressograph

		NIGHT	DAY
NEURO/CEREBRAL	NEURO/CEREBRAL	(Alert) Confused Memory Loss Agitated Oriented x 3 ASKS QUESTIONS ABOUT ULCER CARE	(Alert) Confused Memory Loss Agitated Oriented x 3 NOTES BURNING @ ULCER SITE DURING DRESSING CHANGE
COMFORT/SLEEP	Discomfort Intervention	N/A	
	Sleep Status	Awake (Slept at intervals) Slept	(Awake) Slept at intervals Slept
ACTIVITY/EXERCISE	MOBILITY Limitations/ Devices	(Independent) Assist Dependent	(Independent) Assist Dependent
	ACTIVITY	UP TO BATHROOM x2	UP TO CHAIR IN ROOM x3
SKIN/MUCOSA	Appearance	Warm (Dry) Turgor _____ SKIN INTACT AROUND BONY PROMINENCES	Warm Dry Turgor REDUCED SKIN DRY, INTACT EXCEPT FOR ULCER
	Mattress/ Equipment	Foam Air (Heel Protectors) Aqua K pad Teds	LOTION APPLIED TO BONY PROMINENCES Foam Air (Heel Protectors) Aqua K pad Teds
WOUND	LOCATION Appearance	(L) FOOT ULCER 3CM DIAMETER, DRAINING YELLOW DISCHARGE	(L) FOOT ULCER CONTINUES TO DRAIN YELLOW DISCHARGE, 3CM ULCER INFLAMED ALONG MARGINS
	Dressing Change	X1 WET-TO-DRY SALINE, FINE MESH GAUZE	X2 WET-TO-DRY SALINE AND FINE MESH GAUZE
NUTRI-TION	MEALS Tube Feeding Infusion Device	Continuous Bolus Flush X _____	% Eaten B: 90% (S) A T L: 80% (S) A T Continuous Bolus Flush X _____
ELIMINATION	URINE	(Continent) x2 Incontinent Foley CLEAR, YELLOW URINE	(Continent) x4 Incontinent Foley CLEAR, YELLOW URINE
	BOWEL Bowel Sounds	Continent Incontinent Guaiac _____ Freq X: _____ N/A Absent Present _____ Abdomen _____	(Continent) Incontinent Guaiac _____ Freq X: 1 SOFT FORMED STOOL Absent (Present) ALL QUADRANTS Abdomen SOFT, NON-TENDER
RESPIRATORY	Auscultation	N/A	CLEAR TO AUSCULTATION IN ALL LOBES
		O₂ Cough/Secretion _____	O₂ Cough/Secretion _____
CIRC	CIRCULATION	FEET COOL, DORSALIS PEDIS PULSES WEAK BILATERALLY	PEDAL PULSES WEAK BILATERALLY
OTHER	Specimen	I C Test _____ GLUCOMETER READING AT 10:00 PM - 110	I C Test _____ GLUCOMETER READING AT 8:30 AM - 165 GLUCOMETER READING AT 12:30 PM - 180
	Signature/Status	S. Tucker, RN	Signature/Status
		HYGIENE: (S) A T SAFETY Bath Tub Shower ID Band on ✓ Shave Hair Nails Siderails in Use ✓ (Oral) X1	HYGIENE: (S) A T SAFETY (Bath) Tub Shower ID Band on ✓ Shave (Hair) Nails Siderails in Use ✓ (Oral) x2

Fig. 14-7 Nursing assessment flowsheet.
Courtesy Barnes Hospital, St. Louis.

Nursing Assessment Flowsheet

Date *10/14/88*   C-10b

Instructions: Circle if Present.
           Write in Assessment.
           Indicate N/A if not applicable or not assessed.
Code: S - Self, A - Assist, T - Total
       I - Instructed, C - Collected

EVENING

(Alert)   Confused   Memory Loss   Agitated
Oriented x *3*

BURNING AT ULCER SITE MORE
INTENSE; PRN ANALGESIC AT 7:00 PM
RELIEVED DISCOMFORT

Awake   (Slept at intervals)   Slept

(Independent)   Assist   Dependent

UP TO CHAIR x 2

(Warm)   (Dry)   Turgor

TURNS SELF WELL

Foam   Air   (Heel Protectors)   Aqua K pad   Teds

MINIMAL DRAINAGE NOTED AT ULCER
SITE. WOUND APPEARS CLEAN. SLIGHT
INFLAMMATION ALONG MARGINS
X 1 WET-TO-DRY SALINE, FINE MESH GAUZE

% Eaten D: *90%*   (S) A   T
Continuous   Bolus   Flush X

(Continent) *x 2* Incontinent   Foley
CLEAR, YELLOW URINE

Continent   Incontinent   Guaiac
Freq X: *N/A*
Absent   (Present)   *ALL QUADRANTS*
Abdomen   *SOFT, NON-TENDER*

N/A

O₂
Cough/Secretion

PEDAL PULSES WEAK BILATERALLY

I   C   Test
GLUCOMETER READING AT 5 PM
155

Signature/Status

HYGIENE: (S) A T	SAFETY
Bath Tub Shower	ID Band on ✓
Shave (Hair) Nails	Siderails in Use ✓
(Oral)	

At the time of discharge, the nurse and other health team members summarize the client's condition and review the plan of care for the home. The client's status should be described in relation to planned outcomes or discharge criteria. Discharge summary forms (Fig. 14-9) make the summary concise and instructive. Many forms include a copy that is given to a client, family member, or home health nurse. This transfer of information ensures better continuity of care in the home setting. A summary form reemphasizes what the client or family has already learned. The form may be attached to pamphlets or teaching brochures. In many institutions the social worker also contributes to the discharge summary.

COMPUTERIZED DOCUMENTATION

Computers have been widely used in hospitals and other health care facilities for over a decade. Automated technology improves the integration of informational resources and the accessibility of the information to all health care personnel. The results of a client's laboratory and diagnostic tests can be stored within the computer and displayed on the computer terminal screen with a mere push of a key.

Most hospital information systems have in the past concentrated on ordering programs and communication systems. Nurses have been the primary users of those systems. Supplies, equipment, stock medications, and diagnostic testing are examples of services nurses may order through a computer. Computerized communication systems assist in relaying information about clients quickly and accurately. For example, patient classification data, quality assurance monitoring scores, and diagnostic test results can be organized within the computer for all clients and made accessible when a client's name or identification number is entered.

In the past, most hospital computers had a department-centered focus for computer functions. Even though information could be retrieved by entering a name, most data were organized in separate programs for each service department. For example, for nurses to order equipment, it would be necessary to enter the client's name and department from which the equipment was to be ordered. Today, more information systems are client centered. All of a computer's functions are organized from a client's perspective rather than that of a particular department. Programs that enter and review client identification information to develop assessment histories, care plans, discharge planning profiles, and even vital sign results are available. Client-centered com-

Medical Diagnosis and other pertinent medical information:

10/13/-- DIABETIC, (L) METATARSAL FOOT ULCER

Condition *SATISFACTORY*

Allergies (Drugs, food, other) *PENICILLIN*

Adm. Date 10/13/--	Age 71	Religion *CATHOLIC*	Mode of Travel *WHEELCHAIR*
Service *MEDICINE*	Doctor *WEST*	Resident *TOWNS*	Intern	Stamp Addressograph Plate Here

FREQUENTLY ORDERED ITEMS		Date	Specimens/Daily Lab	Date	Treatments
Temp.		10/13	*ACCUCHEK 07-11-17*	10/14	DRESSING CHANGE (L) METATARSAL
Pulse & Resp.	*VS q 8 HR WHILE AWAKE*				ULCER q 12 HR. CLEAN WITH
BP					NORMAL SALINE AND STERILE
					GAUZE. APPLY COLLAGENASE
I & O					ENZYME LIGHTLY TO ULCER.
Weights					COVER WITH ONE LAYER OF
Spot Checks					MOISTENED SALINE GAUZE,
Chest P.T.					OUTER LAYER OF GAUZE 4 x 4.
Incentive Spirometer					
P.T.					

ACTIVITIES		NUTRITION	Date	Diagnostic Procedures	
Ad lib		Diet			
Ambulate		*1800 CAL. ADA*			
(Chair) (L) FOOT					
BRP *ELEVATED*					
Bedrest					
Bath		Feedings *HS SNACK*			
Self					
Tub		Assist c̄ meals			
Shower		FLUID BALANCE			
Bed *ALPHA*		Force			
(Assist) *KERI*		D E N			
BATH OIL		Restrict			
		D E N			
Orderlies Needed					
Family: *DAUGHTER: SARAH WILSON*					
PHONE: 882: 6010					

NURSING CARE PLAN			
Date	Nursing Diagnosis	Expected Outcomes	Nursing Plan/Orders

Discharge Planning: Destination:	Transportation:	Probable Date:	Referral Agencies:	Appointment:
			Supplies:	

Patient Name

Fig. 14-8 Nursing Kardex.
Courtesy Barnes Hospital, St. Louis.

Barnes Hospital

PATIENT DISCHARGE SUMMARY

C-16

Date __10/17/86__ Time __1030__

MEANS: ☐ Ambulatory ☒ Wheelchair ☐ Stretcher

METHODS: ☒ M.D. order ☐ AMA with release ☐ AMA without release   Addressograph Plate

Afebrile 24 hours? ☒ Yes ☐ No TPR 36^8–72–16 _____ B/P ___124/72_____

☐ Physician notified of irregularities

DISCHARGED TO: ☐ Home ☐ Nursing Home ☒ Home with Home Health Care ☐ Other

    If discharged to Nursing Home or other facility/service:

    Name _____ Address/Phone _____

☐ Release of Information form signed ☐ Chart copied ☐ Transfer form completed ☐ Transportation Arranged

DISCHARGE CONSIDERATIONS:

☐ Valuables from cashier ☐ PTA meds returned ☐ Scripts given
☒ NA ☒ NA ☒ NA

DISCHARGE INSTRUCTIONS

FOR PROBLEMS OR FOLLOW-UP:

    Physician __Dr. Stan Jones_____ Phone __362-5000____ Appt. __10/24/86____

    Other: _____

    _____

Activity: __To remain in bed with Ⓛ foot elevated on two pillows. May be up only to go to the bathroom.__

Diet: __To follow 1800 calorie ADA diet as instructed by the dietitian. For questions about diet, call the dietitian (Sue Marlin) 362-3184.__

Medications: __To take usual dosage of 30 units NPH insulin and 8 units of regular insulin every morning before breakfast.__

Wound Care: __Change dressings to Ⓛ foot daily using moistened fine mesh gauze with dry 4x4 gauze and wrap dressings with 4 kling gauze.__

Teaching Materials Given: __Copy of "Controlling Your Diabetes" and "Diabetic Menu Planning."__

Special Instructions: __Call doctor for increased pain, redness, swelling or drainage from Ⓛ foot wound. Barnes Home Health nurses will be visiting daily to change dressing to Ⓛ foot.__

My discharge instructions have been explained and a copy has been given to me.

Patient/Significant Other __*John Owens*_____ Relation __HUSBAND_____

Nurse __*B. Rand, RN*_____

Fig. 14-9 Discharge summary form.
Courtesy Barnes Hospital, St. Louis.

Steps Used to Select a Computerized Care Plan

Step 1: Nurse Identifies Desired Nursing Diagnosis or Problem Category

- Computer displays a list of all available standard care plans.

Step 2: Nurse Initiates Development of Desired Care Plan

- Computer displays all nursing diagnoses.

Step 3: Nurse Selects Nursing Diagnosis

- Computer displays all desired outcomes.

Step 4: Nurse Selects Specific Desired Outcomes

- Computer displays all available interventions.

Step 5: Nurse Selects Interventions, Including Frequencies

- Computer displays complete individualized care plan.

Step 6: Nurse Reviews Plan and Enters It into Computer System

- Plan can later be displayed on computer screen or printed in a report format.

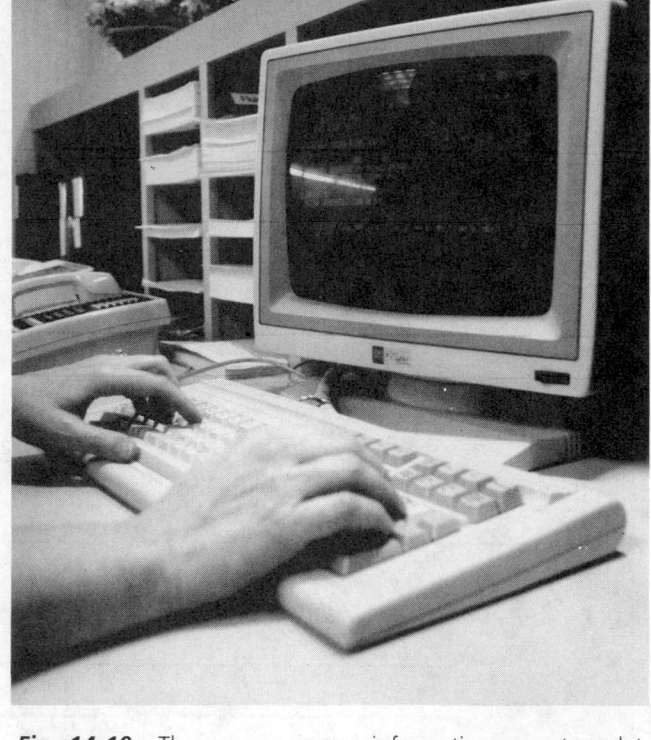

Fig. 14-10 The nurse accesses information or enters data into the computer by using a keyboard.

puter programs also enable nurses to schedule tests and enter information for client billing.

There are many advantages of a well-integrated client-centered information system. Both nurse and physician plans are integrated to make the plan of care more comprehensive. A client's computerized record can be designed so information can be saved as part of a total history or as part of a specific hospital admission. Thus certain information, such as past illnesses or allergies, will appear in a client's record during all subsequent admissions. The data never have to be entered into the computer again.

Automated client care plans can be very useful to nursing staff. The nurse can go to a computer and develop a client-centered plan of care. This is more efficient than selecting plans from a volume of preprinted standardized forms used in a manual system. The box shows steps used to select a care plan within a computer system designed by the Milwaukee County Medical Complex (Albrecht and Lieske, 1985). Although the computerized

plan is organized on the basis of standardized nursing diagnoses, desired outcomes, and nursing interventions, the nurse still uses judgment in selecting an individualized plan for the client. The nurse can modify aspects of the plan at any time. Maintenance of a computerized care plan data base makes quality assurance monitoring easy. Selection of nursing diagnoses can be monitored to determine if standards of care are followed.

Nurses should be familiar with basic computer skills because most hospitals now have some form of automated system. Hospitals have large mainframe computer systems or individualized personal computers. A mainframe system consists of one centrally located computer with a huge memory capacity to power a variety of programs throughout the hospital. Each nursing division or hospital department has a computer screen or cathode-ray tube (CRT) with a keyboard attached to the main computer. Information may be entered or retrieved by using the keyboard (Fig. 14-10) or by pressing a light-sensitive pen directly onto the CRT screen. Most computer programs give the user information that helps to make the proper keyboard or light-pen selections on the screen. More progressive hospitals have small CRTs at each client's bedside. Nurses can enter assessment findings or document interventions that are quickly transmitted for storage. Documentation is timely, and fewer errors occur because the nurse does not have to leave the bedside to record information.

The quality of client care is enhanced when nurses can spend less time on clerical duties. Well-designed computer systems reduce recording errors, save time, and make information readily available to the nurse. Nurses then can focus more directly on the delivery of professional nursing care.

SUMMARY

Recording and reporting are methods of communicating information related to a client's health care management. In any setting the success of a plan of care depends on accurate and complete reporting and precise record documentation. Good reporting and recording create a high level of communication that helps health team members share a common view of the client's problems. Nurses are the primary care providers having the most contact with clients. The use of basic principles for accurate and comprehensive recording and reporting will ensure the delivery of safe and effective nursing care.

KEY CONCEPTS

✓ A client's health care record is a written documentation of the care he receives.

✓ Accurate record keeping requires an objective interpretation of data with precise measurements, correct spelling, and proper use of abbreviations.

✓ A nurse's signature on an entry in a record designates accountability for the contents of that entry.

✓ A concise record or report eliminates nonessential information that can be misleading or confusing.

✓ Any change in a client's condition warrants immediate recording and reporting.

✓ An organized record presents information logically in order of the occurrence of events.

✓ All information pertaining to a client's health care management gathered by examination, observation, conversation, or treatment is confidential.

✓ The major purpose of the nurses' change-of-shift report is to maintain continuity of care.

✓ Any oral report is delivered in a professional manner emphasizing objectivity and a non-judgmental viewpoint.

✓ When information pertinent to care is communicated by telephone, the information must be verified.

✓ Incident reports objectively describe any event not consistent with the routine care of a client.

✓ The client's record serves as a resource to explain and confirm observations or refute interpretations of data.

✓ Because the client's record may become a legal document, only factual information is recorded.

✓ Errors made while recording should never be erased or made illegible.

✓ The regular auditing of documented client care reveals if standards of care are met.

✓ Problem-oriented medical records are organized by the client's health care problems.

✓ Flow sheets eliminate the need to write narrative notes for repeated observations or measurements.

✓ Standardized care plans are preprinted forms the nurse can use to format an individualized plan of care.

✓ Computerized information systems provide information about clients in an organized and easily accessible fashion.

REFERENCES

Albrecht, CA, and Lieske, AM: Automating patient care planning, Nurs Manage 16:21, 1985.

Blake, P: Incident investigation: a complete guide, Nurs Manage 15:37, 1984.

Budziszewski, W: Reports: vital links of communication, Hosp Progr 41:60, 1960.

Gawlinski, A, and Rasmussen, S: Improving documentation through the use of change theory, Focus Crit Care 11:12, 1984.

Hoke, JL: Charting for dollars, Am J Nurs 85:658, 1985.

Riegel, B: A method of giving intershift report based on a conceptual model, Focus Crit Care 12:12, 1985.

Siegrist, LM, et al.: The PIE system: complete planning and documentation of nursing care, QRB 11:186, 1985.

ADDITIONAL READINGS

Atwood, J, et al.: The POR: a system for communication, Nurs Clin North Am 9:229, 1974.

Bergerson, SR: Charting with a jury in mind, Nursing Life 2:30, 1982.

Costello, S, and Summers, BY: Documenting patient care: getting it all together, Nurs Manage 16:31, 1985.

Crews, C, et al.: Computerized central intake: streamlining community health-care admissions, Nurs Econ 4(1):31, 1986.

Dobberstein K: Attaching fuzzy documentation, Am J Nurs 6:599, 1986.

Donaghue, AM, Reiley, PJ: Some do's and dont's for giving report: Sometimes knowing what not to say is as important as knowing what to say, Nurs 81 11:171, 1981.

Gamberg, D, et al.: Outcome charting, Nurs Manage 12:36, 1981.

Georgopoulos, BS, and Sana, JM: Clinical nursing specialization and intershift report behavior, Am J Nurs 71:538, 1971.

Harkins, B: Keep your eye on the patient's problems, RN, 49(12):30, 1986.

Hinson, S, et al.: An automated Kardex and care plan, Nurs Manage 15:35, 1984.

Joint Commission on Accreditation of Healthcare Organizations: Accreditation manual for hospitals, Chicago, 1988, JCAHO.

Kitto, J, and Dale, B: Designing a brief discharge planning screen, Nurs Manage 16:28, 1985.

Napiewocki, JK: Documentation: a nurse's best defense, Prof Nurs 1:321, 1985.

Sanborn, CW, and Blount, M: Standard plans for care and discharge, Am J Nurs 84:1394, 1984.

Vaughan-Wrobel, BD, and Henderson, BS: The problem-oriented system in nursing, ed. 3, St. Louis, 1986, The C.V. Mosby Co.

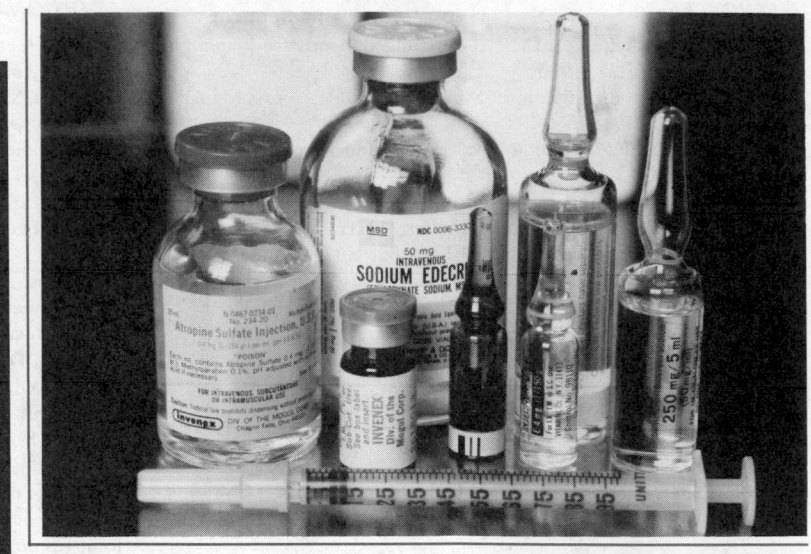

OBJECTIVES

Mastery of content in this chapter will enable the student to:

- Define the key terms listed.
- Discuss the nurse's legal responsibilities in drug prescription and administration.
- Describe the physiological mechanisms of drug action, including absorption, distribution, metabolism, and excretion of medications.
- Differentiate between toxic, idiosyncratic, allergic, and side effects of drugs.
- Discuss developmental factors that influence drug pharmacokinetics.
- Discuss factors that influence drug actions.
- Discuss methods to improve compliance with drug regimens.
- Describe the roles of the pharmacist, physician, and nurse in drug administration.
- Describe factors to consider in choosing routes of drug administration.
- Correctly calculate a prescribed drug dosage.
- Discuss factors to include in assessing needs for and response to drug therapy.
- List the "five rights" of drug administration.
- Correctly prepare and administer subcutaneous, intramuscular, and intradermal injections; insulin injections; oral medications; topical skin preparations; eye, ear, and nose drops; vaginal instillations; rectal suppositories; and inhalants.
- Discuss the purposes of irrigations.

KEY TERMS

Ampule	Intramuscular Injection
Buccal	Intrathecal
Drug Allergy	Intravenous Injection
Drug Dependence	Irrigation
Formulary	Nurse Practice Act
Half-Life	Ophthalmic
Induration	Over-The-Counter Drug
Infusion	Parenteral
Injection	Phlebitis
Instillation	Potentiation
Intraarterial	Prescription
Intraarticular	Subcutaneous Injection
Intracardiac	Synergistic Agent
Intradermal Injection	Topical

Administration of Medications

The safe and accurate administration of medications is one of the nurse's most important responsibilities. Drugs are a primary means of therapy for clients with health alterations, but any drug has the potential for causing harmful effects when administered improperly. The nurse must understand a drug's effects, administer it correctly, monitor the client's response, and help the client self-administer drugs correctly.

In addition to knowing about a specific drug's action, the nurse must also understand the client's previous and current health problems to determine whether a particular medication should be given. The nurse's judgment is critical for proper drug administration.

DRUG NAMES AND FORMS

Medications have always been used in the care of persons suffering illness or disability. A drug or medication is a substance used in the diagnosis, treatment, cure, relief, or prevention of disease. Health care personnel use the term *drugs* and *medications* interchangeably. Lay persons commonly refer to medications as *medicines*.

Physicians and dentists prescribe the majority of medications in the United States and Canada. However, in some states within the United States, nurse practitioners may prescribe medications under a physician's license.

Names

A single drug may have as many as four different names. The *chemical name*, most familiar to the chemist, provides an exact description of the drug's composition. Acetylsalicylic acid, known commonly as aspirin, is a chemical name.

The *generic name* is given by the manufacturer who first develops the drug. Protected by law, the generic name is given before a drug receives official approval. Aspirin and tetracycline hydrochloride (HCl) are examples of generic names.

Federal legislation in 1962 mandated that there be one *official name* for each drug, the name under which the drug is listed in official publications such as the *United States Pharmacopeia* (USP). A drug's generic name often becomes its official name, as with aspirin.

The *trade name, brand name,* or *proprietary name* is the name under which a manufacturer markets a drug. A generic drug may have many different trade names. For example, tetracycline HCl is known by the trade names Achromycin, Panmycin, and Tetracyn V. The trade name has the symbol ® at the upper right of the name, indicating the drug has been registered. So lay persons will recognize trade names readily, manufacturers choose names that are easy to pronounce, spell, and remember. Since many companies may produce the same drug, similarities in trade names can be confusing. Most hospital and clinic pharmacies attempt to dispense medications with the same trade names consistently so nurses can become familiar with them.

Classification

Nurses categorize medications with similar characteristics by their *class*. Drug classification indicates the effect on a body system, the symptoms relieved, or the desired effect. Each class contains drugs prescribed for similar types of health problems. The physical and chemical composition of drugs within a class is not necessarily the same. A drug may also belong to more than one class. For example, aspirin is an analgesic, an antipyretic, and an antiinflammatory drug.

TABLE 15-1 Forms of Medication

Form	Description
Capsule	Solid dosage form for oral use; medication in a powder, liquid, or oil form and encased by a gelatin shell; capsule colored to aid in product identification
Elixir	Clear fluid containing water and alcohol; designed for oral use; usually has a sweetener added
Extract	Concentrated drug form made by removing the active portion of a drug from its other components; for example, a fluid extract is a drug made into a solution from a vegetable source
Glycerite	Solution of drug combined with glycerin for external use; contains at least 50% glycerin
Liniment	Preparation usually containing alcohol, oil, or soapy emollient applied to the skin
Lotion	Drug in liquid suspension applied externally to protect the skin
Ointment (salve)	Semisolid, externally applied preparation, usually containing one or more drugs
Paste	Semisolid preparation, thicker and stiffer than an ointment; absorbed through the skin more slowly than an ointment
Pill	Solid dosage form containing one or more drugs, shaped into globules, ovoids, or oblong shapes; true pills rarely used, since they have been replaced by tablets
Solution	Liquid preparation that may be used orally, parenterally, or externally; can also be instilled into a body organ or cavity (for example, bladder irrigations), contains water with one or more dissolved compounds; must be sterile if for parenteral use
Suppository	Solid dosage form mixed with gelatin and shaped in the form of a pellet for insertion into a body cavity (rectum or vagina); melts when it reaches body temperature, releasing the drug for absorption.
Suspension	Finely divided drug particles dispersed in a liquid medium; when suspension left standing, particles settle to the bottom of the container; commonly an oral medication and is not to be given intravenously
Syrup	Medication dissolved in a concentrated sugar solution; may contain flavoring to make drug more palatable
Tablet	Powdered dosage form compressed into hard disks or cylinders; in addition to primary drug, contains binders (adhesive to allow powder to stick together), disintegrators (to promote tablet dissolution), lubricants (for ease of manufacturing), and fillers (for convenient tablet size)
Enteric-coated	Tablet for oral use coated with materials that do not dissolve in the stomach; coatings dissolve in the intestine where medication is absorbed
Tincture	Alcohol or water-alcohol drug solution
Troche (lozenge)	Flat, round dosage form containing drug, flavoring, sugar, and mucilage; dissolves in mouth to release drug

Nurses should know the general characteristics of medications in each class. Each class has nursing implications for proper administration and monitoring. For example, nursing implications related to diuretic administration include monitoring intake and output, weighing the client daily, assessing the development of edema in body tissues, and monitoring serum electrolyte levels. Nursing implications for all drugs within a class provide guidelines for safe and effective care.

Drug Forms

Drugs are available in a variety of forms or preparations. The form of the drug determines its route of administration. For example, a capsule is taken orally, and a solution may be given intravenously. The composition of a drug is designed to enhance its absorption and metabolism within the body. Many drugs are available in several forms such as tablets, capsules, pediatric elixirs, and suppositories. When administering a medication, the nurse must be certain to give the medication in the proper form (Table 15-1).

DRUG STANDARDS

In 1906, as a result of the Pure Food and Drug Act, the U.S. government set standards for drug quality and purity. Official publications—the *United States Pharmacopeia* (USP) and the *National Formulary*—set standards for drug strength, quality, purity, packaging, safety, labeling, and dosage form. In Canada the *British Pharmacopoeia* (BP) sets similar standards. Physicians, nurses, and pharmacists depend on these standards to ensure that clients receive pure drugs in safe and effective dosages. Accepted standards must be met in five areas:

1. Purity—Manufacturers must meet purity standards for the type and concentration of extraneous substances allowed in drug products.
2. Potency—The concentration of active drug in the preparation affects strength or potency.
3. Bioavailability—The ability of a drug to be released from its dosage form and dissolved, absorbed, and transported by the body to its site of action is its bioavailability.
4. Efficacy—Detailed laboratory studies can help determine a drug's effectiveness.
5. Safety—All drugs should be continually evaluated to determine their side effects.

LEGISLATION AND CONTROL

When clients receive medications, they assume that the drugs will produce the desired effect and will not cause harm and that nurses will administer them correctly. State or provincial (in Canada) and federal legislation governs the production, distribution, prescription, and administration of drugs.

In the United States, drug legislation began with the Pure Food and Drug Act of 1906, which focused attention on the purity of food but also set official standards for drugs. Manufacturers were required to label drugs accurately and to ensure that the strength and purity of drugs conformed to their claims. Since that time, federal law has extended and refined governmental controls on drug sales and distribution; drug testing, naming and labeling; and the regulation of controlled substances (Tables 15-2 and 15-3).

State drug laws must conform with federal legislation. States can also impose additional controls, including control of substances not regulated by the federal government. For example, states vary with regard to the legal sale and use of alcoholic beverages. States also set regulations for punishment of persons found driving while intoxicated or for illicit use of controlled drugs. Local governmental bodies also regulate use of alcohol and tobacco.

Health care institutions establish policies that conform to federal, state, and local regulations. The size of an institution, the types of services it provides, and the types of professional personnel it employs influence policies for drug control, distribution, and administration. Institutional policies are often more restrictive than governmental controls. An institution is primarily concerned with preventing health problems resulting from drug use. For example, a common institutional policy is the automatic discontinuation of antibiotic therapy after a set number of days. Although a physician may reorder an antibiotic, this policy helps to control unnecessarily prolonged drug therapy, which may lead to sensitivity or toxic reactions.

Federal, state, and local legislation governs nursing practice, including the administration of medications. State nurse-practice acts define and set limits on the scope of a nurse's professional functions and responsibilities. These acts are joint policy statements made by nursing, medical, and hospital associations in a state. Institutions and agencies may interpret specific actions allowed under the acts but cannot modify, expand, or restrict the act's intent. The nurse-practice acts protect the public from unskilled, undereducated, and unlicensed nurses.

Nurses must know the regulations affecting drug use in their practice area. When moving from one state to another, a nurse may discover significant differences in the laws governing drug use. For example, laws vary concerning who may prescribe medications and administer drugs intravenously. In the past, only physicians prescribed medications, although it was not unusual for

TABLE 15-2 Federal Drug Laws in the United States

Date	Title of Law	Provisions
1906	Pure Food and Drug Act	Designated official standards for drugs *(United States Pharmacopeia* and the *National Formulary)*; specified standards for drug labeling
1912	Sherley Amendment	Prohibited manufacturers from making fraudulent claims about drug efficacy and therapeutic effects
1914	Harrison Narcotic Act	Legally classified drugs believed to be habit forming as narcotics; regulated importation, manufacture, sale, and use of narcotic substances
1938	Federal Food, Drug, and Cosmetic Act	Added the *Homeopathic Pharmacopeia of the United States* as a third drug standard; required that a drug preparation be approved as safe by the Food and Drug Administration (FDA) before marketing; further outlined criteria for drug labeling
1945	Amendment to the Food and Drug Act	Provided for certification of biological products used as drugs (for example, insulin or antibiotics) on a batch basis; allowed for direct supervision and inspection of drug production
1952	Durham-Humphrey Amendment	Distinguished between prescription ("legend") and nonprescription drugs
1962	Kefauver-Harris Amendment	Authorized the FDA to supervise drug production to ensure safety and efficacy and to establish official drug names; specified greater controls on investigational drugs
1970	Comprehensive Drug Abuse Prevention and Control Act (Controlled Substances Act)	Set strict controls on manufacture and distribution of controlled drugs (possession of controlled substances unlawful without a prescription); established government programs to promote prevention and treatment of drug dependence

TABLE 15-3 Canadian Drug Legislation

Date	Title of Law	Provisions
1908	Proprietary or Patent Medicine Act	Set standards to protect consumers from unsafe and ineffective nonprescription drugs
1953	Canadian Food and Drug Act	Prohibited sale of contaminated, unsafe drugs and of improperly labeled drugs; designated official standards *(Pharmacopoeia Internationalis,* The *British Pharmacopoeia,* The *Canadian Formulary)*; defined certain controlled drugs; prohibited advertising of prescription and controlled drugs to the general public; set standards for labeling
1961	Canadian Narcotic Control Act	Restricted sale, possession, and use of narcotics; set guidelines for reporting loss or theft of narcotics; set standards for labeling and record keeping.

a nurse to request that a client receive a medication. However, several states have recognized the expanding role of the nurse and have revised nurse-practice acts to include prescribing of medications. In most cases, this privilege is limited to licensed nurse practitioners.

Administering medications directly into a vein is a responsibility many nurses now assume. Because the intravenous injection of medications may cause serious adverse effects, previously only physicians were allowed to give such injections. Nurses who perform this function must be qualified through proper training, education, and experience.

The nurse is responsible for following legal provisions in administering controlled substances, which can be dispensed only with a prescription. Violations of the Controlled Substances Act are punishable by fines, imprisonment, and loss of nurse licensure. Hospitals and other health care institutions have policies for the proper storage and distribution of controlled substances (see box).

Nontherapeutic Drug Use

Despite legislative controls, some people use drugs for purposes other than their proper purpose. The indiscriminate use of drugs poses serious health problems for the user, family, and community. In the past, the misuse or abuse of medications was related to use for thera-

Guidelines for Safe Narcotic Administration and Control

- Store all narcotics in a locked secure cabinet or container.
- Nurse(s) in charge carry a set of keys for the narcotics cabinet.
- During an institution's change-of-shift the nurse going off duty counts all narcotics with the nurse coming on duty. Both nurses sign the narcotic record to indicate the count is correct.
- Discrepancies in narcotic counts are reported immediately.
- A special inventory record is used each time a narcotic is dispensed.
- The record is used to document the client's name, the date, time of drug administration, name of drug, dosage, and signature of nurse dispensing the drug.
- The form provides an accurate ongoing count of narcotics used and remaining.
- If only one part of a premeasured dose of a controlled substance is given, a second nurse witnesses disposal of the unused portion and documents such on the record form.

peutic qualities, such as the relief of pain or reduction in anxiety. Today, factors such as peer pressure, curiosity, and the pursuit of pleasure are motivators for drug use. Problems with drug use are not limited to heroin, cocaine, and other "hard" drugs. Millions of people in the United States and Canada consume alcohol daily. It takes only a few minutes of watching television, with its frequent advertisements for pain relievers, decongestants, and antacids, to realize that our society is drug conscious. Table 15-4 lists common terms associated with nontherapeutic use of drugs.

The nurse has an ethical and legal responsibility to understand the problems of persons using drugs improperly. When caring for clients with suspected drug problems, nurses must be aware of their own values and attitudes about those willfully using potentially harmful substances. The nurse cannot develop a therapeutic relationship with clients if personal values interfere with acceptance or understanding of their needs. Knowing the physical, psychological, and social changes resulting from drug abuse allows the nurse to identify clients with drug problems.

A problem involving the misuse of drugs by health professionals also exists. Stress in the work place, personal problems, or the strong desire to perform well are some of the factors that may cause nurses to rely on

TABLE 15-4 Terms Associated with the Nontherapeutic Use of Drugs

Definition	Example
ABUSE	
Use of a chemical substance for nontherapeutic purposes that do not comply with cultural or social standards	A worker ingests alcohol while on the job.
ADDICTION	
Inability to control a drive or craving for a chemical substance	Activities of daily living (for example, socializing with friends, or caring for children) are interrupted by the use of drugs
DRUG DEPENDENCE	
Reliance on the continual use of a substance	A person uses a chemical substance continually throughout the day, often to deal with stressors or problems
PHYSICAL DEPENDENCE	
State characterized by physiological changes that result from frequent use of a chemical substance; failure to take the drug on which one depends leads to withdrawal symptoms	A person experiences lethargy, reduced mental capacity, and inability to make judgments.
PSYCHOLOGICAL DEPENDENCE	
State characterized by an emotional reliance on a drug to attain a sense of well-being	A person may have a mild desire or intense craving for the drug. Feelings of guilt or shame are resolved by taking more drugs.
TOLERANCE	
State developing with the continual ingestion of a chemical substance in which it eventually becomes necessary to increase the dose to produce the same effects achieved from previous doses	Persons taking opiates (for example, morphine or codeine) must continually increase the dosage to feel euphoria and freedom from discomfort

drugs. Nurses must recognize and understand the problems of colleagues who suffer from drug abuse. Chapter 45 describes the nature of health problems related to chemical dependence.

NATURE OF DRUG ACTIONS

Medications act to produce therapeutically useful effects. A drug does not create a function in a tissue or organ but rather *alters* physiological functions. Drugs may protect cells from the influence of other chemical agents, promote cell function, or accelerate or slow cell processes.

Mechanisms of Action

Drugs produce actions by altering body fluids, altering cell membranes, or interacting with receptor sites. The drug aluminum hydroxide gel exerts its effect by altering the chemical properties of a body fluid. Specifically, the stomach's acid contents become neutralized. Drugs, such as general anesthetic gases, interact with cell membranes. After properties of the cells become altered, the drug exerts its effects. The most common mechanism of drug action is binding to a cell's receptor sites. Sites on the receptors interact with drugs because of similar chemical shapes. The drug and receptor bind together much like a lock-and-key fit. When receptors and drugs lock together, the therapeutic effects are realized. Receptors localize drug effects. Each tissue or cell in the body possesses a unique group of receptors. For example, receptors in the myocardial cells respond to digitalis preparations.

Pharmacokinetics

Pharmacokinetics is the study of how drugs enter the body, reach their site of action, are metabolized, and exit from the body. The nurse uses knowledge of pharmacokinetics in timing drug administration, selecting the route of administration, judging the risk for alterations in drug action, and observing client response.

ABSORPTION

Absorption is the passage of drug molecules into the blood. Most drugs, except those applied topically for local effects, must enter the systemic circulation to exert therapeutic effect. Factors influencing absorption include route of administration, ability of the drug to dissolve, and conditions at the site of absorption.

Each route has a different influence on drug absorption, depending on the physical structure of the tissues. The skin is relatively impermeable to chemicals, making absorption slow. The mucous membranes and respiratory airways allow for quick drug absorption because of the high vascularity of mucosal and alveolar-capillary surfaces. Because orally administered drugs must pass through the gastrointestinal tract to be absorbed, the overall rate of absorption may be slow. Intravenous (IV) injection produces more rapid absorption than topical or oral administration, because the IV route provides immediate access to the systemic circulation.

The ability of an oral medication to dissolve after ingestion depends largely on its form or preparation. Solutions and suspensions already in a liquid state are absorbed more readily than tablets or capsules. Solid dosage forms must first disintegrate to expose the chemical to gastric and intestinal secretions. Acidic drugs pass through the gastric mucosa rapidly. Drugs that are basic are not absorbed before reaching the small intestine.

Conditions at the site of absorption influence the ease with which medications enter the systemic circulation. When skin is abraded, topical drugs are absorbed easily. Topical substances normally prescribed for local effect can cause serious reactions when absorbed through the skin's layers. The formation of edema in mucous membranes slows drug absorption because medications take longer to diffuse to blood vessels. The absorption of parenterally administered medications depends on the blood supply of the tissues. Because muscles have a richer blood supply than subcutaneous tissues, a drug given intramuscularly is absorbed more quickly than one injected subcutaneously. In some instances a delayed subcutaneous absorption is preferable to produce long-lasting drug effects. If a client's tissue perfusion is poor, as in the case of circulatory shock, the intravenous route is best. Intravenous administration provides the most rapid and dependable action.

Oral medications are absorbed more easily when administered between meals. When the stomach is filled with food, the contents are emptied slowly into the duodenum, thus slowing drug absorption. Certain foods and antacids cause drugs to bind into complexes that cannot pass through the gastrointestinal tract lining. For example, milk interferes with the absorption of iron and tetracycline. Some drugs are destroyed by the increased acidity of gastric contents and protein digestion during a meal. Enteric coatings on certain tablets resist dissolution in gastric juices and prevent certain medications from being digested in the upper gastrointestinal tract. The coating also protects the stomach lining from irritation by the medication.

The nurse often has little choice about the route of administration. However, knowledge of factors that alter or impair drug absorption helps the nurse administer drugs correctly. Neither food nor antacid drugs should be given within 2 hours before and 1 hour after an orally administered medication. If a person normally eats three meals a day (7 to 8 AM, 12 to 1 PM, 6 to 7 PM), the best administration times are 9 to 10 AM, 2 to 4 PM, and 8 to 10 PM. However, some clients take multiple medications, making such a medication schedule difficult to follow. If a drug (such as aspirin or iron) irritates the gastrointestinal tract, it should be administered immediately after a meal. Before administering a drug by injection, the nurse assesses for local factors (for example, bruising or scarring) that may impair absorption of the drug.

DISTRIBUTION

After a drug is absorbed, it is distributed within the body to tissues and organs and ultimately to its specific site of action. The rate and extent of distribution depend on the physical and chemical properties of drugs and the physiology of the person taking the drug.

BODY SIZE. A direct relationship exists between the amount of drug administration and the amount of body tissue in which it is distributed. Most medications are distributed to body fat or body water (Simonson, 1984). An increase in the percentage of body fat may cause a longer duration of drug action because of slower distribution throughout the body. In obese clients a lower concentration accumulates in the body tissues that are the target for drug action. The less a client weighs, the greater the concentration of a drug in tissues and the more powerful the drug's effects. The elderly experience a reduction in both tissue mass and height and often require lower drug dosages than younger clients.

CIRCULATORY DYNAMICS. Drugs pass more easily from interstitial to intravascular spaces than between body compartments. Blood vessels are permeable to most dissolved substances unless drug particles are large or bound to serum proteins. The concentration of a drug at a specific site depends on (1) the number of blood vessels in tissues (2) the degree of local vasodilation or vasoconstriction, and (3) the rate of blood flow to a tissue site.

Exercise, warming, and chilling alter local circulation. For example, if a client applies a warm compress to an intramuscular injection site, the resultant vasodilation increases drug distribution.

PROTEIN BINDING. The degree to which drugs bind in the bloodstream to the protein albumin affects drug distribution. Most medications bind to this protein to some extent. When drug molecules are bound to albumin, they cannot exert any pharmacological activity. Unbound or "free" drug is the active form of the drug. The elderly have a decrease in albumin in the bloodsteam, probably caused by change in liver function. The same is true for clients with liver disease or malnutrition.

With the potential for more drug being unbound, the elderly may be at risk for an increase in drug activity or toxicity or both. The fraction of unbound meperidine hydrochloride (Demerol) in plasma increases with age (Simonson, 1984) and thus may be the reason for the elderly to be sensitive to this drug.

METABOLISM

After a drug reaches its site of action, it is metabolized into an inactive form that is more easily excreted. Biotransformation occurs under the influence of enzymes that detoxify, degrade, and remove biologically active chemicals. Most biotransformation occurs within the liver, although the lung, kidney, blood, and intestines also metabolize drugs.

The liver is especially important, because its specialized structure oxidizes and transforms many toxic substances. The liver degrades many harmful chemicals before they are distributed to the tissues.

The decrease in liver function that occurs with aging or with liver disease influences the rate at which a drug is eliminated from the body. The resultant slowing of metabolism causes the drug to accumulate in the body. When liver function is impaired, certain drugs may achieve higher-than-normal blood levels. Thus a client would be at greater risk for drug toxicity. Physicians should order lower dosages of drugs for clients with reduced liver function.

EXCRETION

After drugs are metabolized, they exit the body through the kidneys, liver, bowel, lungs, and exocrine glands. The chemical makeup of a drug determines the organ of excretion. Gaseous and volatile compounds such as ether, nitrous oxide, and alcohol exit through the lungs. Deep breathing and coughing (see Chapter 46) help the postoperative client eliminate anesthetic gases more rapidly.

The exocrine glands excrete lipid-soluble drugs. When medications exit through sweat glands, the skin may become irritated. The nurse assists the client in good hygiene practices to promote cleanliness and skin integrity. If a drug exits through the mammary glands, a nursing infant may absorb the chemicals. Mothers should minimize drug use while nursing.

The gastrointestinal tract is another route for drug excretion. Many drugs enter the hepatic circulation to be broken down by the liver and excreted into the bile. Once chemicals enter the intestines through the biliary tract, they may be reabsorbed by the intestines. Factors increasing peristalsis, such as laxatives and enemas, accelerate drug excretion through the feces, whereas factors slowing peristalsis, such as inactivity and improper diet, may prolong a drug's effects.

The kidneys are the main organs for drug excretion.

TABLE 15-5 Drugs Likely to Cause Adverse Reactions in the Elderly

Drug	Reaction or Effect
Digoxin (Lanoxin)	Reduces appetite, alters vision, can cause abnormal heart rhythm
Furosemide (Lasix)	Lowers potassium levels and blood pressure
Warfarin sodium (Coumadin)	Causes bleeding
Theophylline (Elixophyllin)	Causes nausea, seizures, and abnormal heart rhythm
Haloperidol (Haldol)	Causes sedation, restlessness, exaggerated facial movements, and symptoms of parkinsonism

TABLE 15-6 Mild Allergic Reactions

Symptom	Description
Urticaria (hives)	Raised, irregularly shaped skin eruptions with varying sizes and shapes; eruptions have reddened margins and pale centers
Eczema (rash)	Small, raised vesicles that are usually reddened; often distributed over the entire body
Pruritus	Itching of the skin; accompanies most rashes
Rhinitis	Inflammation of mucous membranes lining the nose, causing swelling and a clear watery discharge
Wheezing	Constriction of smooth muscles surrounding bronchioles that decreases diameter of airways; occurs primarily on inspiration because of severely narrowed airways; development of edema in pharynx and larynx that further obstructs airflow

Some drugs escape extensive metabolism and exit unchanged in the urine. Others undergo biotransformation in the liver before they are excreted by the kidney. If renal function declines, a common change in aging, the risk for drug toxicity increases (Table 15-5). If the kidney cannot adequately excrete a drug, it may be necessary to reduce the dosage. Maintenance of a normal fluid intake ensures proper elimination of drugs.

Types of Drug Actions

Because of its chemical makeup and physiological action, a drug may produce more than one effect.

THERAPEUTIC EFFECTS

The therapeutic effect is the intended or predicted physiological response a drug causes. Each drug has a desired or therapeutic effect for which it is prescribed. For example, the nurse administers codeine phosphate to create analgesia and gives theophylline to dilate narrowed respiratory bronchioles. A single medication may have many therapeutic effects. For example, aspirin creates analgesia and reduces inflammation of arthritis.

SIDE EFFECTS

Predictably a drug will cause unintended, secondary effects. Side effects may be harmless or injurious. In the example of codeine phosphate, a client may also experience constipation. Theophylline may cause headache and dizziness. If the side effects are serious enough to negate the beneficial effects of a drug's therapeutic action, the physician may discontinue it. Clients often stop taking medications because of side effects.

TOXIC EFFECTS

After prolonged intake of high doses of medication, or use of drugs intended for external application or when a drug accumulates in the blood because of impaired metabolism or excretion, toxic effects develop. Excess amounts of a drug within the body may have lethal effects, depending on the drug's action. For example, morphine, a narcotic analgesic, relieves pain by depressing the central nervous system. However, toxic levels of morphine cause severe respiratory depression and death.

IDIOSYNCRATIC REACTIONS

Medications may cause unpredictable effects, such as an idiosyncratic reaction in which a client overreacts or underreacts to a drug or has a reaction different from normal. It is impossible to predict which client will have an idiosyncratic response.

ALLERGIC REACTIONS

Allergic reaction is another unpredictable response to a drug. Exposure to an initial dose of a medication may cause an immunological response. The drug acts as an antigen, which causes antibodies to be produced. With repeated administration the client develops an allergic response to the drug, its chemical preservatives, or a metabolite.

An allergic reaction may be mild or severe. Allergic symptoms vary, depending on the individual and the drug. Among the different classes of drugs, antibiotics cause a high incidence of allergic reactions. Common, mild allergy symptoms are summarized in Table 15-6. Severe or anaphylactic reactions are characterized by sudden constriction of bronchiolar muscles, edema of the pharynx, and larynx, and severe wheezing and shortness of breath. The client may also become severely hypotensive, necessitating emergency resuscitation measures. A client with a known history of an allergy to a medication should wear an identification bracelet or medal, which alerts nurses and physicians to the allergy if the client is unconscious when receiving medical care.

DRUG TOLERANCE

Some persons have an unusually low metabolism in response to a drug. An increase in dosage may be needed to cause a therapeutic effect. Opiates and alcohol are common forms of drugs that may cause drug tolerance.

DRUG INTERACTIONS

When one drug modifies the action of another drug, a drug interaction occurs. Drug interactions are common in individuals taking many medications. A drug may potentiate or diminish the action of other drugs and may alter the way in which another drug is absorbed, metabolized, or eliminated from the body.

When two drugs act synergistically, the effect of the two drugs combined is greater than the effect that would be expected if the individual effects of the two drugs acting alone were added together. Alcohol is a central nervous system depressant that has a synergistic effect on antihistamines, antidepressants, and narcotic analgesics.

A drug interaction is not always undesirable. Often a physician orders combination drug therapy to create a drug interaction for therapeutic benefit. For example, a client with moderate hypertension typically receives several drugs, such as diuretics and vasodilators, that act together to keep the blood pressure at a desirable level.

Drug Dose Responses

After the nurse administers a drug, it undergoes absorption, distribution, metabolism, and excretion. Except when administered intravenously, drugs take time to enter the bloodstream. The quantity and distribution of a drug in different body compartments change constantly.

When a medication is prescribed, the goal is to achieve a constant blood level within a safe therapeutic range. Repeated doses are required to achieve a constant therapeutic concentration of a medication because a portion of a drug is always being excreted. When absorption ceases, only metabolism, excretion, and distribution

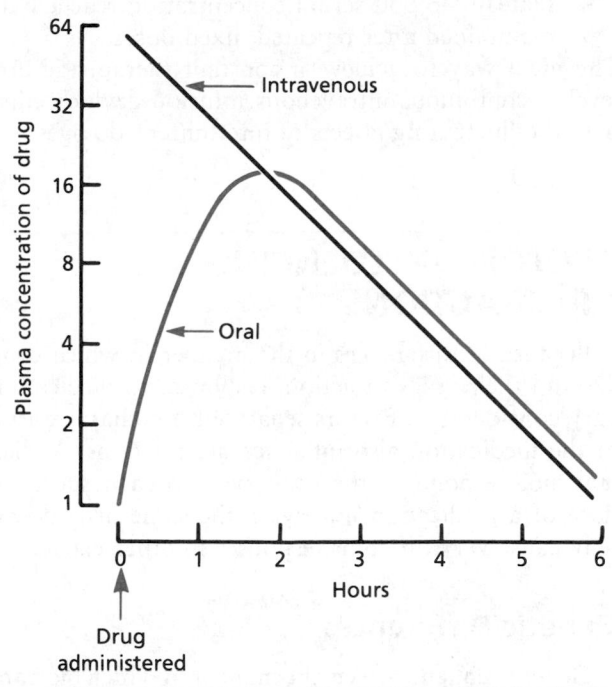

Fig. 15-1   Curve showing therapeutic blood levels.
From Clark, J, Queener, S, and Karb, V: Pharmacological basis of nursing practice, ed. 2, St. Louis, 1986, The C.V. Mosby Co.

continue. The highest serum concentration (peak concentration) of the drug usually occurs just before the last of the drug is absorbed. After peaking, the serum drug concentration falls progressively. With intravenous drug infusions, the peak concentration occurs quickly, but the serum level also begins to fall immediately.

All drugs have a **serum half-life** or the time it takes for excretion processes to lower the serum drug concentration by half. To maintain a therapeutic plateau, the client must receive regular, fixed doses. After an initial medication dose the client receives each successive dose when the previous dose reaches its half-life (Fig. 15-1). In this way an almost constant therapeutic drug concentration is maintained.

The client and nurse must follow regular dosage schedules and adhere to prescribed doses and dosage intervals. Knowledge of the following time intervals of drug action also helps to anticipate a drug's effect:

1. Onset of drug action—Period of time it takes after a drug is administered for it to produce a response
2. Peak action—Time it takes for a drug to reach its highest effective concentration
3. Duration of action—Length of time during which the drug is present in a concentration great enough to produce a response

4. Plateau—Blood serum concentration reached and maintained after repeated, fixed doses

The ideal way to achieve a constant therapeutic drug level is continuous intravenous infusions, which eliminate the fluctuating effects of intermittent dosages.

FACTORS INFLUENCING DRUG ACTIONS

Because of differences in the manner in which drugs act and their types of action, responses to medications vary considerably. Factors separate from characteristics of the medication also influence drug actions. A client may not respond in the same way to each successive dose of a medication. Likewise, the same drug dosage may cause very different responses in other clients.

Genetic Differences

Genetic makeup affects the manner in which biotransformation of drugs occurs. Metabolic patterns are often similar within families. Genetic factors determine whether naturally occurring enzymes are present to assist in drug degradation. As a result, members of a family may share a sensitivity to a medication.

Physiological Variables

Hormonal differences between males and females alter the metabolism of certain drugs. Hormones and drugs compete with each other in biotransformation because they are degraded by the same metabolic processes. Diurnal variations in estrogen secretion may be responsible for cyclic fluctuations in drug reactions experienced by women.

Age has a direct effect on drug action. Infants lack many of the enzymes necessary for normal drug metabolism. Infants and children also require dosages lower than those adults can tolerate.

A number of *physiological changes* accompanying the aging process influence the response to drug therapy (Table 15-7). Body systems undergo functional and structural changes that alter the influence of drugs. The nurse initiates actions that minimize a drug's harmful effects and promote the client's remaining functional capacities.

If a client's *nutritional status* is poor, proper cell function for biotransformation cannot occur. Like all body functions, drug metabolism relies on adequate nutrition for enzyme and protein formation. Most drugs bind with proteins before being distributed to their sites of action.

Any *disease state* that impairs the function of organs responsible for normal pharmacokinetics also impairs drug action. Altered skin integrity, reduced gastrointestinal absorption or motility, and impaired renal or hepatic function are just some of the disease-related conditions that can reduce a drug's efficacy or place a client at risk for drug toxicity.

Environmental Conditions

A client's exposure to severe physical and emotional *stress* triggers a hormonal response that eventually may interfere with drug metabolism. Ionizing *radiation* creates a similar effect by altering the rate of enzyme activity.

Exposure to *heat* and *cold* can affect responses to drugs. Hypertensive clients receive vasodilators to control blood pressure. In hot weather, it may be necessary to reduce vasodilator dosages because the temperature adds to the medication's effects. Cold weather tends to promote vasoconstriction, necessitating an increase in vasodilator dosage.

A reaction to a medication may vary depending on the *setting* in which it is taken. Clients in protective isolation often receive less pain relief from an analgesic than clients in a room where their families can visit them. Similarly, when a person drinks alcohol alone, he may only become sleepy. However, drinking with a group of friends can cause the person to become playful and outgoing.

Psychological Factors

A number of psychological factors influence a client's use of drugs and response to a medication. A person's *attitude* about drugs may stem from early experiences or familial influences. Seeing a parent use medications frequently may cause a child to accept drugs as a normal part of life.

The *meaning* or significance a drug or drug taking has for a client also influences his or her response to therapy. A drug may serve as a means for a person to overcome feelings of insecurity. In this situation the client depends on drugs as a means of coping with life. In contrast, if a client resents his physical condition, anger and hostility may result in adverse reactions to medications. Medications often provide a sense of security. The regular use of over-the-counter drugs such as vitamins, laxatives, and aspirin gives many people a sense of control over their health.

The *nurse's behavior* when administering a drug can have a significant impact on the client's response to a medication. If the nurse conveys a sense that the medication can be helpful, it is more likely the drug will have a positive effect. If the nurse seems uncaring when the client experiences discomfort, the medication administered may prove relatively ineffective.

TABLE 15-7 Influence of Drug Actions in the Elderly

Physiological Change	Drug Action/Client Response	Nursing Interventions
GASTROINTESTINAL TRACT **Oral Cavity**		
Loss of elasticity in oral mucosa, which becomes dry and easily abraded	Difficulty swallowing tablets or capsules; sensitivity to drugs that cause dryness of mouth; susceptibility to gum disease and dental caries	Rinse oral cavity frequently with tepid clear water. Floss daily. Brush gently. Use substitute saliva.
Esophagus		
Delayed esophageal clearance because of weakened contractions and failure of lower esophageal sphincter to relax	Difficulty swallowing large tablets or capsules; tissue erosion caused by drugs such as aspirin and uncoated potassium chloride	Position client upright. Administer full glass of permitted liquid with drug. Crush tablets and mix with food (if gastric pH does not affect absorption).
Stomach		
Decrease in gastric acidity and peristalsis	Potentiation of irritating effects of highly acidic drugs (for example, aspirin); alters solubility of certain drugs	Have client drink full glass of water and take medication with nonfat snack to reduce gastric distress
Large Intestine		
Reduced colon muscle tone; loss of defecation reflex; decreased intestinal blood flow	Slowing of drug excretion; overuse and abuse of laxatives by client; drug absorption delayed	Provide normal fluid intake. Instruct client to eat bulk-forming foods and avoid use of constipating drugs.
SKIN AND VASCULATURE		
Reduced subcutaneous skin fold thickness in extremities (less body fat); reduced elasticity in skin and vasculature	Fragile blood vessels; client prone to easy bleeding after an injection	Avoid using veins in hand for intravenous injections. Apply pressure to injection sites after drug administration. Observe injection sites for bleeding.
LIVER		
Reduced liver size; decline in hepatic blood flow	Longer biotransformation time; longer-than-normal duration of drug action; greater risk for drug sensitivity and toxicity	Monitor for signs of liver impairment (jaundice, pruritus, dark urine). Question dosages for clients with known liver disease
KIDNEY		
Reduced glomerular filtration; decreased tubular function and renal blood flow	Risk of drug accumulation and toxicity	Prevent urinary retention (keep catheters free flowing; observe frequency of urination). Monitor for signs of renal impairment (reduced output, difficulty urinating). Question dosages for clients with renal disease.

Diet

Drug and nutrient interactions can alter a drug's action or the effect of a nutrient. For example, Vitamin K is a nutrient that antagonizes the effect of warfarin sodium (Coumadin), decreasing its effect on clotting mechanisms. Mineral oil decreases the absorption of fat-soluble vitamins. Clients may be required to take nutritional supplements when taking drugs that reduce a nutrient's effect. Similarly, withholding certain nutrients may ensure a drug's therapeutic effect.

ROUTES OF ADMINISTRATION

The route chosen for administering a drug depends on its properties and desired effect and on the client's physical and mental condition (Table 15-8). A nurse must be involved in judging the best route for a medication, as in the following hypothetical situation:

The client, Mr. Bush, has progressively worsened physically. His temperature is 39.2°C. He complains of nausea and is unable to tolerate oral fluids. The nurse checks Mr. Bush's order, which reads, "Aspirin 600 mg orally for temperature above 38.5° C." On the basis of the assessment, the nurse believes Mr. Bush will not be able to tolerate an oral dose of aspirin. By consulting the physician the nurse acquires an order for a rectal suppository instead.

Oral Route

The oral route is the easiest and the most commonly used. Orally administered medications are less expensive than intravenous solutions and many topical preparations. They have a slower onset of action and a more prolonged effect than parenteral medications. Clients generally prefer the oral route because of the discomfort of injections.

SUBLINGUAL ADMINISTRATION

Some drugs are designed to be readily absorbed after being placed under the tongue to dissolve. A drug given sublingually should not be swallowed. Otherwise the desired effect will not be achieved. Nitroglycerine is commonly given sublingually. A drink should not be taken by the client until the drug is completely dissolved.

BUCCAL ADMINISTRATION

Administration of a drug by the buccal route involves placing the solid medication in the mouth and against the mucous membranes of the cheek until the drug dissolves. Clients should be taught to alternate cheeks with each subsequent dose to avoid mucosal irritation. Clients are also warned not to chew or swallow the drug or to take liquids with it. A buccal medication acts locally on the mucosa or systemically as it is swallowed in saliva.

Parenteral Routes

Parenteral administration involves giving a drug by a route other than the gastrointestinal tract.

INJECTION

One form of parenteral administration involves injection. The four major sites of injection are:
1. *Subcutaneous*—injection into tissues just below the dermis of the skin (hypodermic)
2. *Intramuscular (IM)*—injection into a muscle body
3. *Intravenous (IV)*—injection into a vein
4. *Intradermal*—injection into the dermis just under the epidermis

A physician often uses additional routes for parenteral injections, including intrathecal or intraspinal, intracardiac, intrapleural, intraarterial, and intraarticular.

The nurse uses strict sterile technique when preparing medications for parenteral injection. Contamination of medication solutions, syringe needles, or the syringe itself can lead to infection.

Topical Administration

Drugs applied to the skin and mucous membranes principally have local effects. The nurse applies skin medications by applying, painting, or spreading them over an area, applying moist dressings, soaking body parts in a solution, or giving medicated baths.

Some medications (for example, nitroglycerine) can be applied topically via an adhesive disk. The disk secures the medicated ointment to the skin.

Topical applications may cause systemic effects if a client's skin is thin, if the drug concentration is high, or if contact with the skin is prolonged.

The nurse also applies drugs to mucous membranes. They are absorbed quickly. If the drug concentration is high enough, systemic effects may occur.

Mucous membranes differ in their sensitivity to medications. The cornea of the eye and nasal mucous membranes are particularly sensitive. The client may complain of a burning sensation when the nurse administers eye or nose drops. Medications are generally less irritating to vaginal or rectal mucosa.

The nurse uses several methods for applying medications to mucous membranes:
1. Direct application of liquid—eye drops, gargling, swabbing the throat
2. Inserting drug into body cavity—placement of suppository in rectum or vagina, insertion of medicated packing into vagina
3. Instillation of fluid into body cavity—ear drops, nose drops, bladder and rectal instillation (fluid is retained)
4. Irrigation of body cavity—flushing eye, ear, vagina, bladder, or rectum with medicated fluid (fluid is not retained)
5. Spraying—instillation into nose and throat

Inhalation

The deeper passages of the respiratory tract provide a large surface area for drug absorption. The vascular alveolar-capillary network readily absorbs gases and mists introduced through the airways. Medications in-

TABLE 15-8 Factors Influencing Choice of Administration Routes

Route	Advantages	Disadvantages/Contraindications
Oral, buccal, sublingual	Convenient and comfortable to administer; economical; may produce local or systemic effects; rarely causes anxiety	Avoid giving to clients with alterations in gastrointestinal function (for example, nausea and vomiting) reduced motility (after general anesthesia or inflammation of bowel), and surgical resection of portion of gastrointestinal tract. Some drugs are destroyed by gastric secretions. Oral administration is contraindicated in clients unable to swallow (for example, clients with neuromuscular disorders, esophageal strictures, and lesions of the mouth). Oral medications cannot be given when client has gastric suction and are contraindicated in clients before some tests or surgery. An unconscious or confused client is unable or unwilling to swallow or to hold medication under the tongue. Oral medications may irritate lining of gastrointestinal tract, discolor teeth, or have an unpleasant taste.
Subcutaneous, intramuscular, intravenous, intradermal	Provides route of administration when oral drugs are contraindicated; more rapid absorption than with topical or oral drugs; intravenous infusion provides drug delivery when client is critically ill or peripheral perfusion is inadequate	There is a risk of introducing infection, the drugs are expensive, and these routes are to be avoided in clients with bleeding tendencies. There is a risk of tissue damage with subcutaneous injections. Intramuscular and intravenous routes are dangerous because of rapid absorption. These routes cause considerable anxiety in many clients, especially children.
Skin	Primarily provides local effect; painless; limited side effects	Extensive applications may be bulky and cause difficulty in maneuvering. Clients with skin abrasions are at risk for rapid drug absorption and systemic effects.
Mucous membranes: eye, ear, nose, vagina, rectum, buccal, sublingual	Therapeutic effects provided by local application to involved sites; aqueous solutions readily absorbed and capable of causing systemic effects; provides route of administration when oral drugs are contraindicated	Mucous membranes are highly sensitive to some drug concentrations. Insertion of rectal and vaginal medications often causes the client embarrassment. Client with ruptured eardrum cannot receive irrigations. Rectal suppositories are contraindicated if the client has had rectal surgery or if active rectal bleeding is present.
Inhalation	Provides rapid relief for local respiratory problems; provides easy access for introduction of general anesthetic gases; for seriously weakened or unconscious client, oxygen can still be delivered with appropriate respiratory therapy equipment	Some local agents can cause serious systemic effects. Drugs developed to act on body systems other than the lungs cannot be administered by inhalation.

troduced into the lung's airways must not interfere with normal gas exchange such as constricting bronchioles. Inhaled medications may have local effects. Drugs such as oxygen and general anesthetics create general systemic effects. Some medications given by inhalation are designed to produce local effects but have potentially dangerous systemic side effects. The nurse administers oxygen with the appropriate oxygen delivery equipment (see Chapter 36) and administers locally acting medications with hand-operated inhalers.

SYSTEMS OF DRUG MEASUREMENT

The proper administration of medication depends on the nurse's ability to compute drug dosages accurately and measure medications correctly. A careless mistake in placing a decimal point or adding a zero to a dosage can lead to a fatal error. The physician and client depend on the nurse to check the dosage before administering a drug. The nurse is also responsible for teaching clients the dosages prescribed for them.

Three systems of measurement are used in drug therapy: metric, apothecary, and household. Most nations of the world, including Canada, use the metric system as their standard of measurement. Although the U.S. Congress has not officially adopted the metric system, most health professionals in the United States use the metric system as well as the apothecary system. Prescriptions to be self-administered are often written in household measures for clients.

Metric System

As a decimal system, the metric system is the most logically organized of the measurement systems. Metric units can easily be converted and computed through simple multiplication and division. Each basic unit of measurement is organized into units of 10. Multiplying or dividing by 10 forms secondary units. In multiplication, the decimal point moves to the right; in division, the decimal moves to the left. For example:

$$10.0 \text{ mg} \times 10 = 100. \text{ mg}$$
$$10.0 \text{ mg} \div 10 = 1.0 \text{ mg}$$

The basic units of measurement in the metric system are the meter (length), the liter (volume), and the gram (weight). For drug calculations the nurse uses primarily volume and weight units. In the metric system small or large letters are used to designate the basic units:

Gram = g or Gm
Liter = l or L

Small letters are abbreviations for subdivisions of major units:

Milligram = mg
Milliliter = ml

A system of Latin prefixes designates subdivision of the basic units: deci- (1/10 or 0.1), centi- (1/100 or 0.01), and milli- (1/1000 or 0.001). Greek prefixes designate multiples of the basic units: deka- (10), hecto- (100), and kilo- (1000). When writing drug dosages in metric units, physicians and nurses use either fractions or multiples of a unit. Fractions are always in decimal form, for example:

500 mg or 0.5 g, *not* 1/2 g
10 ml or 0.01 L, *not* 1/100 L

When fractions are used, a zero is always placed in front of the decimal to prevent error.

Apothecary System

The apothecary system of measurement is familiar to most people in the United States and Canada. The standards for measurement can be easily seen in the home: milk is bottled in pints and quarts, a yardstick has inches and feet, and a bathroom scale weighs in pounds.

The basic unit of weight is a grain. In colonial days the grain represented the weight of one grain of wheat. Units of weight derived from the grain are the dram, ounce, and pound. The apothecary unit for volume or fluid measurement is the minim. The minim is the approximate quantity of water that weighs a grain. The fluidram, fluid ounce, pint, quart, and gallon are measures derived from the minim.

In the apothecary system, small letters or symbols are used for measurement units:

Grain = gr
Ounce = oz or ℥
Fluid ounce = f℥
Minim = m
Dram = ℥

Lowercase Roman numerals designate the quantities of the apothecary units. The Roman numeral follows the unit of measure:

3 grains = gr iii

Physicians often use fractions as well as symbols, with apothecary units:

2½ fluid ounces = f℥ iiss
½ fluid ounce = f℥ $\frac{1}{2}$ or ℥ ss

Household Measurements

The household unit of measurement is also familiar to most people. The problem with household measures is their inaccuracy. Household utensils such as teaspoons and cups often vary in size. Scales to measure pints or quarts are often not well calibrated. Household measures include drops, teaspoons, tablespoons, and cups for volume, and ounces and pounds for weight. Although pints and quarts are considered household measures, they are also used in the apothecary system.

The advantage of household measurements is their convenience and familiarity for clients. When the accuracy of a drug dosage is not critical, it is safe to use household measures. For example, many over-the-counter drugs, such as laxatives, antacids, and cough syrups, can safely be measured by this method. Table 15-9 gives common equivalents from each of the three measurement units.

TABLE 15-9 Equivalents of Measurement

Metric	Apothecary	Household
1 ml	15 minims (m)	15 drops (gtt)
15 ml	4 fluidrams (f₃)	1 tablespoon (tbsp)
30 ml	1 fluid ounce (f℥)	2 tablespoons (tbsp)
240 ml	8 fluid ounces (f℥)	1 cup (c)
480 ml (approximately 500 ml)	1 pint (pt)	1 pint (pt)
960 ml (approximately 1 L)	1 quart (qt)	1 quart (qt)
3840 ml (approximately 5 L)	1 gallon (gal)	1 gallon (gal)

Solutions

In clinical practice the nurse uses solutions of various concentrations for injections, irrigations, and infusions. The nurse should understand terms that describe concentrations of solutions. A *solution* is a given mass of solid substance dissolved in a known volume of fluid or a given volume of liquid dissolved in a known volume of another fluid. When a solid is dissolved in fluid, the *concentration* is in units of mass per units of volume, for example, g/ml, g/L, mg/ml. A concentration of a solution may also be expressed as a percentage. A 10% solution, for example, is 10 g of solid dissolved in 100 ml of solution. A proportion also expresses concentrations. A 1:1000 solution represents a solution containing 1 g of solid in 1000 ml of liquid or 1 ml of liquid mixed with 1000 ml of another liquid.

CONVERTING MEASUREMENT UNITS

A pharmacist does not always dispense a medication in the unit of measure in which it is ordered. Drug companies package and bottle certain standard equivalents. For example, the physician may order 250 mg of a med-

---

Common Reasons for Drug Conversions

- Converting fluid ounces to milliliters for measurement of intake and output.
- Converting body weight from pounds to kilograms and vice versa.
- Converting volume equivalents to calculate IV flow rates, prepare wound irrigation solutions, enemas, or bladder irrigations.

---

ication that is available only in grams. The nurse is responsible for converting available units of volume and weight to the desired dosages. The nurse must know approximate equivalents in all of the major measurement systems.

Drug administration is not the only function in which nurses use volume and weight conversions (see box). Conversions are used in a variety of nursing activities.

Conversions Within One System

Converting measurements within one system is relatively easy. In the metric system the nurse simply divides or multiplies. To change milligrams to grams the nurse divides by 1000, moving the decimal 3 points to the left.

$$1000 \text{ mg} = 1 \text{ g}$$
$$350 \text{ mg} = 0.35 \text{ g}$$

To convert liters to milliliters the nurse multiplies by 1000 or moves the decimal 3 points to the right.

$$1 \text{ L} = 1000 \text{ ml}$$
$$0.25 \text{ L} = 250 \text{ ml}$$

To convert units of measurement within the apothecary or household system the nurse must consult an equivalent table. For example, when converting fluid ounces to quarts the nurse must first know that 32 ounces is the equivalent of 1 quart. To convert 8 ounces to a quart measurement, for example, the nurse divides 8 by 32 to get the equivalent, ¼ or 0.25 quart.

Conversion between Systems

Frequently the nurse must determine the proper dosage of a medication by converting weights or volumes from one system of measurement to another. Commonly, apothecary and metric units must be converted to equivalent household measures for use at home. When the time comes to make actual drug calculations, it is easier to work with units in the same measurement system.

Tables of equivalent measurements are available in all

health care institutions. The pharmacist is also a good resource.

Before making a conversion the nurse compares the measurement system available with what is ordered. For example, a physician orders morphine gr ⅙ IM. The medication is available only in milligrams. To convert grains to milligrams the nurse must know the equivalents:

$$1 \text{ mg} = \frac{1}{60} \text{ gr}$$
or
$$60 \text{ mg} = 1 \text{ gr}$$

Therefore, by converting gr ⅙ to milligrams, the nurse will have the measurements needed to make the eventual dosage calculation. The nurse divides by 6:

$$60 \text{ mg} \div 6 = \frac{1}{6} \text{ gr}$$
$$10 \text{ mg} = \frac{1}{6} \text{ gr}$$

After calculating that the physician's order for morphine gr ⅙ is the same as 10 mg morphine, the nurse can accurately prepare the medication based on the available dosage.

Dosage Calculations

The nurse can use a simple formula in many types of dosage calculations. The following formula can be applied when preparing solid or liquid forms of medications:

$$\frac{\text{Dose ordered}}{\text{Dose on hand}} \times \text{Amount on hand} = \text{Amount to administer}$$

The dose ordered is the amount of pure drug the physician prescribes for a client. The dose on hand is the weight or volume of drug available in units supplied by the pharmacy. (The dose on hand may be listed on the drug label as the contents of a tablet or capsule or the amount of drug dissolved per unit volume of liquid.) The amount on hand is the basic unit or quantity of the drug containing the dose on hand (for solid drugs the amount on hand may be 1 tablet or capsule). The amount of liquid on hand may be, for example, a milliliter or liter depending on the capacity of the container. Last, the amount to administer is the actual amount of available medication the nurse will give to the client (always expressed in the same unit as the amount on hand).

The following example illustrates how to apply the formula. The physician orders the client to receive Demerol 50 mg IM. Thus the *dose ordered* is 50 mg. The medication is available only in ampules containing 100 mg per 2 milliliters. Thus the *dose on hand* is 100 mg in an *amount on hand* of 2 ml. The formula is applied as follows:

$$\frac{50 \text{ mg}}{100 \text{ mg}} \times 2 \text{ ml} = \text{volume of milliliter to administer}$$

To simplify the fraction, divide numerator and denominator by 50:

$$\frac{1}{2} \times 2 \text{ ml} = 1 \text{ ml to administer}$$

Another example demonstrates how the formula applies with solid dosage forms. The physician orders 0.125 mg PO* of digoxin. The drug is available in tablets containing 0.25 mg.

$$\frac{0.125 \text{ mg}}{0.250 \text{ mg}} \times 1 \text{ tablet} = \text{Number of tablets to administer}$$

The fraction $^{0.125}/_{0.250}$ equals ½ or 0.5. Therefore,

$$0.5 \times 1 \text{ tablet} = 0.5 \text{ or } \frac{1}{2} \text{ tablet to be administered}$$

Many tablets come with scores or indentations across the center of the tablet. A scored tablet is easy to break in half for divided dosages. The nurse should never attempt to estimate the amount of medication in a broken unscored tablet. The potential for giving dangerous doses of medication is high when the nurse must estimate dosage amounts.

Liquid medications often come prepared in volumes greater than 1 ml. In this situation the formula still applies. For example, the medication order is, "Erythromycin suspension 250 mg PO." The pharmacy delivers 100 ml bottles with the labels stating, "5 ml contains 125 mg of erythromycin."

$$\frac{250 \text{ mg}}{125 \text{ mg}} \times 5 \text{ ml} = \text{Volume to administer}$$

The fraction $^{250}/_{125}$ equals 2. Therefore,

$$2 \times 5 \text{ ml} = 10 \text{ ml to administer}$$

In this situation the nurse ignores the total volume of medication available and instead uses the dosage values noted on the label. If the nurse calculated the dosage on the basis of 100 ml available, the following error would occur:

$$\frac{250 \text{ mg}}{125 \text{ mg}} \times 100 \text{ ml} = 200 \text{ ml to administer}$$

On the basis of this calculation the client would receive 20 times the desired dosage.

Pediatric Dosages

Calculating children's drug dosages requires caution. Children are unable to metabolize many drugs as readily as adults. The child's body size also necessitates smaller dosages. In most cases physicians calculate the safe dosage for a child before ordering the medication. However, nurses should be aware of the formulas used to calculate pediatric dosages in order to check dosages that raise suspicion or concern. Most drug references list the normal ranges for pediatric dosages.

---

*PO is the abbreviation for the Latin phrase *per orum,* by mouth.

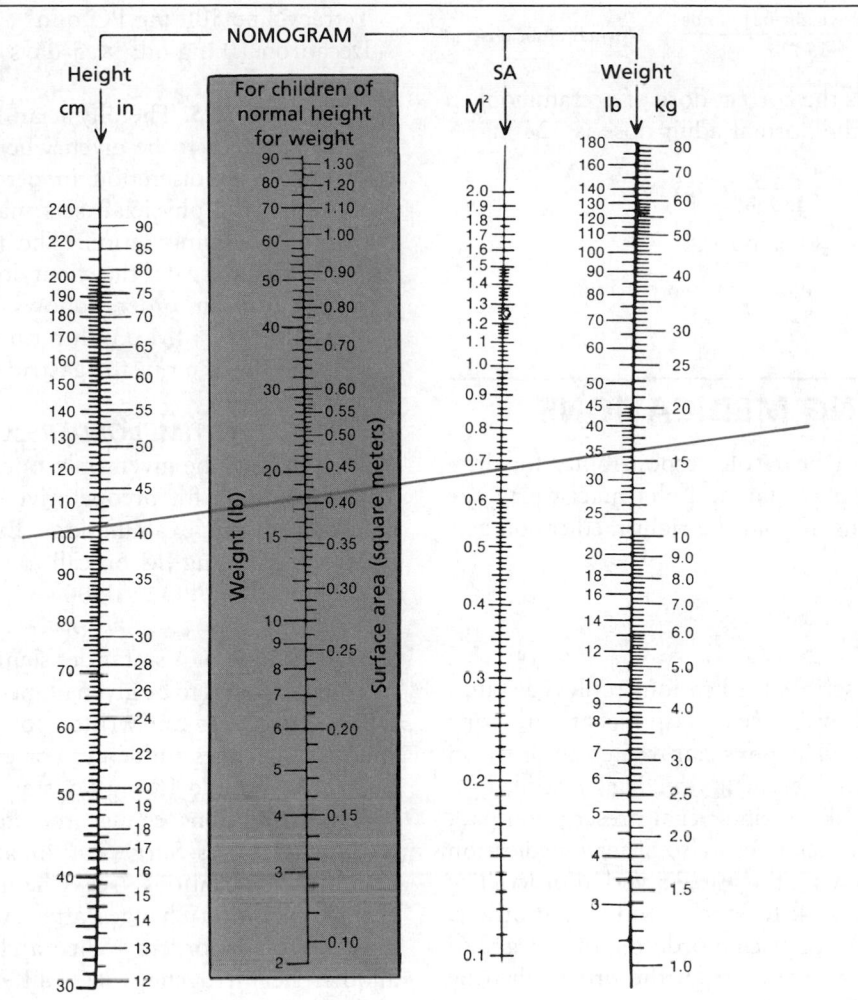

Fig. 15-2 West nomogram for estimation of surface areas in children. A straight line is drawn between height and weight. The point where the line crosses the surface area column is the estimated body surface area.

From Behrman, RE, and Vaughan, VC, editors: Nelson textbook of pediatrics, ed. 13, Philadelphia, 1987, W.B. Saunders Co.; Modified from data of Boyd, E, by West, CD.

BODY SURFACE AREA

The most accurate method of calculating pediatric dosages is based on body surface area. Body surface area is estimated on the basis of weight. Standard nomograms or charts list body surface area by weight and approximate age (Fig. 15-2). The formula is a ratio of the child's body surface area compared with the body surface area of an average adult (1.7 square meters, or 1.7 M^2).

$$\text{Child's dose} = \frac{\text{Surface area of child}}{1.7 \ M^2} \times \text{Normal adult dose}$$

For example, what dose of ampicillin does a child weighing 12 kg require if the normal single adult dose for ampicillin is 250 mg? The nomogram chart shows that a child weighing 12 kg has a surface area of 0.54 M^2.

$$\text{Child's dose} = \frac{0.54 \ M^2}{1.7 \ M^2} \times 250 \ mg$$

The M^2 units cancels out and can be ignored.

$$\text{Child's dose} = \frac{0.54}{1.7} \times 250 \ mg$$

$$\frac{0.54}{1.7} = 0.3$$

$$\text{Child's dose} = 0.3 \times 250 \ mg = 75 \ mg$$

CLARK'S RULE

A less accurate method for calculating pediatric dosages is Clark's rule. Clark's rule compares a child's body weight with the average weight of an adult (68 kg or 150 lb). The formula is applicable to children of all ages.

$$\text{Child's dose} = \frac{\text{Child's weight in pounds}}{150 \text{ lb}} \times \text{Normal adult dose}$$

For example, what is the correct dose of acetaminophen for a 30 lb child if the normal adult dose is 325 mg?

$$\text{Child's dose} = \frac{30 \text{ lb}}{150 \text{ lb}} \times 325 \text{ mg}$$

$$\frac{30}{150} = \frac{1}{5} = 0.2$$

$$\text{Child's dose} = 0.2 \times 325 \text{ mg} = 65 \text{ mg}$$

ADMINISTERING MEDICATIONS

The nurse does not bear sole responsibility for drug administration. The physician and pharmacist play key roles in helping to ensure that the right medication gets to the right client.

Physician's Role

The physician prescribes medications (unless a state's nurse practice act allows nurse practitioners to prescribe in specific situations). The physician writes an order on a designated form in the client's medical record, in a physician's order book, or on a legal prescription pad. In an emergency a physician may also order a medication by telephone or by giving the nurse a verbal order. The nurse enters and signs all telephone and verbal orders, writes the name of the physician ordering the drug, and then has the physician countersign the order when he again becomes available. Most institutions require a physician's signature within 24 hours after the order is made. Institutional policies vary as to which personnel can take verbal or telephone orders. In many institutions nursing students cannot take medication orders. *No medication is to be given without an order.* In some cases a physician's order may allow a drug such as regularly prescribed eye drops to be kept at the client's bedside for self-administration.

Common abbreviations (see end paper) are used when writing orders. The abbreviations indicate dosage frequencies or times, routes of administration, and special information for the nurse to follow in giving the drug.

TYPES OF ORDERS

The four common types of medication orders are based on the frequency of drug administration.

STANDING ORDERS. A standing order is carried out until the physician cancels it by another order or until a prescribed number of days elapse. A standing order may have a final date. Many institutions have policies for automatically discontinuing standing orders. The following are examples of standing orders:

Tetracycline 500 mg PO q6h*
Decadron 10 mg qd† × 5 days

P.R.N. ORDERS. The physician may order a drug on a p.r.n. basis, or to be given when a client requires it. The nurse uses discretion in determining the client's need. Often the physician sets maximum intervals for the time of administration. The nurse may decide to lengthen the interval if the client does not need the drug. Examples of p.r.n. orders follows:

Morphine gr ¼ IM q3-4h p.r.n. for incisional pain.‡
Maalox 30 ml p.r.n. for gastric discomfort.‡

SINGLE (ONE TIME) ORDERS. Often a physician will order a drug to be given only once at a specified time. This is common for preoperative drugs or drugs given before diagnostic examinations. Examples are:

Atropine 0.4 mg IM on call to OR (operating room)
Valium 10 mg PO at 0900

STAT ORDERS. A stat order signifies that a single dose of a medication is to be given immediately and only once. Often stat orders are written for emergencies when a condition changes suddenly. For example:

Give Apresoline 10 mg IM stat

Some conditions change the status of all a client's medication orders. Surgery automatically cancels all preoperative medications (see Chapter 46). Because the client's condition changes after surgery, the physician must write new orders. When a client is transferred to another health agency or a different medical service within a hospital, or is discharged, the new physician orders new medications.

COMPONENTS OF DRUG ORDERS

A medication order is incomplete unless it has seven essential parts:

1. *Client's full name*—The full name distinguishes the client from other persons with the same last name. Hospitals and other agencies may use a nameplate to imprint the name and hospital number on order forms. The imprinter is like a credit card imprinter. Some hospitals use computers to order medications. The computer screen shows a client's identifying information, which must be reviewed before an order is completed.
2. *Date order is written*—The day, month, and year are included. Designating the time an order is written helps to clarify when certain orders are to stop automatically. If an incident occurs involving a medication error (for example, a missed dose), it

---

*PO, by mouth; q, every; h, hour.
†qd, every day.
‡p.r.n., when necessary

is easier to document what happened when the order time is available.

3. *Drug name*—Usually the physician orders a generic or trade-name drug. Correct spelling is important in differentiating names with similar spelling.

4. *Dosage*—The amount or strength of the medication is included.

5. *Route of administration*—The physician uses common abbreviations for drug routes. Accuracy is important because certain drugs are administered by more than one route.

6. *Time and frequency of administration*—The nurse needs to know when to initiate drug therapy. Orders for multiple doses establish a routine schedule for drug administration.

7. *Signature of physician or nurse practitioner*—The signature makes the order a legal request. Insurance companies will not reimburse clients for medications unless a signature accompanies the order.

Prescriptions

The physician writes prescriptions for clients who are to take medications outside the hospital. The prescription includes more detailed information than a regular order because the client must understand how to take the medication and when to refill the prescription if necessary (Fig. 15-3). Parts of a prescription include:

1. *Superscription*—The client's name, address, age, and date are given for identification purposes. The symbol ℞ ("take thou") is at the top of the form.

2. *Inscription*—This is the drug name, strength, and dose.

3. *Subscription*—Directions are given to the pharmacist as to number of tablets or amount to be dispensed.

4. *Signature*—Information to be written on the label, such as directions to the client (for example, take with full glass of water or take between meals), directions for refilling the prescription, and whether the drug name should be on the label, is included.

5. *Personal data*—The physician signs the prescription. If the drug is a controlled substance, the physician includes registration number and address.

Pharmacist's Role

The pharmacist prepares and distributes prescribed drugs. The pharmacist also assumes responsibility for filling prescriptions accurately and for being sure prescriptions are valid. If there is any question that a prescription is forged or that the prescribing physician is unlicensed, the pharmacist should not fill the prescription. The pharmacist calls the physician if an ordered dose seems outside the safe therapeutic range.

The pharmacist in a health care agency rarely has to mix compounds or solutions except in the case of intravenous additive solutions. Most drug companies deliver drugs in a form ready for administration. Dispensing the correct drug in the proper dosage and amount with an accurate label is the pharmacist's chief responsibility. The pharmacist is also a resource for information about drug side effects, toxicity, interactions, and incompatibilities.

DISTRIBUTION SYSTEMS

Systems for the storage and distribution of medications vary among health care agencies. Institutions providing nursing care have a designated area for stocking and dispensing drugs. Special medication rooms, portable locked carts, and individual storage units adjacent to clients' rooms are some of the facilities used. Wherever medications are located, nurses keep close watch on the supply, making sure storage areas are locked when unattended.

STOCK SUPPLY. With a stock system, medications are available in quantity in stock containers. A nurse prepares individual doses from a large stock supply container. The system is time-consuming and costly. Narcotics are usually provided in stock supply.

INDIVIDUAL CLIENT SUPPLY. A separate supply of medications for each client can be kept in specially labeled drawers or storage bins. The pharmacist dispenses only the amount of medication a client will use for a limited period of time. Nurses distribute a client's med-

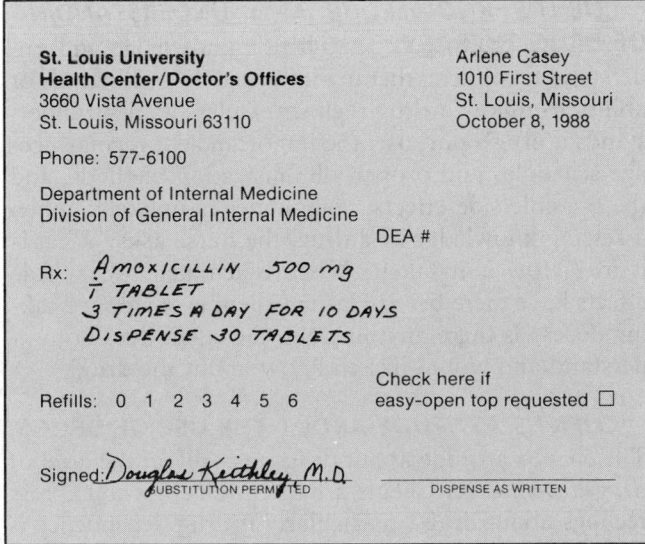

St. Louis University
Health Center/Doctor's Offices
3660 Vista Avenue
St. Louis, Missouri 63110

Arlene Casey
1010 First Street
St. Louis, Missouri
October 8, 1988

Phone: 577-6100

Department of Internal Medicine
Division of General Internal Medicine

DEA #

Rx: Amoxicillin 500 mg
Ī Tablet
3 times a day for 10 days
Dispense 30 tablets

Refills: 0 1 2 3 4 5 6

Check here if
easy-open top requested ☐

Signed: *Douglas Keithley M.D.*
SUBSTITUTION PERMITTED

DISPENSE AS WRITTEN

Fig. 15-3 Example of a medication prescription.
Courtesy St. Louis University Medical Center, St. Louis.

ications only from his own supply. This system reduces the time it takes to dispense medications.

UNIT-DOSE SYSTEM. The unit-dose system uses portable carts containing a drawer with a 24-hour supply of medications for each client. The unit-dose is the ordered dose of medication the client receives at a prescribed hour. At a designated time each day the pharmacist refills the drawers in the cart with a fresh supply of individually wrapped medications. The cart may also contain limited amounts of p.r.n. and stock drugs for special situations such as new drug orders or stat orders.

The nurse takes the medication cart around to each client's room. After administering each drug the nurse charts it immediately on the unit-dose medication form. Use of the unit-dose system reduces the number of medication errors and saves steps in dispensing drugs. When restocking the cart, the pharmacist is more likely to identify missed doses.

Nurse's Role

The nurse's role extends beyond simply giving drugs to a client. The nurse must determine whether a client should receive a drug at a given time, assess the client's ability to self-administer drugs, provide medications at the proper time, and monitor the effects of prescribed medications. Client and family education about proper drug administration and monitoring is also the nurse's role. The nurse uses the nursing process to integrate drug therapy into care.

ASSESSMENT

To determine the need for and potential response to drug therapy, the nurse assesses many factors.

MEDICAL HISTORY. A medical history provides indications or contraindications for drug therapy. Disease or illness may place clients at risk for adverse drug effects. For example, if a client has a gastric ulcer or bleeding tendency, compounds containing aspirin or anticoagulants will increase the likelihood of bleeding. Long-term health problems such as diabetes or arthritis, which require medicinal therapies, suggest to the nurse the type of drugs a client is taking. A client's surgical history may indicate use of medications. For example, after a thyroidectomy a client may require hormone replacement.

HISTORY OF ALLERGIES. Sometimes a physician overlooks a known allergy, or the client fails to discuss an allergy problem. New signs may indicate a reaction to a drug used for long periods without trouble. In a hospital, clients wear identification bands listing medications to which they are allergic. The client's medical record also has a label on the front of the chart that lists allergies. The physician documents medication allergies in the medical progress note.

PURPOSE OF DRUG ORDER. The nurse considers whether a drug is needed. For example, warm milk might eliminate the need for a sedative. If the client had a bowel movement in the morning, a laxative may be unnecessary. Nurses use judgment in administering a p.r.n. order. If a question arises about the need for a standing order, a consultation with the physician should be made.

CLIENT'S CURRENT CONDITION. The ongoing physical or mental status of a client may affect whether a drug is given or how it is administered. The nurse should assess a client carefully before giving any drug. For example, the nurse checks blood pressure before giving an antihypertensive. If the client is nauseated, it is unlikely a tablet can be swallowed. Assessment findings can also serve as a baseline in evaluating the effects of drug therapy.

DIET HISTORY. A diet history reveals normal eating patterns. The nurse can then plan the dosage schedule more effectively.

CLIENT'S PERCEPTUAL OR COORDINATION PROBLEMS. For a client with perceptual or coordination limitations, self-administration may be difficult. The nurse must assess the client's ability to prepare dosages and take medications correctly. If the client is unable to self-administer drugs, the nurse learns whether family members or friends are available to assist.

CLIENT'S KNOWLEDGE AND UNDERSTANDING OF DRUG THERAPY. The client's knowledge and understanding of drug therapy influence the willingness or ability to follow a drug regimen. Unless a client understands a drug's purpose, the importance of regular dosage schedules and proper administration methods, and the possible side effects, compliance is unlikely. When assessing knowledge of a drug, the nurse asks: What is it for? How is it taken? When is it taken? What side effects have there been? Has the client ever stopped taking doses? Is there anything else the client does not understand and would like to know about the drug?

CLIENT'S ATTITUDE ABOUT THE USE OF DRUGS. The client's attitude about drugs may reveal the level of *drug dependence.* Clients are often reluctant to express feelings about drugs, particularly if drug dependence is a problem. To assess attitudes, the nurse may have to observe the client's behavior for evidence of drug dependence.

DRUG DATA. The nurse assesses information about each drug, including action, purpose, normal dosages, routes, side effects, and nursing implications for administration and monitoring. Common questions to ask are: Is the smallest possible dose ordered (a question pertinent to elderly clients)? Can a certain drug interact with other drugs being used? Are there special instructions for administering the drug? Is the drug prescribed for the most effective route of administration, considering the client's condition?

Often, several resources must be consulted to gather needed information. Pharmacology textbooks, nursing journals, the *Physicians' Desk Reference (PDR)*, drug package inserts, and the pharmacist are valuable resources. The nurse is responsible for knowing as much as possible about each drug given. Many nursing students prepare or purchase cards containing drug data to use as a quick resource.

CLIENT'S LEARNING NEEDS. By assessing the client's level of knowledge about a medication, the nurse determines the need for instruction. It may be necessary for the nurse to explain the action and purpose of the drug, expected side effects, correct administration techniques, and ways to help the client to remember the drug regimen. If a client has been placed on a newly prescribed drug, instruction may need to be more involved.

NURSING DIAGNOSIS

Assessment provides data on the client's condition, ability to self-administer drugs, and drug use patterns,

---

Examples of Nursing Diagnoses Related to Drug Therapy

NANDA-APPROVED NURSING DIAGNOSES

Knowledge deficit regarding drug therapy related to:
- Newly prescribed medication
- Cognitive limitations

Noncompliance regarding drug regimen related to:
- Limited economic resources
- Client's health beliefs

Impaired physical mobility related to:
- Upper extremity weakness/paralysis
- Diminished grasp

Sensory/perceptual alterations: visual related to:
- Blurred vision (ophthalmologic alteration)

Anxiety related to:
- Following multiple drug regimens

Impaired swallowing related to:
- Neuromuscular impairment
- Irritated oral cavity

---

which can be used to determine actual or potential problems with drug therapy (see nursing diagnoses box). If the nurse diagnoses knowledge deficit or factors interfering with drug regimen compliance, client education becomes a part of the nursing care plan. If the client has physical limitations that interfere with drug administration, the nurse plans strategies to ensure the client's safety. The identification of appropriate defining characteristics ensures that an accurate diagnosis is made (see sample diagnoses box).

Sample Nursing Diagnoses for Problems Related to Drug Therapy		
Defining Characteristics	**Nursing Diagnoses**	**Related Factors**
Inquires about purpose of medication New drug ordered in the morning No previous history of taking prescribed medication	Knowledge deficit regarding drug therapy	- Newly prescribed medication - Inexperience with drug therapy
Reduced strength in right arm Reduced grasp in right hand Avoids movement of right hand due to pain	Impaired physical mobility	- Upper extremity weakness
Reduced gag reflex Coughs when attempting to swallow capsule Food retained in mouth after eating	Impaired swallowing	- Neuromuscular impairment

Sample Nursing Care Plan for Problems Related to Drug Therapy

Nursing Diagnosis	Goals	Expected Outcomes	Nursing Interventions
Knowledge deficit regarding drug therapy related to inexperience with drug therapy	Client will self-administer medication correctly.	Client takes medication at prescribed intervals.	Establish medication schedule to fit client's daily routine. Offer a daily dose reminder for clients to use at home. Explain when medication is to be taken.
	Client understands purposes and implications of prescribed medication.	Client explains purpose of medication, potential side effects, and toxic effects.	Provide two or three 10-minute discussions about purpose and implications of drug therapy. Offer pharmacy fact sheets about prescribed medication.

PLANNING

Whether a client attempts self-administration of medications or the nurse assumes responsibility for administering medications (see care plan box), the following goals should be met:

1. Avoidance of complications related to the route of administration
2. Achievement of the therapeutic effect of the prescribed medications safely while maintaining the client's comfort
3. Understanding on the part of the client and family members regarding drug therapy
4. Safe self-administration of medications

IMPLEMENTATION

CORRECT TRANSCRIPTION AND COMMUNICATION OF ORDERS. The nurse or a designated unit secretary writes the physician's complete order on the appropriate medication forms or tickets. (Figs. 15-4 and 15-5). The transcribed order includes client's name, room, and bed number, drug name, dosage, and time and route of administration. Each time a drug dosage is prepared the nurse refers to the medication form or ticket. With the unit-dose system, only one transcription is necessary, limiting the opportunity for errors. When transcribing orders, the nurse should be sure names, dosages, and symbols are legible. The nurse rewrites any smudged or illegible transcriptions.

In some institutions a computer printout lists all currently ordered medications with dosage information. Orders are entered directly into the computer, preventing the need for transcription of orders. The same printout may be used to record medications given.

A registered nurse checks all transcribed orders against the original order for accuracy and thoroughness. If an order seems incorrect or inappropriate, the nurse consults the physician. The nurse who gives the wrong medication or an incorrect dosage is legally responsible for the error.

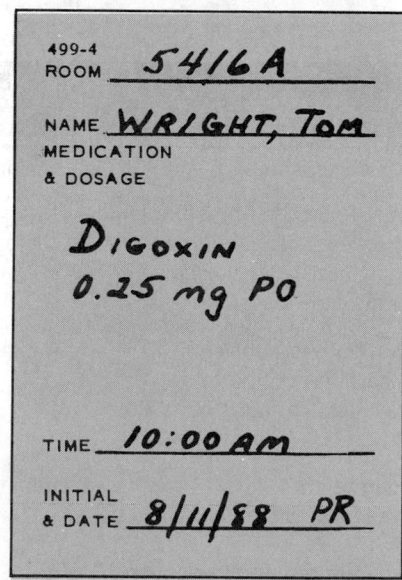

Fig. 15-4 Sample medication ticket.

ACCURATE DOSAGE CALCULATION AND MEASUREMENT. When measuring liquid drugs, the nurse uses standard measuring receptacles. The procedure for drug measurement is systematic to lessen the chance of error. The nurse calculates each dose when preparing the drug, pays close attention to the process of calculation, and avoids interference from other nursing activities.

CORRECT ADMINISTRATION. To administer a medication safely, the nurse uses aseptic technique and proper procedures in handling and giving medications. Promoting comfort such as by positioning increases efficiency. Certain drugs require the nurse to perform assessments at the time of administration, such as assessing heart rate before giving antidysrhythmic medications.

RECORDING DRUG ADMINISTRATION. After administering a drug the nurse records it immediately on the appropriate record form (Fig. 15-5). *The nurse never charts a drug before administering it.* Recording immediately after administration prevents errors. For example, a nurse might give a drug without knowing the client had already received the drug from a nurse on the preceding shift who forgot to record the administration.

The recording of a drug includes the name of the drug, dosage, route, and exact time of administration. Often the drug forms are prepared and the nurse need only record the time. Agency policies may also require that the nurse record the location of an injection.

If a client refuses a drug or is undergoing tests or procedures that result in a missed dose, the nurse explains the reason the drug was not given in the nurse's notes. Some agencies require the nurse to circle the prescribed administration time on the drug record when a dosage is missed.

CLIENT AND FAMILY TEACHING. Unless a client is properly informed about drugs, he may take the drugs incorrectly or not at all. The nurse provides information about the purpose of medications and their actions and effects. Many health care institutions offer easy-to-read leaflets on specific types of drugs. A client must know how to take a drug properly and the effects if he fails to do so. For example, when a client receives a prescription for an antibiotic, he must understand the importance of taking the full prescription. Failure to do this can lead to a worsening of the condition, as well as the development of bacteria resistant to the drug.

Nurses teach proper self-administration of drugs to clients who depend on daily injections. The client learns to prepare and administer an injection correctly using

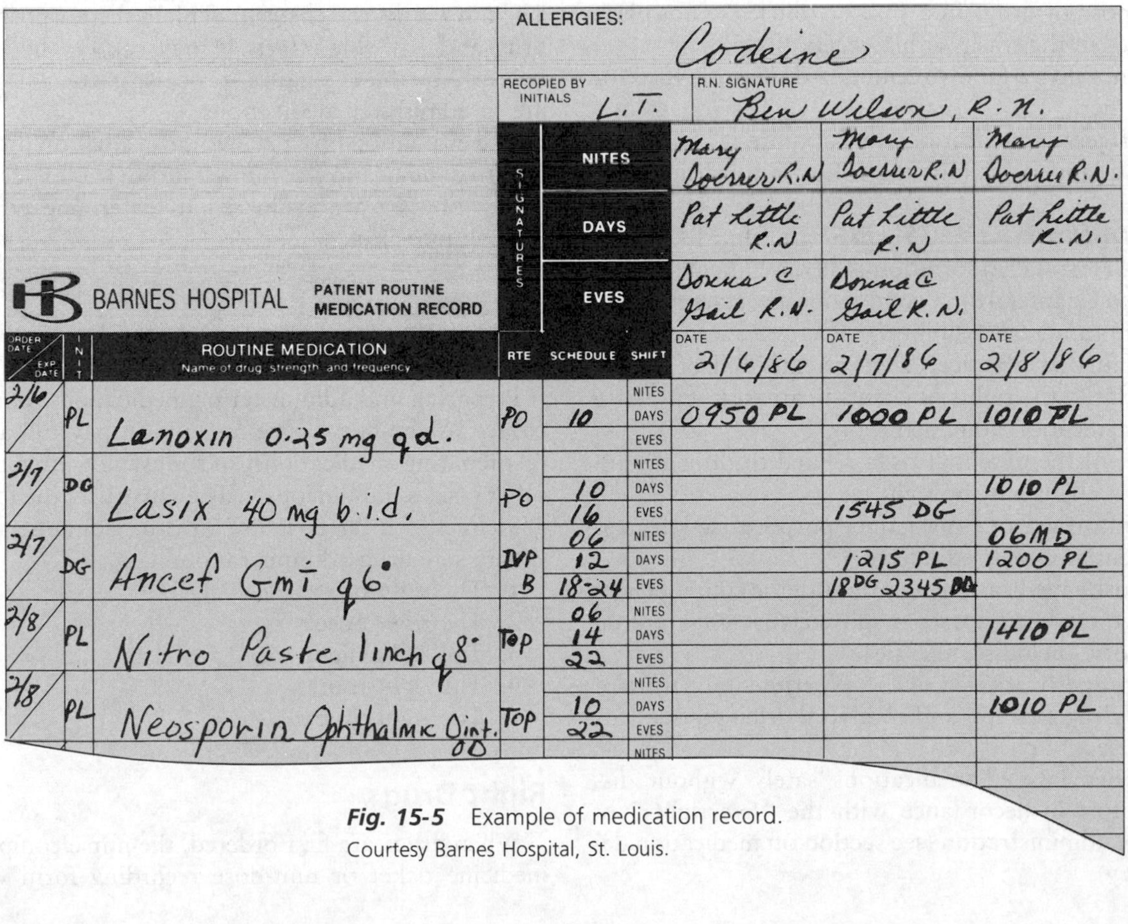
BARNES HOSPITAL PATIENT ROUTINE MEDICATION RECORD

ALLERGIES: Codeine

RECOPIED BY INITIALS: L.T. R.N. SIGNATURE: Ben Wilson, R.N.

SIGNATURES			
NITES	Mary Docrer R.N	Mary Docrer R.N	Mary Docrer R.N.
DAYS	Pat Little R.N	Pat Little R.N	Pat Little R.N.
EVES	Donna C Gail R.N.	Donna C Gail R.N.	

ORDER DATE / EXP DATE	INIT	ROUTINE MEDICATION Name of drug strength and frequency	RTE	SCHEDULE	SHIFT	DATE 2/6/86	DATE 2/7/86	DATE 2/8/86
2/6	PL	Lanoxin 0.25 mg qd.	PO		NITES			
				10	DAYS	0950 PL	1000 PL	1010 PL
					EVES			
2/7	DG	Lasix 40 mg b.i.d.	PO		NITES			
				10	DAYS			1010 PL
				16	EVES		1545 DG	
2/7	DG	Ancef Gm ī q6°	IVP B	06	NITES			06 MD
				12	DAYS		1215 PL	1200 PL
				18-24	EVES		18DG 2345 DG	
2/8	PL	Nitro Paste 1 inch q8°	TOP	06	NITES			
				14	DAYS			1410 PL
				22	EVES			
2/8	PL	Neosporin Ophthalmic Oint. OD	TOP		NITES			
				10	DAYS			1010 PL
				22	EVES			

Fig. 15-5 Example of medication record.
Courtesy Barnes Hospital, St. Louis.

aseptic technique. Family members should be taught to give injections in case the client becomes ill or physically unable to handle a syringe.

Nurses can provide specially designed equipment for clients with visual alterations such as syringes with enlarged calibrated scales for easier reading or braille-labeled medication vials.

Many older clients are responsible for self-medication so instructions should include detailed information about medications and dosage schedules that help them remember to take medications regularly.

Clients must be aware of the symptoms of drug side effects or toxicity. For example, clients taking anticoagulants learn to notify the physician immediately when signs of bleeding develop. Family members should be informed of drug side effects, such as changes in behavior, because they are often the first persons to recognize such effects. Clients are better able to cope with problems caused by drugs if they understand how and when to act.

All clients should learn the basic guidelines for drug safety. These guidelines ensure the proper use and storage of drugs in the home.

1. Keep each drug in its original, labeled container.
2. Be sure labels are legible.
3. Discard any outdated medications.
4. Always finish a prescribed drug unless otherwise instructed. Never save a drug for future illnesses.
5. Dispose of drugs in a sink or toilet. Do not place drugs in the trash within reach of children.
6. Do not give a family member a drug prescribed for another.
7. Refrigerate medications that require it.
8. Read labels carefully and follow all instructions.

MAINTAINING CLIENTS' RIGHTS. In 1973 the American Hospital Association issued a Patient's Bill of Rights (see Chapter 18), a comprehensive statement defining rights and responsibilities for a broad area of medical and nursing practice. The Patient's Bill of Rights helps to clarify the rights of clients in an area of practice such as medication administration.

Because of the potential risks related to drug administration, a client has the right to:

1. Be informed of drug name, purpose, action, and potential undesired effects
2. Refuse a medication regardless of the consequences
3. Have qualified nurses or physicians assess a drug history, including allergies
4. Be properly advised of the experimental nature of any drug therapy and to give written consent for its use
5. Receive labeled medications safely without discomfort in accordance with the "five rights" of drug administration (see section on medication delivery)
6. Receive appropriate supportive therapy in relation to drug therapy
7. Not receive unnecessary medications

The nurse must be aware of these rights and handle all inquiries by clients and families courteously and professionally. A nurse should not become defensive if a client refuses drug therapy. The nurse must have the necessary knowledge and skill to satisfy the responsibilities of safe and effective drug administration.

EVALUATION

The nurse must monitor response to medication. This is easier if the nurse knows the therapeutic action and common side effects of medications. When unpredictable reactions occur, the nurse evaluates the response (for example, assessing vital sign changes and observing any physical alterations). The nurse is alert for reactions in a client with multiple drug allergies or with health alterations that increase sensitivity to a drug.

When the care plan involves teaching the client to self-administer drugs at home, the nurse gives the client ample time to demonstrate understanding. The nurse asks the client to explain when each drug should be taken during the day. If the client is to self-administer injections, the nurse has the client do so under supervision. The nurse asks the client to explain the purpose of each drug and any side effects it may cause. The family is involved in the evaluation process, particularly if they are to administer medications.

The evaluation box reviews the evaluation process for effective medication administration. The expected outcomes of care are evaluated to determine efficacy of nursing measure.

MEDICATION DELIVERY

Preparing and administering medications requires accuracy by the nurse. The nurse must pay full attention to preparing medications and must not attempt to do other tasks simultaneously. The nurse uses the following guidelines, the "five rights" of drug administration, to ensure safe drug administration:

1. The *right* drug
2. The *right* dose
3. The *right* client
4. The *right* route
5. The *right* time

Right Drug

When drugs are first ordered, the nurse compares the medicine ticket or unit-dose recording form with the

Sample Evaluation of Interventions for Problems Related to Drug Therapy

Goals	Evaluative Measures	Expected Outcomes
Client does not experience complication related to route of administration	Inspect injection sites for localized tenderness, inflammation, hardness or bruising.	Injection sites will be clear, without inflammation and with minimal bruising.
	Inspect IV sites for redness, swelling, tenderness, cool or warm skin.	IV site will have no signs of phlebitis or infiltration.
	Question client if gastric distress follows oral intake of medication.	Client denies symptoms of gastric distress.
Client achieves therapeutic effect of prescribed medications.	Nurse or client monitors for desired effect of medication (for example, relief of discomfort after an analgesic, lowering of body temperature after an antipyretic, and lowering or maintenance of blood pressure after an antihypertensive).	Medication exerts measurable therapeutic effect.
Client is safe and comfortable.	Note positioning of client before drug administration (for example, sitting up for oral medication ingestion, or lying on side before ventrogluteal injection).	(When sitting, client is able to swallow oral medications without difficulty, or when lying on side, injection is given correctly in proper tissues).
	Monitor intravenous infusion rate regularly.	Intravenous medication infuses over prescribed time period.
	Observe for potential side effects or toxic effects of medication.	Client denies side effects, and no adverse effects are observed.
Client understands drug therapy.	Ask client or family member to explain purpose of medication and all pertinent information related to drug administration.	Client or family member explains information needed to demonstrate understanding of drug regimen.
Client self-administers medication.	Have client or family member prepare dosage of medication.	Client will prepare correct dosage using proper skills and techniques.

physician's written orders. When administering drugs, the nurse compares the label of the drug container with the form or medicine ticket. The nurse does this three times: (1) before removing the container from the drawer or shelf, (2) as the amount of drug ordered is removed from the container, and (3) before returning the container to storage. With single-dose prepackaged drugs the nurse checks the label with the medicine ticket or form a third time even though there is no permanent container (Fig. 15-6).

Nurses administer only the drugs they prepare. If an error occurs, the nurse administering the drug is responsible for its effects.

If a client questions the medication, the nurse does not ignore these concerns. An alert client will know if a drug is different from those received before. In most cases the drug order has been changed. However, the client's questions might reveal an error. The nurse should withhold the drug until the preparation can be rechecked against physician's orders.

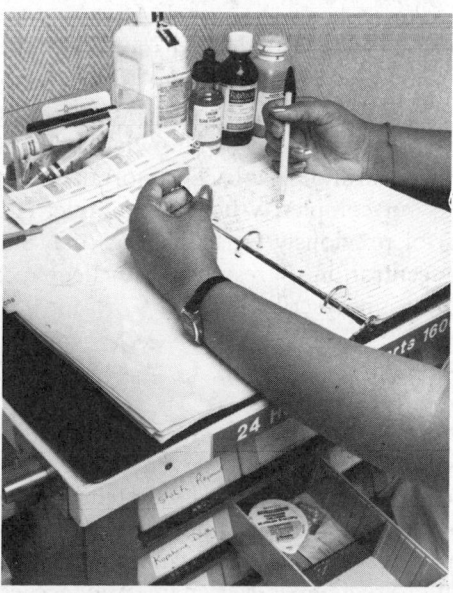

Fig. 15-6   The nurse checks the label of the medication with the transcribed medication order.

Clients who self-administer drugs should keep them in their original labeled containers, separate from other drugs, to avoid confusion.

The nurse never prepares medications from unmarked containers or containers with illegible labels. If a client refuses a drug, the nurse should never return the medication to the original container or transfer the drug to another container (single-dose prepackaged drugs can be returned to storage areas if unopened).

Right Dose

The unit-dose system of drug distribution minimizes errors because most medications come prepared in proper doses. When a medication must be prepared from a larger or smaller volume or strength than needed or when a physician orders a system of measurement different from what the pharmacist supplies, the chance of error increases. When performing drug calculations or conversions, the nurse should have another qualified nurse check the calculated dosages. Most institutions require two nurses to check all insulin and anticoagulant dosages.

After calculating dosages the nurse prepares the medication by using standard measurement devices. For example, many liquid medications come with a scaled dropper. Graduated cups, syringes, and specially designed spoons can be used to measure medications accurately. In the home, clients should use standard kitchen measuring spoons rather than teaspoons and tablespoons, which vary in volume.

To break a scored tablet, the nurse makes sure the break is even. A tablet may be cut in half by using a knife edge or by folding a clean paper towel over the tablet and breaking it with the fingers. Any tablets that do not break evenly are discarded. After a tablet is split, the nurse gives the two halves in successive doses.

Often a nurse prepares a tablet by crushing it in a mortar and pestle so it can be mixed in food, especially when a client has difficulty swallowing and an injection is unnecessary or undesirable. The mortar should always be cleaned out completely before the tablet is crushed. Remnants of previously crushed drugs may increase a drug's concentration or result in the client receiving a portion of an unprescribed drug.

Right Client

An important step in administering drugs safely is being sure the medication is given to the right client. The nurse working in a hospital or extended care setting is frequently responsible for administering drugs to several clients. Clients often have similar last names, and it is difficult to remember every name and face, especially if a nurse has been off duty for several days. To identify

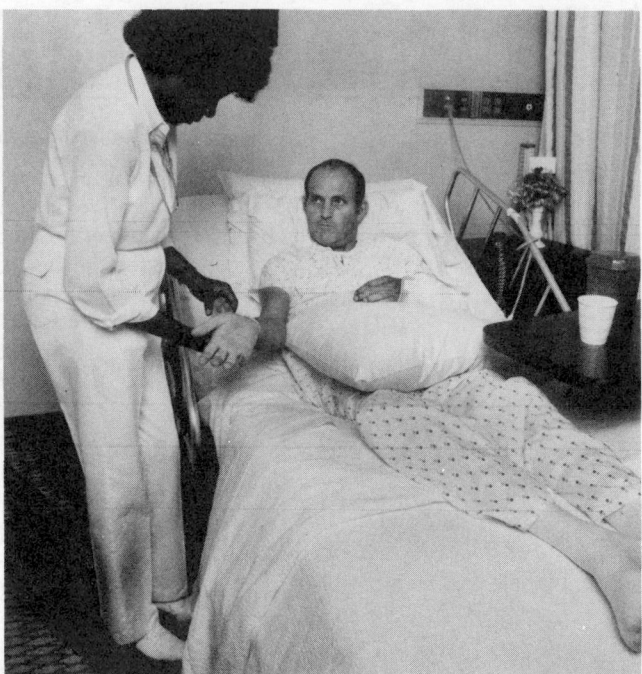

Fig. 15-7 Before administering any medication the nurse checks the client's identification bracelet.

a client correctly, the nurse (1) checks the medicine ticket or form against the client's identification bracelet (Fig. 15-7) and (2) asks the client to state his or her name.

If an identification bracelet becomes smudged or illegible, the nurse acquires a new one. When asking a client's name, the nurse should not speak the name and then assume that the client's response indicates that he or she is the right person. Instead, the nurse asks clients to state their full names. This is vital even if the nurse has been caring for a client for several days and recognizes him or her. To avoid making the client feel uneasy, the nurse simply says that the routine for giving a medication requires identification by name.

Clients who self-administer medications at home should be cautioned never to give a family member one of their medications. A physician should be consulted before one person uses a prescription meant for another because a drug that is safe for one person can be lethal for another.

Right Route

If a physician's order does not designate a route of administration, the nurse consults the physician. Likewise, if the specified route is not the recommended route, the nurse should alert the physician immediately.

When administering injections (see the section on parenteral routes), the nurse ensures that medications are given correctly. It is also important to prepare injections only from preparations designed for parenteral use. The injection of a liquid designed for oral use can produce local complications such as a sterile abscess or fatal systemic effects. Drug companies label parenteral drugs for "injectable use only."

Right Time

The nurse must know why a drug is ordered for certain times of the day and whether the time schedule can be altered. For example, two drugs are ordered, one q8h (every 8 hours) and the other t.i.d. (three times a day). Both medications are to be given three times within a 24-hour period. The physician intends the q8h medication to be given around the clock to maintain therapeutic blood levels of the drug. In contrast, the t.i.d. medication is given during the waking hours. Each institution has a recommended time schedule for medications ordered at frequent intervals, for example, q.i.d. medications may be given at 8 AM, noon, 4 PM, and 8 PM; t.i.d. medications may be given at 8 AM, 2 PM, and 8 PM.

The physician often gives specific instructions about when to administer a medication. A preoperative medication to be given on call means the nurse is to administer the drug when the operating room notifies the nursing division. A drug ordered p.c. (after meals) is to be given within half an hour after a meal, when the client has a full stomach. A stat medication is to be given immediately.

When a nurse is responsible for administering several medications, drugs that must act at certain times are given priority. For example, insulin should be administered at a precise interval before a meal. All routinely ordered medications should be given within 30 minutes of the times ordered.

Some medications require the nurse's clinical judgment in determining the proper time for administration. A p.r.n. sleeping medication should be administered when the client is prepared for bed. Many clients prefer to go to sleep earlier than they might normally at home. However, if the nurse is aware that a procedure might interrupt the client's sleep, it is appropriate to withhold the drug until a time when the client can gain full benefit

TABLE 15-10   Ways to Prevent Drug Administration Errors

Precaution	Rationale	Precaution	Rationale
Read drug labels carefully	Many products come prepared in similar containers.	When a new or unfamiliar drug is ordered, consult a resource.	If the physician is also unfamiliar with the drug, there is greater risk of inaccurate dosages being ordered.
Question the administration of multiple tablets or capsules or vials for a single dose.	Most doses are one or two tablets or capsules or one single-dose vial. Incorrect interpretation of an order may result in an excessively high dose.	Do not administer a drug ordered by a nickname.	Many physicians refer to commonly ordered medications by nicknames. If the nurse or pharmacist is unfamiliar with the name, the wrong drug may be dispensed and administered.
Be aware of drugs with similar names.	Many drug names sound alike (for example, digoxin and digitoxin, Keflex and Keflin, Orinase and Ornade.)		
Check the decimal point.	Some drugs come prepared in quantities that are multiples of one another (for example, Coumadin is available in 2.5 and 25 mg tablets, and Thorazine is available in 30 and 300 mg spansules.)	Do not attempt to decipher illegible writing.	When in doubt, ask the physician. Unless the nurse questions an order that is difficult to read, the chance of misinterpreting the order is great.
		Know clients with the same last names. Also have clients state their full names.	It is common to have two or more clients with the same or similar last names. Special labels on the Kardex or medication book can warn nurses of a potential problem.
Question abrupt and excessive increases in dosages.	Most dosage changes are made gradually so the physician can monitor the therapeutic effect and response.	Do not confuse equivalents.	When in a hurry, it may be easy to misread equivalents (for example, milligram instead of milliliter).

from the medication. A nurse also uses judgment in administering p.r.n. analgesics. When a client's order reads q3-4h, the nurse may give the medication as often as every 3 hours. The nurse assesses the client's level of pain to determine the degree of discomfort. If a client is made to wait until the pain becomes severe, an analgesic is not sufficient. The nurse may need to obtain a stat order from the physician if the client requires a medication before the p.r.n. interval has elapsed.

In the home setting a client may have to take several medications throughout the day. The nurse can help to plan medication schedules based on the preferred drug intervals and the client's daily schedule. For example, the schedule for drugs to be given around mealtime can be easily adjusted to client preferences. For clients who have difficulty remembering when to take medications, the nurse can make a chart that lists the times when each drug is to be taken.

Avoiding Errors

Most medication errors occur when a nurse fails to follow routine procedures (Table 15-10). Unfortunately, many medication errors are never identified.

An error should be acknowledged immediately. The nurse has the ethical and professional responsibility for reporting the error to the physician. Measures to counteract the effects of the error may be necessary, such as administering an antidote when the wrong drug is given, withholding a dose when a medication has been given too soon, or monitoring the effects when an unusually high dosage is given. The nurse is also responsible for completing an incident report describing the nature of the incident. The report is not an admission of guilt or the basis for punishment and is not a part of the client's legal record. The report provides an objective analysis of what went wrong and is a means for the institution's safety personnel to monitor such occurrences. Without incident reports, nursing supervisory personnel have difficulty identifying errors and solving recurrent problems affecting care.

Special Considerations for Age Groups

A client's developmental level is a factor in the way in which nurses administer medications. Knowledge of a client's developmental needs helps the nurse to anticipate responses to drug therapy.

INFANTS AND CHILDREN

Children vary in age, weight, surface area, and the ability to absorb, metabolize, and excrete medications. Children's drug dosages are lower than those of adults, so special caution is needed in preparing drug dosages

for them. Drugs are usually not prepared and packaged in standardized dosage ranges for children. Preparing an ordered dosage from an available amount requires careful calculation.

A child's parents are valuable resources for learning the best way to give a child medications. Sometimes it is less traumatic for the child if a parent gives the drug and the nurse supervises.

All children require special psychological preparation before receiving medications. Supportive care is needed if a child is expected to cooperate. The nurse explains the procedure to a child, using short words and simple language appropriate to the child's level of comprehension. Long explanations may increase a child's anxiety, especially for painful procedures such as an injection. The nurse must approach a child with confidence and act as though the child is expected to cooperate (Whaley and Wong, 1987). If it is possible to involve the child, the nurse may have greater success giving a medication.

Tips for Administering Drugs to Children

ORAL MEDICATIONS

- Liquid forms are safer to swallow to avoid aspiration.
- Offer juice, a soft drink, or frozen juice bar after a drug is swallowed.
- Carbonated beverages poured over finely crushed ice reduce nausea.
- When mixing drugs with palatable flavorings such as syrup or honey, use only a small amount. (The child may refuse to take all of a larger mixture.)
- A plastic disposable syringe is the most accurate device for preparing liquid dosages. (Cups, teaspoons, and droppers are inaccurate.)
- When administering liquid drugs, a spoon, plastic cup, or oral syringe (without needle) are useful.

INJECTIONS

- Be very careful in selecting intramuscular injection sites. Infants and small children have underdeveloped muscles.
- Children can be unpredictable and uncooperative. Have someone available to restrain a child if needed.
- Always awaken a sleeping child before giving an injection.
- Distracting the child with conversation or a toy may reduce pain perception.

For example, saying "It's time to take your pill now. Do you want it with water or juice?" allows a child to make a choice. *Never* give the child the option of taking a medication. After a drug is given, the nurse praises the child and may even offer a simple reward such as a star or token.

Depending on the route of administration, a number of tips exist for effective drug administration for children (see box).

OLDER ADULTS

The elderly also require special consideration during drug administration. Age has an effect on the absorption, distribution, metabolism, and excretion of drugs (see earlier section). In addition to physiological changes of aging, behavioral and economic factors influence an elderly person's use of drugs.

Noncompliance with drug therapy is the failure of clients to follow instructions regarding the use of medication, which is a problem more complicated than simply forgetting to take a medication. Noncompliance may involve failure to take a medication by choice, intentional reduction in drug dosage, failure to take a drug at the right time, increasing the frequency or dosage of medication, or discontinuing use of a drug prematurely. Elderly clients may also deny the presence of an illness and therefore choose not to take a medication.

Although noncompliance may occur in any age group, it is a special problem for the elderly. An older person is more prone to suffer serious physical effects from a particular disease when medications are not taken. Simonson (1984) summarizes the following client-related factors that may cause noncompliance with drug therapy in the elderly:

1. *Lack of understanding of drug therapy*—Elderly clients can easily become confused when prescribed several medications.
2. *Poor self-medication practices*—Clients may consume more nonprescription drugs than needed. These drugs can interfere with the action of prescription drugs.
3. *Lack of social supervision*—Persons living alone are less likely to comply with prescribed drug therapy than those living with another person.
4. *Feeling too ill or tired to take medication*—These feelings may be complicated by an elderly person's difficulty with ambulating and adverse effects of certain drugs.
5. *Sensory losses*—Visual alterations make it difficult to read prescriptions. Hearing problems may alter the ability to understand oral instructions.
6. *Keeping old prescriptions and self-dosing*—These medications may be inappropriate or have little therapeutic effect.

7. *Economic status*—The high costs of certain medications are not affordable for many clients on a fixed income.

Compliance can be improved by offering clients simple, realistic plans for drug therapy. The least possible number of medications and regimens should be prescribed to complement daily habits (for example, meal and bedtime). Eliopoulos (1987) makes the following recommendations for instructing and assisting the elderly with drug regimens:

1. Provide a detailed written and oral description to the client or care giver. Outline the drug's name, dosage schedule, route of administration, action, special precautions, incompatible foods or drugs, and adverse reactions.
2. Offer a color-coded dosage schedule for persons who have visual deficits or are illiterate.
3. Be sure all medication labels are typed in large print.
4. Provide medicine containers with easy-to-remove caps for weak or arthritic hands.
5. Offer memory aids to remind clients of medication schedules (for example, partitioned plastic box containing prescribed doses for one week, labeled plastic baggies holding each timed dose, or a color-coded chart describing each drug and time to be taken).

ORAL DRUG ADMINISTRATION

The most desirable way to administer medications is by mouth (Procedure 15-1). Unless the client has impairment of gastrointestinal functioning or is unable to swallow, an oral medication is the safest and easiest to give.

Most tablets and capsules should be swallowed and administered with an adequate amount of fluid, providing an opportunity for the nurse to increase a client's fluid intake. For clients with nasogastric feeding tubes, liquid medications are preferred but some tablets can be crushed and capsules opened to mix in a solution for administration (see box on p. 391).

When administering medication orally, the nurse must protect the client against possible aspiration. Positioning the client in a sitting or side-lying position will prevent accumulation of liquid or solid medication in the back of the throat. A client who swallows slowly should not be forced to take a large amount of liquid with each swallow. Likewise, a client should swallow only one pill or capsule at a time. If a client begins to cough while taking a medication, the nurse withholds the remaining portion of the drug until the client can breathe easily.

PROCEDURE 15-1

Administering Oral Medications

STEPS	RATIONALE
1. Assess for any contraindications to client receiving oral medication: Is client able to swallow? Is client suffering from nausea or vomiting? Is client diagnosed as having bowel inflammation or reduced peristalsis? Has client had recent gastrointestinal surgery? Does client have gastric suction?	Alterations in gastrointestinal function interfere with drug distribution, absorption, and excretion. Medication can be suctioned from gastrointestinal tract before it can be absorbed.
2. Determine client's preferences for fluids.	Offering fluids during drug administration is excellent way to increase fluid intake.
3. Prepare needed supplies and equipment: a. Medication cards, record form, or computer printout b. Medication cart or tray c. Disposable medication cups d. Glass of water, juice, or preferred liquid e. Drinking straw f. Mortar and pestle (optional) g. Paper towels	Used to crush tablets for clients who have difficulty swallowing.
4. Check accuracy and completeness of each medication card, form, or printout with physician's written medication order. Check client's name, drug name and dosage, route of administration, and time for administration.	Physician's order is most reliable source and only legal record of drugs client is to receive. (Report discrepancy in order to charge nurse or physician.)
5. Prepare drug. a. Wash hands.	Reduces transfer of microorganisms from nurse's hands to medications and equipment.
b. Arrange medication tray and cups in medicine room or move medication cart to position outside client's room.	Organization of equipment saves time and reduces error.
c. Unlock medicine drawer or cart. (Narcotics are stored in a locked box.)	Medications are safeguarded when locked in cabinet or cart.
d. Prepare medications for one client at a time. Keep medication tickets or forms for each client together.	Prevents preparation errors.
e. Select correct drug from stock supply or unit dose drawer. Compare label of medication with medication form, card, or printout.	Reading label against transcribed order reduces error.
f. Calculate correct drug dosage. Take time. Double check calculation.	Calculation is more accurate when information from drug label is at hand.
g. To prepare tablet or capsules from bottle, pour required number into bottle cap and transfer medications to medication cup. Do not touch medicines with fingers. Extra tablets or capsules may be returned to bottle.	Aseptic technique maintains cleanliness of drugs. Drugs are very expensive; avoid waste.
h. To prepare unit dose tablets or capsules, place packaged tablet or capsule directly into medicine cup. (Do not remove wrapper.)	Wrappers maintain cleanliness and identification of medications.
i. All tablets or capsules given to client at same time may be placed in one cup except for those requiring preadministration assessments (for example, pulse rate or blood pressure).	Keeping medications that require preadministration assessments separate from others makes it easier for the nurse to withhold drugs as necessary.
j. If client has difficulty swallowing, grind tablets in mortar with pestle. Place tablet in bottom of mortar and mix. Continue to crush fragments of tablet until smooth powder remains or place tablet between two medication cups and grind with a blunt instrument. Mix tablet in small amount of soft food, such as custard or applesauce.	Large tablets can be difficult to swallow. Ground tablet mixed with palatable soft food is usually easy to swallow.

STEPS	RATIONALE
k. Prepare liquids (see illustration).	
(1) Remove bottle cap from container and place cap upside down.	Prevents contamination of inside of cap.
(2) Hold bottle with label against palm of hand while pouring.	Spilled liquid will not soil or fade label.
(3) Hold medication cup at eye level and fill to desired level on scale. (Scale should be even with fluid level at its surface or base of meniscus, not edges.)	Ensures accuracy of measurement
(4) Discard excess liquid in cup into sink. Wipe lip of bottle with paper towel.	Prevents contamination of bottle's contents and prevents bottle cap from sticking.
l. When preparing narcotic, check narcotic record for previous drug count and compare with supply available.	Controlled substance laws require careful monitoring of dispensed narcotics.
(1) Narcotics are kept in specially designed plastic containers that are sectioned and numbered (see illustration). Remove the next available tablet and drop it in a cup. Complete necessary information on narcotic form and sign.	
m. Compare medication form, card, or printout with prepared drug and container.	Reading label second time reduces error.
n. Return stock containers or unused unit-dose medications to shelf or drawer and read label again.	Third check of label reduces administration errors.
o. Place medications and cards, form, or printout together on tray or cart.	Drugs are labeled at all times for identification.
p. Do not leave drugs unattended.	Nurse is responsible for safekeeping of drugs.
6. Administering medications	
a. Take medications to client at correct time.	Medications are administered within 30 min before or after prescribed time to ensure intended therapeutic effect. Stat or single-order medications should be given at time ordered.
b. Identify client by comparing name on card, printout form, or with name on client's identification bracelet. Ask client to state his full name.	Identification bracelets are made at time of client's admission and are most reliable source of identification. Replace any missing or faded identification bracelets.
c. Perform necessary preadministration assessment for specific medications (for example, blood pressure or pulse).	Assessment data determine whether specific medications should be given at that time.

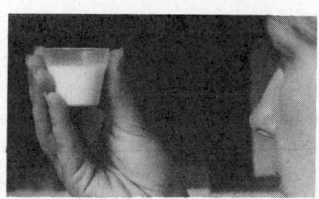

Step 5k

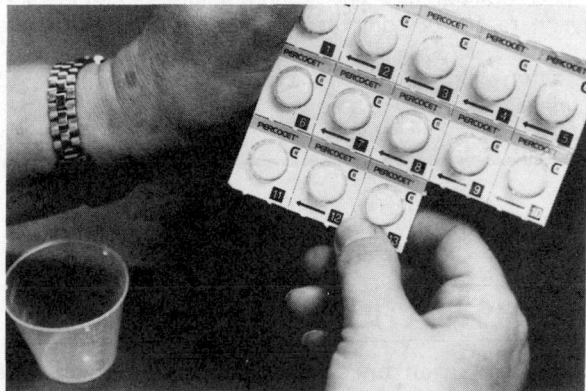

Step 5l (1)

Continued.

PROCEDURE 15-1, cont'd

Administering Oral Medications

STEPS	RATIONALE
d. Explain purpose of each medication and its action to client. Allow client to ask any questions about drugs.	Client has right to be informed, and client's understanding of purpose of each medication will improve compliance with drug therapy.
e. Assist client to sitting or side-lying position.	Sitting position prevents aspiration during swallowing.
f. Administer drugs properly.	
(1) Client may wish to hold solid medications in hand or cup before placing in mouth.	Client can become familiar with medications by seeing each drug.
(2) Offer full glass of water or juice with drugs to be swallowed. Give cold carbonated water if available.	Choice of fluid promotes client's comfort and can improve fluid intake. Carbonated water helps passage of tablet through esophagus (Hasselbalch, 1985).
(3) For sublingual administered drugs, have client place medication under tongue and allow it to dissolve completely. Caution client against swallowing.	Drug is absorbed through blood vessels of undersurface of tongue. If swallowed, drug is destroyed by gastric juices or so rapidly detoxified by liver that therapeutic blood levels are not attained.
(4) Mix powdered medications with liquids at bedside and give to client to drink.	When prepared in advance, powdered drug forms may thicken and even harden, making swallowing difficult.
(5) Caution client against chewing or swallowing lozenges.	Drug acts through slow absorption through oral mucosa, not gastric mucosa.
(6) Give effervescent powders and tablets immediately after dissolving.	Effervescence helps improve unpleasant taste of drug and often has therapeutic value for gastrointestinal problems.
g. If client is unable to hold medications, place medication cup to his lips and gently introduce each drug into his mouth, one at a time. Do not rush.	Prevents contamination of medications. Administering single tablet or capsule eases swallowing and prevents aspiration.
h. If tablet or capsule falls to floor, discard it and repeat preparation.	Drug is contaminated when it touches floor.
i. Stay with client until each medication has been completely swallowed. If uncertain whether client has swallowed medication, ask him to open his mouth.	Nurse assumes responsibility for ensuring that client receives ordered dosage. If left unattended, client may not take dose or may save drugs, causing risk to his health.
j. For highly acidic medications (for example, aspirin) offer client nonfat snack (for example, crackers).	Reduces gastric irritation.
k. Assist client in returning to comfortable position.	Maintains client's comfort
l. Dispose of soiled supplies and wash hands.	Reduces transmission of microorganisms.
m. Return medication cards, forms, or printouts to appropriate file for next administration time.	Cards, forms, and printouts are used as reference for when next dosage is due. Loss can lead to administration error.
n. Replenish stock such as cups and straws, return cart to medicine room, and clean work area.	Clean working space assists other staff in completing duties efficiently.
7. Record actual time each drug administered on medication record or computer. Include initials or signature (see Fig. 15-5).	Prompt documentation prevents errors such as repeated doses. Nurse's signature establishes accountability for administration.
8. Return within 30 min to evaluate client's response to medications.	Nurse assesses drug's therapeutic benefit and can detect onset of side effects or allergic reactions.

ADMINISTRATION OF INJECTIONS

Administering an injection is an invasive procedure that must be performed using aseptic techniques (see box). Once a needle pierces the skin, the risk of infection exists. The nurse administers drugs parenterally by one of the following routes: subcutaneous, intramuscular, intradermal, and intravenous. Each type of injection requires certain skills to ensure that the drug reaches the proper location. The effects of a parenterally administered drug can develop rapidly, depending on the rate

Guidelines for Giving Drugs Through a Nasogastric Tube

- Read medication labels carefully before crushing a tablet or opening a capsule.
- Compressed tablets can almost always be crushed because they are designed to break up in the stomach to release the drug.
- Crush any tablets or capsules into a fine powder for better absorption.
- Buccal or sublingual tablets should *not* be crushed. Give as intended.
- Do not crush enteric-coated tablets.
- Do not crush hard, gelatin capsules. Instead, open the capsule and pour out the contents.
- Do not crush sustained-action capsules because they can cause stomach irritation.
- Soft, gelatin capsules should be dissolved in a cup of water before being given.
- If no contraindications exist for drugs to be taken together orally, mix the powder from several capsules together.
- Place powder in the cup and add 20 to 30 ml warm water.
- Administer medications following agency guidelines for bolus-tube feedings (see Chapter 33).
- Follow medications with at least 60 cc H_2O.
- Medications that cannot be crushed into fine powder should not be given through small-bore feeding tubes because tube will occlude

Preventing Infection During an Injection

- To prevent contamination of solution, draw medication from ampule quickly. Do not allow it to stand open.
- To prevent needle contamination, avoid letting needle touch contaminated surface (for example, outer edges of ampule or vial, outer surface of needle cap, nurse's hands, countertop, or table surface).
- To prevent syringe contamination, avoid touching length of plunger or inner part of barrel. Keep tip of syringe covered with cap or needle.
- To prepare skin, wash skin soiled with dirt, drainage, or feces with soap and water, and dry. Use friction and a circular motion while cleaning with an antiseptic swab. Swab from center of site, and move outward in a 2-inch radius.

of drug absorption. The nurse closely observes the client's response.

Equipment

A variety of syringes and needles are available, each designed to deliver a certain volume of a drug to a specific type of tissue. The nurse uses judgment in determining which syringe or needle will be most effective.

SYRINGES

Syringes consist of a cylindrical barrel with a tip designed to fit the hub of a hypodermic needle and a close-fitting plunger (Fig. 15-8). Most health care institutions use disposable, single-use plastic syringes, which are inexpensive and easy to manipulate. The syringes are packaged separately, with or without a sterile needle in a paper wrapper or rigid plastic container (Fig. 15-9). Glass syringes are also available although they are not commonly used.

The nurse fills a syringe by aspiration, pulling the plunger outward while the needle tip remains immersed in the prepared solution. The nurse may handle the outside of the syringe barrel and the handle of the plunger. To maintain sterility the nurse avoids letting any unsterile object touch the tip or inside of the barrel, the shaft of the plunger, or the needle.

Syringes come in a number of sizes, from 1 to 50 ml. It is unusual to use a syringe larger than 5 ml for an injection. A 2 to 3 ml syringe is adequate for intramuscular and subcutaneous injections. A larger volume creates discomfort. The 2.5 or 3 ml hypodermic syringe often comes prepackaged with a needle attached. However, the nurse may change needle sizes. The hypodermic has two scales along the barrel. One scale is divided into minims and the other into tenths of a milliliter.

An insulin syringe (Fig. 15-9) holds 1 ml and is calibrated in units. Most insulin syringes in the United States and Canada are U-100s, designed for use with U-100 strength insulin. Each milliliter of solution contains 100 units of insulin. In the United States, there are also U-40 and U-500 strengths of insulin preparations.

The tuberculin syringe (Fig. 15-9) has a long, thin barrel with a preattached thin needle. The syringe is calibrated in sixteenths of a minim and hundredths of

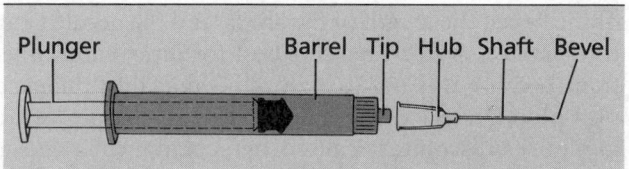

Fig. 15-8 Parts of a syringe and hypodermic needle.

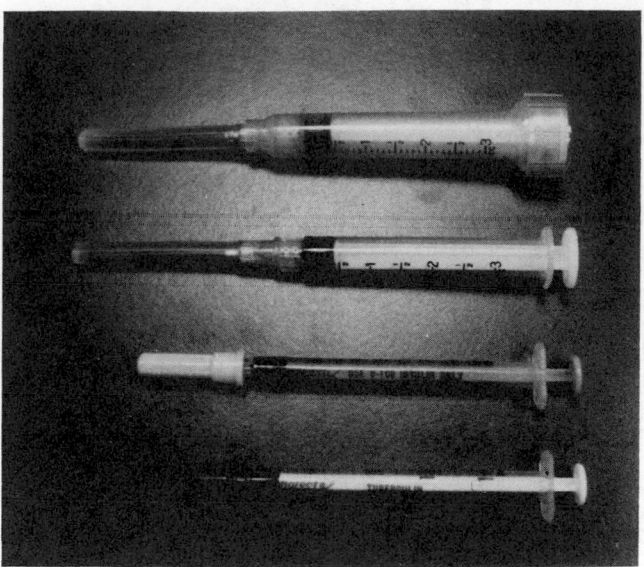

Fig. 15-9 Types of syringes. *From top to bottom:* disposable plastic syringe and needle in case, 3 cc hypodermic syringe, insulin syringe, and Tuberculin syringe.

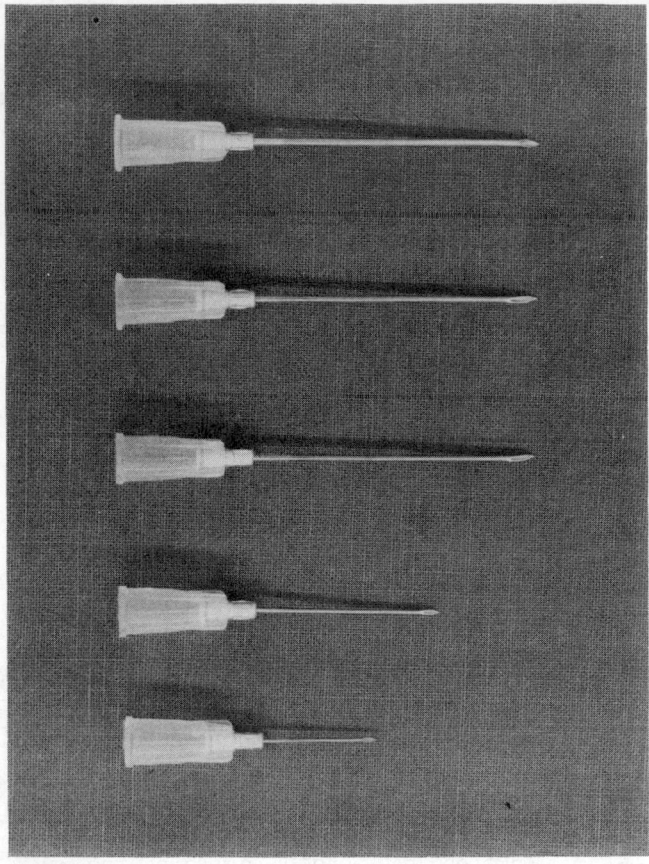

Fig. 15-10 Hypodermic needles arranged in order of gauge. *Top to bottom:* 16-gauge, 19-gauge, 20-gauge, 23-gauge, and 25-gauge.

a milliliter and has a capacity of 1 ml. The nurse uses a tuberculin syringe to prepare small amounts of potent drugs. A tuberculin syringe is also useful in preparing small, precise doses for infants or young children.

The nurse uses large hypodermic syringes to administer certain intravenous drugs, add medications to intravenous solutions, and, with the needle removed, to irrigate wounds or drainage tubes.

NEEDLES

Needles come packaged in individual sheaths to allow flexibility in choosing the right needle for a client. Some needles are preattached to standard-size syringes. Most needles are made of stainless steel, although intravenous catheters are plastic. Needles are disposable, except for those made from surgical steel, which are attached to glass syringes.

The needle has three parts: the hub, which fits onto the tip of a syringe; the shaft, which connects to the hub; and the bevel or slanted tip (see Fig. 15-8). The nurse may handle the needle hub to ensure a tight fit on the syringe. However, the shaft and bevel must remain sterile at all times.

Each needle has three characteristic features: the slant of the bevel, the length of the shaft, and the needle gauge or diameter. A short bevel is best for intravenous injections because it is not easily occluded against the inside of a blood vessel wall. Long bevels are sharper, which minimizes discomfort caused by subcutaneous and intramuscular injections. Needles vary in length from ¼ to 5 inches, although 1½ inches is the maximum length

for injections given by nurses. The nurse chooses needle length according to client size and weight and the type of tissue into which the drug is to be injected. A child or a slender adult generally requires a shorter needle. The nurse uses a longer needle (usually 1 to 1½ inches) for intramuscular injections and a shorter needle (usually ⅜ to ⅝ inch) for subcutaneous injections.

The smaller the gauge, the larger the needle diameter (Fig. 15-10). The selection of a gauge depends on the viscosity of the fluid to be injected or infused. A 16- or 18-gauge large-diameter needle is ideal for infusing blood products because the needle causes less trauma to red blood cells. An intramuscular injection usually requires a 19 to 23- gauge needle, depending on the viscosity of the medication. Subcutaneous injections require smaller-diameter needles, such as a 25-gauge needle, but for an intradermal injection a 26-gauge needle is used.

DISPOSABLE INJECTION UNITS

Disposable, single-dose, prefilled syringes are available for some medications. The nurse checks the dosage and expels any unneeded portion of the drug.

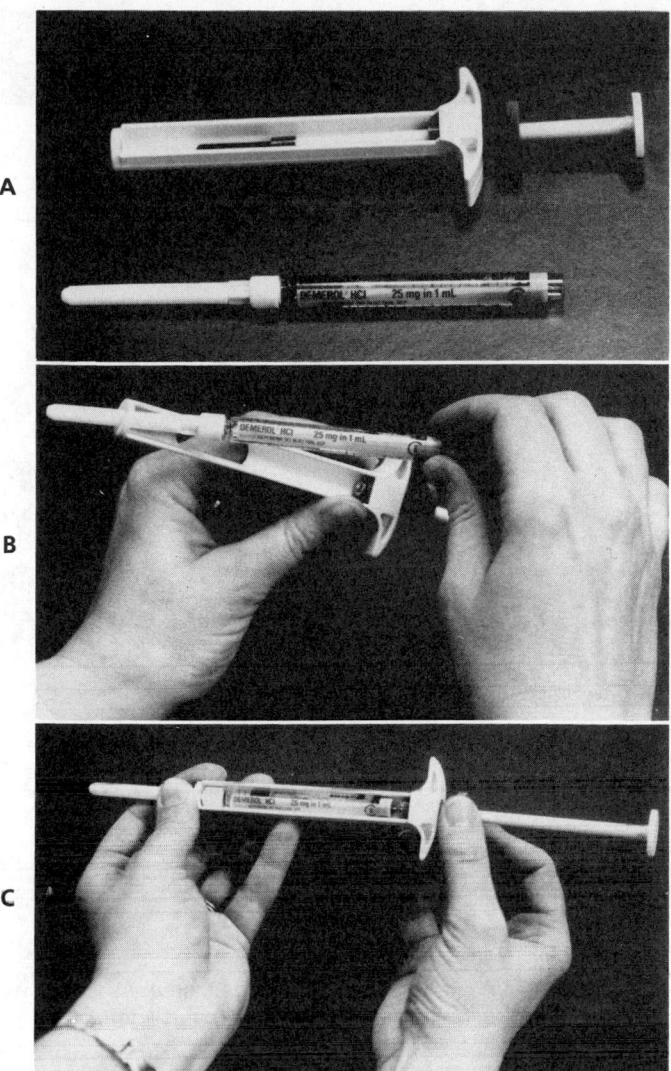

Fig. 15-11 **A,** Carpuject syringe and prefilled sterile cartridge with needle. **B,** Assembling the carpuject. **C,** The cartridge slides into the syringe barrel, turns and locks at the needle end. The plunger then screws into the cartridge end.

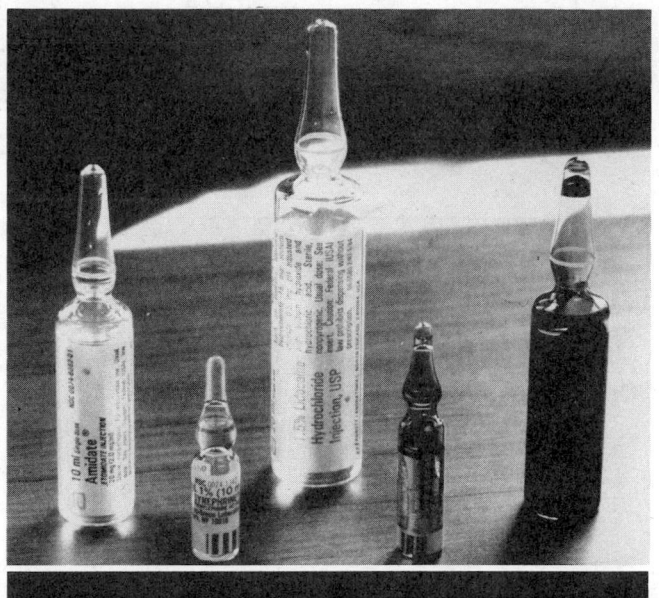

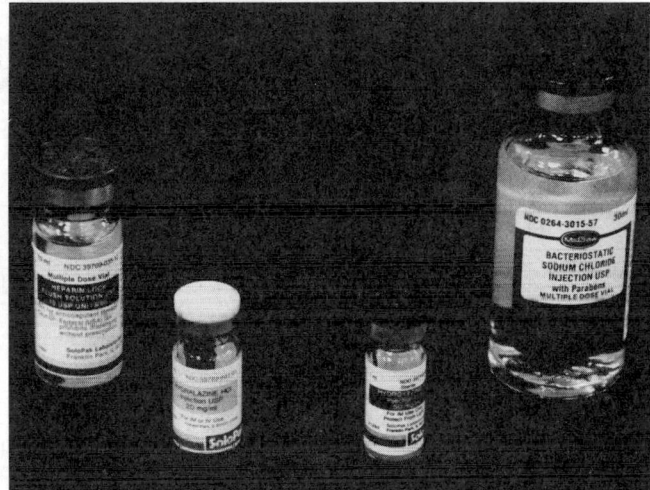

Fig. 15-12 **A,** Ampules. **B,** Vials.

The Tubex and Carpuject injection systems include reusable plastic syringes that hold prefilled, disposable, sterile cartridge-needle units (Fig. 15-11). The nurse slips the cartridge into the syringe, secures it (following package directions), and checks for air bubbles in the syringe. The nurse advances the plunger to expel the medication as in a regular syringe. A new type of injection system involves screwing a plunger-like device into the end of a prefilled vial containing a needle. After the medication is given the entire unit is disposed of in a receptacle.

Preparing an Injection from an Ampule

Ampules contain single doses of medication in a liquid and are available in several sizes, from 1 ml to 10 ml or more (Fig. 15-12, *A*). An ampule is made of clear glass with a constricted neck that must be snapped off to allow access to the medication. A colored ring around the neck indicates where the ampule is prescored to be broken easily. The nurse uses a file to scratch the neck of an ampule that is not prescored. Aspiration of the drug into a syringe occurs easily (Procedure 15-2).

Preparing an Injection from a Vial

A vial is a single-dose or multidose glass container with a rubber seal at the top (Fig. 15-12, *B*). A metal cap protects the seal until it is ready for use. Vials contain liquid or dry forms of medications. Drugs that are unstable in solution are packaged dry. The vial label spec-

PROCEDURE 15-2

Preparing Injections from Ampules and Vials

STEPS	RATIONALE

1. Wash hands.
2. Prepare needed equipment and supplies:
   a. Ampules
      (1) Ampule containing medication
      (2) Syringe and needle
      (3) Small gauze pad or alcohol swab
      (4) Container for disposing of glass
      (5) Small metal file (optional)
   b. Vials
      (1) Vial with medication
      (2) Syringe and needle
      (3) Alcohol swab
      (4) Solvent (for example, normal saline or sterile water)
   c. Medication card, form, or printout.
3. Assemble supplies at work area in medicine room.
4. Check the medication card, form, or printout against the label on the ampule or vial.
5. Ampule
   a. Tap top of ampule lightly and quickly with finger until fluid leaves neck (see illustration).
   b. Partially file neck of ampule if it is not prescored. Place small gauze pad or dry alcohol swab around neck of ampule.
   c. Snap neck of ampule quickly and firmly away from hands (see illustration).
   d. Draw up medication quickly.
      Hold ampule upside down or set it on flat surface. Insert syringe needle into center of ampule opening (see illustration). Do not allow needle tip or shaft to touch rim of ampule
   e. Aspirate medication into syringe by gently pulling back on plunger (see illustration).
   f. Keep needle tip below surface of liquid. Tip ampule to bring all fluid within reach of needle.
   g. If air bubbles are aspirated, do not expel air into ampule.

Reduces transmission of infection.

Used to score or etch cut into ampule's glass neck.

Used to dissolve drugs in dry form.

Verifies order.
Makes procedure orderly.
Ensures right drug and dosage is being prepared.

Dislodges any fluid that collects above the neck. All solution moves into lower chamber.
Filing ensures a clean break. Placing pad or swab around neck protects nurse's fingers from trauma as glass tip is broken off.
Prevents shattering glass toward or in nurse's fingers or face.
System open to airborne contaminants.
Broken rim of ampule is considered contaminated. As long as needle tip or shaft does not touch ampule's rim, solution does not dribble out.

Withdrawal of plunger creates negative pressure within syringe barrel, which pulls fluid into syringe.
Prevents aspiration of air bubbles.

Air pressure may force fluid out of ampule, and medication will be lost.

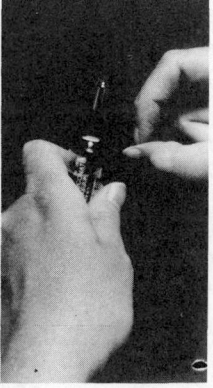

Step 5a

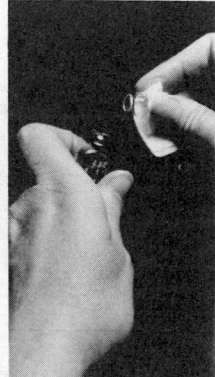

Step 5c

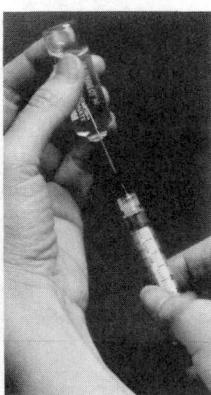

Step 5d

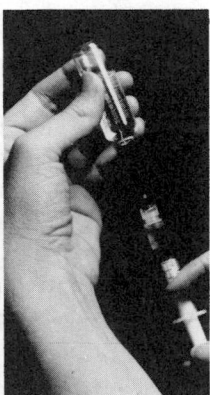

Step 5e

STEPS	RATIONALE
h. To expel excess air bubbles, remove needle from ampule. Hold syringe with needle pointing up. Tap side of syringe to cause bubbles to rise toward needle. Draw back slightly on the plunger, and then push the plunger upward to eject the air. *Do not eject fluid.*	Withdrawing plunger too far will pull it from barrel. Holding syringe vertically allows fluid to settle in bottom of barrel. Pulling back on plunger allows fluid within needle to enter barrel so fluid is not expelled. Air at top of barrel and within needle is then expelled.
i. If syringe contains excess fluid, use sink for disposal. Hold syringe vertically with needle tip up and slanted slightly toward sink. Slowly eject excess fluid into sink. Recheck fluid level in syringe by holding it vertically.	Medication is safely dispersed into sink. Position of needle allows medication to be expelled without it flowing down needle shaft. Rechecking fluid level ensures proper dosage.
j. Cover needle with its sheath or cap. Change needle on syringe.	Prevents contamination of needle and protects nurse from needle stick. Changing needle is required if nurse suspects medication is on needle shaft. New needle prevents tracking medication through skin and subcutaneous tissues.
k. Dispose of soiled supplies. Place broken ampule in special container for glass. Clean work area. Wash hands.	Controls transmission of infection. Proper disposal of glass prevents accidental injury to personnel.
6. Vial	
a. Remove metal cap covering top of unused vial. Expose rubber seal.	Vial comes packaged with cap to prevent contamination of rubber seal.
b. Wipe off surface of rubber seal with alcohol swab.	Removes dust or grease but does not sterilize surface.
c. Take syringe and remove needle cap. Pull back on plunger to draw amount of air into syringe equivalent to volume of medication to be aspirated from vial (see illustration).	To prevent buildup of negative pressure in vial when aspirating medication, air must first be injected into vial.
d. Insert tip of needle, with bevel pointing up, through center of rubber seal (see illustration). Apply pressure to tip of needle during insertion.	Center of seal is thinner and easier to penetrate. Keeping bevel up and using firm pressure prevents cutting rubber core from seal.
e. Inject air into vial, holding on to plunger.	Air must be injected before aspirating fluid. Plunger may be forced backward by air pressure within vial.
f. Invert vial while keeping firm hold on syringe and plunger (see illustration). Hold vial between thumb and middle fingers of nondominant hand. Grasp end of syringe barrel and plunger with thumb and forefinger of dominant hand.	Inverting vial allows fluid to settle in lower half of container. Position of hands prevents movement of plunger and permits easy manipulation of syringe.

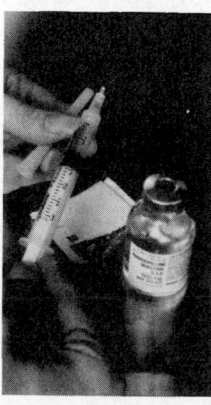
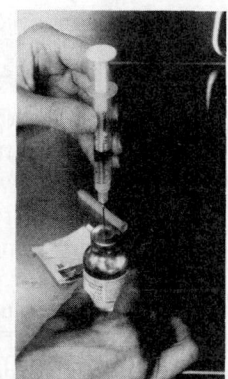
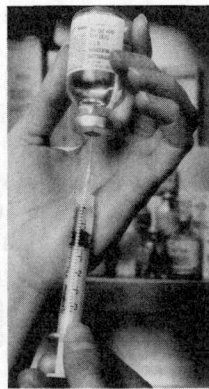
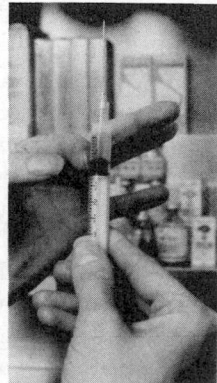

Step 6c   **Step 6d**   **Step 6f**   **Step 6k**

Continued.

PROCEDURE 15-2, cont'd

Preparing Injections from Ampules and Vials

STEPS	RATIONALE
g. Keep tip of needle below fluid level.	Prevents aspiration of air.
h. Allow air pressure to fill syringe gradually with medication. Pull back slightly on plunger if necessary.	Positive pressure within vial forces fluid into syringe.
i. Tap side of syringe barrel carefully to dislodge any air bubbles. Eject any air remaining at top of syringe into vial.	Forcefully striking barrel while needle is inserted in vial may bend needle. Accumulation of air displaces medication and causes dosage errors.
j. Once correct volume is obtained, remove needle from vial by pulling back on barrel of syringe.	Pulling plunger rather than barrel causes separation from barrel and loss of medication.
k. Remove any remaining air from syringe by holding it and needle upright. Tap barrel to dislodge any air bubbles (see illustration). Draw back slightly on plunger, then push plunger upward to eject air. Do not eject fluid.	Holding syringe vertically allows fluid to settle in bottom of barrel. Pulling back on plunger allows fluid within needle to enter barrel so fluid is not expelled. Air at top of barrel and within needle is then expelled.
l. Change needle and cover.	Inserting needle through a rubber stopper may blunt bevel. New needle is sharper, and because no fluid is along shaft, it will not track medication through tissues.
m. For multidose vial, make label that includes date of mixing, concentration of drug per milliliter, and nurse's initials.	Ensures that future doses will be prepared correctly. Certain drugs should be discarded after set number of days after mixing of vial.
n. Dipose of soiled supplies in proper containers. Clean work area.	Prevents transmission of infection.
o. Wash hands.	Reduces transmission of microorganisms.
7. Check fluid level in syringe and compare with desired dosage.	Ensures that accurate dosage has been prepared.

ifies the solvent used to dissolve the drug and the amount of solvent needed to prepare a desired drug concentration. Normal saline and sterile distilled water are solutions commonly used to dissolve drugs.

Unlike the ampule, the vial is a closed system, and air must be injected into it to permit easy withdrawal of the solution. Failure to inject air when withdrawing solution creates a vacuum within the vial that makes withdrawal difficult (Procedure 15-2).

To prepare a powdered drug, the nurse draws up the amount of diluent or solvent recommended on the vial's label. The nurse injects the solvent into the vial in the same manner as injecting air into the vial. Most powdered drugs dissolve easily, but it may be necessary to withdraw the needle to mix the contents thoroughly. Gently shaking or rolling the vial between the hands will dissolve the powdered drug. The needle is reinserted to draw up the dissolved medication. After mixing multidose vials the nurse makes a label that includes the date of mixing and concentration of drug per milliliter. Multidose vials may require refrigeration after contents are reconstituted.

Mixing Medications

If two drugs are compatible, it is possible to mix them together in one injection if the total dosage is within accepted limits. A client will appreciate not having to receive more than one injection at a time. Most nursing units have charts that list common compatible drugs. If there is any uncertainty about drug compatibilities, a pharmacist should be consulted.

MIXING MEDICATIONS FROM TWO VIALS

The nurse follows the following principles when mixing medications from two vials: (1) do not contaminate one medication with another, (2) ensure that the final dosage is accurate, and (3) maintain aseptic technique.

Only one syringe is needed to mix medications from two vials (Fig 15-13). The nurse takes a syringe and aspirates the volume of air equivalent to the first drug's dosage (vial A). The nurse injects air into Vial A, making sure the needle does not touch the solution. The nurse withdraws the needle, aspirates air equivalent to the second drug's dosage (Vial B), then injects the volume of air into vial B. The nurse immediately withdraws the

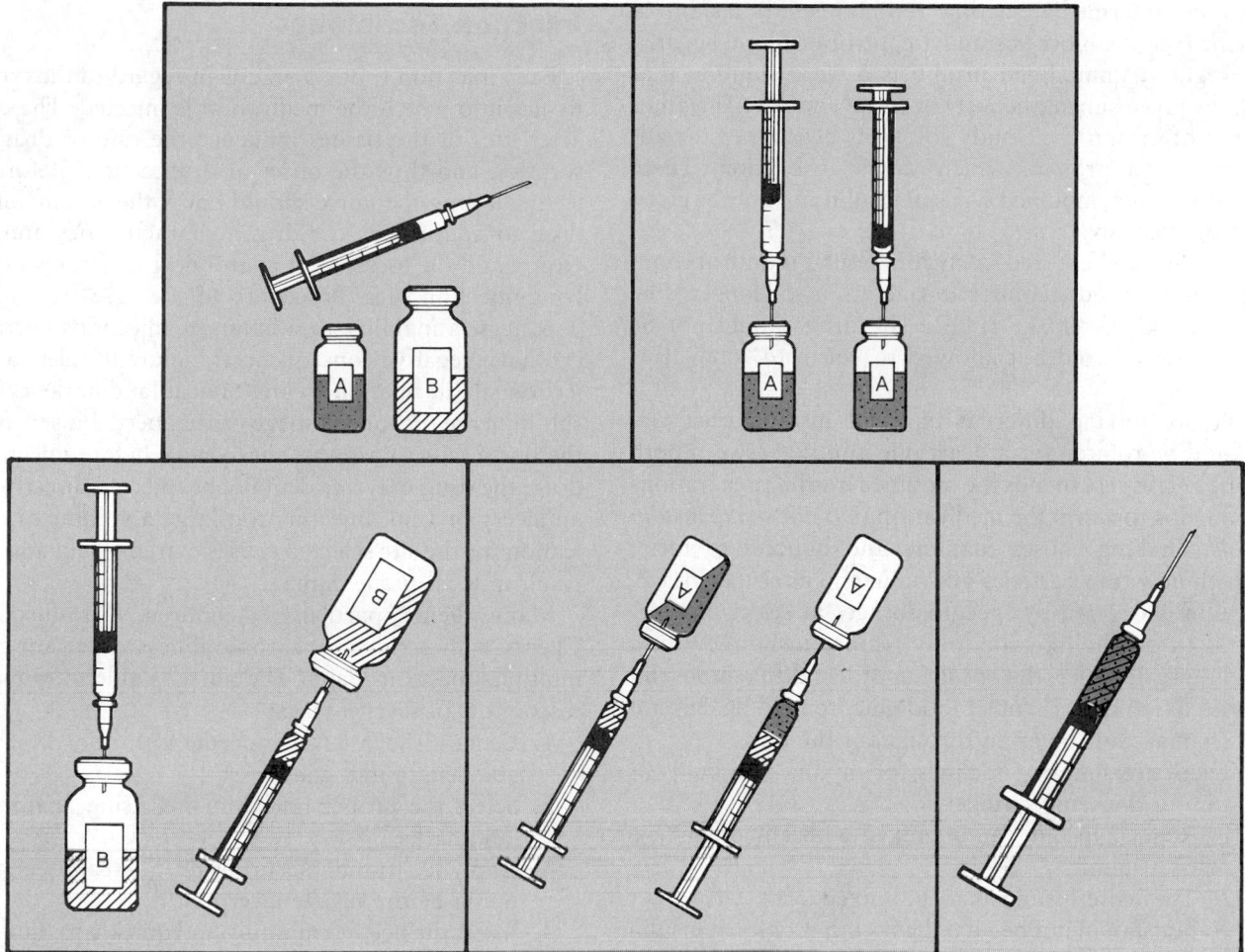

Fig. 15-13 Steps in mixing medications from two vials.

required medication from vial B into the syringe. At this point the drug from vial A has not contaminated vial B.

The nurse applies a new sterile needle to the syringe and inserts it into vial A, being careful not to push the plunger and expel the drug within the syringe into the vial. The nurse then withdraws the desired amount of drug from vial A into the syringe. If a vial has excess positive pressure, the plunger may begin to move before the nurse is ready. This can cause an accidental withdrawal of too much of the drug. After withdrawing the necessary amount of solution, the nurse withdraws the needle, applies a new needle, and sheaths the syringe.

MIXING MEDICATIONS FROM ONE VIAL AND ONE AMPULE

Mixing medications from a vial and an ampule is simple because it is unnecessary to add air to withdraw medication from an ampule. The nurse prepares medication from the vial first and then, using the same syringe and needle, withdraws medication from the ampule.

This technique prevents contamination of solutions and the needle.

INSULIN PREPARATION

Insulin is the hormone used to treat diabetes. The drug must be administered by injection because it is a protein and therefore would be digested and destroyed in the gastrointestinal tract. Most clients with diabetes requiring insulin learn to self-administer injections. In the United States and Canada, the drug is available most commonly in 100 units per milliliter of solution. In the United States, 40 units per milliliter is also available. When preparing insulin, the correct syringe must be used. For example, a 100-unit scaled syringe is used only to prepare 100-unit insulin.

Insulin is classified by rate of action, including rapid, intermediate, and long acting. Each type has a different onset, peak, and duration of action. A client with diabetes may require more than one type of insulin. For example, by receiving a rapid-acting (regular insulin) and an intermediate-acting (NPH insulin) insulin, a client receives more sustained control of blood sugar.

Regular, unmodified insulin is a clear solution that can be given subcutaneously or intravenously. The other types of insulin are cloudy solutions because of the addition of a protein, which slows absorption. These slower-acting, modified types of insulin can only be given subcutaneously.

Insulin can be stored safely for about 1 month at room temperature, but requires refrigeration for longer time periods (Clark et al., 1986). The drug should not be administered cold but allowed to warm to room temperature.

Before mixing different types of insulin, each vial should be rotated for at least one minute between both hands. This resuspends the modified insulin preparations and helps to warm the medication. *Do not shake insulin vials.* Shaking causes foaming and bubbles to form, which may trap particles of insulin and alter the dosage. Insulin is ordered by specific dosages at select time periods or by sliding scale (only regular insulin). With a sliding scale order, the physician orders different insulin doses based on a client's blood glucose reading. Several doses may thus be given throughout the day.

There are simple guidelines for mixing two kinds of insulin in the same syringe:

1. Regular insulin can be mixed with any other type of insulin.
2. The lente insulins can be mixed with each other but should not be mixed with other types of insulin (except regular).

To prepare insulin from two vials the nurse or client follows these steps:

1. With a syringe and needle, inject air, equal to the dose of insulin to be withdrawn, into the vial of modified insulin (cloudy vial). Do not touch tip of needle to the solution.
2. Remove the syringe from the vial of modified insulin.
3. With the same syringe, inject air, equal to the dose of insulin to be withdrawn, into the vial of unmodified (regular) insulin (clear vial). Then withdraw the correct dose.
4. Remove the syringe from the unmodified (regular) insulin. Carefully remove air bubbles in the syringe.
5. Return to the vial of modified insulin, and withdraw the correct dose.
6. Administer mixture of insulins within 5 minutes of preparing it. Regular insulin binds with neutral protamine Hagedorn (NPH), and the action of the regular insulin is reduced.

Always prepare the unmodified (regular) insulin first. This prevents adding unmodified insulin to the modified (regular) vial. If two modified forms are mixed, it makes no difference which vial is prepared first.

Injection Techniques

Each injection route is unique in regard to the type of tissues into which the medication is injected. The characteristics of the tissues influence the rate of drug absorption and thus the onset of drug action. Before injecting a drug the nurse should know the volume of the drug to administer, the drug's characteristics and viscosity, and the location of anatomical structures underlying injection sites (Procedure 15-3).

A nurse's inability to administer injections correctly can have negative consequences. Failure to select an injection site in relation to anatomical landmarks can result in nerve or bone damage during needle insertion. If the nurse fails to aspirate the syringe before injecting a drug, the drug may accidentally be injected directly into an artery or vein. Injecting too large a volume of medication for the site selected causes extreme pain and may result in local tissue damage.

Many clients, particularly children, fear injections. Clients with serious or chronic illness often are given multiple injections daily. The nurse is able to minimize discomfort in several ways:

1. Using a sharp beveled needle in the smallest suitable length and gauge
2. Select the proper injection site, using anatomical landmarks
3. Apply ice to the injection sites to creat local anesthesia before needle insertion
4. Insert the needle smoothly and quickly to minimize tissue pulling
5. Hold the syringe steady while the needle remains in tissues
6. Position the client as comfortably as possible to reduce muscular tension
7. Divert the client's attention from the injection through conversation
8. Massage the injected area gently for several seconds unless contraindicated
9. Increase the duration of injection time, which may reduce pain perception (Perez, 1984).

SUBCUTANEOUS INJECTIONS

Subcutaneous injections involve depositing medication into the loose connective tissue under the dermis (Procedure 15-3). Because subcutaneous tissue is not as richly supplied with blood as the muscles, drug absorption is somewhat slower than with intramuscular injections. However, drugs are absorbed completely if circulatory status is normal. Because subcutaneous tissue contains pain receptors, the client may experience some discomfort during an injection.

The best sites for subcutaneous injections include vascular areas around the outer aspect of the upper arms, the abdomen from below the costal margins to the iliac crests, and the anterior aspect of the thighs. These areas

PROCEDURE 15-3

Administering Injections

STEPS	RATIONALE
1. Assess indications for type of injection to administer (for example, subcutaneous injection chosen when slow drug absorption desired, intramuscular injection chosen if large volume of drug to be given, intradermal route chosen for skin testing).	Ensures proper drug absorption and distribution through tissues to enhance drug action.
2. Assess medical history and history of allergies.	May influence how certain drugs act. Parenteral medications often create sensitivities in form of allergies.
3. Observe verbal and nonverbal responses toward receiving injection.	Injections can be painful. Clients may experience considerable anxiety, which can increase pain.
4. Wash hands.	Reduces transmission of microorganisms.
5. Prepare needed equipment and supplies:	
a. Proper-sized syringe	
(1) Subcutaneous: 1 to 2 ml	
(2) Intramuscular: 2 to 3 ml for adult, 1 to 2 ml for child	Volume injected should be compatible with tissue type.
(3) Intradermal: 1 ml tuberculin	
b. Proper-sized needle	Proper-sized needle avoids added injury to client and ensures proper distribution of drug into tissues.
(1) Subcutaneous: 25- to 27-gauge and ⅜ to ⅝ in in length	
(2) Intramuscular: 19- to 23-gauge and 1 to 1½ in in length for adults; 25- to 27-gauge and ½ to 1 in in length for child	
(3) Intradermal: preattached 26- to 27-gauge	
c. Antiseptic swab (for example, alcohol)	Used to cleanse skin.
d. Medication ampule or vial	
e. Medication card or form	Identifies medication dose ordered and client's name.
6. Check medication order	Ensures accuracy of order.
7. Prepare correct medication dosage from ampule or vial. Check dosage carefully. Be sure all air is expelled.	Ensures medication is sterile. Preparation techniques differ for ampule and vial.
8. For intramuscular injections prepare an air lock. Draw 0.2 cc of air in syringe, being careful not to expel drug dosage. Air moves to end of plunger.	Volume of air will be injected behind bolus of medication to clear needle of medication, preventing tracking of drug through sensitive tissues after needle is withdrawn (Wong, 1982).
9. For intramuscular injection, change needle or syringe if medication is irritating to subcutaneous tissue.	Prevents tracking of irritating substance through tissues as needle passes into muscle.
10. Identify client by checking identification armband and asking client's name.	Ensures correct client is receiving prescribed medication.
11. Explain procedure to client and proceed in calm, confident manner.	Helps client anticipate nurse's actions. Calm approach minimizes client's anxiety.
12. Close room curtains or door.	Provides for client's privacy.
13. Keep sheet or gown draped over body parts not requiring exposure.	Proper selection of injection site may require exposure of body parts.

14. Select appropriate injection site. Inspect skin surface over sites for bruises, inflammation, or edema.
  a. Subcutaneous: palpate sites for masses or tenderness.
  b. Intramuscular: note integrity and size of muscle and palpate for tenderness.
  c. Intradermal: note lesions or discolorations of forearm.
  If injections are given frequently, rotate sites.
	Injection sites should be free of abnormalities that may interfere with drug absorption. An intradermal site should be clear so results of skin test can be seen and interpreted correctly. A site used repeatedly can become hardened from lipohypertrophy.

15. Assist client to comfortable position	
a. Subcutaneous: have client relax arm, leg, or abdomen depending on site chosen.	Relaxation of site minimizes discomfort.
b. Intramuscular: have client lie flat, on his side, or prone, or have him sit, depending on site chosen.	Position that reduces strain on muscle minimizes discomfort of injections.

Continued.

PROCEDURE 15-3, cont'd

Administering Injections

STEPS	RATIONALE
c. Intradermal: have client extend elbow and support it and forearm on flat surface.	Stabilizes site for easiest accessibility.
16. Relocate site using anatomical landmarks.	Accurate injection of medication requires insertion in correct site to avoid injury to underlying tissues, blood vessels, nerves, or bone.
17. Cleanse site with an antiseptic swab. Apply the swab at center of the site and rotate outward in a circular direction for about 5 cm (2 in) (see illustration).	Mechanical action of swab removes secretions containing microorganisms.
18. Hold swab between third and fourth fingers of non-dominant hand.	Swab remains readily accessible when needle is withdrawn.
19. Remove needle cap from needle by pulling it straight off.	Preventing needle from touching sides of cap prevents contamination.
20. Hold syringe correctly between thumb and forefinger of dominant hand.	Quick, smooth injection requires proper manipulation of syringe parts.
a. Subcutaneous: hold as dart, palm up (see illustration) for 45 degree angle, and palm down for 90 degree angle.	
b. Intramuscular: hold as dart, palm down.	
c. Intradermal: hold bevel of needle pointing up.	With bevel up, medication will less likely be deposited into tissues below dermis.
21. Administer injection	
a. Subcutaneous:	
(1) For average-sized client, spread skin tightly across injection site or pinch skin with nondominant hand.	Needle penetrates tight skin easier than loose skin. Pinching skin elevates subcutaneous tissue.
(2) Inject needle quickly and firmly at 45- to 90-degree angle (see illustration). (Then release skin, if pinched.)	Quick, firm insertion minimizes discomfort. (Injecting medication into compressed tissue irritates nerve fibers.)
(3) For obese client, pinch skin at site and inject needle below tissue fold.	Obese clients have fatty layer of tissue above subcutaneous layer.

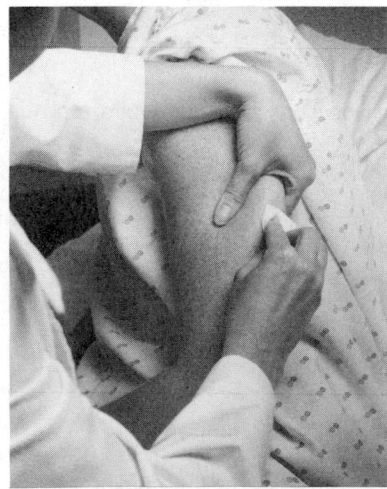

Step 17

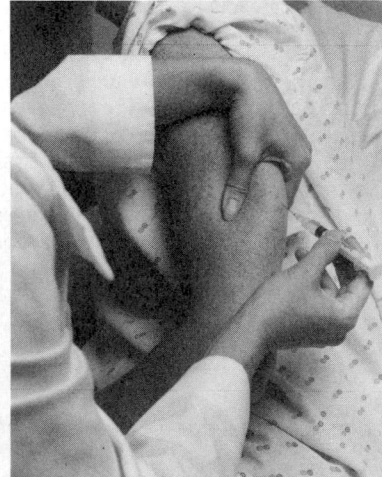

Step 20a

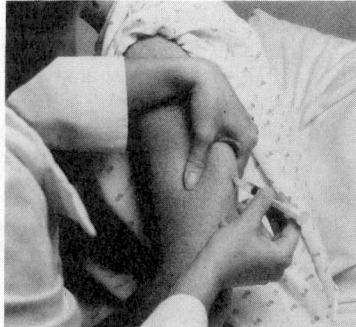

Step 21a

STEPS	RATIONALE

b. Intramuscular:
  (1) Position nondominant hand at proper anatomical landmarks and spread skin tightly. Inject needle quickly at 90-degree angle into muscle.

Speeds insertion and reduces discomfort.

  (2) If client's muscle mass is small, grasp body of muscle between thumb and other fingers.

Ensures that medication reaches muscle mass.

  (3) If medication is irritating, use Z-track method (see section on Z-track method.)

Used to prevent tracking of drug through subcutaneous tissue.

c. Intradermal:
  (1) With nondominant hand, stretch skin over site with forefinger or thumb.

Needle pierces tight skin more easily.

  (2) With needle almost against client's skin, insert it slowly at 5- to 15-degree angle until resistance is felt. Then advance needle through epidermis to approximately 3 mm (⅛ in) below skin surface. Needle tip can be seen through skin.

Ensures needle tip is in dermis.

22. Once needle enters site of subcutaneous or intramuscular injections *only,* grasp lower end of syringe barrel with nondominant hand. Move dominant hand to end of plunger. Avoid moving syringe while slowly pulling back on plunger to aspirate drug (see illustration). If blood appears in syringe, remove needle, discard medication and syringe and repeat procedure.
(It is unnecessary to aspirate an intradermal injection.)

Properly performed injection requires smooth manipulation of syringe parts. Movement of syringe may displace needle and cause discomfort. Aspiration of blood into syringe indicates intravenous placement of needle. Subcutaneous and intramuscular injections are not for intravenous use.

(Dermis is relatively avascular.)

23. Inject medication slowly.
(For intradermal injections it is normal to feel resistance; if not, needle is too deep.)

Minimizes discomfort and trauma at site
(Dermal layer is tight and does not expand easily.)

24. During an intradermal injection, note formation of a small bleb on skin's surface (see illustration).

Bleb indicates medication is deposited into dermis.

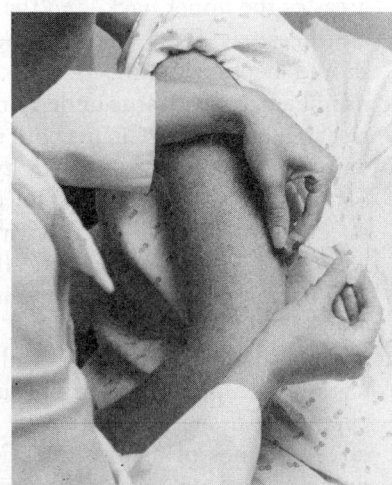

Step 22
(Subcutaneous and intramuscular only)

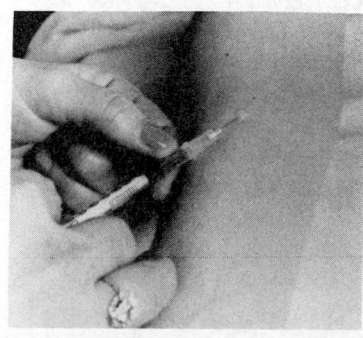

Step 24
(Intradermal only)

Continued.

PROCEDURE 15-3, cont'd

Administering Injections

STEPS	RATIONALE
25. Withdraw needle while applying alcohol swab gently above or over injection site.	Support of tissues around injection site minimizes discomfort during needle withdrawal.
26. For subcutaneous or intramuscular injections, massage skin lightly. It is optional to apply a Band-Aid.	Stimulates circulation and improves drug distribution. (NOTE: Do not massage after subcutaneous heparin injection)
For intradermal injections, *do not massage site.*	Massage may disperse medication into underlying tissue layers and alter test results.
27. Assist client to comfortable position.	Gives client sense of well-being.
28. Discard unsheathed needle and attached syringe into appropriately labeled receptacles.	Prevents injury to clients and health care personnel. CDC no longer recommends capping needles before disposal.
29. Wash hands.	Reduces transmission of microorganisms.
30. Return to room and ask if client feels any acute pain, burning, numbness, or tingling at injection site. Observe for allergic reaction after intradermal injection.	Continued discomfort may indicate injury to underlying bones or nerves. Anaphylactic reaction may occur suddenly after intradermal injection due to drug's toxicity.
31. Return to evaluate response to medication in 10 to 30 min.	Intramuscular medications absorb quickly; undesired effects may also develop rapidly. Nurse's observations determine efficacy of drug action.
32. For intradermal injection, draw circle around perimeter of injection site with skin pencil.	Site must be read at various intervals to determine test results. Pencil mark makes site easier to find.
33. For subcutaneous and intramuscular injections, chart medication dosage, route, and site and time and date given in medication record. Correctly sign according to institutional policy.	Timely documentation prevents future administration errors.
34. For intradermal injections, record area of injection, amount and type of testing substance, and date and time on medication record.	Timely documentation prevents administration errors.

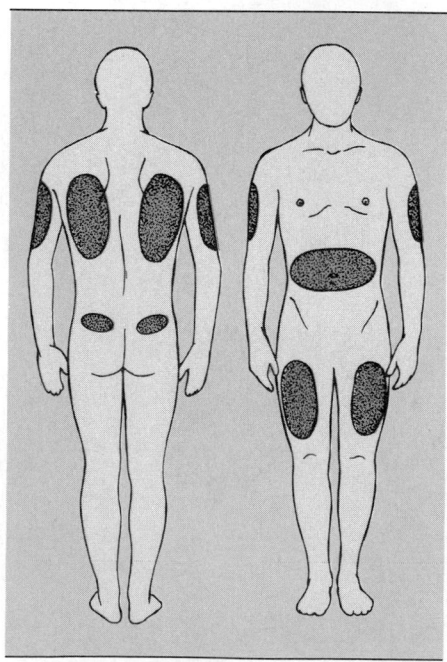

Fig. 15-14 Common sites for subcutaneous injections.

are easily accessible, especially for clients with diabetes who self-administer insulin. The site most frequently recommended for heparin injections is the abdominal wall (Bently et al., 1980). Other sites include the scapular areas of the upper back, and the upper ventral or dorsal gluteal areas (Fig. 15-14). The injection site chosen should be free of infection, skin lesions, scars, bony prominences, and large underlying muscles or nerves (see research highlight). Clients with diabetes regularly rotate daily injection sites to prevent hypertrophy (thickening) of the skin and lipodystrophy (atrophy of tissue). No injection site should be used more than every 6 to 7 weeks. An injection diagram allows nurses and clients to record daily injections to be sure sites are rotated (Fig. 15-15).

Only small doses (0.5 to 1 ml) of water-soluble medication should be given by the subcutaneous route. Subcutaneous tissue is sensitive to irritating solutions and large volumes of medication. Collecting of medication within the tissues can cause sterile abscesses, which appear as hardened, painful lumps under the skin.

Body weight indicates the depth of the subcutaneous

❧ *Research Highlight* ❧

Vanbree et al. studied the effect of techniques for administering subcutaneous, low-dose heparin on the formation of bruises at the injection site. The following variables were held constant for all injections: 1) site (lower abdomen at least 2 inches from umbilicus), 2) preinjection skin preparation (gentle alcohol wipe), 3) grasping a roll of tissue, 4) drug dose and syringe, 5) angle of needle insertion (90 degrees), 6) withdrawal of needle (same angle as inserted), and 7) postinjection skin preparation (press site lightly with alcohol swab for 1 minute).

The following methods were used to study needle manipulation and tracking of medication through tissues: 1) standard subcutaneous injection technique using aspiration, 2) nonaspiration techniques, and 3) use of an air lock technique.

Forty-three patients received 129 injections, 43 injections using each technique. The study revealed that none of the three techniques was clearly superior in ensuring smaller or fewer bruises.

Vanbree, NS, et al.: Clinical evaluation of three techniques for administering low-dose heparin, Nurs Res 33:15, 1984.

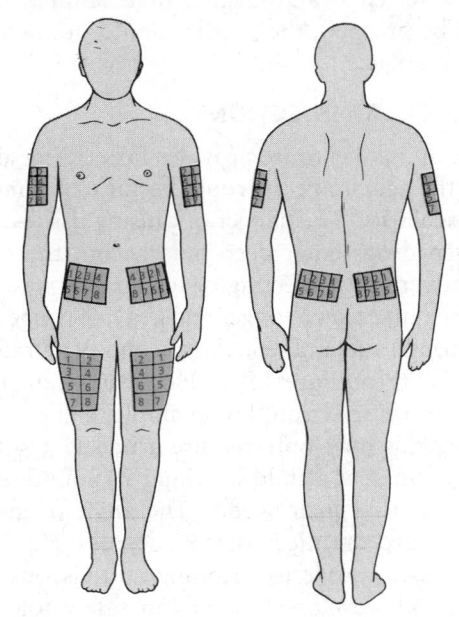

Fig. 15-15 Subcutaneous injection site diagram.

layer. Therefore the nurse must choose the needle length and angle of insertion based on the client's weight. Generally a 25-gauge ⅝-inch needle inserted at a 45-degree angle (Fig. 15-16) deposits medication into the subcutaneous tissue of a normal-sized client. A child may require only a ½-inch needle. If the client is obese, the nurse pinches the tissue and uses a needle long enough to insert through fatty tissue at the base of the skinfold. The preferred needle length is one-half the width of the skinfold. With this method the angle of insertion may be between 45 and 90 degrees.

Thin, cachectic clients may have insufficient tissue for

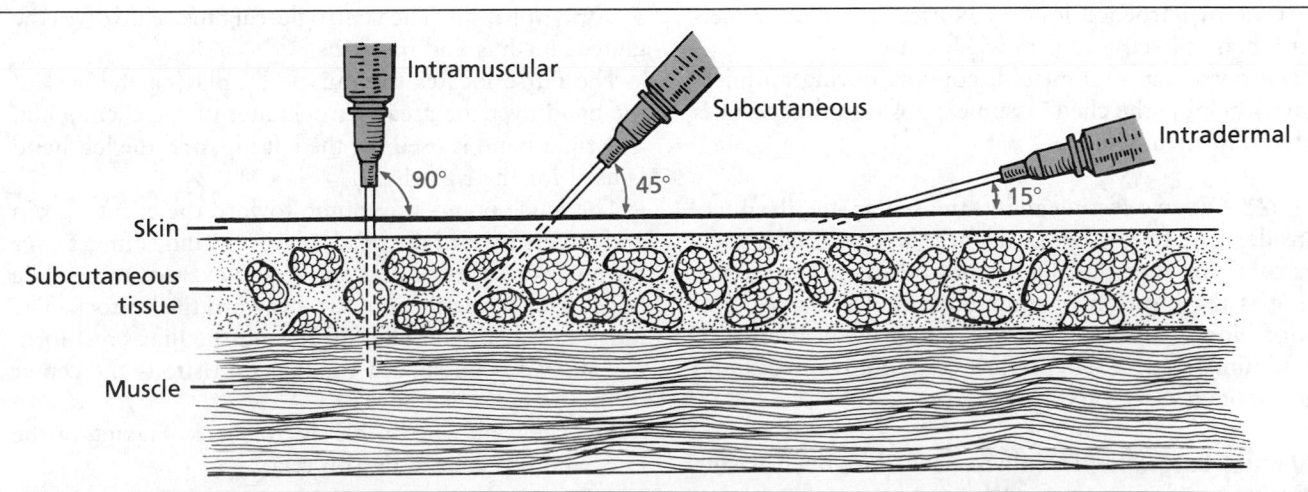

Fig. 15-16 Comparison of the angles of insertion for intramuscular (90 degrees), subcutaneous (45 degrees), and intradermal (15 degrees) injections.

subcutaneous injections. The upper abdomen is the best site for injection with this client. Insulin syringes usually come with 26-gauge needles. To ensure the insulin reaches subcutaneous tissue, a simple rule can be followed: if 2 inches of tissue can be grasped, the needle should be inserted at a 90-degree angle and if 1 inch of tissue can be grasped, the needle should be inserted at a 45-degree angle.

INTRAMUSCULAR INJECTIONS

The intramuscular route provides faster drug absorption than the subcutaneous route because of a muscle's greater vascularity. The danger of causing tissue damage is less when drugs enter deep muscle, but there is the risk of inadvertently injecting drugs directly into blood vessels. The nurse uses a longer and heavier-gauge needle to pass through subcutaneous tissue and penetrate deep muscle tissue (Procedure 15-3). However, weight influences needle size selection. For example, a client weighing 100 pounds may only require a needle 1¼ to 1½ inches long, whereas a child weighing 50 pounds usually requires a ½- to 1-inch needle. The angle of insertion for an intramuscular injection is 90 degrees (Fig. 15-16). Muscle is less sensitive to irritating and viscous drugs. A normal, well-developed client can safely tolerate as much as 3 ml of medication in larger muscles such as the dorsogluteal or vastus lateralis. Smaller muscles can tolerate only smaller amounts of medication without severe muscle discomfort. Children, the elderly, and thin clients tolerate less than 2 ml of medication. Whaley and Wong (1987) recommend giving no more than 1 ml to small children and older infants.

The nurse assesses the integrity of a muscle before giving an injection. The muscle should be free of tenderness. Repeated injections in the same muscle will cause considerable discomfort. By asking the client to relax, the nurse can palpate the muscle to rule out the presence of hardened lesions. Normally a muscle feels soft when relaxed and firm when tense.

The nurse can minimize discomfort during an injection by helping the client assume a position that reduces strain on the muscle.

SITES. When selecting an intramuscular site, the nurse considers the following: Is the area free of infection or necrosis? Are there local areas of bruising or abrasions? What is the location of underlying bones, nerves, and major blood vessels? What volume of medication is to be administered? Each site has certain advantages and disadvantages (see box).

Vastus Lateralis. The thick, well developed vastus lateralis muscle is a preferred injection site for adults, children, and infants. The muscle is located on the anterior lateral aspect of the thigh and extends in an adult

---

Characteristics of Intramuscular Sites

- **Vastus Lateralis.** Lacks major nerves and blood vessels; rapid drug absorption; large developed muscle.
- **Ventrogluteal.** A deep site, situated away from major nerves and blood vessels; less chance of contamination in incontinent clients or infants because it is away from rectum. Easily identified by prominent bony landmark.
- **Dorsogluteal.** Runs risk of striking underlying sciatic nerve, greater trochanter, or major blood vessels; not used with children under 3 years of age. Never use when client is standing. Site must be clean to avoid contamination.
- **Deltoid.** Site easily accessible but muscle not well developed in most clients. Use for small amounts of drugs. Never used in infants or children. Potential for injury to radial and ulnar nerves or brachial artery.

---

from a handbreadth above the knee to a handbreath below the greater trochanter of the femur (Fig. 15-17). The middle third of the muscle is the best site for injection. In width the site extends from the midline of the thigh's top to the midline of the thigh's outer side. See Fig. 15-18 for children.

With young children or cachectic clients, it helps to grasp the body of the muscle during injection to be sure the drug is deposited in muscle tissue. To help relax the muscle, the nurse asks the client to lie flat with the knee slightly flexed or in a sitting position.

Ventrogluteal. The ventrogluteal muscle involves the gluteus medius and minimus.

The nurse locates the muscle by placing the heel of the hand over the greater trochanter of the client's hip. The right hand is used for the left hip, and the left hand is used for the right hip.

The nurse points the thumb toward the client's groin and fingers toward the head, places the index finger over the anterior superior iliac spine, and extends the middle finger back along the iliac crest toward the buttock. The index finger, the middle finger, and the iliac crest form a V-shaped triangle and the injection site is the center of the triangle (Fig. 15-19).

The client may lie on his side or back. Flexing of the knee and hip helps a person relax.

Dorsogluteal. The dorsogluteal muscle has been a traditional site for intramuscular injections. However,

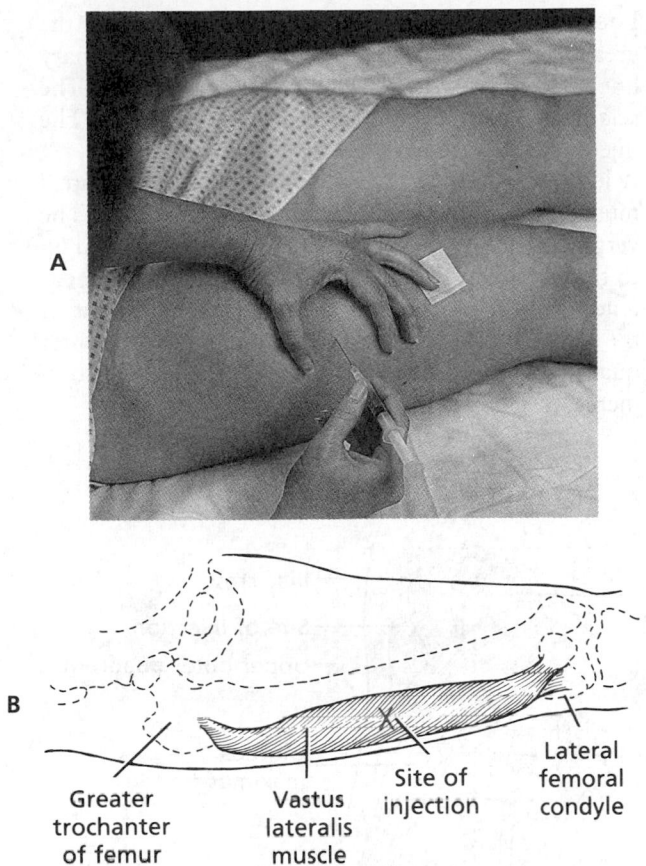

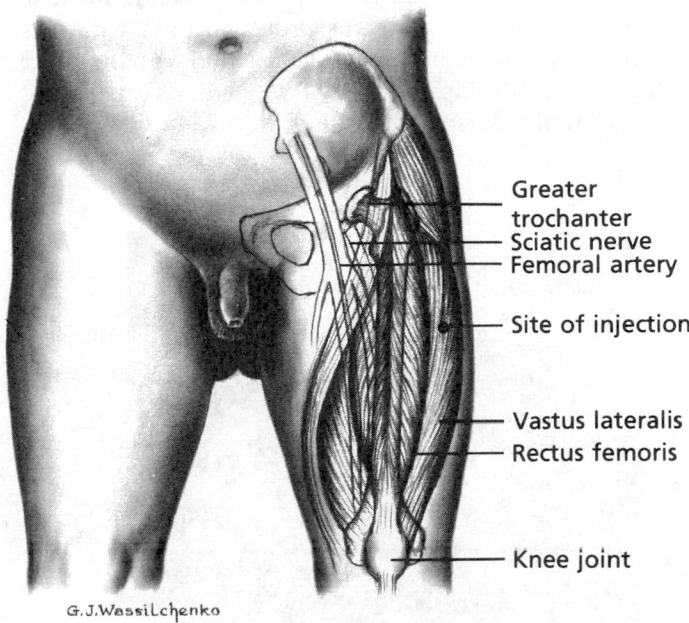

Fig. 15-17 A, Injection site into the vastus lateralis muscle. B, Anatomical view of the site for intramuscular injection into the vastus lateralis muscle.

Fig. 15-18 Acceptable intramuscular site for children, the vastus lateralis.

From Whaley, LF, and Wong, DL: Nursing care of infants and children, ed. 3, St. Louis, 1987, The C.V. Mosby Co.

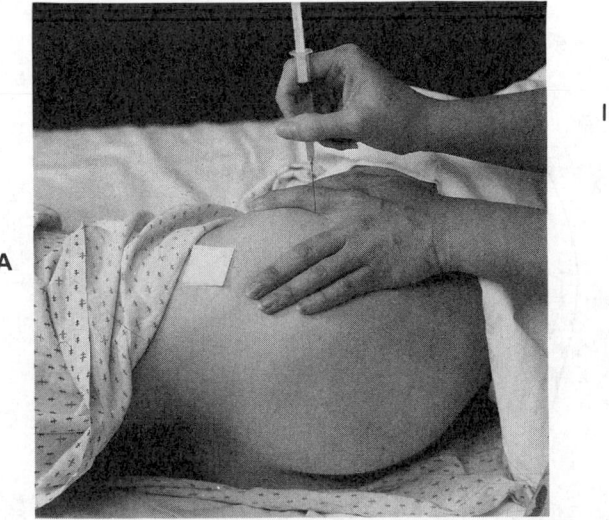

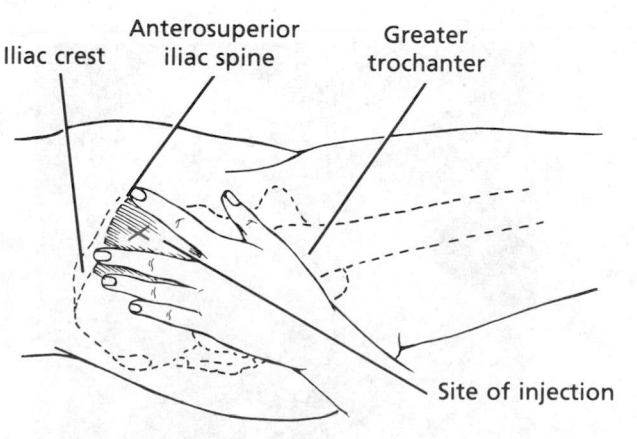

Fig. 15-19 A, Injection site into ventrogluteal muscle avoids major nerves and blood vessels. B, Anatomical view of ventrogluteal muscle injection site.

accidental insertion of a needle into the sciatic nerve can cause permanent or partial paralysis of the involved leg.

Major blood vessels and bone are also near the site. In clients with flabby, sagging tissues, the site is difficult to locate.

The dorsogluteal site is located in the upper outer aspect of the upper outer quadrant of the buttock, approximately 5 to 8 cm (2 to 3 inches) below the iliac crest. Clients may lie in the prone position with toes turned medially or in a side-lying position with the upper leg flexed at the hip and knee. Two methods can be used to locate the dorsogluteal site:

1. Locate the posterior superior iliac spine and the greater trochanter of the femur. Draw an imaginary line between the two anatomical landmarks. The sciatic nerve runs parallel and below the line. The injection site is above and lateral to the line.

2. A less accurate method of locating the dorsogluteal muscle is dividing the buttock into quadrants. The vertical dividing line extends from the gluteal fold up to the iliac crest. The intersecting horizontal line extends from the medial fold to the lateral aspect of the buttock. The injection site is in the upper outer quadrant (Fig. 15-20). This method for site selection increases the risk of injury to the sciatic nerve.

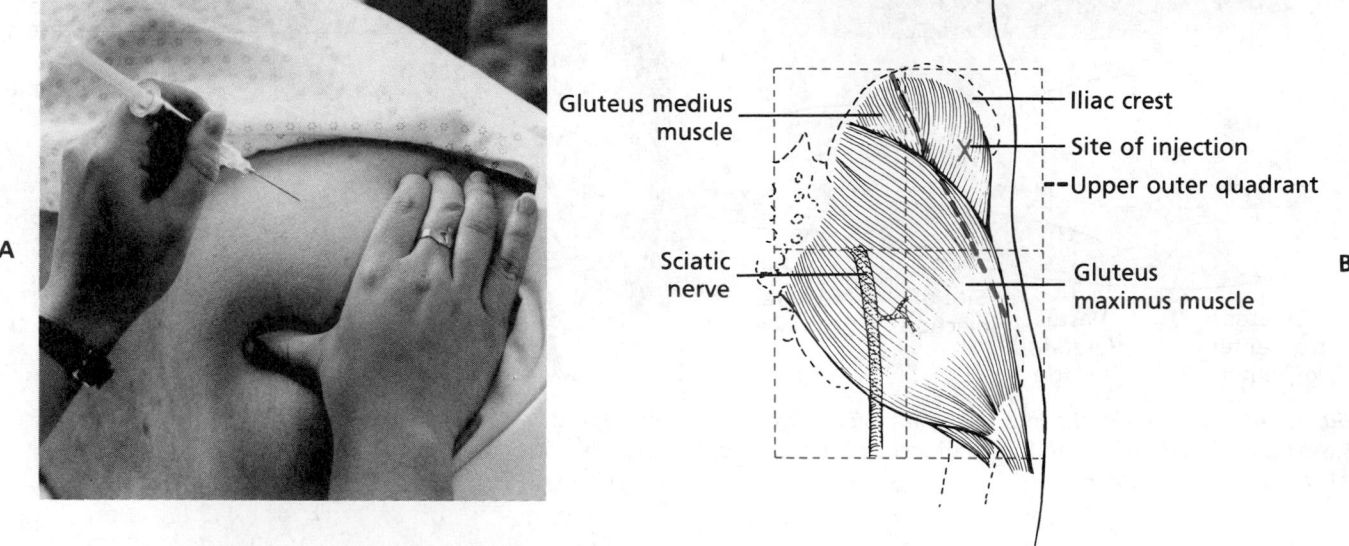

Fig. 15-20 **A**, Site of injection into dorsogluteal muscle. **B**, Imaginary diagonal line extending from the posterior superior iliac spine to the greater trochanter is the landmark for selecting the dorsogluteal injection site. Alternatively, the buttocks may be divided into quadrants for selecting the dorsogluteal injection site.

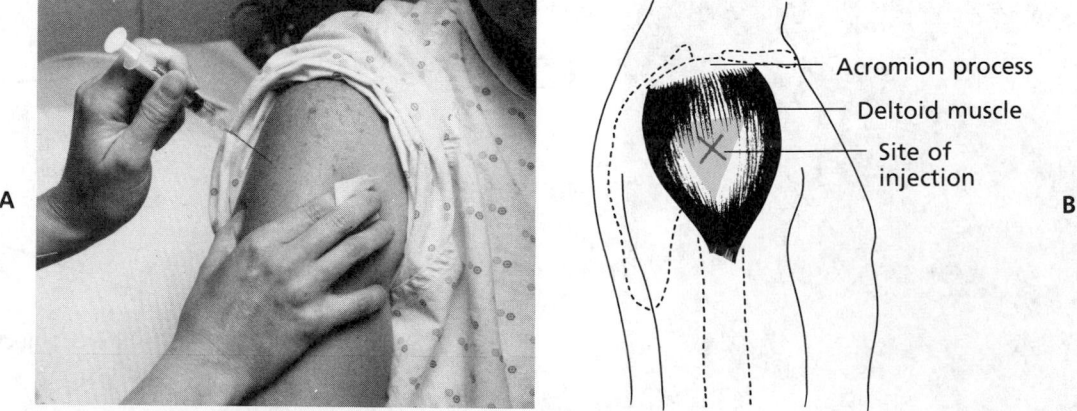

Fig. 15-21 **A**, Site of intramuscular injection into the deltoid muscle. **B**, Site of deltoid muscle injection below acromion process.

Nurses may use the dorsogluteal injection site in adults and children (at least 3 years of age) with well-developed gluteal muscles.

Deltoid. In many adults and most children the deltoid muscle is not well developed. The radial and ulnar nerves and brachial artery lie within the upper arm along the humerus. The nurse uses the deltoid site to administer small volumes of medication or when other injection sites are inaccessible because of dressings, casts, or other obstructions.

To locate the deltoid muscle the nurse has the client expose the upper arm and shoulder fully. A tight-fitting sleeve should not be rolled up. The nurse has the client relax the arm at the side and flex the elbow (Fig. 15-21, *A*). The client may sit, stand, or lie down. The nurse palpates the lower edge of the acromion process, which forms the base of a triangle in line with the midpoint of the lateral aspect of the upper arm (Fig. 15-21, *B*). The injection site is in the center of the triangle, about 2.5 to 5 cm (1 to 2 inches) below the acromion process. The nurse may also locate the site by placing four fingers across the deltoid muscle, with the top finger along the acromion process. The injection site is then 3 finger breadths below the acromion process.

Z-TRACK METHOD. When irritating preparations such as iron or Vistaral are given intramuscularly, the Z-track method of injection minimizes tissue irritation by sealing the drug within the muscle tissues.

The nurse selects an intramuscular site, preferably in larger, deeper muscles such as the ventrogluteal muscle. It is important to apply a new needle to the syringe after preparing the drug so no solution remains on the outside needle shaft. The nurse draws up 0.2 ml of air to create an air lock. After preparing the site with an antiseptic swab, the nurse pulls the overlying skin and subcutaneous tissues approximately 2.5 to 3.5 cm (1 to 1½

inches) laterally to the side. Holding the skin taut with the nondominant hand, the nurse injects the needle deep into the muscle. With practice the nurse learns to hold the syringe and aspirate with one hand. The nurse injects the drug and air slowly if there is no blood return on aspiration. The needle remains inserted for 10 seconds to allow the medication to disperse evenly. The nurse releases the skin after withdrawing the needle, which leaves a zigzag path that seals the needle track wherever tissue planes slide across each other (Fig. 15-22). The drug cannot escape from the muscle tissue.

INTRADERMAL INJECTIONS

The nurse typically gives intradermal injections for skin testing, for example, in tuberculin screening and allergy tests. Because these medications are potent, they are injected into the dermis, where blood supply is reduced and drug absorption occurs slowly. A client may have a severe anaphylactic reaction if the medications enter the client's circulation too rapidly. For clients with a history of numerous allergies the physician often performs skin testing.

Skin testing requires the nurse to be able to clearly see the injection sites for changes in color and tissue integrity. Intradermal sites should be lightly pigmented, free of lesions, and relatively hairless. The inner forearm and upper back are ideal locations.

The nurse uses a tuberculin or small hypodermic syringe for skin testing. The angle of insertion for an intradermal injection is 5 to 15 degrees (Fig. 15-16, p. 403). As the nurse injects the drug, a small bleb resembling a mosquito bite should appear on the skin's surface (Procedure 15-3). If a bleb does not appear or if the site bleeds after needle withdrawal, there is a good chance the medication entered subcutaneous tissues. In this case skin test results will not be valid.

Data from an intradermal injection include a description of the precise location and time of administration. The injected site must be "read" within 48 to 72 hours.

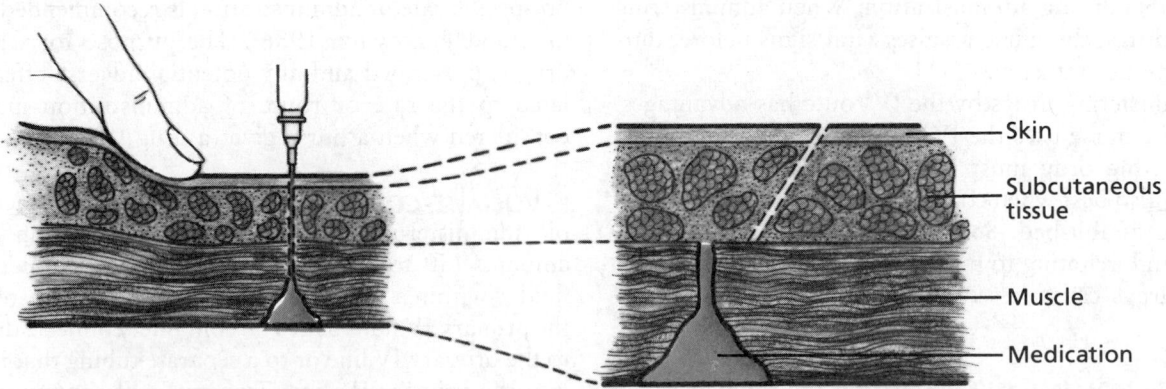

Fig. 15-22 The Z-track method of injection prevents the deposit of medication through sensitive tissues.

If a client has had close contact with a tuberculosis carrier, intradermal skin reactions, including induration measuring 5 mm and larger, are significant. If results are below 5 mm, close contacts are retested in 2 months. Reactions of 10 mm or larger in clients who have not had close contact are also significant. Erythema or bruises from the injection are not significant findings.

INTRAVENOUS ADMINISTRATION

The nurse administers drugs intravenously by three methods:

1. As mixtures within large volumes of intravenous (IV) fluids
2. By injection of a bolus or small volume of medication through an existing intravenous *infusion* line or heparin lock (IV push).
3. By "piggyback" infusion of a solution containing the prescribed drug and a small volume of IV fluid through an adjoining or existing IV line.

In all three methods the client has an existing IV infusion line or an IV access site in the form of a heparin lock. In most institutions, only physicians are allowed to inject drugs directly into a vein through venipuncture. However, nurses working in critical care settings assume more active roles in administering drugs "IV push."

Chapter 37 describes the technique for performing venipuncture and establishing continuous IV fluid infusions. Medication administration is only one reason for supplying IV fluids. IV fluid therapy is used primarily for fluid replacement in clients unable to take oral fluids and as a means of supplying electrolytes and nutrients.

The nurse must observe clients closely for symptoms of adverse reactions when using any method of IV drug administration. After a drug enters the bloodstream, it begins to act immediately, and no way exists to stop its action. Thus the nurse takes special care to avoid errors in dosage calculation and preparation. The nurse should double-check the "five rights" of safe drug administration and know the desired action and potential side effects. If the drug has an antidote, the nurse must have it available during administration. When administering potent drugs, the nurse assesses vital signs before, during, and after infusion.

Administering drugs by the IV route has advantages. Often the nurse uses the IV route in emergencies when a fast-acting drug must be delivered quickly. The IV route is also best when constant therapeutic blood levels must be established. Some medications are highly alkaline and irritating to muscle and subcutaneous tissue. These drugs cause less discomfort when given intravenously.

LARGE VOLUME INFUSIONS. Of the three methods of administering IV medications, mixing drugs in large volumes of fluids is the safest and easiest. Drugs are diluted in large volumes (500 ml or 1000 ml) of compatible IV fluids such as normal saline or lactated Ringer's solution. In most institutions the pharmacist adds drugs to the primary container of IV solution to ensure asepsis. Because the drug is not in a concentrated form, the risk of side effects or fatal reactions is minimal. Vitamins and potassium chloride are two types of drugs commonly added to IV fluids. The danger with continuous infusion is that, if the IV fluid is infused too rapidly, the client may suffer circulatory fluid overload (see Chapter 37 and Procedure 15-4).

INTRAVENOUS BOLUS. An IV bolus involves introducing a concentrated dose of a drug directly into systemic circulation. The IV bolus is used during emergencies, with critically unstable clients, and as a route of administration when rapid and predictable responses are required (Burman and Berkowitz, 1986). An IV bolus may be given directly into a vein, into an existing intravenous line through an injection port, or through a heparin lock.

Because a bolus requires only a small amount of fluid to deliver the drug, it is an advantage when the amount of fluid the client can take is restricted. The IV bolus is the most dangerous method for administering drugs because there is no time to correct errors. In addition, a bolus may cause direct irritation to the lining of blood vessels. Before administering a bolus the nurse confirms placement of the IV line. This involves obtaining a blood return through the IV catheter or needle. The inability to obtain a blood return suggests that the needle or catheter is in tissues or resting against the vein wall. A drug should never be given intravenously if the insertion site appears puffy or edematous or the IV fluid cannot flow at the proper rate. Accidental injection of a medication into the tissues surrounding a vein can cause pain, sloughing of tissues, and abscesses, depending on the drug's composition.

The rate of administration of an IV bolus medication is usually determined by the amount of drug that can be given each minute. The standard rate is 1 ml/min if no specific rate of administration is recommended (Burman and Berkowitz, 1986). The purpose for which a drug is prescribed and any potential adverse effects related to the rate or route of administration must be considered when a nurse gives a drug IV push.

VOLUME-CONTROLLED INFUSIONS. Another way of administering IV medications is through small amounts (50 to 100 ml) of compatible IV fluids. The fluid is within a secondary fluid container separate from the primary IV fluid bag. The container connects directly to the primary IV line or to a separate tubing that inserts into the primary IV line. Two types of containers are: 1) volume control administration sets (for example, Volutrol or Pediatrol) and 2) piggyback sets.

Text continued on p. 417.

PROCEDURE 15-4

Adding Medications to Intravenous Fluid Containers

STEPS	RATIONALE
1. Check physician's order for type of intravenous (IV) solution to use and type of medication and dosage.	Overall physical condition determines type of IV solution to use. Ensures safe and accurate drug administration.
2. When more than one medication is to be added to IV solution, assess for drug compatibility.	Certain drugs are incompatible when mixed. May result in clouding or crystallization of fluids or cause a drug interaction that is not visible.
3. Prepare the following equipment and supplies:	
a. Vial or ampule of prescribed medication	
b. Syringe of appropriate size (5 to 20 ml)	
c. Sterile needle (1 to 1½ in, 19 to 21-gauge) with special filters (optional)	Larger needle gauge ensures easy aspiration of drugs from vial or ampule. Filter prevents solid material from entering syringe and thus avoids transfer to fluid container.
d. Correct diluent (for example, sterile water or normal saline)	Certain IV medications are prepared in dry powder form. Diluent must be added for mixing.
e. Sterile IV fluid container (bag or bottle, 500 to 1000 ml in volume)	IV solution bags are kept sterile by being stored in separate intact plastic bag. IV bottles have plastic or metal seal over bottle cap.
f. Alcohol or antiseptic swab	
g. Label to attach to IV bag or bottle	Continuously infusing medication must be labeled properly for all nurses to observe.
4. Wash hands thoroughly.	Reduces transfer of microorganisms when handling sterile equipment.
5. Assemble supplies in medication room.	Ensures procedure will be orderly with less likelihood of contaminating supplies.
6. Prepare prescribed medication from vial or ampule. (If a filter needle is used, replace it with a regular needle before injecting the medication into the IV fluid container.)	Different techniques used for each type of container.
7. Identify client by reading identification band and asking name.	Ensures correct client receives ordered medication.
8. Prepare client by explaining that medication is to be given through existing IV line or one to be started. Explain that no discomfort should be felt during drug infusion. Encourage client to report symptoms of discomfort.	Allows client to understand procedure and minimizes his anxiety. Most IV medications will not cause discomfort when diluted. However, potassium chloride can be irritating. Pain at insertion site may be early indication of infiltration.
9. Add medication to new container.	
a. Locate medication injection port on IV solution bag.	
(1) Remove plastic cover over port. Port has small rubber stopper at end. Do not select port for the IV tubing insertion or air vent.	Medication injection port is self-sealing to prevent introduction of microorganisms after repeated use.
b. Locate injection site on intravenous solution bottle.	
(1) Remove metal or plastic cap and rubber disk. Place cap upside down on countertop.	Cap seals bottle to maintain its sterility. Inside of cap may remain sterile for reuse.
(2) Locate medication injection site on the bottle's rubber stopper. Site is usually marked by an **X**, circle, or triangle.	Accidental injection of medication through main tubing port or air vent can alter pressure within bottle and cause fluid leaks through air vent.
c. Wipe off port or injection site with alcohol or antiseptic swab.	Reduces risk of introducing microorganisms into bag during needle insertion.
d. Remove needle cap from syringe and carfully insert needle of syringe through center of injection port or site, and inject medication.	Injection of needle into sides of port may produce leak and lead to fluid contamination.
e. Withdraw syringe from bag or bottle. Cover glass bottle top with antiseptic swab and sterile bottle cap.	Open tubing port in bottle provides direct route for microorganisms to enter solution. Bags have self-sealing port.

Continued.

PROCEDURE 15-4, cont'd

Adding Medications to Intravenous Fluid Containers

STEPS	RATIONALE
f. Mix medication and IV solution by holding bag or bottle and turning it gently end to end.	Allows medication to be distributed evenly.
g. Complete medication label with name and dose of medication, date, time, and nurse's initials. Stick it upside down on bottle or bag.	Label can be easily read during infusion of solution. Informs nurses and physicians of contents of bag or bottle.
h. Spike bag or bottle with IV tubing and hang (see Chapter 37). Regulate infusion at ordered rate.	Prevents rapid infusion of fluid.
10. Add medication to existing container.	
a. Prepare vented IV bottle or plastic bag.	
(1) Check volume of solution remaining in bottle.	Proper volume is needed to dilute medication adequately.
(2) Close off IV infusion clamp.	Prevents medication from directly entering circulation as it is injected into bag or bottle.
(3) Wipe off medication port with an alcohol or antiseptic swab.	Mechanically removes microorganisms that could enter container during needle insertion.
(4) Lower bag or bottle from IV pole. Insert syringe needle through injection port and inject medication (see Illustration).	Injection port is self-sealing and prevents fluid leaks.
(5) Gently mix bottle or bag.	Ensures medication is evenly distributed.
(6) Rehang bag and regulate infusion to desired rate.	Prevents rapid infusion of fluid.
b. Complete medication label and stick it to bag or bottle.	Informs nurses and physicians of contents of bag or bottle.
11. Properly dispose of equipment and supplies.	Proper disposal of needle prevents injury to nurse and client.
12. Wash hands.	Reduces transmission of microorganisms.
13. Record solution and medication added to parenteral fluid on appropriate form (see illustration).	Information used to monitor type of solutions client receives and fluid intake over 24 hours.
14. Report any side effects (for example, change in pulse rate, noisy respirations, or change in blood pressure) to nurse in charge or physician.	Reaction may require therapeutic intervention.

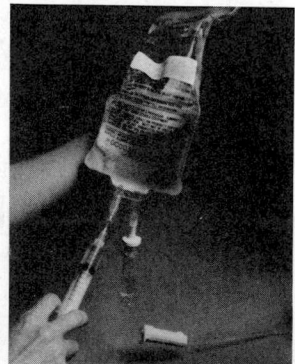

Step 10a (4)

PARENTERAL FLUID

AMT.	TYPE OF FLUID	MEDICATION ADDED	DATE/ HR START	RN INIT	DATE/ HR COMP	RN INIT	AMT. REC'D	SITE	IV SITE CARE DATE/HR	TUBING CHANGE DATE / HR	RN INIT
1L	DSW	20 meq. KCl	1/8 0900	PL	1/8 1800	T.M.	1000 ml	✓	1/8 1000		
1L	LR	20 meq KCl	1/8 1800	T.M.							

Step 13

PROCEDURE 15-5

Administering Intravenous Medications by Piggyback or Volume Administration Sets

STEPS	RATIONALE
1. Check physician's order to determine type of medication and dosage.	Overall physical condition determines type of IV solution used.
	Ensures safe and accurate drug administration.
2. Assess patency of existing IV infusion line (see Chapter 37) by noting infusion rate of main IV line	IV line must be patent and fluids must infuse easily for medication to reach venous circulation effectively.
3. Assess IV insertion site for signs of infiltration or phlebitis (see Chapter 37).	Confirmation of placement of IV needle or catheter and integrity of surrounding tissues ensures medication is administered safely.
4. Prepare following equipment and supplies:	
a. Piggyback	
(1) Medication prepared in a 50 to 100 ml, labeled infusion bag with IV line, microdrip or macrodrip infusion tubing set.	Used for piggyback administration. Most piggybacks are prepared by pharmacies.
(2) Needle (21- or 23-gauge)	Medication is "piggybacked" or connected to client main infusion line by needle inserted through IV line injection port. Larger needle would cause leakage at Y-port connector.
(3) Adhesive tape (optional)	
(4) Antiseptic swab	
(5) Metal hook (optional)	To lower primary infusion bag below smaller infusion bag (used only if tubing is shorter than primary infusion tubing).
b. Volume-control administration set	
(1) Volutrol, Pediatrol, or Burette	Graduated container connects to main IV solution.
(2) Infusion tubing	Connected to administration set used to inject medication into set.
(3) Syringe (5 to 20 ml)	
(4) Needle (1 to 1½ in. 21- or 23-gauge)	
(5) Vial or ampule of ordered medication	
(6) Medication label	
5. Wash hands.	Reduces transmission of microorganisms.
6. Piggyback	
a. Assemble supplies at bedside.	Drug preparation usually not required. May assemble infusion tubing and bag of medication in medication or client's room.
b. Connect infusion tubing to medication bag (see Chapter 37). Allow solution to fill tubing by opening regulator flow clamp.	Infusion tube should be filled with solution and free of air bubbles to prevent air embolus.

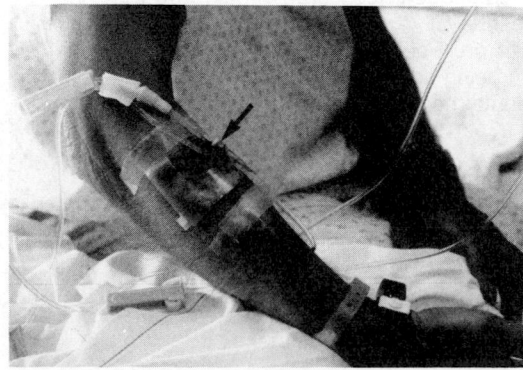

Step 6g

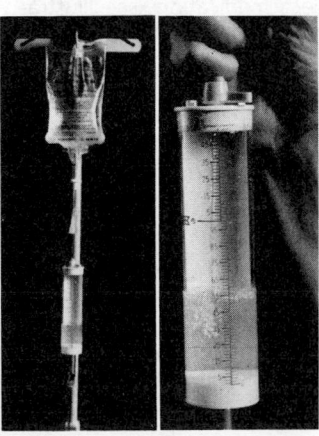

Step 7d

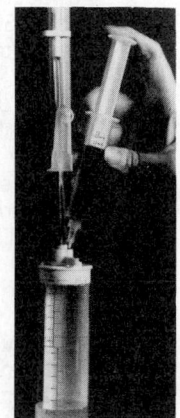

Step 7g

Continued.

Administering Intravenous Medications by Piggyback or Volume Administration Sets

STEPS	RATIONALE
c. Hang medication bag at or above level of main fluid bag. (Hook may be used to lower main bag.)	Height of fluid bag affects rate of flow to client.
d. Connect covered sterile needle to end of infusion tubing.	Cover keeps needle sterile before connecting it to main IV line
e. Check client's identification by looking at armband and asking name.	Ensures drug is administered to correct client.
f. Clean injection Y-port of main IV line with antiseptic swab.	Prevents introduction of microorganisms during needle insertion.
g. Remove cover and insert needle of secondary piggyback line through injection port of main IV line. Secure with strip of adhesive tape if necessary (see illustration).	Establishes route for IV medication to enter main IV line. Tape prevents needle from slipping out of port.
h. Regulate flow rate of medication solution. (Usually medication should infuse within 30 to 60 min)	Provides slow, intermittent infusion of medication infusion in 30 to 60 min maintains therapeutic blood levels.
i. After medication has infused, check flow regulator on primary infusion. A piggyback set hung at the level of the primary bag has a backcheck valve that automatically stops the flow of the primary infusion until the medication infuses. The primary infusion should automatically begin to flow after the piggyback is empty.	Valve prevents backup of medication into main infusion line. Checking flow rate ensures proper administration of IV fluids
j. Regulate main infusion line to desired rate, if necessary.	Infusion of piggyback may interfere with the main line infusion rate.
k. Leave secondary bag, tubing, and inserted needle in place for future drug administration or discard in appropriate containers.	Establishment of secondary line produces route for microorganisms to enter main line. Repeated changes in tubing or needles increase risk of infection transmission.
7. Volume-control administration set (for example, Volutrol)	
a. Assemble supplies in medication room.	Controls risk of contaminating IV solution.
b. Prepare medication from vial or ampule (Procedure 15-2).	
c. Check client's identification by looking at armband and asking name.	Ensures drug administered to correct client.
d. Fill Volutrol with desired amount of fluid (50 to 100 ml) by opening clamp between Volutrol and main IV bag (see illustration).	Small volume of fluid dilutes IV medication and reduces risk of too rapid infusion.
e. Close clamp and check to be sure clamp in air vent of Volutrol chamber is open.	Prevents additional leakage of fluid into Volutrol. Air vent allows fluid in Volutrol to exit at regulated rate.
f. Clean injection port on top of Volutrol with antiseptic swab.	Prevents introduction of microorganisms during needle insertion.
g. Remove needle cap and insert syringe needle through port, then inject medication (see illustration). Gently rotate Volutrol between hands.	Rotating mixes medication with solution in Volutrol to ensure equal distribution.
h. Regulate IV infusion rate to allow medication to infuse in 30 to 60 min.	For optimal therapeutic effect, drug should infuse in prescribed time interval.
i. Label Volutrol with name of drug, dosage, total volume including diluent, and time of administration.	Alerts nurses to drug being infused. Prevents other medications from being added to Volutrol.
j. Dispose of uncapped needle and syringe in proper container.	Prevents accidental needle sticks
8. Wash hands.	Prevents transmission of microorganisms.
9. Observe client for signs of adverse reactions.	IV medications act rapidly.
10. During 30 to 60 min of infusion, periodically check infusion rate and condition of IV site.	IV must remain patent for proper drug administration. Development of infiltration necessitates discontinuing infusion.
11. Record drug, dosage, route, and time administered on medication form (Fig. 15-5). Record volume of fluid in medication bag or Volutrol on intake and output form (see Chapter 37).	Timely documentation prevents medication errors (for example, repeated doses). Fluid balance regulated and monitored on basis of total fluid intake.

There are several advantages to using volume-controlled infusions:

1. Reduces risk of rapid-dose infusion by IV push. IV medications are diluted and infused over longer time intervals (for example, 30 to 60 minutes)
2. Allows administration of drugs that are incompatible with drugs in the primary intravenous solution
3. Allows for administration of drugs (for example, antibiotics) that are stable for a limited time in solution
4. Allows for control of intravenous fluid intake

Volume-control administration sets are small (100 to 150 ml) containers that attach just below the primary infusion bag or bottle (Procedure 15-5). The set is attached and filled in a manner similar to a regular IV infusion (see Chapter 37). However, the priming or filling of the set is different, depending on the type of filter (floating valve or membane) within the set. Package directions should be followed during priming or the set will not function properly.

Piggyback sets are small (50 or 100 ml) IV bags or bottles connected to short tubing lines that connect to the upper Y-part of a primary infusion line or an intermittent venous access. The piggyback tubing is a microdrip or macrodrip system. The sets are called piggyback because in some sets the small bag or bottle is set higher than the primary infusion bottle.

INTERMITTENT VENOUS ACCESS. An intravenous or heparin lock is an IV needle with a small "well"

covered by a rubber diaphragm (Fig. 15-23). Special rubber-seal injection caps serve as "wells" and can be inserted into most IV catheters (see Chapter 37). Advantages to intermittent venous access include:

1. Cost savings resulting from the omission of continuous IV therapy
2. Convenience to the nurse by eliminating constant monitoring of flow rates
3. Increased mobility, safety, and comfort for the client

After an IV bolus or piggyback medication has been administered through a heparin lock, the lock must be flushed with a solution to keep it patent. Disagreement exists as to the type of solution to use to keep heparin locks free of clots. Cyganski et al. (1987) demonstrated that a heparin flush solution (1 ml = 100 units), given after an IV drug, was effective in minimizing phlebitis of IV sites and clotting of IV catheters. However, Dunn and Lenihan (1987) and Harrigan (1985) showed that regular flushes of normal saline were just as effective in keeping heparin locks patent. Agency policies differ.

Normally, checking for a blood return in an IV lock before bolus administration is unnecessary. However, if the needle site becomes puffy or the client complains of discomfort, the "well" must be aspirated for a blood return. Procedure 15-6 describes the technique for administering an IV medication bolus.

DISPOSAL OF EQUIPMENT

After administering injections, the nurse must dispose of used equipment properly (Fig. 15-24). A stray needle can injure the client, nurse, housekeeper, or other health care personnel. A needle stick can be the source of hepatitis or AIDS.

The CDC now recommends that *needles should not be capped before disposal.* Covering a needle may pre-

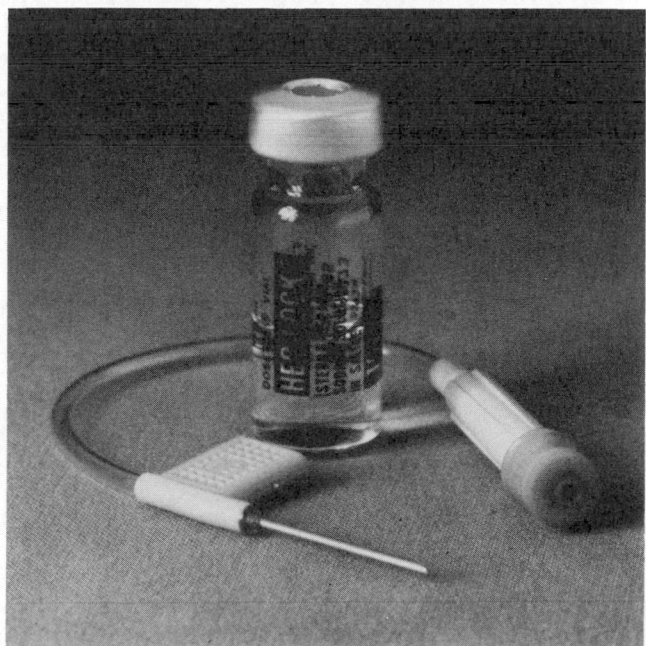

Fig. 15-23 Intravenous lock with vial of flush solution.

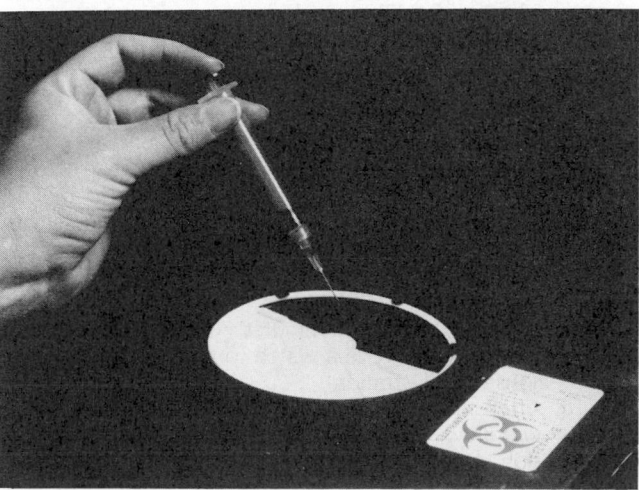

Fig. 15-24 Special containers are available in nursing units for the disposal of contaminated syringes.

PROCEDURE 15-6

Administering Medications by Intravenous Bolus (Push)

STEPS	RATIONALE
1. Check physician's order for type of medication to be administered, dosage, and route.	Ensures safe and accurate drug administration.
2. Assess IV or intravenous (heparin) lock insertion site for signs of infiltration or phlebitis (see Chapter 37).	Confirmation of placement of IV needle or catheter and integrity of surrounding tissues ensures medication is administered safely.
3. If medication is to be pushed into IV line, assess patency of line by noting infusion rate.	IV line must be patent and fluids must infuse easily for medication to reach venous circulation effectively.

4. Prepare the following equipment and supplies:
a. IV push (existing line)
  (1) Medication in vial or ampule
  (2) Syringe (3 to 5 ml)
  (3) Sterile needles (21- and 25-gauge)
	Large-gauge needles used to draw up medication. Small-gauge needles used to insert through Y-port of IV tubing.

(4) Antiseptic swab
  (5) Watch with second hand or digital readout
b. IV push (intravenous lock)
  (1) Medication in vial or ampule
  (2) Syringe (3 to 5 ml)
  (3) Syringe (3 ml)
  (4) Vial of heparin flush solution (1 ml = 100 units or 1 ml = 10 units, depending on agency policy) (optional) or vial of normal saline.
  (5) Sterile needles (21- and 25-gauge)
	Used for medication preparation.
	Used for heparin flush or saline solution.
	Keeps heparin lock patent and free of clots. Studies have not shown clear advantage of using heparin instead of saline (Dunn and Lenihan, 1987; Harringan, 1985).
	Large-gauge needles used to draw up medication. Small-gauge needle used to insert through heparin lock.

(6) Antiseptic swab (7) Watch with second hand or digital readout	
5. Wash hands.	Reduces transmission of infection.
6. Prepare ordered medication from vial or ampule (Procedure 15-2). Read package directions carefully for proper IV dilution of medication.	
7. After preparing medication, apply small-gauge needle to syringe.	Used to insert through IV line or heparin lock.
8. IV push (existing line) a. Check client's identification by looking at armband and asking name.	Ensures drug is administered to correct client.
b. Select injection port of IV tubing closest to client. A circle on port may indicate site for needle insertion.	Allows for easier fluid aspiration to obtain blood return. Injection ports are self-sealing and will not leak.
c. Clean off injection port with the antiseptic swab.	Prevents introduction of microorganisms during needle insertion.
d. Insert small-gauge needle of syringe containing prepared drug through center of port.	Prevents damage to port's diaphragm and subsequent leakage.
e. Occlude the intravenous line by pinching the tubing just above the injection port. Pull back gently on the syringe's plunger to aspirate for a blood return (see illustration).	Final check ensures that medication is being delivered into the bloodstream.
f. After noting blood return, inject the medication slowly over several minutes. (Read directions on drug package.) Use a watch to time the administrations (see illustration).	Ensues safe drug infusion. Rapid injection of an IV drug can prove fatal.
g. After injecting the medication, release the tubing, withdraw the syringe, and recheck the fluid infusion rate.	Injection of a bolus may alter the rate of fluid infusion. Rapid fluid infusion can cause circulatory fluid overload.

STEPS	RATIONALE
9. IV push (intravenous lock)	
a. Check client's identification by looking at armband and asking full name.	Ensures drug is administered to correct client.
b. Heparin flush:	
(1) Prepare a syringe with 1 ml of heparin flush solution.	Flush solution keeps heparin lock patent after drug is administered.
(2) Prepare a syringe with 3 ml of normal saline. Attach 25-gauge needle to syringe.	Used to assess for blood return in heparin lock.
c. Saline only:	
(1) Prepare 2 syringes with 2 ml of normal saline each. Attach 25-gauge needle to each syringe.	Normal saline has been found to be effective in keeping intravenous locks patent.
d. Heparin and saline:	
(1) Clean the lock's rubber diaphragm with the antiseptic swab.	Cleaning prevents introduction of microorganisms during needle insertion.
(2) Insert needle of syringe containing normal saline through center of diaphragm. Pull back gently on syringe plunger and look for blood return.	Determines if IV needle or catheter is positioned in vein. (At times a heparin lock will not yield a blood return even though lock is patent.)
(3) Flush the reservoir with 1 cc saline by pushing slowly on the plunger.	Cleans needle and reservoir of blood.
(4) Remove the needle and saline-filled syringe.	
(5) Clean the lock's diaphragm with the antiseptic swab.	Prevents transmission of infection.
(6) Insert the needle of syringe containing the prepared drug through center of diaphragm.	Using center of diaphragm prevents leakage.
(7) Inject the medication bolus slowly over several minutes. (Each medication has a recommended rate for bolus administration. Check package directions.) Use a watch to time the administration (see illustration).	Rapid injection of an intravenous drug can result in death.

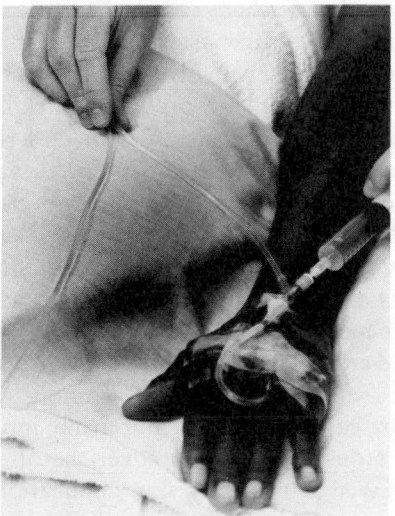

Step 8e

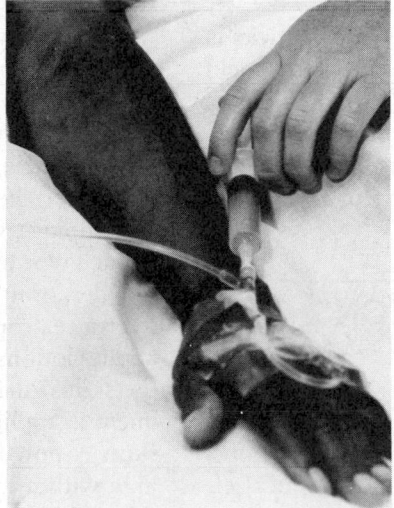

Step 8f

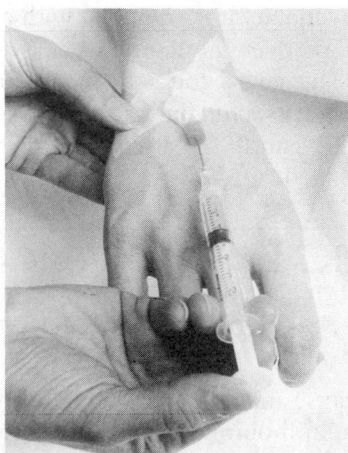

Step 9c (8)

Continued.

PROCEDURE 15-6, cont'd

Administering Medications by Intravenous Bolus (Push)

STEPS	RATIONALE
(8) After administering the bolus, withdraw the syringe.	
(9) Clear the lock's diaphragm with an antiseptic swab.	Prevents transmission of infection.
(10) Repeat the injection of 1 cc normal saline.	Flushes reservoir and needle of medication.
(11) Heparin flush:	Maintains patency of needle by inhibiting clot formation. Diluted heparin avoids anticoagulation.
Insert the needle of syringe containing the heparin through the diaphragm. Inject the heparin slowly, then remove syringe.	
Saline flush:	
If using only saline to flush the reservoir, use 2 cc of saline before and after each use of the intravenous lock.	
10. Wash hands.	Reduces transmission of microorganisms.
11. Observe client closely for adverse reaction as drug is administered, and for several minutes thereafter.	IV medications act rapidly.
12. Dispose of uncapped needles and syringes in proper container.	Prevents accidental needle sticks.
13. Record drug, dosage, route, and time administered on medication form (Fig. 15-5). Also note any adverse reactions.	Timely documentation prevents medication errors.

dispose the nurse to a stick (CDC, 1983). The nurse discards the needle and syringe intact into clearly marked, appropriate containers. Containers should be puncture- and leak-proof. *Needles and plungers should not be broken.* A needle should never be forced into a full needle disposal receptacle. Used needles and syringes should not be placed in wastebaskets, in the nurse's pocket, or at the client's bedside.

A new needle especially designed to prevent sticks is now available. It is equipped with a plastic guard shield that slips over the needle as it is withdrawn from the skin. The guard locks in place, preventing accidental needle sticks and eliminating the need to recap the needle. The guard and needle are disposed of as a single unit (Fig. 15-25).

TOPICAL DRUG APPLICATIONS

Skin Applications

Because many locally applied drugs such as lotions, pastes, and ointments can create systemic and local effects, the nurse should apply these drugs using gloves and applicators. Sterile technique is important, especially if the client has an open wound.

Skin encrustations and dead tissues harbor microorganisms and block contact of medications with the tissues to be treated. Simply applying new medications over previously applied drugs does little to prevent infection or offer therapeutic benefit. The nurse cleans the skin thoroughly before applying medications by washing the area gently with soap and water, soaking an involved site, or locally debriding tissue.

When applying ointments or pastes, the nurse spreads the medication evenly over the involved surface and covers the area well without applying an overly thick layer. Opaque ointments prevent visualization of underlying skin. Physicians often order a gauze dressing to be applied over the medication to prevent soiling of clothes and wiping away of the drug.

Each type of medication, whether an ointment, lotion, powder, or other type, should be applied a specific way to ensure proper penetration and absorption. The nurse applies lotions and creams by smearing them lightly onto the skin's surface. Rubbing may cause irritation. A liniment is applied by rubbing it gently but firmly into the skin. A powder is dusted lightly to cover the affected area with a thin layer. During any skin application the nurse should assess the skin thoroughly. To record administration the area applied, name of medication, and condition of skin should be noted.

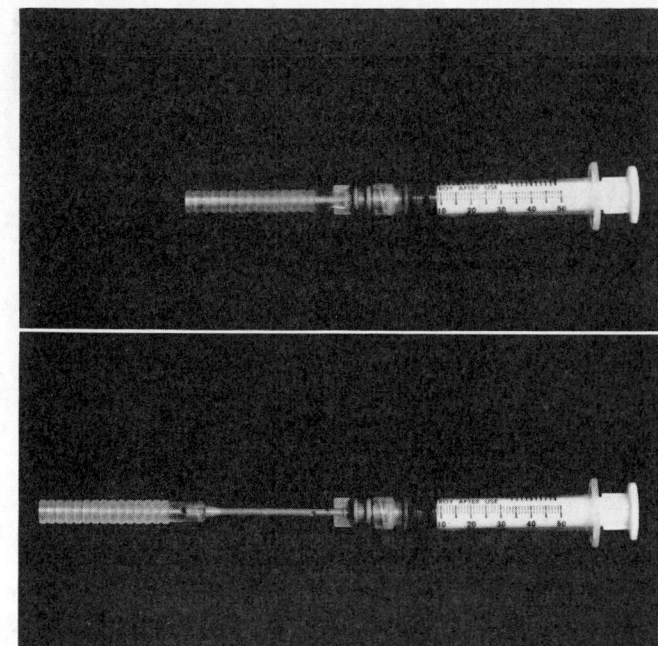

Fig. 15-25 Needle with plastic guard to prevent needle sticks. **A**, Position of guard before injection. **B**, After injection, the guard locks in place covering needle.

Eye Applications

A common medication used by clients is eye drops and ointments, including over-the-counter preparations such as artificial tears, decongestants, and vasoconstrictors (for example, Visine and Murine). However, many clients receive prescribed ophthalmic drugs for eye conditions such as glaucoma and post cataract extraction. A large percentage of clients receiving eye medications are the elderly. Age-related problems, including poor vision, hand tremors, and difficulty grasping or manipulating containers, affect the ease by which the elderly can self-administer eye medications. The nurse instructs clients and family members about the proper techniques for administering eye medications. Donnelly (1987) suggests showing clients each step of the procedure for instilling eye drops to improve their compliance.

The following principles can be followed when administering eye medications:

1) The cornea of the eye is richly supplied with pain fibers and thus very sensitive to anything applied to it. Avoid instilling any form of eye medication directly onto the cornea.
2) Risk of transmiting infection from one eye to the other is high. Avoid touching the eyelids or other eye structures with eye droppers or ointment tubes.
3) Use eye medication only for the affected eye.
4) Never allow a person to use another's eye medications.

Procedure 15-7 reviews the steps for administering eye medications.

Ear Instillations

The internal ear structures are very sensitive to temperature extremes. Failure to instill ear drops or irrigating fluid at room temperature may cause vertigo (severe dizziness) or nausea. Although the structures of the outer ear are not sterile, it is wise to use sterile drops and solutions in case the eardrum is ruptured. Entrance of nonsterile solutions into middle ear structures could result in infection. With ear drainage, the nurse can also check with the physician to be sure the client does not have a ruptured eardrum. A nurse should never occlude the ear canal with the dropper or irrigating syringe. Forcing medication into an occluded ear canal creates pressure that may injure the eardrum.

The external ear structures of children are different from those of adults. When instilling drops or irrigating the canal (Procedure 15-8), the nurse must straighten the ear canal. In infants and young children the nurse straightens the cartilaginous canal by grasping the auricle of the ear and pulling it gently *down* and backward. In adults the ear canal is longer and composed of underlying bone and is straightened by pulling the auricle *upward* and backward. Failure to straighten the canal properly may prevent medicinal solutions from reaching the deeper external ear structures.

Nasal Instillations

Clients with nasal sinus alterations may receive drugs by spray, drops, or tampons (Procedure 15-9). The most commonly administered form of nasal instillation is decongestant spray or drops, used to relieve symptoms of sinus congestion and colds. Clients must be cautioned to avoid abuse of drugs because overuse can lead to a rebound effect in which the nasal congestion worsens. When excess decongestant solution is swallowed, serious systemic effects may also develop, especially in children. Saline drops are safer as a decongestant for children than nasal preparations that contain sympathomimetics (for example, Afrin or Neo-Synephrine).

It is easier to have the client self-administer sprays. In the supine position with head tilted back, the client holds the tip of the container just inside the nares. The client inhales as the spray enters the nasal passages. For clients who use nasal sprays repeatedly, the nurse checks the nares for irritation. In children, nasal sprays should be given with the head in upright position so excess spray will drip anteriorly from the nostrils and not be swallowed (Nurses Drug Alert, 1984).

Nasal drops are effective in treating sinus infections. The nurse learns the proper way of positioning clients to permit the medication to reach the affected sinus.

Text continued on p. 423.

PROCEDURE 15-7

Administering Eyedrops and Ointment

STEPS	RATIONALE
1. Review physician's medication order, including client's name, drug name, concentration, number of drops (if a liquid), time, and eye (right or left) to receive medication.	Ensures correct administration of medication.
2. Wash hands.	Reduces transmission of microorganisms.

3. Prepare following equipment and supplies:
  a. Medication bottle with sterile eye dropper or ointment tube
  b. Medication card, form, or printout
  c. Cotton ball or tissue
  d. Wash basin filled with warm water and wash-cloth
  e. Eye patch and tape (optional)
	Ophthalmic drops come in plastic or glass bottles. Ointments are prepared in small tubes.

4. Check client's identification by looking at identification bracelet and asking name.	Ensures correct client receives medication.
5. Assess condition of external eye structures (see chapter 13).	Provides baseline to later determine if local response to medications occurs. Also indicates need to clean eye before drug application.
6. Explain procedure to client.	Client often becomes anxious about medication being instilled into eye because of potential for discomfort.
7. Arrange supplies at bedside.	Ensures a smooth orderly procedure.
8. Ask client to lie supine or sit back in chair with head slightly hyperextended.	Position provides easy access to eye for medication instillation and minimizes drainage of medication through tear duct.
9. If crusts or drainage are present along eyelid margins or inner canthus, gently wash away. Soak any crusts that are dried and difficult to remove by applying damp washcloth or cotton ball over eye for few minutes. Always wipe clean from inner to outer canthus.	Crusts or drainage harbor microorganisms. Soaking allows easy removal, thus preventing pressure from being applied directly over eye. Cleansing from inner to outer canthus avoids entrance of microorganisms into lacrimal duct.
10. Hold cotton ball or clean tissue in nondominant hand on client's checkbone just below lower eyelid.	Cotton or tissue absorbs medication that escapes eye.

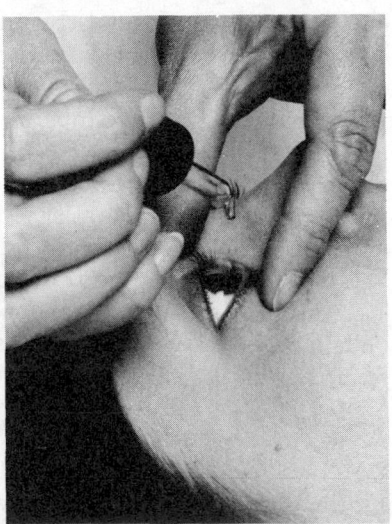

Step 13a

STEPS	RATIONALE
11. With tissue or cotton resting below lower lid, gently press downward with thumb or forefinger against bony orbit.	Technique exposes lower conjunctival sac. Retraction against bony orbit prevents pressure and trauma to eyeball and prevents fingers from touching eye.
12. Ask client to look at ceiling.	Action retracts sensitive cornea up and away from conjunctival sac and reduces stimulation of blink reflex.
13. Instill eyedrops.	
a. With dominant hand resting on client's forehead, hold filled medication eye dropper approximately 1 to 2 cm (½ to ¾ in) above conjunctival sac (see illustration).	Helps prevent accidental contact of eyedropper with eye structures, thus reducing risk of injury to eye and transfer of infection to dropper. Ophthalmic medications are sterilized.
b. Drop prescribed number of medication drops into conjunctival sac.	Conjunctival sac normally holds 1 to 2 drops. Applying drops to sac provides even distribution of medication across eye.
c. If client blinks or closes eye or if drops land on outer lid margins, repeat procedure.	Therapeutic effect of drug obtained only when drops enter conjunctival sac.
d. When administering drugs that cause systemic effects, protect your finger with clean tissue and apply gentle pressure to client's nasolacrimal duct for 30 to 60 sec.	Prevents overflow of medication into nasal and pharyngeal passages. Prevents absorption into systemic circulation.
e. After instilling drops, ask client to close eye gently.	Helps to distribute medication. Squinting or squeezing of eyelids forces medication from conjunctival sac.
14. Instill eye ointment.	
a. Holding ointment applicator above lid margin, apply thin stream of ointment evenly along inside edge of lower eyelid on conjunctiva.	Distributes medication evenly across eye and lid margin.
b. Ask client to look down.	Reduces blinking reflex during ointment application.
c. Apply thin stream of ointment along upper lid margin on inner conjunctiva.	Distributes medication evenly across eye and lid margin.
d. Have client close eye and rub lid lightly in circular motion with cotton ball.	Further distributes medication without traumatizing eye.
15. If excess medication is on eyelid, gently wipe it from inner to outer canthus.	Promotes comfort and prevents trauma to eye.
16. If client had eye patch, apply clean one by placing it over affected eye so entire eye is covered. Tape securely without applying pressure to eye.	Clean eye patch reduces chance of infection.
17. Dispose of soiled supplies in proper receptacle and wash hands.	Maintains neat environment at bedside and reduces transmission of microorganisms.
18. Observe response to medication, noting signs and symptoms of potential systemic effects and condition of eye.	Evaluates reaction to medication.
19. Record drug, concentration, number of drops, time of administration, and eye (left, right, or both) that received medication record.	Timely documentation prevents drug errors (for example, repeated or missed doses).

Administering Eardrops

STEPS	RATIONALE
1. Review physician's medication order for client's name, drug name, concentration, time of administration, number of drops to instill, and ear (right or left) to receive medication.	Ensures safe and correct administration of medication.
2. Wash hands.	Reduces transmission of microorganisms.
3. Prepare following equipment and supplies:	
a. Medication bottle and dropper	
b. Medication card, form, or printout	
c. Cotton-tipped applicator	Used to remove cerumen or drainage.
d. Tissue	
e. Cotton ball (optional)	
4. Identify client by reading identification bracelet and asking name.	Ensures correct client receives medication.
5. Assess condition of external ear structures and canal (see Chapter 13).	Provides baseline to determine later if local response to medication occurs, whether client's condition improves, or whether it will be necessary to clean ear before instilling medication.
6. Explain procedure to client.	Reduces client's anxiety.
7. Arrange supplies at bedside.	Helps nurse perform procedure smoothly.
8. Have client assume side-lying position with ear to be treated facing up.	Position provides easy access to ear for instillation of medication. Ear canal is in position to receive medication.
9. If cerumen or drainage occludes outermost portion of ear canal, wipe out gently with cotton tipped applicator (see illustration). *Do not force wax inward to block or occlude canal.*	Cerumen and drainage habor microorganisms and can block distribution of medication into canal. Occlusion of canal interferes with normal sound conduction.
10. Straighten ear canal by pulling auricle down and back (children) or upward and outward (adult).	Straightening of ear canal provides for direct access to deeper external ear structures.
11. Instill prescribed drops holding dropper 1 cm (½ in) above ear canal (see illustration).	Forcing drops into occluded canal can cause injury to eardrum.
12. Ask client to remain in side-lying position 2 to 3 min. Apply gentle massage or pressure to tragus of ear with finger (see illustration).	Allows complete distribution of medication. Pressure and massage moves medication inward.
13. At times physician orders insertion of portion of cotton ball into outermost part of canal. Do not press cotton into canal.	Inserting cotton into outer canal prevents escape of medication when client sits or stands. Cotton should not block canal to impair hearing.
14. Remove cotton in 15 min.	Time period promotes drug distribution and absorption.
15. Dispose of soiled supplies and wash hands.	Keeps bedside neat. Reduces transmission of infection.
16. Assist client to comfortable position after drops are absorbed.	Restores comfort.
17. Evaluate condition of external ear between drug instillations.	Determines response to medication.
18. Record drug, concentration, number of drops, time administered, and ear into which drops instilled on medication form.	Timely documentation prevents drug errors (for example, repeated doses).
19. Record condition of ear canal in nurse's notes.	Documents client's status and response to therapy.

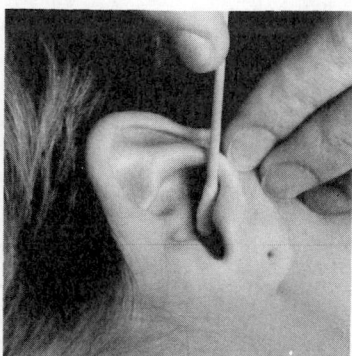

Step 9

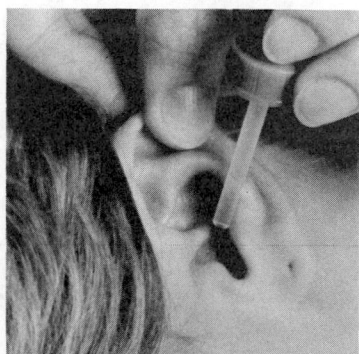

Step 11

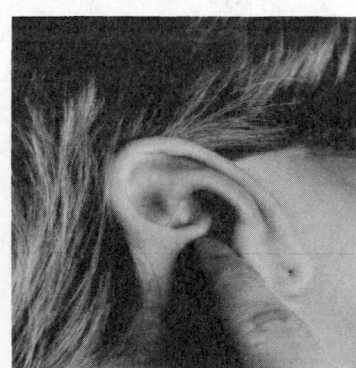

Step 12

Administering Nasal Drops

STEPS	RATIONALE
1. Review physician's medication order for client's name, drug name, concentration of solution, number of drops, and time of administration.	Ensures safe and correct administration of medication.
2. Refer to the medical record to determine which sinus is affected.	Will affect positioning that client assumes during drug instillation.
3. Wash hands.	Reduces transmission of microorganisms.
4. Prepare following equipment and supplies:	
a. Prepared medication with clean dropper.	Dropper or applicator need not be sterile but should be clean.
b. Medication card, form, or printout	
c. Facial tissue	
d. Small pillow (optional)	Used in positioning client.
e. Washcloth (optional)	Used to clean nares.
5. Check client's identification by reading identification bracelet and asking name.	Ensures correct client receives medication.
6. Inspect condition of nose and sinuses (see Chapter 13). Palpate sinuses for tenderness.	Findings provide baseline to monitor effect of medication. Discharge will interfere with drug absorption.
7. Explain procedure regarding positioning and sensations to expect, such as burning or stinging of mucosa or choking sensation as medication trickles into throat.	Helps to reduce anxiety.
8. Arrange supplies and medications at bedside.	Ensures smooth, orderly procedure.
9. Instruct client to blow his nose unless contraindicated (for example, risk of increased intracranial pressure or nose bleeds).	Removes mucus and secretions that can block distribution of medication.
10. Administer nasal drops.	
a. Assist client to supine position	Position provides access to nasal passages.
b. Position head properly:	Position allows medication to drain into affected sinus.
(1) Posterior pharynx—tilt client's head backward.	
(2) Ethmoid or sphenoid sinus—tilt head back over edge of bed or place small pillow under client's shoulder and tilt head back (see illustration).	
(3) Frontal and maxillary sinus—tilt head back over edge of bed or pillow with head turned toward side to be treated (see illustration).	

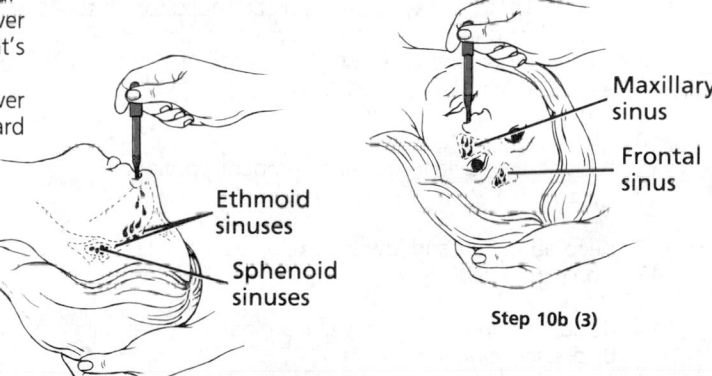

Step 10b (2)   Ethmoid sinuses   Sphenoid sinuses

Maxillary sinus   Frontal sinus   Step 10b (3)

STEPS	RATIONALE
Support client's head with nondominant hand.	Prevents straining of neck muscles.
c. Instruct client to breathe through mouth.	Mouth breathing reduces chance of aspirating nasal drops into trachea and lungs.
d. Hold dropper 1 cm (½ in) above nares and instill prescribed number of drops toward midline of ethmoid bone.	Avoids contamination of dropper. Instilling toward ethmoid bone facilitates distribution of medication over nasal mucosa
e. Have client remain in supine position 5 min.	Prevents premature loss of medication through nares.
f. Offer facial tissue to blot runny nose, but caution client against blowing nose for several minutes.	Allows maximum amount of medication to be absorbed.
11. Assist client to a comfortable position after drug absorbed.	Restores comfort.
12. Dispose of soiled supplies in proper container and wash hands.	Maintains neat, orderly environment. Reduces spread of microorganisms.
13. Record medication administration, including drug name, concentration, number of drops, nostril into which drug was instilled, and time of administration.	Timely documentation prevents drug errors (for example, repeated doses).
14. Observe client for side effects 15 to 30 min after administration.	Drugs absorbed through mucosa can cause systemic reaction.

PROCEDURE 15-10

Administering Vaginal Instillations

STEPS	RATIONALE
1. Review physician's order including client's name, drug name, form (cream or suppository), route, dosage, and time of administration.	Ensures safe and correct administration of medication.
2. Wash hands.	Reduces transfer of microorganisms.

3. Prepare following supplies for suppository insertion:
  a. Vaginal suppository
  b. Clean, disposable gloves
  c. Lubricating jelly
  d. Clean facial tissues
  e. Perineal pad (optional)
  f. Medication ticket, form, or printout
	These are stored in refrigerator to maintain solid shape.
	
	Eases insertion of suppository.

4. Prepare following supplies for cream or foam instillation:
  a. Vaginal cream or foam
  b. Plastic applicator
  c. Clean, disposable gloves
  d. Paper towel
  e. Perineal pad (optional)
  f. Medication ticket, form, or printout
	Prepared in plastic tube or can.

5. Check client's identification by reading identification bracelet and asking name.	Ensures correct client receives medication.
6. Inspect condition of external genitalia and vaginal canal (see Chapter 13).	Findings provide baseline to monitor effect of medication.
7. Assess client's ability to manipulate applicator or suppository and to position self to insert medication.	Mobility restriction will indicate level of assistance required from nurse.
8. Explain procedure to client. Be specific if client plans on self-administering medication.	Promotes understanding. Will enable client to self-administer drug if physically able.
9. Arrange supplies at bedside.	Helps nurse perform procedure smoothly.
10. Close room curtain or door.	Provides for privacy.
11. Assist client to lie in dorsal recumbent position.	Position provides easy access to and good exposure of vaginal canal. Dependent position also allows suppository to dissolve in vagina without escaping through orifice.
12. Keep abdomen and lower extremities draped.	Minimizes client's embarrassment.
13. Apply disposable gloves.	Prevents transmission of infection between nurse and client.
14. Be sure vaginal orifice is well-illuminated by room light or gooseneck lamp.	Proper insertion requires visualization of external genitalia.
15. For suppository insertion with gloved hand: a. Remove suppository from foil wrapper and apply liberal amount of petroleum jelly to smooth or rounded end. Lubricate gloved index finger of dominant hand.	Lubrication reduces friction against mucosal surfaces during insertion.
b. With nondominant gloved hand, gently retract labial folds.	Exposes vaginal orifice.
c. Insert rounded end of suppository along posterior wall of vaginal canal entire length of finger (7.5 to 10 cm or 3 to 4 in) (see illustration).	Proper placement of suppository ensures equal distribution of medication along walls of vaginal cavity.
d. Withdraw finger and wipe away remaining lubricant from around orifice and labia.	Maintains comfort.
16. For application of cream or foam: a. Fill cream or foam applicator following package directions.	Dosage is prescribed by volume in applicator.
b. With nondominant gloved hand, gently retract labial folds.	Exposes vaginal orifice.

STEPS	RATIONALE
c. With dominant gloved hand, insert applicator approximately 5 to 7.5 cm (2 to 3 in). Push applicator plunger to deposit medication into vagina (see illustration).	Allows for equal distribution of medication along vaginal walls.
d. Withdraw applicator and place on paper towel. Wipe off residual cream from labia or vaginal orifice.	Residual cream on applicator may contain microorganisms.
17. Remove gloves by pulling them inside out and discard in appropriate receptacle. Wash hands.	Reduces transfer of microorganisms.
18. Instruct client to remain on her back for at least 10 min.	Medication will be distributed and absorbed evenly throughout vaginal cavity and not be lost through orifice.
19. If applicator is used, wash with soap and warm water, rinse, and store for future use.	Vaginal cavity is not sterile. Soap and water assist in removal of bacteria and residual cream.
20. Offer client perineal pad when she resumes ambulation.	Provides client comfort.
21. Inspect condition of vaginal canal and external genitalia between applications.	Determines whether vaginal medication effectively reduced irritation or inflammation of tissues.
22. Record drug name, dosage, route, and time of administration on medication record.	Timely recording prevents drug errors.

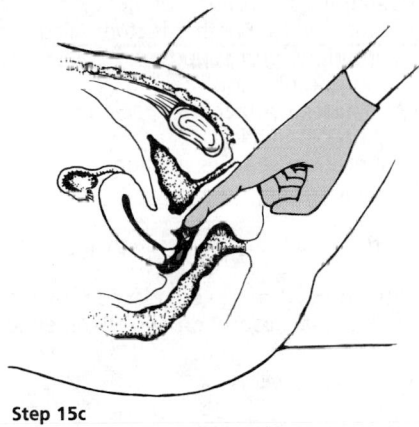

Step 15c

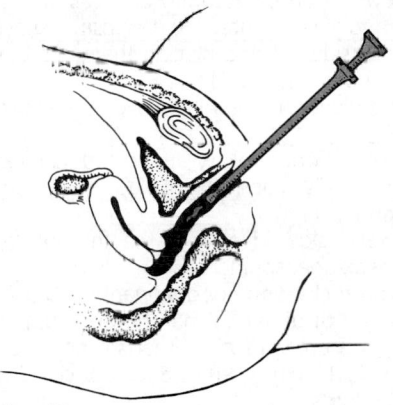

Step 16c

Severe nose bleeds are usually treated with packing or tampons. Tampons are treated with epinephrine, to reduce blood flow. Usually a physician places nasal tampons.

Vaginal Instillations

Vaginal medications are available as suppositories, foam, jellies, or creams. Suppositories come individually packaged in foil wrappers. Storage in a refrigerator prevents the solid, oval-shaped suppositories from melting. After a suppository is inserted into the vaginal cavity, body temperature causes the suppository to melt and be distributed. Foam, jellies, and creams are administered with an inserter or applicator (Procedure 15-10). A suppository is given with a gloved hand. Clients often prefer administering their own vaginal medications and should be given privacy. After instillation of the drug she may wish to wear a perineal pad to collect excess drainage. Because vaginal medications are frequently given to treat infection, any discharge may be foul smelling. Good aseptic technique should be followed and the client should be offered frequent opportunities to maintain perineal hygiene (see Chapter 32).

PROCEDURE 15-11

Administering Rectal Suppositories

STEPS	RATIONALE
1. Review physician's order, including client's name, drug name, form, route, and time of administration.	Ensures safe and correct administration of medication.
2. Review medical record for history of rectal surgery or bleeding.	Conditions contraindicate use of suppository.
3. Wash hands.	Reduces transfer of microorganisms.

4. Prepare following equipment and supplies:
  a. Rectal suppository
  b. Lubricating jelly
  c. Clean, disposable gloves
  d. Tissue
  e. Medication ticket, form, or printout.	

5. Apply disposable gloves.	Prevents contact with infected material.
6. Check client's identification by reading identification bracelet and asking name.	Ensures correct client receives medication.
7. Explain procedure. Be specific if client wishes to self-administer drug.	Promotes understanding and cooperation. Will enable client to self-administer drug if physically able.
8. Arrange supplies at bedside.	Helps nurse perform procedure smoothly.
9. Close room curtain or door.	Maintains privacy and minimizes embarrassment.
10. Assist client in assuming a side-lying Sims' position with upper leg flexed upward. Keep client draped with only anal area exposed.	Position exposes anus and helps client to relax external anal sphincter. Maintains privacy and facilitates relaxation.
11. Examine condition of anus externally and palpate rectal walls as needed (see Chapter 13). Dispose of gloves by turning them inside out and placing them in proper receptacle if they become soiled.	Determines presence of active rectal bleeding. Palpation determines whether rectum filled with feces, which may interfere with suppository placement. Reduces transmission of infection.
12. Apply disposable gloves (if previous gloves were soiled and discarded).	Minimizes contact with fecal material to reduce transmission of infection.
13. Remove suppository from foil wrapper and lubricate rounded end with jelly. Lubricate gloved index finger of dominant hand.	Lubrication reduces friction as suppository enters rectal canal.
14. Ask client to take slow deep breaths through the mouth and to relax anal sphincter.	Forcing suppository through constricted sphincter causes pain.
15. Retract client's buttocks with nondominant hand. With gloved index finger of dominant hand, insert suppository gently through anus, past internal sphincter, and against rectal wall, 10 cm (4 in) in adults, 5 cm (2 in) in children and infants.	Suppository must be placed against rectal mucosa for eventual absorption and therapeutic action.
16. Withdraw your finger and wipe client's anal area.	Provides for comfort.
17. Discard gloves by turning them inside out, and dispose of them in appropriate receptacle.	Reduces transfer of microorganisms.
18. Ask client to remain flat or on his side for 5 min.	Prevents expulsion of suppository.
19. If suppository contains laxative or fecal softener, place call light within client's reach so he can obtain assistance to reach bedpan or toilet.	Being able to call for assistnce provides client with sense of control over elimination.
20. Wash hands.	Reduces risk of transfer of infection.
21. Return within 5 min to determine if suppository expelled.	Reinsertion may be necessary.
22. Record drug name, dosage, route, and time of administration on medication record.	Timely recording prevents errors.

PROCEDURE 15-12

Using Metered Dose Inhalers

STEPS	RATIONALE
1. Review physician's medication order, including client name, drug name, dosage, number of inhalations, and time of administration.	Ensures safe and correct administration of medication.
2. Assess client's ability to hold and manipulate inhaler.	Any impairment of grasp or presence of tremors of hands will interfere with client's ability to depress canister within inhaler.
3. Assess drug schedule and number of inhalations prescribed for each dose.	Influences explanations nurse provides for use of inhaler.
4. Have client prepare following equipment and supplies:	
a. Metered dose inhaler with medication canister (see illustration)	
b. Facial tissues (optional)	
c. Wash basin or sink with warm water.	Water is used to clean inhaler.
d. Paper towel	
5. Instruct client in comfortable environment by sitting in chair in hospital room, or sitting at kitchen table in home.	Client will be more likely to remain perceptive of nurse's explanations.
6. Allow client opportunity to manipulate inhaler and canister. Explain and demonstrate how canister fits into inhaler.	Client must be familiar with how to use equipment.
7. Explain what metered dose is, and warn client about overuse of inhaler, including drug side effects.	Client must not arbitrarily decide to administer excessive inhalations because of risk of serious side effects. If given in recommended doses, side effects are uncommon.
8. Explain steps used to administer inhaled dose of medication. (Demonstrate steps when possible).	Use of simple, step-by-step explanations allows client to ask questions at any point during procedure. Nurse demonstrates actual depression of canister without self-administering drug dose.
a. Remove mouthpiece cover from inhaler.	
b. Open lips and place inhaler in mouth with opening toward back of throat.	
c. Exhale fully, then grasp mouthpiece with teeth and lips while holding inhaler with thumb at the mouthpiece and the index finger and middle finger at the top (see illustration).	Medication should not escape through mouth.
d. While inhaling slowly and deeply through mouth, depress medication canister fully.	Medication is distributed to airways during inhalation. Inhalation through mouth rather than nose draws medication more effectively into airways.

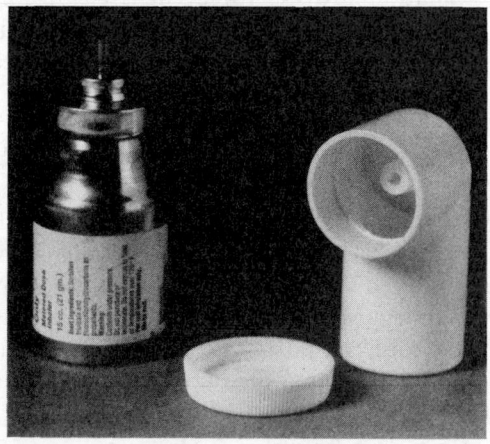

Step 4a

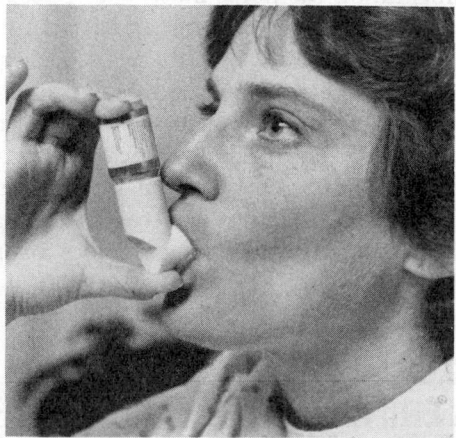

Step 8c

Continued.

Using Metered Dose Inhalers

STEPS	RATIONALE
e. Hold breath for approximately 10 sec.	Allows tiny drops of aerosol spray to reach deeper branches of airways.
f. Exhale through pursed lips.	Pursed lip breathing keeps small airways open during exhalation.
9. Instruct client to wait 5 to 10 min between inhalations or as ordered by physician.	Drugs must be inhaled sequentially. First inhalation opens airways and reduces inflammation. Second or third inhalations penetrate deeper airways.
10. Instruct client against repeating inhalations before next scheduled dose.	Drugs are prescribed at intervals during day to provide constant bronchodilation and minimize side effects.
11. Explain to client that he may feel gagging sensation in throat caused by droplets of medication on pharynx or tongue.	Results when inhalant is sprayed and inhaled incorrectly.
12. Instruct client in removing medication canister and cleaning inhaler in warm water.	Accumulation of spray around mouthpiece can interfere with proper distribution during use.
13. Ask client if he has any questions.	Provides opportunity to clarify misconceptions or misunderstanding.
14. Have client demonstrate use of inhaler and explain drug schedule.	Return demonstration provides feedback for measuring learning. Improves likelihood of compliance with therapy.
15. Describe in nurses' notes content of skills taught and client's ability to perform skill.	Information provides continuity to teaching plan so other members of nursing staff will not teach same material.

Rectal Instillations

Rectal suppositories differ in shape from vaginal suppositories, being thinner and bullet shaped. The rounded end prevents anal trauma during insertion. Rectal suppositories contain medications that exert local effects, such as promoting defecation, or systemic effects, such as reducing nausea. Rectal suppositories are stored in the refrigerator until administered.

During administration the nurse must place the suppository past the internal anal sphincter and against the rectal mucosa (Procedure 15-11). Otherwise the suppository may be expelled before it can dissolve and be absorbed into the mucosa. With practice a nurse learns to recognize the sensation of the sphincter relaxing around the finger. The suppository should not be forced into a mass of fecal material. It may be necessary to clear the rectum with a small cleansing enema before a suppository can be inserted.

ADMINISTERING DRUGS BY INHALATION

Drugs administered with hand-held *inhalers* are dispersed through an aerosol spray, mist, or powder that penetrates lung airways. The alveolar-capillary network absorbs medications rapidly. Inhaled medications are usually designed to produce local effects such as bronchodilators. However, some medications can create serious systemic side effects.

Clients who receive drugs by inhalation frequently suffer chronic respiratory disease such as chronic asthma, emphysema, or bronchitis. Drugs given by inhalation provide these clients with control of airway obstruction, and because these clients depend on medications for disease control, they must learn about them and how to administer them safely.

A metered dose inhaler (Procedure 15-12) delivers a measured dose of drug with each push of a canister. Approximately 5 to 10 pounds of pressure must be used to activate the aerosol (Statz, 1984). However, hand strength diminishes with age and from chronic respiratory disease. Statz (1984) found that metered dose inhalers work best when clients use a three-point or lateral hand position to activate canisters. Manufacturers indicate that the two-point position is least effective.

IRRIGATIONS

Medications may be used to irrigate or wash out a body cavity and are delivered through a stream of so-

PROCEDURE 15-13

Ear Irrigations

STEPS	RATIONALE
1. Review the physician's order for client name, purpose of irrigation, type of irrigant ordered, and time of administration.	Ensures safe and correct administration of irrigation.
2. Check client's identification by reading identification bracelet and asking name.	Ensures correct client receives irrigation.
3. Wash hands.	Reduces transfer of microorganisms.
4. Assess condition of external ear structures and canal for redness, swelling, and discharge (see Chapter 13).	Evidence of signs of infection serves as baseline data in determining effectiveness of irrigation.
5. Determine if client is experiencing localized tenderness or discomfort.	Indicates inflammation of outer ear structures.
6. Prepare the following equipment and supplies:	
a. Container of sterile irrigating solution warmed to room temperature	Warmed solution minimizes chance of causing client to feel dizzy when solution comes in contact with tympanic membrane.
b. Irrigating syringe (rubber bulb or Asepto)	Used to introduce solution under low pressure.
c. Kidney-shaped basin	Used to collect irrigating solution.
d. Towel	
e. Applicator swab and cotton balls	Used to clean and dry ear canal.
7. Explain procedure. Warn that the irrigation may cause sensation of dizziness, fullness, and warmth.	Prepares client to anticipate effects of irrigation, and promotes cooperation.
8. Arrange supplies at bedside.	Helps nurse to perform procedure smoothly.
9. Close curtain or room door.	Maintains privacy.
10. Assist client to assume a sitting or lying position with head turned toward the affected ear. Place towel under client's head and shoulder and have client hold basin under affected ear.	Position minimizes leakage of fluids around neck and facial area for comfort. Solution will flow from ear canal to basin.
11. Gently clean the auricle and ear canal with cotton applicator. Do *not* force drainage or cerumen into the ear canal.	Prevents infected material from reentering ear canal.
12. Fill the irrigating syringe with solution (approximately 50 cc).	Enough fluid is needed to provide a steady irrigating stream.
13. Gently grasp the auricle of the ear and straighten the ear canal by pulling it down and back (children) or upward and outward (adult).	Allows fluid to flow length of the canal.
14. Slowly instill the irrigating solution by holding the tip of the syringe 1 cm (½ inch) above the opening to the ear canal. Allow the fluid to drain out during instillation. Continue until canal is cleansed or all solution is used.	Slow instillation prevents buildup of pressure in the ear canal and ensures contact of the medication with all of the canal surfaces.
15. Do *not* occlude the canal with the tip of the syringe.	Buildup of fluid in canal under forced pressure could cause rupture of the tympanic membrane.
16. Dry off outer ear canal with cotton ball. Leave cotton loosely in place for 5 to 10 minutes.	Maintains comfort. Absorbs excess moisture in ear canal.
17. Assist client to a sitting position.	Maintains comfort.
18. Wash hands and dispose of supplies.	Reduces transmission of infection.
19. Record and report irrigation solution used, character of ear structures, appearance of fluid return or discharge, and client's response.	Documents response to therapy.

lution. Irrigations are most commonly performed with sterile water, saline, or antiseptic solutions on the eye, ear, throat, vagina, and urinary tract (see Chapter 38). When there is a break in the skin or mucosa, the nurse uses aseptic technique to perform an irrigation. When the cavity to be irrigated is not sterile, as in the case with the ear canal (Procedure 15-13), vagina, or eye, clean technique is acceptable. In health care settings, however, sterile solutions are always used. An irrigation can serve to cleanse an area or apply a medication or heat or cold to injured tissue. When performing irrigations, the nurse follows the following principles:

1) Avoid further injury to tissue
2) Prevent the transmission of infection
3) Maintain the client's comfort

SUMMARY

The nurse is responsible for safely and effectively administering medications, which requires understanding of legal guidelines affecting drug prescription and administration. The nurse's care of clients also involves making decisions about the need for drug therapy.

The nurse must have detailed knowledge about a drug and the client receiving it. A thorough assessment of the client's physical condition, medical history, allergies, diet, and medication history ensures that accurate judgments will be made about drug therapy.

Preparation of drugs requires accurate calculation and a methodical approach. Application of physiological, anatomical, and aseptic principles ensure safe administration of drugs. When monitoring a response to medications, the nurse uses physical assessment skills and knowledge of expected drug effects. The nurse also teaches clients and families to administer drugs safely and to follow schedules for drug therapy.

If medications are given incorrectly, they can injure the client. A client's well-being depends on the nurse's application of all principles of drug administration.

KEY CONCEPTS

- ✓ Learning drug classifications improves understanding of nursing implications for administering drugs with similar characteristics.
- ✓ Nurse practice acts define and set limits on the scope of a nurse's professional functions and responsibilities in giving medications.
- ✓ All controlled substances are handled according to strict procedures that account for each drug.
- ✓ The nurse applies understanding of the physiology of drug action when timing administration, selecting routes, initiating actions to promote drug efficacy, and observing responses to drugs.
- ✓ Clients with alterations in organs that excrete drugs are at risk for drug toxicity.
- ✓ The elderly client's body undergoes structural and functional changes that alter drug actions and influence the manner in which nurses provide drug therapy.
- ✓ Children's drug dosages are computed on the basis of body surface area or weight.
- ✓ Repeated doses of a drug are required to achieve constant therapeutic blood levels.
- ✓ Drugs given parenterally are absorbed more quickly than drugs administered by other routes.
- ✓ The metric system is the standard system for drug measurement in most countries of the world.
- ✓ Each drug order should include the client's name, the order date, the drug name, dosage, and route and time of administration, and the physician's signature.
- ✓ A teaching plan for drug therapy should include guidelines for drug safety.
- ✓ The "five rights" of drug administration ensure accurate preparation and administration of drug dosages.
- ✓ Nurses administer only medications they prepare.
- ✓ The nurse never administers a drug without accurately identifying a client.
- ✓ Drugs should be charted immediately after administration.
- ✓ A nurse uses clinical judgment in determining the best time to administer p.r.n.-ordered medications.

✓ The nurse reports a drug error immediately.

✓ When preparing medications, the nurse checks the drug container label against the medication card or form three times.

✓ The nurse never leaves a prepared medication unattended.

✓ The nurse rotates injection sites when giving repeated parenteral administrations.

✓ Failure to select injection sites by anatomical landmarks may lead to tissue, bone, or nerve damage.

REFERENCES

Burman, R, and Berkowitz, H: IV bolus: effective but potentially hazardous, Crit Care Nurs 6(1):22, 1986.

Centers for Disease Control: Guidelines for isolation procedures, Atlanta, 1983.

Clark, JB, et al.: Pharmacological basis of nursing practice, ed. 2, St. Louis, 1986, The C.V. Mosby Co.

Cyganski, JM, et al.: The case for the heparin flush, Am J Nurs 87:796, 1987.

Donnelly, D: Instilling eye drops: difficulties experienced by patients following cataract surgery, J Adv Nurs 12:235, 1987.

Dunn, DL, and Lenihan, SF: The case for the saline flush, Am J Nurs 87:798, 1987.

Eliopoulos, C: Geriatric pharmacology. In Eliopoulos, C: Gerontological nursing, ed. 2, Philadelphia, 1987, J.B. Lippincott Co.

Harrigan, CA: Intermittent IV therapy without heparin: a study, NITA 8:519, 1985.

Hasselbalch, H, et al.: Alternative to optimal administration of tablets, Acta Med Scand 217:527, 1985.

Nurses Drug Alert: Hazards of nasal decongestants in young children, Am J Nurs 84:1265, 1984.

Simonson, W: Medications and the elderly: a guide for promoting proper use, Rockville, Md., 1984, Aspen Publishers, Inc.

Whaley, LF, and Wong, DL: Nursing care of infants and children, ed. 3, St. Louis, 1987, The C.V. Mosby Co.

Wong, DL: Significance of dead space in syringes, Am J Nurs 82:1237, 1982.

Research Articles

Perez, S: Reducing injection pain, Am J Nurs 84:7, 1984.

Statz, E: Hand strength and metered dose inhalers, Am J Nurs 84:800, 1984.

ADDITIONAL READINGS

Allen, MD: Drug therapy in the elderly, Am J Nurs 80:1474, 1980.

Bauer, LA: Clinical pharmacokinetics, Nurse Pract 7:42, 1982.

Birdsall, C, and Uretsky, S: How do I administer medication by NG? Am J Nurs 84:1259, 1984.

Brock, A: Self-administration of drugs in the elderly: nursing responsibilities, J Gerontol Nurs 6:402, 1980.

Clayton, M: The right way to prevent medication errors, RN 50(6):30, 1987.

Cushing, M: Drug errors can be bitter pills, Am J Nurs 86:895, 1986.

Davis, NM, and Cohen, MR: Learning from mistakes: 20 tips for avoiding medication errors, Nurs 82 12:65, 1982.

Hayes, JE: Normal changes in aging and nursing implications of drug therapy, Nurs Clin North Am 17:253, 1982.

Keen, MF: Comparison of intramuscular injection techniques to reduce site discomfort and lesions, Nurs Res 35:207, 1986.

Keithley, JK, and O'Donnell, J: Look out for these drug-nutrient interactions, Nurs 86, 16(2):42, 1986.

Labar, C: Filling in the blanks of prescription writing. Am J Nurs 86:30, 1986.

Lent-Wunderlich, E, and Ott, MJ: Helping your patient through eye surgery, RN 49:43, 1986.

LeSage, J: Drug therapy in long term care facilities, Nurs Clin North Am 17:331, 1982.

McCaffery, M: Narcotic analgesia for the elderly, Am J Nurs 85:296, 1985.

McConnell, EA: The subtle art of really good injections, RN 45:24, 1982.

McGovern, K: Ten steps for preventing medication errors, Nurs 86: 16(12): 36, 1986.

Miyares, MV: Medication aids your elderly patient will love, RN 48:44, 1985.

Moree, NA: Nurses speak out on patients and drug regimens, Am J Nurs 85:51, 1985.

Rettig, FM, and Southby, JR: Using different body positions to reduce discomfort from dorsogluteal injection, Nurs Res, 31:219, 1982.

Sandroff, R: Booby-trapped orders, RN 44:26, 1981.

Scharf, L: Safe needle disposal: a timely reminder, RN 49:42, 1986.

Shepherd, MJ, and Swearingen, P: Z-track injections, Am J Nurs 84:746, 1984.

Smith, JB: The patient who can't remember to take her meds, RN 49(9):38, 1986.

Tanner, S: IV bolus leaves no room for error, RN 44:54, 1981.

Thatcher, G: Insulin injections: the case against random rotation, Am J Nurs 85:690, 1985.

Thompson, DA: Teaching the client about anticoagulants, Am J Nurs 82:278, 1982.

Todd, B: Drugs and the elderly: using eye drops and ointments safely, Geriatr Nurs 4(1):55, 1983.

Vanbree, NS, et al.: Clinical evaluation of three techniques for administering low-dose heparin, Nurs Res 33:15, 1984.

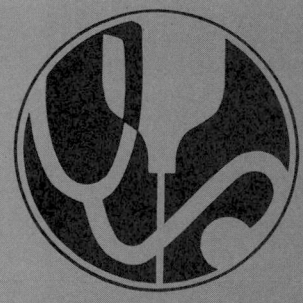

UNIT *4*

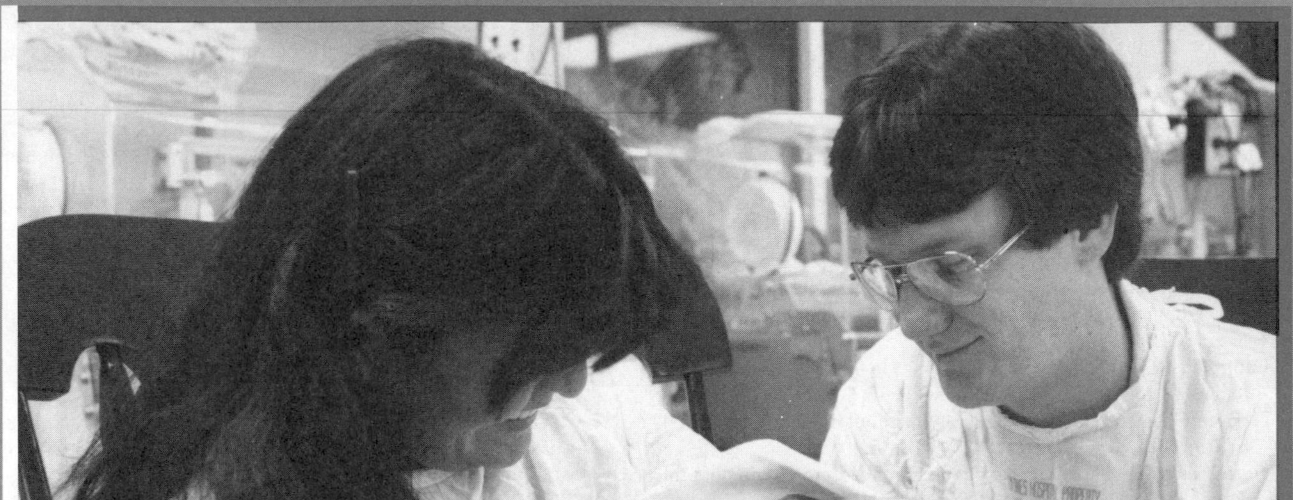

Professional Nursing Concepts

The five chapters in Unit 4 focus on concepts of professional nursing practice important in all health care areas. These concepts involve the following aspects of the nurse-client relationship: values, ethics, legal issues, communication, and teaching and learning process.

Values clarification helps the nurse and client understand their values and the effects of those values on attitudes and health practices so they can work together effectively to meet the client's health care goals. Because nurses are responsible and accountable for their actions, they must understand the profession's code of ethics and ethical issues. Because of the legal complexities of the health care system, nurses must be aware of the potential legal implications of their actions. Because nurses continually communicate with clients and other professionals, they use the principles of communication to provide successful care. Client teaching is also an essential aspect of nursing, requiring the nurse to individualize methods and apply basic teaching principles throughout the nursing process.

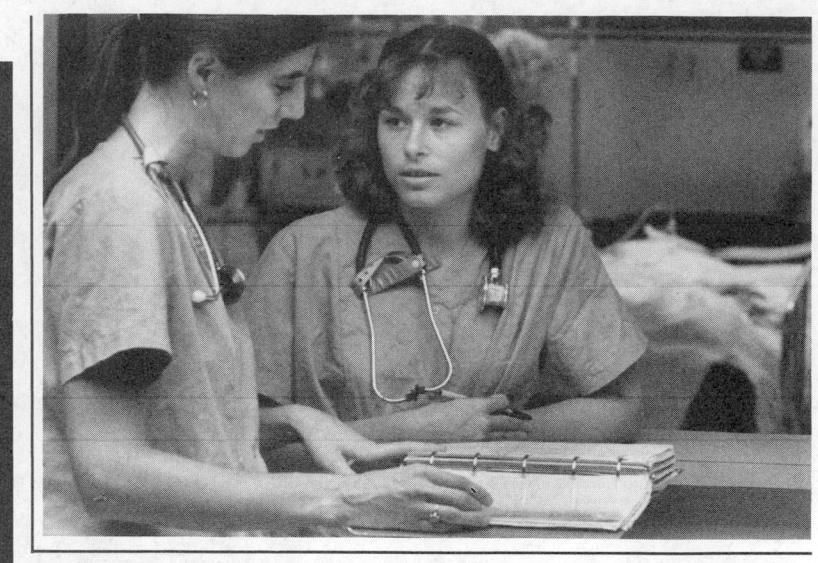

OBJECTIVES

Mastery of content in this chapter will enable the student to:

- Define the key terms listed.
- Describe how values influence behavior and attitudes.
- Discuss the ways in which values are learned.
- Contrast and compare modes of value transmission.
- Compare how values are formed at different stages of development.
- Discuss the influence of ethnicity on value formation.
- Explain the relationship between nurse's values and clinical decision making.
- Describe the process of values clarification.
- Discuss the advantages of values clarification in nursing.
- Use a values clarification strategy to examine personal values.
- Discuss the techniques used to help clients clarify values.
- Analyze personal values as a student of nursing.

KEY TERMS

Autonomy

Industry

Initiative

Laissez-Faire

Modeling

Moralize

Value

Values Clarification

Values Clarification Strategy

Values

Facing decisions with a clear perspective and purpose is no simple task. Every day brings situations that require thought, decision making, and action. Frequently the person deciding is confused over the many options involved in a decision. How is a decision made? Who will be affected by the decision? What influences a person's thoughts when deciding? What are the implications of the decision? A decision is based in part on the person's conscious or unconscious values. A value is a personal belief about the worth of a given idea or behavior. Values are standards that influence our behavior. The values an individual holds reflect his personal needs, the culture and society in which he lives, and the significant others to whom he relates. Values vary from person to person, developing and changing as a person grows and matures.

Nurses practice under a personal and professional set of values. As persons, nurses have the right to express and act on their beliefs (Bernal, 1985). Each client also has a value system unique to his own needs and preferences. Many values a nurse holds (for example, a belief about the prolongation of life for cancer clients) can influence a client's care. Conflict between a nurse's values and the clients served ultimately may lead to ethical dilemmas (see Chapter 17). It is important for nurses to understand their own values, as well as those of their clients. An objective analysis of value systems helps nurses to act in a more professional and knowledgeable way.

In the health care setting, the values of the nurse, health team, client, and society interact. Clients often find themselves dependent on the nurse in a role inconsistent with their valued independence. Society expects clients to conform to the behaviors of the sick role (see Chapter 2). The nurse attempts to minimize the effect of his or her personal values on the client's recovery. However, the nurse's values that are consistent with a client's improved health status should be enforced to help clients assume a more functional and improved level of health.

The threats posed by illness cause individuals to reassess their health-related values. The frequency and intensity with which a person practices health-promoting behaviors depend on the value placed on reducing the threat of illness and promoting health. The nurse helps the client clarify personal values, reorder value priorities, minimize conflict, and achieve consistency among values and behaviors related to illness prevention and health promotion. The nurse helps clients understand themselves and the impact of certain behaviors on their well-being.

NATURE AND FUNCTION OF VALUES

The values a person chooses as important are a part of his or her identity. Values represent a way of life. Rokeach (1973) has made the following observations about values:

1. The total number of values a person possesses is relatively small.
2. Values are organized into value systems.
3. The origin of human values can be traced to culture, society, institutions, and personality.
4. The consequences of human values will be manifested in all phenomena social scientists might consider worth studying and understanding.

The values a person consciously acknowledges as important and most significant in influencing one's life are few. It is easy to identify a large number of values: justice, fairness, beneficence, equality, independence, and responsibility. However, only a few values have a consistent and predictable impact on a person's behavior. No two individuals give equal importance to the same values. The values that hold the greatest importance in shaping a person's thoughts and actions are a part of his unique identity.

Values related to one another form a value system. Examples of value systems are those related to religion, health, and self-respect. Rokeach (1973) described value systems as learned principles and rules to allow choice and to guide decisions. A person's values about health will determine the choices made about health promotion. For example, eating a balanced diet, exercising and seeking early medical attention during illness are the result of a person's value of staying fit. It is important

that the behaviors a person assumes as a result of personal values are realistic. A young man with severe heart disease cannot set unrealistic expectations for the maintenance of his physical strength and endurance. A realistic value system allows the person to be flexible and to attain greater satisfaction from the attitudes, behaviors, and feelings that are influenced by his values.

Values may be classified as intrinsic or extrinsic (Steele, 1986). Intrinsic values are related to the maintenance of life such as the value of food or love. Values categorized as extrinsic originate from outside a person and are not essential to the maintenance of life. For example, values associated with the choice of an occupation are extrinsic. Some values will appear less important than others depending on the type of choices a person must make or the priority of the values held.

A person's perceptions of other individuals are influenced by his or her values. When meeting someone for the first time, how does the person act? What aspect of his personality does he choose to show? What behaviors does she look for in another individual? Values direct people's responses toward one another. The nurse who grasps the outstretched hand of a dying client values the subtleties of interpersonal communication and the importance of compassion. The nurse also perceives the dying client's value of being able to maintain courage during a time of suffering. The nurse's values guide how he or she present themselves to others and form a basis for their evaluation of themselves and others.

Values are the basis for a person's positions on personal, professional, social, political, or philosophical issues. In health care, values influence the way nurses attain high-quality care for all clients. For example, if a nurse values humanistic, individualized, and coordinated efforts at providing nursing care, it is likely that the care she or he provides will be of high quality. These values will establish standards of excellence for the profession. Nurses make decisions about the care of their clients on the basis of their personal and professional values.

A value is not the same as an attitude. Attitudes are feelings toward a person, object, or idea (Steele, 1986). A person's attitudes are relatively constant. With any attitude a person evaluates whether the person, object, or idea is good or bad, positive or negative. A person may have an attitude about certain ideas without valuing them. Values have a strong motivational component that directs a person's conduct. Attitudes can also influence behavior. However, values become the standards for guiding a person's actions, developing and maintaining attitudes toward relevant objects, for morally judging self and others, and for comparing self and others (Rokeach, 1973).

Values give meaning to life, guiding the behavior and to fulfill the need for self-esteem and self-actualization (the understanding and achievement of a person's potential in life). Values involve a search for meaning and a desire for self-understanding. What makes people happy? How do they become satisfied with a choice or a decision? What ideas do they share with others or defend? As people form and test values, they retain those that provide the most reliable and satisfying solutions to problems.

FORMATION OF VALUES

Values are learned through observation and experience. An individual observes not only behavior but also the setting in which it occurs and the response it evokes. He repeats and values behavior that he observes as being successful or productive. For example, a beginning nursing student closely observes a clinical instructor's actions at the client's bedside. The student watches the client's reactions as the instructor demonstrates nursing skill. If the client remains relaxed and accepting as the instructor administers care, the student learns to value being a competent and caring nurse. The instructor's competence and caring as a professional nurse are incorporated into the student's value system.

Values are also acquired through experience. After repeatedly experiencing the same situations, a person is wise to look back on personal successes and failures. What behaviors led to desirable effects? How did other people respond to those behaviors? The nature of the response a person receives after acting a certain way determines whether he acquires the behavior permanently. The nursing student who receives an instructor's praise after performing a task well will probably continue to set high standards of achievement. Repeated reinforcement and positive guidance result in the student becoming a skilled clinician.

Brill (1973) has summarized the manner in which values are learned or acquired:

1. A particular circumstance demands a reaction from an individual.

2. The individual responds on a trial-and-error basis or on the basis of principle.

3. The individual selects an effective response.

4. The individual comes to believe that this is the "right" response because it works for him or her.

5. The individual believes that people who respond differently in the same situation are "wrong."

People learn or acquire values by observing and interacting with others. Each person holds values believed to be important for a satisfying life. People often transmit their values to others in an effort to influence the attitudes and behaviors of those with whom they live.

Modes of Value Transmission

Values are learned in childhood. This is not a deliberate process whereby individuals consciously choose the values they wish to have throughout life. Values become a part of an individual during socialization in the family, school, church, and other social groups. As children observe parents, family, and friends, they internalize behaviors that become a part of their value system (Fig. 16-1). A child may not know why he behaves in a certain way in a given situation, but often his response becomes invested with an almost ritualistic and emotional significance. For example, a child observes his father saying prayers in church and offering a prayer of thanks at the dinner table. If feelings of happiness are conveyed by family members during these times, the child may begin to value religious activities. Saying a simple bedtime prayer may become the child's way of incorporating the father's religious values.

The people who influence a child are generally unaware of the way they transmit their values. For example, if a parent consistently demonstrates honesty in his dealings with others, his child will likely see the value of telling the truth. The child becomes honest without his father's insistence or threat. However, the process of imposing values can be deliberate, as when a parent says to a child who has lied, "You should be ashamed of yourself. Good boys don't lie."

There are four traditional modes of value transmission: modeling, moralizing, laissez-faire, and responsible choice. Table 16-1 demonstrates the way these four modes may lead to widely varying effects.

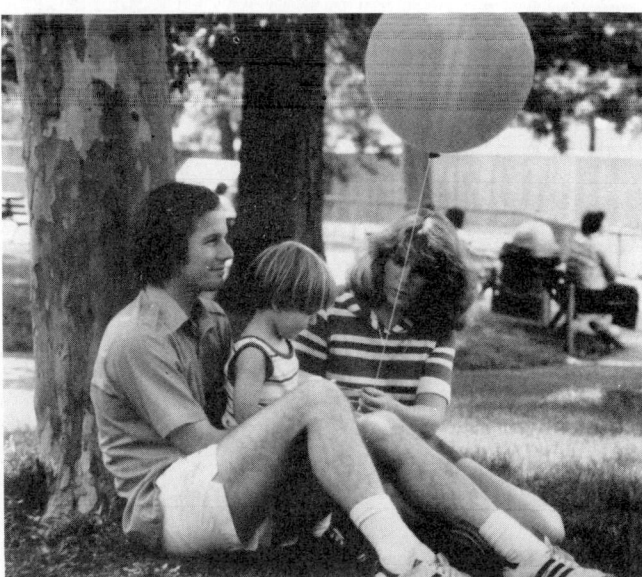

Fig. 16-1 A child's relationship with his parents can influence the values he forms as an adult.
Courtesy Tom Morton.

TABLE 16-1 Modes of Value Transmission

Description	Implications
MODELING	
Persons act in a way to show others the preferred way to behave. People acquire values from a variety of role models.	Children initially wish to be like their parents, and thus parents can model values they perceive as significant. Modeling may not lead to socially acceptable behavior (for example, viewing another person's aggressive behavior). Unless parents point out which values are most desirable, children can follow any role model.
MORALIZING	
Parents and teachers hold standards for what is right and wrong and rigidly enforce children to conform to their set of values.	Approach can be very authoritarian. A moralizing parent may be unwilling to consider alternative values for a child. One way is often the only way. Young persons reared by moralizing adults often have difficulty making independent choices.
LAISSEZ-FAIRE	
Acquiring values by behaving informally without restrictions or limitations. No one value system is right for everyone, and a child forms values without parent's rigid guidelines.	Parents want children to be free to explore a variety of life experiences. Children are encouraged to be inquisitive and learn from experiences. Parents may refrain from discipline. A limitation is that no one assumes responsibility for the child's behavior. Conflict and confusion may arise if a child has no direction.
RESPONSIBLE CHOICE	
A balance of freedom and restriction allows children to select values that lead to personal satisfaction and parental support. A child's choices are more limited as compared with the laissez-faire approach.	Values are not strictly imposed by parents. As a child chooses values, parents, other family, and teachers, allow him to explore within boundaries new behaviors and their consequences. A child who can freely discuss his behavior and its effects will learn to understand his own values.

Influence of Development

The formation, modification, and reinforcement of values take place throughout life. A person's cognitive and emotional development influences the way he acquires and learns values and his response to the different modes of value transmission. The nurse who is familiar with a client's developmental level and corresponding needs is better able to help clients identify values, understand the effect illness has on values, and modify values as needs arise.

INFANT

The newborn seeks emotional and physical security from parents. Although an infant possesses no real ability to reason, he or she senses the emotions and behaviors of people around him. The manner in which parents react to their children is often a function of their values.

For example, a parent who values being in control or having a "perfect" child may reward a baby who does not cry with a smile or a hug. If the child becomes irritable, such a parent may become angry, shout at the child, and frighten him. When the parents' values regarding methods of discipline conflict with the child's needs for security, the child may ultimately express fear, anger, or mistrust. The infant gains emotional security through prompt, predictable, and consistent responses to personal needs.

TODDLER

The toddler learns through imitating others and gaining the approval of others when he engages in acceptable behavior. The child's experiments and exploration of his environment lead to an understanding of the world around him. As he strives for a sense of autonomy (self-direction), he begins to form an identity, shaped by the values of the people with whom he associates.

Parents who do not overly criticize or restrict the child's behavior help him attain a healthy independence. As the child is helped to achieve new physical skills, such as walking up stairs, he learns to value his parents' direction and becomes more assertive.

The parents must balance the child's need for independence against the necessity for protecting him. A toddler is too young to judge what behaviors are safe. When parents fail to provide sufficient supervision, the child can easily injure himself. A child needs a safe environment in which to explore. However, every new encounter is a valuable learning experience, and restrictions imposed by parents who value a highly protective environment inhibit the child's testing of normal behaviors.

PRESCHOOL CHILD

The preschool child is at the stage of cognitive development when concept formation begins. Concepts are objects, events, and experiences that have acquired meaningful labels: dogs bark, trees have leaves, a mother holds and comforts. The preschooler begins to think concretely but not yet abstractly; that is, the child can name what he sees or hears, but hearing the name does not conjure up a mental image of the object. The words "right" and "wrong" do not elicit thoughts of an array of acceptable or unacceptable behavior. What is right or wrong can only be associated with single acts. If the child is repeatedly told not to put toys in his mouth, he learns that this act is wrong, but he does not yet have an abstract awareness of all "wrong" behaviors.

The preschool child strives for a sense of initiative, or the ability to set goals independently and act on them. Play allows the child to demonstrate initiative. The preschooler uses imagination to act out fantasies in play. Parents who value a child's need for creative and imaginative play are less likely to instill guilt in the child when he fails.

Consistent, fair, and kind limits for behavior let the child know that his parents care about him. The preschool stage of development is a suitable time for parents to begin directing the child toward behaviors they value. The child learns kindness when the parent encourages him to share toys and accept playmates. When the child initiates a behavior that reflects a desirable personality characteristic, the parents reinforce it so that the behavior becomes valued.

The nurse is particularly challenged by preschool children who are chronically ill. The parents and siblings of a chronically ill child frequently envelop him, preventing him from asserting initiative. The nurse shows ways in which the preschooler can be independent within his physical limitations.

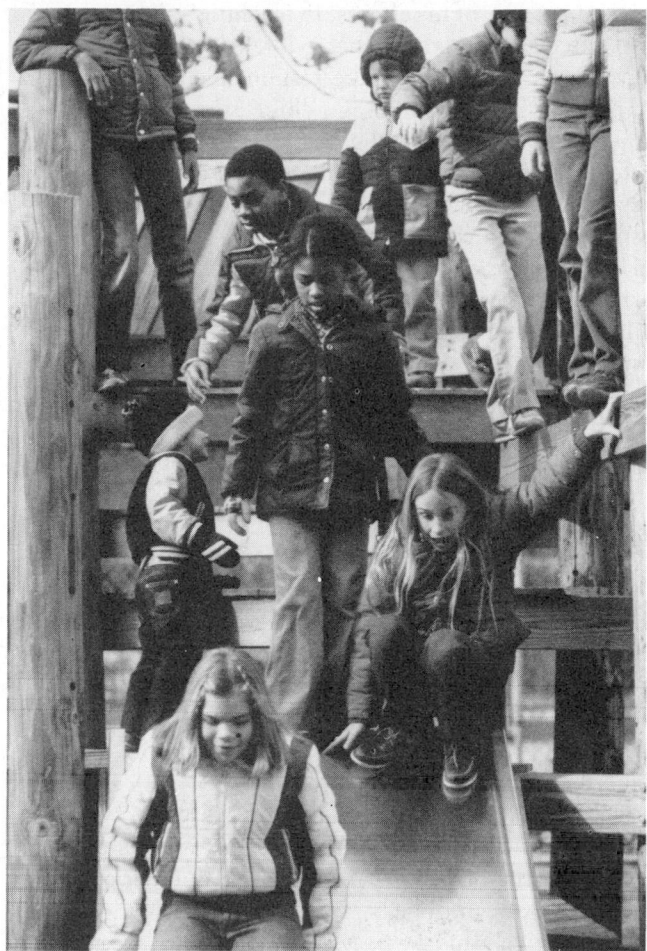

Fig. 16-2 The school-age child learns the values of children his own age through socialized play.
Courtesy Richard Benkof.

SCHOOL-AGE CHILD

The school-age child is influenced by people holding diverse values, such as school personnel and peers in his neighborhood, school, and church. As the school-ager becomes socialized with other children, he becomes less self-centered and more aware of the group (Fig. 16-2). The child is involved in a competitive environment, motivated by peer pressure and a desire to satisfy the adults in his life. It is important for the child to acquire a sense of industry and to feel that he contributes to his peer group and family. As the school-ager matures, he comes to value self-motivation and productiveness rather than being manipulated by his peer group.

Parents and teachers promote a sense of industry by providing the school-age child with constructive guidance. Planning specific school activities, setting aside times for study, and allowing a variety of activities with the child's peer group give the school-ager opportunities to compare his behaviors with those of his peers and to see the products of his efforts. In teaching values, parents who offer alternatives of behavior help the child learn to solve problems and make responsible decisions. For example, when a school-age child asks his father for money to buy a radio, the father might refuse to give the child money or might challenge the child to think of ways to earn the money. As the child seeks opportunities to perform chores around the home, he gains the experience of working toward a meaningful goal. Once he earns the money for the radio, he will value the product of his efforts and realize the benefits of hard work and commitment.

ADOLESCENT

Adolescence is a critical development period during which the youth gains greater freedom and responsibility. It is also a time of rapid learning, with the adolescent being exposed to a multitude of new ideas and values. The adolescent undergoes dramatic physical changes that may affect his ability to develop a stable self-concept. The parents of an adolescent must be patient, supportive, and understanding of their child's need for independence. If the adolescent feels free to be himself and is also able to rely on his parents for support, he will value the family's relationship.

The adolescent's primary concern is to develop an identity that conveys his uniqueness, as well as conformity with peers. He experiments with a number of roles, often aimlessly, until he begins to acquire behaviors that are distinctively his own. Most adolescents are unable to identify the specific values or attitudes that comprise their identity. However, as the adolescent matures, he gradually develops a workable philosophy of life, a personally meaningful set of values, and worthy ideals. The adolescent often adopts the values of his parents, but they are no longer the only source of direction and support.

ADULT

The mature adult ideally is able to test values and freely determine which ones are acceptable. At each level of adulthood (young, middle aged, and elderly) the adult has certain experiences that lead to confrontations over the most desirable values.

Marrying, rearing children, and choosing a career often require the young adult to redefine his values.

The middle-aged adult begins to redefine his self-concept to suit the needs of later life. Middle-aged adults whose values have been reinforced through time have a growing sense of security. However, the onset of aging may pose a threat to adults who value youth and vitality. During middle age an insecure adult may sacrifice previously held values in an effort to regain lost years. For example, a married man might flirt with younger women to prove his virility. In contrast, the well-adjusted adult

values each year of his life for the pleasures gained and the opportunities afforded. As old age approaches, an individual suffers less emotional turmoil if he is satisfied with his life and his values.

During late adulthood an individual faces significant changes in life including retirement from work, the physical alterations of aging, and the loss of close friends and family. It is important for the older adult to remain active and independent so that life continues to be enriching. Maintaining social relationships beyond the immediate family helps the older adult fulfill many of the values he holds significant, such as friendship, love, and an active way of life. The older adult may see many of his values threatened as he becomes inactive and less able to maintain meaningful interpersonal relationships. It is therefore essential for the adult to remain open to new ideas and values so that the opportunity for growth and satisfaction exists despite advancing age.

Sociocultural Influences

Values are formed in social settings where the educational, socioeconomic, spiritual, and cultural backgrounds of people vary. Leininger (1978) describes culture as "a way of life belonging to a designated group of people." A culture can have subcultures—small groups that assume an identity of their own—that have similarities to the larger culture (Steele, 1986). In America, there are many subcultures, for example, American Indians, Italians, or Germans, that share some values with the larger American culture while adopting some values unique to their subculture.

It is difficult to establish norms for any subculture, since no absolute agreement about what values are acceptable exists within a particular culture. The nurse is expected to respect the values of clients even when his or her cultural background is different from theirs.

A particular culture's value orientation will influence the way in which members pursue health care. Human beings face a certain number of problems as social groups, and there are a finite number of solutions to those problems. Kluckhohn (1950, 1951) believed that it is the ordering of these solutions that makes a distinctive profile of a culture. Persons in certain cultural groups may seek health care for the slightest problems, whereas those in other groups seek care only when their condition is serious. For example, clients from lower socioeconomic levels tend to value health promotion behaviors less than clients from higher socioeconomic levels. Individuals who belong to a lower socioeconomic subculture are often less motivated to seek health care early and thus may have a lower level of overall health.

For nurses to give effective care, they must understand the influence cultural traditions have on a person's health behaviors, response to stress, use of health care services, and adjustment to illness. The professional care giver's value system may differ from that of the client. However, the nurse must also realize that no single culture agrees on what is "right" or "wrong." The nurse must respect a person's cultural orientation but also look further into the individual's uniqueness.

CHANGING VALUES

As individuals mature and experience new situations, their values change. It would be unusual if any one value remained the primary motivating factor throughout a person's life. Value changes may involve a reordering of values or the replacement of old values with new ones. As a result of changing values, the person modifies his or her attitudes and behavior. The willingness to change shows a healthy attitude toward life and the ability to adapt to new experiences.

Personal and Professional Values in Nursing

The person entering the profession of nursing has a set of personal values that guide actions. These values are the result of personal choice or habit. Examples of values that influence a person's selection of the nursing profession as a career include serving others, respect, health education, or responsibility. Young people may choose nursing because they respect and see nurses as members of a helping profession that commands respect from others. A student who values drama or excitement may see the life-and-death situations nurses face as a reason for this career choice. Young adults entering nursing will find that they are unable at first to identify themselves with all the attributes of a professional nurse. As they become socialized into the nursing profession, they soon find the personal and professional values interacting.

Two primary values that Hall (1973) identifies are self-value and equal worth. Self-value is one's belief that one is of worth to significant others. Self-value is related to trust, the expression of emotions, and the ability to become involved with other people. The value of equal worth is a belief that other people are equal in worth to oneself. Hall suggests that the two primary values must exist together. Having a positive feeling for others requires that a person first value self. These two primary values are guiding forces in a nurse's personal and professional life. A nurse has difficulty helping and caring for others when she does not feel good about herself.

When a nurse's personal and professional values are similar, the professional role is assumed with little difficulty. When personal and professional values are in-

consistent, the nurse may become frustrated and dissatisfied. A commitment to professional values, for example, competence, influences the way peers and society view a nurse. A competent nurse must be knowledgeable and able to perform nursing care skills efficiently and effectively. If a nurse fails to remain current and competent in the application of nursing knowledge, his or her effectiveness as a professional declines.

Society's Health Values

The health care needs of society have recently undergone significant change. In the past, most health care services were delivered in an acute care hospital setting. Because of changes in health care reimbursement and a reorientation by many members of society to a wellness model, questions must be raised as to how to prepare professional nurses. A conflict in values may arise, particularly in hospitals. A nurse educator who values a highly competent, skilled clinician may not place as much emphasis on teaching students about self-care activities such as relaxation or exercise as on more advanced clinical skills. Nursing education that is futuristic and designed to prepare nurses for nontraditional self-care or wellness models may not meet all of society's needs. Steele (1986) suggests that the growing interest in wellness by many members of society indicates that part of society is shifting to a wellness model instead of the traditional illness model of health care. The nursing profession is obligated to prepare its members to understand the values that are consistent with the way nursing is practiced in all settings.

VALUES AND CLINICAL DECISION MAKING

Nurses identify diagnoses and make clinical judgments on the basis of subjective and objective information they collect about clients. The decision-making process is an important responsibility of the nurse. Each client's unique needs are analyzed so that the correct decisions are made about their care.

A nurse's values also influence clinical decision making. When a nurse values physical aspects of care, he or she is more likely to administer an analgesic and position a client comfortably before spending time talking with the client. When a nurse faces life and death decisions regarding a client's care, it is important that the nurse consistently apply a set of values in decision making (Taylor, 1985). Persons who believe in the sanctity of life support the concept that life is a paramount right that must be protected at all costs. A nurse who values sanctity of life may not be able to assist with an abortion.

In contrast, persons supporting the value of quality of life, believe that no life at all is better than a life with suffering or deficits (Taylor, 1985). A nurse may be better able to withhold treatment from a terminally ill client if he or she values quality of life. When quality of life becomes a criteria in health care, Taylor (1985) warns that decision making can become biased. Differences in social and economic class can define quality of life in a variety of ways. For example, an intelligent, socially accomplished and technically skilled person may become biased as to the type of care an uneducated, illiterate, or physically handicapped person would seek.

Nurses care for clients who possess their own values about life and the human experience. To make intelligent and thoughtful decisions, nurses must know their own values, how they interact with the values of clients, and the influence values have in client care decisions.

VALUES CLARIFICATION

For individuals to change their values in a manner that suits their needs and preferences, they must be aware of what they value. In addition, individuals must realize the implications their values have for their own behavior. Yet a person does not suddenly become aware of his values, and many people are unable to define their values clearly and meaningfully. To achieve an awareness of one's personal values, a cognitive process of values clarification is helpful.

Values clarification, or valuing, is a process of self-discovery that helps a person gain a clearer insight into his or her values. It is not a set of rules that interferes with conscientious decision making. The process of values clarification does not imply that a specific set of values should be accepted by all persons. It is also not a method of indoctrination to religious, moral, or cultural standards. As a person clarifies values in a given situation, he or she learns what choices to make when alternatives are presented and how to determine whether choices are rationally made. The result of valuing is greater self-awareness and personal insight.

Raths, Harmin, and Simon (1979) pioneered values clarification as an approach to an individual's appraisal of values. Valuing involves three steps: choosing, prizing, and acting (see box). By using the values clarification process the person ranks his values in a hierarchical order that provides a guide for personal conduct, lifestyle, and interpersonal interactions.

The person must choose personal values freely. The freedom to select among alternatives allows a person to cherish his or her final choice. However, the individual must understand what alternatives exist. For example, an older woman may experience the sudden loss of her husband. As she shares her concerns with a community health nurse, it is clear that she has several choices. She can continue to live alone and grieve for her husband, become active in a senior citizens' group, or begin to socialize with male and female companions. The nurse helps the woman examine her choices without passing judgment or offering advice. A clear understanding of all alternatives and their consequences will ensure that the woman's final choice is the right one for her.

Prizing is showing private and public satisfaction with the value chosen. A person holds a value in esteem, feeling good about his or her choice. When a nurse helps a client use values clarification, the client reaches a point in the process when he is able to affirm his values in the presence of significant others. When a terminally ill client chooses to die without emergency resuscitation, he prizes his decision by being able to share it with family members. By announcing his values a person reaffirms their importance or relevance.

Acting on a chosen value solidifies its acceptance. Acting requires a translation of values into behavior. A young man permanently disabled by a serious injury to his leg chooses to retain his independence by living alone. He acts further on his choice by entering a rehabilitation program to learn to use an artificial leg. Raths, Harmin, and Simon (1979) suggest that persons should act consistently and regularly on their chosen values. The young man who values independence would thus continue to act independently in work and social life. It may, however, be difficult to act consistently on a chosen value. For example, a client who values independence may be too disabled by illness to safely function alone. The client may be able to at least make decisions for himself. The

---

The Three Steps in Values Clarification

- Choosing one's beliefs and behaviors
  - Choosing from alternatives
  - Choosing freely
  - Considering all consequences
- Prizing one's beliefs and behaviors
  - Prizing and cherishing the choice
  - Publicly affirming the choice
- Acting on one's beliefs
  - Making the choice part of one's behavior
  - Acting with a pattern of consistency and repetition

Modified from Raths, LE, Harmin, M, and Simon, SB: Values and teaching, ed. 2, Columbus, Ohio, 1966, Charles E. Merrill Publishing Co.

nurse carefully clarifies alternatives for clients so that the best possible choice can be acted on.

Values Clarification Versus Ethical Decision Making

Values clarification is inadequate as a guide for solving ethical dilemmas (Bernal, 1985). There are often conflicts in values among health care professionals and clients that lead to ethical dilemmas (see Chapter 17). For example, a client may decide not to have surgery for lung cancer. The physician believes that surgery is the client's only choice. The nurse may believe in a client's autonomy but is unsure if this client has made a rational decision.

When many different values are expressed in a situation, values clarification will likely not resolve the dilemma. Each person may benefit from knowing the other's values, yet they may not agree on the final decision. Ethical decisions require a clear analysis of all facts with the nurse assuming a client advocate role. It must be assumed that some values are better than others. Until health care professionals and clients can jointly agree on one value, such as client autonomy, ethical decisions cannot be easily made.

Strategies for Values Clarification

A system of strategies can be used to make valuing more insightful, practical, and meaningful for the person whose values are unclear. These strategies are exercises to help an individual clarify personal values using the three steps of valuing. The nurse can use the strategies with clients or to clarify his or her own values. For example, the strategy of completing unfinished sentences (see box) helps nurses determine and explore their own attitudes, beliefs, interests, and goals, which are indicators of their professional values. The finished sentences can be shared with a group to give nurses an opportunity to affirm their choices.

The strategy of rank ordering (see box) requires the selection of priorities among different values. The nurse in practice can develop a similar exercise to help clients order their values in specific situations. This strategy demonstrates that many issues require more consideration of values than is usually given in decision making.

Sentence Completion

- Complete the following sentences. Use them to examine your feelings and values.
- I believe I succeed as a nurse when . . .
- A patient has a right to . . .
- I wish the director of nursing would . . .
- Physicians and nurses work together best when . . .
- I fail as a nurse if I cannot . . .
- The most difficult patient is one who . . .

Modified from Simon, SB, et al.: Values clarification: a handbook of practical strategies for teachers and students, New York, 1978, Hart Publishing Co.

Rank Ordering

The following questions require you to make value judgments. Rank the choices to the questions below according to your value preferences. Write the number "1" to the left for the most important value. Continue in the same manner until all four values are ranked. Share your feelings with a colleague and examine the available alternatives.

If you had the time, money, and skill to solve problems of nurses on your division, you would
___ Increase nurses' salaries
___ Enhance staff education
___ Increase the number of nurses to staff the division
___ Give staff more positive feedback

In developing a professional relationship with a physician, the nurse should
___ Respond promptly to all requests
___ Demonstrate knowledge of the patients assigned to the physician
___ Look attractive and be neatly dressed
___ Share ideas about the clients' needs

When assigned to a client's care, it is most important to
___ Make him as physically comfortable as possible
___ Let him know you are interested in his ideas and feelings
___ Be competent and skilled in the performance of all procedures
___ Allow the client to make decisions about his care

What would you prefer to have happen to you if you had a serious health problem?
___ Not be told
___ Be told immediately by the physician
___ Learn by accident
___ Keep it secret from your family

Modified from Uustal, DB: Am J Nurs 78:2058, 1978.

The health value scale (see box) is an exercise for setting value priorities. It consists of 10 values that a client ranks in order of importance. The client is asked to rank items in a way that accurately reflects his value hierarchy. If health is ranked in one of the top four positions, the client places a high value on health. The value placed on health is moderate if ranked 5, 6, or 7 and low if ranked 8, 9, or 10. Information obtained from this exercise can help the nurse plan health care teaching methods.

Nurses' Values Clarification

When a nurse uses values clarification for personal benefit, personal growth and professional satisfaction are gained. During contacts with clients, peers, physicians, and other health care professionals, the nurse's values are challenged and tested. How does the nurse show a willingness to be accountable for actions as a professional? How do the nurse's attitudes about a client influence the care provided? When another nurse performs some action unsafely, what should be done? What are the nurse's beliefs about the quality of life? The nurse has difficulty assuming the role of a professional when personal values are poorly conceived and unclear. Values clarification helps nurses explore their values and decide whether to act on their beliefs (see box on p. 440). The nurse is able to establish more effective relationships with clients and better meet their needs once the nurse's own values are clearly defined. Values clarification facilitates decision making and problem solving for nurses in their professional roles.

The purpose of values clarification can be used between nurses and other health care workers who daily face similar value conflicts. In working relationships it can be valuable for staff to understand those values that influence decisions about client care. What type of client frustrates a nurse? What makes nurses feel more satisfied about their job? When frustration with a fellow staff member arises, what is the cause? Sharing values about clients, their families, and colleagues with peers assists nurses in recognizing their commonly held values. This sharing helps nurses understand the behavior of colleagues. Communication lines become more open when dealing with controversial issues.

Clients' Values Clarification

Valuing is a useful tool in helping clients and their families adapt to the stress of illness and other health-related problems. The nurse helps the client sort out emotions to clarify their meaning and significance. Values clarification helps clients gain an awareness of personal priorities, identify ambiguities in values, and resolve major conflicts between values and behavior. Communication with a client becomes more effective, since the nurse is able to focus attention on what the client is expressing and why. The client becomes more willing to express problems and true feelings, and thus the nurse is able to establish an individualized plan of care (Fig. 16-3).

A nurse is responsible for educating clients about health-promoting behaviors. The nurse's goal is to help the client establish health-protecting or -promoting behaviors. Frequently clients are taught facts and concepts about their condition but their health behavior remains unchanged. The nurse who learns what the client values and wants to know is able to devise a successful teaching program. Giving clients meaningful and practical information increases the likelihood that they will assume behaviors that promote their well-being.

Behaviors Reflecting the Need for Values Clarification

Sometimes it is difficult for the nurse to determine when a client might benefit from values clarification. Not all clients share socially preferable values such as the desire to maintain one's health, a willingness to work hard, or the importance of having a successful career. For example, a client may not worry about his health

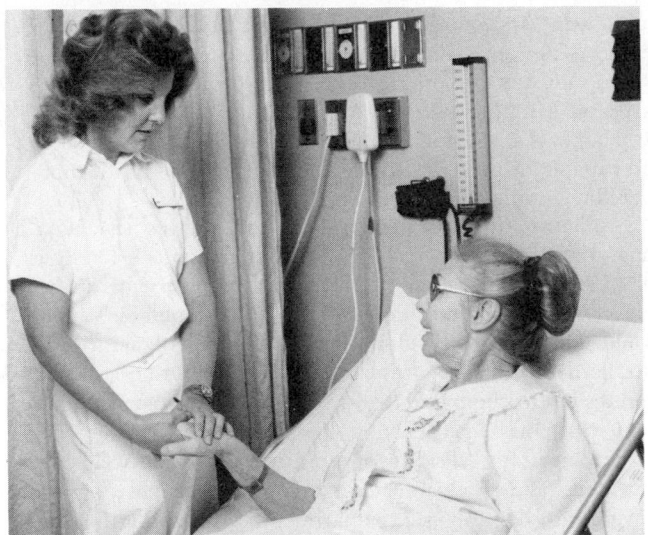

Fig. 16-3 Through values clarification the nurse helps the client become more aware of personal values and their influence on the client's behavior.

and may ignore his physician's orders. Any attempts at changing his values would be rejected. Also, the nurse should never coerce clients to change their values. Yet in some cases a client's behaviors suggest to the nurse that his values are unclear. Such behaviors could ultimately interfere with the nurse's efforts at promoting good health care. The nurse's role in each of the following situations should be to determine if the client is unhappy with or unsure of his value system or is experiencing a conflict of values that could be detrimental to his health. In such cases, values clarification might be appropriate for the client.

Apathy. Mr Smith has reentered the hospital numerous times for the same health problem. His wife reports that he will not consistently follow his diet restrictions. During a discussion with the nurse, Mr. Smith cannot remember when he should take his medications. He does not seem to care about health promotion activities. When asked if he understands his physician's orders, Mr. Smith replies, "Oh, I suppose so. I just have trouble remembering sometimes. It's hard to always do the right thing."

Flightiness. Mrs. Jones is visited at home by a public health nurse, who is giving advice on the care of Mrs. Jones' newborn infant. Mrs. Jones tells the nurse, "I'm so glad you are here; I have questions about the baby." Before the nurse is able to answer questions about breast feeding, Mrs. Jones changes the subject and discusses her new kitchen curtains. Even Mrs. Jones' actions seem poorly directed. She places the infant in bed but returns in a moment and picks the child up again.

Uncertainty. Ms. Nelson has been suffering a gradual loss of vision. Her physician has proposed a new type of experimental surgery. Ms. Nelson has not been able to decide whether to follow the physician's recommendations. She has

asked her family and friends for their opinions. She asks each nurse who cares for her whether surgery is the right choice.

Inconsistency. Mr. Wall has had serious heart disease for 3 years. He rarely follows the exercise plan prescribed by his physician. In a conversation with a nurse, Mr. Wall remarks that people should become more concerned about maintaining their health.

Drifting. Mr. Rush has had back pain for 3 years. His first physician recommended surgery to correct his problem. Since that time Mr. Rush has also visited a chiropractor and an osteopath. He believes in physical fitness and wants to find a cure for his pain. However, he tries each remedy for only a short time.

Overconforming. Mrs. Wade has gone to a physician for advice on weight reduction. The physician has ordered a diet of 1500 calories per day and a program of regular exercise. Mrs. Wade has bought four diet books to help her count calories and a scale to weigh foods. She keeps a chart on the refrigerator door to record each day's meals. Once Mrs. Wade eats the limit of 1500 calories, she refuses to eat for the remainder of the day, even if it means missing dinner. Each day she runs a mile at 7:15 AM and 5:45 PM.

Role Playing. Mrs. James might be called the "perfect" client. She always has a smile for the nurses, never talks about her predicament, and rarely complains about pain. This is despite the fact that Mrs. James, age 24 and mother of three children, is dying of cancer.

Values Clarification as a Tool in Client Care

Merely encouraging clients to express their feelings may provide inadequate information if the real problem is a conflict in values. For example, a middle-aged man has a diagnosed terminal disease. His values of health, economic security, and family unity are threatened. When encouraged to discuss his feelings, he may be unable to describe clearly how he feels. The nurse who is familiar with values clarification can help the client define values, clarify goals, and seek solutions.

Helping clients clarify values is not an attempt at psychoanalysis. The nurse's role is to shape responses to the client's questions or statements in a manner that stimulates the client's introspection. The nurse's clarifying verbal response comes from the awareness that the valuing process will motivate the client to examine his thoughts and actions. Such responses can help the client choose a value freely, consider alternatives, prize the choice, affirm the choice with others, act on the choice, and incorporate into his life the behaviors that reflect the value selected.

When the nurse makes a clarifying response, it should be: (1) brief, (2) selective, (3) nonjudgmental, (4) thought provoking, and (5) spontaneous. A good clarifying exchange between nurse and client lasts only a short time. The nurse's response makes the client think about his values after the exchange is over. Clarifying responses are used only when values conflict is the issue. For example, when the nurse explains a medical procedure, an attempt at values clarification is not needed. A nurse makes a clarifying response only for situations in which no right or wrong answer exists. Situations lacking answers are those involving beliefs, aspirations, feelings, and attitudes.

The nurse's response does not judge the client's values. A client will be unable to find comfort in his values if the nurse moralizes or advises on choices. The nurse's response must evoke the client's creative thinking. For example, a client might be undecided whether to seek another physician's opinion about his medical problem. It would be simple (although unethical) for the nurse to advise the client as to which physician is the most skillful in a given area. Likewise, the nurse could easily explain the hazards of proposed surgery. However, it is the client who must live with his choice; the focus must be on the client and what he views as the possible outcomes of any decision.

A nurse's spontaneity helps a client think creatively. The nurse often has little warning when the client seeks solutions to his values dilemma. With experience, a nurse can learn to make clarifying responses without advanced planning. Although the response is consciously and deliberately designed to stimulate thought, it should not appear contrived.

Values clarification can occur in any setting. The client's bedside, a clinic office, or the client's home is a suitable place for the client to express his feelings. Valuing is often more successful when the nurse has the opportunity for repeated contact with the client. It is difficult for the nurse to help the client meaningfully achieve each step of the valuing process when she spends little time with him.

Ultimately the client gains a perception of how valuing provides personal satisfaction. Values clarification promotes effective reasoning and decision making. The client becomes more aware of how his values influence his actions, and this awareness is an essential component of problem solving.

CASE STUDY

Mrs. James is a 73-year-old woman who fractured her ankle in a fall at home. Mrs. James' daughter is concerned about her mother's welfare and wants Mrs. James to live with her family. The daughter has voiced concern to the nurse that Mrs. James is incapable of caring for herself. Mrs. James' rehabilitation has progressed well. One day Mrs. James asks the nurse, Ms. Fryer, "What should I do? I know my daughter worries about me, but I don't want to be cared for like a child."

Ms. Fryer realizes that Mrs. James is experiencing a conflict in her values for her independence, her love for her daughter, and her health. The nurse thinks the values clarification process would help Mrs. James make her choice. Ms. Fryer begins by helping Mrs. James choose from the alternatives available.

Choosing from Alternatives. The nurse's response depends partly on Mrs. James' age, education, and level of maturity. Mrs. James is an alert woman, knowledgeable about her needs and capable of making decisions for herself. She has demonstrated motivation in her rehabilitation.

Examining All Consequences. Mrs. James loves her daughter and knows that the offer to join the daughter's family is genuine. Mrs. James says that she has many friends in her apartment building and that moving to her daughter's home would make it very difficult for her to socialize with her friends. Mrs. James' present apartment is on the second floor, which requires her to climb two flights of stairs. A downstairs apartment will soon be vacant.

The nurse says, "Perhaps it would be helpful to weigh the advantages and disadvantages of joining your daughter against moving into the downstairs apartment." In making this suggestion the nurse carefully avoids letting her own values influence Mrs. James' thinking, even though she has a close relationship with her own daughter and has been very happy when they shared her house on extended visits.

Choosing Freely. The next day, Ms. Fryer enters Mrs. James' room during breakfast. The nurse's goal is to determine if Mrs. James was able to make a decision of her own. Mrs. James says, "I've decided to move into the downstairs apartment," Ms. Fryer asks, "Was this a difficult choice to make?"

Prizing the Choice. Mrs. James acknowledges that she does not want to hurt her daughter's feelings; however, she knows her decision was the best one. "I still have many friends and they have encouraged me to stay in the apartment. I still feel spry and able to take care of myself." The nurse recognizes that it is important for Mrs. James to be satisfied with her choice.

Affirming the Choice. It is important that Mrs. James be able to speak out in support of her decision. She may need assistance from the nurse in thinking of ways to affirm the choice. An appropriate response by Ms. Fryer is, "What will be the best way to share your decision with your daughter?" Mrs. James replies, "My daughter and son-in-law are coming by to visit this evening. I've decided to let them know tonight."

Acting on the Choice. Mrs. James has made the decision to retain her independence. She is able to share her choice and the rationale for it with her daughter. The nurse using values clarification recognizes Mrs. James' need to act on her decision. She asks, "What can you do to begin planning for your move?"

Mrs. James calls the apartment manager to arrange for her new home. She is going to stay with her daughter for a week after discharge from the hospital. Meanwhile, she will have the opportunity to select new paint and wallpaper for the apartment. Mrs. James' value of independence remains alive in the measures she has taken to accomplish her move.

Acting with a Pattern. A month after discharge, Mrs. James returns to her physician's office for a checkup. She stops by the nursing division to say hello to Ms. Fryer. Ms. Fryer is interested in learning if Mrs. James has continued to retain her independence. A value must be kept alive. For independence to be meaningful to Mrs. James, it must become integrated into her life-style. Ms. Fryer asks, "Was your choice to remain in the apartment the right one?" Mrs. James responds, "For now, yes. I am feeling much better and there are many friends to help me. My daughter visits every week. You know, though, I do have to be cautious in the way I walk around. I know someday I may have to live with my daughter."

As Mrs. James becomes more physically dependent, a conflict will arise between the independence she prizes and her ability to act on that value. The value of the genuine love and concern expressed by Mrs. James' daughter may become a higher priority than the value of independence. Mrs. James' maturity will be reflected in her eventual ability to modify her values. As she becomes more physically dependent, she must adapt her values accordingly. Mrs. James will still be alert and capable of making decisions. The daughter's ability to provide a safe environment for her mother without compromising Mrs. James' ability to make her own decisions should prove to be mutually satisfying.

As in the preceding case study, it takes time for the nurse to develop values clarification as a tool for a client's care. The nurse cannot attempt to help clients explore their values unless he or she has insight into her own. Values clarification can be a valuable means of helping clients sort out their true feelings and beliefs and gain a better awareness of their goals in life.

SUMMARY

A person's unique set of values influences personal decisions and actions and in part determines his or her identity. Although values may be acquired and held unconsciously, a person's conscious awareness of values helps in reaching decisions and avoiding conflicts. Clients who are conscious of their values related to health and health behaviors are able to participate fully in health care, and nurses conscious of their own values are better able to help clients clarify values and make decisions.

People form values through observation and experience, noting the responses evoked by their own and others' behaviors. Values are acquired from parents, family and significant others in a continuous process that begins in infancy. Values are transmitted through one or more modes: modeling, moralizing, laissez-faire, and responsible choice.

Nurses have both personal and professional values. The personal values of a student nurse may already be similar to the professional values of a nurse in practice, such as respect for clients as individuals and the value of health. With socialization into the nursing profession these two sets of values may converge into one. The process of values clarification can be valuable in increasing the nurse's awareness of the impact of personal values on professional behavior and in avoiding conflicts within the nurse's value system or between the nurse's and the client's values.

Values clarification is the use of various strategies to explore the meaning of one's values and behaviors. The valuing process involves choosing, prizing, and acting on one's beliefs. When values are clearly detailed and positively affirmed, the client is more capable of making objective decisions about health care.

KEY CONCEPTS

✓ When nurses can clearly differentiate their personal values from their professional values, they are better able to help clients understand their values.

✓ A person's perceptions of others are shaped by his values.

✓ Values provide a standard for acceptable behavior.

✓ A person acquires values after observing behaviors that prove successful or productive for others.

✓ A child acquires values from parents, other family members, school, church, and other social institutions.

✓ Restrictions that parents set for a child should be balanced with opportunities for the child to explore behaviors and their consequences.

✓ Value formation begins in the early developmental stages and continues through the life span.

✓ A person's sociocultural background influences values toward health and health care.

✓ Values clarification is not an indoctrination method but a process that promotes an individual's understanding of what his values are.

✓ A person must be able to choose values freely from available alternatives and understand the consequences of his choice.

✓ A person may have an attitude about a certain idea, without valuing it.

✓ A nurse's values influence decisions made about a client's care.

✓ Nursing is obligated to prepare its members to understand the values that are consistent with the ways nursing is practiced in all settings.

✓ Values clarification helps a nurse explore personal values and feelings and decide whether to act on personal beliefs.

✓ The nurse who learns about what a client values is better prepared to help the client assume health-protecting or -promoting behaviors.

✓ Values clarification strategies are useful tools to help clients understand their own values.

✓ Nurses who use values clarification with clients offer clarifying responses that stimulate the clients' introspection about their values and behavior.

✓ Values clarification promotes effective reasoning and decision making.

REFERENCES

Bernal, EW: Values clarification: a critique, J Nurs Educ 24:174, 1985.

Brill, NI: Working with people, the helping process, Philadelphia, 1973, J.B. Lippincott Co.

Hall, BP: Value clarification as learning process, New York, 1973, Paulist Press.

Leininger, M: Transcultural nursing: concepts, theories, and practices, New York, 1978, John Wiley & Sons, Inc.

Raths, LE, Harmin, M, and Simon, SB: Values and teaching, ed. 2, Columbus, Ohio, 1979, Charles E. Merrill Publishing Co.

Rokeach, M: The nature of human values, New York, 1973, The Free Press.

Steele, SM: AIDS: clarifying values to close in on ethical questions, Nurs Health Care, 7(5):246, 1986.

Taylor, SG: The effect of quality of life and sanctity of life on clinical decision making, AORN 41:924, 1985.

Research Articles

Kluckhohn, FR: Dominant and substitute profiles of cultural orientations, Social Forces 28:375, 1950.

Kluckhohn, FR: Dominant and variant cultural value orientations, Social Welfare Forum 1951, p. 97.

ADDITIONAL READINGS

Brink, PJ: Value orientation as an assessment tool in cultural diversity, Nurs Res 33:198, 1984.

Cannon, RB, et al.: A values clarification approach to cultural diversity, Nurs Health Care 5:161, 1984.

Coletta, SS: Values clarification in nursing: why? Am J Nurs 78:2057, 1978.

Ford, JG, Trygstad-Durland, LN and Nelms, BC: Applied decision making for nurses, St. Louis, 1979, The C.V. Mosby Co.

Gortner, SR, et al.: Appraisal of values in the choice of treatment, Nurs Res 33:319, 1984.

Kirschbaum, H: Advanced values clarification, La Jolla, Calif., 1977, University Associates.

McNally, JM: Values: part I, Superv Nurse 11:27, 1980.

Uustal, DB: Values clarification in nursing: application to practice, Am J Nurs 78:2058, 1978.

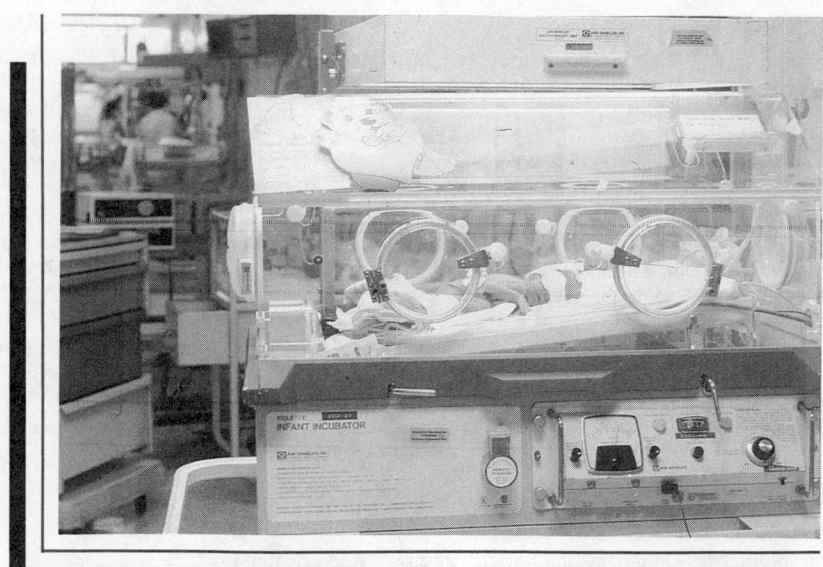

OBJECTIVES

Mastery of content in this chapter will enable the student to:

- Define the key terms listed.
- Describe the influence of ethics on nursing practice.
- Differentiate ethical issues from moral and legal issues.
- Explain the influence of historical changes in health care on nursing ethics.
- Describe the influence of personal and professional values on ethical decisions.
- Contrast and compare responsibility and accountability.
- Explain the relationship between accountability and ethics.
- Identify the purposes of a professional code of ethics.
- Explain the ethical implications of client advocacy.
- Discuss the type of ethical conflicts confronted by nurses.
- Discuss the process used to resolve ethical problems.

KEY TERMS

Abortion

Accountability

Advocacy

Autonomy

Bioethics

Brain Death

Code of Ethics

Confidentiality

Contraception

Ethics

Legal Right

Living Will

Morality

Profession

Psychosurgery

Psychotherapy

Responsibility

Resuscitation

Sterilization

Terminal Illness

Transplantation

Ethics in Nursing

In health care today, professional nurses face a larger variety of ethical problems than ever before. Some of the conflicts arise from the nurse's complex role in the health care delivery system. Nurses are well educated, more independent, and have considerable responsibility for making ongoing clinical decisions. Advanced technology has expanded the scope of their duties. With clients becoming more aware of their rights to high-quality health care, the nurse acts as a liaison between clients and other health professionals to ensure that clients' rights are honored. The nurse is often faced with difficult responsibilities requiring a high level of knowledge, skill, and decision making.

The daily close contact with clients puts nurses in a unique position compared with other health care professionals. The nurse is present during the simplest of human activities such as bathing, eating, ambulation, and elimination. The nurse also performs specific care activities such as medication administration, dressing changes, and physical assessment. The nurse also gives psychological support to clients experiencing pain, fear, joy, or grief. Thus the nurse has a special relationship with clients, a relationship built on trust. This relationship is the foundation for nursing ethics.

Dilemmas in health care cause nurses to be unsure of their relationships with clients, physicians, and other health care professionals. Questions will be asked of the nurse. Physicians will order treatments the nurse is responsible for implementing. The nurse soon becomes faced with difficult issues. Who decides what is best for a client? What should clients know about their health? What is the nurse's responsibility when client's rights become threatened?

449

Value conflicts associated with these dilemmas often add to a nurse's confusion. An understanding of ethical decision making can help nurses make proper clinical decisions. Nurses can also learn to help clients deal with their own dilemmas and grow while solving them.

DEFINITION OF ETHICS

Ethics is the principles or standards governing proper conduct as applied to professional problems. The term originates from the Greek word, *ethos,* meaning custom. Simply, ethics indicates what a person ought to do. Ethics addresses how human beings relate to each other in a philosophy of fairness. Characteristic of all professions, ethics serves to protect the rights of human beings.

Nurses deal with many types of ethical dilemmas in situations that may seem ordinary or routine. Consider the following case examples:

Ms. Torrez has a serious neurological disease requiring routine oral medications, but she refuses the medications. She states, "Those pills are dangerous. I don't have to take them if I don't want to." Should the nurse, Mr. Wagner, attempt to force Ms. Torrez to take the medication?

Ms. Stein, RN, is responsible for making a request for organ donation from Ms. Adams, whose father has just died. Ms. Stein states, "Organ donation is an option you have. Is this something your father has ever discussed?"

Ms. Adams replies "Everything is such a shock. The doctor just told me yesterday that my father was getting better. He hasn't even come by to tell me what happened." Ms. Stein knows the physician is not in the hospital. Should she continue the request for organ donation or help Ms. Adams find the answer about the cause of her father's death?

Mr. Jacobs has suffered a massive stroke. He is completely paralyzed on both sides and does not respond to painful stimulation. A mechanical ventilator maintains his respirations, and intravenous medications maintain his blood pressure. His doctor has ordered, "Do not resuscitate," which means cardiopulmonary resuscitation should not be used if Mr. Jacobs' heart ceases to beat. The nurse, Ms. Martin, prepares to enter Mr. Jacobs' room to administer hygiene. An intern walks by and states, "Don't go to so much trouble over that man. He's going to die anyway." How should Ms. Martin respond?

Each of these situations represents a typical ethical dilemma in which conflicts arise over philosophies, values, and professional duties. A dilemma is a situation requiring a choice between what appear to be equally desirable or undesirable alternatives (Curtin and Flaherty, 1982). In an ethical dilemma, there is a conflict in values, and a person is unsure of what constitutes proper conduct. No absolute right or wrong exists.

Clients receiving health care expect a nurse to be knowledgeable, skillful, and supportive of their rights.

Curtin and Flaherty (1982) defines human rights as "a person's just due." Similar to a client's actions, a nurse's actions are guided by personal and professional beliefs and values, a philosophy of life and of nursing, and cultural and emotional variables. The many factors shaping a nurse's ethical standards make it difficult for the nurse to perceive ethical dilemmas clearly. Some basic questions can help to clarify ethical perspective. What should be the philosophy of nursing? What constitutes good nursing practice? How should personal values influence professional decision making? Nurses study ethics in order to prepare themselves to behave ethically when confronted with dilemmas and to function in ways consistent with what they believe.

Ethical, moral, and legal values are not necessarily related. A moral belief is the personal conviction that something is absolutely right or wrong in all situations. A person is generally unwilling to change personal opinions on issues of a moral nature. To one person, for example, abortion may be an absolute moral wrong—in other words, there are no acceptable reasons for any woman to attempt to terminate her pregnancy prematurely. If this person holds morally consistent views, he or she may also believe that capital punishment is a moral wrong. Not all persons hold the same moral views, and something that is a moral issue for one can be an ethical dilemma for another. In regard to the example of abortion, another person may be willing to accept abortion under certain situations. The values of the woman undergoing the abortion or the expected nature of the future life of the unborn child may make a difference in regard to whether abortion is acceptable. A moral issue becomes an ethical one when the choice is no longer clear between right and wrong.

A difference also exists between ethical and legal issues. Frequently the two are closely related, as in the case of a family's willingness to halt life-support measures for a terminally ill child. The parents have the legal right to stop all efforts to keep their child alive when physicians agree therapy is no longer beneficial. However, they must struggle with the ethical issue of whether it is right to end the life of such a young human being. Both ethics and the law refer to rules of conduct based on understanding principles of right and wrong. A legal right is that which a person is entitled to have, to do, or to receive from another person, whose duty is imposed within the limits of the law (Creighton, 1986). Legal and ethical overtones accompany a person's rights. The legal view implies that legal obligations coexist with rights.

In contrast, an ethical right involves no legal guarantees, as in the example of the right to health care. If it is assumed that health care is a right, it must be assumed that ethical obligations are involved. But if health care is a right, who is obligated to provide it? The right to health care is not legally enforceable because it is not a legal right. Health professionals do, however, feel obliged to provide health care to those seeking it. They are motivated to provide health care as through it were a legal right.

The profession of nursing is practiced within certain legal constraints (see Chapter 18) that ensure safe and effective care. However, ethical considerations are also involved in the nurse's daily performance of care. Ethics provides standards governing nursing decisions and actions. Nursing ethics must keep pace with the diversity in nursing practice to remain relevant to that practice.

HISTORICAL PERSPECTIVES

Society's image of nursing has changed throughout history. During primitive times a folk image existed of a nurse as a mother who cared for the young, sick, or injured. The nurse's image in medieval times was a religious image of care giver for the sick. It was not until the nineteenth century that the foundation for professional nursing was laid. Florence Nightingale saw the need for well-educated nurses trained in the skills necessary to care for the ill.

As recently as the turn of the twentieth century the nurse's role focused primarily on tending a person's basic needs. The nurse functioned in a dependent role under the watchful eye of the physician. Nursing ethics was simple when all nurses had to do was follow physician's orders.

By the end of World War II, however, an evolution of nursing's professional identity began. The ANA Code for Nurses (1950) was the first formal attempt to define nurses' professional accountability. Clients instead of physicians became the focus of nurses' commitment. Nursing schools slowly began to teach scientific theory supporting nursing care. Nurses struggled to identify a distinct body of knowledge for their profession.

Even with a professional code of ethics, change occurred slowly. The majority of nurses still worked in bureaucratic hospital settings. The role and social position of physicians dominated the way ethical decisions were made. Nurses continued to have little voice in decisions affecting clients' care.

The 1980s have seen a dramatic change in nursing education. The scope of nursing involves caring for all aspects of a person's health care needs, not just care during illness. Nursing theories guide nurses in the practice of helping clients and families adjust to health alterations. Nurses are no longer subservient to physicians. They are professionals who play a major role in identifying the client's total health care plan. Nurses practice in new, more independent roles such as home health nurses, nurse specialists, and school nurses. As the profession expands its roles and responsibilities, nurses face a larger variety of ethical dilemmas.

Unfortunately, a gap still exists between nursing education and practice. Nurses have difficulty in meeting their ethical commitments to clients in the practice setting. Often it seems that a nurse's commitment to clients is limited by the rules or regulations of an institution. There are risks when nurses choose to act on behalf of clients whose rights are in conflict with the interests of a hospital.

Nurses may not yet have the total freedom needed to meet their commitment to clients. However, the importance of ethical accountability among health professionals is growing. The new field of bioethics deals with the complex ethical problems health care professionals face daily. Advances in medicine and technology create rapid social change, resulting in new ethical dilemmas. Nurses must be informed about current ethical issues and feel comfortable in making ethical choices.

FOUNDATIONS OF ETHICAL DECISION MAKING

The purpose of nursing is the welfare of other human beings (Curtin, 1986). For nurses to gain the knowledge to make ethical decisions for clients' welfare, the relationship between values, professional ethics, and accountability must be clarified.

Personal Values

Values underlie all ethical decision making. Values are a person's beliefs about the worth of ideas or behavior (see Chapter 16). It is impossible to separate oneself from value orientation when ethical dilemmas occur. Each person's values are unique. One person may consider the quality of life most important and prefer death to suffering and pain. Another person may believe every possible effort should be taken to maintain life, even if it means enduring pain. Values are standards that influence behavior. Understanding personal values helps a nurse recognize how they affect professional development and nursing practice.

Professional values are a reflection of personal values. The ability of a nurse to protect a client's right to privacy or accept responsibility for maintaining nursing skills depends on the nurse's personal view of the importance of confidentiality and professional development. When persons enter the nursing profession, they do not suddenly develop values, nor do they abruptly change them to meet life circumstances. In time, experience helps nurses to adapt personal values to professional experiences and expectations. It benefits a beginning nurse to know and understand differences between personal and professional values. Most nursing students begin professional socialization after personal values have become clear. However, since their health care experiences are limited, nursing students have many opportunities for growth when applying values to new experiences. Once a nurse's personal values complement and reinforce professional values, it becomes easier to practice nursing as an ethically responsible person. The nurse also gains the ability to help clients clarify their own values.

Professional Ethics

The characteristics of professional nurses are similar to those of other professionals. However, the manner in which each characteristic is exercised makes nursing unique from other professionals. Curtin and Flaherty (1982) describe the following characteristics of professional nurses:

1. Education—general and specific. General education gives nurses the ability to think and reason and to understand their world. Specific education provides the theoretical framework for nursing practice, as well as the technical skills needed for delivering nursing care.
2. Acceptance of a code of ethics—The code ensures integrity on the part of members of the profession. Basic to the code is the value placed on the worth and dignity of human beings.
3. Dedication to master craftsmanship in their work—Mastery of nursing is an ongoing process. Nurses must continually add to their skills to expand the body of knowledge for nursing.
4. Informed membership and involvement in the organized profession—Nurses are responsible for the growth of their own profession.
5. Accountability—Nurses participate in decision making and assume responsibility for their own behavior.

A professional nurse makes a commitment to clients and the nursing profession to provide high-quality health care. Nurses as professionals must refine their own practice and adjust to the changing demands of the health care system to grow professionally.

CODES OF ETHICS

The nursing profession has codes of ethics affirming professional regard for high ideals of conduct. A profession's ethical code is a collective statement about the group's expectations, a standard of behavior. An ethical code for nurses summarizes the special responsibilities assumed by those who care for the ill. Nurses deal with people who, because of illness or injury, are often vulnerable and dependent on the professional's knowledge and skill. The nursing profession formulates and adheres

---

American Nurses' Association Code of Ethics

1. The nurse provides services with respect for human dignity and the uniqueness of the client unrestricted by considerations of social or economic status, personal attributes, or the nature of health problems.
2. The nurse safeguards the client's right to privacy by judiciously protecting information of a confidential nature.
3. The nurse acts to safeguard the client and the public when health care and safety are affected by the incompetent, unethical, or illegal practice of any person.
4. The nurse assumes responsibility and accountability for individual nursing judgments and actions.
5. The nurse maintains competence in nursing.
6. The nurse exercises informed judgment and uses individual competence and qualifications as criteria in seeking consultation, accepting responsibilities, and delegating nursing activities to others.
7. The nurse participates in activities that contribute to the ongoing development of the profession's body of knowledge.
8. The nurse participates in the profession's efforts to implement and improve standards of nursing.
9. The nurse participates in the profession's efforts to establish and maintain conditions of employment conducive to high quality nursing care.
10. The nurse participates in the profession's effort to protect the public from misinformation and misrepresentation and to maintain the integrity of nursing.
11. The nurse collaborates with members of the health professions and other citizens in promoting community and national efforts to meet the health needs of the public.

From American Nurses' Association: Code for nurses with interpretive statements, Kansas City, Mo., 1985, The Association.

---

to high ideals of conduct to assure the public and society that individual nurses will not exploit their positions.

Ethical codes provide standards of conduct and thus allow a profession to discipline its members. These standards indicate some of the factors nurses must take into consideration when determining proper conduct. Ethical codes also provide a common foundation for professional nursing curricula.

Ethical dilemmas are not always easy to resolve. A useful code of ethics must be brief, yet detailed enough to offer clear guidance and attain widespread accep-

Canadian Nurses Association Code of Ethics

The body of the code is divided into the following sources of nursing obligations:

CLIENTS

- A nurse is obliged to treat clients with respect for their individual needs and values.
- Based on respect for clients and regard for their rights to control their own care, nursing care should reflect respect for clients' right of choice.
- The nurse is obliged to hold confidential all information about a client learned in the health care setting.
- The nurse has an obligation to be guided by consideration for the dignity of clients.
- The nurse is obligated to provide competent care to clients.
- The nurse is obliged to represent the ethics of nursing before colleagues and others.
- The nurse is obligated to advocate clients' interests.
- In all professional settings, including education, research, and administration, the nurse retains a commitment to the welfare of clients. The nurse has an obligation to act in a fashion that will maintain trust in nurses and nursing.

HEALTH TEAM

- Client care should represent a cooperative effort, drawing on the expertise of nursing and other health professions. By acknowledging personal or professional limitations, the nurse recognizes the perspective and expertise of colleagues from other disciplines.
- The nurse, as a member of the health care team, is obliged to take steps to ensure that the client recives competent and ethical care.

SOCIAL CONTEXT OF NURSING

- Conditions of employment should contribute to client care and to the professional satisfaction of nurses. Nurses are obliged to work toward securing and maintaining conditions of employment that satisfy these goals.

RESPONSIBILITIES OF THE PROFESSION

- Professional nurses' organizations recognize a responsibility to clarify, secure, and sustain ethical nursing conduct. The fulfillment of these tasks requires professional organizations to remian responsive to the rights, needs, and interests of clients and nurses.

From Canadian Nurses Association: Code of Ethics for Nursing, 1985.

tance. The ANA and CNA have established widely accepted codes the professional nurse should attempt to follow (see boxes). Although these codes differ somewhat in specific emphasis, they reflect the same underlying principles.

Accountability and Responsibility

A nurse assumes responsibility and accountability for nursing care personally delivered. Responsibility refers to the execution of duties associated with a particular role assumed by the nurse (ANA, 1985). When administering a medication, a nurse is responsible for assessing the client's need for the drug, giving it safely and correctly, and evaluating the response to it. Professionally the nurse is responsible for using the nursing process to help clients promote, maintain, or restore health. A responsible nurse is competent in knowledge and skills. The responsibility of a nurse also involves a willingness to perform ethically within the guidelines of the profession.

Whenever nurses perform care, they must be accountable. Accountability refers to being answerable for one's

Maintaining Professional Accountability

SELF

- Report any personal conduct that endangers clients.
- Stay informed of current nursing practice theory and issues.
- Make judgments based on facts.

CLIENT

- Provide clients with accurate information about care.
- Conduct nursing care in a manner that ensures client safety and well-being.

PROFESSION

- Maintain ethical standards in practice.
- Encourage other professional peers to follow the same ethical standards.
- Report a colleague's unethical behavior.

EMPLOYING INSTITUTION

- Follow policy and procedures defined by the institution.

SOCIETY

- Maintain ethical conduct in the care of all clients in all settings.

own actions. A nurse is accountable to self, the client, the profession, the employing institution, and to society (see box). If a wrong dose is given during administration of medication, the nurse is accountable to the client who received it, the physician who ordered it, the nursing service that set standards of expected performance, and society, which demands professional excellence. To be accountable, a nurse acts under an ethical code. Thus, when an error is made, the nurse reports it and initiates care to prevent further injury to the client. Accountability calls for an evaluation of a nurse's effectiveness in practice.

Professional accountability serves the following basic purposes:

1. To evaluate new professional practices and reassess existing ones
2. To maintain standards of health care
3. To facilitate personal reflection, ethical thought, and personal growth on the part of health professionals.
4. To provide a basis for ethical decision making

It is essential for nurses to be accountable for nursing care and not to let members of other disciplines assume that responsibility. Therefore nurses must be actively involved in the ethical decisions made. Accountability is achieved when a nurse assumes responsibility for professional competence and uses a systematic process to resolve ethical dilemmas.

NURSE AS ADVOCATE

Ethical standards provide general guidelines for the behavior of professionals and institutions toward clients. In real-life situations, nurses must also remember moral principles, such as autonomy, self-determination for clients, avoidance of harm, doing good, telling the truth, and ensuring justice when caring for clients. However, these principles may be threatened in situations that involve caring for the terminally ill, acquiring informed consent, obtaining organ donations, and using life-support measures or expensive diagnostic procedures. Nurses may face situations in which it seems difficult to maintain and promote the health of clients, as well as to respect the client's worth and dignity. Curtin (1986) describes nursing as a moral art, one that involves the search for good during relationships with other human beings.

A nurse can only behave ethically when the rights of all clients are respected. The nurse-client relationship is the foundation on which the nurse and client can freely determine the form of that relationship (for example, client and counselor and friend and friend) (Curtin, 1986).

The human relationship existing between nurse and client allows the nurse to be the client's advocate. Advocacy involves giving clients the information they need to make decisions and then supporting those decisions. A nurse's legal responsibilities are met by properly informing clients, and the ethical standard of honoring the right to self-determination is met by supporting them.

In a health care setting, clients can become very vulnerable. Illness interferes with clients' independence, forcing them to go to nurses or physicians for assistance. Illness can also cause loss of freedom of action. Clients may no longer be able to express themselves fully because of altered movement, communication, or intellectual capacity. An illness may also interfere with a clients' abilities to make choices. For clients' rights to be preserved, health professionals cannot make decisions for them. Client advocacy respects the unique human needs of each client and ensures that each client is properly informed in making decisions.

The two primary functions of advocacy are to inform and to support. To inform a client properly, a nurse must have accurate information or know where to get it. The nurse may rely on other health professionals as resources for correct information. A nurse advocate must also *want* the client to have the information. Frequently, nurses and physicians are fearful that clients may question or even refuse needed care if they know too much. However, clients also have the right *not* to know. A nurse advocate presents information in a way that is meaningful to the client, which involves providing information when clients request it and when they are prepared for it. The nurse may provide basic explanations or plan several short discussions. A nurse advocate also recognizes that many persons, such as family members, physicians, and health care administrators, may not want clients to have information. This situation makes advocacy very difficult. In this case, the role of advocate becomes a careful balancing act between telling clients what they need to know and not threatening their relationship with the physician or family.

The supportive aspect of advocacy requires a nurse to support a client without falling into a defensive or rescuing position. The responsibility for decision making rests with the client and not the advocate. The nurse advocate does not give advice, pass judgment, or offer approval. Advocacy is not an easy task. The nurse is well aware of the risks if clients make a wrong decision about health care. For example, a client may refuse a treatment or refuse to participate in care. Either decision could seriously impede his recovery and rehabilitation. A nurse gives clients the knowledge they need, thereby placing them in a position to make their own decision. If the decision is wrong, the nurse teaches the client how to accept it and how to make a better one in the future.

The beginning nursing student will frequently encounter clients asking for help in decision making: "Should I take my bath now, before I go to x-ray?" and "Do you think I need this medication?" Simple questions may be significant to a client who is ill. However, they provide excellent opportunities for the nurse to help clients learn to make decisions for themselves so the client will be more capable of making bigger decisions when they arise. In helping clients to make seemingly small decisions, a nurse gains practice in the advocate's role.

Consider the following hypothetical situation:

Mr. Tate is preparing for discharge from the hospital after removal of a cataract. He tells a nurse, "My doctor said I shouldn't bend over or lift heavy weights for 6 weeks. Do you think it's OK to pick up my 1-year-old little boy if I'm careful?"

The nurse could simply tell Mr. Tate to avoid picking up anything weighing more than 10 pounds. However, to help Mr. Tate make his own decision, the nurse first explains why the lifting restriction is made and the effects lifting would have on his eye. The nurse clarifies with Mr. Tate how heavy his son actually is. The nurse and the client also discuss whether there is anyone at home during the day to watch the infant, since Mrs. Tate works.

At the end of the discussion the nurse says, "Well, Mr. Tate, I really can't tell you what to do. We've talked about the pros and cons of restrictions related to your surgery. What do you think is best?"

Mr. Tate still has a choice. He can avoid lifting his son for 6 weeks or risk injuring his eye by ignoring the physician's and nurse's warnings. What if Mr. Tate chooses to ignore the restrictions? The nurse might feel guilty for not insisting that the client make the safer decision. However, even then the nurse would have no assurance that the client would follow the restrictions at home. Using an advocate's approach places the responsibility for decision making with the client. The nurse fulfills ethical responsibility by providing the client with a means to choose his own course of action.

There is one key point to remember when a nurse pursues an advocacy role. Not all clients require an advocate. Many clients are capable of making their own decisions without a nurse's support. However, it is always appropriate for a nurse to share pertinent and meaningful information with a client.

ETHICAL PROBLEMS IN NURSING

Diverse ethical issues are involved in health care today. Issues may arise in any of the five areas in which the nurse is accountable: self, profession, client and family, employing institution, and society. In addition a nurse will face ethical issues unique to nursing practice in any area or specialty (see box).

Community Health Nursing

AIDS is a fatal and transmittable disease. Persons diagnosed with this disease often have histories of homosexual or heterosexual relationships with several partners, intravenous drug abuse, or blood transfusions. AIDS is viewed by society as a catastrophic health problem. Many nurses have values incongruent with caring for clients with AIDS. The general public is often confused about the risks involved when coming in contact with persons with AIDS.

For example, as a head nurse in a community health clinic, Mrs. Jamison has distributed to staff members the Centers for Disease Control (CDC) guidelines for caring for AIDS clients. The clinic has several AIDS clients who visit for a variety of health problems. The nurses who staff the clinic are concerned about exposing themselves to the disease. One nurse has requested not to be assigned to the specific clinic visited by an AIDS client. Mrs. Jamison knows the nurse is not at great risk for exposure to the AIDS virus. Should Mrs. Jamison change the nurse's assignment? How many other nurses will also make the same request? Will AIDS clients recognize the staff's reluctance to care for them?

Home Health Nursing

Prospective reimbursement in health care has created the incentive for hospitals to discharge clients in a timely and efficient manner. As a result, nurses in hospitals often have less time to educate or prepare clients and families for continued care needed in the home setting. More clients return home with pain, ambulation restrictions, new medications, and incompletely healed surgical incisions. Nurses working in the home health care setting face the dilemma of clients who have limited financial resources and who need care that is not reimbursable.

Mr. Evers is a 41-year-old man who has had diabetes for over 10 years. The home health care nurse visits Mr. Evers to change the dressing on a healing foot ulcer. This dressing care is reimbursable. However, during a visit, the nurse finds that Mrs. Evers also has been diagnosed with diabetes. Mrs. Evers apparently has limited knowledge about diet control and is unable to explain common complications of the disease. The nurse has an ethical responsibility to give clients information they need for self-care. Several visits to Mrs. Evers' home would be needed for proper instruction. Regulations prohibit reimbursement for client education if it is the only service offered by the home health nurse. What should the nurse do to help the Evers family? Diabetic persons having a

---

Ethical Issues in Nursing Practice

COMMUNITY HEALTH NURSING

- Abortion
- Artificial insemination by a donor
- Blood donors tested for AIDS
- Contraception
- Genetic counseling
- Rights to health care

HOME HEALTH NURSING

- Reimbursement restrictions for home health care
- Undertreatment of terminally ill with analgesic medications
- Client's refusal to be hospitalized
- Treatments administered by family members

MEDICAL-SURGICAL NURSING

- Artificial heart transplantation
- Brain death protocols
- Disclosure of diagnosis to terminally ill clients
- Inadequate staffing
- Living wills
- Termination of life support
- Organ transplants
- Client abuse

NURSING HOMES

- Elderly abuse
- Research involving residents
- Loss of residents' autonomy

NURSING OF CHILDREN

- Allowing severely ill neonates to die
- Child abuse
- Organ donation

MENTAL HEALTH NURSING

- Behavior control
- Psychotherapy
- Involuntary hospitalization
- Solitary confinement
- Informed consent

NURSING RESEARCH

- Confidentiality
- Informed consent
- Rights of human subjects
- Identification of risks

NURSE-PHYSICIAN-CLIENT RELATIONSHIPS

- Confidentiality
- Informed consent
- Role conflicts
- Verbal or telephone orders
- Impaired physicians

NURSE-NURSE RELATIONSHIPS

- Reporting nurses who are impaired or observing incorrect nursing practice
- Interdependent roles
- Staffing

---

poor understanding of the disease often experience complications.

Medical-Surgical Nursing

Transplantation of organs and tissues is now a realistic option for persons suffering chronic and disabling diseases. Surgeons today can transplant the heart, kidneys, liver, lungs, corneas, and bone marrow. Organ and tissue recipients are able to resume a productive life-style after surgery, and their life expectancy may be extended several years.

With the success of organ transplants, ethical concerns have increased. The availability of organs from donors is limited, making transplantation an expensive procedure. What criteria should be used to determine who should be a recipient? Should a transplant be withheld if a client cannot afford it? Nurses care for the donors and the recipients, and the issues of organ transplantation can become very emotional.

For example, a 14-year-old boy has suffered brain death as a result of injuries sustained in an automobile accident. Mechanical life support is the only thing keeping his body alive. Meanwhile, a 58-year-old man suffering from renal failure lies in a hospital bed waiting for a kidney donor. Should attempts to preserve the boy's life be halted in order to use his kidneys? Should the family feel obligated to donate the boy's kidneys? The nurse faces a difficult ethical dilemma when in this situation.

Most states now have "Required Request" laws making it mandatory for trained staff to inform families of the option for organ donation when the decreased person is a potential organ or tissue donor. The option of organ donation raises many questions. Will the body be disfigured because of organ or tissue removal? Are there donor costs related to organ recovery? Will burial be delayed? (The answer to all of these questions is "No.") The nurse learns to be an advocate, giving families the information needed to decide if organ donation is desirable. If the families decide against donation, their decision should be respected and supported.

Nursing Homes

The number of elderly in the United States and Canada is increasing every year, due in part to medical cures for some diseases, better treatment for chronic illness, and more interest in health promotion. A relatively small percentage of the elderly population lives in nursing homes. Unfortunately, an alarming number of elderly entering nursing homes are victims of abuse from family members.

The types of harm experienced by the elderly are physical and psychological abuse, financial and personal exploitation, and neglect. Unreasonable confinement to a nursing home is also a form of abuse. Certain symptoms may point to physical abuse, including skin bruising, bleeding, malnutrition, sexual molestation, burns, fractured bones, and soft tissue swelling. These symptoms are especially significant if they are not a part of the client's past history. A nurse may see the symptoms of abuse when a client is first admitted to a nursing home or after he returns from a short visit with his family.

In 1986, 37 states required nurses and other health care professionals to report abuse of older adults by family members (Gilbert, 1986). Most states require nurses to report cases when abuse is suspected, regardless of whether the older adult wishes a report to be made. To comply with the law, nurses may feel as though they are intruding into the older adult's life. Nurses may also fear their assessment of abuse is wrong. Making any wrong conclusions can seriously threaten the relationship with the client and family. Many older adults who are victims of abuse are able to make their own decisions, but state laws support the false idea that most elderly people are incompetent.

Nurses who obey the laws often face an ethical conflict that the elderly client's right to autonomy is violated. It is important to assess the capacity of older adults to make their own decisions. If nurses believe in autonomy, it will be the option of the older adult, rather than the option of the nurses, to decide if they have been abused.

Nursing of Children

The question of whether a person should be allowed to die is one of the most difficult dilemmas faced by health care professionals and society. The issue is even more value laden when it involves children because it is difficult to understand why a young child must lose his life without having had the opportunity to experience life. If a child suffers from a terminal illness, parents and family members may have to decide between preserving life artificially and allowing the child to die. Advocates

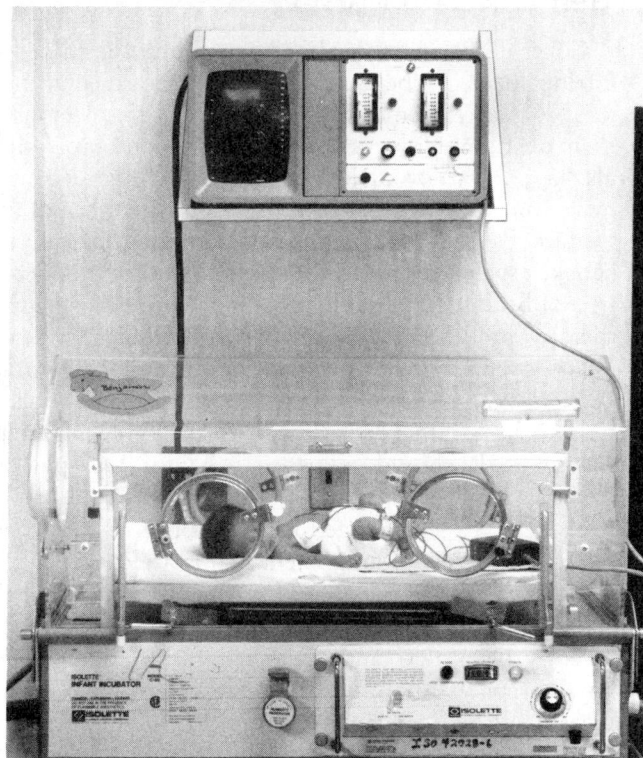

Fig. 17-1 A difficult ethical issue for a nurse to face is whether a child should be allowed to die peacefully, without aggressive medical care.

of "death with dignity" believe that persons should not be forced to endure pain, suffering, or humiliation, and that the persons have the right to choose relief by dying. Those who support the "right to life" attitude, however, believe that hope should never be discarded. They argue that no individual has the right to determine when life is over and that only God can decide such a matter.

The physician, bound by the Hippocratic Oath, is committed to preserving life. The nurse has the responsibility to support any measures ordered by the physician, as well as to maintain the dignity of the dying person.

Parents and other family members experience fear, guilt, and anger when the question of death is raised. The infant or child facing death cannot make a choice. The responsibility rests entirely with the parents. If the child is an only child, if the illness occurred suddenly, or if the parents have never been faced with the death of a family member, a decision will be especially difficult. The parents will often seek the nurse's advice. The nurse, aware of the influence of personal emotions and values, must help the parents clarify their own values. As a client advocate, the nurse helps the parents to understand their child's predicament and supports them in the difficult decision they face (Fig. 17-1).

Mental Health Nursing

Controlling a person's behavior can be considered an infringement of liberty. Confinement in a mental institution is an extreme example of depriving persons of their freedom. However, mental health care professionals have a variety of less extreme methods to control behavior in the interest of the person's own health and welfare and the welfare of society. Tranquilizers, electric shock, psychosurgery (removal or destruction of a portion of brain tissue that controls behavior), and psychotherapy are examples. Many ethical dilemmas arise: Who decides whether behavior is normal or desirable? Who is expert enough to identify normal behavior? If persons have difficulty adjusting to their role in society, whose goals should influence behavior therapy—the client's, family's, therapist's, or society's? Should a person's behavior be changed if he does not wish it to be?

For example, a young client is hospitalized in a psychiatric unit for depression. The nurse has cared for the client over the course of a 2-week period. The client has recently been alert and rational. One morning as the nurse prepares to administer medications, the client refuses the drug, remarking, "These drugs are experimental. I have the right not to take them anymore." Is the client capable of making a decision? Will the failure to take the medication cause the client to become depressed or even self-destructive? When ethical dilemmas develop, the nurse's relationship with a client can help determine to what extent a client is acting appropriately.

Nursing Research

Many opportunities exist in nursing practice when researching the effectiveness of nursing interventions. For example, staff nurses may wish to compare two methods for decubitus ulcer care or two different teaching methods on a group of clients. The studies may prove that one form of care is measurably better than the other. Nursing research can contribute to the body of knowledge influencing nursing practice.

Research involving human subjects can be useful and beneficial to the common good. The nurse is ethically responsible for obtaining free and informed (voluntary) consent from persons participating in a research study. Informed consent means that all study subjects understand the purpose of the study, the research methods (for example, application of a new type of ulcer dressing) used, and the possible risks or benefits. The nurse who identifies the type of study and plans all research methods is responsible for acquiring informed consent.

For example, the nurse, Mr. Wills, is seeking cancer clients to participate in a survey measuring attitudes about pain control. Mr. Wills is on a tight time schedule and must have 30 clients' agreement to participate in the study. Mr. Wills approaches a client, Mrs. Sims, who has a history of being confused at times. He explains the purpose of his study and hands Mrs. Sims a letter of consent to sign. Mrs. Sims remarks, "I'm not sure what you want, but I guess it's ok," and signs the consent form. Should Mr. Wills include Mrs. Sims in the study? Does the client understand the purpose and implications of the study? Clients involved in research have the right to ask any questions about the study at any time. If a client is unable to understand the implications of a research study because of disease, illness, or injury, the nurse should not involve the client in the study.

Nurse-Physician-Client Relationships

Client advocacy requires a commitment to the needs of all clients. This commitment may be difficult to fulfill because nurses are accountable to clients, as well as to families, physicians, and health care administrators. A nurse strongly committed to serving client interests may come in conflict with the physician or with the interests of the hospital.

Smith and Davis (1980) summarize the following factors influencing a nurse's ability to make ethical decisions within institutional settings:

1. Nurses, as employees, work under policies established by others.
2. Conflicts arise between the professional model of nursing education and the bureaucratic model of health care institutions.
3. Nurses are often given responsibility and accountability but not authority.
4. Nurses experience role conflicts with other health care professionals.
5. Nurses experience conflicts between meeting a client's needs and following institutional procedures.
6. Nurses often have either limited or no input into decisions that they are responsible for implementing.

For example, a nurse cares for a client who is seriously weakened and feels discomfort. Throughout the morning, several physicians visit to ask questions and examine the client. Just as the client relaxes and falls asleep, an x-ray technician arrives to announce that the client must be taken away for a test. The nurse calls the radiology department to reschedule the test for later in the day but learns rescheduling is impossible unless the test is postponed until the next day. The nurse knows the hospital is under pressure not to hospitalize clients longer than necessary. What is the best decision for the client? What are the implications if the test is postponed? How can the nurse resolve an ethical dilemma so the client's welfare is maintained?

Nurse-Nurse Relationships

In most areas of nursing practice, several nurses work together. Because of the interdependent relationships of nurses, one nurse's practice affects and is affected by the practice of others. When one nurse acts unethically, questions may be raised about the entire nursing team.

Several factors add to the complexity of ethical issues between nurses. Levels of experience among nurses vary widely. A nurse experienced in one area of practice and informed about current developments in nursing is likely to be more clinically qualified than a recent graduate. Nurses place differing degrees of importance on theoretical models of nursing, as well as on activities involved in the nursing process. It is not uncommon to find two nurses correctly performing the same procedure in two entirely different ways.

Regardless of educational preparation and experience, nurses are expected to perform competently. Ethical conflicts between nurses may arise when a nurse's competence is questioned. For example, Mary and Ruth have worked together on the evening shift for over 3 years. Ruth notices that, over the course of the last month, Mary's behavior has been inconsistent. Mary has been slow in following through with orders and seems more temperamental. One client complains to Ruth about Mary's slow response to requests. One evening Ruth smells alcohol on Mary's breath. Should Ruth report the incident or ignore it?

Situations that raise ethical questions involving other nurses will always exist. Nurses can be ethically responsible if they ignore unethical conduct of colleagues. Careful judgment and methodical decision making help a nurse to make sound ethical decisions.

PROCESS FOR RESOLVING ETHICAL PROBLEMS

Decision making based on ethical reasoning is similar to the nursing process because it requires deliberate, systematic thinking (Fig. 17-2). The nurse first distinguishes ethical problems from communication or legal problems (Aroskar, 1985). To distinguish an ethical problem from other problems Curtin and Flaherty (1982) recommend that the nurse decide whether the problem has one or more of the following characteristics:

1. It cannot be resolved solely through a review of scientific data.
2. It is perplexing. One cannot easily think logically or make a decision about the problem.
3. The final answer to the problem will have a profound relevance for several areas of human concern.

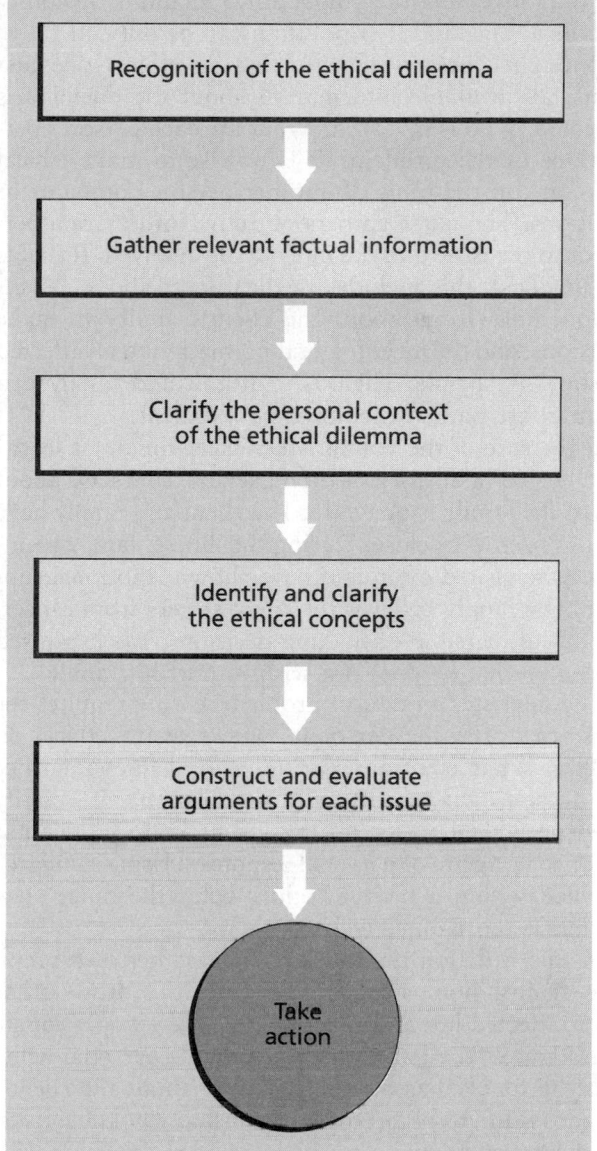

Fig. 17-2 Process for resolution of ethical dilemmas.

For example, a nurse learns that a young client, diagnosed as having AIDS, is being discharged. The client has requested that his family not be informed of his disease, but family members will be involved in the client's care. Should the client be forced to inform his family of his condition? Which branch of science or what source of data can clearly answer the question? The client has the right to confidentiality. It also seems unfair to expose the family unknowingly to any potential risks during care of the client. Obviously a conflict in values makes a decision difficult. Finally, it is obvious that, whatever the decision about the client, there will be a significant effect on the relationship of the client with his family and their relationship to others in society. The dilemma involving the young AIDS victim is obviously an ethical one, and its resolution can be difficult.

Once the nurse recognizes that an ethical dilemma exists, all available information about the dilemma is collected. Who is involved? What are each person's perceptions of the problem? It is unwise to make ethical decisions on the basis of another person's opinions or emotions. The nurse gathers objective information pertinent to the issue and the individuals involved. If clients are involved, this includes medical facts about the situation, knowledge about the client's ability to make decisions, and the meaning of the situation to all affected persons. A client's religious, cultural, and family orientation are part of the nurse's assessment.

In the case of the young AIDS client the nurse learns that he has a history of homosexual contacts, about which the family is unaware. The client and family have always been very close. During the illness, family members have visited often and have shown emotional support. The family believes the client suffers from cancer. The client, capable of making decisions, has expressed a concern that he does not wish to hurt his family.

The next step in ethical problem solving requires the nurse to clarify the personal context of the ethical dilemma. What emotions, attitudes, or values influence the nurse's own perception of the dilemma? To clarify the true ethical issues in any given situation, a nurse needs to be aware of personal responses. Using standards clarified within a code of ethics helps the nurse view dilemmas more objectively.

In this situation the nurse recognizes her own prejudice against homosexuals. However, this attitude has never affected her ability to be kind and compassionate to homosexual clients. The nurse has a personal belief that the family has a right to know about the client's diagnosis and to be protected against any possible risks. Furthermore the nurse has had a good relationship with the family and believes they will be understanding. Despite her feelings the nurse clearly recognizes that the client has the right to keep any information about his condition confidential.

Ethical decision making can be complex. Any decision has consequences. Ethical issues must be clear so decisions are not made solely on an emotional level. The nurse must know the implications of any decision and know if the client's rights have been jeopardized. A careful, ethical decision-making process will help the nurse take a defensible and intelligent position on the issue.

The young client with AIDS has the right to choose his course of therapy and to refrain from informing the family about his disease. Human freedom consists of the right to one's domain, whether it is the body, life, property, or privacy (Bandman, 1978). AIDS can be transmitted through contact with blood or body fluids. It is possible that during the care of the client, especially during its terminal stages, the family can become unknowingly exposed to the AIDS virus. The family members have the right to be reasonably protected from physical harm. The client's freedom should not endanger the life of someone else. The nurse must consider to what extent the family may be at risk.

Once the nurse has a clear perception of the ethical problem it is time to list all options to determine which action will maintain the client's rights and the nurse's professional integrity. The nurse constructs and reviews arguments for each possible action to find the best solution. The ethical principles and values involved must be considered. Weighing all sides of a dilemma helps the nurse anticipate outcomes and know whether reasons for action are valid or sound. An ethical code helps to evaluate the priorities of the situation.

The nurse knows that the client loves and respects his family and is trying to protect them from further emotional harm. If the client informs the family about his disease the family can become educated as to how to safely care for the client. A well-educated family can also anticipate the client's needs more effectively. There is a risk, however, that the client's acknowledgment of his condition may cause the family to reject him. The client has already expressed the desire to be cared for in the home. As the client becomes more critically ill, the family might become exposed to body fluids. The nurse considers whether there are ways to protect the family from harm if they are uninformed.

The nurse acts after evaluating all alternative courses of action and is thus able to respond to objections or arguments from others. Regardless of how careful a person is in resolving ethical dilemmas, others may very well reject the solution or opinion. Involvement of all informed health team members can prove a useful resource.

In the case of the young AIDS client, the nurse decides to talk with the client about the feelings and beliefs affecting his decision. The nurse realizes the client may be unaware of the risks to which he may be exposing the family. The nurse explains to the client the way his condition will progress over time and the extent to which the family should be protected. If the client still chooses not to inform the family, the nurse assures him that his right will be respected and works with the family and a home health care nurse to be sure the family learns about good infection control techniques. These techniques can be explained without revealing the client's true diagnosis.

No two ethical dilemmas are the same. Without a systematic approach to ethical decision making, a nurse cannot resolve ethical issues in a consistent, objective, and professional manner.

SUMMARY

Ethics consists of the principles governing proper professional conduct. The professional nurse is in a unique relationship with clients and other health care professionals by being in the forefront of ethical decision making. Rapid social and technological advancement have changed the roles of nurses. Likewise, the ethical principles governing nursing practice have changed to become compatible with a growing profession.

Nurses face a variety of ethical problems in connection with professional experiences. To resolve these ethical problems, nurses use a systematic process to understand the nature of the problem and to plan a responsible course of action. No ethical problem is easy to resolve. A nurse must be willing to spend time and personal commitment to arrive at logical, fair, and human ethical decisions.

KEY CONCEPTS

✓ Technological advances in health care have created many types of ethical dilemmas.

✓ The nurse's role has become multifaceted, a situation that has increased the number and diversity of ethical dilemmas a nurse encounters in practice.

✓ The special relationship between nurse and client is the foundation for nursing ethics.

✓ A moral belief is the conviction that something is absolutely right or wrong.

✓ An ethical dilemma results from conflicts in values, causing uncertainty in decision making.

✓ Clients have the legal right to safe and effective nursing care.

✓ Experiences in nursing practice help nurses adapt personal values to professional values.

✓ Personal values make the ethical commitment to avoid value judgments difficult for the nurse.

✓ A code of ethics is a set of shared ethical principles accepted by the members of a profession.

✓ A professional nursing code of ethics protects the vulnerable and dependent members of society.

✓ Professional nurses have a commitment to clients, the profession, and society to provide high-quality health care.

✓ An ethical nurse maintains skill competency and assumes responsibility for nursing judgments.

✓ "Responsibility" refers to the scope of functions and duties a nurse is required to perform.

✓ A nurse is accountable when demonstrating a willingness to assume responsibility for nursing care.

✓ When nurses witness acts that may endanger clients, they are obligated to report them.

✓ The primary functions of advocacy are to inform and to support.

✓ Client advocacy requires a nurse to present a client with accurate, meaningful information without jeopardizing the client's relationship with physician or family.

✓ There are ethical issues unique to each area of nursing practice.

✓ The supportive role of advocacy protects a client's right to self-determination.

✓ A methodical approach to the resolution of ethical dilemmas requires the nurse to clarify personal values.

✓ Taking a stance in an ethical dilemma is easier when both sides of the dilemma are evaluated.

REFERENCES

American Nurses' Association: Code for nurses, Am J Nurs 50:196, 1950.

American Nurses' Association: Code for nurses with interpretative statements, Kansas City, Mo., 1985, The Association.

Aroskar, MA: Nurses as decision makers: ethical dimensions, Imprint 32:29, 1985.

Bandman, B: Option rights and subsistence rights. In Bandman, EL, and Bandman, B, editors: Bioethics and human rights, Boston, 1978, Little, Brown & Co., Inc.

Creighton, H: Law every nurse should know, ed. 5, Philadelphia, 1986, W.B. Saunders Co.

Curtin, LL: The nurse as advocate: a philosophical foundation for nursing, In Chinn, P, editor: Ethical issues in nursing, Rockville, Md., 1986, Aspen Publishers, Inc.

Curtin, L, and Flaherty, MJ: Nursing ethics: theories and pragmatics, Bowie, Md., 1982, Brady.

Gilbert, DA: The ethics of mandatory elder abuse reporting statutes, ANS 8:51, 1986.

Smith, SJ, and Davis, AJ: Ethical dilemmas: conflicts among rights, duties, and obligations, Am J Nurs 80:1463, 1980.

ADDITIONAL READINGS

Annas, GJ: Rules for research in nursing homes, N Engl J Med 315:1157, 1986.

Applegate, ML, and Entrekin, NM: Teaching ethics in nursing, New York, 1984, The National League for Nursing.

Aroskar, MA: Anatomy of an ethical dilemma: the theory, Am J Nurs 80:658, 1980.

Aroskar, MA: Anatomy of an ethical dilemma: the practice, Am J Nurs 80:661, 1980.

Aroskar, MA: Ethics of nurse-patient relationships, Nurse Educ 5:18, 1980.

Creighton, H: The nurse and artificial insemination, Nurs Manage 16:1802, 1985.

Creighton, H: The maintenance of life: 1983-1985. II. Nurs Manage 17:12, 1986.

Curtin, LL: Ethical issues in nursing practice and nursing education. In National League for Nursing: Ethical issues in nursing and nursing education, New York, 1980, The League.

French, DG: Ethics: nurse, am I going to live? Nurs Manage 15:43, 1984.

Fromer, MJ: Ethical issues in health care, St. Louis, 1981, The C.V. Mosby Co.

International Council of Nurses: ICN code for nurses: ethical concepts applied to nursing, Geneva, 1973, Imprimeries Populaires.

Kloosterman, N, et al.: Statement on ethics in critical care research. I. Focus Crit Care 12(3):47, 1985.

Kloosterman, N, et al.: Statement on ethics in critical care research, II. Focus Crit Care 12(4):58, 1985.

Kohnke, MF: Advocacy: risk and reality, St. Louis, 1982, The C.V. Mosby Co.

MacMillan-Scattergood, D: Ethical conflicts in a prospective payment home health environment, Nurs Econ 4(4):165, 1986.

O'Rourke, KD: Ethics of research on human subjects, Parameters: publication of Saint Louis University, p. 16, Spring-Summer, 1986.

Parent, B: Moral, ethical, and legal aspects of infection control, Am J Infect Control, 13:278, 1985.

Robinson, A: Genetic screening's medical progress prompts ethical questions, AORN 43(5):1137, 1986.

Scott, RS: When it isn't life or death, Am J Nurs 85:19, 1985.

Steele, SM: AIDS: clarifying values to close in on ethical questions, Nurs Health Care 7(5):247, 1986.

Thompson, HO, et al.: Code of ethics for nurse-midwives, J Nurse Midwife, 31:(2)99, 1986.

Vaughan-Cole, B, and Kee, HK: A heart decision, Am J Nurs 85:535, 1985.

Wax, J: Solving ethical problems, AORN 43(3):608, 1986.

Yarling, RR, and McElmurry, BJ: The moral foundation of nursing, ANS 8:63, 1986.

Younger, SJ, et al.: Psychosocial and ethical implications of organ retrieval, N Engl J Med 313:321, 1985.

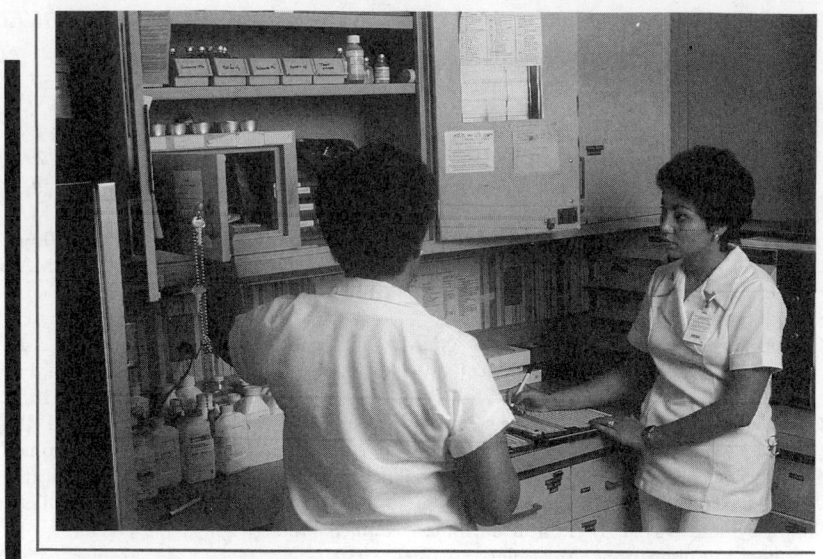

OBJECTIVES

Mastery of content in this chapter will enable the student to:

- Define the key terms listed.
- Understand legal concepts that apply to nursing practice.
- Describe legal responsibilities, obligations and legal parameters of nursing practice.
- List sources for standards of care for nurses.
- Understand areas of potential legal liability.
- Define legal aspects of nurse-client, nurse-physician, nurse-nurse, and nurse-employer relationships.

KEY TERMS

Assault

Battery

Crime

Libel

Malpractice

Negligence

Slander

Tort

Witness

Legal Issues in Nursing

Contemporary law is a composite of all the rules and regulations by which society governs itself. Without law, society could not deal with disputes and problems in an orderly fashion. The laws of any society are flexible and ever changing through either legislative process or judicial decisions.

The general public is better informed than in the past about health and illness. Through reports in newspapers and magazines and on television, more information is available to consumers of health services. Many clients are knowledgeable about their rights, and nurses are challenged to become advocates for clients. In 1972 the American Hospital Association developed and adopted a Patient's Bill of Rights. In 1974 the Dying Person's Bill of Rights was completed, and in 1975 the Pregnant Patient's Bill of Rights was written. Although these documents are not considered legally binding, many hospitals use them to provide guidelines for care.

Many nurses view the law with apprehension because they fear being named in a malpractice lawsuit. With increased emphasis on clients' rights, nurses today must understand their legal obligations and responsibilities to clients. Nurses who give competent care based on their education will seldom need to worry about a malpractice lawsuit.

The law serves many valuable functions when applied to nursing practice. It differentiates nursing practice from the practice of other health care professions. It also describes and protects the rights of clients and nurses. For these reasons, nurses should understand basic legal concepts as they relate to nursing practice.

GENERAL LEGAL CONCEPTS

Two basic sources exist for contemporary law. Statutory law is created by elected legislative bodies such as state or provincial legislatures, the U.S. Congress, or the Parliament of Canada. Common law is created by judicial decisions made in courts when cases are decided. From these two sources two categories of law are defined, civil law and criminal law.

Civil law is concerned with the protection of a person's rights. Although violations of civil law might cause harm to an individual or his property, no grave threat to society as a whole usually exists. For example, defamatory statements made about a person might lead to personal problems but do not threaten society in general. Civil law is also considered the portion of law that does not pertain to crimes.

Criminal law is concerned with acts that threaten society and its order but may involve only an individual. Misuse of controlled substances is an example of criminal conduct for nurses.

From a legal standpoint nurses providing care assume three roles: providers of service, employees of institutions (or occasionally independent contractors for service), and private citizens. They perform these roles as they care for clients and work with physicians and for employing institutions. If nurses do not adhere to standards of care, they may face legal consequences.

LEGAL LIMITS OF NURSING

Standards of Care

Nursing standards of care establish the boundaries within which nurses practice. Many standards apply generally or specifically, depending on the nurse's specific field of practice. All U.S. state legislatures and Canadian provincial parliaments have passed *nursing practice acts* defining the scope of nursing practice in that state or province. These acts, which vary among states and provinces, set educational requirements for nurses, distinguish between nursing and medical practice, and generally define the ways in which a nurse should practice. All nurses are responsible for knowing the provisions of the act for the state or province in which they work.

Professional organizations are another source for standards of care. The ANA and CNA have developed standards for nursing practice, policy statements, and similar resolutions. These standards are general and include recommendations such as the obligation of nursing service departments to provide continuing education programs.

The written policies and procedures of the employing institution detail how the nurses are to perform their duties. These policies are usually quite specific and are set down in procedure manuals found in most nursing units. For example, a procedure policy outlining the steps that should be taken when changing a dressing or administering medication gives specific information about how nurses are to perform these tasks. These policies provide another definition of standards of care.

Standards of care are very important. If a nurse is a defendant in a malpractice lawsuit, these standards may be used to determine if he or she has acted as any reasonably prudent nurse with the same level of education and experience would. In other words, standards of care serve as guidelines for determining whether a nurse performed duties in an appropriate manner. If a nurse is named as a defendant in a malpractice lawsuit and it is shown that neither the accepted standards of care outlined by the state or province nursing practice act, nor the policies of the employing institution were followed, the nurse's legal defense would be tenuous.

A 1966 case, *Darling v. Charleston Community Memorial Hospital,* involved an 18-year-old man with a fractured leg. When the cast was applied to his leg, the physician placed insufficient padding under the plaster. The man's toes became swollen and discolored, and he had decreased sensation in them. He complained to the nursing staff many times. Although nurses recognized his symptoms as signs of impaired circulation, they failed to tell their supervisor that the physician did not respond to their calls or the patient's needs. During the next 4 days, gangrene developed, and the man's leg had to be amputated. The physician in the emergency room was liable for incorrectly applying the cast. The nursing staff was also liable because they had not adhered to the standards of care appropriate to the client's symptoms (Rocereto and Maleski, 1982).

Another issue in this case was inadequate nurse staffing in the emergency room. Since the JCAHO standard for the number of staff was not met, the institution was also liable in this lawsuit.

Standards of care basically concern a nurse's accountability for nursing care. A general duty nurse is legally responsible for meeting the same standards as other general duty nurses in a similar setting. However, specialized nurses such as nurse anesthetists, intensive care nurses, certified nurse-midwives, or operating room nurses are held to standards of care and skill exercised by those in the same specialty as defined by applicable standards. All nurses should know the standards of care they are expected to meet.

Standards of care are guidelines by which nurses should practice. If nurses do not perform duties within accepted standards of care, they may place themselves in jeopardy of legal action.

Licensure

Requirements for licensure vary among states in the United States and provinces in Canada, but in most nurse licensing acts, requirements exist for education and the nurse must pass an examination. All states use the National Council Licensure Examinations (NCLEX) for registered nurse and licensed practical nurse examinations. Nurse licensing statutes usually require that nurses be 21 years of age, be citizens or have work permits, and exhibit good moral character (Cazalas, 1978).

A license can be suspended or revoked by the board of nursing if conduct violates provisions contained in the licensing statute. For example, nurses who perform illegal acts such as selling or taking controlled substances, jeopardize their licensed status. Before a nurse's license is revoked, he or she must be notified of the charges and permitted to attend a hearing in which evidence can be presented on his or her behalf. These hearings are not court proceedings but are usually conducted by the state or provincial board of nursing. Some states and provinces do provide for judicial review of such cases if the nurse has exhausted all other forms of appeal (Cazalas, 1978).

Student Nurses

If a client suffers harm as a direct result of a nursing student's action or lack of action, the liability for the incorrect action is generally shared by the student, the instructor, the hospital or health care facility and the university or educational institution. Student nurses should never be assigned to tasks for which they are unprepared and should be carefully supervised by instructors as they learn new procedures. Although student nurses are not considered employees of the hospital, the institution does have a responsibility to monitor the acts of nursing students. Student nurses are expected to perform as professional nurses would at that point in their experience. Faculty members are usually responsible for instructing and observing students, but in some situations, staff nurses may share these responsibilities. Every nursing school should provide clear definitions of responsibility (Cazalas, 1978).

Sometimes student nurses are employed as nursing assistants or nurse's aides when not attending classes. If student nurses are employed in this capacity, they should not perform tasks that do not appear in a job description for a nurse's aide or assistant. For example, even if a student has learned to administer intramuscular medications in class, this task may not be performed as a nurse's aide.

LEGAL LIABILITY IN NURSING

Crimes

A crime is an offense against society that violates a law. Criminal acts are prosecuted in the criminal justice system. A felony is a crime of a serious nature that carries a penalty of imprisonment. A misdemeanor is a crime of a less serious nature, and the penalty is usually a fine or imprisonment for less than a year. In nursing there are few crimes nurses would commit if they practiced within accepted standards of care. For the purpose of this chapter, flagrant criminal activity such as murder and illegally dispensing controlled substances will not be discussed. Laws pertaining to such offenses apply to nurses as to all individuals.

Torts

A tort is a civil wrong committed against a person or property. Torts may be subtle and difficult to define. Unintentional torts such as negligence and intentional torts are willful acts that violate another's rights (for example, assault and battery). If a nurse performs an act that could be considered a tort, the case is tried in a civil (not a criminal) court to assess fair compensation for the client (plaintiff) who brought suit. The purpose of the judgment is not to punish the nurse, as it would be in a criminal proceeding.

NEGLIGENCE

If nurses give care that does not meet appropriate standards, they may be held liable for negligence. Negligence may involve carelessness such as not checking an armband and consequently administering the wrong medication. However, carelessness is not always the cause. If nurses perform procedures for which they have not been trained and do it carefully but still harm the patient, a claim of negligence could be made (Hemelt and Mackert, 1982).

Nurses have been involved in several common negligent acts. Errors in sponge counts in surgical cases are among the most common. In these cases a sponge is left inside the client by mistake. If an infection or another problem develops because of the sponge, a claim of negligence and liability against the physician, nurse, or both, would be justified.

Another common negligent act is causing a burn. If a nurse applies a heating device that is too hot and the client sustains a burn, the nurse is legally liable for negligence. Cases also exist in which electronic equipment malfunctioned and the client sustained an electrical burn from a monitor probe. Nurses should never use equipment they know is malfunctioning and must ensure that electrical equipment is grounded to prevent the chance of shock.

Many negligent acts can occur when administering medications. Incorrect dosages, mixups that result in the wrong medication being given to a client, incorrectly administered medication, and inaccurate computations of dosages are among the most common errors. Nurses must use extreme care when involved in administration of medications because the possibility for error is great.

A claim of negligence could also be made when infection can be traced to an action or failure to use aseptic technique. Therefore nurses must be concerned with the cleanliness of the client's environment, as well as with accepted standards of care regarding prevention of cross-contamination. For example, nurses must follow accepted practice for handling blood and other body fluids from patients with AIDS.

Nurses are responsible for performing all procedures correctly and for exercising professional judgment as they carry out physicians' orders and duties not ordered but for which they have authority. Any nurse who does not meet accepted standards of care or who performs duties in a careless fashion runs a risk of being found negligent.

INVASION OF PRIVACY

A claim of invasion of privacy also might be brought against a nurse. A client is entitled to confidential health care. All aspects of a client's care should be free from unwanted publicity or exposure to public scrutiny.

One form of invasion of privacy is the release of information to an unauthorized person. In an Alabama case in 1973, *Horne v. Patton,* a physician revealed medical information about a client's condition to the client's employer. The client lost his job. A lawsuit found the physician liable for releasing information to the employer, who did not have a legitimate interest in the client's health history (Hemelt and Mackert, 1982).

Gossiping about a client's activities is another form of invasion of privacy and could lead to a charge of slander. If a client has a venereal disease, for example, the nurse should not discuss that information except as it directly relates to care and treatment. Nurses are required in some areas to report certain communicable diseases and are immune from prosecution when they make reports.

A nurse's unwanted intrusion in private family matters is another example of invasion of privacy. For example, if a client is terminally ill and does not want his family to know, the nurse could try to persuade him to inform his family because it would be in his best interest and beneficial to them, but the nurse should not tell them without the client's permission.

An individual's right to privacy may conflict with the public's right to information. For example, a threat or benefit to public health may override the individual's right to privacy. Disclosures of private information were made about individuals who had toxic shock syndrome and in the Tylenol poisoning cases. Sometimes the client is a public figure whose physical condition is considered newsworthy. There are also cases in which information is released about a scientific discovery or a major medical breakthrough, as with the first heart transplant cases or the first artificial heart recipient. If an event falls into any of these categories, information should be channeled through the public relations department of the institution to ensure invasion of privacy does not occur. The nurse should not attempt personally to decide the legality of disclosing information.

DEFAMATION OF CHARACTER

Any communication that injures an individual's reputation and is disclosed by another person is considered libel (written) or slander (oral). For example, if a nurse tells a client that his physician is incompetent, the nurse could be held liable for slander. The nurse who writes such a comment could be sued for libel. The important issue in a claim of defamation of character is whether harm is done to the reputation of the plaintiff (Cazalas, 1978).

ASSAULT AND BATTERY

Although assault and battery might be considered criminal in the context of this chapter, only the civil aspects will be discussed. If a nurse is accused of assault and battery, the client could bring a civil lawsuit against the nurse to recover damages. Such a case would be tried in a civil (not a criminal) court.

Assault is an act intended to provoke fear in a victim. The victim believes harm will come to him as a result of the threat. Assault may be subtle. For example, a nurse might attempt to coerce a client into taking a medication the client does not wish to take. A more blatant example might involve a nurse handling an uncooperative client in the emergency room. If the exasperated nurse yells, "If you don't take off those filthy clothes, I'm going to rip them off you!" and moves toward the client, a claim of assault could be made.

Battery is willful touching of another's body, anything he is wearing or holding, or anything attached to him, without his consent (Northrop and Kelly, 1987). There have been instances of abuse of confined clients in mental institutions. In addition, if a nurse attaches fetal electrodes during labor without the consent of the mother, a claim of battery could be made. The important issue is the client's informed consent. In some situations consent is implied. For example, if a nurse says, "I have your injection for you, Mr. Jones," and he holds out his arm, he is giving implied consent to the injection. In Canada, the term *battery* is not used, but there are three classifications of assault.

It is unimportant that the procedure that constitutes

battery (without consent) helps the client. In a case in 1905, *Mohr v. Williams,* the client gave written consent for surgery on his right ear. Once the client was anesthetized, the physician discovered that the left ear was more seriously affected and operated on that ear. The client sued because surgery was performed on the "wrong" ear (Cazalas, 1978).

Procedure in a Malpractice Lawsuit

In a malpractice lawsuit against a nurse the following criteria must be established: (1) the nurse (defendant) owed a duty to the client (the plaintiff), (2) the nurse did not perform that duty, (3) the client (plaintiff) was injured, and (4) the client's injury was a result of the nurse's failure to perform the duty. The best way for a nurse to avoid being named in a lawsuit is to follow standards of care, give competent health care, and develop empathetic rapport with the client. A client who believes the nurse did everything possible is unlikely to initiate a lawsuit.

Malpractice Insurance

Feutz (1987) recommends that "nurses should ascertain before practicing nursing that they are adequately protected in all aspects of their professional practice, either under their employer's liability insurance or their own individual policy." Since an institution's policy is designed primarily to protect the institution, nurses should not assume they are equally protected. Although each nurse must consider individual risks and benefits, most nurses should carry personal liability insurance. Malpractice insurance is also available for nursing students practicing in assigned clinical areas. When student nurses work as nursing assistants within an agency, they should determine before starting that the institution provides insurance coverage or that student malpractice insurance provides liability coverage. If the employing institution does not cover a nurse's legal expenses, it may be very costly "to prove innocence," according to Grace Barbee, former attorney for the California Nurses' Association (Creighton, 1986). The uninsured nurse must also finance his or her defense.

LEGAL CONCEPTS AND THE NURSE-CLIENT RELATIONSHIP

The nurse deals with many people, including the client and family, physicians, other nurses, and other health care professionals, as well as the employing institution. In nurse-client interactions, several legal issues may arise. The Patient's Bill of Rights, adopted by the American Hospital Association, is a statement of guidelines related to nurse-client interaction (see box).

The Patient's Bill of Rights

1. The patient has the right to considerate and respectful care.
2. The patient has the right to obtain from his physician complete current information concerning his diagnosis, treatment and prognosis in terms the patient can be reasonably expected to understand.
3. The patient has the right to receive from his physician information necessary to give informed consent prior to the start of any procedure and/or treatment. . . . Where medically significant alternatives for care or treatment exist, or when the the patient requests information concerning medical alternatives, the patient has the right to such information (and) to know the name of the person responsible for the procedures and/or treatment.
4. The patient has the right to refuse treatment to the extent permitted by law, and to be informed of the medical consequences of his action.
5. The patient has the right to every consideration of his privacy concerning his own medical care program.
6. The patient has the right to expect that all communications and records pertaining to his care should be treated as confidential.
7. The patient has the right to expect that within its capacity a hospital must make reasonable response to the request of a patient for services.
8. The patient has the right to obtain information as to any relationship of his hospital to other health care and educational institutions insofar as his care is concerned (and) any professional relationships among individuals, by name, who are treating him.
9. The patient has the right to be advised if the hospital proposes to engage in or perform human experimentation affecting his care or treatment (and) has the right to refuse to participate.
10. The patient has the right to expect reasonable continuity of care.
11. The patient has the right to examine and receive an explanation of his bill regardless of source of payment.
12. The patient has the right to know what hospital rules and regulations apply to his conduct as a patient.

THE CHILDREN'S MERCY HOSPITAL
Kansas City, Missouri

TERMS AND CONDITIONS OF ADMISSION

NECESSARY MEDICAL TREATMENT:
Recognizing the need for hospital care for the child whose name appears herein, consent is hereby given to The Children's Mercy Hospital for hospital services rendered under the general and specific instructions of the attending physician and treatment to be necessary for the safety, welfare and health of the child.

PROFESSIONAL CARE:
The patient is under the professional care of an attending physician who arranges for services for the care and treatment of the patient. The attending physician is usually selected by the patient's parent or guardian, but may when not designated or under emergency circumstances be otherwise selected.

RELEASE OF INFORMATION:
The Hospital is authorized to furnish information from the patient's medical record to any insurer, compensation carrier or welfare agency who may be providing financial assistance for hospital care.

PHOTOGRAPHS:
Photographs of the patient may be taken under the supervision of The Children's Mercy Hospital by members of the Staff or other persons for teaching, medical research purposes or for publicity as deemed proper by the Hospital and the taking of pictures, unless specifically denied in writing, shall not be deemed an invasion of privacy.

PERSONAL VALUABLES:
The Hospital shall not be liable for loss or damage to any personal property of the patient brought into The Children's Mercy Hospital.

PAYMENT FOR HOSPITAL CARE:
I/We do hereby assume financial responsibility for and agree to make payment in full to The Children's Mercy Hospital for all charges for services or medical supplies furnished the above patient. Payment is to be made within 30 days as bills are presented with settlement in full, or arrangements for same to be made in the Financial Counseling Department before departure of the patient.

I/We do certify that the financial information given is true, accurate and complete to the best of my/our knowledge, and further authorize The Children's Mercy Hospital to investigate any and all financial information given on this admission under their normal investigative procedures.

I/We do hereby assign and authorize payment directly to the above named Hospital and physician(s) of all hospitalization or insurance benefits and physician fee benefits and guarantee to pay any balance, with the understanding that the account is not settled or closed until after the insurance benefits are received by the Hospital and if there is a remaining balance I/we agree to pay the same. I/We are aware of the above contents.

I/We hereby certify that I/we have read all parts of this Admission Form and agree and accept all terms and conditions hereon and state that all representations made by me are true.

I am aware of the above contents.

A photocopy of this agreement shall be considered as valid and effective as the original.

SIGNED	ADDRESS	PHONE
RELATION TO PATIENT	DATE	
WITNESS	DATE	
SECOND WITNESS (TELEPHONE CONSENTS)	DATE	

Fig. 18-1 Sample consent form for admission to the hospital.
Courtesy The Children's Mercy Hospital, Kansas City, Mo.

Informed Consent

A signed consent form is required for potentially hazardous procedures such as surgery, for some treatment programs such as chemotherapy, and for research involving clients. For a consent to be valid (1) the person giving consent must be mentally and physically competent and be legally an adult, (2) the consent must be given voluntarily—no coercive measures may be used to obtain it, (3) the person giving consent must thoroughly understand the procedure, its risks and benefits and alternative procedures, and (4) the person giving consent must have the opportunity to have all questions answered satisfactorily. If a client is deaf or has some other impediment in communication (such as speaking a foreign language), an interpreter should be available to explain the terms of consent. Fig. 18-1 is an example of a consent form for admission to the hospital.

Because nurses do not perform surgery or direct the medical procedure, obtaining client consent does not fall within the nursing duty. However, in many institutions the nurse assumes responsibility for confirming consent. When a nurse takes a consent form for the client to sign, the nurse should ask if the client understands the procedure for which consent is being given. If he answers that he does not understand or the nurse realizes he does not understand even though he states he does, the nurse is obligated to notify the physician or nursing supervisor and to make certain that the client is informed before signing (Northrop and Kelly, 1987). The court says a client's right to self-determination gives the client the right to clear information with which to make a decision for informed consent (Hemelt and Mackert, 1982). Fig. 18-2 is a sample consent form for a special procedure that is similar to some consent forms for surgery. Notice that possible complications are listed to make certain the client understands them as part of *informed consent*. The consent form for immunizations has even become more detailed (Fig. 18-3).

If a client participates in an experimental treatment program, or submits to use of experimental drugs or treatments, an even more detailed and stringently regulated informed consent form is used (Fig. 18-4). The Federal Food and Drug Administration and the institutional review board reviews the information in the consent form for research involving human subjects. The client is always given the option of withdrawing from the experiment at any time.

A client refusing surgery or other medical treatment must be informed about any harmful consequences. If the client persists in refusing the treatment, the rejection should be written, signed, and witnessed.

Parents are usually the legal guardians of pediatric clients and therefore are the persons who must sign consent forms. Occasionally a parent or guardian refuses treatment for a child. For example, in a recent Texas case a child whose parents were Jehovah's Witnesses refused a lifesaving blood transfusion for the child. The child was made a ward of the court, and the blood transfusion was administered. The court ruled that although parents are adults and may choose to become martyrs, they cannot make a martyr of their child (Creighton, 1986). The practice of making a child a ward of the court, administering necessary treatment, and then returning legal guardianship to the parents is relatively common in such cases. If such a case occurs, the nurse should inform the nursing supervisor, who will enlist the aid of the appropriate hospital administrator to handle the problem.

In some instances, obtaining informed consent is difficult. If the client is unconscious, for example, consent must be obtained from a person legally authorized to give consent on the client's behalf (Cazalas, 1978). If a person has been declared legally incompetent in a judicial proceeding, consent must be obtained from the person's legal guardian. In emergency situations, if it is impossible to obtain consent from the client or an authorized person, the procedure required to benefit the client (or perhaps save his or her life) may be undertaken without liability for failure to obtain consent (Cazalas, 1978).

Death and Dying

Many legal issues surround the events of death, including a basic definition of the actual point at which a person is considered dead. A definition of death becomes very important in organ donation and transplantation or when questions exist about whether to continue life support. Nurses must be aware of legal definitions of death because they must document all events that occur during the time the client is in their care.

The point of death was traditionally described as the time at which heart beat and respirations cease. However, modern technology, which includes the use of cardiopulmonary resuscitation and cardioventilatory support, has made this definition obsolete. In 1968, the Harvard Medical School Ad Hoc Committee to Examine the Definition of Brain Death introduced irreversible coma into the discussion of death. Since then, some states have passed statutes to further define death. Most definitions state that the most important issue in determining death is the judgement of absence of brainstem function made by an attending physician, a neurologist, a neurosurgeon, or a specialist in reading electroencephalograms. The actual pronouncement of death is usually the legal responsibility of the physician.

The Dying Person's Bill of Rights is a set of guidelines used in many settings in the care of dying clients (see Chapter 26). *Text continued on p. 479.*

INFORMED CONSENT FOR AMNIOCENTESIS

I. I hereby request and authorize Doctor _____ to perform a diagnostic amniocentesis (pass a needle through the abdominal wall and withdraw some of the amniotic fluid). I further request that an attempt be made to perform the following test(s) on my unborn child:

A. Chromosome analysis _____ (Initial)

B. Alpha-fetoprotein _____ (Initial)

C. Acetylcholinesterase _____ (Initial)
(If indicated)

D. _____ _____ (Initial)

II. I consent to the performance of an ultrasound examination for the purpose of dating the pregnancy, locating the placenta and selecting a site for placement of the needle.

III. I understand that:

A. the procedure of amniocentesis involves a small risk to both mother and fetus and that these risks include; discomfort at the site where the needle was inserted, cramping, bloody spotting, leakage of amniotic fluid, intrauterine infection and miscarriage.

B. there is a possibility that growing the fetal cells may not be successful and that repeat amniocentesis would then be required.

C. although the liklihood of an error is considered to be extremely small, a complete and correct diagnosis of the condition of the fetus based on the test(s) performed cannot be guaranteed.

D. the results provided of normal chromosomes or normal biochemical status of the fetus does not eliminate the possibility that the child may have birth defects and/or mental retardation because of other disorders.

E. in the case of twins, the results may apply to only one of the pair.

F. in some Rh negative mothers Rh sensitization has occurred following amniocentesis.

IV. I have had my questions answered and understand and accept the risks and limitations of this test.

Signed: _____ (Patient)

_____ (Spouse)

_____ (Witness)

Date: _____

Fig. 18-2 Sample consent form for a special procedure.
Courtesy The Children's Mercy Hospital, Kansas City, Mo.

THE CHILDREN'S MERCY HOSPITAL
Kansas City, Missouri

IMPORTANT INFORMATION
ABOUT POLIO AND ORAL POLIO VACCINE

Page 1

Please read this carefully

WHAT IS POLIO? Polio is a virus disease that often causes permanent crippling (paralysis). One person out of every 10 who get polio disease dies from it. There used to be thousands of cases and hundreds of deaths from polio every year in the United States. Since polio vaccine became available in the mid-1950's, polio has nearly been eliminated. In the last five years, fewer than 25 cases have been reported each year. It's hard to say exactly what the risk is of getting polio at the present. Even for someone who is not vaccinated, the risk is very low. However, if we do not keep our children protected by vaccination the risk of polio will go back up again.

ORAL LIVE POLIO VACCINE: Immunization with oral live polio vaccine is one of the best ways to prevent polio. It is given by mouth starting in early infancy. Several doses are needed to provide good protection. Young children should get two doses in the first year of life and another dose at about 18 months of age. A booster dose is important for children when they enter school or when there is a high risk of polio, for example, during an epidemic or when traveling to a place where polio is common. The vaccine is easy to take, effective in preventing the spread of polio, and, in over 90% of people, gives protection for a long time, probably for life.

POSSIBLE SIDE EFFECTS FROM THE VACCINE: Oral live polio vaccine rarely produces side effects. However, once in about every 4 million vaccinations, persons who have been vaccinated or who come in close contact with those who have recently been vaccinated are permanently crippled and may die. Even though these risks are very low, they should be recognized. The risk of side effects from the vaccine must be balanced against the risk of the disease, both now and in the future.

PREGNANCY: Polio vaccine experts do not think oral polio vaccine can cause special problems for pregnant women or their unborn babies. However, doctors usually avoid giving any drugs or vaccines to pregnant women unless there is a specific need. Pregnant women should check with a doctor before taking oral polio vaccine.

WARNING - SOME PERSONS SHOULD NOT TAKE ORAL POLIO VACCINE WITHOUT CHECKING WITH A DOCTOR:

* Those with cancer or leukemia or lymphoma.

* Those with diseases that lower the body's resistance to infection.

* Those taking drugs that lower the body's resistance to infection, such as cortisone or prednisone.

* Those who live in the same household with any of the above persons.

* Those who are sick right now with something more serious than a cold.

* Pregnant women.

Fig. 18-3 Sample consent form for immunizations.
Courtesy The Children's Mercy Hospital, Kansas City, Mo.

Continued.

＊ Most persons over the age of 18 because adults have a slightly bigger risk of developing paralysis from oral polio vaccine than children. (However, if the risk of polio is increased - as may occur, for example, when there is an outbreak in your community - polio experts recommend that unprotected persons receive oral polio vaccine regardless of age.)

NOTE ON INJECTABLE (KILLED) POLIO VACCINE: Besides the oral polio vaccine, there is also a killed polio vaccine given by injection which protects against polio after several shots. It has no known risk of causing paralysis. Many polio experts feel that oral vaccine is more effective for controlling polio in the United States. Injectable polio vaccine is recommended for persons needing polio vaccination who have low resistance to infections or who live with persons with low resistance to infections. It may also be recommended for unprotected adults who plan to travel to a place where polio is common. It is not widely used in this country at the present time, but it is available. If you would like to know more about this type of polio vaccine, please ask us.

QUESTIONS: If you have any questions about polio or polio vaccination, please ask us now or call your doctor or health department before you sign this form.

REACTIONS: If the person who received the vaccine gets sick and visits a doctor, hospital, or clinic in the 4 weeks after vaccination, please report it to:

THE CHILDREN'S MERCY HOSPITAL

I have read the information on this form about polio and the oral vaccine. I have had a chance to ask questions which were answered to my satisfaction. I believe I understand the benefits and risks of oral polio vaccine and request that it be given to me or to the person named above for whom I am authorized to make this request.

_____   _____

Signature of parent or guardian or adult person   Date
authorized to make the request

Reprinted with permission of Department of Social Services - Missouri Division of Health

Fig. 18-3, cont'd Sample consent form for immunizations.

INFORMED CONSENT - CHORIONIC VILLI SAMPLING

1. STATEMENT OF CONSENT:

I, _____, voluntarily agree to participate in an investigational program which studies the experimental medical procedure of chorionic villi sampling as a method of prenatal diagnosis of genetic disease in a developing fetus. This program will investigate specifically:

a. the risks of this new medical procedure, and
b. its accuracy as a diagnostic method.

I understand that "chorionic villi sampling" means using a small plastic catheter to withdraw a tiny sample of placental tissue from within the womb. The sample is obtained when I am 9-11 weeks pregnant.

I have been offered participation in this investigation because there is a significant risk of disease in the fetus which I carry. I understand that this medical procedure is indicated, because I am at risk for a genetic or biochemical abnormality, namely: _____.

2. PROCEDURES:

I hereby authorize Dr._____ to perform the following medical procedure on me: introduction of a small catheter into the uterus through the cervix and attempted withdrawal of a sample of placental tissue.

I understand that this procedure is occasionally accompanied by a little discomfort or cramping and that the procedure will be completed in 15-20 minutes.

I understand that up to three individual samplings for the placental tissue may be attempted but that there is no guarantee that chorionic villi will be obtained from any of the attempts.

I understand that an attempt to obtain a tissue culture from cells of any particular sample of chorionic villi may be unsuccessful, or that the chromosome preparation may be of poor quality and unusable, or that a DNA or biochemical study being performed may be unsuccessful due to technical difficulties, or may be difficult to interpret. If this occurs I will be offered the opportunity to repeat the chorionic villi sampling in subsequent weeks if the length of gestation permits or I will be offered amniocentesis in the second trimester.

I understand that amniocentesis is available for the verification of chromosomal or biochemical test results if difficulty in interpretation is present, or if failure to obtain chorionic villi occurs. The reliability of diagnosis by amniocentesis has been well established and I have received an information sheet concerning amniocentesis and its specific risks.

I understand that although the likelihood of a misinterpretation of the chromosomal, DNA, or biochemical study from this procedure is considered to be very small, not enough experience has been accumulated to assure me that it is as reliable as fetal diagnosis by amniocentesis. However, from either of these fetal diagnostic procedures (CVS or amniocentesis) a complete and correct diagnosis of the condition of the fetus based on the karyotype (chromosome content) or biochemical analysis cannot be guaranteed.

I understand that in the event of my being Rh negative and therefore at potential risk for developing Rh disease, as may also occur following amniocentesis, Rh immune globulin (such as Rho-gam) will be administered following the procedure (and possibly every 12 weeks thereafter if felt appropriate by Dr._____). This is done to reduce the possibility of the development of Rh isoimmunization.

I understand that an assay for alpha-fetoprotein will be made available to us at our request. This will be done, if requested, at 16 weeks gestation from a maternal blood sample. This test may help determine the risk of bearing a child with an open spinal defect (spina bifida).

Fig. 18-4   Sample consent form for experiments on human subjects.
Courtesy The Children's Mercy Hospital, Kansas City, Mo.

Continued.

I understand that under certain circumstances, such as the presence of vaginal infection, abnormal or unusual configuration or position of the uterus, unusual or difficult positioning of the developing placenta, inability to obtain adequate tissue after three catheter passes, or other unusual problems or unforeseen circumstances, the doctor may determine it is not in the best interest of my pregnancy to perform or continue the procedure. In such a circumstance I understand that the chorionic villi sampling will not be done, but that amniocentesis will still be available to me for prenatal diagnosis if I so desire.

3. RISKS AND BENEFITS:

Although chorionic villi sampling is an investigational technique which has been used in over 30,000 cases worldwide, the hazard (risks) to the mother and fetus is currently considered to be uncertain. The range of loss of the pregnancy in various world centers is from 2.5 to 10%, with most being around 2-3%. It cannot be guaranteed that the procedure will not cause damage to the mother or fetus which could result in one of the following problems.

a. Infection: There is a small risk of infection as a result of sampling. I understand a culture will be done for gonorrhea and that if present, I will be informed as to the results and appropriate treatment. I also understand that a serious infection can result that can start with flu-like symptoms, accompanied by low to high grade fever and general malaise. This could result in loss of the pregnancy and if severe enough could require hospitalization, intravenous antibiotics, or even complete hysterectomy (complete removal of the womb). I also understand that this problem has, on rare occasions resulted in death. I understand that if I have any of the above symptoms I am to contact my personal physician or Dr._____ immediately.

b. Maternal Bleeding: I understand that following the procedure there may be internal bleeding, or spotting for up to two weeks.

c. Fetal Bleeding: I understand that there is a small chance for fetal bleeding which may be monitored by a blood test taken before and after the procedure.

d. Fetal Death: I understand that there is a risk of the fetus dying as a result of this procedure, which would result in a miscarriage or necessitate a D&C for removal of the pregnancy from the womb.

e. Placental Abruption: I understand there is a risk of separation of the placenta from the wall of the uterus as a consequence of this procedure. If this is severe it could lead to fetal death and miscarriage or if less severe could lead to retarded growth of the baby due to decreased placental nourishment.

f. Rupture of the Bag of Waters: I understand there is a small risk of rupture of the fetal membranes which could lead to infection or miscarriage.

g. Birth Defects: I understand that there is a theoretical chance that the procedure could cause an injury to the developing fetus.

h. Intrauterine Growth Retardation: I understand that there is a theoretical risk that removal of part of the placenta could result in decreased growth of the fetus.

i. Uterine Cramping: I understand that this procedure could cause irritation of the womb and could result in menstrual like cramping pain of a few hours duration.

In comparison, the alternative procedure of amniocentesis has well defined risks which have been similar in all reporting medical centers throughout the world. The accepted risk associated with amniocentesis is 1/2%, or one pregnancy loss in every two hundred procedures. As far as benefits are concerned, CVS is completed in the first trimester (prior to 13 weeks) of pregnancy. Therefore, if as a result of the evaluation I elect to terminate the pregnancy, I may experience less physical and emotional side effects. It is also possible that I may derive no direct benefits from participation in this investigation. However, information obtained through my participation may benefit other women with similar problems.

Fig. 18-4, cont'd Sample consent form for experiments on human subjects.

4. ALTERNATIVE PROCEDURES:

I understand that amniocentesis is an alternative means by which prenatal diagnostic information may be obtained. I have been furnished with information about this procedure, including an Amniocentesis Fact Sheet. My questions regarding this alternative have been answered.

5. ADDITIONAL INFORMATION ABOUT CHORIONIC VILLI SAMPLING:

I have been provided additional information concerning the performance of prenatal genetic diagnostic studies in the first trimester. This includes the material entitled, 'First Trimester Prenatal Diagnosis Information Sheet' and 'Patient Instructions:Chorionic Villi Sampling Procedure'. I have read this information and have had any questions answered by the doctor or the counselor. In addition, I understand the following:

a. That every effort will be made to obtain results of prenatal diagnostic studies as soon as possible. Generally results will be available in 10 to 14 days from the date of the sampling procedure, assuming that sampling, growth, and analysis are successful. During the first six months of 1986, the cytogenetic laboratory was able to obtain a successful diagnosis for seven out of seven (100%) trial samples. (A chromosomal abnormality was diagnosed in one of the trial samples). As soon as results are available my physician and I will be notified.

b. That the chromosomal and biochemical abnormalities that may be diagnosed by means of this test are not curable. If test results indicate the abnormalities are present, it will be my decision whether or not to continue the pregnancy.

c. That a normal genetic result, either chromosomal or for a possible biochemical disease, does not guarantee a normal, or healthy infant; it does not eliminate the possibility of birth defects and/or mental retardation due to other disorders or unknown causes.

d. That if the results are not completed by 13 weeks, I will have to decide whether to continue the pregnancy into the second trimester without results.

e. That there is a small chance that the tissue obtained does not represent the genetic makeup of the fetus, either due to chromosomal mosaicism (two or more cell types) or maternal cell contamination.

6. DURATION OF THE STUDY:

I understand that this technique is still investigational and that information on the progress and outcome of pregnancies tested with this technique is essential to learning more about its safety and accuracy. I therefore agree to ultrasound examination of the fetus and uterus one week following the procedure and at 16-18 weeks of gestation. I also agree to cooperate with attempts to follow up on the remainder of the pregnancy, delivery, and development of the infant over the first year of life.

7. CONFIDENTIALITY OF DATA:

I understand that since the CVS procedure is still investigational my medical records, without identifying information, may be used to learn more about the safety and accuracy of the CVS procedure. These records may be inspected by representatives of the Food and Drug Administration as part of the investigation. All records will otherwise be kept strictly confidential, and all identifying information can only be released with my written permission.

8. LIABILITY:

The University of Missouri and Truman Medical Center, in fulfilling their public responsibilities have individually and separately provided professional and general liability insurance coverage for any physical injury in the event such injury is caused by the negligence of the University of Missouri, its faculty and staff or Truman Medical Center and its employees, respectively. In the event I believe that I have suffered any physical injury as the result of my participation in the research program, I may contact Dr._____, telephone number_____ at the University of Missouri-Kansas City School of Medicine or the Clinical Research Review Board, telephone number_____, at Truman Medical Center who can review the matter with me and provide further information on how to proceed.

Fig. 18-4, cont'd   Sample consent form for experiments on human subjects.

Continued.

9. RIGHT TO WITHDRAW:

I understand that any questions I have regarding this study will be fully answered. I understand I may withdraw at any time, without consequences, by notifying my physician, the genetic counselor or Dr._____, and that I will not be charged for procedures not performed. I understand that if I decide to withdraw, amniocentesis will still be available to me for prenatal diagnosis if I so desire.

10. COSTS FOR THE STUDY:

The total cost for this study has a package price of $684.50. I understand that this is the entire cost; whether I go through CVS, or amniocentesis, or for reasons listed above I will need both CVS and amniocentesis. (The package price is broken down as follows: Physician fees, $200.00; Truman Hospital facility usage fees, $84.50; and Counseling and Cytogenetic fees, $400.00). If I want to have alpha fetoprotein analysis determined I understand this will be an additional $35.00 charge. (Please note: these prices may change).

11. MISCELLANEOUS:

Dr._____ has not made or represented any guarantee to me as to the results that I may expect from participation in this study.

I have received a copy of this informed consent for my permanent records.

In full recognition of the possible hazards and limitations of the techniques and interpretation involved in the chromosomal or biochemical analysis of my unborn child, as outlined above, I elect to have the analysis attempted and hereby voluntarily request same.

12. WHOM TO CONTACT FOR QUESTIONS:

I understand that this is an experimental procedure and if I have any questions about the study I should contact one of the following people. I also understand that I am to contact one of these people if I have any questions about my rights as the subject of an experimental study.

Dr._____

Section of Genetics
(The Children's Mercy Hospital)

13. SIGNATURES:

_____   _____
Signature of Patient   Date

_____   _____
Signature of Spouse   Date

_____   _____
Signature of Witness   Date

Fig. 18-4, cont'd   Sample consent form for experiments on human subjects.

Handling of Bodies

Nurses are legally obligated to treat a deceased person's remains with dignity and care. Wrongful handling could cause emotional harm to the survivors. In one case, for example, survivors sued when a mislabeling of bodies led to an Orthodox Jew's body being prepared for a Roman Catholic funeral and a Roman Catholic's body being prepared for a Jewish burial.

Autopsy and Organ Donation

Consent for autopsy must be given by the decedent (before his death) or a close family member. Laws in many states and provinces give an order of priority for family members who may give consent. For an adult male, for example, his wife, then his children, then any other family member may give consent.

Autopsies may resolve legal and medical questions and are required in certain circumstances such as death resulting from suspected child abuse or other criminal activity. Sometimes an autopsy consent stipulates exclusions (such as no studies involving the brain). As with any consent, the physician should not use coercion to obtain consent for autopsy.

A legally competent person is free to donate his or her body or organs for medical use. Consent forms are available for this purpose. A nurse may serve as a witness when a person wishes to give consent for the donation of organs or body.

In most states, required request laws stipulate that, at the time of a person's death, a qualified health care giver must ask family members to consider organ or tissue donation. In the past, this option has not been offered to the family.

The Uniform Anatomical Gift Acts address many problems of organ donation and stipulates that the physician who certifies death shall not be involved in removal or transplant of organs. The National Organ Transplantation Act prohibits selling or purchasing organs and facilitates this area of medical and nursing practice (42 U.S.C. § 274e).

Wills

A will legally declares a person's intentions after death. It usually contains provisions for property division, guardianship of children, and estate administration. A nurse should be knowledgeable about wills because he or she may be asked to be a witness. A witness must watch the person sign the will, know it was voluntarily signed, and, using the best judgment, know that the person was of sound mind and memory at the time of signing.

Most wills are written, and the number of witnesses required varies from one to three, depending on the state or province in which the person resides. If a client wishes to make an oral will, the nurse should write the statements and send a written memorandum to the hospital administrator. A client might declare several wills during a prolonged illness, and the nurse should follow the same procedure each time (Cazalas, 1978).

■ ■ ■

Many possible legal questions are involved in nurse-client interactions. If a nurse is confounded by some particularly difficult legal question, help is always available. Hospitals generally have the benefit of legal counsel, and someone should be able to address particular problems.

LEGAL CONCEPTS AND NURSING PRACTICE

In addition to encountering legal problems in the care of clients, nurses may share liability for errors made by physicians and other health care personnel or for inadequate care provided by the employing institution.

Physician Orders

The physician is responsible for directing medical treatment. Nurses are obligated to follow physicians' orders unless they believe the orders are in error or would be detrimental to clients. Therefore all orders must be assessed, and if one is determined to be erroneous or harmful, further clarification from the physician should be sought. If the physician confirms the order, and the nurse still believes it is inappropriate, the supervising nurse should be informed. A written memorandum to the supervisor detailing the events in chronological order and the reasons for refusing to carry out the order should protect the nurse from disciplinary action (Hemelt and Mackert, 1982). The supervising nurse should help resolve the questionable order. A nurse carrying out an inaccurate order may be legally responsible for any harm suffered by the client.

The physician should write all orders, and the nurse should transcribe them carefully. Oral orders are not recommended because they leave possibilities for error. If an oral order is necessary, during an emergency, for example, it should be written and signed by the physician as soon as possible, usually within 24 hours.

A difficult area regarding physician orders involves an order of "no code" or "do not resuscitate" (DNR) for a terminally ill client. Many physicians are reluctant to write such an order because they fear legal repercussions for "abandoning" clients. Cushing (1981) suggests that if a physician has documented in progress notes that the client's condition is deteriorating and that the decison not to administer cardiopulmonary resuscitation has been made, the physician is perfectly justified in writing a "no code" order. Many sources suggest that guidelines for DNR orders include written documentation of those orders, specific description of treatment to be withheld, discussion of DNR orders with the client or family, discussion with nurses and other staff to withhold CPR, and regular review of DNR orders in case the client's condition warrants a change in the order (Younger, 1987).

According to guidelines adopted by the American Heart Association, cardiopulmonary resuscitation is not intended for use when a client has an irreversible illness in which death is expected (Cushing, 1981). Partial code or "slow code" verbal instructions have occasionally been suggested as a way for a physician to avoid writing a "no code" order. "Slow code" may be defined differently by various institutions but usually means resuscitative procedures should be performed more slowly than recommended by the American Heart Association. If a nurse assists in a "slow code," however, this may be interpreted as not performing resuscitative procedures as a competent person would and therefore be the basis for a lawsuit.

Short Staffing

The JCAHO has established guidelines to determine the number (staffing ratios) of nurses required to give care to a specific number of clients. Legal problems may arise if there are not enough nurses to provide competent care. If a nurse is assigned to care for more clients than is reasonable, he or she should attempt to reject the assignment by informing the nursing supervisor that it is inappropriate. If the nurse is required to accept the assignment, a written protest should be made to nursing administrators. Although the nurse's protest would not relieve him or her of responsibility if a client suffered because of inattention, it would show that the nurse was attempting to act in good faith. A nurse should not walk out when staffing is inadequate, since a charge of abandonment could be made (Horsley, 1981).

Controlled Substances

In 1970 the Comprehensive Drug Abuse Prevention and Control Act was passed in the United States. It covers substances such as narcotics, depressants, stimulants, and hallucinogens. The act regulates hospital distribution systems, rehabilitation programs for drug abuse, and research into the medical treatment of addiction. Canadian law similarly regulates controlled substances. Nurses may administer controlled substances only under the direction of a licensed physician.

Controlled substances should be kept securely locked and only authorized personnel should have access to them. Criminal penalties exist for misuse of controlled substances. There have been cases in which physicians illegally prescribed and dispensed controlled substances, and if nurses employed by such physicians fail to report these activities, they are legally accountable for aiding and abetting the physicians (Cazalas, 1978).

"Floating"

Nurses are sometimes required to "float" from the area in which they normally practice to another nursing unit. Creighton (1986) reports a case in which a nurse in obstetrics was assigned to an emergency room. A client entered the emergency room and complained of chest pain. The client was given a markedly incorrect increased dosage of lidocaine by the obstetrical nurse and died after cardiac arrest and subsequent irreversible brain damage. The nurse lost the malpractice lawsuit against her and the hospital.

A nurse who is floated should inform the supervisor of any lack of experience in the new nursing unit. The nurse should also request and be given orientation to the unit (Creighton, 1986).

Incident Reports

An incident report (Fig. 18-5) is filed in any unusual situation in which there is a possibility that a lawsuit might be filed. For example, if a nurse administers an incorrect dose of medication, a client falls out of bed, or an intravenous solution infiltrates the skin causing sloughing and scar formation, the nurse should complete an incident report. Most institutions provide a specific form for this purpose. The nurse records all the details of the incident, and the physician examines the details of the incident, and the physician examines the client and indicates any adverse effects the error might have.

Many nurses are reluctant to file incident reports because they believe these reports are detrimental to their employment record. Actually, incident reports are used by the institution administration for quality assurance and risk management. By reviewing incident reports, administrators can determine areas of client risk. For example, if a certain kind of problem has occurred repeatedly, educational methods can be used to prevent the problem in the future. In addition, the insurance carrier for a hospital or other institution relies on incident reports to assess liability and possible future claims. A system of quality assurance helps ensure provision of high-quality care. With this system, several steps are taken to identify and correct problems that could compromise care.

The Children's Mercy Hospital
INCIDENT REPORT
*An incident is any happening which is
not consistent with routine operation
of the hospital or care of a particular
patient. It may be an accident or a
situation which might result in an
accident.*

Person(s) involved _____

Complete as applicable if possible injury

☐ Patient → ☐ Inpatient   Diagnosis _____ Age _____
                ☐ Outpatient Who was supervising patient? _____

☐ Employee → Department _____ Job title _____
             Length of time on job _____ Age _____ Home phone _____

☐ Other → Home address & phone _____
          Reason for being at hospital _____

Exact location of incident _____ Date of incident _____ Time _____

Names & addresses } _____
of witnesses } _____

INCIDENT FACTS _____
_____
_____
_____
_____
_____
_____
_____
_____

(Use reverse side if necessary.)

Was person involved seen by CMH physician because of incident?
                    ☐ No   ☐ Yes   Date _____ Time _____
Signature of person reporting _____ Date written _____

PHYSICIAN'S STATEMENT (Clinical information on patients must ALSO be charted.)

Description of any injury _____
_____

Treatment given or recommended _____
_____

If employee involved, when is return to work permitted? _____
Signature of physician _____ Date _____ Time _____

If patient, parent, or nursing personnel involved, send to Nursing Supervisor. Send all
others to Administration.

Fig. 18-5 Sample incident report.
Courtesy The Children's Mercy Hospital, Kansas City, Mo.

Continued.

The Children's Mercy Hospital
    INCIDENT REPORT

INCIDENT FACTS (continued from reverse side) _____

_____
_____
_____
_____
_____
_____
_____
_____
_____
_____
_____
_____
_____
_____
_____
_____
_____
_____
_____
_____

                                 DO NOT WRITE BELOW THIS LINE

Incident report number _____
Reviewers and dates of review

_____ _/_ _/_   _____ _/_ _/_

_____ _/_ _/_   _____ _/_ _/_

_____ _/_ _/_   _____ _/_ _/_

Fig. 18-5, cont'd   Sample incident report.

Risk management is a system of ensuring appropriate nursing care. Steps involved in risk management include identifying possible risks, analyzing them, acting to reduce them, and evaluating steps taken. One tool used in risk management is an incident report.

For nurses in practice, the underlying rationale for quality assurance and risk management programs is the highest possible quality of care. Some insurance companies, medical and nursing organizations, and the JCAHO encourage the use of quality assurance and risk management procedures.

Reporting Obligations

In some situations, nurses are required to report certain communicable diseases or criminal activities, such as abuse, gunshot wounds, attempted suicide, or rape, to the appropriate authority. For example, most states require health care professionals to report suspicions of child abuse. Because cases that must be reported vary among states and provinces, the nurse should be familiar with local statutes.

Good Samaritan Laws

Good Samaritan laws have been enacted in almost every state and province to encourage health care professionals to assist in emergency situations. These laws limit liability and offer legal immunity for people helping in an emergency, providing they give reasonable care under the conditions of the emergency (Hemelt and Mackert, 1982). If a nurse stops at the scene of an automobile accident and gives appropriate emergency care (for example, using caution when moving the injured person in case there is a spinal injury, or applying pressure to stop hemorrhage), the nurse is acting within accepted standards, even though proper equipment was not available.

Contracts

A contract is a written or oral agreement between two people in which goods or services are exchanged. An oral contract is as legally binding as a written one but may be more difficult to prove. A breach of contract occurs if either party fails to carry out agreed obligations.

By accepting a job, a nurse enters into an agreement with an employer. The nurse will perform professional duties competently, adhering to the policies and procedures of the institution. In return, the employer not only pays for the nurse's services but also furnishes the facilities and equipment in proper working order to enable the nurse to provide efficient and competent care (Hemelt and Mackert, 1982).

Nurses also enter into contractual agreements with clients. The nurse agrees to give competent care, and the client agrees to pay for the service. When a client signs an admission form on entering the hospital or agrees to nursing care in any health agency, the contract is initiated. Private duty nurses have specific written contracts with their clients.

LEGAL ISSUES IN PRACTICE AREAS

Many possible legal liabilities exist in all areas of nursing practice. Any nurse working in a specialized field should study the legal issues pertaining to that area of practice.

Perinatal Nursing

Perinatal nursing involves care of women before, during, and immediately after pregnancy, as well as care of newborn infants. Many legal issues are involved in the care of a mother and her infant.

Some of the ethical issues involved in contraceptive counseling are discussed in Chapter 17. From a legal standpoint, persons receiving sexual counseling or treatment for venereal disease have a right to privacy and confidentiality. However, some states have passed laws requiring that parents of minors be informed if a minor seeks contraceptive information or treatment for venereal disease or if a minor girl becomes pregnant.

Infertility of couples desiring to have a child may pose legal questions that usually arise from the solution the couple chooses to solve their problem. One solution is the artificial insemination of a woman with sperm from a donor other than her husband. Because of the potential legal problems, the mother, her husband, and the donor must given written consent to the procedure. Preferably the husband and wife are not told the identity of the donor and vice versa.

Another solution to the problem of infertility is the use of a "surrogate mother." The husband donates sperm to be artificially inseminated into a woman who is not his wife. The woman bears the child and then relinquishes it to the husband and wife. Legal questions arise if the surrogate mother receives monetary compensation because this might be defined as illegal "baby selling" (Annas, 1981). Kentucky has equated mother-surrogate arrangements to the sale of infants and has made the practice illegal in that state. Legal problems may also occur if the surrogate mother changes her mind and wants to keep the baby.

The highly publicized Stern-Whitehead Baby M case in New Jersey illustrates some of the legal problems inherent in the practice of using surrogate mothers. Annas (1986) describes the use of commercial mother surrogates (in which the woman is paid for her services) as exploitative of women and dehumanizing to infants.

Abortion is one of the most emotionally charged issues confronting perinatal nurses. After the Supreme Court ruling on *Roe v. Wade* in 1973, which legalized abortion, two conflicting groups formed, those who support the woman's right to make decisions about her own body and those who support the fetus' right to life. Legal decisions, including other United States Supreme Court cases, continue the debate. For example, in *Planned Parenthood Association of Kansas City, Missouri v. Ashcroft* in 1983, the Supreme Court declared as unconstitutional the provision in a Missouri statute that required that all second-trimester abortions be performed in a hospital. In the *City of Akron v. Akron Center for Reproductive Health, Inc.,* a similar provision was declared unconstitutional. Provisions dealing with parental consent, 24-hour waiting periods for informed consent, and disposal of fetal remains were also declared unconstitutional in this case.

Improved medical and nursing knowledge about neonates has pushed the standard of viability of abortion from 28 weeks to 22 or 23 weeks, bringing new legal questions to bear on the abortion issue. Opinions of legal experts and court decisions that use this new scientific and medical evidence have begun to alter the legal status of the fetus (Callahan, 1986). Nurses working in the perinatal setting should know the laws that apply to this area of practice.

In most states and provinces, laws concerning abortion include provisions known as *conscience clauses.* These clauses allow nurses, physicians, and institutions to refuse to assist in abortions, without fear of reprisal, if it is against their ethical, moral, or religious principles (Harris, 1985). If nurses are ethically or morally opposed to assisting in abortions, they should exercise the right provided by conscience clauses. However, the nurses should never impose their values on clients (see Chapter 16).

Nurses have legal responsibilities regarding fetal monitoring during labor (Wiley, 1976). A claim of battery may be made if the nurse does not obtain client consent before attaching monitor leads. The nurse is also responsible for recognizing ominous fetal monitor patterns. If signs of fetal distress are noted, the nurse must notify the physician and the nursing supervisor and prepare for emergency treatment such as an immediate cesarean section.

There are legal requirements in providing nursing care for newborns, such as properly identifying the infant-mother pair as soon as possible with fingerprints, footprints, and wrist bands or obtaining a blood sample for phenylketonuria (PKU) testing when required by law. Standards of care for the infant immediately after delivery include providing a clear airway, clamping the umbilical cord, applying antibiotics or silver nitrate to the eyes and minimizing stress by drying the infant and keeping the infant warm. Resuscitation equipment must be in the delivery room.

When a stillborn infant is delivered, the nurse must record all events about the delivery. Although the atmosphere in a delivery room is disquieting, the nurse must complete legal requirements by careful documentation.

When an infant requiring intensive care is born, the nurse has many legal responsibilities similar to those in other intensive care settings. Ethical problems involved in removing infants from ventilatory support are discussed in Chapter 17.

An important legal issue that has surfaced in neonatal practice has surrounded "Baby Doe Regulations." The original 1982 case involved an infant born in Indiana with Down's syndrome complicated by esophageal atresia. The infant's parents refused permission for surgical repair of the esophageal defect, and the infant died.

An ongoing debate, complete with court decisions and federal statutes regulating the treatment of handicapped infants, began. Most authorities agree that a compromise supporting the rights of disabled infants yet not imposing governmental interference on parent and physician decisions is necessary. In a 1986 Supreme Court ruling, *Bowen v. American Hospital Association,* the court ruled that section 504 of the 1973 Rehabilitation Act did not apply to Baby Doe situations (Moskop and Saldanha, 1986).

The most recent Baby Doe legislation, The Child Abuse and Neglect Amendment of 1984, was passed by the U.S. Congress. This legislation requires states to establish programs that would respond to any reports of medical neglect, including possible withholding of medical treatment from handicapped infants with life-threatening conditions. This law does not mandate that all disabled infants be treated but promotes parent and physician decision making in these cases. There are many medical centers that use "ethics committees" to help the decision-making process (Weil, 1986).

Iatrogenic disease in a critically ill infant in a neonatal intensive care unit (NICU) may have legal consequences for those involved in the infant's care. An iatrogenic disease results from treatment administered. For example, retrolental fibroplasia, a form of blindness caused by too much oxygen, is an iatrogenic disease. Frequent monitoring of the inspired oxygen concentration and frequent blood gas determinations are standards of care that must be met by nurses working in an NICU.

Pediatric Nursing

Every state and province with child abuse legislation requires that suspected child abuse or neglect be reported. Health care professionals such as nurses are among those mandated to report suspected cases. To encourage persons to report suspected cases, states and provinces provide legal immunity for the reporter if the report is made in good faith and without malice. A health care professional who does *not* report suspected child abuse or neglect may be held liable for civil or criminal legal action (Kreitzer, 1981).

As in all areas of nursing practice, negligence involving pediatric patients is possible. A $450,000 settlement was recently awarded in a New York case, *Beardsley v. Wyoming County Community Hospital*. A 6-year-old boy was taken to the hospital after a sledding accident. Although his prognosis was good after a splenectomy, the nurses administered D5W as his only intravenous fluid instead of alternating it with isotonic saline solution as ordered. Brain damage occurred, and although the boy's condition improved during the next 10 months, he was left with permanent residual damage. The monetary award was large because the boy had lost future earnings because of the nurses' negligent acts, which clearly did not meet appropriate standards of care. Regan (1981) suggests that monetary awards in future cases involving permanent injury to minors will probably be even higher.

Pediatric nurses are responsible for preventing children in their care from accidentally harming themselves. Cribs, which sometimes have a restraining device over the top, are designed to keep infants and toddlers from climbing out of bed and injuring themselves. All poisonous substances and sharp objects should be kept out of the reach of small children. Whenever possible, small children should be kept under constant surveillance to minimize opportunities for accidental harm.

Medical-Surgical Nursing

As in the case of pediatric clients, disoriented adults may require some form of restraint to prevent accidental self-injury. Standards of care, laws, and regulations about the use of restraints and supervision apply to nursing practice with medical-surgical and other clients. Side rails are available on most hospital beds for adult clients. Some disoriented elderly clients may also require belt restraints to prevent them from falling out of bed. If a client falls out of bed and injures himself, he may bring a lawsuit against the nurses and institution.

Critical Care Units

Nurses working in critical care settings are also legally accountable for performing their duties. Critical care nurses require additional training and ongoing in-service education to provide them with information about advances in care methods.

The staffing ratio in an intensive care setting should be one nurse for each client or at most 1:2½, depending on the severity of clients' conditions. The JCAHO recommends these ratios because of the intensity of care required by such clients. These clients usually require careful observation and assessment of their condition and many treatment procedures and medications. If a nurse is assigned to three or four intensive care clients and is unable to give appropriate care and a client suffers harm, the nurse is liable for accepting the client assignment.

Possible legal problems for critical care nurses are associated with the use of electronic monitoring devices. No monitor can be considered totally reliable, and the nurse must not be completely dependent on it. There may also be electrical hazards. The equipment should be checked routinely by engineers to ensure that a client will not receive an electrical shock.

Psychiatric Nursing

The primary purpose for hospitalizing a client with mental illness is rehabilitation so he or she may return to society as a useful and healthy citizen. Current principles of treatment suggest a mentally ill client should be given as much freedom as possible. One problem arising from this freedom is the possibility that the client will slip away, or elope. If a client should be under close scrutiny because of his mental condition and the nurse fails to take due care to prevent his walking out of the health facility, the nurse and the employer would be held liable for any injuries the client sustains or inflicts as a result of the elopement.

Another concern for nurses who care for psychiatric clients is the possibility of client suicide. If a client's history and medical records indicate that the client has suicidal tendencies, he or she must be kept under close surveillance.

Home Health Nursing

An evolving trend in nursing is an increased provision of nursing services in the home. Although community nursing programs have existed for years, the model of nursing care in the home has expanded to include more hours per day, up to full-time, 24-hour care. Many hospitals are dismissing clients with more complex problems requiring sophisticated physical care such as those who need continuous intravenous therapy, or clients with increased oxygen requirements, including ventilatory support. Families are taught to perform some tasks, but some clients need nurses to provide care.

Nurses functioning in this area of practice must provide reasonable care within guidelines and standards of care governing home health care. Legal exposure exists in this area of practice, as in more traditional settings, and nurses should review their need for malpractice insurance.

AIDS

The mention of AIDS causes fear and panic in many members of our society. This lethal disease is found in clients in virtually every segment of nursing practice, from AIDS victims on medical-surgical units, to mothers and infants in perinatal units, to young children with hemophilia in pediatric settings.

Legal questions surround this disease in relation to the civil liberties of the victim. For example, does a client with AIDS have the right to withhold information about the diagnosis from the family members who are to care for him? Rights of the individual versus protection of public health are debated (Levine et al., 1986). In the future, new laws enacted by the legislature and many court cases addressing this problem will arise. (Levine et al., 1986)

SUMMARY

Legal issues confronting practicing nurses today are many, but the nurse should view the law not with apprehension but as a helpful adjunct to defining nursing practice. Competent nursing care is an important part of all health care delivery systems. Nurses aware of legal rights and obligations will be better prepared to care for clients.

Nursing standards of care serve to delineate and define appropriate nursing care. Some standards are stated in general terms such as those enacted in nursing practice statutes and those provided by professional nursing organizations. More specific standards are defined by the employing institution. If nurses act within the accepted standards of care, their chances of being involved in a malpractice lawsuit are reduced.

Some legal issues, such as the necessity for informed consent, avoiding negligence, and the legal obligation when reporting unusual incidents, are involved in almost every branch of nursing. Some of these issues are confined to specific areas of nursing practice, such as conscience clauses for perinatal nurses asked to assist in abortions. However, regardless of the situation, nurses are responsible for knowing the laws that apply to their areas of nursing practice.

Nurses rendering health care to clients must understand the legal significance of their acts. Knowledge of the law is necessary for all nurses.

KEY CONCEPTS

✓ With increased emphasis on client rights, nurses in practice today must understand their legal obligations and responsibilities to clients.

✓ The civil law system is concerned with the protection of a person's private rights, and the criminal law system deals with the rights of individuals and society as defined by legislative statutes.

✓ Under the law, practicing nurses must follow standards of care, which originate in nurse practice acts, the guidelines of professional organizations, and written policies and procedures of employing institutions.

✓ Registered nurses and licensed practical nurses are licensed by the state or province in which they practice, based on educational requirements, the passing of an examination, and other criteria.

✓ Student nurses are expected to perform as professional nurses, should be assigned only to tasks for which they are prepared, and should be carefully supervised.

✓ A tort is a civil wrong committed against a person or property, including unintentional torts such as negligence and intentional torts such as assault and battery.

✓ Nurses are responsible for performing all procedures correctly and exercising professional judgment as they carry out physician orders. Otherwise they may be guilty of negligence.

✓ All clients are entitled to confidential health care and freedom from unauthorized release of information. Otherwise nurses may be guilty of invasion of privacy, slander, or libel.

✓ Assault is an act intended to coerce or provoke fear. Nurses should act and speak carefully to avoid frightening, coercing, or physically intimidating clients.

✓ Battery is a willful or angry touching of another's body or property in contact with the person. Informed consent allows physical procedures to be carried out in a lawful manner.

✓ A nurse can be found guilty of malpractice if the following criteria are established: (1) the nurse (defendant) owed a duty to the client (plaintiff), (2) the nurse did not carry out that duty, (3) the client was injured, and (4) the client's injury resulted from the nurse's failure to carry the duty.

✓ Nurses are responsible for confirming that informed consent has been given for any surgery or other medical procedure before the procedure is performed.

✓ In emergency situations, informed consent is not necessary if it is impossible to obtain consent from the client or an authorized person.

✓ Legal issues involving death include documenting all events surrounding the death, treating a deceased person with dignity (wrongful handling is grounds for a lawsuit), and obtaining consent for an autopsy from the decedent (before death) or a close family member.

✓ A competent adult can legally give consent to donate specific organs, and nurses may serve as witnesses to this decision.

✓ Nurses may be witnesses for clients' wills, which must meet certain legal criteria.

✓ Nurses are obligated to follow physicians' orders unless they believe the orders are in error or could be detrimental to clients, in which case the nurses must make formal reports explaining the refusal.

✓ Staffing standards have been set for the ratio of nurses to clients, and if the nurse is required to care for more clients than is reasonable, a formal protest should be made to the nursing administration.

✓ Nurses must file incident reports in unusual situations when there is a possibility of a lawsuit. These reports are also used for quality assurance and risk management.

✓ Depending on state and province laws, nurses are required to report possible criminal activities, such as child abuse, gunshot wounds, attempted suicide, or rape, and certain communicable diseases.

✓ Conscience clauses in most state and province laws allow any health care professional or institution to refuse to assist in abortions without fear of reprisal if it is against their ethical, moral, or religious principles.

✓ Nurses practicing in specialized areas such as critical care are legally accountable for performing specialized duties and therefore require additional training and ongoing in-service education.

✓ All nurses should know the laws that apply to their area of practice.

REFERENCES

Annas, GJ: Contracts to bear a child: compassion or commercialism? Harvey Lect, Hastings Center Report 11(2):23, 1981.

Annas, GJ: The baby broker boom, Hastings Cent Rep, 16(3):30, 1986.

Callahan, D: How technology is reframing the abortion debate, Hastings Cent Rep 16(1):33, 1986.

Cazalas, MW: Nursing and the law, ed. 3, Rockville, Md., 1978, Aspen Publishers, Inc.

Creighton, H: Law every nurse should know, ed. 5, Philadelphia, 1986, W.B. Saunders Co.

Cushing, M: Verbal no-code orders, Am J Nurs 81:1215, 1981.

Feutz, SA: Professional liability insurance. In Northrop, CE, and Kelly, ME: Legal issues in nursing, St. Louis, 1987, The C.V. Mosby Co.

Harris, CH: Legal and ethical aspects of maternity nursing. In Jensen, M, and Bobak, I, editors: Maternity and gynecology care: the nurse and the family, ed. 3, St. Louis, 1985, The C.V. Mosby Co.

Hemelt, MD, and Mackert, ME: Dynamics of law in nursing and health care, ed. 2, Reston, Va., 1982, Reston Publishing Co., Inc.

Horsley, JE: Short-staffing means increased liability for you, RN 44:73, 1981.

Kreitzer, M: Legal aspects of child abuse: guidelines for the nurse, Nurs Clin North Am 16(1):149, 1981.

Levine, C, et al.: AIDS: public health and civil liberties, Hastings Cent Rep 16(6):9, 1986.

Moskop JC, and Saldanha, RL: The Baby Doe rule: still a threat, Hastings Cent Rep, 16(2):8, 1986.

Northrop, CE, and Kelly ME: Legal issues in nursing, St. Louis, 1987, The C.V. Mosby Co.

Regan, WA: Nursing malpractice: a giant leap in damages, RN 44:69, 1981.

Rocereto, LR, and Maleski, CM: The legal dimensions of nursing practice, New York, 1982, Springer Publishing Co., Inc.

Weil, WB: The Baby Doe regulations: another view of change, Hastings Cent Rep, 16(2):12, 1986.

Wiley, J: The nurse's legal responsibility in obstetric monitoring, JOGN Nurs 5(suppl.):77s, 1976.

Younger, SJ: Do-not-resuscitate orders: no longer secret, but still a problem, Hastings Cent Rep, 17(1):17, 1987.

ADDITIONAL READINGS

Bowen v American Hospital Association, 106 S Ct. 2101 (19), 1986.

Fenner, K: Ethics and law in nursing: professional perspectives, New York, 1980, Van Nostrand Reinhold Co., Inc.

Rothman, DA, and Rothman, NL: The professional nurse and the law, Boston, 1977, Little, Brown & Co., Inc.

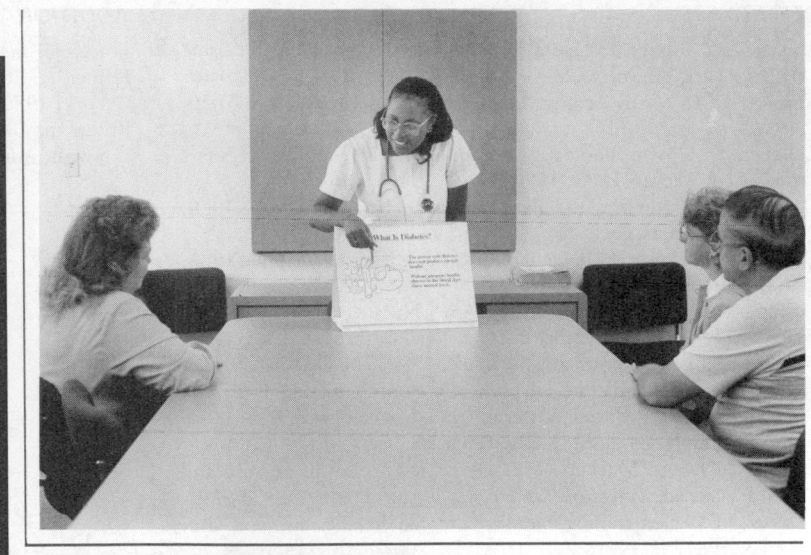

OBJECTIVES

Mastery of content in this chapter will enable the student to:

- Define the key terms listed.
- Describe differences between the three levels of communication.
- Identify characteristics of verbal and nonverbal communication.
- Discuss the importance communication skills play in the nurse-client relationship.
- Describe each element of the communication process.
- Identify factors that influence communication.
- Give examples of techniques that promote therapeutic communication.
- List and discuss the phases of a therapeutic helping relationship.
- Explain the dimensions of a helping relationship.
- Discuss nursing care measures for clients with communication alterations.

KEY TERMS

Auditory
Change Agent
Communication
Dysarthria
Interpersonal Communication
Intonation
Intrapersonal Communication
Message
Paraphrasing
Perception
Public Communication
Receiver
Referent
Sender
Tactile
Territoriality
Therapeutic
Visual

Communication Skills in Nursing

Communication is a basic element of human interactions. The definition of communication relates to its purpose. Webster defines it as "the act or action of imparting or transmitting." People transmit messages to others through talking, writing, or singing. Communication may also occur through dancing or even the clothes worn. Another definition of communication is nonverbal and verbal behavior in a social context (Satir, 1967). This definition refers to feelings and emotions that two people may convey in a relationship. A nurse listening to an anguished husband whose wife has died is an example of communication.

Because of the many dimensions of communication, a useful definition is the ongoing, dynamic series of events that involves transmission of information or feelings between two or more people. Communication is unique because of the individual qualities of each person communicating and the time when communication occurs (Sundeen et al., 1988). Not only does communication convey information and influence a relationship, it is a means to establish relationships.

An important component of nursing practice is the ability to communicate. A nurse uses a wide range of communication techniques with clients. Fritz et al. (1984) point out several advantages to nurses who use effective communication skills. They help generate trust between nurse and client, prevent legal problems in practice, and provide nurses with professional satisfaction. Communication is also a means for nurses to bring about change. The nurse speaks and acts to initiate change that promotes a client's well-being. Failure to communicate can lead to serious problems for the nurse and client and can threaten the nurse's professional credibility. The process of communication cannot be simply memorized and put into practice. It is complex and requires a careful application of principles.

LEVELS OF COMMUNICATION

Communication occurs at three levels: intrapersonal, interpersonal, and public. Intrapersonal communication occurs within an individual. When a nurse walks into the client's room and thinks, "He looks uncomfortable. I'd better turn him on his side," the communication is intrapersonal. Communication occurs constantly within our consciousness. Intrapersonal communication helps us remain alert to events around us. By considering our thoughts internally, we can better express ourselves to others.

Interpersonal communication is face-to-face interactions between two people or a small group. Those communicating are continually aware of one another. Healthy interpersonal communication allows problem solving, sharing of ideas, decision making, and personal growth.

In nursing there are many situations that challenge interpersonal communication skills. Each encounter with a client, such as collecting a blood specimen or taking a medical history, requires exchange of information. Meetings with staff members, physicians, social workers, and therapists test the nurse's communication skills with people who may have different opinions and experiences. Being a member of a nursing committee challenges the nurse's ability to express ideas clearly and decisively. Interpersonal communication is the heart of nursing practice. A nurse can assist a client only by communicating at a meaningful interpersonal level.

Public communication is interaction with large groups of people. Giving a lecture to a roomful of students and speaking to a consumer group on health education are examples of public communication. Being a competent communicator with an audience requires being able to envision oneself speaking to a group. Special platform skills such as use of posture, body movements, and tone of voice to express a point are helpful.

ELEMENTS OF THE COMMUNICATION PROCESS

Examination of the communication process components helps the understanding of communication. A model can simply and graphically demonstrate complex processes, but it can also oversimplify. A model provides the nursing student with a framework for observing,

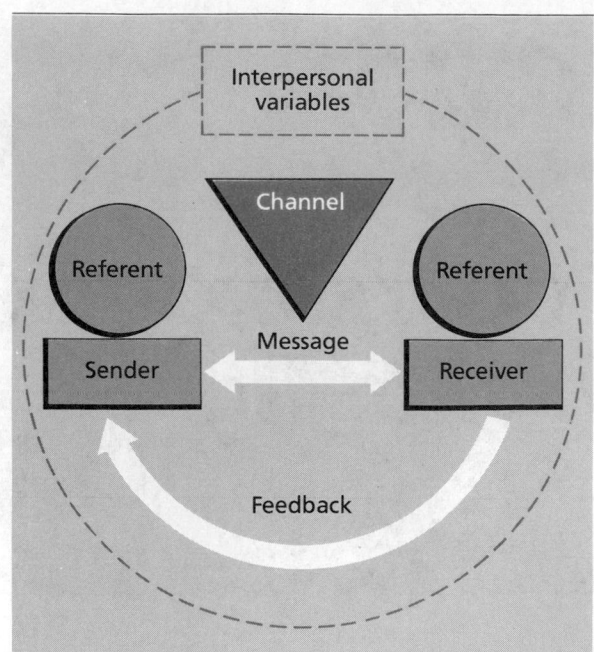

Fig. 19-1 Communication as an active process between sender and receiver.

understanding, and predicting what occurs as two people communicate.

A communication model must incorporate several principles. Communication is complex, involving many verbal and nonverbal symbols and messages exchanged between persons. Communication is a process. Once a client and nurse begin to communicate, each subsequent message or thought has its base in what was said before (Fritz et al., 1984). Messages may be sent intentionally or unintentionally. Often messages are conveyed about personality or attitude without being aware of it. Communication is a response between two or more persons as they send and receive stimuli or messages.

The basic elements of communication are shown in Fig. 19-1. Communication occurs on a social level with participants engaged in intrapersonal and interpersonal contact. The process is dynamic, with the meaning of messages negotiated by participants. During communication, the person may or may not be aware of each element of communication. During casual conversation participants do not bother to analyze the meaning of every gesture or word. For example, a person may become quite animated using hands to express an idea, without consciously thinking, "I'll wave my hand to stress this point." The nurse, however, learns to be conscious of each element of the communication process. In this way the nurse can control interactions effectively with clients and remain aware of how communication affects them. Each element described in the following paragraphs can be considered from the perspectives of both natural, uninhibited communication and consciously controlled communication.

Referent

The referent is what motivates a person to communicate with another. It may be an object, experience, emotion, idea, or act. If the individual consciously considers the referent during an intrapersonal interaction, he or she can carefully develop and organize the message.

Sender

The sender is the person who initiates the interpersonal communication. The sender puts the referent such as an idea into a form that can be transmitted. The role of sender may switch back and forth between participants at any time when information is transmitted.

Message

The message is the information that is sent or expressed by the sender. The most effective message is clear, organized, and expressed in a manner familiar to the person receiving it. The message may be comprised of verbal and nonverbal information, for example, spoken words and facial expressions.

Channels

The message is sent along a channel of communication. Channels are means of conveying messages such as through visual, auditory, and tactile senses. The sender's facial expression visually conveys a message. The spoken word travels via auditory channels. Placing a hand on an individual while communicating uses the channel of touch. Generally, the more channels the nurse uses to send a message, the better the client will understand it. For example, when attempting to relieve a client's pain, the nurse verbalizes concern, expresses a sense of compassion, and moves a client gently to lessen the pain.

Receiver

The receiver is the person to whom the message is sent. For communication to be effective the receiver must perceive or become aware of the message. The message generated by the sender then acts as one of the receiver's referents. It prompts the receiver to respond to the sender's message. The nurse learns to engage in intrapersonal communication to analyze and interpret what the client has to say.

The process of communication is ongoing. The receiver returns a message in the form of feedback to the sender. Feedback helps to reveal whether the meaning of the message was received. Mere intent to communicate is insufficient to ensure that a message is accurately received. The receiver's verbal and nonverbal response sends feedback to the sender to reveal the receiver's understanding of the message. The nurse must be open to feedback from a client to be sure explanations are understood.

The roles of sender and receiver are dynamic. The first sender assumes the role of receiver when a message is transmitted back. Because of the reciprocal relationship involved in communication, the model tends to oversimplify a complex process.

Intrapersonal Variables

The sender and receiver are influenced by several intrapersonal variables (see pp. 497 to 498). Perceptions, values, cultural background, knowledge, and roles and the setting of interaction come into play to influence the content of a message and the manner in which it is shared. Interpersonal communication is made more complex because each person is influenced differently by these intrapersonal variables. Intrapersonal variables make each interpersonal communication unique.

Each element of the communication process is crucial. Information and meaning can be gained or lost if any element is altered. By understanding each element and the factors influencing it, a nurse can communicate more effectively.

MODES OF COMMUNICATION

People send messages in two modes: verbal and nonverbal. These are closely bound together during interpersonal interaction. As we speak, we express ourselves through movements, tone of voice, facial expressions, and general appearance. These modes can convey the same or different messages. The nurse learning skills of communication masters techniques of each mode.

Verbal Communication

Verbal communication involves the spoken or written word. Language is a code that conveys meaning. The addition of a single word can change the meaning of a phrase or sentence. Language is effective only when each of the persons communicating understands a message clearly.

A nurse encounters clients of various cultures who speak different languages. Also, some clients speak the same language as the nurse but use subcultural variations of certain words. For example, the word "dinner" may mean a midday meal to one person and the last meal of the day to another. Often a nurse works with clients who speak the same language but interpret messages differently from the way the nurse intended. To make a message clear, the nurse uses effective verbal communication techniques.

CLARITY AND BREVITY

Effective communication is simple, short, and to the point. Fewer words spoken result in less confusion. Because of the intrapersonal variables involved, human communication is imprecise in many ways. Ambiguous phrases such as "you know" add little to clarity of a message. Clarity is achieved through speaking slowly and enunciating clearly. Using examples can make an explanation easier to understand. For instance, instructing an arthritic client on self-care measures at home is more meaningful when the nurse provides specific examples.

Repeating important parts of a message also makes communication clearer. The receiver should know the what, why, how, when, who, and where of ideas communicated.

Brevity is best achieved by using words that express an idea simply. "Tell me where your pain is" is better than "I would like you to describe for me the location of your discomfort." A simple, clear phrase communicates more effectively.

VOCABULARY

Communication is unsuccessful if the receiver is unable to translate the sender's words and phrases. In nursing and medicine there are many technical terms. If the nurse often uses technical terms, the client may become confused and unable to follow instructions or learn important information. Rather than telling the client, "Sit up while your lungs are auscultated," it might be better to say, "Sit up while I listen to your lungs." The first statement might make the client feel anxious. A message spoken in terms the client understands makes communication more effective.

DENOTATIVE AND CONNOTATIVE MEANING

A single word can have several meanings. A denotative meaning is one shared by individuals who use a common language. For example, the word "baseball" has the same meaning for all individuals who speak English, and the word "code" denotes cardiac arrest to nurses. The denotative meaning is what is used to define a word so it means about the same to everyone.

The connotative meaning of a word is the thought, feelings, or ideas that people have about the word (Duldt et al., 1984). Using the word "serious" to describe a client's condition may suggest to his family that he is close to death, but nurses may not consider him to be

near death unless the word "critical" is used. Connotations are shades or interpretations of a word's meaning rather than different definitions.

When nurses communicate with clients they carefully select words that cannot be easily misinterpreted. This is important when explaining a client's condition, therapy the client receives, or the purpose of therapies.

PACING

Verbal communication is more successful when expressed at an appropriate speed or pace. Talking rapidly, using awkward pauses, or speaking too slowly and deliberately can convey an unintended message. Consider the nurse who uses awkward pauses during an explanation to a client.

Client: Do you know if the doctor found anything wrong?
Nurse: No (pause), but I'm sure if he did (longer pause) he would have come to explain things to you. (then very rapidly) Now let's get back to where we were.

Long pauses and rapid shift to another subject may give the client the impression that the truth is being hidden.

The speed with which a message is verbalized, in addition to the presence, absence, and length of pauses, can determine the degree to which communication satisfies the listener. The nurse should not talk so quickly that enunciation is unclear. Pauses should be used to accentuate or stress a particular point, giving the listener time to digest and comprehend the meaning of words. Proper pacing is achieved by thinking through what to say before speaking. Looking for nonverbal cues from the listener that might suggest confusion or misunderstanding is also useful. Ask a listener if the pace is too fast or too slow.

TIMING AND RELEVANCE

Timing is critical to reception of a message. If the boss is in a bad mood, the time is wrong to ask for a raise. If a client is crying in pain, the time is wrong to explain the risks of surgery. Even though a message is clearly and concisely stated, poor timing can prevent it from being accurately received. Therefore the nurse must be sensitive to the appropriate time for discussions with clients. Often the best time for interaction is when a client expresses an interest in communicating. By asking a simple question such as "Would you like to talk about your surgery?" the nurse can avoid wasting time and energy if the client does not.

A person is more likely to communicate when a message holds importance. For example, when a client is facing open-heart surgery the next day, a discussion of the risks of cigarette smoking has less relevance than a review of preoperative procedures. An explanation of the side effects of birth control pills is relevant to the young woman who has received her first prescription for the medication. Verbal communication is more likely to have impact when messages pertain to an individual's interests and needs.

Nonverbal Communication

Actions often speak louder than words. Nonverbal communication is transmission of messages without the use of words. It is one of the most powerful ways people convey messages to others. We continually communicate nonverbally in every face-to-face encounter. Gestures impart meanings that are more significant than words. Ekman (1965) describes the ways in which nonverbal communication and verbal communication are interrelated. Nonverbal cues add meaning to what is being said in verbal communication (Table 19-1).

A nurse needs to be aware of verbal and nonverbal messages sent to clients. Even the phrase "Good morning, how are you?" can convey a number of meanings. A verbal message should be reinforced or complemented by nonverbal cues. Clients may sense a lack of trust or anxiety when a mismatch exists between what a nurse verbally and nonverbally communicates.

It is part of the nurse's assessment to observe client's verbal and nonverbal messages. A client who says he or she feels fine but grimaces with each movement is communicating two different messages. Becoming a good observer of nonverbal behavior requires time and practice. The nurse who perceives nonverbal messages is better able to understand clients, detect changes in conditions, and determine nursing care needs.

PERSONAL APPEARANCE

The general impression formed of another person influences response to that person (Zunin and Zunin, 1973). A person's appearance is one of the first things noticed during an interpersonal encounter. Physical characteristics, dress and grooming, and the presence of jewelry and adornment provide clues to the person's physical well-being, personality, social status, occupation, religion, culture, and self-concept.

Clothing, cosmetics, and jewelry that are not part of a professional uniform represent a personal choice and are taken as clues to the way people want others to respond to them. How a person dresses can also influence their behavior. Knapp (1978) notes that clothes fulfill functions of decoration, protection (psychological and physical), sexual attraction, self-assertion, group identity, and role display.

Nurses can help clients maintain a sense of worth by allowing them to wear their own clothes. Hospital gowns are drab and ill-fitting. Personal clothes give a sense of physical recovery and mental alertness.

Physical characteristics, such as the condition of hair, color of skin, weight, energy level, and presence of a physical deformity, also communicate information about the level of health. There are no established standards for physical characteristics that demonstrate good health. Each individual displays combinations of physical characteristics. The nurse remains alert for changes in a person's physical appearance, since they can be significant signs of disease.

Physical appearance often leads to impressions about personality and self-concept. Unfortunately, stereotyped views regarding the "perfect body" influence the image

TABLE 19-1 Relationships Between Verbal and Nonverbal Communication

Relationship	Example
Repeating—verbal and nonverbal cues saying the same thing but in different ways	When a mother describes how tall her son is, she also holds her hands at a distance above the floor equal to the child's height.
Contradicting—verbal and nonverbal cues conveying different messages	The nurse tells the client that obtaining a blood specimen "won't hurt a bit," but her sarcastic grin delivers a different message.
Complementing—nonverbal messages adding to verbal messages	A client says she is afraid to be admitted to the hospital, and her anxious expression and trembling hands leave little doubt of her fear.
Accenting—nonverbal cues emphasizing what is stated verbally	A wave of the hand while saying hello accentuates the word spoken.
Relating and regulating—nonverbal cues indicating when to begin or stop talking	A client who continually opens and closes her mouth briefly as her physician is talking is seeking an opportunity to speak.
Substituting—a nonverbal cue being used instead of words	The nurse nods vigorously to show approval of the client's decision.

that body features communicate. The nurse should assess the importance physical appearance holds for a client that is threatened with loss of body parts or body function.

The nurse's physical appearance influences the client's perception of care received. Each client has a preconceived image of what a nurse should look like. The traditional nurse's white uniform can be a symbol of purity and cleanliness. Although the uniform is not a reflection of the nurse's abilities, it may become more difficult to establish a sense of trust and reliability if the nurse fails to meet the clients' image. Professional nurses today wear uniforms, scrubsuits, and laboratory coats, as well as street clothes, to perform their duties. A neat, well-tailored look conveys the message of a competent professional.

INTONATION

Tone of a speaker's voice can have a dramatic impact on a message's meaning. Depending on intonation, the simple phrase "How are you?" can express enthusiasm, concern, indifference, and even annoyance. A person's emotions can directly influence tone of voice. Often this effect is unconscious, and the words send one message while voice tone conveys the opposite. The nurse must be aware of emotions when interacting with clients. Intention to convey sincere interest in a client's welfare can be blocked if the nurse's tone of voice gives a different mood or meaning. Clients may question a nurse's credibility if his or her voice is not sincere and pleasing. Voice tone can be a cue to a client's emotional state. Fear, anger, and grief can be expressed through intonation and voice pitch. Similarly, voice tone may indicate a client's energy level. A rested, alert person usually has a voice full of variations and inflections in tone and rapidity, whereas a fatigued person tends to talk in a mumbled monotone with incomplete sentences (Duldt et al., 1984).

FACIAL EXPRESSION

The face is rich in communication potential. A mutual glance or meeting of eyes between two people set the tone for an interpersonal encounter. The face and eyes send overt and subtle cues that assist in interpretation of messages. Studies show that the face reveals six primary emotions: surprise, fear, anger, disgust, happiness, and sadness (Knapp, 1978). Facial expressions often become the basis for important interpersonal judgments. Because of diversity in facial expressions, their meanings may be difficult to judge. The face may reveal genuine emotions, contradict true emotions, or facial expressions may be suppressed. Often people are unaware of the messages their expressions convey. Providing clear feedback helps lessen confusion created by conflicting messages and expressions. When facial expressions fail to reveal clear messages, verbal feedback should be sought to be sure of the speaker's intent.

For example, nurses are frequently watched by clients. Consider the impact a nurse's facial expression might have on a client who asks, "Am I going to die?" The slightest change of expression can reveal the nurse's true feelings. It is difficult to control all facial expressions. However, the nurse learns to be aware of what expressions can reveal. For example, when caring for a debilitated or deformed client, the nurse should avoid expressions of disgust.

Eye contact is an important part of facial expressions conveyed by eye movements. Wide eyes are associated with frankness, terror, and naiveté; downward glances reflect modesty; raised upper eyelids reveal displeasure; and a stare is often associated with hatred and coldness. When two people confront each other, eye contact often prefaces a message. Initiating eye contact shows a willingness to communicate. Persons who maintain eye contact during a conversation are perceived as believable. Maintaining eye contact allows one to become a good observer of another individual. It has been suggested that the level at which eye contact occurs significantly influences communication. The nurse should avoid looking down at a client during a discussion. The nurse appears less dominant and threatening sitting near the client at the same eye level.

POSTURE AND GAIT

The way people stand and move is a visible form of self-expression. Posture and gait reflect one's attitudes, emotions, self-concept, and physical wellness. Leaning forward or toward a person conveys attention to that person. Leaning backward in a more relaxed manner shows less interest and caution.

An erect posture and a quick, purposeful gait communicate a sense of well-being and assuredness. A slumped posture and slow, shuffling gait may indicate depression or discomfort. A bent-over posture may be a protective response to physical disease and injury. Nurses can collect useful information by observing clients' posture and gait. Specific illnesses cause identifiable gaits such as the shuffle of parkinsonism. Gait may be altered by many physical factors such as pain, drugs, or fractures.

GESTURES

A wave of the hand, a salute, and shifting of feet are gestures. They are visual italics, which emphasize, punctuate, and clarify the spoken word. Duldt et al. (1984) identify three functions of gestures: illustrating an idea, expressing an emotional state, and signaling by use of an agreed on sign. Gestures alone may reveal specific meanings, or they may send messages in conjunction with other communication cues.

Gestures are used to illustrate an idea that is difficult or inconvenient to describe in words. A client who points to an area of pain may be more accurate than describing the pain's location. Gestures may be used to convey emotions toward oneself or others. Covering the eyes, touching a part of the face, or pointing an accusing finger can reveal a client's inner feelings.

TOUCH

Touch is a personal form of nonverbal communication. Persons engaged in communication must be close to each other when touch is used. Because touch is more spontaneous than verbal communication, it generally seems more authentic. Various messages are conveyed through touch such as affection, emotional support, encouragement, tenderness, and personal attention (Fig. 19-2). Touch is an important part of the nurse-client relationship, but it must be used with discrimination because strong social norms govern its use. Who, when, why, and where people touch are determined by unwritten sociocultural guidelines. Many persons mistakenly perceive touch as having only sexual implications.

Nurses rely on touch when carrying out interventions. Nurses can touch clients while performing physical assessments, giving baths, providing backrubs, and assisting with dressing. The nurse who is unaccustomed to touching or being touched may feel uncomfortable when performing interventions.

Similarly, the person who is sick must permit closer physical contact than normally tolerated. Illness places a person in a dependent role that calls for the nurse to initiate and maintain closer interpersonal contact. It is important to remain sensitive to the client's disposition toward touching. If the client shies away from the nurse's touch or refuses to hold the nurse's hand during pain, the client is probably uncomfortable with being touched. Finally, touch can be a useful therapeutic tool. Holding the hand of a grieving client can often convey understanding better than words or other gestures. Nurses must be sure to use touch purposefully during interactions. Although touch can be helpful to a client, its use must be clearly understood and accepted.

FACTORS INFLUENCING COMMUNICATION

Each person is unique and makes different associations and interpretations of messages communicated. Factors influencing communication are many, thus making each interpersonal interaction different. An understanding of these factors helps a nurse know why a client may have difficulty communicating and the strategies needed to help.

Development

Children are born with the physical mechanisms and capacity to develop speech and language skills. The rate of speech development varies among children and is directly related to neurological competence and intellectual development (Whaley and Wong, 1987). A child's environment must also offer stimulation for normal speech and language development. The quality of the learning environment provided by parents will affect a child's ability to communicate. The nurse uses special techniques to communicate with children of different developmental stages (see later section).

Perceptions

Each person senses, interprets, and understands events differently. Perception is a person's personal view of events occurring around him. A nurse might state "I've noticed you have been quiet since your family left. Would you like to talk about it?" The client's perception of the nurse's intent will affect his or her willingness to talk. Perceptions are formed by expectations and experiences. Differences in perceptions between people interacting can be a barrier to communication.

Values

Values are standards that influence our behavior (see Chapter 16). They represent what is considered impor-

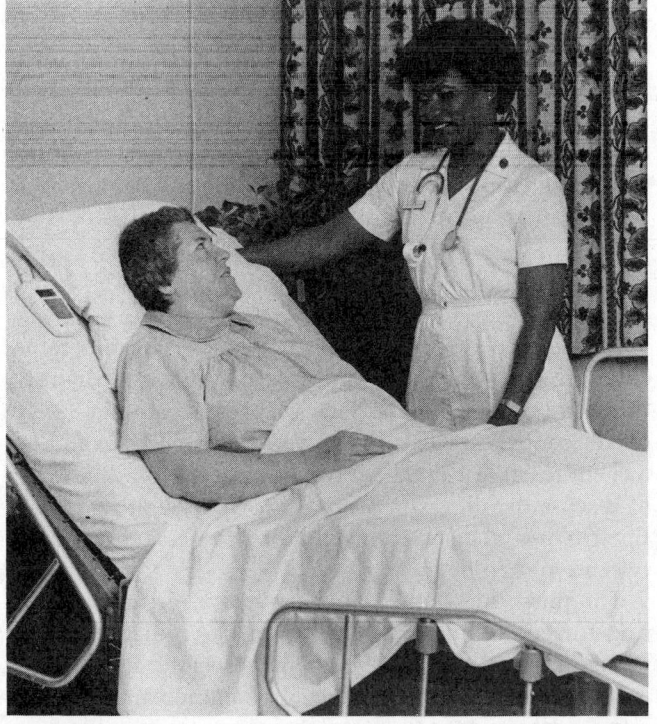

Fig. 19-2   Nurse and client communicating.

tant in life and thus influence expression of thoughts and ideas. Values also affect interpretation of messages. A nurse avoids allowing personal values to interfere with professional relationships. Judgmental attitudes will destroy trust with clients and block effective communication.

Emotions

Emotions are a person's subjective feelings about events. The way a person relates or communicates with others is influenced by emotions. A client who is angry may react to a nurse's instructions differently than one who is frightened. Emotions a person is experiencing will influence the ability to successfully receive a message. Emotions can cause a person to misinterpret or not hear a message. A nurse can assess clients' emotions by observing them interact with family, physicians, or other nurses.

When nurses care for clients they must be aware of their emotions. It is difficult to hide emotions. Clients are perceptive and can sense when a nurse is angry, frustrated, or depressed. It is not appropriate for the nurse to discuss personal emotions with the client. A social support system of colleagues allows nurses to express emotions.

Sociocultural Background

Language, gestures, values, and attitudes reflect a person's cultural origin. Often nurses care for clients who speak a different language. Culture, however, influences more than language or accent. Winkler and Doherty (1983) believe that communication style is highly dependent on cultural factors. For example, their research showed that American couples tend to be more calm and reasonable in communicating with one another than Israeli couples, who are verbally more aggressive. The influence of culture sets limits for the way we act and communicate.

When a nurse cares for a client who speaks another language an interpreter may be necessary. If a family member serves as an interpreter, it may be easier for the nurse to devise ways to communicate with the client. The nurse learns key words such as "water," "pain," or "bathroom" to ensure the client's basic needs are assessed and understood.

Knowledge

Communication can be difficult when those communicating have different levels of knowledge. A message will not be clear if the words or phrases are not part of the listener's vocabulary. "The incision is well approximated without drainage" means the same as "The incision is clean and healing fine," but the latter would be understood by a greater number of people.

Nurses communicate with clients and professionals who have different levels of knowledge. A common language is essential in communicating across different knowledge levels. The nurse assesses clients' knowledge by noting their response to questions, their ability to discuss health problems, and the questions they ask of the nurse. After assessment the nurse uses terms and phrases clients understand to promote attention and interest.

Roles and Relationships

We communicate in a style appropriate to our roles and relationships. A student talks with a friend in a different way than with an instructor, physician, or minister. Words, facial expressions, tone of voice, and gestures used to convey an idea depend on the person receiving the communication.

A nurse may feel comfortable communicating with colleagues, joking about daily events, and sharing amusing stories. However, communicating with a client entering a clinic for the first time requires a different role. Anticipating that the client may be apprehensive, the nurse avoids humor until it can be determined how the client relates to him or her. The client is probably looking for support rather than funny stories. Later, when the relationship between the nurse and client is stronger, casual conversation may be appropriate.

The better we know an individual, the more liberty we can take in expressing ideas. We feel more comfortable in expressing ideas to individuals with whom we have developed positive, satisfying relationships. As a nurse-client relationship develops, both the nurse and the client gain confidence in relating ideas and feelings. Communication is more effective when the participants remain aware of their roles in a relationship.

Environment

People tend to communicate better in a comfortable environment. A warm room, free of noise and distractions, is best. Noise and lack of privacy or space may create confusion, tension, or discomfort. For example, a client fearful of the diagnosis of cancer would hesitate to discuss the illness in a busy, crowded waiting room. Environmental distractions can distort messages sent between two people.

The nurse has some control when selecting the setting for communicating with clients. A quiet office or lounge is ideal. When the client is visited at home, a bedroom or den may be best. It is important that the nurse's efforts to convey information are not blocked by environmental distractions.

Space and Territoriality

Territoriality is the drive to gain, maintain, and defend one's exclusive right to an area of space (Pluckhan, 1978). During social interaction, people consciously maintain a distance between themselves. Personal space is invisible and mobile—it goes with a person. Territory can be separated and made visible to others, such as a fenced-in yard, a towel on the beach, or the hospital bed. Whenever personal space becomes threatened by intrusion, a defensive response occurs, preventing effective communication. Nurses often work with clients in situations where space and territory are important. As with touch, the distance separating nurse from client must be judged by the situation. Physically restraining a client in danger of self-injury, giving mouth-to-mouth resuscitation, holding a crying infant, and facilitating the excretory functions of an incontinent client require that an intimate distance be maintained. Hein (1973) describes *intimate distance* as 18 inches or less. The client receiving care is sensitive about how the nurse uses distance. The nurse must convey confidence and gentleness.

As the distance becomes greater, both the client and nurse feel more at ease. Greater flexibility is afforded when intimate contact is not required. Sitting with a client is an example of a nursing measure in which *personal distance* (18 inches to 4 feet) provides the closeness needed. Increasing the physical distance makes it easier for the client and nurse to communicate because the nurse becomes less imposing. *Social distance* (4 to 12 feet) is needed when dealing with groups. Making rounds with physicians is an example of group interaction. Communication at a social distance is less threatening than communication in an intimate or personal space because intimate sharing of thoughts and feelings is less likely to occur.

THERAPEUTIC COMMUNICATION

Beginning nursing students are often told to "get to know your client" as they establish interpersonal relationships with clients. This is not easy, and sometimes becomes the only barrier to an effective relationship. A nurse cannot "get to know" a client without being able to appreciate the client's uniqueness. Without knowing this, the nurse is unable to help the client cope with health problems. Therapeutic communication helps form a working relationship with the client and fulfills the purposes of the nursing process.

Therapeutic communication is not casual. Instead, it is a planned, deliberate, professional act. However, preoccupation with the techniques of communication can cause the nurse to forget the client as a person. When the nurse first uses theraputic communication tech-

niques, the communication process may seem artificial and contrived. It is more helpful to perceive each client interaction as an opportunity to achieve a positive relationship that results in attainment of nursing care goals.

Social Interaction

The first attempt at communicating with a client usually consists of a brief social interaction. The messages conveyed are superficial in that neither the nurse nor client discusses deeply personal matters of concern. Interpersonal exchange tends to be based on intuitive, unthinking, and automatic responses. Superficial interaction makes participants feel safe because the discussion holds no hidden intent for personal disclosures.

A nurse often uses superficial social interaction at the beginning of a conversation with a client to lay a foundation for a closer relationship. For example, the nurse might greet a client by saying, "Good morning, Mrs. Sears, it's nice to see you today," or "Hi, Mr. Simpson, how do you like the great weather we're having?"

The skillful nurse does not allow social interaction to dominate a conversation, but does maintain a congenial and warm style to build the client's trust. The goal is to help the client feel comfortable in sharing attitudes and feelings.

Therapeutic Communication Techniques

The nurse uses communication skills while establishing a therapeutic relationship. There is no formula for forming a relationship with a client. Each person communicates uniquely, and each client requires different communication techniques. The nurse should be flexible in techniques used to foster communication with individual clients.

LISTENING ATTENTIVELY

Listening is one of the most effective therapeutic communication techniques. It requires a nurse's complete attention. Attentive listening involves an attempt to understand the entire message a person is communicating verbally and nonverbally. Although hearing is considered a passive, neurological process of receiving information, listening is an active, learned process. An attentive listener conveys nonverbally to a speaker that "You are a person of worth. I am interested in what you have to say."

Listening effectively may at first seem awkward and time consuming. An effective listener, however, gains satisfaction from working with people and understanding their deeper health concerns.

To be an attentive listener the nurse will use the following skills:

1. Face the client while he or she is speaking.
2. Maintain natural eye contact to show willingness to listen.
3. Assume a relaxed posture. Avoid crossing legs and arms, since it conveys a defensive posture.
4. Avoid distracting body movements, such as wringing hands or tapping feet.
5. Nod in acknowledgment when the client talks about an important point or looks for feedback.
6. Lean toward the speaker to communicate involvement.

The nurse must appear natural while listening to clients. Nonverbal cues, such as leaning toward the speaker, should not become overbearing or threaten the client's intimate space. Listening skillfully during a nursing procedure is beneficial and an efficient use of time. For example, much can be learned and conveyed by the nurse who listens while giving the client a bath. The client becomes the center of attention and not the bath procedure.

CONVEYING ACCEPTANCE

To show acceptance means being nonjudgmental of another person. This is difficult at times. Because a nurse meets clients of diverse backgrounds and interests, often client's values and ideas conflict with those of the nurse. Acceptance is not the same as agreement. Acceptance is a willingness to hear the person without conveying doubt or disagreement.

Certainly a nurse does not accept all aspects of a client's behavior or illness. The nurse works to bring about change that improves a client's level of health. Acceptance is tolerance toward others that fosters a relationship between nurse and client.

To show acceptance the nurse remains aware of personal nonverbal expressions. The nurse avoids facial expressions and gestures that suggest disapproval, such as frowning, rolling the eyes upward, or shaking the head in disbelief. The following show a client that the nurse accepts what he or she has to say:

1. Listening without interrupting
2. Providing verbal feedback that demonstrates understanding
3. Being sure nonverbal cues match verbal communication
4. Avoiding arguing, expressing doubts, or attempting to change the client's mind

ASKING RELATED QUESTIONS

Questioning is a direct method of communicating. The nurse's aim is to gain specific information about the client. Questions used during a conversation set the tone of the verbal interaction and control its direction. Questions are most effective when they relate to the topic or subject being discussed.

During an assessment of the client's health status, questions follow a logical sequence.

Nurse: Mr. James, can you tell me where you are having pain?
Client: Well, it seems to be in my back.
Nurse: What part of your back?
Client: Here, in the lower part.
Nurse: How would you describe the pain?
Client: It feels like a knife went through me.

The nurse's line of questioning helps the client tell a story. Each question focuses on a specific aspect of the story. The nurse is careful not to move on to another subject until the current topic is adequately explored. The nurse selects a question on the basis of the client's previous response so that information discussed flows logically.

If the nurse wants the client to elaborate, open-ended questions are most effective. They give a client a chance to talk more completely about problems or concerns. Such questions cannot be answered with a "yes" or "no". Examples of open-ended questions include: "Would you describe the pain you have been feeling?" "What seems to be the problem?" "Could you explain how your family feels about your illness?"

Asking the client open-ended questions allows the nurse to assess a number of factors. How the client responds verbally and nonverbally can reveal real emotions. The nurse may be able to judge the level of the client's vocabulary and understanding of health by the response. Often the nurse seeks details of physical signs and symptoms, and the open-ended question elicits more accurate and detailed descriptions. Since an open-ended question prompts a lengthy response, the nurse can assess gaps or discrepancies.

PARAPHRASING

Paraphrasing is restating the client's message in the nurse's own words. Usually a paraphrased statement uses fewer words than the original statement. Through paraphrasing the nurse sends feedback that lets the client know if his or her message was understood and prompts further communication.

Client: I've had it. My doctor won't tell me what is going on. He doesn't seem to care what I think.
Nurse: You're saying that you're angry with your doctor?
Client: Yes, he obviously doesn't know what it's like to be sick.

Practice is required to paraphrase accurately. If the meaning of a message is changed or distorted through paraphrasing, communication may become ineffective. For example, a client may say, "I've been overweight all my life and never had any problems. I can't understand why I need to be on a diet." Paraphrasing this statement by saying, "You mean you don't care if you're overweight or not?" is incorrect. "It seems that you're not convinced you need a diet, since you've remained healthy," is a proper way of paraphrasing the statement.

CLARIFYING

Despite efforts at paraphrasing, the nurse may not understand the client's message. When a misunderstanding occurs, the nurse momentarily stops the discussion to clarify meaning. Without clarification valuable information can be lost. Information critical to the client's care plan can be incomplete unless confusing or conflicting data are clarified. The nurse can either attempt to repeat the message or admit confusion and ask the client to restate the message. For example, a client has come to the clinic for a checkup:

Client: I knew I might have a problem. It seems to be in my family. The last time I was here, though, it wasn't bad so I didn't mention it.
Nurse: Excuse me, Mr. Brewer, can you tell me what type of problem you're having?

It is also important for the nurse to clarify messages. Examples can be used to clarify a vague, abstract idea. When using examples, the nurse describes ideas or situations to which the client can easily relate. In the following dialog a nurse is explaining activity restrictions to a client who has had eye surgery:

Nurse: Now, Mr. Lee, once you go home you are not supposed to place stress on your eye.
Client: I'm not sure I know what you mean.
Nurse: Well, you're not allowed to stoop or bend over with your head down. For example, if you want to pick up your slippers off the floor or pick up a basket of laundry, don't bend over. Instead, bend your knees and keep your head up.
Client: I have a dog at home. I guess I can't bend over to pick him up?
Nurse: That's right. Bend your knees to lower yourself down if you want to pet your dog.

The more specific a clarifying message, the more likely it will be understood. Clients who are easily confused by the complex terms and jargon of medicine appreciate a simple, down-to-earth explanation that uses familiar examples.

FOCUSING

As the client discusses topics related to his health, the messages often become vague. A client may say to the nurse, "Well, I've just been feeling funny lately. It doesn't really bother me that much. It's just this feeling I'm having in my head." The client's description tells little except that he does not feel well. If the nurse does not help focus specifically on the physical complaint, the client will likely continue vague descriptions.

Focusing helps to limit the area of discussion to which the client can respond. The nurse might respond to the client by saying, "You said you've been feeling funny lately. Tell me when this feeling first started," or "Describe the feeling in your head." As in clarifying, the nurse seeks meaning in the client's message. In the case of focusing, however, the nurse understands the client's message but realizes it is nonspecific or vague.

The nurse does not use focusing if it interrupts the client while discussing an important issue. If the conversation begins to drag on without new information or the client begins to repeat himself, focusing is useful.

STATING OBSERVATIONS

When communicating, a person is often unaware how his messages are received. Feedback from others tells him if he communicated the intended message. One way the nurse can provide feedback is by sharing with the client observations of his or her behavior during communication. The nurse describes impressions created by the client's nonverbal cues.

Miss Tucker is sitting in the waiting room of her physician's office. She is slumped in the chair, her body movements are slow, and she yawns while speaking with the nurse. The nurse says, "Miss Tucker, you appear to be quite tired."

If the client's verbal message conflicts with nonverbal cues, the nurse's observation may help convey a clearer message. Stating observations often leads the client to communicate more clearly without the need for extensive questioning, focusing, or clarifying by the nurse.

The nurse does not state observations that might embarrass or anger the client. The nurse in the preceding example would not say, "Miss Tucker, you look a mess." Even if such an observation is made with humor, the client can become resentful.

OFFERING INFORMATION

When two people communicate, the process is rarely one sided. In an interaction with a client the nurse frequently offers information that gives the client additional data or insight. The client in the following dialog is scheduled to have surgery the next day for an abdominal tumor removal.

Client: My doctor has told me I'm first on the schedule for surgery tomorrow.
Nurse: Yes, we'll be awakening you about 6:00 AM.
Client: My family would like to be here then.
Nurse: That's no problem. They are free to come at 6:00 and we'll show them where to wait for you once you've left for the operating room.

Providing the client with additional information encourages him to respond further. Offering information on an ongoing, timely basis not only facilitates communication but also promotes health teaching.

It is not helpful to withhold information from the client, particularly when he seeks it. If the nurse avoids sharing information or gives only partial information, the client may lose trust in the nurse. The nurse cannot share information that the physician chooses to withhold. However, there is a wide range of information the nurse can share (see Chapter 16). The nurse must avoid advising a client when giving information. Information can facilitate a client's decision making, but the nurse should not make the decision.

MAINTAINING SILENCE

Silence allows the nurse and client to organize their thoughts. The use of silence can be effective but is difficult, since pauses in conversation that last several seconds or minutes can make the client and nurse uneasy.

The use of silence requires skill and timing. Silence allows the client an opportunity to communicate intrapersonally, to organize thoughts, and to process information. It gives the client time to search for words or feelings. Silence is particularly useful when the client is confronted with a difficult decision that he or she is not sure how to share with the nurse. For example, silence may help a client gain the confidence needed to share the decision to refuse medical treatment.

Silence also allows the nurse to observe clients unobtrusively. The nurse pays particular attention to nonverbal messages, as a worried expression or loss of eye contact. Remaining silent demonstrates the nurse's willingness to wait for a response. Often the nurse has many questions to raise with clients, but some, especially the elderly, are unable to reply quickly. Impatience expressed by the nurse frustrates the client's efforts at communicating. Silence shows that the nurse is interested and will accept any response the client can express.

When clients become emotionally upset, silence helps them gather thoughts. A quiet period may diffuse an emotionally tense situation. A nurse's silence acknowledges the client's need for a few moments of privacy. Once the client is ready to talk again, he or she will more likely express feelings clearly.

USING ASSERTIVENESS

Assertiveness means standing up for one's rights without violating those of others (Stanhope and Lancaster, 1988). Through assertive techniques, a person expresses feelings and emotions confidently, spontaneously, and honestly. Assertive persons make choices and decisions and are able to control their lives more effectively than nonassertive individuals. A nurse can teach clients assertiveness skills and use them to promote their own health.

Examples of assertiveness skills include speaking clearly, dealing with manipulation, and protecting against criticism (see box). A clear message is complete and specific and includes all information a client needs to understand. To avoid being manipulated, nurses ac-

---

Assertiveness Skills

SPEAKING CLEARLY
Incorrect Technique

Nurse: Your recovery depends on your ability to exercise right.
Client: Does that mean I can begin running?

Complete Message

Nurse: Your recovery will involve walking daily, progressing to about a mile a day within a month. Your therapist should be consulted before you begin to run.

DEALING WITH MANIPULATION
Learning To Say "No"

Staff member: Listen, I'm really in a rush. Can you help me get this report completed?
Nurse: I've planned a home visit this morning. Perhaps my schedule will permit it tomorrow. I'll let you know.

PROTECTING AGAINST CRITICISM

Supervisor: Nancy, I've been concerned about your performance lately.
Nurse: What have your concerns been?
Supervisor: I see you've been involved in two separate incidents with medication errors.
Nurse: Can you suggest ways I might avoid errors next time?

---

quire skills to protect themselves from others who consciously or unconsciously use them. Learning to say "no" and resisting guilt imposed intentionally by others are two helpful techniques.

Constructive criticism can promote growth, but manipulative criticism makes people vulnerable (Stanhope and Lancaster, 1988). Negative inquiry is a skill that involves asking for more information when a criticism has been made. The person remains unemotional and low-key when asking for information and avoids sounding angry or sarcastic. Using criticism for growth helps nurses feel good about themselves.

SUMMARIZING

Summarization is a concise review of main ideas that have been discussed. It sets the tone for further interactions between the nurse and client. Beginning a new interaction by summarizing a previous one helps the client recall topics discussed and shows the client how the nurse has analyzed their communication.

Ms. Spier has been working for several days to help Mrs. Ramos learn about diabetes. Ms. Spier enters the client's room and says, "Good morning, Mrs. Ramos. I've come to talk with you more about your diabetes. If you recall, yesterday we discussed the purpose of insulin, its side effects, and how to give an injection."

Summarizing helps the nurse review key aspects of an interaction. Further communication can then focus on relevant issues. The client will be able to sense whether the nurse understood his part of the message. With a summary the client is able to review information and make additions or corrections.

Nontherapeutic Communication Techniques

There are communication techniques or styles that cause interpersonal interactions to be nontherapeutic. These barriers can be damaging when a nurse is building a client relationship. Many techniques that normally promote effective communication can be detrimental if used improperly.

GIVING AN OPINION

Giving an opinion takes decision making away from the client. It inhibits spontaneity, stalls problem solving, and creates doubt. Consider the following example:

Nurse: Mr. Jones, you look like you're deep in thought.
Client: Oh, no, not really. I was just thinking about whether my daughter is coming to see me.
Nurse: Well, if you ask me, she should have been here before now. It would mean so much to you.

Often the client simply needs an opportunity to express feelings. Giving an opinion prevents the client from developing solutions to problems.

There may be times when clients require suggestions. For example, when a client is selecting a special diet, the nurse's help may be needed to choose the right food. Suggestions are best presented to clients as options, since the final decision rests with the client.

OFFERING FALSE REASSURANCE

When a client is seriously ill, the nurse is tempted to offer hope to the client with statements such as "You'll be fine" or "There's nothing to worry about." When a client is reaching out for understanding, false reassurance from the nurse may discourage open communication. For example:

Client: I'm so afraid of becoming dependent on my wife. I feel I'm never going to get any better.
Nurse: There's no reason to be so afraid. Things will get better.

Bradley and Edinberg (1982) have identified six conditions about which a client can safely be reassured:

1. There is hope
2. The nurse is listening
3. Care is available
4. Certain undesirable changes can be expected
5. The client will be treated like a person
6. The client's problem is understood

The following example shows how the nurse conveys a willingness to understand a client's concerns without falsely reassuring the client that the illness is minor.

Mrs. Stevens is a 58-year-old woman with terminal cancer. Her nurse, Ms. Fry, is sitting by her side.
Mrs. Stevens: I sometimes think this isn't happening to me. It seems so unfair . . . .Oh, I'm sorry. You don't want to hear my problems.
Ms. Fry: No, please, Mrs. Stevens, I do want to hear how you feel.

BEING DEFENSIVE

Defensiveness in response to criticism suggests that the client has no right to an opinion. When a nurse becomes defensive the client's concerns are often ignored.

Mr. Locke has been a regular visitor to the health clinic for several years. The last time he visited the clinic Mr. Locke had symptoms that resulted in his hospitalization. He now is returning to the clinic for a checkup 1 week after his discharge from the hospital.
Mr. Locke: Well, I hope I don't have to see Dr. Warren today.
Nurse: I don't understand, Mr. Locke, is something wrong? Dr. Warren has been your doctor here for some time.
Mr. Locke: I don't care. He was the one who put me in the hospital and that was a waste of time.
Nurse: That's silly. Dr. Warren is an excellent physician.
Mr. Locke: You think so, huh? He hasn't put you in the hospital for no reason.
Nurse: You were very ill, Mr. Locke. I know Dr. Warren made the right decision.

The nurse has threatened her relationship with Mr. Locke. He will probably not trust the nurse to keep his concerns confidential. She is ignoring the client's feelings and will probably not take any action to remedy his problem. After this conversation the nurse will have difficulty continuing a rapport that will prompt the client to discuss additional problems.

When a client expresses criticism, the nurse should listen to what he has to say. Listening does not imply agreement. The nurse avoids becoming defensive in order to learn the reasons behind the client's criticism. There are two sides to any story, and the nurse attempts to learn why the client has become angry or dissatisfied.

Mr. Locke: Well, I hope I don't have to see Dr. Warren today.
Nurse: You seem upset, would you like to talk about it?
Mr. Locke: I just don't think he should have put me in the hospital.
Nurse: You believe hospitalization was unnecessary?

Mr. Locke: Yes, they really didn't do much of anything. They took a few tests and did some x-rays.

Nurse: Mr. Locke, did your doctors tell you what the tests showed?

Mr. Locke: No, not really. That's why I'm, so angry.

The nurse's patience led to an identification of the client's real concern, not knowing the results of his diagnostic tests. By avoiding defensiveness the nurse defused Mr. Locke's anger so he could describe his concerns.

SHOWING APPROVAL OR DISAPPROVAL

Expressing excessive approval can be as harmful to a nurse-client relationship as stating disapproval. Offering excessive praise implies that the behavior being praised is the only acceptable one. Often the client shares a decision with the nurse not in an effort to seek approval, but to provide a means to discuss feelings.

Client: I've decided that when I leave the hospital I'll stay with my son. He doesn't want me to go home and be alone.

Nurse: Oh, I'm so glad to hear that. I think you definitely made the right decision. It's best for you to be with your son.

This nurse's comment will likely end further discussion of the topic. The client may perceive the nurse agrees with the son. Perhaps the client would be better off with his son. On the other hand, the client may have a strong desire to remain independent, and now that has been repressed. The nurse's excessive approval did not allow the client to think or act freely and inhibited potential for decision making.

Disapproval implies that the client must meet the nurse's expectations or standards.

Client: Oh, I feel good, I was able to get up in the chair once today.

Nurse: Only once? You're going to have to get up more often than that!

It would have been better for the nurse to say, "You're making fine progress. Your doctor would like you to try to be up at least three times today. Do you think you'd like to sit up just before going to bed?"

A disapproving statement causes the client to feel rejected. The client may avoid further interaction with the nurse, thus potentially slowing recovery.

STEREOTYPING

Everyone is unique. However, stereotyped responses inhibit uniqueness and oversimplify the situation. Stereotypes are generalized beliefs held about people. The use of stereotypes inhibits communication and can threaten a nurse-client relationship. Stereotyping statements such as "Elderly people are always confused" or "Clients with back problems cannot tolerate pain" seriously impair interpersonal communication.

Another nontherapeutic communication is the use of meaningless, stereotyped responses. Their use minimizes the importance of a person's message. For example:

Client: I slept poorly last night. My incision seemed to be pulling.

Nurse: You can't win them all. At least the incision is healing well.

ASKING WHY

Whenever one disagrees with or fails to understand another person, the temptation is to ask why he believes or has acted in such a way. A client frequently interprets a "why" question as an accusation. The client may also think the nurse knows why and is simply testing him. Regardless of what the client perceives the nurse's motivation to be, "why" questions can cause resentment, insecurity, and mistrust.

If the nurse wants additional information, there are more effective ways of phrasing questions than beginning with "why." For example, rather than asking "Why didn't you do your exercises?" the nurse could say, "You didn't do your exercises. Is something wrong?" Rather than asking "Why are you so anxious?" the nurse could say, "You appear upset. Would you like to talk about it?"

CHANGING THE SUBJECT INAPPROPRIATELY

A nurse might inadvertently stop a client from discussing a subject of importance by changing the subject. Abruptly interrupting conversation is rude and shows a lack of empathy.

Nurse: Good morning, Mr. Jones. How are you feeling?"

Mr. Jones: (facial expression shows discomfort) Oh, not so good. My incision is rather sore.

Nurse: Well, let's get you up in a chair. We need to discuss your exercises.

The nurse's comment shows an unwillingness to discuss Mr. Jones' discomfort. The chance for a therapeutic assessment of his discomfort is lost. In this example changing the subject was nontherapeutic, since the nurse ignored a potentially serious problem.

Changing the subject stalls progress of a therapeutic communication. The client's thoughts and spontaneity are interrupted, ideas become tangled, and as a result, the information provided may be inadequate. It is particularly important to avoid changing the subject during an assessment. If the client has the opportunity to complete a message, the information shared will be more thorough and useful.

HELPING RELATIONSHIPS

The nurse-client relationship is more than a mutual partnership. Travelbee (1971) calls it a human-to-human relationship. King (1971) calls the nurse-client relationship "learning experiences whereby two people interact to face an immediate health problem, to share, if possible, in resolving it, and to discover ways to adapt to the situation."

The nurse uses skills of interpersonal communication to develop a relationship with the client that allows understanding of the client as a total person. The relationship is therapeutic, promoting a psychological climate that brings positive change and growth in the client. The relationship also focuses on meeting the client's needs. Although the nurse may gain much satisfaction from the relationship, the client should be the primary recipient of benefits.

Creation of a therapeutic environment rests on the nurse's ability to provide physical and psychosocial comfort to the client. Basic to the nurse's role is assurance that the client's physiological needs are satisfied. For example, the nurse positions the client so breathing is normal for comfortable sleep. The nurse's actions consider the client's preferences. The nurse and client mutually determine how needs are met.

Mrs. Greer is a 63-year-old widow who is hospitalized for lung cancer. She makes frequent requests for pain medication before a dose is due. When a nurse delivers the medication, Mrs. Greer criticizes her for being late. Nothing the nurses do seems to satisfy Mrs. Greer.

Ms. Edwards has cared for Mrs. Greer for the past 2 days. She could easily be tired of Mrs. Greer but chooses to be assigned to her for another day. Ms. Edwards enters her client's room and begins to straighten out the bed linen. Ms. Edwards asks, "Are you comfortable in that position, Mrs. Greer? Would you like a pain shot now?" Mrs. Greer accepts the offer and begins to relax in Ms. Edwards' presence. The nurse helps Mrs. Greer assume a more comfortable position on her side.

Once the client's pain has diminished, Ms. Edwards sits by her bed and says, "I know you've been experiencing much discomfort. Over the past few days we have not always been able to help you feel better. Can you help me to know the best way to make you feel comfortable?"

Efforts at improving Mrs. Greer's comfort make her more willing to discuss problems. The nurse soon learns of Mrs. Greer's great fear of death. The client has made frequent requests of the nurses to avoid feeling lonely. By discussing Mrs. Greer's fears, the nurse and client are able to find ways to minimize loneliness. The nurse's concern for Mrs. Greer leads to solutions to the client's problems.

A helping relationship between nurse and client does not just "happen." It is built with care as the nurse uses therapeutic communication techniques.

Dimensions of Helping Relationships

Characteristics of any helping relationship are trust, empathy, caring, autonomy, and mutuality (Sundeen et al., 1988). These are essential if the nurse is to establish a positive and supportive relationship with clients.

TRUST

With respect to helping relationships Travelbee defines trust as "the assured belief that other individuals are capable of assisting in times of distress and will probably do so." Unless a client believes a nurse wishes to care for his or her needs, a trusting relationship cannot develop. Trust fosters open, therapeutic communication. Previous experiences may affect a client's willingness to trust a nurse. Lack of previous health care experience or a traumatic experience causes clients to hesitate trusting care-givers. To foster trust the nurse acts consistently, reliably, and competently. Honesty in sharing information with clients also builds trust. Without trust a nurse-client relationship will not progress beyond social interaction and tending superficial needs.

EMPATHY

Empathy is the ability to understand and accept the life of another person and to accurately perceive feelings. It is a fair, sensitive, and objective look at what another person experiences. In contrast, sympathy is thinking or feeling as another person does. Sympathy is subjective.

Empathy helps clients explain and explore their feelings so problem solving might occur. It takes time for empathy to develop in a relationship. A nurse cannot automatically understand what a client feels or experiences. Being open and receptive helps the nurse learn to be empathetic.

Ms. Vincent has been caring for Mr. Pierce since his admission to the hospital 2 days ago. Mr. Pierce is scheduled to have open-heart surgery tomorrow. Ms. Vincent enters the client's room, makes eye contact with him, and sits in the chair beside his bed. The following conversation occurs:

Ms. Vincent: Hello, Mr. Pierce. You look as though you're rather deep in thought.

Mr. Pierce: Oh, I suppose I do. It's just that I can't help but think about what tomorrow will bring.

Ms. Vincent: Would you like to talk about your surgery? I imagine you have a lot of questions.

Mr. Pierce: Yes, I would like to know more.

The nurse could easily have avoided Mr. Pierce's true concerns and even attempted to change the subject. An unhelpful remark would be, "Don't worry about tomorrow, Mr. Pierce. Would you like me to get you something to read?" Such a comment would ignore Mr. Pierce's fears about surgery and prevent development of a meaningful relationship between the nurse and client. The skillful nurse moves the conversation forward to learn more about the client.

CARING

Caring is having a positive regard for another person. It is basic to a helping relationship. Most clients will directly or indirectly express a need to be cared for at some time. Nurses show caring by accepting clients for who they are and respecting them as individuals. When clients feel cared for they feel secure in threatening or anxiety-producing situations. Caring also promotes trust. Touching is an effective way for nurses to communicate care.

AUTONOMY AND MUTUALITY

Autonomy refers to an ability to be self-directed. Mutuality involves sharing with another. These are important in any helping relationship. The nurse and client work as a team, with both participating in the care process. Nurses offer clients opportunities to make decisions, even if it is as simple as choosing bath time. As a client becomes more independent, the nurse offers more opportunities for decision making. The nurse also acts as an advocate to keep clients informed of health care alternatives and to give support in decision making.

Phases of a Helping Relationship

The helping relationship is established and maintained by the professional nurse. The relationship is reciprocal; nurse and client relate to each other as they progress to therapeutic rapport. A helping relationship progresses over time as the nurse and client interact, but the helping relationship is not the same as the nursing process. The nursing process is a series of steps taken to manage a client's health problems. A helping relationship is a bond that allows the nurse to be more effective in carrying out the nursing process. The nurse is responsible for directing the client through the helping relationship to ensure that the client's needs are met.

Chapter 6 discusses the interview as a method for obtaining a nursing health history and identifying changes in the client's level of wellness and living patterns. Although the three phases of an interview and of a helping relationship are the same, communication patterns are different. The interview can initiate a nurse-client relationship because it may be their first encounter. However, the interview is not the mechanism for maintaining a long-term therapeutic relationship. A helping relationship goes beyond the scope of an interview to establish rapport that is the basis for an ongoing resolution of the client's health problems. The boxes on pp. 506 to 511 provide examples of therapeutic communication throughout all phases of the helping relationship.

PREINTERACTION PHASE

Before a first meeting with a client, the nurse reviews information pertaining to the client. Such information may include the medical or nursing history, an entry in the nurse's notes of the medical record, or a discussion with another nurse who cared for the client. By this review the nurse thinks about concerns that may develop. For example, before entering a relationship with a young cancer client the nurse considers how the client is adjusting and whether death may be discussed. The preinteraction phase is a time when the nurse plans an approach. This process helps avoid stereotyping clients and allows the nurse to think about personal values or feelings. Although the nurse may feel anxious about a client, this sharpens mental processes and helps planning. The beginning nursing student should seek assistance from instructors if anxiety becomes intense.

A final step to the preinteraction phase is to choose a location and setting for the first meeting with a client. A comfortable, private, and attractive setting fosters interpersonal interaction. The nurse also plans sufficient time for this discussion.

ORIENTATION

The orientation phase begins when the nurse and the client first meet. It sets the tone for the rest of the nurse-client relationship. The orientation phase is superficial and is often marked by uncertainty and exploration.

During any initial encounter both participants closely observe each other. The nurse and client make inferences and form judgments about each other's behaviors. Therapeutic communication will be more effective if the nurse is genuine, emphathetic, and caring.

The nurse and client meet and identify each other by name. It is wise to address the client formally by using last names, for example, "Good morning, Mr. Spencer. My name is Ms. Tucker. I am a student nurse assigned to take care of you today." As the therapeutic relationship develops a client may ask the nurse to be more

---

Communication to Place Client at Ease

Nurse: It certainly is a lovely day, Mrs. Spier.
Client: Yes, isn't it? If I were home and feeling better, I'd be planting my garden.
Nurse: You're a gardener? What types of plants do you enjoy growing?
Client: Oh, a little of everything. I like some tomatoes, lettuce, radishes, and maybe some squash.

The nurse directs the conversation so that she and Mrs. Spier feel at ease. If the nurse had rushed into a therapeutically oriented discussion with Mrs. Spier feeling uncomfortable, then no purpose would have been served. The nurse and Mrs. Spier can come to know each other better and begin to develop a meaningful relationship if the social interaction is directed properly.

informal. Failure of the nurse to identify herself or himself can create uncertainty because the client often encounters many personnel when seeking health care.

At the beginning of the relationship, neither individual is able to perceive the other's uniqueness. The nurse perceives a person who has a health-related problem. The client perceives the nurse as one of many health care professionals whose job is to help. Engaging in a social interaction initially helps the nurse and client to become relaxed (see box).

TESTING. The client often tests the nurse during the orientation phase. This is caused by the client's difficulty in acknowledging a need for help, fear of expressing true feelings, and anxiety over the need to change. The nurse

---

Communication Involving Testing

Mr. Miles is a 52-year-old businessman who has been hospitalized for treatment of a bleeding stomach ulcer. He is very independent and is accustomed to making decisions for himself. Ms. Rains, the nurse, enters the client's room.

Ms. Rains: Good morning, Mr. Miles. My name is Ms. Rains and I will be caring for you today.

Mr. Miles: You will, huh? Tell me, how long have you been a nurse?

Ms. Rains: About 2 years. I have worked in this hospital since graduating from nursing school.

Mr. Miles: Well, you won't have to worry about me. I can take care of myself.

Ms. Rains: I can imagine it's frustrating to be very independent one minute and then suddenly become ill and feel as though everyone is telling you what to do.

Mr. Miles: You can say that again. I'm just not used to needing help.

Ms. Rains: Mr. Miles, I'm not here to take away your independence. There are a number of things I need to do for you, but there are also many things I want you to be able to do for yourself. Let me explain some of the procedures I will be doing.

Mr. Miles: OK, I appreciate that.

Ms. Rains recognizes Mr. Miles' attempt to test her competence. Mr. Miles is fearful of losing his independence. If Ms. Rains has had minimal experience in developing relationships with clients, she may feel the need to remain superficial and nondirective. The client will sense the nurse's superficiality during testing and avoid meaningful discussion. In Mr. Miles' case Ms. Rains acknowledges concerns and acts to eliminate his fears.

---

who is aware of the client's concerns attempts to display confidence and competence. The nurse should not be defensive during testing but should be open and interested in the client's concerns. The client may use silence to avoid communicating. The nurse can show a desire to help by explaining the actions taken and performing care smoothly (see box).

BUILDING TRUST. Trust is relying on someone without doubt or question. Confidence, dependability, confidentiality, and credibility result in a trusting relationship. It is not easy for a client to perceive the need for help or to ask for it. Often a client trusts the nurse but is incapable of asking for assistance. Trust provides the foundation for effective communication as individuals become more open in expressing feelings and thoughts.

Trusting another person involves risk. As the client begins to share feelings and attitudes with the nurse, he becomes vulnerable. The client must become comfortable in revealing personal information. The nurse who is insecure with clients may choose superficial methods to build trust: sharing secrets, telling private jokes, or encouraging the client to establish the relationship on a first name basis. Some clients accept such behaviors, but others may resent being treated differently. Instead of enjoying the nurse's extra attention, they become distrustful.

Genuine caring is a powerful method for acquiring the client's trust. The nurse shows sensitivity and understanding of the client's needs. Expressing concern is one way to establish trust. By showing concern the nurse encourages the client's growth and progress (see box on p. 508).

IDENTIFYING PROBLEMS AND GOALS. At the initial encounter, the nurse begins assessing the client's health status. Through observations and interaction the nurse begins to make diagnostic conclusions. The client's health problems may be simple, such as moving without discomfort, choosing foods that will be easily tolerated, or getting out of bed safely. The relationship with the client is strengthened if the nurse discovers what problems are important. Also, the client may not be able to recognize problems. During the orientation phase the nurse uses communication techniques to direct the client toward an awareness of problems, focus on the nature of the problems, and explore potential solutions. As problems are identified, the nurse and client mutually set goals. When the client is able to participate in goal setting and see the desired benefits, nursing interventions are more effective.

Identification of problems uses attentive listening, open-ended questioning, paraphrasing, and clarifying. Initially the nurse avoids identifying a large number of actual or potential problems. Bombarding the client with

Communication to Build Trust

Mr. Squires: I've been home now for 4 days and I just don't know what to do.

Ms. Ramsey: You're obviously upset. Tell me what the problem is. I'd like to help.

Mr. Squires: The doctor put me on that new diet. It seemed easy in the hospital but I'm afraid I'm not eating right.

Ms. Ramsey: You've improved so much since your hospitalization. Let's sit down together and see what kinds of foods you should eat. Then we'll look at the types of foods you like that are allowed in your new diet.

Mr. Squires begins to trust Ms. Ramsey, who shows a willingness to help, not out of duty but out of a desire to meet his needs.

Mr. Squires: You shouldn't have to go to so much trouble for me.

Mr. Ramsey: You're not causing me trouble at all. An important part of my job is to help you stay healthy. Helping you to understand your diet better is part of my job.

Mr. Squires: Well, if I can learn to fix and eat the right foods, my doctor says I may stay out of the hospital longer this time.

Ms. Ramsey: Your doctor is right. Now let's go over what you know so far.

Another element that aids establishment of trust is recognizing Mr. Squires' individuality. He realizes that Ms. Ramsey respects him as a unique person.

Mr. Squires: The doctor said I should eat more vegetables and fruits. I really don't like many vegetables.

Ms. Ramsey: Well, let's make a list of what you do like. You know there are different ways to prepare the same kinds of foods. If you're able to eat the things you like, you'll be able to follow the diet more easily.

Mr. Squires: That sounds good. Before I left the hospital, I didn't think I would have much choice in what I ate.

Ms. Ramsey: Sure you do. I'll show you that you can have a lot of variety in your diet and even enjoy it. It's important that the diet be planned for you and not someone else.

Trust develops on a foundation of caring. Ms. Ramsey's time, patience, and conscientiousness show her concern for Mr. Squires' welfare.

Communication to Identify Problems and Goals

Mr. Sachs is a 58-year-old man who has suffered a partial paralysis of his right side. Mr. Sachs needs to regain function in his right hand to retain his job as a telephone repairman. He is also fearful of damage to his self-image. He feels deformed and unable to live normally again.

Mr. Sachs: So much has happened to me. I know I may never again be able to do the things I once enjoyed.

Nurse: I know it's a difficult time for you now, but there are many things we can do to help you regain normal function.

Mr. Sachs: But there are so many things wrong with me.

Nurse: Let's take one at a time. What is most important to you?

Mr. Sachs: If only I could use my hand.

Nurse: Your doctor has ordered some exercises to increase the strength in your hand. I'll show you how to do each one. Are you willing to try them?

Mr. Sachs: You bet I am. If only I could use my hand again to work.

Nurse: Let's start with some simple goals. First we'll help you gain strength in your fingers so you can grasp eating utensils, a comb, or a razor. After that we'll try some more strenuous exercises.

Mr. Sachs: OK, that sounds reasonable. Show me what I need to do.

too many questions can result in emotional and physical fatigue. Also, it makes the client less trusting and more suspicious of the nurse's intentions. Limiting problem identification facilitates the client's understanding of what the client's and nurse's roles will be (see box).

CLARIFYING ROLES. Once a helping relationship is initiated, roles must be clarified. This occurs through a sharing of information: what the nurse has assessed as the client's immediate needs, how the client perceives those needs, when various nursing care measures are to be instituted, and how the client can participate in this care. The helping relationship requires participation from both parties, but the nurse assumes the leadership role. Leadership does not mean control in the manipulative sense. Instead, the nurse takes the initiative in determining the client's point of view. The client assumes a role as receiver of care, but also assumes an ongoing role as a participant in care.

Communication to Form a Contract

Nurse: Mr. Reed, I'll be seeing you each morning for the next 4 days. After we practice your exercises together, I'd like you to do them on your own. Practice the exercises as often as you can without feeling pain or fatigue. On Friday I'll introduce you to the nurse who will work with you next week. I'll be sure she knows the types of exercises you're doing.

FORMING CONTRACTS. Once goals and roles are clearly defined, the nurse establishes a contract with the client. Generally, this involves a brief verbal interchange. Elements of the contract include location, frequency, and length of contacts with the client and duration of the relationship. The nurse should not present the contract in an overly formal way, but should outline a contractual agreement in a way that clarifies expectations. The nurse thus informs the client of what they both must do to facilitate progress toward health (see box).

It is important to let the client know when the relationship will be terminated. If the relationship is successful, the nurse and client frequently share close bonds of respect and concern. The closer the nurse and client become in working together, the more difficult it is to end the relationship. If the client can anticipate how long the relationship will last, termination will be less stressful. A student nurse often spends time with only one or two clients, often resulting in close relationships. Clients must be prepared for the end of the student's clinical experience, otherwise the client may become angered or disappointed.

WORKING PHASE

During the working phase of a helping relationship, the nurse strives to meet goals set during the orientation phase. The nurse and client work together. The relationship broadens and becomes more flexible as the nurse and client are more willing to share feelings and discuss problems.

The nurse encourages the client's open expression of feelings. This may best be achieved by listening and attending. If a client is unaccustomed to sharing feelings, the nurse is patient and understanding. The nurse's empathy and respect helps explore the client's true thoughts and feelings.

As the relationship progresses the client participates in more self-exploration and is better able to discuss relevant issues. The nurse helps clients understand their feelings so that change can occur when necessary. Sun-

Communication Skills

CONFRONTATION

Ms. Perkins is a 60-year-old client with a history of obesity and high blood pressure. She has been returning to the clinic monthly for checkups:

Ms. Perkins: I feel frustrated and I'm tired of being fat.

Nurse: When I saw you last month you told me you had lost 10 pounds and your clothes fit better. I can tell the difference.

Ms. Perkins: You're right, but it takes so much time to lose weight. I just get down on myself.

IMMEDIACY

Nurse: As we've talked, you've seemed distant.

Client: Um-hm.

Nurse: Perhaps you are upset since I was not able to come talk with you as soon as I had promised.

SELF-DISCLOSURE

Ms. Wells' mother died just a month ago. Since then, she has had difficulty following her diet.

Nurse: This has been a difficult time for you.

Ms. Wells: It seems as though my world's collapsed.

Nurse: Three years ago I lost my mother. It was a very difficult time. I came to realize though that her death was a part of life and that she would want me to continue living life to its fullest.

deen et al. (1985) describe three communication skills that will help clients gain self-understanding (see box):

1. *Confrontation*—The nurse makes the client aware of inconsistencies in behavior or thoughts that interfere with self-understanding. The technique helps clients recognize growth or deal with important issues.

2. *Immediacy*—The nurse focuses interaction on the present situation between nurse and client. The client learns to understand how he or she interacts with others. This involves drawing attention to the client's behavior or statements.

3. *Self-disclosure*—The nurse reveals personal experiences, thoughts, ideas, values, or feelings in context of the relationship. This is not therapy for the nurse. It shows the client that his or her experiences can be understood.

If the working phase is successful the client is able to act on ideas and feelings. This often requires risk and the nurse must remain supportive. Clients must deal with success and failure as they make decisions and resolve

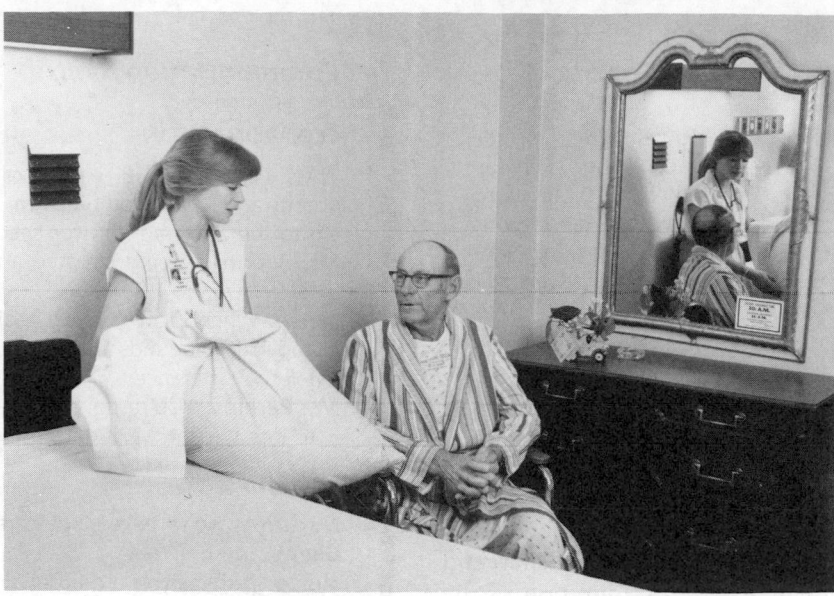

Fig. 19-3 The nurse integrates therapeutic communication skills into all aspects of care.

problems. Any attempt at change should be within the client's abilities. Change becomes less of a threat when clients express feelings about change and accept temporary setbacks. The nurse should encourage even the slightest progress.

INTEGRATING COMMUNICATION WITH NURSING ACTIONS. Nursing actions can generally be divided into four groups: physiological, psychological, spiritual, and socioeconomic. Bradley and Edinberg (1982) categorize the groups by their visibility. Physiological actions that attend to a client's physical needs, such as nutrition, elimination, and comfort, have high visibility. Most physiological actions are nonverbal and routinely performed. Traditionally, emphasis has been placed on a nurse's ability to perform physiological actions. Their high visibility allows the client to recognize the nurse as a good practitioner.

In contrast, psychological, socioeconomic, and spiritual nursing actions have low visibility. Psychological actions serve emotional needs. Socioeconomic actions such as referring clients to community health agencies assist clients in adapting to an environment. Spiritual actions help clients gain support for their belief system. Low-visibility tasks are not readily observed or measured by others. Psychological, socioeconomic, and spiritual actions require cognitive and affective skills that are not routine and have traditionally led to less reward for the nurse.

Communication is important in performing both high- and low-visibility tasks (Fig. 19-3). Giving emotional support or educating the client's family obviously require effective communication, but so do basic nursing care procedures, as shown in the boxed examples of communication.

TERMINATION

During orientation the nurse tells the client when to expect the relationship to end. When termination occurs, the client should not be surprised. By remaining aware of goals of the relationship, the client should be prepared to function effectively without the nurse's support. Termination can nonetheless be difficult and painful. The primary objective at the end of any helping relationship is termination in a planned and satisfying manner.

EVALUATION OF GOAL ACHIEVEMENT. Vital to termination is evaluation of goals. The nurse encourages assessment of the appropriateness and outcome of goals established (see box).

SEPARATION. Depending on the relationship between nurse and client, the client may have feelings of anxiety or ambivalence as termination nears. Ideally the client expresses feelings regarding termination. The nurse plans time to allow the client to share concerns or fears.

If the client remains in the health care setting and the nurse is the one leaving as a result of a scheduled day off or vacation, the client may feel abandoned. The nurse makes sure the client's care is uninterrupted by introducing the new nurse or communicating the client's needs with a written care plan. The nurse shares information that might foster the development of a helping relationship between other nurses and the client.

Communication to Facilitate Nursing Care

The nurse, Ms. Thomas, silently enters Mr. Richards' room. She tells him, "It's time for your pain shot." He is mildly startled and grimaces as he turns to see Ms. Thomas. As Mr. Richards starts to ask a question, she quickly reaches for his arm and prepares to inject the needle.

In contrast, a second nurse, Mr. Ives, enters Mr. Richards' room and says, "I have that pain medication you requested. Are you still feeling uncomfortable?" He turns and replies, "Yes, my back feels like a knife went through it. Will the pain ever go away?" Mr. Ives lays the syringe on the table, sits down next to Mr. Richards, and says, "It's normal to have pain the first few days after surgery. Let me give you that shot and then I can show you how to move more carefully in bed to avoid worsening the pain."

Mr. Richards would welcome Mr. Ives for his nurse but would want to bar the door if Ms. Thomas appeared. A few words of concern and reassurance (low-visibility communication skills) make receiving an injection more acceptable and encourage Mr. Richards to express his feelings.

Communication facilitates all nursing care measures. Integrating high- and low-visibility tasks allows Mr. Ives to accomplish several goals simultaneously. He quickly and efficiently assesses Mr. Richards' pain, provides a reassuring explanation, and demonstrates an alternative way of relieving pain. Therapeutic communication during high-visibility tasks increases the client's acceptance and understanding of procedures, lessens anxiety, and improves the client's willingness to cooperate.

Communication to Evaluate Goals

Ms. Garner has worked with the client, Mr. Adams, during his 4-week stay in the hospital. Mr. Adams had surgery for repair of a fractured leg. Together Ms. Garner and Mr. Adams set goals for his physical rehabilitation and return home.

Ms. Garner: Well, Mr. Adams, your doctor has discharged you for tomorrow morning. How do you feel about going home?

Mr. Adams: Oh, I'll be glad to get out of here. My leg feels pretty good.

Ms. Garner: Do you feel comfortable walking with the crutches?

Mr. Adams: Yes, I do. As you suggested, I practiced climbing stairs quite a bit in physical therapy. As you know, I have five stairs to climb up to my front door. I can climb now without losing my balance.

Ms. Garner: You've also worked hard on learning to transfer from the bed and chair to a standing position with the crutches.

Mr. Adams: It's a lot easier now. All the practice you suggested helped. Since you've explained all of the right ways to hold the crutches, they feel like a natural part of me. I do hope I can get rid of them soon.

Ms. Garner: Well, it sounds like you're ready to leave. Continue your leg exercises as you've done them here and soon you won't need those crutches.

Mr. Adams: Thanks again for your help. I didn't think I'd ever be able to walk with these things, but now the crutches are no problem.

Both Ms. Garner and Mr. Adams experience satisfaction in meeting goals, particularly because the goals are mutually set. If goals are left unaccomplished, the reasons are examined and plans are made for attainment in the future. Mr. Adams has not achieved the ability to walk without his crutches. Ms. Garner encourages him to continue his exercise regimen so he will become strong enough to walk independently.

COMMUNICATION AND THE NURSING PROCESS

Communication is important to the nursing process. A nurse uses communication skills during each step of the process (see box). Assessment, nursing diagnosis, planning, implementation, and evaluation of a client's care depends on effective communication between the nurse, client, client's family, and health care team.

Communication is also important when caring for clients with communication problems. If a client is unable to interact with people because of illness, developmental delay, physical limitations imposed by therapy, or emotional reasons the nurse's role is to encourage communication. The nurse uses the nursing process to ensure that clients communicate in a meaningful and effective way.

ASSESSMENT

Assessment can begin with a review of factors influencing communication. The client's developmental level, perceptions, emotions, cultural orientation, and knowledge are just a few the nurse must understand before planning ways to promote communication. It may be difficult to assess all of these factors if a client has phys-

Communication Through the Nursing Process

- **Assessment.** Interviewing and history taking, physical examination (use of visual, auditory, tactile channels), observing nonverbal behavior, reviewing medical records, literature, diagnostic tests.
- **Nursing Diagnosis.** Written analysis of assessment findings, discussing health care needs and priorities with client and family.
- **Planning.** Written care plans, health team planning sessions, discussions with client and family to determine methods of implementation.
- **Implementation.** Discussion with other health professionals, health teaching, providing therapeutic support, contacting other health resources, recording client's progress in care plan and nurse's notes.
- **Evaluation.** Acquiring verbal and nonverbal feedback, writing results of expected outcomes, updating written plan of care, explaining revisions to clients.

TABLE 19-2 Assessment of Physical Communication Barriers

Physical Speech or Language Mechanisms	Alterations Affecting Speech
Respiratory system	Extreme dyspnea or shortness of breath
	Artificial airways: endotracheal tube or tracheostomy
	Laryngectomy
Oral and nasal cavities	Cleft palate
	Loose fitting dentures
	Neurological disease affecting articulation (for example, parkinsonism)
Speech center	Aphasia related to stroke (cerebrovascular accident) or brain tumor
Auditory system	Conduction or nerve deafness

ization of the same words or phrases, or a loose association of ideas. The nurse must isolate psychological causes of speech problems from possible neurological causes.

NURSING DIAGNOSIS

The inability to communicate effectively influences a client's ability to express needs or react to the environment. The nurse's success in identifying the client's communication problem will ensure the formulation of an accurate nursing diagnosis (see sample nursing diagnoses box). The diagnosis should focus on the cause of the communication disorder so appropriate interventions are chosen.

The nurse may also diagnose clients who have difficulty interacting with other persons. In these situations the client's difficulty of expression or a change in the client's communication patterns leads the nurse to make a diagnosis.

The nursing diagnoses box lists examples of diagnoses for clients with communication alterations.

ical barriers to communication. Family or friends then may become important for the nurse's assessment.

PHYSICAL AND PSYCHOLOGICAL BARRIERS TO COMMUNICATION

A client may suffer physical or psychological alterations that impair communication. In order to speak spontaneously and clearly one must have an intact respiratory system, normal oral and nasal cavities, and a functioning speech center in the cerebral cortex. Normal acquisition of language requires an intact auditory system. In the case of a child, the nurse assesses a child's ability to communicate, including the observation of sounds, gestures, and vocabulary expressed. If an adult client develops hearing problems later in life, the ability to receive and understand messages is impaired. Review of a client's medical history, as well as the physical assessment, provides clues to the client's physical ability to communicate (Table 19-2). Physical barriers cause loss of speech, impaired articulation, or inability to find or name words.

The nurse should also consider whether clients are taking medication that impairs speech. Some medications, such as antidepressants, neuroleptics, or sedatives, may cause a client to slur words or use incomplete sentences. The nurse should be familiar with common side effects of such medications.

Some psychological illnesses such as psychosis or depression influence the ability to communicate. The client may demonstrate flight of ideas, constant verbal-

PLANNING

For each diagnosis the nurse develops a plan of care individualized to the client's needs (see care plan box). The nurse considers ways to help a client communicate more effectively. It is especially important to have the client make decisions about the plan of care. A person must feel comfortable and willing to communicate. If the nurse sets unrealistic expectations or fails to be sensitive to the client's communication problems an effective plan of care will not be established.

Sample Nursing Diagnoses for Communication Alterations

Defining Characteristics	Nursing Diagnoses	Related Factors
Unable to speak dominant language Does not or cannot speak Stuttering; slurring Impaired articulation Inability to name or find words	Impaired verbal communication	▪ Decreased circulation to brain ▪ Tracheostomy ▪ Cultural difference ▪ Cleft palate
Change in usual communication pattern Verbal manipulation Verbalization of inability to cope or ask for help Alteration in societal participation	Ineffective individual coping	▪ Situational crises ▪ Life changes ▪ Inadequate support systems
Verbalized discomfort in social situations Observed use of unsuccessful social interaction behaviors	Impaired social interaction	▪ Communication barriers

Examples of Nursing Diagnoses Related to Communication Alterations

NANDA-APPROVED NURSING DIAGNOSES

Impaired verbal communication related to:
▪ Physical barrier or tracheostomy
▪ Cultural difference
▪ Developmental deficit
Ineffective individual coping related to:
▪ Situational crises
▪ Maturational crises
Impaired social interaction related to:
▪ Communication barriers

Success of promoting a client's ability to communicate depends on the nurse's style of communication and the ability to establish a helping relationship. Use of therapeutic communication skills allows the nurse to perceive, react to, and respect the client's uniqueness. Successful interpersonal interaction meets the following goals of care for a client:

1. Transmit clear, concise, and understandable messages.
2. Gain a sense of trust in the nurse as a care giver.
3. Send and receive feedback.

Sample Nursing Care Plan for Communication Alterations

Nursing Diagnosis	Goal	Expected Outcomes	Nursing Interventions
Impaired verbal communication related to difficulty in speaking English	Client will express needs clearly.	Client will try to use simple English phrases. Client will speak in Spanish when use of English is unclear.	Do not rush client as he attempts to ask questions or express ideas. Use attentive listening. Ask simple short questions. Use a communication board with key words spelled in English and the client's language (Spanish). Use an interpreter (Mrs. Santiago, Lab dept., ext. 5444) as needed.

Communication Aids

- Pad and felt-tipped pen or magic slate
- Communication board with words, letters, or pictures denoting basic needs (for example, water, bedpan, pain medication)
- Call bells or alarms
- Sign language
- Use of eye blinks or movement of fingers for simple responses (for example, "yes" or "no")
- Flash cards with common words or phrases the client may use
- Language cards for non-English-speaking clients

IMPLEMENTATION

With all clients the nurse tries to develop a helping therapeutic relationship. Clients will then feel more comfortable in interaction despite communication alterations.

DEVELOPING SOCIAL SKILLS

If ineffective coping or impaired social interaction is present, the nurse's interventions focus on helping clients:

1. Express feelings and needs.
2. Develop conversational skills.
3. Communicate thoughts and feelings clearly (verbally and nonverbally).
4. Demonstrate assertiveness.
5. Problem solve.
6. Facilitate conversation with peers and staff.

A nurse who has more exerience with communication skills and interpersonal dynamics may assist clients through role playing. This allows clients to practice situations in which they have difficulty communicating.

There are also simple interventions that can be used to reinforce attempts at interaction:

1. Encourage participation in normal social activities.
2. Discuss neutral topics or subjects in which the client has an interest.
3. Give positive reinforcement for acceptable social interactions.
4. Help clients identify persons with whom they feel comfortable and encourage activities with them.
5. Change bed or room assignments (in hospital) to encourage friendships or associates with same interests.
6. Minimize the client's idle time.

PROVIDING ALTERNATE COMMUNICATION METHODS

Clients with physical communication barriers may be unable to speak or clarity of speech is so poor that alternate methods of communication are needed (see box). For these clients it is important to provide methods that are simple to use. Anything complicated can be frustrating and make communication more difficult. The nurse is patient as the client tries to communicate. The client must be able to physically use whatever method the nurse provides. Clients must have communication boards or pencil and pad nearby. A client who is unable to speak can be at risk for injury unless personal needs can be quickly communicated.

CONTROLLING THE ENVIRONMENT

If an environment is uncomfortable or distracting a client will have difficulty communicating regardless of the problem. The nurse can control the environment so that it is conducive to interpersonal interactions. Methods of environmental control include:

1. Regulating room temperature to a comfortable level
2. Eliminating or reducing loud noises in the room (for example, radio, equipment alarm)
3. Making the client comfortable
4. Asking other staff or family (if appropriate) not to enter room during interaction
5. Reducing bright or glaring light

COMMUNICATING WITH A CHILD

Communication with a child requires special considerations so the nurse can develop a working relationship with both the child and his or her family. The nurse receives much information from parents. Because contact between parent and child is usually close, information communicated by parents can be assumed to be reliable. However, some parents may exaggerate. If the client is a young child, it helps to offer toys or materials for play so the parent can give full attention to the nurse. The nurse gives periodic attention to infants and younger children as they play to make them participants. An older child can be actively involved in communication.

To communicate effectively with children, the nurse must understand the influence of development on language and thought processes. Both affect the way a child communicates and the manner in which the nurse can successfully interact.

Children, particularly the young, are especially responsive to nonverbal messages. Sudden movements or threatening gestures can frighten a child. The nurse walking into an examination room with a broad grin and animated hand movements might inhibit formation of a relationship. The nurse should remain calm and gentle. It

Communicating with Sensorially or Motor Impaired Clients

HEARING IMPAIRED

- Be sure hearing aid is clean, inserted properly, and has a functioning battery.
- Adjust volume of hearing aid to a comfortable level.
- Speak slowly and articulate clearly.
- Stand in front of client to provide opportunity for lip reading.
- Talk toward client's best ear.
- Reduce background noise.

VISUALLY IMPAIRED

- Keep eyeglasses clean and intact (allows client to see nonverbal communication).

APHASIA

- Ask simple questions that require "yes" or "no" answers.
- Allow time for understanding and a response.
- Use visual cues (for example, words, pictures, objects) when possible.
- Only one person should talk at a time.
- Do not shout or speak too loudly.

DYSARTHRIA

- Listen attentively, be patient, and do not interrupt.
- Encourage client to converse.
- Refer to speech therapist as needed.

helps to let the child make the first move in interpersonal contacts. A quiet, friendly, confident tone of voice is best.

Children dislike being stared at. Adults looking down on them make them feel vulnerable. While communicating with a young child, the nurse should meet the child at eye level. The child feels helpless in most situations involving health care personnel.

Whenever it is necessary to give explanations or directions, the nurse uses simple, direct language. The nurse must be honest with children. Deceiving a child into thinking a painful procedure is painless will only make the child angry. To minimize fear and anxiety a child should always be told what to expect immediately before a procedure begins.

Drawing and play are two effective ways to communicate with young children. Drawing provides an opportunity for the child to communicate nonverbally (by making the drawing) and verbally (by explaining the picture). The nurse can use a child's drawing as a basis for initiating a conversation.

COMMUNICATING WITH ELDERLY CLIENTS

Because of sensory disturbances and motor disabilities, the elderly often have communication problems. Sensory alterations prevent the elderly from receiving messages clearly. Motor disturbances such as dysarthria interfere with clarity of pronunciation. Many of the elderly adapt to sensory losses (see Chapter 44) and can learn to communicate effectively. When obvious deficits exist, the nurse maximizes existing motor and sensory function so the client can communicate more effectively (see box).

Sample Evaluation of Interventions for Communication Alterations

Goals	Evaluative Measures	Expected Outcomes
Client transmits clear concise, and understandable messages.	Observe client's interactions with nurse and others.	Client uses effective communication techniques (including communication aids as needed).
	Confirm meaning of message the client intended to send.	Client uses appropriate language. Client expresses feelings appropriately.
Client gains a sense of trust in the nurse as caregiver.	Observe client's openness and willingness to discuss personal thoughts or feelings.	Client spontaneously discusses thoughts or feelings with the nurse. Client expresses accomplishment of goals or relationship. Client shares feelings about termination of helping relationship.
Client sends and receives feedback.	Observe client's interactions.	Client listens carefully. Client asks for and receives feedback. Client uses appropriate nonverbal cues to match verbal messages.

EVALUATION

Successful communication is evaluated by the nurse's observations of client interactions. It is important not only if communication exists, but whether the client appears satisfied the message was received. The nurse is effective in promoting communication if goals of care are met. The nurse uses evaluative criteria in determining the outcome of interventions (see evaluation box).

SUMMARY

Communication is one of the most important skills for a nurse. It allows nurses to better understand clients' needs and develop relationships that will help clients attain healthy behaviors. A nurse's competence depends on the ability to send timely and intelligent messages as the client's needs dictate and on the ability to understand the client's communications. Communication is affected by many factors and is a complex process that includes both verbal and nonverbal communication.

Therapeutic communication with the client involves planned, deliberate interactions that foster a helping relationship. Throughout the relationship the nurse uses skills that promote communication and avoids words and actions that inhibit communication. Through effective communication the nurse helps clients adapt to changes resulting from health alterations.

There are clients with special communication problems. The nurse acts to help them communicate effectively in spite of physical, emotional, or developmental limitations.

KEY CONCEPTS

- ✓ Effective communication is the process that allows nurses to establish working relationships with clients.
- ✓ Successful communication requires the message intended by the speaker to be similar or identical to the meaning acquired by the receiver.
- ✓ The way a person receives a message depends on past experiences, sensory function, and personal expectations.
- ✓ Words that have different connotative meanings can be easily misinterpreted by the person receiving the message.
- ✓ Effective verbal communication requires clear and concise phrasing of words, a proper pacing of statements, and an understandable vocabulary.
- ✓ When the sender's verbal and nonverbal communications complement each other, a receiver is unlikely to misinterpret a message.
- ✓ Communication aids the nurse in performing nursing care measures effectively and efficiently.
- ✓ Communication is a means for the nurse to help clients adjust to changes imposed by illness.
- ✓ A nurse does not use all of the skills that promote effective communication for every client.
- ✓ Many skills that normally promote communication can be detrimental to nurse-client relationships if used improperly.
- ✓ Ineffective communication skills tend to inhibit the client's willingness to express ideas or concerns openly.

✓ Trust, empathy, caring, autonomy, and mutuality are basic dimensions of a helping nurse-client relationship.

✓ The working phase of a helping relationship involves nurse and client working together so that a client can express thoughts and feelings freely and constructively.

✓ Clients with physical communication barriers may be able to express themselves more effectively with communication aids.

✓ Clients with ineffective social skills may benefit from positive reinforcement and encouragement to participate in interactions.

REFERENCES

Bradley, J, and Edinberg, MA: Communication in the nursing context, New York, 1982, Appleton-Century-Crofts.

Duldt, BW, et al.: Interpersonal communication in nursing, Philadelphia, 1984, F.A. Davis Co.

Ekman, P: Communication through nonverbal behavior: a source of information about an interpersonal relationship. In Tomkins, SS, and Izard, CE, editors: Affect, cognition, and personality, New York, 1965, Springer Publishing Co.

Fritz, P, et al.: Intrapersonal communication in nursing: an interactionist approach, East Norwalk, Conn., 1984, Appleton & Lange.

Hein, EC: Communication in nursing practice, Boston, 1973, Little, Brown & Co., Inc.

King, I: Toward a theory for nursing, New York, 1971, John Wiley & Sons, Inc.

Knapp, M: Nonverbal communication in human interaction, New York, 1978, Holt, Rinehart & Winston.

Pluckhan, ML: Human communication: the matrix of nursing, New York, 1978, McGraw-Hill Book Co.

Satir, V: Conjoint family therapy, rev. ed, Palo Alto, Calif., 1967, Science & Behavior Books.

Stanhope, M, and Lancaster, J: Community health nursing: process and practice for promoting health, ed. 2, St. Louis, 1988, The C.V. Mosby Co.

Sundeen, SJ, et al.: Nurse-client interaction: implementing the nursing process, ed. 4, St. Louis, 1988, The C.V. Mosby Co.

Travelbee, J: Interpersonal aspects of nursing, ed. 2, Philadelphia, 1971, F.A. Davis Co.

Whaley, LF, and Wong, DL: Nursing care of infants and children, ed. 3, St. Louis, 1987, The C.V. Mosby Co.

Winkler, I, and Doherty, WJ: Communication styles and marital satisfaction in Isreali and American couples, Fam Proc 22:221, 1983.

Zunin, L, and Zunin, N: Contract: the first four minutes, New York, 1973, Ballatine Books.

ADDITIONAL READINGS

Beck, C, Rawlins, R, and Williams, S: Mental health–psychiatric nursing: a holistic life-cycle approach, St. Louis, 1988, The C.V. Mosby Co.

Bermosk, LS: Interviewing: a key to therapeutic communication in nursing practice, Nurs Clin North Am 1(2):205, 1966.

Bird, B: Talking with patients, Philadelphia, 1973, J.B. Lippincott Co.

Cameron, JE: Giant leap forward begins with the nursing interview, Aust Nurses J 12(2):47, 1982.

Coad-Denton, A: Therapeutic superficiality and intimacy. In Longo, D, and Williams, R: Clinical practice in psychosocial nursing, New York, 1978, Appleton-Century-Crofts.

Doona, ME: Traveller's interventions in psychiatric nursing, ed. 2, Philadelphia, 1979, F.A. Davis Co.

Ebersole, P, and Hess, P: Toward healthy aging, ed. 3, St. Louis, 1987, The C.V. Mosby Co.

Egan, G: The skilled helper, Monterey, Calif., 1975, Brooks/Cole Publishing Co.

Enelow, A, and Scott, S: Interviewing and patient care, ed. 2, New York, 1979, Oxford University Press.

Goda, S: Speech development in children, Am J Nurs 70:276, 1970.

Kemp, CG: Perspectives on the group process, Boston, 1964, Houghton-Mifflin Co.

Knowles, RD: Building rapport through neuro-linguistic programming, Am J Nurs 83:1011, 1983.

Loweree, F, et al.: Admitting an intoxicated patient, Am J Nurs 84:617, May 1984.

McKay, M, Davis, M, and Fanning, P: Messages: the communication book, Oakland, Calif., 1983, New Harbinger Publications.

Murray, RB: Therapeutic communication for emotional care. In Murray, RB, and Huelskoetter, MM: Psychiatric mental health nursing: giving emotional care, Englewood Cliffs, N.J., 1983, Prentice-Hall, Inc.

Purtilo, R: Health professionals-patient interaction, ed. 2, Philadelphia, 1978, W.B. Saunders Co.

Raudseff, E: 7 ways to cure communication breakdowns, Nurs Life 4:51, 1984.

Rogers, CR: On becoming a person: a therapist's view of psychotherapy, Boston, 1961, Houghton-Mifflin Co.

Satir, V: Peoplemaking, Palo Alto, Calif., 1972, Science & Behavior Books.

Walker, R: Effective listening, Am J Med Technol 35:8, 1969.

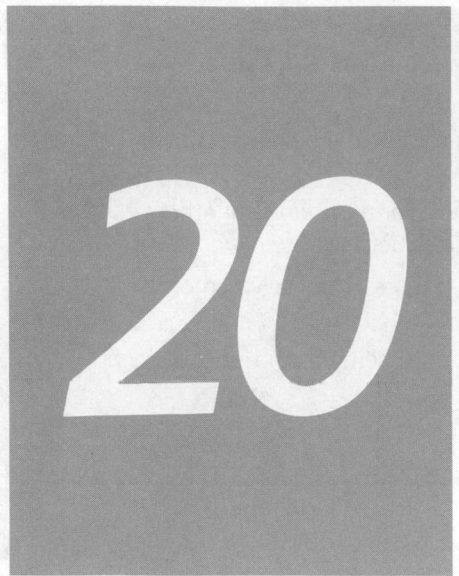

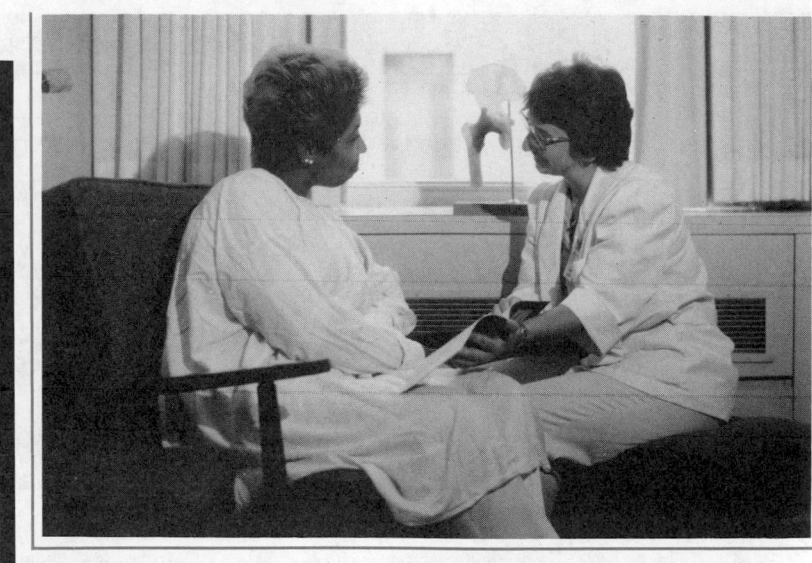

OBJECTIVES

Mastery of content in this chapter will enable the student to:

- Define the key terms listed.
- Describe the similarities and differences between teaching and learning.
- Identify the purposes of client teaching.
- Compare the communication process with the teaching process.
- Describe the domains of learning.
- Differentiate factors that determine readiness to learn from those that determine ability to learn.
- Explain the importance of learner participation in teaching and learning.
- Discuss factors that contribute to a positive learning environment.
- Develop a client's teaching plan.
- Write a learning objective.
- Describe ways to incorporate teaching with routine nursing care.
- Identify methods for evaluating learning.
- Identify principles of effective teaching.

KEY TERMS

Analogy
Cognitive Learning
Compliance
Domains of Learning
Illiterate
Learning
Learning Objectives
Motivation
Psychomotor Learning
Reinforcement
Teaching

Teaching-Learning Process

Client education has become one of the more important roles for nurses. Shorter hospital stays, increased demands on nurses' time, and the need to give seriously ill clients technical information as soon as possible emphasizes the importance of quality client education. Providing clients with needed information for self-care is necessary to assure continuity of care from the hospital to the home. A well-designed, comprehensive teaching plan that fits a client's learning needs can reduce health care costs, improve the quality of care, and help clients gain more independence.

It is impossible to separate teaching from learning. *Teaching* is an interactive process that promotes learning. It consists of a deliberate set of actions that helps individuals either gain knowledge or perform new skills. Redman (1988) defines teaching as an "interpersonal" influence aimed at changing the way persons can or will behave. With regard to health care, Bartlett (1984) defines client education as a process of informing clients and their families about illness, treatment, and other health related matters, including how to stay on treatment plans and helping them change behavior. Teaching is most effective when it is responsive to a learner's needs. The teacher is responsible for identifying these by fielding questions and inquiring into the learner's interests. The process of teaching thus relies on principles of interpersonal communication to send messages of significance to the learner and to receive the learner's feedback.

To learn is to acquire knowledge or skills through reinforced practice and experience. A diabetic client demonstrates the technique for preparing insulin in a

519

Client Education Standards

STRUCTURE

Standards in regard to structure relate to human and material resources, including administration and management of the health care agency. Nurses in both staff and administrative roles should contribute to their development and implementation.

Standard 1

The health care agency has a philosophy, goals, and objectives that reflect its mandate and provide direction for client education.

Guidelines

The philosophy includes:

- recognition of individuality of the client, the client's right to information and planned education, and the value of client education as an integral part of quality health care.
- identification of the relationship between the client, the nurse, and other members of the health care team
- consideration of the society and community in which client education is provided
- collaboration with members of the health care team and client representatives
- a written format that is interpreted at the time of staff orientation and as necessary

Standard 2

Client education is integrated into all areas of nursing practice in the health care system.

Guidelines

1. Client education responsibilities are outlined in all nursing job descriptions and evaluated in performance appraisals.
2. Nursing personnel serve as members of committees involved in client education within the health care agency and the community.

Standard 3

The nursing department of the health care agency is active in developing a comprehensive plan for client education.

Guidelines

The plan includes:

- specific objectives for client education and the systematic process that will ensure they are achieved
- expectations for the client, health care agency, departments within the agency, and personnel

From the Alberta Association of Registered Nurses: Client education: position statement and guidelines, 1985, Edmonton, Alberta, Canada, 1986, The Association.

- identification of nursing personnel responsible for client education within the agency
- agency support of individual professional development in client education
- a report of the material, human, and financial resources in terms of needs, availability, and implications
- a mechanism for periodic review and evaluation

Standard 4

An individual/department is responsible for facilitating and coordinating matters of client education.

Guidelines

1. There is rationale given for identification of the individual/department responsible for client education.
2. The individual/department should have educational and experiential background in client education.
3. The individual/department has responsibility for decision making with regard to client education in collaboration with professionals involved.
4. The individual/department is responsible for assisting in interpreting the agency's philosophy of client education to members of the health care team.
5. The individual/department assists in and directs planning, implementation, and evaluation of client education within the agency.
6. The individual/department provides continuing education for nursing personnel in such areas as principles of teaching-learning and adult education.

PROCESS

Process standards outline criteria by which client education is delivered. The educational process includes the same steps as the nursing process.

Standard 1

The primary focus of the educational process is the client.

Guidelines

The educational process:

- provides for client participation
- assists clients to understand their lifestyle, condition, treatment, and care
- assists clients to understand their responsibility for participation in self-care to achieve and/or maintain optimal well-being.

Standard 2

An educational assessment is done by the nurse in collaboration with the client.

Guidelines

1. The collection of data is systematic and continuous.
2. Assessment data are communicated to appropriate members of the health care team.

3. To complete an education assessment, the following should be considered:
   - client's beliefs, attitudes, cultural/ethnic influences, and experiences regarding health and illness
   - client's language preference
   - client's physical or mental limitations to learning
   - client's existing knowledge and self-assessed health status
   - client's level of literacy and comprehension
   - client's motivation and readiness to learn
   - client's acceptance of and adjustment to the condition
   - what the client wants to learn
4. Findings of the assessment are validated with the client.
5. On the basis of the data, a nursing diagnosis of the knowledge deficit(s) is formulated (NANDA).
6. In conjunction with the client the educational needs are given priorities.

Standard 3

The nurse demonstrates planning in the educational process.

Guidelines
1. The plan for client education will:
   - establish specific measurable, realistic objectives with expected outcomes
   - provide a list of objectives in order based on priorities and increasing complexity
   - identify approved material resources
   - identify appropriate educational method(s)
   - identify personnel to implement the teaching process
2. The educational plan is individualized to meet needs of the client.
3. The educational plan includes goals formulated with other health care team members.
4. The educational plan is validated with the client and other members of the health care team.
5. The proposed educational plan will be recorded in the permanent health care record.

Standard 4

The nurse applies principles of the educational process in implementation of client education.

Guidelines
The implementation of client education:
- provides a climate conducive to learning
- is initiated according to the client's readiness and receptivity
- provides a means for the client and nurse to assess learning that has occurred
- provides a means to reinforce what is taught
- provides opportunities for additional learning for the client
- demonstrates that principles of adult learning are applied in the educational process.

Standard 5

A written outline of the educational process is available as a communication tool, a resource to health professionals, and as a record.

Guidelines
1. Documentation includes the educational plan.
2. Communication with appropriate family members, health care team members, and agencies includes recommendations to ensure continuity of the educational process.

OUTCOME

Outcome standards are the criteria to measure results of the educational process.

Standard 1

The nurse evaluates the educational process.

Guidelines
1. The evaluation of client education:
   - identifies what has been learned by providing opportunities for client feedback
   - provides opportunities for the client to indicate the level of satisfaction with the educational experience
   - assesses the format, content, teaching-learning activities, environment, media, client satisfaction, time, cost, and resources of the educational plan
2. The evaluation of the educational plan is documented in the permanent health record.
3. The client's progress directs reassessment, reordering of priorities, new goal setting, and revision of the teaching plan.

Standard 2

The client participates in evaluating the educational process.

Guidelines
1. The client indicates the level of satisfaction with the educational experience.
2. The client demonstrates the extent to which learning has occurred.
3. The client and nurse discuss specific aspects of the educational experience, such as media used and environment.
4. The client has the opportunity to request additional learning.

syringe. A surgical client discusses with the nurse preoperatively ways to relieve pain postoperatively. Newly acquired knowledge or skill gained by a client reflects the teacher's success. Nurses use several teaching methods that assist clients and family members to become participants in health care. Client education is a key to health maintenance and illness prevention. It is the nurse's responsibility to be aware of information clients and their families need. Although the physician is ultimately responsible for providing information about a client's diagnosis, treatment, and prognosis, the nurse can clarify that information as well as become the primary source of information about nursing care.

STANDARDS FOR CLIENT EDUCATION

Accrediting agencies in the United States and Canada set guidelines for provision of client education within health care institutions. The guidelines ensure clients and their families receive information necessary to maintain the client's optimal level of health. In the United States, the JCAHO (1987) cites two standards relating to client education:

1. Education and knowledge of self-care are given special consideration for the patient and family in the nursing plan.

2. As appropriate, patients who leave the hospital still requiring nursing care receive instructions and individual counseling prior to discharge.

In 1986, the Alberta Association of Registered Nurses developed a set of client education standards (see box). They address the educational process related to adult learners. The broad usefulness of the standards helps direct nurses in client education.

PURPOSES FOR CLIENT TEACHING

Health care today calls for comprehensive nursing practice. The emphasis is more on maintaining health than on simply treating disease. Clients are more knowledgeable about health and seek involvement in their health maintenance. Comprehensive client education includes three important purposes, each involving a separate phase of health care, described in the following sections and listed in the box.

Maintenance of Health and Illness Prevention

The public has become more health conscious in recent years. Participation in fitness clubs, diet programs, regular exercise activities, and health-screening pro-

---

Topics for Health Teaching

HEALTH PROMOTION/ILLNESS PREVENTION

- First aid
- Avoidance of risk factors: smoking, alcohol
- Growth and development
- Hygiene
- Immunizations
- Normal childbearing
- Nutrition
- Exercise
- Safety (in home and hospital)
- Sceening (blood pressure, vision, cholesterol levels)

RESTORATION OF HEALTH

- Client's disease or condition
  - Anatomy and physiology of body system affected
  - Cause of disease
  - Origin of symptoms
  - Expected effects on other body systems
  - Prognosis
- Rationale for treatment
  - Medications
  - Tests and therapies

- Nursing measures
  - Surgical intervention
- Expected duration of care
- Hospital/clinic environment
- Hospital/clinic staff
- Methods for client participation in care
- Limitations posed by disease or surgery

COPING WITH IMPAIRED FUNCTIONS

- Home care
  - Medications
  - Diet
  - Activity
  - Self-help devices
- Rehabilitation of remaining function
  - Physical therapy
  - Occupational therapy
- Prevention of complications
  - Knowledge of risk factors
  - Implications of noncompliance with therapy
  - Environmental alterations

grams are examples of ways people pay more attention to their health.

The nurse is a convenient resource for clients who want to improve their physical and psychological well-being. In the school, home, clinic, or workplace the nurse provides information and skills that will allow clients to assume healthier behaviors (see box on p. 522). For example, in childbearing classes, nurses teach expectant parents what to anticipate and do during pregnancy. The expectant parents learn about the stages of fetal (unborn child) development and factors that can alter normal growth. Physical and psychological changes the woman undergoes during pregnancy also are a part of the class. After learning about normal childbearing the mother is more likely to eat healthy foods, get physical exercise, and avoid drugs or other substances that might harm the fetus. Promoting healthy behavior through education increases clients' self-esteem by allowing them to assume more responsibility for their health. With greater knowledge a person can maintain better health habits. When clients become more health conscious, they are more likely to seek early diagnosis of health problems.

Restoration of Health

Clients who are injured or ill need information or skills that will help them regain improved levels of health (see box on p. 522). Clients recovering from stress of illness or injury and accepting the associated limitations often seek information about their conditions. However, clients who find it difficult to adapt to illness may become uninterested in learning. The nurse learns to identify clients' receptivity to acquiring knowledge and institutes methods to motivate interest.

The family is often a vital part of a client's return to health and needs to know as much as the client. If the nurse excludes the family from a teaching plan, conflicts may arise. For example, if the family does not understand a client's need to regain independent function, their efforts may cause the client to become unnecessarily dependent and retard progress.

Coping with Impaired Functioning

Not all clients fully recover from illness or injury. Many must learn to cope with permanent health alterations. Knowledge and skills are often necessary for clients to continue activities of daily living (see box on p. 522). For example, the client whose ability to speak is lost following surgery of the larynx learns new ways of communicating, and the client with severe heart disease learns to avoid physical activities that pose risk for further heart damage.

In the case of serious disability the client's role within the family may change, making understanding and ac-

ceptance by family members necessary. The family's ability to provide support is a result of education. Education begins as soon as the client's needs are identified and the family displays a willingness to help. The nurse teaches family members how to assist clients with health care management. This would include, for example, giving medications and baths and applying dressings. Families of clients with other kinds of alterations, such as alcoholism, mental retardation, or drug dependence, learn to adapt to their emotional effects.

A nurse learns to recognize what information to teach clients at different levels of wellness. To do this, the nurse must consider their needs in relation to their ability to meet them. Learning occurs when information is practical and useful. Comparing the client's desired level of health with the actual state enables the nurse to plan a meaningful teaching program.

TEACHING AS A FORM OF COMMUNICATION

The teaching process closely parallels the communication process (see Chapter 19). In fact, teaching is a form of interpersonal communication. A teacher applies each element of the communication process while imparting information to students. As in the case of a sender and receiver communicating, the teacher and student become involved in a process that increases the student's knowledge and skills.

In a therapeutic nurse-client relationship, change results from trust and understanding formed between the nurse and client. In a teacher-learner relationship, learning also evolves from trust and understanding. The nurse builds trust by teaching information the client perceives as important and is able to understand. Teaching takes time, and the nurse must adapt to the client's learning speed. A client will sense the nurse's commitment and become more receptive to teaching endeavors.

The steps of the teaching process can be compared to those of the communication process (Table 20-1). In teaching, the referent represents the need to provide the client with information. The client may request information, or the nurse may perceive a need for it. The nurse then identifies specific learning objectives. A learning objective describes what the learner will be able to do after successful instruction.

The nurse as a teacher is the sender, whose aim is to convey a message to the client. The nurse promotes learning by communicating in language recognizable to the learner. Many intrapersonal variables influence the nurse's style and approach. The nurse's attitudes, values, emotions, and knowledge influence the way the nurse sends messages. Past experiences with teaching help the

TABLE 20-1 Comparison of Terms Used in Teaching and Communication

Communication	Teaching
REFERENT	
An idea that initiates the reason for communication	Perceived need to provide a person with information; teacher establishes relevant learning objectives
SENDER	
Person who conveys the message to another	Teacher who performs activities aimed at assisting the other person to learn
INTRAPERSONAL VARIABLES (SENDER)	
Knowledge, values, emotions, and sociocultural influences that affect the sender's thoughts	Teacher's philosophy of education (based upon learning theory); knowledge of teaching content; teaching approach; experiences in teaching; the teacher's own emotions and values
MESSAGE	
That which is expressed or transmitted by the sender	Content or information taught
CHANNELS	
Methods used to transmit a message: visual, auditory, touch	Methods used to present content: visual, auditory, touch, taste, smell
RECEIVER	
Person to whom the message is transmitted	The learner
INTRAPERSONAL VARIABLES (RECEIVER)	
Knowledge, values, emotions, and sociocultural influences that affect the receiver's thoughts	Willingness and capability to learn: physical and emotional health, education, experience, developmental level
FEEDBACK	
Information revealing that the true meaning of a message was received	Determination of whether learning objectives were achieved

nurse choose the best way to present information to a client.

As is the case with communication, the message or content to be taught is delivered clearly and precisely. The nurse organizes information to be taught in a logical sequence so the client will more easily understand skills or ideas. Each lesson is presented in a meaningful progression from simple to more complex skills or ideas.

The nurse may use several channels to present teaching content. All the senses are channels for presenting information. The auditory channel is the simplest, as in a lecture or discussion. But the learning process becomes more stimulating when several sensory channels are used.

The receiver in the teaching-learning process is the learner. As with communication, a number of intrapersonal variables affect the client's willingness and ability to learn. The client is ready to learn when expressing a desire to learn and is more likely to receive the message when perceiving and understanding the content. The client's attitudes, anxiety, and values are a few factors influencing ability to perceive a message. The ability to learn depends on the client's emotional and physical health, education, stage of development, and previous knowledge.

An effective teacher provides a mechanism for evaluating whether a teaching plan was successful. Having a client demonstrate a newly learned skill and asking the client to describe the correct dosage schedule for a medication are ways to gather feedback. Whatever form of feedback the nurse uses, it must show the success of the learner in achieving objectives; that is, the learner displays or relates what was intended to be learned.

DOMAINS OF LEARNING

Learning occurs in three areas or domains: cognitive, affective, and psychomotor. Any topic to be learned may involve all or any one learning domain. The nurse works with clients who need to learn in each domain. The characteristics of learning within each domain affect the teaching approach and methods used by a nurse as well as the method for evaluating learning.

Cognitive Learning

This domain includes learning intellectual behaviors. Bloom (1956) classified cognitive behaviors in an ordered hierarchy. The simplest behavior is acquiring knowledge, whereas the most complex is evaluation.

KNOWLEDGE

Using knowledge is acquiring new facts or information and being able to recall them. For example, a client learns about a prescribed medication and is able to describe its purpose and potential side effects.

COMPREHENSION

Comprehension is the ability to understand the meaning of learned material. For example, the client is able to explain specifically how the new medication will improve physical condition.

Application involves using abstract, newly learned ideas in concrete situations. For example, the client learns to self-administer the medication according to a meal schedule to minimize side effects.

ANALYSIS

Analysis involves relating ideas in an organized way. This allows a person to distinguish important information from unimportant information. For example, the client is able to distinguish which side effects are more likely to be experienced from the medication and to compare them with the effects experienced by another person.

SYNTHESIS

Synthesis is the ability to recognize parts of information as a whole. For example, the client experiences side effects from a medication and is able to take appropriate preventive steps.

EVALUATION

Evaluation is a judgement of the worth of a body of information for a given purpose. For example, a client is able to recognize a symptom associated with the medication.

Affective Learning

Affective learning deals with expression of feelings and acceptance toward attitudes, opinions, or values. Values clarification (see Chapter 16) is an example of affective learning. The simplest behavior in the hierarchy is receiving and the most complex is characterizing (Krathwohl, 1964).

RECEIVING

Receiving is being willing to attend to another persons' words. For example, a female client shows a willingness to listen to a nurse explain the surgical procedure for removal of the client's breast.

RESPONDING

Responding involves active participation through listening and in reacting, both verbally and nonverbally. The person feels satisfied from the response. For ex-

ample, the client asks the nurse about the appearance of the incision she will have.

VALUING

Valuing means attaching worth to an object or behavior. This is shown through the learner's behavior. The person is motivated to act out the behavior. For example, the client expresses a concern about how surgery will change her appearance. After surgery, the client refuses to look at the incision and wears a gown with a high neck.

ORGANIZING

Organizing is developing a value system by identifying and organizing values and resolving conflicts. For example, the client learns to accept changes created by surgery and is willing to participate in social activities.

CHARACTERIZING

Characterizing involves acting and responding with a consistent value system. The person behaves consistently when values are tested or challenged. For example, the client assumes a normal life-style after having breast surgery. She is able to discuss with others her positive feelings about herself.

Psychomotor Learning

The psychomotor learning domain involves acquiring skills that require the integration of mental and muscular activity such as the ability to walk or to use an eating utensil. The simplest behavior in the hierarchy is perception, whereas the most complex is origination (Simpson, 1972).

PERCEPTION

Perception is being aware of objects or qualities through the use of sense organs. A person associates a sensory cue with the task to perform. For example, when a person hears the siren of an ambulance he considers driving to the curb to avoid a collision.

SET

A set is a preparatory readiness to take a particular action. There are three sets: mental, physical, and emotional. For example, a person uses judgment to decide which is the best way to perform a motor act (mental readiness). Before performing the act, such as rising from a wheelchair, the person aligns and postures himself properly (physical readiness).

GUIDED RESPONSE

A guided response is a performance of an act under the guidance of an instructor. This involves imitation on trial and error. For example, a client fills a syringe after watching a nurse's demonstration.

MECHANISM

A mechanism is a higher level of behavior whereby a person has gained confidence and skill in performing the behavior. Usually the skill is more complex or involves several more steps than a guided response. For example, a client is able to fill a syringe for different drug doses.

COMPLEX OVERT RESPONSE

A complex overt response involves performing a motor skill involving a complex movement pattern. The person performs the skill smoothly and accurately without hesitation. For example, a client is able to self-administer an insulin injection using several sites.

ADAPTATION

Adaptation occurs when a person is able to change a motor response when unexpected problems arise. For example, as a nurse administers an injection, the appearance of blood during aspiration results in changing the way the syringe is handled.

ORIGINATION

Origination is highly complex motor act that involves creating new movement patterns. A person acts on the basis of existing psychomotor skills and abilities. For example, a nurse uses a different method of venipuncture on a client whose arm is swollen.

∎ ∎ ∎

Understanding each learning domain prepares the nurse to select proper teaching techniques. However, the nurse needs to also be able to apply basic principles of learning to any teaching method.

BASIC LEARNING PRINCIPLES

To teach effectively and efficiently the nurse must first understand how people learn. Learning depends on three conditions: the readiness to learn, the ability to learn, and the learning environment. A person's emotional readiness to learn is a reflection of a desire to learn. Readiness means that a person is willing to take necessary action to become involved in learning. Previous knowledge, attitudes, and sociocultural influences combine to form a person's experiential readiness.

The ability to learn depends on the learner's physical and cognitive attributes. Developmental level, physical wellness, and intellectual thought processes determine whether a person is capable of learning. If a person's learning ability is impaired, a teacher postpones teaching

activities or modifies strategies to better meet the learner's needs.

The environment has a significant impact on a person's ability to learn. One of the teacher's major tasks is to manipulate environmental conditions to facilitate learning.

Readiness to Learn

ATTENTIONAL SET

Our minds generally function with mental pictures. While a teacher explains how to give support to a dying client, we might envision grasping the fragile hand of a person taking a last breath. Before we can learn, we must give attention to, or concentrate on, information to be learned. An attentional set is an internal state of the learner that allows focusing and comprehension. A number of factors influence a learner's ability to attend: physical discomfort, anxiety, and environmental distractions.

Any physical condition that impairs a person's ability to concentrate interferes with learning. Pain, fatigue, hunger, thirst, and even the urge to urinate or defecate create barriers to learning.

Anxiety may increase or decrease the ability of a person to attend. Anxiety is uneasiness from anticipation of threat or danger. Anytime a person faces change or the need to act differently, anxiety normally results. Learning requires a change in behavior and thus produces anxiety. A mild level of anxiety may motivate a person to learn. If a student did not become anxious about an upcoming examination, study is unlikely. However, a high level of anxiety prevents learning. Severe anxiety incapacitates a person, creating an inability to attend to anything other than its immediate relief.

Environmental distractions (discussed in a later section) interfere with the ability to attend to a teacher and to learning activities. Unplanned interruptions or an uncomfortable environment are not conducive to learning.

MOTIVATION

Motivation is an internal impulse that causes a person to take action. The motivation to learn is the desire to learn. A person may become motivated to learn by an idea, emotion, or physical need. If a person does not want to learn, it is unlikely that learning will occur.

There are three types of motives that stimulate a person to learn: social, task mastery, and physical. Social motives are a need for affiliation, social approval, or self-esteem. For example, often a student works hard to win praise from a teacher. Task mastery motives are based on needs such as achievement and competence. A nursing student repeatedly works in a laboratory to learn the technique for giving an injection because of the motivation to master the task or skill. Once success is gained, there is usually greater motivation to achieve more.

Often the motives of a health care client are of a physical nature. If a client suffers a physical change in function, that change may become a motivator for learning. When a client is in pain, for example, there is great motivation to learn methods for pain relief.

Not everyone is interested in maintaining health. A person with lung disease may continue to smoke. A woman whose obesity worsens her heart condition may refuse to follow her diet. All the therapies in the world will have little effect unless a person is motivated by the belief that health is important. The trend in health care is to treat clients in their homes after they recover from the acute phase of illness. Treatment in the home can be successful only if the client complies with recommendations of the physician and health care team. The obese woman will not reduce her weight unless she becomes motivated by the benefits of weight loss. Compliance is the client's fulfillment of the prescribed course of therapy and the nurse's ultimate goal in any health teaching plan.

A person's *health beliefs* can be powerful motivators, and they are influenced by a number of variables (see Chapter 2). Four health beliefs are critical to a client taking a health action (Rosenstock, 1960):

1. The person believes he or she is susceptible to the disease in question.
2. The person believes the disease would have serious effects on his or her life.
3. The person believes that actions can be taken to reduce the likelihood of contracting the disease or lessen its severity.
4. The person believes the threat of taking these actions is not as great as the threat of the disease.

The nurse's knowledge of a client's health beliefs helps determine what factors will motivate learning. However, there is no standard method for motivating a person with a given health belief. Health teaching often involves a changing of attitudes and values that are not altered by simple teaching of facts. Therefore the nurse gives attention to ideas or beliefs that motivate a person to learn, and applies the motivating factor to the teaching plan. For example:

TABLE 20-2   Relationship Between Psychosocial Adaptation to Illness and Learning

Stage of Grieving	Clients' Behavior	Learning Implications	Rationale
Denial	Client avoids discussion of illness ("There's nothing wrong with me"), withdraws from others, and disregards physical restrictions.	Provide support, empathy, and careful explanations of all procedures while they are being done. Let the client know you are available for discussion when he or she is ready. Explain to the family what is happening. Teach in the present tense (for example, explain current therapy).	Any attempt to convince or tell the client he or she is ill will result in further anger or withdrawal (client is not prepared to deal with his problem). Provide only information he pursues or absolutely requires.
Anger	Client blames and complains and often directs anger toward the nurse.	Do not argue with the client. Listen to concerns, and teach in the present tense. Reassure the family of the client's normality.	Client needs opportunity to express feelings and anger; he or she is still not prepared to face the future.
Bargaining	Client offers to live a better life in exchange for promise of better health ("If God lets me live, I promise to be more careful").	Continue to introduce only reality. Teaching remains in present tense.	Client is still unwilling to accept limitations.
Resolution	Client begins to express emotions openly, realizes illness has created changes, and begins to ask questions.	Encourage expression of feelings. Begin to share information needed for the future, and set aside formal times for discussion.	Client begins to perceive the need for assistance and is ready to accept responsibility for learning.
Acceptance	Client recognizes the reality of his or her condition, actively pursues information, and strives for independence.	Focus teaching on future skills and knowledge required. Continue to teach about present occurrences. Involve family in teaching information for discharge.	Client is more easily motivated to learn. Acceptance of his illness reflects a willingness to deal with implications.

Mr. James is a 42-year-old businessman with high blood pressure. The nurse recognizes that Mr. James needs to learn about his condition, the type of treatment, and implications of his illness for his busy life-style. Mr. James is a highly motivated man who works hard for success. He admits that he has always felt himself invincible to any physical malady. Now he tells the nurse that he knows he cannot continue his hectic work pace unless he regains his health.

The nurse's teaching plan will integrate two principal motivators that Mr. James has acknowledged: the desire to succeed and the concern that high blood pressure will seriously affect his work life. The nurse will use Mr. James' motivation for success as the means to help him acquire better health habits. Mr. James will learn how high blood pressure impairs physical function and the ways in which he can avoid factors in his work environment that can aggravate blood pressure problems.

PSYCHOSOCIAL ADAPTATION TO ILLNESS

A loss of health, whether temporary or permanent, is difficult for a person to accept. The process of grieving allows the person time to adapt psychologically to the emotional and physical implications of illness. The stages of grieving (see Chapter 26) are a series of responses clients experience during illness. People experience the stages at different rates and sequences; some people fail to complete all stages. The implication for learning is that a person's readiness to learn is significantly related to his stage of grieving (Table 20-2, p. 527). Learning will not occur when a client is unwilling or unable to accept the reality of illness. The nurse identifies the client's stage of grieving on the basis of typical behaviors. When the client enters the stage of acceptance, which is compatible with learning, the nurse presents a teaching plan. Continuous assessment of the client's behaviors determines what stages of grieving the client is in. Teaching continues as long as the client remains in a stage conducive to learning.

ACTIVE PARTICIPATION

A client's involvement in learning implies an eagerness to acquire knowledge or skills. It also improves the likelihood that the client will have the opportunity for decision making during teaching sessions. For example, a client diagnosed as a diabetic must learn how diet and exercise can control the disease. Through participation with the nurse and dietitian the client learns to adapt a new diet and exercise routine to his or her personal life-style. The client helps decide what type of meal plan will work best.

Roter (1987) describes a partnership model for health education between nurse and client. The model stresses the value of clients collaborating with nurses during any educational activity. In learning through participation, there is a greater transfer of knowledge and a learner gains confidence in the ability to solve problems. In ad-dition the client gains knowledge and skills that will be useful and meaningful in day-to-day experiences.

Ability to Learn
DEVELOPMENTAL CAPABILITY

A person's cognitive level of development influences ability to learn. A nurse can be a competent teacher, but if the client's intellectual abilities are not considered, teaching will be unsuccessful. A teaching booklet will not be useful if a client is found to be illiterate. A client who is unable to perform simple mathematical calculations will have difficulty learning to measure medication dosages.

Learning is an evolving process, as is developmental growth. The nurse must know the client's level of knowledge and intellectual skills before beginning a teaching plan. Table 20-3 shows the types of learning problems clients may have when their intellectual skills are not fully developed.

There is a requisite level of maturation and cognitive development before an individual becomes capable of learning. The nurse is wrong to assume the client has a certain level of knowledge. The client's level of knowledge should be assessed before starting any teaching plan. Learning occurs more readily when new information complements existing knowledge.

AGE GROUP. Age reflects the developmental capability for learning and learning behavior that can be acquired (Table 20-4). Without proper biological, motor, language, and personal-social developmental, many types of learning cannot take place (Fig. 20-1, p. 530).

TABLE 20-3 Cognitive Skills and Learning Implications

Intellectual Skill	Examples of Potential Learning Problems
Math calculation	Computing drug dosages; measuring liquid or solid food allotments; reading a thermometer or syringe calibrations
Reading	Reading directions and instructions in teaching booklets and on medication labels
Problem solving	Learning how to regulate insulin dosages on the basis of signs and symptoms
Comprehension and application	Understanding physical restrictions imposed by illness; following directions in performing self-care in accordance with limitations

TABLE 20-4 Developmental Capacities for Learning

Learning Capacity	Teaching Methods
INFANT	
Relies on parents for basic needs. Learns to trust adults when they convey love and compassion. Explores the environment through the senses.	Keep routines (e.g. feeding, bathing) consistent. Hold an infant firmly while smiling and speaking softly to convey a sense of trust.
TODDLER	
Learns to understand words and to express feelings verbally. Also learns by associating words with objects. Likes to explore the environment through play.	Use play to teach a toddler a procedure or activity (for example, handling examination equipment, applying a bandage to a doll). Offer picture books that describe the story of children in a hospital or clinic. Use simple words such as "cut" instead of "laceration" to promote understanding.
PRESCHOOLER	
Vocabulary grows. Preschoolers use language without comprehending meaning of words, especially concepts (for example, right or left and time). During play the child expresses feelings more through actions than words. Preschoolers ask questions and imitate adults.	Role playing, imitation, and play make it fun for preschoolers to learn. Encourage questions and offer explanations. Simple explanations and demonstrations work well. Preschools encourage children to learn together through pictures and short stories of how to perform hygiene.
SCHOOL-AGE CHILD	
Interacts with adults and peers outside the immediate family. Begins to acquire the ability to relate a series of events and actions to mental representations that can be expressed verbally and symbolically. Are able to make judgments on what they reason. Child matures physically. Play becomes more formal and imaginative. Is inquisitive and asks many questions about health.	Can learn psychomotor skills needed to maintain health. Complicated skills, such as learning to use a syringe, may take considerable practice. Offer opportunities to discuss health problems and answer questions.
ADOLESCENT	
Struggles between childlike feelings of dependence and the independence of adults. Wants to be in control but during illness, fears loss of self-concept or body image. Is able to solve abstract problems and hypothesize relationships. Learn best when an immediate benefit is gained.	Help adolescents learn about their feelings and the need for self-expression. Teaching must be a collaborative activity. Allow adolescents to make decisions about health and health promotion (for example, safety, sex education, substance abuse). Problem solving helps adolescents make choices.
YOUNG AND MIDDLE ADULT	
Adult clients comply with health teaching because they either fear the results if they do not, are trying to gain approval, are responding to the nurses' attitude toward them, or know it is in their best interest (Woodard, 1983.) Learning occurs when adults value information being taught.	Encourage adults to participate in the teaching plan by setting mutual goals. Independent learning can be successful. Offer information so adult can understand effects of health problem.
OLDER ADULT	
Many elderly have sensory alterations, mobility limitations, and physical coordination problems that affect the capacity to learn. The elderly take pride in being independent and caring for themselves. There is no decline in intelligence with age.	Teach when clients are alert and rested. Older adult learners enjoy being involved in discussion or activity. Focus on wellness and the person's strengths. Use approaches that enhance a sensorially impaired client's communication (see Chapter 44). Keep teaching sessions short.

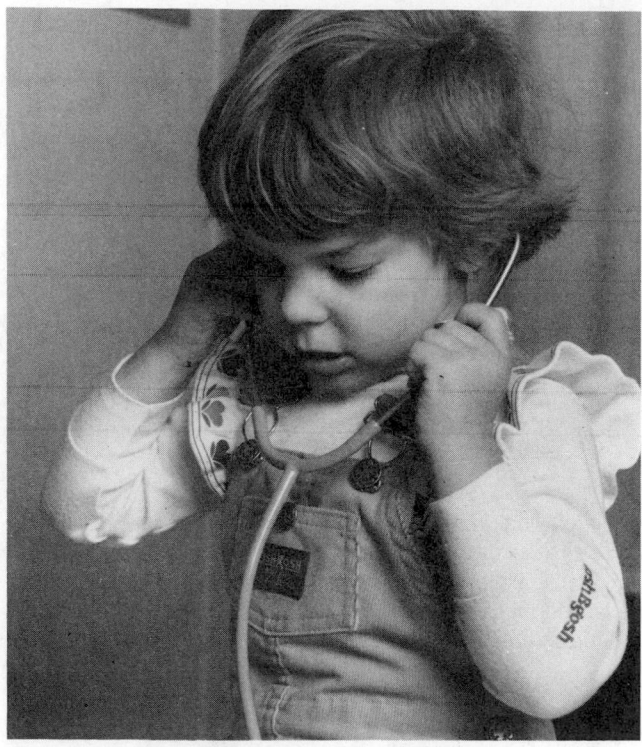

Fig. 20-1 The preschool child learns not to be afraid of medical equipment by being allowed to handle the stethoscope and imitating its use.

Learning occurs when behavior changes as a result of experience or growth (Whaley and Wong, 1987).

PHYSICAL CAPABILITY

Ability to learn often depends on the level of physical development and overall physical health. To learn psychomotor skills, a client must possess the necessary level of strength, coordination, and sensory acuity. For example, it will be useless to teach a client how to transfer from a bed to a wheelchair unless he or she has sufficient upper body strength. An elderly client cannot learn to apply an elastic bandage if his eyesight is poor and his fingers cannot grasp the bandage tightly. Therefore the nurse should not overestimate the client's physical development. The following physical attributes are required to learn psychomotor skills:

1. Size (height and weight match the task to perform or the equipment to use; for example, crutch walking)
2. Strength (ability to follow strenuous exercise program)
3. Coordination (dexterity needed for complicated motor skills, such as using utensils or changing a bandage)
4. Sensory acuity (visual, auditory, touch, taste, and smell: sensory modalities needed to receive and respond to messages taught)

The nurse assesses a client's physical capabilities before beginning instruction.

Mrs. Lyon is a 68-year-old woman who received a prescription from her physician for a heart medication that slows the heart's rate. It is important that Mrs. Lyon learn how to check her pulse to be sure her heart does not beat too slowly. The nurse's assessment reveals that Mrs. Lyon is unable to feel an arterial pulse because her fingers are stiff and callused. No one who lives with Mrs. Lyon can check her pulse for her. However, Mrs. Lyon's hearing is still good. The nurse chooses an alternative: teaching Mrs. Lyon how to listen to her heartbeat with a stethoscope.

In larger hospitals, clinics, or community health agencies the services of physical therapists can be valuable in assessing a client's physical capabilities. The therapist can measure a client's activity tolerance and determine if assistive devices are needed.

Any condition (for example, pain) that depletes a person's energy will also impair ability to learn. A client who spends a morning undergoing a rigorous schedule of studies and tests will unlikely be capable of a learning discussion. When a client's illness becomes aggravated by complications, such as a high fever or respiratory difficulty, teaching should be postponed. The nurse assesses a client's energy level by noting the willingness to communicate, amount of activity initiated, and responsiveness toward questions. The nurse may halt teaching temporarily if a client needs rest. The nurse achieves greater teaching success when the client is an active participant in learning.

Learning Environment

The physical environment where teaching takes place makes learning either pleasant or difficult. The nurse chooses a setting that helps the client focus on the learning task. The following factors are important when choosing the setting:

1. Number of persons being taught
2. Need for privacy
3. Temperature
4. Lighting
5. Noise
6. Ventilation
7. Furniture

The ideal environment for learning is a room with good lighting, good ventilation, appropriate furniture, and a comfortable temperature (Fig. 20-2). A darkened room will interfere with the client's ability to see, especially during demonstrations and use of visual aids. A room that is cold, hot, or humid and stuffy will make

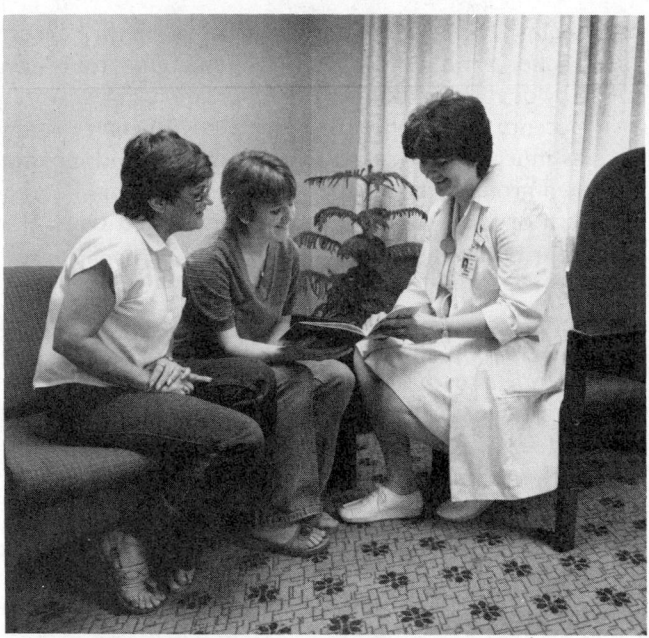

Fig. 20-2 Choosing a comfortable, pleasant environment enhances the learning experience. This nurse is using a teaching booklet to explain health care principles to the client and a family member.

the client too uncomfortable to attend to the nurse's activities. Comfortable furniture helps eliminate distractions, such as the need to continually change position or shift body weight.

It is also important to choose a quiet setting. In a hospital the nurses' station has constant activity, with telephones ringing and several conversations occurring at the same time. In a client's home the sounds of the television prevent a person from listening attentively. These sounds, instead of the teacher, become the focus of attention.

When a nurse is working with only one client, the best setting is a quiet one that offers privacy. The nurse can provide privacy even in a busy hospital by closing cubicle curtains or taking the client to a quiet spot. In a client's home a bedroom might separate the client from household activities. If the client desires, family members might share in discussions. However, some clients are reluctant to discuss their illness when others, even close family members, are in the room.

Teaching a group of clients requires a room that allows everyone to be seated comfortably and within hearing distance of the teacher. The size of the room should not overwhelm the group, tempting participants to sit outside the group along the room's perimeter. Arranging the group to allow participants to observe one another further enhances learning. More effective communica-

tion occurs as learners observe others' verbal and nonverbal interactions.

BASIC TEACHING PRINCIPLES

Teaching is the process of leading someone to learn. Just as there are basic principles that promote learning, there are also principles that improve a teacher's effectiveness. The realm of teaching deals with the (1) teacher's behavior, (2) reason teachers behave the way they do, and (3) effects of their behavior on students. There is no single way to teach correctly. Each learning situation has different implications for the best way to teach. The principles of teaching are basically techniques of the principles of learning.

Timing

When is the right time to teach? When a client first enters a clinic or hospital? At the time of discharge? Each may be appropriate since clients continue to have learning needs and opportunities as long as they stay in the health care system. Teaching must be timed to coincide with the client's readiness to learn. This can be difficult, since emphasis is placed on a client's early discharge from a hospital. For example, following surgery, it may take several days for a client to become free of discomfort so that he can attend to learning. By the time the client feels ready to learn, discharge may already be scheduled. The nurse should plan teaching activities for a time when the client is most attentive, receptive, and alert. Many hospitals are providing information to clients before their admission. The client's activities should be organized to provide time for rest as well as time for teaching-learning interactions. The client who receives drugs that cause drowsiness or impair concentration should be taught before the drugs are given.

The length of teaching sessions also influences learning ability. Prolonged sessions cause clients to lose concentration and attentiveness. Frequent sessions lasting 20 to 30 minutes are more easily tolerated and retain the client's interest. The nurse can assess a client's loss of concentration by observing for nonverbal cues, such as poor eye contact or slumped posture. Once loss of concentration is noted, the session should be stopped. However, teaching sessions should not be too brief. The client needs time during each session to comprehend the information and to give feedback regarding understanding.

Teaching sessions should be held frequently enough to document the client's learning. The frequency of sessions depends on the learner's abilities and the complexity of the material. Intervals between teaching sessions should not be so long that the client might forget information. For clients discharged home early, it is essential that home health nurses reinforce learning.

Organizing Teaching Material

A good teacher carefully considers the order in which to present information. An outline helps organize information into a logical sequence. Material should progress from simple to complex ideas because a person must learn the basics before making associations or complex interpretations of ideas. For example, to teach a client how to calculate a 1200-calorie diet, the nurse teaches what calories, proteins, and carbohydrates are, and then uses simple math to help the client learn to calculate amounts.

It is also helpful to begin instruction with essential content. Clients are more likely to remember information that is taught during the first third of a teaching session (Miller, 1985). For example, after removal of a cancerous lung tumor, the client's risk for recurrence makes learning the warning signs of cancer crucial. Start with essential information and then complete a teaching session with informative but less critical content.

It also helps to summarize important points. Repetition reinforces learning. A concise summary of key topics will help the learner know the most important information.

Speaking the Client's Language

It is important to use words a client can understand. The nurse defines unfamiliar medical or nursing terms and uses them consistently throughout a teaching session. Medical jargon can be confusing.

Byrne and Edeani (1984) found that clients understand fewer medical words than health professionals predict. The problem of functional illiteracy is also real. Kozol (1985) reports that in the United States 44% of black adults, 33% of Hispanic adults and 16% of white adults are functionally or marginally illiterate.

The nurse uses simple terminology to enhance clients' understanding. Frequently asking clients for feedback determines if clients comprehend.

Maintaining Learner Attention and Participation

Active participation is a key learning principle. However, it is the teacher's responsibility to find ways to keep learners interested and involved. Learning is improved when more than one of the body's senses are stimulated. Audiovisual aids, drawings, and printed materials stimulate learner attention.

A teacher's actions can also increase learner attention and interest. When conducting a discussion with a client, the teacher should stay active by changing tone and intensity of voice, making eye contact, and using gestures that accentuate key points. An effective teacher often uses as much energy as the learner, talking and moving among a group rather than remaining stationary behind a lectern or table. A client remains interested when the teacher is enthusiastic.

Building on Existing Knowledge

A client learns best on the basis of preexisting cognitive abilities and knowledge. Thus a teacher will be more effective by building on a learner's knowledge. The key to this is finding out how much the learner knows about the topic.

Teaching must be individualized on the basis of the client's learning needs. Clients will quickly lose interest if a nurse begins with familiar information.

Reinforcing

The principle of reinforcement applies to the process of learning; however, it is often the teacher who must be the source of reinforcement. *Reinforcement* is using a stimulus that increases probability of a response. A learner who receives reinforcement before or after a desired learning behavior will likely repeat the behavior. Feedback is a common form of reinforcement.

Reinforcers are either positive or negative. Positive reinforcement, such as a smile or approval, produces desired responses. A reinforcement is negative if its removal from a situation following a response produces the desired behavior. Threatening, complaining, and criticizing are examples of negative reinforcers. People usually respond better to positive reinforcement. The effects of negative reinforcement are less predictable and often undesirable.

There are three types of reinforcers: social, material, and activity. When a nurse works with a client, most reinforcers are social—a smile, compliment, word of encouragement, or physical contact. A nurse uses verbal and nonverbal communication when acknowledging that a skill has been learned well. Examples of material reinforcers are food, toys, and music. These work best with young children.

Activity reinforcers rely on the principle that a person is motivated to engage in an activity if promised that, after its completion, he will be able to do something else he likes better. A client will more likely perform a painful exercise if given the chance to take a nap afterwards.

Choosing an appropriate reinforcer involves careful thought and attention to preferences. Observing a client's behavior often helps reveal the best one to use. Reinforcers should never be used as a threat, and reinforcement is not always effective with every client. Young children tend to respond more to social reinforcers than older children or adults. An adult with whom the nurse has a good relationship is more effectively reinforced than an adult with whom the nurse has a poor relationship. Thus trusting relationship with a client yields results when attempting to provide positive reinforcers for learning.

Matching Teaching Methods with Learners' Needs

The effectiveness of a teaching method depends in part on the client's learning need. Clients with psychomotor deficits learn best through demonstrations and supervised practice. The client masters skills by manipulating equipment and practicing manual skills. Discussions, question-and-answer sessions, and formal lectures are effective for promoting cognitive learning. Clients with intellectual deficits are given the opportunity to explore new ideas, recognize new relationships, and apply knowledge to their unique needs. A highly effective method for stimulating affective learning is group discussion. Clients learn to share ideas and values with one another, realizing there are alternative ways to view the world. Whatever the method, it should complement the client's needs.

NURSING PROCESS IN TEACHING

Teaching can become habitual for a nurse experienced in a specialty area of nursing. A nurse working in an orthopedic unit will be much more comfortable teaching a client how to use crutches than will a nurse who works in a gynecologist's office. Achieving spontaneity in teaching does not eliminate the need for a methodical approach toward teaching, however. Spontaneity has the benefit of making both the nurse and client more at ease during the teaching process, but regardless of a nurse's familiarity with certain educational topics, each learner is different. Thus an individualized approach toward the teaching process ensures that the nurse will meet a client's learning needs.

The nursing process provides a useful framework for individualizing the teaching process. The two processes are not the same. The nursing process requires an assessment of all sources of data to determine a client's total health care needs. The teaching process focuses primarily on the client's learning needs in addition to the willingness and capability to learn. Table 20-5 compares the teaching and nursing processes.

ASSESSMENT

Success in teaching a client requires the nurse to assess what influences the content to be taught, the client's ability to learn, and methods and resources for instruction. The client, family members, and the health care team are resources for the nurse's assessment.

LEARNING NEEDS

What information is critical for the client to learn? The client's learning needs determine the choice of teaching content.

TABLE 20-5   Comparison of the Nursing Process and the Teaching Process

Basic Steps	Nursing Process	Teaching Process
Assessment	Collect data about the client's physical, psychological, social, cultural, developmental, and spiritual needs. Sources of data are the client, family, diagnostic tests, medical record, nursing history, and literature.	Gather data about the client's learning needs, willingness to learn, ability to learn, and teaching resources. Sources of data are the client, family, learning environment, medical record, nursing history, and literature.
Diagnosis	Identify appropriate nursing diagnoses.	Identify client's learning needs on the basis of the three domains of learning.
Planning	Develop an individualized plan of care. Set diagnosis priorities on the basis of client's immediate needs. Nurse and client collaborate on plan of care.	Establish learning objectives, stated in behavioral terms. Identify priorities regarding client's learning needs. Nurse and client collaborate on teaching plan. Identify type of teaching method to use.
Implementation	Perform nursing care therapies. Include client as an active participant in care. Involve family in client's care as appropriate.	Implement teaching methods. Actively involve client in learning activities. Include family participation as appropriate.
Evaluation	Identify success in meeting desired outcomes of nursing care.	Determine outcomes of teaching-learning process. Measure client's ability to achieve learning objectives.

The nurse assesses:

1. Questions raised by the client or family about health issues.
2. The client's level of understanding of current health status, implications of illness, types of therapy, and prognosis.
3. Information or skills needed by the client to perform self-care and to understand his condition and its implications. (Health care members anticipate learning needs related to specific health problems. For example, a newly diagnosed diabetic will obviously need to learn about dietary control. A client who has had major surgery must learn the physical restrictions imposed by the procedure).
4. The client's experiences that influence the need to learn. For example, a client who has had surgery before is more likely to be familiar with preoperative procedures.
5. Information family members require to support the client's needs. This will depend on the extent of the family's role in helping the client.

READINESS TO LEARN

Is the client prepared and willing to learn? The nurse assesses:

1. Client behavior (attention span, tendency to ask questions, memory, and ability to concentrate during questioning).
2. Presence of pain, fatigue, anxiety, or other symptoms that can interfere with a client's ability to attend and participate.
3. Factors that motivate the client to learn (social, task mastery, or physical).
4. Client's sociocultural background. A client's beliefs and values about health and various therapies may influence willingness to learn.

ABILITY TO LEARN

What physical and cognitive capabilities does the client possess for learning? The nurse assesses:

1. Physical strength, movement, and coordination. The nurse determines to what extent the client can perform skills to be taught.
2. Presence of sensory deficits that may affect the client's ability to understand or follow instruction.
3. The client's reading level. This can be difficult to assess since functionally illiterate clients are often able to conceal it. Ask a client to read instructions from a teaching brochure and then explain its meaning.
4. The client's developmental level.

TEACHING ENVIRONMENT

The environment for a teaching session must be conducive to learning. The nurse assesses:

1. Presence of distractions. A quiet area should be set aside for teaching.
2. Comfort of the room including ventilation and temperature.
3. Room facilities and available equipment.

RESOURCES FOR LEARNING

The family may become directly involved in caring for the client. The nurse needs to understand the home environment in which the client lives. Resources also include teaching aids available. The nurse assesses:

1. Family members' perceptions and understanding of the client's illness and its implications. Family perceptions should match those of the client, otherwise conflicts may arise in the teaching plan.
2. The client's willingness to have family members involved in the teaching plan. Information about the client's health care is confidential unless the client chooses to share it.
3. Resources within the home. These include persons willing to assist the client with procedures such as bathing or taking medications; financial or material resources such as health care equipment; and architectural resources such as arrangement of rooms or stairways.
4. Teaching aids including printed materials, audiovisual aids, or charts. Printed material should match the client's reading level and present subject material clearly and logically. Brochures or booklets must be current.

NURSING DIAGNOSIS

After assessing information related to the client's ability and need to learn, the nurse uses it to form diagnoses that reflect learning needs. This ensures the nurse's teaching will be goal directed or individualized. If a client has several learning needs, nursing diagnoses allow for setting priorities.

Each diagnostic statement describes the specific learning need and its cause. Classifying diagnoses by the three learning domains helps focus on what and how to teach. Examples of diagnoses related to clients' learning needs are shown in the nursing diagnoses box.

Some health care problems can be managed or eliminated through education. In these situations the related factor stated in the diagnostic statement is knowledge deficit (see sample nursing diagnosis box). For example, a client may have difficulty interacting socially caused by a lack of effective communication skills.

There are also nursing diagnoses that indicate teaching may be inappropriate. The nurse may identify conditions that can cause barriers to effective learning (for example, pain or activity intolerance).

Examples of Nursing Diagnoses Related to Learning Needs

NANDA-APPROVED NURSING DIAGNOSES

Altered health maintenance related to:
- Lack of knowledge about health practices
- Lack of fine motor skills

Knowledge deficit: affective related to:
- Misunderstanding of prognosis

Knowledge deficit: cognitive related to:
- Newly diagnosed disease
- Newly prescribed therapy

Knowledge deficit: psychomotor related to:
- Inexperience with crutchwalking
- Lack of interest in learning

Noncompliance with medications related to:
- Poor understanding of therapies

Impaired social interaction related to:
- Altered affective knowledge

PLANNING

During development of a teaching plan the nurse determines expected outcomes and involves the client in selecting learning experiences. A teacher must know what a student should accomplish. Expected outcomes of the plan guide the choice of teaching strategies and approaches with clients. Client participation ensures a more relevant and meaningful teaching plan.

TEACHING PRIORITIES

Teaching priorities are set reflecting the priorities of a client's nursing diagnoses. A client's learning needs must be prioritized to conserve time and energy of both the client and nurse. For example, a client with a permanent leg injury has a knowledge deficit regarding the nature of the injury and its implications, as well as the types of skills needed to resume normal life at home. The client will benefit most from first learning about the injury and the resultant physical changes before learning how to cope with the disability.

LEARNING OBJECTIVES

A learning objective identifies the expected outcome of a learning experience. Objectives are either short or long term. Short-term objectives relate to the client's immediate learning needs, such as knowing the nature of gallbladder disease to understand an upcoming test. Long-term objectives have been met—for example, learning to plan a diet within restrictions imposed by gallbladder disease.

The nurse and client develop learning objectives to-

Sample Nursing Diagnoses for Learning Needs		
Defining Characteristics	**Nursing Diagnoses**	**Related Factors**
Newly diagnosed as having diabetes Inability to explain or discuss nature of disease Questions asked about meaning of diabetes and its implications Client previously very healthy.	Knowledge deficit: cognitive	- Newly diagnosed disease - Unfamiliarity with disease process
Fractured right leg placed in cast Physician order of non-weight-bearing crutch stance Good upper body strength Crutches not used before	Knowledge deficit: psychomotor	- Inexperience with crutchwalking
Demonstrated lack of knowledge regarding basic health practices Expressed interest in improving health behaviors Reported or observed lack of resources (financial or equipment) Inability to take responsibility for health practices	Altered health maintenance	- Lack of fine motor skills - Ineffective individual coping - Lack of knowledge about health practices

gether. Learning objectives should be specific, indicating what behavior the learner should master, under what conditions, and under what standards. Learning objectives make the teacher and learner more comfortable in knowing what to expect from the teaching-learning process, and specific objectives clarify these expectations.

Each learning objective involves three aspects: statement of a behavior and content, identification of the conditions for learning, and identification of criteria for achieving the behavior.

Each objective points to a *behavior,* reflecting the learner's ability to do something after a learning experience. A behavioral objective contains an active verb describing what the learner will do once the objective is met, such as *to walk* with crutches or *to identify* drug dosages. These are measurable and observable. The nurse observes for behavioral changes in the client as a result of the teaching plan.

If content is missing, the objective cannot guide teaching and learning. A behavioral objective also indicates the content to be learned, for example: "to perform the *three-point crutch gait.*" The objectives describe precise behaviors and content. This becomes the standard for feedback that reflects a client's learning and forms the basis for evaluation of the teaching plan.

An objective is more precise when it also describes *conditions* under which the behavior occurs. Conditions should be realistic and designed for the learner's needs. It is also helpful to consider conditions under which the client or family will typically perform the learning behavior; for example, "to walk from bedroom to bath using crutches."

The criteria for acceptable performance set a standard by which achievement of an objective is measured. A teacher sets criteria on the basis of a desired level of accuracy, success, or satisfaction. For example, a client undergoing therapy for a fractured leg will walk on crutches *to the end of the hall within 3 days.* Criteria are more acceptable when established jointly by the teacher and learner. However, the nurse serves as a resource in setting the minimal criteria for success. Mutually agreed on criteria help to define expected behaviors and quality of performance. The client uses the criteria as a form of self-evaluation, which is a powerful motivator of behavior.

TABLE 20-6 Teaching Methods

Teaching Method	Description
COGNITIVE	
Discussion (one-on-one or group)	May involve nurse and client only or nurse with several clients. Promote active participation and focusing on topics of interest to client. Group discussions lend peer support.
Lecture	More formal method of instruction, controlled by teacher.
Question-and-answer session	Designed specifically to address client's concerns. Assists client in application of knowledge.
Teaching booklets, visual aids, computerized instructional programs	Learners use material independently at their own speed. Instructor reinforces or clarifies information. Material must be at client's reading level.
Role playing	Client can actively apply knowledge in a controlled situation.
AFFECTIVE	
Role playing	Client's active participation in acting out a role allows for expression of values, feelings, and attitudes.
Discussion (group)	Client can acquire support from others in a group. Learns from other clients' experiences.
Discussion (one-on-one)	Client can discuss personal, sensitive topics of interest or concern.
PSYCHOMOTOR	
Demonstration	Nurse performs procedures or skill in same manner in which client will later perform it. The client can incorporate modeling of nurses' behavior. Nurse controls questioning during demonstration.
Practice	Client has opportunity to perform skill using actual equipment. Provides for repetition.
Return demonstration	Client performs skill as nurse observes. Excellent source of feedback and reinforcement.

SELECTION OF TEACHING METHODS

During planning the nurse chooses appropriate teaching methods and encourages the client to offer suggestions. A teaching method is the way the teacher delivers information. The teaching method chosen depends on the client's knowledge deficit: cognitive, affective, or psychomotor (Table 20-6). More than one method may be used for instruction. A client's fear or anxiety affects the initial selection of a teaching method. For example, a client who has recently undergone a mastectomy will likely feel anxious about her appearance. A private discussion with the nurse about incisional care will be more acceptable than a group discussion.

TIMING

The nurse and client collaborate to set the best time for a teaching session. The client is often the best resource for acknowledging fatigue, pain, or other discomfort. In a hospital setting the nurse knows the time of tests and procedures the client must undergo during the day. A teaching session is ideally conducted without interruptions. In the home setting a client will prefer a teaching session that does not interfere with important daily routines. For example, if a home health nurse plans to teach a client the way to bathe an infant, it will be best at a time convenient to the mother and when the infant is less likely to be asleep.

WRITTEN TEACHING PLANS

In all health care settings nurses develop written teaching plans for use by colleagues. The written plan includes topics to include in instruction, optional resources (for example, equipment or teaching booklets) and expected outcomes or goals of the teaching plan. A plan may be extensive or in outline format. When several nurses are involved, the written plan should be specific to ensure continuity. Changes in the plan are communicated to the client and health care team. Health team members such as dietitians or social workers may contribute to the plan. A step-by-step description of teaching content is useful if several teaching sessions are needed. It is easier to implement a teaching plan when the nurse knows at what point the last teaching session ended to avoid unnecessary duplication. The care plan box is an example of a written teaching plan.

Sample Nursing Care Plan for Learning Needs

Nursing Diagnosis	Goal	Expected Outcomes	Nursing Interventions
Knowledge deficit: cognitive related to newly diagnosed disease	Client will attain self-care of diabetes.	Client will identify the signs and symptoms of hypoglycemia.	Conduct a one-to-one discussion with client and wife on diabetes pathophysiology and symptomatology.
		Client will describe the disease process of diabetes.	Provide teaching booklet, *Know Your Diabetes.* Use flip chart containing diagrams of diabetic signs and symptoms and related causes. Offer opportunity during mid-morning and early afternoon for client to ask questions.
		Client selects a daily meal plan containing correct dietary sources.	Conduct two to three short lectures on the importance of diet in diabetes control. Provide pamphlets on food exchanges and sample menus. Have client select a menu for each meal of the day.

IMPLEMENTATION

Implementation of a teaching plan involves application of all teaching and learning principles:

1. Know the client's learning needs.
2. Select a time that coincides with the client's readiness and ability to learn.
3. Know the client's ability to comprehend (see research highlight).
4. Select a teaching method that fits the learning domain.
5. Involve the client and/or family actively in the teaching plan.
6. Be aware of personal teaching abilities (knowledgeable of content, interested in the learner, aware of personal behavior and motives).
7. Use a teaching approach that fits the task and relationship behaviors. (Table 20-6).
8. Use appropriate teaching aids .
9. Control the environment so it is conducive to learning.
10. Use repetition and reinforcement appropriately.
11. Give the client feedback.
12. Select and prioritize content.

Implementation involves anticipating each interaction with a client as an opportunity for effective learning; watching for behaviors during a teaching session that suggest the client is losing interest or the ability to attend;

✄ *Research Highlight* ✄

Streiff (1986) understood that the problem of functional illiteracy is growing in the United States. Nurses often rely on educational pamphlets or brochures as teaching aids for clients. However, most are written at well above the eighth grade level. A reading level below fifth grade is considered functional illiteracy.

Streiff conducted a study to determine if clients in an ambulatory care setting read at a level allowing them to comprehend educational material. Streiff interviewed 106 adults and their reported and actual reading levels were compared. Reported reading levels, indicated by the client's last grade completed in school, were significantly higher (mean = 3.1 grades) than actual reading level. The majority of clients (54.7%) read at levels that did not allow them to comprehend any educational materials available at their site of primary care.

Streiff, LD: Can clients understand our instructions? Image J Nurs Sch 18(2):48, 1986.

---

and using a diversified approach to create an active student-teacher exchange of ideas.

TEACHING APPROACHES

A nurse's approach in teaching is different from methodology. Approach involves the nurses' task and relationship behaviors (Paulish, 1987). Some situations require a teacher to be directive while others require a non directive approach. An effective teacher concentrates on the task and recognizes that the approach may change based on the learner's response.

A client's needs and motives can change. Thus, the nurse must always be aware of the need to change teaching approaches. Paulish (1987) suggests a model for teaching approaches based upon situational leadership theory (see Chapter 48).

TELLING. This approach (high task - low relationship behavior) is appropriate when limited information or instructions must be conveyed. If a client is highly anxious, but it is vital for information to be shared, telling can be effective. Paulish (1987) warns that telling may not be an effective approach to teaching. When using telling the nurse outlines the task (cognitive or psychomotor) to be done by the client and gives explicit instructions. There is little client participation and little or no opportunity for feedback.

SELLING. Although the nurse still provides structure and instruction in this approach, (high task - high relationship) two-way communication is adopted. The nurse paces instruction on the basis of client response. Specific feedback is given to the client who shows success at learning. For example, a client learns the step-by-step procedure for a dressing change. The nurse uses how the client feels about performing the procedure to adapt the teaching approach.

PARTICIPATING. This approach (high relationship - low task behaviors) involves the nurse and client setting objectives and participating in the learning process together. The client helps decide content to be taught. The nurse guides and counsels the client with pertinent information. For example, a client with cancer must learn about diet, pain control, and hygiene needs in order to remain functional in the home setting.

ENTRUSTING. With this approach (low relationship - low task behaviors) the client shows the ability to manage self care. Responsibilities are accepted and tasks are performed well. The nurse observes the client's progress and remains available to assist without introducing a lot of new information. For example, a diabetic client has been self-administering insulin for over 3 months. Injections are performed correctly and the client can explain signs and symptoms of low blood sugar levels.

INCORPORATING TEACHING WITH NURSING CARE

Many nurses find that they can teach more effectively while delivering nursing care. For example, while bathing a diabetic the nurse discusses foot care or while administering drugs the nurse may explain a medication's side effects. An informal, unstructured style relies on the positive therapeutic relationship between nurse and client, which fosters spontaneity in the teaching-learning process. This does not suggest that teaching should occur without a formal plan. When the nurse follows a teaching plan in an informal way, the client feels less pressure to perform, and learning becomes more of a shared activity. A nurse generally feels comfortable when delivering routine care. Therefore this is a good time for the teaching-learning process.

GROUP TEACHING

When a nurse teaches groups of clients or families, a more formal teaching method is appropriate. Group discussions allow open sharing of ideas and attitudes among participants. Clients and families learn from each other as they review common experiences. A productive group discussion helps participants solve problems and arrive at solutions toward improving each member's health. To be an effective group leader, the nurse must be able to guide participation. Acknowledging a group member's look of interest, asking questions, and summarizing key issues foster group involvement. However, not all clients benefit from group discussions, and a client's physical or emotional level of wellness may prohibit participation.

PREPARATORY INSTRUCTION

Frequently clients face unfamiliar tests or procedures that create significant anxiety. Providing information about procedures helps the client form a realistic image of what to anticipate. When the actual experience matches expectations, the client is more apt to attend to the nurse's future explanations. A nurse gains authority and respect when preparatory explanations prove useful.

There are three guidelines for preparatory explanations:

1. Physical sensations during the procedure are described but not evaluated. For example, Mr. Reynolds is to have blood drawn as a routine admission test. The nurse explains that he will feel a sticking sensation as the needle punctures the skin. The nurse does *not* say, "It won't hurt very much."
2. The cause of the sensation is described, preventing misinterpretation of the experience. For example, the nurse tells Mr. Reynolds that often a needle insertion burns because alcohol used to clean the skin enters the puncture site.
3. Clients are prepared only for aspects of the experience that have commonly been noticed by other clients. For example, the nurse explains that while blood is being drawn, often the tight tourniquet causes the hand to tingle and feel numb.

The client finds comfort in knowing what to expect. When the nurse's descriptions are accurate, the client copes more effectively with stress of procedures and therapies. The known is less threatening than the unknown.

DEMONSTRATIONS

A demonstration is useful for teaching psychomotor skills. The client is able to observe a skill before practicing it. Before the demonstration the nurse follows these steps:

1. Review the rationale and steps of the procedure.
2. Assemble and organize equipment.
3. Perform each step in sequence while analyzing knowledge and skills involved.
4. Determine at what step explanations are to be given, considering the client's learning needs.
5. Judge proper speed and timing of the demonstration.

The nurse demonstrates a skill in the same order in which the client will perform it. The demonstration involves:

1. Performing each step slowly and accurately.
2. Encouraging the client to ask questions so that each step is understood.
3. Explaining the rationale for each step.
4. Allowing the client to observe each step.
5. Avoiding a hurried approach.
6. Allowing the client to handle equipment and practice the skill under the nurse's supervision.

The client demonstrates the procedure independently to ensure acquisition of the skill. The independent demonstration should occur under the same conditions found at home. For example, if a client is learning to walk with crutches, the nurse simulates the home environment. If short, narrow steps lead to the client's bedroom, the client should learn to climb similar stairs in the hospital.

USING ANALOGIES

Learning occurs when a teacher translates complex language or ideas into words or concepts the client understands. In addition, the client benefits by integrating new information into daily routines.

Analogies supplement verbal instruction with familiar images that make complex information more real and understandable (Elsberry and Sorensen, 1986). For example, when explaining intestinal peristalsis to a client, an analogy would be the movement of an earthworm as the wave moves down the length of the worm. Another is comparing arterial blood pressure to the flow of water

Sample Evaluation of Interventions for Learning Needs		
Goal	**Evaluative Measures**	**Expected Outcomes**
Client attains self-care of diabetes.	Have client discuss the pathophysiological process of diabetes.	Client will describe the disease process of diabetes in basic terms.
	Ask client to identify the signs and symptoms that develop from hypoglycemia.	Client will describe the signs and symptoms of hypoglycemia.
	Give the client models or pictures of different foods and have the client plan a menu for a day.	Client will select a meal plan for a day containing correct dietary sources.
	Have the client prepare a meal (in the home).	

through a hose. To use analogies the nurse follows these principles:

1. Be familiar with the concept.
2. Know the client's background, experience, and culture.
3. Keep an analogy simple and clear.

DOCUMENTATION OF CLIENT TEACHING

Because client teaching often occurs informally between nurse and client (for example, during medication administration or physical examination), it is difficult to document client education consistently. Nurses often fail to take the time to write down what has been taught. However, because a nurse is legally responsible for providing accurate and timely information to clients, quality documentation is essential.

Barron (1987) suggests the following for documenting client education:

1. *Specific content.* Describe what was taught specifically so that other nursing staff can follow up and reinforce teaching (for example, "Insulin injection demonstrated" or "Explained side effects of Inderal"). Avoid generalizations, such as "medications taught," that leave staff confused.
2. *Evaluation of learning.* Document evidence of the client's learning (for example, a return demonstration, or the attempt to evaluate learning). This informs staff about the client's progress and determines what still needs to be taught.
3. *Method of teaching.* Describe how teaching was done. Knowing methods used in instruction (for example, demonstrations or discussion) helps staff follow up more efficiently or offer alternate teaching methods if learning does not occur. When resources such as pamphlets or audiovisual materials are used the nurse documents it in the client's record. Many institutions have special forms that allow easy documentation.

EVALUATION

Client education is not complete until the nurse evaluates outcomes of the teaching-learning process (see evaluation box). Did the client learn what was intended? The nurse evaluates the client's success at meeting each learning objective by observing performance of each expected behavior under the desired conditions. Success depends on the client's ability to meet established performance criteria.

Return demonstrations, use of questions, observing client behaviors, role playing, and discussions can be methods for evaluating clients. For example, the client who is to use a three-point crutch gait while walking to the end of the hall must demonstrate the actual crutch-walking technique. A client who is to identify five signs and symptoms of hypertension must be able to do so when questioned or during a discussion of the disease.

If the evaluation process continues to indicate a knowledge or skill deficit, the nurse repeats or modifies the teaching plan. Alternative teaching methods often help to clarify information or skills the client was unable to comprehend or perform originally.

Evaluation may reveal the presence of new learning needs or existence of new factors that may interfere with the client's ability to learn. The nurse reassesses those to update the teaching plan and make it relevant. As with the nursing process, the teaching process is continuous and changing.

SUMMARY

More than ever, an emphasis in health care today is to provide patients and families information about health and management of health problems. During interaction with a client the nurse has an opportunity to teach. The nurse teaches clients to function more independently. Client education focuses on the client's unique needs and capacity for learning. The most effective teaching plan is one in which the nurse and client work together to define information and skills the client needs to learn.

A nurse cannot teach effectively without understanding the basic learning domains: cognitive, affective, and psychomotor. The characteristics of each domain affect selection of the teaching methods and manner in which learning is evaluated. A good teacher uses basic teaching principles to promote a student's participation in learning. Teaching sessions convene when the learner is most receptive. A teacher organizes teaching material in a format that progresses from simple to more complex ideas. The teacher's actions and use of instructional resources help to stimulate a student's interest in learning.

The nursing process provides a useful framework for organizing the teaching process. The nurse conducts a thorough assessment to identify clients' learning needs, readiness and ability to learn, the teaching environment, and resources for learning.

Nursing diagnoses focus on specific types of learning needs. The teaching plan involves the nurse and client in a collaborative effort, setting realistic learning objectives. The nurse also selects the teaching methods based on the client's learning priorities.

During implementation the nurse uses a variety of teaching methods to engage the client actively in learning. To determine whether a client has gained necessary knowledge or skills, the nurse evaluates success of the plan on the basis of expected learning outcomes.

KEY CONCEPTS

✓ Teaching is most effective when it is responsive to learners' needs.

✓ With the emphasis in health care on the maintenance of health, client education is a primary responsibility of the nurse.

✓ Teaching is a form of interpersonal communication with teacher and student actively involved in a process that increases the student's knowledge and skills.

✓ Teaching a client a specific behavior can involve incorporation of behaviors from all three learning domains.

✓ The client's ability to attend to the learning process depends on physical comfort and anxiety and the presence of environmental distraction.

✓ Because it is unlikely that clients will learn unless they want to, the nurse applies principles of motivation when teaching.

✓ A person's health beliefs influence the willingness to gain knowledge and skills necessary to maintain health.

✓ Active participation in learning promotes the learner's ability to problem solve and make decisions.

✓ Teaching must be timed to coincide with the client's readiness to learn.

✓ Learning objectives describe in behavioral terms what a person is to learn.

✓ Evaluation of the teaching-learning process is based on fulfillment of teaching goals.

✓ Clients of different ages require different teaching strategies as a result of developmental capabilities.

✓ The ideal environment for promoting learning is a room that is well lit and free of distractions and that has good ventilation, appropriate furniture, and a comfortable temperature.

✓ Presentation of content should progress from simple to more complex ideas.

✓ The use of instructional resources involves the principles of promoting active learner participation.

✓ A combination of teaching methods improves the learner's attentiveness and involvement.

✓ A teacher is more effective when presenting information that builds on a learner's existing knowledge.

✓ Teaching methodologies should match the client's learning need.

✓ An informal teaching style fosters spontaneity between teacher and learner.

✓ A teacher's approach with a student may change based upon the learner's needs and response.

✓ A nurse evaluates a client's learning by observing performance of expected learning behaviors under desired conditions.

REFERENCES

Barron, S: Documentation of patient education, Patient Educ Couns 9:81, 1987.

Bartlett, EE: Assessing benefits of patient education under prospective pricing, Patient Education Newsletter, University of Alabama, 1984.

Bloom, BS, editor: Taxonomy of educational objectives. I. Cognitive domain, New York, 1956, Longman, Inc.

Elsberry, NL, and Sorensen, ME: Using analogies in patient teaching, Am J Nurs 86:1171, 1986

Joint Commission on Accreditation of Hospitals: Accreditation manual of hospitals. Chicago, Ill., 1987, The Commission.

Kozol, J: Illiterate America, Garden City, N.Y., 1985, Doubleday.

Krathwohl, DR, et al.: Taxonomy of educational objectives: the classification of educational goals, Handbook II: Affective domain, New York, 1964, David McKay Co., Inc.

Miller, A: When is the time ripe for teaching? Am J Nurs 85:801, 1985.

Paulish, C: A model for situational patient teaching, J Contin Educ Nurs 18:163, 1987.

Redman, BK: The process of patient education, ed. 6, St. Louis, 1988, The C.V. Mosby Co.

Rosenstock, IM: What research in motivation suggests for public health, Am J Public Health 50:295, 1960.

Roter, D: An exploration of health education's responsibility for a partnership model of client-provider relations, Patient Educ Couns, 9:25, 1987.

Simpson, EJ: The classification of educational objectives in the psychomotor domain. In Contributions of behavioral science to instructional technology: the psychomotor domain, Mr. Rainer, Md., 1972, Gryphon Press.

Whaley, LF, and Wong, DL: Nursing care of infants and children, ed. 3, St. Louis, 1987, The C.V. Mosby Co.

Woodard, S: Preoperative patient education seminar presentation, Denver, 1983, Resource Applications, Inc.

Research Article

Byrne, TJ, and Edeani, D: Knowledge of medical terminology among hospitalized patients, Nurs Res 33:178, 1984.

ADDITIONAL READINGS

Anderson, WF: Is health education for the middle-aged and elderly a waste of time? In Wells, T, editor: Aging and health promotion, Rockville, Md., 1982, Aspen Systems Corp.

Bartlett, EE: Advocacy skills and strategies for patient education managers, Patient Educ Couns 8:397, 1986.

Bennett, HL: Why patients don't follow instructions, RN 49:45, March 1986.

Berg, BK, and Leisner, B: Developing a geriatric patient education program, Patient Educ Couns 8:201, 1986

Bille, DA: Educational strategies for teaching the elderly patient, Nurs Health Care 5:256, 1980

Bille, DA: Practical approaches to patient teaching, Boston, 1981, Little, Brown & Co.

Boyd, CW: Patient education promotes transition from hospital to home, Patient Educ Couns 8:295, 1986.

Cunningham, MA, and Baker, D: How to teach patients better and faster, RN 50:52, 1986.

Cushing, M: Legal lessons on patient teaching, Am J Nurs 84:721, 1984.

Foster, SD: An innovative documentation tool, MCN 11:419, 1986.

Fox, V: Patient teaching: understanding the needs of the adult learner, AORN J 44:234, 1986.

Hindelang, M: Aging: a positive experience of growth, Patient Educ Couns 9:209, 1987.

Huckabay, LMD: Conditions of learning and instruction in nursing, St. Louis, 1980, The C.V. Mosby Co.

Joyce, B, and Weil, M: Models of teaching, ed. 2, Englewood Cliffs, N.J., 1980, Prentice-Hall, Inc.

Leff, EW: Ethics and patient teaching, MCN 11:375, 1986.

McHatton, M: A theory for timely teaching, Am J Nurs 85:798, 1985.

McHugh, NG, Christman, NJ, and Johnson, JE: Preparatory information: what helps and why, Am J Nurs 82:780, 1982.

Morrison, JL: The special needs of the special patient, RN, 49(7):49, 1986.

Moss, R.C.: Overcoming fear: a review of research on patient, family instruction, AORN J 43:1107, May 1986.

Pohl, ML: The teaching function of the nursing practitioner, ed. 2, Dubuque, Iowa, 1973, William C. Brown Group.

Smith, CE: Patient teaching: it's the law, Nurs 87, 1987.

Streiff, LD: Can clients understand our instructions? Image J Nurs Sch 18(2):48, 1986.

Ward, DB: Why patient teaching fails, RN 49:45, 1986.

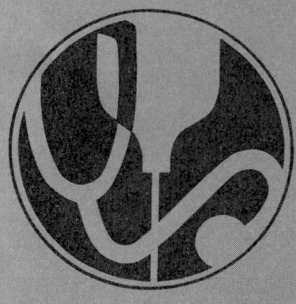

UNIT 5

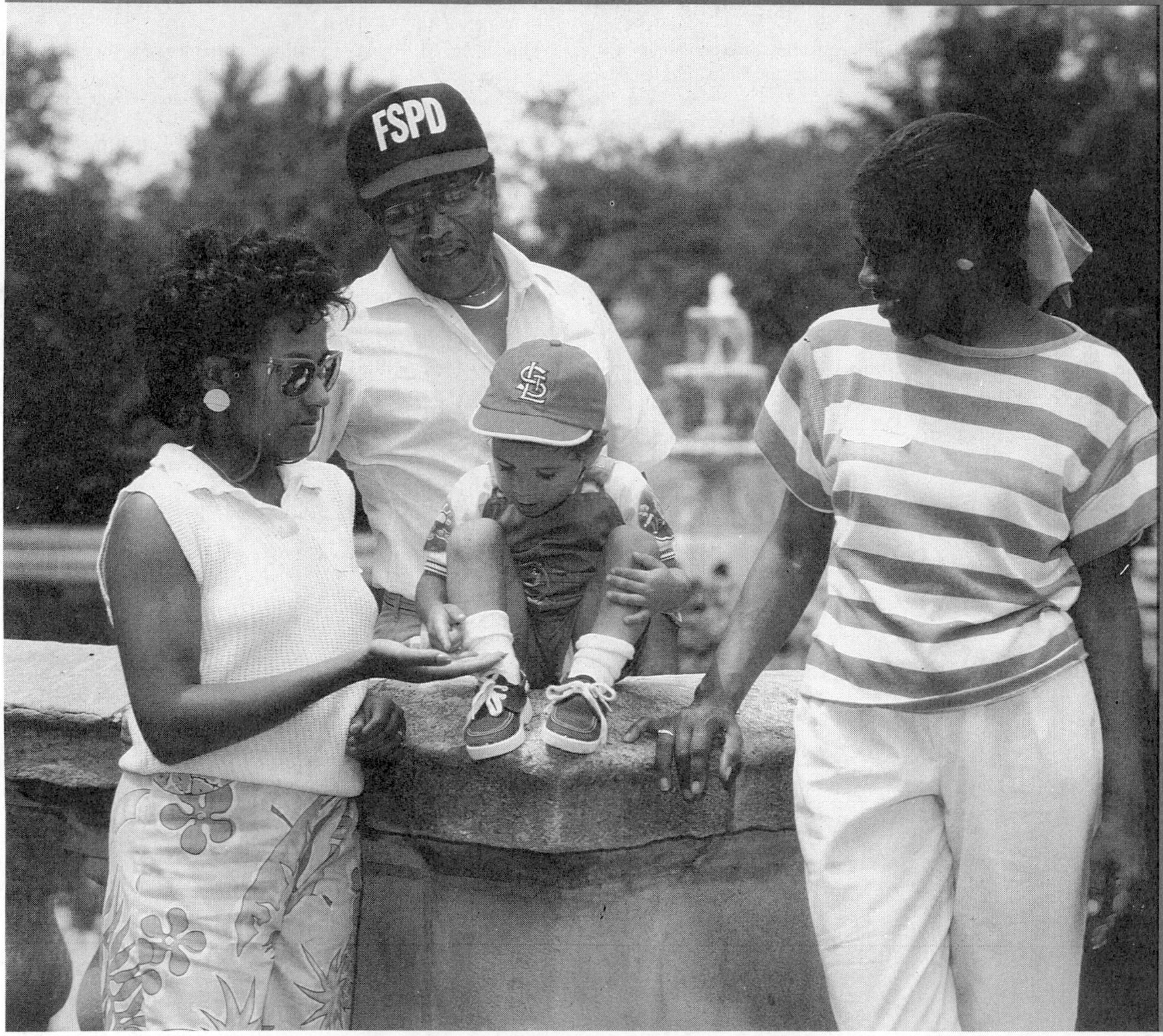

Growth and Development for the Individual and Family

Human growth and development involve many complex changes in all dimensions throughout the life span. The nurse can assess the client's current status and intervene when necessary to promote healthy development only by understanding the normal ranges of growth and development within each developmental stage. Each stage is associated with certain physiological and psychosocial health needs and risk factors, and the nurse's awareness of these elements is important when providing care for any kind of health problem. Similarly, each developmental stage involves unique resources and coping mechanisms that the nurse can use to help clients adapt to the problems of illness. By incorporating a developmental perspective in nursing care, the nurse can more effectively address all the client's health needs. The chapters in Unit 5 promote this perspective by examining important theories of growth and development and the appropriate health issues for each stage. One chapter discusses the health of the family as it grows and develops and the relationship of the family to the individual's health. The last chapter, on death, loss, and the grieving process, focuses on the special needs of clients related to this last stage of growth and development.

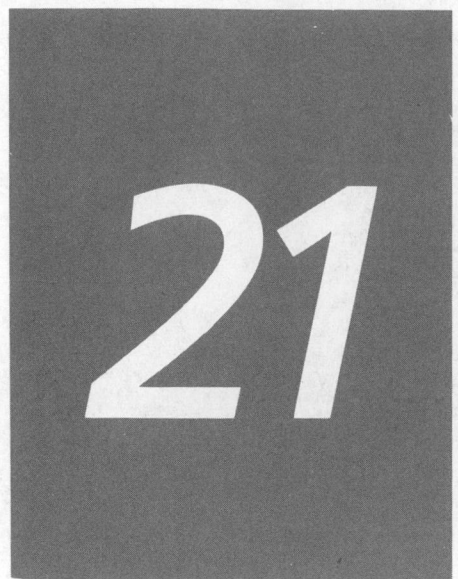

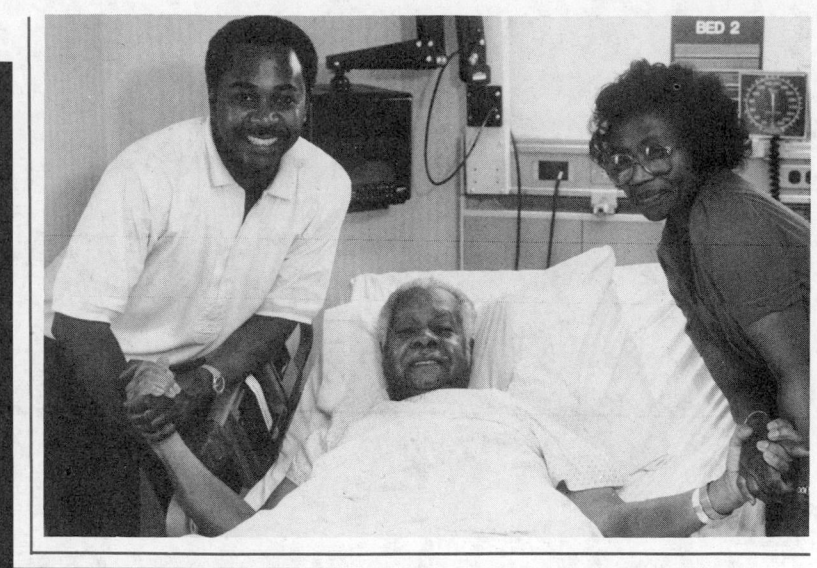

OBJECTIVES

Mastery of content in this chapter will enable the student to:

- Define the key terms listed.
- Discuss the way family members influence one another's health.
- Describe current trends in the American family.
- Define the family in terms applicable to all family forms.
- Describe five common family forms and discuss the relevant health concerns of each.
- Explain the way family structure and pattern of functioning affect the health of family members and the family as a whole.
- Compare family as environment to family as client, and explain the way these perspectives influence nursing practice.
- Describe the family nursing process in terms of assessment, nursing diagnosis, planning, intervention, and evaluation.
- Describe the attributes of effective and ineffective families.

KEY TERMS

Blended Family

Communal Family

Extended Family

Family

Family as Client

Family as Environment

Family Functions

Family Health

Family of Origin

Family of Procreation

Family Structure

Nuclear Family

Single-Parent Family

The Family

Despite many challenges, the family remains the central institution in society. Within this social unit, individuals grow and develop and seek health. Twenty years ago, many people felt the family was an endangered species. Some social scientists predicted that family influence on individual members would decline. Rapid social change and a mobile population were anticipated to cause psychological and physical distancing of family members. However, although family members today may be geographically farther from each other than in the past and may be living in nontraditional families, family ties remain strong. Wattenburg found in a 1985 study that most families get together several times a month. Although the elderly are often portrayed as isolated and alone, this is not the reality for most of America's elderly. More than two thirds of elderly persons see their children or communicate with them by telephone or letter at least once a week.

The influence of the family is important in American society, and this must always be considered in interactions with clients. The family shapes early health beliefs and values, and family members have an impact on each other's health practices and status. The nurse views the client as an individual and as a person who is an integral part of a family. All members need to be incorporated into the nursing process whenever possible because the family environment significantly influences health outcomes.

CURRENT TRENDS

Although the institution of the family remains strong, the family itself is changing, and the emerging patterns are having a major impact on society. Many recent statistics reveal fundamental changes from the traditional family form. Families are smaller. People are marrying later, women are delaying childbearing, and couples are choosing to have fewer children. Although most American women say they want to have two children, the total fertility rate has remained approximately 1.7 children per woman for white women and only slightly higher for women of other races. Divorce rates have tripled since the 1950s, and if current rates continue, one half of all first marriages will end in divorce. The number of female-headed households have increased dramatically, not only because of divorce but also because of an increase in the number of children born to single mothers. Although divorce occurs often, marriage is valued. In the 1980s, five out of six divorced men and three out of four divorced women will remarry, usually within a few years after divorcing (Skolnick, 1987). Remarriage often results in a blended family, with a complex set of relationships between stepparents and stepchildren and half brothers and half sisters.

The majority of women are in the work force. Approximately 51% of married mothers with children under age 6 work outside the home (Cancellier, 1984). Division of labor within the home and the need for child care are major issues facing many families today. The number of "one-person households" is growing rapidly. Although some people choose a single life-style, singlehood is not always a matter of choice. Demography and culture have created a "marriage squeeze," a shortage of men compared with the number of women in the prime marrying ages (Zinn and Eitzen, 1987).

The fastest-growing age group is 65 and over. This "graying" of America has an impact on families and society as a whole. Although it is often assumed that a large number of elderly live in nursing homes, this is not the case. Most retirees live with spouses or alone. Only about 6% reside in a health care institution. Because of the increased life span of most adults and decreased birth rate, couples are often together for 20 to 30 years after their children have left home. Although most researchers agree that the departure of the last child from the home does not precipitate a prolonged or particularly difficult period, it does necessitate a redefinition of the how the married couple relate to each other.

CONCEPT OF FAMILY

A popular conception exists about what the family is or at least what it should be. This "ideal" model dictates that the family (1) is a nuclear unit, (2) consists of a mother, father, and their children, and (3) exhibits a sexual division of labor (that is, the mother cooks, cleans, and is responsible for child-rearing, and the father works outside the home). Family evokes a visual impression, a mental image of adults and children living together in a satisfying, harmonious fashion (Zinn and Eitzen, 1987). Families are, however, as diverse as the individuals that compose them. Nurses, like all people, have feelings and values rooted deeply in their own family experiences, which influence their ideas of what a family *should* be. Unless nurses recognize these values as their own, they may inhibit their understanding and acceptance of clients' perspectives of their families.

Clients have widely varying concepts of family. Some clients consider the family to include only persons related by marriage, birth, or adoption. Other clients consider aunts, uncles, close friends, and cohabitating persons to be family. To accept all clients' concepts of family, the nurse can define the family as a group of interacting individuals composing a basic unit of society (Fawcett, 1975). This definition is broad and flexible and recognizes widely divergent conceptions. It accepts differences in family structure and function arising from social circumstances and cultural and individual differences. Client attitudes about family are deeply ingrained and deserve respect.

The nurse's personal beliefs about the appropriate composition of a family need not agree with those of the client. The essential goal is to recognize and accept the client's view. The attitudes of many clients are based on common family forms. The nurse should be knowledgeable about these forms and their health implications.

FAMILY FORMS

Family forms are patterns of people considered by family members to be included in the family. Although all families have some things in common, each family form has unique problems and strengths. The nurse needs to have an open mind about what constitutes a family so potential resources and concerns are not overlooked.

Nuclear Family

Although the nuclear family is not the dominant family form in North America, health care professionals often consider it to be the usual and ideal form. The nuclear family consists of the husband, wife, and perhaps one or more children. For the children, this family is often referred to as the family of origin. For the parents, it is the family of procreation. Many couples in American society choose to not have children. Others are unable to have children because of infertility. The presence or absence of children affects a family's health concerns and goals.

Extended Family

The extended family includes relatives, as well as members of the nuclear family. Aunts, uncles, grandparents, and cousins are all part of the extended family. The extended family can be psychologically and geographically close or separated. The closer the extended family, the greater the influence on the client and the greater the importance of incorporating them into the health care plans. Extended families often provide a larger range of experience and talents and therefore a more diverse support base than the nuclear family. After the birth of a child with a physical deformity, for example, the grandparents may be capable of providing comfort to the parents at a time when they feel extremely vulnerable and unable to give each other emotional support. Other relatives can be recruited to cook meals to give the parents more time together or with their child.

Single-Parent Family

Single-parent families can be formed when one parent leaves the nuclear family because of death, divorce, or desertion. The circumstances of the separation influence its impact on the family. In the past, most single-parent families existed because of the death of one parent. Today, these families are most commonly the result of divorce or the decision of a single person to have or adopt a child. Reduced financial resources accompanying the loss of one spouse can affect the health of single-parent families. Children are most often placed in the custody of the mother, which contributes to the fact that female-headed households are the fastest growing type of family today (Zinn and Eitzen, 1987). Many unwed mothers choose to live on their own. Because women earn 40% less than males and do not often receive child support, divorce constitutes a major cause of poverty among women and children (Cancellier, 1984). Extended families and a social network can provide financial and emotional support and are particularly important for single-parent families. Single-parent families are also formed when a single person has or adopts a child.

Specific health concerns of single-parent families include the following:

1. Adequate income to provide the essentials for a healthy life-style, including food, clothing, and recreation.
2. Availability and access to medical care in the event of illness, and child care arrangements during episodes of routine illness.

3. Emotional health of family members, the remaining parent carrying the extra burden of accomplishing all tasks of child rearing and nurturing alone, which puts additional stress on all family members.

Blended Family

Blended families are formed when parents bring unrelated children from prior marriages into a new, joint-living situation because of remarriage or cohabitation. With the rate of divorce and remarriage, one out of every five children belong to a blended family (Romanczuk, 1987). Although studies have in general failed to demonstrate that divorce and remarriage have long-term negative effects on children, subtle changes appear to occur in children's relationships with fathers, mothers, siblings, and other family members (see research highlight). The nature of the prior living situations and rapidity with which the family members must adapt to changes can influence health. Multiple, rapid changes severely tax the family's coping resources. The stress experienced during the earlier family dissolution, the length of time in which each family functioned with one parent, and the extent of the new family members' familiarity with one another also influence the blended family's coping capabilities.

⚔ *Research Highlight* ⚒

Amato investigated the effects of divorce and remarriage on the adjustment and development of children in three types of families: mother-custody one-parent, mother-custody stepparent, and intact families. Interviews were conducted with 402 children (195 primary and 207 secondary) at school and with the children's parents in the home. The interviews dealt with family relationships and activities and contained open-ended and close-ended questions. The author concludes that children in one-parent homes have more demands placed on them but also have corresponding privileges, resulting in an egalitarian family environment. Children in stepparent families also had many household responsibilities but no more autonomy than in intact families. In one-parent and stepparent families, the author perceived low cohesion in family life.

Amato, P: Family processes in one-parent, stepparent, and intact families: the child's point of view, Journal of Marriage and the Family 49(2):327, 1987.

The key to healthy stepfamily functioning is establishment of a strong couple bond, which provides the foundation of the new family unit (Engebretson, 1982). The mental health of family members during adjustment to the new family pattern is of primary interest. This adjustment period can last up to 2 years. The long-term impact of stress on the health of the individual members and of the family as a whole during this extended period requires assessment. The nurse can assure families that this period is a normal developmental phase and can help the family assess its resources to prevent or lessen stressful situations.

Communal Family

The communal family is not a recent development. Communal living reached its peak in numbers of members and rate of success in the 1940s. Although communal living may never again be so popular, economic pressures and shifting social attitudes could foster a substantial return to this form of family life. Membership of communal families varies. Members may share religious affiliation, economic commodities, ideology, goals of self-sufficiency, or the desire for an extended family arrangement.

The health concerns of communal families involve two major issues: the stability of relationships within the family and the nature of child-rearing practices. Because stable relationships appear to bolster the mental health of family members, concern exists that relationships in communal families shift or are unstable and that less psychological support is provided to individual family members. The degree to which child-rearing is shared between males and females also varies in different communes. In most communal living arrangements, however, females continue to provide the majority of child care. Specific child care practices vary from authoritarian to quite liberal. The nature of these practices is not as great a risk to children's emotional and mental health as changes in child-rearing practices that occur if communal family membership changes rapidly. Changing membership can, on the other hand, expose the child to a wide range of supportive, loving adults.

Other Family Forms

The "typical" family has become a rarity. In 1983, only 6.2 percent of American families consisted of a bread-winning husband, a full-time housewife, and two children (Skolnick, 1987). The diversity in life-styles and new living arrangements is an outgrowth of economic and family trends. This rise in alternatives is associated with new patterns of divorce and remarriage and new expectations about individual fulfillment and personal life (Zinn and Eitzen, 1987). Many individuals structure their lives differently than their parents did.

☒ *Research Highlight* ☒

Sund and Ostwald investigated personal and life-style–related variables and stress levels in dual-earner families in the preschool stage of development. In a sample consisting of 92 families, family stress levels were measured by The Family Inventory of Life Events and Changes. The conclusion that dual-earner families in this study had only a moderate amount of family stress compared to national stress level norms contraindicated the notion that mother's employment outside the home increases stress. The authors suggest that the advantages resulting from a dual-earner life-style help maintain equilibrium within the family.

Sund, K, and Ostwald, SK: Dual-earner families' stress levels and personal life-style–related variables, Nurs Res 34(6):357, 1985.

In the early 1980s an estimated 1.8 million couples cohabitated, and the figure is expected to increase (Cherlin, 1983). Some who choose to live together view cohabitation as an alternative to marriage. However, the majority see it as a temporary arrangement and as a pretrial for marriage.

Approximately half of all gay male couples live together, compared to three fourths of lesbian couples. Although unable to marry by law, many homosexual couples define their relationship in family terms. They have become more open about their sexual preferences and more vocal about their legal rights. Less controversial but more significant departures from the past include dual-earner families, commuter marriages, and couples who are voluntarily childless. It has been suggested that these departures from the more traditional form of family can result in added stress. However, evidence exists that this is not the case and that certain life-styles do not threaten the family health (see research highlight).

STRUCTURE AND FUNCTION

Families have both a structure and a way of functioning. Structure and function are closely related and continually interact with one another. Structure is based on organization (that is, the ongoing membership of the family and the pattern of relationships). Relationships can be numerous and complex. For example, a woman's relationships may include wife-husband, mother-son, and mother-daughter, each with different demands, roles, and expectations. Although the definitions of structure vary, the nurse asks the following questions:

Support Functions of the Family
<ul><li>Collects and disseminates information to family members</li><li>Provides feedback to family members to guide them in interaction with the larger society</li><li>Transmits to family members beliefs, values, attitudes, and coping mechanisms</li><li>Guides family members in problem solving</li><li>Provides practical services and concrete assistance such as financial aid</li><li>Provides a safe, comfortable environment when family members need rest and recuperation</li><li>Provides standards of behavior and attitudes against which family members can judge themselves</li><li>Helps family members establish an identity and reinforces identity in times of stress</li><li>Assists family members in controlling or working through negative emotions</li></ul>

Provides heritage + status [handwritten annotation]

quence. These symptoms include emotional responses such as anger, delinquent behavior, somatic complaints and depression (Friedman, 1981). Caplan (1975) suggests that the family has nine support functions for its individual members (see box). The emphasis on one or more functions varies from family to family. Within the same family, individual members may differentially emphasize specific functions, and shifts in emphasis occur from time to time.

Goals are more easily achieved when communication is clear and direct. Clear communication enhances problem solving and resolution of conflict. Another family process facilitating goal achievement is the ability to nurture and promote growth. Families need to have available and must be able to use internal and external resources. A social network is useful as an external support system. Social relationships act as buffers, particularly during times of stress, and reduce a family's vulnerability.

"Who is included in the family?" "Who performs which tasks?" and "Who makes which decisions?" Structure may enhance or detract from the family's ability to respond to the expected and unexpected stressors that are realities of daily life. Very rigid or very flexible structures can be detrimental to the functioning of the family. A rigid structure specifically dictates who is permitted to accomplish a task and may also limit the number of persons outside the immediate family allowed to assume these tasks. For example, the mother might be considered the only acceptable person to provide emotional support for the children or the husband the only one to provide financial support. A change in the health status of the person responsible for a task places a burden on the family because no other person is available or considered acceptable to assume that task. An extremely open structure can also present problems for the family. An underlying stability that otherwise leads to automatic action during a crisis or rapid change is often absent.

Friedman (1981) describes functioning as what the family does. Family functioning involves the processes used by the family to achieve its goals. These processes include communication among family members, goal setting, conflict resolution, nurturing, and use of internal and external resources. The reproductive, sexual, economic, and educational goals that were once considered central family goals no longer apply to all families. Although many families pursue these goals at various times during their development, they provide psychological support to their members throughout the life span. When the psychological needs of family members are not met, symptoms of family dysfunction are the usual conse-

DEVELOPMENTAL STAGES

Families, like individuals, change and grow over time. Although families are far from identical to one another, they do have a basic pattern and similarity in experiences resulting in predictable stages. Each of these developmental stages has its own challenges, needs, and resources and includes tasks that need to be completed before the family can successfully move on to the next stage. McGoldrick and Carter (1985) have developed a model of family life stages based on expansion, contraction, and realignment of family relationships that support the entry, exit, and development of the members. This model provides the nurse with the emotional aspects of transition, as well as the changes and tasks necessary for the family to proceed developmentally (Table 21-1). Consequently, the nurse can promote behaviors consistent with achievement of the essential tasks and help families prepare for later transitions. This model does not take into account diverse family forms. However, other researchers suggest alternative models. For example, Aldous, as reported in McCubbin and Dahl, has devised a six-stage system for single-mother families resulting from divorce. The initial stage is the establishment of the single-parent family, and the final stage is retirement of women from their work-life or from the responsibilities of parenthood.

FAMILY AND HEALTH

The health status of family members influences family functioning, and family functioning, in turn, influences its own and society's perceptions of its health. When the family satisfactorily meets its goals through adequate

TABLE 21-1 Stages of the Family Life Cycle

Family Life Cycle Stage	Emotional Process of Transition: Key Principles	Changes in Family Status Required to Proceed Developmentally
Between families: The unattached young adult	Accepting parent-offspring separation	Differentiation of self in relation to family of origin Development of intimate peer relationships Establishment of self in work
The joining of families through marriage: The newly married couple	Commitment to new system	Formation of marital system Realignment of relationships with extended families and friends to include spouse
The family with young children	Accepting new generation of members into the system	Adjusting marital system to make space for child(ren) Taking on parenting roles Realignment of relationships with extended family to include parenting and grandparenting roles
The family with adolescents	Increasing flexibility of family boundaries to include children's independence	Shifting of parent-child relationships to permit adolescents to move in and out of system Refocus on midlife marital and career issues Beginning shift toward concerns for older generation
Launching children and moving on	Accepting a multitude of exits from and entries into the family system	Renegotiation of marital system as a dyad Development of adult to adult relationships between grown children and their parents Realignment of relationships to include in-laws and grandchildren Dealing with disabilities and death of parents (grandparents)
The family in later life	Accepting the shifting of generational roles	Maintaining own and/or couple functioning and interests in face of physiological decline; exploration of new familial and social role options Support for a more central role for middle generation Making room in the system for the wisdom and experience of the elderly; supporting the older generation without overfunctioning for them Dealing with loss of spouse, siblings, and other peers, and preparation for own death. Life review and integration

From McGoldrick, M, and Carter, E: The stages of the family life cycle. In Henslin, J, editor: Marriage and family in a changing society, New York, 1985, The Free Press; in Walsh, F: Normal family processes, New York, 1982, The Guilford Press.

functioning, its members tend to feel positive about themselves and their family. Conversely, when they do not meet goals, families view themselves as ineffective. Constant stress resulting from inadequate functioning can also adversely affect an individual family member's health. Constant stress may disrupt cardiovascular function, blood pressure, and circulating neuroendocrine substances, and these disruptions are suspected precursors of poor health (see Chapter 28). Maladaptive behaviors within the family negatively impact on the health of its members and the overall ability of the family to meet its goals. A lack of communication or poor communication inhibits the family's ability to make decisions and solve problems. Good health may not be highly

valued, and, in fact, detrimental practices may be accepted. In some cases a family member may provide mixed messages about health. For example, a parent may continue to smoke while telling children that smoking is bad for them. Family environment is crucial because health behavior reinforced in early life has a strong influence on later health practices.

Pratt (1976) assessed the effectiveness of alternate forms of family structure. Families fostering health encourage (1) autonomy of family members, (2) varied and regular communication, (3) active coping, and (4) social ties within the community. Rueben Hill noted nearly 30 years ago that it is possible to explain the reactions of crisis-proof and crises-prone families by the factors of integration and adaptability (Adams, 1986). The crisis-proof or effective family is able to integrate the need for stability with the need for growth and change and has a flexible structure allowing adaptable performance of tasks and acceptance of help from outside the family system. The structure is flexible enough to allow for adaptability but not so flexible that the family lacks cohesiveness and a sense of stability. The effective family has control over the environment and exerts influence on the immediate environs of home, neighborhood, or school. The ineffective family may lack, or believe that it lacks, control over these environs.

The health of the family is influenced by its relative position in society. Although American families share the same culture, they live in very different ways. The structure and function of any family is a reflection and a result of its social class, its economic resources, and its racial and ethnic background. For some minority groups and the poor, patterned differences in family living are consequences of inequalities deeply rooted in our society. Class and ethnicity can produce differences in the access of families to society's resources and re-wards, and this access creates differences in family life and most significantly in different life chances for its members (Zinn and Eitzen, 1987). Distribution of wealth greatly affects the capacity to maintain health. Economic stability creates more opportunity for sound nutrition, rest, education, lack of stress, and better access to health care (Estes et al., 1984). The higher infant mortality rates and shortened life span of the poor and some minority groups demonstrate how inequality impacts health status (See Chapter 2).

FAMILY NURSING: FAMILY AS ENVIRONMENT AND AS CLIENT

The family can be approached as the environment within which the individual client strives for health or as the client itself. The approach depends on the situation. If only one family member is receptive to nursing care, it is realistic and practical to view the family as environment. When all family members are involved in the day-to-day care of one another, nursing intervention with one individual necessitates some change in the activities of the others. Both approaches—family as environment and family as client—can be useful in providing effective nursing care. Friedman (1981) suggests that nursing care must be directed to the family as a whole, as well as to individual members.

When the family is viewed as environment, the primary focus is the health and development of an individual member existing within a specific environment (that is, the client's family). Although assessment, nurs-

---

✂ *Research Highlight* ✂

Gilliss explored stress in the family during and after coronary artery bypass surgery. The purpose was to (1) examine the relationship of the client's stress to that of the spouse's stress, (2) report the major sources of stress, and (3) examine the couple's social process of recovery. To determine whether a difference existed compared to subjective stress, 71 clients' scores were compared with their spouses' scores. The spouses reported higher stress levels than the clients. The author concluded that it is essential to include the family in nursing intervention.

Gilliss, CL: Reducing family stress during and after coronary artery bypass surgery, Nurs Clin North Am 19(1):103, 1984.

---

ing diagnosis, planning, implementation, and evaluation concentrate on the individual's health status, the nurse also assesses the extent to which the family provides the individual's basic needs (see Chapter 27). These needs vary, depending on the individual's developmental level and situation. Families provide more than just material essentials, so their ability to help the client meet psychological needs must also be considered. Family members may also need intervention. This is particularly true in the case of acutely ill clients. For example, the hospitalized child's parents feel a great deal of stress, as does a spouse whose partner is undergoing surgery (see research highlight).

Although nurses have cared for families for years, it is only recently that nurse researchers have begun to study the family as a whole (Murphy, 1986). The family is viewed as more than the sum of its individual members, and the family unit is the primary focus of nursing care because any nursing intervention with one member ultimately influences all members. Family patterns versus individual characteristics are studied. For example, a single, 25-year-old man lives at home with his parents and two younger siblings. He requests the assistance of the nurse in altering his diet and developing stress management techniques to help him cope with his borderline hypertension, which is thought to be related to high-sodium intake, a stressful job, and continuing expectations by his family for participation in their activities. If the family is viewed as environment, the nurse focuses on the client as an individual. The nurse might assess the client's knowledge of high-sodium foods, strategies for reducing the number of high-sodium foods in the diet, realistic opportunities to reduce the number and extent of perceived stressors in work and family environments, and knowledge and skill in stress management such as relaxation or biofeedback techniques. If the family is viewed as client, the nurse would assess the family's current dietary patterns and its desire and resources for changing the patterns. The nurse also determines the demands placed on the hypertensive family member and explores the potential for redistribution of the demands among other family members. The family's capabilities to support the hypertensive member's development and use of stress management are also assessed. The structure of the American health care system can make it difficult to provide effective nursing care to the family as a whole, because the system focuses on individual health. However, the nurse must always be aware that clients are affected by their families whether their members are present or not, and that clients, in turn, affect their families.

NURSING PROCESS FOR THE FAMILY

Family nursing process is the same, whether the focus is family as client or family as environment. The nursing process used is the same as that used with individuals (that is, assessment, nursing diagnosis, planning, intervention, and evaluation). Friedman (1981) notes that the only difference is that both the individual and the family receive care. Assumptions underlying the family approach to the nursing process is that all individuals must be viewed within their family context and that families impact on individuals and individuals impact on families.

ASSESSMENT

Family assessment is an essential component of the nursing process (see box). Although the family as a whole differs from individual members, the measure of family health must be more than a summation of the health of all members. Areas included in family assessment are the form, structure, and function of the family, its developmental stage, and its progress toward or accomplishment of developmental tasks. Cultural background is an important variable when assessing the family because race and ethnicity impact on structure and function and influence health beliefs and values. The nurse begins assessment by determining who composes the client's family, the client's attitude toward family, and the extent to which the family can be incorporated into the nursing process. To determine the family form and membership, the nurse can ask the client, "Whom do you consider your family?" or ask with whom the client shares strong emotional feelings. If the client is

unable to express a concept of family, the nurse can ask with whom the client lives, spends time, and shares confidences, and then ask the client to validate this observation: "Do you consider the person to be family or like family to you?" To further assess the family structure, the nurse asks questions that determine the power structure and patterning of roles and tasks. For example, "How are the tasks divided in your family?" "Who does the laundry?" "Who mows the lawn?" "Who decides on where to go on vacation?" Since a moderately flexible structure is generally most beneficial to the family, nursing interventions therefore may involve modulating the family patterns away from extremely rigid or flexible structures if either extreme causes problems related to the health of an individual or the family as a whole. In general, however, the nurse attempts to work within the family structure when providing care and does not attempt to change the structure.

The nurse assesses family functions such as the ability to provide emotional support for members, the ability to cope with its current health problem or situation, and the appropriateness of its goal setting (that is, whether or not the goals are realistic and obtainable considering its current status and developmental stage). Although families' goals vary, measures of family health care must be flexible. The nurse also assesses whether the family is able to provide and allocate sufficient economic resources and if its social network is extensive enough to provide support. Additional criteria for family health include the opportunity to attain a satisfactory identity and worth and whether its life-style minimizes risks and promotes active coping to achieve family goals (O'Brien, 1979). Attainment of family developmental tasks is also a useful criterion of family health. Few clinical measures of family health are currently available, but family nursing is an exciting and rapidly growing area of research. It seems reasonable that a true measure of family health will incorporate aspects of the health of all family members, as well as aspects of total family health. New research developments of family health criteria include determination of consensus and discrepancies between family members, use of diaries that address health concerns, and active coping efforts of members. Roberts and Feetham (1982) suggest the use of the Feetham Family Functioning Survey for research and clinical practice. This instrument measures relationships between the family and community, within the family, and of the subsystems of the family.

NURSING DIAGNOSIS

Nursing assessment results in clustering pertinent data that support the nursing diagnosis and identifies where functioning is inadequate or deficient and intervention

Assessment Tool

The family assessment tool is used when the beginning student interviews family members and observes family interaction. It is a *guideline* only and is not meant to be all inclusive. The student must also assume that individual health histories accompany this assessment.

FAMILY FORM AND STRUCTURE

Family name _____

Woman _____ Man _____

Relationship _____

(Single, married, divorced, separated, cohabitating)

Names of children   Ages

_____

_____

_____

Others living in home (include age, sex, relationship) _____

_____

Cultural background (include any pertinent health beliefs, child-rearing practices, related health concerns)

_____

Developmental stage _____

Progress toward accomplishment of developmental tasks _____

Concerns related to developmental stage _____

RESOURCES

Significant relatives and friends not occupying immediate residence _____

Strengths and coping skills _____

How does the family obtain health services? _____

Membership in community groups (for example, church affiliation) _____

Education (formal and informal) _____

Finances (ability to meet current and future needs) _____

FAMILY PATTERNS

Persons working outside the home _____

Type of work _____ Number of hours _____

Satisfaction with work _____

How are the housekeeping tasks accomplished? _____

Are family members satisfied with the way tasks are divided? _____

How are child-rearing responsibilities divided? _____

Who makes the major decisions in the family? _____

Who makes day-to-day decisions? _____

Are family members satisfied with the way decisions are made? _____

FAMILY FUNCTION
Goals

Long term _____

Short term _____

Individual family member's goals _____

Are individual and family goals appropriate, considering their current health problem and status? _____

How are individual family members and the family as a whole coping with their current health problem and status?

_____

Communication

Do husband and wife communicate regularly and effectively with each other? _____

Are family members able to communicate openly and honestly with each other? _____

Is conflict openly expressed and discussed? _____

Do family members respect each other's point of view? _____

Do family members offer emotional support to each other? _____

is needed. The diagnosic label may include the family's health needs, current and potential health problems, level of wellness, or a combination of the above. In addition the diagnosic statement should indicate possible causes and etiologies. Friedman (1981) notes the difficulty in defining discrete nursing diagnoses because information about the family is interrelated (see nursing diagnoses and sample nursing diagnoses boxes).

The nursing diagnosis often focuses on the family's ability to cope with its current situation, whether it is an acute illness or an anticipated developmental transition. Coping strategies can be adaptive or maladaptive. Appropriate use of external and internal resources allows the family to cope with day-to-day stressors and with unexpected occurrences that threaten its equilibrium and health. Families unable to mobilize strengths can experience defeat (Miller and Janosik, 1980). To cope effectively, the family needs to coordinate its member's positive adaptive responses. A health crisis can potentially be a growth experience and can result in greater family cohesiveness. Barbarin et al. (1985) identify the following copying techniques used by parents of children with cancer: information seeking, problem solving, help seeking, maintenance of emotional balance, reliance on religion, optimism, denial, and acceptance. They suggest that parents' coping styles determine whether the experience of childhood cancer is destructive or growth producing.

PLANNING

When nursing diagnoses have been formulated, the next step is to plan a course of action with the family. Planning includes goal setting, identification of potential internal and external resources, choosing effective approaches, and setting priorities. It is imperative that the plan of care be clearly understood by the family and that they agree to it. Goal setting must be a mutual endeavor, and the goals must be concrete, realistic, and acceptable to family members. For example, Mr. and Mrs. Venoy are newlyweds. Both have been divorced. Mrs. Venoy is childless, and Mr. Venoy has custody of three teenage children, a boy and two girls. This blended family is adjusting to new roles and family patterns, and all feel a great deal of tension. The daughters are doing poorly in school and are misbehaving in the classroom and at home. The son is verbally abusive to his sisters and often stays out late at night, refusing to tell his parents where he goes. The new wife describes the children in very negative terms such as "worthless" and "obnoxious." She openly acknowledges that her problems with the children are having a negative impact on

---

> ### Examples of Nursing Diagnoses for a Family with a Hospitalized Adult Member
>
> **NANDA-APPROVED NURSING DIAGNOSES**
>
> *Altered family processes* related to:
> - Sudden, unexpected illness
> - Financial concerns
> - Inability to problem-solve
> - Inadequate communication
>
> *Fear* (individual family members) related to:
> - Hospitalization
> - Knowledge deficit
>
> *Powerlessness* (individual family members) related to:
> - Hospitalization
> - Knowledge deficit
>
> *Ineffective family coping* related to:
> - Chronic illness
> - Family disorganization
>
> *Impaired home maintenance management* related to:
> - Dysfunctional grieving
> - Alteration in communication skills

her relationship with her husband. She also feels that none of the family member's psychological needs are being met and that, although she always wanted to have children, she does "not know how to deal with them." During goal setting, Mrs. Venoy agreed to gain more knowledge about teenage development and behavior. The care plan box provides a sample nursing care plan for this goal.

IMPLEMENTATION

Once the goals and actions have been defined, implementation begins. Interventions are strategies that help families adjust goals or are the processes by which the family attains them. Family interventions include nursing actions that increase members' ability in a certain area, remove barriers to health care, and do things that the family cannot do for itself (Friedman, 1981). The nurse guides family members in problem solving and provides practical service and concrete aid. In the above example, the nurse's role is that of educator. By providing appropriate information, it is possible that Mrs. Venoy's ability to understand and parent teenagers will increase. The problem is, of course, very complex, and this intervention will only be part of the overall nursing care plan. It is often necessary for the nurse to refer the family to other members of the health care team such as social workers or family therapists.

One approach for meeting goals is the use of family

Sample Nursing Diagnoses for Families

Defining Characteristics	Nursing Diagnoses	Related Factors
Physical, spiritual, social and emotional needs of family members not being met Ineffective communication between family members Family failing to meet developmental tasks	Altered family processes	▪ Situational transition or crisis ▪ Developmental transition or crisis
Family unable to maintain home and care for family member(s) Poor hygiene Impaired care giver Substance abuse	Impaired home maintenance management	▪ Debilitating, chronic disease ▪ Insufficient knowledge ▪ Gain or loss of a family member ▪ Lack of a support system
Neglect of family member(s) Complaints of abuse Emotional outbursts Helplessness and dependency	Ineffective family coping	▪ Chronic illness ▪ Family disorganization: parents are single, mentally disturbed, alcoholic, abusive; child or children are physically or mentally handicapped, unwanted, terminally ill ▪ Economic difficulties ▪ Change in family unit

Sample Nursing Care Plan for Families

Nursing Diagnosis	Goal	Expected Outcome	Nursing Interventions
Knowledge deficit (stepmother lacking necessary information for effective parenting of teenagers) related to lack of exposure to appropriate information	Stepmother will gain appropriate knowledge about teenage development and behavior.	Stepmother will be able to verbalize correct information about teenage development and behavior	Discuss with stepmother the developmental needs and tasks of adolescents. Provide and encourage appropriate reading material (for example, *Parent Effectiveness Training*).

strengths. Families often do not realize resources inherent in their own system. Otto (1973) uses this approach when counseling families. He identifies strengths and shares them with the family, thereby increasing the family's awareness of its own potentials and capabilities. Family strengths include clear communication, healthy child-rearing practices, support and nurturing among family members, active community participation, flexi-

bility in roles and functioning, and the use of crisis for growth. The nurse can expand on the idea of family strengths and help the family focus on its strengths instead of its problems and weaknesses. For example, the nurse could point out to the Venoys that their willingness to seek help during a difficult period is a strength in itself and that all the members are physically healthy and therefore have the energy to work out their problems.

Sample Evaluation of Interventions for Families

Goal	Evaluative Measures	Expected Outcome
Stepmother will gain appropriate knowledge about teenage development and behavior.	Record stepmother's verbal expression of appropriate knowledge. Record stepmother's description of behavior expected from teenagers. Ask father to describe stepmother's reaction to teenagers' behavior. Observe interactions between stepmother and children.	Stepmother will be able to verbalize correct information about teenage development and behavior.

EVALUATION

The final phase of the nursing process is evaluation. The response of the family and its members is appraised against the predetermined expected outcomes. The nurse evaluates the family's change in functioning and its satisfaction with the new level of functioning. Evaluation is an ongoing process. Goals and interventions are modified as needed, based on evaluation (see sample evaluation box).

SUMMARY

Although the structure and form of the American family is changing, the institution remains central in American society and strongly influences the client's health practices, beliefs, and values. The family's impact on health is as significant now as ever, and each family member can influence the health of other family members, as well as the health of the family as a unit. Since the concept of family varies, the nurse begins family assessment by determining the client's definition of and attitude toward family.

Different family forms often have many health concerns and resources for resolving those concerns. When the family faces health problems, the nurse assesses its structure and function to plan effective interventions. At times family structure and functioning may require alteration before a specific health problem is managed.

The nurse can apply the nursing process, whether the family is viewed as a highly significant environment within which the client seeks to maintain health or whether it is viewed as the client itself. If the family is viewed as the client's environment, the nursing focus is on the individual member's health. If the family as a whole is viewed as the client, the nurse focuses on the family's health, which is more than a summation of the health of its individual members. Using either perspective, the nurse maximizes therapeutic effectiveness by recognizing the family's influence and using its resources to promote individual and family health.

KEY CONCEPTS

✓ The family has a significant impact on the lives of its members.

✓ Family members mutually influence one another's health beliefs, practices, and status.

✓ Because the concept of family is highly individual, the nurse should base care on the client's attitude toward family rather than on an inflexible definition of the family.

✓ Specific family forms tend to have typical family health problems with which the nurse should be familiar.

✓ The family's structure and functioning significantly influence its health and ability to respond to health problems.

✓ The nurse can view the family as an important environment for the individual family member or can view the family unit as the client. The approach for any family depends in part on the situation.

✓ Measures of family health involve more than a summation of individual members' health.

REFERENCES

Adams, BN: The family: a sociological interpretation, New York, 1986, Harcourt Brace Jovanovich, Inc.

Barbarin O, et al.: Stress, coping, and marital functioning among parents of children with cancer, Journal of Marriage and the Family 47:473, 1985.

Cancellier, P: The American family: changes and challenges, Washington, D.C., 1984, Population Reference Bureau.

Caplan, G: The family as a support system. In Caplan, G, and Killilea, M: editors: Support systems and mutual help: multidisciplinary exploration, New York, 1975, Grune & Stratton, Inc.

Cherlin, A, and Furstenberg, F: The American family in the year 2000, The Futurist 17:7, 1983.

Engebretson, JC: Stepmothers as first-time parents: their needs and problems, Pediatr Nurs 8:387, 1982.

Estes, C, et al.: Political economy, health, and aging, Boston, 1984, Little, Brown & Co., Inc.

Fawcett, J: The family as a living open system: an emerging conceptual framework for nursing, Int Nurs Rev 22:113, 1975.

Friedman, M: Family nursing: theory and assessment, New York, 1981, Appleton-Century-Crofts.

McCubbin, H, and Dahl B: Marriage and family: individuals and life cycles, New York, 1985, The Free Press.

McGoldrick, M, and Carter, E: The stage of the family life cycle. In Henslin, J, editor: Marriage and family in a changing society, New York, 1985, The Free Press.

Miller, J, and Janosik, E: Family focused care, New York, 1980, Gardner Press, Inc.

Murphy, S: Family study and nursing research, Image: J Nurs Sch 18(4):170, 1986.

O'Brien, R: A conceptualization of family health. Paper presented in clinical and scientific sessions of the American Nurses' Association, Nashville, Tenn., Nov. 8-11, 1979.

Otto, H: A framework for assessing family strengths. In Reinhart, A, and Quinn, M, editors: Family centered community nursing, St. Louis, 1973, The C.V. Mosby Co.

Pratt, L: Family structure and effective health behavior: the energized family, Boston, 1976, Houghton Mifflin Co.

Roberts, C, and Feetham, S: Assessing family functioning across three areas of relationships, Nurs Res 31:231, 1982.

Skolnick, A: The intimate environment: explaining marriage and the family, 1987, Little, Brown & Co.

Wattenburg, BJ: The good news is the bad news is wrong, New York, 1985, Simon and Schuster, Inc.

Zinn, MB, and Eitzen, DS: Diversity in American families, New York, 1987, Harper & Row, Publishers, Inc.

ADDITIONAL READINGS

Amato, P: Family processes in one-parent, stepparent, and intact families: the child's point of view, Journal of Marriage and the Family 49(2):327, 1987.

Blumstein, P, and Schwartz, P: American couples, New York, 1983, William Morrow & Co., Inc.

Carpenito, L: Nursing diagnosis: application to practice, Philadelphia, 1983, J.B. Lippincott Co.

Croog, S, Lipson, A, and Levine, S: Help patterns in severe illness: the roles of kin networks, nonfamily resources and institutions, Journal of Marriage and the Family 34:34, 1972.

Gilliss, CL: Reducing family stress during and after coronary artery bypass surgery, Nurs Clin North Am 19(1):103, 1984.

Knafl, KA, and Grace, HK: Families across the life cycle, Boston, 1978, Little, Brown & Co.

Romanzuk, A: Helping the stepparent parent, Matern Child Nurs J 12:106, 1987.

Sund, K, and Ostwald, SK: Dual-earner families' stress levels and personal and life-style–related variables, Nurs Res 34(6):357, 1985.

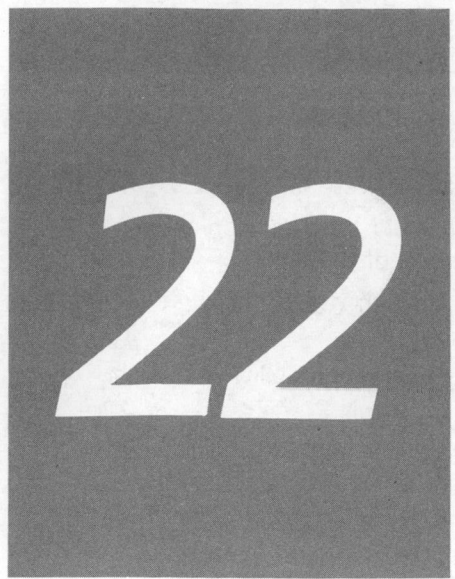

22

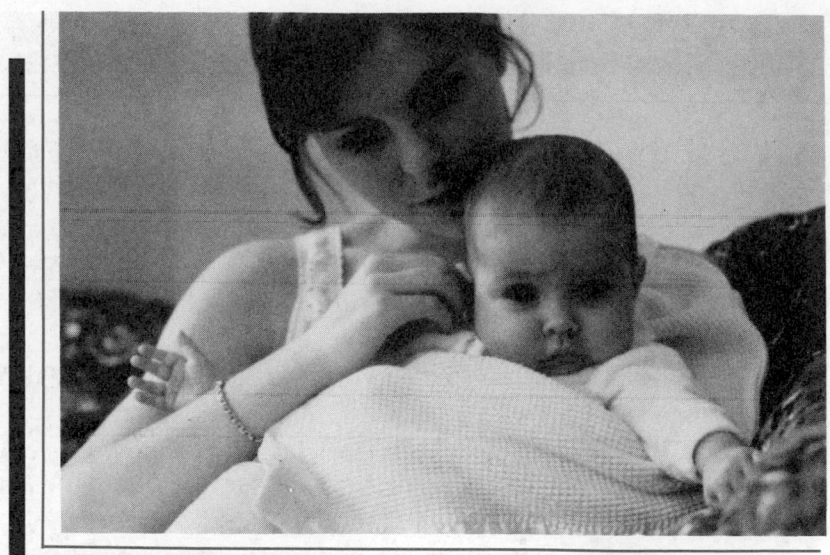

OBJECTIVES

Mastery of content in this chapter will enable the student to:

- Define the key terms listed.
- Describe three commonalities in human development and the six principles of growth and development related to them.
- Discuss the major factors influencing growth and development.
- Compare and discuss the theories of development related to nursing.
- Describe ways in which the nurse can provide support to the woman during pregnancy.
- Discuss physiological and psychosocial health concerns during the transition from intrauterine to extrauterine life.
- Describe the physical growth characteristics of the unborn child, infant, and toddler.
- Identify factors important for normal cognitive development through infancy and toddlerhood.
- Explain the importance of parent-child attachment and list factors that may impede the attachment process.
- Describe variables influencing how a child learns about and perceives his health status.
- Discuss ways the nurse can assist parents in promoting the child's health in all dimensions.
- Discuss the nursing process for the hospitalized child.

KEY TERMS

Accommodation	Maturation
Apgar Score	Molding
Assimilation	Morula
Attachment	Neonate
Blastocyst	Placenta
Chromosomes	Prenatal
Development	Preschooler
Embryo	Separation Anxiety
Fetus	Teratogen
Growth	Toddlerhood
Heredity	Vernix Caseosa
Infancy	Zygote
Lanugo	

Conception Through Preschool

Children are the future, and their health is the well-being of society. Understanding children and their growth and development is essential to promoting health and establishing healthful patterns for the entire life span. The nurse must have a clear understanding of normal or expected growth and behavior in early developmental stages to guide and promote normalcy and to prevent abnormalities. For example, without the knowledge that the average 2½- to 3-year old child is toilet trained, the nurse cannot promote learning of this skill at an appropriate earlier age.

Nursing practice based on principles of growth and development is organized and directed toward helping individuals adapt to changing internal and external conditions.

This chapter discusses principles and concepts related to the growth and development process and to the application of these principles in health promotion and nursing. It also discusses the growth and development characteristics from conception through preschool, as related to the nursing process.

GROWTH AND DEVELOPMENT THEORY

Human growth and development are orderly, predictable processes beginning with conception and continuing until death. Each person progresses through definite phases of growth and development, but the pace and behavior of this progression are highly individual. A child must learn to walk before he can run, for example, but one child may walk at 10 months and another may not walk until 15 months. Both children progress through the same developmental phase and both demonstrate normal, healthy behaviors, but each accomplishes the task at his own pace.

The ability to progress through each developmental phase influences a person's level of health. The success or failure experienced within a given phase affects the ability to complete subsequent phases. If an individual repeatedly fails to develop, inadequacies that may threaten health result, but if the individual experiences repeated successes, competencies that help maintain and promote health result. A child not learning to walk by 18 or 20 months, for example, demonstrates delayed gross motor ability that slows exploration and manipulation of the environment, which are essential to learning. A child walking by 10 months is able to explore and find stimulation in the environment, thereby enhancing his or her learning.

Because nursing promotes the health of individuals of all ages, the nurse must (1) understand the growth and development process, (2) understand the theories and principles of growth and development, (3) be able to identify the stages of growth and development, (4) be able to identify factors influencing the developmental progress, and (5) assess the individual's ability to respond in a healthy manner to the process. Knowledge and understanding of these basic concepts provide a foundation for delivering health care. A developmental approach allows the nurse to organize knowledge about human behavior into common patterns that can be applied to individuals.

A developmental perspective helps the nurse understand *why* commonalities and variations exist and the influence they have on health. With this knowledge the nurse can intervene in a manner consistent with the client's unique needs and in the context of his or her general developmental level.

Definitions

Growth and development are synchronous processes, which are interdependent in the healthy individual. A person experiences quantitative and qualitative changes in growth and development.

PHYSICAL GROWTH

Physical growth is the quantitative or measurable aspect of an individual's increase in physical measurements (Whaley and Wong, 1987). Measurable growth indicators include height, weight, and the indices of dental, skeletal, and sexual age. Increases in these indicators demonstrate growth. For example, infants generally double their birth weight by 6 months of age and double

their height by 36 months. Also, females experience rapid sexual growth during puberty, beginning with breast budding at an average of 10 years, followed by the onset of menses at the average age of 12.

DEVELOPMENT

The qualitative or behavioral aspects of progressive adaption to the environment are called *development*. An example of these qualitative changes is increased functioning capacity resulting from mastery of several smaller skills. For instance, a significant qualitative and observable change for toddlers is saying "please" when asking for something. However, before toddlers develop this social skill, they must master several other skills, including recognizing specific objects (such as a cookie), speaking coherently, and identifying sensations (such as appetite or hunger).

MATURATION

Maturation is the process of becoming fully developed and grown. It involves the individual's biology, physiology, and desire to learn more mature behaviors. To mature, the individual may have to relinquish previous behaviors and learning, integrate new patterns into existing behaviors, or both. The process of maturation influences the sequence and timing of the qualitative and quantitative changes associated with growth and development. For example, the infant relinquishes crawling for walking because it permits more extensive investigation of his environment and more learning. However, he cannot walk until he has developed the biological ability and structures to perform the action (that is, increased muscle cells and tone).

CRITICAL PERIODS OF DEVELOPMENT

Stages of growth and development involve the concept of "critical periods of development." A critical period is a specific span of time during which the environment has its greatest impact on the individual (Behrman and Vaughan, 1987). During these critical periods, some form of sensory stimulation is necessary for developmental progression. Without stimulation, task completion is difficult or unattainable. For example, the toddler who has not been encouraged to learn to walk during a set time period may have difficulty learning to walk at another time. Therefore an individual's developmental progression depends on the timing and degree of stimulation, as well as on his readiness to be stimulated by the environment. A stimulus provided too early may not be useful. For example, an 18-month-old child cannot learn to write, regardless of the intensity of the stimuli, whereas a 6-year-old has the readiness and ability to learn and write if stimulated to do so.

PRINCIPLES OF GROWTH AND DEVELOPMENT

Growth and development involve certain commonalities true of all people. These commonalities are expressed by the following concepts:

1. An individual has adaptive potential for qualitative and quantitative changes by receiving stimuli from and giving stimuli to the environment.
2. An individual derives uniqueness from the interaction and heredity and environment.
3. The primary goal of development is achievement of potential (self-realization or self-actualization).

The basic principles of growth and development follow:

1. *Development has direction,* proceeding in an orderly way and in a set sequence.
2. *Development is complex yet predictable,* occurring with a consistent pattern and chronology.
3. *Development is unique* to individuals and their genetic potential, and each individual tends to seek a maximal potential for development.
4. *Development occurs through conflict and adaptation,* and different aspects develop at different rates, creating periods of equilibrium and disequilibrium.
5. *Development involves challenges* for the individual, in the form of certain tasks specific to age and ability.
6. *Developmental tasks require practice and energy,* the focus of which varies with each developmental stage and task accomplished.

STAGES OF GROWTH AND DEVELOPMENT

Human growth and development are intricate, complex processes. Although these processes are continuous, they are often divided into stages organized by age group. Although this chronological division is arbitrary, it is based on the timing and sequence of developmental tasks the individual must accomplish to progress to another stage. The chronology of growth and development is listed in Table 22-1.

Major Factors Influencing Growth and Development

The human being is a complex, open system influenced by natural forces from within and by forces from the environment. Interaction between these forces ultimately affects development. In general, natural factors set the potential limits for development, whereas external factors present opportunities for achieving that potential. The most influential forces of nature are heredity and temperament, whereas family and peers are the primary external forces (Table 22-2).

THEORIES OF HUMAN DEVELOPMENT

Since the beginning of this century, research into human growth and development has led to a number of developmental theories. These theories vary in the way humans are viewed and in the aspect of development emphasized. Some theories view development as a continuous process, moving from the simple to the more complex. Others consider it as discontinuous, with alternating periods of relative equilibrium and disequilibrium. Health care professionals often use different theoretical frameworks when providing care, which may complicate communication between them. Therefore the nurse needs to be familiar with the more common theories to communicate effectively with other health professionals when planning, implementing, and evaluating coordinated health care. In addition, knowledge of these theories is essential for comprehensive nursing care because no one framework addresses all developmental areas. A review of the most common developmental theories appears in Table 22-3.

SELECTING A DEVELOPMENTAL FRAMEWORK FOR NURSING

Providing nursing care to clients of all developmental stages is easier when planning is based on a theoretical framework. An organized, systematic approach ensures that client needs are assessed and met by the care plan. If nursing care is delivered only as a series of isolated actions, one or more of the client's developmental needs may be overlooked. A developmental approach encourages organized care directed toward the client's current level of functioning to motivate self-direction and health promotion. For example, understanding an adolescent's need to be independent should prompt the nurse to establish with a teenage client a contract about the plan of care and its implementation.

The developmental approach also has advantages for clients. Their capabilities are used, and they are actively involved in their own care. Total health is also promoted because the nurse is aware of the clients' present developmental stages and the directions in which they are

Text continued on p. 568.

TABLE 22-1 Chronology of Growth and Development

Stage	Age Span	Significant Behavioral Milestones
Prenatal	Conception–birth	Maternal physical and psychosocial adjustment and progression through pregnancy Health and growth of fetus
Neonatal	Birth–1 month	Infant attachment behaviors: rooting, sucking, grasping, clinging Visual fixation: objects, face Equality of body movements
Infancy	1 month–1 year	Physical: lifts head, rolls, sits, crawls, pulls to stand, walks, grasps, rakes, transfers hand objects, uses pincer grasp Psychosocial: smiles, vocalizes, laughs, feeds self finger foods, says "Da-Da" and "Ma-Ma," plays peek-a-boo and pat-a-cake
Toddlerhood	1–3 years	Physical: walks well forward and backward, stoops and recovers, climbs, runs, jumps in place, throws overhand, voluntarily releases hand, uses spoon, drinks from cup, scribbles, builds two- then four-block tower Psychosocial: indicates wants by behaviors other than crying, increases vocabulary, imitates, helps with household chores, points to body parts, recognizes animals, engages in solitary play
Preschool	3–6 years	Physical: rides tricycle, walks up then down stairs alternating feet, hops on one foot, tandem walks, draws circle, then cross, then triangle, dresses with assistance, then with supervision, then alone Psychosocial: knows first name, then age, then last name, engages in parallel play progressing to interaction play, uses plurals and three-word sentences progressing to complex sentences, follows directions, counts
School age	6–11 years	Physical: skips, skates, tumbles, tandem walks backward, prints progressing to script, ties knots, then bows Psychosocial: engages in interactive play with rules progressing to organized sports or activities, has significant peer relationships, enjoys hobbies, assumes complete responsibility for personal care
Adolescence	11–21 years	Physical: undergoes cognitive growth spurt, develops secondary sex characteristics, increases cognitive ability and formal operational thought Psychosocial: develops sense of identity and sex role, establishes independence, develops peer relationships with both sexes, develops life philosophy (values, beliefs), makes occupational decisions
Young and middle adulthood	21–65 years	Physical/cognitive: has established physical growth state and functioning, undergoes menopause, begins physical/physiological degeneration, refines formal operational abilities Psychosocial: develops self-sufficiency, pursues vocation/occupation, has intense interpersonal relationships (most frequently marriage and children)
Older adulthood	65 years–death	Physical cognitive: has general slowing of physical and cognitive functioning Psychosocial: needs to establish highest degree of independence (self-sufficiency) physically possible by adapting environment to ability, reflects on life accomplishments, events, and experiences, continues interpersonal relationships

TABLE 22-2 Major Factors Influencing Growth and Development

Factors	Relevant Influences
FORCES OF NATURE	
Heredity	Genetic endowment includes sex, race, hair and eye color, physical growth, and stature.
	Biologically inherited psychological uniqueness includes easy, slow to warm, and difficult temperaments.
EXTERNAL FORCES	
Family	Family purpose is to protect its members.
	Family functions include means for survival, security, assistance with emotional and social development, assistance with maintenance of relationships, instruction about society and world, and assistance in learning roles and behaviors.
	Family influences through its values, beliefs, customs, and specific patterns of interaction and communication.
	Ordinal position and sex influence an individual's interaction and communication in family
Peer group	Peer group provides a new and different learning environment.
	Peer group provides different patterns and structures of interaction and communication necessitating a different style of behavior.
	Functions of peer group include allowing the individual to learn about success and failure; to validate and challenge his thoughts, feelings, and concepts; to receive acceptance, support, and rejection as a unique person apart from the family; and to achieve group purposes by meeting demands, pressures, and expectations.
Life experiences	Life experiences and learning processes allow the individual to develop by applying what has been learned to what needs to be learned.
	Learning process involves a series of steps: recognition of need to know a task; mastery of skills to perform task; mastery of task; expertise in performing task, which expands capabilities; integration into the whole functioning; use of accumulated skills and experiences to develop a repertoire of effective behavior.
Health environment	Level of health affects individual's responsiveness to environment.
Prenatal health	Preconception (for example, genetic and chromosomal factors, maternal age and health) and postconception (for example, nutrition, weight gain, use of tobacco and alcohol, medical problems, use of prenatal services) factors affect fetal growth and development.
Nutrition	Growth is regulated by dietary factors. Adequacy of nutrients influences whether and how physiological needs, as well as subsequent growth and development needs, are met.
Rest, sleep, and exercise	Balance between rest or sleep and exercise is essential to rejuvenating the body. Imbalances diminish growth, whereas equilibrium reinforces physiological and psychological health.
State of health	Illness or injury potentially hampers growth and development. The nature and duration of the health problem influence its impact. Prolonged injury or illness leaves the individual less able to cope and respond to the demands and tasks of the developmental stage.
Living environment	Factors affecting growth and development include season, climate, housing, and socioeconomic status.

TABLE 22-3 Overview of Development Theories

Theory	Stages	Characteristics	Strengths	Limitations
Freudian psychoanalytical theory	Oral—birth-1 years Anal—2-3 years Phallic—4-5 years Latent—6-12 years Genital—13-death	Basis of inner drives; psychosexual focus	Recognizes importance of instinctual needs; defines id, ego, superego as personality; defines conscious and unconscious mind.	Heavy emphasis on sexual behaviors; does not deal with adult cognitive or moral development; based on data from psychiatric clients, hence not easily applied to normal clients.
Erikson's psychosocial development theory	Basic trust versus mistrust—birth-1 year Autonomy versus shame—2-4 years Initiative versus guilt—4-8 years Industry versus inferiority—8-12 years Identity versus role confusion—13-20 years Intimacy versus solidarity versus isolation—20-30 years Generativity versus self-absorption and stagnation—30-60 years Integrity versus despair—60 years-death	Socialization focus; ongoing process throughout life directed toward balance; stages with positive and negative components that individual must balance	Recognizes role of social, biological, and environmental factors in development; relates specific tasks to appropriate age; well organized; includes all ages.	Broad age ranges; does not include cognitive or moral development; tasks within stages are not absolute and may overlap.
Maslow's theory of human need	Physiological needs—birth-1½ years Safety—2-5 years Love and belonging—all ages Self-esteem—6-19 years Self-actualization—young adult-older adult	Human need focus; ongoing process directed toward homeostasis	Identifies human needs; recognizes physical and psychosocial aspects of person; emphasizes meeting of needs, not accomplishment of stage.	Does not identify age chronologically, making assessment difficult; last stage/goal not generally attainable in absolute sense; does not fully explain the complex nature of human beings.

Theory	Stages	Characteristics	Strengths	Limitations
Piaget's theory of cognitive development	Sensorimotor—birth-2 years, divided into 6 substages Preoperational—2-7 years, divided into 2 substages Concrete operations—7-11 years Formal operations—11-death	Cognitive focus; defines process in terms of assimilation, accommodation, and adaptation.	Accounts for heredity and environmental interaction; well defined; incorporates language concepts.	Does not deal with psychosocial aspects; does not account for individual differences and variability in progression; strict hierarchical progress questionable.
Havighurst's developmental tasks	Infancy and early childhood Middle childhood Adolescence Early adulthood Middle age Later maturity	Learning to develop is focus; ascribes a certain set of socially defined tasks to each age group	Specific definition of tasks needing completion; goal-oriented development; practical and organized by age; recognizes the importance of timing to development	Some tasks not reflective of changes in today's society; overemphasis on learning and somewhat inflexible in outcome (that is, no adaptation); does not deal with cognition.
Social learning theory	No stages—views human development as a continuous process of learning and changing behavior.	Based on drives, cues, responses, and reinforcement; behavior oriented; imitation major source of learned behavior	Achieves behavioral results; stimulus-response pattern well defined; applicable to all age groups without restraint.	Does not recognize natural forces in humans; little recognition of psychosocial needs; little recognition of individuality and may not promote self-direction.
Kohlberg's theory of moral development	Premoral: Obedience and punishment orientation—4-6 years Hedonistic orientation—6 to 9 years Conventional: "Good-boy" orientation—9-10 years Authority maintains morality—10-12 years Self-accepted moral principles: Contractual morality—adolescence-death Principles of conscience—adolescence-death	Follows a sequence corresponding to cognition; morality developed when cognitively prepared	Assigns order and definition to moral code development; serves as a basis for assessment of morality.	Levels and stages are not absolute—variability probably does exist; final level difficult to achieve; does not address psychosocial issues.

headed. Therefore the nurse can focus health activities that promote developmental task completion. For example, the nurse might encourage a young adult client to apply for a job promotion because both nurse and client recognize that he needs to establish his career, that he is motivated, and that he desires to succeed.

Although a developmental approach facilitates nursing practice, no single theory addresses all needs relevant to nursing. All theories have advantages and disadvantages. These theories are useful in guiding assessment, nursing diagnosis, planning, intervention, and evaluation of care. An ideal framework would be applicable to clients of all ages in a variety of settings and would consider the physical, psychosocial, and cognitive processes. No theory meets all these criteria. Therefore the nurse must combine the most useful aspects of several theories into a practical approach.

If the nurse integrates the stage theories into a life span perspective, care can be focused on the aspect of development that demonstrates needs. For example, nursing activities for a client with acute pneumonia would be based on meeting physical and psychosocial needs related to the illness. The nurse would be concerned with care that returns the client to a healthy state and that helps him deal with treatment, hospitalization, and recovery.

A general age-stage developmental framework for nursing practice allows for individuality, even though most people share common experiences in the general developmental processes. Because individuals respond differently to common experiences and needs, movement within and between stages is highly individualized. Therefore the nurse should not rigidly apply the age stages of any developmental theory but should rather plan individualized care. Practicality and flexibility are the basis for successful nursing care.

CONCEPTION

From the moment of conception, human development proceeds at a rapid rate. Most intrauterine health problems are caused by a combination of genetic and environmental factors. During the prenatal period, the embryo grows from a single cell to a zygote, a complex, physiological being. All major organ systems develop in utero, with some functioning before birth. The psychosocial being also begins to emerge during the gestation period.

Intrauterine Life

Intrauterine life generally lasts 9 calendar or 10 lunar months. The organism's life begins when the ovum is penetrated by one sperm. Fertilization most often takes place in the fallopian tube, usually within 12 to 24 hours after the ovum is released from the ovary and sexual intercourse has occurred. The ovum and sperm fuse, and the material from both cell nuclei unite. The organism then has its full genetic complement in one pair of sex chromosomes and 22 pairs of autosomal chromosomes. The ovum and the sperm each contribute one chromosome to each pair. It is through this mechanism that genetically programmed diseases (such as Down's syndrome) and genetically determined characteristics (such as eye color) are transmitted from parent to child.

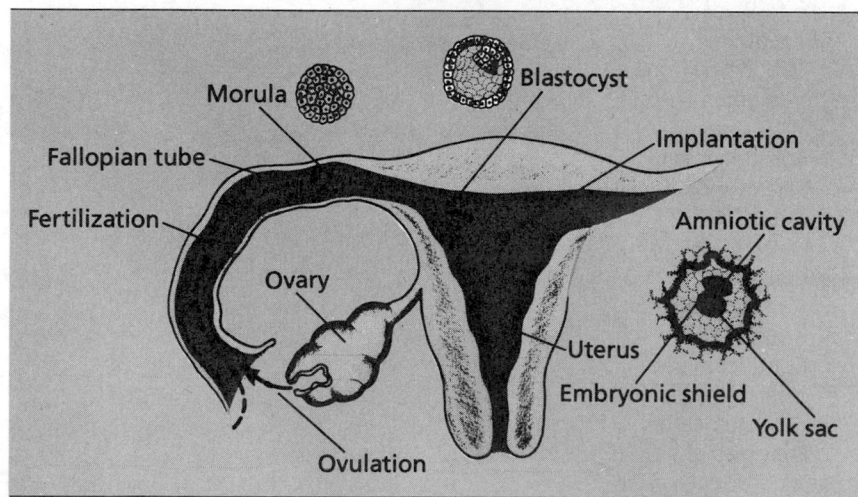

Fig. 22-1 The fertilization cycle.
From Nelms, BC, and Mullins, RG: Growth and development: a primary health care approach, © 1982, p. 137. Reprinted by permission of Prentice-Hall, Inc., Englewood Cliffs, N.J.

The fertilized ovum, or zygote, passes through the fallopian tube to the uterus within 4 days. During this time the zygote continues to divide. By the third day a solid ball of cells, the morula, has formed. This solid ball soon develops a central cavity, or blastocyst. Even at this early stage, cells begin to differentiate in structure and function. Cells at one end of the blastocyst develop into the embryo, and those at the opposite end form the placenta. By day 4 the embryo has traveled through the fallopian tube into the uterus and is implanted in the uterine wall (Fig. 22-1).

Before implantation the embryo is relatively protected from the external environment, but with implantation, it becomes more vulnerable to the larger maternal environment via exchange of materials through the placenta. The placenta produces essential hormones that help maintain the pregnancy and that permit transfer of material between the embryo and mother, including oxygen, carbon dioxide, nutrients, and waste products. Because the placenta is extremely porous, noxious materials such as viruses and drugs can also pass from mother to child. The effect of noxious agents on the unborn child depends on the developmental stage in which exposure takes place.

The period of gestation is frequently divided into three time periods called trimesters. Because the developing fetus is in a different stage of development in each trimes-ter, interference with the development process has different outcomes in each.

Physical Development
FIRST TRIMESTER

The first trimester is the first 3 calendar months. After implantation, fetal cells continue to differentiate and develop into essential organ systems. These processes of cellular change (differentiation) and staged organ change (development) occur at different rates and times, and each organ is extremely vulnerable to environmental insult during its time of most rapid growth. Interference with growth can cause the congenital absence of an organ system or extensive structural or functional alterations. Fig. 22-2 shows the time periods for differentiation of major organ systems.

Because several organ systems develop at the same time, disruption of one system is often associated with disruption of others. The nurse should consider this simultaneous development when conducting the initial newborn nursing assessment.

HEALTH CONCERNS Agents capable of producing adverse effects in the fetus are called *teratogens*. Some teratogens produce defects only if the fetus is exposed to the agent at a critical time when the vulnerable organ

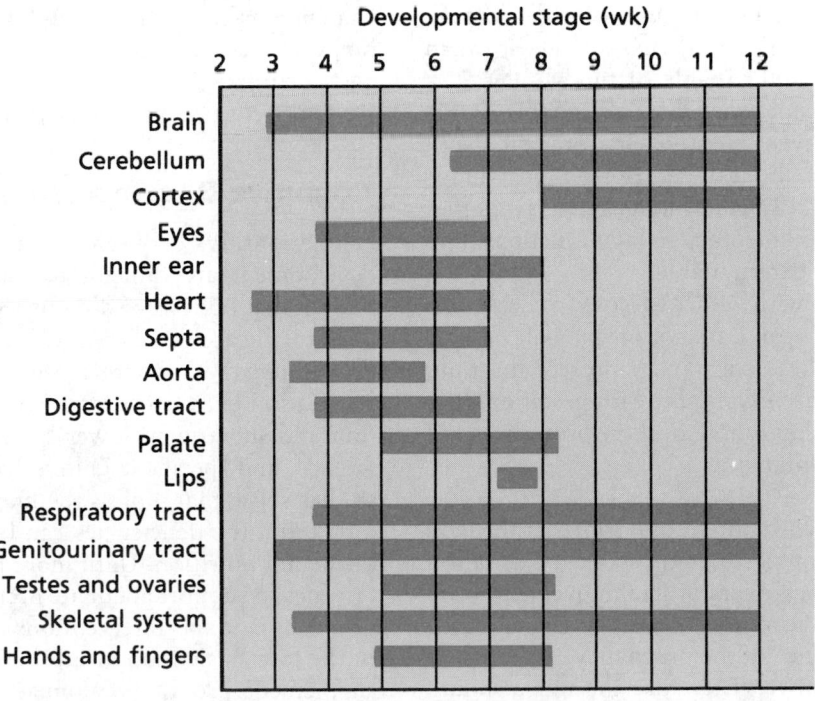

Fig. 22-2 Periods of organ differentiation.
From Whaley, LF, and Wong, DL: Nursing care of infants and children, ed.1, St. Louis, 1979, The C.V. Mosby Co.

is developing. One such teratogen is the rubella or measles virus, which can cause abortion, stillbirth, or defects of the eyes, ears, and heart, primarily when exposure is in the first trimester. Other infectious agents such as those causing syphilis and herpes are also known to adversely affect fetal health.

Many drugs are teratogenic during rapid organ growth (organogenesis) in the first trimester. Barbiturates, alcohol, hydantoins, anticonvulsants, and anticoagulants are only a few of the chemical agents associated with fetal abnormalities, and many other agents are under investigation. Benefits of any drug needed to maintain the mother's health must be weighed against potential harm to the fetus. Drug abuse results in infants with low birth weight and congenital abnormalities. In addition, studies show that mothers who smoke deliver infants with lower birth weights than infants delivered by nonsmoking mothers (Warshaw, 1986; Williams, 1986).

With this knowledge, the nurse should explore lifestyle changes that can help the woman maintain abstinence from tobacco, alcohol, and medications. For example, nonpharmacological relaxation techniques of progressive muscle relaxation are preferred for relieving tension. The nurse also provides emotional support as the woman tries to implement new strategies.

SECOND TRIMESTER

During the second trimester, the third through the sixth month, some organ systems continue basic development and the functional capabilities of others are refined. By the end of the second trimester, most organ systems are complete and capable of functioning. The fetus is therefore considered viable, or capable of life outside the uterus if given intensive environmental support. The fetus weighs about 0.7 kg (1½ pounds) and is approximately 30 cm (12 inches) long. Fingers and toes are differentiated, a rudimentary kidney functions, and the sex of the fetus is determinable.

The fetus is covered with vernix caseosa, a cheese-like substance coating the skin. Lanugo, or fine hair, is over most of the body. These substances protect the thin, fragile skin and decrease in amount with gestation. Prematurely born infants have more of these protective coverings than full-term infants.

HEALTH CONCERNS. In the second trimester the fetal heartbeat becomes audible to stethoscope auscultation and the mother becomes aware of fetal movement. Both events are highly significant to the mother, because they provide tangible evidence of the pregnancy and reassure her that the fetus is alive. Therefore the nurse should focus on these events during prenatal care.

Changes in maternal behavior during this period include planning for the birth, concern for personal safety, and preoccupation with health and appearance. The nurse can help the woman adapt to these changes and plan for the impending birth. This is often a good time for education about gestational events and appropriate maternal rest and nutrition. Discussing birth alternatives and providing support and reassurance about the pregnancy's progression are appropriate nursing actions at this stage.

THIRD TRIMESTER

During the last 3 months of intrauterine life the fetus grows to approximately 50 cm (19 to 20 inches) in length. Subcutaneous fat is stored, and weight increases to between 3.2 and 3.4 kg (7 to 7½ pounds). The skin thickens, lanugo begins to disappear, and the fetal body becomes rounder and fuller.

A tremendous spurt in brain growth begins during the third trimester and lasts well into the first few years of postnatal life. The central nervous system has established its total number of neurons and connections between neurons, and myelination of nerve fibers progresses at a rapid rate. Exposure to noxious agents and the absence of essential nutrients are the most common causes of damage to the central nervous system during this trimester. The nurse can teach the woman about these factors, particularly nutritional counseling.

At the end of the third trimester the normal fetus is physically able to make the transition from intrauterine to extrauterine life. The cardiac system is capable of changing its circulation to end bypassing the lungs. The lungs are capable of maintaining the inflated state for gas exchange, and primitive temperature maintenance systems, reflexes, and sensory organs are ready for use.

Cognitive Development

Relationships between prenatal events and cognitive development are difficult to establish. However, it is known that periods of diminished oxygen (anoxia) during fetal life are associated with deficits in later cognitive functioning (Westwood, 1983). Some research shows an association between severely inadequate prenatal nutrition and subsequent lower brain weight, head circumference, and specific cognitive abilities. However, other studies show that, unless the malnutrition is severe and long term, the deficiencies can be averted by later supplemental nutrition. Until more is known, the nurse intervenes to support adequate prenatal nutrition and prevent fetal anoxia. Interventions can include discussions of the four basic food groups, enrollment in a nutrition supplement program (Women, Infants, and Children [WIC] Program), and discussion of activities associated with low blood oxygen levels.

Psychosocial Development

Little information is available about the relationship between prenatal experiences and the child's psychosocial development. Some authorities believe that the biochemical environment of the uterus can significantly influence later psychosocial development. Because the biochemical environment is influenced by the mother's emotional state, her emotional and physical states may have significant psychosocial consequences for the unborn child. Furthermore, the mother's emotional state may influence her behavior after childbirth, which in turn influences the child's psychosocial development. The nurse therefore assesses the family's response to the pregnancy and the sources of family stress so she can intervene to minimize potential adverse effects on the child's psychosocial development.

TABLE 22-4 Apgar Scoring

Sign	Score 0	Score 1	Score 2
Heart rate	Absent	Slow (below 100)	Over 100
Respiratory effort	Absent	Slow, irregular, hypoventilation	Good, crying lustily
Muscle tone	Flaccid	Some flexion of extremities	Active motion, well flexed
Reflex irritability	No response	Cry, some motion	Vigorous cry
Color	Blue, pale	Body pink, hands and feet blue	Completely pink

From Korones, S: High-risk newborn infants: the basis for intensive nursing care, St. Louis, ed. 4, 1986, The C.V. Mosby Co.

TRANSITION FROM INTRAUTERINE TO EXTRAUTERINE LIFE

The transition from intrauterine to extrauterine life requires rapid changes in the neonate. The nurse assesses the neonate's ability to make these changes and intervenes if necessary to ensure success. Gestational age, exposure to depressant drugs before or during labor, and the neonate's own behavioral style influence adjustment to the external environment. Therefore the initial assessment encompasses a variety of physical and psychosocial elements. The nurse also provides opportunities for the parents and child to develop close emotional ties.

Physical Health Concerns

An immediate assessment of the neonate's condition is performed because the nurse's first concern is the physiological functioning of the major organ systems. Nursing care is then directed toward maintaining an open airway, stabilizing body temperature, and protecting the neonate from infection.

Patency of the airway is best ensured by removing nasooropharyngeal secretions with a bulb syringe. Once the airway is open, the nurse directs efforts toward stabilization of body temperature. Wrapping the neonate in small, soft blankets usually provides adequate heat preservation. For neonates unable to sustain body temperatures, Isolettes and incubators, which supply radiant heat, can be used. Proper handwashing and clean gloves during diaper changes help protect the neonate, the nurse, and other neonates from infection and should be performed before and between handling neonates. Fric-

tion is the most important element of the handwashing technique. Additional infection-prevention measures include the instillation of antibiotics or 2 drops of 1% silver nitrate solution into the eyes to prevent *Neisseria gonorrhoeae* infections, which can be transmitted to the neonate during passage through an infected vaginal canal. A drying antiseptic agent, such as alcohol, should be applied daily to the umbilicus to prevent infection.

Most institutions require immediate identification of the neonate. The nurse usually attaches identification bands to the mother and neonate and secures foot and hand prints for birth records. In addition, the nurse records the neonate's vital signs and measurements.

The nurse is frequently responsible for assessing the neonate's physiological functioning at birth. The most widely used assessment tool is the Apgar score, which rates five physiological characteristics. The newborn's heart rate, respiratory effort, muscle tone, reflex irritability, and color are rated to determine the overall status. The Apgar assessment is generally conducted at 1 and 5 minutes after birth and may be repeated until the newborn's condition stabilizes. Table 22-4 outlines the scoring criteria of physiological functioning. A total score of 0 to 3 signifies severe distress, a score of 4 to 6 represents moderate difficulty, and a score of 7 to 10 indicates little difficulty in adjusting to extrauterine life. The nurse can use the Apgar score to determine areas requiring further assessment and careful observation.

Psychosocial Concerns

After immediate physical evaluation the nurse assesses the parent's and newborn's needs for close physical contact. Early parent-child interaction has been found to encourage later close parent-child attachment. Physical factors, such as the parent's fatigue, hunger, and health, and emotional factors, such as being happy about the birth and needing to be affectionate and to touch, see and be close to the infant, are assessed.

Merely placing the family together does not promote closeness or acquaintance. Parents and neonate must be capable and desirous of exploring and responding to each other. Most healthy neonates are awake and alert for the first half hour after birth, and if the parents are receptive, this is an opportune time for parent-child acquaintance to begin. Close body contact, often including breast feeding, is a satisfying way for most families to start. If immediate contact is not possible, the nurse incorporates it into the care plan as early as possible, which may mean bringing the newborn to an ill parent or bringing the parents to an ill or premature child.

Attachment occurs when parent and newborn elicit reciprocal and complementary behaviors. Parental attachment behaviors include attentiveness and physical contact. Neonate attachment behavior involves maintenance of contact with the parent. Preterm and ill neonates and their parents have more difficulty forming this attachment if separation is prolonged. The attachment process is further complicated if parents are unable to care for the usual infant needs. The nurse should give

the parents support throughout the early attachment process, particularly if the newborn is ill or separated from the parents.

NEONATE

The neonatal period is the first 28 days of life. During this stage the newborn's physical functioning is mostly reflexive, and stabilization of major organ systems is the body's primary task. The newborn's behavior greatly influences interaction between him and his environment and care givers. For example, the average 2-week-old smiles spontaneously and is able to regard his mother's face. The impact of these reflexive behaviors is generally a surge of maternal feelings of love that prompt the mother to cuddle the baby.

Nurses can apply their knowledge of this stage of growth and development to promote newborn and parental health. If the nurse understands, for example, that the newborn's cry is generally a reflexive response to an unmet need (such as hunger), parents can be assisted in identifying ways to meet those needs, such as counseling the parents to feed their baby on demand rather than on a rigid schedule.

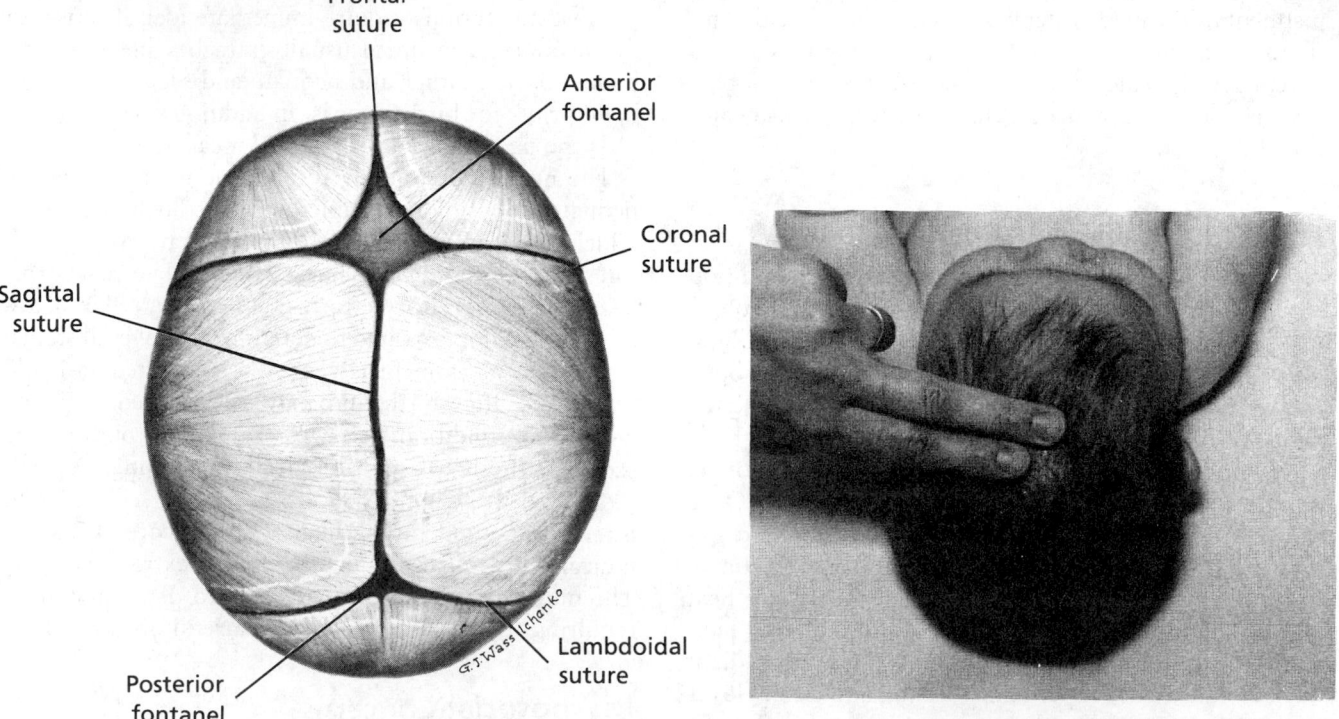

Fig. 22-3   Fontanels and suture lines.
From Whaley, LF, and Wong, DL: Nursing care of infants and children, ed. 3, St. Louis, 1987, The C.V. Mosby Co.

Physical Development

A comprehensive nursing assessment is performed as soon as the neonate's physiological functioning is stable, generally within a few hours after birth. At this time the nurse measures height, weight, head circumference, temperature, pulse, and respirations and observes general appearance, body functions, sensory capabilities, and responsiveness. In addition, the nurse coordinates screening tests and other laboratory tests as indicated by the neonate's state of health. Blood tests such as those for hypothyroidism and phenylketonuria (PKU) allow early detection and treatment, thereby preventing permanent central nervous system damage. These and other screening tests are required by law in many states.

The average newborn weighs 3200 g (7 pounds, 1 ounce), is 50 cm (20 inches) in length, and has a head circumference of 35 cm (14 inches). Up to 10% of birth weight is lost in the first few days of life, primarily through fluid losses by respiration, urination, defecation, and decreased intake. Birth weight is usually regained by the second week of life, and a gradual pattern of increase in weight, height, and head circumference is evident by 1 month. These increases average 4 to 7 ounces in weight per week, 0.6 to 1.2 cm (¼ to ½ inch) in length per month, and 2 cm in head circumference per month.

The neonate's heart rate gradually decreases from the fetal rate of 130 to 160 beats per minute to 120 to 140 beats per minute. Systole and diastole are of shorter duration, greater intensity, and higher pitch. The newborn's respiratory movements are primarily abdominal and vary in rate and rhythm. The average rate is 30 to 50 respirations per minute. The axillary temperature ranges from 36.5° to 37° C and generally stabilizes within 24 hours after birth.

Normal physical characteristics include the continued presence of lanugo on the skin of the back, cyanosis of the hands and feet, especially during activity, and a soft protuberant abdomen. Skin color varies according to racial and genetic heritage. Molding, or overlapping of the soft skull bones, is common during birth. The bones readjust in a few weeks, producing a more rounded appearance. Linear breaks, sutures, and small diamond-shaped spaces, the fontanels, are palpable between the unfused skull bones (Fig. 22-3). The anterior and the posterior fontanels are usually palpable at birth.

Normal behavioral characteristics of the newborn include periods of sucking, crying, sleeping, and activity. Movements are generally sporadic, but they are symmetrical and involve all four extremities. The relatively flexed position of intrauterine life continues as the neonate attempts to maintain an enclosed, secure feeling. Newborns normally watch the care giver's face, reflexively smile and respond to sensory stimuli, particularly the primary care giver's face, voice, and touch.

Neurological function is assessed by observing the neonate's level of activity, alertness, irritability, and responsiveness to stimuli, and the presence and strength of reflexes. Normal reflexes include blinking in response to bright lights and startling in response to sudden, loud noises. Table 22-5 lists other commonly evaluated neonatal reflexes. Their absence indicates possible trauma or central nervous system complications. Because the newborn depends largely on reflexes for response to environment, assessment of these response characteristics is vital.

Cognitive Development

Early cognitive development begins with the neonate's innate behaviors, reflexes, and sensory functions. During this time the newborn initiates reflex activities, assimilates new objects into behavior, and accommodates these behaviors to achieve his desire. For example, the neonate learns to turn to the nipple. Although the infant behaves of his own volition, activities learned are limited to reflex and sensory function (Nelms and Mullins, 1982).

Sensory functions contribute to cognitive development in the newborn. At birth the newborn can focus on objects about 8 to 10 inches from the face and can perceive forms. A preference for the human face is apparent. Auditory and vestibular systems function from birth. These sensory capabilities allow the neonate to elicit stimulation actively rather than simply receive stimuli passively. The nurse should teach the new mother the importance of providing sensory stimulation, such as talking to her baby and holding the newborn so he can see her face. This allows the infant to seek or take in stimuli, thereby enhancing learning and promoting cognitive development.

Whether infant crying is the precursor of refined language is debatable. However, crying does elicit a response and care givers do discriminate cry patterns. Crying therefore has significance to the newborn and the parents. For the neonate, crying is a means of communication. They cry for a reason, although at times this reason is difficult to determine. Some babies cry because they are wet or hungry or want to be held. Others cry just to make noise. An infant's crying may frustrate the parents if they cannot see an apparent cause. With the nurse's help, parents can learn to define their infant's cry patterns to take appropriate action when necessary.

Psychosocial Development

During the first 28 days of life, parents and infants normally develop a deep attachment. Parent-child in-

TABLE 22-5 Infant Reflexes

Reflex	Stimulus	Response
Babinski	Using a blunt object, stroke lateral aspect of the plantar surface of foot from heel to toes.	Hyperextension or fanning of toes occurs. As myelinization is completed, the normal response becomes flexion (downward curling) of all toes; the positive (pathological) sign is hyperextension (dorsiflexion) of the great toe with or without fanning of the remaining toes.
Blinking	Shine a light suddenly at the infant's open eyes.	Eyelids close in response to light (disappears after first year).
Landau	Suspend infant carefully in prone position by supporting infant's abdomen with hand.	By 3 months of age the expected response consists of extension of head, trunk, and hips. Head is slightly above horizontal plane. (Reflex disappears by 2 years of age).
Moro	With infant in supine position, gently support head and lift it a few centimeters off the surface. As soon as neck relaxes, suddenly release the head and let it drop back to the surface. **or** Produce sudden, loud noise or jar the table or crib suddenly.	Normal response is present at birth. The arms extend outward, the hands open, and then are brought together in midline. The legs flex slightly. Infant may cry. (Reflex usually disappears by 3 to 4 months).
Neck righting	With infant in supine position, turn head to one side.	Infant's trunk rotates in direction in which head is turned (appears at 4 to 6 months and disappears at 24 months).
Palmar grasp	With infant's head positioned in midline, place index fingers from ulnar side into infant's palm and press against palm.	Normal response is flexion of all fingers around examiner's fingers (present at birth and disappears by 4 months when infant is ready to reach).
Placing	Hold infant erect, with the dorsum of one foot touching the undersurface of the examining table top.	Infant flexes hip and knee and places stimulated foot on top of the table (present at birth and disappears by 6 weeks or variable).
Plantar grasp	Place finger firmly across base of infant's toes.	Toes curl downward (present at birth and disappears by 10 to 12 months).
Rooting	Hold infant in supine position with head in midline and hands against chest. Stroke perioral skin at corner of mouth or cheek.	Infant opens mouth and turns head toward stimulated side (present at birth and disappears by 3 to 4 months [awake]; by 7 months [asleep]).

Modified from Chow M, et al.: Handbook of pediatric primary care, ed.2, Somerset, N.J., 1984, John Wiley & Sons, Inc.

teractions during routine care enhance or detract from the attachment process. Feeding and brief periods of play consume much of the infant's waking hours. These interactive experiences provide a foundation from which later attachments form. The neonate is an active participant in the process.

If the parent or child experiences health complications after birth, attachment may be compromised. The infant's behavioral cues may be weak or absent. Care and care giving are less mutually satisfying. The tired, ill mother has difficulty interpreting and responding to her infant. Children who have congenital anomalies, who are too weak to be responsive to parental cues, and who require special care need supportive nursing care. For example, a child born with a heart defect may tire easily during feeding. He may rest frequently after several

bursts of sucking and fall asleep after taking 1 to 1½ ounces. This child may awaken after 1½ hours, crying because he is hungry again. The mother, not understanding that the crying is a physiologically dictated sequence of events, may think the child is being fussy or that she is inadequate. Both infant and mother derive decreasing pleasure from feeding experiences. Attachment is not enhanced and may even be reduced unless nursing intervention breaks the sequence of events.

INFANT

Infancy is the period from 1 month to 1 year of age. Rapid physical growth and change characterize this stage. Psychosocial development, facilitated by the progression from reflexive to more purposeful behavior, advances. Interaction between the infant and environment is greater and more meaningful. The infant who purposefully giggles and rolls over in response to his father's tickling is interacting more with his social environment and is receiving a greater response than when he merely smiled in response to a hug.

During this phase of growth and development the nurse can observe adaptive potential, because both qualitative and quantitative changes occur rapidly.

Physical Development

Steady and proportional growth of the infant is more important than absolute growth values. Charts of normal age- and sex-related growth measurements enable the nurse to compare growth with norms for a child's age. With growth charts the nurse can also evaluate growth pattern by recording measurements of weight, length, and head circumference at intervals. Repeated measurements recorded over time are the best way to monitor growth and identify problems. For example, an infant with a growth problem may be generally below the expected norms at all intervals or may experience an acute, brief interference with growth in any one or all of the parameters.

GROWTH

Infants usually double their birth weight by 6 months and triple it by 12 months. Infants grow 10 to 12 inches by the end of the first year.

Physiological functioning stabilizes and, by the end of the first year, the heart rate is 80 to 130 beats per minute, and the respiratory rate is 30 to 35 breaths per minute.

Patterns of body function also stabilize, as evidenced by predictable sleep, elimination, and feeding routines.

NUTRITION

The quality and quantity of nutrition influence the infant's growth and development. The nurse's role in promoting good nutrition and dietary habits is to help parents select and provide a nutritionally adequate diet for their infant. The nurse therefore must have a sound knowledge base about nutrition. The nurse must also understand that nutrition is influenced by many variables (such as food preferences, slow eating, or food allergies) and that no diet is effective for all children or for one age group.

FEEDING ALTERNATIVES. Supplying essential nutrients to the infant is the nurse and parents' goal. Breast feeding is recommended for infants because it contains the essential nutrients of protein, fats, carbohydrates, and immunoreactive proteins that bolster the ability to resist infection. However, milk other than human milk may be successfully used. Commercially prepared formulas are popular because they are convenient, contain standard ingredients, and are fortified with vitamins and minerals. It is the nurse's responsibility to support and reassure the parents' choice of feeding methods and help them feed the infant successfully.

The 1-month-old infant takes *approximately* 28 ounces of milk per day. This amount increases slightly during the first 6 months and drops to about 24 ounces per day by the end of the first year. Cereals, fruits, vegetables, and meats are important sources of nutrients during the second 6 months of life. The nurse must be aware, however, that the amount and frequency of feedings vary among infants. The nurse must teach parents about differences in feeding patterns. Table 22-6 provides feeding guidelines for the first year of life.

SUPPLEMENTATION. The need for dietary vitamin and mineral supplements is variable and depends on the infant's diet. Full-term infants are born with some iron stores. The breast-fed infant absorbs adequate iron from breast milk during the first 4 to 6 months of life. After 6 months, iron-fortified cereal is generally considered an adequate supplemental source. Because iron in formula is less readily absorbed than that in breast milk, formula-fed infants should receive iron-fortified formula throughout the first year. Adequate concentrations of fluoride to protect against dental caries are not available in human milk, and therefore fluoridated water or supplemental fluoride is generally recommended. The presence of fluoride in formula depends on the type of formula and the source of water used in preparing the concentrated forms, and supplementation may be necessary. In general, cow's milk is not recommended in the first year of life because of inadequate amounts of the essential nutrients, particularly fats and carbohydrates.

The association between overfeeding, infant obesity, and later adult obesity is still controversial. However, early feeding experiences can influence later eating habits. The nurse should therefore emphasize balanced nutrition and good dietary habits through feeding experiences mutually satisfying for the parents and infant.

Cognitive Development

The infant learns much by experiencing and manipulating the environment. Developing motor skills and increasing mobility expand an infant's environment and, in combination with developing visual and auditory skills, enhance cognitive development. For example, a 1-month-old infant can visually follow the path of a moving object. Improved vision acuity and eye-hand coordination allow grasping and exploration of objects. In addition, rudimentary color vision begins by 2 months

TABLE 22-6 Guidelines for Feeding during the First Year

Age	Type of Feeding	Specific Recommendations
Birth-6 months	Breast feeding	This is most desirable complete diet for first half year.* Infant requires supplements of fluoride (0.25 mg), regardless of the fluoride content of the local water supply, iron by 6 months of age, and vitamin D (400 units) if mother's diet is inadequate or if infant is not exposed to sufficient sunlight.
	Formula	Iron-fortified commercial formula is a complete food for the first half year.* Fluoride supplements (0.25 mg) are required when the concentration of fluoride in the drinking water is below 0.3 parts per million. Evaporated milk formula requires supplements of vitamin C, iron, and fluoride (in accordance with the fluoride content of the local water supply).
6-12 months	Solid foods	Solids may be added by 5 to 6 months of age; earlier introduction tends to contribute to overfeeding. First foods are strained, pureed, or finely mashed. "Finger foods" such as teething crackers, raw fruit, or vegetables can be introduced by 6 to 7 months. Chopped table food or commercially prepared junior foods can be started by 9 to 12 months. With the exception of cereal, the order of introducing foods is variable; a recommended sequence is weekly introduction of other foods, beginning with fruit, followed by vegetables, and then meat. Breast-fed infants require more high-protein foods than formula-fed infants. As the quantity of solids increases, the amount of formula should be limited to approximately 900 ml (30 ounces) daily.
	Cereal	Introduce commercially prepared iron-fortified infant cereals and administer daily until 18 months of age. Rice cereal is usually introduced first because of its low allergenic potential. Supplemental iron can be discontinued once cereal is given.
	Fruits and vegetables	Applesauce, bananas, and pears are usually well tolerated. Avoid fruits and vegetables marked in cans that are not specifically designed for infants because of variable and sometimes high lead content and addition of salt, sugar, and preservatives. Offer fruit juice only from a cup, not a bottle, to reduce "nursing bottle caries."
	Meat, fish, and poultry	Avoid fatty meats. Prepare by baking, broiling, steaming, or poaching. Include organ meats such as liver, which has a high iron, vitamin A, and vitamin B complex content. If soup is given, be sure all ingredients are familiar to child's diet.
	Eggs and cheese	Serve egg yolk hard boiled and mashed, soft cooked, or poached. Introduce egg white in small quantities (1 teaspoon) toward end of first year to detect any allergic manifestation. Use cheese as a substitute for meat and as a "finger food."

Modified from Whaley, LD and Wong, DL: Nursing care of infants and children, ed. 3, St. Louis, 1987, the C.V. Mosby Co.
*The American Academy of Pediatrics recommends breast-feeding or commercial formula feeding for up to 12 months of age. After 1 year, whole cow's milk can be used.

and improves throughout the first year, making the environment more interesting to see and explore. The infant's hearing also progresses, allowing localization and discrimination of sounds. By 1 year the infant typically knows the meaning of several different sounds such as "Ma-Ma," "Da-Da," and "no."

Speech is another aspect of cognition that develops during the first year. The infant proceeds from crying, cooing, and laughing to imitating sounds, comprehending the meaning of simple commands, and repeating words with knowledge of their meaning. By 12 months the infant begins to name objects in the environment, which is essential to later cognitive development.

The infant needs opportunities to develop and use the senses. Nurses must evaluate the appropriateness and adequacy of these opportunities. For example, an ill or hospitalized infant may lack the energy to interact with the environment, thereby slowing his cognitive development. On the other hand, continuous stimulation can overwhelm and confuse the infant. The infant needs to be stimulated according to his temperament, energy, and age capabilities. Visual, sensory, and tactile stimulation is as necessary for healthy development as food. The nurse uses stimulation strategies that maximize the infant's development while conserving his energy and orientation.

Psychosocial Development

During the first year the infant begins to differentiate himself from others as a separate being capable of acting on his own. Initially the infant is unaware of the boundaries of self but through repeated experiences with the environment, he learns where the self ends and the external world begins. This process of differentiation is slow, and the infant occasionally experiences brief frustrations with more frequent and consistent satisfactions. As the infant determines his physical boundaries, he begins to respond to the presence of others. The 2- to 3-month old infant begins to smile responsively rather than reflexively. Similarly, he can recognize differences in people when his sensory and cognitive capabilities improve. By 8 months, most infants can differentiate a stranger from a familiar person and respond differently to the two. Close attachment to the primary care giver, most often a parent, is usually established by this age. The infant seeks out this person for support and comfort during times of stress. The ability to distinguish self from others allows the infant to interact and socialize more within his environment. By 9 months, for example, the infant plays simple social games such as pat-a-cake and peek-a-boo. More complex interactive games such as hide-and-seek are possible by age 1.

The nurse assesses the availability and appropriateness of experiences contributing to psychosocial development. Hospitalized infants may have difficulty establishing physical boundaries because of repeated bodily intrusions and painful sensations. Limiting these negative experiences and providing pleasurable sensations are interventions that support early psychosocial development. Extended separations from parents complicate the attachment process and increase the number of care givers with whom the infant must interact. Unless the parents continue to provide the majority of care during hospitalization, the infant's needs will be satisfied inconsistently. These inconsistencies overwhelm the infant. Therefore, when feasible, the nurse should encourage the parents to provide routine daily care to their infant during hospitalization. When this is impossible, it is advisable to limit the number of people providing daily care. Use of detailed nursing care plans for daily routine and needs can minimize inconsistencies between staff members.

Perception of Health

The foundation for a child's perception of his own health status is laid early in life. Internal body sensations and experiences with the outside world affect self-perceptions. The nature of this influence and the value of nursing interventions to alter later perceptions are unknown. It is known, however, that parents tend to label children who are ill in early life as more vulnerable than their siblings and that this labeling may affect the child's perceptions of his own health. In addition, because infants and children depend on others for their health care, their experiences with care givers influence their health attitudes and behaviors. The nurse has a responsibility to educate parents and other care givers about health promotion behaviors that will positively affect the child's perception of health and self.

TODDLER

The toddler period ranges from the first to the third year of life. Toddlerhood is characterized by increasing independence bolstered by greater physical mobility and cognitive abilities. The toddler is increasingly aware of his ability to control and is pleased with successful efforts with this new skill. This success leads him to repeated attempts to control his environment. Unsuccessful attempts at control may result in negative behaviors and temper tantrums. These behaviors are most common when parents thwart the initial independent action. Parents cite these as the most problematic behaviors during the toddler years and at times express frustration with trying to set consistent and firm limits while simultaneously encouraging independence. Parents often seek the guidance of health care professionals for assistance in learning these essential parenting tasks.

Physical Development

Many characteristics of physical development become obvious in the toddler years. The child walks in an upright position with a broad-stanced gait, protuberant abdomen, and arms flung out to the side for balance. Gross motor skills develop rapidly, as evidenced by the ability to walk up and down stairs, kick a ball, jump, and stand on one foot for several seconds. By the end of the third year, most toddlers can ride a tricycle and run well. Fine motor capabilities move from scribbling spontaneously to drawing circles and crosses accurately. By 3 years the child draws simple stick people and can usually stack a tower of small blocks. Improved mobility, the ability to undress, and development of sphincter control allow toilet training if the toddler has developed the necessary cognitive abilities. Parents often consult nurses for an assessment of readiness for toilet training. The nurse needs to remind parents that patience, consistency, and a nonjudgmental attitude, in addition to the child's readiness, are essential components of successful training.

The cardiopulmonary system becomes stable in the toddler years. The heart and respiratory rates slow to 110 beats and 24 breaths per minute. Many health care professionals begin routine blood pressure measurement at age 3 to establish baseline values. Standardized values for toddlers are still controversial, but normal readings are about 110/60 mm Hg.

The anterior fontanel closes between 12 and 18 months of age, ending the period of most rapid growth of the skull and brain. Routine measurement of head circumference is usually not continued past this age.

The rate of increase in both weight and length slows. By 2 years the child weighs four times his birth weight. Height during toddlerhood increases 3 to 5 inches a year, mainly as a result of increases in leg length. Slowed growth rates are accompanied by decreased caloric need and smaller food intake, which leads some parents to worry about the adequacy of dietary intake. The nurse can reassure parents by confirming the child's continued proportional growth pattern with growth charts.

Most toddlers change from breast milk or formula to milk, consuming three to four glasses per day. Nutritional requirements are increasingly met by solid foods in the remaining three basic food groups. Because the consumption of more than a quart of milk per day decreases the child's appetite for these essential solid foods, the nurse should advise parents to limit milk intake to 28 ounces per day. The healthy toddler requires the daily intake of the foods in Table 22-7. Because parents frequently overestimate the size of a normal serving for their child, the nurse can reduce their anxiety about inadequate intake by pointing out the normal serving size.

TABLE 22-7 Daily Dietary Requirements of the Healthy Toddler

Food	Number of Servings	Size of Serving
Milk	3-4	6-8 ounces
Meat	2-3	3 tablespoons
Vegetables and fruits	4	4 ounces
Cereals and breads	4 or more	½ slice bread ½ cup rice or cereal

Children who are ill, who are undergoing surgery, or who have diseases involving ingestion, absorption, or utilization of nutrients require special dietary considerations. Alterations in the type of foods and calorie requirements may be necessary. Children on strict vegetarian diets also require careful planning to ensure adequate, balanced intake.

Regardless of the child's health status, several basic principles of nutrition apply. Mealtime has psychosocial and physical significance. If the parents struggle to control the toddler's dietary intake, problem behaviors and conflicts may result. The nurse should encourage parents to offer a variety of nutritious foods at meals and to provide only nutritious snacks between meals. Serving finger foods to the todder allows him to eat by himself and to satisfy his need for independence and control. Small *reasonable* servings allow the toddler to eat all his meal.

Cognitive Development

The toddler moves from the sensorimotor to the preconceptual stage of cognitive development. In this stage the child learns the permanency of objects, develops a memory of events, and begins to understand cause and effect. Thought has an egocentric focus, and the toddler is unable to assume the view of another. The toddler becomes increasingly capable of symbolic interaction and frequently expresses fantasy and magical thinking.

Because moral development is closely associated with cognitive ability, the moral development of a toddler is only beginning and is also egocentric. Toddlers do not understand concepts of right and wrong. However, they do grasp the fact that some behaviors bring pleasant results (positive reinforcement) and others elicit unpleasant results (negative reinforcement). Therefore, until the toddler achieves a higher level of cognitive function, he behaves simply to avoid the unpleasant and seek out the pleasant.

The 18-month-old child uses approximately 10 words. The 24-month-old child has a vocabulary of up to 300 words and is generally able to speak in short sentences. By 36 months, most toddlers talk incessantly. They ask endless questions, can give their full name, follow and give simple commands, and use appropriate pronouns. Despite the large vocabulary of older toddlers, most parents comment that their child's favorite word remains "no" until well into the third year.

Psychosocial Development

During toddlerhood the child develops autonomy. Although toddlers move out to explore their immediate environment, they continue to return at periodic intervals for encouragement and emotional support of parents. This process, called *refueling,* is illustrated by the toddler who can play alone in his bedroom but calls out at intervals to make sure that the parent is still in the house. Parents usually remain the most significant persons in the toddler's life.

The toddler is also capable of parallel play with others. Although two toddlers play in close proximity, true sharing or systematic turn taking is rare. The children play *next to* rather than *with* one another. Toddlers share toys inconsistently and rarely. Learning to control one's possessions, as well as oneself, is a primary task of toddlers. Learning to share is a later development.

Because a toddler is extremely active yet unable to limit his own behavior, parents must set limits. This inevitably causes conflict between the parents and child. Parents appreciate professional reassurance that this conflict lessens as the child grows older and internalizes behavior limits. Firm, consistent limit setting enhances this process.

Limit setting is extremely important for the toddler's safety. Automobile safety requires the toddler to remain in a car seat, even though he says (often loudly) he would prefer to move freely about the car. Poisoning is another hazard. The toddler's exploratory capabilities can lead him to open and taste noxious materials. The wise parent removes or locks up all possible poisons, including plants, cleaning materials, and medications (see Chapter 40). In this way the parent creates a safer environment for exploratory behavior.

Perception of Health

The toddler's perception of his own health is limited by his cognitive capabilities. The child increasingly recognizes internal body sensations but has difficulty pinpointing their location. Therefore the child often associates generalized responses with illness. The child who deviates radically from his usual pattern of eating, sleeping, or playing requires assessment to determine if these alterations result from illness.

During this stage the child begins to internalize the labels that parents or health professionals give to the somatic states. That is, if the parents label particular sensations, such as abdominal discomfort, an "illness," the child begins to label related sensations similarly. At the same time the child observes and mimics parents' health care practices. Health beliefs and practices are therefore being significantly shaped, even in these early years.

PRESCHOOLER

The preschool years are a transition between toddlerhood and the school-age years. The period spans the ages between 3 and 6. Many people consider these the most intriguing years of parenting because the child is less negative, can more accurately share his thoughts and can more effectively interact and communicate. Physical development continues to slow, and cognitive and psychosocial development is rapid.

Physical Development

Several aspects of physical development continue to stabilize in the preschool years. Heart and respiratory rates decrease only slightly to approximately 90 beats per minute and 24 breaths per minute. Blood pressure remains stable at about 90/60 mm Hg. Weight increases approximately 5 pounds per year, making the child's average weight about 45 pounds by age 5. Height increases approximately 2 inches per year. Leg growth continues to account for most of the increase in height. Birth length is generally doubled by age 4, making the average height 42 inches. Nutritional needs remain relatively stable.

Large and fine muscle coordination improves. The preschooler runs well, walks up and down steps with ease, and learns to hop. By 6 years he can usually skip and throw and catch a ball. Improving fine motor skills allow intricate manipulations. The child can copy circles, crosses, squares, and triangles. These skills make printing of letters and numbers possible.

The child needs opportunities to learn and practice these physical skills. Nursing care of healthy and ill children includes an assessment of the availability of these opportunities. Although children with acute illnesses benefit from rest and exclusion from usual daily activities, children who have chronic conditions or who have been hospitalized for long periods need ongoing exposure to developmental opportunities. The parents and nurse weave these opportunities into the child's daily experiences, depending on abilities, needs, and energy level.

Cognitive Development

The preschooler continues to master the preoperational stage of cognition. The continued egocentricity of early thinking makes it difficult to suggest acceptable alternatives to the preschooler. With maturation, experience, and increased use of symbolic thinking, the child is able to consider the views of another, and his thinking becomes less egocentric.

By 6 years, egocentric thinking is partially replaced by intuitive thought. The preschooler can increasingly solve a problem intuitively on the basis of only one aspect of a situation.

The preschooler's knowledge of the world remains closely linked to concrete experiences. Even the rich fantasy life of a preschooler is grounded in the perception of reality. The mixing of the two aspects by the child can lead to many childhood fears and may be misinterpreted by adults as lying when the child is actually presenting reality from his perspective.

Early causal thinking develops in the preschool years. Thought is transductive (that is, reasoning occurs from one particular to another). If two events are related in time or space, the child links them in a causal fashion. The hospitalized child, for example, may reason, "I cried last night, and that's why the nurse gave me the shot." As children near age 5, they begin to use or can be taught to use sets of rules to understand causation. The child then begins to reason from the general to the particular. This forms the basis for more formal logical thought. The child can now reason, "I get a shot twice a day, and that's why I got one last night."

The preschooler's moral development expands to include a beginning understanding of behaviors considered socially right or wrong. The child continues to be motivated, however, by the wish to avoid punishment or the desire to obtain a reward. The primary difference between this stage of moral development and that of the toddler is that the preschooler is better able to identify behaviors that elicit rewards or punishment and that he begins to label these behaviors as right or wrong.

The child's improving language skills facilitate symbolic thought. Vocabulary increases greatly. By age 5 the child has more than 2000 words with which he can express himself. The child can name colors and body parts, and he can define familiar objects. However, the child may confuse phonetically similar words, such as "die" and "dye." Because of this limitation and literal interpretation of words, the preschooler may misunderstand things that are said to him. It is important for the nurse to assess the preschooler's ability to understand what is being told to him, especially when preparing him for treatment. Grammatical refinement also occurs during these years. The 5-year-old child uses longer sentences and appropriate adjectives.

Psychosocial Development

The preschooler relies heavily on the support of parents or primary care givers for security but increasingly ventures out to initiate contact with other children and adults. The preschooler is less afraid of strangers and may ask a new adult acquaintance a seemingly unending stream of questions. The child seeks out experiences with peers and seems to enjoy this contact.

During times of stress or illness, however, the preschool child relies more on parents. This return to an earlier pattern of behavior, called *regression,* is not limited to the preschool years. It can occur anytime in a person's life, occurring most often when a person ex-

periences stress he is unable to relieve with prior coping behaviors. Regression involves stepping back to a more comfortable behavior, one that may have required less energy to maintain. Often these behaviors were helpful in the past, and the person consciously or unconsciously anticipates they will help in the current situation.

Regression is obvious in the preschooler because the regressive, dependent behavior contrasts markedly with the usual independent behavior. Parents are often confused and embarrassed by the regression and can benefit from the nurse's reassurance that it is a normal coping behavior. The nurse should accept regressive behavior yet help the child understand and gain control of the new situation. The nurse should provide experiences the child can master with his current behaviors. These successes give the child the motivation and strength to return to his prior level of independent functioning.

Interactive play with peers begins in the preschool years. Parallel play moves to associative play, and, as the child nears school age, associative play becomes cooperative play. In associative play, children play with others in a similar activity, but very little organization or division of responsibility exists. As they develop, children engage in cooperative play and not only take turns but join efforts to produce desired outcomes. For example, preschoolers can work together to build a play store or take roles in a short play or skit. A sense of group initiative and self-initiative develops during these play activities.

In many play activities the preschooler displays an awareness of social context. Sex role identification is strengthening, and children most often assume roles of persons of their own sex. Children frequently mimic or repeat social experiences. This tendency is especially significant for the nurse working with hospitalized children. Through play the child may express questions, fears, anger, and misunderstanding about his illness and care. The nurse should be alert to clues the child gives during spontaneous play and ensure that every child has the opportunity to play within his energy limits. The nurse can also use play to provide new information or clear up misunderstandings. Incorporating play techniques into care is essential for all pediatric clients.

Perception of Health

Little research has explored the preschooler's perceptions of his own health. Although parents' beliefs about health are important in the child's developing sense of his health status, so are his bodily sensations and his ability to perform usual daily activities. The preschooler is usually quite independent in washing, dressing, and feeding. Alterations in this independence can influence his feelings about his own health.

ASSESSMENT

For children, hospitalization and illness are stressful experiences, primarily because of separation from the normal environment and significant others, a limited selection of coping behaviors, and an altered state of health. A child's reaction to illness and hospitalization is based on developmental age, previous experiences with hospitalization, available support persons, coping skills, and the seriousness of the diagnosis (Whaley and Wong, 1987). These factors should be the focus of the assessment. Table 22-8 lists relevant assessment areas for a hospitalized child and an information goal for each.

Developmental Assessment

The objective of a developmental assessment is to evaluate the child's ability to complete certain age-appropriate tasks. The Denver Developmental Screening Test (DDST) is the most widely used developmental screening tool. The DDST is applicable for children from birth through 6 years and assesses personal-social, fine motor adaptive, language, and gross motor skills. Such a tool allows the nurse to identify and assess the hospitalized child's current level of developmental function to plan care that maintains the developmental level and promotes further development. For example, a developmental assessment might reveal that a 4-year-old child is toilet-trained and attends nursery school, separating easily from his mother. The accomplishment of these tasks signify that the child has achieved a sense of trust, can maintain control over bodily functions, and has

TABLE 22-8 Assessment of Hospitalized Child

Assessment Area	Informational Goals
Development	Identify current developmental level and skills achieved.
Observation of response to hospitalization	Identify current coping behaviors and their intensity.
History of previous illness, hospitalization, and separation	Identify previous patterns of coping and their effects.
Medical history	Identify level of seriousness of problem and its effect on developmental abilities.
Available support systems	Identify availability and willingness of significant others to participate in care and provide support.

achieved a degree of autonomy. Accordingly, the nurse can provide opportunities for the child to (1) maintain his sense of trust by assigning the same nursing personnel for his care and encouraging parents to room-in, (2) promote control of bodily functions by integrating his usual toileting and self-care routines into his hospital care, and (3) promote a sense of autonomy by allowing the child to make choices and preparing him for therapies.

Observation of Response to Hospitalization

Separation anxiety, loss of control, and fear of bodily injury and pain are the primary causes of behavioral reactions of hospitalized children. The age of the child dictates the specific manifestation, as evidenced by the infant who loudly cries and protests separation from parents and the toddler who may kick, bite, or hit. Loss of control behaviors are more apparent in the toddler or preschooler, who may have frequent temper tantrums or exhibit regressive behaviors. Fear of bodily injury and pain reactions occur in all children, including newborns. An infant reacts to pain with body rigidity, thrashing, and facial grimacing, whereas the preschooler loudly protests and possibly becomes physically and verbally aggressive (Whaley and Wong, 1987).

Observing behavioral reaction to hospitalization allows the nurse to identify current coping behaviors and plan care accordingly. For example, knowing a 4-year-old has achieved a sense of trust and autonomy, the nurse can intervene when behavior indicates these achievements have been disrupted. Behaviors such as crying for his parents, being uncooperative, and regressing in toileting habits are reactions to an interruption in achieved developmental tasks created by hospitalization. The nurse can minimize this interruption by activities such as providing favorite toys from home, encouraging sibling visits, providing a warm, accepting attitude and environment, and encouraging parents to provide care. Minimizing separation from parents, modifying care and procedure to reduce discomfort, and facilitating control over care and therapies are goals for the hospitalized child (see care plan box on p. 584).

History of Previous Illness, Hospitalization, and Separation

The way a child coped with a previous hospitalization (specific behavior reactions [for example, protests, withdrawal, aggression, regression]) and the effect the hospitalization had on subsequent behavior (negative behaviors after discharge [for example, nightmares, aloofness, clinging, temper tantrums]) is relevant data for the nurse to gather when assessing a current hos-

Examples of Nursing Diagnoses for a Hospitalized Child

NANDA-APPROVED NURSING DIAGNOSES

Altered nutrition: less than body requirements related to:
- Response to hospitalization
- Separation from family
- Effect of illness
- Pain

Potential for infection related to:
- Procedures, therapies
- Illness
- Decreased body defenses
- Insufficient knowledge to avoid pathogens

Potential for injury related to:
- Change in environment
- Mode of transporting
- Mode of restraining

Social isolation related to:
- Separation from significant others
- Effects of illness
- Interruption of developmental task progress
- Hospitalization and routines

Altered family processes related to:
- Hospitalization
- Chronic illness

Activity intolerance related to:
- Conditions of illness
- Hospitalization

Sleep pattern disturbance related to:
- Unfamiliar environment
- Separation
- Procedure and therapies
- Pain
- Illness

Diversional activity deficit related to:
- Hospitalization
- Effects of illness
- Pain

Altered growth and development related to:
- Hospitalization and response
- Illness
- Pain
- Separation
- Multiple care givers

Powerlessness related to:
- Unfamiliar environment
- Illness

Pain related to:
- Illness
- Procedures and therapies

Anxiety related to:
- Unfamiliar environment
- Separation from significant others

pitalization response. Recognizing previous behavioral patterns will facilitate the nurse's plan of care. For example, allowing a preschooler to select a colorful bandage to put on after an injection and praising him for cooperating may reduce the reoccurrence of a biting and kicking response.

Medical History

From the medical history the nurse should determine the seriousness of health problem and the effect it will have on development and nursing care. She should also determine the effects of therapies on developmental achievements. For example, the toddler whose activity is severely restricted because of his illness or therapy will have difficulty maintaining his independence. Restricting or limiting movement interferes with exploration needed to develop a sense of autonomy. The nurse needs to provide opportunities for the toddler to explore within the limits of his illness by allowing him to use manipulative toys, taking him for a ride in a wheelchair or wagon, or reading to him.

Available Support Persons

The availability and willingness of significant others to provide support for the hospitalized child is valuable information. For example, separation behaviors are minimized for the child whose parents can be with him around the clock versus the child whose family can only visit sporadically during the day. Identifying the child's resources and support system (for example, parents, grandparents, aunts, uncles, and siblings), using these support persons when implementing care by helping them arrange a schedule for being with the child, and assigning the same nursing personnel to the child will facilitate adjustment to the hospital.

NURSING DIAGNOSIS

The nurse's assessment will reveal how the child copes with hospitalization and if hospitalization has created other health problems (see sample nursing diagnoses box, opposite). In addition, data that will assist in potentially solving problems associated with hospitalization may be gathered. For example, an assessment finds a 4-year-old crying for his parents, hitting when nursing personnel approach, not eating, and relinquishing his normal toilet habits after a few days. The parents work and are having difficulty securing time off during the day. Further data reveals that the maternal grandparents live nearby and are willing to stay with the child during

Sample Nursing Diagnoses for a Hospitalized Child		
Defining Characteristics	**Nursing Diagnoses**	**Related Factors**
Weight loss Refusal to eat Lack of interest in food	Altered nutrition: less than body requirements	▪ Pain ▪ Pathological process of illness ▪ Separation from support system
Attempts to climb out of crib Pulling at IV or tubes Uncooperative during procedures	Potential for injury	▪ Unfamiliar environment ▪ Fear of procedures or therapies ▪ Mode of restraining ▪ Discomfort ▪ Lack of ability to understand directions
Parents unable to stay with child Child separated from parents and siblings Parents reluctant to express feelings	Altered family processes	▪ Hospitalization of child ▪ Illness of child ▪ Lack of coping strategies

the day. The defining characteristics of difficulty in performing skills typical of the age group and inability to self-control age-appropriate activities indicate a nursing diagnosis of "growth and development, altered."

The nursing diagnosis also identifies the probable cause of the problem, such as separation anxiety, pain, or disruption of normal life-style. Indentification of the cause allows the nurse to plan interventions. For example, the hospitalized 4-year-old responds behaviorally to being separated from parents and family. The nurse can alleviate the problem by assisting family in making arrangements for grandparents to stay during the day and parents during evening and night.

Hospitalization may affect the child in other ways. For example, the child may not eat because he may be upset over being separated or may be experiencing discomfort. The nursing diagnosis, "nutrition, altered: less than body requirements," indicates that the nurse must closely monitor fluid and solid intake and offer small, frequent meals incorporating favorite foods.

Appropriate defining characteristics need to be identified when choosing a nursing diagnosis to ensure individuality of care. The nursing diagnoses box (opposite) illustrates nursing diagnoses for the hospitalized child.

PLANNING

Once nursing diagnoses have been established, the nurse develops a plan of care (see care plan box on p. 584). Individualized care can be developed after the

nurse recognizes the child's coping behaviors, identifies significant others and objects, and realizes the impact of hospitalization on development. Because the child is unable to articulate his feelings and needs, the family (frequently the parents) acts as his spokesperson. Their involvement in care is essential because the best approaches and solutions for helping the child often come from the parents.

Goals of care for a hospitalized child should include:
1. Minimal separation anxiety
2. Establishing trust
3. Reducing fear
4. Minimal physical discomfort
5. Achieving maximum or normal growth and development
6. Participating in diversional activities

IMPLEMENTATION

Nursing interventions can be implemented by nursing personnel, the child, and the family. Interventions should focus on the provision of quality care, resolution of stresses created by hospitalization, and positive growth outcomes for the child and family.

Minimizing Separation Anxiety

Being separated from his family in an unfamiliar environment when not feeling well is possibly the greatest stress a child faces in the hospital. The primary goal of nursing interventions is to prevent separation and, in the event of its occurrence, minimize its effect.

Sample Nursing Care Plan for a Hospitalized Child

Nursing Diagnosis	Goals	Expected Outcomes	Nursing Interventions
Anxiety related to separation from family	Minimal or no separation.	Child displays fewer separation behaviors.	Encourage parents or family members to room-in when possible.
			Provide consistent care givers.
			Assist family in arranging a schedule of visiting or staying with child.
			Allow siblings to visit.
			Assign same nursing personnel, including a primary nurse.
			Assign consistent volunteer to spend 1 to 2 hours with child a day.
			Instruct parents in appropriate techniques of care.
			Teach parents important signs and symptoms they should observe.
			Encourage parents to express feelings about involvement with care.
		Parents understand separation behaviors.	Reassure parents that child's behaviors are normal.
			Encourage parents to cuddle, hold, and demonstrate affection.
			Encourage parents to visit for frequent short intervals.
			Encourage parents to tell child when leaving, when they will return, and why they have to leave.
	Freedom to express feelings.	Child verbalizes or plays out fears, feelings, or concerns.	Accept feelings and be verbally or behaviorally expressive.
			Provide opportunity for expression.
			Use toys, dolls, and drawing as a means of expressing feelings.
	Freedom for regression.	Child resolves regressive behaviors.	Provide a routine as close to that at home as possible.
			Recognize and accept regressive behavior as a normal part of illness.
	Alleviation of fear of unknown.	Child understands information about therapies and illness.	Give age-appropriate explanation, using visual aids for therapies, procedures, hospitalizations, and routines.
			Allow child to handle and touch equipment.
			Reassure child.
			Allow parents to participate in care.
			Use play therapy.

Nursing Interventions for Physical Discomfort

- Prepare for procedures and therapies, using age-appropriate language, dolls, puppets, books, or drawings.
- Allow parent(s) to accompany child to procedures and therapies if appropriate.
- Allow child to see and handle procedural or therapy equipment or to use it on a doll.
- Alter procedural techniques if possible (for examples take axillary versus rectal temperature or oral versus intravenous medication).
- Allow expression of feelings.
- Use reassuring measure (for example, a bandage, sticker, or praise).
- Use correct technique for procedures.
- Avoid delays and limit use of restraints.
- Allow child to sit rather than lie.
- Assess pain through observation and questions.

Nursing Interventions for Promotion of Growth and Development

- Allow and accept regressive behavior.
- Deal with and teach parents to handle regressive behavior with firm, consistent approach.
- Incorporate usual feeding, bathing, toileting, and bedtime routines into hospital care (for example, allow child to wear own pajamas, eat at a table, and use his own terms for body functions).
- Allow for opportunities to continue current developmental skills (for example, permit walking, and dressing and feeding self if the child is learning these skills).
- Provide a safe environment.
- Allow child to make choices when possible.
- Limit use of restraints.
- Transport child in wagon or wheelchair for change of scenery.
- Explain routines, procedures, and therapies in age-appropriate language.
- Use nonpharmacological pain management (for example, distraction, relaxation, guided imagery techniques, thought stopping, cutaneous stimulation, and behavioral contracting) to reduce discomfort.
- Use pharmacological agents to prevent pain and to provide maximum comfort.

Modified from Whaley, LF, and Wong, DL: Nursing care of infants and children, ed. 3, St. Louis, 1987, The C.V. Mosby Co.

Minimizing Physical Discomfort

All children fear bodily injury and pain, and recent studies demonstrate newborn and infant reaction to painful stimuli. The nurse must be aware of the child's fears and reactions to physical discomfort and plan appropriate nursing interventions (see box above).

Promoting Growth and Development

Normal developmental progression is affected by hospitalization. Contributing to the disruption of this process is the feeling of loss of control that may result from separation, physical restriction, changed routine, enforced dependency, magical thinking, and altered roles (Whaley and Wong, 1987). The nurse can minimize these barriers, thereby promoting growth and development (see box above right).

Providing Diversional Activities

Play is a child's work and can be one of the most effective tools for managing a hospitalized child. Play in the hospital allows the child to work out fears and meet his developmental need for stimulation. Play can be used as a diversion, a security, a release of tension, a promotion of development, a teaching tool, or a communication technique. Because play is vital to development, nursing interventions should be implemented to provide diversional activities (see box at right).

Nursing Interventions for Diversional Activity

- Provide safe, age-appropriate toys for child (for example, bring toys to child or take child to playroom).
- Allow adequate time for play.
- Allow toys from home.
- Provide play materials compatible with health problem.
- Use play as a stress reducer.
- Use play as a teaching tool.
- Encourage interaction with other children (for example, place another child in room or take child visiting with children of the same age).
- Monitor TV time.
- Encourage creative or interactive activities.
- Read to child.

Sample Evaluation of Interventions for a Hospitalized Child

Goals	Evaluative Measures	Expected Outcomes
Prevent or minimize separation.	Observe child when sleeping and eating with parents rooming-in.	Child is more responsive to environment, cries less, has less aggression or regression.
	Observe for parents telling child when they are leaving and returning.	Child is less upset when parent takes a break.
Establish trusting relationship with child.	Observe child's behaviors with primary nurse.	Child participates in care.
		Child is cooperative with procedures.
		Child demonstrates trusting behaviors.
Allow expression of feeling.	Observe child's expressions of fear.	Child uses dolls to act out fears.
		Child draws pictures that express fears.
		Child talks about his fears.

EVALUATION

Each child responds differently to hospitalization, making it necessary to evaluate nursing therapies to determine if each child's needs have been met. For example, in an attempt to minimize separation, the nurse may suggest allowing siblings to visit, but the hospitalized child may prefer to have a friend or grandparents visit.

The nurse evaluates interventions to determine whether the goals have been met. For example, separation behaviors may not be minimized by a sibling visit. The child may become upset and miss home and his usual life-style, so a friend's visit may serve as a diversion and not a reminder of home. Using evaluative criteria in determining the outcome of therapies is generally most effective (see evaluation box).

SUMMARY

Providing nursing care is a highly complex and individualized process. The nurse must first understand the individual and his growth and development. The nurse must assess the factors in the individual's life that have or will have an influence on growth and development. Only then can the nurse and client or family make decisions about developmental needs and plan and implement nursing activities (interventions) that promote health.

The complexities of growth and development are interrelated processes influenced by many factors. Developmental theories can be applied by the nurse to assess strengths and weaknesses and in planning care accordingly.

A developmental approach is used to individually examine the different stages of growth and development. The physical, psychosocial, and cognitive dimensions of development, as well as how developmental factors function, are relevant in the steps of the nursing process of assessment, nursing diagnosis, planning, implementation, and evaluation.

KEY CONCEPTS

✓ Growth and development are orderly, predictable, interdependent processes that continue throughout the life span.

✓ People progress through similar stages of growth and development but at an individual pace and with individual behaviors.

✓ A person's ability to progress through each developmental stage influences the person's health in that stage and thereafter.

✓ A developmental perspective helps the nurse understand both commonalities and variations in each stage and the impact they have on the client's health.

✓ Development depends on progressive adaptation to the environment.

✓ Maturation is the process of altering previous functions and learning more mature behaviors, involving environmental opportunities and biological abilities.

✓ During critical periods of development a person faces certain tasks necessary for successful developmental progression.

✓ Development has direction, is complex but predictable, is unique for each individual, involves conflict and adaptation, presents challenges, and requires practice and energy.

✓ Growth and development can be understood in terms of chronological stages involving tasks and changes.

✓ Growth and development are influenced by the inner forces of heredity and temperament and the outer forces of family, peers, life experiences, and elements in the environment.

✓ The developmental theories of Freud, Erikson, Maslow, Piaget, Havighurst, and Kohlberg help explain the aspects of development and can be used to form a individualized perspective for each client.

✓ Since the embryo and fetus grow and develop throughout the intrauterine period, impairments in any body system may occur in utero.

✓ Health risks for the unborn child include genetic impairments and environmental factors (teratogens).

✓ Physiological health concerns during childbirth include adequate functioning of all systems and prevention of infection.

✓ A psychosocial health concern that begins at childbirth is the establishment of parent-child attachment.

✓ Physiological, cognitive, and psychosocial development continues throughout the neonate, infant, toddler, and preschool periods, and the nurse must be familiar with normal parameters to determine potential problems and promote normal development.

✓ The nurse recognizes that the child's perception of health and health behaviors begins early and assists the parent and child to establish healthful patterns that will continue for the entire life span.

✓ The nurse educates the parents about risk factors and the child's health needs, provides emotional support to the parents in the prenatal period, and helps them understand the changes and needs of the developing child.

✓ Nursing interventions for an ill and hospitalized child encourage the child's continued cognitive and psychosocial development.

✓ Developmental assessment and nursing care help the infant and child adapt to internal and external changes.

✓ The hospitalized child requires assessment of his development, response to hospitalization, previous experiences with separation, medical history, and available support systems.

✓ The nursing process for the hospitalized child should focus on minimizing separation anxiety, promoting growth and development, minimizing physical discomfort, and providing diversional activities.

REFERENCES

Behrman, RE, and Vaughan, VC: Nelson textbook of pediatrics, ed. 13, Philadelphia, 1987, W.B. Saunders Co.

Chow, MP, et al.: Handbook of pediatric primary care, ed. 2, New York, 1984, John Wiley & Sons, Inc.

Korones, S: High-risk newborn infants: the basis for intensive nursing care, ed. 4, St. Louis, 1986, The C.V. Mosby Co.

Nelms, BC, and Mullins, R: Growth and development: a primary health care approach, Englewood Cliffs, N.J., 1982, Prentice Hall, Inc.

Warshaw, JB: Intrauterine growth retardation, Pediatr Rev 8:107, 1986.

Westwood, M, et al.: Growth and development of full term nonasphyxiated small-for-gestational-age newborns: follow-up through adolescence, Pediatrics 71:376, 1983.

Whaley, LD, and Wong, DL: Nursing care of infants and children, ed. 3, St. Louis, 1987, The C.V. Mosby Co.

Williams, JK: Counseling adolescents about environmental teratogens, Pediatr Nurs 12:292, 1986.

ADDITIONAL READINGS

Adzick, NS, Flake, AW, and Harrison, MR: Recent advances in prenatal diagnosis and treatment, Pediatr Clin North Am 32:1103, 1985.

Birchfield MD: Nursing care for hospitalized children based on different stages of illness, Matern Child Nurs J 6(1):46, 1981.

Brown, M, and Murphy, M: Ambulatory pediatrics for nurses, ed. 2, New York, 1981, McGraw-Hill Book Co.

Chernoff, GF, and Jones, KL: Fetal preventive medicine: teratogens and the unborn baby, Pediatr Ann 10:210, 1981.

Chess, S, and Thomas, A: Individuality: dynamics of individual behavioral development. In Levine, MD, et al., editors: Developmental-behavioral pediatrics, Philadelphia, 1983, W.B. Saunders Co.

Chess, S, and Thomas, A: Temperamental differences: a critical concept in child health care, Pediatr Nurs 11(3):167, 1985.

Clatworthy, S: Therapeutic play: effects on hospitalized children, Child Health Care 9(4):108, 1981.

Committee on Nutrition: Pediatric nutrition handbook, ed. 2, Elk Grove Village, Ill., 1985, American Academy of Pediatrics.

Conway, BL: Pediatric neurological nursing, Philadelphia, 1977, J.B. Lippincott Co.

Craft, MJ, and Wyatt, N: Effect of visitation of siblings on hospitalized children, Matern Child Nurs J 15(1):47, 1986.

Dole, JC: A multidimensional study of infants' response to painful stimuli, Pediatr Nurs 12(1):27, 1986.

Duvall, E: Marriage and family development, Philadelphia, 1977, J.B. Lippincott Co.

Erickson, ML: Assessment and management of developmental changes in children, ed. 2, St. Louis, 1980, The C.V. Mosby Co.

Erikson, E: Childhood and society, New York, 1963, W.W. Norton & Co., Inc.

Feinstein, JM, et al.: Factors related to early termination of breast feeding in an urban population, Pediatrics 78(2):210, 1986.

Frankenburg, WK, et al.: The newly abbreviated and revised Denver Developmental Screening Test, J Pediatr 106(2):343, 1985.

Furstenberg, F: Unplanned pregnancy: the social consequences of teenage pregnancy, New York, 1981, The Free Press.

Garot, PA: Therapeutic play: work of both child and nurse, J Pediatr Nurs 1(2):111, 1986.

Hall, C: A primer of Freudian psychology, New York, 1954, World Publishing Co.

Havighurst, R: Developmental tasks and education, ed. 2, New York, 1964, David McKay Co., Inc.

Jackson, RL: Long term consequences of suboptimal nutritional practices in early life, Pediatr Clin North Am 24:63, 1977.

Knutson, MG, Biro, PJ, and Padgett, D: Tracking infants at risk: Washington State's high priority infant tracking system, J Pediatr Health Care 1(4):180, 1987.

Kohlberg, L: Stages and sequence: the cognitive-developmental approach to socialization. In Goslin, DA, editor: Handbook of socialization theory and research, Chicago, 1969, Rand McNally & Co.

LaMontagne, LL: Children's locus of control beliefs as predictors of preoperative coping behavior, Nurs Res 33(2):76, 1984.

Lowery, GH: Growth and development of children, ed. 8, Chicago, 1986, Year Book Medical Publishers, Inc.

Maslow, A: Toward a psychology of being, New York, 1968, Van Nostrand Reinhold Co., Inc.

Moore, ML, and Galloway, K: Newborn family and nurse, ed. 2, Philadelphia, 1981, W.B. Saunders Co.

Neumann, CG, and Alpaugh, M: Birth weight doubling time: a fresh look, Pediatrics 57(3):469, 1976.

Scipien, G, et al.: Comprehensive pediatric nursing, ed. 2, New York, 1979, McGraw-Hill Book Co.

Suskind, R, editor: Textbook of pediatric nutrition, New York, 1981, Raven Press.

Tanner, JM, and Davies, PSW: Clinical longitudinal standards for height and height velocity of North American children, J Pediatr 107:317, 1985.

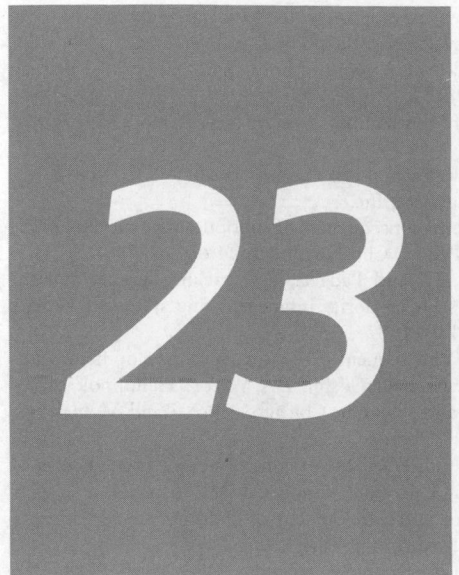

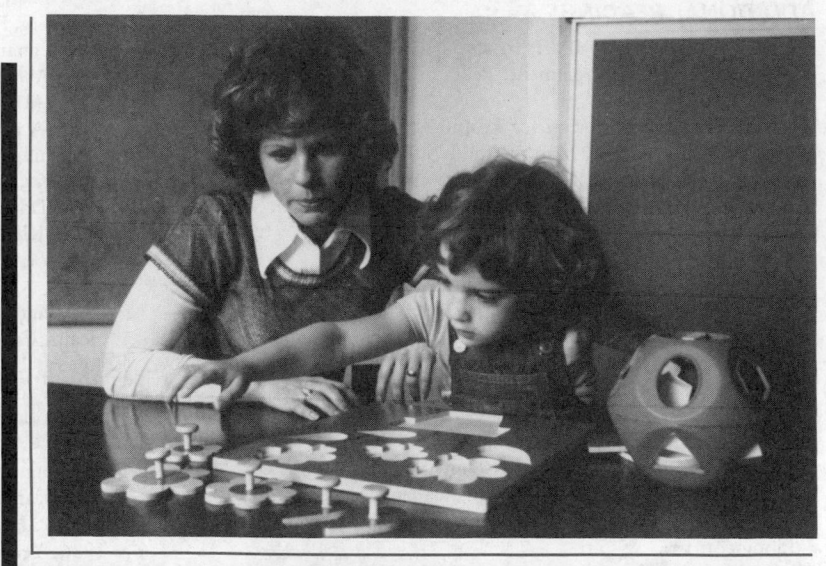

OBJECTIVES

Mastery of content in this chapter will enable the student to:

- Define the key terms listed.
- Describe the influence of the school environment on the cognitive psychosocial development of the school-age child and adolescent.
- Discuss ways in which the nurse can help parents adjust to their child's developmental needs.
- Describe the normal physical changes that occur during the school-age years and adolescence.
- Discuss behavior reflecting cognitive development of the school-age child and adolescent.
- List nursing interventions for health concerns specific to the school-age child and adolescent.
- Compare and contrast the ways by which a school-age child and an adolescent develop moral values.
- Discuss ways in which an adolescent gains a sexual, group, and personal identity.

KEY TERMS

Abstract Thought

Adolescence

Concrete Thought

Estrogen

Gonadotropic Hormones

Menses

Metacognition

Puberty

Sexually Transmitted Disease

Syntax

Testosterone

School-Age Child to Adolescent

School-age children and adolescents lead demanding, challenging lives. The developmental changes of individuals between age 6 and 18 are diverse and span all areas of growth and development. Physical, psychosocial, cognitive, and moral skills are developed, expanded, refined, and synchronized so the individual may become an accepted and productive member of society. The environment in which the individual develops skills also expands and diversifies. Instead of the principal limits of family and close friends, the environment may encompass the school, community, and church. Because of expectations for development, increasing skill and knowledge base, and environmental expansion, the individual experiences new difficulties and dilemmas. The nurse must know the appropriate developmental expectations for each age group to carry out assessment. For example, before assessing risk-taking behaviors, the nurse must know that adolescents normally strive to achieve a sense of identity while developing a moral code compatible with society. The nurse needs to direct the school-age child or adolescent toward normal developmental behaviors, assisting him to maximize his abilities and use them to cope. By helping children and adolescents achieve a necessary developmental balance, the nurse promotes health. Table 23-1 provides an overview of developmental behaviors typical of school-age children and adolescents. The nurse must also increasingly involve the child or adolescent in charting a developmental course. Because school-age children have increased cognitive and social skills, they are better able to participate in development. Not only can they describe their feelings about the changes, but they can think through these changes, eventually learn-

TABLE 23-1 Developmental Behaviors of School-Age Children and Adolescents

	School-Age Child	Adolescent
Interpersonal relations	Learns that parents can be wrong; continually appraises parent action and values; can sometimes be disillusioned with own parents and would like to trade them in or is certain he is adopted; learns to share some of his own thoughts only with peers; returns to parents and home for companionship, comfort, and security	Is ambivalent about expanding relationships; alternately believes parents are wonderful, wise, understanding, or deceitful, dishonest, stupid; has intense and unstable relationships with peers; has idealistic and shallow perception of world; strives for emotional independence
Fears		Worries about loss of identity (bodily, emotional) and failure (in school, career, friendship); is uncertain
Play	Gradually becomes more sensitive to others; shows superstitions, teasing, and insults in games; plays cooperatively—baseball, jacks, hopscotch; finds peers of the same sex and conformity to a group important; demonstrates hoarding by making collections	Develops skills in individual and group games, sports, and activities; joins clubs, groups, and sports teams; is part of a clique that involves peers of the same sex but shares activities with the opposite sex
Dependence	Rejects some ideas of parents and tries own ideas but usually returns to home base; reduces need for dependency by using rituals—bedtime, mealtime, bathtime; becomes responsible, reasonable, and dependable	Is highly ambivalent about wanting limits and needing freedom; discovers responsibility that comes with freedom; makes decisions on own
Morality	May cheat, especially in early years; thinks of own needs first and is out to satisfy them; can think of relationship between an act and its consequences; begins to develop an idea of what it means to live by a label (good boy, good girl, bad boy, bad girl); has a strict literal conscience; begins to be influenced morally by peer group with fixed rules and rituals; becomes concerned about right and wrong	Begins to see that own actions affect a large group of individuals rather than just self; begins logical thought about own principles, rights, and justice as compared with rest of community; establishes a moral code by internalizing principles
Self-image	Begins to see self as labeled by others (boy, girl, mean, nice, bully, cute); has increasing awareness of sexuality and reproduction, but is modest; is self-critical and anxious to do things right; recognizes individual differences	Learns through group contact; desires to be just like everyone else but more so; tries many different roles; worries excessively about body and bodily functions
Habits	Eating: eats with family and can sit through entire meal; has definite likes and dislikes, but may change suddenly; has rituals about mealtime—same location at table, same silverware, same food Bowels: needs no help from adults Sleeping: may spend night away from home Dressing: can decide on own clothing and dress self but may ask for help and then ignore it; can comb own hair Behavior: may develop annoying habits (hair twirling, nail biting)	Eating: tries many food fads; eats constantly because of worry over bodily functions, tries fad diets to correct specific problems; would rather eat with peers than family Sleeping: may be so wound up in activities that he sleeps very little; may have trouble going to bed and getting up in morning Dressing: conforms to peers in clothing, hair, makeup, jewelry
Physical	Has increased gross motor ability—rides two-wheel bicycle, climbs trees; has increased manual dexterity, visual perception, and hand-eye coordination; can do multiple physical activities at one time (hold books, ride bicycle); has improved balance	Has completed major gross and fine motor development; expands experiences with physical capabilities
Cognitive	Is talkative; uses expressive language; begins to understand time and money; has increasing intellectual curiosity; develops favorite subjects to explore; can plan and see a project to completion	Develops adult intellectual skills and concepts; uses abstract logic: constructs hypotheses, and tests them through deductive reasoning

Modified from Brown, M, and Murphy, M: Ambulatory pediatrics for nurses, ed. 2, New York, 1981, McGraw-Hill Book Co.

ing to solve problems on their own and achieve the outcomes they desire. This paced, active participation may initiate a style of involvement in lifelong self-care.

School-age children and adolescents must cope with changes involving all areas of development and frequently occurring at the same time. For example the 6-year-old child must learn to (1) play with a group of children, following a set of rules, (2) distinguish right from wrong, (3) develop reasoning ability, and (4) read and write. Because of the stress of these changes, a child may develop physical and psychosocial health problems (for example, increasing susceptibility to upper respiratory infections, school maladjustment, inadequate peer relationships, or learning disorders). The nurse's role is to help the child or adolescent avoid or minimize health problems while supporting developmental growth.

SCHOOL-AGE CHILD

Calling the years between 6 and 12 the "school-age years" reflects a cultural bias, but most cultures provide some systematic, structured learning experiences during these years, to assist children in becoming productive, functioning members of the society. For children in the United States and other industrialized countries, this means formal schooling. In some other cultures, children acquire agricultural or hunting skills necessary for survival. These learning experiences can be interpreted as schooling and will be treated as such in this chapter. The provision of learning experiences occurring in all cultures during later childhood and adolescence takes advantage of children's increasing physical, cognitive, and psychosocial abilities. Although some educational authorities advocate early childhood learning programs, it is generally accepted that optimal learning occurs after, not before, 6 years of age.

The school or educational experience expands the child's world and is a transition from a life of relatively free play to a life of structured play, learning and work. Both the school environment and the home influence growth and development, requiring adjustment by the parents and child. The child must learn to cope with rules and expectations presented by the school and peers. Parents must learn to allow their child to make decisions, accept responsibility, and learn from life's experiences.

The role of the nurse in this adjustment process is to promote health. The nurse can help the parents and child identify stresses before they occur and plan to minimize stress and the child's reaction to it. This intervention must include parent, child, and teacher for maximal success. Table 23-2 provides an overview of stressors commonly encountered by school-age children and the appropriate nursing interventions.

Physical Development
HEIGHT AND WEIGHT

Gradual and steady physical growth and development occur between 6 and 12 years. Height increases 1 to 2 inches per year. Weight increase is more variable, averaging 3 to 6 pounds per year. Children generally have a slimmer, long-legged look.

Continued evaluation of the height and weight curve on a growth chart is essential. Alterations in growth provide a clue to the onset of many childhood disease processes. Thus monitoring of growth indices and vital signs is an important tool of assessment.

Until approximately ages 9 to 10, boys are an average of 1 inch taller and 2 pounds heavier than girls. Then girls begin a rapid growth period and by age 12 are generally 2 pounds heavier and 1 inch taller than boys. The prepubertal physical changes and growth spurts can occur between 9 and 14 years for girls and 12 and 16 years for boys (Tanner, 1974). Until this time, sexual growth and development of secondary sex characteristics, such as the growth of pubic hair, enlargement of the penis, and onset of menses, are minimal.

CARDIOVASCULAR FUNCTIONING

Cardiovascular functioning is refined and stabilized during the school-age years. The heart rate averages 65 to 90 beats per minute, the blood pressure normalizes at 110/70 mm Hg, and the respiratory rate stabilizes to 16 to 18 breaths per minute. Lung growth is minimal. However, by the end of this period the heart is six times the size it was at birth and has generally reached its adult size.

GROSS MOTOR COORDINATION

During the 7 years of the school-age period, children gain control over their bodies. Strength doubles and large muscle coordination improves. Refinement of neuromuscular function is a major accomplishment during these years. These developments make school-age children appear more skillful in their body movements. They can successfully participate in activities and games requiring coordinated muscle movements. Individual differences in the rate of mastering skills and ultimate skill achievement become apparent. Exposure to a variety of experiences, as well as innate ability, plays a role in individual differences of motor skills ultimately achieved.

FINE MOTOR COORDINATION

Fine motor coordination improves between 6 and 12 years. Most 6-year-old children can hold a pencil adeptly and print letters and words, but by age 12 the child can make detailed drawings and write sentences in script. Painting, drawing, playing computer games, and model

TABLE 23-2 Potential School-Related Stressors

Age (years)	Stressor	Nursing intervention
6-8	Adjusting to teacher's disciplinary approach	Promote parent-teacher-nurse communication through conferences aimed toward identifying expectations, encouraging parental involvement in school or classroom activities, and mediating in conflicts or difficult situations.
	Meeting teacher's behavioral expectations	Encourage communication between child and parent about school expectations, happenings, and adjustments.
	Competing with peers for teacher's attention	Promote fair and equal treatment of children in the classroom. Discourage favoritism and performance comparisons and encourage appropriate individual attention and praise.
	Maintaining self-concept	Evaluate parent-child relationship for interaction problems that may transfer to classroom; communicate these to the teacher.
	Coping with hurtful honesty of peers	Promote close supervision of peer activities and behaviors. Discuss peer relationships, their nature, and characteristics with parents and teacher.
	Testing out new ideas and behaviors at home	Set limits on destructive or antisocial behaviors. Allow exploration of new behaviors and ideas with guidance.
	Coping with being away from home for extended period of time; adjusting to school rules and routines	Assist child to identify physical setup of school and daily routines in first few days.
8-10	Concentrating on cognitive pursuits; meeting cognitive expectations of school; meeting own and family's cognitive expectations to best of ability	Encourage communication about the child's performance between the parent, child, and teacher. Assist in identifying skills mastered and those in need of mastery. Assist in identifying early problems. Assess level of health, particularly sensory function, as it may relate to school difficulties. Accept the child and his performance and behaviors as individual when considered within the norm.
	Integrating peer values into behavior without interference with family values	Observe peer activities and interactions. Reinforce positive behaviors and performance. Provide education for parents and teachers regarding normal behaviors of age.
10-12	Assuming responsibility for own learning	Encourage the allocation of learning responsibilities and allow child to carry them out. Encourage the child's participation in identifying learning needs.
	Deriving satisfaction from own cognitive performance	Positively reinforce good performance and guide the child when performance is optimal; do not punish.
	Participating in organized school or peer activity	Assist child in identifying school or peer group activity that he enjoys and in which he can potentially be successful. Assist parents in realizing need for extracurricular activities and encouraging the child's appropriate participation (avoid excessive demands to win and promote honest, fair play). Encourage teachers to recognize importance of after-school activities and avoid overloading children with homework.
	Beginning to develop a set of behavioral standards that reflect being in control and requiring little or no adult supervision	Promote good conduct through praise and example. Encourage parents to trust child, recognizing that not all behaviors will be "perfect."

Modified from Laige, J: The school age child and his family. In Hymovich, D, and Barnard, M, editors: Family health care: developmental and situational crises, New York, 1973, McGraw-Hill Book Co.; and McElroy, E, and Tackett, JJ: Growth and development needs of the family with school age children: maintaining wellness. In Tackett, JJ, and Hunsberger, M, editors: Family centered care of children and adolescents, Philadelphia, 1981, W.B. Saunders Co.

making provide vehicles for children to practice and improve newly refined skills. Nurses should encourage children and have parents encourage them to pursue these activities.

Assessment of neurological development is often based on fine motor coordination. This assessment may include penmanship, stacking ability, and performance of sequential rapid, alternating movements such as touching the finger to the nose and then to the examiner's finger (smooth movement without tremors is the normal response). Fine motor coordination is critical to success in the typical American school, where children must be able to hold pencils and crayons and use scissors and rulers. Teachers frequently ask the school nurse to conduct fine motor assessment of a child with questionable ability. Nurses need to know what constitutes normal fine motor functioning to perform this neurological screening. The nurse should refer children with deviations from normal function for more comprehensive assessments.

NUTRITIONAL NEEDS

Nutritional requirements remain relatively stable in the school-age years. Children need a balanced diet that includes the four basic food groups. Promotion of good nutrition and eating habits is an important part of the nurse's role. Nurses should encourage parents to provide a variety of foods for children, in adequate amounts to support both growth and energy for play. Because play activities vary from day to day, energy requirements also vary. Children of this age do not usually eat a large amount of food at one time. Providing nutritious snacks is often the best way for a parent to ensure adequate nutritional intake. Small servings of fruit, vegetables, and high-protein foods should be made available to encourage nutritious snacking.

OTHER CHANGES

Other physical changes take place during the school-age years. A steady skeletal growth in the trunk and extremities occurs, and small and long bone ossification

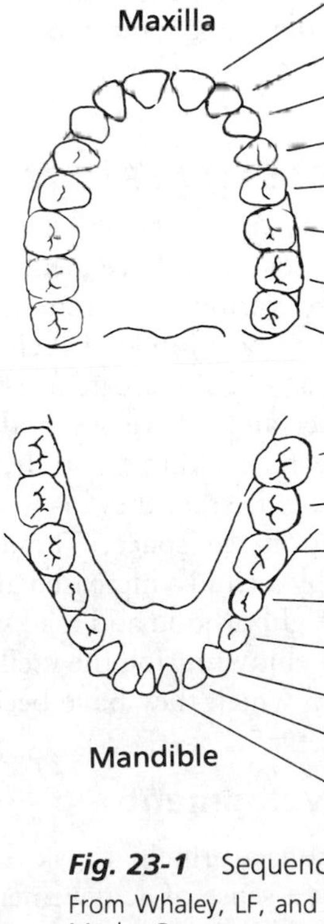

	Average age (months) of eruption of primary teeth	Average age (years) of shedding of primary teeth	Average age (years) of eruption of secondary teeth
Maxilla			
Central incisor	9.6	7.5	7.5
Lateral incisor	12.4	8.0	8.5
Canine	18.3	11.5	11.5
First premolar	15.7	10.5	10.5
Second premolar	26.3	10.5	11.1
First molar			6.3
Second molar			12.4
Third molar			17.0-21.0
Third molar			
Second molar			11.5
First molar			6.0
Second premolar	26.0	11.0	11.2
First premolar	15.1	10.0	10.3
Canine	18.2	9.5	10.1
Lateral incisor	11.5	7.0	7.5
Mandible Central incisor	7.8	6.0	6.4

Fig. 23-1 Sequence of eruption of secondary teeth.
From Whaley, LF, and Wong, DL: Nursing care of infants and children, ed. 3, St. Louis, 1987, The C.V. Mosby Company.

is present but not complete by age 12. Facial bones grow and remodel, as indicated by the presence of frontal sinuses by age 8 or 9. Dental growth is prominent during the school-age years. By 12 years, all primary teeth have been shed and the majority of permanent teeth have erupted. Fig. 23-1 illustrates the pattern and timing of dental shedding and eruption. Infrequent or inadequate dental care remains a persistent need of many American children.

As skeletal growth progresses, overall body appearance and posture change. Earlier posture, which was characterized by a stoop-shouldered, slightly lordotic stance and prominent abdomen, changes to a more erect posture.

Eye shape alters because of skeletal growth. This improves visual acuity, and normal adult 20/20 vision is achievable. Screening for vision and hearing problems is easier, and results are more reliable because school-age children can more fully understand and cooperate with the test directions. The school nurse typically assesses the dental, visual, and auditory status of school-age children biannually and refers those with possible deviations to a pediatrician.

Cognitive Development

Cognitive changes provide the school-age child with powerful capabilities for exploring, understanding, and communicating an understanding of the world. The ability to think abstractly, use past information, and plan for the future develops or improves during the years between 6 and 12. According to Piaget's theory, during these years, children move toward the stage of formal operations, in which thought processes are abstract. Between 5 and 7, children learn to organize facts by classifying, sorting, and ordering. This process remains quite concrete, however, and is based on perceptions. As experience increases, children consolidate new skills and increasingly move from concrete thinking to inductive logic. Children can group objects, identify general similarities and differences, and solve problems. By understanding principles of combination, they can add, subtract, and count objects. This is evident in the common school-age pastime of collecting items such as stamps, rocks, or buttons. The manner in which the child groups items in a collection can serve as a clue to his understanding of objects and their uses.

Between 7 and 12, children become able to carry out many cognitive processes without physically going through the motions or manipulating objects. Cognitive function extends beyond past and potential concrete experiences. The child considers the views of others, and his thinking is more socialized.

Children now begin metacognition, or thinking about their own thought processes. Metacognition allows a person to plan and initiate strategies to improve his learning processes. Some cognitive theorists consider metacognition the underlying principle responsible for cognitive growth (Siegler, 1978). The cognitive processes involved in short-term memory illustrate children's developing use of metacognition. Young children of 4 or 5 years are able to remember short lists of meaningful items. In a play situation, if given a list of items to obtain from a play store, the preschool child may aid his memory by repeating the list aloud to himself. If asked how he remembered the items, however, he is likely to be unable to respond. In contrast, school-age children *consciously* develop strategies for remembering the desired items. They may classify the items alphabetically or phonetically. If asked how they remembered, school-age children can describe their strategy. They can think about their thinking, employing metacognitive processes.

LANGUAGE DEVELOPMENT

Language development also continues during the school years. Children learn the language of peers and adults. Vocabulary increases with exposure to new words. Children are less bound by the restrictions of their family's language. They become more aware of the rules of syntax (that is, the rules for linking words into phrases and sentences). School-age children can identify generalizations and exceptions to rules. They accept language as a means for representing the world in a subjective manner and come to realize that words have arbitrary, rather than absolute, meanings. They can use different words for the same object or concept, and they understand that a single word may have many meanings.

UNDERSTANDING OF SPATIAL RELATIONSHIPS

During the school-age years the child's ability to understand spatial representation is refined. Children are now able to visualize various positions in space and evaluate how changes in position alter their perspective. For example, a 10-year-old can create a mental picture of how he would feel and where his body would be placed on a roller coaster making a 360-degree loop. In addition, children recognize that they, as well as objects, assume relative positions in space. These developing abilities are reflected by a child's increased ability to find his way around the neighborhood and read simple maps. Hospitalized children enjoy touring the facility, locating all the departments to which they have been.

Psychosocial Development

According to Erikson, a principal task of school-age children is developing a sense of achievement versus inferiority. A sense of achievement comes from success with effort. The child's psychosocial development is influenced by his physical and cognitive skill development. For example, improved fine motor capabilities, such as buttoning and tying, allow the school-age child to dress himself and take care of his personal needs. Most school-age children demand and are capable of independence in activities of daily living because of increased skill level. They develop strong preferences in the way their needs are met. An adult's introduction or suggestion of new practices, styles of clothing, or food can meet with strong resistance, which is a reflection of the school-age child's need to maintain control. The nurse recommending changes to parents or attempting to implement changes in the school-age child's activities of daily living needs to consider the child's need for independence. The child should therefore be involved in any decisions about changes and the specific actions for implementing the changes.

PEER RELATIONSHIPS

Group and personal achievements become important to the school-age child. Success is important in physical and cognitive activities. Play involves peers and the pursuit of group goals. Although solitary activities are not eliminated, they are overshadowed by group play. Learning to contribute, collaborate, and work cooperatively toward a common goal becomes a measure of success.

The school-age child prefers same-sex peers to opposite-sex peers. This strong gender identity is evidenced by the close network of same-sex companions a child maintains. In general, girls and boys view the opposite sex negatively. Peer influence becomes quite diverse during this stage of development. Mannerisms, clothing styles, and speech patterns are reinforced and influenced by contact with peers. Group identity increases as the school-age child approaches adolescence.

MORAL DEVELOPMENT

The need for a moral code and social rules becomes more evident to the school-age child as his or her cognitive ability and social experiences increase. For example, the 12-year-old child is able to consider what society would be like without rules because of his ability to reason logically and his experiences with group play. The child views rules as necessary principles of life, not just dictates from authorities. In the early school years, children strictly interpret and adhere to rules. As they develop, they make more flexible judgments and evaluate rules for applicability to a given situation. School-age children consider motivations and the actual behavior when making judgments about the way their behavior will affect themselves and others. The ability to be flexible when applying rules and to take the perspective of others is essential in developing moral judgments.

These abilities are present at times in earlier years but are more consistently displayed in later school years.

SELF-CONCEPT AND HEALTH

During the school-age years, identity and self-concept become stronger and more individualized. A child's perception of wellness is based on readily observable facts such as presence or absence of illness and adequacy of eating or sleeping. Functional ability is the standard by which a child judges his or her own health and the health of others.

Promotion of good health practices is a nursing responsibility. Programs directed toward health education are frequently organized and conducted in the school. The nurse's goal for such programs should be the development of behaviors that positively affect children's health status. Examples of program topics that encourage positive behaviors are dental health, good nutrition and eating habits, and treatment for a cold.

Specific Health Concerns

Accidents and injuries are a major health problem affecting school-age children. Motor vehicle accidents and accidents related to recreational activities or equipment are the leading causes of death or injury for school-age children. Nurses should promote health through accident prevention and safety education to individuals and groups (see Chapter 40). Involvement with social reform or environmental change may also be needed.

School-age children are also significantly affected by cancer, birth defects, influenza, and pneumonia (Department of Health, Education and Welfare, 1979). In this age group, these problems have a relatively low mortality but a high morbidity compared with accidents (see research highlight). Cognitive and psychomotor

---

⚕ *Research Highlight* ⚕

Miller et al. cite the most recent epidemiological studies in the United States to identify key indicators of health in school-age children and adolescents. For children, key indicators include immunization status, growth levels, blood lead levels, and non-motor-vehicle accident fatalities. For adolescents, key indicators include births to school-age mothers, suicides, and motor vehicle accidents. Iron deficiency anemia and child abuse and neglect are presented as relevant to all children.

Miller, C, et al.: Monitoring children's health: key indicators, Washington, D.C., 1986, Printing of the American Public Health Association.

skills allow increased participation by the child in management of a chronic illness.

School-age children face other significant health problems, including learning and school difficulties, behavioral disturbances, infectious diseases, and speech, hearing, or vision problems. To promote normal and healthy growth and development, the nurse must be aware of the risks and direct nursing actions toward reducing them. The nurse must also integrate an understanding of normal growth and development into all phases of the nursing process when providing health or illness care to a child.

ADOLESCENT

Adolescence is the stage of development marking the transition from childhood to adulthood. The term *adolescence* refers to psychological maturation of the individual. Puberty is the biological maturation that makes reproduction possible (Tackett and Hunsberger, 1981).

The period of life between 13 and 18 years is characterized by a steady progression of physical, social, cognitive, psychological, and moral changes. Adaptations required by these changes push the adolescent to develop coping mechanisms and styles of behaviors, which he will continue to use or adapt throughout life.

During this stage of development an adolescent must establish his own identity, make major decisions about his life and vocation, develop and refine adult cognitive skills, and establish a code of morality by which all of these tasks are ordered. With so much to accomplish, adolescents may at times be moody and difficult to live and work with.

The nurse's understanding of development provides a unique perspective for helping teenagers and parents anticipate and cope with the stresses of adolescence. Nursing activities, particularly education, can promote healthy development. These activities occur in a variety of settings and can be directed toward the adolescent, the parents, or the adolescent and parents together. For example, the nurse can conduct seminars in a high school to provide practical suggestions for solving problems of concern to a large group of students, such as treating acne or making responsible decisions about drugs or alcohol use. Similarly, a group education program for parents about how to cope with teenage children would promote parental understanding of adolescent development. These programs can be held in the school, clinic, private office, or community center. The nurse must identify needs and desires to learn more about specific topics or problems. Involving participants when identifying the topic and developing the activities produces more active, interest learners.

Physical Changes and Sexual Maturation

Physical changes occur rapidly in both males and females. Sexual maturation occurs with the development of primary and secondary sexual characteristics. Primary characteristics are physical and hormonal changes necessary for reproduction, and secondary characteristics externally differentiate males from females. Four main focuses of the physical changes are summarized by Tanner (1974):

1. Increased growth rate of skeleton, muscle, and viscera
2. Sex-specific changes, such as changes in shoulder and hip width
3. Alteration in distribution of muscle and fat
4. Development of the reproductive system and secondary sex characteristics

A wide variation exists in the timing of physical changes associated with puberty, and girls tend to begin their physical changes earlier than boys.

WEIGHT AND SKELETAL CHANGES

The majority of height and weight increases occur during the prepubertal growth spurt, which generally precedes adult maturity by 1 to 2 years. The growth spurt for girls generally begins between 10 and 14. Height increases 2 to 8 inches, and weight increases by 15 to 50 pounds. The male growth spurt usually takes place between 12 and 16. Height increases approximately 4 to 12 inches, and weight increases by 15 to 60 pounds. Fat is redistributed into adult proportions as height and weight increase, and gradually the adolescent torso takes on an adult appearance. Although individual differences and differences between sexes do occur, growth follows a similar pattern for both sexes. The legs lengthen first, followed by widening of thighs, broadening of shoulders, and trunk growth. Hips then widen in females and shoulders continue to widen in males.

Personal growth curves continue to be meaningful in assessing physical development. The individual's sustained progression along the curve, however, is more important than how the measurements correspond to the norm. The nurse continues to chart growth measurements during routine health assessments to evaluate growth changes in relation to past growth patterns.

EFFECTS OF PHYSICAL CHANGES ON PEER INTERACTION

Adolescents are sensitive about physical changes that make them different from peers. For this reason, they are generally interested in the normal pattern of growth and their personal growth curves. Consequently, the nurse should share this information to reassure adolescents that their own patterns are normal. The number of eating disorders is on the rise in adolescent girls (see research highlight), and knowledge of growth progression may be a way to discourage radical weight-reduction activities. If an adolescent deviates radically from the usual pattern, further assessment is necessary to identify the cause. Weight extremes resulting from excessive or inadequate caloric intake are common nursing diagnoses for the adolescent years. Allowing the adolescent to see when and how the weight curve changed can be a first step in identifying the problem and implementing dietary changes.

PUBERTY

TIMING. A wide variation exists between the sexes and within the same sex as to when the physical changes of puberty begin. This variation is more pronounced in males (Tanner and Whitehouse, 1982). In American males, the time of onset of pubertal changes appears to have a significant effect on psychosocial development. Early physical development has been found advantageous in later psychosocial interactions because early-developing males, who are more successful in group activities and peer relationships, gain an early sense of desirability that is maintained throughout later life. Less information is available about the impact of timing of physical development in females.

SEQUENCE. Despite the wide variation in timing, the sequence of pubertal growth changes is the same in most individuals. This stability is the basis of the most widely recognized and used systems for rating sexual maturity (Tanner and Whitehouse, 1982). Fig. 23-2 presents the criteria for this categorization. The wide ranges of *normal* progression are stressed. As with increases in height and weight, the pattern of sexual changes is more significant than their time of onset. Large deviations from the normal time frames require investigation. For ex-

ample, a 17-year-old girl who has not menstruated requires further assessment and referral.

Being like peers is extremely important for adolescents. Any deviation in the timing of the physical changes can be extremely difficult for them to accept. The nurse should therefore provide emotional support for adolescents undergoing assessment of early or delayed puberty. Even adolescents whose physical changes are occurring at the normal times may seek confirmation of and reassurance about their normalcy.

HORMONAL CHANGES. Visible and invisible changes take place during puberty. Among these are hormonal changes.

All pubertal events are created by hormonal changes within the body when the hypothalamus begins to produce gonadotropin-releasing hormones, which signal the pituitary to secrete gonadotropic hormones. The gonadotropic hormones stimulate ovarian cells to produce estrogen and testicular cells to produce testosterone. These hormones contribute to the development of secondary sex characteristics such as hair growth and voice changes and play an essential role in reproduction. The changing concentrations of these hormones are also linked to problems of concern to adolescents, such as acne and body odor. Understanding this hormonal physiology enables the nurse to reassure adolescent clients and educate them about changing body care needs.

Cognitive Development

School-age children can think logically about problems involving concrete situations. In adolescence the range of problems that can be addressed is extended, as is the ability to reason abstractly. Adolescents are capable of formal operations in which they must think about thinking and separate the real from the possible. This means that adolescents can use deductive reasoning, even in situations beyond their concrete experiences. Abstractions from hypothetical situations can be processed and understood. Adolescents can consider the logic of a problem, regardless of its contents. They can even solve problems requiring simultaneous manipulation of several abstract concepts. Development of this ability is important in the pursuit of an identity. For example, the newly acquired cognitive skills allow the teenager to decide which sex role behaviors are appropriate, effective, and comfortable, and to consider their potential impact on peers, family, and society. The ability to think logically about these behaviors and their outcomes encourages adolescents to develop their own thoughts and means of expressing sexual identity. In addition, a higher level of cognitive functioning makes the adolescent receptive to more detailed and diverse information about

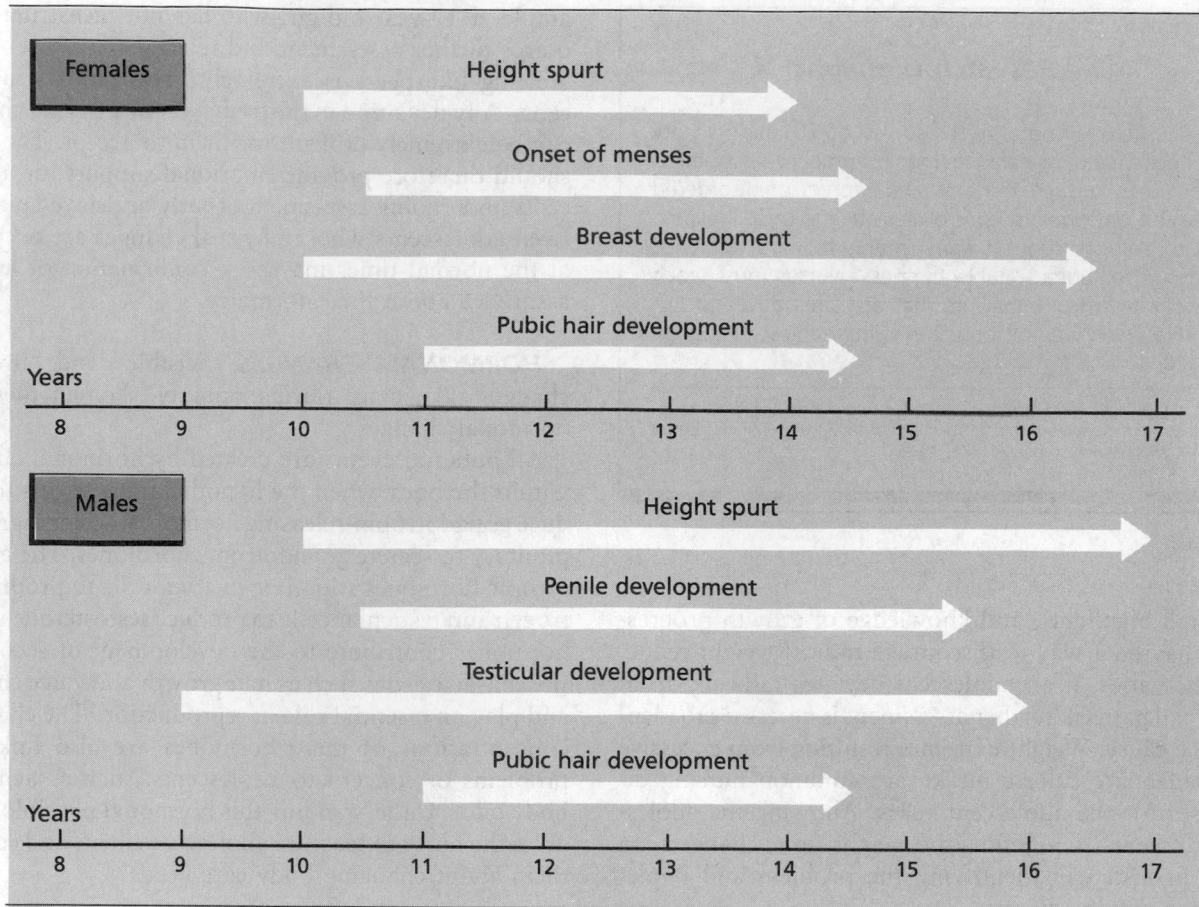

Fig. 23-2   Criteria for rating sexual maturity and growth.
Modified from Marshall, W, and Tanner, J: Arch Dis Child, 44:291, 1969, and 45:13, 1970.

sexuality and sexual behaviors. For example, sex education can include an explanation of the physiology of sexual changes and a detailed outline of how birth control measures work to prevent normal physiological events.

However, the potential to function at this cognitive level does not ensure corresponding performance. Cognitive abilities and performance vary greatly among adolescents. In fact, an adolescent may perform at different cognitive levels in different situations. Past stimulation, experiences, formal education, and motivation in the use of logic and effective deductive strategies, as well as the individual situation, influence the expression of cognitive abilities.

LANGUAGE SKILLS

Language development is fairly complete by adolescence, although vocabulary continues to expand. The primary focus becomes the development of communication skills that can be used effectively in various sit-

uations. The adolescent needs to communicate thoughts, feelings, and facts to peers, parents, teachers, and other persons of authority. The skills used in these diverse communication situations are varied. The adolescent must select the person with whom to communicate, decide how much to say, and choose the way he will transmit the message. For example, the way a teenager tells parents about a failing grade is not the same as the way he tells friends. The adolescent develops different skills and styles of communication and learns how and when to use them most effectively. These diverse communication skills are used and refined throughout life. Good communication skills may be critical for adolescents to overcome peer pressures to participate in nonhealthy behaviors.

Psychosocial Development

As adulthood approaches, teenagers must establish close peer relationships or remain socially isolated. An emotional independence from and equilibrium with families must be established, and they must adjust to and master their own sexuality.

Identity is consolidated during adolescence. Choices about vocation and life-style are also made. Evolving from all these tasks is a sexual, group, and personal identity unique to the individual.

SEXUAL IDENTITY

Achievement of sexual identity is enhanced by the physical changes of puberty. The physical evidence of being a mature male or female encourages the development of masculine and feminine behaviors. If these physical changes involve deviations, the person has more difficulty developing a comfortable sexual identity. Adolescents depend on these physical clues because they want assurance of maleness or femaleness and because they do not wish to be different from peers. Without these physical characteristics the process of achieving sexual identity is difficult. Other influences are cultural attitudes and expectations of sex role behavior and available role models. The masculine and feminine behaviors teenagers see and the expectations they perceive for behaving as a man or woman affect the way they express sexuality. The adolescent masters age-appropriate sexuality after feeling comfortable with sexual behaviors, choices, and relationships.

GROUP IDENTITY

Adolescents seek a group identity because they need esteem and acceptance. Similarity in dress or speech is common in teenage groups. Popularity is a major concern. Trends in the desire for popularity have not changed much in recent years. Females of middle-class status, more than any other group, regard popularity as particularly important. Conforming to group activities, being friendly, being oneself, and having a good personality are considered by teenagers to be the most important factors in gaining popularity (Padin, Lerner, and Spiro, 1981). Popularity with opposite sex and same-sex peers is important. The strong need for group identity seems to conflict at times with the adolescent's strive for personal identity. It is as though the adolescent requires a close bond with peers to later redefine himself against this group identity.

FAMILY RELATIONSHIPS

The movement toward stronger peer relationships is contrasted with the adolescent's movement away from parents. Although financial independence for adolescents is not the norm in American society, many adolescents work part-time, using their income to bolster independence. The adolescent has more control over purchases and social activities if parents are not the only financial resource.

Some adolescents and families have more difficulty during these years than others. The differences can result from the number, extent, and nature of the adolescent's usual cyclical movements from periods of independence to relative dependence. Adolescents need to make choices, act independently, and experience the consequences of actions. This testing, however, is best done against a firm, supportive, family foundation. The family needs to allow independence while providing a haven in which adolescents can contemplate actions. Families unable to provide this support complicate movement toward identity formation. Support to the family and adolescent may be essential to their success.

PERSONAL IDENTITY

One component of personal identity involves selecting an occupational or vocational direction in life. Because of society's changing needs, adolescents must be somewhat future oriented when making these choices. However, because the jobs that will be available or that adolescents will find rewarding 10 or 20 years in the future are not clear, selecting a livelihood is a complicated task. The nurse should provide emotional support during this process and should help adolescents select courses of action that promote self-satisfaction, identity, and continual opportunity for growth.

Another part of an adolescent's personal identity is his perception of his health. This component is of specific interest to health care providers. Healthy adolescents evaluate their own health according to feelings of well-being, ability to function normally, and absence of symptoms. Interventions to improve health perception might therefore concentrate on these areas. Health problems causing severe or long-term alteration of these factors may permanently alter self-identity.

MORAL DEVELOPMENT

The development of moral judgement depends heavily on cognitive and communication skills and peer interaction. Although moral development begins in early childhood, it is consolidated in adolescence because of the presence of these skills. Adolescents learn to understand rules as cooperative agreements that can be modified to fit the situation, rather than as absolutes. Adolescents learn to apply rules by using their own judgment rather than simply to avoid punishment as in the earlier years.

Kohlberg (1964) explains moral developments in terms of stages (see Chapter 22). Adolescents can achieve the highest level of moral judgment. At this level, morality is derived from individual principles of conscience. Adolescents judge themselves by internatilized ideals, often leading to conflict between personal and group values. Group values become less significant in later adolescence.

Not all adolescents attain the same level of moral development. There is, however, a general forward movement through the stages of moral development, and the sequence of the stages is similar for all individuals, even when time of achievement varies.

Specific Health Concerns

The leading cause of death in adolescence is accidents (Shen, 1980), with motor vehicle accidents being the most common. Such accidents are often associated with alcohol or drug abuse, depression, and stress. In addition, alcohol and drug abuse, depression, and stress increase the risk of suicide. Nurses educate adolescents to recognize these factors in themselves and their peers. Educational interventions can reduce the potential for accidents.

Another area of concern to adolescent health is the formation of healthy habits of daily living. Emphasis on exercise, sleep, nutrition, and stress-reduction habits is increasing. It is the nurse's responsibility to recognize the importance of these habits and to identify ways to adapt them to the individual. To do this the nurse must assess the individual's positive and negative habits and attitudes about health. Accidents and the formation of healthy habits have psychological and physical components and effects. Extensive and long-term follow-up is required if individualized interventions are to succeed. The nurse needs to be aware of the prevalence of these problems and make assessments accordingly.

Sexual experimentation is common among adolescents. Peer pressure, physiological and emotional changes, and societal expectations all contribute to early heterosexual and homosexual relations. The nurse must provide sex education and counseling. The degree of sexual activity among teenagers may not change significantly, but the degree of informed, consenting participation can. Two prominent consequences of adolescent sexual activity are sexually transmitted disease and pregnancy.

Sexually transmitted diseases are the most common communicable diseases among adolescents. The combined incidence of gonorrhea, syphilis, and genital herpes simplex has increased to over 12 million cases a year (DHEW, 1979). Nurses should encourage early recognition and prompt reporting and treatment to reduce this incidence. Extensive educational efforts to prevent the spread of AIDS in this age group has been advocated by the U.S. Secretary of Health. Some states have mandated these educational efforts, with nurses playing key roles in planning, implementation, and evaluation.

NURSING PROCESS

The nursing process can be readily applied to the care of children, regardless of age. To illustrate the use of the nursing process in organizing and documenting the care of children and adolescents, an example will be provided from the case of a 10-year-old boy with an acute attack of asthma requiring emergency room treatment.

ASSESSMENT

As with care provided to all children, the nursing assessment of the school-age child and adolescent includes developmental level, response to care, history of prior health care, medical history, and available support persons.

Assessment of the developmental level provides information about the ability of the child to understand, cooperate with, and possibly assume limited responsibility for immediate and long-term care needs. Assessment focuses on cognitive, motor, and psychosocial abilities and limitations. In an emergency situation (such as the child with an asthma attack), cognitive and psychosocial information might initially be assessed indirectly from parental report. Information can be confirmed directly with the child when dyspnea(difficulty breathing) lessens and the child becomes more verbal. Motor abilities can be assessed by observing the child unbuttoning a coat or removing pieces of clothing in preparation for the physical examination. Cognitive assessment might be based on the report of school grades, favorite activities, and responses to questions from parents and health care providers.

A history of prior health care will enlighten the nurse's understanding of the child's response to current care. In the example, the 10-year-old child had been diagnosed with asthma 6 years before and has had multiple exacerbations in the last 6 months. The boy has been on daily cromolyn sodium for 1 year but took no other medications. For the past 3 days the entire family had been "fighting off a cold." At 8 pm the child's cough increased, he felt tired, and he decided to go to bed. At 1:30 am, he woke with audible wheezing and complaints of a "tight chest, like a brick laid on top of me." Shortness of breath continued to increase rapidly, so the parents took the child to the nearest emergency room. During the ride to the hospital the boy began to cry.

Knowing that the child had three exacerbations of asthma in the past 6 months, two of which required hospitalization, assists the nurse in interpreting the child's insistence that he is feeling better, despite objective physiological signs and symptoms of a worsening condition. Knowing that the child told his parents he "hated the hospital" and begged them not to "leave me at the hospital this time" emphasizes the importance of not minimizing deteriorating physiological parameters. It also stresses the importance of reassuring the child that hospitalization is not planned and that he will be informed of any change in this decision.

Assessment data may also guide long-term planning that will assist the child in learning to replace his wish for improvement with realistic assessment of his own status so he might take self-care actions earlier in the course of the exacerbation. Earlier action might then minimize the exacerbation and avert the need for hospital treatment.

Data about the availability of supportive significant others and the child's ability to utilize this support is critical. For example, the nurse may observe the child reaching for the father's hand for providing physical comfort but responding best to the mother's firm directions for cooperating with nebulizer treatment. This information will guide the selection of strategies that can maximize the support each parent can offer. Sharing these observations with the parents can lessen their feelings of helplessness, which are related to the child's ability to cooperate with therapies. It is also useful to identify the internal supports the child believes effective. For example, the child might find reading, listening to soft music, or using guided relaxation therapies helpful. School-age children and adolescents can often be helped to identify their internal support systems and taught to use them at appropriate times.

NURSING DIAGNOSIS

The nursing diagnoses box lists examples of potentially relevant nursing diagnoses. Any or all of the nursing diagnoses may be applicable to a particular child. The sample nursing diagnoses box selects three of these diag-

---

Examples of Nursing Diagnoses for School-Age Child Having an Acute Episode of Asthma

NANDA-APPROVED NURSING DIAGNOSES

Anxiety related to:
- Unknown progressive nature of the exacerbation
- Unknown personal response to treatment

Fear related to
- Potential treatments (that is, injections, hospitalization)
- Recurrence of exacerbation

Impaired gas exchange related to:
- Airway hyperreactivity
- Increased airway secretions
- Swelling of airway tissues

Impaired verbal communication related to:
- Shortness of breath
- Treatment regimen (that is, O_2, nebulizer mask)

Ineffective airway clearance related to:
- Airway constriction
- Thickened secretions
- Reduced force of cough

Ineffective breathing pattern related to
- O_2 and CO_2 alterations
- Weakening breathing muscles

Powerlessness related to:
- Inability to terminate exacerbation without assistance of health care team
- Inability to prevent exacerbations, past and future

Sample Nursing Diagnoses for School-Age Child Having an Acute Episode of Asthma

Defining Characteristics	Nursing Diagnoses	Related Factors
Wheezing Weak or absent cough without sputum Dyspnea	Ineffective airway clearance	- Fatigue
Speaks with difficulty Inability to express needs or wishes about care Speech limited to single words	Impaired verbal communication	- Dyspnea - Interference of treatment equipment
Dread of specific, identifiable objects (for example, hospital equipment) and abstract feelings (for example, fear of dying)	Fear	- Dread of injections, hospitalizations, and recurrence of exacerbation

noses and gives examples of defining characteristics and related factors. Ineffective airway clearance, impaired verbal communication, and fear represent primary physiological, social, and psychological concerns. In the example the nurse noted the child had a weak, ineffective cough but a large amount of thick secretions. Wheezes (abnormal lung sounds) were bilateral and loud throughout an initial nebulizer treatment. The sensation of dyspnea was identified after observing the child's use of accessory breathing muscles and flared nostrils and from the words the child used to describe how he felt ("like a brick laid on top of me"). These characteristics led to the nursing diagnosis of ineffective airway clearance.

Verbal communication is impaired because of the dyspnea and the medical therapeutic equipment, which includes a nebulizer and mask. In planning care the nurse will need to structure verbal communication to require only brief responses from the child or devise an alternative communication system. Writing responses is an alternative for the adolescent, whereas drawing may provide a means of communication for the school-age child.

Fear of hospitalization is quite evident in the child in the example. Dread of injections is also a common fear

in children with asthma because treatment often includes repetitive injections of epinephrine. In this example, repeated exacerbations in the prior 6 months could cause fear of continued recurrences.

PLANNING

The care plan box demonstrates further application of the nursing process for ineffective airway clearance and provides the related sample nursing care plan for achieving two outcomes. The diagnosis, the goal to be achieved, expected outcomes, and interventions are shown. This plan is based on the nurse's prior knowledge of nursing care, physiology, pathophysiology, human development, and the assessment of the child and family. Airway clearance is essential to improvement of the child's health. Thus the nurse planned interventions to reduce this problem after an initial, medically prescribed, 15-minute nebulizer treatment. The nurse waits until after the treatment so the medication given by the neb-

---

Sample Nursing Care Plan for School-Age Child Having an Acute Episode of Asthma

Nursing Diagnosis	Goal	Expected Outcomes	Nursing Interventions
Ineffective airway clearance related to thick secretions and weak cough	Airway is clear of thick mucus secretions.	Adequate hydration is maintained.	Offer 3-4 ounces of favorite liquid every 30 minutes. Monitor mucus membranes, urine output, and skin turgor for signs of severe dehydration. Inform medical staff of results of the above interventions, so prompt initiation of IV fluids can be begun, if needed.
		Cough is strong enough to move secretions.	Allow rest periods between clearance attempts and discourage frequent ineffective coughing. Demonstrate and monitor performance of preferable coughing attempts (that is, sitting, 1 or 2 deep breaths before coughing, expectoration of sputum). Perform postural drainage or chest percussion if medically prescribed.

Sample Evaluation of Interventions for School-Age Child Having an Acute Episode of Asthma		
Goal	**Evaluative Measures**	**Expected Outcomes**
Airway is clear of thick mucus secretions.	Observe skin turgor, mucous membranes, and urinary output.	Adequate hydration maintained, as evidenced by child consuming 6-8 ounces of liquid every hour, moist mucous membranes, normal skin turgor, and adequate urinary output
	Observe for forceful cough and productive sputum	Cough is strong enough to move secretions
	Auscultate lungs.	Lungs are clear to auscultation with normal adventitious sounds
	Obtain blood gas values.	Blood gas values are normal

ulizer can relax the smooth muscles of the respiratory system and so the child can rest before the clearing efforts, which require his active cooperation. The plan to improve the airway also incorporates actions to maintain adequate hydration and to structure coughing sessions that actively involve the child, teach the most effective techniques, and provide supplemental passive drainage.

IMPLEMENTATION

Implementation of the care plan must be highly individualized. The fluids offered will depend on the child's preference and will probably change during therapy. Having the child add up his own intake contributes to active involvement and a potential sense of personal mastery over at least one aspect of his illness. Thus this intervention and its outcome could also contribute to improvement of a related nursing diagnosis included in the box of nursing diagnoses: powerlessness.

EVALUATION

The nursing process is incomplete unless a continuing evaluation is performed as a basis for revision of the care plan. The success of the interventions to improve airway clearance can be evaluated based on factors shown in the evaluation box. Proper timing of the nursing clearance efforts, presence of a productive cough, reduction of wheezing, decreased dyspnea, improved blood gas values, moist mucus membranes, and proper skin tugor and urinary output are used to evaluate the effectiveness of interventions to achieve desired outcomes and goals.

SUMMARY

The school-age child and adolescent grows and develops significantly. At the beginning of the school-age years the child is a slightly egocentric, inquisitive, reality-oriented person whose physical and cognitive abilities do not always measure up to his psychosocial needs and desires. By age 12, the child has become intellectually and physically adept, has established a social sphere, has begun to develop a moral code, and has started to mature sexually.

Further developmental advances are made during the adolescent years. By age 18, most adolescents have made the transition to adulthood. They are well on their way to becoming socially responsible, productive human beings capable of sustaining interpersonal relationships and a vocation and demonstrating formal cognitive abilities and moral judgment, all with a firmly developed individual identity.

A nurse must guide and counsel individuals through the school-age and adolescent stages, which are particularly challenging because of the diversity and simultaneous development of changes in all spheres. The ability to examine and assess all components of these and other developmental stages is an essential skill of nursing.

KEY CONCEPTS

✓ A developmental task of the school-age child is the formation of a sense of achievement.

✓ The prepubertal growth spurt usually affects girls at an earlier age than boys.

✓ Changes in growth pattern may indicate the onset of disease.

✓ During the school-age years, a child gains the muscle strength and coordination needed to participate in complex gross and fine motor activities.

✓ The school-age child moves toward the ability to think abstractly, reflect on thought processes, and plan for the future.

✓ During the school-age years, the child learns the rules of language development.

✓ The school-age child develops a sense of what is morally right and wrong and respects the role of authority.

✓ The extent to which the school-age child develops physically and cognitively will influence his psychosocial development.

✓ The school-age child needs to exert control and make personal decisions.

✓ The school-age child learns to develop cognitively and psychosocially through peer relationships.

✓ The adolescent must adapt to significant stressors to gain a sense of identity and achieve psychological maturity.

✓ During adolescence, primary and secondary sexual characteristics develop.

✓ The adolescent is concerned about patterns of growth because of the fear of being different from peers.

✓ A wide variation exists among members of the same sex as to when physical changes of puberty occur.

✓ Physical changes of puberty are linked to hormonal changes.

✓ The adolescent is capable of abstract thought and deductive reasoning.

✓ Although the adolescent's use of language is well developed, he must acquire effective communication skills.

✓ The adolescent's sense of right and wrong evolves from the application of moral rules to daily decision making.

✓ The formation of a meaningful identity depends on an adolescent's needs for normal physical development, acceptance from peers, independence from family, and choice of a future occupation.

✓ Sexually transmitted diseases are the most common communicable diseases among adolescents.

REFERENCES

Department of Health, Education, and Welfare: Healthy people, Washington D.C., 1979, U.S. Government Printing Office.

Kohlberg, L: Development of moral character and moral ideology. In Hoffman, ML and Hoffman, LNW editors: Review of child development research, vol. I, New York, 1964, Russell Sage Foundation.

Padin, M, Lerner, R, and Spiro, A: Stability of body attitudes and self esteem in late adolescence, Adolescence 61:371, 1981.

Shen, J, editor: The clinical practice of adolescent medicine, New York, 1980, Appleton-Century-Crofts.

Siegler, R: Children's thinking: what develops? Hillsdale, N.J., 1978, Lawrence Erlbaum Associates, Inc.

Tackett, JJ and Hunsberger, M, editors: Family centered care of children and adolescents, Philadelphia, 1981, W.B. Saunders Co.

Tanner, JM: Sequence and tempo in the somatic changes of puberty. In Grumbach, MM, et al., editors: Control of the onset of puberty, New York, 1974, John Wiley & Sons, Inc.

Tanner, JM and Whitehouse RH: Atlas of children's growth: normal variation and growth diseases, New York, 1982, Academic Press, Inc.

ADDITIONAL READINGS

Brown, MS and Murphy, MA: Ambulatory pediatrics for nurses, ed. 2, New York, 1981, McGraw-Hill Book Co.

Chow, M, et al.: Handbook of pediatric primary care, ed. 2, New York, 1984, John Wiley & Sons, Inc.

Dickey, S: A guide to the nursing of children: clinical nursing diagnosis series, Baltimore, 1987, Williams & Wilkins.

Falkner, E, and Tanner, M, editors: Human growth: a comprehensive treatise, ed. 2, New York, 1986, Plenum Publishing Corp.

Laige, J: The school aged child and his family. In Hymovich, D, and Barnard, M, editors: Family health care: developmental and situational crises, New York, 1973, McGraw-Hill Book Co.

Lundholm, K, and Littrett, J: Desire for thinness among high school cheerleaders: relationship to disordered eating and weight control behaviors, Adolescence 21:573, 1986.

Marshall, W, and Tanner, J: Variations in the patterns of pubertal changes in girls, Arch Dis Child 44:291, 1969.

Marshall, W, and Tanner, J: Variations in the patterns of pubertal changes in boys, Arch Dis Child 45:13, 1970.

McElroy, E, and Tackett, JJ: Growth and development needs of the family with school age children: maintaining wellness. In Tackett, JJ, and Hunsberger, M, editors: Family centered care of children and adolescents, Philadelphia, 1981, W.B. Saunders Co.

Miller, C, et al.: Monitoring children's health: key indicators. Washington, D.C., 1986, American Public Health Association.

Whaley, LF, and Wong, DL: Nursing care of infants and children, ed. 3, St. Louis, 1987, The C.V. Mosby Co.

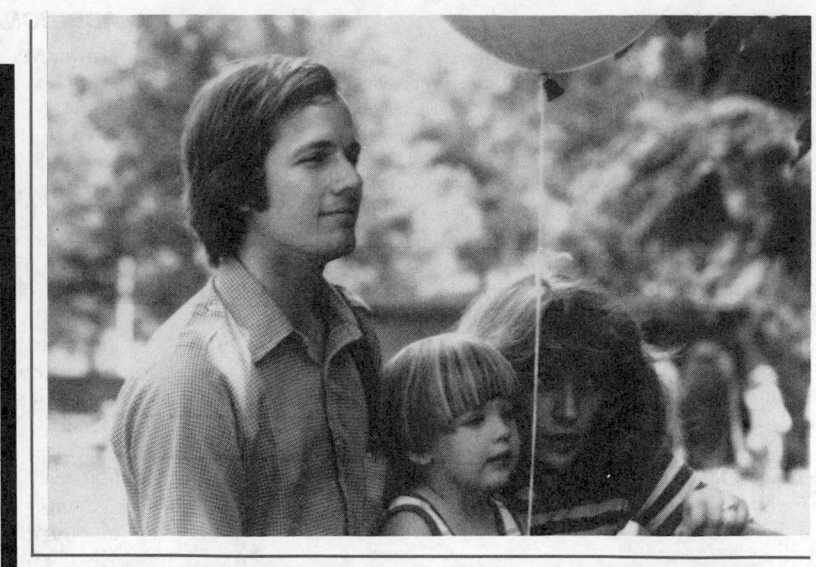

OBJECTIVES

Mastery of content in this chapter will enable the student to:

- Define key terms listed.
- Discuss developmental theories of the young and middle adult.
- List and discuss major life events of the young and middle adult and the childbearing family.
- Describe developmental tasks of the young adult, the childbearing family, and the middle adult.
- Discuss the significance of family in the life of the adult.
- Describe normal physiological changes in young and middle adulthood and in pregnancy.
- Discuss cognitive and psychosocial changes occurring during the adult years.
- Describe health concerns of the young adult, the childbearing family, and the middle adult.
- List nursing diagnoses appropriate for the young and middle adult.
- Use the nursing process to administer care to young- and middle-adult clients.

KEY TERMS

Climacteric
Family Stress
Infertility
Lactation
Maturity
Morning Sickness
Orgasmic Maturity
Proactive Decision
Puerperium
Reactive Decision

Young and Middle Adult

Young and middle adulthood is a period of challenges, rewards, and crises. Adults have the challenge of entering the work force, the reward of a job well done, and the crises associated with caring for parents and rearing a family or remaining single.

Adult development involves orderly changes in characteristics and attitudes. Developmental changes are based on earlier characteristics that help shape subsequent behavior and characteristics (Beck, Rawlins, and Williams, 1984). The changes experienced by the young adult include the natural processes of maturation and socialization. The young adult passes through alternating periods of stability and change. During periods of stability the person makes certain choices and builds a structure around them. In periods of change the individual reevaluates these choices and considers new alternatives (Levinson et al., 1978).

Young adulthood is the period between the early twenties and the late thirties or early forties. During this time the person increasingly separates from his family of origin, establishes career goals, and decides whether to marry and begin a family or remain single. The young adult is active and must adapt to new experiences.

The person's entry into middle age depends on events that generally signify transition into this time of life. The midlife transition occurs when a person becomes aware that changes in reproductive and physical abilities signify the beginning of another stage in life. During this transition period individuals may reassess their goals in life and add new goals.

MATURITY AND ADULTHOOD

People can be said to have reached maturity when they have attained a balance of growth in physiological, psychosocial, and cognitive areas. Mature individuals feel comfortable with the abilities, knowledge, and responses they have developed over the years. They look at the world with a broad perspective, based on a blend of insight, emotion, and imagination. They take on problems that can be solved but recognize and learn to live with unsolvable problems.

Mature people are open to suggestions and can accept constructive criticism without a major loss of self-esteem. They weigh other persons' input and recommendations when making a decision but are not overly influenced or intimidated by others. Above all, mature people develop by learning from their own and other's experiences.

Other characteristics of maturity are related to interpersonal communication and behavior. The mature person acknowledges both accomplishments and shortcomings. When a mistake is made the ego is not crushed and blame is not transferred to others.

The pleasure principle—the drive for immediate gratification of a need so dominant in infancy and early childhood—is much less active in adult behavior. In fact, it is the ability to set long-range goals and direct energy toward a distant objective that is often the crucial element in a person's self-actualization. The stresses inherent in developing maturity and judgment are greatly increased in times of change. High levels of stress can have adverse effects on a person's health status. The nurse can help a young or middle adult maintain health by understanding that finding a place in society is a developmental task in this stage of life.

YOUNG ADULT

Theories of Young Adulthood

Many theorists have attempted to describe the phases of young adulthood and related developmental tasks. Levinson has identified four phases of young adult development (Levinson et al., 1978): (1) early adult transition (ages 18 to 20), when the person separates from the family and desires independence; (2) entrance into the adult world (ages 21 to 27), when the person tries out careers and life-styles; (3) transition (ages 28 to 32), when the person may modify life activities greatly; and (4) settling down (ages 33 to 39), when the person experiences greater stability.

A second theory for young adult development has been developed by Diekelmann (1976). Diekelmann proposes that young adults experience five developmental tasks: (1) the young adults achieve independence from parental controls; (2) they begin to develop strong friendships and intimate relationships outside the family; (3) they establish a personal set of values; (4) they develop a sense of personal identity; (5) they prepare for life work and develop the capacity for intimacy.

These theories provide the nurse with a basis for understanding the life events and developmental tasks of young adults. Each young adult, however, brings unique characteristics and needs to this developmental stage. Clients in this developmental stage present challenges to nurses who themselves are young adults and who are coping with the demands of this period. Young adult nurses must be careful to recognize the needs of their young adult clients even if they themselves are not experiencing the same challenges and events.

ASSESSMENT

PHYSIOLOGICAL DEVELOPMENT

Unlike the adolescent, the young adult experiences few maturational changes in body shape or physical structures. An exception to this is the pregnant or lactating woman. The physical, cognitive, and psychosocial changes and the health concerns of the pregnant woman and the childbearing family are extensive and are detailed in a later section.

Young adults are usually quite active, experience severe illnesses less commonly than other age groups, tend to ignore physical symptoms, and often postpone seeking health care. The physical characteristics of the young adult begins to change as middle age approaches. Unless the client has an illness, the physical assessment findings are generally within normal limits.

Nonetheless, clients in this developmental stage may benefit from a personal life-style assessment (see Chapter 2). The personal life-style assessment developed by Stanhope and Lancaster (1984) can help the nurse and the client identify habits that increase the risk for cardiac, malignant, pulmonary, renal, or other chronic diseases.

COGNITIVE DEVELOPMENT

Rational thinking habits increase steadily through the young and middle adult years. Formal and informal educational experiences, general life experiences, and occupational opportunities dramatically increase the individual's conceptual and problem-solving skills, as well as motor skills.

Identifying a preferred occupational area is a major task of the young adult. When people know their educational preparation, skills, talents, and personality characteristics, occupational choices are easier, and they are generally more satisfied with their choices. In the young and middle adult years, job satisfaction has been found to be a major factor in achievement and responsibility.

An understanding of how young adults learn assists the nurse in developing teaching plans for the client. The adult comes to the teaching-learning situation with a background of unique life experiences. The nurse, therefore, always views a young adult, like other clients, as a unique individual. The adult's compliance with a particular regimen, such as medications, treatments, or lifestyle changes, involves a decision-making process. The teaching process should present the client with as much information as is needed to make a decision about the prescribed course.

Because young adults are continually evolving and adjusting to changes in the home, workplace, and personal lives, the decision-making process ideally should be flexible. The more secure young adults are in their roles, the more flexible and open to change they are. The insecure person tends to be more rigid in making decisions.

PSYCHOSOCIAL DEVELOPMENT

Emotional health of the young adult is related to the individual's ability to address and resolve personal and social tasks. Certain patterns or trends are relatively predictable. Between the ages of 23 to 28, the person refines self-perception and ability for intimacy. From ages 29 to 34 the person directs enormous energy toward achievement and mastery of the surrounding world. The years from 35 to 43 are a time of vigorous examination of life goals and relationships. Alterations are made in the adult's personal, social, and occupational lives. Often the stresses of this reexamination result in a "midlife crisis" where the outcome may be changes in a marital partner, life-style, and occupation.

In the young adult years the person generally gives more attention to occupational and social pursuits. During this period, indivudals attempt to improve their socioeconomic status. Upward mobility is possible through career choices. However, many career choices require special educational preparation, and success may depend on family or social associations. Career and personal counseling can help the individual identify career choices and set realistic goals.

Ethnic factors and sex differences also have a sociological and psychological influence in an adult's life. A frank understanding of the expectations and limitations imposed by social stereotyping or on the basis of ethnicity, race, or gender enables the adult to understand and cope with boundaries in interactions with others.

Support from the nurse, access to information, anticipatory guidance, and appropriate referrals open a world of possibilities for achievement of the adult's full potential. Because health is not merely the absence of disease but involves wellness in all human dimensions, the holistic, humanistic nurse acknowledges the importance of the young adult's psychosocial needs as well as those in other dimensions.

The young adult must make major decisions concerning a career, marriage, and parenthood. Although each individual makes these decisions based on individual factors, the nurse should understand the general principles involved in these aspects of psychosocial development in order to assess the young adult's psychosocial status.

CAREER

Many adults devote a major portion of their energy and interest to their chosen career. Therefore, a successful vocational adjustment is important in the lives of most men and women. Successful employment not only ensures economic security but also leads to friendships, social activities, support, and respect from coworkers. In addition, in North America a person's occupation and achievements are major determinants of social status and self-esteem (Kaluger and Kaluger, 1984).

Two-career marriages are increasing. The two-career marriage has benefits as well as liabilities. In addition to increasing the family's financial base, the woman who works outside the home is able to expand friendships, activities, and interests. Stresses may occur in a two-career family. These stressors result from a job change to a new city, increased expenditures of physical, mental or emotional energy, child care demands, or household needs (see research highlight).

Male and female stereotypes of the past are decreasing. Men are becoming more involved in childrearing and homemaking duties. Women are becoming active in house and automobile maintenance. The major principle for avoiding stress in a two-career family is that neither partner can assume all responsibilities. For some families a solution may be to limit recreational expenses and instead hire someone to do routine housework. Others may set up an equal division of house, shopping, and cooking duties.

SEXUALITY

The development of secondary sexual characteristics occurs during the adolescent years (see Chapter 23). Physical development is accompanied by the ability to perform sexual acts. The young adult usually has emotional maturity to complement the physical ability and is therefore able to develop mature sexual relationships.

ORGASMIC MATURITY. Masters and Johnson (1970) have contributed much important information

⚮ *Research Highlight* ⚮

Sund and Ostwald investigated personal and life-style related variables and stress levels in 92 dual-earner families having preschool-aged children. The findings from the sample were based according to national stress norms calculated for families in the preschool stage of development. Major reductions in stress were identified. First was parental age and age of children; the older the couple and the older the average age of children, the lower the family stress. Second, income and satisfaction with income; families with a higher income and satisfaction with that income reported less family stress. Third, families with flexibility in scheduling vacations reported less stress. Last, satisfaction with child-care arrangements resulted in reduced reports of family stress.

Sund, K, and Ostwald, SK: Dual-earner families' stress levels and personal life-style related variables, Nurs Res 34:357, 1985.

about the physiology of the adult sexual response. Orgasmic maturity in sexual response occurs in four phases: excitement, plateau, orgasm, and resolution (see Chapter 30).

More important than either the individual's type or frequency of sexual intercourse is the psychodynamic aspect of sexual activity. The person's psychological beliefs and expectations give feelings of pleasure and satisfaction to the young as well as the middle adult. To maintain total wellness, adults should be encouraged to explore various aspects of their sexuality.

CHILDBEARING CYCLE. Conception, pregnancy, birth, and lactation are the major phases of the childbearing cycle. The changes during these phases are complex. Fawcett et al. (1986) demonstrated significant changes in perception of body image during the second trimester of pregnancy and immediately postpartum for the woman without a corresponding significant change in perception on the part of her spouse. The nurse can assist the couple to prepare for this cycle through health teaching in such areas as nutrition, anatomy, and physiology and discussions of feelings and attitudes toward childbearing and child rearing. Education such as Lamaze classes can prepare the couple to participate in the birthing process. Brown (1986) reported that the presence of social support and stressors have an impact on the health of the expectant mother and father. Partner support appeared to be the most important variable in understanding the expectant father's health, but the

larger context of spousal support along with social support was an important variable for the expectant woman. Last, chronic illness and stress had a greater impact on the health of the expectant mother than on the father.

The personal and social changes occurring in the lives of a couple following the birth of a baby cannot be underestimated. The nursing assessment of the couple's response to the birthing experience and parent-child bonding are detailed in a later section of the chapter.

FAMILY

SINGLEHOOD. Social pressure to get married is not as great as it once was (Table 24-1). Today it is socially acceptable for a young adult to leave home and live in an apartment or to own a home without first marrying.

Another cause for the increased single population is the expanding career opportunities for women. Women enter the job market with greater career potential and have greater opportunities for financial independence. It is also becoming more socially acceptable for single individuals to live together outside of marriage. In North America an estimated 2% to 3% of two-income households are singles living together. Similarly, it has become more socially acceptable for married couples to separate or divorce if they find their marital situation unsatisfactory.

MARRIAGE. Every couple's relationship is unique. While there are no rules that guarantee a successful marriage, some guidelines are useful for building a happy marriage. Before marriage the couple ideally should complete five tasks. First, they should make certain their emotions are based on love rather than physical or sexual attraction. Early in a relationship, each is physically or sexually attracted to the other, but these feelings do not necessarily provide a basis for a marriage or other long-term commitment. When one or both partners begin to think of the other as "a person I need to be with" or "a friend and a lover," the relationship may be progressing beyond physical and sexual attraction.

Second, both partners should explore their motivation for wanting to marry. Is the desire to marry a result of family and social pressure? Do they wish to marry because they hear the "biological clock" ticking? Does the man desire marriage because having a wife is good for his career?

Third, the couple considering marriage should focus on developing clear communication. Several questions should be discussed. If both partners want children, how many and when? How are finances to be managed, and will both partners participate in financial decisions and management? If either partner has an ill or elderly parent, how will the married couple cope with the inevitable future needs of the parent? What are the career goals of

TABLE 24-1   Factors Influencing Choice of Singlehood or Marriage

Singlehood		Marriage	
Pushes Toward	**Pulls Toward**	**Pushes Toward**	**Pulls Toward**
Limitations (suffocating one-to-one relationships, feeling trapped, monotony)	Career opportunities and mobility	Financial security	Parental influence
	Variety of experiences	Influence from mass media	Desire for children
Obstacles to self-development and self-expression	Self-sufficiency and self-expression	Expectation of partners	Peer pressure
		Unhappy home life	Romantic image of marriage
Boredom, unhappiness, and anger	Sexual availability and variety	Interpersonal and personal reasons	Love (physical attraction, emotional attachment)
Role playing and conformity to expectations	Exciting life-style and experience	Fear of independence	Security, social status, prestige
Poor communication with mate	Freedom to change and experiment	Loneliness	Social stability
	Mobility	Alternatives that did not seem feasible	
Feelings of sexual frustration	Sustaining friendships	Social and cultural influences	
Limited friends, isolation, loneliness	Support groups such as men's and women's groups, group living arrangements, specialized groups	Regular sex	
Limitation of mobility and available experience		Guilt over singlehood	
Influence of and participation in women's movement and other social movements			

Modified from Stein, PJ: Family Coordinator 24:4, 1975.

both partners before and after children? If the future husband wants his wife to quit her job and remain home with the children, does that goal complement his wife's plans? How does the couple anticipate the resolution of common marital stressors, such as financial pressures, household chores, and job pressure? Research has demonstrated a high correlation among clear communication patterns and power-sharing couples (Hurley, 1981).

Fourth, the couple planning marriage should understand that any annoying behavior patterns and habits are unlikely to change after marriage. The person who is compulsive is likely to remain so after marriage. Likewise, the disorganized individual also retains this behavior.

Last, the couple should determine their compatibility in important beliefs and values. For example, if one partner places a high value on fidelity and the other does not, their marriage is headed for conflict. Religious values and needs, such as church affiliations, should also be considered.

Stages of Marriage. Like an individual life, a marriage relationship generally passes through developmental stages.

The *establishment stage* begins at the wedding and continues as the couple attempts to function as a dyad. They learn patterns of sexual expression and how to live intimately with each other. They must learn styles of

conflict resolution, decision making, and role patterns. In addition, each partner may experience a sense of loss of individuality and self in the transition from "me" to "we." Together the married partners help each other achieve seven goals:

1. Seeking mutual self-growth and well-being
2. Practicing open communication techniques
3. Being tolerant of each other
4. Responding appropriately to each other's moods
5. Being kind and issue centered during arguments
6. Being each other's best friend
7. Bargaining openly regarding duties, obligations, and privileges

The *family orientation stage* is directed toward childbearing and child-rearing activities. Parenting roles must be defined and practiced. Nurturing and socialization needs of the children can put pressure on the couple's intimate relationship. Each parent's image of the "perfect parent" conflicts with reality. Parent-child relationships can become stressful as the child pulls away and experiments or if the parents disagree on child rearing.

A couple who cannot or chooses not to have children may direct their energies to their careers or to participation in the lives of other families with children.

In the middle adult years, as children depart from the household, the family enters the *postparental family stage*. Time and financial demands on the parents decrease, and they face the task of redefining their own relationship. As grandchildren arrive, grandparenting styles must be chosen.

Dyad Responsibility of the Married Couple. When establishing a household and family, the married couple has important work to do as a team. They have the following tasks:

1. Establishing an intimate relationship
2. Deciding on and working toward material and economic goals
3. Establishing guidelines for power and decision-making issues
4. Setting standards for extrafamily interactions
5. Finding companionship with other couples for a social life
6. Choosing mores, values, and ideologies acceptable to both

These major tasks of adults require considerable maturity and self-esteem. When faced and carried out, however, they provide the foundation for a stable relationship.

Growth in marriage extends over many years. Success in solving the formidable problems that occur in any marriage offers marital partners insight into each other.

PARENTHOOD. The availability of contraception makes it easier for today's couples to decide when to start a family. One factor influencing that decision is the reason for wanting a child. Social pressures may encourage a couple to have a child or may influence them to limit the number of children they have. Economic considerations frequently enter into the decision-making process, since having and bringing up children is expensive. The later average age for first marriages and postponed pregnancies because of career goals mean that general health status and age are also considerations in decisions about parenthood.

Phases of Parenthood. Parenthood is a process during which the parent assumes several roles. The psychological adjustment to parenting begins with the adoption of a parental self-image. A nurturing role emerges to meet the needs of the newborn. The authoritative role is added as the toddler begins to test the world around him and the parent must offer guidance.

Through the later school years and adolescence the parent functions in an integrative role, permitting the freedom for personal growth while offering safety and guidance.

In the departure phase the parent must relinquish the parent role as the young person is launched into adulthood. At this time parent and child must establish a new relationship as fellow adults.

HALLMARKS OF EMOTIONAL HEALTH

Most young adults have the physical and emotional resources and support systems to meet the many challenges, tasks, and responsibilities they face. During a psychosocial assessment of a young adult, the nurse can assess for 10 hallmarks of emotional health (see box), which indicate that the young adult has successfully matured in this developmental stage.

HEALTH CONCERNS

PHYSIOLOGICAL CONCERNS. The average young adult is active and without major health problems. However, young adults' fast-paced life-styles may put them at risk for the development of illnesses or disabilities during middle or older adult years. In addition, infertility is a problem for many young adults.

Risk Factors. Risk factors for the young adult's health originate in the community, life-style, and family history. These risk factors fall into five general categories: (1) violent death and injury, (2) substance abuse, (3) unwanted pregnancies, (4) sexually transmitted diseases, and (5) environmental or occupational factors. Life-style habits such as smoking, stress, lack of exercise, and poor personal hygiene also increase the risk of future illness, as does family history of cardiovascular, renal, endocrine, or neoplastic disease.

Violence is the greatest cause of mortality and morbidity in the young adult population. Death and injury can occur from physical assaults, motor vehicle or other accidents, and suicide attempts. Recent statistics show that homicides account for approximately 10% of deaths, motor vehicle accidents for 48.7 deaths per

---

Ten Hallmarks of Emotional Health

- A sense of meaning and direction in life
- Successful negotiation through transitions
- Absence of feelings of being cheated or disappointed by life
- Attainment of several long-term goals
- Satisfaction with personal growth and development
- When married, feelings of mutual love for partner; when single, satisfaction with social interactions
- Satisfaction with friendships
- Generally cheerful attitude
- Not sensitive to criticism
- No unrealistic fears

Modified from Stanhope, M, and Lancaster, J: Community health nursing: process and practice for promoting health, ed. 2, St. Louis, 1987, The C.V. Mosby Co.

100,000, and suicides for 32.5 deaths per 100,000 in the 20- to 48-year-old group (Stanhope and Lancaster, 1987).

Substance abuse, the use of alcohol or drugs, directly or indirectly contributes to mortality and morbidity in young adults. Even if intoxicated young adults are not severely injured in a motor vehicle accident they have caused, the accident may well result in death or permanent disability to another young adult.

Dependence on stimulant or depressant drugs can result in death. Overdose of a stimulant drug ("upper") can stress the cardiovascular and nervous systems to the extent that death occurs. The use of depressants ("downers") can lead to an accidental or intentional overdose and death.

It is a misconception that drug abuse occurs only among adolescents. Cocaine is increasingly used by young adults who have families and responsible jobs. Chapter 45 discusses the many physiological and psychosocial problems resulting from substance abuse.

A young adult who has recovered from substance abuse is still at risk for long-term effects that surface in middle or older adult years. These include hepatitis, cardiovascular and pulmonary disease, chromosome damage, hepatic cirrhosis, and recurrent infections.

Unwanted pregnancies, although more common among adolescents, can also have long-term physical and emotional effects if they occur in the young adult years. For example, a 25-year-old woman with an unplanned pregnancy may choose to terminate the pregnancy. If she is unable to resolve her feelings about the loss, she may require long-term counseling. Another woman may choose to have the baby and give it up for adoption but similarly be unable to accept the loss. Still another may decide to keep the child but, because of the emotional, financial, and other burdens, suffer severe emotional stress, lose weight, and find herself unable to cope.

Sexually transmitted diseases include syphilis, gonorrhea, genital herpes, and acquired immune deficiency syndrome (AIDS). These diseases may occur in any sexually active person. Recently sexual activities with multiple partners have decreased. Many young adults are seeking to establish meaningful relationships before engaging in sexual activity.

Sexually transmitted diseases have immediate effects such as discharge, discomfort, and infection. They may also lead to chronic disorders as with genital herpes; infertility, which is a common sequela of gonorrhea; or even death as with AIDS.

A common *environmental or occupational risk factor* is exposure to airborne particles, which may cause lung diseases and cancer. Such lung diseases include silicosis from inhalation of talcum and silicon dust, pneumoconiosis from inhalation of coal dust, and emphysema from inhalation of smoke. Cancers resulting from oc-

TABLE 24-2 Occupational Hazards Associated with Cancers

Occupational Chemical	Cancer
Asbestos	Mesothelioma (pleural and peritoneal)
	Lung
Vinyl chloride (plastics)	Liver (hemangiosarcoma) (200 times at risk)
	Brain (4 times at risk)
	Lung (2 times at risk)
Benzene	Leukemia, predominantly acute myelogenous
Bischloromethane ether	Oat cell carcinoma
Chromium	Nasal or paranasal sinus, lung, larynx
Arsenic	Lung
Coal tar pitch, coke oven emissions	Lung, larynx, skin
Iron oxide	Lung, larynx
Nickel	Lung
Petroleum distillates	Lung, larynx

From Stanhope, M, and Lancaster, J: Community health nursing: process and practice for promoting health, ed. 2, St. Louis, 1987, The C.V. Mosby Co.

cupational exposures may involve the lung, liver, brain, blood, or skin (Table 24-2).

Life-Style. Life-style habits, particularly those that activate the stress response (see Chapter 28), have been documented to increase the risk of illness.

Smoking is a well-documented risk factor for pulmonary, cardiac, and vascular diseases. Inhaled cigarette pollutants increase the risk of lung cancer, emphysema, and chronic bronchitis. The nicotine in tobacco is a vasoconstrictor that acts on the coronary arteries, increasing the risk of angina, myocardial infarction, and coronary artery disease. Nicotine also causes peripheral vasoconstriction and may lead to vascular problems such as Raynaud's disease or Buerger's disease.

Prolonged *stress* increases wear and tear on the body's adaptive capacities. Stress-related diseases such as ulcers, emotional disorders, and infections can occur (see Chapter 28).

Exercise patterns can affect a person's present and future health status. Research has demonstrated that exercise producing a sustained increase in pulse rate for 15 to 20 minutes three times a week improves cardiopulmonary function by decreasing blood pressure and heart rate. In addition, exercise decreases fatigability, insomnia, tension, and irritability.

Personal hygiene habits can be risk factors. Sharing eating utensils with a person who has a contagious illness obviously increases the risk of illness. Poor dental hygiene increases the risk of periodontal disease. These diseases—gingivitis, or inflammation of the gums, and periodontitis, or loss of tooth support—can be avoided through routine brushing and flossing (see Chapter 32).

A *familial history* of a disease may put a young adult at risk for developing the disease in his middle or older adult years. For example, a young man whose father and paternal grandfather had a myocardial infarction (heart attack) in their fifth decade of life has a risk for a future myocardial infarction. As noted in Chapter 6, the presence of certain chronic illnesses in the family increases the family members' risk of developing a disease. This family risk is distinct from hereditary disease.

TABLE 24-3 Classification and Causes of Infertility

Classification	Possible Causes	Classification	Possible Causes
WOMEN		**MEN**	
Tubal obstruction or dysfunction	Pelvic inflammatory disease Tuberculosis Puerperal infection Endometriosis Congenital anomalies Peritonitis	Decreased spermatozoa	Varicocele Testicular failure Endocrine disorders Cryptorchidism Other causes—stress, smoking, heat, systemic infections
Ovulation factors	Anovulation Inadequate corpus luteum Amenorrhea with low estrogen production Production of pathological ova Ovarian tumors, Stein-Leventhal syndrome Ovarian endometriosis Genetic absence of follicular tissue	Abnormal semen	Low volume Necrospermia and agglutination High viscosity Autoimmunity
Uterine factors	Myomas, polyps Developmental anomalies of the endometrial cavity Synechiae Congenital absence of uterus Endometritis Endometriosis Insufficient transformation of endometrium Neoplasms Infections Pelvic inflammatory disease	Ductal obstructions	Epididymis, postinfection Congenital absence of vas deferens Postvasectomy Ejaculation duct, postinfection
Cervical factors	Obstruction or stenosis of cervix from surgery or neoplasms Destruction of endocervical glands from surgery Chronic cervicitis Inadequate cervical mucus	Failure to transport spermatozoa to vagina	Ejaculatory disturbances Hypospadias Sexual problems such as impotence Spinal cord injury
Vaginal factors	Congenital absence of vagina Imperforate hymen Vaginismus Vaginitis Hyperacidity of vaginal secretions		

*Modified from Fogel, CI, and Woods, NF: Health care of women: a nursing perspective, St. Louis, 1981, The C.V. Mosby Co.

Infertility. Infertility is the man's, woman's, or couple's involuntary inability to conceive. Most health professionals define it as the inability to conceive after a year or more of regular sexual intercourse. An estimated 10% to 15% of all couples are infertile. About half of the couples who are evaluated and treated in major infertility clinics, however, become pregnant (Fogel and Woods, 1981). In about 10% to 20% of couples the cause of the infertility is unknown and the couple will remain infertile. The remaining 30% have the cause of their infertility diagnosed, but they remain infertile owing to endometriosis, blocked fallopian tubes, or decreased sperm motility.

Infertility occurs in both men and women (Table 24-3). Infertility in women can result from endocrine or nutritional imbalances, lack of ovulation, congenital abnormalities, or infections.

In men, infertility is due to interference with the development of sperm, decreased motility of sperm, obstruction in transport of sperm from the testicles to the urethra, and interference with ejaculation of the sperm.

For some infertile couples, the nurse may be the first resource identified. Particularly in a community or clinic setting where the nurse-client relationship has developed over an extended period, the couple may feel more comfortable discussing their fertility problems with the nurse. To effectively intervene with a couple who have a fertility problem, the nurse should be familiar with fertility centers to which the couple can be referred.

PSYCHOSOCIAL CONCERNS

The psychosocial health concerns of the young adult often are related to stress, such as job stress or family stress. As noted in Chapter 28, stress can be valuable in motivating a client to change and move ahead. However, if the stress is prolonged and the client is unable to adapt to the stressor, health problems can develop.

JOB STRESS. Job stress can occur every day or from time to time. Most young adults are able to handle day-to-day crises. Situational job stress may occur when a new boss enters the workplace, a deadline is approaching, or the worker is given new responsibilities. Job stress also occurs when a person becomes dissatisfied with a job or responsibilities. Because individuals perceive jobs differently, the types of job stressors vary from client to client.

FAMILY STRESS. Family stressors can occur at any time in family life. Family life has peaks, when everyone in the family works together, and valleys, when everyone appears to pull apart. Situational stressors occur in a family with birth, death, illnesses,, marriage, job loss, etc.

As with all groups, each family has certain predictable roles or jobs for members. These roles enable the family to function and be an effective part of society. One necessary role is the family leader. In most families one parent is the leader or both parents act as co-leaders. In single parent families the one parent or occasionally a member of the extended family is the family leader.

PREGNANT WOMAN AND CHILDBEARING FAMILY

A developmental task for most young adult couples is the decision to begin a family. Although the physiological changes of pregnancy and childbirth occur only in the woman, cognitive and psychosocial changes and health concerns affect the entire childbearing family, including the husband, siblings, and grandparents.

PHYSIOLOGICAL CHANGES. Women anticipating pregnancy will benefit from good health practices, such as a balanced diet, exercise, dental checkups, avoidance of alcohol, and cessation of smoking before conception. Women trying to become pregnant should not try weight reduction diets. The physiological changes and needs of the pregnant woman vary with each trimester.

First Trimester. All woman experience some physiological changes in the first trimester, but some changes affect only certain women. The nurse must be familiar with these physiological changes, their cause, and helpful interventions for the pregnant woman (Table 24-4).

During this period usually no signs of pregnancy are observable by others. If a woman frequently has morning sickness, however, her family, friends, and co-workers may be able to guess that she is pregnant.

The newly pregnant woman needs routine prenatal care. The first visit includes a pelvic examination. After the thirteenth week of pregnancy, pelvic examinations are not done. Instead the physician or certified nurse-midwife measures fetal growth by palpating the abdomen to determine the size of the uterine fundus.

Second Trimester. In the second trimester, growth of the uterus and fetus results in some of the physical signs of pregnancy (Table 24-5). Morning sickness has usually disappeared, and the woman's energy level is restored if her nutritional intake has caught up with her metabolic demands. The urinary frequency ceases and she is able to sleep through the night.

If this is the woman's first pregnancy, she may be able to see and feel the enlarged uterus. However, it is common for her abdomen to stay relatively flat. In subsequent pregnancies she may "show" as early as the beginning of the second trimester.

Third Trimester. During the third trimester an increase in Braxton-Hicks contractions, fatigue, and urinary frequency occurs. The uterus continues to grow

TABLE 24-4 Physiological Changes in the First Trimester

Symptom	Cause	Appropriate Nursing Interventions
Amenorrhea (one or two missed periods)	Fertilization of the egg by the sperm	Instruct woman to have a pregnancy test
Positive pregnancy test done at home or in laboratory	Presence of human chorionic gonadotropin (HCG) in first voided urine specimen of day	Instruct woman to obtain prenatal care, avoid all medications, avoid alcohol intake, and maintain good nutritional habits.
Morning sickness—nausea and/or vomiting from sixth week to end of fourth month; may occur in the morning, evening, or all day	Increased serum hormone levels	Instruct client to eat dry crackers, cold fluids, such as ice and popsicles, and small frequent meals to reduce nausea. Have client inform her doctor if prolonged vomiting results in a weight loss of 5 or more pounds, abdominal pain, or tenderness (Fogel and Woods, 1981).
Breast enlargement and tenderness; nipples darkened and enlarged	Increased estrogen levels	Instruct woman to wear a supportive bra at all times, even while asleep. Application of ice packs will decrease tenderness.
Urinary frequency	Pressure of uterus on bladder	Reassure client that frequency decreases as the enlarging uterus moves from the pelvis upward to the abdominal region. Prepare client for return of frequency as the head of the fetus moves into the pelvis in the middle to late third trimester.
Fatigue	Hormonal increases	Ensure that client has proper nutrition, sleep patterns, and rest periods to help decrease fatigue.
	Increased nutritional demands on the woman	
	Decreased nutritional intake resulting from morning sickness	Instruct client to take prenatal vitamins as prescribed.
Chadwick's sign on pelvic examination (6-8 weeks): bluish violet hue of mucous membranes of the vulva, vagina, and cervix	Vascular congestion	Instruct client to have prenatal pelvic examination to confirm changes in the cervix.

Data from Jones, DA, Lepley, MK, and Baker, BA: Health assessment across the life span, New York, 1984, McGraw-Hill Book Co.

(Table 24-6). Close to the time of the onset of labor, the woman may experience a burst of energy during which she cleans house and prepares for the baby by shopping for baby clothes, food, and diapers. This period is called "nesting." Many experts in obstetrics and seasoned veterans of pregnancy believe that "nesting" indicates a rapidly approaching time of delivery.

Puerperium. The puerperium is a period of approximately 6 weeks following delivery. During this time the uterus involutes, returning to approximate prepregnancy size. In addition, the uterine lining regenerates. The top layer of lining is sloughed off and the endometrium reforms. The sloughed-off layer, referred to as "lochia," is excreted via the vagina. Lochial discharge is present in all women who have delivered a fetus, whether the delivery is vaginal or via caesarian section. Lochia is also present when the woman has delivered a stillborn infant.

Three stages of lochia occur: lochia rubra, bright red to pink drainage; lochia serosa, pink to brownish discharge; and lochia alba, white to yellow discharge. Lochia increases with nursing because sucking on the breasts causes uterine contraction. Lochia discharge may last anywhere from 2 to 6 weeks.

Breast changes occur about the third or fourth postpartum day. The breast becomes firm and tender, indicating that milk is available for the infant. The tenderness is relieved by nursing. The mother should be instructed to begin nursing slowly, usually starting with 2 minutes a side and working up to 10 minutes. The

TABLE 24-5 Physiological Changes in the Second Trimester

Symptom	Cause	Appropriate Nursing Interventions
Integument: pigmented nipple and breast, hyperpigmentation of abdominal line (linea nigra), mottling of cheeks or forehead (chloasma or "mask of pregnancy"), local or generalized pruritus	Melanocyte-stimulating hormone	Reassure client that skin color changes are normal and temporary. Instruct client to avoid hot baths and use of soap or lotions, which can dry skin and increase itching.
Mouth: hypertrophy of gums (pregnancy epulis), causing gingival swelling and bleeding	Proliferation of interdental papillary blood vessels, resulting in local inflammation and hyperplasia	Teach client good "flossing" technique. Instruct client to get routine dental checkups during second trimester.
Lungs: increased respiratory rate	Increase in oxygen consumption by 20%	
Heartburn	Increased hydrochloric acid, decreased gastric mobility, and esophageal reflux	Instruct client to avoid foods that precipitate heartburn. Check with her physician about use of antacids. Have client sleep in high Fowler's position.\nGenitalia: pelvic examination not routinely performed from the first prenatal visit until the last month of pregnancy to avoid trauma to the developing fetus and placenta
Neck: enlarged thyroid, goiter of pregnancy	Response of thyroid to increased metabolic demands	Reassure client that this is a normal finding in some women.
Breasts: hyperplasia and tenderness	Gradual development of glandular tissue	Instruct client to increase her bra size as needed.
Abdomen: increasing size of uterine fundus—at level of symphysis at 9 weeks, at intraabdominal organs at 12 weeks, between symphysis and umbilicus at 16 weeks, at umbilicus at 20-22 weeks	Growth of fetus	Reinforce nutrition.
Sensation of movement or gaslike movements (quickening)	Fetal motion	Instruct client to notify physician if these movements are absent or decline.
Braxton-Hicks contractions	Expanding uterus and preparation of uterus for labor	Instruct client that these are irregular short contractions, not early labor, and will continue periodically throughout the pregnancy. Instruct client to notify her physician if contractions become regular and increased in frequency and duration.
Fetal heartbeat with Doppler or Fetoscope; rate of 120-140 beats per minute, with points of maximal intensity determined by fetal position		Allow mother to hear heartbeat.

Data from Jones, DA, Lepley MJ, and, Baker, BA: Health assessment across the life span, New York, 1984, McGraw-Hill Book Co.

TABLE 24-6 Physiological Changes in the Third Trimester

Symptom	Cause	Appropriate Nursing Interventions
Lungs: dyspnea	Pressure of fetus against diaphragm, decreasing lung expansion	Instruct client to sit upright. Use of two pillows at night may ease breathing during sleep.
Heart: cardiac displacement with counterclockwise rotation and lateral upward displacement of heart	Elevation of diaphragm by enlarging uterus, displacing heart	Reassure client that changes are temporary.
Increased pulse rate and palpitations	Increased metabolic rate and increased plasma blood volume	
Breasts: increased colostrum, the precursor of true milk	Preparation of breasts for lactation by hormones	Instruct client to express colostrum to prevent clogged milk ducts. If client chooses to breast feed, instruct her to "toughen" her nipples using lanolin cream and vigorous drying with a towel after bathing. This will decrease the risk of cracked nipples during the initial nursing phase.
Abdomen: fundus at xiphoid at 36 weeks; baby's head down by ninth month as determined by palpation; mother may feel that baby has "dropped" and that pressure on xiphoid, diaphragm, and stomach is relieved.	Descent of baby's head into pelvis (engagement), which may occur at any point from thirty-sixth week to onset of labor	Reassure client of baby's growth. Reassure client that baby can be safely repositioned in utero if needed. Reassure client that her pregnancy is coming to an end.
Elimination system: increased urinary frequency, constipation	Pressure on bladder from enlarged fetus; pressure and displacement of colon and decreased gastric motility	Instruct client to reduce fluid intake after 8 PM and increase roughage in diet.
Extremities: pedal edema (increased in hot, humid weather)	Fluid retention and decreased venous return	Unless edema is accompanied by elevated blood pressure and protein in urine, reassure client that this is normal. Instruct her to elevate her feet whenever possible.
Musculoskeletal system: waddling gait	Altered center of gravity in pregnancy	Instruct client to wear low, comfortable shoes. High heels may cause her to lose her balance and fall.

Data from Jones, DA, Lepley, MK, and Baker, BA: Health assessment across the life span, New York, 1984, McGraw-Hill Book Co.

woman should also be instructed to alternate the beginning side at each nursing period because the infant sucks more vigorously at the beginning of the nursing period.

The greater the quantity of milk consumed, the greater the quantity of milk produced. When the mother decides to decrease the number of breast feedings or the infant's needs decrease, the quantity of milk production decreases.

COGNITIVE CHANGES. Cognitive changes during pregnancy, primarily involving sensory perception and needs for education, affect both parents and occur gradually or quickly.

Sensory Perception. The pregnant woman generally experiences changes in sensory perception. Temporary changes occur in visual and hearing acuity, taste, and smell. Many pregnant women frequently stroke the abdomen, possibly because of a change in the sensation of touch or other sensory need. The woman may be using the sensation of touch to initiate bonding with her child (Jones, Lepley, and Baker, 1984).

Needs for Education. The entire childbearing family needs education about pregnancy, labor, delivery, breastfeeding, and integration of the newborn into the family structure.

Childbirth classes help the parents plan for the birth of the child. Such classes focus on the normal physiological changes of pregnancy and the processes of labor and delivery. The classes prepare the expectant parents for natural childbirth or childbirth with anesthesia. Other types of classes may emphasize newer advances in obstetrics, such as birthing rooms.

Many health care centers also have sibling preparation classes. These classes explain to children in the family, at their level of comprehension, the processes of pregnancy, birth, and integration of the baby into the family structure.

PSYCHOSOCIAL CHANGES. Like the cognitive changes of pregnancy, psychosocial changes may occur at various times during the 9 months of pregnancy and in the puerperium. The major categories of psychosocial changes involve body image, role, sexuality, coping mechanisms, and stresses during the puerperium.

Body Image. Although the physical changes of pregnancy are not obvious to others until the second trimester, the woman generally perceives changes in her body during the first 3 months.

One change that some women consider positive is an increase in breast size, which may make the woman feel more feminine and sexually appealing. Also, because she is pregnant, the woman may take extra time with her hygiene and grooming, trying new hairstyles and makeup.

The woman having difficulty with morning sickness and fatigue may have a poor body image. She may be too tired and ill to care about her appearance. Her major goal is often just getting through the phase of morning sickness and fatigue.

Most women, particularly those who are pregnant for the first time, enjoy the second trimester. They are beginning to "show" and start planning their maternity wardrobe. Their energy level has returned to normal and they have a general feeling of well-being. Because they are able to feel the baby move and hear the heartbeat, the baby becomes real to them and they are able to fantasize about the infant's features.

During the third trimester the fetus grows more rapidly. Toward the end of the pregnancy the woman may feel big, awkward, and unattractive. It is important that her family and support group help the pregnant woman feel more attractive. This may also be a good time for the woman to buy a comfortable nightgown and robe for the postpartum period. If she plans to breast feed the infant, she should select a nightgown that can easily accommodate breast feeding. She should also be counseled not to anticipate wearing her prepregnancy clothes home from the hospital. Because the uterus takes time to involute completely, she will need to wear loose clothing for a bit longer.

Role Changes. As the pregnancy advances, both partners think about their role changes. It is normal for expectant parents to feel ambivalent about the upcoming event and to wonder if this is the right time to begin or to enlarge a family. Both partners may also be concerned about their ability to be parents. They may observe the interactions between parents and children in their friends' families and wonder if they can cope. The nurse can help the future parents overcome their insecurities about parenting by emphasizing that the infant and the parent grow together, learning about each other's habits, moods, and behaviors.

Another role change can involve the choice to remain employed or to stay home after the baby's birth. This is no longer solely a woman's decision. An increasing number of men are becoming househusbands. This is occurring because some wives make more money than their husbands and therefore need to remain in the workforce. In addition, a husband may choose to remain home or may be laid off or become unemployed near the time of the child's birth.

Sexuality. Pregnancy does not alter a woman's basic sexual response, nor is sexual activity harmful to a normally developing fetus. Often the pregnant woman and her partner need to be reassured about these facts.

However, the woman's perception of her body image influences her desire for sexual activity. Some women may feel more attractive and sexually desirable. Others perceive the changes in their bodies as unattractive. A woman may desire cuddling and holding rather than sexual intercourse (Jones, Lepley, and Baker, 1984).

Coping Mechanisms. Pregnancy requires many adjustments. The pregnant woman and her partner need to remember that, while childbirth and child rearing are wonderful, they are also stressful. Many times the parents are unable to cope with a particular stressor such as finding new housing, preparing the nursery, or participating in childbirth classes.

Stresses During the Puerperium. It is not uncommon for the new mother to bring the baby home from the hospital, place him in his crib, sit down, and wonder, "Now what do I do?" A visiting nurse can help the new parents during the transition from hospital to home. Many child-care books are available that can help prepare parents for their baby's needs and for their own emotional and social adjustments. A new mother needs to know, for example, that on a rainy day when the baby has rarely stopped crying, she may also find relief in a good cry. The mother can hand the baby to her husband as he walks in the door from work and take a long bath while enjoying a glass of wine or iced tea. Neither of these behaviors indicates poor parenting. On the contrary, they may be good coping practices.

A second stressor during the puerperium may be the mother's return to work. She may feel guilt, worry, relief, or a sense of freedom. Even when a return to work is necessary, as in the case of a single parent, the mother has mixed emotions about leaving her child. Parents selecting child care need assistance in obtaining references of reliable care givers and agencies. Community organizations and churches can be a good beginning for parents needing child care.

HEALTH CONCERNS. The pregnant woman and her partner have many health questions. Will the pregnancy be normal? Will the baby be normal? Where will the baby be born? The majority of the health needs related to pregnancy can be met with proper prenatal care.

Prenatal Care. Prenatal care is routine examination of the pregnant woman by an obstetrician, a nurse practitioner, or a certified nurse-midwife. During the prenatal visit the pregnant woman's weight and blood pressure are taken, her urine is checked for glucose, acetone, and protein, and the fundus is measured. Regular health care can address common health concerns such as preeclampsia, eclampsia, excessive weight gain, and the high-risk infant.

Preeclampsia is an abnormal condition of pregnancy characterized by the onset of acute hypertension after the twenty-fourth week of gestation. The classic triad of preeclampsia includes hypertension, proteinuria, and edema. Eclampsia is a complication of pregnancy characterized by grand mal seizures, coma, hypertension, proteinuria, and edema.

Excessive weight gain increases the woman's risk for salt and water retention, which may result in hypertension. Depending on the pregnant woman's body build and pregnancy weight and fetal growth, the ideal weight gain is 9 to 13 kg (19 to 30 pounds). Rapid weight gain with corresponding rapid growth of the uterus can also indicate a possible multiple birth.

MIDDLE ADULT

In middle adulthood, the adult makes lasting contributions through involvement with others. Personal and career achievements have often already been experienced, and the person has socioeconomic stability. Many find particular joy in assisting their children and other young people to become productive and responsible adults. This period is also a time of helping aging parents

progress through the later years of life. Using leisure time in satisfying and creative ways is a challenge that, if met satisfactorily, will enable the individual to prepare for retirement.

Both men and women must adjust to inevitable biological changes. As in adolescence, the middle-aged adult uses considerable energy to adapt self-concept and body image to physiological realities and changes in physical appearance. High self-esteem, a favorable body image, and a positive attitude toward physiological changes are fostered when the adult engages in physical exercise, a balanced diet, adequate sleep, and good hygiene practices, promoting a vigorous, healthy body.

Theories of Middle Adulthood
ERIKSON'S THEORY

According to Erikson's developmental theory, the primary developmental task of the middle years, the seventh stage of life, is to achieve generativity. Generativity is the willingness to care for and guide others. Middle adults can achieve generativity with their own children or the children of close friends, or through guidance in social interactions with the next generation. If middle adults fail to achieve generativity, stagnation occurs, which is manifested by excessive concern with self or destructive behavior toward their children and the community.

HAVIGHURST'S THEORY

Havighurst's developmental theory has been summarized in terms of the following seven developmental tasks for the middle adult (Beck, Rawlins, and Williams, 1987):
1. Achieving adult civic social responsibility
2. Establishing and maintaining a standard of living
3. Helping teenage children become responsible and happy adults
4. Developing leisure activities
5. Relating to one's spouse as a person
6. Accepting and adjusting to the physiological changes of middle age
7. Adjusting to aging parents

BUHLER'S THEORY

Another theorist, Buhler, emphasizes goal formation and achievement during the middle adult years. The ability to achieve one's goals depends on four factors: the satisfaction of needs, the ability to expand creatively, personal adjustment to limitations, and consistency in the inner self. Middle-aged adults who believe that the majority of their life goals have not been achieved may be depressed, even to the point of suicide (Beck, Rawlins, and Williams, 1987).

ASSESSMENT

PHYSIOLOGICAL DEVELOPMENT

Major physiological changes occur between 45 and 65 years of age. Table 24-7 summarizes these normal developmental changes, as noted on physical assessment.

The most visible changes are graying of the hair, wrinkling of the skin, and thickening of the waist. Balding commonly begins during the middle years, but it may also occur in the young adult. Often these physiological changes have an impact on the person's self-concept and body image. The most significant physiological changes during middle age are menopause in women and the climacteric in men.

MENOPAUSE. Menstruation and ovulation occur in a cyclical rhythm in the female body from adolescence into middle adulthood. Menopause is the disruption of this cycle, primarily because of the inability of the neurohumoral system to maintain its periodic stimulation of the endocrine system. The ovaries no longer produce estrogen and progesterone, and the blood level of these hormones drop markedly. Menopause typically occurs between 45 and 60 years of age.

CLIMACTERIC. The climacteric or andropause, so named because of the decreased level of androgens, occurs in men in their late forties or early fifties. Throughout this period and thereafter, a man is still capable of producing fertile sperm and fathering a child. After the male climacteric, however, penile erection is less firm, ejaculation is less frequent, and the refractory period is longer (Beck, Rawlins, and Williams, 1987).

COGNITIVE DEVELOPMENT

Changes in the cognitive function of middle adults are rare except in the presence of illness or trauma. The middle adult is able to continue learning new skills and information. Some middle-aged adults enter educational or vocational programs to prepare themselves for entering the job market or changing jobs.

PSYCHOSOCIAL DEVELOPMENT

The psychosocial changes in the middle adult may involve expected events, such as children moving away from home, or unexpected events, such as a marital separation or the death of a spouse. These changes may result in stress that can affect the middle adult's overall level of health.

TABLE 24-7 Physiological Changes in the Middle Adult as Found During Physical Assessment

Body System	Findings
Integument	Intact; appropriate distribution of pigmentation; slow progressive decrease in skin turgor; graying and loss of hair (Baldness patterns in males are established by age 55. Hair loss after this time might have other causes.)
Head and neck	Symmetry of scalp, skull, and face; normal accessory organs of vision
Eyes	Visual acuity by Snellen chart <20/50; pupillary reaction to light and accommodation; normal visual fields and extraocular movements; normal retinal structures
Ears	Normal auditory structures and acuity
Nose, sinuses, and throat	Patent nares and intact sinuses, mouth, and pharynx; trachea at midline; lateral thyroid lobes nonpalpable
Thorax and lungs	Anterior-posterior (A-P) diameter increased; respiratory rate 16 to 21 breaths per minute and regular; ratio of respiratory rate to heart 1:4; normal tactile fremitus, resonance, and breath sounds heard throughout
Heart and vascular system	Normal heart sounds: systole—$S_1<S_2$ at the base, diastole—$S_1>S_2$ at the apex; point of maximal impulse at fifth intercostal space in the midclavicular line and 2 cm or less in diameter
	Vital signs: temperature 36.7° to 37.6° C (97° to 99.6° F); pulse 60-100 (conditioned athlete $\cong$ 50); blood pressure: systolic—95-140 mm Hg, diastolic—60-90 mm Hg; all pulses palpable
Breasts	Decreased size owing to decreased muscle mass; normal nipples
Abdomen	No tenderness or organomegaly; decreased strength of abdominal muscles
Female reproductive system	Change in menstrual cycle and in duration and quantity of menstrual flow; "hot flashes"; change in cervical mucosa
Male reproductive system	Normal penis and scrotum; prostatic enlargement in some individuals
Musculoskeletal system	Decreased muscle mass; decreased range of joint motion
Neurological system	Appropriate affect, appearance, and behavior, lucidity and appropriate level of cognitive ability; intact cranial nerves; adequate motor responses; responsive sensory system

CAREER TRANSITION. Career changes may occur by choice or as a result of changes in the workplace or society as a whole. In recent decades middle-aged adults are more often changing occupations because they find themselves bored with their present employment after a long period in the same field. In some cases technological advances or other changes force the middle-aged adult to seek a new job. Such changes, particularly when unanticipated, may result in stress that can affect the person's health, as well as family relationships, self-concept, and other dimensions.

SEXUALITY. The onset of menopause and the climacteric can affect the sexual health of the middle adult. Menopause results in cessation of ovulation and the ability to conceive. A woman may desire more sexual activity because pregnancy is no longer possible. Although menopause does not decrease libido or sexual response, the menopausal woman may feel less sexually attractive. The middle-aged man may notice changes in the strength of his erection and a decrease in his ability to experience repeated orgasm. Both the middle-aged woman and man may experience stresses related to sexual changes or a conflict between their sexual needs and self-perceptions and social attitudes or expectations.

MARITAL CHANGES. Marital changes that may occur during middle age include death of a spouse, separation, divorce, and the choice of remarrying or remaining single. A widowed, separated, or divorced client goes through a period of grief and loss in which it is necessary to adapt to the change in marital status (see Chapter 25).

If single middle adults decide to marry, the stressors of marriage are similar to those for the young adult. In addition, the couple may have to cope with the social expectations and pressures related to middle-age marriage.

FAMILY TRANSITIONS. The departure of the last child from the home of the middle-aged parents may or may not be a stressor. Many parents welcome freedom from child-rearing responsibilities, whereas others feel lonely or directionless because of this change. Eventually the parents usually reassess their marriage and are able to resolve conflicts and plan future goals. Occasionally this readjustment phase may lead to marital conflicts for which no resolution can be achieved, resulting in separation and divorce (Beck, Rawlins, and Williams, 1987).

CARE OF AGING PARENTS. Increasing life span in the United States and Canada has led to increased numbers of older adults in the population. Therefore, greater numbers of middle-aged adults must address the personal and social issues confronting their aging parents.

Housing, employment, health, and economic realities have altered the traditional social expectations between generations in families. The middle-aged adult and the older adult parent may have conflicting priorities related to their relationship. Negotiations and compromises are useful in defining and resolving such problems. Nurses deal with both middle and older adults in the community, long-term care facilities, and hospitals. The nurse can help identify the health needs of both groups and can assist the multigenerational family in determining the health and community resources available to them as they make decisions and plans.

HEALTH CONCERNS

PHYSIOLOGICAL CONCERNS

Stress. Because middle-aged adults are experiencing physiological changes and face certain health realities, their perceptions of health and health behaviors are often important factors in maintaining health. Today's complex world makes individuals more prone to stress-related illnesses such as heart attacks, hypertension, migraine headaches, ulcers, colitis, autoimmune disease, backache, tension, arthritis, and cancer.

When middle-aged adults seek health care, the nurse's focus on the goal of wellness can guide clients to evaluate health behaviors, life-style, and environment. Attention to risk factors that can be altered to improve the client's health can increase the quality of life and add years to it.

Levels of Wellness. The nurse must be able to assess the health status of the middle adult client. Such assessment offers direction for planning nursing care and is useful in evaluating the effectiveness of nursing interventions. Table 24-7, showing the physiological changes of the middle-aged adult, can also be used as a guide for physical assessment, along with other standard assessment techniques (see Chapter 6).

Forming Positive Health Habits. A habit is a person's usual practice or manner of behavior. This behavior pattern is reinforced by frequent repetition until it becomes the individual's customary way of behaving. Some habits support health, such as exercise and brushing and flossing the teeth each day. Other habits involve risk factors to health, such as smoking or eating foods with little or no nutritional value.

In the assessment phase of the nursing process, the nurse frequently obtains data indicating both positive and negative health behaviors of the client. In the planning, implementation, and evaluation phases, the nurse helps the client maintain habits that protect health and offers healthier alternatives to poor habits.

TABLE 24-8   Risk Factors for Depression in the Middle Years

Risk Factor	Characteristics
Sex	Female
Age	Declines for women after early fifties; increases for men after late fifties
Social isolation	Absence of intimate, confiding relationships following a change in the nature of the relationship with parents, children, and spouse
Losses	Parental deprivation or loss of a mother before age 14; other losses during midlife such as job loss, career difficulties, marital problems, and physical changes; departure of last child from home
Family history	History of depression in the family of origin

From Beck, CM, Rawlins, RP, and Williams, SR: Mental health-psychiatric nursing: a holistic life-cycle approach, ed. 2, St. Louis, 1987, The C.V. Mosby Co.

PSYCHOSOCIAL CONCERNS. Two common psychosocial health concerns of the middle adult are anxiety and depression.

Anxiety. Adults often experience anxiety in response to physiological and psychosocial changes that show they are entering middle age. Such anxiety can motivate the adult to rethink life goals and can stimulate productivity. For some adults, however, this anxiety precipitates psychosomatic illness and preoccupation with death. In this case the middle adult views life as being half or more over and thinks in terms of the time left to live (Beck, Rawlins, and Williams, 1987).

Clearly the presence of a life-threatening illness, marital transition, or job stressor increases the anxiety of the client and family. The nurse may need to use crisis intervention or stress management techniques to help the client adapt to the changes of the middle adult years (see Chapter 28).

Depression. Depression is common among adults after entrance into the middle years and may have many causes. The risk factors for depression are listed in Table 24-8. Menopause is no longer believed to be a sole cause of depression. Depression that occurs during the middle years, often referred to as agitated depression, is characterized by moderate to high anxiety, bizarre physical complaints, and paranoid ideation. Depression may be worsened by the abuse of alcohol or other substances.

The nurse may need to refer a severely depressed middle-aged client for specialized psychological therapy.

NURSING DIAGNOSIS

The nursing assessment of the young or middle-aged adult will reveal clusters of data that indicate potential or actual nursing diagnoses (see nursing diagnoses box). The nursing diagnostic statement should include expected or anticipated causes or etiologies for the statement. For example, the assessment of two middle-aged clients and their families resulted in the identification of Coping, ineffective in individual. However, in one family the stressor was the death of a spouse, but in the second family the stressor was a new baby within the home. The inclusion of the etiology statement enables the nurse quickly to target specific goals and interventions of causative factors for each diagnostic statement.

The diagnostic statements require appropriate defining characteristics that provide the rationale for the diagnosis. The defining characteristics are identified from the pertinent assessment data obtained by the nurse. The sample nursing diagnoses box includes examples of nursing diagnoses and the appropriate defining characteristics with related factors.

Examples of Nursing Diagnoses for the Young and Middle Adult

NANDA-APPROVED NURSING DIAGNOSES

Impaired adjustment related to:
- Changes in physical appearance
- Changes in body image

Ineffective family or individual coping related to:
- Infertility
- Death of a spouse
- Adjustment to new baby
- Loss of job

Altered family processes related to:
- Chronic or acute illness
- Death of spouse
- Marital problems
- Financial problems

Altered sexuality patterns related to:
- Infertility
- Pregnancy
- Menopause or climacteric

Altered health maintenance related to:
- Risk factors, (for example, smoking, substance abuse)
- Lack of knowledge for positive health behaviors

Sample Nursing Diagnoses for the Young and Middle Adult

Defining Characteristics	Nursing Diagnoses	Related Factors
Inability to solve problems Inability to meet basic needs Inability to meet role expectations Increased rate of accidents Increased rate of illness	Ineffective individual or family coping	• Infertility • Death of spouse • Adjustment to new baby • Loss of job
Family system unable to meet physical, emotional, social, or spiritual needs of members Family unable to adapt to stressors Poor communication	Altered family processes	• Chronic or acute illness • Death of spouse • Marital problems • Financial stressors

PLANNING

The identification and formulation of nursing diagnoses are followed by the development of a nursing care plan (see care plan box). In providing nursing care for the young or middle-aged adult, the nurse must recognize that clients are also part of a family or community and that their needs can be affected by or can have a direct impact on the needs of that family or community. Nursing interventions are individualized for the client and are modified accordingly for home-based or hospital-based nursing care.

General goals for young or middle adult clients are those that reflect the clients' reactions to day-to-day life events as opposed to nursing goals that are the result of the clients' response to a specific illness, physiological need, psychosocial need, emotional need or spiritual need. The goals of nursing for the young or middle aged adult can include:

1. Improved knowledge about the impact of risk factors on a person's level of health.
2. Improved health promotional activities.
3. Improved communication within family structure.
4. Fewer experiences of illnesses, inability to problem-solve, etc.

Sample Nursing Care Plan for Young and Middle Adult

Nursing Diagnosis	Goal	Expected Outcomes	Nursing Interventions
Altered health maintenance related to excessive use of alcohol.	Client will understand the impact of alcohol excess on level of health.	Client will state physiological, emotional, and psychosocial effects of alcohol excess. Client will supply verified and documented reports of abstinence for alcohol.	Provide instruction about the hazard of alcohol excess at each nightly session for first week. Have client keep a daily log of activities, stressors, etc., for 3 days. After second session, provide client with a support group of recovered alcohol abusers.

IMPLEMENTATION

The nursing interventions for the young or middle-aged adult are generalized into changing health habits, health promotion, and stress management.

Changing Health Habits

Health teaching and health counseling are often directed at improving health habits (see Chapter 20). The more fully the nurse understands the dynamics of behavior and habits, the more likely interventions will help the client to bring about or reinforce health-promoting behaviors (see box).

The nurse's role in helping the client form positive health habits is that of teacher and facilitator. By providing information about how the body functions and how habits are formed and changed, the nurse raises the client's level of knowledge regarding the potential impact of behavior on health. No person can change a habit for another person. Clients have control of and are responsible for their own behavior. The nurse can explain psychological principles of changing a habit and offer information about health risks. The nurse can also offer positive reinforcement (such as praise and rewards) for health-directed behaviors and decisions. Such reinforcement increases the likelihood that the behavior will be repeated. Ultimately, however, the client decides which behaviors will become habits of daily living.

Barriers to change do exist (see box). Unless those barriers are minimized or eliminated, it is futile to encourage the client to take actions that are going to be blocked.

Health Promotion

Community health programs for young and middle adults are designed to prevent illness and promote health, as well as to detect disease in the early stages. Nurses can make valuable contributions to community health by taking an active part in the planning of screening and teaching programs (see Chapter 2).

Family planning, birthing, and parenting skills are program topics in which adults might be interested. Health screening for diabetes, hypertension, eye disease, and cancer is a good opportunity for the nurse to perform assessment and provide health teaching and health counseling.

Health education programs can promote changes in behavior and life-style. The nurse as health teacher offers information that will enable the client to make wise decisions about health practices. With health counseling the nurse and client design a plan of action addressing the client's health and well-being. Through objective problem solving, the nurse assists the client to grow and change.

Regardless of the age of family members and the structure of the family, they face certain health tasks. The nurse as health teacher and health counselor understands the autonomy of the family and supports it while promoting family health.

Nursing roles include community-centered care, hospital-based acute care, and care of the chronically ill. Participation in community health programs for the adult or family often requires the full extent of nursing roles and skills.

Stress Reduction

At any point in people's lives, they may be exposed to many actual or potential stressors (see Chapter 28).

Dynamics of Behavior and Habits

- Habits are frequently repeated behaviors.
- The more often a behavior is repeated, the more likely it will be repeated thereafter.
- Habits can be a stress reduction mechanism for the individual (for example, nail biting) but may be simultaneously detrimental to health (for example, alcohol consumption).
- Habits often meet some basic need for the person.
- Changing a habit requires a significant motivation by the client. Changing the habit must provide greater pleasure or satisfaction than the habit itself.
- Any change in habits or behavior patterns creates stress.

Barriers to Change

EXTERNAL

- Lack of facilities
- Lack of materials
- Lack of social supports

INTERNAL

- Lack of knowledge
- Lack of motivation
- Insufficient skills to affect change in health habits
- Undefined short- and long-term goals

Following the identification of specific stressors, the client and nurse can work together to intervene and modify the stress response. Specific interventions for stress reduction can fall into three categories (Pender, 1987). First, minimize the frequency of stress-producing situations. Together the nurse and client identify approaches to prevent stressful situations such as habituation, change avoidance, time blocking, time management, and environmental modification (Pender, 1987). The second category is psychophysiological preparation to increase stress resistance such as increasing the client's self-esteem, improving assertiveness, redirecting goal alternatives, and reorienting cognitive appraisal (Pender, 1987). Last, avoid the psysiological response to stress. The nurse uses relaxation techniques, imagery, and biofeedback to recondition the client's response to stress. Chapter 28 explains in greater detail these general interventions.

EVALUATION

Each young or middle-aged client has different health goals. The success of the nurse and client in achieving these goals is determined in the evaluation component. While it is not practical to describe all the evaluation techniques for the care of the young or middle-aged client, the evaluation box includes some of these measures.

SUMMARY

Transitional periods and developmental tasks of the young and middle adult and family members can be a source of stress and conflict that can threaten health. Often several family members are facing different developmental issues at the same time, increasing the strain on the family.

The nurse who understands the interrelationship of physiological, cognitive, and psychosocial needs and their influence on overall health, assesses life changes as a part of the nursing history of a young or middle adult. Anticipatory guidance can provide the client with insight into normal life cycle events within a family. The nurse can inform the client about normal growth and development patterns of young and middle adulthood. In addition, the nurse providing care for the young or middle adult may teach the client about marriage stages and the challenges, conflicts, and stresses associated with marriage.

With an understanding of the norms and common problems faced by others in the same developmental period, young adult and middle-aged clients are better able to put health-related events into perspective. When the client experiences more complex difficulties, the nurse can refer the client for the appropriate professional counseling.

Sample of Evaluation of Interventions for the Young and Middle Adult

Goals	Evaluative Measures	Expected Outcomes
Improved knowledge about the impact of risk factors on a person's level of health	Client reports previous 24-hour nutritional intake.	Client will reduce daily intake of sodium, fat, and cholesterol.
Improved health promotional activities	Client reports exercise activities.	Client will begin an exercise program of a minimum of 3 times a week.
	Weigh client each Friday to document weight loss.	Client loses weight at a rate of 2-3 pounds per week.
Improved communication within family structure	Client and family reports on problem-solving activities.	Reduction in conflicts over problem-solving measures.
		Clearer understanding of family members' needs and expectations.
Experienced fewer periods of illness	Client keeps an activity log for 1 month, including work attendance and social functions.	Decreased frequency of illness-related absences from work or social events.

KEY CONCEPTS

✓ Adult development involves orderly and sequential changes in characteristics and attitudes that adults experience over a period of time.

✓ Many changes experienced by the young adult are related to the natural process of maturation and socialization.

✓ Maturity is reached when the young adult attains a balance of growth in the physiological, psychosocial, and cognitive areas.

✓ Young adults are in a stable period of physical development, except for changes related to pregnancy.

✓ Cognitive development continues throughout the young and middle adult years.

✓ Emotional health of young adults is correlated with the ability to address and resolve personal and social problems.

✓ Young adults must choose a career and decide whether to remain single or marry and begin a family.

✓ Pregnant women need to understand physiological changes occurring in each trimester.

✓ Cognitive and psychosocial changes and health concerns during pregnancy and the puerperium affect the parents, the siblings, and often the extended family.

✓ Prenatal care reduces maternal and fetal mortality and morbidity.

✓ Midlife transition begins when a person becomes aware that physiological and psychosocial changes signify passage to another stage in life.

✓ Erikson, Havighurst, and Buhler have described the primary developmental tasks of the middle adult.

✓ Two significant physiological changes of the middle years are menopause in women and the climacteric in men.

✓ Cognitive changes are rare in middle age except in cases of illness or physical trauma.

✓ Psychosocial changes for middle adults may be related to career transition, sexuality, marital changes, family transition, and care of the aging parent.

✓ Health concerns of middle adults commonly involve stress-related illnesses, health assessment, and adoption of positive health habits.

REFERENCES

Beck, CM, Rawlins, RP, and Williams, SR: Mental health-psychiatric nursing: a holistic life-cycle approach, ed. 2, St. Louis, 1987, The C.V. Mosby Co.

Diekelmann, JL: The young adult: the choice is health or illness, Am J Nurs 76:1276, 1976.

Fogel, CI, and Woods, NF: Health care of women: a nursing perspective, St. Louis, 1981, The C.V. Mosby Co.

Jones, DA, Lepley, MK, and Baker, BA: Health assessment across the life span, New York, 1984, McGraw-Hill Book Co.

Kaluger, G, and Kaluger, MF: Human development: the span of life, ed. 3, St. Louis, 1984, The C.V. Mosby Co.

Levinson, D, et al.: The seasons of a man's life, New York, 1978, Alfred A. Knopf, Inc.

Masters, WH, and Johnson, VE: Human sexual response, Boston, 1970, Little, Brown & Co.

Pender, NJ: Health promotion in nursing practice, ed. 2, Norwalk Conn., 1987, Appleton-Lange.

Stanhope, M, and Lancaster, J: Community health nursing: process and practice for promoting health, ed. 2, St. Louis, 1987, The C.V. Mosby Co.

Research Articles

Brown, MA: Social support, stress, and health: a comparison of expectant mothers and fathers, Nurs Res 35:72, 1986.

Hurley, PM: Communication pattern and conflict in marital dyads, Nurs Res 30:38, 1981.

ADDITIONAL READINGS

Edelman, C and Mandle, CL: Health promotion throughout the lifespan, St. Louis, 1986, The C.V. Mosby Co.

Fawcett, J, et al.: Spouses' body image changes during and after pregnancy: a replication and extension, Nurs Res 35:220, 1986.

Fife, B: A model for predicting the adaptation of families to medical crises: an analysis of role integration, Image: J Nurs Sch, 17(4):108, 1985.

Laffrey, SC: Normal and overweight adults: perceived weight and health behavior characteristics, Nurs Res 35:173, 1986.

McLane, AM: Classification of nursing diagnoses: proceedings from the seventh conference (NANDA), St. Louis, 1987, The C.V. Mosby Co.

Sandelowski, M, and Pottock, C: Women's experiences of infertility, Image: J Nurs Sch 18(40):140, 1986.

Sund, K and Ostwald, SK: Dual-earner families' stress levels and personal and life-style related variables, Nurs Res 34:357, 1985.

Walker, LO, Crain, H, and Thompson, E: Maternal role attainment and identity in the postpartum period: stability and change, Nurs Res 35:68, 1986.

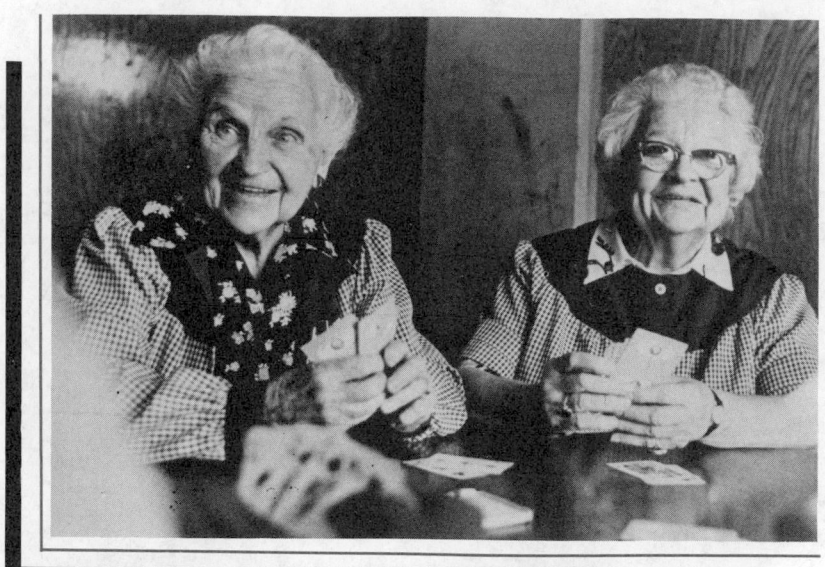

OBJECTIVES

Mastery of content in this chapter will enable the student to:

- Define the key terms listed.
- Describe common myths and stereotypes about older adults.
- Discuss nurses' attitudes toward older adults.
- Discuss three physiological theories of aging.
- Discuss three psychosocial theories of aging.
- State and discuss developmental tasks of the older adult.
- Describe physiological changes of aging.
- Describe cognitive changes of dementia and delerium found in some older adults.
- Describe common causes of dementia and delerium.
- Discuss psychosocial changes of retirement, social isolation, sexuality, housing, and death to which older adults must adjust.
- Discuss physical and psychosocial health concerns of older adults and related nursing interventions.
- Describe community and institutional health care services available to older adults.

KEY TERMS

Ageism
Alzheimer's Disease
Attitudinal Isolation
Behavioral Isolation
Confabulation
Delirium
Dementia
Geographical Isolation
Geriatrics
Gerontology
Korsakoff's Syndrome
Presbycusis
Presbyopia
Presentational Isolation
Reality Orientation
Reminiscence
Resocialization
Respite
Sundown Syndrome
Wernicke's Syndrome

Older Adult

The older adult is in the last developmental stage of life. This stage traditionally begins after retirement, usually between 65 and 75 years of age. No other population group is increasing as rapidly as older adults. Therefore, health care professionals must focus on identifying and meeting their special needs. Older adults are seeking greater participation in identification, definition, and resolution of issues affecting them. A greater incidence of chronic health problems, technological advances, and contemporary economic, social, ethical, and health issues have prompted health care professionals to focus on improving not only the duration of life, but its quality as well (Stanhope and Lancaster, 1984).

Increased life expectancy and decreased birth rate have contributed to a "graying" population. Demographers project a continuing increase in the older adult population well into the next century (Table 25-1). The life expectancy for persons born in 1983 is 71 years for men and 78.3 years for women (US Bureau of the Census, 1985). The older adult population is expanding in all cultural and ethnic groups in the United States and Canada. In the United States, blacks compose approximately 8% of persons 65 years and older. This is expected to increase to 11% by 2000 (Stanhope and Lancaster, 1987). Asians and Pacific islanders account for 6% of the older adult population, and Native Americans and Hispanics account for 4% (Office of Human Development Services, 1981). Older adults are distributed among the states in the same pattern as the total population. However, concentrations are found in some larger states, as well as the Northeast and Northcentral regions (Yurick et al., 1984).

TABLE 25-1 Population Growth and Projections for Older Adults

Year	Total Number (in millions)	Percent of Total Population
1900	3.0	4.1
1940	9.0	6.8
1980	25.5	11.3
1990	30.2	12.1
2000	32.4	12.2
2010	35.4	12.6
2020	45.6	15.4
2030	55.8	18.2

From Office of Human Development Services: Facts about older Americans, 1980-81, Washington, D.C., Department of Health and Human Services.

Nursing care of older adults poses special challenges because of the diversity in client's physiological, cognitive, and psychosocial health. Older adults vary in their level of function and productivity as members of society. Many are physically active, intelligent, socially engaging, and productive members of their communities. On the other end of the scale are those who have lost the physical capacity to care for themselves, are confused or withdrawn, and are unable to make decisions concerning their needs.

Before making a health assessment the nurse should be aware of the expected findings of physical and psychosocial assessment for an older adult. Normal changes of aging should also be considered. A comparison of expected and actual findings prevents the nurse from focusing on abnormal assessment data. In other words, the nurse should not assume that all older adults have signs, symptoms, or behaviors representative of the lower end of the health continuum. By remembering that each older adult is an individual, the nurse avoids stereotyping this age group.

MYTHS AND STEREOTYPES

In recent years a health specialty has been developed for older adults. Geriatrics deals with the physiology and psychology of aging and with diagnosis and treatment of diseases affecting the aged. Gerontology is the study of all aspects of the aging process and its consequence in humans and animals. Gerontologic nursing applies nursing process to older adults to achieve a level of wellness consistent with limitations imposed by aging (Yurick et al., 1984). The term *gerontological nursing* is used because geriatrics is concerned with diseases of old age. Also nurses working with older adults have a broader focus of assisting them to maximize their capabilities.

Although health-related research on aging is rapidly increasing and scientific knowledge has expanded, many false stereotypes persist. Some depict older persons as lacking understanding, forgetful, rigid, bored, and unpleasant. Furthermore, the aged are often stereotyped as ill, crippled, hard of hearing, and bald.

Many people believe that most of the elderly are institutionalized. In fact, only about 5% of the aged population resides in institutional settings (Public Health Service, 1976-1977).

While financial constraints on the aged are significant, 85% of persons 65 years and older have incomes above poverty level (Office of Human Development Services, 1981). However, the incomes of most older persons are fixed or do not rise as quickly as inflationary increases in the cost of basic necessities.

Many people incorrectly believe that the aged have decreased learning ability. As a result, health care professionals often fail to provide health education opportunities for the aged, since they wrongly assume that older clients cannot learn to care for themselves (Stanhope and Lancaster, 1987).

There are many misconceptions concerning older adults and sex. Older adults are thought to have no sexual desire for a variety of reasons (see box). In reality the older adult experiences sexual drive and activity, although altered owing to physiological changes and sociocultural expectations. Health problems, medications, availability of a mate, privacy, and living arrangements all may alter sexual activity.

Our society values attractiveness, energy, and youth. As people age, their contributions become less appreciated. After leaving the workforce because of age, an individual is sometimes viewed as no longer possessing worth.

These notions have led to the concept of ageism, which is discrimination against people because of increasing age, just as people who are racists and sexists discriminate because of skin color and gender. However, sexists or racists never become concerned about changing their attitudes because neither their own gender nor skin color will change. In contrast, an ageist will eventually become old. This realization produces anxiety and a reluctance to accept aging as a normal process.

Unfortunately, when a youth image dominates society, the most diversified segment of our population is ignored. Older adults have a unique perspective on social, economic, and technological developments. In 100 years society has progressed from riding horse-drawn carriages to space shuttle flights. Older adults may have experienced two world wars, the Spanish Civil War, the Korean War, and the Vietnam War and now live with the threat of nuclear war.

> ### Common Myths and Misconceptions about Sex and Aging
>
> - Sex does not matter. The later years are supposed to be (and usually are) sexless.
> - Interest in sex is abnormal for older people.
> - Remarriage after the loss of a spouse should be discouraged.
> - It is all right for older men to seek younger women as sex partners, but it is ridiculous for older women to be sexually involved with younger men.
> - In institutions, older people should be separated according to sex to avoid problems for the staff and criticism by families and the community.
> - Emission of semen during sexual activity weakens men and therefore should be avoided in old age.
> - Masturbation is a childish activity that should not continue after adolescence.

In regard to health care, older adults have lived from the era of the family doctor into the age of specialization. They have seen the establishment of our first national health insurance, the Medicare and Medicaid systems.

It should be clear that older adults are valuable to society, even though society fails to take advantage of their potential. The dramatic increases in older adult numbers, however, may mean a change in their impact.

A nurse may enter the profession with preconceptions about older adults. To provide appropriate nursing care for these clients, one may first need to clarify personal values about the elderly (see Chapter 16). The nurse must learn to distinguish between myth and reality and be able to identify the clients' strengths and limitations.

NURSES' ATTITUDES TOWARD OLDER ADULTS

Why is it important for nurses to assess their attitudes toward aging? How do nurses' attitudes influence nursing care? How can nurses foster positive attitudes toward the aged?

These are important questions for the nurse. Negative attitudes displayed by the nurse toward older adult clients may result in a reduction in the client's sense of security, adequacy, and well-being. Furthermore, such attitudes may lead to a decline in the quality of care. Clients in long-term care facilities present a special challenge for the nurse. They are often considered losers by themselves or society or both. How can the nurse promote independence and self-esteem of a client who feels life is not worth living?

The nurse must clarify personal attitudes and values about older adult clients to provide the most effective care. Research has shown that a nurse's age, education, employment experience, and type of agency where employed influence the nurse's stereotypes. The nurse's personal experiences with older adults such as family members can also affect attitudes. Chapter 16 discusses techniques to assist the nurse in clarifying personal and professional values. Since older adults are becoming more prevalent in health care settings where nurses work, it becomes imperative for the nurse to perform a critical self-examination of ageist attitudes.

Nurses who work with older adults must collect complete assessment data, including the client's strengths and resources as well as limitations. For example, the nurse should consider the client's hobbies, work history, and methods of dealing with stress. Information about such resources helps the nurse engage in meaningful interactions with the client. The client will sense the nurse's interest in him as a unique individual.

The nurse's interventions should attempt to incorporate the client's routines or rituals. The older adult often feels more secure when familiar rituals are continued in a hospital or institution. For example, if the nurse learns that the client follows certain practices at bedtime, including these in the care plan will alleviate the client's anxiety and provide him with the opportunity to remain independent.

Gerontological nursing has expanded to provide nurses with creative approaches for maximizing the potential of older adult clients. With knowledge that is available regarding the elderly's needs and problems, nurses working in this specialty can better maintain their clients' physical abilities and create an environment for psychosocial health.

THEORIES OF AGING

A number of attempts have been made by theorists to describe the complex biopsychosocial process of aging. Proposed theories provide clues but also raise questions. No theory fully explains the aging process; all are in various stages of development and have limitations. However, nurses can use these theories to understand phenomena affecting the health and well-being of aged clients.

Biological Theories
FREE RADICAL THEORY

The free radical theory emphasizes the mechanism of oxygen use at the cellular level. Free radicals are molecules with an extracellular charge. This charge creates a reaction that alters the structure or function of the cell membrane. Oxidation of fat, protein, and carbohydrates within the body produces free radicals. Environmental pollutants are external sources of free radicals (Ebersole and Hess, 1985). Research is being conducted on the role free radical scavengers and antioxidants play in aging.

CROSS-LINK THEORY

The cross-link or collagen theory postulates that collagen, a connective tissue component, becomes cross-linked, rigid, and less permeable with age. Cross-linkage is thought to result from chemical reactions that create bonds between normally separate molecules (Ebersole and Hess, 1985). Research efforts are directed at what causes, reduces, and impedes cross-linkage.

IMMUNOLOGICAL THEORY

One group of theories suggests that the immune system is responsible for aging. Erratic cellular mechanisms are thought to cause attacks on body tissues through either autoaggression or immunodeficiencies (Ebersole and Hess, 1985). Investigation in immunoengineering attempts to control, moderate, or eliminate the effects of autoimmunity and immunodeficiency.

Psychosocial Theories

In the past, psychosocial theories of development have focused primarily on the child and adolescent. There are theories about aspects of psychosocial aging, but there is no adequate evidence to support a single theory. Researchers have demonstrated that genetics is not the primary determinant of longevity. Life-style, personality, and environmental factors are also influences (Murray, Huelskoetter, and O'Driscoll, 1980).

DISENGAGEMENT THEORY

The disengagement theory formulated by Cummings and Henry (1961) postulates that aging people withdraw from customary roles and engage in more introspective, self-focused activities. This theory includes four basic concepts: (1) the aging person and society mutually withdraw from each other; (2) disengagement is biologically and psychologically intrinsic and inevitable; (3) disengagement is considered necessary for successful aging; and (4) disengagement is beneficial for both the elderly and society (Maddox, 1974). Disengagement theory remains controversial, since it does not indicate whether society or the aging person initiates disengagement or whether personality, health, culture, and other factors influence disengagement.

ACTIVITY THEORY

The activity theory disagrees with the disengagement theory and holds that the continuation of middle-adult activities is the criterion of successful aging. Most members of the aging population maintain a high level of activity. The individual's level of activity is influenced by past life-style and by present social and economic forces. According to this perspective, the maintenance of optimal physical, mental, and social activity is necessary for successful aging (Havighurst, 1963). This theory assumes that older adults have the same needs as middle-aged persons. Activity theory does not address the impact of biopsychosocial changes or the presence of multiple losses on the ability of the older person to continue or replace activities.

CONTINUITY THEORY

The continuity or developmental theory (Neugarten, 1964) states that as people age their personality remains the same and behavior becomes more predictable. Personality and behavior patterns developed during a lifetime determine the degree of engagement and activity in old age. This is a promising psychosocial theory because it addresses the complexities of aging, as well as a person's adaptive ability.

■　■　■

These theories demonstrate that aging is not a simple progression and that there is no universally accepted theory that can predict and explain the complexities of older adults. The nurse must be aware of uncertainties about the aging process, the scientific attempts to explain these phenomena, and the many environmental factors involved.

GROWTH AND DEVELOPMENT

As in other stages of life, older adults have specific developmental tasks. These are described by Burnside (1979), Duvall (1977), and Havighurst (1953) and include seven major categories (see box).

First, the older adult must adjust to physical changes. As each body system ages, changes in appearance and functioning occur. These are not associated with a disease but are normal. Structural and functional changes associated with aging are described in the following section on physiological development.

Second, older adults are commonly retired from full-time employment and therefore must adjust to boredom, decreased socialization, and reduced or fixed income. However, since retirement is usually anticipated, a person may plan ahead to participate in consultation or volunteer activities. Most older adults, while above the poverty level, are on fixed incomes and find it difficult to meet basic needs.

Third, the majority of older adults are faced with the

<table>
<tr><td>

**Developmental Tasks
of the Older Adult**

- Adjusting to decreasing health and physical strength
- Adjusting to retirement and reduced or fixed income
- Adjusting to the death of a spouse
- Accepting oneself as an aging person
- Maintaining satisfactory living arrangements
- Realigning relationships with adult children
- Finding meaning in life

</td></tr>
</table>

These seven developmental tasks are common to older adults. How an older adult adjusts to the changes of aging, however, depends on the individual. For some the adaptation and adjustment are easy and without stress. For others, each developmental task requires nursing intervention. Many of these tasks are associated with loss. Loss occurs throughout life, but it occurs more often in old age. Those losses most commonly linked with aging are loss of health, income, usefulness, socialization, loved ones, and independent living. The nurse must be sensitive to the effect of such losses on older adult clients and be prepared to offer support.

ASSESSMENT

Physiological Changes

An older adult's concept of health generally depends on personal perceptions of functional ability. Therefore older adults engaged in activities of daily living consider themselves healthy, while those whose activities are limited by physical, emotional, or social impairments may perceive themselves as ill.

Physiological changes that occur with advancing age vary with each client. Table 25-2 describes general physiological changes anticipated in older adults.

Physiological changes of aging are not pathological processes. They occur in all persons but at different rates and depend on circumstances in an individual's life. The nurse should become knowledgeable about these changes to provide correct care for older adults and to assist them in adapting to the changes.

The nurse assessing older adults should also consider the potential for sensory changes that may influence data gathering. For example, if a client has visual problems from cataracts or hearing impairments from nerve deafness, the nurse must consider these in choosing communication techniques. If a client is unable to pick up on the nurse's visual or auditory cues, assessment data may be inaccurate. For example, if a client has difficulty hearing the nurse's questions, an inappropriate response may lead the nurse to believe the client is confused.

GENERAL SURVEY

In an initial inspection of an older adult, the nurse may observe facial wrinkles, gray hair, loss of tissue on the extremities, and an increase in tissue and fat in the truncal region. Older clients are often encountered during a health fair or a health promotion or illness prevention program, such as hypertension screening, rather than in an institutional setting.

INTEGUMENTARY SYSTEM

The skin loses resilience and moisture in old age. The epithelial layer thins, and elastic collagen fibers shrink

death of their spouse, friends, and sometimes children. This loss is often difficult to resolve. Assisting the older adult through grief can enable adjustment to the loss (see Chapter 46). When the grieving process has ended, the person may need help to identify resources to fill the void.

Fourth, it is often difficult to perceive oneself as an aging person. Some older adults may demonstrate their inability to cope by denying upcoming retirement, requesting that their grandchildren not call them "Grandma" or "Grandpa," or choosing to live like a young or middle aged adult. This is different from merely remaining active and can pose a threat to the client's health if physical limitations are exceeded.

Fifth, an older adult may be required to change living arrangements. For example, physical impairments may necessitate relocation to a smaller home with all the rooms on one floor. Severe health problems may require the older adult to live with relatives or friends for a time or permanently. A change in living arrangements may require an extended period of adjustment during which assistance and support from health care professionals and family are needed.

Sixth, older adults often need to redefine relationships with adult children. The issues of role reversal, dependence, conflict, guilt, and loss require recognition and resolution. Frequently adult children must cope with guilt feelings if they feel that they should have "come sooner" or made an elderly parent move into their home. Often adult children must realize that some behaviors of a parent are symptoms rather than meanness or stubbornness.

Last, older adults must learn to acquire new activities and interests to maintain quality of life. A person who was socially active throughout life may find it relatively easy to meet new people and acquire new interests. However, a person who was somewhat introverted, with limited socialization, may have difficulty meeting new people during retirement.

TABLE 25-2 Normal Physical Changes of Aging

System	Normal Findings
Integumentary	
Skin color	Spotty pigmentation in areas exposed to the sun; pallor even in the absence of anemia
Moisture	Dry, scaly
Temperature	Extremities cooler; perspiration decreased
Texture	Decreased elasticity; wrinkles; folding; sagging
Fat distribution	Decreased on extremities; increased on abdomen
Hair	Thinning and graying on scalp; axillary and pubic hair and hair on extremities may be decreased; facial hair in men decreased; chin and upper lip hair may be present in women
Nails	Decreased growth rate
Head and Neck	
Head	Nasal and facial bones sharp and angular; loss of eyebrow hair in women; men's eyebrows become bushier
Eyes	Decreased visual acuity; decreased accommodation; reduced adaptation to darkness; sensitivity to glare
Ears	Decreased pitch discrimination; diminished light reflex; diminished hearing acuity
Nose and sinuses	Increased nasal hair; decreased sense of smell
Mouth and pharynx	Use of bridges or dentures; decreased sense of taste; atrophy of the papillae of the lateral edges of the tongue
Neck	Thyroid gland nodular; slight tracheal deviation resulting from muscle atrophy
Thorax and Lungs	Increased anterior-posterior diameter; increased chest rigidity; increased respiratory rate with decreased lung expansion
Heart and Vascular	Significant increase in systolic pressure with slight increase in diastolic pressure; changes in heart rate at rest are usually not significant; peripheral pulses easily palpated; pedal pulses weaker and lower extremities colder, especially at night
Breasts	Diminished breast tissue; pendulous; flabby
Gastrointestinal	Decreased salivary secretions, which make swallowing more difficult; decreased peristalsis; decreased production of digestive enzymes: hydrochloric acid, pepsin, and pancreatic enzymes; constipation
Reproductive	
Female	Decreased estrogen; decreased uterine size; decreased secretions; atrophy of epithelial lining of the vagina; decreased frequency of intercourse
Male	Decreased testosterone; decreased frequency of intercourse; decreased sperm count; decreased testicular size
Urinary	Decreased renal filtration and renal efficiency; subsequent loss of protein from kidney; nocturia in both men and women; decreased bladder capacity
Female	Urgency and stress incontinence resulting from decrease in perineal muscle tone
Male	Urinary frequency and retention resulting from prostatic enlargement
Musculoskeletal	Decreased muscle mass and strength; bone demineralization (more pronounced in women); shortening of trunk as a result of intervertebral space narrowing; decreased joint mobility; decreased range of joint motion
Neurological	Decreased rate of voluntary or automatic reflexes; decreased ability to respond to multiple stimuli; insomnia, shorter sleeping periods

Modified from Ebersole, P, and Hess, P: Toward healthy aging: human needs and nursing response, ed. 2, St. Louis, 1985, The C.V. Mosby Co.

and become rigid. Wrinkles of the face and neck reflect lifetime patterns of muscle activity and facial expressions, the pull of gravity on tissue, and diminished elasticity.

Spots and lesions may also be present on skin. Smooth, brown, irregularly shaped spots (age spots or senile lentigo) initially appear on the backs of the hands and on forearms. Small, round, red or brown "cherry angiomas" may be found on the trunk. Seborrheic lesions or keratosis may appear as irregular, round or oval, brown, watery lesions.

HEAD AND NECK

The facial features of the older adult become more pronounced from loss of fat and skin elasticity. Facial features may appear asymmetrical because of missing teeth or improperly fitting dentures. In addition, changes in voice pitch (usually a rise) occur from decline in power and range.

The older adult's visual acuity declines. This may be the result of retinal damage, a reduction in pupillary diameter, a reduction in opacity of the lens, or loss of lens elasticity. Presbyopia, a decline in the ability of the eyes to accommodate for close and detailed work, is common. Presbyopia begins early in the fourth decade and continues throughout life. The older adult also has a reduced ability to see in darkness.

Auditory changes are subtle and may first be noted as difficulty hearing speech. Age-related changes in auditory acuity are called presbycusis. It affects ability to hear high-pitched sounds and sibilant consonants such as "s," "sh," and "ch." The assessment of an older client's hearing is best accomplished using a 202 8Hz frequency tuning fork to screen for high-frequency losses (Forbes and Fitzsimmons, 1981).

Taste buds atrophy and lose efficiency. The older adult is able to discern salty, sweet, sour, and bitter tastes but less acutely. Sense of smell is also decreased, further reducing taste.

THORAX AND LUNGS

Because of changes in the musculoskeletal system, the configuration of the thorax sometimes changes. There is an increase in the anterior-posterior diameter. Kyphosis is a subtle, progressive change in the vertebral structure that is permanent when accompanied by osteoporosis. Calcification of the costal cartilage can cause decreased mobility of the ribs (Forbes and Fitzsimmons, 1981).

Decreased muscle mass and muscle tone lead to decreased lung expansion. Decreased elasticity of lung alveoli results in emphysematous changes in the lungs, and hyperresonance may be present on percussion. If kyphosis or chronic obstructive lung disease is present, breath sounds are distant.

HEART AND VASCULAR SYSTEM

Decreased contractile strength of the myocardium results in a decreased cardiac output. The decrease is significant when the older adult is stressed by anxiety, excitement, illness, or strenuous activity. The body tries to compensate for decreased cardiac output by increasing the heart rate during exercise. However, after exercise it takes longer for the client's rate to return to the baseline rate.

Frequently the older adult's baseline blood pressure rises. This is the result of vascular changes and the accumulation of sclerotic plaques along the walls of the vessels. Peripheral pulses are palpable but frequently weaker in the lower extremities. The lower extremities are cold, particularly at night.

BREASTS

Decreased muscle mass, tone, and elasticity result in smaller breasts in older women. In addition, the breasts sag. Atrophy of glandular tissue, coupled with more fat deposits, results in a slightly smaller, less dense, and less nodular breast.

GASTROINTESTINAL SYSTEM AND ABDOMEN

The aging process leads to an increase in the amount of tissue in the trunk and abdomen. As a result, the abdomen increases in size. Because muscle tone and elasticity are decreased, it also becomes more protuberant.

The older adult also experiences changes in gastrointestinal function. Some may be slight, such as the sudden development of intolerance to certain foods. Because of decreased peristalsis an older adult experiences delayed gastric emptying and may be unable to consume large meals. Decreased peristalsis also affects emptying of the colon, resulting in constipation.

REPRODUCTIVE SYSTEM

Changes in structure and function of the reproductive system occur as the result of hormonal alterations. Female menopause is related to a reduced responsiveness of the ovaries to pituitary hormones and a resultant decrease in estrogen and progesterone levels. In males, there is no definite cessation of fertility associated with aging. Spermatogenesis begins to decline during the fourth decade but continues into the ninth. Most men experience a climacteric, or "male menopause," but it may result from underlying illness.

The changes in reproductive structure and function do not affect libido. Less frequency of sexual activity can be a result of illness, death of a sexual partner, decreased socialization, or loss of sexual interest.

URINARY SYSTEM

Hypertrophy of the prostate gland may develop in older men. This hypertrophy enlarges the gland, and pressure is displaced to the neck of the bladder. As a result, the older man may experience urinary tract infections, frequency, incontinence, and retention of urine. In addition, prostatic hypertrophy can result in difficulty initiating and maintaining a stream.

Older women, particularly those who have had children, can experience stress incontinence, in which an involuntary release of urine occurs when she coughs, sneezes, or lifts an object. This is a result of a weakening of the perineal and bladder muscles. In addition, older women notice an urgency in voiding.

MUSCULOSKELETAL SYSTEM

The older adult who exercises regularly does not lose as much bone and muscle mass or tone as those who are inactive. Muscle fibers are reduced in size, and muscle strength diminishes in proportion to the decline in muscle mass.

The postmenopausal woman has a greater rate of bone demineralization than an older man. Women who maintain calcium intake throughout life and into menopause have less bone demineralization than those who do not.

NEUROLOGICAL SYSTEM

The number of neurons in the nervous system begins to decrease at about the middle of the second decade (Ebersole and Hess, 1985). These neurons do not regenerate, and decrease or damage in neurons can lead to functional changes. The changes can affect the special senses described earlier. In addition, the client may experience a decreased sense of balance or uncoordinated motor responses.

The sleep-wake cycle is also influenced by the brain. Characteristically, older adults do not sleep through the night. This disruption has three causes. First, the sleep cycle is shortened. Second, sleep disruption can be the result of frequent bladder emptying, pain, or psychological upsets. Third, medication may affect the sleep-wake cycle.

■ ■ ■

The physiological changes of aging described here are common and can be anticipated. Some older clients may experience all of these changes, and others only a few. The body changes continually with age, but how this change affects the client depends on health, life-style, stressors, and environmental conditions.

Cognitive Changes

Much of the psychological and emotional trauma of old age arises from the misconception that older adults have cognitive impairments—that all elderly people are senile. Gerontologists have documented that structural and physiological changes occurring in the brain during aging do not necessarily affect adaptive and functional abilities (Ebersole and Hess, 1985).

Neurophysiological cellular changes vary among individuals, and even with obvious cellular loss some older adults do not demonstrate mental deterioration. Furthermore, some clients with significant cerebral cell loss respond well to therapy.

Occasionally when cerebral dysfunction is present, the client's preexisting behavioral tendencies are magnified. Therefore a person who was compulsive as a young and middle-age adult becomes more compulsive when older. Cognitive changes occur in the older adult when cerebral dysfunction or trauma is present. It is helpful for the nurse to understand these so clients can be helped to maintain optimal functioning.

DEMENTIA

Dementia is a syndrome involving progressive impairment of memory and other cognitive abilities (that is, thinking and judgment) and personality change, which can have a variety of causes (Zarit, Orr, and Zarit, 1985). Senile dementia of the Alzheimer type (SDAT), or Alzheimer's disease, is the most frequent cause of irreversible dementia. Causes of reversible dementia include infection, drug reactions, a variety of metabolic disorders, and even depression. These conditions are often mistaken for irreversible dementia in the older adult. Consequently, aged clients with such disorders may not be appropriately assessed and treated, and a reversible dementia may become irreversible.

DELIRIUM

Delirium is a syndrome resembling both irreversible and reversible dementia but is distinguished by clouding of consciousness (American Psychiatric Association, 1987). Other features include attentional deficits, illusions, hallucinations, occasional incoherent speech, disturbed sleep-wake cycle and disorientation. The onset of delirium is typically sudden, and there are rapid fluctuations in symptoms and severity. Delirium and reversible dementia both resemble irreversible dementia. However, their causes can usually be treated, and recovery is possible. Table 25-3 summarizes frequent causes of delirium and reversible dementia.

The nurse must be aware that cognitive changes in an older adult are not normal, expected outcomes of aging. There are several causes of mental change frequently assumed to be irreversible dementia that respond to treatment. Making the distinction between irreversible dementia and delirium and reversible dementia is necessary to plan nursing care for promotion of functional ability.

CHRONIC DISORDERS

Chronic brain disorders are irreversible and usually progressive. However, with careful and supportive nurs-

TABLE 25-3   Reversible Causes of Dementia Symptoms and Delirium

	Dementia	Delirium	Either or Both
Therapeutic drug intoxication			Yes
Depression	Yes		
Metabolic			
Azotemia or renal failure (dehydration, diuretics, obstruction, hypokalemia)			Yes
Hyponatremia (diuretics, excess ADH, salt wasting, IV fluids)			Yes
Hypernatremia (dehydration, IV saline)		Yes	
Volume depletion (diuretics, bleeding, inadequate fluids)			Yes
Acid-base disturbance		Yes	
Hypoglycemia (insulin, oral hypoglycemics, starvation)			Yes
Hyperglycemia (diabetic ketoacidosis, hyperosmolar coma)		Yes	
Hepatic failure			Yes
Hypothyroidism			Yes
Hyperthyroidism (especially apathetic)			Yes
Hypercalcemia			Yes
Cushing's syndrome	Yes		
Hypopituitarism			Yes
Infection, fever, or both			
Viral			Yes
Bacterial			
Pneumonia		Yes	
Pyelonephritis		Yes	
Cholecystitis		Yes	
Diverticulitis		Yes	
Tuberculosis			Yes
Endocarditis			Yes
Cardiovascular			
Acute myocardial infarct		Yes	
Congestive heart failure			Yes
Dysrhythmia			Yes
Vascular occlusion			Yes
Pulmonary embolus		Yes	
Brain disorders			
Vascular insufficiency			
Transient ischemia		Yes	
Stroke			Yes
Trauma			
Subdural hematoma			Yes
Concussion/contusion		Yes	
Intracerebral hemorrhage		Yes	
Epidural hematoma		Yes	
Infection			
Acute meningitis (pyogenic, viral)		Yes	
Chronic meningitis (tuberculous, fungal)			Yes
Neurosyphilis			Yes
Subdural empyema			Yes
Brain abscess			Yes
Tumors			
Metastatic to brain			Yes
Primary in brain			Yes
Normal pressure hydrocephalus	Yes		

From NIA Task Force: Senility reconsidered, JAMA, Oct. 1980.

Continued.

TABLE 25-3 Reversible Causes of Dementia Symptoms and Delirium—cont'd

	Dementia	Delirium	Either or Both
Pain			
Fecal impaction			Yes
Urinary retention		Yes	
Fracture		Yes	
Surgical abdomen		Yes	
Sensory deprivation states such as blindness or deafness			Yes
Hospitalization			
Anesthesia or surgery			Yes
Environmental change and isolation			Yes
Alcohol toxic reactions			
Lifelong alcoholism	Yes		
Alcoholism new in old age			Yes
Decreased tolerance with age producing increasing intoxication			Yes
Acute hallucinosis		Yes	
Delirium tremens		Yes	
Anemia			Yes
Tumor—systemic effects of nonmetastatic malignant neoplasm			Yes
Chronic lung disease with hypoxia or hypercapnia			Yes
Deficiencies of nutrients such as vitamin B_{12}, folic acid, or niacin	Yes		
Accidental hypothermia		Yes	
Chemical intoxications			
Heavy metals such as arsenic, lead, or mercury			Yes
Consciousness-altering agents			Yes
Carbon monoxide			Yes

ing management, clients with chronic brain disorders can be helped to maintain function.

ALZHEIMER'S DISEASE. Alzheimer's disease is a disorder of brain cells characterized by changes in the brain: senile plaques, neurofibrillary tangles, and an overall loss of neurons (Zarit, Orr, and Zarit, 1985). These tissue changes occur mainly in the cortex and hippocampus. The cause is not known and although several theories are being investigated, none are definitive.

Alzheimer's disease involves a gradual, progressive deterioration in functioning. Symptoms have been grouped according to the stage of dementia (see box) (Wolanin and Phillips, 1981).

Nursing management of clients with Alzheimer's disease is complex. The limited mobility of these clients increases their risk for the hazards of immobility. Therefore the nurse must continually meet the client's physical needs (see Chapter 42). The client's confusion usually increases at night, and he may wander through his home or hospital. As the client progresses through the three stages, communication becomes more difficult. The client may easily misperceive his environment and feel threatened. Typical behavior responses of the client with Alzheimer's disease who feels threatened include aggressive gestures or acts, increased voice volume, restlessness, agitation, and hostility (Bartol, 1979). Nursing care objectives are individualized to help the client with Alzheimer's disease use his capacities to the maximum (see box).

MULTI-INFARCT DEMENTIA. Multi-infarct dementia is the second most common cause of dementia, accounting for 10% to 20% of cases (Terry, 1978; Heyman, 1978). Although clients with this form of dementia may display symptoms of SDAT, multi-infarct dementia is distinguished by periods of remission, preservation of personality, insight, lability of emotion, and epileptoid attacks. Multi-infarct dementia is thought to be related to vascular disorders within the brain and may result from the following:

1. Arteriosclerotic plaques blocking cerebral circulation
2. Cerebrovascular accident (stroke)
3. Systemic emboli lodging in cerebrovascular pathways

Stages of Irreversible Dementia

EARLY

- Attention difficulties
- Decreasing interest in life
- Indifference to ceremony and courtesy
- Forgetting nouns in speech
- Vague, uncertain, and hesitant

ADVANCED

- Deficits in memory, retention, and recall
- Hesitant response to questions
- Time disorientation, day/night confusion
- Misplaced belongings, forgets regular responsibilities
- Forgets dates and appointments
- Difficulty remembering simple directions
- Neglects personal health and hygiene

LATER

- Disoriented to place; wanders
- Loses possessions
- Forgets and misidentifies people
- Immodesty
- No sense of time; short-term memory loss
- Communication difficulties

FINAL OR TERMINAL

- Urinary and fecal incontinence
- Severe motor impairments; loss of ability to walk; extreme psychomotor retardation
- Unable to communicate; little or no response to stimuli
- Overall marked physical deterioration

Modified from Wolanin, MO, and Phillips, LR: Confusion: prevention and care, St. Louis, 1981, The C.V. Mosby Co.

Comprehensive Nursing Care Objectives for the Client with Alzheimer's Disease

- Keep ambulatory as long as possible.
- Protect from physical injuries.
- Maintain daily exercise program.
- Maintain optimal nutritional status.
- Maintain integrity of gums and mucous membranes to preserve dental function.
- Assess and evaluate the need for psychotropic medications.
- Provide cognitive stimuli.
- Provide regular social interaction.
- Maintain self-esteem through involvement with activities of daily living.
- Maintain reality orientation.
- Maintain a structured milieu.
- Avoid translocation.
- Maintain nonverbal and verbal communication patterns.
- Reduce negative behavior through behavior modification.
- Provide ongoing support for family members.
- Protect from infection.
- Prevent the hazards of immobility.

Modified from Bartol, M: J Gerontol Nurs 5:21, 1979.

4. Transient ischemic attacks
5. Decreased cerebral circulation resulting from decreased cardiac output or rupture of cerebral aneurysm
6. Severe hypertension

The causes of multi-infarct dementia are not known, but it is believed that the same risk factors are involved as in heart disease and stroke. These include high blood pressure, high cholesterol diet, overweight, smoking, and lack of exercise. The client with cognitive impairment resulting from multi-infarct dementia usually has a history of hypertension, diabetes mellitus, blackouts, falls, or seizures. In addition, a physical impairment such as hemiplegia or hemiparesis may be present. Nursing management of clients with multi-infarct dementia is similar to that described in the above box.

SUBSTANCE ABUSE AND COGNITIVE IMPAIRMENT. Long-term abuse of alcohol and drugs can affect cognitive functioning. After 15 to 20 years of alcohol abuse, tolerance for drinking declines. Prolonged use of large amounts of alcohol creates cerebral, cerebellar, sensory, and peripheral nervous system damage. Many chronic alcoholics also have vitamin B_1 deficiency. A prolonged deficiency can cause neuropathy, myopathy, and encephalopathy, exhibited as Wernicke's syndrome or Korsakoff's syndrome. Wernicke's syndrome is present in more advanced stages of vitamin B_1 depletion and is characterized by nystagmus, pupillary abnormalities, ataxia, tremor, and stupor. Korsakoff's syndrome is a psychosis characterized by disorientation of time, place, and person, amnesia for recent events, and confabulation. Confabulation is a defense mechanism in which the person fabricates experiences or situations and recounts them in a detailed and plausible way to fill in memory gaps.

The effects of prolonged drug abuse on the older adult have not been clearly described, but cognitive impairments may occur similar to those associated with alcohol abuse. In addition, a drug overdose may cause cerebral impairment. In this case cognitive impairment may result from decrease of oxygen delivery to the brain.

■ ■ ■

A nurse who cares for an older adult with cognitive impairments is challenged to meet the physical needs of the client and to improve or maintain cognitive functioning. To achieve this, the nurse may use three types of interventions: reality orientation, resocialization, and remotivation. These are described later in the chapter.

Psychosocial Changes

The older adult must adapt to psychosocial changes that occur with aging. Although these vary among clients, there are some common to the majority of older adults.

RETIREMENT

Retirement often carries associations of passivity and seclusion and often leads to psychosocial stresses. These include role changes with the spouse or family and problems of social isolation (see next section).

Mandatory retirement age varies. For example, in a state civil service job it may be 65, whereas a federal employee may not be required to retire until 70. In private industry the mandatory retirement age is usually between 62 and 70. More companies are developing early retirement plans to provide advancement for younger employees. One popular program is the "30 and out" plan, which allows workers to retire with full pension, and in some cases large bonuses, after 30 years.

Preretirement planning is advisable during middle age and essential in late middle age (see Chapter 24). People who plan retirement activities generally make a better adjustment. For example, an individual may plan volunteer work, home remodeling, travel, or other activities.

Retirement also has an impact on a spouse not working outside the home. Tension can occur because of role changes in the relationship and because the homemaker may feel that the workload is increased.

The most powerful factors that influence the retired person's satisfaction with life are health status, the option to continue working, and sufficient income. Those who retire unwillingly are at risk for alcoholism, depression, and suicide (Ebersole and Hess, 1985).

The nurse can help clients and their families prepare for retirement. The most effective assistance can usually be given to clients known through a long-term relationship, as in a community or outpatient setting.

Counseling of older adults for retirement should focus on six issues (Diekelman, 1978). First, what provisions have the client and family made for retirement income? Will these financial resources be enough to meet necessities. How long will these resources meet the needs— 5 years, 10 years, or indefinitely?

Second, what postretirement activities are available? On what abilities, skills, and interests can the client draw? Will any of these be a source of income?

Third, what living arrangements may be needed? Is the present house too large, difficult, or expensive to maintain? Relocation should be considered. Ideally the client should spend several months in a new location before making a permanent commitment.

Fourth, what preparations have been made for role changes? Have the marriage partners discussed how they will spend time together? Will they divide household tasks, spend more time with grandchildren, or become involved in volunteer activities?

Fifth, what provisions have been made to meet health care needs? How will the retired couple meet exercise, nutrition, and other health needs?

Last, how will the retired person attend to legal affairs? Estate planning, education in legal affairs, and ability to cope with bureaucratic procedures are essential. Community colleges, offices on aging, and legal aid services may provide guidance.

SOCIAL ISOLATION

Many older adults experience social isolation, which increases as they age. There are four types of social isolation: attitudinal, presentation, behavioral, and geographic. Some older adults may be affected by all four and others by only one (Ebersole and Hess, 1985).

Attitudinal isolation occurs because of personal or cultural values. Ageism is a prevailing attitude that stigmatizes the older adult. It is a bias against and rejection of people of advanced age. Therefore attitudinal social isolation occurs when the older adult is not easily accepted into social interactions because of society's bias. A vicious circle may result. As the older adult is increasingly rejected, self-esteem may diminish, leading to fewer attempts to socialize.

Presentation isolation results from a person's unacceptable appearance or other factors involved in presenting oneself to others. Contributing factors are body image, hygiene, and visible signs of illness or functional loss (Ebersole and Hess, 1985). The person becomes isolated because of rejection by others or because little interaction is sought as a result of self-consciousness.

Behavioral isolation results from the person's unacceptable behaviors. In all age groups and particularly with older adults, socially unacceptable behaviors cause others to withdraw. Behaviors commonly associated with isolation of the older adult include confusion, de-

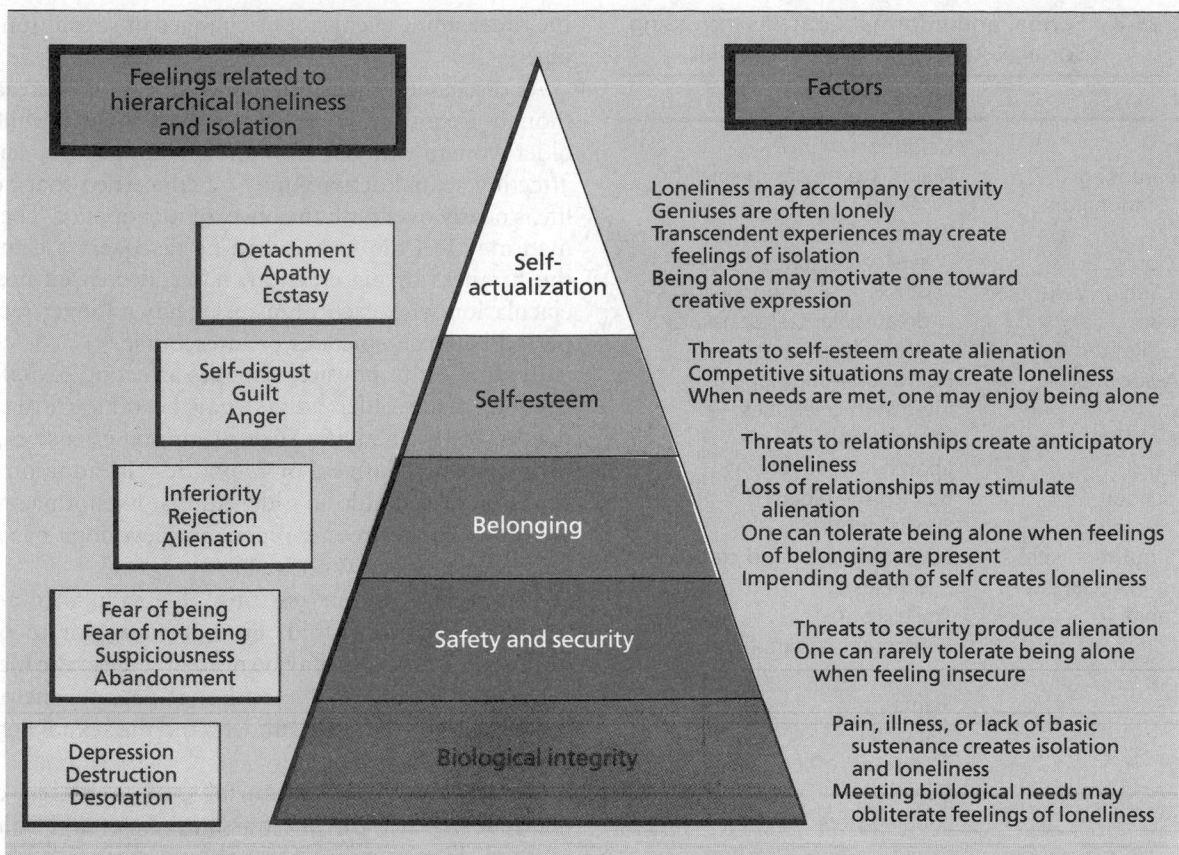

Fig. 25-1   Loneliness in relation to Maslow's hierarchy.
From Ebersole, P, and Hess, P: Toward healthy aging: human needs and nursing response, ed. 2, St. Louis, 1985, The C.V. Mosby Co.

mentia, alcoholism, eccentricity, egocentricity, incontinence, and deviant behavior. The nurse can use behavior modification techniques to help decrease the frequency of these behaviors in older adults (Ebersole and Hess, 1985).

Geographic isolation occurs because of distance from family, urban crime, and institutional barriers. In today's mobile society it is common for children to live great distances from parents. As parents begin to have physical limitations or experience the death of a spouse, the opportunity to visit children decreases. This leads to further isolation.

In urban areas a high crime rate can deter older adults from socializing. Living in a high-crime area may result in unwillingness to leave home, since it might be vandalized or robbed while unoccupied.

One institutional barrier is lack of easy access for wheelchairs, dependent older adults, or those who require the use of walkers, canes, or crutches. Also, when an older adult requires institutional care, segregation from friends and family outside the institution occurs. Social interaction depends largely on those who come to visit.

Nurses need to determine if clients who are alone are lonely or merely prefer to be alone. The effects of loneliness and social isolation depend on how the person is able to meet basic human needs. Fig. 25-1 shows the relationship of basic human needs to loneliness and isolation. Loneliness is often associated with poor health, dissatisfaction with housing and other environmental factors, and the loss of a spouse.

The nurse can assist lonely older adults in rebuilding a social network. One resource is outreach programs designed to make contact with isolated older adults. It may be planned to meet nutritional needs, such as Meals on Wheels; socialization needs, such as daily telephone calls by volunteers; or need for activities, such as outings to cultural events or a park. In addition, the nurse can investigate networks within the older adult's community (Table 25-4). These increase the opportunity to meet people with similar activities, interests, and needs.

SEXUALITY

Sexuality is increasingly recognized as important in the care of older adults. Any older adult, whether healthy or frail, has the need to express sexual feelings. Sexuality

TABLE 25-4 Formal and Informal Contacts Increasing Social Networks of the Older Adult

Formal	Informal
Church	Neighbors
Grandparenting	Maids, waitresses in small hotels
Foster Grandparents	
Vista	Beauty salons, restaurants, bars, service personnel, shops
Peace Corps	
Retired Senior Volunteer Program	Psychological withdrawal—dreams, fantasies, hallucinations, daydreams
National Retired Teachers Association	Fictive kin—soap operas
Unions	Interest in celebrities
Friends of the Library	Laundromats
Volunteers	Sports
Public school	Bus for the elderly
Senior centers	Special tours
Title VII nutrition sites	Education, arts, and crafts courses
Involved in social issues for seniors	Trailer courts
	Retirement communities
	Pets
	Plants
	Dancing
	Physicians' office
	Clinics
	Lobby gazers
	Vicarious participation
	Surrogate families—nurses, aides
	Nursing home—social corridor
	General social touching
	Radio shows
	Nostalgia
	Phone lines

From Ebersole, P, and Hess, P: Toward healthy aging: human needs and nursing response, St. Louis, 1985, The C.V. Mosby Co.

is linked with a person's identity and validates the person's belief that he can give to others and have the gift appreciated. Sexuality involves love, warmth, sharing, and touching, not just the act of intercouse.

When caring for the older adult, the nurse must ensure that care is directed toward helping the client maintain sexual health. It requires integration of somatic, emotional, intellectual, and social aspects of sexual being. Success will enhance personality, communication, and love (Woods, 1983).

To help the older adult achieve or maintain sexual health, the nurse needs to understand the physical changes in sexual response. Knowledge of those changes described in Table 25-5, as well as the physical changes in male and female genitalia, enables the nurse to educate the older adult client about changes in sexual functioning.

As discussed earlier, the libido does not decrease, although frequency of sexual activity may decline. An older woman who does not understand physical changes affecting sexual activity may be concerned that her sex life is nearly over with the onset of menopause. The older man may feel the same when he discovers a change in the firmness of his erection, has a decreased need for ejaculation with each orgasm, or has a longer recovery period between episodes of intercourse.

In addition to physical changes affecting sexual functioning, many older adults may be taking drugs that depress sexual activity, such as antihypertensives, antidepressants, sedatives, or hypnotics. In addition some drugs increase libido in older adults. Phenothiazines increase sexual desire in women, and levodopa has a similar effect in men (Woods, 1983).

The nurse's role in assisting older adults to achieve sexual health is twofold. First, a counselor to one or both sexual partners may be needed to describe methods for sexual satisfaction. Second, the nurse may help other health care professionals understand the sexual behavior of older adults.

Not all nurses feel comfortable in counseling clients about sexual health. The nurse need not feel obligated to do so. However, the nurse should recognize when the client requires assistance. If the nurse is uncomfortable in discussing sexuality, another health care professional should be consulted.

The nursing student needs to recognize that knowledge of client's sexual needs will increase with professional growth. As information is gained, the nurse will be able to incorporate this information into the nursing care plan (see Chapter 8).

HOUSING AND ENVIRONMENT

Changes in social roles, family responsibilities, and health status influence the older client's living arrangements. Some choose to live in a household with family members. Others prefer their own home or apartment near members of the family. Leisure or retirement communities provide older people with living and social opportunities in a one-generation setting. Federally subsidized housing, where available, offers apartments with communal social and, in some cases, eating arrangements. Housing most appropriate for older adults depends on their level of independence (Fig. 25-2).

In assisting older adults with housing needs, the nurse should assess their activity level, financial status, accessibility of public transportation and community activities, environmental hazards, and support systems. In addition, the nurse should help the client determine how long the arrangement will be appropriate. For example, an older adult with recently diagnosed angina may not

TABLE 25-5 Physical Changes in Sexual Response in the Older Adult

Phase	Female	Male
Excitation	Diminished vaginal lubrication (1 to 3 minutes may be required for adequate amounts to appear); diminished flattening and separation of labia majora; disappearance of elevation of labia majora; decreased vasocongestion of labia minora; decreased elastic expansion of vagina (depth and breadth); slower and less prominent uterine elevation or tenting; decreased muscle tension	Less intense and slower erection (but can be maintained longer without ejaculation); less vasocongestion of scrotal sac; less pronounced elevation and congestion of testicles; decreased muscle tension
Plateau	Decreased capacity for vasocongestion; decreased areolar engorgement; labial color change less evident; less intense swelling or orgasmic platform; decreased secretions of Bartholin's glands	Nipple erection and sexual flush less often; no color change at coronal ridge of penis; decrease or absence of secretory activity (lubrication) by Cowper's gland before ejaculation
Orgasm	Fewer contractions of orgasmic platform; rectal sphincter contractions with severe tension only	Fewer penile contractions; fewer rectal sphincter contractions; decreased force of ejaculation with decreased amount of semen (if long ejaculation, seepage of semen occurs)
Resolution	Observably slower subsidence of nipple erection; quicker subsidence of vasocongestion of clitoris and orgasmic platform	Slow subsidence of vasocongestion of nipples and scrotum; loss of erection and descent of testicles shortly after ejaculation; refractory time extended (time required before another erection ranges from several to 24 hours, occasionally longer)

Modified from Ebersole, P, and Hess, P: Toward healthy aging: human needs and nursing response, St. Louis, 1985, The C.V. Mosby Co.

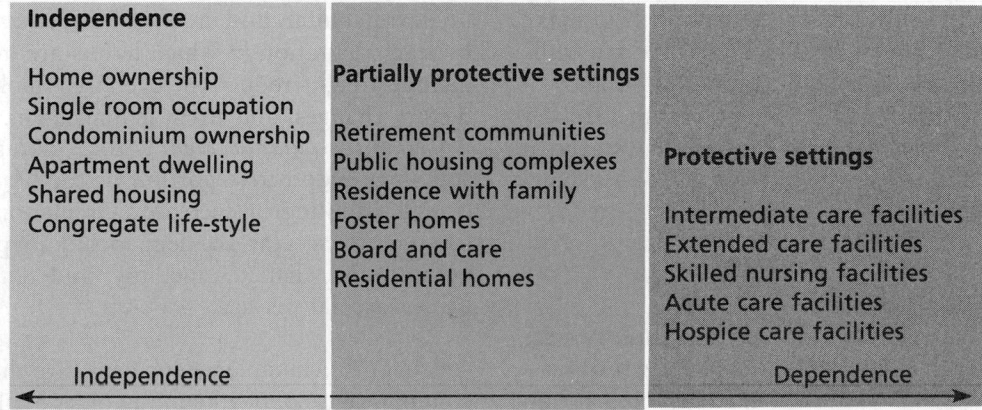

Independence

Home ownership
Single room occupation
Condominium ownership
Apartment dwelling
Shared housing
Congregate life-style

Independence ⟷

Partially protective settings

Retirement communities
Public housing complexes
Residence with family
Foster homes
Board and care
Residential homes

Protective settings

Intermediate care facilities
Extended care facilities
Skilled nursing facilities
Acute care facilities
Hospice care facilities

Dependence ⟶

Fig. 25-2 Continuum of housing security.

From Ebersole, P, and Hess, P: Toward healthy aging: human needs and nursing response, ed. 2, St. Louis, 1985, The C.V. Mosby Co.

be able to live in a second-floor apartment and should be advised to find one on the first floor.

Housing and environment are important because they can have a major impact on the health of older adults. The environment can support or hinder physical and social functioning, enhance or drain the individual's energy, and complement or tax existing physical changes such as vision and hearing. For example, red, orange, and yellow are easiest for the elderly to see. Pastels, green, blue, violet, white, and dark colors are the most difficult. Some older adults in health care settings have difficulty finding their room, but painting the door frame a bright color to contrast with the wall helps an older person to see it at a distance. Painting a stripe along the bottom of a wall makes the boundaries of a hall or room visible. The glare of highly polished floors should be eliminated.

Furniture should be comfortable and address musculoskeletal changes of the elderly. It should be easy to get into or out of and provide back support. A dining room chair should be tested for comfort during meals and height in relation to the table. An elderly client should examine furniture carefully for size, comfort, and function before purchasing.

The nurse has the challenge of assessing environmental needs of older adults in the home and institutional setting. The environment should be modified to increase independence and functional ability, and thus the quality of life, for older adults.

DEATH

Birth and death are universal yet unique events in life. Death of a young or middle aged person is viewed as tragic because life goals are uncompleted. A common misconception is that the death of an older adult is a blessing and the culmination of a full life. Many dying older adults still have goals, and they are not emotionally prepared to die. Families and friends are often unable to cope with dying and loss of a loved one.

With knowledge and skills the nurse can help make the dying process a time of fulfillment and growth while enlisting the support, understanding, and assistance of family and friends of the dying client. Chapter 26 describes the work of Kübler-Ross and the five stages of dying. It also describes nursing interventions for a dying client and the family.

Health Concerns

Older adults particularly value good health. A state of wellness provides energy, vitality, and a zest of life.

The nurse is in a unique position to establish health maintenance programs that promote the older adult's wellness. Senior citizens' centers, churches, schools, shopping malls, libraries, and hospital lobbies can be used to conduct screening tests and present information to older adults on health topics. Using creative approaches, the nurse can include health promotion activities in assessments for older adults.

PHYSIOLOGICAL HEALTH CONCERNS

Approximately 80% of adults over 65 have at least one chronic health problem. The effect of the problem on mobility and independence depends on the individual. The nurse should be familiar with chronic health problems common in the older adult population.

CARDIOVASCULAR PROBLEMS. Cardiovascular problems frequently associated with aging are hypertension, angina pectoris, myocardial infarction, and cerebrovascular accident.

Hypertension is diagnosed when repeated blood pressure measurements of 95 mm Hg diastolic and 160 mm Hg systolic are present. Risk factors for hypertension include smoking, obesity, lack of exercise, and stress. Blacks are at a greater risk than whites, and men are at greater risk than women. Treatment of hypertension includes weight reduction, decreased salt intake, exercise, stress management, and drugs (Stanhope and Lancaster, 1984).

Angina pectoris is a coronary artery disease in which chest pain is induced by exercise or stress. Risk factors for angina include family history of heart disease, obesity, hyperlipidemia, smoking, and stress. Treatment usually includes vasodilator therapy, an exercise program, smoking cessation, weight reduction, and stress management.

Myocardial infarction (heart attack) is a disease in which the coronary artery becomes occluded, thus depriving the myocardium of oxygen and blood supply. Myocardial ischemia then occurs. Risk factors include a family history of cardiac disease, angina pectoris, diabetes mellitus, smoking, obesity, hypertension, hyperlipidemia, lack of exercise, and stress. Treatment of a myocardial infarction involves hospitalization, followed by a rehabilitation in which habits are modified. These include weight reduction, exercise, smoking cessation, dietary changes, and stress management.

Cerebrovascular accident (stroke) occurs when vessels supplying blood to a portion of the brain become occluded, resulting in decreased circulation. Risk factors for cerebrovascular accident include hypertension, hyperlipidemia, diabetes mellitus, and family history of cardiovascular disease.

CANCER. Malignant neoplasms are the second most common cause of death among older adults. Along with early detection and treatment, the nurse can develop programs to decrease the risk. Examples include smoking cessation, teaching female clients to perform BSE and have routine Pap smears, and teaching male clients to perform testicular self-examination. It is also important to educate clients about the seven danger signals of cancer. Detection of cancer is not always easy because symptoms of malignancy may be mistakenly identified as part of the normal aging process. The nurse caring for older persons must be aware of their similarities. Careful assessment is necessary before assuming the problem is a normal result of aging.

ARTHRITIS. Approximately 44% of older adults have arthritis. It is more common in women than in men (Stanhope and Lancaster, 1987). The degree to which mobility of older adults is impaired depends on the extent of the disease and joints affected. Arthritis has no cure, but recently developed pharmacological agents can decrease pain and swelling and therefore increase joint motion.

SENSORY IMPAIRMENTS. The older adult usually has changes in vision, hearing, taste, and smell. These are often the result of normal aging. The nurse can help the older adult client identify resources to help correct visual and auditory problems (see Chapter 44). Seasonings can help make food more palatable.

DENTAL PROBLEMS. Dental problems are common in older adults. When present, there can also be changes in the client's taste and a decrease in nutritional intake. Because of missing teeth or poorly fitting dentures, the older adult may restrict the diet to soft foods.

The nurse can help to prevent dental and gum disease through education about routine dental care (see Chapter 32). The nurse can also help the client find dental services that offer reduced rates to older adults.

MORTALITY

The four major causes of death in older adults are heart disease, malignant neoplasms, cerebrovascular disease, and influenza or pneumonia (Table 25-6).

Health screenings and health fairs can identify older adults at risk so that prevention activities can be initi-

TABLE 25-6 Mortality of Older Adults, 1978

Disease	Percent
Heart disease	44
Malignant neoplasms	19
Cerebrovascular disease	12
Influenza and pneumonia	3

Modified from Office of Human Development Services: Facts about older Americans, 1980-81, Washington, D.C., 1981, Department of Health and Human Services.

ated. In addition, the older adult, especially one with a chronic disease, should be encouraged to obtain a yearly flu shot. An older adult with a history of pneumonia should be encouraged to get a Pneumovax vaccination, which provides lifelong immunity against pneumococcal pneumonia.

DRUG EFFECTS

As a group, adults over 65 are the greatest users of prescription medications. The most frequently prescribed medications are for heart and vascular disease, hypertension, mental health disorders, diabetes mellitus, respiratory diseases, and gastrointestinal disorders (Ebersole and Hess, 1985).

Medications may interact with one another, either potentiating or negating the effect of another drug. In addition, frequently prescribed medications increase confusion, affect balance, cause dizziness, nausea, and vomiting, or promote constipation or urinary frequency. Some older adults are unwilling to take prescribed drugs because of side effects.

Sedatives and tranquilizers in particular may increase nighttime confusion. Ironically, these are drugs frequently administered to confused older clients. Confusion that varies with time is referred to as sundown syndrome and occurs most frequently in an institutional setting. Older clients with clear mental status by day suddenly become disoriented at night when institutional tempo changes. Drugs used to manage this behavior should be carefully administered, taking into account age-related changes in body systems that can affect the pharmacokinetic activity of drugs. Additionally the nurse can use creative measures, such as making the environment more meaningful, providing adequate light, encouraging use of prostheses, or even making a telephone call to a friend or family member to let the client hear a reassuring voice (Wolanin and Phillips, 1981).

NUTRITION

Minimum nutritional needs for the older adult are the same as those of younger adults except that greater amounts of calcium, vitamin C, and vitamin A are required. Total caloric intake usually declines in response to illness, changes in metabolic rate, and physical activity. Nutritional needs of older adults are described in Chapter 33.

EXERCISE

The older adult should be encouraged to maintain physical exercise and activity. Before beginning an exercise program the client should have a physical examination, which may include a stress cardiogram or stress test. This provides information about cardiovascular function during sustained exercise.

When the older adult begins an exercise program, the

nurse should plan one that meets physical needs while allowing for physical impairments.

■ ■ ■

Most older adults are interested in their health and are capable of taking charge of their lives. They like to remain independent and prevent disability. Initial screenings by nurses establish baseline data that can be used to determine wellness, identify health needs, and design health maintenance programs to prevent later problems.

Nursing students will find it challenging to test their knowledge and skills in screening sessions. Under the direction of an instructor, students make presentations on nutrition, arthritis, hypertension, foot and skin care, Heimlich's maneuver, medications, and exercise. Other topics, such as consumer affairs, safety precautions, and Medicare reimbursement policies, are also of interest. Nurses can significantly improve the quality of life and health of the elderly by health promotion, teaching, advising, and counseling. The use of self-help strategies is appropriate for the aged because of their limited financial and social resources. Many older adults monitor their own or their spouse's blood pressure, attend health fairs, plan special diets, and care for a spouse with a chronic disease. The self-help network of older adults is extensive. For example, while shopping, older adults may exchange information about the best physician for cataract surgery, a hospital that provides the best care, and what nursing homes to stay away from. They have a "gray grapevine" of information.

As part of health screening, the nurse should encourage older adults to complete a stress inventory scale. Individuals at high risk for illness resulting from stress should receive health teaching from the nurse. The nurse needs to be knowledgeable about relaxation and stress reduction techniques to assist the client in selecting the best one.

PSYCHOSOCIAL HEALTH CONCERNS

Psychosocial health concerns vary among older adults. Many role transitions occur between middle age and older adulthood. Because of this and the cognitive, social, and physical effects of aging, many older adults require nursing assistance to maintain psychosocial health.

Interventions for psychosocial health of older adults resemble those of other age groups. However, some interventions are more crucial for the older adult who is experiencing social isolation, cognitive impairment, or other psychosocial problems. These interventions include therapeutic communication, touch, reality orientation, resocialization, reminiscence, and interventions to improve body image.

THERAPEUTIC COMMUNICATION. With therapeutic communication the nurse perceives and respects the client's uniqueness. The nurse who communicates effectively with an older adult client will be accepted as one who shares a genuine concern for his welfare.

The nurse cannot simply enter a client's environment and immediately establish a therapeutic relationship. She must first be knowledgeable and skilled in communication techniques. The nursing student can practice these techniques with other students (see Chapter 19).

TOUCH. Touch is the first sense to become functional. It provides knowledge about others throughout life. In all cultures, gentle touch conveys affection and friendliness. Often older adults who are victims of social isolation are deprived of the touching that was an important part of earlier life.

Touch is a therapeutic tool that nurses can use to help comfort the older adult. It can provide sensory stimulation, reduce anxiety, orient the person to reality, relieve physiological and emotional pain, and give comfort during the dying process (Barnett, 1972).

An older adult who is isolated, dependent, ill, fears death, or lacks self-esteem has a greater need for touch. The client may invite touch by reaching for a nurse's hand. Too often elderly men are wrongly accused of sexual advances when they demonstrate this need. The nurse should recognize that the client may be suffering from touch deprivation. Nurses should not use touch in a condescending way, however, such as a pat on the head or a gentle pinch. Touch should convey respect and sensitivity. The nurse should not be surprised if the client reciprocates with touch because of an unmet neet for intimacy.

REALITY ORIENTATION. Reality orientation was first described by Taulbee and Folsom in 1966. It is a communication modality used to make a client aware of time, place, and person. The major purposes of reality orientation include (1) restoring sense of reality, (2) improving level of awareness, (3) promoting socialization, (4) elevating the client's independent functioning, and (5) minimizing confusion, disorientation, and physical regression.

The nurse can use reality orientation techniques anywhere. When an older adult experiences a change in environment, surgery, illness, or emotional stress, he is at risk for becoming disoriented. Environmental changes, such as the bright lights and lack of windows in specialized units of a hospital, often lead to disorientation and confusion. The client's environment and the nursing personnel often change in a hospital and the client's environment is unstable. This makes adaptation difficult. It is no wonder that many older clients lose track of time and become confused while in the hospital.

Guidelines for Reality Orientation

REALISM

- Use reality information such as time, date, place, and name in conversation.
- Refer to clocks and other reality orientation props when necessary.
- Do not reinforce delusions or hallucinations.
- Direct back to reality-oriented endeavors if they ramble in conversation or talk unrealistically.
- If erratic behavior is shown, such as picking at clothes, give purposeful things to do.

INDEPENDENCE

- Express confidence in the person's ability to be self-directing.
- Encourage him to perform tasks and make decisions, assisting only when necessary.
- Make sure the person has needed aids, such as glasses, dentures, and hearing aids, and that they work.
- Provide bowel and bladder training when necessary.
- Provide speech or physical therapy when necessary.
- Reduce medication to a minimum.

INDIVIDUALIZATION

- Keep reality orientation classes small to permit individual attention.
- Allow the person to keep familiar treasures and objects.
- Encourage meaningful object relationships.

REINFORCEMENT

- Watch for small changes in behavior that indicate progress, and reward them.
- Reward correct behavior with verbal praise, touch, or smiles.
- Reinforce achievement with increased responsibility.
- Encourage special talents or interests.

REPETITION

- Repeat information, directions, statements, and questions as necessary.
- Be patient and allow time for a response or reply.
- Give clues to the answer when asking a question; if he is unable to answer, provide the correct response and let him repeat it.

CLARITY

- Enunciate clearly and speak slowly.
- Reword statements and questions if necessary.
- Give directions in clear, simple, short statements.

CONSISTENCY

- Maintain continuity of care.
- Adhere to scheduling.
- Use the same personnel when possible.

From Beck, CM, Rawlins, RP, and Williams, SR: Mental health—psychiatric nursing: a holistic life-cycle approach, ed. 2, St. Louis, 1987, The C.V. Mosby Co.

The problem is compounded by sedatives, tranquilizers, anesthesia, and restraints that take away his dignity.

The nurse should anticipate disorientation and confusion as a consequence of hospitalization, relocation, surgery, loss, or illness and incorporate reality orientation interventions into the nursing care plan. These interventions are based on seven principles (see box). Though not a panacea, reality orientation can diminish moderate confusional states when used with other therapies (Burnside, 1984).

RESOCIALIZATION. Resocialization is an intervention that assists the older adult to expand his social network. It is especially beneficial to older adults whose previous social interaction depended on employment. Once retired they find themselves without social contact. Similarly, resocialization is important for older adults whose spouse or close friends have died.

The key to resocialization is knowing resources easily available to the client. Many older adults eagerly participate in senior citizen groups, foster grandparent programs, or hospital volunteer work. However, they may not know how to make the initial contact. The nurse can provide the older adult with names or can personally contact the agency. The nurse and client must work together for effective resocialization.

Developing Secondary Relationships. Just as socialization is important for older adults at risk for isolation, secondary relationships are important for those who maintain primary relationships. Family and friends provide long-term support for many older adults. However, it is important that reliable secondary relationships with peers be developed to provide a social group not bound by emotions frequently experienced in families. For example, elderly persons in a day-care center enjoy socializing with peers and younger staff. They share experiences and concerns but are related only by common feelings or ideas.

The nurse can help to form secondary relationships by promoting discussion on topics of mutual interest at day-care centers, nutrition program sites, or long-term care centers. For example, clients with arthritis may benefit from discussing ways to maintain activity. The following are some guidelines for conducting discussion sessions:

1. Select a small, quiet room that is well lit and has comfortable furniture. Be sure to consider visual, hearing, or musculoskeletal impairments.
2. Keep meetings short enough to promote learning while not becoming exhausting (20 minutes).
3. Choose participants who are able to participate.
4. Consider the older adults' sensory deficits when using visual aids (such as brightly colored posters with large print).
5. Present one topic for discussion at each meeting.
6. Make it clear that participation is voluntary.

Establishing peer group meetings for the older adult allows the participants to develop secondary relationships independently. The older adult learns to share ideas

and solve problems without dwelling on physical ailments or feelings of hopelessness.

REMINISCENCE. Reminiscence is recalling the past to assign new meanings to experiences (Beck, Rawlins, and Williams, 1987). It is an adaptive function of older adults. As a therapy, reminiscence is an elaboration of the natural way older adults revive their past to give meaning or reconcile conflicts and disappointments as they prepare for death (Butler, 1963). Reminiscing contributes to successful old-age adaptation by maintaining self-esteem, reaffirming identity, and working through loss.

Reminiscence can be used for impaired, disturbed, or depressed older adults. The nurse organizes the group and selects strategies for reminiscence. This is done by adapting the group's size, structure, process, and goals, as well as activities, to meet the group members' needs. Table 25-7 details the techniques of reminiscence.

BODY IMAGE INTERVENTIONS. The way an older adult presents himself has a significant impact on body image and feelings of isolation. Some physical characteristics of old age are socially desirable, such as distin-

TABLE 25-7   Reminiscence Group Strategies

	Cognitively Impaired	Psychologically Disturbed	Depressed
Patient selection	No more than five members; age cohorts, both sexes	10 members; varied ages; both sexes	Eight to 10 members; those with similar problems, for example, grieving, retired; both sexes
Structure	Consistent place and time; frequent, 20-minute meetings; coleaders	Consistent place and time; biweekly, 1-hour meetings; one leader consistently	Varied meeting places; weekly, 1-hour meeting; variable leadership
Process	Connect specific events, things, and places common to group.	Connect members through shared feelings and survival strategies	Focus members on successful coping during life span; encourage mutuality.
Goals	Stimulate memory, enhance identity, raise self-esteem, increase socialization skills	Recognize feelings and meaning of suppressed conflicts, enlarge coping strategies, integrate self-view, promote universality	Reduce feelings of hopelessness, restore personal control, increase affectual responsiveness, develop a sense of integrity and acceptance of life as lived, promote caring between members
Nurse's function	Provide a comfortable, mildly stimulating environment. Select props that will stimulate memories. Assist members by giving specific information, reminders, and clues. Give praise and recognition for participation.	Establish a private meeting and a closed group. Plan to focus on specific developmental stages or critical life events. Accept and validate all expressions of feeling. Clarify multiple meanings of events. Reduce anxiety	Provide a comfortable, stimulating environment. Appeal to sensory memories. Focus members' attention on evidence of caring and sharing. Demonstrate a caring attitude. Allow time to complain.

From Ebersole, P, and Hess, P: Toward healthy aging: human needs and nursing response, ed. 2, St. Louis, 1985, The C.V. Mosby Co.

guished-looking gray hair. Other features are also impressive, such as a lined face that displays character or wrinkled hands that convey a lifetime of hard work. Too often, however, society sees elderly people as incapacitated, deaf, obese, or shrunken in stature. When an older adult has an acute or chronic illness, the related physical dependence makes it difficult for maintenance of body image. A nurse with stereotypes about the appearance of older adults may give little attention to grooming or hygiene.

Consequences of illness and aging that threaten the older adult's body image include invasive diagnostic procedures, pain, surgery, prostheses, loss of sensation in a body part, skin changes, dependence on life-sustaining medication, denture odor, loss of scalp hair, and incontinence.

The nurse has direct influence on the client's appearance. The importance to the older adult of presenting a socially acceptable image must be considered. It takes little effort to assist the client with combing hair, cleaning dentures, shaving, or changing clothing. The older adult does not choose an objectionable appearance. The nurse should also be sensitive to odors in the client's environment. Odors created by urine and some illnesses are often present. By controlling sources of offending odors, the nurse may prevent visitors from shortening their stay or not coming at all.

COMMUNITY AND INSTITUTIONAL HEALTH CARE SERVICES

Health care services generally available are described in Chapter 3. However, there are five services that are used more frequently by the older population.

Home Care

Home health care and homemaker services prevent or delay institutionalization for older adults who need assistance with daily living. These agencies may be governmental, private, or voluntary.

Home health care is covered by Medicare and health insurance. Care is provided by professional nurses or nonprofessional staff, such as homemaker aides.

Hospice

Hospice is a resource for the terminally ill. A hospice can be an independent unit within the community or may be contained within an institution. The program focuses on meeting the needs of the dying client and the family. It provides pain control and maintains the client's quality of life. The hospice does not attempt to prolong life.

Day Care

Day care provides an alternative to institutionalization, offering health and rehabilitative services. Day-care center clients are usually not seriously ill, although they may have chronic conditions or disabilities that limit independence. A typical participant lives with a family member who must be away during the day. Day care thus enables the client's family to maintain employment and other activities (Stanhope and Lancaster, 1987).

Respite Care

Respite care is temporary relief for the primary care giver of a dependent older adult. Service is provided in the home or an institution. Respite care enables the permanent caretaker to be away from home for a few days.

The continual demand for care of a seriously ill or dependent family member can create emotional and physical stress. Studies indicate that respite services reduces stress of the care giver.

Long-Term Care

Declining health, decreased physical and human resources, and increased dependence may require an older adult to stay in a long-term care facility. Such a facility provides extended nursing care, medical care, and personal or psychosocial services.

The decision for such care is not easily made, and the family requires much support. In addition, a nurse's help may be needed in locating a proper facility. When possible the facility should be close to the client's and family's home to make visiting easier.

NURSING DIAGNOSIS

Data are systematically collected in the assessment phase of nursing (see Chapter 6). Assessment is essential in gerontological nursing, where client status changes often. Data regarding the physiological, cognitive, and psychosocial status of the older adult yield actual or potential problems (see nursing diagnoses box). Obviously, any nursing diagnosis can have a variety of related factors. Identification of the related factor or probable cause for each diagnosis will give direction in developing nursing interventions. For example, interventions for a client with constipation would be different

Examples of Nursing Diagnoses Related to the Older Adult

NANDA-APPROVED NURSING DIAGNOSES

Altered nutrition: less than body requirements related to:
- Altered sense of taste
- Social isolation

Altered thought processes related to:
- Loss (for example, of control, routine, familiar surroundings)
- Progressive cognitive impairment

Anxiety related to:
- Impending retirement
- Hospitalization

Constipation related to:
- Medication side effect
- Immobility

Sexual dysfunction related to:
- Decreased vaginal lubrication
- Joint pain

if the probable cause was a medication side effect rather than immobility.

Analysis of assessment data requires consideration of individual strengths and limitations, as well as the older client's perception of health status. Validations of data with family, friends, nursing colleagues, other health professionals, and client records may be necessary.

Assessment data contain subjective and objective characteristics necessary for validation of a nursing diagnosis. Accurate assessment is essential since this is the foundation upon which care is built. The sample nursing diagnoses box includes examples with defining characteristics and related factors.

PLANNING

The older adult client often has multiple physical and psychosocial problems. Accurate identification of these in a nursing diagnosis is followed by development of a nursing care plan (see care plan box).

A care plan for the older adult client prescribes activities to prevent, improve, reduce, or eliminate problems. Priorities of care are established, client goals determined, and interventions selected. This is done with the client's participation so that they are understood and conflicts in approaches or priorities can be avoided. Consideration by the nurse of the experiences of a lifetime, as well as values and sociocultural patterns developed, should serve as the basis for planning individual care.

Goals of care established with the older adult client should (1) reflect consideration of factors that influence normal aging, (2) maintain independence as much as possible, and (3) facilitate an optimal level of comfort and coping.

Although more time consuming and difficult, including the older client in the care planning process and allowing maximum independence in self-care activities can promote physical and psychosocial health.

IMPLEMENTATION

Nursing interventions for older adults can encompass health maintenance, recovery, restoration, adaptation, adjustment, and preservation. Interventions generally are aimed at facilitating independence and supporting abilities. Care activities require more time because of slower responses, the number of problems, and the close relationship between physical and psychosocial aspects of aging.

Sample Nursing Diagnoses for the Older Adult

Defining Characteristics	Nursing Diagnoses	Related Factors
Disorientation Agitation Memory loss Poor judgment Rambling conversation	Altered thought processes	- Progressive cognitive impairment
15 pound weight loss in 3 months Lives alone in home Limited mobility Self-report of "not hungry any more"	Altered nutrition: less than body requirements	- Social isolation

Sample Nursing Care Plan for the Older Adult

Nursing Diagnosis	Goals	Expected Outcomes	Nursing Interventions
Altered nutrition: less than body requirements related to social isolation	Client will improve nutritional intake to meet metabolic demands.	Client will participate in social activities that include meals two times a week.	Assist client in identifying resources and barriers to social contact. Assist client in identifying strategies to expand social participation and initiate necessary referrals.
		Client will demonstrate adequate nutrition through oral intake as demonstrated by 7-day diet log.	Contract with client to keep record for 1 week of: <ul><li>What foods eaten and when and where</li><li>Others present</li><li>Feelings associated with meals</li></ul>
		Client will gain 2 pounds in 2 weeks.	

EVALUATION

Evaluation measures the degree to which the plan and interventions were effective in meeting the expected outcomes. The frequency of evaluation with an older adult is highly individual. Change is often slow and subtle. Thus one could argue for either infrequent or frequent evaluations (Yurick et al., 1984). The type of problems, goals established, and interventions used determine frequency of evaluations. For example, if the goal is for the client to be free from skin complications of immobility, evaluation should be frequent and regular. If the intervention is a weight reduction diet, evaluation should be weekly. The nurse plays a major role in encouraging older adult clients to be a participant in evaluating the plan, interventions, and progress. The evaluation box includes measures.

Sample Evaluation of Interventions for the Older Adult Client

Goals	Evaluative Measures	Expected Outcomes
Episodes of confusion are reduced or eliminated.	Client will achieve a passing score on the mental status examination.	Client oriented to person, place, and time. Client demonstrates meaningful contact with reality. Client participates in self-care activities.
Bowel elimination is improved.	Client keeps 7-day diet log to include intake of fiber-rich foods and fluids. Client reports daily stool pattern for 1 week.	Clients eats four servings/day of whole-grain cereals, fruits, and vegetables. Client drinks at least 2 liters of fluid daily. Client's bowel elimination pattern returns to baseline.
Client experiences satisfying sexual activity.	Client reports pain-free intercourse.	Client uses water-soluble lubricant. Client uses relaxation technique of choice before sexual activity.

SUMMARY

Nursing care for the older adult is challenging and rewarding. The older adult must learn to adapt to physical, cognitive, and social changes. The degree of these changes varies from one person to another. Likewise, adaptive capacities are different for each client.

Nurses must develop care plans to meet the individual needs of the older adult, while trying to maintain an optimal level of physical and cognitive function. The nurse also incorporates family and community resources to assist in the care of the older adult.

The older adult's independence depends on physical health, cognitive abilities, and social support network. When any are absent or dysfunctional, the older adult's ability to maintain independence decreases and more extensive health care services are needed.

KEY CONCEPTS

✓ Myths and stereotypes portray the elderly as ill, rigid in thinking, institutionalized, poor, unable to learn, and without sexual needs.

✓ A nurse's attitudes toward older adults affects the quality and level of care.

✓ Physiological and biological theories of aging rely on physiological explanations for the aging process; these include the free radical theory, cross-link theory, and immunological theory.

✓ The psychosocial theories of aging, which include the disengagement, activity, and continuity theories, attempt to describe the effects of life-style, personality, and environmental factors on longevity.

✓ The older adult must adjust to physical changes in body systems.

✓ The older adult must adjust to retirement.

✓ The death of a spouse, a friend, or children affects adaptation to aging.

✓ Many older adults have difficulty perceiving themselves as old.

✓ Some older adults require a change in living arrangements.

✓ Realignment of relationships between older adults and their children is necessary.

✓ The older adult must acquire new activities and interests to maintain quality of life.

✓ Physiological changes are a normal part of aging and not the result of illness.

✓ Structural and physiological changes that occur in the brain during aging do not necessarily impair the older adult's adaptation and functional ability.

✓ Cerebral dysfunction can magnify preexisting behavioral tendencies.

✓ Characteristics of dementia include decreased intellectual function, personality change, impaired judgment, and change in affect.

✓ Cognitive impairment includes acute, potentially reversible disorders and chronic, irreversible, progressive disorders.

✓ Classic symptoms of dementia and delerium include decreases in attention span, learning, and memory. Some clients have hallucinations, illusions, aphasias, emotional lability, and depression.

✓ Chronic brain disorders include Alzheimer's disease and multi-infarct dementia.

✓ Cognitive impairment can result from chemical substance abuse.

✓ Psychosocial changes affecting the older adult include retirement, social isolation, change in housing, death, and sexual changes.

✓ Sexuality is linked with a person's identity and validates the person's belief that he can give to others and have the gift appreciated.

✓ In addition to physical changes, drugs prescribed for the older adult may affect sexual functioning.

✓ Changes in social roles, family responsibility, and health status influence the choice of living arrangements appropriate for the older adult.

✓ The older adult and his family require nursing interventions to help them cope with the dying process.

✓ The major health problems of the older adult include hypertension, angina pectoris, myocardial infarction, cerebrovascular accident, cancer, arthritis, sensory impairments, and dental problems.

✓ The four leading causes of death in the older population are heart disease, malignant neoplasms, cerebrovascular disease, and influenza and pneumonia.

✓ Nursing interventions for psychosocial problems should be individualized; they include the technique of therapeutic communication, touch, reality orientation, resocialization, and reminiscence.

✓ Health care services for older adults are available in the community and institutional settings.

REFERENCES

American Psychiatric Association: Diagnostic and statistical manual of mental disorders (DSM-III-R), Washington, D.C., 1987.

Barnett, K: A survey of the current utilization of touch by health team personnel with hospitalized patients, Int J Nurs Stud 9:195, 1972.

Bartol, M: Dialogue with dementia: non-verbal communication in patients with Alzheimer's disease, J Gerontol Nurs 5:21, 1979.

Beck, CM, Rawlins, RP, and Williams, SR: Mental health—psychiatric nursing: a holistic life-cycle approach, ed. 2, St. Louis, 1987, The C.V. Mosby Co.

Burnside, IM: Transition to later life: developmental theories and research. In Burnside, IM, Ebersole, P, and Monea, HE, editors: Psychosocial caring through the life span, New York, 1979, McGraw-Hill Book Co.

Burnside, IM: Working with the elderly: group process and techniques, ed. 2, Belmont, Calif., 1984, Wadsworth, Inc.

Butler, R: Life review: an interpretation of reminiscence in the aged, Psychiatry 26:65, 1963.

Cummings, E, and Henry, WE: Growing old: the process of disengagement, New York, 1961, Basic Books, Inc.

Diekelman, N: Pre-retirement counseling, Am J Nurs 78:1337, 1978.

Duvall, EM: Family development, ed. 5, Philadelphia, 1977, J.B. Lippincott Co.

Ebersole, P, and Hess, P: Toward healthy aging: human needs and nursing responses, ed. 2, St. Louis, 1985, The C.V. Mosby Co.

Forbes, EJ, and Fitzsimmons, VM: The older adult: a process for wellness, St. Louis, 1981, The C.V. Mosby Co.

Havighurst, RJ: Human development and education, New York, 1953, David McKay Co., Inc.

Havighurst, RJ: Successful aging. In Williams, RH, Tibbits, C, and Donahue, W, editors: Process of aging, vol. 1, New York, 1963, Atherton Press.

Heyman, A: Differentiation of Alzheimer's disease from multi-infarct dementia. In Katzman, R, Terry, RD, and Bick, KL, editors: Alzheimer's disease: senile dementia and related disorders, New York, 1978, Raven Press.

Maddox, GL: Disengagement theory: a critical evaluation, Gerontologist 4:80, 1974.

Murray, RB, Huelskoetter, MMW, and O'Driscoll, DL: The nursing process in later maturity, Englewood Cliffs, N.J., 1980, Prentice-Hall, Inc.

Neugarten, BL: Personality in middle and late life, New York, 1964, Atherton Press.

Office of Human Development Services: Need for long-term care: information and issues, Washington, D.C., 1981, Department of Health and Human Services.

Public Health Service: Health United States, 1976-1977, Washington, D.C., 1976-1977, Health Resources Administration, National Center for Health Statistics, Department of Health, Education and Welfare.

Stanhope, M, and Lancaster, J: Community health nursing: process and practice for promoting health, ed. 2, St. Louis, 1987, The C.V. Mosby Co.

Taulbee, LA, and Folsom, JC: Reality orientation for geriatric patients, Hospital and Community Psychiatry 17(5):1966.

Terry, RD: Aging, senile dementia, and Alzheimer's disease. In Katzman, R, Terry, RD, and Bick, KL, editors: Alzheimer's disease: senile dementia and related disorders, New York, 1978, Raven Press.

United States Bureau of the Census, Statistical Abstract of the United States, 1985.

Wolanin, MO, and Phillips, LR: Confusion: prevention and care, St. Louis, 1981, The C.V. Mosby Co.

Woods, NF: Human sexuality in health and illness, ed. 3, St. Louis, 1983, The C.V. Mosby Co.

Yurick, AG, et al.: The aged person and the nursing process, ed. 2, Norwalk, Conn. 1984, Appleton-Century-Crofts.

Zarit, SH, Orr, NK, and Zarit, JM: The hidden victims of Alzheimer's disease: families under stress, New York, 1985, New York University Press.

ADDITIONAL READINGS

Adams, M: Aging: gerontological nursing research, Ann Rev Nurs Res 4:77, 1986.

Butler, FR, et al.: Neuroleptics and behavior: a comparative study, J Gerontol Nurs 13:15, June 1987.

Chang, BL, et al.: Adherence to health care regimens among elderly women, Nurs Res 34:27, 1985.

Department of Health and Human Services: Final report: the 1981 White House Conference on Aging, Washington, D.C., 1981, The Department.

Foreman, MD: Acute confusional states in hospitalized elderly: a research dilemma, Nurs Res 35:34, 1986.

Greenhill, ED, and Baker, MF: The effects of a well older adult clinical experience on students' knowledge and attitudes, J Nurs Educ 25:145, 1986.

Groër, MW, and Shekleton, MT: Basic pathophysiology: a conceptual approach, ed. 2, St. Louis, 1983, The C.V. Mosby Co.

Gropper-Katz, EI: Reality orientation research, J Gerontol Nurs 13:13, August, 1987.

Langland, R, et al.: Change in basic nursing students' attitudes toward the elderly after a nursing home experience, J Nurs Educ 25:31-33, 1986.

Lappe, JM: Reminiscing: the life review therapy, J Gerontol Nurs 13:12, 1987.

Morgan, DL: Nurse's perceptions of mental confusion in the elderly: influence of resident and setting characteristics, J Health Soc Behav 26:102, 1985.

Nagley, SJ: Predicting and preventing confusion in your patients, J Gerontol Nurs 12:27, March 1986.

Newman, MA, and Gaudiano, JK: Depression as an explanation for decreased subjective time in the elderly, Nurs Res 33:137, 1984.

Slimmer, LW, et al.: Perceptions of learned helplessness, J Gerontol Nurs 13:33, 1987.

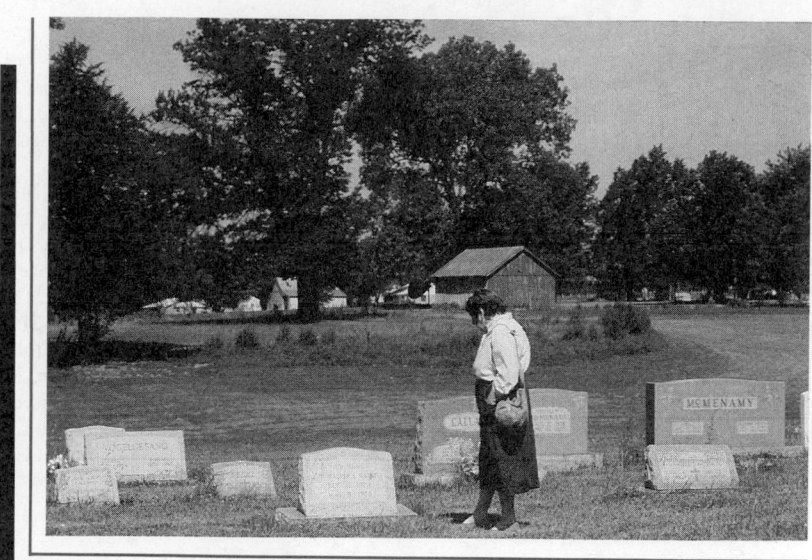

OBJECTIVES

Mastery of content in this chapter will enable the student to:

- Define the key terms listed.
- Identify the nurse's role in assisting clients with problems related to loss, death, and grief.
- Describe and compare the phases of grieving from Engel, Kübler-Ross, and Martocchio.
- List and discuss the five basic categories of loss.
- Describe the six dimensions of hope.
- Assess a client's reaction to grief and ability to cope.
- Describe characteristics of a person experiencing grief.
- Compare and contrast grief after loss, anticipatory grief, and resolved grief.
- Develop a care plan for a client or family experiencing grief.
- Implement interventions for grieving clients to provide therapeutic communication, maintain self-esteem, and promote a return to normal activities.
- Describe how the nurse helps meet the dying client's needs for comfort.
- Explain ways for the nurse to assist a family in caring for a dying client.
- Discuss the purposes of a hospice.
- List and discuss important factors in caring for the body after death.

KEY TERMS

Algor Mortis
Anticipatory Grief
Antiemetic
Autopsy
Bereavement
Enucleation
Grief
Grieving Process
Hope
Hospice
Livor Mortis
Maturational Loss
Mortician
Palliative Therapy
Rigor Mortis
Situational Loss
Unresolved Grief

Loss, Death, and Grieving

Birth, loss, and death are universal and individually unique events of the human experience. Life is a series of losses and gains. A child beginning to walk gains independence with mobility. An elderly person with visual and hearing changes loses self-reliance. Illness and hospitalization frequently cause losses.

A nurse works with many clients who experience different types of loss. The coping mechanisms a person learns have much to do with that person's ability to face and accept loss. The nurse's role is to assist clients in understanding and accepting loss so that life can continue.

Humans are able to anticipate personal death. This causes anxiety, planning, denial, love, loneliness, achievement, and lack of achievement. Death is an overwhelming experience that affects the dying person, as well as family, friends, and care givers. When a person becomes terminally ill, others are reminded of their mortality. The style of dying reflects a person's style of living, and a person's attitudes about death depend on the beliefs and emotional strengths that person brings to dying.

LOSS, DEATH, GRIEF, AND NURSING

The nurse needs to understand loss, death, and grief. Nursing by its nature is involved in all processes of life from birth to death. The nurse interacts daily with clients and families experiencing loss and grief. At the same time, the nurse is experiencing personal loss as the client-family-nurse relationship ends through transfer, discharge, recovery, or death of the client. The nurse is accustomed to dealing with the client's biological and physical care. The nurse may find it easy and nonthreatening to relieve physical symptoms associated with illness and death, but becoming involved in meaningful interpersonal relationships to support a person who is suffering or dying is difficult. Feelings, values, and experiences influence the extent to which nurses can support clients and families during a loss or death. Self-assessment—exploring personal attitudes, feelings, and values—is necessary before the nurse can use a sensitive, therapeutic approach with others. Developing the art of being with the grieving and dying requires an inner strength that arises from the nurse's positive belief in self. Formulation of a philosophy of life helps the nurse function during difficult times. Knowledge of the concepts of loss and the grieving process enables the nurse to use creative interventions to promote health, prevent illness, and support dying clients.

Loss

A person experiences loss in the absence of an object, person, body part or function, or emotion that was formerly present. Losses may be actual or perceived. Actual losses are easily identified, as with the child whose playmate moves away, or the adult who loses a marriage partner through divorce. Perceived losses are less tangible and are easily misunderstood, such as the loss of confidence or prestige. The more that is invested in what is lost, the greater the feeling of loss. Loss may be maturational, situational, or both. The child learning to walk loses the infantlike body image, the woman experiencing menopause loses the ability to bear children, the unemployed man loses self-esteem.

Personal loss is any significant loss that requires adaptation through the grieving process. Loss occurs when something or someone can no longer be seen, felt, heard, known, or experienced. The type of loss influences the degree of stress. For example, it might be assumed that the loss of an object would not generate the same stress as the loss of a significant other. However, individuals respond to loss differently. The death of a family member would be expected to cause more stress than the loss of a pet. But for an elderly woman living alone, death of a pet that has been a constant companion would likely cause more emotional stress than that of a cousin she had not seen for years. The type of loss is significant to the grieving process, yet the nurse must recognize each person's interpretation of a loss.

There are five categories of loss: loss of external objects, loss of a known environment, loss of a significant other, loss of an aspect of self, and loss of life. Nurses may encounter clients who experience more than one type. For the hospitalized chronically ill adult, Lewis

---

Losses Faced by the Chronically Ill

* Health
* Independence
* Sense of control over life
* Privacy
* Modesty
* Body image
* Relationships
* Established roles inside and outside the home
* Social status
* Self-confidence
* Possessions
* Financial security
* Means of productivity and self-fulfillment
* Life-style
* Plans or fantasies for the future
* Fantasy of immortality
* Money
* Daily routine
* Sleep
* Sexual functioning
* Leisure activities

Modified from Lewis, K: J Rehabil 49:8, 1983.

(1983) describes many potential permanent losses (see box). The losses a client faces threaten self-concept, self-esteem, and sense of worth. The nurse must recognize each loss' meaning to a client and its impact on physical and psychological functioning.

LOSS OF EXTERNAL OBJECTS

Loss of an external object involves any possession that is worn out, misplaced, stolen, or ruined by disaster. For a child the object may be a toy or a blanket; for an adult it may be jewelry or an article of clothing. The extent of grieving a person feels for a lost object depends on its value, the sentiment the person attaches to it, and the object's usefulness.

LOSS OF A KNOWN ENVIRONMENT

The loss associated with separation from a known environment includes leaving a familiar setting for a period or relocating permanently. Examples include moving to a new neighborhood or city, taking a new job, or hospitalization. Loss through separation from a known environment may occur through maturational or situational circumstances and through injury or illness.

When a person becomes hospitalized, confinement within an institution results in isolation from routine events. The rules of a hospital create an environment that is often impersonal and demoralizing. The loneliness of an unfamiliar setting threatens a person's self-esteem and makes grieving more difficult.

LOSS OF A SIGNIFICANT OTHER

A significant other may be family, friends, or acquaintances. Significant others include parents, spouses, children, siblings, teachers, clergy, friends, neighbors, and work associates. Entertainment figures and well-known athletes may be significant others for young people. Research shows that many people regard pets as significant others. Loss occurs as a result of separation, moving, running away, promotion at work, and death.

LOSS OF AN ASPECT OF SELF

The loss of an aspect of self may include a body part, physiological function, or psychological function. Such a loss lessens the individual's well-being. Physical loss includes loss of a body part such as a limb, an eye, hair, teeth, or a breast. Loss of physiological function includes loss of urinary or bowel control, mobility, strength, or sensory function. Loss of psychological function includes loss of memory, humor, self-esteem, self-confidence, power, respect, or love. Illness, injury, or developmental and situational changes result in loss of an aspect of self. A person not only experiences grief over loss but may experience permanent changes in body image and self-concept (see Chapter 29).

LOSS OF LIFE

Persons who face death live, feel, think, and respond to events and people around them until the moment of death. A person's concern is often not about death itself but about pain and loss of control. Each person responds differently to impending death. For the aged who have lived alone and suffered long terminal illness, death sometimes is a relief. Some perceive death as an entry into an afterlife to be reunited with loved ones in paradise. Others fear death and displace the emotion to other anxieties such as fear of separation, abandonment, loneliness, or mutilation. The threat of death often causes individuals to become dependent. The helplessness and shame of dependence create a challenge for the nurse.

Grief and Bereavement

Martocchio (1985) defines bereavement as the response to loss caused by death. It is a subjective experience that occurs after the loss of a person with whom there has been a loving relationship (Schowalter, 1975). Grief is a form of sorrow involving thoughts, feelings, and behaviors. The purpose of grieving is to achieve more effective functioning. Grieving is a crisis that requires time for adjustment. The grieving person tries a variety of strategies to cope. Worden (1982) describes the following four tasks that must be accomplished:

1. Accept reality of the loss
2. Accept grief as painful
3. Adjust to an environment that no longer includes the person who has died
4. Reinvest emotional energy into new relationships

In the past, our society discouraged openness during grief. The unhappy child was told not to cry when a playmate moved away; the awkward adolescent was told not to be embarrassed about a sudden growth spurt; the dying person was told to remain calm and dignified. Changes in attitudes, beliefs, and values have promoted more open expressions of grief. For example, nurses learn to seek support from peers in expressing their concerns about dealing with terminal clients. Similarly, family members seek support from care givers to express anger and fear over loss of a loved one. Grieving can lead to new understanding that can promote growth. A person can grow from experiences of loss through openness, encouragement of others and adequate support.

Concepts and Theories of the Grieving Process

Behaviors and feelings associated with the grieving process occur in individuals suffering such losses as a physical deformity or the death of a close friend. They also occur in individuals facing their own death. Both the person undergoing loss and the significant others in that person's life experience grief. The concept and theories of grief are tools for the nurse. They can be used to anticipate emotional needs of clients and families and plan interventions to help them understand their grief and deal with it.

A dying person should not be stereotyped as experiencing a certain phase of grief. Similarly all those involved in the care of the dying individual will experience different aspects of the grieving process. The nurse's role is to assess grieving behaviors, recognize how grief is influencing behavior, and provide empathetic support.

ENGEL'S THEORY

The classic work of Engel (1964) proposes that the grieving process has three phases (Table 26-1). The phase theory helps understand the concept of grief. The framework can be applied to grieving, as well as dying, persons. Engel's framework is process oriented and has three steps.

In step one the individual denies reality of the loss and may withdraw, sit motionless, or wander aimlessly. It may seem to observers that the full impact has not hit the person. Physical reactions may include fainting, diaphoresis, nausea, diarrhea, rapid heart rate, restlessness, insomnia, and fatigue.

TABLE 26-1 Comparison of Two Theories of the Grieving Process

Engel (1964)	Kübler-Ross (1969)
Shock and disbelief	Denial
	Anger
Developing awareness	Bargaining
	Depression
Reorganization and restitution	Acceptance

In step two, the individual begins to feel the loss acutely and may experience desperation. Suddenly anger, guilt, frustration, depression, and emptiness occurs. Engel believes that crying is typical in this stage as the individual becomes preoccupied with the loss. Crying seems to involve "both an acknowledgement of the loss of the regression to a more helpless and childlike status" (Engel, 1964).

In step three, inevitability of the loss is acknowledged. Anger or depression is no longer needed. The loss is clear to the individual, who begins to reorganize life. By experiencing the three steps a person moves from a low to a higher level of emotional and intellectual integration. New self-awareness is also developed.

KÜBLER-ROSS' STAGES OF DYING

The framework provided by Kübler-Ross (1969) is behavior oriented and includes five stages: denial, anger, bargaining, depression, and acceptance (Table 26-2).

In the denial stage the individual acts as though nothing has happened and may refuse to believe a loss has occurred. Statements such as "No, that can't be so," and "It can't be happening to me!" are common (Table 26-2).

In the anger stage the individual resists the loss and may "act out" to everyone and everything in the environment. In the bargaining stage there is postponement of the reality of the loss. The individual may attempt to make a deal in a subtle or overt way to prevent the loss. The client frequently seeks opinions of others during the bargaining stage. A hospitalized client may show model behavior because he is convinced the staff will make him well if he is a "good patient."

The depression stage occurs when the loss is realized and the full impact of its significance is apparent. This fourth stage may be accompanied by overwhelming loneliness and withdrawal. The depression stage provides an opportunity to work through the loss and begin problem solving. In the fifth stage acceptance is reached. Physiological reactions cease and social interactions resume. Kübler-Ross stresses that acceptance is coming to terms with the situation rather than submitting to resignation or hopelessness.

MARTOCCHIO'S PHASES OF GRIEVING

Although the grieving process has a predictable course and distinctive symptoms, no two persons progress through it in the same way or over the same time. A person will progress and then regress until the loss is finally resolved. Martocchio (1985) describes *five phases* of grief that have overlapping boundaries and no expected order (Table 26-3). Remember that while a client is passing through phases of grief, family and friends also experience grief in their way and at their pace. This is why the nurse's role in supporting grieving clients and their families can become complicated. It is common for people to work through grief over 1 to 2 years or longer.

TABLE 26-2 Behaviors Representative of Kübler-Ross' Stages of Dying

Stage	Behaviors
Denial	Avoids reality, cannot deal with decisions about treatment; may attempt activities of which one is no longer physically capable; isolates self from sources of accurate information; fails to comply with medical therapy; uses considerable emotional energy to deny truth; may appear artificially happy
Anger	May retaliate against family members, nursing staff, or physicians; becomes demanding and accusing; anger may arouse guilt because client knows he depends on care givers; guilt may foster feelings of anxiety and low self-esteem
Bargaining	Is fearful of losing body functions, experiencing uncontrollable pain, and losing control; is willing to do anything to change prognosis or fate; accepts new forms of therapies
Depression	Recognizes potential loss of loved ones; may withdraw from important relationships to avoid painful feelings; may become quiet and noncommunicative when feeling loss of control; may express feelings of loneliness; does little to maintain appearance; may become suicidal when unrealistic hopes of a cure fade
Acceptance	Accepts terms of death; begins to make plans for death (e.g., writes a will, completes financial arrangements for the family, gives up personal possessions); is able to discuss feelings about death; reminisces about the past

Hope

The concept of hope is a multidimensional, changing life force. It is characterized by a confident yet uncertain expectation of achieving a future goal (Dufault and Martocchio, 1985). Hope is not a single act but a complex series of thoughts, feelings, and actions that change often. Clients facing terminal illness or serious loss and their families will experience different dimensions of hope. Dufault and Martocchio define the concept of hope as having six dimensions: affective, cognitive, behavioral, affiliative, temporal, and contextual (Fig. 26-

TABLE 26-3 Martocchio's Phases of Grief

Stage	Client Behaviors	Nursing Implications
Shock and disbelief	A person's immediate response after death or serious loss.	Do not share client's denial.
	Physiologic responses may include muscular weakness, tremors, deep sighs, diaphoresis, flushed or cold and clammy sensations, anorexia, discomfort.	Be accepting.
	Mood swings common.	Do not discuss reasons for client's behavior or the need to cope.
	Offers of comfort and support are often rejected.	
	Person disbelieves and searches for evidence that death or loss has not occurred.	
Yearning and protest	Bereaved person experiences anger toward the deceased for dying.	Assure client that anger is normal.
	Anger expressed toward God and care givers.	Do not take anger personally.
	Bereaved person may feel jealous or resentful of others who still have loved one.	Meet those needs that cause the angry response.
	Bereaved person may be reluctant to share thoughts and feelings with others.	
Anguish, disorganization, and despair	Reality and permanence of loss becomes recognized.	Show support and understanding during crying episode, be empathetic.
	Bereaved person becomes confused, unmotivated, disinterested, and indecisive.	
	Crying is common.	Listen attentively.
	Withdrawal from activities and social relationships.	Use touch to communicate caring.
	Reminiscent about lost loved one.	
	Gains new awareness of value of life, but may cope by following unhealthy behaviors such as excess drinking.	
Identification in bereavement	The bereaved takes on the behavior, qualities, habits and goals of the lost loved one.	Must carefully assess symptoms to rule out presence of physical illness.
	May experience symptoms of the same illness the deceased suffered.	Do not ignore client's complaints.
Reorganization and restitution	Process begins about 6 months after the loss and lasts 1 or more years.	Offer person opportunity to discuss feelings about loss.
	Recurring episodes of depression mixed with periods of well-being.	Show acceptance during episodes of depression.
	Life begins to stabilize.	Assist client in discussing plans for the future.

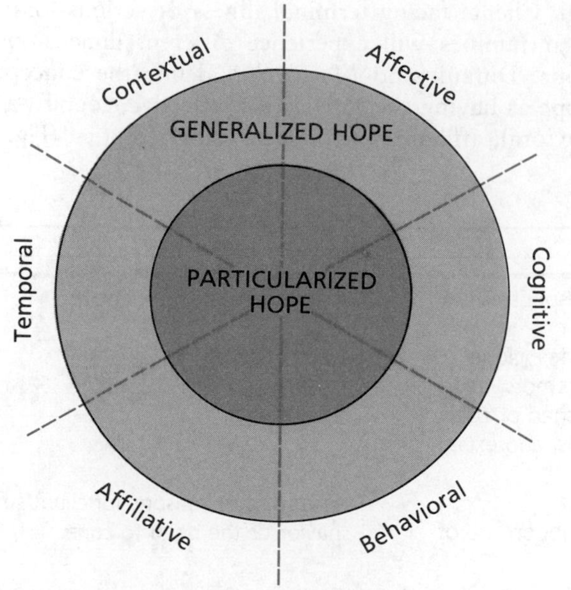

Fig. 26-1 Spheres and dimensions of hope.

From Dufault, K, and Martocchio, BC: Hope: its spheres and dimensions, Nurs Clin North Am 20:379, June 1985.

1). The process of hoping involves moving through the various dimensions. Dufault and Martocchio also describe two spheres of hope, generalized and particularized. Generalized hope is broad and directed toward a future beneficial development. For example, a person with generalized hope may often express "I always hope for the better." Particularized hope is concerned with a specific outcome or state of being (for example, living until a couple's anniversary or a loved one's birthday). A person with particularized hope perceives what is important and is motivated to cope with obstacles that interfere with it.

Awareness of the dimensions of hope (see box) helps the nurse support a client's hope. This can help relieve the grieving associated with terminal illness.

ASSESSMENT

Assessment of the grieving client and family begins with exploring the meaning of the loss through collecting objective and subjective data. With listening, empathy, open communication, and alertness to nonverbal cues, the nurse can draw inferences from the client's responses and behavior. These inferences must then be validated with the client to develop a diagnosis and plan effective interventions. The grieving process may be viewed as a sequence of responses and behaviors. An understanding

---

Dimensions of Hope

AFFECTIVE

- Sensations and emotions (for example, feelings of confidence or an attraction to the desirable outcome) that are part of hoping.

COGNITIVE

- The processes by which persons wish, imagine, perceive, think, learn, or judge in relation to hope.

BEHAVIORAL

- The actions a person takes to directly achieve hope. Actions may be physiological, psychosocial, cultural or spiritual.

AFFILIATIVE

- A person's sense of involvement beyond self. Social interaction, mutuality, attachment, and intimacy compose affiliation. There is a relationship with others.

TEMPORAL

- The person's experience of time (past, present, and future) in relation to hoping.

CONTEXTUAL

- Hope is perceived within the context of life as interpreted by the person. Life situations influence and are a part of hope. An actual or potential loss may be the context in which hope arises.

---

of this sequence is beneficial for planning nursing interventions.

A major consideration for the nurse is to assess not how the client should be reacting but how the client is actually reacting. Sequences or phases may occur in order, a phase may be skipped or a phase may recur. Through assessment, the nurse considers many variables affecting a client's grief reaction.

Age

A person's age plays a role in the recognition and reaction to loss. An infant is not generally able to understand loss and death. Loss, separation, and death have little meaning to infants until they are able to recognize familiar persons, form an attachment to a consistent care giver (usually the mother), and demonstrate anxiety concerning strangers. Once a trust bond forms between parent and child, even a temporary loss can cause profound anxiety and resistance in the child.

A toddler's cognition is still not sufficiently developed to understand death. The child's self-centeredness and difficulty in separating fact from fantasy prevent comprehending an absence of life. The toddler experiences anxiety over loss of objects, such as a favorite toy, and separation from parents or the familiar setting of the home.

The preschooler has heard the word "death" and perceives it as a kind of sleep or temporary departure. Since the preschooler's concept of time is immature, the finality of death is not comprehended. A preschooler strongly identifies with the parent of the opposite sex and may wish to take the place of the same-sex parent. This Oedipus or Electra complex eventually resolves, with the child identifying with the role of the same-sex parent. However, if the same-sex parent dies during the child's unresolved psychosexual conflict, the preschooler may feel guilt and shame over the death.

School-age children are aware of their bodies and will suffer grief over loss of a body part or function. At this age children are conscious of differences in themselves and others and are strongly affected by such a loss. The school-age child associates misdeeds or bad thoughts with causing death and may feel intense guilt over loss of a significant other. Unlike younger children, however, the school-age child is able to understand logical explanations about death. The child's concept of death is one of destruction. At the age of 6 or 7 the child associates death with "ghosts" or "evil spirits." By 9 or 10 the child recognizes the universality of death. The child may acquire an unusual fear of the unknown when a death in the family occurs or when faced with a terminal illness.

For the adolescent physical attributes and strength are essential for a healthy self-concept. Acute grief is felt when loss of a body part or function occurs. The adolescent fears rejection by peers and views such a loss as interfering with future plans. Adolescents have an adult comprehension of the concept of death. Yet they are the least likely of any age group to accept the loss of life, particularly their own. The rejection of death is related to the adolescent's developmental task of establishing identity and purpose in life.

The young adult relates loss to its significance for status, role, and life-style. A loss of job or economic well-being, divorce, or a physical impairment causes considerable grief and threatens success. A young adult's concept of death is largely a product of religious and cultural beliefs. The death of a young adult is perceived as especially tragic by society, since it is the loss of a life not fully lived.

During middle age a person begins to realize that youthfulness and physical fitness cannot be taken for granted. The middle-aged adult begins to reexamine life to consider what options are available to gain fulfillment.

The person becomes sensitive to the physical changes of aging. Any loss in physical function can create grief. Middle-aged people usually associate actively with friends, since their children are at an age to move away. Loss of significant others creates a significant threat to the middle-aged person's life-style. The career-oriented adult has usually reached a professional peak. Any loss of job or ability to perform a job will cause considerable grief. The middle-aged adult knows that time is at a premium and life is finite. Adults often take time to consider what the rest of life will be like and how death will occur.

The elderly experience anticipatory grief as a result of physical changes accompanying aging and fear of losing capabilities for self-care. The loss of independence is perhaps the greatest source of grief in the elderly. In contrast to stereotype, most elderly people are able to meet their needs and continue socializing. The way an elderly person reacts to death is a reflection of the sense of fulfillment and the contributions made to others. Whether an elderly person can accept death depends on personality traits, feelings of self-worth, and the amount of functional ability retained. The aged often fear events surrounding death more than death itself. They may perceive loneliness, isolation, loss of social role, prolonged illness, and loss of self-determination and dignity as worse than death (Gonda, 1971; McGrory, 1978).

Nature of Relationships

The quality and type of relationship lost influences the survivor's reaction to grief. Martocchio (1985) notes different grief reactions when a spouse, child, or parent dies.

SPOUSE

One of the most stressful events in life is loss of a spouse. If marital partners usually shared household responsibilities, the death of one leaves the other with incomplete skills and total responsibility. If children are in the home, the surviving parent may become emotionally overloaded with the extra responsibilities. The loss of a sexual partner may affect the surviving spouse's perception of sexuality and desire for sex.

Last, the death of a spouse makes it difficult for the survivor to establish new friendships. Hampe (1975) studied needs of spouses when attempting to cope with their mate's impending death. The spouse's needs identified include:

1. Need to be with the dying person
2. Need to be helpful to the dying person
3. Need for assurance of the spouse's comfort
4. Need to be informed of the spouse's condition
5. Need to be informed of the impending death
6. Need to ventilate emotions

7. Need for comfort and support of family
8. Need for acceptance, support, and comfort from health professionals

CHILD

A child's death is traumatic because it is premature. Parents often feel guilt and blame themselves.

PARENTS

The reaction to loss of a parent depends on the quality of the relationship. Death of the parent who was the most nurturing will likely cause the greatest grief for a child.

■ ■ ■

The nurse who is able to anticipate a spouse's or significant other's needs during loss and grief, and to assess how surviving family members adjust to their loss, is better equipped to provide emotional support. The nurse must also obtain from physicians the information sought by families about their loved one's condition.

Nature of the Death

A person's ability to recover from bereavement depends on the meaning of death and factors surrounding the death. A death that is sudden and unanticipated leads to slower recovery from bereavement. Deaths by violence through suicide, homicide, or self-neglect are more difficult to accept. When death is painful or prolonged the survivor may become impatient for the death and suffer less grief.

Cultural and Spiritual Beliefs

Values, attitudes, beliefs, and customs are cultural aspects that influence reaction to loss, grief, and death. The expression of grief generally arises from cultural background and family dynamics. Culture influences each person differently, and it is essential that the client's uniqueness be considered. A nurse avoids stereotyping clients by cultural or ethnic origins. Expectations of how a person should react in situations of loss are learned throughout life. Chapter 4 explores the aspects of culture and ethnic background. It also stresses the need for self-assessment by the nurse to provide an assessment model of clients' values and attitudes and to avoid judgmental or prejudicial reactions. A bereaved person may suppress feelings and emotions in an attempt to protect others from grief. Cultural expectations influence the acceptability of expressing grief.

Spiritual or religious beliefs include practices, rites, and rituals directed toward loss experiences and the grieving process. Individuals may find solace and meaning in losses through spiritual beliefs. Frequently a griev-

> ### ✃ *Research Highlight* ✄
>
> One of the most notable characteristics of the last years of life is the spiritual or religious dimension of human experience. Reed examined religious perspectives of terminally ill adults who were ambulatory and not in need of hospitalization. The researcher hypothesized that terminally ill adults report a greater religiousness than healthy adults. Reed also studied the sense of well-being perceived by the terminally ill.
>
> Fifty-seven terminally ill adults and 57 healthy adults, matched by age, gender, education, and religious affiliation were studied. Each completed a Religious Perspective Scale and an Index of Well-Being. Terminally ill subjects rated themselves considerably poorer on health status than did the healthy group. The terminally ill also indicated awareness of having a shorter life span than did the healthy group. The study also found that the terminally ill indicated significantly greater religiousness than the healthy group. Subjects who were both female and terminally ill contributed significantly to greater religiousness.
>
> Reed, PG: Religiousness among terminally ill and healthy adults, Res Nurs Health 9:35, 1986.

ing person turns to religion for strength and support. The nurse should be alert to the significance of religious practices, not only for the client but for the family as well (see research highlight). By words and actions the nurse can indicate sensitivity to these needs. Through openness in responses, the nurse can verify who or what sustains the client and family to plan appropriate interventions. For example, members of the Jewish faith remain in a dying person's presence to witness death and be assured everything possible was done. If a dying client is Catholic, a priest performs last rites to ensure the person's resurrection. The nurse must be familiar with rituals surrounding death because the nurse usually has the most contact with a dying client and the family.

For some clients the experience of loss triggers questions about the meaning of life, personal values, and beliefs. Typically this is shown by the "why me?" response. Internal conflict concerning religious beliefs may occur.

Sex Roles

Reaction to loss is influenced by the social expectations of male and female roles. In the U.S. and Canada, it is generally more difficult for men than women to express grief openly. The nurse must be alert to this and

---

Characteristics of People Experiencing Dysfunctional Grief

- Verbal expression of distress
- Denial of loss
- Expression of guilt
- Expression of unresolved issues
- Anger
- Sadness
- Crying
- Difficulty in expressing loss
- Alterations in eating habits
- Alterations in sleep
- Alterations in dream patterns
- Alterations in activity level
- Alterations in libido
- Idealization of the lost object
- Reliving of past experiences
- Interference with life functioning
- Developmental regression
- Labile affect
- Alterations in concentration and pursuit of tasks

---

verify with the client feelings, reactions, and the personal meaning attached to a loss. Men and women attach different significance to body parts, functions, interpersonal relationships, and objects. The nurse assesses personal thoughts and feelings in regard to sex roles and considers these while relating to clients.

A self-assessment of expectations about how men and women should react to loss will help a nurse be more supportive.

Socioeconomic Status

Loss is universal, experienced by everyone regardless of socioeconomic status. The poor react to loss in the same way as the rich and middle class. Emotional investment is not tied to "station in life" but is experienced by everyone. However, assessment of the client's socioeconomic status is essential because it influences the family's ability to use resources and support mechanisms to cope with the loss. The family's financial resources determine their options. In all instances the nurse can identify options and provide resource information.

Phase of Grief

Observation of a grieving client allows the nurse to make inferences about effects of the loss. This will help predict the phase of grief a client is experiencing.

People do not grieve exactly the same. However, there are distinct patterns. A person in shock and disbelief will act differently from one who achieves reorganization and restitution. A client moves back and forth through phases of grief until final resolution.

The ability to recognize behaviors characteristic of grieving will help the nurse formulate nursing diagnoses and identify means of communicating with and supporting clients and their families. The box lists characteristics of dysfunctional grief for an actual or perceived loss.

A Dying Person's Grief

The meaning of death varies widely for individuals as a result of many variables, including the setting in which death occurs. Most nurses care for dying clients in a hospital. However, as hospice organizations develop, nurses also work with the terminally ill in their home. Nurses observe client behaviors toward staff and families. A client's response to death will influence the nurse's choice of therapies.

The intensity of coping and the rate at which the client and family pass through the stages of grief are influenced by the time between the client's first awareness that he is going to die and the moment of death. In an intensive care unit clients generally either recover or die quickly. The unit often has an aura of death. Death is sudden and unexpected, and the client and family have little time for expressing grief. In contrast, the process of dying is usually gradual in units for terminally ill clients. Clients have time to go through the phases of grief and generally can accept death more easily.

A client experiences many emotions depending on the stage of dying or grief. The nurse must recognize that each emotion serves a purpose. The nurse must not identify the client's grief phase on the basis of a single behavior or emotion. However, the client's responses determine techniques used by the nurse to relate to the client. For example, in the acceptance stage of death the nurse can encourage a client to discuss feelings about leaving family members behind. This would not work if the client is in the anguish and despair phase.

Risk Factors in Survivors

What risk factors predict whether a person in grief will suffer psychological or physical illness during bereavement? If a nurse is aware of these risks, individuals can be targeted for specific nursing interventions. Early identification of risks can improve a survivor's outcome from grief. Martocchio (1985) lists the following nine risk factors:

1. low socioeconomic status
2. poor health
3. sudden death or short illness

4. perceived lack of available social support
5. lack of support from religious beliefs
6. lack of a supportive family or one which discourages grief expressions
7. strong tendency to cling to the person before death or preoccupation with the deceased's image
8. strong reactions of distress, anger, and self-reproach
9. history of psychiatric illness or suicidal intention

Physical Symptoms of Grief

The nurse observes for behaviors that may indicate grief. Physical symptoms of grief should also be noted. Gastrointestinal disturbances such as indigestion, nausea and vomiting, anorexia, or a recent change in weight may indicate the emotional stress of grieving. Persons experiencing bereavement also may complain of sleep difficulty. Fatigue and a reduced activity level may also be present. A single physical symptom does not lead to a nursing diagnosis related to grief.

NURSING DIAGNOSIS

The nurse gathers various data to make a definitive nursing diagnosis regarding grief or a client's reaction to it. Clustering of client or family behaviors, charac-

---

Examples of Nursing Diagnoses Related to Grieving

NANDA-APPROVED NURSING DIAGNOSES

Anticipatory grieving related to:
- Perceived potential loss of spouse
- Perceived potential loss of employment

Dysfunctional grieving related to:
- Death of a spouse
- Chronic fatal illness
- Loss of body part

Impaired adjustment related to:
- Incomplete grieving

Ineffective family coping: compromised related to:
- Significant person's preoccupation with anticipatory grief
- Inadequate family support

Altered family processes related to:
- Loss of spouse, child, or parent

Hopelessness related to:
- Failing physical condition
- Long-term stress

Social isolation related to:
- Loss of significant others

Sleep pattern disturbance related to:
- Stress of grief response

Altered nutrition: less than body requirements related to:
- Depressed grief response

Sample Nursing Diagnoses for Grieving

Defining Characteristics	Nursing Diagnoses	Related Factors
Guilt Changes in eating habits Alterations in sleep patterns Expressed distress over potential loss Anger Altered libido	Anticipatory grieving	- Perceived potential loss of spouse - Perceived potential loss of employment
Denial of loss Sadness, guilt Crying Alterations in sleep patterns Difficulty in expressing loss Reliving past experiences Altered concentration	Dysfunctional grieving	- Chronic fatal illness - Loss of body part - Loss of spouse
Absence of supportive significant other Sad affect Withdrawal socially Expresses feelings of loneliness	Social isolation	- Loss of significant other

teristics, and data involving the loss leads to an individualized nursing diagnosis (see nursing diagnoses box). Identification of defining characteristics assumes interventions will be developed in the nurse's plan of care (see sample nursing diagnoses box).

The diagnosis of anticipatory grief refers to accomplishing part of the grief work before actual loss. For example, a hospitalized woman scheduled for a mastectomy may have begun the grieving process from the moment a breast mass was discovered. Before admission she may have worked through the phases of disbelief and anger. When the nurse meets her, she may be developing awareness of the loss significance. In the same way, a family member commonly experiences anticipatory grief before the loss of a love one. Nurses also feel anticipatory grief while caring for their clients during the stages of dying. Anticipatory grief can be beneficial if it helps progression to a healthier emotional state after the loss.

Dysfunctional grieving involves **actual or perceived** loss of a meaningful person or material **object**. The nurse must recognize that while a person **moves through** the grieving process to resolution of a loss, **there** may be recurring feelings of sorrow. If resolution **does** not occur in a reasonable time, unresolved grief **may** become chronic and be expressed through depression (Werner-Beland, 1980).

In addition to a diagnosis of grief, **the nurse** may also diagnose health problems common to a **grieving client,** (for example, sleep pattern disturbance). **These** may be significant enough to require the nurse's **close attention.**

The dying client requires special consideration when nursing diagnoses are formulated. The need to grieve is one of many problems presented by such a client. A client with a terminal illness that causes deformity or physical disabilities is likely to undergo alterations in body image or self-concept. Examples are a client with leukemia who receives drugs that cause loss of hair, or a client with bone cancer who becomes disabled because of chronic pain. As a dying client's condition worsens, the nurse makes diagnoses relevant to basic needs such as alterations in comfort, alterations in elimination, ineffective breathing, or sensory alterations. Because of the nature and severity of terminal illness, physical assessment data are collected frequently and can be used to validate diagnoses.

PLANNING

Grieving is the natural response to loss. Grieving has a therapeutic value, enabling people to think through their loss, recollect their thoughts, and resume life with new insights and direction. In addition, physiological, emotional, developmental, and spiritual needs of the client must be met.

The goals for a client are to resolve grief, accept the reality of the loss, regain a sense of self-esteem, and renew normal activities or relationships. In planning, the nurse has several resources including family members, other team members and community support groups. The care plan box outlines a sample care plan.

When caring for dying clients, the nurse's responsibilities extend to the dying clients' physical needs and unique psychological and social problems. The nurse must be tolerant and willing to spend more time with dying clients, to listen to expressions of grief, and to maintain their quality of life. Additional goals for dying clients include:

1. Gaining comfort
2. Maintaining independence in daily activities
3. Maintaining hope
4. Achieving spiritual comfort
5. Gaining relief from loneliness and isolation

The nurse must support the grieving family and provide opportunities for them to support the client.

IMPLEMENTATION

Therapeutic Communication

Nursing care of the grieving client begins with establishing the significance of the loss. This is difficult if the client is unwilling to express feelings or is in a phase of shock or denial. The nurse observes response to the loss and then attempts to identify the client's strengths in dealing with it. To identify strengths the nurse uses open-ended questions and reflective statements such as "You appear concerned about your brother's condition" or "When the doctor informed you about the test results, you appeared frightened." These responses are respectful and give importance to the person's feelings. The nurse must schedule adequate time with the client and family to promote open communication in a private location. The nurse should convey acceptance of all grief reactions. For example, if a client begins to cry, the nurse quietly remains ready to offer comfort, rather than abandoning the client at the time of greatest need. Acknowledging grief through touch and concern promotes trust.

If a client chooses not to share feelings, the nurse conveys a willingness to be available when needed. When the nurse acknowledges the client's beliefs and values, a therapeutic relationship may evolve. Sometimes clients need to begin resolving grief before they can discuss the loss.

When considering a client's potential reactions to loss, the nurse is alert to expressions of denial, anger, depression, or guilt. An initial denial of the loss is normal. If

Sample Nursing Care Plan for Grieving

Nursing Dianoses	Goals	Expected Outcomes	Nursing Interventions
Dysfunctional grieving related to chronic fatal illness	Client resolves grief.	Client discusses feelings related to death.	Acknowledge client's grief. Be empathetic.
		Client expresses emotions (for example, crying openly).	Listen to client during discussions about the illness.
		Client expresses realistic hope.	Encourage client to express anger, guilt, and sense of loss.
			Offer time for discussions daily when client is not fatigued.
			Offer to read to the client.
		Client remains involved with daily care activities.	Offer family members opportunity to visit client regularly and assist with feeding and bathing.
			Encourage client to make decisions about care.
Hopelessness related to failing physical condition	Client will express a realistic sense of hope.	Client will express confidence in chosen therapies.	Reinforce client's strength in being able to cope with pain.
			Provide information about chemotherapy and radiation.
		Client will participate in self-care.	Allow client to assist with self-care activities.
		Client will communicate appropriately with others.	Arrange meeting to meet volunteer from SHARE support group.
			Encourage visitation with wife and sister.
			Offer time for client to discuss successes in life and meaning illness has for him.

the nurse encourages the client to face the reality of loss too soon, the nurse may become the target of anger or fear once denial is resolved. Because it is difficult not to take anger personally, the nurse may avoid expressions of anger or guilt. In an effective relationship the nurse must deal with personal feelings before encouraging the client's expression of anger. The nurse must let the client and family know that such expressions are normal. For example, the nurse might say, "You are obviously upset, but so are most people in this situation. I just want to let you know I'm available to talk if you'd like."

It is important that the nurse not erect barriers to communication (Chapter 19). This is done by denying the client's grief, providing false reassurance, or avoiding discussion of the problem. For example, when a client is expressing anger about a terminal illness, the nurse avoids making statements such as "Don't worry, you'll probably outlive us all" or "Since you're upset, why don't we discuss something else?"

The nurse also does not give advice or analyze causes for a client's loss or behavior. Statements such as "It was God's will" or "You'd feel better if you interacted more with others" show little sensitivity. The nurse must be careful in giving reassurance and support. Although the purpose is encouragement, a statement such as "At least you still have your mother" may discount a client's true feelings.

When a client demonstrates a readiness to move on to the awareness or reorganization phase, the nurse might explain the recognized grief reactions. Effective listening techniques, as well as communication of concern and understanding, also help the client move through the grieving process.

No topic should be avoided that a dying client wishes to discuss. The client will be more likely to talk about death with a person who listens. The client may initially test the nurse by offering a statement that does not express true concerns. For example, the client may make an open-ended statement such as "My doctor talked with me today. . .," hoping the nurse will respond.

If the nurse senses the client's desire to talk, it is important to let the client discuss *his* concerns. The nurse responds to questions as honestly and positively as possible. The nurse may use several strategies to support a client's or family member's hope (see box). The ones chosen depend on the client's dimensions of hope (Dufault and Martocchio, 1985).

When a client's condition is terminal, the nurse should not encourage expressions of denial. However, the nurse can help develop a hopeful attitude while the client is still physically strong. It is easy for the dying client to become depressed. If the nursing staff can instill feelings of hope and cheer during treatment, the client will be better able to participate in the treatment.

Refusal to die or accept the feeling of helplessness is a motivator. Clients who remain confident and determined despite severe illness are better able to tolerate side effects of treatment, make fewer demands on staff, serve as models for other clients, and often live longer than predicted. By teaching clients and families the early signs of hopelessness and despair (such as asking few questions about treatment, avoiding discussions of the client's condition, refusing to eat, or ignoring efforts to maintain personal hygiene), the nurse can help the client assume healthier behaviors.

As the grieving client moves to the resolution or reorganization phase, the nurse can encourage discussion of how the loss has affected the client's life and perceptions of the situation. The nurse may share with the client and family the signs of resolution. When the client is ready to loosen ties with the past and begin to look ahead, the nurse should encourage these efforts

The nurse should recognize limitations in being able to provide appropraite interventions for a grieving client. When other professionals are needed, the nurse explores with the client and family alternatives in selecting resource persons, community agencies, or groups to enhance grief work. Available in some communities are self-help, bereavement, widow-to-widow, and parent

---

Nursing Implications for Promoting Hope

AFFECTIVE DIMENSION

- Convey an empathetic understanding of client's worries, fears, and doubts. Reduce degree to which client becomes immobilized by concerns; build on client and family strengths of patience and courage.

COGNITIVE DIMENSION

- Clarify or modify the hoping person's reality perceptions; offer information about illness or treatment, correct misinformation, share experiences of others as a basis of comparison.

BEHAVIORAL DIMENSION

- Assist client to use own resources and those of others in relation to hope. Balance levels of independence, interdependence, and dependence when planning care.
- Enhance person's self-esteem and capabilities; give praise and encouragement appropriately.

AFFILIATIVE DIMENSION

- Strength or foster those relationships with others that are consistent with hope.
- Help clients know they are loved, cared for, and important to others.

TEMPORAL DIMENSION

- Attend to a client's experience of time. Use client's insights from past experiences and apply to the present.

CONTEXTUAL DIMENSION

- Provide opportunity to communicate about life situations that have an influence on hope.
- Encourage discussion about desired goals, reminiscing, reviewing values, and reflecting on the meaning of suffering, life, or death.

---

groups. Signs of unresolved grief and pathological grieving reactions may require referral to a psychologist, psychiatrist, or counselor.

Maintenance of Self-Esteem

Nursing interventions with the grieving client and family focus on promoting the client's sense of identity, dignity, and self-esteem (see Chapter 29). The nurse can help by listening, responding quickly and positively to requests, maintaining confidentiality, and providing comfort and support. The quality and quantity of time spent with the client are important in creating a therapeutic environment for the grieving process. Davitz and Davitz (1980) explored the characteristics of nurses with a "highly refined" empathy to their clients. They identified the nurse's relationship with the client as the core of nursing.

Measures that provide comfort and support should be implemented in a caring, nonhurried manner to reinforce the client's feelings of self-worth and dignity and to decrease the fear of rejection, isolation, and sense of hopelessness.

Self-esteem and dignity complement each other. Dignity is the person's ability to maintain a self-concept. The disabilities of a dying client may threaten dignity. Care givers often take control of the client's life. Taking away the right to make decisions about care will foster hopelessness and feelings of despair. The client loses the will to live. To maintain self-esteem the client must believe that opinions are valuable in decisions that affect his or her dying.

The nurse can promote self-esteem by giving attention to the client's appearance. Cleanliness, a lack of body odors, attractive clothing, and personal grooming (shaving or well groomed hair) promote a sense of worth. The nurse who manages the client's body functions must show an attitude of respect and helpfulness rather than encourage dependence or guilt.

Promotion of Return-to-Life Activities

As clients begin to accept their loss, it is important for the nurse to encourage a return to a normal lifestyle. If clients and families are able to express grief openly and to progress through the grief process with support and understanding, resolution of grief is easier. Depending on the nature of a client's loss, many demands may be placed on the family's resources.

The nurse can help by encouraging clients to participate in decisions about relationships and resources for the future. The identification of usual life-style practices helps bring a sense of closure to the loss. For example, if a woman has begun to accept the loss from a mastectomy, the nurse introduces her to a member of Reach for Recovery who explains breast prostheses, talks about clothing, and discusses ways to resume normal activities.

The Dying Client

Nursing care of the terminally ill can be demanding and stressful. However, helping a dying person retain dignity is one of nursing's greatest rewards. A client may experience many symptoms for months before death occurs. The nurse can share the dying client's suffering and intervene in a way that improves the quality of life. A

The Dying Person's Bill of Rights

I have the right to be treated as a living human being until I die.

I have the right to maintain a sense of hopefulness, however changing its focus may be.

I have the right to be cared for by those who can maintain a sense of hopefulness, however changing this might be.

I have the right to express my feelings and emotions about my approaching death in my own way.

I have the right to participate in decisions concerning my care.

I have the right to expect continuing medical and nursing attention even though "cure" goals must be changed to "comfort" goals.

I have the right not to die alone.

I have the right to be free from pain.

I have the right to have my questions answered honestly.

I have the right not be deceived.

I have the right to have help from and for my family in accepting my death.

I have the right to die in peace and dignity.

I have the right to retain my individuality and not be judged for my decisions which may be contrary to beliefs of others.

I have the right to discuss and enlarge my religious and/or spiritual experiences, whatever these may mean to others.

I have the right to expect that the sanctity of the human body will be respected after death.

I have the right to be cared for by caring, sensitive, knowledgeable people who will attempt to understand my needs and will be able to gain some satisfaction in helping me face my death.

From Barbus, AJ: The dying person's bill of rights, © 1975, American Journal of Nursing Company. Reprinted with permission from the American Journal of Nursing, 75:99, Jan. 1975.

---

dying client must be cared for with respect and concern. The dying person's bill of rights (see box) assures comprehensive and compassionate care.

PROMOTION OF COMFORT

Comfort for a dying client includes relief of psychobiologic distress (Oncology Nursing Society and the ANA, 1979). The nurse provides a variety of comfort measures for the terminally ill (Table 26-4). Pain control is important, since pain alters sleep, appetite, mobility, and psychologic function. Fear of pain is common in cancer clients. However, research suggests that only

TABLE 26-4 Promoting Comfort in the Terminally Ill Client

Symptoms	Characteristics or Causes	Nursing Implications
Pain	Acute or chronic.	Administer narcotic analgesics on a regular schedule and not prn (see Chapter 35).
	Pain from progressive cancer is usually chronic and constant.	Relaxation, guided imagery, distraction, and peripheral nerve stimulators provide relief.
		Use combinations of analgesics or other therapies as client's needs change.
		Oral route for narcotics is preferred, but rectal suppositories, injections, continuous intravenous infusions, and intrathecal infusions are available.
	Any source of physical irritation may worsen pain.	Thorough skin care including daily baths, lubrication of skin, massage to potential pressure sites, and dry and clean bed linens minimize irritants.
	As a client approaches death the mouth remains open, the tongue becomes dry and edematous, and the lips become dry and cracked.	Provide frequent oral care every 2 to 4 hours. Use soft toothbrushes or foam swabs for frequent mouth care. Apply a light film of petroleum jelly to lips and tongue (see Chapter 32).
	Blinking reflexes diminish near death causing drying of cornea.	Eye care removes crusts from eyelid margins. Artificial tears will reduce corneal drying.
Nausea and vomiting	Results from disease process (for example, gastric cancer), complications (for example, bowel obstruction), or medications.	Confer with physician about changing medications when possible. Administer antiemetics before meals. Bowel decompression with insertion of a nasogastric tube may provide relief from obstruction. Provide mouth care and promptly clean up emesis.
Fatigue	Metabolic demands of a cancerous tumor cause weakness and fatigue.	Set mutual goals with client after identifying valued or desired tasks, then conserve energy for only those tasks. Frequent rest periods in a quiet environment. Time and pace nursing care activities to conserve client's energy.
Constipation	Narcotic medications and immobility slow peristalsis. Lack of bulk in diet or reduced fluid intake may occur with appetite changes. Constipation can add to discomfort.	Preventive care is most effective: increase fluid intake, include bran, whole grain products, and fresh vegetables in diet, and encourage exercise. Administer prophylactic stool softeners.
Diarrhea	Results from disease process (for example, colon cancer) and complications of treatment or medications.	Assess for presence of a fecal impaction. Confer with physician to change medication if possible. Provide low residue diet.
Urinary incontinence	Results of progressive disease (for example, involvement of spinal cord or reduced level of consciousness).	Protect skin from irritation or breakdown using absorbent pads and clean linen. Indwelling urinary catheter or condom catheters may be used.
Inadequate nutrition	Nausea and vomiting can decrease appetite. Depression from grieving may cause anorexia.	Smaller portions and bland foods may be more palatable (Marino, 1981). Home cooked meals may be preferred by client and gives the family a chance to participate.

Continued.

TABLE 26-4 Promoting Comfort in the Terminally Ill Client—cont'd

Symptoms	Characteristics or Causes	Nursing Implications
Dehydration	As disease progresses client is less willing or able to maintain oral fluid intake.	Provide relief of thirst by using ice chips, sips of fluids, or moist cloth to lips.
	Certain forms of cancer cause obstruction to portions of gastrointestinal tract.	Provide frequent mouth care.
Ineffective breathing patterns	Causes include disease progression involving lung tissue capacity, pneumonia, and pulmonary edema.	Position upright to improve breathing capacity. Administer supplemental oxygen as ordered. Administer bronchodilator as ordered.
	Clients may also be severely anemic, causing reduced oxygen carrying capacity.	Narcotics can suppress cough and ease breathing and apprehension. Suction accumulated secretions from the mouth and throat.

50% of cancer victims experience pain (Anderson, 1982). The sooner a dying client obtains pain relief, the more energy becomes available for maintaining quality life activities. Providing comfort for the terminally ill also involves controlling symptoms of disease or therapies administered.

Personal hygiene is a routine part of keeping the terminally ill comfortable. The client eventually depends on the nurse or family for basic needs. Clients may be embarrassed by their dependence. When possible, let clients make decisions about their care.

MAINTENANCE OF INDEPENDENCE

The ultimate choice for a dying client is choosing a location of care. There are options other than the acute care hospital. Hospice care (see later section) allows comprehensive care in the home. The nurse must inform clients about options for care.

The dying client gains satisfaction from being as self-sufficient as possible. Allowing the client to perform simple tasks such as washing, putting on eyeglasses, or eating maintains dignity and sense of worth. When a client becomes physically unable to perform self-care, the nurse encourages participation in decision making to give a sense of control. The nurse looks for nonverbal cues that suggest unwillingness to participate in care. The nurse should not force participation, particularly if physical limitations make it difficult. The family must also learn to encourage the client to make decisions, since they often have a tendency to take over. When clients are cared for in the home, normal routines can be reestablished to help create a sense of control.

PREVENTION OF LONELINESS AND ISOLATION

When the nurse is detached and avoids discussion of the situation, the dying client experiences an overwhelming loneliness. It takes experience for a nurse to react positively toward dying clients. Nurses are oriented to the cure of clients and may find it difficult to provide the necessary support for those who die. Death symbolizes failure for many health care providers. Furthermore, the process of dying may cause a client to be unpleasant. If the client's condition causes offensive odors, incontinence, confusion, or combativeness, nurses may avoid the client. In a hospital the dying person is often confined to a private room to avoid exposing others to suffering. The room may be dimly lit, curtains drawn, and sounds reduced. Without meaningful sensory stimulation the dying person feels abandoned and isolated.

To prevent loneliness and sensory deprivation the nurse intervenes to improve the quality of the client's environment. Dying clients should not be routinely placed in private rooms in out-of-the-way locations. Clients feel a sense of involvement when sharing a room and watching the nurse's activities. The client can then also share conversation and companionship with roommates and visitors. When the client dies, however, the nurse should give attention to the roommate, because watching a person die can be frightening.

Providing meaningful environmental stimulation comforts the client. Rooms in the hospital or home should be well lit, attractively decorated, and offer a stimulating view. Pictures, cherished objects, cards or letters from family members, and live plants console the client.

Perhaps most important in preventing loneliness is involvement with family members and friends. In the home setting family and friends can more easily interact with the client. In a hospital or extended care facility visitors should be allowed to remain with dying clients at any time. If the client shares a room, however, the nurse should be sure the visitors will not disturb the roommate. If several family members visit, a private room may be necessary. The elderly client becomes particularly lonely at night and may feel more secure if someone stays at the bedside. The nurse should know how to contact family members at any time if a visit is requested or the client's condition worsens.

It is important for the client to have someone who can share the dying experience. Nurses should not feel guilty if they cannot provide this support. However, care may require long intervals of time with the client. It is the nurse's responsibility to stay with dying clients when needed and to show concern and compassion.

PROMOTION OF SPIRITUAL COMFORT

Providing a client with spiritual comfort means much more than asking clergy to visit. The nurse must support the client in the expression of a philosophy of life. As death approaches, the client will often seek comfort by analyzing values and beliefs related to life and death. A dying client seeks to find purpose and meaning to life before surrendering to death (Conrad, 1985). A dying client often feels guilt if life is perceived as unfulfilled. Therefore the client will often ask for forgiveness, either from God or people around him or her. Additional spiritual needs are hope and love (Conrad, 1985). The nurse and family can assist in understanding and expressing hope. Love can best be expressed through kind, compassionate care.

Ways the nurse or family can provide spiritual comfort include therapeutic communication skills, expressing empathy, praying with the client, reading inspirational literature, and playing music. Prayer should not be used to avoid the client or the dying process. Reciting prayers or praying as a means to close a discussion does not address the client's feelings (Conrad, 1985).

It is important for the nurse to feel comfortable about personal spiritual beliefs and values before offering support to the client. Attentive listening encourages the client to express feelings, clarify them and accept death. When clients seek clergy and do not have their own, the nurse makes referrals.

SUPPORT FOR THE GRIEVING FAMILY

Family members must be supported through the dying and death of the client and, at the same time, be encouraged to provide support to the client. In an institutional setting the family has greater difficulty giving support. The nurse must recognize the value of family members as resources and assist them in working with the dying person.

In the home the family becomes closely involved in the client's care. A terminal illness places heavy demands on a family's social and financial resources. The emotional strain often disrupts normal communication channels. The family may become afraid to interact with the client. Benoliel (1985) describes circumstances that make

---

Suggestions for Involving the Family in the Care of a Dying Client

- Assist in planning a visitation schedule for family members to prevent client and family from becoming fatigued.
- Allow young children to visit a dying parent when the client is able to communicate.
- Be willing to listen to family complaints about the client's care, as well as positive or negative feelings about the client.
- Help family members learn how to interact with the dying person (for example, using attentive listening, avoiding false reassurances, conducting conversations about normal family activities or problems).
- Allow family members to help with simple care measures such as feeding, bathing, and straightening bed linen. Family members are often more successful than nursing staff in persuading the client to eat.
- When the family becomes fatigued with care activities, relieve them from their duties so they can acquire needed rest and support. Refer them to resources for meals and lodging.
- Support the act of grieving between client and family. Provide privacy when preferred. Do not discourage open expression of grief between family and client.
- Provide information daily with regard to the client's condition. Prepare the family for sudden changes in the client's appearance and behavior.
- Communicate news of impending death when the family is together if possible. Members can provide support for one another. Convey the news in a private area and be willing to stay with the family.
- At the time of death, help the family stay in communication with the dying person through short visits, caring silence, touch, and telling the client of their love for him.
- After death assist the family with decision making, such as selection of a mortician, transportation of family members, and collection of the client's belongings.

---

it difficult for families to cope with demands of terminal illness. These include a lengthy period of dying, symptoms that are difficult to control, unpleasant sights and smells, limited coping resources, poor relationships with care givers, and a dying child.

Acknowledging a family's grief is the nurse's first step in helping to develop a supportive relationship with families. The family will sense the nurse's concern and be more willing to share feelings. When the client is in a hospital the nurse can ease family anxieties and fears by explaining equipment used in the client's care. Most families want to know where a tube or equipment is located in the body, if it hurts, why is it needed, and when it is to be removed (Johnson, 1986).

Before using family members as resources the nurse must determine if the family wants to be involved. Some will not. The nurse assesses what the family's role will be: observer, comforter, or caregiver. Their roles may change often. The box offers recommendations for family involvement.

HOSPICE CARE

A desire to change traditional care for the dying led to hospice programs. A hospice program is family-centered care designed to assist the terminally ill to be comfortable and maintain a satisfactory life-style through the phases of dying. Most clients in hospice programs have 6 months or less to live. Hospice programs began in England and reached the United States and Canada in the 1970s.

There are several hospice programs. Acute care hospitals and long term care facilities often have separate units or dedicated beds for hospice care. A trained interdisciplinary team works with clients and families. The home care component of a hospice is operated either by a hospital or separate home health agency. There are also independent hospices that care only for the terminally ill. Home health agencies and skilled nursing facilities also operate hospice programs.

Pitorak (1985) describes the following nine components of hospice care:

1. Coordinated home care with available inpatient beds under hospital administration
2. Control of symptoms (physical, sociological, psychological, and spiritual)
3. Physician-directed services
4. Provision of an interdisciplinary care team composed of physicians, nurses, clergy, social workers, and counselors
5. Medical and nursing services available at all times
6. Client and family are the unit of care
7. Bereavement follow-up after a client's death
8. Use of trained volunteers as a part of the team
9. Clients accepted into the program on basis of health care needs rather than ability to pay

A hospice program emphasizes palliative treatment and the control of symptoms rather than curative treatment of disease (Aroskar, 1985). The client and family participate in care. Client care is well coordinated between the home and inpatient setting. Efforts are directed at keeping the client at home as much as possible. The family becomes the care giver, administering med-

---

Tissues and Organs Used for Transplant

NONVITAL TISSUES

- Corneas, skin, long bones, middle ear bones

VITAL ORGANS

- Heart, liver, lung, kidney, pancreas (Recovered after a client is pronounced clinically dead or brain dead, circulatory and ventilatory support is maintained to perfuse the organs before removal.)

---

ication and treatment, while the interdisciplinary team provides psychological and physical resources needed for family support.

Care After Death

The physician is responsible for certifying a client's death in the medical record. The time of death and a description of therapies or actions taken are described in the medical record. The physician may request permission from the family for an autopsy. Autopsies are required in circumstances of unusual death (for example, violent trauma or unexpected death in the home). A trained staff member, often a nurse, asks the family or guardian for organ or tissue donation when the client is a suitable donor (see box). State laws govern the procedure for documenting tissue and organ requests.

The nurse may be the best person to care for the client's body after death because of the therapeutic nurse-client relationship and therefore may be more sensitive to the need of caring for the body with dignity and sensitivity. After death the body undergoes many physical changes (Table 26-5). The body should be cared for as soon as possible after death to prevent tissue damage or disfigurement of body parts. If the family requests organ donation, correct measures must be taken immediately. For example, small ice packs placed over the client's closed eyelids help preserve corneal tissues before enucleation.

If family members ask to view the body, the nurse prepares the room and body to minimize the stress of the experience. The nurse removes supplies and equipment from sight. Tubes remaining in the body are either removed, clamped, or cut to within 2.5 cm (1 inch) of the skin and taped in place. Care of tubes and specimens depends on whether an autopsy is to be performed and agency policy. Dirty linen and other clutter should be

TABLE 26-5 Physiological Changes after Death

Change	Related Interventions
Stiffening of body (rigor mortis), developing in 2 to 4 hours after death; involves contraction of skeletal and smooth muscle owing to lack of Adenosinetriphosphate (ATP).	Before rigor mortis develops, position body in normal anatomical alignment, close eyelids and mouth, insert dentures in mouth.
Reduction in body temperature with loss of skin elasticity (algor mortis).	Remove tape and dressings gently to avoid tissue breakdown. Avoid pulling on skin or body parts.
Purple discoloration of skin (livor mortis) in dependent areas owing to breakdown of red blood cells.	Elevate head to prevent discoloration.
Body tissues soften and liquify by bacterial fermentation.	Store body in cool place in hospital morgue or other designated area.

removed. A spray deodorizer will eliminate unpleasant odors in the room.

The nurse prepares the body by making it look as natural and comfortable as possible. If it is placed in a supine position with arms at the sides, palms down, or across the abdomen, a mortician can better prepare the body for interment. The nurse places a small pillow or folded towel under the head to prevent discoloration from blood pooling. The eyelids will usually remain closed, if gently held down for a few seconds. If this does not work, a moistened cotton ball will hold the eyelids in place.

The nurse inserts the client's dentures to maintain normal facial features. A rolled-up towel under the chin will help keep the mouth closed.

The nurse washes soiled body parts, dresses the body in a clean gown, combs or brushes the hair, and covers the body to the shoulders with clean linen. Most shroud kits contain absorbent pads that are placed under the perineal and rectal area to collect oozing feces or urine from relaxed sphincter muscles. The nurse removes jewelry and presents it and other valuables to the family. In some agencies a single wedding band may be left in place as long as it is taped securely to the finger. After the body is prepared, the family is allowed into the room. When possible, the nurse should not allow a single family member to enter alone. The nurse or another family member should be there to provide emotional support. It is important not to rush the family while they spend time with the deceased.

After the family leaves, the nurse places tags containing name and other information on the client's wrist and ankle or toe. The gown is removed, and the body is wrapped completely in a shroud, a large rectangular piece of plastic or cotton material. Another identification tag is placed on the shroud. If a client had transmissible infection, special labeling may be used to alert those who move and store the remains. The body is then either transported to the morgue for cooling, or the mortician picks it up from the client's room. Methods for transporting the body through hallways vary between institutions.

Nursing personnel are also responsible for disposition of the deceased's personal belongings and noting this in the medical record. The nurse can check with the client's family about taking the belongings or ensure that they are transported with the deceased. If the family or friends have left, contact a supervisor. Do not discard any clothing, dentures, plants, gifts, hair pieces, or other personal items.

EVALUATION

Although resolution of grief may require months or even years, most clients are under a nurse's care only a short time. The nurse may become frustrated when, just as the client or family begins to express grief, the client leaves the health care institution or dies. Greiving is an individual process, and resolution of loss does not follow a set schedule. To evaluate nursing care for a greiving client or family, it is important for the client to discuss and share the experience with significant others. The nurse also observes the quality of interactions (see evaluation box).

The care of the dying client requires that the nurse evaluate whether the client has accepted fate and whether the nurse was able to sustain the quality of life. The success of the nurse's evaluation will partly depend on the bond formed with the client. Unless the client trusts the nurse, expression of true feelings and concerns is unlikely. The client's level of comfort is evaluated on the basis of physiologic outcomes such as a reduction in pain, control of symptoms, and maintenance of functioning body systems.

Sample Evaluation of Interventions for Grieving

Goals	Evaluative Measures	Expected Outcomes
Client resolves grief and accepts reality of loss.	Observe client discussing loss with a significant other.	Client discusses feelings related to loss.
	Observe client's behaviors.	Client expresses emotions of sorrow, anger.
	Ask client to talk about feelings of loss.	Client describes meaning the loss has for him or her.
Client gains sense of self-esteem.	Observe client's personal appearance and grooming habits.	Client maintains neat, well-groomed appearance.
	Observe client's willingness to interact with others.	Client initiates discussion with nurse and significant others about the future.
Client returns to routines of daily living.	Observe client's involvement in self-care activities.	Client resumes self-care activities.
	Ask client to discuss future plans.	Client verbalizes decisions about care.
		Client discusses or makes plans to return to work or school, as appropriate.
	Evaluate with family members the client's level of participation in social activities.	Client participates in more social activities.

SUMMARY

Categories of loss include loss of an aspect of self, external objects, a significant other, that experienced in separation from a known environment, and loss of life. Nurses interact daily with clients and families experiencing loss. Knowledge of the concepts and theories concerning loss, death, and the grieving process provides a framework for the nursing process. The nurse's responses and interactions with the grieving client and family create the climate for openness in expressing grief. The nurse explores the strengths of the client and support systems available through listening, being available when needed, and conveying respect for the client's values and beliefs. A trust relationship creates a therapeutic environment that encourages expression of grief and fosters the client's sense of dignity and self-esteem. The nurse's understanding promotes growth and paves the way for effective nursing care of grieving or dying clients and their families.

KEY CONCEPTS

✓ A loss is the absence of an object, person, body part or function, or emotion.

✓ The grieving process involves a set of emotional, cognitive, and behavioral responses to an actual or perceived loss.

✓ The purpose of grieving is to achieve more effective functioning.

✓ Individuals experience different aspects of the grieving process at different times.

✓ The phases of the grieving process vary among theories but progress from distress and shock to resolution and acceptance.

✓ Dying may lead to a grief response similar to that with other kinds of losses.

✓ A nurse's support of a client's hope can help relieve grieving associated with a loss.

✓ The individual's loss reaction is influenced by many factors including developmental stage, beliefs, roles, relationships, and socioeconomic status.

✓ Assessment of the grieving client considers behavioral characteristics that suggest the client's stage of grieving.

✓ There are risk factors that predict whether a person in grief will suffer psychological or physical illness during bereavement.

✓ Nursing diagnoses focus on the type of grief experienced by clients or health-related problems common to grieving clients.

✓ Therapeutic communication is an important nursing intervention to assist both the grieving and the dying client in coping with loss.

✓ Nursing care of the grieving and dying client should promote the client's sense of identity, dignity, and self-esteem.

✓ Nursing interventions to promote a return to life activities assist the client in resolving grief and accepting the loss.

✓ Nursing care of the terminally ill client focuses on promoting comfort and improving the quality of remaining life.

✓ As death approaches, a client reviews and analyzes values and beliefs pertinent to the meaning of life and death.

✓ A nurse must assess whether a family member is willing to be involved in a dying client's care before using the family member as a resource.

✓ Care after death involves caring for the body with dignity and sensitivity.

✓ The evaluation of nursing care for the grieving and dying client is ongoing and based on identifiable behavioral changes through the grieving process.

REFERENCES

Anderson, J: Nursing management of the cancer patient in pain: a review of the literature, Canc Nurs 5:33, 1982.

Aroskar, MA: Access to hospice—ethical dimensions, Nurs Clin North Am 20:299, 1985.

Benoliel, JQ: Loss and terminal illness, Nurs Clin North Am 20:439, 1985.

Conrad, NL: Spiritual support for the dying, Nurs Clin North Am 20:415, 1985.

Davitz, L, and Davitz, J: Nurses' responses to patients' suffering, New York, 1980, Springer Publishing Co.

Dufault, K, and Martocchio, BC: Hope: its spheres and dimensions, Nurs Clin North Am 20:379, 1985.

Engel, GL: Grief and grieving, Am J Nurs 64:93, 1964.

Gonda, TA: Coping with dying and death, Geriatrics 26:71, 1971.

Johnson, SH: 10 ways to help the family of a critically ill patient, Nurs 86 16:50, 1986.

Kübler-Ross, E: On death and dying, New York, 1969, Macmillan, Inc.

Lewis, K: Grief in chronic illness and disability, J Rehabil 49:8, 1983.

Martocchio, BC: Grief and bereavement: healing through hurt, Nurs Clin North Am 20:327, 1985.

McGrory, A: A well model approach to care of the dying client, New York, 1978, McGraw-Hill Book Co.

Oncology Nursing Society and the American Nurses' Association: Outcome standards for cancer nursing practice, Kansas City, Mo., 1979, American Nurses' Association.

Pitorak, EF: Establishing a medicare-certified inpatient unit, Nurs Clin North Am 20:311, 1985.

Schowalter, JE: Parent death and child bereavement. In Schoenberg B, et al.: Bereavement: Its psychosocial aspects, New York, 1975, Columbia University Press.

Werner-Beland, JA: Grief response of long term illness and disability, Reston, Va., 1980, Reston Publishing Co., Inc.

Worden, JW: Grief counseling and grief therapy, New York, 1982, Springer Publishing Co.

Research Article

Hampe, SO: Needs of the grieving spouse in a hospital setting, Nurs Res 24:113, 1975.

ADDITIONAL READINGS

Ames, B: Art and a dying patient, Am J Nurs 80:1094, 1980.

Buturusis, B, et al.: Assessing health needs: the well elderly, J Gerontol Nurs 12(6):11-14, 1986.

Castles, MR, and Murray, RB: Dying in an institution: nurse patient perspectives, New York, 1979, Appleton-Century-Crofts.

Ebersole, P, and Hess, P: Toward healthy aging: human needs and nursing responses, ed. 2, St. Louis, 1986, The C.V. Mosby Co.

Engel, GL: Psychological development in health and disease, Philadelphia, 1962, W.B. Saunders Co.

Evans, MA, Esbenson, M, and Jaffe, C: Expect the unexpected when you care for a dying patient, Nurs 81 11:55, 1981.

Fairbairn, W: Synoposis of an object-relations theory of the personality, Int J Psychoanal 44:244, 1963.

Groves, J: Differentiating grief, mourning and bereavement, Am J Psychiatry 135:(7):875, 1978.

Kalish, RA: Death, grief, and caring relationships, ed. 2, Monterey, Calif., 1985, Brooks-Cole Publishing Co.

Kim, MJ, et al.: Pocket guide to nursing diagnoses, St. Louis, 1987, The C.V. Mosby Co.

Lee, R: Object loss and counseling the bereaved. In Fruehling, J, editor: Sourcebook on death and dying, Chicago, Ill., 1982, Marquis Professional Publications.

Lindemann, E: Symptomatology and management of acute grief. In Parad, H, editor: Crisis intervention, New York, 1965, Family Association of America.

Marino, L: Cancer nursing, St. Louis, 1981, The C.V. Mosby Co.

Miles, HS, and Hays, DR: Widowhood, Am J Nurs 75:280, 1975.

Moseley, JR: Alterations in comfort, Nurs Clin North Am 20:427 1985.

Mulhern, RM: When there's no treatment left but the truth, RN, 49:26, 1986.

Musgrave, CF: The ethical and legal implications of hospice care: an international overview, Canc Nurs 10:183, 1987.

Reed, PG: Religiousness among terminally ill and healthy adults, Res Nurs Health 9:35, 1986.

Rothman, DA, and Rothman, NL: The professional nurse and the law, Boston, 1977, Little, Brown & Co.

Smith, S, and Duell, D: Nursing skills and evaluation: a nursing process approach, Los Altos, Calif., 1982, National Nursing Review.

Stickney, SK, and Gardner, ER: Companions in suffering, Am J Nurs 84:1491, 1984.

Stockdale, L, and Hutzenbiler, T: How you can comfort a grieving family, Nurs Life 23, 1986.

Taylor, PB, and Gideon, MD: Holding out hope to your dying patient, Nursing 82 12:42, 1982.

Tyner, R: Elements of empathetic care for dying patients and their families, Nurs Clin North Am 20:393, 1985.

Wegmann, JA: Hospice home death, hospital death, and coping abilities of widows, Canc Nurs 10:148, 1987.

Zach, MV: Loneliness: A concept relevant to the care of dying persons, Nurs Clin North Am 20:403, 1985.

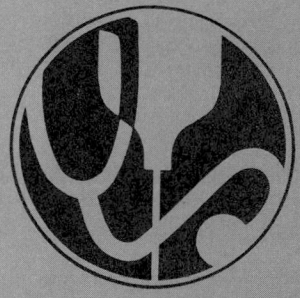

UNIT 6

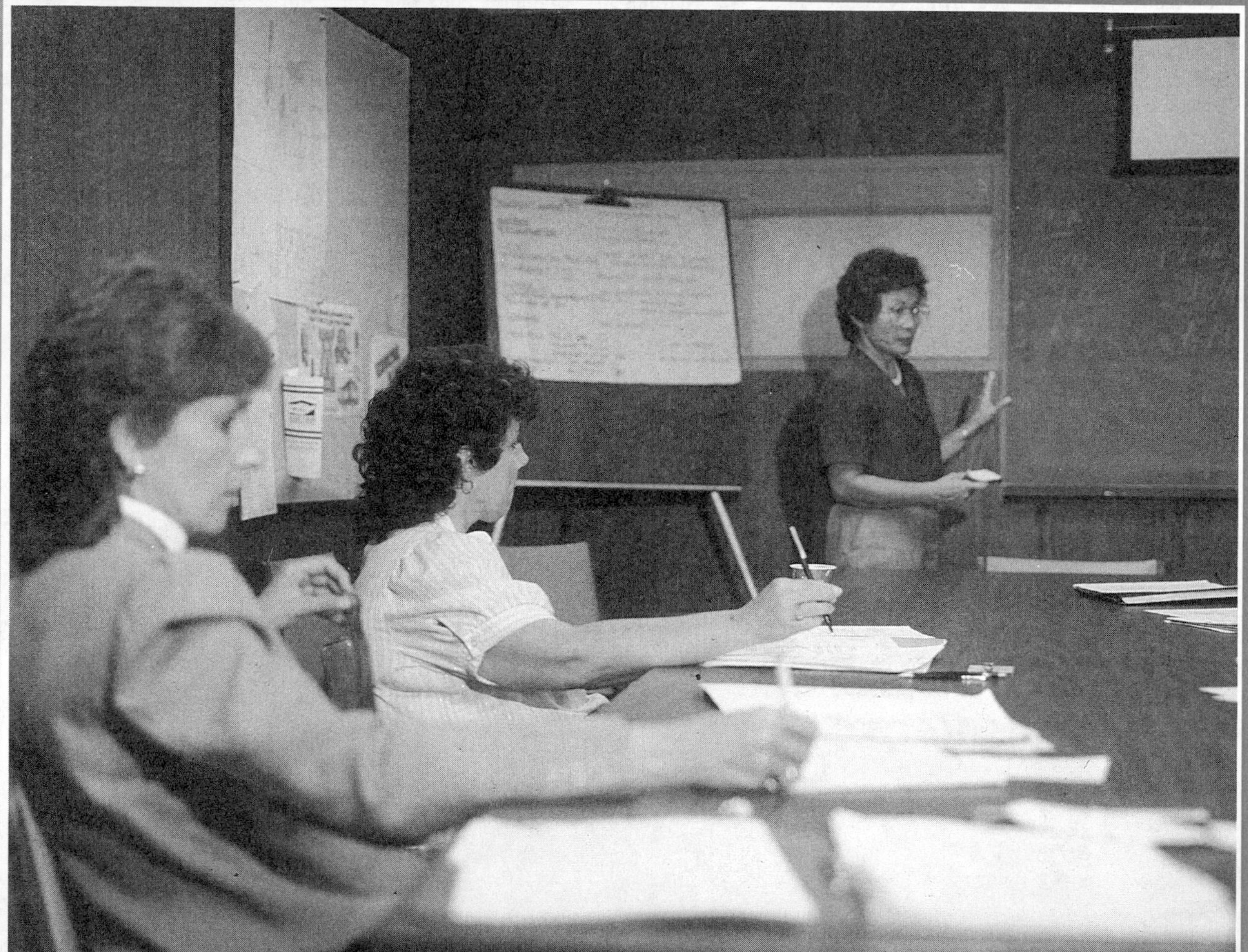

Human Needs in Health and Illness

Nurses have the opportunity to address clients' human needs, including psychosocial and physiological, on all levels. By recognizing that clients are complex, multidimensional individuals, nurses can provide holistic health care in these areas by using the nursing process.

The five chapters in Unit 6 consider the human needs frequently encountered in nursing practice. The nurse's knowledge of basic needs and the person's response and adaptation to stress is fundamental in helping clients maintain or regain good health. Illness or other problems may also result in alterations in self-concept or body image or may adversely affect the sexual dimension. Similarly, illness may threaten the client's spirituality, or the client's spiritual resources may help in coping with the stresses of illness.

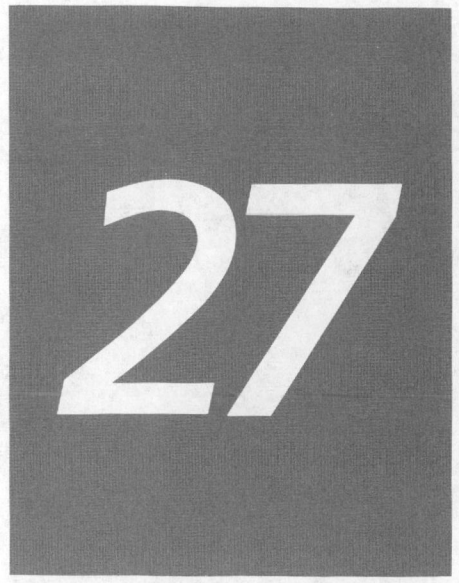

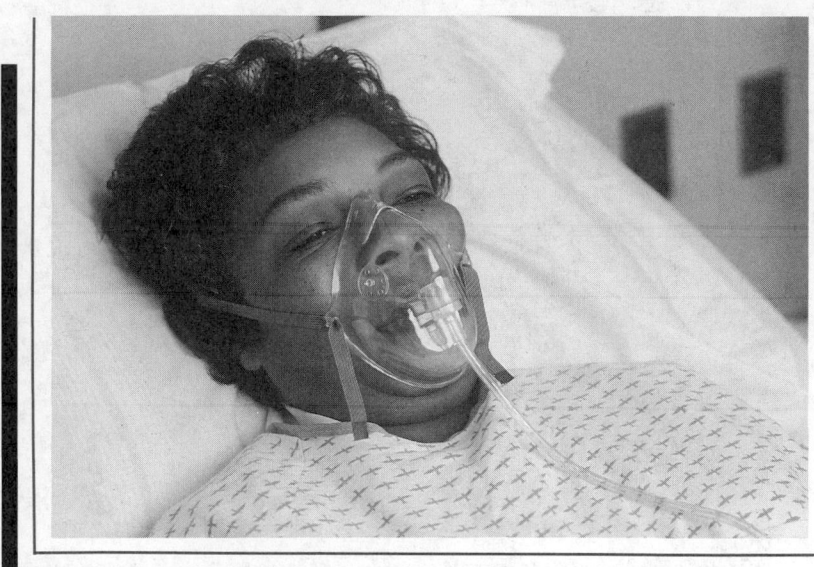

OBJECTIVES

Mastery of content in this chapter will enable the student to:

- Define the key terms listed.
- Discuss each component of Maslow's hierarchy of needs.
- Describe assessment techniques for identifying unmet needs.
- Identify actual or potential conditions that threaten fulfillment of a client's needs.
- Identify nursing diagnoses appropriate for unmet basic needs.
- Describe the basic nursing implications concerning unmet needs.
- Describe relationships among the different levels of needs.
- State factors that influence the individual client's need priorities.

KEY TERMS

Aerobic Metabolism

Anaerobic Metabolism

Basic Human Needs

Carbon Dioxide

Cyanosis

Dehydration

Edema

Frostbite

Hierarchy of Basic Human Needs

Physiological Needs

Safety and Security Needs

Self-Actualization

Self-Esteem

Basic Human Needs

Basic human needs are those things, such as food, water, safety, and love, that are necessary for survival and health. Although each person has other, unique needs, these are shared by all. The extent to which a person's basic needs are met is a major factor in determining level of health and position on the health-illness continuum (see Chapter 2). Nurses are therefore concerned that the basic human needs of clients are being met.

Abraham Maslow's hierarchy of needs is a theory nurses can use to understand the relationships among basic human needs when providing nursing care. Maslow assigned priorities to basic needs. According to his theory, certain human needs are more basic than others; that is, some needs must be met before the individual directs attention to meeting others. For example, a starving person is more likely to seek food than to engage in activities that increase self-esteem. The hierarchy of human needs arranges the basic needs in five levels of priority (Fig. 27-1). On the most basic, or first, level are physiological needs such as air, water, and food. On the second level are safety and security needs, including the need for both physical and psychological security. On the third level are needs for love and a sense of belonging, including needs for friendship, social relationships, and sexual love. On the fourth level is the need for self-esteem, self-confidence, usefulness, achievement, and self-worth. The final level is the need for what Maslow calls self-actualization, the state of fully achieving one's potential and having the ability to solve problems and cope realistically with life's situations.

At any time an individual's basic human needs may

687

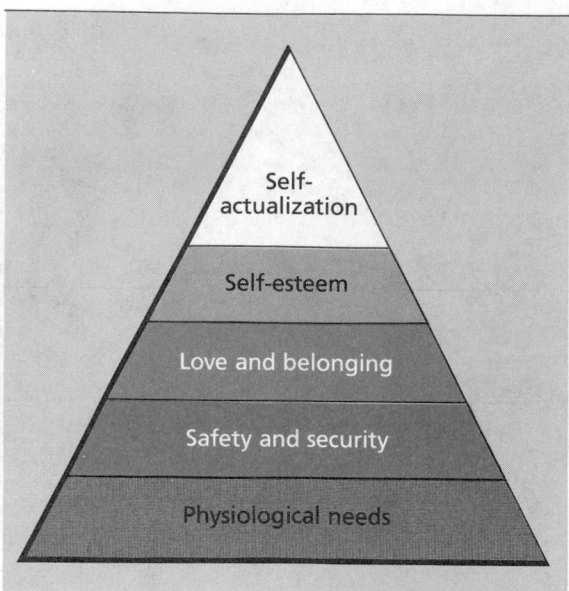

Fig. 27-1 Maslow's hierarchy of needs.

be unmet, partially met, or wholly fulfilled. According to this theory, a person whose needs are all met is healthy, and a person with one or more unmet needs is at risk for illness or may be unhealthy in one or more of the human dimensions.

The hierarchy of needs is a theoretical model; that is, the priorities given human needs are *generally* true of people but not necessarily true of all individuals. Thus the hierarchy of needs can still be applied to individuals who seem to have different priorities. In providing care to those with unmet needs, the nurse should always take into account the individual's priorities, as well as other factors, such as environment and social interactions, that influence how well needs can be met.

Clients entering the health care system generally have unmet needs or may be unable to continue meeting their needs. A person brought to an emergency room with a cardiac arrest has an unmet need for air, the most basic physiological need. An elderly female client in a high crime neighborhood may be concerned about physical safety and while hospitalized may have a need for psychological security from fear that her home will be burglarized. A widowed homemaker whose children have moved away may feel that she does not belong or is not loved. Nurses in all practice settings encounter clients whose needs are actually or potentially unmet. Nursing care includes helping clients, and often the family, meet these needs.

The hierarchy of needs is a useful way for nurses to evaluate and understand the needs and behaviors of clients. Although one need may take priority and the nurse often must first be concerned with it (such as re-

storing an adequate airway before helping the client adjust to an emotional conflict), the nurse simultaneously assesses needs on different levels. An example is assisting a client meet the need for social belonging while also helping achieve adequate nutrition. The nurse assesses the client's needs and then considers how nursing care can best help meet them.

PHYSIOLOGICAL NEEDS

Physiological needs have the highest priority in Maslow's hierarchy. An individual who has several unmet needs generally seeks first to fulfill physiological needs (Maslow, 1970). For example, a person who lacks food, safety, and love usually searches for food before seeking love.

Physiological needs are for things necessary or important for survival. Humans have eight such needs; oxygen, fluid, nutrition, temperature, elimination, shelter, rest, and sex.

An infant requires someone to meet its needs for food, shelter, fluids, adequate temperature, and elimination. As the individual grows and progresses developmentally, the ability to satisfy physiological needs is increased. A 2-year-old who wants a drink of water usually knows where water is and how to get it. Although the child's efforts may not be very efficient, if the motivation is great enough and no one else will meet the need, the need will be met. Healthy adults are usually able to meet physiological needs without assistance.

The very young, very old, poor, ill, and handicapped frequently depend on others for meeting basic physiological needs. The nurse often has a role in helping the client meet physiological needs.

Oxygen

Oxygen is the most essential physiological need. The body depends on oxygen for moment-to-moment survival. Some tissues, such as skeletal muscles, can survive for a time without oxygen through anaerobic metabolism, a process by which these tissues provide their own energy in the absence of oxygen. In long-distance running, for example, the runner's skeletal muscles undergo anaerobic metabolism so that the available oxygen can be used by more vital organs—the heart, brain, and lungs.

Tissues that carry out only aerobic metabolism, the process of providing energy in the presence of oxygen, depend totally on oxygen for survival. The brain, for example, cannot function without oxygen for longer than 4 to 5 minutes.

Oxygen must be adequately delivered from the environment to the lungs, the bloodstream, and finally the tissues. At any point in the life span, clients are at risk for not meeting their oxygen needs. The need can be acute, as with a cardiac arrest, or chronic, as with the disease emphysema.

ASSESSMENT

Nurses continually evaluate clients' oxygenation to determine if this need is being met. This assessment is basically the same in chronic and acute situations (see Chapter 13). The client may be confused or lethargic because the level of oxygen in blood and tissues is decreased. When oxygen needs are unmet, a person is unable to lie flat because of air hunger and is forced to remain upright so gravity can assist in lung expansion. The client breathes quickly to deliver more oxygen to the lungs, and respirations are usually shallow. Frequently, this effort fatigues the client rather than meets the need for oxygenation. Other signs of inadequate oxygenation include nasal flaring and sternal, substernal, and suprasternal retractions, so that the client appears to be tugging for air.

Clients with a progressive long-term decrease in tissue oxygen show cyanosis, a bluish discoloration of skin and mucous membranes caused by decreased oxygen in the blood. Cyanosis is a late sign of poor oxygenation, so the nurse should be aware of the earlier, more subtle indicators.

NURSING IMPLICATIONS

Because many organs such as the brain and heart cannot survive without oxygen, oxygen has the highest priority of all physiological needs. The nurse must be able to identify a client's need for oxygen and to assist in meeting this need. The problem can be corrected in some instances by controlling anxiety, which causes a tendency to hyperventilate. This decreases the intake of oxygen and increases the expiration of carbon dioxide. The person will become more anxious and confused and feel a tingling of the hands and feet, numbness around the lips, and dizziness. The nurse helps control the imbalance of respiratory gases by having a client breathe into a paper bag, which will cause the client to rebreathe carbon dioxide and slow the respiratory rate. Once the client has adequate oxygen, the nurse may use reassurance, teaching, and counseling to help control anxiety.

In other instances the nurse uses specific techniques to help the client meet oxygen needs. For example, a 50-year-old man has a long smoking history and a medical diagnosis of chronic obstructive pulmonary disease. He has chronic breathlessness and requires 1 liter per minute of oxygen every night administered through nasal cannulae. Because of the client's frequent breathlessness, the nurse first helps plan daily care activities so that there is adequate opportunity to meet needs for hygiene, nutrition, and rest. The nurse also teaches the client how

to rest in a position that increases respiratory volume and thus the level of oxygen.

Nursing measures to meet the oxygen needs range from emergency cardiopulmonary resuscitation for cardiac arrest to supportive measures such as administering oxygen to clients with pulmonary disease during exercise. Chapter 36 discusses in detail measures necessary for meeting oxygen needs of clients.

Fluids

The human body requires a balance between intake and output of fluids. Fluids are taken in by mouth or parenterally and fluids leave the body from the intestines, lungs, and skin and as urine from the kidney. Clients of any age can have unmet fluid needs, but the very young and very old have the greatest risk. Severely ill, traumatized, or handicapped clients are also more likely to have unmet fluid needs.

Two conditions indicate unmet fluid needs: dehydration and edema. Dehydration is the excessive loss of water from body tissues and is accompanied by a disturbance of body electrolytes. Dehydration may result from excessive and prolonged fever, vomiting, diarrhea, trauma, or any condition that causes a rapid fluid loss. Edema is the abnormal accumulation of fluid in interstitial spaces of tissues, the pericardial sac, the intrapleural space, the peritoneal cavity, or joint capsules. Edema is also accompanied by a disturbance of electrolytes and may occur in a nutritional, cardiovascular, renal, malignant, traumatic, or other disorder that results in a rapid accumulation of fluids.

ASSESSMENT

The nurse examines clients for actual or potential fluid imbalance. A number of signs and symptoms can reveal dehydration: poor skin turgor, flushed dry skin, decreased tearing or salivation, coated tongue, decreased urine output, confusion, and irritability. Skin turgor is the normal elasticity of the skin, which becomes lax with dehydration; when grasped and raised between two fingers, the skin only slowly returns to its former position (see Chapter 13).

The dehydrated client's skin is dry because the body transfers fluid that is present to the circulation and more vital organs. The skin may be flushed because of an elevated body temperature that can accompany dehydration. The tongue is coated and dry. A person may cry but not have tears. Oliguria, a diminished ability of the kidneys to form and excrete urine, is frequently caused by dehydration.

Because of the fluid and associated electrolyte imbalances, mental status is altered, and the client may be irritable and confused. In cases of severe dehydration the client may even be comatose.

Excessive body fluids is most commonly manifest as edema. Edema may be caused by decreased serum protein, severe burns, altered functioning of the cardiovascular, renal, or hepatic system, or drugs. Edema is first observed in lower body regions; when the person is standing, the edema is seen in feet and legs. The client with edema may also have a daily weight gain, shortness of breath, or an increased heart rate.

NURSING IMPLICATIONS

The overall nursing goal for clients with unmet fluid needs is to restore body fluid and electrolyte balances. The nurse uses simple or complex measures to meet this goal. For example, if the client has diarrhea without vomiting, an appropriate nursing intervention is to increase the client's oral intake of fluids. If fluid loss is greater, as with a severe burn, nursing interventions are more complex and include intravenous administration of fluids.

If the client has excess fluids, nursing actions restrict the client's fluid intake and facilitate elimination of fluids from the body. In addition, the skin of a client with excessive body fluids is smooth and shiny and susceptible to skin breakdown. The nurse must provide meticulous skin care and establish an appropriate turning schedule to reduce the risk of breakdown.

Chapter 37 describes in detail the knowledge and techniques the nurse needs for restoring fluid, electrolyte, and acid-base balances.

Nutrition

The human body has an essential need for nutrients, although it can survive without food longer than without oxygen and fluids. Like other physiological needs, nutritional needs may be unmet in a person of any age.

The body's metabolic processes control digestion, storage of nutrients, and elimination of waste products. Digestion and storage of nutrients are essential in meeting the body's nutritional demands.

After food is eaten, digestive processes break down nutrients into usable compounds such as glucose, amino acids, and fatty acids, which meet immediate nutritional needs. Glucose is a body sugar that satisfies immediate energy requirements. Nutrients not needed immediately are stored as glycogen, protein, or fat.

When a person skips a meal, eats insufficiently or sporadically, or fasts, the body uses its stored reserves to meet nutritional needs. Glycogen, stored in the liver and muscles, is used first because it is readily available and can be quickly converted to glucose. If the person still has not eaten when glycogen is depleted, the body begins to use stored protein and fat.

The body also needs vitamins and minerals to function with full efficiency. For example, deficiencies in vitamin C impair wound healing. Deficiencies in calcium and vitamin D retard bone growth and bone metabolism.

ASSESSMENT

To determine whether a client is meeting nutritional needs, the nurse considers many factors in addition to body weight. Clients with appropriate body weight may still have nutritional deficits. Nutritional assessment should include measurement of body muscle mass, laboratory data, food intake patterns, as well as the client's weight.

Signs and symptoms indicating that a client is not meeting nutritional needs include failure to grow or gain weight, unplanned weight loss, fatigue, pallor, and recurring mouth and gum sores.

NURSING IMPLICATIONS

Clients require adequate nutrition to carry out activities of daily living, promote wound healing, and maintain wellness. In some cases the nurse takes a direct role in meeting the client's nutritional needs. For example, when caring for an infant with the syndrome known as the failure to thrive, the nurse and the health care team assume total responsibility for the child's nutrition.

Sometimes a nurse assists in meeting nutritional needs through a teaching role. An adult with recently diagnosed insulin-dependent diabetes mellitus, for example, needs to be taught to balance nutritional needs, insulin intake, and exercise habits.

To help clients meet their nutritional needs, the nurse must understand digestive and metabolic processes of the body. The nurse may use various nutritional supplements and techniques to correct nutritional deficits. Chapter 33 discusses in detail nursing measures related to the nutritional needs of clients.

Temperature

The body can function normally within only a narrow temperature range, between 35° C (97° F) and 41° C (106° F) (Mountcastle, 1980). Body temperatures outside this range can result in injuries, and permanent effects such as brain damage, or death.

The body can temporarily regulate temperature by certain mechanisms. For example, a person shivers when moving from a warm environment to one of 55° F. This adaptive response can temporarily increase body temperature. Chapter 12 discusses other responses.

ASSESSMENT

The body has a physiological response to extreme temperatures. Prolonged exposure to cold decreases the body's rate of metabolism and use of oxygen. If body temperature is lowered beyond the point at which the body can adapt, vital signs decrease, consciousness decreases, the person is more difficult to arouse, skin is pale and cold, and urinary output decreases. A localized exposure to cold, as occurs when hands are bare in the winter, leads to frostbite (see Chapter 12). Frostbite is a traumatic effect of extreme cold on the skin and subcutaneous tissues and is first displayed as distinct pallor. Blood circulation in the area is impaired, leading to decreased oxygen in tissues. This may cause tissue death.

Prolonged exposure to heat increases the body's metabolic activity and increases tissue oxygen demand. Extreme or prolonged heat exposure can also have specific physiological effects. Local exposure to heat can result in first-, second-, or third-degree burns. Overexposure to sun can lead to sunstroke, which is characterized by high fever, convulsions, and coma (see Chapter 12). Elderly persons living in poorly ventilated homes without air conditioning are at risk for heatstroke during prolonged hot weather. Symptoms are an elevated body temperature, dehydration, and fluid and electrolyte imbalances. If untreated the person becomes disoriented and confused, enters a coma, and dies.

NURSING IMPLICATIONS

Nursing care for clients exposed to extreme heat or cold is directed toward restoring normal body temperature. In addition, the nurse helps clients avoid exposure to heat or cold.

To treat frostbite, the nurse gently warms the affected area. Do not rub the area in an attempt to increase circulation, since this can further damage skin and underlying tissues.

A client with sunstroke needs emergency treatment to reduce body temperature. Nursing measures include a tepid sponge bath, fluid replacements, and medications.

Elimination

The elimination of waste materials is one of the body's metabolic processes. Waste products are eliminated by the lungs, skin, kidneys, and intestines.

The lungs primarily eliminate carbon dioxide (CO_2). This is gas formed during tissue metabolism. Most CO_2 formed by tissue metabolism is carried to the lungs by the venous system and excreted through breathing. If a client has difficulty eliminating CO_2, as with acidbase imbalances that originate in the respiratory system, nursing measures are needed to prevent severe impairment or death (see Chapter 36). The water eliminated by the lungs daily amounts to about 200 ml. The nurse considers this in calculating fluid needs of a dehydrated client.

Skin eliminates water and sodium, most noticeably as sweat. This also assists in temperature regulation because evaporation of sweat lowers the body temperature. Sweat cannot always be seen, but the skin excretes water continuously, about 200 ml a day. A client with fever or prolonged exposure to hot humid weather has an increased water loss from skin. The nurse considers water loss from skin when caring for a client with actual or potential dehydration.

The kidneys are the body's primary means of excreting excess body fluids, electrolytes, hydrogen ions, and acids. Urinary elimination normally depends on fluid intake and circulatory blood volume; if either is decreased, urinary output decreases. Urinary output is also changed in persons with kidney disease, which affects both the quantity of urine and the content of waste products within the urine. Kidney disease can be life threatening (see Chapter 38).

The intestines eliminate solid waste products and some fluid from the body. The elimination of solid waste by bowel evacuation usually becomes a pattern at 30 to 36 months of age (see Chapter 39).

ASSESSMENT

A client whose urinary elimination needs are unmet may be incontinent. Incontinence can occur becuse the person is unable to perceive the urge to void, as when waking from general anesthesia or after severe head injury or spinal cord injury. Urinary incontinence may also occur if an immobilized person is unable to reach a bedpan or obtain assistance.

Unmet urinary elimination needs also result in fluid and electrolyte imbalances. A fluid volume loss such as that occurring with dehydration or shock may lead to an imbalance in waste products eliminated by the kidneys. Electrolyte imbalance may result from an acute or chronic kidney disorder.

A client's unmet needs for bowel elimination may lead to changes in the pattern of elimination or diet intake. Changes in bowel elimination patterns include incontinence, constipation, and diarrhea. Altering the diet intake of fluids and foods can also change elimination patterns and needs.

NURSING IMPLICATIONS

Nursing care assists the client in meeting elimination needs. Nursing intervention may be simple, such as providing privacy or changing the diet, or complex, such as inserting a catheter or administering an enema. In helping clients meet urinary and bowel elimination needs, a nurse uses knowledge of anatomy and physiology along with specific skills and techniques. Chapters 38 and 39 describe in detail the knowledge and skills needed to meet urinary and bowel elimination needs of clients.

Shelter

All humans need shelter. Although most people have some kind of shelter, sometimes it is substandard and does not offer full protection from the elements. Disasters such as floods, fire, and tornadoes can render an entire community homeless. Disaster agencies such as the Red Cross are resources in helping clients obtain shelter.

ASSESSMENT

Often the nurse can identify environmental risk factors in a client's home that could lead to shelter needs not being meet. These include exposure to temperature extremes, as in a poorly insulated, drafty home or a poorly ventilated home without air conditioning. Others may involve physical safety of the home and its environment. A home with a leaky roof is inadequate shelter, as is an unprotected home in a high-crime neighborhood.

Clients at risk for unmet shelter needs include those with limited financial, social, and family resources. Frequently such clients are elderly, handicapped, or have limited job skills. Often they feel trapped in their environment because they are unaware of resources that can help them relocate.

In assessing whether a client is meeting shelter needs, the nurse identifies conditions that risk illness or injury. Environments that are dirty may attract insects or rodents which can increase the risk for illness. If a home is poorly lighted or cluttered, there is an increased risk of accidental injury.

NURSING IMPLICATIONS

In many situations it is unrealistic for a nurse to seek new shelter for a client and family. However, the nurse makes referrals to community agencies that can help. Community agencies can establish standards for rental housing and help a client pay utility bills or make home repairs. Such agencies can also help the client identify alternatives for shelter.

The nurse can help the client make changes within the home to make it healthier. For example, grab rails can be installed in a bathroom for a client who has difficulty ambulating and maneuvering. Health promotion often involves teaching clients about the relationship between home environment and health.

Rest

Every person has a basic physiological need for regular rest. The amount of sleep needed varies, depending on the person's quality of sleep, health status, activity patterns, life-style, and age.

A client with chronic disease requires more rest than a healthy person of the same age. Pregnancy and lactation increase the need for rest, as do health status changes such as surgery.

Physical and emotional stress may also increase a client's need for rest. Rest and sleep often provide temporary relief from stress, which can be therapeutic in helping cope with it. But rest can also provide an escape that a client may depend on as a nonproductive method for resolving stress.

ASSESSMENT

With insufficient sleep, a person's appearance and behavior change. Circles under the eyes, pale skin, and disheveled appearance are signs of such change. The person may also have less energy, seem less motivated, be more irritable or withdrawn, stare into space, have difficulty concentrating, and be restless.

NURSING IMPLICATIONS

When possible, the nurse should plan care to fit the client's usual sleep-wake cycle. If the client has habits before retiring, such as walking, bathing, reading, or drinking milk, this should be incorporated into the plan of care.

Frequently a client's pattern of rest is changed by illness or pain. The nurse uses specific methods to promote comfort and relieve pain so that the client's need for rest can be anticipated and met (see Chapters 34 and 35). If the client is unable to sleep and rest because of other factors, such as life-style or chronic stress, the nurse directs care toward resolving the cause while helping meet these needs.

Sex

Sex is considered by Maslow (1970) to be a basic physiological need that generally takes priority over higher-level needs. Sexual needs and the manner in which they are met are influenced by age, sociocultural background, ethics, values, self-esteem, and level of wellness.

Health professions are giving increasing attention to sexuality as a component of health. As nurses become more knowledgeable about clients' sexual needs, nursing care takes them into consideration. Sexuality involves more than physical sex. It may be emotional, social, and spiritual needs. Sexuality can be affected by illness, chronic conditions, and hospitalization.

ASSESSMENT

A client unable to meet sexual needs may, through behavior, indicate that these needs are unmet. Some clients seek alternatives which may not meet sexual needs or may lead to other conflicts, such as excessive sexual language, excessive masturbation, or exposing sexual organs. Other clients flirt or redirect sexual need to physical exercise, overeating, or overwork.

Paralysis, mastectomy, or colostomy are physical conditions that can affect how a person feels about sexuality and the ability to fulfill sexual needs because of a change in physical appearance. This must be accepted by the client and the client's sexual partner. Their sexual behavior, including activities other than those involving sexual organs, may require readjustment.

Clients experiencing depression, grief, or life-style changes are at risk for having unmet sexual needs. For some clients the meeting of sexual needs is only temporarily interrupted. For others, especially those with severe depression, sexual needs are unmet longer and may resolve only with professional counseling.

NURSING IMPLICATIONS

Nursing care designed to help meet needs related to sexuality must consider the client's age, maturity, developmental level, values, habits, level of health, sexual partner, and sexual practices. The nurse must be comfortable discussing sexuality.

Not all nurses feel competent to discuss sexuality with clients, but it is important to recognize when a client is unable to meet sexual needs so that another nurse, physician, or social worker can help. Chapter 30 discusses sexuality in detail.

NURSING DIAGNOSIS

The nurse assesses specific physiological needs, as well as other basic needs. From the assessment, nursing diagnoses are developed by clustering defining and relevant characteristics. For ease of presentation the nursing diagnoses box provides examples of nursing diagnoses for clients with unmet needs. Identification of related factors further specifies the diagnostic statement, thus individualizing it for each client.

The subsequent sections of this chapter describe basic needs and provide general assessment and nursing implications.

SAFETY AND SECURITY NEEDS

Next in priority after physiological needs are needs for physical and psychological safety and security.

Physical Safety

An infant enters the world totally dependent on others for needs and physical safety. As the infant grows and develops, greater independence is gradually achieved. Adults are generally able to provide for their physical safety, but the ill, handicapped, and elderly may need help.

Maintaining physical safety involves reducing or eliminating threats to body or life. The threat may be illness, accident, danger, or environmental exposure. When ill, a client may be vulnerable to complications, such as infection, and therefore depends on professionals in the health care system for protection.

Meeting physical safety needs sometimes takes precedence over a physiological need. For example, a nurse may need to protect a disoriented client from falling out of bed before providing care to meet nutritional needs.

ASSESSMENT

When assessing physical safety needs of a client, the nurse considers actual and potential threats. Clients with limited movement or total immobilization of an extremity are at risk for developing joint contractures, skin breakdown, and muscle atrophy. Clients taking medication are at risk for side effects. Clients with indwelling intravenous lines or Foley catheters are at risk for secondary infections.

Clients with acute or chronic illnesses, disability, or handicaps may need help meeting safety needs. The nurse assesses the total environment, whether it is the client's home or a hospital setting, to identify potential or actual threats.

Health problems in other dimensions may also present a safety risk to a client. A client under emotional stress, for example, may behave in a manner that would potentially threaten his safety. A socially isolated client may be unaware of environmental factors that threaten physical safety.

> ## Examples of Nursing Diagnoses Related to Unmet Needs
>
> ### NANDA-APPROVED NURSING DIAGNOSES
>
> *Impaired gas exchange* related to:
> - Physiological change resulting from escaping gas
> - Slow adaptation to a high-altitude climate
>
> *Potential fluid volume deficit* related to:
> - Excessive water loss
>
> *Altered nutrition: less than body requirements* related to:
> - Lack of finances
> - Poor access to grocery stores
>
> *Activity intolerance* related to:
> - Inadequate nutrition
> - Lack of rest
>
> *Potential for injury* related to:
> - Inadequate safe housing
> - Lack of protection from environmental elements
>
> *Ineffective individual coping* related to:
> - Feelings of loss and loneliness
> - Loss of friends or loved one

NURSING IMPLICATIONS

The early identification of potential threats to a client's physical safety is perhaps the best way to maintain the client's safety. For example, nurses teach parents about common risks to their children through the developmental stages (see Chapters 22, 23, and 40).

The nurse teaches clients receiving medication or therapy about side effects, interaction effects, and potential hazards of treatments, as well as the desired effects. The nurse individualizes education for clients and families to best assist in meeting their needs.

In addition, the nurse increases the client's physical safety in a health care setting by maintaining electric beds in the low position, side rails up, and call light within easy reach. The hospital or home bedroom is uncluttered so that the client can easily move about without risk of injury. Last, frequent observation of the client by the nurse maintains continual assessment of physiological and psychosocial status and complications or threats that can be reduced.

Psychological Safety

To be safe and secure psychologically, a person must understand what to expect from others, including family members and health care professionals. The person must also know what to expect from procedures, new experiences, and encounters within the environment. Everyone feels some threat to psychological safety with new and unfamiliar experiences. A student entering college may feel insecure, a person starting a new job may feel threatened by having to interact with unfamiliar people, and a client about to undergo a diagnostic test may be threatened by the technology involved. In such cases people generally do not directly state that their psychological safety is threatened, but their conversation may indirectly reveal their feelings.

ASSESSMENT

Assessment of psychological safety needs is often difficult because the nurse may have to interpret the client's language and behaviors. Because a perceived threat causes stress, the client may act in various ways to adapt to the stress (see Chapter 28). The client's behavior may change radically. For example, an outgoing, active person may become withdrawn, or a previously cooperative client may suddenly refuse to participate in care. Most clients want to be active and cooperative, and a drastic change in behavior is a clue that some threat to psychological safety may be felt.

NURSING IMPLICATIONS

The nurse can use teaching methods with the client and family to reduce a threat to psychological safety, particularly when the potential threat includes a change in role, a change in body image or an invasive diagnostic or surgical procedure. Because people often fear or have unrealistic expectations about the unknown, telling clients and their families what to expect greatly reduces anxiety and increases their participation in health care.

Healthy adults are generally able to meet physical and physiological safety needs without help from health care professionals. But a person who is ill or handicapped is more susceptible to threats to physical and emotional well-being, so the nurse intervenes to help protect the client from harm.

LOVE AND BELONGING NEEDS

The next priority after physiological and safety needs is the need for love and belonging. People generally need to feel they are loved by their family and that they are accepted by peers and the community. This need generally arises after physiological and safety needs are met, because only when the individual feels safe and secure does he have time and energy to seek love and belonging and to share that love with others (Rogers, 1961).

Even a person who is generally able to meet needs for love and a sense of belonging is often unable to fulfill them when illness or injury occurs. It becomes even more difficult in the hospital. The client is forced to adapt to aspects of the health care delivery system such as organization, routines, environmental limitations, and visiting hours. As a result, there is little time or energy left to meet the needs for love and belonging with family or significant others.

ASSESSMENT

A client of any age in any health care setting may have difficulty meeting love and belonging needs. The ways in which these unmet needs are manifested depend on the client. The client's behavior may be similar to the adaptive behaviors of a person responding to stress.

Discussion with the family and significant others is important as the nurse compares the client's needs for love and belonging with how he normally meets these needs. The nurse may identify changes in the family or in the client's relationship with a significant other that can provide insight into the client's needs for love and belonging.

Physical and behavioral changes may indicate that a client is unable to meet love and belonging needs. The client's appearance and hygiene habits may change. A normally well-groomed person may seem uncaring about appearance. The client may complain of physical ailments such as headaches or gastrointestinal problems when separated from family and significant others. Sleep and eating habits may also change.

A person's conversation often demonstrates that needs for love and belonging are not being met. A hospitalized client may speak often of family or friends expected to visit. Or, a client who becomes anxious because family or friends have not yet visited may attempt to cope with unmet needs by insisting it does not matter. A child separated from parents because of illness or injury may seem to adopt the nurse as surrogate parent. A client may attempt to interact with the nurse as with a close friend or may even become possessive about the amount of time spent with the nurse. All these are manifestations of the normal human need for love and affection.

If a person's need persists for a long period without being met, behavior may change in more noticeable ways. A usually mild-tempered person may become easily irritated. An outgoing person may withdraw from interaction with co-workers and friends. The person's work habits may change, leading to increased absenteeism or overcommitment to the job.

NURSING IMPLICATIONS

The nursing care plan for clients should include means by which needs for love and belonging can be met. For example, if the client is a young child hospitalized for some time, the nursing care plan should include specific opportunities for the child and family to interact. In some cases it may be important for the mother or father to remain overnight.

A client isolated from family and others by illness or injury cannot meet needs for love and belonging in usual ways. If opportunities for social interaction are limited, the client may have a sense of not belonging and begin to withdraw. The nurse can take specific actions to help the client maintain social contacts and thus meet love and belonging needs. A hospitalized client may benefit from short social visits by members of the health care team. Resources in the community may help. For example, an elderly client can be helped to meet the need for contact with others through a senior citizens' center.

Finally, the nurse works with the client and family to adapt the nursing care plan in any way to help the client meet needs for love and belonging. The more actively involved the client is in developing the plan of care, and the more control he has over the environment while receiving care, the easier it will be for him to meet his needs.

ESTEEM AND SELF-ESTEEM NEEDS

People need a stable sense of self-esteem, as well as the feeling that they are held in regard by others. The need for self-esteem is linked to the desire for strength, achievement, adequacy, competence, confidence when facing the world, and independence. People also need recognition or appreciation from others. When both of these needs are met, a person feels self-confident and useful. If a person's needs for self-esteem and esteem of others are unfulfilled, he may feel helpless and inferior (Maslow, 1970).

ASSESSMENT

A change in a person's roles may threaten self-esteem. The change may be anticipated, such as retirement, or sudden, as with an injury. With the change in role comes a change in the person's independence and relationship with others. People who were formerly independent may become more dependent, and strains are put on relationships with others. A person may become more dependent on family members, social agencies, or health care professionals and may begin to question his usefulness and importance—he may lose self-esteem. If no longer functioning in a former role, such as that of a worker, a person may feel the esteem of others is lost as well.

Changes in a person's body image, such as those caused by illness or injury, may also influence self-esteem. Body image changes include both obvious changes such as the amputation of a leg, and unobservable changes such as a hysterectomy. Normal developmental changes such as puberty or menopause can change a person's image.

It is not the magnitude of a change in body image or role that affects a person's self-esteem, but rather how the person perceives himself after the change. A person's sense of self-esteem and the esteem of others therefore depends on values and beliefs, support from others, and self-concept.

There are many indications that a client has unmet needs for self-esteem or the esteem of others. A client who feels helpless or inferior may defer all decisions to the nurse rather than expressing wishes. The client may become self-critical or seem unusually lethargic or apathetic about anything involving himself, including appearance. The person's general attitude may be summed up as a feeling of hopelessness. In some cases a client with low self-esteem may avoid or ignore opportunities for actions that could increase self-esteem because of the possibility of failure. The loss of self-esteem can thus become a self-fulfilling prophecy.

A client feeling the lack of esteem of other people may test others by making statements that call for their approval or praise. Conversely, he may act in a way that prevents such approval if he has little self-esteem and is certain of failure.

NURSING IMPLICATIONS

Helping meet needs for self-esteem begins with the first contact between client and nurse. The nurse from the beginning must convey respect for the client as an individual. Even though the client may have different beliefs and values, the nurse needs to accept, not judge, the client's values.

If the client's self-concept is changed by illness or injury, nursing care involves improving self-concept and body image. Specific nursing actions depend on the client's support system and personality, the cause of altered self-concept, and available resources (see Chapter 29). If the client's level of self-esteem is so low that he fails to care for himself, the nurse may have to help meet other needs, such as those for nutrition and safety, while taking steps to increase self-esteem.

NEED FOR SELF-ACTUALIZATION

Self-actualization is the highest level need in Maslow's hierarchy of human needs. Theoretically, when people have met all the lower-level needs, it is by self-actualization that they achieve their fullest potential (Maslow, 1970).

Self-actualized people have multiple characteristics (see box). They have a mature multidimensional personality, frequently they are able to assume and complete multiple tasks, and they achieve fulfillment from the pleasure of a job well done. They are not totally dependent on the opinions of others about appearance, quality of work, or how they solve problems. Although they may have failings and doubts, they generally deal with them realistically.

How well people meet their need for self-actualization depends on present needs, environment, and stressors. Self-actualization is possible when there is a balance

---

Assessment Characteristics for Self-Actualization

- Solves own problems
- Assists others in problem solving
- Accepts suggestions of others
- Broad interests in work and social related topics
- Possesses good communication skills both as a listener and as a communicator
- Manages stress and assists others in managing stress
- Enjoys privacy
- Seeks new experiences and knowledge
- Confident in abilities and decisions
- Anticipates problems and successes
- Likes self

---

among the clients' needs, stressors, and ability to adapt to changes of the body and environment.

ASSESSMENT

Illness, injury, loss of loved one, change in role, change in status can threaten or disturb a client's self-actualization. A loss of self-actualization occurs when a client can no longer achieve the fullest potential because of the limitations imposed by the illness or injury. This loss may result in behavioral changes. The client may feel frustrated because the illness prevents decision making, creativity, and independent problem solving. Instead, because of the illness, the client is forced to be more self-centered, more dependent on others, and motivated more by external factors.

NURSING IMPLICATIONS

The major focus for nursing care is to restore the client as much as possible to a self-actualized state. Nursing care is planned to encourage the client to make decisions when possible, particularly in regard to health care. Thus the nurse seeks the involvement of the client in the planning and delivery of nursing care.

Because the self-actualized person tends to be creative and highly individual in many ways, nursing care should include the opportunity for the client to fulfill creative needs. The client should be encouraged to continue with specific projects, and if he is hospitalized, time should be set aside for them. Frequently, hospital routines leaves little free time for relaxing activities.

The client's need for privacy must be respected and met. When in good health the self-actualized person generally has a strong need for privacy. An illness, especially in a hospital setting, can greatly reduce a person's privacy. Nurses can help meet this need by planning health care so that the client's privacy will not be interrupted during specific times.

APPLICATION OF BASIC NEEDS THEORY

Maslow's theory of human needs can provide a basis for nursing care of clients of all ages and health settings. When the nurse applies this theory in practice, however, the focus is on needs of the individual rather than rigid adherence to Maslow's hierarchy. Maslow's hierarchy is a generalization about the need priorities of most people—not all people. In all cases an emergency physiological need takes precedence over a higher-level need. With one client the need for self-esteem may be a higher priority than a long-term nutritional need, whereas for another client this may be reversed. To provide the most effective care, the nurse needs to understand relationships among different needs for the individual client and the factors that determine their priorities. Furthermore, although the hierarchy of needs suggests that one should be met before another, nursing care often addresses two or more at the same time.

Relationships among Needs

In some nursing situations it is unrealistic to expect a client's basic needs to occur in the fixed hierarchical order. For example, a client enters the health care system with a chronic respiratory infection. While providing care, the nurse learns that he has not eaten adequately, slept well, or maintained social relationships since his wife died 2 years ago. In this case the client has several unmet needs, including the physiological needs for nutrition and rest and needs for love and a sense of belonging. For the client these separate needs are closely related. Nursing care in this situation would not simply be directed to helping the client meet the higher-priority needs for nutrition and rest, because these needs in part occurred because the client was not meeting lower-priority needs. Nursing care for this client focuses also on assisting him through the grief process (see Chapter 26) so that, once he has resolved feelings of grief and loneliness, he is able to regain former eating and sleeping habits and thus meet these physiological needs.

An opposite relationship among similar needs may be true of a different client. For example, a woman is receiving treatment for severe arthritis and often feels pain or discomfort during certain activities. Because of this, she has changed her habits and no longer visits family members and friends. The nurse realizes that the woman also has unmet needs for love and belonging. As with the client in the preceding example, these two sets of needs are clearly related and the nurse provides care directed to meeting both. In this situation, however, the priority is to provide relief from pain, which will then allow the woman to return to former activities that meet the lower-priority needs.

For different individuals, needs on different levels may be related in different ways. One person may give sexual need higher priority than the need for love, whereas for another person sexual need is deferred until the need for love is met, so that the sexual relationship follows love. Similarly, a person with an unmet need for self-esteem may be unable to seek fulfillment of his need for love if his level of self-esteem is so low that he feels inferior and fears rejection. In these and many other ways, needs on different levels may be closely related for an individual client. The nurse in assessing needs and planning care must be careful not to assume that a lower-level need always takes priority. As with all other aspects of providing care, the nurse individualizes the nursing care plan to provide for unique needs and desires.

Simultaneous Meeting of Needs

The nurse provides care for clients with many needs, because illness often disrupts the ability to meet needs on different levels. After identifying the client's specific needs, the nurse generally has to set priorities to help the client meet these needs. However, setting priorities does not mean that the nurse provides care for only one need at a time. The nurse does not, for example, simply begin with the first need in the hierarchy and move up only after the first has been met. In emergency situations, of course, physiological needs take precedence, but even then the nurse is aware of the client's other needs. Even in an emergency case the nurse considers the client's higher-level needs and treats the client with respect.

A young man who is hospitalized with paraplegia resulting from a severed spinal cord, for example, certainly needs assistance in meeting physiological needs. But he may also have low self-esteem related to his condition. The nurse is faced with the challenge of simultaneously meeting his physiological needs and need for self-esteem because, if the client does not feel good about himself, he may not eat properly or participate in physical care. The nurse should not offer the client false hope about future recovery. However, while planning care to meet physiological needs the nurse can include measures that will help restore self-esteem.

Factors Influencing Need Priorities

Ideally, nursing care can be directed toward the simultaneous meeting of several needs. In practice, though, one need often takes precedence over another and priorities must be determined so that care can be more focused and effective. Life-threatening situations always take first priority, and unmet physiological needs that pose a threat to life certainly have a high priority. In other situations the nurse has to consider factors that influence which needs take priority over others for the individual client.

First, a person's personality and mood affect how the perception of and ability to meet a particular need. A depressed person may react negatively to a suggestion for an activity that could increase self-esteem, although in another mood the person might respond with enthusiasm. Thus, when providing care to help meet several needs, the nurse can adjust the care plan to correspond most effectively to the client's personality and mood.

Second, some needs must be deferred until the client is in better health. A client recovering from an acute gastrointestinal infection should not be encouraged to resume physical activities related to need for self-esteem until needs for physical safety and security have been met by achieving full health. Similarly, a diabetic client whose condition is unstable may have to defer other needs until nutritional needs related to insulin therapy are satisfied.

Third, the client's perception of needs varies among socioeconomic and cultural groups (see Chapter 4). In addition, the client's perception of some needs, such as sexual needs, varies between the sexes and among different developmental levels. The nurse considers the client's perception of needs when planning care and does not impose personal perceptions about the client's need priorities.

Fourth, the client's family structure can influence the way needs are satisfied (see Chapter 21). A mother may, for example, place the needs of an infant before her own needs, such as by interrupting a meal or sleep to feed the child.

Last, and perhaps most important, when setting need priorities the nurse considers that basic needs are interrelated. Physiological functioning is closely related to a person's body systems, environment, values, ethics, and culture. One need does not occur independently of others. For example, if a person's nutritional need is unmet for a long time, he begins to show signs of malnutrition, his body deteriorates, he becomes weak, and he is unable to recognize or meet the lower-priority needs of safety, love, and self-esteem. Needs are interrelated in unique ways for each person, and the nurse considers such relationships in planning care. The nurse involves the client and family in this planning so that need priorities of the client are neglected rather than simply following the hierarchy of the human needs theory.

SUMMARY

Healthy adults are usually able to meet most of their basic needs. But as an adult ages or becomes ill or handicapped, the risk of not being able to meet basic needs increases.

Maslow's theory postulates a hierarchical relationship among different levels of human needs. A client entering the health care system may have one or more unmet needs at different levels. Nursing care addresses all the client's needs. Essential, life-sustaining needs generally take priority over others. The client's different needs may be interrelated in unique ways, and the nurse considers the client's priorities. Nursing care may be directed toward meeting several needs simultaneously. The nursing care plan is based on the nurse's assessment of the extent to which the client is meeting, and is able to meet, all needs.

Nursing involves providing care for the whole person. The nurse applies knowledge about the body systems and also about the client's family, social system, emotions, values, ethics, and goals of health care. In this way the theory of human needs corresponds to nursing's holistic perspective by addressing the client's needs in his physiological, psychological, sociocultural, developmental, and spiritual dimensions. Basic needs theory is appropriate and applicable in community health, psychiatric, outpatient, and institutional settings, including critical care units and rehabilitation centers. This theory can provide a basis for nursing care for clients of all ages and developmental stages, from the neonate to the geriatric client. Human needs theory is therefore a set of concepts important for the nurse's understanding of health and illness and the client's position on the health-illness continuum.

KEY CONCEPTS

✓ Basic human needs are the needs for things such as oxygen, food, water, safety, and love required to survive and be healthy.

✓ Some human needs are more necessary to survival than others and must be met first.

✓ Maslow's hierarchy is a theoretical representation of the levels of basic needs.

✓ The very young, very old, chronically ill, and handicapped are generally less able than others to meet needs without assistance.

✓ The highest priority is given to physiological needs: oxygen, fluid, nutrition, temperature, elimination, shelter, rest, and sexuality.

✓ Oxygen is the most essential physiological need. A chronic or acute oxygen need can be identified by confusion, lethargy, rapid shallow respirations, an inability to lie flat, nasal flaring, retractions, a decreased level of consciousness, and cyanosis.

✓ Fluid needs require a balance between the intake and output of fluids. Dehydration or edema indicates unmet fluid needs.

✓ Dehydration may result in flushed, dry skin, poor skin turgor, coated tongue, dry mucous membranes, decreased saliva, decreased tears, and oliguria.

✓ Edema may result in the swelling of a dependent body part, weight gain, shortness of breath, increased heart rate, and smooth, shiny skin.

✓ Nutritional needs require an adequate intake of foods to allow the body to carry on metabolic processes. Unmet nutritional needs may be indicated by weight loss or failure to grow or gain weight, fatigue, pallor, and recurring sores in the mouth and gums.

✓ The body is able to function within only a small temperature range, 35° C (97° F) to 41° C (106° F). Unmet temperature needs may result from exposure to cold or heat.

✓ Elimination needs involve the body's removal of excess fluids and wastes. The body meets these needs by elimination through the skin, lungs, kidneys, and intestines.

✓ The need for shelter is a physiological need. Unmet needs can be identified through assessment of a client's environment.

✓ Sleep and rest needs vary depending on the individual's quality of sleep, age, health status, activity patterns, and life-style. Unmet needs may result in a decreased level of energy, disheveled appearance, irritability, decreased concentration, and restlessness.

✓ People have different needs related to sexuality at different times in life, and the manifestation of unmet sexual needs can take many forms.

✓ Safety and security needs include both physical and psychological safety and the need to prevent complications.

✓ Clients in the health care system may be unable to meet their needs for love and belonging because of changes in relationships with others and the separation often imposed by illness.

✓ People need stable self-esteem as well as the esteem of others. Illness, role changes, or changes in body image may threaten a person's ability to meet these needs.

✓ The self-actualized person is autonomous, easily motivated, and not self-centered. The need for self-actualization can be threatened by changes that occur with illness or injury.

✓ To apply basic needs theory in practice, the nurse considers the relationships among the client's specific needs, sets priorities for meeting needs by considering the client's priorities, and when possible and necessary assists the client in meeting needs on different levels simultaneously.

REFERENCES

Maslow, AH: Motivation and personality, ed. 2, New York, 1970, Harper & Row, Publishers, Inc.

Mountcastle, VR: Medical physiology, ed. 14, St. Louis, 1980, The C.V. Mosby Co.

Rogers, C: On becoming a person, Boston, 1961, Houghton Mifflin Co.

ADDITIONAL READINGS

Maslow, AH: Toward a psychology of being, ed. 2, New York, 1968, Van Nostrand Reinhold Co.

Maslow, AH: Toward a humanistic biology, Am Psychol 24:724, 1969.

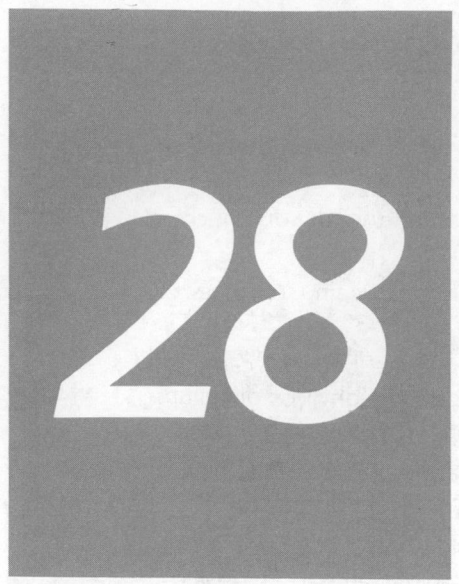

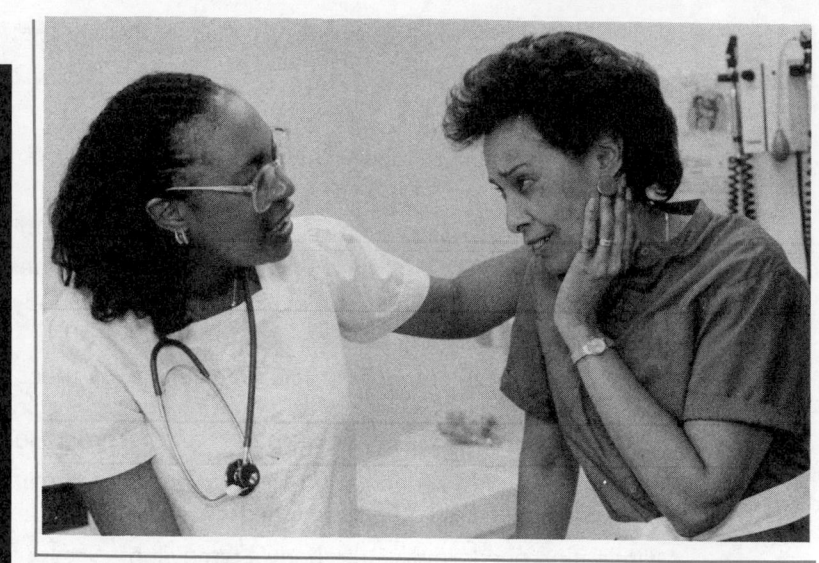

OBJECTIVES

Mastery of content in this chapter will enable the student to:

- Define the key terms listed.
- Discuss the limitations of homeostatic control.
- Discuss four models of stress as they relate to nursing practice.
- Describe how adaptation occurs in each of the five dimensions.
- Describe two forms of local physiological adaptation.
- Describe the three phases of the general adaptation syndrome.
- List and discuss behaviors that are responses to stress.
- List and discuss the most common ego-defense mechanisms that are responses to stress.
- Discuss the effects of prolonged stress on each of the five dimensions of a person's functioning.
- Describe stress management techniques that nurses can help clients use.
- Discuss techniques of crisis intervention.
- Describe stress management techniques that can benefit nurses themselves.

KEY TERMS

Adaptation
Coping mechanism
Crisis
Crisis Intervention
Ego-Defense Mechanism
External Stressor
Flight-or-Fight Syndrome
General Adaptation Syndrome
Identification
Internal Stressor
Job Stress
Local Adaptation Syndrome
Medulla Oblongata
Mild Stress Situation
Moderate Stress Situation
Pituitary Gland
Reticular Formation
Severe Stress Syndrome
Situational Crisis
Stress
Stress Behaviors
Stressor

Adaptation to Stress

Every person experiences forms of stress throughout life. Stress can provide the stimulus for change and growth, and in this respect some stress can be positive. However, too much can result in poor judgment, physical illness, and inability to cope with the stressor.

The term *stress* is derived from the Latin word *stringere*, which means "to draw tight." Claude Bernard, in 1867, was one of the first physiologists to recognize potential consequences of stress for an organism. He proposed that changes in the internal and external environments disrupted the functioning of an organism and that it is essential for an organism to adapt to a stressor to survive. In 1920, Walter Cannon introduced the term "homeostasis" to describe how an organism successfully responds to stress. Cannon studied specific mechanisms that organisms use to adapt to stress and in turn to maintain a balance (homeostasis) within the internal environment.

Hans Selye developed a biochemical model of stress known as the general adaptation syndrome (GAS). The GAS model clearly describes what occurs in the human body during a stress response. Selye also introduced the concept of stressors, those internal or external stimuli that cause stress (Selye, 1976). Selye's research into stress and stressors has been important for health care professions and is the primary focus of this chapter. The GAS model is readily applicable to nursing practice.

CONCEPTS OF STRESS

Stress and Stressors

Everyone experiences stress from time to time, and normally a healthy person is able to adapt to long-term stress or cope with short-term stress until it passes. Stress can place heavy demands on a person, and if unable to adapt, illness can result.

Stress can be defined as a state in which any nonspecific demand requires an individual to respond or take action (Numerof, 1983; Sundeen et al., 1985). Stress involves both physiological and psychological responses. Stress can lead to negative or counterproductive feelings or threaten emotional well-being. Stress can threaten the way a person normally perceives reality, solves problems, or thinks in general. It can threaten relationships with others and sense of belonging. In addition, stress can threaten a person's general outlook on life and attitude toward loved ones.

A major change that an individual perceives or experiences initiates the stress response. The stimuli preceding or precipitating the change are called stressors. Stressors may be physiological, psychological, developmental, spiritual, or cultural and represent an unmet need. Stressors can generally be classified as internal or external. Internal stressors originate inside a person, such as a fever, a condition such as pregnancy or menopause, or an emotion such as guilt. External stressors originate outside a person, such as a marked change in environmental temperature, a change in family or social role, or peer rejection.

Homeostasis

Homeostasis is the body's tendency to maintain itself in a state of relative constancy. Homeostasis is a dynamic form of equilibrium in the body's internal environment. The internal environment is constantly changing and the body's adaptive mechanisms are continually functioning to adjust to these changes and thus to maintain equilibrium.

Homeostasis is maintained by physiological mechanisms that control body functions and monitor body organs. For the most part these mechanisms are controlled by the nervous system and do not involve conscious behavior. The body makes adjustments in heart rate, respiratory rate, blood pressure, temperature, fluid and electrolyte balances, hormone secretions, and level of consciousness—all directed toward maintaining homeostasis.

MECHANISMS

When a person becomes aware of an unmet physiological need, such as for food or warmth, deliberate actions can meet the need. For the most part, however, homeostasis involves adjustments the body makes automatically to maintain equilibrium. These homeostatic mechanisms are self-regulatory, in the sense that they are automatic in a healthy person. In a person with an illness or injury, however, the mechanisms may not be able to maintain homeostasis. Homeostatic mechanisms function also through a process of negative feedback, a process by which the controlling mechanism senses an abnormal state, such as a lowered body temperature, and makes an adaptive response, such as initiating shivering to generate heat.

Three of the major homeostatic mechanisms are controlled by the medulla oblongata, the reticular formation, and the pituitary gland.

MEDULLA OBLONGATA. The medulla oblongata controls vital functions—such as heart rate, blood pressure, and respiration—that are necessary to survival. Impulses traveling to and from the medulla oblongata can either increase or decrease these vital functions. For example, regulation of the heartbeat is the result of sympathetic or parasympathetic nervous system impulses traveling from the medulla oblongata to the heart. The heart rate increases in response to impulses from sympathetic fibers and decreases with impulses from parasympathetic fibers.

RETICULAR FORMATION. The reticular formation is a small cluster of neurons in the brainstem and spinal cord. It controls vital functions as well but also continuously monitors the physiological status of the body through connections with sensory and motor tracts. For example, certain cells within the reticular formation can cause a sleeping person to regain consciousness or increase the level of consciousness when a need arises.

PITUITARY GLAND. The pituitary gland, a small gland attached to the hypothalamus, supplies hormones that control vital functions. The pituitary gland produces hormones that are necessary for adaptation to stresses, as well as growth hormones. In addition, the pituitary gland regulates the secretion of thyroid, gonadal, and parathyroid hormones. Hormone secretion, like other homeostatic mechanisms, is normally regulated by a feedback mechanism, which continuously monitors hormone levels in the blood. When hormone levels drop, the pituitary gland receives a message to increase hormone secretion. When hormone levels rise, the pituitary gland decreases hormone production.

LIMITATIONS OF HOMEOSTATIC CONTROL

Homeostatic control mechanisms work together through complex relationships in the nervous system, hormone levels, and other body systems to maintain relative constancy within the body. In a healthy person these mechanisms are effective in maintaining homeostasis so that physiological needs are met. However, homeostatic mechanisms can provide only short-term control over the body's equilibrium. These mechanisms cannot adapt to long-term changes in hormone secretion or vital functions. Thus illness, injury, or prolonged stress can decrease the adaptive capacity of homeostatic functions. Decreased functioning can take two forms: continued but inadequate homeostatic control or breakdown of the feedback mechanism that allows control. Either results in illness or death.

In severe stress situations, for example, the pituitary gland continues to supply the body with necessary hormones to cope. However, these hormones may be insufficient in quantity to provide the physiological energy necessary for the person to cope with the stressor, in which case the person's condition deteriorates and functioning declines. The feedback mechanism of homeostatic control may break down because of an organ abnormality.

For clients with homeostatic limitations, the health care professional directs therapeutic interventions toward restoring physiological balance. Often such interventions are successful. If ineffective, however, the body may no longer be able to function properly, resulting in illness or death.

Models of Stress

The origins and effects of stress can be understood in terms of various medical and behavioral theoretical models. A stress model is used to predict what constitutes stressors for an individual, how the person will respond, and to understand how stressors and the individual interact. For the nurse, the purpose of any stress model is to help a client cope with unhealthy, nonproductive responses to stressors. This chapter focuses primarily on the psychophysiological response to stress described by Selye. The four alternative stress models described in the following sections are useful in gaining an understanding of stress and responses to stress in all dimensions.

PSYCHOSOMATIC MODEL

The psychosomatic model is based on the premise that stressors in one dimension can have pathological effects in other dimensions. Frequently, for example, stressors that arise in the emotional dimension are manifested in physiological ways. A freshman may enter a university fearful of "failing." Even after studying hard, completing assignments satisfactorily, and meeting deadlines, the freshman is preoccupied with fear of failure. At midsemester, the symptoms of stomach pains, headaches, and inability to sleep can be traced directly to fear of failing. Thus physical symptoms are the result of a psy-

chosomatic response to stress. Once the student is able to control emotional responses to the stressor of college, fear of failure is controlled, and the physical symptoms subside.

In the psychosomatic model of stress, as in other models, it is important for a person to control response to a stressor. Many kinds of stressors cannot be avoided, but response to a stressor can be controlled.

ADAPTATION MODEL

The adaptation model of stress proposes that four factors determine whether a situation is stressful (Mechanic, 1962). The first is the ability to cope with stress. This ability usually depends on the person's experience with similar stressors, support systems, and overall perception of the stressor.

The second factor comprises the practices and norms of the person's peer group. If the peer group considers it normal to talk about the stress of the upcoming test, the student may respond by complaining or worrying aloud. This response may help adaptation to the stress, or the student may respond in this way simply because of trying to conform to the peer group behavior.

The third factor in the adaptation model is the means the social environment provides an individual to adapt to a stressor. For example, a college freshman who suspects having a sexually transmitted disease may confide this fear to an upperclassman, who may then refer him or her to a student health service. In this example the resources of both the older student and the student health service offer the means to reduce severity of the stressor.

The last factor in the adaptation model is the nature of the process that determines where and how an individual can use resources in the social environment to deal with stress. In the example just given, the student needs only a valid identification card to use the prepaid health benefits, and the health service is open 7 days a week from 9 AM to 9 PM. Both of these factors make the resource easily accessible to help the student cope with the stress.

The adaptation model of stress is based on the understanding that when people feel unprepared to cope with a stressful situation they are uncomfortable and experience anxiety and often increased stress. This concept is essential for members of the health professions. With appropriate interventions, nurses can help clients and their families to reduce the effects of stress in all human dimensions.

SOCIAL ENVIRONMENT MODEL

The social environment model of stress is concerned with the effects of a person's work role on health (French and Kahn, 1962). The model focuses on six variables that determine how a person's work role interacts with

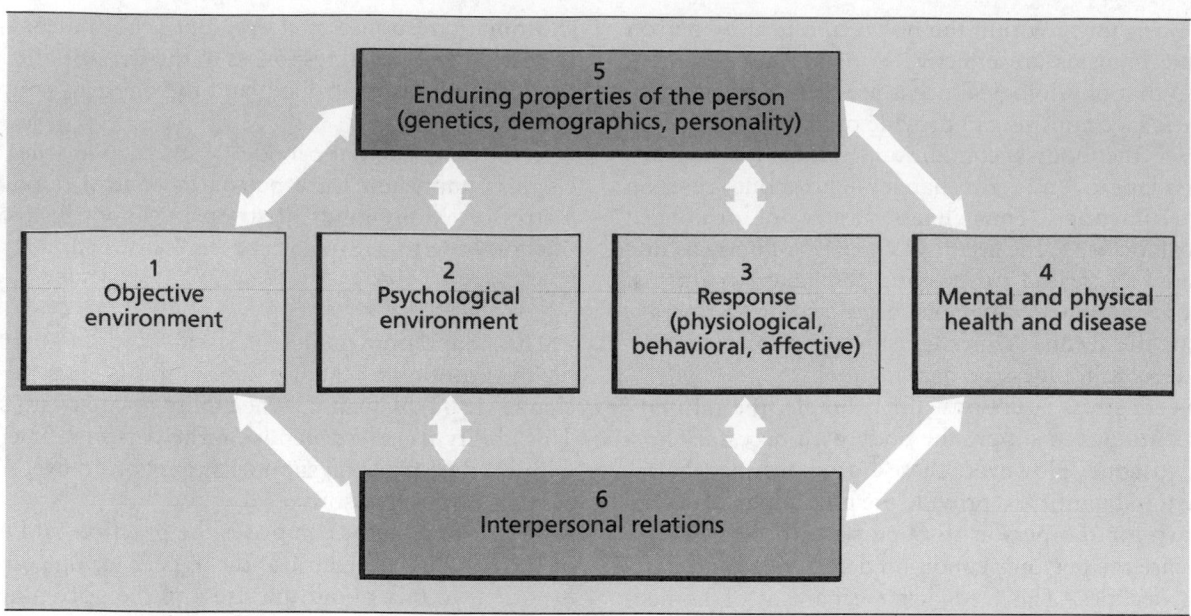

Fig. 28-1 Social environment stress model.
From Katz, D, and Kahn, RL: The social psychology of organizations, ed. 2, New York, 1978, John Wiley & Sons, Inc.

health (Fig. 28-1). The model explains the way a person's personality, external and internal environments, individual responses to stressors, and interpersonal relationships influence how he or she responds to the stresses of work and ultimately affect physical and mental health.

When assessing clients' levels of wellness, nurses should identify actual and potential stressors in clients' work environments. Although nurses may not be able to remove stressors, they can plan nursing interventions directed toward helping clients change their responses.

PROCESS MODEL

The process model of stress is concerned with how a person chooses responses to stress with the overall goal of changing the situation and thus reducing the stress (McGrath, 1976). The process model describes a stress situation as a four-stage, closed-cycle set of processes. As shown in Fig. 28-2, the four stages are linked by four processes: cognitive appraisal, decision, performance, and outcome. In the first stage, the person encounters the stress situation. The individual's thought processes, previous experiences with similar stressors, and coping mechanisms all affect what and how he or she thinks of the situation. Thus, the person either does or does not perceive the situation as a stressor. If stress is perceived (the second stage) the person then decides how to respond to the stressor (the third stage). The person then acts in some way, the fourth stage, and finally assesses the situation again to determine whether it has changed and whether stress is reduced. If the level of stress re-

mains high, the person moves through the process again and attempts new responses.

The process model of stress is useful in understanding stress situations within organizations, and it is helpful for nurses caring for clients with disabilities or chronic illnesses. Such clients must continually evaluate their levels of health and modify daily activities to maintain

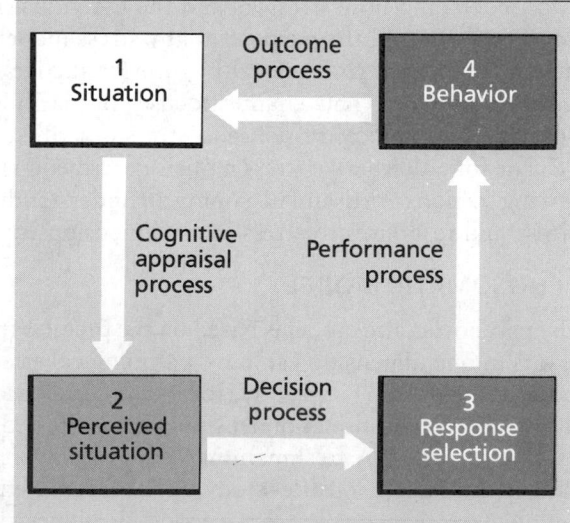

Fig. 28-2 Process model of stress.
From Stress and work: A managerial perspective, by John M. Ivancevich and Michael T. Matteson. Glenview, Ill., Copyright © 1980 by Scott, Foresman & Company. Reprinted with permission.

optimal levels of wellness. The nurse can use the process model of stress to teach clients with chronic diseases and their families how to adapt to changes in functioning and life-style. Application of the process model in nursing situations requires active participation by clients' families and therefore is not effective in all cases. The individual needs of each client will determine which model of stress can be effective.

COMPARISON OF MODELS

Each of the four models of stress emphasizes a different aspect of stress. However, all are concerned with *how* stress affects individuals. Because of their differences in emphasis, these models can be applied in different practice settings, according to which is most appropriate. Thus, as with other aspects of nursing care, the nurse's care plan is individualized.

Despite differences in emphasis, all four models agree on the primary principle of stress management. This principle recognizes that because stressors themselves cannot always be controlled, persons experiencing stress must learn to change their response to the stressor.

Factors Influencing Response to Stressors

A person's response to any stressor depends on the personality and behavioral characteristics of the person and on the nature of the stressor. The nature of the stressor involves four factors, each influencing how a person responds:

1. Intensity of the stressor
2. Scope of the stressor
3. Duration of the stressor
4. Number and nature of other stressors

A person may perceive the intensity or magnitude of a stressor as minimal, severe, or somewhere in between. Obviously, the greater the magnitude of the stressor, the greater the stress response.

Likewise, the scope of a stressor can be described as limited, medium, or extensive (Sundeen et al., 1985). The greater the scope of a stressor, the greater the stress response. The greater the duration of the stressor, the greater the response. The presence of other stressors may increase the person's response.

CONCEPTS OF ADAPTATION

Adaptation is the process by which a person in one or more dimensions changes in response to stress. Because many stressors cannot be avoided, the focus in health care is often on how a person, family, or community adapts to stress.

Adaptation to stress has many forms. Homeostatic mechanisms make possible a continuous physiological adaptation to the constant changes and stresses in the body's internal environment. A similar process of adaptation, however, may occur in all of a person's dimensions, as well as in those of a family, group, or community.

An adaptive response occurs when a stimulus from the internal or external environment causes a departure from the balanced state of the organism. Adaptation thus is an attempt to maintain optimal functioning. Included in adaptation are reflexes, automatic body mechanisms for protection, coping mechanisms, and instincts (Coelho, Hamburg, and Adams, 1974). A stressor that stimulates adaptation may be short term, such as a fever, or long term, such as paralysis of a limb. To function optimally, a person must be able to respond to such stressors and adapt to the required demands or changes. Adaptation requires an active response from the whole person.

Like an individual, a family or group may need to adapt to a stressor. Family adaptation is the process by which a family maintains a balance so that it can fulfill its purposes and tasks, deal with stress, and promote the growth of individual family members. For a family to adapt successfully, there must be (1) good communication skills, (2) mutual respect for all family members, (3) adequate resources available for adaptation, and (4) previous experience with stressors.

The adaptive response of a group is similar to that of a family. Groups vary according to purpose, size, and complexity. When a group encounters a stressor, the group as a whole must adapt, usually by change in tasks or purpose. Such change is necessary to maintain an equilibrium within the group.

Dimensions of Adaptation

Any stress can have effects in any of the human dimensions—physical, emotional, intellectual, social, and spiritual. Adaptive resources exist in each of these dimensions. Therefore, when evaluating how a client is adapting to the stress of illness or any type of stress, a nurse must consider the total person. Responses in dimensions other than the physical often influence how a person adapts to the stress of physical illness.

PHYSICAL-DEVELOPMENTAL DIMENSION

Physiological adaptation is the process by which the body responds to a stressor in order to maintain functioning compatible with survival. Physiological adaptive responses are stimulated by demands either in the internal environment, such as fever or inflammation, or in the external environment, such as changes in altitude or ambient temperature. A physiological response to stress may be limited to a particular body area, or it may involve the entire body. The sections on local and general adaptation syndromes, later in this chapter, will discuss physiological adaptive responses in more detail.

Each developmental stage poses particular tasks and thus involves particular potential stressors. A young adult, for example, may have to adapt to such stressors as establishing a career and rearing children. At the same time, each developmental stage is characterized by certain potential adaptive resources by which an individual can respond to stress. An older adult, because of greater past experience with certain stressors, may be better able to adapt than a young adult. The chapters in Unit 5 discuss such developmental differences in detail.

EMOTIONAL DIMENSION

Adaptation in the emotional dimension involves use of normal psychological coping mechanisms to resolve stress. Because every client has a different personality, every client copes with stress in a different way, although certain basic forms of psychological adaptation are common. Adaptive behavior is most successful when it leads to a sense of discovery and creativity. A person may not always be happy and content in adapting to stress, but the goal of adaptation is to live constructively.

INTELLECTUAL DIMENSION

A person's intellectual dimension includes not only development and education, but also perceptions of other people and the world in general, problem-solving ability, communication patterns, and past coping strategies. Intellectual adaptive responses to stress include gathering information, solving problems, and communicating with others to adjust.

Intellectual adaptation can be strongly influenced by a person's emotions. If a person is unable to adapt emotionally to the changes necessitated by an illness, for example, he or she may be less able to adapt intellectually by learning more about the illness. Similarly, helping a client to adapt emotionally can lead to more effective intellectual adaptation. Nurses are often in a unique position to assist clients in intellectual adaptation to stress.

SOCIAL DIMENSION

Everyone has social relationships with others, including spouse, family members, co-workers, and peers. This network can be important in helping a person adapt to stresses. The social group may provide psychological support and can help direct a person to resources for coping with stress. For example, friends often can help a person adjust to the death of a loved one by encouraging the person to express feelings. In addition, organized social groups, such as Alcoholics Anonymous, can help people adapt to specific stresses in the social dimension.

A client's social dimension is often closely interrelated with other dimensions. A client unable to cope emotionally with stress may, for example, withdraw from contact with people who could assist in adapting.

SPIRITUAL DIMENSION

A person's spiritual dimension can include beliefs about a Supreme Being, a feeling of oneness with nature and the world as a whole, and a positive sense of life's meaning and purpose. These beliefs or attitudes can be a powerful resource for adapting to stress. Chapter 31 discusses ways in which nurses can help clients meet their spiritual needs and use their spiritual strength to cope with the effects of illness and other stressors.

RESPONSE TO STRESS

The discussion of adaptation emphasized that the total person is involved in responding and adapting to stresses. Most research into stress responses, however, has focused on the psychological or emotional and physiological responses, even though these dimensions overlap and interact with the other dimensions of functioning.

When stress occurs, a person uses both psychological and physiological energy to respond and adapt. The amount of energy required, as well as the effectiveness of the attempt to adapt, depends on the intensity, scope, and duration of the stressor and on the number of other stressors.

Physiological Response

The two physiological responses to stress are the local adaptation syndrome (LAS) and the general adaptation syndrome (GAS). The LAS is a response of body tissue, an organ, or a part of the body to the stress of trauma, illness, or other physiological change. The GAS is a defense response of the whole body to stress.

LOCAL ADAPTATION SYNDROME

The body produces many localized responses to stress. These include blood clotting, wound healing (see Chapter 47), accommodation of the eye to light, and response to pressure (see Chapter 42). Two localized responses, the reflex pain response and the inflammatory response, are described here as examples of the local adaptation syndrome. Nurses encounter these responses in many health care settings.

All forms of the LAS share four characteristics. First, the response is localized; it does not involve entire body systems. Second, it is an adaptive response, meaning that a stressor is necessary to stimulate the response. Third, it is a short-term response. It does not persist indefinitely.

Fourth, it is a restorative response, meaning that the LAS assists in restoring homeostasis to the body region or body part.

REFLEX PAIN RESPONSE. The reflex pain response is a localized response of the central nervous system to pain (see Chapter 35). It is an adaptive response and serves to protect the tissue from further damage. The response involves five physiological components: (1) a sensory receptor, (2) a sensory nerve to the spinal cord, (3) a connector neuron within the spinal cord, (4) a motor nerve from the spinal cord, and (5) an effector muscle. An example would be the unconscious, reflex removal of one's hand from a hot surface.

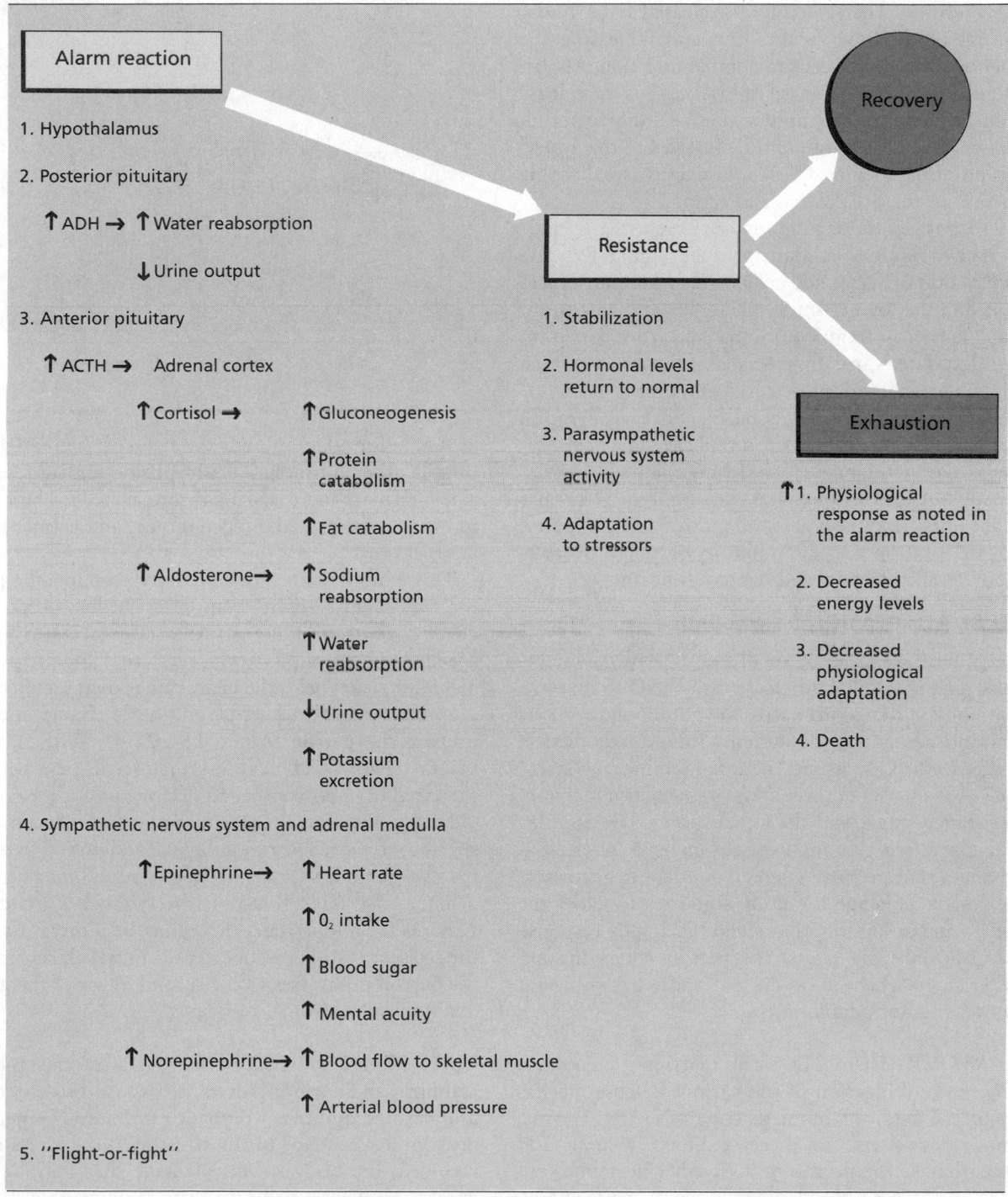

Fig. 28-3 General adaptation syndrome.

INFLAMMATORY RESPONSE. The inflammatory response is stimulated by trauma or infection. The purposes of the inflammatory response are to localize the inflammation, thus preventing its spread, and to promote healing. The inflammatory response may produce localized pain, swelling, heat, redness, and changes in functioning. It occurs in three phases. The first phase involves changes in cells and the circulatory system. Initially, narrowing of blood vessels occurs at the injury to control bleeding. Then histamine is released at the injury, increasing blood flow to the area and increasing the number of white blood cells to combat infection. Almost simultaneous with the release of histamine is the release of kinins, which increase capillary permeability to permit the flow of proteins, fluid, and leukocytes to the injury. At this point the localized blood flow decreases, keeping leukocytes in the area to fight infection.

The second phase of inflammatory response is characterized by release of exudate from the wound. Exudate is a combination of fluid, cells, and other substances produced in the area of injury. The type and amount of exudate vary from injury to injury and from person to person. Exudate is usually released at the injury, which may be a cut, laceration, or surgical incision.

The last phase is repair of tissue, by either regeneration or scar formation. Regeneration replaces damaged cells by identical or similar cells; scar formation replaces original tissue but is not functional. Inflammatory response alerts the nurse that the body is adapting to a local injury. During adaptation the inflammatory response protects the body from infection and promotes healing.

GENERAL ADAPTATION SYNDROME

The general adaptation syndrome is a physiological response of the whole body to stress. The GAS involves several body systems, primarily the autonomic nervous system and the endocrine system. Some textbooks, in fact, refer to the GAS as the "neuroendocrine response."

The GAS consists of three stages—the alarm reaction, the resistance stage, and the exhaustion stage (Fig. 28-3). The alarm reaction involves a number of physiological changes that prepare a person to adapt to a stressor. In the resistance stage the body stabilizes to allow the person to make an adaptive response. If this response fails to alleviate the stress, the person enters the exhaustion stage when he or she no longer has sufficient energy to attempt adaptation.

ALARM REACTION. The alarm reaction is characterized by the mobilization of the various defense mechanisms of the body or mind to cope with the stressor. Hormone levels rise to increase blood volume and thereby prepare the person to act. Other hormones are released to increase blood sugar levels to make energy

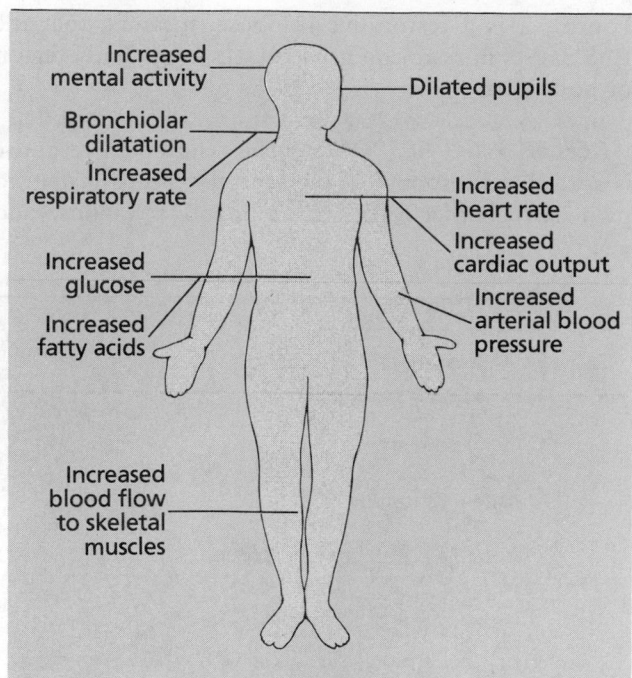

Fig. 28-4 Flight-or-fight response.

available for adaptation to the stressor. Increased levels of still other hormones—epinephrine and norepinephrine—result in increased heart rate, increased blood flow to muscles, increased oxygen intake, and greater mental alertness.

This extensive hormonal activity prepares the person for the "flight-or-fight" response. Cardiac output is increased, oxygen intake is increased, respiratory rate is speeded up, the pupils of the eyes are dilated to produce a greater visual field, the heart rate is increased for more muscular and other energy, and other changes occur to prepare the person to act (Fig. 28-4). With increased mental energy and alertness that result, the person is prepared to choose either to flee or to fight the stressor.

During the alarm reaction the person is faced with a specific stressor. The physiological response is extensive, involving major systems of the body, and may last from a minute to many hours. If the stressor is extreme or remains for a long time, there may be a threat to life. If the stressor is still present after the initial alarm reaction, the person progresses to the second phase of the general adaptation syndrome, resistance.

RESISTANCE STAGE. In the resistance stage the body stabilizes and hormone levels, heart rate, blood pressure, and cardiac output all return to normal. The person is attempting to adapt to the stressor. If the stress can be resolved, the body repairs damage that may have occurred. However, if the stressor remains present, as in continued blood loss, debilitating disease, or long-term severe mental illness, and the person is unable to adapt, he or she enters the third phase of the general adaptation syndrome, exhaustion.

EXHAUSTION STAGE. The exhaustion stage occurs when the body can no longer resist stress, when the energy necessary to maintain adaptation is depleted. The physiological response is intensified, but the person's energy level is compromised and adaptation to the stressor diminishes. The body is unable to defend itself against the impact of the stressor, physiological regulation diminishes; and, if the stress continues, death may result.

Psychological Response

Exposure to a stressor results in psychological as well as physiological adaptive responses. Healthy individuals, as they encounter life stressors, develop psychological adaptative behaviors to cope with them. These behaviors are efforts directed at stress management and are acquired through learning and experience, as a person learns which are acceptable and successful.

Psychological adaptive behaviors can be constructive or destructive. Constructive behaviors help an individual accept the challenge to resolve conflict that is causing stress. Even anxiety can be constructive, when it signals that a threat is present so that a person can take measures to reduce its severity.

Destructive behaviors are those that do not help a person cope with a stressor. Destructive behaviors affect an individual's reality orientation, problem-solving abilities, personality, and, in severe circumstances, ability to function. Anxiety can be destructive, for example, if a person is so overcome as to be unable to act to remove the stressor. Another example is abuse of alcohol or drugs, which may seem an adaptive behavior to an individual, when in reality it may increase rather than decrease the stress.

Psychological adaptive behaviors are also referred to as coping mechanisms. Such mechanisms can be task oriented, involving the use of direct problem-solving techniques to cope with the threats, or they can be ego-defense mechanisms, whose purpose is to regulate emotional distress and thus give protection from anxiety and stress. Ego-defense mechanisms are indirect methods of coping with stress.

TASK-ORIENTED BEHAVIORS

Task-oriented behaviors involve a person's cognitive abilities in an attempt to reduce stress, solve problems, resolve conflicts, and gratify needs (Stuart and Sundeen, 1987). The goal of task-oriented behaviors is to enable

---

Psychological Adaptive Behaviors

TASK-ORIENTED BEHAVIORS

- **Attack Behavior.** Acting to remove or overcome a stressor or to satisfy a need.
- **Withdrawal Behavior.** Removing oneself physically or emotionally from the stressor.
- **Compromise Behavior.** Changing the usual method of operating, substituting goals, or omitting the satisfaction of needs to meet other needs or to avoid stress.

EXAMPLES OF EGO-DEFENSE MECHANISMS

- **Compensation.** Making up for a deficiency in one aspect of self-image by strongly emphasizing a feature considered an asset.
- **Conversion.** Unconsciously repressing an anxiety-producing emotional conflict and transforming it into nonorganic symptoms.
- **Denial.** Avoiding emotional conflicts by refusing to acknowledge consciously anything that might cause intolerable emotional pain.
- **Displacement.** Transferring emotions, ideas, or wishes from a stressful situation to a less anxiety-producing substitute.
- **Identification.** Patterning one's behavior after that of another person and assuming that person's qualities, characteristics, and actions.
- **Regression.** Coping with a stressor through actions and behaviors associated with an earlier developmental period.

---

a person to cope realistically with demands of a stressor. Three general types of task-oriented behavior are attack behavior, withdrawal behavior, and compromise (see box).

EGO-DEFENSE MECHANISMS

Ego-defense mechanisms, first described by Sigmund Freud, are unconscious behaviors that offer psychological protection from a stressful event. These are used by everyone, and help protect against feelings of worthlessness and anxiety. Occasionally a defense mechanism can become distorted and no longer able to assist in adapting to a stressor.

There are many ego-defense mechanisms (see box above). The mechanisms described in this section are ones commonly observed. These are frequently activated by short-term stressors and usually do not result in psychiatric disorders. This section is meant to serve as an orientation to these mechanisms, not as a guide to psychiatric nursing.

NURSING PROCESS AND ADAPTATION TO STRESS

ASSESSMENT

Each client has specific perceptions and responses to stress. How a stressor is perceived is based on beliefs and norms, life experiences, life patterns, environmental factors, family structure and function, developmental stage, past experiences with stress, and coping mechanisms.

Because nurses are able to spend a great deal of time with clients and their families or friends, nurses are in a unique position to help clients cope with stress. Nurses also provide care for clients in various settings, and thus nurses are often able to assess how clients react to stress. The nurse assesses for indicators of stress in all dimensions of adaptation.

PHYSIOLOGICAL INDICATORS

Physiological indicators of stress are objective and more readily identified (see box). The client's vital signs are usually elevated and he or she may appear restless and be unable to rest or concentrate. These indicators can appear at any stage of stress. The symptom's duration and intensity can also be directly related to duration and intensity of the stressor.

Health care professionals are becoming increasingly aware of the relationship between psychological stress and medical illness. The link between psychological stress and disease is frequently called the mind-body

---

Physiological Indicators of Stress

- Elevated blood pressure
- Increased muscle tension (neck, shoulders, back)
- Elevated pulse and/or increased respiration
- "Sweaty" palms
- Cold hands and feet
- Slumped posture
- Tension headache
- Upset stomach
- Higher pitched voice
- Change in appetite
- Changes in urinary frequency
- Restlessness—difficulty in falling asleep or frequent awakening
- Dilated pupils
- Increased glucose

---

interaction. Research has increasingly shown that stress can affect illness and disease patterns. At the turn of the century, infectious diseases were the leading causes of death, but since then, antibiotics, improved living conditions, increased knowledge of nutrition, and better sanitation methods have lowered the death rate from infection. Now the leading causes of death are diseases highly correlated with life-style stressors.

During any of the three stages, there may be physical complaints such as nausea, vomiting, diarrhea, or headache. Last, physical appearance is changed; posture may be slumped, hygiene and grooming are poor, and style of dress differs. Prolonged stress has been linked with cardiovascular and gastrointestinal diseases. Some cancers and immunological disorders, as well as fatigue, burnout, and irritability, are associated with prolonged, unresolved stressors (Carr and Powers, 1986; Bargagliotti and Trygstd, 1987).

Mild stress situations do not usually produce long-lasting physiological damage, but moderate and severe stress can create risk for medical illness. Mild stress situations are stressors that everyone encounters regularly, such as oversleeping, traffic jams, a flat tire, or criticism from a superior. Such situations usually last from a few minutes to a few hours. These short-term, isolated stress situations are not likely to increase the risk of illness, unless a person experiences them on a continuous basis (Ivancevich and Matteson, 1980).

Moderate stress situations last longer, from several hours to a number of days. For example, an unresolved disagreement with a co-worker, work overload, new job expectations, and the prolonged absence of a family member are moderate stress situations. These can be significant because they increase the risk of a physical illness in a person with a predisposition to that illness. The relationship between illness and moderate stress situations has been documented in cases of myocardial infarction in men who are predisposed to coronary disease (Ivancevich and Matteson, 1980).

Severe stress situations are chronic ones which may last several weeks to several years, such as continual marital disagreements, prolonged financial difficulties, and long-term physical illness (Ivancevich and Matteson, 1980). The more intense and longer the stress situation, the higher the health risk.

Response to stress is unique, because of various factors in the person's different dimensions (Sutterly, 1979). How an illness develops in cases of a stress-related disease can be understood in terms of the health-illness continuum (Fig. 28-5). As a person's stress increases, stress behaviors increase gradually, which decreases energy and adaptive responses.

Understanding the mind-body interaction is crucial for predicting whether a person is at risk for stress-related illness. A nurse can often consider the effects on a client

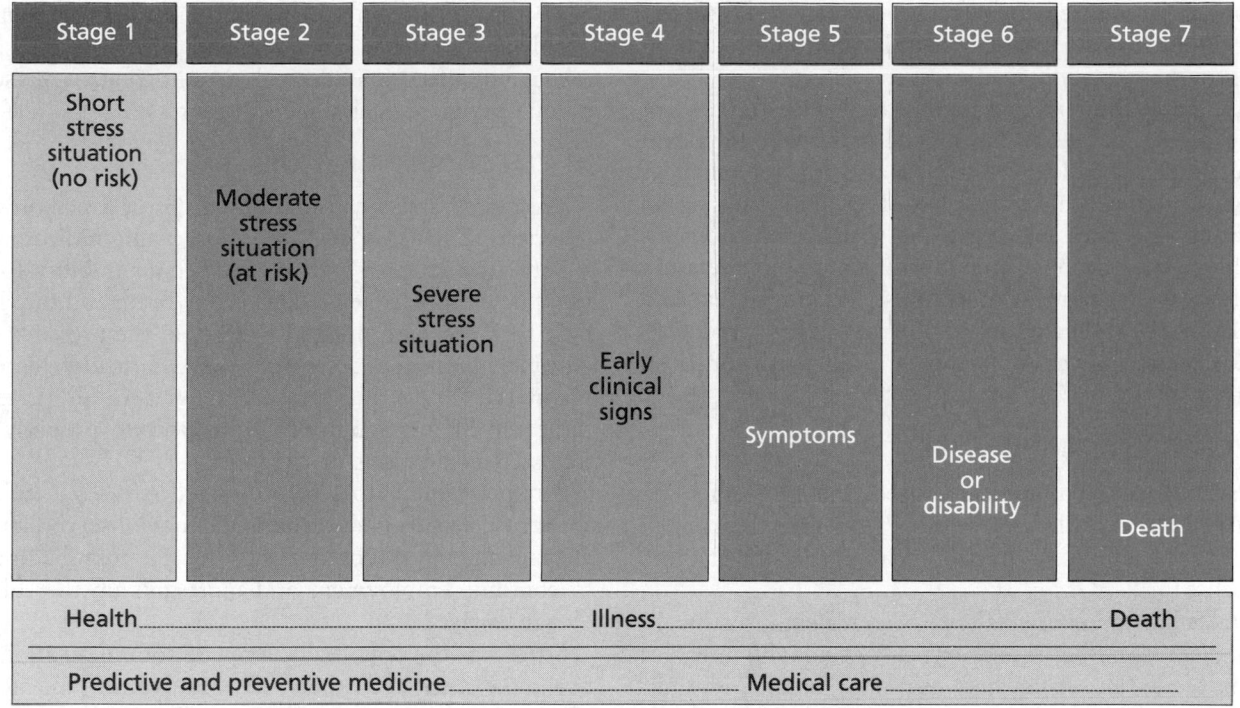

Stage 1	Stage 2	Stage 3	Stage 4	Stage 5	Stage 6	Stage 7
Short stress situation (no risk)	Moderate stress situation (at risk)	Severe stress situation	Early clinical signs	Symptoms	Disease or disability	Death

Health_____ Illness_____ Death

Predictive and preventive medicine_____ Medical care_____

Fig. 28-5   Stages of illness development in stress-related diseases.

of a stressful life-style or events and assess how well the client is able to adapt.

DEVELOPMENTAL INDICATORS

A person in any developmental stage can experience prolonged stress, which can result in observable indicators of stress that affect a particular stage. In any developmental stage a person normally encounters tasks and engages in behaviors characterstic of the stage. Prolonged stress can interrupt or impede passage through the stage. In extreme forms, prolonged stress can lead to maturational crises, which can generate stress.

An infant or young child generally encounters stressors within the home environment. For example, an infant must learn trust through the relationship with parents. However, if parental figures are absent or fail to provide the infant with the security needed to develop a sense of trust, this void can become a stressor for the infant. In later life there may be chronic distrust, resulting in withdrawal and limited interpersonal relationships.

As the infant progresses into childhood, he normally develops a sense of autonomy. If parents or the environment prevent this, he may experience stress. An indicator of this stress may be too much dependence on others.

A preschool child normally develops through exploring surroundings, exploring differences between males and females, and developing a conscience. The child is ashamed when he is caught being "bad" and wants to be told when he is being "good." An indicator of stress at this stage may be passive, inactive behavior toward the environment.

A school-age child normally develops a sense of adequacy. The child begins to realize he can accumulate knowledge and master skills to accomplish goals, and self-esteem develops through friendships and sharing with peers. At this stage, stress is indicated by the child's inability or unwillingness to develop friendships.

An adolescent normally develops a strong sense of identity and at the same time has a need to be accepted by peers. There are many stressors in this age group, including conflicts involving sexual drive and expected standards of behavior. Prolonged conflict may indicate indecision and confusion, rebelliousness, depression, or anxiety, which if not resolved can remain troublesome in later years.

A young adult is in transition from youthful experiences to adult responsibilities. The young adult must prepare for a career, for living alone, and perhaps for forming a family. Conflicts may develop between work and family responsibilities and the desire to maintain an active social life. Stressors in this stage include conflicts between expectations and desires.

Middle-age adults are usually involved in family building, creating stable careers, and perhaps caring for elderly parents. Middle-age adults are generally able to control desires, and in some cases substitute the needs of spouses, children, or parents for their needs. Stress can result, however, if they feel that too many responsibilities have been placed on them.

An older adult is commonly faced with the task of adapting to changes in family and perhaps to the death of a spouse. The older adult must also adjust to changes in physical appearance and physiological functioning. In addition, the stress of decreasing social interactions, as friends die or become unable to maintain contact, and retirement often brings more stress. Prolonged fear and stress can be indicated in an older adult by overdependence, which may cause further stress on family or social relationships.

PSYCHOSOCIAL INDICATORS

Psychosocial changes are a direct and sometimes obvious result of prolonged stress. Frequently a nurse can observe the emotional impact of stress through changes in behavior.

Stress has many effects on a person's emotional wellbeing (see box). Because everyone's personality involves a complex relationship between many factors, an individual's reaction to prolonged stress depends on support systems, prior experience with stressors, coping mechanisms, and overall stress response. A change in behavior should alert a nurse, family members, or friends that the

---

Behavioral and Emotional Indicators

- Anxiety
- Depression
- Burnout
- Increased use of chemical substances
- Changes in eating habits
- Changes in sleep and activity patterns
- Mental exhaustion
- Feelings of inadequacy
- Loss of self-esteem
- Increased irritability
- Loss of motivation
- Emotional outbursts and crying
- Decreased productivity and quality of job performance
- Tendency to make mistakes—poor judgment
- Forgetfulness and blocking
- Diminished attention to detail
- Preoccupation—daydreaming or "spacing out"
- Inability to concentrate on tasks
- Increased absenteeism and illness
- Lethargy
- Loss of interest
- Accident proneness

---

person needs help in adapting to stress. Ideally, coping problems should be anticipated and preventive measures taken, but often it is difficult to anticipate a person's unique psychological reaction to stress.

INTELLECTUAL INDICATORS

Prolonged stress can manifest itself in a person's intellectual dimension and have observable indicators of a particular stressor's effects. A person's ability to acquire new knowledge or skills is impaired, and the client may be faced with unemployment. In the presence of a chronic illness the client may have difficulty learning about the illness and treatment. As a result, stress is indicated by an inability to learn how to properly administer medications or treatments.

There are indicators of prolonged stress on the person's role performance. The nurse may observe that the client is having difficulty parenting. He may be unable to continue employment and must give up the role of "wage earner."

Stress has the potential to impede communication between the client and others. The family may indicate the effect of stress by an inability to resolve conflicts. In addition, the client's ability to effectively solve problems is reduced and is indicated by increased dependence on others.

SPIRITUAL INDICATORS

People use spiritual resources to adapt to stress in many ways, but stress can also threaten a person in the spiritual dimension. Severe stress may result in a person becoming angry at God or a Supreme Being, or the person may view the stressor as punishment. Stressors such as acute illness or the death of a loved one may threaten a person's meaning of life and can lead to spiritual depression. In providing care to a client who is affected spiritually, a nurse should not judge the appropriateness of religious feelings or practices but should assist the client in using spiritual resources to adapt to the stress.

NURSING DIAGNOSIS

A review of the assessment provides the nurse with the opportunity to cluster data that indicate a potential or actual stressor and the client's response. These data clusters ultimately result in the listing of nursing diagnoses occurring from stress (see nursing diagnoses box).

The nursing diagnosis should also identify the probable etiology for the problem. Incorrect identification of the cause of a nursing diagnosis can result in an inappropriate care plan and selected interventions.

The nurse must also be aware that stress can result in

Examples of Nursing Diagnoses Related to Stress

NANDA-APPROVED NURSING DIAGNOSES

Activity intolerance related to:
- Physiological stress (for example, illness)
- Emotional or situational crisis

Altered growth and development related to:
- Unresolved maturational stress (for example, delayed onset of menses)
- Situational crises (for example, unplanned pregnancy)

Fatigue related to:
- Physiological response to stress
- Impaired coping strategies

Hopelessness related to:
- Inability to resolve conflict (stress)
- Inability to control response to stress
- Lost belief in values

Ineffective family coping: compromised or *disabled*, or *ineffective individual coping* related to:
- Impaired coping strategies
- Prolonged stress (physiological, psychosocial, situational)

Potential for injury related to:
- Anxiety
- Impaired problem-solving abilities

Sleep pattern disturbance related to:
- Emotional or situational crises
- Anxiety

multiple diagnostic statements. Examples selected here are representative and not a conclusive list. Units 7 and 8 contain additional nursing diagnoses that occur when an individual has unmet physiological or environmental needs resulting from stress. Chapters 29 and 31 include nursing diagnoses associated with unmet self-concept and spiritual and sociocultural needs.

Identification of a nursing diagnostic label requires the presence of appropriate defining characteristics. These defining characteristics must be present in the assessment data base for the diagnostic label to be supported. The sample nursing diagnoses box provides examples of stress-related nursing diagnoses with appropriate defining characteristics and possible causes.

PLANNING

The formulation of nursing diagnoses initiates a plan for care (see care plan box). The care plan is individualized to the client's perception of both the stressor and response to stress. It is helpful for the nurse and client to develop realistic goals and interventions that are designed to assist the client with coping with the stressor. Whenever possible, it is important that a friend or family member be involved in care planning.

In most situations stress management plans are long term and are conducted in the client's home environment. Therefore the nurse must also be knowledgeable about the availability and cost of resources in the client's community.

Sample Nursing Diagnoses for Stress

Defining Characteristics	Nursing Diagnoses	Related Factors
Fatigue Weakness Dyspnea Change in vital signs	Activity intolerance	• Physiological stress (illness) • Emotional or situational crisis
Passivity Decreased affect Decreased response to stimuli Change in appetite Lack of involvement	Hopelessness	• Inability to resolve conflict • Inability to control response to stress • Lost belief in values
Random activities Restlessness Inability to concentrate Expression of fears	Potential for injury	• Anxiety • Impaired problem-solving abilities

Sample Nursing Care Plan for Stress			
Nursing Diagnosis	**Goal**	**Expected Outcomes**	**Nursing Interventions**
Activity intolerance related to situational crises	Client reports decrease in physiological indicators of stress.	Client's heart rate returns to a range of 70 to 90 beats per minute. Client no longer experiences dyspnea at rest or on exertion. Client reports falling asleep within 30 minutes of going to bed. Client reports physical tolerance to activity.	Encourage client to use progressive relaxation techniques for 20 minutes, twice a day. Client gradually increases activities Client schedules activities to allow for rest and sleep.

Stress management is designed to match the client's actual and potential stressors. The general goals for clients requiring stress management include:

1. Reduction in frequency of stress-inducing situations
2. Decreased physiological response to stress
3. Improved behavioral and emotional responses to stress

IMPLEMENTATION

A person is subjected to a variety of stressors every day. For some the stressors are minimal and do not pose a threat to physical or emotional well-being. In other situations, multiple stressors can combine synergistically resulting in prolonged stress and the need for stress management techniques. There are three areas for stress management: (1) reducing stressful situations, (2) decreasing physiological response to stress, and (3) improving behavioral and emotional responses to stress.

REDUCING STRESSFUL SITUATIONS

It is unrealistic, if not impossible, to try to eliminate all stressors. However, some can be reduced and thereby provide the client with a greater sense of control. Pender (1987) identifies five methods to assist in reducing stressful situations.

HABITUATION. Each client has unique habits and routines that are helpful in accomplishing day-to-day activities. "Routines reduce the need for expenditure of physical and psychological energy, resist change, and thus serve as a stabilizing force" (Pender, 1987). Ill-

nesses, crises, or hospitalization disturbs a client's routine, thereby disturbing his or her pattern of living and resulting in greater energy expenditure.

During actual or potential stress an established routine is effective in supporting energy conservation. For example, a woman who has chosen to stay at home to raise children is now sending her youngest child to school. While she anticipated this change, she was unable to obtain a job in her field. Presently she verbalizes fear about being "unable to get anything done at home." In this situation the client's habituation has been disrupted, and a new routine has not been developed. A plan that assists the client in developing a new routine consistent with her goals can reduce the stress.

CHANGE AVOIDANCE. Change avoidance is merely limiting unnecessary and avoidable changes. For example, Mary Jane, a mother of two school-age children, is divorcing her husband and is experiencing stress-related symptoms. A college roommate is pressuring her to relocate. Mary Jane and her children are experiencing a change in family structure, therefore this is not the time to consider a move.

Tension created by multiple changes increases the individual's response to stress. Each time a distressing change occurs the power of previous changes for upsetting well-being is increased. Deliberately reducing or postponing changes that result in tension assists the client to deal more constructively with unavoidable change.

Changes occurring during stress that are controlled or self-initiated provide a challenge for the client. The client is then able to turn the challenge into personal growth such as increased coping strategies or increased self-confidence as opposed to the production of more tension.

TIME BLOCKING. Time blocking is a technique in which an individual has a specific period of time to focus on and adapt to stressors. The major advantage of time blocking is that the client establishes a period of time to address specific goals or concerns and reduce the sense of time urgency. In addition, the client uses time and resources more effectively because the level of anxiety is reduced (Pender, 1987; Girdano and Everly, 1979).

TIME MANAGEMENT. A person who uses time efficiently generally experiences less stress related to social, family, and job activities. For some clients, time management techniques may include developing a list of tasks to be performed in order of priority. This technique can be beneficial for a client who is unable to get anything done because there seems to be too much to do.

Another time management measure is learning to say "no" to potential disruptions. Time management may also include scheduling appointments realistically to avoid rushing from task to task, meeting to meeting, or errand to errand.

Controlling demands of others is essential for effective time management. Few people are able to meet all requests made by others. It is important for a client, or a nurse, to learn to recognize which requests can be realistically met, which are impossible to meet, and which are negotiable.

ENVIRONMENTAL MODIFICATION. Changes in a client's environment that are realistic can reduce stressful situations. For example, job-related stress can be reduced by avoiding situations and people that are stress producing. Changing factors in the client's home to reduce housework or to light up a walkway around the house reduces stress. Eliminating committee work or club memberships that induce stress also helps.

When clients have realistic control over their environment, stress is mediated. Once the minimal or moderate stressors are mediated then the client is better able to resolve severe stressors.

DECREASING PHYSIOLOGICAL RESPONSE TO STRESS

In general, stress management techniques involve health-enhancing habits that can reduce the impact of stress on physical and mental health. These are often common-sense approaches that provide a basis for low-stress living. General prerequisites for stress management include regular exercise, good nutrition and diet, adequate rest, and relaxation techniques.

REGULAR EXERCISE. It has been shown that a regular exercise program improves muscle tone and posture, controls weight, reduces tension, and promotes relaxation. In addition, exercise reduces the risk of cardio-vascular disease and improves cardiopulmonary functioning.

Clients who have a history of a chronic illness, who are at risk for developing an illness, or who are over the age of 35 should begin a physical exercise program only after discussing the plan with a physician. In general, for a fitness program to have positive physical effects, a person should exercise at least three times a week for 30 to 40 minutes.

Everyone should use warm-up exercises prior to vigorous exercise such as jogging, aerobic dancing, or tennis. Warm-up exercises stimulate blood flow to the muscles and increase flexibility. Their goal is to reduce the risk of damage to the musculoskeletal system during exercise. Similarly, after vigorous exercise it is recommended that a person do a series of cool-down exercises rather than stop abruptly. For example, after jogging or aerobic dancing a person should walk around at a moderate pace, gradually slowing down and stopping. Cool-down exercises allow the cardiovascular, pulmonary, musculoskeletal, and metabolic systems to gradually return to their resting states.

Exercise programs are effective in decreasing the severity of such stress-related conditions as hypertension, overweight, tension headaches, fatigue, mental exhaustion, irritability, and depression. Adults, particularly, need routine exercise plans. They are occupied with rearing children, developing careers, and establishing homes, so their life-styles are often sedentary.

NUTRITION AND DIET. Nutrition and exercise are closely related. Food provides the body with fuel for activity and increased exercise improves circulation and delivery of nutrients to body tissues.

Everyone is encouraged to maintain weight according to standard ranges for sex, age, and body build. In addition to avoiding overeating or undereating, one should be aware of the nutritional quality of the foods. Too much caffeine, salt, or sugar can upset the body's metabolic functioning, as can deficiencies in vitamins, minerals, and nutrients.

Poor dietary habits can exacerbate a stress response and make a person irritable, hyperactive, and anxious. This impairs the ability to meet personal, family, and job responsibilities. Nursing measures for helping clients meet their nutritional needs are detailed in Chapter 33. In general, dietary goals should be based on the following three objectives endorsed by the U.S. Senate Committee on Nutrition and Human Needs:

1. Reduce consumption of salt, refined sugar, fat, and cholesterol.
2. Increase consumption of fruit, vegetables, and whole grains.
3. Limit meat consumption, substituting poultry and fish.

Changes Resulting from Relaxation Techniques

- Lowered blood pressure (baseline)
- Lowered heart rate (baseline)
- Decreased cardiac dysrhythmias
- Decreased oxygen demands and oxygen consumption
- Decreased muscle tension
- Lowered metabolic rate
- Increased alpha brain waves
- Increased reports of restfulness
- Improved concentration
- Improved ability to cope with stressors

REST. An established, habitual pattern of sufficient rest and sleep is also important to stress management. A person experiencing stress may need to be encouraged to allow time for rest and sleep. They not only refresh the body but also help a person become mentally relaxed. A client may need specific help in learning to relax in order to fall asleep.

RELAXATION TECHNIQUES. Techniques of progressive relaxation with muscle tension, progressive relaxation without muscle tension, and imagery reduce the physiological and emotional components of the stress response. Relaxation techniques are learned behaviors and require training and practice sessions (see Chapter 35). Once the client is skilled at these techniques, tension is reduced and physiological parameters are changed (see box).

IMPROVED BEHAVIORAL AND EMOTIONAL RESPONSES TO STRESS

Behavioral and emotional responses to stress can be mediated by the use of support systems, crisis interventions, and enhancing self-esteem.

SUPPORT SYSTEMS. The saying "No man is an island" is of particular importance for stress management. A support system of family, friends, and colleagues who will listen and offer advice and emotional support is beneficial to a person experiencing stress. Support systems can reduce stress reactions and promote physical and mental well-being. Thus a person experiencing stress should be encouraged to expand social and personal contacts.

Nurses can use various methods to help clients build their support systems, such as encouraging family or significant others to visit, making support groups available, encouraging involvement in church groups, and encouraging recreational activities. Nurses can use therapeutic communication skills to encourage clients to express their feelings and begin to identify causes of stress. When stress is the result of confusion or wrong information, a nurse can use teaching techniques to help relieve clients' stress. If stress results from differences between the expectations and realities, a nurse can use methods to help the client gain a stronger self-concept or body image. All these methods generally help clients indirectly to build stronger support systems. If stress is the result of social isolation, nursing strategies are aimed at helping the person develop a new social network.

CRISIS INTERVENTION. Crisis intervention is a therapeutic technique for helping a client resolve a particular, immediate stress problem. Crisis intervention does not involve an indepth analysis of a client's situation but addresses the immediate, urgent need for stress reduction. The goal is to restore the person as quickly as possible to the precrisis level of functioning in all dimensions.

A crisis occurs when a person encounters a problem or stress situation that he or she is unable to cope with in usual ways. Behavior tends to be disorganized, and a person may make only abortive attempts at resolving the problem (Aguilera and Messick, 1986).

Both clients and nurses are at risk for two types of crises, situational and developmental. A situational crisis arises suddenly in response to an external event or conflict involving a specific circumstance. Symptoms associated with situational crises are transient, and the episode is brief. Situational crises include giving birth, major role changes, acute physical illness, physical assault or rape, family changes such as remarriage or the death of a family member, and unexpected unemployment.

Developmental crises occur when a person is unable to complete developmental tasks of a psychosocial stage and is therefore unable to continue developing. A developmental crisis can occur at any point in life, if circumstances prevent a person from meeting the challenge of a particular stage.

When a nurse assesses that a client is experiencing a crisis, the nurse plans and implements specific measures to help resolve the crisis. Aguilera and Messick (1986) have developed an approach to intervention that can be used for both types of crises (Fig. 28-6). This approach enables the nurse to understand how a stressful event has lead to a state of disequilibrium, or crisis. Resolution of the crisis depends on the person's perceiving the stressful event realistically, having adequate support, and using adequate coping mechanisms. If the client is lacking in one or more of these areas, the nurse and client plan specific methods to restore equilibrium. If the crisis has

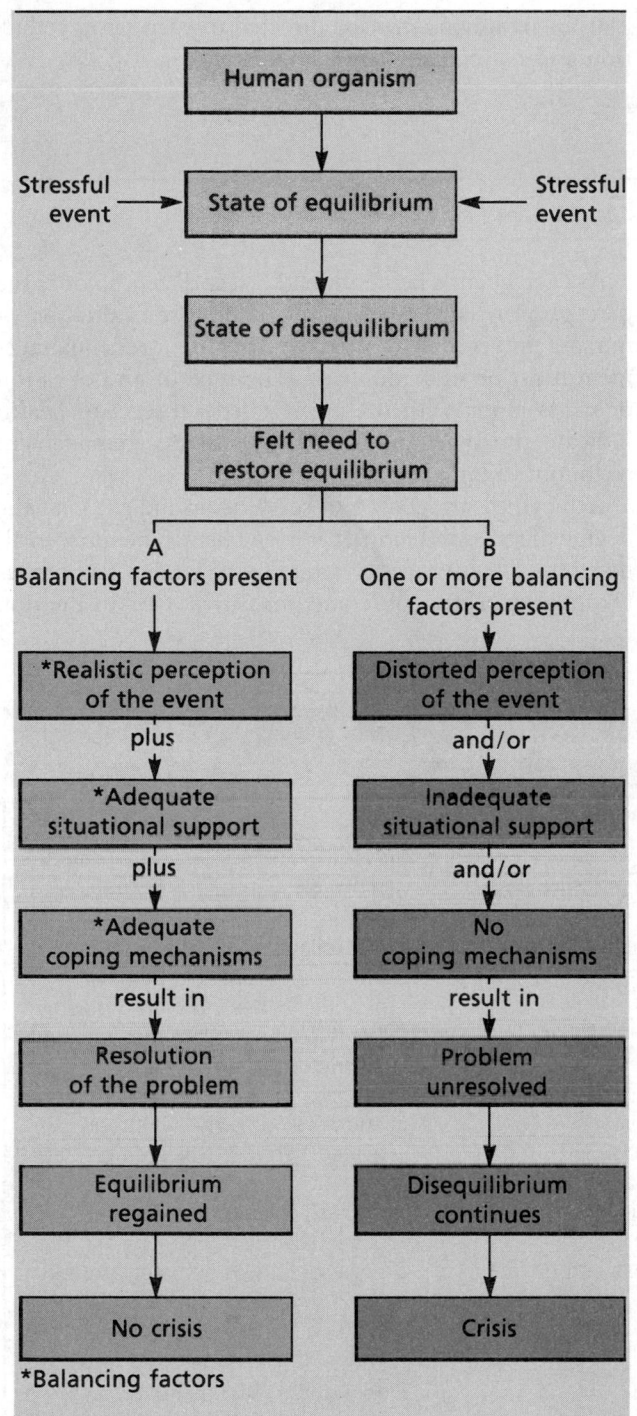

Fig. 28-6 Crisis intervention model.
From Aguilera, DC, and Messick, JM: Crisis intervention: theory and methodology, ed. 5, St. Louis, 1986, The C.V. Mosby Co.

arisen because perception of the event is distorted, then the nurse uses techniques to help the client perceive the stressful event realistically. If the crisis has arisen because of a lack of situational support or coping mechanisms, then the nurse initiates measures to assist the client in

these areas by maximizing available coping mechanisms and developing additional supports. The nurse then evaluates the extent to which the client is able to resolve the crisis with these means.

ENHANCING SELF-ESTEEM. Improvement in a client's self-esteem can assist in positive stress-reduction strategies (see Chapter 29). When clients identify positive characteristics, they can focus attention on attributes that others admire. This increased positive self-awareness will result in behavior that reflects the client's positive characteristics (Pender, 1987).

STRESS MANAGEMENT FOR NURSES

Rapid changes in society, health care technology, and health care knowledge, as well as changes in the nursing profession, can all place stress on nurses. Job stress is "the condition in which some factor or combination of factors at work interact with the worker to disrupt his or her psychological or physiological balance" (Margolis and Kroes, 1974).

Most nurses experience stress in their work environments. Stressors can be related to rotation of shifts, floating to different units, severity of clients' illnesses, number of clients per nurse, interactions with other nurses and other health care workers, and institutional policies. Reaction to a job-related stressor depends on the nurse's personality, health status, previous experience with stress, and coping mechanisms.

Job stress is frequently associated with a condition called "burnout," which is characterized by emotional, physical, and spiritual exhaustion. In the work setting an individual experiencing burnout may withdraw from others, exhibit negative feelings toward others, have increased absences from work, and perform work tasks less effectively than previously (Claus and Bailey, 1980).

Nurses are at risk for job stress as a result of three factors. First, new graduates generally have high expectations, which may not be accomplished in the work setting, leading to feelings of frustration. Second, nurses usually work in close interaction with others, specifically, clients and other health care professionals. Such continuous interaction can lead to conflicts and other stresses. Finally, the work setting itself increases the risk for job stresses. Most nurses work in institutional settings that are frequently unable to meet all the individual needs of either clients or nurses.

Nurses can reduce these stresses by using the stress management techniques used for clients. Those common-sense techniques improve the nurses' physical and mental well-being, enabling them to cope more successfully with stressors. In addition, nurses should identify specific stressors in their work environments and if possible eliminate or minimize them. Finally, nurses can use

---

Problem-Solving Process for Reducing Stress in the Work Environment

- Define overall needs, purposes, and goals.
- Define the problem.
- Analyze capabilities, constraints, and interest groups.
- Specify an approach to problem solving.
- State behavioral objectives.
- Generate alternative solutions.
- Analyze alternatives.
- Choose the best alternative.
- Implement and control the action chosen.
- Evaluate the effectiveness of the action.

Modified from Bailey, JT, and Claus, KE: Decision making in nursing: tools for change, St. Louis, 1975, The C.V. Mosby Co.

a problem-solving process directed toward stress reduction and conflict resolution (see box).

EVALUATION

As each client's perception of stress differs so does the perception of stress reduction. Therefore evaluation of nursing interventions directed toward stress management must be individualized. The type of and duration of stress along with the client's general level of health indicate the type and intensity of stress management techniques required.

Achieving care goals can serve as an indicator of the degree of stress reduction for each client. The nurse evaluates the effectiveness of stress management techniques through expected outcome measures (see evaluation box).

Sample Evaluation of Interventions for Stress

Goals	Evaluative Measures	Expected Outcomes
Frequency of stress-inducing situations is reduced.	Observe client self-reporting stressful events.	Client reports decrease in stressors.
	Obtain information about stressful events from client's family or friends.	Client follows new routine. Client reports scheduled time periods for dealing with problems. Client implements time management techniques at home, work, and in school.
Physiological response to stress is decreased.	Observe client's verbal and nonverbal interaction.	Client does not carry out stress-related behavior (for example, excessive frowning, smoking).
	Obtain client's vital signs.	Heart rate decreases to 70 to 90 beats per minute.
	Review client's exercise and dietary patterns.	Client exercises three times a week for 20 minutes. Dietary patterns show decrease intake of salt, sugar, and fat with increased intake of fruits, vegetables, and whole grains. Client successfully demonstrates relaxation techniques.
Behavioral and emotional responses to stress improve.	Observe client's verbal and nonverbal cues about stress.	Client reports use of support system.
	Obtain information from family and friends about client's behavioral and emotional response to stress.	Client states more positive attributes about self. Client gives more attention to hygiene and grooming. Excessive crying, anger, and aggression are absent.

SUMMARY

Stress is present to some degree in everyone's life. Each person reacts to stress differently, according to perception of the stressor, personality, prior experience with stress, and use of coping mechanisms. Various models of stress—and Selye's general adaptation syndrome, the most commonly used model—help the nurse understand causes and responses to stress.

Stress can be positive if it results in necessary changes in a person's life-style and work environment. However, prolonged stress can affect a person's level of health, resulting in physical or mental illness. Stress management techniques are directed toward changing how a person reacts to a stressor. Many of the techniques presented in this chapter are common-sense approaches to coping with stress and developing healthy personal habits.

A nurse, like anyone else, is exposed to stressors, but the practice of nursing exposes a person to additional stressors. Management of job stress requires an ability to solve problems and thus avoid job burnout.

Stress is a fact of life, but it need not control life. How a person responds to stress can be controlled and changed. Through the use of health promotion and maintenance strategies, nurses can help clients manage stress successfully.

KEY CONCEPTS

✓ Homeostasis is a state of relative constancy in the internal environment.

✓ Key homeostatic mechanisms are controlled by the medulla oblongata, the reticular formation, and the pituitary gland.

✓ Prolonged stress decreases the adaptive capacity of homeostatic mechanisms.

✓ Stress is a physiological or psychological tension that can affect a person in any or all of the human dimensions.

✓ Stressors are events, situations, or other stimuli that an individual may encounter in the internal or external environment.

✓ Stressors necessitate change or adaptation so that a state of equilibrium can be maintained.

✓ A person's response to stress is influenced by the intensity, duration, and scope of the stressor and by the number of stressors present at one time.

✓ Adaptation is the process through which a person changes in response to stress.

✓ A person adapts to stress by using resources in all dimensions—physical and developmental, emotional, intellectual, social, and spiritual.

✓ Physiological adaptation is the body's attempt to maintain optimal functioning.

✓ The two forms of physiological response to stress are the local adaptation syndrome and the general adaptation syndrome.

✓ The local adaptation syndrome involves several specific responses to stress, including the reflex pain response and the inflammatory response.

✓ The general adaptation syndrome is a multisystem physiological response to stress.

✓ The three stages of the GAS are the alarm reaction, the resistance stage, and the exhaustion stage.

✓ Psychological responses to stress include task-oriented behaviors and ego-defense mechanisms.

✓ Task-oriented behaviors include attack behavior, withdrawal, and compromise.

✓ Ego-defense mechanisms are unconscious behaviors that offer a person psychological protection from stressful feelings or events.

✓ Stress has been shown to have an impact on the onset, course, and outcome of illness.

✓ Prolonged stress decreases a person's ability to adapt to the stress and affects the person in all five dimensions.

✓ People generally learn to use both short- and long-term strategies to cope with stress.

✓ Stress management techniques include health-enhancing habits, crisis intervention, and methods of reducing job stress.

REFERENCES

Aguilera, DC, and Messick, JM: Crisis intervention: theory and methodology, ed. 5, St. Louis, 1986, The C.V. Mosby Co.

Claus, KE, and Bailey, JT: Living with stress and promoting well-being: a handbook for nurses, St. Louis, 1980, The C.V. Mosby Co.

Coelho, G, Hamburg, D, and Adams, J, editors: Coping and adaptation, New York, 1974, Basic Books, Inc., Publishers.

French, JRP, and Kahn, RL: A programmatic approach to studying the industrial environment and mental health, J Soc Issues 18:1, 1962.

Girdano, D, and Everly, G: Controlling stress and tension, Englewood Cliffs, N.J., 1979, Prentice-Hall.

Ivancevich, JM, and Matteson, MT: Stress and work: a managerial perspective, Glenview, Ill., 1980, Scott, Foresman & Co.

Margolis, B, and Kroes, W: Occupational stress and strain. In McLean, A, editor: Occupational stress, Springfield, Ill., 1974, Charles C Thomas, Publisher.

McGrath, JE: Stress and behavior in organizations. In Dannette, MD, editor: Handbook of industrial and organizational psychology, Chicago, 1976, Rand McNally & Co.

Mechanic, D: Students under stress, Glencoe, Ill., 1962, The Free Press.

Numerof, RE: Managing stress: a guide for health professionals, Rockville, Md., 1983, Aspen Systems Corporation.

Pelletier, K: Mind as health, mind as slayer, New York, 1977, Dell Publishing Co., Inc.

Pender, NJ: Health promotion in nursing practice, ed. 2, Norwalk, Conn., 1987, Appleton & Lange.

Selye, H: The stress of life, ed. 2, New York, 1976, McGraw-Hill Book Co.

Stuart, GW, and Sundeen, SJ: Principles and practice of psychiatric nursing, ed. 3, St. Louis, 1987, The C.V. Mosby Co.

Sundeen, S, et al.: Nurse-client interaction: implementing the nursing process, ed. 3, St. Louis, 1985, The C.V. Mosby Co.

Sutterly, DC: Stress and health: a survey of self-regulation modalities, Top Clin Nurs 1:1, 1979.

Research Articles

Bargagliottli, CA, and Trygstad, LN: Differences in stress and coping findings: a reflection of social realities or methodologies, Nurs Res 36:170, 1987.

Carr, JA, and Powers, MJ: Stressors associated with coronary bypass surgery, Nurs Res 35:243, 1986.

ADDITIONAL READINGS

Edelman, C, and Mandle, CC: Health promotion throughout the life span, St. Louis, 1986, The C.V. Mosby Co.

Gherman, EM: Stress and the bottom line, New York, 1981, American Medical Association Communication.

Hurst, MW, Jenkins, CD, and Rose, RM: The relation of psychological stress to onset of medical illness. In Garfield, CA, editor: Stress and survival: the emotional realities of life-threatening illness, St. Louis, 1979, The C.V. Mosby Co.

MacNeil, JM, and Weisz, GM: Critical care nursing stress, Heart and Lung, 16:274, 1987.

Norbeck JS: Types and sources of social support for managing job stress in critical care nursing, Nurs Res 34:225, 1985.

Qamar, SL: The stress-carative model of nursing practice, Focus Crit Care 13(6):15, 1986.

Roberts, JG, et al.: Analysis of coping responses and adjustment: stability of conclusions, Nurs Res 36:94, 1987.

Selye, H: The general adaptation syndrome and the diseases of adaptation, Clin Endocrinol 6:117, 1946.

Sund, K, and Ostwald, SK: Dual-earner families' stress levels and personal and life-style–related variables, Nurs Res 34:357, 1985.

Thomas, SP, and Groër, M: Relationship of demographic, life-style, and stress variables to blood pressure in adolescents, Nurs Res 35:169, 1986.

Wilson, VS: Identification of stressors related to patients' psychologic responses to the surgical intensive care unit, Heart Lung 16:267, 1987.

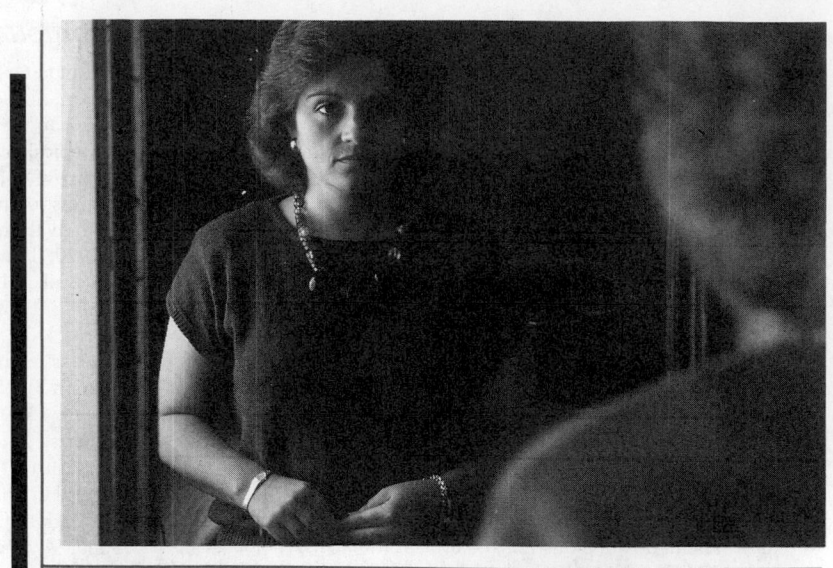

OBJECTIVES

Mastery of content in this chapter will enable the student to:

- Define the key terms listed.
- Describe development of self-concept, relating Erikson's psychosocial stages and Piaget's cognitive stages.
- Discuss factors that influence each of the four components of self-concept: identity, body image, self-esteem, and roles.
- Describe the five processes of socialization.
- Identify stressors that affect each of the four components of self-concept.
- Explain the processes that can lead to role conflict, role ambiguity, and role strain.
- Discuss identity confusion as a developmental aspect of adolescence and as a problem of self-concept.
- Discuss ways in which the nurse's self-concept and nursing activities can affect the client's self-concept.
- Describe behavior or defining characteristics that may indicate each of the following: identity confusion, disturbed body image, low self-esteem, and role conflict.
- List, for each of the four components of self-concept, a common nursing diagnosis related to self-concept disturbance and related factors.
- Describe goals of care, specific nursing interventions and outcome/evaluation measures for a client with self-concept disturbance.

KEY TERMS

Body Image
Depersonalization
Identification
Identity
Identity Confusion
Inhibition
Reinforcement-Extinction
Role
Role Ambiguity
Role Conflict
Role Overload
Role Strain
Self-Concept
Self-Esteem
Self-Ideal
Socialization

Self-Concept

A person's self-concept represents a complex integration of conscious and unconscious feelings, attitudes, and perceptions about the total self, the body, a sense of worth, and roles. It reflects interpretations of past experiences, social interactions, and sensations. Self-concept is what one believes about oneself as a separate and distinct entity. Self-concept is based in part on how we believe others see us (Cooley, 1956).

Self-concept is not the same as the self. The self includes the total subjective and objective qualities of a person as seen personally and by others. For example, the self includes the person's actual appearance, values, ideas, and knowledge, as well as self-perceptions and the perceptions of others. Self-concept is the person's subjective image of the self—the perception of physical, emotional, and social attributes or qualities. Self-concept is a frame of reference that affects how the person deals with situations and relates to others. An individual's self-image may or may not be accurate, and while aspects of the person may constantly undergo change, a person's self-concept is slow to change (Yamamoto, 1972). Discrepancies between certain aspects of the person and the self-concept may become a source of stress or conflict.

Hospitalization, illness, surgery, separation from family, and other health factors can affect self-concept. For example, amputation of an extremity results in an altered body image. Adaptation to the amputation includes integrating the bodily change into the physical concept of self—that is, body image. Chronic illness may affect a person's ability to provide financial support for the family, thereby affecting the sense of self-worth and the role within the family. These changes will also alter self-concept. In each of these two examples, the altered self-concept would be readily apparent to a nurse. But many changes in clients' self-concepts may not be as apparent; therefore, a nurse must understand how stressors affect self-concept and be able to recognize behaviors that show that a client is in need of nursing interventions.

This chapter provides an overview of the development of self-concept, stressors affecting self-concept, and the role of the nurse in relation to the client's self-concept. To provide nursing care for a client with a self-concept disturbance, the nurse uses the nursing process—assessing the client's condition, determining the nursing diagnosis, and planning, implementing, and evaluating care.

DEVELOPMENT OF SELF-CONCEPT

The development and maintenance of self-concept constitute a complex process involving many variables. Self-concept, body image, and self-esteem are interrelated concepts. The following includes definitions, application of the concepts to nursing, and a description of the development of self-concept throughout the life span.

Self-concept is the psychic representation or identity of an individual, the central core of "I" around which all perceptions and experiences are organized. Self-concept is a dynamic combination formulated over a period of years based on the following sources: (1) reactions of others to the infant's/child's body and behavior; (2) ongoing perceptions of others' reactions to the self; (3) experiences with self and others; (4) personality structure; (5) perceptions of physiological and sensory stimuli that impinge on the self; (6) prior and new experiences; (7) present feelings about physical, emotional, and social self; and (8) expectations about the self. Self-concept gives a sense of continuity, wholeness, and consistency to the person. It has a high degree of stability and represents the person's general feelings toward the self, either positive or negative. Self-concept is expressed through behavior, words, intellect, goals, attitudes, and values (Cooley, 1956; Coopersmith, 1967; Jacobsen, 1964; Murray, 1982).

Each person has numerous perceptions of self based on gender, age, family roles and background, occupational and social roles, and use of leisure activity. Normally, these various facets of the self, the various "masks" the person may wear when in different situations, are not too diverse or different from each other. A consistency remains even though the person feels dif-

ferently about the self from time to time or is perceived in different ways by others. The ill person not only experiences negative feelings about self but also may feel a lack of wholeness, a sense of distortion, and discontinuity because of pain, surgery, disease in a specific organ or body system, or emotional illness.

Body image is the mental picture of one's body, including the external, internal, and postural image of the body. The mental image held by the person is not necessarily consistent with the actual body structure or appearance. The image of the body includes attitudes, emotions, and personality reactions toward the body as an object in space, with a distinct boundary and separate from all others and the general environment (Schilder, 1951). Body image develops gradually over several years as the person learns more about the body, its structure, functions, abilities, and limitations. Body image may change within a few hours, days, weeks, or months, depending on external stimuli on the body and actual changes in appearance, structure, or function. Other people's responses to the individual, positive or negative, may also create a change in body image (Fisher and Cleveland, 1968). For example, if the nurse shows acceptance of a mastectomy scar, the woman will be assisted in reconstructing a more positive, whole view of self. If a family member reacts with disgust, avoidance, or repugnance to a person with a deformed or amputated limb, the individual may construct a negative or distorted body image that lacks a sense of a whole or unified being, or the individual may be more helpless than is warranted by the actual change in structure or function.

Self-esteem is the evaluation that individuals customarily maintain of themselves and convey to others by verbal reports or overt behavioral expressions. This judgmental feeling about self includes a sense of approval or disapproval and indicates the extent to which the person believes the self capable, significant, valued, successful, and worthy (Coopersmith, 1967). Self-esteem refers to the acceptance of self because of basic worth, in spite of weaknesses, limitations, or deficiencies. The person who values self and feels valued by others usually has a positive self-concept. The person who feels worthless, does not feel respected by others, and does not respect the self usually has a negative self-concept.

An ill person may feel inferior, less valued, unaccepted by others, and unacceptable to self. The client may need considerable assistance to overcome limitations, weaknesses, or deficiencies. The nurse avoids judgment or criticism while assisting, teaching, or supporting to help the client overcome problems. The nurse's acceptance of the client's behavior and appearance and of the client as a person with worth and dignity is crucial in helping the client regain positive self-esteem.

Developmental Sequence of Self-Concept and Body Image

INFANT

At first newborn babies can barely discriminate between their own pleasurable sensations and the objects from which the sensations are derived. They have diffuse feelings of hunger, pain, rage, and comfort. They do not differentiate the self from the environment. The external world is an extension of self. Only as perceptive and sensory functions mature do infants gradually learn about their bodies. Babies gradually distinguish themselves from other objects as they are fed, diapered, touched, or as they bang their heads, bite their hands, and mouth objects. The process of defining self begins when children act reflexively, such as when they suck or grasp an object. The act itself is important, and so is the significance attributed to it by parents, since they reinforce behavior. Gradually the child experiences visceral, visual, auditory, kinesthetic, and motor sensations (Anthony, 1968; Schilder, 1951).

Weaning, contact with others, and exploration of the environment also heightens self-awareness. As the child approaches the first birthday, coordination of these sensory experiences is being internalized into the motor body image. The child is aware that some body parts give greater pleasure than other parts and that differences in sensation occur when the body or when another object is touched (Anthony, 1968; Murray and Zentner, 1985; Schilder, 1951).

Without adequate stimulation of both the motor abilities and the senses, body image and self-concept development are impaired, as shown by studies of infants in premature incubators who lacked rocking, stroking, and cuddling (Kramer et al., 1975). The infant's initial experiences with his body, determined largely by maternal care and attitudes, are the basis for developing body images and how he later accepts and handles the body and react to others (Murray and Zentner, 1985).

TODDLER

As children move into the toddler stage (1 to 3 years of age), they are more mobile and able to interact with others. They are gaining skill with feeding themselves and with basic tasks of hygiene. They are learning to coordinate movements and to imitate others. They are learning control of their bodies through locomotion, toilet training, speech, and socialization skills.

Young children are not always aware of the whole body and might even consider distal parts such as hands and feet as something apart from themselves. They do not always know when they are ill, fatigued, too cold, thirsty, or have wet pants. They are simply aware of general feelings and are increasingly aware of others' reactions to themselves and their behavior. For example, when toddlers are playing with toys or interacting happily with people, they feel good and in control. When things are not going well, if they can't succeed or are punished excessively, they feel bad and shameful (Anthony, 1968). Gradually they become more aware of body sensations and movements and their ability to control these to some degree.

PRESCHOOLER

The preschool years (3 to 5 years of age) help children to realize what they are capable of. Body boundaries, sense of self, and gender become more definite to preschoolers because of a developing sexual curiosity and awareness of how they differ from others of the same and opposite gender. Increased motor skills with precision of movement and maturing sense of balance, improved spatial orientation, maturing cognitive and language abilities, ongoing play activities, and relationship and identification with parents add to self-concept and body image development (Anthony, 1968).

Learning about the body, where it begins and ends, what it looks like, and what it can do, is basic to self-concept and body image formation. Growing self-awareness includes discovery of feelings in the sense that preschoolers are now learning names for feelings. They are beginning to learn how they affect others and how others respond to them. They are also learning the rudiments of control over feelings and behavior. The concept of body is reflected in the way the child talks, moves, draws pictures, and plays. The child who has no frame of reference in relation to self experiences increased anxiety and misperception of self and others.

Parental and cultural attitudes about appropriate behavior for boys and girls may contribute to body image confusion, especially if behavior and appearance does not match the expectations of others. Children begin to test roles they have seen and continue to imitate as they identify with the same-sexed parent or significant other.

Although children still feel small in relation to adults, they now have established basically a positive or negative view of self. Children hear and experience emotions and pronouncements of others, especially parents, about themselves as people, as well as about things and events around them. When these expressions are repeated many times they begin to form a predictable pattern, so that the child internalizes the views of others and begins to see them as part of the self. The child then behaves to match those views. This incorporated self-view begins as a judgment made by another. For example, Johnny's parents consider him to be mechanically inclined. This behavior was not a part of Johnny at birth, but as he develops, and corresponding experiences are given him, the perception becomes a part of him and he acts accordingly. Children learn to value what their parents value. The appraisal by a significant other becomes self-appraisal. A positive self-concept is imperative for happiness and personality unity. Negative self-concepts cause children to feel defensive toward others and about themselves. A negative self-concept hinders adjustment to school, academic progress, peer relationships, and developmental tasks.

SCHOOL-AGE CHILD

Until the child attends school, self-concept and body-image development is based primarily on parental attitudes. Now others contribute to self-concept and body image.

As the child enters the school years, growth is steady and more motor, social, and intellectual skills are acquired. The physique is changing, and sexual identity is strengthening. The child is now a part of a new group—teachers, peers, and school-age society. Attention span has increased, and reading allows expansion of self-concept through imagination into other roles, behaviors, places. Games become a major portion of the school-child's activity. Through games, the child interacts with peers, develops additional motor and intellectual skills, and thereby expands self-concept and body image. As children learn and follow rules, they also learn about their acceptability to others, strengthening a positive self-concept. Games also expand understanding and awareness of other people and other places. Children express feelings through games, literature, drawing, and music. The child who has a positive and realistic image of self tends to express this as behavior movements, drawings, and music, as well as in statements and games. With increased problem solving, a greater self-awareness of personal strengths and limitations develops. Self-concept and body image are quite fluid, for the child is changing physically, emotionally, mentally, and socially. While children are not able accurately to name body organs, they are increasingly aware of their bodies as well as of their abilities.

ADOLESCENT

Puberty, with hormonal changes and growth spurts, is a critical period in the development of self-concept. Adolescence brings upheaval physically, emotionally, and socially. As the child matures sexually, new feelings, roles, and values must be integrated. The rapid growth of this period, noticed by the adolescent and others is an important factor in body-image revision.

Adolescent girls and boys are sometimes said to be "all legs." They are often clumsy and awkward. Because growth changes cannot be denied, the adolescent is forced to alter the mental picture of self to function. Physical changes in size and appearance cause a change in self-perception as well as in use of the body. The adolescent spends a great deal of time in front of the mirror for hygiene, grooming, and clothing. Age, maturation, gender, size, shape, and even the person's name are emphasized in behavior, music, dance, or sports—all normal ways for the adolescent to integrate a changing body image.

Development of self-concept and body image is closely akin to identity formation (Erikson, 1963). The adolescent must be studied in the context of the present as well as the past. Earlier experiences continue to have important affects. Those experiences that were positive enable the adolescent to feel good about self. Negative experiences may result in a poor self-concept. If children enter adolescence with negative feelings, they will find this a difficult period.

Growth, appearance, and functional changes draw adolescents' attention to changing body parts, and they become more sensitive about it, causing a distorted view of self. They may overemphasize perceived defects, such as a pointed nose, too large ears, short stature, or a large body frame, and consequently under-evaluate themselves. The body acts as the basic source of acceptance or rejection from others. The adolescent is idealistic but may not be able to achieve an ideal body. If adolescents do not feel accepted for themselves or their bodies, they may try to compensate through sports, vocational or academic success, a religious commitment, use of alcohol or drugs, or by seeking a date or group of friends to enhance prestige. Thus, identification with the same sexed parent, harmonious relationships with other adults and peers, and having ideals as well as realistic goals to strive for are essential.

If the adolescent does have a disability or defect, peers and adults may react with fear, pity, repulsion, or curiosity. The adolescent may retain and later reflect these impressions because people tend to perceive themselves as others perceive them. If the adolescent develops a negative self-image, his motivation, behvior, and eventual life style may lack harmony and be out of step with social expectations.

Adolescents begin to relate to the opposite sex in new ways and with increasing interest. They sample various behavioral roles as they establish a sense of identity, who they are, what life means, and where they are going. Self-esteem becomes closely related to self-concept as the person gets older. All of this sets the stage for adulthood.

YOUNG ADULT

Although physical growth has stopped by this stage, cognitive, social, and behavioral changes continue for the rest of life. Young adulthood (early 20s to mid 40s) is a period of choice, with settling in so that there is stability in the establishment of employment, an intimate relationship, and family, whether family includes having children or is limited to friends who are as significant as close family members. Self-concept and body image are established. Self-expectations, reactions of others, perceived abilities and limitations, values, attitudes, knowledge, and habits have been integrated into a functioning, adaptive, unified whole.

The young adult's search for self-definition is complicated by confusion in society over gender behavior, the meaning of maleness and femaleness, and the variety of roles and occupations from which to choose. Masculine and feminine roles are becoming diffuse. The stereotypes that once characterized these roles are disappearing. Self-concept and body image are social creations, and approval and acceptance are given for normal appearance and proper behavior according to societal standards. Self-image continually influences and enlarges the person's world, mastery of interaction with it, and the ability to respond to the many experiences it offers. Self-concept is constantly evolving and can be identified in the person's values, attitudes, and feelings about self. Experiences with the body, whether on the job, in dance, sports, or leisure activity, or by the reflection in the mirror, are interpreted in terms of feelings, earlier self-views, and group or cultural norms (Coopersmith, 1967; Schilder, 1951).

In the young adult, a close interdependence between body image and personality, self-concept, and identity exists. Therefore self-concept is an important determinant of behavior. A positive, realistic self-concept, mature body image, and mature behavior depend on having met the changing demands of each previous developmental era. In particular, the time for development of dominant body parts such as the mouth in infancy, the limbs in preschool and school years, and the genitals at puberty are important eras. If each of these body zones, their functioning and related social expectations, are not integrated into a total self-image, the adult's self-concept and body image will remain immature in some aspects. The immature self-image may interfere with securing adult satisfactions and may be evidenced by personality disturbance. However, mature young adults can accept their bodies without undue preoccupation with appearance, function, or control of these functions, so that they are free to focus on other experiences (Cleveland and Morton, 1967).

MIDDLE ADULT

Gradually occurring physical changes confront the middle adult and are mirrored in others. These changes may include additional fat deposits, baldness, gray hair, wrinkles, varicosities, prominent veins, tissue atrophy, and sagging tissue. This developmental stage, resulting from changing hormone production, causes appearance changes, as well as realignment of attitudes about the self that cuts into the personality and its definition. Cultural values about youth, negative attitudes about age,

and other life stresses cause people to view themselves and their bodies differently. The person realizes he looks older, and subjectively feels older as well. Work may be stressful if middle-age people feel they have less stamina, endurance, and vigor to cope with the task at hand. This decrease in energy often is the result of a lower basal metabolic rate, decreasing muscle tone, and sensory changes. The illness or death of loved ones can create concerns about one's own health. These concerns can become excessive, and thoughts of death become more frequent. The person can feel inferior to youth as the previous self-image of a strong and healthy body with boundless energy is replaced with a self-image reflecting the changes of aging. The person's previous personality largely influences the intensity of these feelings and the symptomatology of body-image changes. Difficulties in accepting the loss of youth are also caused by fear of the effects of the climacteric, folklore about sexuality, social and advertising pressures describing the virtues of youth, and emphasis on obsolescence.

Most people gradually adjust to their slowly changing body and accept the changes as part of maturity. Emotionally mature people realize they cannot return to youth and acknowledge that their own pasts and experiences are valid and valuable in their own right. Excitement in the middle years is achieved by using past experiences, insights, and values. Middle-age people who are content with their ages and have no desire to relive the youthful years exhibit a healthy self-concept.

OLDER ADULT

Physical changes that accompany aging, changes in the appearance and function of the older individual, combine negatively to influence self-image. Loss of muscle strength and tone result in reduced ability to perform tasks requiring strength. Elderly people see themselves as weaker and less worthwhile than workers in tasks necessary for survival or in the use of energy for recreational activities. Not only biological changes but also changes in self-regard have an impact on self-concept.

In a society that values youth and beauty, loss of skin tone, with accompanying wrinkles and appearance changes, causes the aging person to feel stigmatized. Changing body contours, whether in the sagging breasts, bulging abdomen, or the "dowager's hump" caused by osteoporosis, produce an appearance change that may have a negative effect. Societal stigma can also affect the sexual response. Changes in body image may be an important deterrent to sexual activity because of anticipated or perceived rejection by a partner or because of anticipated or feared inability to perform, even though most research indicates that no physical barriers exist.

Loss of sensory acuity also prevents the elderly from interacting with the environment (see Chapter 44). Although eyeglasses and good illumination are helpful, the elderly are affected by an inability to read fine print or to do handwork requiring good vision for small objects. The inability to adjust to rapid changes in lighting, the inability to tolerate glare or inadequate light emphasizes an awareness of sensory changes and a changing self. The danger of injury because of failure to see obstacles in their paths and a sense of incoordination or unsteadiness make the elderly insecure about the relationship of their bodies to the environment. A fear of cataracts resulting in loss of vision plagues the elderly. They often seek help too late because they do not understand the implications of the diagnosis or of the chances for successful correction.

Hearing loss can cause negative personality changes as older people realize they no longer are aware of all that is happening or all that is said around them. Suspiciousness, irritability, impatience, or withdrawal may develop because hearing is impaired. Again the aged may be afraid to admit the problem or may hesitate to seek treatment, especially if they are unaware of the possibilities of help through the use of hearing aids or corrective surgery. Often the elderly view the hearing aid as another threat to body image, although it is now possible to obtain aids that are hardly noticeable. Yet to many older adults, eyeglasses are more socially acceptable because they are worn by all age groups, but a hearing aid is perceived as direct evidence of age. Adjustment to the use of a hearing aid may be difficult; if motivation is low, the hearing aid may be rejected.

Jourard (1964) speaks of "spirit-titre," suggesting the term *spirit* be used to express the titre or concentration of purpose that may be encouraged in the aged to produce a well-integrated "personality-health." Certainly the way an individual perceives the body determines to a large degree whether or not the person remains active or maintains the highest possible level of energy. The older adult with a positive self-concept and body image is best equipped to adjust to the decrease in energy.

Psychosocial Theories

Erikson describes eight stages of psychosocial development, the completion of each of which is important to the evolution of a person's self-concept (Erikson, 1963). Piaget and Inhelder (1969) describe four stages of cognitive development. These two theories do not conflict but rather represent different ways of looking at one aspect of the development of self-concept.

In each stage of psychosocial development, an individual faces certain tasks that, if not positively completed, may lead to psychological problems. Through social and cultural reinforcement, an individual learns the relevance of concepts, the cultural connotations of concepts, and the emotional significance of concepts. Erikson's theory demonstrates the influence of society on the development of self-concept. For example, infants need to develop a sense of trust if they are to be psychologically healthy. Infants who learn through parental reinforcement to trust their worlds will feel secure as adults. Mistrust arises from uncertainty, frustration, discomfort, or physical harm. If people do not develop a sense of trust as infants, they may have difficulty with later psychosocial development (Erikson, 1963). If they become ill as adults, for example, they may experience a sense of physical and psychosocial vulnerability and a distrust of the environment, especially a hospital environment. With an insecure self-concept, they may have more difficulty with the changes caused by illness or therapy than the average person would have.

COMPONENTS OF SELF-CONCEPT

A person's self-concept has four aspects: identity, body image, self-esteem, and roles. Each aspect develops from birth onward and reflects the changes taking place throughout the life span. Although these four components can be considered as separate aspects of a person's self-concept, they overlap and are interrelated. Thus, a person's self-concept can be described in terms of a continuum from strong to weak, or positive to negative, depending on the individual strengths of the four components.

Identity

"Identity" is derived from the Latin word *idem*, which means "the same." Identity involves the internal sense of individuality, unity, and sameness of a person over time and in various circumstances. Identity thus includes a level of consistency and continuity. It implies a consciousness of being oneself, distinct and separate from others, a sense of wholeness and maintenance of solidarity with the ideals of one's social group while expressing individuality and uniqueness (Erikson, 1963).

Adolescence, Erikson's fifth stage of development, is a particularly crucial time for the development of sense of self, or identity. Adolescence is a time of physical, emotional, cognitive, and social changes; peer pressure; and preparation for future independence. If people are unable to meet personal and social expectations and define themselves, they experience identity diffusion or identity confusion resulting from a sense of distortion, fragmentation, and unclear roles. An adolescent has an obvious need to belong and to be accepted by a peer group. The ability to form an identity is also related to cognitive development, for people must be able to label themselves and perceive labeling by others. A person with a sense of identity will feel integrated rather than diffuse, fragmented, or out of touch with self or others (Erikson, 1963).

During socialization, children experience the identification process and thereby learn culturally accepted behaviors and roles. A child identifies first with parenting figures and later with teachers, peers, and cultural heroes. To form an identity, the person must have the ability to synthesize these learned behaviors into a coherent, consistent, and unique whole (Erikson, 1963). This synthesizing process is particularly characteristic of adolescence. A person's sense of identity is continually evolving and is influenced by circumstances throughout life. The achievement of identity is necessary for involvement in intimate relationships, since much of a person's identity is expressed in relationships with others.

Sexual identity is a part of a person's general sense of identity. Sexual identity is the image a person has of himself or herself as a male or a female and the meaning that this has for the person. This image and its meaning depend on standards learned through the socialization process.

When people behave in ways that conform to their self-concepts, they reinforce their sense of identity. But when they behave in ways that contradict their self-concept, they may experience anxiety, apprehension, and identity conflict.

Body Image

Body image is an individual's psychological and mental image and experience of the internal and external body. It includes the person's feelings and attitudes toward the body. A person's body image is influenced by their own view of physical characteristics and physical abilities, as well as by their perception of how others view them. Body image is an important factor in self-concept. The reverse is also true: a person's self-concept influences body image.

Body image is also affected by cognitive growth and by physical development. Any physical stimulus, whether internal or external, affects the mental image or concept that people have of their bodies. Normal developmental changes, such as growth and aging, have a more apparent effect on a person's body image than on other aspects of self-concept. For example, a 2-year-old's body image is very different from an infant's, because of the ability to walk. This physical change, walking, depends on physical maturation.

Somatic, kinesthetic, behavioral, and topological elements or stimuli also play a part in the development and maturation of body image. Somatic elements include neurological, metabolic, endocrine, and hormonal factors. Hormonal changes occur during adolescence and in later stages of life (for example, menopause), influencing a person's body image. Aging involves a decrease

in visual acuity, hearing, mobility, and perception, all of which may affect body image.

Kinesthetic elements include neuromuscular functions, whether walking, dancing, or engaging in sports or gymnastics, and conscious recognition of the orientation of different parts of the body with respect to each other, as well as the rates of movement of different parts of the body (Schilder, 1951).

Behavioral elements include experiences related to a person's cognitive, motor, and perceptual experiences and development. Topological stimuli are superficial sensations and physical characteristics of the body surface. Topological stimuli are particularly important during adolescence, when significant physical changes occur. During aging, topological stimuli are again important, as a person recognizes physical signs of old age.

Cultural and societal attitudes and values influence a person's body image. Youth, beauty, and wholeness are emphasized in American society, a fact that is apparent in television programs, movies, and advertisements. These attitudes and values affect how people perceive their physical bodies, because body image is a combination of the ideal and the real.

Since a person's body image depends only partly on the reality of the body, people generally do not adapt quickly to changes in the physical body. As with the total self-concept, a physical change may not be incorporated into the image one has of one's body. Studies have shown, for example, that even people who have experienced significant weight loss do not readily perceive themselves as thin; in some cases such people continue dieting to an extreme in an effort to become thin, because they still have their old body images. The client who has a limb amputated may experience the phantom limb syndrome. The limb can be "felt," and pain in the limb is perceived. Another example where a person's body image does not adapt to physical change is normal aging. People often report they do not feel different, but when they look in the mirror they are surprised by the wrinkled older face or the gray hair.

Self-Esteem

Like body image, self-esteem is based on many internal and external factors. Self-esteem is an individual's sense of self-worth, an evaluation that an individual makes and maintains about self. According to Erikson, young children begin to develop a sense of usefulness or industry by learning to act on their own initiative. Self-esteem is often related to individual evaluation of effectiveness at school, at work, within the family, and in other situations. Society and family generally set the standards by which individuals evaluate themselves.

Self-evaluation is an ongoing mental process. Self-

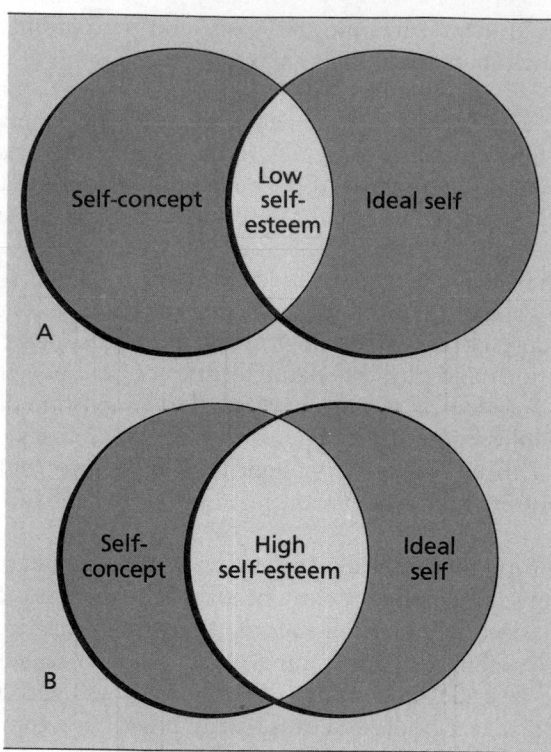

Fig. 29-1 **A,** Individual with a large discrepancy between self-concept and ideal self, resulting in a low level of self-esteem. **B,** Person with greater conformity of self-concept and ideal self and therefore with a high level of self-esteem.

Modified from Sundeen, SJ, et al.: Nurse-client interaction, ed. 3, St. Louis, 1986, The C.V. Mosby Co.

worth or self-esteem is a basic human need, according to Maslow's hierarchy (see Chapter 27). A person has an imperative need to feel competent and worthy of living. Self-esteem thus is involved in the enhancement and maintenance of self-concept. A person's level of self-esteem is an important factor in psychosocial development and motivations (Gibson, 1980).

Self-esteem can be understood in terms of the relationship of a person's self-concept to the ideal self or ego ideal. The ideal self or ego ideal consists of the aspirations, goals, values, and standards of behavior that the person considers ideal and strives to attain. The ideal self or ego ideal originates in the preschool years and develops throughout life; it is influenced by societal norms and the expectations and demands of parents and significant others. In general, a person whose self-concept comes close to matching the ideal self or ego ideal has a high level of self-esteem, whereas a person whose self-concept varies widely from the ego ideal or ideal self has a low level of self-esteem (Fig. 29-1). Studies have shown that negative self-concept or an extreme difference between ideal self and self-concept is characteristic of many persons with mental illness.

Roles

A role is a set of behaviors by which a person participates in a social group. Roles involve expectations or standards of behavior that have been accepted by society or the person's social group, such as family or community. A person's behavior is based on patterns established through the process of socialization. Socialization is the "acquisition of the requisite orientation for satisfactory functioning in a role" (Parsons, 1951). The process of socialization begins just after birth, when an infant responds to an adult and the adult responds to the behavior of the infant. Parsons (1951, 1972) considers the value-orientation patterns established in childhood to be a basic personality structure. The patterns are stable and change only minimally during adulthood. There are five methods through which the child learns behaviors approved by society:

1. *Reinforcement-extinction*—certain behaviors that become common or are avoided, depending on whether they are approved and reinforced, or discouraged and punished.
2. *Inhibition*—a person learns to refrain from a behavior even when motivated to engage in the behavior because of each reinforcement
3. *Substitution*—replacement of one behavior by another that provides the same gratification
4. *Imitation*—a person acquires knowledge, skills, or behaviors from members of one's social or cultural group
5. *Identification*—internalization of the beliefs, behavior, and values of a role model into the person's unique expression overtly.

During the socialization process a person generally develops the skills necessary for satisfactory functioning in many different roles. Unsuccessful socialization may lead to an inability to function acceptably according to society's values.

Brim and Wheeler (1966) differentiate between socialization of children and socialization of adults. Adults are more concerned with the actual behavior appropriate to roles than with learning the basic values implicit in roles. Adults are also expected to distinguish between ideal role expectations and realistic expectations. In addition, adults experience many roles and role expectations and increased role specificity. The self-other relationship is important to adults. In other words, adults are concerned about their relationships with other persons in their lives. The success of relationships in various roles contributes to the adult's sense of well-being or self-esteem. In contrast, the I-me relationship predominates in children. Children learn about their own physical being and their immediate environment. Only after children become comfortable with their physical selves and have established trust in parents can they begin to socialize with other children. School-age children and adolescents are influenced by this socialization as they develop and learn role behaviors.

An individual learns behaviors appropriate to a given role through interactions with people who hold beliefs about appropriate behaviors and who reward or punish the individual on the basis of their beliefs. To function effectively in a role, a person must know the expected behavior and values, must desire to conform to them, and must be able to meet the role requirements.

Roles involve three components: the individual, or actor; the behavior, or action; and the relationships between the individual and the behavior (Biddle and Thomas, 1966). Most individuals have more than one role. Common roles include mother or father, wife or husband, daughter or son, employee, friend, or boss. Each role involves meeting certain expectations of others. Fulfillment of these expectations leads to rewards. Failure to comply with them leads to disapproval.

STRESSORS AFFECTING SELF-CONCEPT

A self-concept stressor is any factor or change, real or perceived, that threatens an individual's identity, body image, self-esteem, or role behavior. Stressors challenge the adaptive capacities of a person. Stress is not unique to any one age group or to any cultural or economic group (see Chapter 28). Selye (1956) states that stress is the normal wear-and-tear of life, not the specific result of any one action or typical response to any one thing acting on us. Whether internal or external, the influencing factor affects an individual's equilibrium.

Different individuals react to the same situation with varying degrees of stress. A variety of responses to stress may be observed, including anxiety, frustration, anger, inability to adjust to a situation, difficulty with making decisions, and various physical or mental changes. Perception of stress is an important factor that influences the person's response. People do not have to understand a specific stressor to feel stress, as long as they perceive the stressor. Each person has learned a pattern of behavior that usually provides means for coping with or adapting to stressors, thus providing a method for coping with future stressors. However, some people are immobilized by perceived threats and require help from other people. Prolonged stress can deplete an individual's adaptive ability.

Stressors can affect any or all of the components of a person's self-concept. Hospitalization, illness, and surgery are stressors that can have interrelated effects on self-concept. The nurse must understand the effects of these stressors on clients and provide appropriate support and intervention. A physical change in the body leads to an altered body image, but the person's identity and self-esteem may also be affected. Certain chronic illnesses alter a person's roles, which may change identity and self-esteem. The following example illustrates how the four components of self-concept are interrelated:

A young man is injured in a diving accident and is paralyzed from the waist down, causing an altered body image. The man had been a construction worker but can no longer function in that job, resulting in an altered role. His self-esteem may be diminished because he can no longer support himself, and his identity as a self-supporting, active man will change. Because he no longer has the same self-concept and body image he had before the accident, a disparity between the prior self-concept and his present reality leads to stress and anxiety. His previous life experiences, sense of identity, unconscious use of defense mechanisms, mental coping strategies, and family and societal resources will influence how he adapts to this stressful change.

A crisis is an imbalance occurring when a person cannot overcome obstacles with usual methods of problem-solving and adapting. Any crisis requires change and thus threatens the self-concept. Some crises directly assault the self-concept, identity, or body image. During a self-concept crisis, as with other kinds of crises, supportive resources are necessary to help the person learn new ways of coping with and responding to the event or situation and to maintain a positive self-esteem and self-concept.

For example, becoming paralyzed involves a major crisis. This client requires help in adapting, and time is required for interventions to succeed. Rehabilitation and restoration of a positive self-concept usually do occur following traumatic events. An understanding of the relationships among a person's sense of identity, body image, self-esteem, and roles is essential to the planning of appropriate nursing interventions.

Identity Stressors

A person's identity is affected by stressors throughout life. Adolescence, in particular, is a critical period for the development of identity. Many stressors during this stage may affect a person's sense of identity. Adolescence is a time of change, causing insecurity and anxiety. Adolescents are trying to adjust to the physical, emotional, and mental changes of an increasing maturity. They are preparing for a vocation, seeking economic independence, forming close relationships, and coping with emerging sexuality. Stressors may arise in any of these areas or as a result of conflicts between them.

An adult generally has a more stable identity and a more firmly held self-image. Cultural and social, rather than personal, stressors may have more impact on an adult's identity. Cultural and social stressors may challenge an adult's values. Examples include finding oneself in the position of having to decide between career and marriage, cooperation and competition, or dependence and independence in a relationship (Stuart and Sundeen, 1987).

Menopause, retirement, decreasing physical abilities, and other factors associated with aging will also affect a person's sense of identity. Identity, like body image, is closely related to how one looks or what one can do. Changes in appearance and physical capabilities require adaptation. Another potential stressor during middle and later life involves achievement of life goals. Retirement may mean the loss of an important means of achievement and continued success. People may begin to question who they are and what they have accomplished. Physical and emotional isolation may add additional stress as significant others die. Identity confusion, a form of altered self-concept in which a person does not maintain a clear, consistent, and continuous consciousness of personal identity, may result if the person is unable to adapt to identity stressors. Finally, in old age, self-despair rather than ego integrity may result (Erikson, 1963). In extreme cases an individual may experience depersonalization, a state in which inner and outer realities or the differences between self and others are indistinguishable.

Body-Image Stressors

Changes in the appearance, structure, or function of a body part or feature will require change in the person's body image. Changes in the appearance of the body, such as amputation or facial disfigurement, are obvious stressors affecting body image. Mastectomy, colostomy or ileostomy also alters the appearance and function of the body but the changes are not apparent when the person is dressed. Body image stressors involving a change in function include renal disease and cardiac disease, where the body no longer functions at an optimal level and the person is physically limited. Even the "normal" body changes resulting from developmental tasks of aging are stressors that can affect a person's body image. Pregnancy affects body image, as does any significant weight gain or loss. Stressors affecting body image can be related to injuries, diseases involving sensorimotor change, physical alterations from surgical intervention, or toxic or metabolic disorders that may slowly alter a body function or require changes in such areas as diet and activity level.

The significance of changes in appearance of the body or a loss of structure or function varies among individuals, families, and cultures. Paralysis caused by a war injury may be considered acceptable; the person may be treated as a hero and praised for bravery and strength, and governmental resources will be available to assist in rehabilitation. However, a young man who has an automobile accident while drunk and suffers severe injuries and paralysis may receive a different response from society. Society will likely be less accepting of his situation, and financial resources may be more difficult to obtain.

The significance of loss of function or structure or a change in appearance is affected by the individual's *perception of* the alteration, because body image consists of both ideal and real elements. For example, femininity is sometimes associated with the size of the breasts, and if a woman's body image incorporates this as the ideal, the loss of a breast by mastectomy may be a very significant alteration. Another consideration is the importance of the body to a person's self-concept. The greater the importance of the body or a specific body part, the greater the threat felt from a change in body image.

Many people associate success with a specific body part or function. For example, athletes may consider their bodies and their physical activities to be the focus of personal success. What happens if an accident occurs and they can never again participate in physical activities? How will they adapt or become rehabilitated? How do they revise long-accepted assumptions about themselves and alter their life-styles, including sexual functioning? In order to regain positive self-concept, and self-esteem, and maintain good health, they must adapt to the body-image stressor.

Studies have shown that after head and neck surgery people generally participate less in social interaction (Dropkin, 1979). A person who has had facial alterations may feel isolated, excluded, stigmatized, or helpless. The feeling of social isolation is often based in reality, because people are afraid of embarrassing or offending a person who is badly burned or "deformed," and thus they avoid contact with the person. A person with an altered body image may fear rejection and isolation or may have actually experienced it.

There have been and continue to be positive social changes with regard to illness and altered body image. The news media more frequently present positive stories about persons who have had major body-altering surgery. For example, accounts of a Canadian runner who was struck by a car and paralyzed showed this young man in a realistic but positive light. Recovery after mastectomy and procedures for performing breast self-examination have been presented on television. Movies have documented the amazing rehabilitation of young people after severe trauma. These stories presenting real people coping and adapting provide role models for persons undergoing unusual stressors, and for families, friends, and society. This social change may be helpful in eliminating much of the stigma associated with altered physical appearance or functioning, thereby reducing stressors to body image.

Self-help groups are available in most communities

for persons who have had ostomies (United Ostomy Association), mastectomies (Reach to Recovery), or laryngectomies (Laryngectomy Club). Self-help groups assist people who are trying to lose weight, parents of children with spina bifida, and people with cancer. These groups provide a special kind of support. Someone who has experienced a particular stressor and who has adapted to it can be instrumental in helping a client adapt to a body image change. Such a person can be a special role model, and his family or significant other can help the family assist in the adaptation.

Self-Esteem Stressors

Self-esteem is a person's sense of being respected, accepted, competent, and worthy. Self-esteem begins to develop in infancy, when perceived acceptance or rejection by parents is an important factor. Persons with high self-esteem are generally happier and more able to cope with demands and stressors than persons with low self-esteem (Gibson, 1980). Persons with low self-esteem tend to feel unloved and often experience depression and anxiety. Self-esteem fluctuates with surrounding conditions, although a basic core of positive or negative feeling is maintained.

Many stressors may affect the self-esteem of the infant, toddler, preschooler, or adolescent. Inability to meet parental expectations, harsh criticism, inconsistent punishment, sibling rivalry, or repeated defeats may reduce the level of self-worth. Stressors affecting the self-esteem of adults include perceived lessened ability in comparison to spouse, friend, or work colleague; failures in relationships; divorce; and loss of a job.

Illness, surgery, or accidents that interrupt or change life patterns may also decrease feelings of self-worth. Chronic illnesses such as diabetes, arthritis, and cardiac dysfunction require changes in a person's accepted and long-assumed behavioral patterns. When a change is slow and progressive, the person has an opportunity for anticipatory mourning, and adaptation occurs along with the change. However, the more a chronic illness interferes with a person's ability to engage in activities contributing to a feeling of worth or success, the more it will affect self-esteem.

An individual's self-evaluation is based on relationships with others and on activities. How an individual defines success or failure influences whether a change is a stressor in terms of self-concept. Many people, for example, consider success at work to be important to a sense of achievement and worth. Chronic illness, surgery, or severe trauma may necessitate a change in a person's life work and thus may be a self-esteem stressor.

Societal standards and the responses of significant others also affect the importance of a stressor and its impact on self-esteem. Dyk and Sutherland (1956), in a classic study of ostomy patients, found that a husband generally accepted his wife's colostomy more readily than a wife accepted her husband's, apparently because society expects men to be strong, healthy, and working. Wives tended to view a colostomy as an indication that a man was now sick, in need of physical help, and unable to reenter the work force, even when the colostomy did not alter his ability to work.

Role Stressors

Throughout life a person undergoes numerous role changes. Both change within the same role and the adoption of new roles require the incorporation of new expectations and standards for behavior. Meleis (1975) identifies three categories of role transition: developmental, situational, and health-illness. Normal changes associated with growth and maturation result in developmental transitions. Situational transitions occur when one loses a parent, spouse, or close friend, moves, marries, divorces, or changes jobs. A health-illness transition is movement from a state of health or well-being to one of illness. Any of these types of role transitions may threaten a person's self-concept, resulting in role conflict, role ambiguity, or role strain.

ROLE CONFLICTS

Role conflict is a lack of compatible role expectations (Broadwell, 1983). When a person is required to simultaneously assume two or more roles that are inconsistent, contradictory, or mutually exclusive, role conflict may occur. For example, a woman's professional role may include the expectation that she make decisions on her own, while her role as a spouse may include the husband's expectation that he has responsibility for all major decisions. Role conflict could result unless she can accept the contradictory expectations. The importance of each of the conflicting roles influences the degree of conflict experienced. A major role is a significant frame of reference. It influences how a person evaluates other role situations. Role conflict usually involves situations in which an inconsistency between two or more expected and sanctioned behaviors exists, and the person's major role does not eliminate this inconsistency.

There are four basic kinds of role conflict based on the source of conflicting expectations: interpersonal, interrole, person-role, and role overload. Interpersonal conflict occurs when one or more persons have opposing or incompatible expectations for an individual in a particular role. For example, a woman's friends and her mother may have very different expectations of how she should care for her children. Interrole conflict occurs when pressures or expectations associated with one role oppose pressures or expectations associated with another role. A man who works 10 to 12 hours a day at his job may have problems if his wife expects him to be home with the family. Person-role conflict occurs when role requirements violate an individual's values. For example, a nurse who values the preservation of life will have conflict when faced with assisting a woman undergoing an abortion. Role overload occurs when an excessive number of demands and a conflict of priorities results in an individual being unable to decide with which pressures to comply. Role overload is a complex type of conflict involving both internal and external conflicts. People may be expected to comply with role expectations of one or more persons. They attempt to establish priorities. However, if it is impossible to deny any of the pressures, role overload develops. The expectations of the various roles become overwhelming, and the person does not have the physical, intellectual, economic, emotional, and other resources to adapt to or perform them.

ROLE AMBIGUITY

Role ambiguity involves unclear role expectations and an inability to predict the reactions of others to one's behavior (Broadwell, 1983). When there are unclear expectations, people are unsure of what they are to do, how they are to do it, or both. Such a situation is often stressful and confusing. Role ambiguity is common in adolescence. Adolescents are pressured by parents, peers, and the media to assume adultlike roles. They may be expected to work, yet employment opportunities may be severely limited. Their parents may emphasize one set of expectations, yet not meet them themselves. For example, parents may demand that an adolescent not drink alcoholic beverages and drive, yet the adolescent may observe that they drink and drive themselves. Role ambiguity is also common in employment situations. In complex, rapidly changing, or highly specialized organizations, employees often become unsure of what is expected of them.

TABLE 29-1 Self-Concept Stressors

Component of Self-Concept	Stressors	Component of Self-Concept	Stressors
Identity	School entry (elementary, secondary, college)	Self-Esteem	Lack of advancement in job
	Developmental tasks of adolescence		Loss of job
	Peer pressure		Marital stress, separation or divorce
	Parent-child conflicts		Doing less well than expected
	Relationship concerns		Repeated failures
	Sexual concerns		Unrealistically high aspirations for self
	Alcohol or drug abuse		Dependency on others
	Death of spouse or significant others		Abuse or battering from parent or spouse
	Employer-employee conflicts		Neglect by parents
	Appearance changes in mid- and late life		Victim of assault, rape
	Burglary of home		Sexuality concerns, infertility
	Rape	Roles	Child having to assume adult responsibilities
	Assault		Unemployment in family
Body Image	Impaired sensory function (deaf, blind, chronic pain)		Marital role conflict
	Altered motor and sensory-perceptive function after CVA		Conflict with employer or colleagues
	Alteration in or loss of body structure or function (hysterectomy, mastectomy, ileostomy, ileo-bladder, colostomy, tracheostomy)		Incompatible role expectations
			Lack of preparation for role
			Unclear role expectations
	Arthritis, musculoskeletal disease		Inability to adequately perform and cope with multiple roles
	Normal growth and developmental changes (puberty, pregnancy, menopause, aging)		Societal attitudes of ageism related to elderly
	Anorexia nervosa		Imposed social isolation
	Diabetes mellitus or diabetes insipidus		Excessive competition in relationships with others
	Incontinence		Not allowed to perform role for which prepared
	Dermatitis		
	Obesity		

ROLE STRAIN

Role strain is a general term incorporating role conflict and role ambiguity. Role strain may be expressed as a feeling of frustration when a person feels inadequate or unsuited to a role. Role strain is often associated with sex role stereotypes (Stuart and Sundeen, 1987). Women in positions typically held by men may be perceived by others as less competent, less objective, or less knowledgeable than their male counterparts. Thus, many women in such situations feel they must work harder and be better than average in order to compete. Men in typically female roles also encounter bias. In addition, a person's femininity or masculinity may be questioned, resulting in further stress.

Chapter 2 describes the sick role as an aspect of illness behavior. This role involves the expectations of others and society and thus role strain may occur in association with the sick role. A person is expected to seek health care, to be ill only temporarily, to acknowledge that illness is undesirable, and to be dependent on health care providers. Role conflict may occur between any of these general societal expectations and the expectations of co-workers, family members, and others. For example, even though people with cardiac illness are expected to reduce their participation in physically stressful activities, friends may after a month or two expect the person to again participate in such activities, producing stress for the person.

The sick role may also involve role ambiguity. People are expected to be dependent and yet, simultaneously, to participate actively so they can be well and leave the sick role quickly. What then is expected of a chronically ill person? The sick role is supposed to be temporary, yet compliance with therapy may be necessary for the remainder of life. At what point is the sick role no longer acceptable? How much dependence, submission, and undemanding behavior is required?

Clients who bring work to the hospital, keep in close contact with business associates, ask questions, and so on, may be considered "bad" clients by some health care workers, but then so are clients who will not help themselves, who are too dependent, or who do not resume social roles. In addition, sick role behaviors and expectations are based on societal standards. The standards adopted by health care providers may change more quickly than those accepted by clients, resulting in role strain.

■ ■ ■

A person's self-concept can be altered by stressors affecting identity, body image, self-esteem, or roles. Examples of stressors that may affect the self-concept and each of its components are described in Table 29-1.

Self-concept may also be affected by physical stressors, which can temporarily alter a person's perceptions or level of consciousness. Lack of oxygen, hyperventilation, biochemical imbalances, endocrine and metabolic disorders, and sensory deprivation for example, will alter how one perceives the world and oneself. Alcohol, drugs, radiotherapy, chemotherapy, and exposure to other toxic substances may also distort these perceptions or the level of consciousness.

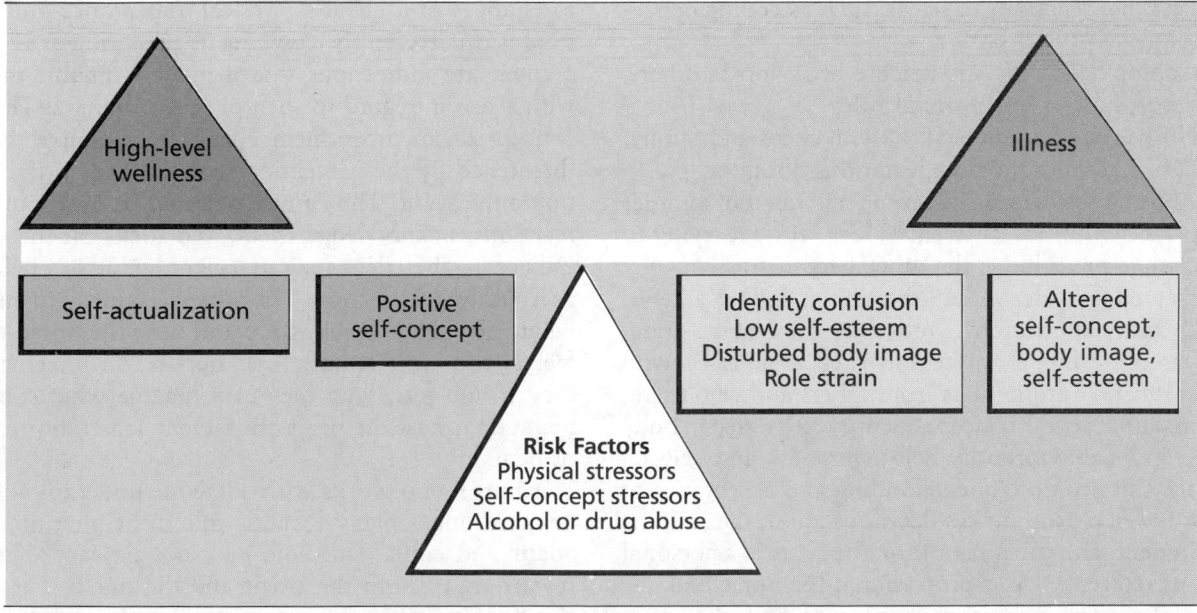

Fig. 29-2   Self-concept health-illness continuum.

Stressors potentially affecting a person's self-concept are also risk factors in regard to the person's health. If a person is unable to adapt to such a stressor, the level of health may be lowered, and if the resulting identity confusion, disturbed body image, low self-esteem, or role conflict, strain, or ambiguity is not relieved, illness may result (Fig. 29-2).

NURSE'S EFFECT ON CLIENT'S SELF-CONCEPT

Impact of Nurse's Self-Concept

The nurse may be the first role model met by a client who is undergoing changes in self-concept. The nurse's acceptance of a client with an altered self-concept may be the factor that stimulates positive rehabilitative results. In the case of a client whose physical appearance has changed and who must adapt to a new body image, both the client and the family may look to the nurse and observe responses and reactions to the client's new situation. To be an effective role model, nurses should acknowledge that they can have a significant impact on the client. The feelings and expectations of the nurse will be communicated both nonverbally and verbally to the client, family, and friends, and to other health care providers. Nursing plans formulated to help a client with an altered self-concept can be either enhanced or defeated by the nurse's unconsciously communicated values and feelings. Thus the nurse should try to understand the following:

1. Personal feelings regarding health and illness.
2. Personal reactions to stress, such as coping behaviors.
3. Coping behaviors and defense behaviors in others.
4. Perception of professional role.
5. Nonverbal communication with client and family.
6. Personal values and expectations about people.
7. Ability to positively intervene on behalf of another person who has different values without trying to change or to judge the other person.

Nurses cannot deny that they have feelings, ideas, values, and expectations, and that they make judgments. In providing care, the nurse acts as a person who is separate and autonomous from others and who therefore has a unique self-concept, identity, self-esteem, body image, and behavior role. Self-awareness and self-acceptance can promote understanding and acceptance of others. Every person makes decisions about the self, the environment, and other people on the basis of a personal frame of reference. As a professional the nurse must be prepared to work with other people who have their own frames of reference. Nurses must develop an awareness of their own reactions to various situations and stressors.

Nurses' reactions to a client's illness are influenced by their own self-concept and can have a significant impact on the client's self-concept. Clients with low self-esteem, for example, may be particularly sensitive to how a nurse involves them in therapy. If nurses lack self-confidence, they may be hesitant in making suggestions, thus inadvertently implying that the client might be unable to follow suggestions. They may insist that clients assume too much responsibility for their own care, thus frightening them. In either case the client's self-esteem may be additionally threatened, rather than strengthened. If, however, the nurse demontrates confidence in the client's abilities and is self-confident, the client's sense of worth will be reinforced. A similar principle operates in regard to identity. Nurses who are secure in their own identity can more readily accept and thus reinforce the client's identity, whereas nurses who are not sure of their own identity may be unable to accept the client and may react as if the client should be something or someone else, thus threatening the sense of identity.

The nurse's impact is also significant in the area of body image. A client who must adapt to a changed body image caused by illness or surgery needs support, as does the client's family. If the nurse feels, for example, that an ostomy or a mastectomy is a horrible thing, that opinion should not be expressed to the client. The nurse should talk with someone who has more experience in the care and rehabilitation of such clients. Meeting people who have had such surgery and who have recuperated and have been rehabilitated can do wonders for a nurse's perspective. If nurses feel insecure about their own body image, they are likely to react more strongly to changes in a client's physical appearance and functioning. Inadvertently frowning or grimacing or avoiding a client are indications that a nurse is unable to cope with stress in regard to such physical changes. The self-concept of an incontinent client, for example, can be threatened by the perception that others find the situation unpleasant. Thus a nurse should be aware of these reactions, acknowledge them, and focus on the client. Otherwise the client may perceive the nurse's behavior as isolation or rejection. The nurse should try to imagine what the client's feelings are and how the nurse would feel in the same situation. If nurses can imagine how they would feel, then they can imagine what someone might do to ease their embarrassment, frustration, anger, or denial.

A nurse who works with someone undergoing body-image changes plays a major role in helping the client adapt and cope. This role may not be easy, but it is rewarding to both the client and the nurse. The nurse can be a valuable resource to the family and the client making this adjustment.

Impact of Nursing Activities

We all perceive some aspects of human experience as stressful, frightening, frustrating, anger provoking, or saddening. The stressors associated with illness and the treatment of illness affect an individual's self-concept in various ways. Clients need an environment that is safe, nonjudgmental, and supportive. Sultenfuss (1982) has specified three messages a nurse should convey to the client to provide a therapeutic environment that does not threaten the client's self-concept:

1. Whatever the client communicates is normal and acceptable.
2. The communciation is not threatening or frightening to the nurse.
3. The nurse will not reject or isolate the client because of anything communicated.

Conveying these messages may sound like an easy task; however, consider them one at a time. The first message is that all communications are normal and acceptable. Is it all right if the client prefers relationships with someone of the same sex? Is it all right if the significant other is not a wife, husband, sister, or daughter? Is it all right if the client is looking forward to surgery? If the nurse, while providing care, implies that the client's values are in any way unacceptable, the client's sense of identity or self-esteem may be threatened.

The second message is that the nurse does not feel threatened by the client's communications. Not reacting to anger with anger is an example. Clients who are angry at themselves, at their disease, or at someone else, may direct their anger toward nurses, other health care providers, or even their families. It is often difficult for the nurse not to react, to recognize that the client's anger may be related to loss of control or to an inability to act as usual. Reactions revealing that the nurse is frightened or threatened can become stressors for the client's self-concept.

To convey the third message, nurses must assess and evaluate their own actions and reactions. In addition, they must notice if other nurses or other health care personnel are avoiding a client. Isolation and rejection, real or imagined, will negatively affect the client's self-concept.

The nurse should be aware that many health care activities in and of themselves can have an adverse effect on a client's self-concept unless the nurse takes action to prevent it. A hospitalized client, for example, almost always experiences role changes and lowered self-esteem as a result of dependence on those who are providing care. In addition, physical examination of the client's body, drawing blood samples for laboratory analysis, and many other routine actions can threaten the client's body and his or her privacy. Because such nursing activities are far from routine for most clients, as is the health care environment itself, the client often feels alienated, out of place, and vulnerable, and these feelings affect self-concept. The nurse can do much, however, to minimize these feelings and to assist the client in maintaining a positive self-concept. Encouraging visits by family members, for example, helps the client maintain a usual role within the family. Discussing all procedures with the client and encouraging participation in the nursing care plan are examples of ways in which a nurse can respect the client's identity as a person capable of making decisions. If the client feels merely like a body being manipulated by health care professionals, a loss of self-esteem may occur. In general, the nurse's goal is to assist the client in carrying on as usual—as much as possible— with activities and relationships that support self-concept. If clients' self-concepts have depended on activities in which they are no longer able to participate, as in the case of athletes who have experienced paralysis, the nurse can help them adapt to change through other kinds of activities that rebuild a strong self-concept and a sense of normality.

The nurse's role and impact will be different with each client. The primary role, perhaps, is as a caring person who is a role model. The nurse provides an example for the client and the family. Acceptance of the client as a

---

⚔ *Research Highlight* ⚔

Muhlenkamp and Sayles determined relationships between perceived social support, self-esteem scores, and positive health practices among adults living in a large apartment complex in a southwestern city. The sample consisted of 98 volunteers, 55 men and 43 women, between the ages of 18 and 67 years, with a mean age of 29. The majority were white and single with a median income in the $10,000 to $14,999 range. The Coopersmith Self-Esteem Inventory was used to measure self-esteem, the Personal Resources Questionnaire was used to measure social support, and the Personal Lifestyle Questionnaire was used to measure positive health practices in the areas of nutrition, exercise, relaxation, safety, substance abuse, and health promotion. A simple correlation matrix determined positive association between the variables of self-esteem, social support, and life-style. Other statistical techniques supported the findings that self-esteem and social support are positive indicators of life-style. Social support was found to exert influence indirectly through its effects on self-esteem.

Muhlenkamp, A, and Sayles, J: Self-esteem, social support, and positive health practices, Nurs Res 35(6):334, 1986.

TABLE 29-2 Assessment of Characteristics for Self-Concept Disturbance

Identity Confusion	Body Image	Self-Esteem	Role Function
Verbalizations of distortion, fragmentation and feeling mixed up: "I didn't feel like myself" "I don't feel like the same person."	Verbalizations of distorted sense of body: "I feel like I don't know myself when I look in the mirror" "I can't stand how I look" "I get so mad that I can't move like I used to."	Verbalization of negative feelings: "I hate myself" "I wish I were dead—I'm good for nothing" "I can't do anything right."	Verbalizations of feeling inadequate in performance: "I can't do budgeting as well as Mary" "I can't manage the household anymore" "They expect too much of me" "He (spouse, child) never does his share of the work" "I don't get a chance to do the things I enjoy and that I used to do" "I'm just a bad person."
Expresses sense of life-style change related to illness	Perceives machines (oxygen, monitor) as part of self.	Expresses shame or guilt about changes in appearance, structure, or function.	Expresses dissatisfaction or frustration over inability to perform previous tasks/activities.
Expresses feelings of hopelessness, helplessness, or powerlessness in relation to self or life.	Unable to distinguish self from others.	Expresses feeling of being unloved, unlovable, or unable to love.	Demonstrates lack of initiative in activities or roles.
Does not answer to own name, calls self by an impersonal pronoun, or calls self the name of an object.	Expresses feelings of depression about physical deterioration.	Demonstrates lack of confidence in self-care, performance of activities of daily living, managing body, role performance.	Demonstrates change in social involvement or relationships with others.
Expresses feelings of inability to be either autonomous or intimate with another.	Does not participate in or has difficulty with self-care.	Demonstrates lack of eye contact with others, stooped posture, change in personal hygiene habits.	Expresses mistrust of caretakers and their performance.
Demonstrates same defense mechanism(s) in a variety of situations.	Expresses fear of rejection from others as a result of illness, surgery, or trauma.	Does not acknowledge encouragement, realistic praise, or positive reinforcement.	Expresses uselessness of efforts at expressing will and self-direction.
Expresses feelings of aloneness, alienation from others, or is suspicious about others' behavior to self.	Refuses to acknowledge or look at actual changes in body structure, appearance, or function.	Is not able to communicate feelings, needs, or ideas.	Expresses excessively high expectations of self in self-care, performance of activities of daily living, or other roles.
Demonstrates inability to make decisions about self or own life-style or inability to act on suggestions.	Is unable to or inaccurate in estimating spatial relationship of body in bed, wheelchair, or environment.	Demonstrates anxiety, apathy, or irritability when asked to engage in self-care or role performance.	Demonstrates inability to relate effectively with family, friends, or caretakers.
Expresses feelings of depersonalization, of being someone else, or that part of body does not belong to self.	Overexposes or conceals parts of or all of body.	Repeats stories about negative experiences or feelings about self.	Demonstrates excessive dependence on or independence from others in relation to health care, activities of daily living, or other roles.
Refusal to engage in self-care or daily living activities, for example, eating, sleeping, elimination.	Expresses grief about body changes (weeping, anger, despair, sadness).	Expresses the expectation of a bad outcome in the situation.	Changes usual patterns of life-style or responsibility.
Demonstrates self-destructive acts (alcohol or drug abuse, accident prone).	Refuses to participate in nursing or medical therapies or rehabilitative activities.	Demonstrates regressive behavior.	
Demonstrates or expresses exaggerated emotional responses.		Expresses excessive criticism of self or others.	
		Expresses excessive worry or fear about situation.	
		Minimizes strengths or abilities; exaggerates limits or weakness.	
		Expresses sense of self-defeat, fragility, inadequacy, self-contempt.	
		Disregards opinion of others; hesitates to offer own opinions.	

human being who has ideas, feelings, and values, and who is worthy and whole despite illness or physical alterations, is important. The client's feelings of insecurity, fears of rejection, or loss of self-worth can be lessened through sensitive, knowledgeable nursing care.

ALTERED SELF-CONCEPT AND THE NURSING PROCESS

ASSESSMENT

Assessment should focus on actual and potential self-concept stressors and on behaviors associated with altered self-concept (see research highlight)

The nursing assessment also reviews the client's previous coping behaviors, the nature of the stressors, the number and intensity of the stressors, and the client's internal and external adaptive resources. Clients may perceive threats to themselves, for example, as threats to a significant other. In addition, the nursing assessment should include the significant other if that person is to be a support and resource for the client.

Table 29-2 gives examples of defining characteristics that may be assessed with self-concept disturbance.

NURSING DIAGNOSIS

Clients with self-concept disturbance may have a number of nursing diagnoses that are pertinent to identity,

---

Examples of Nursing Diagnoses Related to Disturbance in Self-Concept

NANDA-APPROVED NURSING DIAGNOSES

Actual altered parenting related to:
- Identity confusion subsequent to earlier conflicts with own parents
- Lack of preparation for role

Altered role performance related to:
- Demands on time as result of entry into college
- Perceptions about ageist attitudes encountered in work setting
- Perception about abilities after myocardial infarction

Anticipatory grieving related to:
- Planned surgery for malignancy
- Planned geographical move
- Terminal illness of offspring

Anxiety related to:
- Perception of mid-life aging changes and implication for job security
- Marital role conflicts
- Concerns about sexuality

Body-image disturbance related to:
- Perception of self after hysterectomy
- Visual impairment

Dysfunctional grieving related to:
- Unemployment of two months
- Unresolved crisis of divorce

Fear related to:
- Recent burglary of home
- Unresolved crisis of being assaulted

Impaired social interaction related to:
- Recent widowhood
- Recent admission to extended care facility

Impaired verbal communication related to:
- Low self-esteem
- Hearing impairment

Ineffective individual coping related to:
- Low self-esteem
- Previous neglect by parents
- Unclear role expectations

Pain related to:
- Phantom limb syndrome after amputation
- Keloid formation at site of mastectomy

Personal identity disturbance related to:
- Rapid loss of weight
- Value conflicts aroused by peer group
- Death of spouse

Potential for violence: self-directed related to:
- Identity confusion in adolescence
- Inability to cope with multiple role expectations
- Low self-esteem after abuse from spouse

Powerlessness related to:
- Incompatible role expectations at home and work
- Previous neglect from parents

Rape-trauma syndrome related to
- Unresolved crisis of being assaulted sexually

Self-esteem disturbance to:
- Inability to secure job promotion
- Perception of sexuality after infertility problems
- Role conflict with colleagues

Social isolation related to:
- Perception of disfigurement after accidental injury
- Low self-esteem after abuse from parents
- Marital role conflicts

Spiritual distress related to:
- Identity confusion in mid-life
- Altered body image from accidental paralysis
- Alcohol and drug abuse

Sample Nursing Diagnoses for Disturbance in Self-Concept

Defining Characteristics	Nursing Diagnoses	Related Factors
Rigid posture Wringing hands Crying intermittently Rapid, urgent speech	Anxiety (moderate level)	▪ Preoperative concerns ▪ Job termination ▪ School entry ▪ Unplanned pregnancy
Rationalization about lack of role performance Does not participate in self-care Projects negative feelings on caretakers Unable to manage activities of daily living	Ineffective individual coping	▪ Inability to perform role expectations ▪ Disturbed body image after colostomy ▪ Low self-esteem ▪ Feelings about loss of vision
Drastic life-style change Belief that left side of body in bed belongs to roommate Repeated suicidal attempts Emotional lability	Personal identity disturbance	▪ Mid-life crisis ▪ Abuse by spouse ▪ Alcohol/drug abuse

body image, self-esteem, or role performance disturbance. The nursing diagnoses box lists examples of pertinent nursing diagnoses and related etiologies. The diagnostic label is validated by defining characteristics of behaviors, observed signs, expressed symptoms, feelings, or beliefs. Examples of defining characteristics and related factors for three of the nursing diagnoses are presented in the sample nursing diagnoses box.

PLANNING

After determining the nursing diagnosis, the nurse and the client plan care directed toward helping the client regain a healthy self-concept. Interventions center on helping the client adapt to the stressors that led to the disturbance of self-concept and on supporting and reinforcing the development of coping methods (see care plan box).

In planning interventions, the nurse considers the client's present level of adaptation. The client's level of adaptation can be located on a continuum in each of the following five areas (Bernstein and Cope, 1976):

Active coping ↔ Passive surrender
Leading and co-managing treatment ↔ Resisting treatment
Loving exchange ↔ Rage
Awarenes ↔ Denial
Adaptive defenses ↔ Maladaptive defenses

Planning should take into account the client's position on each continuum. For example, a client may perceive the situation as overwhelming, and thus may passively surrender to circumstances rather than attempting to cope. The nursing care plan should show acceptance, use open-ended questions and active listening, and provide understanding and support as the client explores self-concept and expresses feelings (crying, anger, depression). Clients need time to adapt to changes. The nurse must validate a client's strengths and provide resources and education to turn limitations into strengths. Client education should be actively planned, and the client should be included throughout the planning phase.

The nurse should plan for a therapeutic environment that supports the client through the stages of adaptation. Chapter 26 describes the stages of grieving. These stages also occur when a person is faced with the crisis of self-concept or body-image disturbance or change. Sometimes a person appears to adapt to a change in the body but still does not emotionally accept the fact that a change has occurred. Clients may need a great deal of time to accept some changes.

In the case of a client who must adapt to an altered body image as a result of surgery or another physical change, a visit by a rehabilitated person is often helpful. However, the timing of such a visit is important. If the client is still denying that the problem exists, the visit will not be constructive.

Sample Nursing Care Plan for Disturbance in Self-Concept

Nursing Diagnosis	Goal	Expected Outcome	Nursing Interventions
Anxiety related to preoperative concerns about cholecystectomy	Client achieves sense of calm before surgery.	Client demonstrates relaxed posture and facial expression and verbalizes acceptance of surgery and confidence in health care team.	Use open-ended questions to explore feelings and concerns about planned surgery. Show acceptance of feelings, listen carefully. Answer questions about preoperative and postoperative care measures. Indicate who will provide postoperative nursing care.

IMPLEMENTATION

Critical to intervening with the client with a self-concept problem is the ability to establish a therapeutic relationship. The first step in establishing a helping relationship with the client is to establish rapport, that is, to create a sense of harmony by a warm, friendly manner, appropriate smile, and eye contact. The following behaviors are involved in establishing rapport:

1. Relate to the client as an equal to eliminate social barriers, convey acceptance, and promote a sense of trust.
2. Find a common interest or experience for initiating conversation.
3. Establish a smooth, easy pattern of conversation.
4. Convey a keen, sympathetic interest in the other person, give full attention, listen carefully, and indicate that there is time to listen.
5. Adopt the client's terminology and conventions and meet him on his own ground to the extent possible.

Trust is essential to any helping relationship. Trust is the firm belief on the part of the client in the honesty, integrity, reliability, and justice of the nurse. Thus, a trusting relationship depends on the attitude, flexibility, consistency in response, maturity, and reliability of the nurse (Murray, 1982). Empathy or feeling with the person, understanding behavior, and being motivated to act on the client's behalf are other essential characteristics for establishing a helping relationship. Empathy enables the nurse to sense the client's private world and feelings (Peplau, 1952).

Various interventions are useful within the nurse-client relationship to assist the client in reintegrating a positive self-concept and realistic body image. These interventions include the following:

1. Establish rapport and trust.
2. Convey acceptance and empathy, establishing a therapeutic nurse-client relationship.
3. Use therapeutic communication and effective interviewing techniques.
4. Encourage venting of anger.
5. Use interventions to help client work through feelings of hopelessness, sadness, and grieving.
6. Give positive reinforcement to behavior frequently, as appropriate.
7. Maintain a therapeutic nurse-client relationship.
8. Encourage understanding of behavior and feelings; teach as indicated to promote self-care.
9. Present courses of action and ideas on how to cope with situations and how to change behavior to be more adaptive.
10. Assist the client (and family) in identifying resources or support systems.
11. Reduce actual or perceived threats or hindrances as much as possible, in alliance with the client and family.
12. Introduce changes gradually, one at a time if possible, to allow adequate time for adjustment and avoid further threats to the self-concept.
13. Encourage the client to express self-affirmations ("I can").
14. Consult with other health care team members and refer to community support groups as indicated, encourage client participation as appropriate.
15. Validate strengths, potentials and appropriate ideas, behavior and choices of alternatives in self-care, and rehabilitation.
16. Summarize and reinforce progress in behavior or

TABLE 29-3 Sequential Levels of Nursing Interventions for Self-Concept Disturbance

Principle	Rationale	Nursing Actions
LEVEL ONE **Goal: Expand the Client's Self-Awareness**		
Establish an open trusting relationship.	This reduces the threat that the nurse poses to the client and helps to broaden and accept all aspects of personality.	Offer unconditional acceptance. Listen to the client. Encourage discussion of thoughts and feelings. Respond nonjudgmentally. Convey to individuals that they are valued people who are responsible for themselves and able to help themselves.
Work with whatever resources the client possesses.	Some resources, such as self-control and self-perception, are needed as a foundation for later nursing care.	Guidelines for the client with limited resources are as follows: 1. Begin by confirming identity. 2. Provide support measures to reduce the level of anxiety. 3. Approach the client in an undemanding way. 4. Accept and attempt to clarify any verbal or nonverbal communication. 5. Prevent the client from isolation. 6. Help to estabish a simple routine. 7. Help set limits on inappropriate behavior. 8. Orient the client to reality. 9. Reinforce appropriate behavior. 10. Gradually increase activities and tasks that provide positive experiences. 11. Assist in personal hygiene and grooming. 12. Encourage the client to care for self.
Maximize the client's participation in the therapeutic relationship.	Mutuality is necessary in order for the client to assume ultimate responsibility for behavior and coping responses.	Gradually increase the client's participation in decisions that affect care. Convey that the client is a responsible individual.
LEVEL TWO **Goal: Encourage the Client's Self-Exploration**		
Show interest in and accept the client's feelings and thoughts.	When the nurse shows interest in and accepts the client's feelings and thoughts, the nurse is helping the client to do so also.	Attend to and encourage the client's expression of emotions, beliefs, behavior, and thoughts—verbally, nonverbally, symbolically, or directly. Utilize therapeutic communication skills and empathic responses. Note the use of logical and illogical thinking and the reported and observed emotional responses.
Help the client to clarify self-concept and relationships to others through self-disclosure.	Self-disclosure and understanding one's self-perceptions are prerequisites to bringing about future change; this may, in itself, bring about a reduction in anxiety.	Elicit the client's perceptions of strengths and weaknesses. Help to describe a self-ideal. Identify self-criticisms. Help to describe how the client perceives relations to other people and events.
Be aware and have control of your own feelings.	Self-awareness allows the nurse to model authentic behavior.	Be open to your own feelings. Accept both positive and negative feelings of your own. Therapeutic use of self: 1. Share your own feelings with the client. 2. Describe how another might have felt. 3. Mirror your perception of the client's feelings.

TABLE 29-3—cont'd

Principle	Rationale	Nursing Actions
Respond empathically, not sympathetically, emphasizing that the power to change lies with the client.	Sympathy can reinforce the client's self-pity; rather, the nurse should communicate that the client's life situation is subject to one's own control.	Use empathic responses and monitor yourself for feelings of sympathy or pity. Reaffirm to clients that they are not helpless or powerless in the face of problems. Convey verbally and behaviorally that clients are responsible for their own behavior, including the choice of maladaptive or adaptive coping responses. Discuss with the client the scope of choices, areas of strength, and coping resources that are available.

LEVEL THREE

Goal: Assist the Client in Self-Evaluation

Help the client to clearly define the problem.	Only after the problem is accurately defined can alternative choices be proposed.	Identify relevant stressors with the client and ask for appraisal of them. Clarify to the client that one's beliefs influence both feelings and behaviors. Mutually identify faulty beliefs, misperceptions, distortions, illusions, and unrealistic goals. Mutually identify areas of strength. Place the concepts of success and failure in proper perspective. Explore with the client the use of coping resources.
Explore the client's adaptive and maladaptive coping responses to the problem.	Examination of client's choices made during coping will help define successful and unsuccessful responses.	Describe to the client how all coping responses are freely chosen and have both positive and negative consequences. Contrast adaptive and maladaptive responses. Mutually identify the disadvantages of the client's maladaptive coping responses. Mutually identify the advantages or "payoffs" of the client's maladaptive coping responses. Discuss how these payoffs have perpetuated the maladaptive response.

LEVEL FOUR

Goal: Assist the Client in the Formulation of Realistic Goals

Help the client identify alternative solutions.	Only when all possible alternatives have been evaluated can change be effected.	Help the client understand that one can only change oneself, not others. If the client holds inconsistent perceptions, show that the following can change: 1. Beliefs or ideals, to bring them closer to reality. 2. Environment, to make it consistent with beliefs. If self-concept is not consistent with behavior, the client can change the following: 1. Behavior, to conform to self-concept 2. The beliefs underlying self-concept, to include behavior 3. Self-ideal Mutually review how the client can use coping resources.

TABLE 29-3, cont'd Sequential Levels of Nursing Interventions for Self-Concept Disturbance

Principle	Rationale	Nursing Actions
Help the client conceptualize realistic goals.	Goal setting that includes a clear definition of the expected change is necessary.	Encourage the client to formulate personal (not the nurse's) goals. Mutually discuss the emotional and practical consequences of each goal. Help the client clearly define the concrete change to be made. Encourage the client to enter new experiences for their growth potential. Utilize role rehearsal, role modeling, and role playing when appropriate.
LEVEL FIVE **Goal: Assist the Client in Becoming Committed to a Decision and in Achieving Goals**		
Help the client take the necessary action to change maladaptive coping responses and maintain adaptive ones.	The ultimate objective in promoting the client's insight is to replace the maladaptive coping responses with more adaptive ones.	Provide opportunity for the client to experience success. Reinforce the strengths, skills, and healthy aspects of the client's personality. Assist the client in gaining the assistance needed (vocational, financial, and social services). Use family and groups to enhance the client's self-esteem. Allow the client sufficient time to change. Provide the appropriate amount of support and positive reinforcement for the client to maintain progress.

Modified from Stuart, GW, and Sundeen, SJ: Principles and practice of psychiatric nursing, ed. 3, St. Louis, 1987, The C.V. Mosby Co.

self-care and improving self-image as appropriate.

17. Encourage mutual evaluation of progress.
18. Terminate the nurse-client relationship after working through feelings of separation and termination.

In providing care to a client who is experiencing stress that affects self-esteem and identity, it is important that the nurse include activities in which the client will achieve success. Tasks should not be so difficult that the client cannot succeed. Ensuring a small success is better than risking a defeat at a larger task. Sequential tasks enable the client to build on each success, continuously reinforcing achievement.

The nurse should keep other nurses and other health care professionals up to date on the client's progress, because they can be involved in offering support and reinforcement for the client. If a body alteration is particularly severe, staff conferences are useful in helping nurses to handle their own feelings and emotions.

The specific nursing care plan for a client with an altered self-concept should be based on both short- and long-term goals of adaptation. For a client who is beginning to receive chemotherapy and is experiencing body image stressors, for example, the short-term goals might include encouraging the client to describe the physical effects of the medication and to express feelings about the illness and treatment. The long-term goal might be to help the client adapt successfully and accept a new body image.

Interventions designed to help a client reach the long-term goal of adapting to changes in self-concept or attaining a positive self-concept are based on the premise that the client first develops insight and self-awareness concerning problems and stressors and then acts to solve the problems and cope with the stressors. This approach involves five specific levels of intervention (Stuart and Sundeen, 1987):

1. Increased self-awareness
2. Self-exploration
3. Self-evaluation
4. Formulation of realistic goals
5. Commitment to goals and achievement through action

Each level includes specific nursing goals and actions. The nurse helps the client proceed step by step through the five levels. The extent of nursing actions for each level should be individualized. If the alteration in self-concept is severe, the nurse should seek assistance from other professionals, such as mental health nurses, or

Sample Evaluation of Interventions for Disturbance in Self-Concept		
Goal	**Evaluative Measures**	**Expected Outcome**
Client achieves sense of calm before surgery.	Observe client for appropriate posture, facial expression, and movements. Observe client talking with others. Have client discuss readiness for surgery and willingness, participate in preoperative preparation.	Client demonstrates relaxes posture and facial expression, verbalizes acceptance of surgery and confidence in health care team.

should refer the client for specialized care. Table 29-3 (p. 742) describes in more detail the nursing interventions involved in each of the five levels.

EVALUATION

Evaluation determines how well the client's response to nursing therapies or the behavioral outcomes have met the goals of nursing care. Effective use of the evaluation step of the nursing process also includes determining the effectiveness of the nurse's approach with the client. Each of the goals and categories of interventions on the nursing care plan include objective evaluation criteria. The evaluation box presents evaluation measures for expected outcomes for one of the goals of care presented in the care plan box. Desired outcomes for a client with self-concept disturbance includes statements of self-acceptance, acceptance of change in client's appearance or function conveyed by significant others, social interaction, adequate self-care, acceptance of use of prosthetic devices, positive attitudes toward rehabilitation, movement toward independence, and return to preexisting roles at work or at home. The establishment of a therapeutic nurse-client relationship early in the treatment and rehabilitative process is essential to involve the client in evaluation.

The nurse should continually evaluate the approach to the client to determine if effective communication methods have been used and if the main verbal and nonverbal messages have met positive responses. The nurse should examine personal feelings and responses to the client and those feelings conveyed by the client. Periodic meetings with a supervisor can help the nurse to validate feelings and therapy approaches. The nurse's self-awareness serves as a basis for promoting the client's self-awareness. Care of the client with a self-concept disturbance can be a rewarding experience.

The client's adaptation to major changes may take a year or longer, but the fact that this period is long does not signify maladaptation. The nurse should look for signs that the client has reduced some stressors, though perhaps not all. A person's reorganization of self-concept takes time. The self-concept took years to develop to its pre-illness state, and additional change and development also require substantial time.

SUMMARY

The self-concept is a complex, dynamic entity. Many variables—including illness, injury, hospitalization, childbirth, and surgery—can affect any or all of the components of self-concept—self-worth, body image, identity, and roles. A person's self-concept is a combination of both the real self and the ideal self. The ideal self is based on social and cultural standards that an individual accepts and attempts to incorporate into the self-concept. A discrepancy between the real and the ideal self can be a source of stress. A positive self-concept is important to a person's developmental and cognitive maturation throughout life, and numerous variables in each stage of life affect the self-concept.

The nurse's role in providing care for a client with a self-concept disturbance depends on the severity, intensity, or suddenness of the change. Even an apparently minor loss of function, change in appearance, or role change can create a severe self-concept problem. A loss or change not apparent to others can also result in alteration of a client's self-esteem or identity. The nurse's own self-concept and nursing actions can have positive or negative effects on a client's self-concept.

Everyone who is admitted to a hospital or seen by a health care provider should be assessed for stressors that may affect self-concept in any of its components. Although most people can adapt to stressful situations, a client may need assistance in learning to cope with a new situation. Using the nursing process, the nurse identifies self-concept stressors and plans and implements care to encourage the client's self-awareness, self-exploration, and self-evaluation, which lead to the client's formulating realistic goals for coping with changes and then acting to achieve them.

KEY CONCEPTS

✓ Self-concept, the total awareness of self, is first formed based on others' reactions to the person, and then by the person's interpretations of others' reactions to the self, and total life experiences—physiologically, emotionally, and socially.

✓ Self-concept is the sense of continuity and unity, the general positive or negative feelings about self that maintains its general direction, and includes body image and self-esteem.

✓ Self-concept is influenced by gender, age, body structure and function, family experiences, social and occupational roles, and intellectual and leisure activities.

✓ The components of self-concept are identity, body image, self-esteem, and roles.

✓ Self-concept develops as a normal part of growth and maturation, and each developmental stage involves factors important to the development of a healthy, positive self-concept.

✓ Identity is a consistent and persistent sense of self as a person who is distinct from others.

✓ Body image is the mental picture of one's body, including external, internal, and postural aspects of the body, and is not necessarily consistent with actual structure or appearance.

✓ Body image includes the mental picture of body, as well as attitudes, emotions, and personality reactions of the person toward the body as an object in space.

✓ Body image changes when the person experiences disease; change in structure, function, or appearance; pain; or emotional illness.

✓ Body image is influenced by growth and development, cultural and societal values and attitudes, as well as by individual perceptions of the body.

✓ Body-image stressors include changes in physical appearance, structure, or functioning caused by normal developmental changes or by illness.

✓ Self-esteem is a person's sense of self-worth; it depends on a person's self-ideal, or ego ideal, which is influenced by societal values, and on the person's behavior in the family, work, and other activities.

✓ Self-esteem stressors include developmental and relationship changes, illness (particularly chronic illness involving changes in normal activities), surgery, and accidents, as well as the responses of other individuals to changes resulting from these events.

✓ Roles are learned through socialization; they involve the expectations of others about how one should behave in particular positions (family member, employee, and so on).

✓ Role stressors include role conflict, role ambiguity, and role strain, which may originate in unclear or conflicting role expectations and be aggravated by the effects of illness.

✓ One's identity is particularly vulnerable during adolescence. Identity stressors during this time include the expectations of others to prepare for a career and independence, to cope with one's sexuality, and to make choices about relationships and roles; such stressors may lead to identity confusion or sense of depersonalization.

✓ The nurse's self-concept and nursing actions can affect a client's self-concept.

✓ A nursing assessment should include consideration of actual and potential self-concept stressors and observation for behaviors indicative of self-concept disturbance.

✓ Nursing diagnoses in regard to self-concept disturbance include changes in any or all of the four components of self-concept.

✓ Planning and implementing nursing interventions for self-concept disturbance involve expanding the client's self-awareness, encouraging self-exploration, aiding in self-evaluation, helping formulate goals in regard to adaptation, and assisting in acting to achieve goals.

REFERENCES

Anthony, EJ: The child's discovery of his body, Physical Therapy 48, (6), 1103, 1968.

Bernstein, NR, and Cope, O: Emotional care of the facially burned and disfigured, Boston, 1976, Little, Brown & Co.

Biddle, BJ, and Thomas, EJ, editors: Role theory: concepts and research, New York, 1966, John Wiley & Sons, Inc.

Brim, OG, and Wheeler, S: Socialization after childhood: two essays, New York, 1966, John Wiley & Sons, Inc.

Broadwell, DC: Validation of a role conflict, role ambiguity, and role predictability instrument, doctoral dissertation, Atlanta, 1983, Georgia State University.

Cleveland, S, and Morton, R: Group behavior and body image, Human Relations 15 (1):77, 1967.

Cooley, CH: Human nature and the social order, New York, 1956, The Free Press.

Coopersmith, S: The antecedents of self-esteem, San Francisco, 1967, Freeman Publishing Co.

Dropkin, NJ: Compliance in postoperative head and neck patients, Canc Nurs 2(5):379, 1979.

Dyk, RB, and Sutherland, A: Adaptation of the spouse and other family members to the colostomy patient, CA 9:123, 1956.

Erikson, EH: Childhood and society, New York, ed. 2, 1963, W.W. Norton & Co., Inc.

Fink, S: Crisis and motivation: a theoretical model, Arch Phys Med Rehabil 48 (11):592, 1967.

Fisher, S, and Cleveland, S: Body image and personality, New York, 1968, Dover Publications.

Gibson, DE: Reminiscence, self-esteem, and self-other satisfaction in adult male alcoholics, J Psychiatr Nurs, March 1980.

Jacobsen, E: The self and the object world, New York, 1964, International Universities Press, Inc.

Jourard, S: The transparent self, Princeton, N.J., 1964, D. Van Nostrand.

Kramer, M, et al.: Extra tactile stimulation of the premature infant, Nurs Res 24 (5):324, 1975.

Meleis, A: Role insufficiency and role supplementation: a conceptual framework, Nurs Res 24:264, 1975.

Murray, R: Model for psychiatric and mental health nursing. In Carlson C, Craft, C, and McGuire, A, editors: Nursing diagnoses, Philadelphia, 1982, W.B. Saunders Co.

Murray, R, and Zentner, J: Nursing assessment and health promotion through the life span, ed. 3, Englewood Cliffs, N.J., 1985, Prentice-Hall.

Parsons, T: Illness and the role of physician: a sociological perspective, Am J Orthopsychiatry 21:452, 1951.

Parsons, T: Definitions of health and illness in light of American values and social structures. In Jaco, EG, editor: Patients, physicians, and illness, 1972, ed. 2, New York, The Free Press.

Peplau, H: Interpersonal relations in nursing, New York, 1952, G.P. Putnam's Sons.

Piaget, J, and Inhelder, B: The psychology of the child, New York, 1969, Basic Books, Inc.

Schilder, P: Image and appearance of the human body, New York, 1951, International Universities Press.

Selye, H: The stress of life, New York, 1956, McGraw-Hill Book Co.

Stuart, GW, and Sundeen, SJ: Principles and practice of psychiatric nursing, ed. 3, St. Louis, 1987, The C.V. Mosby Co.

Sultenfuss, SR: Psychosocial issues and therapeutic intervention. In Broadwell, DC, and Jackson, BS, editors: Principles of ostomy care, St. Louis, 1982, The C.V. Mosby Co.

Yamamoto, K: The child and his image, Boston, 1972, Houghton Mifflin Co.

ADDITIONAL READINGS

Argyle, M: The psychology of interpersonal behavior, Baltimore, 1967, Penguin Books.

Biddle, BJ: Role therapy: expectations, identities, and behaviors, New York, 1979, Academic Press, Inc.

Blaesing, S, and Brockhuas, J: The development of body image in the child, Nurs Clin North Am 7(4):597, 1982.

Brundage, DJ, and Broadwell, DC: Altered body image. In Phipps, WJ, Long, BC, and Woods, NF, editors: Medical-surgical nursing: concepts and clinical practice, ed. 3, St. Louis, 1987, The C.V. Mosby Co.

Carpeninto, L: Handbook of nursing diagnosis, Philadelphia, 1984, J.B. Lippincott.

Dempsey, M: The development of body image in the adolescent, Nurs Clin North Am 7(4):609, 1972.

Duespohl, T: Nursing diagnosis manual for the well and ill client, Philadelphia, 1986, W.B. Saunders.

Fisher, S: "Sex differences in body perception," Psychol Monogr 78:1, 1964.

Gordon, M: Manual of nursing diagnosis 1984-1985, New York, 1985, McGraw-Hill Book Co.

Jourard, S, and Secord, P: Body cathexis and the ideal female figure, J Abnorm Soc Psychol 50:243, 1955.

Kim, M, McFarland, G, and McLane, A, editors: Classification of nursing diagnoses: proceedings of the seventh conference, (NANDA), St. Louis, 1987, The C.V. Mosby Co.

McFarland, G, and Wasli, E: Nursing diagnoses and process in psychiatric-mental health nursing, Philadelphia, 1986, J.B. Lippincott.

Katchadourian, HE, editor: Human sexuality, Berkeley, 1979, University of California Press.

Maslow, AH: Motivation and personality, New York, 1970, Harper & Row, Publishers, Inc.

Molla, PM: Self-concept in children with and without physical disability, J Psychiatr Nurs 19(6):22, 1981.

Morris, C: Self-concept as altered by diagnosis of cancer, Nurs Clin North Am 20(4), 611, 1985.

Murray, R: Body image development in adulthood, Nurs Clin North Am, 7(4), 617, 1972.

Murray, R: Principles of nursing intervention for the adult patient with body image changes, Nurs Clin North Am 7(4), 697, 1972.

Murray, R, Huelskoetter, M, and O'Driscoll, D: The nursing process in later maturity, Englewood Cliffs, N.J., 1980, Prentice-Hall, Inc.

Norris, J, and Kunes-Connell, M: Self-esteem disturbance, Nurs Clin North Am 20(4):745, 1985.

Oldaker, S: Identity confusion: nursing diagnosis for adolescents, Nurs Clin North Am 20(4):763, 1985.

Rubin, R: Body image and self-esteem, Nurs Outlook 16(6):20, 1968.

Sundeen, SJ, et al.: Nurse-client interaction, ed. 3, St. Louis, 1986, The C.V. Mosby Co.

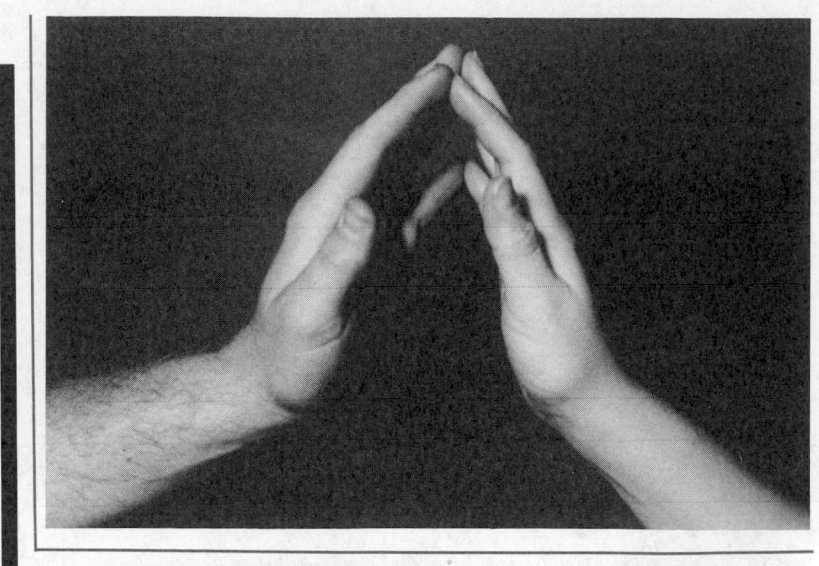

OBJECTIVES

Mastery of content in this chapter will enable the student to:

- Define the key terms listed.
- Identify personal attitudes, beliefs, and biases related to sexuality.
- Discuss the nurse's role in maintaining or enhancing a client's sexual health.
- Define sexuality as a component of personality.
- Describe key concepts of sexual development during infancy, childhood, adolescence, and adulthood.
- Identify male and female genitalia and describe functions related to sexual stimulation/response and reproduction.
- Describe the sexual response cycle (Masters and Johnson model).
- Describe physical, therapeutic, and psychological issues affecting sexuality.
- Identify potential causes of sexual dysfunction.
- Assess a client's sexuality.
- Define appropriate nursing diagnoses on sexuality.
- Identify and describe nursing interventions to promote sexual health.
- Evaluate a client's sexual health.
- Identify sexual concerns outside the nurse's level of expertise, and identify potential referral resources.

KEY TERMS

Ambiguous Genitalia
Anlingus
Biological Identity (Sex)
Bisexual
Coitus Interruptus
Contraception
Corpus Luteum
Cunnilingus
Dyspareunia
Erectile Dysfunction
Fellatio
Female Genitalia
Follicular Phase
Gender Identity
Gender Role (Sex Role)
Graafian Follicle
Heterosexual
Homosexual
Lesbian
Libido
Luteal Phase
Male Genitalia

Masturbation
Menarche
Menopause
Menstrual Cycle
Menstruation
Orgasm
Ovulation
Premenstrual Syndrome
Puberty
Refractory Period
Secondary Sex Characteristics
Sensate Exercises
Sex
Sex Skin
Sexual Dysfunction
Sexual Orientation
Sexual Response Cycle
Sexuality
STDs
Transsexual
Transvestism
Tumescence

Sexuality

S ex is a topic that was long considered taboo for proper adult conversation. Gradually, over the last 30 to 50 years, knowledge about sex and discussion of issues of sexuality have come to be recognized as important and necessary for human development. During the past 20 years health care professionals have finally recognized the relevance of sexual health as a component of all individuals' well-being. Even with this recognition, a lack of knowledge regarding human sexuality remains among many adults, including health care providers. More significantly, care givers lack comfort and confidence in addressing these issues with their clients.

Sexual issues are relevant to nursing assessment and intervention. The nurse omits an integral system when sexuality is ignored during history taking. While providing intimate physical care of bathing and toileting, the nurse establishes a relationship that may foster an environment conducive to discussion of sensitive issues.

Sexual issues must be included in client education. Often, clients are reluctant to raise questions related to sexual issues. Client's concerns may include postpartum resumption of sexual intercourse, adolescent concerns about normalcy of development, or anxiety over the effects of antihypertensive medication on sexual function. The nurse must assume the responsibility of initiating relevant sexual topics on the client's current developmental and health status. The client then may feel more comfortable and relate additional concerns. To address issues of sexuality in practice, the care provider must have the necessary knowledge base and assessment and communication skills.

Because sexual issues can be so value-laden, it is also critical that care givers recognize personal attitudes and beliefs. Religious teachings, culturally prescribed sex roles, ethical beliefs toward homosexuals, and all the other past and present social and environmental influences affect our values systems. Health professionals must acknowledge where biases exist so they recognize when biases and attitudes may potentially interfere with client interaction. Gaining knowledge and desensitization toward sexual issues may also broaden an individual's understanding of the vast range of normal sexual behavior. This enables health care providers to become nonjudgmental and more effective in working with the vast array of clients they will encounter over years of practice.

CONCEPTS OF SEXUALITY

Sexuality and sex are two different things. Sexuality is often described as a person's sense of being female or male. It has biological, psychological, social, and ethical components. Present from birth to death, it is a shaper of life experiences and in turn is shaped by those experiences. The word "sex" has a more limited meaning. It usually describes the biological aspects of sexuality such as genital sexual activity. Sex may be used for both pleasure and procreation. As a result of life's changes or by choice, sexual activity may be absent from a person's life for brief or prolonged periods of time.

The process by which people come to know themselves as females or males is not clearly understood. That a person is born with female or male genitalia and subsequently learns female or male social roles seems to be a key ingredient, yet this does not explain all of the variations of sexuality and sexual behavior. This diversity is more understandable when we remember that sexuality is intertwined with all aspects of self and of learning to be a person. The Sex Information and Education Council of the United States (1980) has defined sexuality in holistic terms as

a function of the total personality . . . concerned with the biological, psychological, sociological, spiritual and cultural variables of life which, by their effects on personality development and interpersonal relations, can in turn affect social structure.

Biological Identity

Biological differences between males and females are determined at conception. Female fetuses have received two X chromosomes, one from each parent, and male fetuses have received an X chromosome from the mother and a Y chromosome from the father. Initially the gen-

italia of the fetus are undifferentiated. It is not until the sex hormones begin to cue fetal tissues that the genitalia assume male or female characteristics. The male fetus is genetically programmed to produce testosterone, which causes the growth of some sexual parts and the inhibition of others, at about 7 weeks after conception. The corresponding sex hormone in females, estrogen, does not seem to be essential for the development of female genitalia. Thus, in the absence of significant amounts of testosterone, the fetus continues to develop female reproductive anatomy. Hormones will continue to influence the individual at critical stages of fetal development and again at puberty. Barring any malfunction in the growth process, females will develop a cyclical menstrual cycle and female secondary sex characteristics. Males will develop a relatively constant production of sperm and male secondary sex characteristics.

Gender Identity

Gender identity is the individual's sense of being feminine or masculine. As soon as an infant is born (and perhaps sooner with use of amniocentesis or other antenatal testing) the parents and community label the child as girl or boy. Often the first words of the birth helper begin this process. Once a label is attached to an infant, adults adjust their behavior to relate to a female or male being. Different patterns of interaction influence the infant's developing sense of gender identity.

As children begin to explore and understand their own bodies, they combine this information with the way society treats them to create an image of themselves as girls or boys. By the age of three, children are aware that they will remain girls or boys and that changes in outward appearance will not alter their gender. This recognition is part of the development of self-concept.

Gender Role or Sex Role

Much research and writing in the last decade has been produced on the origin of gender role behavior—the way people act as females and males. Social learning theorists believe that societal influences shape female and male behavior and are thus the primary source of a person's sense of femaleness or maleness. Since gender role behavior is encouraged by parents, peers, and the media, differences among individuals' sexual behavior develop.

Environmental factors alone do not satisfactorily explain the differences and similarities between female and male sexual behavior. Some researchers believe that sex hormones influence the development of fetal brain tissue, contributing to the differences in female and male sexual behavior. Most likely, as with other human behaviors, sexual behavior is a combination of many interacting biological and environmental factors.

Cultural factors can be key elements in defining sex roles. Culture may tightly prescribe roles as feminine or masculine, for example, the role of breadwinner and home finance coordinator as masculine roles and child care provider and cook as feminine roles. Other cultural groups may be more flexible in role definition and encourage women or men to explore a variety of roles or behaviors without labeling the behavior as sex-linked. The Women's Liberation Movement of the 1970s did much to expand the North American cultural definition of appropriate feminine behavior, for example, primary breadwinner and mother. Ripple effects of this movement have also offered men a broader range of socially acceptable behavior, allowing them open expressions of emotion and increased involvement in child care. These expanded options have created dilemmas, particularly for women. Conflicts may arise in choosing between or juggling a career with childbearing and rearing. Biological reproductive time frames and family attitudes and values also cause conflict.

Sexual Orientation

Sexual orientation is the clear, persistent, erotic preference of a person for one sex or the other. The Kinsey studies of human sexuality in the 1940s and 1950s showed a continuum between heterosexuality and homosexuality. Few, if any, individuals are totally confined to one end of the continuum throughout their life span regarding interests or desires. Most people cluster near the heterosexual (straight) end of the continuum, with a smaller percentage at the homosexual (gay or lesbian) end, but some people are bisexual (bi) and feel comfortable having sexual relations with either sex. It is not unusual for an individual to have occasional erotic feelings toward someone of the same sex without acting on these feelings. Likewise, it is not uncommon to have a same-sex encounter during adolescence without settling at the homosexual end of the continuum. People may change their sexual orientation during their lifetime (Haeberle, 1978).

The origins of sexual orientation are still not understood. Biological theories describe heterosexuality and homosexuality in genetic terms and thus as determined at the time of conception. These theories attribute sexual orientation to the genetic composition of the individual. Psychological theories emphasize early learning experiences and cognitive processes as determining sexual orientation. Still other theories acknowledge the influence of genetics and environment in the development of sexual-partner preference.

Incongruence in Sexual Self-Conduct

For some people the inner sense of sexual identity does not match the biological body. Such people are known as transsexuals. A man may think of himself as a female in a male body, or a female may describe herself as a man trapped in a woman's body. No clear understanding exists of how this mismatch occurs. These people do not see their sexual identity as a matter of choice. Their identification of self as a sexual and social female or male is as clear and persistent, often from early childhood, as it is for people whose inner and outer identities match. Through counseling and perhaps rehabilitative sex reassignment surgery, such individuals may gain the relief they seek and deserve.

Homosexuality and transvestism are separate phenomena. Society sometimes thinks of homosexual men as somehow feminized and wishing to be like women and of lesbians as desiring to be like men. This is a pervasive myth. Although there are some effeminate-behaving men and masculine-behaving women in the homosexual population, most homosexual men and women define themselves as quite satisfied with their gender and social role. They simply have a persistent desire for their own sex. A transvestite is usually a heterosexual man who periodically dresses like a woman for psychic and sexual relief. Transvestites generally do this in private and their behavior is sometimes kept secret even from the people closest to them.

Sexual Ethics

Since sexuality is linked to every aspect of living, any sexual decision involves personal, family, cultural, religious, and social standards of conduct. A person's ideas about ethical sexual conduct and emotions related to sexuality form the basis for sexual decision making. The spectrum of attitudes toward sexuality ranges from the traditional view of sex only within marriage to an attitude that each individual must decide what is right. Sexual decisions that transgress a person's ethical code may result in internal conflict. The person may feel guilty or feel a sense of wrong doing and may even experience sexual dysfunction. The behavior will either stop to reduce negative feelings or the ethical code will be adjusted to include the behavior.

Several general approaches to ethical sexual decision making are suggested by Masters, Johnson, and Kolodny (1982). In one approach, sexual decisions are based solely on religion. Another approach views any sexual act between consenting adults in private as moral. Some people believe that moral sexuality is that which enhances personal growth and interpersonal relationships. Others believe that the morality of a sexual act must be decided on the basis of the situation in which it occurs. No matter what one believes about sexual ethics, others will have opposing points of view.

The split between conservative and liberal thinking concerning sexuality does not seem to be diminishing.

The debate over sexuality-related issues such as abortion, contraception, sources of sex education, sexual variations, and premarital or extramarital intercourse continues. In the absence of a universally accepted moral code, each person must make sexual decisions thoughtfully, with the best interests of the individual and the community in mind.

ATTITUDES TOWARD SEXUALITY

Each person learns a set of behaviors that represents femininity or masculinity. Individuals reveal themselves as females or males by their gestures, mannerisms, clothing, vocabulary, and patterns of sexual activity. A person's attitudes toward sexual feelings and behaviors change as the person grows older and passes through life stages. These changes may become more traditional or more liberal. Societal changes, feedback from others, and involvement in religious all-community groups contribute to the ongoing modifications an individual makes in expressions of femininity or masculinity. Nurses' and clients' attitudes toward sexuality and sexual bahavior significantly affect how health care is provided. Attitudes can show themselves openly and dramatically. Clients may overhear disparaging remarks about their sexuality made by nurses or physicians. Nurses may refuse to deal with a client because of the client's sexual attitudes or behavior. On a more subtle level, the invasion of a client's privacy, lack of regard for a hospitalized client's need for time alone with a sexual partner, or even the way a nurse touches a client reflects attitudes toward sexuality.

Since good health includes sexual health, a client's sexuality should be part of a health care program. Yet sexual assessment and interventions are not always included in health care. The area of sexuality can be emotionally loaded for both nurses and clients. Lack of information, conflicting value systems, anxiety, or guilt feelings of the client or nurse may cancel the best intentions of nurses to promote sexual health. Clients may not discuss certain sexual concerns out of fear that the nurse will be judgmental. Nurses may ignore clients' hints about sexual concerns because they are uncomfortable with the whole topic of sexuality. Such words as masturbation, homosexuality, abortion, and orgasm may have emotional overtones far out of proportion to the reality of the behavior.

Factors Influencing Attitudes

Biology and personality help to shape attitudes and behaviors, but other powerful factors are involved. Sexual attitudes can be the result of religious beliefs. A striking characteristic of contemporary religious thinking is the lack of agreement about sexual values and behavior. Not only are there differences among Catholic, Jewish, and Protestant teachings about sex, but within each faith there is often a lack of uniformity (Hogan, 1982). In addition, discrepancies exist between professed belief and actual behavior. People may publicly say they believe in a particular sexual value system but behave quite differently in private.

Society plays a powerful role in shaping sexual values and attitudes. Each social group has its own set of rules that guide the behavior of group members. These rules become an integral part of an individual's thinking. In the traditional, conservative value system the bias is toward sex as a reproductive function, and masturbation and sexual variations may be condemned because they do not serve the reproductive role. Sexual behavior is seen as binding the couple closer together in the reproductive role. Sex strengthens the monogamous, heterosexual partnership and becomes the ultimate expression of love between partners. This traditional view encompasses fixed roles for female and male sexual behavior.

A more individualistic morality became widespread in the 1960s and 1970s. Many people reevaluated their moral codes and came to see sexuality as a mode of self-expression. Many women asserted their right to control pregnancy and the expression of their sexual feelings. This new morality emphasized ownership of one's own body and feelings, free choice, and self-actualization. The 1980s and 1990s may see a return to more conservative, monogamous expressions of sexuality because of fear of sexual transmission of disease, particularly AIDS.

Sexual bias of nurses as feminine and subservient may arise from the traditional nursing role. The historical image of the nurse is one of discipline, purity, and cleanliness. Because nurses had the right to touch hospitalized clients' bodies and carry out clients' personal hygiene, they were expected to suppress their own sexuality (Hogan, 1980). Although these traditional attitudes have almost vanished from nursing practice, the bias involving traditional nursing roles may be evident to male nurses as they move into a historically female profession.

Clients' Sexual Attitudes

Each person has a sexual value system acquired over a lifetime of experiences. All people have personal beliefs and preferences concerning sexuality. These experiences either make it easy for a client to deal with sexual concerns in a health care setting or act as roadblocks. Some clients may be confused about their own sexual value systems and thus experience ambiguous or distressing feelings when they deal with their sexuality.

The most common concern people have about their

sexuality is whether their sexual attitudes, feelings, and actions are normal. Given the fact that society has not encouraged open talk about sexuality, such anxiety is understandable. Religion, society, the media, family, peers, and experience have all sent messages about sexual normalcy.

Clients may be concerned about how nursing interventions will affect their self-care abilities and sexual activities. This is most clear when dealing with masturbation and sexual fantasy. Traditionally, strong societal and religious prohibitions exist against both, especially for women. In most hospital settings, however, they are the only sexual outlets available to clients who feel well enough to engage in them. Yet the attitude of the nursing staff may prevent these activities. Nurses who do suggest fantasy or masturbation as part of an intervention may also bring the client into conflict with personal beliefs and prohibitions.

Nurses' Attitudes Toward Sexuality

Since health care professionals represent society with its diverse sexual attitudes and behaviors, diversity is understandable and expected among health care professionals. A nurse can deal with personal attitudes by accepting their existence, exploring their sources, and finding ways to work with them. Professional behavior need not compromise the personal sexual ethics of nurse or client. Professional behavior must guarantee that the client is provided with the best health care possible without diminishing the sense of self-worth.

Nurses may find it difficult to be nonjudgmental about a client's sexuality when the client's orientation or values are different from their own. What seems strange or wrong to the nurse might seem normal and acceptable to the client as a result of the diversity of cultural and societal norms with which we live. Attempting to change a client's sexual attitudes and behaviors ignores the fundamental differences in attitudes among people. Promotion of sex education and honest examination of one's own sexual values and beliefs can be helpful in reducing sexual bias. Such a process would emphasize the following for the nurse (Hogan, 1980):

1. Awareness of beliefs, attitudes, and values about sexuality
2. Awareness of how beliefs and attitudes affect nursing practice
3. Knowledge of subject matter
4. Skill in assessment, intervention, and communication

Giving clients information about sexuality does not imply advocacy. Clients need accurate and honest information about how their illness may affect their sexuality and how sexuality can contribute to their wellness. Nurses need to provide that information so their own or clients' normal biases do not get in the way of the ability to care for the client.

SEXUAL ANATOMY AND PHYSIOLOGY

Female Sex Organs

The female genitalia are comprised of external and internal sex organs. The external sex organs, referred to collectively as the vulva, include the mons veneris, labia majora, labia minora, clitoris, and vaginal opening or introitus (Fig. 30-1). The vagina, uterus, fallopian tubes, and ovaries comprise the internal sex organs (Fig. 30-2).

EXTERNAL SEX ORGANS

MONS VENERIS. The mons veneris (mons pubis) is a layer of fatty tissue that covers the pubic bone and is covered by pubic hair in the postpubescent female.

LABIA. The two labia majora are fatty folds of skin whose outer surfaces are covered with pubic hair and whose inner surfaces are smooth and hairless. The labia majora extend down from the mons veneris and form the outer boundaries of the vulva. The function of the labia majora is to cover and thereby protect the vaginal and urinary openings. They have sensory receptors that are sensitive to touch, pressure, pain, and temperature.

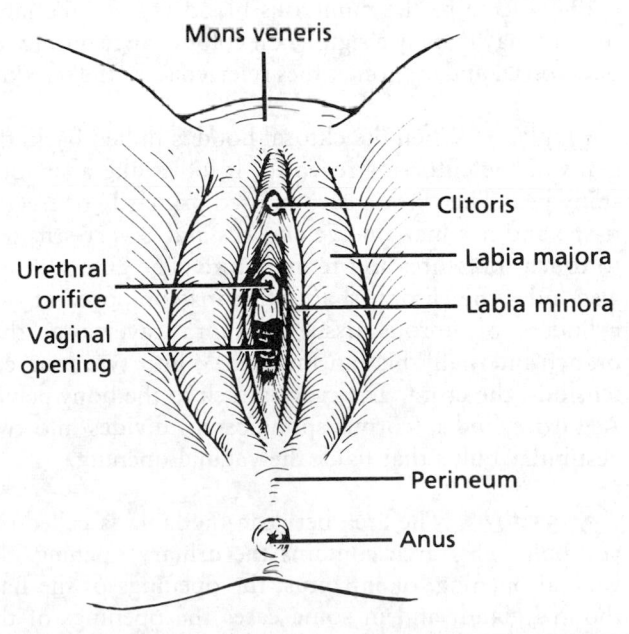

Fig. 30-1 External female sex organs.

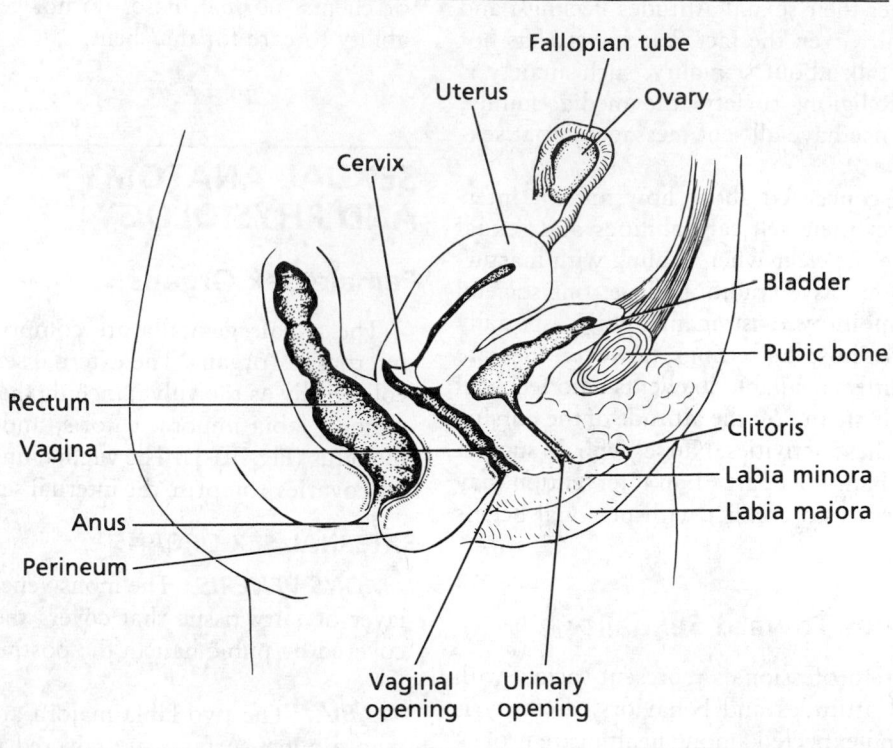

Fig. 30-2   Internal female sex organs.

The two labia minora, which are just inside the labia majora, are thin folds of pigmented skin that extend upward to form the clitoral hood. These inner folds possess many blood vessels and have many sensory nerve endings. Due to the numerous blood vessels, the labia minora may display a significant color change during sexual arousal and are sometimes referred to as the sex skin.

CLITORIS. When the clitoral hood is pulled back, the glans of the clitoris is revealed. It looks like a smooth, shiny pea. The clitoris is composed primarily of erectile tissue and has many nerve endings and is very sensitive to touch, pressure, and temperature. The clitoral hood also hides the clitoral shaft, which is composed of two cylinders of fibrous tissue (corpora cavernosa) that branch internally like an inverted V into two long extensions, the crura. The crura attach to the bony pelvis. A third cylinder (corpus spongiosum) divides into two vestibular bulbs that flank the vaginal opening.

VESTIBULE. The area between the labia is called the vestibule. This area contains the urinary opening, the vaginal opening, or introitus, the openings of the Bartholin's gland, and in some cases the openings of the paraurethral or Skene's glands.

The urinary meatus lies midline in the vestibule be-

tween the clitoris and the vaginal opening. It is not considered to be a sex organ. The paraurethral ducts, or Skene's ducts, open on either side of the urethra usually into the vestibule, although in some women they open just inside the meatus on the posterior wall of the urethra. The paraurethral gland may contribute slightly to vaginal lubrication.

The Bartholin's glands are two small ducts that open on the vestibule next to the vaginal opening. The Bartholin's glands secrete a small amount of lubrication fluid. This fluid contributes minimally to lubrication of the introitus and vagina during sexual arousal, as most of the lubrication comes from the walls of the vagina.

The vaginal opening or introitus is between the urethra and the anus. The hymen is a membranous fold of tissue that partially covers the introitus and has no known function. It usually remains intact until the first intercourse. At times the hyman in a virgin may be torn because of an athletic injury or, rarely, tampon insertion. Some women will maintain an intact hymen even after repeated intercourse, although this is also rare. In some cases, an infant is born with an imperforated hymen completely occluding the vagina. In these cases, without surgical rupture of the hymen, menstrual discharge is retained within the vagina and internal examination and sexual intercourse is impossible.

INTERNAL SEX ORGANS

VAGINA. The vagina is a thin-walled, muscular organ that tilts upward at a 45-degree angle toward the small of the back (Masters, Johnson, and Kolodny, 1982). The walls of the vagina consist of a thin outer serosa, which is part of the membrane that lines the body cavity and covers its organs; a middle layer of smooth, involuntary muscle that is continuous with the muscle of the uterus; and an inner layer of moist mucous membrane called mucosa (Goldstein, 1976). The muscle layer is extremely distensible to allow for sexual intercourse and childbirth. The mucosal layer, during sexual excitement, sweats with vasocongestion providing vaginal lubrication. The vagina serves as a passageway for menstrual flow, childbirth, and sexual pleasure.

UTERUS. The uterus is a thick-walled muscular organ located between the urinary bladder and rectum. It is about 7.6 cm (3 inches) long and looks like a small pear turned upside down. The fallopian tubes enter the uterus on either side near the top (Haeberle, 1978). The wide upper part of the uterus is known as the body. The bottom part, called the cervix, protrudes into the vagina. The inner lining of the cervix contains many glands, which secrete varying amounts of mucus that plug the opening to the uterus. Changes in the cervical mucus indicate when ovulation is taking place. The mucus is more readily penetrable by sperm at the time of ovulation.

The uterus is composed of three layers: the thin external connective tissue layer called the perimetrium, the middle layer of smooth muscle called the myometrium, and the inner mucous membrane called the endometrium.

Muscle fibers of the myometrial layer enlarge during pregnancy to allow for fetal growth. Contractions of these intertwining muscles and pressure from the presenting part of the fetus cause cervical effacement and dilation. Uterine muscle contractions and bearing-down movements forcefully expel the fetus. Contraction of uterine muscles also occurs during orgasm.

Every month the endometrium thickens and prepares for possible implantation of a fertilized ovum. If no implantation occurs, the endometrium deteriorates and is discharged through the cervix and vagina during menstruation.

FALLOPIAN TUBES. The two fallopian tubes begin at the uterus and end in long fingerlike fibriae near the ovaries. Fallopian tubes function as a conduit for the passage of both egg and sperm so fertilization can take place. Muscles and cilia of the fallopian tubes facilitate sperm transport toward the ovary and ova transport toward the uterus. Fertilization usually occurs in the upper part (ovarian portion) of one of the fallopian tubes.

OVARIES. The two walnut-sized ovaries, one on each side of the uterus, have two functions. They produce eggs that are released and transported through the fallopian tubes, and they secrete female hormones, including small amounts of androgen, directly into the bloodstream. The process of egg production begins in the female fetus and ends before birth. Every female is born with a total complement of ova. These eggs continue to undergo atresia so that at puberty approximately 400,000 remain. One egg undergoes maturation each month with the cycle continuing until ovarian function ceases with menopause.

BREASTS

The breasts are not a part of the external or internal sex organs but rather are considered secondary sex characteristics—physical characteristics other than genitals that distinguish females from males. The breasts are composed internally of fatty tissue and milk-producing glands. Variations in breast size are due mainly to the amount of adipose tissue around the milk glands. Breasts are often not symmetrical in size or shape. Visible changes in a woman's breasts occur in conjunction with her physical development. During adolescence both the fatty tissue and the glandular tissue develop markedly. With adulthood the breasts become conical or hemispherical. Breasts show size variations at different phases of the menstrual cycle and when influenced by pregnancy, nursing, or birth control pills (Crooks and Baur, 1983).

Each breast contains 15 to 20 lobes of glandular tissue, with each lobe drained by a duct opening onto the nipple surface. The lobes are surrounded by fatty and fibrous tissue, giving a soft consistency to the breast. The pink or brown pigment area surrounding the nipple is called the areola. The areola pigment and size vary from woman to woman. The nipples are pigmented and protuberant. Their size and shape vary among women. The nipples consist of smooth muscle fibers and a network of nerve endings that make them sensitive to touch and temperature.

MENSTRUAL CYCLE

Menstruation is the process by which the ovaries and the uterus prepare for the development and implantation of a fertilized egg. It is a cycle lasting an average of 28 days. Menarche, the onset of a girl's first menstruation, usually occurs between 9 and 16 years of age. Menopause, the cessation of menstruation, usually takes place between the ages of 45 and 60.

The menstrual cycle is controlled through a feedback loop involving hormones of the hypothalamus, pituitary,

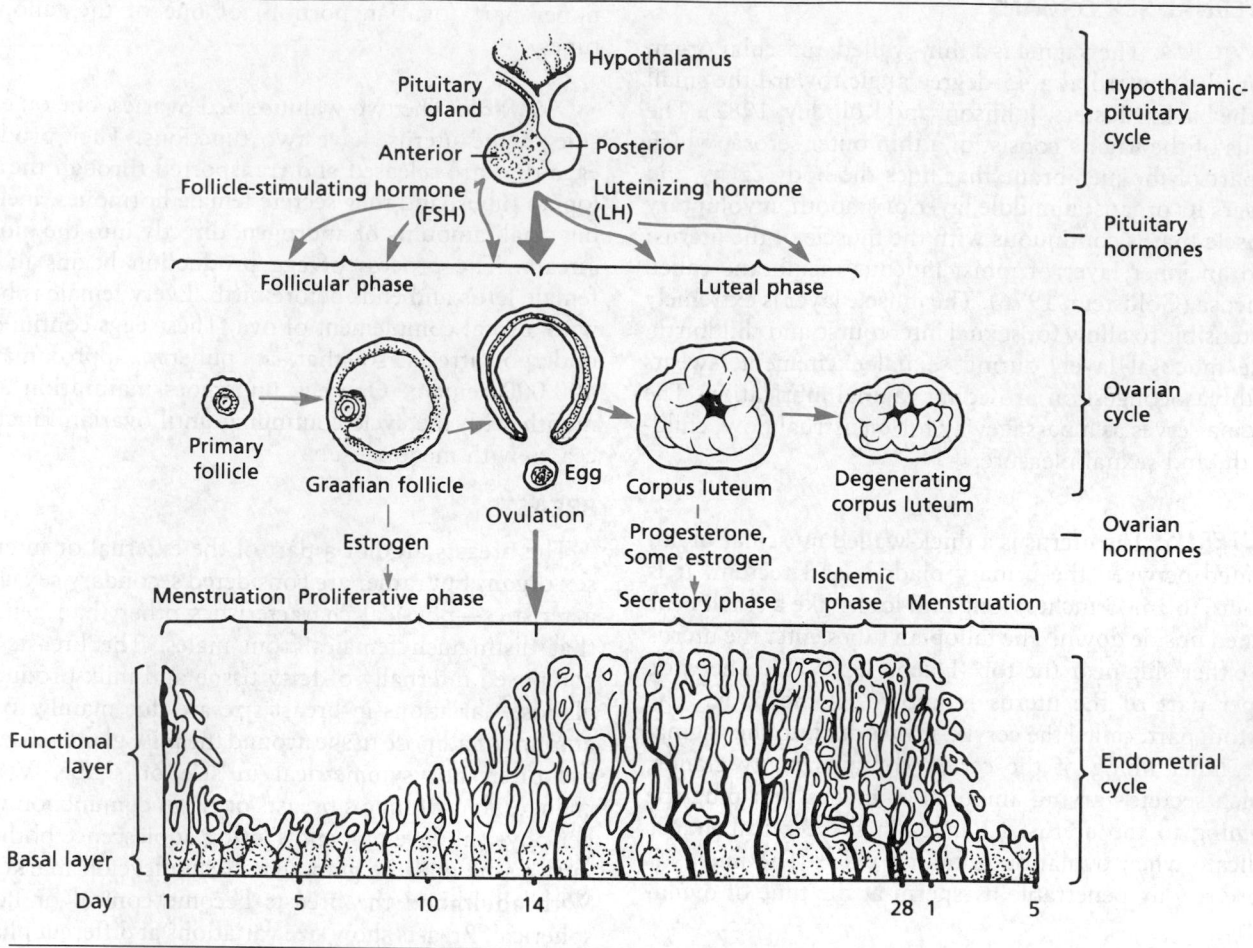

Fig. 30-3   Hormonal control of the menstrual cycle.
From Bobak, IM, Jensen, MD, and Zalar, M: Maternity and gynecologic care, ed. 4, St. Louis, 1989, The
C.V. Mosby Co.

and ovaries. The hormones produce changes in the ovaries and uterine endometrium (Fig. 30-3). The hypothalamus regulates the pituitary hormones through gonadotropin releasing hormone (GnRH) at the beginning of the cycle. GnRH stimulates the pituitary to release large amounts of follicle-stimulating hormone (FSH) and small amounts of luteinizing hormone (LH). These hormones travel through the blood stream and affect the ovaries. Under this influence, several ovarian primary follicles (immature eggs) are stimulated to begin maturation. The ovaries produce increasing amounts of estrogen, which provides a negative feedback loop to the hypothalamus-pituitary level to inhibit further FSH production. This process is the follicular phase of the menstrual cycle.

A few days before ovulation all but one follicle begins to regress. The one follicle (occasionally more than one), under the estrogen influence, continues to grow rapidly and is known as the Graafian follicle. The estrogen influences the pituitary to increase LH release, which surges about 24 hours before ovulation. Ovulation occurs about day 14 of an average 28 day menstrual cycle as the ovum ruptures from the Graafian follicle. The ova then is picked up by the fallopian tube and proceeds to the uterus over the next few days.

After ovulation the ruptured follicle becomes known as the corpus luteum. The corpus luteum produces large amounts of progesterone, peaking about 5 to 7 days after ovulation. The corpus luteum is maintained in part by continued circulating levels of LH. If pregnancy does not occur, LH levels decrease and progesterone levels decrease about 10 to 11 days postovulation. The luteal phase of the cycle ends as menstrual flow begins about 14 days after ovulation.

The hormones that stimulate ovarian activities also cause uterine changes. The uterine phases of the menstrual cycle are known as the proliferative and secretory phases. The proliferative phase is the period before ovulation. High levels of estrogen influence the uterine endometrium to become thick. The cervical mucous becomes more clear and slippery and very stretchable. These qualities of the mucous peak at the time of ovulation and produce an environment receptive to the entrance of sperm for fertilization. (Noting these changes in the quality of cervical mucous is a helpful aid in fertility awareness for planning or prevention of conception.)

The secretory phase of the menstrual cycle occurs postovulation. Under the influence of high levels of progesterone and continued estrogen production, the endometrium continues to thicken in preparation to nourish a fertilized egg. If pregnancy does not occur, the built up endometrium begins to slough with the decreased LH and progesterone. A new menstrual cycle begins with the shedding of the endometrium while the hypothalamus and pituitary kick in to repeat hormonal stimulation.

The average length of a complete cycle is 28 days. Women vary in the average length of the menstrual cycle, and each woman will have some variation in length from one menstrual cycle to the next. Normal cycle lengths may range from 21 to almost 40 days. Menstrual flow consists of blood, mucous, and tissue particles. Average blood loss is about 3 ounces during menstrual flow lasting 3 to 7 days. Again, individuals vary from the average and from cycle to cycle.

PREMENSTRUAL SYMPTOMS. Many women experience symptoms at the time of ovulation or during the postovulatory phase of their menstrual cycle. Some symptoms are partly due to the effects of estrogen or progesterone and may include lower abdominal pain or discomfort at the time of ovulation, breast fullness or tenderness, weight gain of about 3 pounds, fluid retention, irritability, or depression. For some women these symptoms are more consistent and severe and cluster into the premenstrual syndrome (PMS). Although PMS is not a definite diagnosis and the physiology is unclear, it is a real, documented disorder. PMS is a cluster of symptoms including somatic complaints and psychological concerns.

SEX DURING MENSTRUATION. There is no physiological reason for a woman to abstain from sexual activity during menstruation. The uterine contractions that occur during orgasm may even ease the discomfort of pelvic congestion and cramping. Excessive menstrual flow or physical discomfort may however discourage a woman from sex while she is menstruating. Cultural attitudes or other factors may also inhibit sexual activity during menstruation. If a couple does decide to abstain from genital sexual activity during menstruation, they can learn other ways of sharing intimacy until the woman is ready to resume sexual activity.

MENOPAUSE. One of the physiological responses to aging is the cessation of menstruation and fertility. Menopause takes place at around 45 to 60 years of age. The ovaries cease production of estrogen and progesterone, although low levels of these hormones remain in the bloodstream from the continued activity of the adrenal glands. Each woman's body responds to menopause in its own way. For some women the only symptom is the disappearance of menstruation. Other women report headaches, hot flashes, insomnia, and changes in breast and vaginal tissue (Crooks and Baur, 1983). Hot flashes occur when the blood vessels rapidly dilate as a result of fluctuating hormone levels. The decrease in hormone levels also may affect the skin, breasts, and genitalia, causing the tissue to thin. The resulting decrease in the length and elasticity of the vagina and decrease in vaginal lubrication, may make intercourse uncomfortable or painful.

Menopause should not interfere with a woman's sexual capacity, and many women continue to be sexually active. Some women find that the lack of concern about pregnancy enhances their enjoyment of sex. Physical discomfort during penetration owing to reduced lubrication can be eased by using a waterbased lubricant. A waterbased lubricant is necessary so it can easily be removed with soap and water, thus removing a medium for bacterial growth and subsequent vaginitis and urethritis.

Male Sex Organs

The male sex organs produce sperm and hormones and provide a system for conveying sperm from the testicles to outside the body. The external male genitalia are the penis and scrotum. The male internal sex organs include the testicles, which produce hormones and sperm; the epididymis and vas deferens, a system of ducts that transport sperm; and the prostate gland, seminal vesicles, and Cowper's glands, whose secretions become part of the ejaculated semen (Haeberle, 1978) (Fig. 30-4).

EXTERNAL SEX ORGANS

PENIS. The penis consists of the shaft, which is composed primarily of erectile tissue, and the glans, which has both erectile and sensory tissue. The penile shaft comprises three parallel tubes: two corpora cavernosa, which lie side by side, and beneath them a single corpus spongiosum, which surrounds the urethra. All three fibrous tubes of the penile shaft are spongelike. The large vascular spaces between arteries and veins can become engorged with blood, causing the penis to become stiff and erect. The three tubes extend backward, each corpus

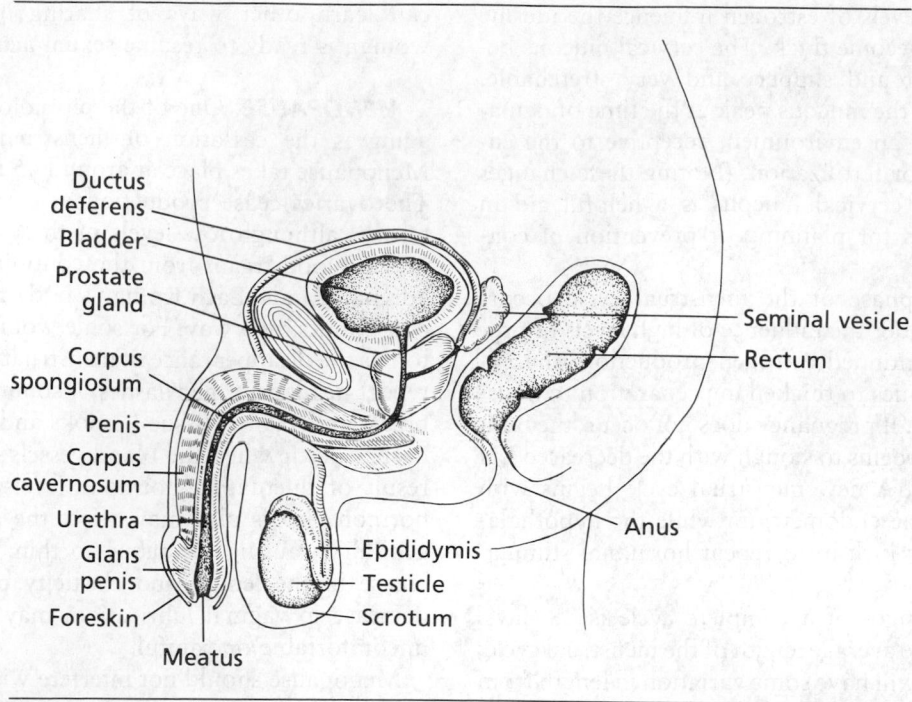

Ductus deferens
Bladder
Prostate gland
Corpus spongiosum
Penis
Corpus cavernosum
Urethra
Glans penis
Foreskin
Meatus
Epididymis
Testicle
Scrotum
Seminal vesicle
Rectum
Anus

Fig. 30-4 External and internal male sex organs.

cavernosum attaching to an arch of the pubic bone and the corpus spongiosum extending into the urethral bulb.

The anterior end of the corpus spongiosum fits over the corpora cavernosa and is called the glans. The glans resembles an acorn. The area where the glans arises abruptly from the shaft is called the corona, meaning crown. The glans and especially the corona, which contains many nerve endings, are the most sensitive parts of the penis. If the male is uncircumcised, the skin of the shaft continues forward and forms a loose-fitting hood over the glans. This hood is called the foreskin or prepuce. On the undersurface the glans is attached to the prepuce by a thin fold of skin called the frenulum, which is also very sensitive to touch. Circumcision is the removal of the foreskin.

SCROTUM. The scrotum is a thin, loose sac of skin that protects the two testicles. It is located at the base of the penis. The scrotum is divided into two compartments, each containing a testis, epididymis, and part of the vas deferens and are considered internal organs even though they are outside the body cavity. The scrotum is responsive to temperature changes; cold temperatures cause it to contract, pulling the testicles closer to the body. The temperature in the scrotum is slightly lower than body temperature so sperm can be produced (Goldstein, 1976).

INTERNAL SEX ORGANS

The male internal sex organs are the testicles (or testes); the system of ducts called the epididymis, the vas deferens, and the urethra; and some accessory organs (seminal vesicles, prostate gland, and bulbourethral glands) (Haeberle, 1978). The left testicle usually hangs lower than the right. The testicles have two main functions: to produce sperm and to produce hormones. Sperm is produced in the seminiferous tubules inside each testicle. The hormones produced in the testicles are called androgens, of which testosterone is most important. Testosterone stimulates growth and development of the genital organs and contributes to growth and development of bones and muscles.

The sperm drain into the epididymis, a duct that lies just outside the testicle. Sperm take 2 to 4 weeks to travel from the epididymis to the vas deferens. The vas deferens is a long tube from each testicle that goes up and out of the scrotum. It curves around the urinary bladder and then turns downward and opens into an enlargement 10 cm (4 inches) long called the ampulla. The ampulla is a reservoir for the sperm before they are discharged into the ejaculatory duct, which carries them through the prostate into the posterior urethra. The ejaculatory ducts result from the fusion of each seminal vesicle with the ampulla of its respective vas deferens. The urethra goes from the bladder to the penis tip and carries urine or semen, but not simultaneously because of an internal bladder sphincter.

The function of the seminal vesicles and prostate is to secrete seminal plasma. Their secretions serve primarily to dilute and carry the sperm. The secretions give the ejaculate its characteristic odor. The paired seminal vesicles, about 5 cm (2 inches) long, are glands secreting a portion of the ejaculate that contributes to the nutrition of the sperm. The prostate is about the size of a chestnut and is located beneath the bladder. The ejaculatory ducts and a portion of the urethra pass through it. In the prostate, prostatic secretions unite with the sperm and fluid from the seminal vesicles. This combined fluid is called *seminal fluid* and provides nutrients to the sperm passing into the urethra. The seminal fluid also buffers vaginal acidity to aid fertility. Even when a male is not ejaculating, small amounts of prostatic secretions are discharged into the urethra and eliminated in the urine.

The bulbourethral glands are pea-sized structures sometimes referred to as the Cowper's glands. They are located below the prostate on either side of the penile urethra. They secrete a clear, alkaline lubricating fluid that sometimes appears at the tip of the penis soon after sexual arousal. The function of this fluid is uncertain, but it is thought to neutralize the acidity of the urethra and make it a suitable environment for sperm. The fluid from this gland may contain sperm.

MALE CLIMACTERIC

Males do not experience a true counterpart to female menopause. They do experience changes in sexual response. The male does not experience the dramatic hormone changes nor loss of fertility experienced by menopausal women. Although at 90, a male may be capable of spermatogenesis, the delayed erectile and ejaculatory ability experienced at 50 or 60 may cause significant concerns about potency and masculinity.

Males who are 50, 60, and 70 years old experience a gradual increase in the length of time it takes to achieve full erection. The older male will maintain erection for a longer period than in his younger days. This results in delayed ejaculation. The ejaculatory phase usually becomes shorter and less intense. The refractory period (time until the male is able to achieve another erection) is lengthened, and the penis returns to its flaccid state much more quickly than in men younger than 60.

The aging male may continue to have a satisfying sex life. The changes in delayed erection and ejaculation may bring about a more mutually satisfying sexual relationship between male and female partners. Both older partners may benefit from extended foreplay, which may increase the woman's vaginal lubrication and aid the male's full erection. Psychological influences may play a significant role in sexual satisfaction in later years. This will be addressed in more detail later in the chapter.

SEXUAL DEVELOPMENT

Infancy

At birth the infant is given a gender assignment of female or male. Rarely, infants are born with ambiguous genitalia and may be assigned a gender that seems consistent with external genitalia but is incongruous with internal sex organs and hormones. As discussed earlier, the self-perception of feminine or masculine (gender identity) is not firmly established until about three. Obviously, for the least emotional trauma to the parents and child, the earlier that accurate gender can be assigned the better.

Psychologically the infant is in a stage of developing trust in parents, the environment, and herself or himself (Erikson, 1963). This trust is established through learning that needs (for example, food, warmth, and affection) are promptly and predictably met by the care giver. The infant also learns to trust his or her own body to respond in predictable ways (for example, certain movements or actions result in predictable responses: "If I move these muscles, I will turn over;" "If I am cuddled, it feels good;" "If I am fed, my stomach doesn't hurt anymore"). The learning process involves exploration and experimentation to define body limits, actions and responses, and pleasant from unpleasant sensations. Exploration includes the discovery of self-soothing behaviors such as thumb sucking and other pleasant forms of self-stimulation such as touching the genital area.

Infant genitalia are sensitive to touch from birth. With stimulation the male infant will respond with a penile erection and the female with vaginal lubrication. (Males will also experience spontaneous nocturnal erections without stimulation.) These behaviors and responses are not associated with erotic psychological contact as in puberty or adulthood but rather are normal learning behaviors in forming a sense of self. Parental response to these exploratory behaviors may set the tone for the child's sexual development, education, and comfort for dealing with sexuality in the home.

Parents should be encouraged to accept the infant's exploratory behavior as a positive step toward development of a positive self-identity. Providing other forms of tactile stimulation through sucking, cuddling, and touching or stroking aids the infant in defining pleasant and comforting experiences through human interaction and from body contact. Touch and the human body begin to acquire a definition as "good."

Toddlerhood and Preschool

The child from age 1 to 5 or 6 continues to solidify the sense of gender identity and to differentiate socially defined, gender-appropriate behavior. This learning process occurs in the course of normal adult-child inter-actions, from the toys given to the child, clothing worn, games played, and responses encouraged. Children also observe adult behavior, begin to imitate actions of the same-sex parent, and maintain or modify their behavior based on parental feedback.

Children reared in single-parent families need exposure to adults of both sexes. Particular attention should be given to the opposite-sex child of a single-parent household. Same-sex role modeling may occur through exposure to visitation periods in cases of divorce or through time with relatives, church, or community groups, and organizations such as "Big Brothers" or "Big Sisters." These interactions are very important in the development of gender identity. Equally important are the messages the single parent conveys about the opposite sex and more specifically, the missing parent. Storybooks and television and movie content may also be used to discuss various family models and gender-appropriate roles.

Body exploration continues at this age. Exploration may include self-stroking, genital manipulation, cuddling of dolls, pets or people, and other sensual experimentation. Concepts of pleasant and unpleasant are thus reinforced. During this stage the child may extend exploration to others as part of gaining a sense of autonomy and initiative (Erikson, 1963). Children may role play games of doctor or mommy and daddy and explore each others bodies in various stages of undress. Questions regarding anatomical differences between female and male and where babies come from often arise at this age.

The child must begin to learn about socially acceptable behavior in an environment that is open to questioning about sex and that enhances self-worth. While learning that the body is good and certain stimulation is pleasant, the child can also be taught the differences in private versus public behavior. Playmate sex games can be handled in a matter-of-fact manner. The parent can interpret the curiosity exhibited as an indication that the child is ready to learn the differences in and proper names for female and male genitalia. This information may be provided at bath time, with anatomically correct dolls, or through the use of many excellent books.

Questions about where babies come from or sexual behavior the child observes should be addressed openly, honestly, and simply. If children wish more information than the answer provided, they should be encouraged to ask and a more detailed response given. Even if questions are not asked, learning opportunities should be offered through pointing out pregnant women, animal behavior at the zoo, or discussions of sexuality as a follow-up to stories or television programs that touch on these topics. Information should not be forced on the child, but through presenting opportunities for discussion, the adult gives the child permission to question.

Childhood

Children from 6 to 10 years of age, or prepuberty, expand their horizons from home to include school and the community. Learning and reinforcement of gender-appropriate behavior come from parents and teachers but more significantly from the peer group. North American society today defines a broad range of behavior acceptable to girls and boys (for example, both sexes participate in cooking and woodworking activities). Less sex stereotyping is seen in elementary school textbooks. Children are exposed to various professional and job options through career days and school counselors. Local, cultural, religious, and peer influences may more narrowly define these behaviors. Parents should encourage socially acceptable behaviors without applying labels of feminine or masculine. Health care personnel must take their cues from the child, family, and community and should remain nonjudgmental in labeling behavior unless it is overtly gender inappropriate.

School-aged children will likely continue self-stimulating behavior. Again, cultural and religious values become more strongly ingrained and must be respected. Parents and children can be informed that masturbation does not have any harmful physical or emotional effects. Acceptance of this behavior may, however, be contrary to the family's religious beliefs. If parents view masturbation as wrong, they should be encouraged to convey to the child who masturbates the disapproval of the behavior without identifying the child as bad. Explanations of times, places, and relationships appropriate for sexual expression should also be provided and should be given in the context of values and rationale on which these beliefs are based.

Children in this age continue to have questions about sex and will assert their independence by testing the limits of appropriate behavior. Limit testing may be displayed by using dirty words or telling jokes with sexual connotations while watching adult reaction. Limit testing is an important part of developing a sense of independence from the family. The testing of sexual limits is also a means of identifying appropriate expressions of sexuality and an opportunity the parents should use to explore questions and concerns.

Children also have a desire and need for privacy. As body changes preparing for puberty begin to occur, the child will experience an increased sense of modesty. Questions about sex may or may not be asked of parents, depending on communication patterns established earlier. Even in a very open, expressive household, the child may develop strange perceptions of sexual behavior because of misinformation and fantasies shared by peers. The child may also learn that questions about sex cause uncomfortable responses from adults. This may limit the child's freedom in pursuing knowledge.

The child should receive accurate information from

home and school about the impending changes to the body that will occur during puberty. This timing for education allows the child to gain information and ask questions before these become personal concerns regarding normalcy and therefore too threatening to ask. The knowledge may also decrease some of the potential anxieties of puberty when an uninformed child may fear menstruation or nocturnal emission and view these as evidence of some dreadful disease. By the age of 10, many girls and some boys are already beginning some of the changes of puberty.

By early school age, the child should also be given information to guard against sexual abuse potential. Many schools are beginning to include this content in their curriculum. Parents should be encouraged to view this material to approve of the content, as well as to be able to provide home follow-up with their children. Very young children can be taught the differences between good touch and bad touch and that certain body parts are not ordinarily touched by adults except at bath time or during physical examination. Children should be told that if they feel uncomfortable about how they are touched, they should say no and tell a trusted adult about the incident. Preschoolers and young children rarely make up stories about sexual abuse and should always be believed. Other ways to limit the potential for abuse include teaching children that families should not keep secrets (other than birthday surprises or other time-limited events), that adults are not always right, and that all people should have control over their bodies and can decide who may or may not hug them.

If abuse does occur, a child who knows the proper anatomical terms for genitalia will be able to describe what occurred accurately. At these times the child should be assured that the adult abuser is the one who was wrong or did something bad and that the child is not responsible for what occurred. Another factor that can be critical to how a child copes with the aftereffects of abuse is how the parents respond. Parents should be encouraged to attempt controlled emotional expressions in front of the child and, as necessary, use other adults to vent anger, frustration, and find support.

Puberty and Adolescence

The onset of puberty in girls is usually signaled by the development of the breasts. After an initial growth of breast tissue, the nipple and areola increase in size. This process, which is in part controlled by heredity, may begin as early as 8 and may not be complete until the late teen years. Rising levels of estrogen are also beginning to affect the genitals. The uterus begins to enlarge, and increased vaginal lubrication occurs, either spontaneously or as a result of sexual arousal. The vagina lengthens, and pubic and axillary hair appears. Menarche varies widely. It may occur as early as 8 or not

until 16 or later. Although the menstrual cycle is initially irregular and ovulation may not occur at first, fertility should always be assumed unless proved otherwise.

Rising testosterone levels in boys during puberty are marked by an increase in size of the penis, testicles, prostate, and seminal vesicles. Both boys and girls may experience orgasm before puberty, but ejaculation in boys does not occur until the sex organs begin to mature, around the age of 12 or 14. Ejaculation may first occur during sleep (nocturnal emission). This may be interpreted as an episode of bed-wetting and even in knowledgable boys can be very embarrassing. About the time genital development takes place, pubic, facial, and body hair begins to grow. The voice changes as the larynx increases in size. This also occurs in girls, but in boys the more dramatic shifts or "cracking" of the voice may be a source of embarrassment. Boys must understand that, although they may not produce sperm with their first ejaculations, they will soon be fertile 24 hours a day.

The emotional changes during puberty and adolescence are as dramatic as the physical ones. The adolescent confronts a powerful peer group with the almost constant anxiety of "Am I normal?" and "Will I be accepted?" Same-sex peers remain influential in defining appropriate behavior, but now comes the added task of establishing a relationship with the opposite sex. Adolescence is a very self-centered, egocentric stage. The degree of introspection is probably necessary to establish a sense of self within the context of family, community, and emotional relationships. Assurance of normalcy in physical and emotional development should be given honestly and often. Because of the concerns of normalcy, body changes and normal introspection of adolescents' modesty and privacy become increasingly important.

The adolescent is faced with many decisions and thus needs accurate information on topics such as body changes, sexual relationships and activity, sexually transmitted diseases (STDs), and pregnancy. This factual information may come from home, school, books, or peers. Even with this information, the adolescent may or may not integrate this knowledge into a life-style. Adolescents have a present orientation and a sense of invulnerability. These characteristics may cause adolescents to believe pregnancy or disease cannot happen to them, and therefore precautions are not necessary. Health education must be provided within this developmental context. More significant than the factual content is guidance in establishing a personal value or beliefs system to use as a framework for decision making. Much of this guidance has already been conveyed by parents in the course of childrearing. Values are expressed verbally and nonverbally as the parents respond to infant self-exploratory behavior, preschool questioning about childbirth, family discussions of media topics such as rape, parental public expression of affection, and so on.

Attitudes of parents regarding gender appropriate roles and behaviors will also influence the adolescent's career and family choices and may affect decisions regarding sexual activity and parenting.

School incidents such as a classmate's pregnancy, television and newspaper issues on abortion, or popular music content can all be used as a basis for discussing family, religious, and personal values. This kind of discussion is difficult even when two-way communication channels are well-established throughout childhood. Parents must accept the responsibility to provide information, share their values, and promote sound decision-making styles but they must be aware that the ultimate decision can only be made by the adolescent. Sexual issues that should be addressed from a knowledge and attitudinal standpoint include dating issues such as appropriate age, curfew, and dating activities: masturbation; emotional commitment in relationships; virginity versus premarital sexual behavior; contraception; teen pregnancy and issues of adoption, abortion, or single parenthood; and risks of STDs. Ideally these discussions should be held in the context of mutual respect of beliefs to promote positive self-esteem.

If not recognized earlier this may be the age of identifying a same-sex sexual partner preference. Many adolescents will have at least one homosexual experience with an individual or in a group. Adolescents may fear that this experience defines their total sexuality as homosexual. This is not true, as many individuals continue with a strictly heterosexual orientation following such experiences. However, some teens may recognize their preference as distinctly homosexual. This can be a frightening and confusing recognition for the adolescent and family requiring a great deal of support. Support may come from a variety of sources such as school counselors, clergy, family, or mental health professionals.

Adolescence may be the first time the child seeks health care without parental accompaniment. The health care provider will need to establish an environment of trust and a willingness to listen to be effective in interventions with this age group. Issues of confidentiality must be clarified and respected. Nurses will need to sort out personal values regarding teen sexuality before they can be effective. Whether an adolescent may be given contraceptives or an abortion without parental consent may be a legal issue in some states, but it is always an ethical issue. Those providing adolescent or reproductive health care must deal with the practitioners' ethical concerns and be knowledgeable of the legal ones and have an in-depth knowledge of adolescent development.

Regardless of the laws, the nurse should provide information where it is lacking. Health care should include suggestions for good health maintenance practices that include self-breast and testicular examination and more general issues such as nutrition and hygiene. Care pro-

viders should encourage discussion of fears and concerns, and should ease communication between adolescent and parents regarding issues such as contraception, STDs, or pregnancy. If the health care provider believes confidentiality must be breached for the welfare of the adolescent, this information should be shared with the teen. The teen should be informed out of respect for the client relationship with the adolescent while recognizing safety concerns. This is a decision that cannot be taken lightly as it may be necessary, for example, to prevent a suicide, but the decision must be weighed against possible perceptions of mistrust of the health care system that may remain throughout adulthood.

Adulthood

The adult has gained physical maturation but is continuing to explore and define emotional maturation in relationships. Young adults are traditionally viewed in roles of childbearing and childrearing. This model does represent the vast majority of adults. Intimacy and sexuality are also issues for adults who choose to abstain from sex, remain single by choice or circumstance while desiring sexual activity, are again single after leaving a relationship, are homosexual, or are unable to bear children. For all individuals, sexuality should be defined and integrated into the self-image and sense of worth.

Sexual health has been defined as "the integration of the somatic, emotional, intellectual, and social aspects of sexual being, in ways that are positively enriching and that enhance personality, communication, and love." (World Health Organization, 1975). All adults can and should strive for sexual health regardless of how they choose to express their sexuality. Adults abstaining from interpersonal sexual activity must decide if autoerotic behavior is appropriate to their value system and lifestyle. It must also be appreciated that although sexual activity is often defined as a basic need, it is one that can be denied and channeled into other forms of intimacy throughout a lifetime. The single individual desiring sexual activity must decide on contraception, single parenthood, and risks of STDs. Gender roles and self-concept may need redefinition for women still single at 40 who desire motherhood. Self-worth can be maintained and nurturing roles fulfilled through community volunteer activities with children. The divorced individual may need to assume the added role of primary breadwinner while learning adult dating behavior. Homosexual adults confront the individual task of developing satisfactory intimate relationships while confronting community and possible career prejudice because of sexual orientation.

All sexually active adults, as they develop intimate relationships, must learn techniques of stimulation and sexual response that are satisfying to members of the opposite sex and their partner specifically. Some adults may only need permission to experiment with alternate behaviors or assurance that sexual expression other than penile-vaginal intercourse is normal. Religious teaching, family values, and earlier-formed attitudes will influence acceptance of some forms of stimulation or may carry residual emotional effects that may exhibit as guilt, anxiety, or sexual dysfunction.

Adults should also be encouraged to verbalize to their partners those types of stimuli and sexual or affectionate acts perceived as pleasant. To enhance sexual enjoyment, individuals should try to gather information about their partners' preferences. Mutual recognition of desires and preferences and negotiation of sexual practices will provoke more positive sexual expression. Knowledge of sexual options can provide the necessary foundation to prompt this experimentation.

Later in the adult years, the individual adjusts to social and emotional changes as children move out. Renewed intimacy may be possible or needed between partners. A potential problem is that one spouse may experience a threat to self-image as the body ages and may attempt to regain youth through sexual relationships with a much younger partner. Couples can be helped to find novelty and new excitement in a long-standing, monogamous relationship through experimentation with sexual positions, techniques, use of fantasy, and so on.

Actual physical changes occur in the course of aging. Because of decreased hormonal influences the postmenopausal woman has diminished vaginal lubrication and elasticity. The aging man experiences an increased ejaculation length in the postejaculatory refractory period, delayed ejaculation, and other changes. The reasons for these changes should be explained before they occur to prevent fears of performance failure rather than normal physiological changes. Aging adults will also need to adjust sexual action and response to chronic illness, medications, aches and pains, or other health concerns. The health care professional can again provide guidance on stimulation techniques to enhance sexual enjoyment.

Older Adulthood

The capacity for sexuality is lifelong. Theoretically people can engage in sex as far into old age as they choose. The best indicator for continued sexual satisfaction with aging is a regularly active sex life during adulthood and into later life. However, older people face health concerns and societal attitudes that may make it difficult for them to continue sexual activity. Although declining physical abilities may make sex as they knew it painful or impossible, with sympathetic intervention they can experiment with and learn alternative ways of sexual expression. The decreasing vaginal lubrication that occurs with aging may make a supplemental lubri-

cant necessary. Decreases in the fat pads that surround the clitoris may make it hypersensitive even to clothing rubbing on it. Cushions and bolsters can be used to support the limbs and torso to ease the strain on the body during sexual activity. An erect penis is not necessary for sexual pleasure. If erectile capacity is diminished or absent, men can be encouraged to continue to express their sexual feelings through touch. If erection is not possible or is long-delayed, the flaccid penis can also be used in touch to stimulate the partner.

The aging male may experience social and emotional concerns that affect sexual functioning. Masters and Johnson (1966) have identified six general areas of concern: monotony in sexual relationships, career and financial concern, mental or physical fatigue, overindulgence in alcohol, illness, and fear of failure. Aging individuals, particularly women, face a real concern over lack of sexual partners. The women may be widowed and as age increases, the number of available men decreases.

Perhaps the most difficult obstacle for the elderly is the myth that sex is for the young. Some older people stop having sexual activity because they feel it is inappropriate for their age group. Hospitals, nursing homes, and other health care institutions may discourage sexual behavior among clients, although some nursing homes now give clients the opportunity and privacy to meet their needs for intimacy. Finding a partner may be a problem for some elderly persons. The need to touch, be touched, and be sexual must not be left out of the aging equation.

SEXUAL RESPONSE

Sexual Response Cycle

Masters and Johnson (1966) have defined a sexual response cycle with the following phases: excitement, plateau, orgasm, and resolution. These phases are the result of vasocongestion and myotonia, which are the basic physiological responses of sexual arousal (Table 30-1). Vasocongestion is the pooling of blood in the genitals and female breasts during sexual arousal. In women this reaction leads to vaginal lubrication, tumescence of the clitoris and the labia minora and majora, and engorgement of the outer third of the vagina (orgasmic platform). In men, vasocongestion leads to erection of the penis. Myotonia, or neuromuscular tension, gradually increases throughout the body during the excitement and plateau phases. Myotonia peaks during orgasm, resulting in involuntary contractions of the woman's vagina and the man's vas deferens and urethra. Both women and men experience contractions of the

TABLE 30-1 Comparison of Sexual Response Cycle in Women and Men

Phase	Women	Men
Excitement	Vaginal lubrication—"sweating" of vaginal walls Expansion of inner two thirds of vaginal barrel Increased sensitivity and engorgement of clitoris and labia Nipple erection and increase in breast size	Penile erection Thickening and elevation of scrotum Moderate enlargement of testicles
Plateau	Retraction of clitoris under clitoral hood Formation of orgasmic platform—swelling of outer one third of vagina and labia minora Elevation of cervix and uterus—"tenting" effect "Sex skin": vivid color change in labia minora Areolar engorgement Increase in muscle tension and breathing	Increase in size of glans (tip) of penis Glans may become intense in color Elevation and 50% increase in size of testicles Mucoid emission from Cowper's glands, possibly with sperm Increase in muscle tension and breathing
Orgasm	Involuntary contractions of orgasmic platform, uterus, rectal and urethral sphincters, and other muscle groups Hyperventilation and increase in heart rate	Internal urinary sphincter closes Sensation of ejaculatory inevitability Contractions of vas deferens, seminal vesicles, prostate, and ejaculatory duct Relaxation of external bladder sphincter Contractions of urethral and rectal sphincter muscles Hyperventilation and increase in heart rate Ejaculation—sperm mostly in first part
Resolution	Gradual relaxation of vaginal walls Rapid color change of labia minora Sweating reaction Breathing, heart beat, and muscle tension gradually return to normal Often ability to return to orgasm, since women do not experience a refractory period as men often do	Loss of penile erection Refractory period when continued stimulation is uncomfortable Sweating reaction Descent of testicles Breathing, heart rate, and muscle tension gradually return to prearousal level

arm and leg muscles, facial muscles, and gluteal muscles. Carpopedal spasms, or spastic contractions of the muscles of the hands and feet, may occur. After orgasm, both vasocongestion and myotonia return to prearousal levels.

The phases described by Masters and Johnson are not absolute. Although phases vary in duration and intensity, the female and male response patterns are more similar than different. They are strongly influenced by psychological and environmental factors such as fatigue or alcohol intake, and the timing and intensity of the phases vary among individuals.

EXCITEMENT

The excitement phase involves a gradual increase in sexual arousal. The earliest signs of sexual arousal are vaginal lubrication and penile erection. The vaginal barrel begins to elongate and increase in size, and the labia majora, nipples, and breasts become congested with blood. The vaginal wall "sweats" to produce lubrication. In men, the testicles become elevated and enlarged and the scrotum becomes elevated and thickened. In some men nipple erection and tumescence occur late in this phase.

PLATEAU

The responses of the excitement phase are heightened in the plateau phase. Vasocongestion and myotonia increase, as do heart rate, blood pressure, pulse rate, and respiration. In some women the breasts enlarge. The areolae become engorged, and slight flush develops in the skin. There are marked color changes in the labia minora (sex skin); as they swell, the color deepens from pink to a deep red. The clitoris moves upward and inward under the hood. The cervix and uterus pull back and up, causing a "tenting" of the cervical os while the vaginal barrel elongates.

In men the coronal ridge increases in circumference and deepens in color. The penis becomes congested and extends to its maximum size. The testicles enlarge by 50% and elevate closer to the perineum. Drops of fluid secreted from the Cowper's glands may appear at the urethral opening (Goldstein, 1976). This fluid may contain spermatazoa, which is a major risk of using coitus interruptus as a contraceptive technique.

ORGASM

Orgasm is the sudden release of the pooled blood and tension in the muscles at the climax of sexual excitement.

TABLE 30-2 Comparison of Sexual Response Cycle in Older Women and Men

Phase	Older Women	Older Men
Excitement	Decrease in amount of vaginal lubrication Slower lubrication of vagina Slower reaction of clitoris to stimulation Much less engorgement of labia majora Only slight engorgement of labia minora Less enlargement of breasts	Takes longer to attain an erection but can be maintained for long periods of time Less enlargement of scrotum Less elevation of testes
Plateau	Orgasmic platform reduced by half Less expansive capacity of vaginal walls Loss of consistency of "sex skin" (labial color change) Less engorgement of areolae	Less likely to have intensity of color change of glans Phase likely to be prolonged owing to better ejaculatory control Penis becomes fully erect just before ejaculation
Orgasm	Less tension from muscle contraction Less frequent rectal contractions Shortened vaginal contraction phase Shorter orgasm time	Feeling of ejaculatory inevitability is eliminated Penile contractions are fewer in number and intensity Rectal contractions are less frequent Ejaculation lacks the same force and duration Less volume of semen
Resolution	Vaginal changes returning quickly to prearousal state Clitoral swelling lost Slower loss of nipple erection	Rapid loss of erection Refractory period (time it takes for stimulation to cause another erection) may be greatly extended Rapid descent of testicles

It can be a highly pleasurable event involving the feeling of physiological and psychological release. A series of involuntary, reflex contractions, varying in intensity, occurs in the genitals and limbs. In women the outer one third of the vagina (orgasmic platform), uterine muscles, and anal sphincter contract rapidly. At the onset of ejaculation the internal bladder sphincter closes, preventing retrograde ejaculation into the bladder. Rhythmical contractions of the urethra, epididymis, seminal vesicles, prostate, and anal sphincter occur in men. The hands and feet may clutch and grasp. Heart rate, blood pressure, and respiratory rate all reach peak levels during orgasm. The clitoris and glans penis may be so sensitive at the moment of orgasm that further stimulation is uncomfortable or painful.

RESOLUTION

Resolution involves a physiological and psychological return to an unaroused state. During the resolution phase there is a rapid loss of genital vasocongestion, nipple erection, and the sex flush. As vital signs return to normal, the palms or soles may start to sweat. The person experiences a feeling of relaxation.

In women the clitoris and vaginal barrel return to their prearousal state. The labia minora and majora fade to their usual pink color. All women have the capacity for multiple orgasms if they continue to receive effective sexual stimulation.

During the resolution phase there is a rapid loss of vasocongestion in the penis and scrotum. Immediately after orgasm most men experience reduced sensitivity to continued erotic stimulation. This so-called refractory period is a recovery time during which further orgasm or ejaculation is physiologically impossible. The refractory period, lasting from a few minutes to several hours, varies in duration and is a major difference in sexual response between the sexes. Most men are incapable of experiencing multiple orgasms in the same cycle. Women do not experience a refractory period.

Aging and Sexual Response

Given reasonably good health and the acceptance of sexual capacity, there is no reason why people cannot remain sexually active as long as they choose. This can most effectively be accomplished by maintaining regular sexual activity (sexual intercourse once or twice per week) through life. Particularly for the woman, regular intercourse helps maintain vaginal elasticity, prevent atrophy, and maintain the ability to lubricate. Nonetheless, the aging process does have an effect on sexual behavior (Table 30-2).

PREGNANCY AND SEXUALITY

As with menstruation, cultural attitudes and old wives' tales may inhibit sexual activity during pregnancy. Pregnancy does not present any physiological contraindication to intercourse. Contraindications that may occur during pregnancy include bleeding, experiencing or being at risk for preterm labor, or after rupture of membranes. Even in the presence of contraindications or maternal or paternal fears of miscarriage or fetal injury, the couple should be encouraged to continue expressions of sexual affection. These activities may include cuddling, kissing, hand holding, and massage. Cautions regarding noncoital sexual activity should be taken, since often when intercourse is contraindicated, female orgasm should also be avoided, and if the couple practices cunnilingus, blowing air into the vagina should be avoided because air emboli are possible.

Women and men experience a variety of emotions with impending parenthood. Fear of injury may be a major concern limiting sexual activity. Conversely, some couples are relieved because they no longer fear an untimely pregnancy and sexual desire is increased. Women, during the first trimester, may have a decreased interest in sex because of nausea, vomiting, and fatigue. Often an increased interest and responsivity during intercourse occurs in the second trimester because of a general sense of health and well-being. In addition, the pelvic and vulvar vasocongestion of pregnancy induces an almost constant state of semiarousal. Multiple orgasm may occur for the first time. During the third trimester, sexual intercourse often will decrease, in part because of fatigue, size, position, and discomfort of pressure on the cervix from the penis and the fetal-presenting part. Intercourse continued past the second half of pregnancy should use positions that avoid having the women flat on her back and placing uterine weight on the major blood vessels, causing decreased maternal blood flow and therefore potential fetal hypoxia.

Couples may need to be informed that sexual intercourse or nipple stimulation may prompt labor to begin or to accelerate. Semen contains some prostaglandins and may encourage uterine contractions. Breast stimulation induces the release of natural oxytocin, which also stimulates uterine contraction. It is for this reason that some health care providers may warn against intercourse late in pregnancy.

Changes in sexuality also continue in the postpartum period. Hormonal changes, particularly decreased estrogen, will decrease the amount of vaginal lubrication and may necessitate use of water-soluble lubricants. Fatigue caused by feedings and sleep interruption and general changes in household chores and routines may negatively influence sexual desire in both partners. Fear of pain becuse of vaginal or episiotomy discomfort can also deter sexual activity. Physiologically, the couple should refrain from sexual intercourse until bleeding has stopped and episiotomy and vaginal discomfort subsides. This often occurs 2 to 3 weeks postpartum. Even during this early period and even with breastfeeding, the couple must consider contraceptives. Condoms are effective at this time. Some women may remain disinterested in or have diminished sexual responses for 6 months or longer. Expressions of sexuality and affection should still be encouraged.

ISSUES RELATED TO SEXUALITY

Whether acknowledged or not, potential fertility is always an issue for premenopausal women having sexual intercourse. Most often the concern is prevention of conception through biological, chemical, mechanical, or surgical methods. At times the choice consciously or unconsciously may be to not use contraception. The issue then is primarily emotional anxiety until the next menstrual period occurs. For a smaller percentage of couples, the issue may be continued infertility in a relationship where children are desired.

An additional issue for sexually active individuals is safe sex. Practicing safe sex has gained increasing recognition in the late 1980s as the fear of AIDS has risen.

Sexual intercourse and manipulation, although intended to provide pleasure for the participants, may be abusive in dysfunctional situations. Sexual abuse may include rape, pedophilia (sexual activity with children), child pornography, and incest.

The nurse's major roles related to these issues are teaching and support. Nurses may also be involved in administering therapies and medications, providing assessment and evaluation of effectiveness, or providing public education regarding the facts, fiction, and importance of dealing with these issues in the family, school, and community.

Contraception

The ability to prevent a pregnancy or to plan the time between pregnancies should be part of a client's health care plan. An unwanted pregnancy can affect health on many levels. The health of the parent, the child, and ultimately the community in which they live depends on the presence of adequate physical, emotional, and financial resources to care for the child. A client who is burdened with an unwanted child often enters the health care system with stress-related complaints. The unwanted child may suffer neglect or even abuse.

Ways of preventing unwanted pregnancy have been developed. Each woman's right to choose if and when to become pregnant is generally acknowledged. It would seem a simple process then to control pregnancy with an appropriate method of contraception. Yet the number of pregnancies among teenagers, abortions in all age groups, and unwanted children indicate that the decision to use or not use contraceptives is much more complex.

FACTORS INFLUENCING USE OF CONTRACEPTION

The nurse considers three major factors when exploring why a client is not using contraception effectively: the client, the client's environment, and the appropriateness of the contraception technique (Fogel and Woods, 1981).

The first factor involves the client's ability to take meaningful action. For several reasons clients might not act in their own best interests in using contraception techniques. Some clients truly do not believe that they can control conception and often view themselves as controlled by events or people outside themselves. A client may also fail to use contraceptive measures because of a lack of knowledge about contraception or about the potential danger of a pregnancy to health or life-style. Shame, guilt, and denial can affect a client's ability to use contraception effectively. When a client uses contraception, he or she must acknowledge that sexual behavior is likely. This may be difficult for the client to admit. If the client has to deal with a pharmacist or health care provider to obtain contraceptives, the embarrassment or sense of personal risk may be too high for the client to act.

Adolescents fail to use contraceptives for a variety of reasons including lack of knowledge and issues of self-concept, for example, difficulty acknowledging self as a sexually active individual, or insecurity in the relationship. Reasons identified for contraceptive nonuse include lack of awareness that pregnancy could occur with first intercourse, lack of knowledge on availability of contraceptives, partner objected to use or fear of losing partner, perceived as unromantic, did not plan to have intercourse or did not have contraceptive available at the time, perceived that contraception is a woman's problem, or trusted that the partner would take care of it (Zelnik and Kantner, 1979). Many of these issues relate to the adolescent's developmental level of establishing a sense of sexual self-concept, appropriate sex-role behavior related to sexual activity, egocentricity, orientation to the here and now, and a sense of invincibility and therefore risk-taking behavior. Characteristics of adolescents who use contraceptives effectively include high socioeconomic status, having a parent or sibling who uses contraceptives, older age, and having a personal experience or a close friend experience a pregnancy scare (Flick, 1986).

A second factor influencing the effective use of contraception is the client's environment. The client's family, community, or religion may disapprove of or prohibit contraception. A woman may have been reared in a family environment in which she was taught that sex for pleasure rather than procreation is wrong. A partner who is not knowledgeable about contraception or does not cooperate in its use increases the risk of contraception failure. People learn about contraception from peers, health care providers, or public health agencies. Good contraception education requires a health care system and an educational system that can deliver such education to the community, but not all communities can afford or support that kind of education.

Finally, the method of contraception must be appropriate for the client. The effectiveness of contraception is related to its safety, comfort, expense, availability, and ease of use. The nurse should remember in discussing contraception with clients that each method has a theoretical effectiveness and an actual effectiveness. The former is based on the ideal circumstances under which the method could be used. The latter considers all personal and environmental factors and may be considerably lower if the client does not use the method regularly or properly.

The decision to use or not use a contraceptive method must be made by the client. The nurse can play an effective role in the decision-making process by helping the client clarify values about contraception and by providing accurate information. The discussion between nurse and client might include questions such as the following:

1. How does the method work?
2. What are the risks involved in using the method?
3. Are there contraindications that rule out particular methods?
4. How will it affect lovemaking?
5. Does the partner object to it?
6. Will it cause any discomfort?
7. Is it readily available, affordable, and easy to use?
8. Will either partner feel embarrassed using it?
9. Is the risk of pregnancy acceptable?
10. Are there other alternatives?

BIOLOGICAL METHODS

For the purpose of this chapter, biological methods of contraception are considered to include any method not using chemical, mechanical, or surgical means to prevent pregnancy. The most effective means of preventing pregnancy is abstinence. This method is often overlooked when discussing options for pregnancy prevention with young, unmarried individuals. Because of the national campaigns promoting "say no" to smoking, alcohol, and drugs, and the fear of AIDS, abstinence may become more common and socially acceptable for adolescents.

Coitus interruptus or withdrawal is a method of contraception often used by adolescents, but this is one of the least effective means of pregnancy prevention. Although the penis is withdrawn from the vagina before ejaculation, sperm is usually present in the preejaculation fluid discharged. A smaller but potential risk also exists that sperm ejaculated just outside the vagina may still travel up the vagina and result in pregnancy. An intent to use withdrawal may not be effective as the male in the plateau phase may choose personal pleasure over pregnancy prevention. Consistent use of coitus interruptus may also cause later sexual dysfunction in the form of premature ejaculation (Masters and Johnson, 1970). Douching immediately after intercourse is also an ineffective means to prevent conception sometimes used by adolescents. Sperm travel into the cervix far too rapidly for postintercourse douching to wash away all possibility of pregnancy.

More scientific biological methods of contraception involve the timing of sexual intercourse to periods in the menstrual cycle when conception is least likely. Contraceptive methods based on the menstrual cycle include the calendar method, the mucus method, and the basal body temperature method. Such methods are popular among clients who reject the idea of putting anything foreign into their bodies, who want a method with no side effects or health risks, or whose religious practices and beliefs prohibit the use of contraceptive agents.

All three of the methods require that the client thoroughly understand the reproductive cycle of the body and be aware of the subtle signs and signals the body gives during the cycle.

Effective use of these methods requires consistent, accurate record keeping for 6 or more months before use as contraception and to determine least fertile days. All methods are not practical for women with irregular or recently established menstrual cycles. Last, these methods necessitate a degree of control as intercourse must be postponed during likely fertile days, whenever they occur. The degree of predictability and control does not correspond with certain life-styles and therefore limits the individuals for whom these methods are appropriate.

The calendar method, also known as the rhythm method, calculates likely fertile days based on usual length of the menstrual cycle. One method recommends recording cycles for 8 months. Fertile days are calculated by subtracting 18 days from the length of the shortest cycle and 11 days from the longest cycle. These numbers then are the days one should avoid intercourse during each cycle (Example: shortest cycle of 27 days and longest cycle of 33 days. $27 - 18 = 9$ and $33 - 11 = 22$. With these cycles the woman would avoid intercourse from day 9 through day 22 of each menstrual cycle). To increase effectiveness the woman should refrain from intercourse from the beginning of each cycle through the last calculated fertile day (Reeder, 1987).

Somewhat more accurate methods of predicting ovulation are based on the body changes produced by hormones. One method records basal body temperature (BBT) the first thing each morning. Just after ovulation the body temperature rises 0.4 to 0.8 degrees Farenheit because of the progesterone influence. The woman is no longer considered fertile after 2 to 3 full days of increased temperature. Because sperm survive several days, the individual may conceive if she has sexual intercourse 1, 2, or more days before the temperature rise. The effectiveness of the BBT method is also reduced when temperature fluctuates because of illness, schedule changes, and so on.

A method often combined with the BBT system monitors the quality of cervical mucus to predict ovulation. Just before ovulation the amount of mucus increases, and just after ovulation the cervical mucus becomes more clear, viscous, and stringy or elastic. Days of wet, abundant, slippery, stretchable, clear cervical mucus are the most fertile. Use of spermicidal gels or creams, lubricants, douching, or checking mucus just after intercourse may affect the perceived quality of cervical mucus and decrease effectiveness.

Other than withdrawal or douching, these three methods of contraception based on monitoring symptoms and cycle regularity are the least effective means of contraception. Actual effectiveness can exceed 80% if used conscientiously. Pregnancy prevention rates are even higher if intercourse is avoided from the first day of the menstrual period until after the last calculated fertile day. The disadvantage is that intercourse may be limited to 1 to 2 weeks at the end of each cycle. If these methods are to be used successfully the couple may need to learn other means of expressing affection and attaining sexual satisfaction.

CHEMICAL METHODS

The most effective method of pregnancy prevention available is the oral contraceptive pill (OCP). The OCP combines various concentrations of estrogen and progestin. Recently a progestin-only "mini-pill" was developed. OCPs suppress the release of FSH and LH, thereby preventing ovulation. The pills must be prescribed and may be contraindicated for women with a history of thrombophlebitis, liver disease, hypertension, diabetes, or for those who smoke and are over 35 years of age. The pills are costly and should be prescribed only under ongoing health supervision which includes an annual physical examination and Papanicolaou's (Pap) test.

Side effects of OCPs include weight gain, spotting between periods, headaches, nausea, breast tenderness, depression, and vaginal yeast infections. Side effects are mostly related to estrogen concentrations and may be minimized by adjusting the prescription to determine the pill with the proper combination of hormones for each patient. Serious reactions that should be promptly reported to the health care provider are severe chest pain, abdominal or leg pain, shortness of breath, severe headaches, blurred vision, or loss of vision.

The OCP is started on the fifth day of the menstrual cycle and is taken daily for 21 days. A menstrual period occurs usually within 2 or 3 days of stopping the hormones. Some packages of OCPs include an additional 7 pills containing an inert substance. This system provides a pill for every day and does not require the woman to count seven days and remember to begin her next cycle of pills. OCPs should be taken at the same time every day to provide maximal effectiveness. If a pill is missed, the woman should take two doses the next day. When 2 or more pills are missed in one cycle, the woman should use another form of contraception, for example, condoms, for the remainder of that cycle.

Spermidical creams and jellies used alone are not as effective as when combined with a barrier method of condom or diaphragm. The vaginal sponge combines the two approaches into one. Spermicidal products are sold over the counter and are relatively inexpensive. The spermicidal products act by providing a barrier at the cervical opening to prevent ejaculate from entering the uterus. A disadvantage is that the spermicide needs to be inserted into the vagina close to the time of intercourse and therefore may interrupt foreplay. Some women object to the contact with their genital area necessary to use these products, while others may object to the messiness. Dermal irritation may occur to the vagina or penis of some individuals with some products.

Spermicidal creams, jellies, or foams are used by inserting the product into the vagina a half hour or less before intercourse. A second act of intercourse requires another dose of spermicide to provide protection. Spermicidal suppositories must dissolve and foam to be effective. The woman should not douche or use tampons for 6 hours after intercourse.

The vaginal sponge is a sponge saturated with spermicide inserted into the vagina to provide a barrier. The sponge may be left in place for 24 to 30 hours and does not necessitate additional doses of spermicide for repeated intercourse during this period. The disadvantage of the sponge, which is different from other spermicides, is the risk of toxic shock syndrome (TSS). The risk of TSS can be decreased if women do not use the sponge while menstruating.

MECHANICAL METHODS

Other forms of contraception, which ideally combine barrier and spermicide, are condoms and diphragm. The diaphragm provides a barrier by covering the cervical os. It must be fitted and prescribed by a health care provider. The diaphragm should be replaced yearly and must be refitted after weight change of 10 pounds and after childbirth. Before each use the woman should check the diaphragm for tears and punctures.

The diaphragm should be used by placing spermicidal gel on the diaphragm, inserting the diaphragm over the cervix, and inserting additional spermicidal gel into the vagina. The process should take place 30 minutes or less before intercourse and the diaphragm should be left in place 6 to 8 hours after intercourse but not more than 24 hours. The risk of TSS is present with this method. Potential disadvantages included the need for genital manipulation, which may be disagreeable, and the interruption of sexual spontaneity. Allergic reactions to the rubber of the diaphragm or the spermicide may occur. Effectiveness is less than that of oral contraceptive pills but more than that of spermicide or diaphragm alone. Diaphragms provide the added benefit of some protection against STDs.

The condom provides the most effective protection against STDs for men and women while providing a contraceptive alternative to abstinence. Condoms are latex sheaths that cover the penis and contain the ejaculate. The condom should be placed on the erect penis with a pocket or reservoir at the tip to collect the ejaculate. To prevent leakage, the base end of the condom should be held in place as the penis is removed from the vagina. Use with spermicide increases the effectiveness. Condoms interfere with the spontaneity of sex.

Condoms are the only readily available form of contraception used by men. With the increased awareness of STDs, sexually active women are beginning to carry condoms to ensure availability and personal protection during intercourse.

Intrauterine devices (IUDs) are less available as of the late 1980s because of fear of litigation related to manufacturers' product liability from side effects. These products are addressed here because a progesterone-containing IUD is still available and some women may have other IUDs in place. The IUD is an object, which may or may not contain hormones or copper, that is inserted into and retained in the uterus. The IUD is inserted by health care personnel. The woman does not need to think about contraception other than to ensure that the IUD remains in place by periodically feeling inside the vagina for the placement of the string at the end of the device.

It is not known exactly how an IUD functions as a contraceptive but is thought that this foreign body causes endometrial inflammation, which prevents implantation. The progesterone in some IUDs also provide hormonal contraceptive protection. At the time of insertion IUDs may cause cramping pain. Some women experience an increased menstrual flow and dysmenorrhea with an IUD in place. More serious risk associated with, IUDs are pelvic infections and uterine perforations. A woman should be instructed to contact her health care provider if she misses a period, experiences unusually heavy periods with clots, severe abdominal pain, or notices signs of infections such as a elevated temperature or foul-smelling vaginal discharge.

SURGICAL METHODS

The two surgical methods of contraception are male and female sterilization. Sterilization has become more popular owing to improved surgical methods and increased societal approval. It is the most effective contraception method other than abstinence, and it is permanent. Female sterilization or tubal ligation involves cutting the fallopian tubes. It is done usually with a laparoscope through a surgical incision in the abdominal wall, usually at the navel. The procedure involves only the fallopian tubes; no other part of the woman's sexual or hormonal system is affected.

In male sterilization or vasectomy, the vas deferens that carries the sperm away from the testicles is cut and tied. Using a local anesthetic, the surgeon makes an opening in the scrotal sac and removes a segment of the vas deferens, tying off or cauterizing the ends to prevent them from rejoining. Because sperm are still traveling up through the vans deferens, the client should be considered fertile for some time after the procedure. Sperm are usually absent from the ejaculate 6 to 8 weeks after the procedure (Crooks and Baur, 1983).

Infertility

When one thinks of family planning, it is generally in terms of pregnancy prevention. One group with special needs that receives little public attention is adults who want to conceive but cannot. In a society that places great value on contraception, adults who cannot conceive are faced with emotional pain and frustration. They may experience a sense of failure as women or men and may feel that their bodies are somehow defective. They may direct every waking moment toward creating the right timing for conception. With advances in reproductive technology, the dilemmas infertile couples face are multifaceted and can involve religious and ethical values and financial constraints. The decision to pursue adoption, medical assistance with fertilization, or to adapt to the probability of remaining childless are options a couple must weigh.

Infertility is generally thought of as a female problem. In reality, an equal percentage of women and men have problems that contribute to difficulties bearing children. The evaluation of fertility must include both partners. Health care evaluation is usually recommended if pregnancy does not occur after 1 year of regular, unprotected intercourse. In couples over 30, this evaluation may be recommended if pregnancy does not occur in 6 months.

Evaluation of potentially infertile couples includes physical examinations to determine general health, review of sexual activity, and understanding of the physiology of conception. Specific procedures related to infertility include semen analysis for men, postcoital testing for mucus and sperm compatibility, endometrial biopsy, hysterosalpingogram (x-ray study) to evaluate uterine and tubal anatomy, and possible laparoscopy.

Causes of infertility may be altered levels of sperm motility and quantity or abnormal formation. The woman may have reduced tubal patency because of endometriosis or pelvic infections, abnormal uterine anatomy, or hormonal alterations that affect endometrial changes during the menstrual cycle or the quality of the cervical mucus. Depending on the causes of infertility, treatment may be hormonal to stimulate ovulation or surgical to restore tubal patency through microsurgery. Other forms of treatment that are available through more controversial methods include artificial insemination using the husband's sperm or donor sperm, in vitro fertilization, and surrogate motherhood and embryo transfer.

The stress of fertility testing, the pain and continuing routine of therapies, and excessive cost produce a tense environment. Support groups are available for couples coping with these stressors. A percentage of couples will remain infertile regardless of treatments used. These individuals need to work through a grief process for the loss of their potential, dreamed-of children. Couples also need to be able to deal with the adverse misconceptions of friends and family. Support groups such as RESOLVE can assist. Contrary to community beliefs, recommendations such as "just relax" or "adopt a child then you'll get pregnant" are not means of increasing fertility.

The decision to adopt or remain childless is one the couple must make based on values regarding family and parenthood. The number of children available for adoption has decreased because of improved contraceptive technology and increased abortions. Couples deciding on adoption may require support to decide to parent children who have physical handicaps or are of multiple ethnic origin. Adoptions of South or Central American or Korean children have been a satisfying decision made by many couples. Support groups are available to assist these couples in continued integration of multiethnic families. North American infants are also available for adoption, although in fewer numbers.

Abortion

Abortion remains an issue that stimulates heated discussions of morality, women's rights to body control, and when life begins. Abortions have been performed since ancient times. The increased safety and availability of abortions in the United States has improved since the Supreme Court Roe vs. Wade, 1973, decision has removed the stigma of illegality. Abortions are also safer and less costly when performed in the early weeks of pregnancy. This is possible with improved pregnancy testing and more accurate early diagnosis.

Methods of abortion include dilation and curettage procedure (D & C) or vacuum aspiration, induction of cervical dilatation and uterine contraction with prostaglandins and oxytocin, and saline injected into the amniotic sac to stimulate expulsion of the fetus. Rationales for abortion are varied and may include a decision to terminate an untimely pregnancy or a choice to abort a fetus known to have a defect incompatible with life. Clients who decide to abort a pregnancy may experience guilt over this decision. The guilt may surface immediately after the procedure or may be more covert and manifest by sexual dysfunction or inappropriate perceptions (for example, a woman who later develops cervical cancer, viewing the condition as punishment for this wrong doing). Some of these beliefs may be assessed before the procedures and should be evaluated by those counseling women experiencing unwanted pregnancies. The woman who has an abortion will experience a sense of loss and should be prepared for and supported through the necessary grief. The male partner may also experience this loss and grief.

Health care providers must sort out personal values related to methods and rationale for abortion. The health care provider is entitled to personal opinions and should not be forced to participate in procedures or counseling that is contrary to beliefs and values. Nurses should choose specialities or places of employment so their personal values are not compromised and the care of a client in need of health care is not jeopardized.

Sexually Transmitted Diseases

A major problem in dealing with STDs is finding and treating the people who have them. Sometimes people do not seek treatment because they are embarrassed about how they became infected. Some people may not even know they are infected because symptoms are absent or go unnoticed. Since sexual behavior may include the whole body rather than just the genitalia, many parts of the body are potential sites for an STD. The ears, mouth, throat, tongue, nose, and eyelids can be used for sexual pleasure. The entire surface of the skin can be thought of as having sexual potential. Although the perineum, anus, and rectum are rarely discussed in terms of sexual pleasuring, they are frequently included in sexual activity by both women and men. Furthermore, any contact with another person's body fluids, around the head, open lesion on the skin, anus, or genitals has the potential to transmit an STD.

Clients may be hesitant to talk about their sexual behavior if they feel it is not normal, normal usually being whatever they believe society approves. Oral-genital sex, anal sex, or any sexual behavior that embarrasses the client may hinder the detection of an STD. Specific STDs of the throat and intestine can thus go undetected at great cost to the client.

The most valuable tool the nurse can develop for providing care in areas of sexuality is communication skills. By questioning and talking with the client in a nonjudgmental manner that evokes trust, the nurse can pick up valuable clues about the presence of an STD that the client may have missed. The nurse can also begin to assess the client's attitudes toward sexuality and adjust the intervention to make it acceptable to the client's sexual value system.

Clients should understand the signs and symptoms of STDs so they can seek treatment and inform sexual partners. Gonorrhea and *Chlamydia* exhibit similar symptoms and often occur together. Both diseases are more often symptomatic in men, while more than half of the women with gonorrhea or *Chlamydia* may not have symptoms. In men, symptoms generally occur about a week after contact and include burning or itching when urinating and a whitish discharge from the penis. Women who do experience symptoms may experience burning urination and/or vaginal discharge. *Chlamydia* symptoms occur within about the same time frame after contact and are the same as for gonorrhea. Problems with genital discharge or urination are manifestations of the disease when contracted through genital sexual activity. The disease can also be spread through anal-genital and oral-genital contact. Untreated disease may cause sterility in the male or female. Gonorrhea and *Chlamydia* are both treated with antibiotics.

Syphilis is another long-known STD. Transmission is usually through sexual intercourse, but the disease may also be contracted through oral and anal routes. Syphilis may take as long as 3 months before symptoms are exhibited. The initial symptom is a lesion (chancre) that occurs at the site of entry for the organism. The chancre is usually a clean, round, and painless lesion. This sore heals in 1 to 3 months. The untreated organisms, however, continue to produce a systemic affect. Secondary syphilis includes a rash and sore throat. If untreated, years later, tertiary syphilis causes cardiac and central nervous system damage. Until the tertiary phase, syphilis is treatable with antibiotics.

Herpes simplex virus II is an STD that is treatable but not curable. The site of contact is usually penis and vagina, and symptoms take a few days to weeks to appear. A small cluster of painful blisters at the site of infection is the initial symptom. These symptoms will disappear in several weeks but usually recur. The disease, however, does not progress like syphilis but continues to recur as local sores. Herpes can only be transmitted when lesions are present.

AIDS is another disease transmitted through sexual contact. Transmission occurs through exchange of body fluids as may occur with anal-genital, genital-genital, oral-genital, oral-oral, and oral-anal contact. Much is still not known about the HIV virus and AIDS. Evidence of AIDS may take 6 months to 7 years to show up. Symptoms include persistent fever, diarrhea, swollen glands, fatigue, and weight loss. The disease is not curable and is fatal. The ultimate course of the HIV virus in the body in individuals without symptoms of AIDS is not known. It is thought that those carrying the HIV virus will ultimately develop the disease of AIDS. Those positive for HIV may transmit this virus through sexual contact as described.

All five sexually transmitted diseases may cause serious problems to infants born to mothers when the disease is active. Syphilis and AIDS may be transmitted in utero. Sexually active clients should understand symptoms that need reporting and be aware that most STDs, if untreated, may cause serious health consequences for the individual. They should also understand that because they were once infected and cured they do not have immunity, and the diseases may recur with additional contact with an infected partner.

SAFE SEX

Safe sex is a phrase used to describe responsible sexual practices aimed at minimizing sexual disease transmission, particularly AIDS. Safe sex is responsible sex and includes knowing one's sex partners, having a relationship with open communication that enables the partners to discuss current health status and disease exposure, and using protective devices. Additional measures include limiting the number of sex partners, avoiding sexual contact with intravenous drug users, and using condoms properly. Condoms provide the barrier between body fluids only with sexual activity involving the penis. No protection would be provided for oral-anal contact, for example, and therefore these practices should be avoided. The only 100% effective method to avoid sexually contracting a disease is abstinence.

A controversial issue related to safe sex for adolescents is the placement of condom dispensers in public restrooms in places frequented by teenagers, particularly in schools. Those in favor of this program state that one cannot stop teens from having sex, therefore adults should promote their health through ensuring a means to minimize pregnancy and STDs. Those opposed believe that providing condoms implies approval for teen sexual activity. The fact is that the rate of adolescent pregnancy and STD incidence continues to increase.

Sexual Abuse

Sexual abuse occurs far more often than reported. The known cases of rape, incest, or child molestation probably only represent the tip of an iceberg. Incidents such as these have a traumatic effect on the victim, which may cause psychological problems and later sexual dysfunction. Physical injury, STD, and pregnancy may be the result of sexual abuse. The covert nature of some forms of abuse is one rationale for assessing sexuality in all ages.

Evidence of sexual abuse in children may be uncovered during history taking or physical examination. In children under 6 years of age, the child may exhibit behavioral changes such as excessive nail biting, thumb sucking, or excessively clinging to parent or others. The child may have sleep disturbances or enuresis or encopresis (bed wetting or bowel movements). School-age children may display similar behaviors or symptoms along with excessive fears and anxieties as tics, phobias, and

truancy. The child may fear close contact with others. The adolescent more than 12 years of age may exhibit antisocial or socially unacceptable behavior (for example, sexual promiscuity, drug abuse, or running away from home). A daughter may be seen assuming much of the mother's role behaviors. Low self-esteem and depression may be present. Often the adolescent will avoid close contact with adults. Specific symptoms raising questions of abuse include a child showing an early, exaggerated awareness of sex or exhibiting seductive behavior toward adults; and swollen anus, vagina, or penis; bruises on or around breasts, buttocks, vagina, or penis; lacerations of or foreign substance in vagina or anus; and STD in child under 15 years of age.

When abuse is recognized, support needs to be mobilized for the victim and the family. All family members may require therapy in situations of incest to promote healthy interactions and relationships. Rape victims may need to work through the crisis before feeling comfortable with intimate expressions of affection. The partner may need support in understanding this process and how to assist the victim. Children who have been sexually molested need to understand they are not at fault for the incident. The parents must understand how critical their response is to how the child reacts and adapts. The nurse may come in contact with clients confronting any of these stressors. At the least, nurses should be aware of sources for referral and support in the community and refrain from applying personal values to the individuals and families.

Effects of Illness on Sexuality

Healthy sexuality involves all human dimensions, and illness can directly or indirectly influence any or all of these dimensions. Although illness and the healing process do indeed influence established living patterns, the idea that health is a matter of degree rather than a matter of being either sick or well may be a new one for the client. Viewing sexuality in terms of a continuum rather than as being present or absent may also be a new concept for the client. The nurse's task is to help the client integrate the physical, psychological, and social systems during the course of the illness. The degree to which any nursing intervention involving sex is successful depends on the attitudes and beliefs of both nurse and client and their understanding of the effects of the illness and its treatment on sexual functioning.

The media's treatment of sexuality suggests that only the young and fit are sexual. Eroticized images and descriptions of ill or disabled people are rare. Because of this, most people seldom think about or imagine how ill people feel or behave sexually. A dynamic approach to total health care, however, considers all the ways in which an illness might affect a client's sexuality.

PHYSIOLOGICAL AND PSYCHOLOGICAL CHANGES AND ILLNESS

Sexual behavior depends on intact neural, vascular, and hormonal systems. The genitals and other soft body tissues that respond to sexual arousal require uninterrupted neural pathways and an adequate supply of blood. Hormones influence both sexual moods and physiological functioning in sexual expression. Joints and muscles must bend and stretch as the body gives expression to sexual feelings. Any change in any one of these systems can have a ripple effect on the others. To accommodate to changes in these systems, the client may have to learn new sexual behaviors. Changes in body functions and structures as a result of illness may not directly influence sexuality but may affect feelings of desirability and arousal. In this case it is the client's perception of self as sexually capable and sexually desirable that is being influenced.

Chronic illness interferes with sexuality because of the extended period of care and attention involved. A client or partner providing home care may have little energy left for sexual feelings or activity. For a client with a highly debilitating illness such as chronic lung disease, only very limited sexual activity may be possible. There are no therapies for reversing sexual impairment resulting from neurological or vascular disease (Unsain, Goodwin, and Schuster, 1982). Diseases such as diabetes not only necessitate changes in daily habits but also may lead to reduced sexual desire. Vascular and neurological changes of diabetes may cause lack of or change in orgasmic response and erectile dysfunction. Spinal cord injuries not only may sever nerve pathways and remove genital sensation but may also psychologically affect sexuality. Self-esteem is usually lowered with the accompanying change in body image, gender identity, and altered ability to perform sex-role behaviors (Weinberg, 1982). Chronic pain and limited range of movement present obstacles to sexual activity. To adjust to these limitations, the client must learn effective communication skills and be willing to experiment with new positions for sexual activity. The nurse has an essential role in easing these adjustments, particularly when the client's background does not encourage open discussion of sexual topics.

Cancer can also interfere with sexuality. Medical and surgical treatments alter body image. Alopecia from chemotherapy along with severe nausea and fatigue may temporarily remove all sexual desires. However, individuals with cancer or any terminal illness continue to remain sexual beings. As stated above, altered expression of affection and sexual stimualation may need to be explored to adjust to pain, radiation effects, and so on. Even when death is imminent, the ill individual may wish to affirm what remains of life through intercourse. The client's spouse or partner will need to deal with grief and beliefs to respond sexually. The nurse's role may be to acknowledge these desires as normal and healthy means of communication. Nurses may need to initiate discussion of these issues and support the partner in grief.

EFFECTS OF MEDICATION ON SEXUALITY

The effect of medications on sexual feelings and functioning is an enormously complex topic, simply because of the number of medications in use and the variable individual response. Medications can interfere with sexual desire as well as all phases of the sexual response cycle.

Antihypertensives such as methyldopa, propranolol, and clonidine often cause erectile dysfunction. Controversy exists as to whether the client should be told this when treatment is initiated for fear of generating significant performance anxiety and a self-fulfilling prophecy. Methyldopa has been known to decrease libido in women and men. Thiazide diuretics, used to treat hypertension, are also known to cause erectile dysfunction. Depression usually negatively affects sexuality with diminished desire. Antidepressant medication may produce an increased libido but may also cause delayed female orgasms and delayed or failed ejaculation. Chemotherapeutic agents, along with the psychological effects caused by alopecia and nausea may also result in decreased libido, impotence, and amenorrhea, decreased spermatogenesis and sterility. Young men interested in future child bearing can freeze sperm before chemotherapy or radiation treatment. Medication is perceived to have an effect on sexuality and is a significant area of assessment.

HOSPITALIZATION

Being hospitalized can have a powerful symbolic meaning to clients. Clients tend to think their situation is serious if a hospital is involved. The procedures of hospital health care may take on a mystery that is beyond a client's capacity to understand. The need to have some power over life and the powerlessness of being hospitalized may become crucial issues for a hospitalized client. The client has left the home environment with its security and privacy and entered a much more public and intrusive environment. The hospital room is open to the nurse day and night, and privacy is represented only by a cubicle curtain. Hospital clothing is notoriously scant. Even carrying out activities of personal hygiene may be beyond the client's ability. Add to this feelings of illness and anxiety, and it is no wonder that sexual behavior and feelings may diminish or vanish.

Nurses can assist clients in learning to meet sexual needs in the hospital setting. Simply acknowledging the openness of the setting lets a client know that the nurse understands. Knocking or signaling before entering the client's space is a basic courtesy and provides a needed sense of privacy. The use of a do-not-disturb sign offers the client some feeling of control over the privacy of the environment.

Some hospitalized clients may act out sexually through use of obscene language, pinching or other suggestive contact with the nurse, or consistent nudity or exposure of genitals when the nurse enters the room. This behavior may be a means of exerting control over the clinical environment or an attempt to validate continued identity as a sexual being. It may also be a means of attracting needed attention or limit testing (Woods, 1984). Assessment and intervention to deal with persistent sexual acting out is a nursing challenge that benefits from the psychiatric nurse specialist's expertise. Consistency in approach to the client, and attention and reinforcement for desirable behavior, is essential to minimize the acting out.

Surgery not only changes body structures and functions but also influences the client's body image (Dickman and Livingston, 1982). Surgical clients may experience loss of self-esteem and feelings of loss involving their masculinity or femininity (Lion, 1982). They may blame themselves for needing surgery and consider the surgical consequences their just punishment. Alteration or removal of the internal or external genitalia can make conventional and accustomed sexual activities uncomfortable or impossible. The client is then faced not only with the loss or alteration of body parts but also with the necessity of having to learn new sexual behaviors that may seem strange or repugnant. Prostatectomies, hysterectomies, mastectomies, and ostomies can be expected to creat sexual problems for clients.

After a heart attack or heart surgery, clients often have a decline in sexual activity (Lion, 1982). This is true even after they are evaluated as fit and able to resume normal activities of daily living. These clients typically fear having another attack or dying while masturbating or having intercourse. The client's partner is often anxious about initiating sex because of fear of contributing to another attack. Such anxieties are cultivated through misunderstanding, misinformation, or lack of information on the client's part (Shuman and Bohachick, 1987). Clearly, accurate and honest information is needed at every stage of the rehabilitation process.

Sexual Dysfunction

The causes of sexual dysfunction may be physiological or psychological. Sometimes the cause of a dysfunction cannot be identified or is a combination of several factors. An estimated 10% to 20% of sexual dysfunctions are caused by physiological factors (Kolodny, Masters, and Johnson, 1979). In another 15% of cases, physiological problems contribute to the sexual dysfunction without being its sole cause (Masters et al., 1982). In

most instances a sexual assessment should include a complete physical examination to identify or rule out physiological conditions that might be contributing to sexual dysfunction.

PSYCHOLOGICAL FACTORS

In many instances sexual dysfunction can be traced to a lack of knowledge about sexuality, ignorance of sexual techniques, or general misinformation about sexuality. For example, unsatisfactory lovemaking can be the result of a lack of information about sexual anatomy. Some segments of society still place strong prohibitions on discussions of sexual behavior. Children may receive some information at home and in school, although word of mouth sharing among peers may still be a major source of misinformation. Open discussion of sex, even between partners, traditionally has not been encouraged, and the result has been feelings of distance or alienation.

Another psychological factor is the destructive belief that the ability to perform sexually is inherently developed by the time a person reaches adulthood. Sexual performance is often perceived as instinctual and mysteriously understood when a person comes of age. Thus ignorance and silence about sexual matters prevail, because a person who lacks knowledge about sexual function seldom realizes that one needs to be taught this information. Myths and outright misinformation about sexuality add to the problem of lack of knowledge for many individuals.

It is important for the nurse to understand how the phenomena of ignorance and avoidance of sexual issues have developed in our society. Human sexuality is a basic drive frequently accompanied by intense and conflicting emotions. Society has therefore developed standards for sexual behavior, which serve to minimize fears and confusion about how a person should act. Unfortunately, they an also create unrealistic expectations, demands, and restrictions that are internalized by individuals and become a part of their value systems.

The psychological forces that prevent violation of sexual rules in many cultures are guilt and anxiety. When guilt and anxiety become associated with early sexual learning, the person develops a pattern of inhibited sexual response and carries this through to adulthood. For instance, a woman may be actively discouraged from sexual stimulation in early childhood and as an adult may find that she not only has to learn to enjoy sexual stimulation, but also has to overcome negative feelings associated with her sexual self-concept.

Other sources of sexual anxiety, such as fear of failure, demand for performance, and rejection, can be destructive to sexual functioning. Anticipation of the inability to perform is a cause of erectile dysfunction, and perhaps to some extent, of orgasmic dysfunction. A person who has experienced an episode of failure may have an increased fear of its recurrence. Anticipatory anxiety related to sexual performance can start a self-defeating cycle of fear that escalates from a single failure into a state of serious chronic dysfunction. In "spectatoring," the phenomenon that maintains this cycle, one remains outside oneself and observes one's sexual responses. This results in poor performance, which then reconfirms one's anxieties and fear of failure (Masters and Johnson, 1970).

Fear of rejection by one's partner or an excessive need to please may also generate anxiety. To wish to give enjoyment and share pleasure with a partner is desirable

TABLE 30-3   Common Female Sexual Dysfunctions

Description	Possible Causes	Interventions
Preorgasmic (primary orgasmic dysfunction): a woman who has never had an orgasm	Religious prohibitions Restrictive learning environment Fear of losing control Poor communication with partner Inadequate clitoral stimulation Excessive drug or alcohol use Past negative sexual experiences	Information on sexual prohibitions and restrictions Sensate focus exercises* Genital play Kegel exercises† Directed masturbation Nondemand intercourse Referral to a preorgasmic support group
Secondary orgasmic dysfunction: a woman who has experienced orgasm in the past but does not currently	Low sexual interest Attitude toward partner Causes listed for primary orgasmic dysfunction	Discussion of attitude toward partner Information on sexual prohibitions Sensate focus exercises* Nondemand intercourse Genital play Kegel exercises† Directed masturbation Partner communication
Vaginismus: a woman who experiences involuntary constriction of the outer one third of the vagina, making vaginal penetration impossible	Religious prohibitions Sexual prohibitions Experience of sexual assault Painful intercourse Painful pelvic examinations Alcohol abuse Traumatic early experiences with sex Fear of pregnancy, venereal disease, or cancer	Legitimization of existence of spasm Use of vaginal dilators in graduated sizes Kegel exercises† Improvement of partner communication
Dyspareunia: painful intercourse	Negative attitude toward partner Strong religious prohibitions Sexual prohibitions Genital sensitivity Physical problems (tears, infections, trauma, spasms, lack of lubrication) Roughness during intercourse Lack of arousal	Thorough and detailed examination of sex organs Treatment of physical problems Provision of sufficient lubrication Discussion of sexual attitudes Discussion of comfortable positions
Lack of desire: a woman who has lost interest in being sexual	Preorgasmia Strong netative emotions Illness Drug or alcohol use Avoidance response because of feeling sexually pressured Unresolved anger or fear Depression History of sexual abuse or incest Pain associated with intercourse	Discussion of attitude toward partner Information on sexual prohibitions and restrictions Sensate focus exercises* Kegel exercises† Genital play Resolution of any conflicts between partners

*Series of pleasurable touching exercises that are focused on sensual (not sexual) activities with a partner.
†Exercises for the pubococcygeus (PC) muscle to increase sensation and maintain muscle tone of the pelvic floor.

and healthy. It is when this becomes a compulsive need to please, to perform, to serve, and to not disappoint that the emotion becomes dysfunctional.

Poor communication is frequently associated with sexual dysfunction. A person with communication problems may be unable to discuss sex and thus may have limited knowledge and restrictive standards of acceptable sexual behavior. In this self-defeating cycle, partners perpetuate ignorance, lack of understanding, and misinformation about their sexual and emotional needs. To communicate effectively about sex, they must openly share information about their interests, desires, and wishes. Negotiation and compromise result from effective communication patterns.

Other relationship issues often play a large part in sexual dysfunction. Anger, power struggles, and unresolved conflict within the relationship are important causes of sexual dissatisfaction that lead to dysfunction. Fear of pregnancy is a factor that may make it difficult for a woman to relax.

TABLE 30-4   Common Male Sexual Dysfunctions

Description	Possible Causes	Intervention
Primary erectile dysfunction: a male who cannot penetrate during sexual contact, has never been able to sustain an erection to the point of penetration, and may masturbate to ejaculation.	Not well understood Extreme religious prohibitions Traumatic initial failure Performance anxiety and fears	Relieving pressure of goal-oriented sexual performance Discussing sexual prohibitions and restrictions Providing accurate information Sensate focus exercises Reducing "spectatoring" Restricting intercourse Encouraging female superior position with lubrication Encouraging options to intercourse, manual stimulation, oral-genital sex
Secondary erectile dysfunction: a male who cannot maintain or perhaps even experience an erection but has succeeded at penetration at least one time; has experienced erectile failure during at least 25% of his sexual opportunities.	Interference with central nervous system caused by drugs, alcohol, stress, fatigue, diseases, or surgical procedures Performance anxiety Poor communication with partner Depression	Relieving pressure of goal-oriented sexual performance Discussing sexual prohibitions and restrictions Providing accurate information Sensate focus exercises Kegel exercises Reducing "spectatoring"
Premature ejaculation: a male who consistently ejaculates sooner than he would desire	Adolescent fast ejaculation patterning Failure to attend to internal cues of approaching ejaculation Lack of sensual self-awareness Performance anxiety	Providing accurate information Encouraging communication with partner Sensate focus exercises Kegel exercises Stop-start technique Encouraging different positions Retraining ejaculatory response Relieving pressure of performance anxiety Changing tempo of thrusting during intercourse
Delayed ejaculation: a male who cannot ejaculate during penetration	Religious restrictions Fear of impregnating Lack of physical interest Active dislike for partner Past traumatic sexual event Infidelity Punishment for masturbation as a child Excessive drug or alcohol use	Relieving pressure of goal-oriented sexual performance Discussing sexual prohibitions and restrictions Providing accurate information Sensate focus exercises Kegel exercises Encouraging communication with partner

A history of sexual abuse may have an impact on sexual functioning. Anger, guilt, and a need for control are emotional sequelae to abuse and often underlie the development of sexual problems, including inhibited desire and avoidance of sexual contact. Researchers have begun to examine the variables associated with molestation that contribute to adult sexual adjustment. These include the person's age at the time of molestation, the frequency and duration of molestation, and the person's negative feelings associated with molestation. These findings help explain variations in sexual functioning that exist among people with histories of abuse. Further investigation is needed to help us understand and effectively treat the population of abused persons who seek counseling for sexual difficulties (Livingston, McIntyre, and Fogel, 1984).

Tables 30-3 (p. 777) and 30-4 (p. 778) summarize the most common female and male sexual dysfunctions, their possible causes, and intervention strategies.

PHYSIOLOGICAL FACTORS

Orgasmic dysfunction in women is seldom caused by physiological factors. However, diabetes, alcoholism (Livingston, McIntyre, and Fogel, 1984), neurological problems, hormone deficiencies, and some pelvic disorders resulting from infections or surgery may impair or hinder orgasmic response. Vaginismus, or involuntary vaginal contraction, is most often caused by psychological factors, while dyspareunia, or painful intercourse, is more likely the result of physical disorders such as infections, surgical scarring, diabetes, or use of drugs (for example, antihistamines, tranquilizers, or marijuana). Physiological causes for lack of sexual desire include hormone deficiencies, alcoholism, kidney failure, drug abuse, and severe chronic illness (Masters, Johnson, and Kolodny, 1982).

Physiological factors that may cause erectile dysfunction in men include neurological disorders such as spinal cord injury or multiple sclerosis, vascular insufficiency problems, hormonal deficiencies, and genital infections or injuries. Diabetes and alcoholism are the two most common physiological causes of erectile dysfunction. Both prescription medications and street drugs sometimes cause erection problems. Physiological problems rarely cause premature ejaculation, but delayed ejaculation is sometimes the result of neurological disorders. About 10% of cases of delayed ejaculation are due to drug and alcoholism (Masters, Johnson, and Kolodny, 1982).

The distinction between physiological and psychological causes of sexual dysfunction is not always clear. Physiological interventions sometimes clear up the problem. At other times psychological concerns have been masked by a physiological condition. It is important to monitor the client's progress carefully even when it seems that only a physiological condition is involved. An understanding of the possible psychological and physiological causes of sexual dysfunction is needed before the nurse can determine what further assessment and intervention is necessary in a given case.

SEXUALITY AND THE NURSING PROCESS

ASSESSMENT

Ideally, sex is a natural, spontaneous act that passes easily through a number of recognizable physiological stages and culminates in satisfaction for both partners. Following sexual activity, there should be a period of "afterglow" in which both partners experience a sense of warmth, well-being, and closeness. In reality, this sequence of events is often the exception rather than the rule, as demonstrated by the number of self-help sexual enhancement books available in bookstores. Nurses can expect to encounter clients who have problems with one or more of the stages of sexual behavior, including the feeling of wanting sex, the physiology and emotions of having sex, and the feelings experienced after sex. Clients may unconsciously provide the nurse with clues to their sexual problems. The nurse's role includes the promotion of the client's sexual health as a component of overall wellness. The nurse can promote sexual health by helping the client to gain insight into the problem and explore methods to deal with it effectively. The nurse must provide the opportunity for clients to discuss sex and can provide permission by initiating the topic at the time of assessment.

Many nurses find that they are uncomfortable talking about sexuality with their clients, but they can reduce their discomfort with several methods. First, nurses should build a sound knowledge base and understanding of healthy sexuality and the most common areas of sexual alteration or dysfunction. The nurse must understand how sexual orientation, culture, and religious beliefs influence sexuality. Second, nurses can assess their own comfort level and limitations in discussing sexuality and sexual functioning (see Chapter 16). Finally, they can learn to recognize sexual problems that are outside the realm of their expertise and to refer the client for help.

FACTORS AFFECTING SEXUALITY

Sexual desire is an appetite that waxes and wanes. Furthermore, appetites vary among individuals: some people want and enjoy sex every day, whereas others want sex only once a month, and still others have no sexual desire and are quite comfortable with that fact. Sexual desire becomes an issue if the client simply wants to feel sexier more often, if the client believes it is necessary to measure up to some perceived cultural norm, or if a discrepancy in the sexual desires of the partners in a relationship appears to be causing conflict. Clients may bring up such sexual problems by saying that they "just don't feel turned on sexually" as they used to, or that their partners seem demanding about sexual issues in the relationship. The client should be assured that almost any change in one's environment or sense of self may lead to sexual changes, ranging from mild, transient emotional discomfort to a sexual dysfunction that requires professional counseling or therapy.

PHYSICAL FACTORS. A client may experience a decrease in sexual desire for physical reasons. Sexual activity may bring on pain or discomfort. Even imagining that sex could hurt can lessen one's sexual desire. Minor illness or simply feeling tired is a reason why a person may not feel sexual. Medications can affect sexual desire. Even the prescribing physician may not be able to predict the effects of a given medication on the client's sexual feelings and behavior. Poor body image, particularly when magnified by feelings of rejection or by body-altering surgery, can turn off clients sexually.

RELATIONSHIP FACTORS. Issues in a relationship can distract a person from wanting sex. Just as there is an ebb and flow of sexual appetite in an individual, so sexual desire ebbs and flows in a relationship. Couples often find after the initial glow of the relationship has faded that they are faced with major differences in their values or life-styles. The degree to which they still feel close to each other and interact on an intimate level will depend on their ability to negotiate and compromise. Thus, communication skills play a crucial role when dealing with sexual desire in a relationship. Decreased interest in sexual activity can result just from the anxiety of having to tell a partner what sexual behavior is acceptable or pleasurable.

LIFE-STYLE FACTORS. Life-style factors, such as the use or abuse of alcohol and the lack of time to devote to a relationship, can influence sexual desire. Traditionally associated with sexual behavior, particularly in advertisements, alcohol can induce a false sense of well-being or seductiveness in the initial stages of sex. However, ample evidence now shows that alcohol's negative effects on sexuality far outweigh the euphoria it may initially produce. Finding the time for sexual activity is another life-style factor. Some clients do not know how to structure their working and home time to include

sexual behavior. Working parents, for example, may feel so overburdened that they perceive sexual advances from a partner as one more demand on them. Such clients often describe their need to be alone to think and rest as more important than sex.

SELF-ESTEEM FACTORS. The client's level of self-esteem can also lead to personal and emotional conflicts involving sexuality. The degree of a client's sexual desire may depend on the client's sense of personal value and learned sexual skills. If sexual self-esteem has not been nurtured by encouraging the development of a strong sense of a sexual self and the learning of sexual skills, sexuality may bring forth negative feelings or lead to the suppression of sexual feelings. Sexual self-esteem can be lowered in many ways. Rape, incest, and physical or emotional abuse leave deep scars. Lowered sexual self-esteem can also result from lack of adequate sex education, negative role models, or attempts to live up to unrealistic personal or cultural expectations.

SEXUAL HEALTH HISTORY

Every nursing history, whether taken in a clinic or hospital, should include a few sex-related questions to determine initially if the client has any sexual concerns. These questions should be incorporated in the review of systems and addressed in a routine manner. As with any aspect of assessment, the nurse must understand why the question is being asked, understand what will be done with the information gained, and be able to provide this rationale to the client on request. Gaining information for the sake of curiosity is never appropriate. An opening statement such as "Sex is an important part of life and can be affected by our health status or vice versa. To better understand your health, it is useful to know . . ." is a good example to use. Other questions for adults are the following:

1. How do you feel about the sexual part of your life?
2. Have you noticed any changes in the way you feel about yourself as a man, woman, husband, wife, and so on?
3. How has your illness, medication, or impending surgery affected your sex life?
4. It is not unusual for people with your condition to be experiencing some sexual problems. Has that been a concern to you at all?

Questions that may be addressed to a child's parents include the following:

1. Have you noticed your child exploring his body, for example, touching his penis?
2. Has your child begun to ask questions about where babies come from?
3. Have you talked with your child about sex, pregnancy, or contraception?

Adolescents may best respond to a question such as:

1. Many adolescents have questions about STDs or whether their body is developing at the right rate. Do you have any questions about sex or other things?

It may be appropriate to explore physical, relationship, life-style or self-esteem factors in more depth depending on other aspects of the assessment.

Some clients may be too embarrassed or not know how to ask the nurse sexual questions directly. Thus they may be very subtle in asking for information. The nurse must be aware of cues from the client that indicate a question or problem in the area of sexuality. Such cues might include the following (Siemens and Brandzel, 1982):

1. Talking about going home from the hospital and being afraid of what their partner will think or expect of them
2. Asking direct easy questions and then seeming hesitant about the next question
3. Joking of a sexual nature
4. Asking questions that suggest concerns about achieving orgasms such as "When my episiotomy was repaired, could the doctor have sewn it up too tight?"
5. Making self-conscious comments such as, "Well, I'm just not as young as I used to be."
6. Using euphemisms such as, "I just want to be a good partner."
7. Looking down when asked a question about sexuality, blushing, and changing the topic
8. Asking questions about normal behavior such as, "Is it normal for a man not to ejaculate when he gets older?"

Observing and listening to client's concerns about sexuality takes practice. It is up to the nurse to clarify and paraphrase or ask questions that will help clients be more direct about sexual concerns. If sexual concerns are identified, the nurse may wish to pursue a sexual health history in more detail. By including sexuality in the discussion, the nurse indicates that sexuality is an important component of health care and acknowledges the need for the client to discuss these concerns.

In pursuing sexual history, several interview strategies such as the following can help to enhance the client's and nurse's comfort (see Chapter 19):

1. Allow adequate time to conduct an uninterrupted interview.
2. Assure confidentiality and privacy.
3. Use a warm, empathetic approach.
4. Assume that all clients are uncomfortable talking about their sexuality.
5. Listen carefully, and notice nonverbal cues of the client.
6. Adapt the interview to the client's life-style and

attempt to overcome cultural and language barriers.

7. Have a rationale for each question and be willing to share this with the client.
8. Assume that all clients are sexually experienced unless they tell you otherwise.
9. Avoid pressuring clients to respond to questions about their sexuality.
10. Move through questions from least sensitive to more sensitive.
11. Use open-ended questions that encourage more than a yes-or-no response. It is sometimes useful to ask how or when questions rather than "do you" questions.
12. Focus attention on the client, not on documenting responses.

A helpful guide for a brief sex history would include answers to the following questions (Annon, 1975):

1. What does the client see as the sexual concerns?
2. When did these sexual concerns begin and how have they changed over time?
3. What does the client see as the cause of the concerns?
4. What sorts of treatment has the client sought to help alleviate this concern?
5. How would the client like this concern to be resolved, and what are the client's goals for treatment?

A detailed assessment of long-standing sexual problems or concerns such as erectile dysfunction or vaginismus is outside the realm of general nursing practice. These clients should be referred to health providers specializing in areas of sex therapy. Often, however, the nurse may identify a sex concern related to medication, lack of knowledge, or fear that the client's fantasies or desires are abnormal. Interventions aimed at these concerns are appropriate to nursing practice in any setting.

PHYSICAL ASSESSMENT

The physical examination is important in evaluating the cause of sexual concerns or problems or may be the best opportunity to teach the client about sexuality. The techniques of inspection and palpation are used in this examination (see Chapter 13). The nurse will have the opportunity to assess the client's reaction, answer questions, and provide information about the examination or anatomy and physiology.

EXAMINATION OF WOMEN. Examination of a woman begins with inspection of the genitalia. The inspection includes the secondary sex characteristics: breast development, hair distribution, and the development of the external genitalia. The breasts are inspected to determine size, symmetry, contour, and appearance of the skin. Although often one breast is smaller than the other, the breasts usually are relatively symmetrical. Variations in breast contour may include the presence of masses, dimpling, or flattening. The color of the skin of the breasts, presence of thickened areas, and abnormalities of the venous pattern may be indicative of pathological processes. The nipples may be inverted, but this is usually not pathological. However, the direction in which the nipples are pointing may provide a clue to masses when there is asymmetry. Discharge from the nipples may indicate disease or may merely occur with the hormonal fluctuation of the menstrual cycle. Ulcerated areas and other nipple lesions require further exploration.

During the physical examination, women can also be encouraged to examine their breasts each month. The conclusion of the menstrual period or a few days thereafter is the best time for this, since premenstrual engorgement of the breasts may cause them to be lumpy or tender. Because of the cyclical changes in the consistency of breast tissue, it is recommended that the self-examination be performed at a consistent point in the menstrual cycle. Breast self-examination is described in Chapter 13.

Examination of the genitalia of women and men is performed with a gloved hand. The external genitalia, including the labia majora and minora, mons, vulva, clitoris, urethral opening, and vaginal introitus, are examined before doing the internal pelvic examination. Inflammatory processes, ulcerations, congenital or surgical absence of structures, lesions, nodules, and discharge are noted. The labia minora, clitoris, and urethral opening can be inspected by separating the labia majora. While the labia are separated with the middle and index finger, the woman can be requested to strain down. Any bulging of the vaginal walls or gaping of the introitus is noted. The former may be indicative of cystocele and rectocele, and the latter of injury to the pubococcygeus muscle surrounding the vaginal outlet. Presence of surgical scarring, such as an episiotomy site, may also be noted at this time. This part of the examination affords the practitioner the opportunity to teach the woman Kegel's exercises if she does not already know how to do them (see box). These exercises strengthen the pubococcygeus muscle. Toning of this muscle decreases due to stretching with childbirth and due to loss of general elasticity and muscle tone in aging. Maintaining good tone decreases the chances of a bladder or rectal prolapse into the postpartum vagina (cystocele or rectocele), minimizes problems with later urinary incontinence, and can lead to increased sexual enjoyment through and beyond menopause.

A pelvic examination is customarily performed as part of a total health assessment for women. It consists of two primary components: the speculum examination of the cervix and vagina and the manual palpation of the

---

Kegel's Exercises for the Pubococcygeus Muscle

To identify the pubococcygeus muscle, sit on the toilet seat with your knees as far apart as possible. Start and stop the flow of urine. This should not be done as an ongoing exercise. Begin exercising this muscle gradually, at intervals throughout the day. The following exercises can be done each day:

1. Contracting the pubococcygeus muscle and holding for 3 seconds (this feels the same as it did when you stopped the flow of urine)
2. Contracting the pubococcygeus muscle rapidly
3. Breathing deeply and tightening the pubococcygeus muscle as you inhale
4. Bearing down, then relaxing, and as you relax, tightening the pubococcygeus muscle

Ten to 25 contractions each day is usually sufficient to maintain good muscle tone.

---

uterus and ovaries (see Chapter 13). The pelvic examination can be an educational experience for the woman, as well as an experience that validates her sexuality. The practitioner should avoid making an assumption about whether the woman is sexually active or with whom, as well as any assumption about her desire for fertility control. The examination should begin with the woman in a sitting position rather than in the lithotomy position (which usually causes poor eye contact and a feeling of inferiority). The woman should be offered a drape. Since some women prefer to see what is happening, the woman should be asked whether she would like a mirror. This often enables the woman to see her cervix or even her genitals for the first time. Many examiners use a lighted speculum to facilitate the woman's viewing of her own anatomy.

By explaining the steps of the examination, the examiner can validate the woman's sexuality and health. For example, the examiner might say "I'm going to look at your labia and clitoris now. . . They look very healthy." When preparing to insert the speculum, the examiner can inform the woman of any noise the speculum might make (plastic speculums are especially noisy) and also advise her of what will be done, for example, "Now I'm going to put two fingers in your vagina. I'm going to put the speculum into your vagina, and I'll open it up so you can see your cervix. Your vagina looks very healthy. Can you see your cervix?" Insertion of the speculum is facilitated by using warm tap water as a lubricant. Some practitioners advocate inserting the speculum blades at a slight oblique angle, whereas others prefer to insert the blades horizontally. The primary concern is avoiding painful pressure on the urethra. When removing the speculum, the practitioner closes the blades after the cervix is cleared to avoid pinching the cervix between the speculum blades.

The woman can participate in the bimanual examination. For example, she may wish to palpate her ovaries. This orientation to the pelvic examination affords many opportunities for teaching that sexuality is a wholesome, positive phenomenon.

EXAMINATION OF MEN. Inspection of the penis, scrotum, testicles, and breasts of the male is usually part of the general physical examination. As these structures are examined, the practitioner notes the hair distribution pattern over the axillary and pelvic areas.

The breasts are inspected for deviations in contour, symmetry, abnormalities in the skin, and irregularities of the nipple. Although breast cancers in men are rare, abnormal discharges or lesions should be noted and further addressed. The examiner looks for gynecomastia, an enlargement of breast tissue that often occurs during normal puberty and at other times during the life cycle.

Inspection of the penis includes observations of the skin for ulcers or lesions. The shaft is observed for deviations in shape and size or symmetry. The foreskin may be present in uncircumcised males, and the client may be asked to retract it to facilitate inspection of the glans area for lesions. Abnormalities of the glans and urethral meatus may also be noted, including deviations in the location of the urethra, ulcerations of the glans, and discharge from the urethral meatus.

The scrotal skin is inspected next for the presence of nodules or inflammation and to check contour. Usually the left testicle is somewhat lower in the scrotal sac than the right. Absence or atrophy of the testicles may also be identified by inspection. During the examination, males should be taught and encouraged to perform testicular self-examination for lumps that may indicate testicular cancer. The penis, scrotal sac and contents, prostate gland, and rectum may be palpated.

Explanations similar to those provided to women can be used when examining men. Some men may elect to use a mirror to see their genitals.

NURSING DIAGNOSIS

Altered sexuality patterns and sexual dysfunction are recognized as approved nursing diagnoses (McLane, 1987) (see nursing diagnoses box). The difference in diagnosing sexual dysfunction or altered patterns of sexuality depends on whether the client perceives problems

---

Examples of Nursing Diagnoses for Altered Sexuality

NANDA-APPROVED NURSING DIAGNOSES

Sexual dysfunction related to:
- Spinal cord injury
- Chronic illness
- Pain

Altered sexuality patterns related to:
- Death of spouse
- Illness of spouse
- Depression
- Decreased self-esteem

Impaired adjustment related to:
- New role as parent
- Diagnosis of life-threatening illness
- Change in body image

Rape-trauma syndrome related to:
- Forceful sexual activity with stranger
- Date rape

Knowledge deficit related to:
- Unfamiliarity with birth control
- Sexual inexperience

Body-image disturbance related to:
- Surgical mutilation
- Sexual dysfunction
- STD

---

in achieving sexual satisfaction or expresses concern regarding sexuality. In making diagnoses of sexual problems, the nurse must assess anatomical, physiological, sociocultural, ethical, and situational issues that may be related factors (see sample nursing diagnoses box).

Nursing diagnoses include altered sexuality patterns or sexual dysfunction—related to postpartum, hormonal, and life-style changes; anxiety (of cardiac affect during sexual intercourse) postmyocardial infarction; lack of knowledge of physiological changes associated with aging; or values conflict between partners.

Other nursing diagnoses may be integrally related to sexuality. Changes in body image from surgery such as mastectomy, ostomy, or amputation may alter one's self-concept and therefore inhibit sexuality.

Altered body image relates to surgical mutilation. In this example, discussions of sexual issues and potential concerns is an appropriate area for assessment, intervention, and evaluation.

Sample Nursing Diagnoses for Sexual Dysfunction or Altered Sexual Patterns

Defining Characteristics	Nursing Diagnosis	Related Factors
Change in desire or sexual activity Decreased sexual satisfaction Painful intercourse Expressions of concern over normalcy of physical sexual development Lack of sexual partner	Sexual dysfunction or altered sexuality patterns	• Medications (prescribed) • Medication (abuse) • Alcohol use • Decreased self-esteem • Neurological injury • Chronic illness • Infidelity • Decreased love for partner • Death of partner • Depression • Obesity • Delayed development of secondary sexual characteristics

Sample Nursing Care Plan for Enhancing Sexuality/Sexual Functioning in a 50-Year-Old Male with Diabetes

Nursing Diagnosis	Goal	Expected Outcomes	Nursing Interventions
Sexual dysfunction related to diabetic complications	Client and wife will attain satisfaction in their sexual expression.	Client describes reasons for diminished sexual response. Client and wife establish discussion of sexual behaviors that each find satisfying. Client and wife define mutually satisfying methods of stimulation through experimentation. Client and wife verbalize satisfaction with their sexual activity expression within reality of diabetic complications.	Encourage client to define methods and satisfaction with sexual activity before complications. Provide client and wife information on neurological and vascular changes of diabetes and the effect on sexual response. Describe to client and wife changes in sexual response that occur with aging. Discuss with client and wife various methods of sexual expression (for example, hugging, french kissing, massage, oral genital sex, mutual masturbation). Facilitate discussion between client and wife of acceptable and satisfying sex practices. Encourage playful approach to sexual experimentation with open discussion of preferences. Provide for individual and couple follow-up discussion of sexual satisfaction. Refer to urologist to discuss penile prothesis.

Sample Nursing Care Plan for Enhancing Sexuality/Sexuality in a 30-Year-Old Female after Treatment for Cervical Cancer

Nursing Diagnosis	Goals	Expected Outcomes	Nursing Interventions
Altered sexuality patterns related to physical and emotional effects of cervical cancer	Client will acknowledge physical changes and integrate them into a positive self-image. Client and husband will continue positive expressions of sexuality.	Client will describe methods to prevent vaginal atrophy after radiation and hysterectomy/oophorectomy. Client will initiate grief process for loss of childbearing. Client and husband will discuss fears of prognosis and begin to resume intimate expressions of affection.	Instruct client on use of vaginal dilators, finger manipulation, or sexual intercourse twice per week to maintain vaginal tone. Encourage client and husband to verbalize previous plans for children and encourage expressions of anger and grief for loss of these potential children. Facilitate client's expression of femininty through use of makeup, hair care, and nightgowns. Ascertain client and husband understand prognosis and proposed treatment. Provide 1 hour of uninterrupted privacy for client and husband each evening.

Lack of knowledge about sexual development may be an appropriate diagnosis for a parent expressing concerns about a preschooler's genital manipulation and that parent's inability to respond to questions of anatomy or the reasons for these behaviors.

Lack of knowledge related to safe sexual practices may apply to an adolescent who confirms sexual activity. Interventions should relate to knowledge and attitudinal issues about risks of pregnancy, STD, and emotional involvement.

Based on the definition of sexuality, anything affecting one's physical or psychological or emotional health or one's sociocultural, or ethical attitudes and beliefs may have an impact on sexual functioning. These are areas for assessment, potential diagnosis of alterations or dysfunction, and intervention.

PLANNING

The goals for the client experiencing actual or potential alterations in sexual functioning include:

1. Obtaining knowledge of sexual development and functioning of women and men
2. Attaining or maintaining biologically and emotionally healthy sexual practices
3. Establishing or maintaining sexual satisfaction for self and partner if appropriate
4. Attaining, maintaining, or enhancing positive self-esteem with integration of cultural/religious/ethical beliefs, sexual practices, past and present, and situational realities

In planning interventions appropriate to the client's needs, the nurse must determine the appropriate diagnosis, related factors, and mutually agreed on goals for meeting these needs. To plan interventions concurring with the client's self-concept, the client, and with permission, the sex partner should be involved in the planning process. Sample care plans are provided in the care plan boxes. Expression and recognition of the values and preferences of both partners are critical to achieving successful interventions. Goals will not be achieved if recommended interventions are incongruous with the client's sexuality, that is, gender identity, sex roles, partner preferences, and so on. Because expressions of sexuality are often interpersonal activities, the partner's participation and value system must also be considered.

IMPLEMENTATION

Nursing interventions that address client alterations in sexual patterns or sexual dysfunction are generally in the category of awareness raising, assisting a client to clarify issues or concerns, and information giving. Nurses who have pursued specialized education in sexual functioning and counseling may provide more intensive sex therapy. As in any area of practice, nurses should recognize when a client's needs exceed their levels of expertise and provide appropriate referral. Most clients encountered in clinics or hospital settings may benefit from the discussion and teaching provided by the nurse generalist.

The initial intervention often includes exploring present sexual practices with the client. The client should be encouraged to investigate and acknowledge social and ethical values and analyze how sexuality fits into self-concept. When there is significant discrepancy between values and past or present practices, the client may need referral for more intensive counseling.

Providing the opportunity to explore and discuss values and levels of satisfaction, and to provide sex education requires good communication skills. The environment and timing should be structured to provide privacy, uninterrupted time, and client comfort. For example, when discussing methods of contraception with a woman, provide comfortable chairs in an office setting rather than holding this discussion in the examination room with the client only partially clothed.

Areas of education will vary depending on the defining characteristics and related factors that prompted the diagnosis. Education may provide guidelines for normal development as when talking to a toddler's mother regarding a new baby coming, a school-aged child regarding appearance of pubic hair, or a 60-year-old male regarding more delayed ejaculation. Details of physiological changes should be provided as a part of general health care. This also gives permission for clients to raise questions or concerns regarding personal functioning.

As major developmental crises, for example, puberty or climacteric/menopause, should prompt education about effects on sexuality, so should situational crises. A life change such as pregnancy, illness, extreme financial stress, placement of a spouse in a nursing home, or loss and grief will affect sexuality. The effect may last for days, months, years or even generate performance anxieties that lead to continued sexual dysfunction. If a client is prepared for possible changes in sexual functioning, performance anxieties may be minimized. A

professional relationship may also be established in which the client feels comfortable raising concerns about sexuality as they occur.

Illness and surgery are situational stressors that nurses will confront frequently. Clients may experience major physical changes, effects of drugs or treatments, and the emotional stress of prognosis, future functioning, and separation/hospitalization. Sexuality, as a component of personality, may be affected by all components of illness. It should never be assumed that sexual functioning is not a concern merely because of an individual's age or severity of prognosis. Once concerns are assessed and identified, they can be addressed in the context of the individual's value system.

In response to identified concerns, the nurse may initiate discussion of methods of sexual stimulation, the sexual response cycle or the use of creativity and fantasy in sexual relations. It may be appropriate to discuss sexual practices such as oral-genital sex or mutual masturbation as methods of expressing intimate affection when penile-vaginal intercourse is contraindicated. A partner experiencing joint pain may appreciate a discussion of various positions for intercourse. Use of fantasy or a sense of playfulness may add new romance or stimulation to a long-term relationship. A couple may need confirmation or assurance that the thoughts and acting out of nonharmful fantasy is normal and healthy.

Discussions of healthy sex should always include contraception when talking with women and men of childbearing age. Men should not be excluded from discussions of contraception. The discussion may include future desires for children, usual sexual practices, and acceptable methods of contraception. Factors that need to be considered when educating clients about contraceptives include scheduling or frequency of sex, comfort with genital touching, and comfort with interruption of sexual acts. All methods of contraception should be reviewed to provide necessary information for an informed client choice. The best method is the one the client will use consistently.

All individuals having more than one sex partner or whose partner has other sexual experiences should learn more about safe-sex practices. As discussed earlier, information should be provided on STD transmission and symptoms, use of condoms, and risky sexual activities, for example the trauma of penile-anal sex. Safe sex may also consider what the client can emotionally risk in a relationship. Role play may be a useful educational tool for the client to learn to say no or to request a partner to use a condom.

When sexual dysfunctions are identified as ongoing premature ejaculation, vaginismus, or concerns over transsexual dressing, the nurse should provide appropriate referrals. Clients may still require support to follow through with a referral and reinforcement of explanations of procedures, treatments or exercises. The nurse must be comfortable with her sexuality and aware of her values and biases to be effective with any intervention. Referral may also be necessary when a client's values or needs are in significant conflict with those of the nurse.

EVALUATION

Individuals have a right to understand how their bodies function and to predict changes occurring as one develops. Clients should understand development of the body, the manner of male and female sexual response,

and changes that normally occur with aging and life stresses.

Resolution of sexual concerns must meet the client's perceptions of improvement. Sexuality is not an absolute. An individual must define what is acceptable and satisfying. The client's partner's level of sexual satisfaction must also be considered. To effectively resolve concerns, the client must also perceive positive self-esteem. To again state the World Health Organization's definition of sexual health, it is "the integration of the somatic, emotional, intellectual, and social aspects of sexual being, in ways that are positively enriching and that enhance personality, communication and love" (1975). A sample evaluation of interventions is provided in the evaluation box.

Sample Evaluation of Interventions for Enhancing Sexuality-Sexual Functioning

Goals	Evaluative Measures	Expected Outcomes
Client obtains knowledge of sexual development and functioning of women and men.	Have client (or parent) describe normal ranges of sexual development.	Young children—parents verbalize understanding of normal childhood sexual behavior (for example, self-genital manipulation, sex play with peers, questions regarding male and female anatomy, sex and childbirth).
	Ask client (or parent) to state where they (or child) are in process of sexual development.	Adolescents—client states age ranges and basic physiology of development of secondary sexual characteristics and menarche or nocturnal emissions. Adult—client describes male and female sexual response patterns. Older adult—client describes physiological changes with aging and effect on sexual response for self and partner.
Client attains or maintains biologically and emotionally healthy sexual practices.	Ask client to describe physiology of conception and probable fertile period of menstrual cycle.	Client correctly describes act of intercourse and fertilization of sperm and ova in fallopian tubes with implantation in uterus. Client correctly identifies probable fertile period by date from last menstrual period and other symptoms.
	Request client to demonstrate use of condom or contraceptive method.	Client demonstrates application of condom on model and verbalizes correct timing of application and need to hold base of condom when removing penis from vagina. Client demonstrates proper insertion and removal of diaphragm and describes timing of insertion, removal, and reapplication of spermicide.

Continued.

Sample Evaluation of Interventions for Enhancing Sexuality-Sexual Functioning—cont'd

Goals	Evaluative Measures	Expected Outcomes
	Have client produce charts of basal body temperature.	Client restricts intercourse to "safe" days. Pregnancy is prevented until client verbalizes readiness for childbearing.
	Ask client to describe symptoms of STD and risky sex practices.	Client identifies symptoms that require health care evaluation (for example, dysuria, vaginal itching, penile discharge, sore on genitals).
	Have client use role play communication skills to describe sensitive sexual issues.	Client is able to demonstrate communication with partner (for example, request partner to use condom, say no to sex). Client reports successful communication with partner and verbalizes positive self-worth from interaction.
Client establishes or maintains sexual satisfaction for self and partner.	Have client verbalize satisfaction with level of sexual activity and responsibility. Ask client to report level of sexual satisfaction. Have client use role play communication of sexual issues.	Client describes actual or proposed sexual activities to produce satisfaction. Client verbalizes activities that provide sexual stimulation for self and partner. Client is able to role play discussion with partner methods to enhance sexual excitement. Client reports successful interaction with partner regarding sexually stimulating activities.
Client attains, maintains, or enhances positive self-esteem with integration of cultural, religious, and ethical beliefs, sexual practices, past and present, and situational realities.	Determine if client expresses positive perceptions of self and sex life. Determine if client is able to acknowledge cultural, religious, and ethical beliefs regarding sexuality. Ask client to report level of sexual satisfaction within limits of physical conditions, interpersonal relationships, and life stresses.	Client describes self in positive terms. Client describes biases/beliefs. Client accepts sexual practices, biases, and beliefs of others. Client describes alternate methods of sexual stimulation consistent with physical limitations. Client and partner report resumption of intimate expressions of affection as stresses resolve. Client and partner report satisfaction with present level of sexual activity.

SUMMARY

Sexuality is an integral component of personhood and therefore may impact on or be affected by health status. The nurse, as a provider of intimate care and education, will confront issues of client sexuality. The individual's cultural, religious, and ethical beliefs significantly influence sexual values and practices. This is true for the health care provider, as well as the client. These beliefs must be recognized, acknowledged, and should never compromise meeting of a client's health needs.

Sex will always remain a controversial issue because of ethical value systems. Facts of conception, development, contraception, and sexual disease transmission may be taught but cannot be totally divorced from intermingled ethical issues. Issues such as appropriate age for first intercourse, homosexuality, and oral-genital sex will continue to polarize opinions and complicate care and education. With sensitivity and insight, nurses can assist their clients in assuming responsibility for decisions about sexuality, thus enhancing their total health.

KEY CONCEPTS

- ✓ Sexuality is related to all dimensions of a person's health; therefore sexual concerns or problems should be addressed as a part of nursing care.

- ✓ Sexuality is a component of personality and includes biological sex, gender identity, gender role, and sexual partner preference.

- ✓ Gender identity and gender role vary widely among individuals and result from the interaction of many biological and environmental factors.

- ✓ Sexual orientation, a person's erotic attraction to others, exists on a continuum between heterosexuality and homosexuality.

- ✓ Attitudes toward sexuality vary widely and are influenced by religious beliefs, society's values, the media, the family, and other factors.

- ✓ Nurses' attitudes toward sexuality also vary and may differ from the client's attitudes, and a nurse should be nonjudgmental about a client's sexual preferences and needs.

- ✓ Sexual stimulation varies among individuals but generally involves erotic fantasy and touching and the other senses.

- ✓ The range of sexual behavior includes manual stimulation, oral-genital stimulation, anal stimulation, and coitus.

- ✓ The four-phase sexual response cycle is a way of understanding the physiological changes of sexual response during excitement, the plateau phase, orgasm, and resolution.

- ✓ Sexual development is a process beginning in infancy and involves some kind of sexual behavior or growth in all developmental stages.

- ✓ The physiological sexual response changes with aging for both men and women, but aging need not lead to diminished sexuality.

- ✓ Sexual health involves physical and psychosocial aspects and contributes to an individual's sense of self-worth and positive interpersonal relationships.

- ✓ Clients' problems involving sexuality include personal and emotional conflicts, the effects of illness on sexuality, and sexual dysfunction.

- ✓ Personal and emotional conflicts leading to sexual problems may originate in differences in sexual desires, physical factors, relationship problems, life-style factors, or low self-esteem.

- ✓ Specific sexual dysfunctions for both men and women result from psychological and physiological factors.

✓ Interventions for sexual dysfunctions depend on the condition and the client; interventions often include giving information, use of specific exercises, improving communication between partners, and specific techniques of the sexuality counselor.

✓ Sexuality is affected by physiological changes or chronic illness, hospitalization, fertility, and sexually transmitted diseases, and the nurse helps the client adapt to the situation and maintain healthy sexuality.

✓ Concerns regarding AIDS should promote the use of condoms, but sexual transmission can only be prevented by abstinence.

✓ Individuals in any state of health or illness continue to be sexual beings and may desire and be positively affected by sexual stimulation or expressions of sexuality.

✓ Choice and use of effective contraception methods are affected by sexual biases, comfort with touching genitalia, desire for future fertility, financial status, ability to be future oriented and plan sexual contact, and the ability to communicate with one's sex partner regarding sensitive issues.

✓ A brief review of sexuality should be included in every nursing assessment of a client's level of wellness.

✓ The nurse is accountable to obtain only information that will be acted on through nursing interventions and referral.

✓ Most nursing interventions to enhance a client's sexual health will involve providing information and education.

✓ In-depth sexual counseling requires professional expertise and may be provided by qualified nurse specialists.

✓ Evaluation of intervention is primarily determined through client and partner expressions of satisfaction in meeting personal goals for sexual functioning that can be validated by nursing observations of nonverbal communication.

REFERENCES

Annon, J: The behavioral treatment of sexual problems, vol. 1, Brief therapy, Honolulu, 1975, Enabling Systems, Inc.

Crooks, R, and Baur, K: Our sexuality, Menlo Park, Calif., 1983, The Benjamin-Cummings Publishing Co., Inc.

Dickman, G, and Livingston, C: Sex and the female ostomate, Los Angeles, 1982, United Ostomy Association, Inc.

Erikson, E: Childhood and society, New York, 1963, W.W. Norton & Co., Inc.

Flick, LH: Paths to adolescent parenthood: implications for prevention, Public Health Rep 101(2):132, 1986.

Fogel, C, and Woods, NF: Health care of women, St. Louis, 1981, The C.V. Mosby Co.

Goldstein, B: Human sexuality, New York, 1976, McGraw-Hill Book Co.

Haeberle, E: The sex atlas, New York, 1978, The Seabury Press.

Hogan, R: Human sexuality: a nursing perspective, New York, 1980, Appleton-Century-Crofts.

Hogan, R: Influences of culture on sexuality, Nurs Clin North Am 17(3):365, 1982.

Kolodny, R, Masters, W, and Johnson, V: Textbook for sexual medicine, Boston, 1979, Little, Brown & Co.

Lion, EM: Human sexuality in nursing process, New York, 1982, John Wiley & Sons, Inc.

Livingston, C, McIntyre, M, and Fogel, C: Sexual dysfunction: etiology and treatment. In Woods, NF, editor: Human sexuality in health and illness, ed. 3, St. Louis, 1984, The C.V. Mosby Co.

Masters, W, and Johnson, V: Human sexual response, Boston, 1966, Little, Brown & Co.

Masters, W, and Johnson, V: Human sexual inadequacy, Boston, 1970, Little, Brown & Co.

Masters, W, Johnson, V, and Kolodny, R: Human sexuality, Boston, 1982, Little, Brown & Co.

McLane, AM, editor: Classification of nursing diagnoses: proceedings of the seventh conference (NANDA), St. Louis, 1987, The C.V. Mosby Co.

Sex Information and Education Council of the United States: the SIECUS/New York University/Uppsala principles basic to education for sexuality, SIECUS Report 8:8, 1980.

Siemens, S, and Brandzel, R: Sexuality: nursing assessment and intervention, Philadelphia, 1982, J.B. Lippincott Co.

Unsain, L, Goodwin, M, and Schuster, E: Diabetes and sexual functioning, Nurs Clin North Am 17(3):387, 1982.

Weinberg, JS: Human sexuality and spinal cord injury, Nurs Clin North Am 17(3):407, 1982.

Woods, NF: Human sexuality in health and illness, ed. 3, St. Louis, 1984, The C.V. Mosby Co.

World Health Organization: education and treatment in human sexuality: the training of health professionals, WHO Tech Rep Ser, 572, Geneva, 1975, WHO.

Research Articles

Shuman, NA, and Bohachick, P: Nurse's attitudes toward sexual counseling, DCCN 6(2):75, 1987.

Zelnik, M, and Kantner, JF: Reasons for nonuse of contraception by sexually active women aged 15-19, Fam Plan Perspec 11(3):289, 1979.

ADDITIONAL READINGS

Boyle, CA, Berkowitz, GS, and Kelsey, JL: Epidemiology of premenstrual symptoms, Am J Public Health 77(3):349, 1987.

Brosnan, CA: Long term results of an elementary sexuality program, Ped Nurs 13(2):130, 1987.

Brown, MA, and Zimmer, PA: Personal and family impact of premenstrual symptoms, J Obstet Gynecol Neonatal Nurse 15(1):31, 1986.

Calderone, M, and Johnson, E: The family book about sexuality, New York, 1981, Harper & Row Publishers, Inc.

Fischman, SH, et al.: Changes in sexual relationships in postpartum couples, J Obstet Gynecol Neonatal Nurs 15(1):58, 1986.

Hatcher, RA, et al.: Contraceptive technology 1986-1987, 13th ed., New York, 1986, Irvington Publishers, Inc.

Jain, H, Shamoian, CA, and Mobarak, A: Sexual disorders in the elderly, Med Aspects of Human Sexuality-special issue 21(3):14, 1987.

Kisker, EE: Teenagers talk about sex, pregnancy and contraception, Fam Plan Perspect 17(2):83, 1985.

Krajicek, MJ: Developmental disability and human sexuality, Nurs Clin North Am 17(3):377, 1982.

Madaras, L, with Madaras, A: The what's happening to my body book for girls, New York, 1983, Newmarket Press.

Madaras, L, with Saavedra, D: The what's happening to my body book for boys, New York, 1984, Newmarket Press.

Mims, F, and Swenson, M: Sexuality: a nursing perspective, New York, 1980, McGraw-Hill Book Co.

Muscari, ME: Obtaining the adolescent sexual history, Ped Nurs 13(5):307, 1987.

Planned Parenthood: How to talk with your child about sexuality, Garden City, New York, 1986, Doubleday & Co, Inc.

Reeder, SJ, and Martin, LL: Maternity nursing: family, newborn and women's health, ed. 16, Philadelphia, 1987, J.B. Lippincott Co.

Rondon, N: KID-ABILITY: taking action against sexual abuse, Child Today 15(4):22, 1986.

Schuster, EA, Unsain, IC, and Goodwin, MH: Nursing practice in human sexuality, Nurs Clin North Am 17(3):345, 1982.

Shipes, E: Sexual functioning following ostomy surgery, Nurse Clin North Am 22(2):303, 1987.

Shipes, E, and Lehr, S: Sexuality and the male cancer patient, Canc Nurse 5(5):375, 1982.

Woods, NF, Most, A, and Dery, GK: Prevalence of premenstrual symptoms, Am J Pub Health 72(11):1257, 1982.

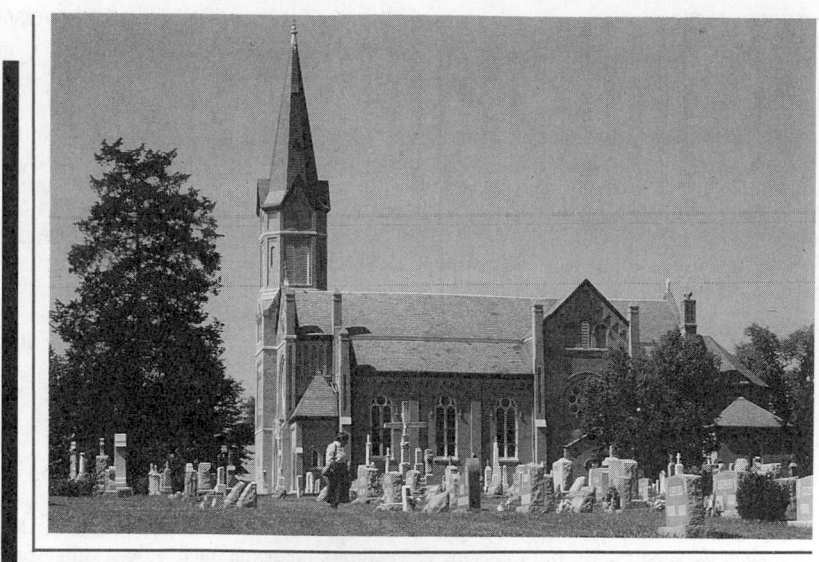

OBJECTIVES

Mastery of content in this chapter will enable the student to:

- Define the key terms listed.
- Discuss the relationship of spiritual health to physiological and psychosocial health.
- Contrast spiritual and religious aspects of health.
- Assess components of spiritual health.
- Describe a spiritually healthy person.
- Describe the signs of unmet spiritual needs.
- List interventions in the nursing plan for spiritual care.
- Evaluate attainment of spiritual health.
- Identify resources that can help clients attain spiritual health.

KEY TERMS

Religious
Spiritual Distress
Spiritual Health
Spirituality

Spiritual Health

Human nature has a spiritual component just as it has physiological, psychological and sociocultural components. Living fully requires spiritual health, as well as mental and physical well-being. As with other dimensions of health, the perception of spiritual health is highly individualized, and spiritual health changes as other dimensions of health fluctuate. The ultimate state of health would seem to be a delicate balance of all dimensions—physical, developmental, psychological, sociocultural, and spiritual.

The spiritual dimensions of nursing care may take on particular significance for the client with a physical health problem. Physically unhealthy clients may not be able to manage their spiritual needs. The nurse giving holistic care seeks to determine all needs, including those within the spiritual realm. Just as psychological or sociocultural needs may sometimes take precedence, spiritual needs are sometimes of the most concern to the client and nurse.

This chapter focuses on the Christian approach to spirituality but discusses the tenets of other major religions in regard to general health beliefs, birth, diet, health crises, and death.

Although in the past there was a dearth of material on the spiritual dimension of nursing care, nurses' need for information about applying standards of care in the spiritual realm has prompted authors and educators to address this topic in more depth. The NANDA classification of nursing diagnoses has included spiritual diagnoses under the classification "spiritual distress" (Kim and Moritz, 1986). Several researchers have compiled descriptions of the practices of different religions to help nurses understand and provide for religious practices.

DEFINITION OF SPIRITUAL HEALTH

Spiritual health can be considered an awareness of and openness to a system of beliefs, Supreme Being, or God or a presence with or in each person and in the world. The response to the Supreme Being or God is faith or a belief system.

Faith is defined by Studzinski (1986) as more than a set of beliefs. He calls it "a way of relating to self, others, and God and integrating our past, present, and future with God as center." Hanley (1985) describes the six stages of faith based on 400 interviews with believing persons of several traditions. The author indicates that some adults remain in early stages of spiritual development with such weaknesses as legalism, provincialism, and narcissism. Thus all clients must be treated with gentleness and respect. The nurse must respond personally and flexibly to each client's state of faith.

Peck (1981) uses examples from the Bible to illustrate faith healing. For example, piles of crutches at Lourdes demonstrate the therapeutic effect of faith. She describes the elaborate ceremonies of Taiwanese shamans and the belief in psychic energy of Egyptian pyramid power. She also reviews the destructive power of black magic, voodoo, the curse, and the hex.

Meeks (1977) discusses belief systems and suggests the following questions for the individual's consideration in achieving high-level wellness:

1. What do I believe?
2. What gives meaning to my life?
3. How is my belief system working for me?
4. Is my behavior compatible with my belief system?
5. How does my belief system relate to my future?
6. Is there a relationship between my belief system and my health behavior?

In many belief systems, disease is viewed as part of a divine plan to test faith in a Supreme Being or God or to make him an example of patience or restitution. Thus meaning can be found in suffering. The goal of nursing, within this framework, is to help healthy or ill clients to use their faith. Exploring the symbolic beliefs and spiritual support of clients, providing the spiritual resources they request, and suggesting alternatives or sharing beliefs without imposing values are ways nurses can help meet clients' spiritual needs.

RELATIONSHIP OF SPIRITUAL TO OTHER DIMENSIONS OF HEALTH

The interrelatedness of the physiological, psychological, sociocultural, and spiritual dimensions is demonstrated by the great number of clients with psychosomatic diseases. The insistence of health care providers on a body-mind-spirit conceptual model of human nature results in their concern with the moral, ethical, and spiritual dimensions of personality and character development. The nurse's goal in holistic health care is to help the client achieve a balanced, dynamic integration of body, mind, and spirit. Holistic health care includes meeting the client's physiological needs, promoting psychological development, fostering sociocultural relationships, and supporting the fulfillment of spiritual aspirations.

Nurses should realize the interdependence of the physiological, the psychosocial, and the spiritual aspects of development. Just as unexpressed anger and resentment can cause diseases referred to as psychosomatic, forms of spiritual distress such as guilt, irascibility, and lack of forgiveness of self or others, and vindictiveness can lead to illness.

SPIRITUAL AND RELIGIOUS ASPECTS OF HEALTH

In this chapter the word *spiritual* means a belief in a system of beliefs, a Supreme Being or God, and the presence of that being in the world. Religion is an affiliation with a denomination or sect. The word *religious* is the specific practices, rites, and rituals of a religion.

Religion can make sense of sickness, according to Sevensky (1981). Using the Book of Job, this author illustrates how suffering can be seen as educational, in some sense a purification, for others, sacrificial, and finally, as a mystery. Although recognizing the potential misuse of religion in fostering guilt and negative attitudes toward sexuality and emotions, Sevensky reviews the resources available to a religious person. Some of these resources include prayer, support from a caring, religious community, and religious rituals such as forgiveness, communion, anointing with oil, and laying on of hands.

The nurse should be aware of the client's general spiritual needs and should assist the client in meeting those needs. Information about religions and sects is available from a number of sources. Hindu, Buddhist, Moslem, Jewish, and Christian beliefs and practices regarding birth, dietary restrictions, procedures in health crises, and death are described in the following sections and in Tables 31-1, 31-2, and 31-3. Nurses should keep in mind that the spiritual dimension of health care is not limited to the practices and dogma of organized religion. The client's individual needs must be identified and addressed.

Beliefs about Health

Hindus believe that praying for health is the lowest form of prayer; thus they tend to dismiss or be uncon-

TABLE 31-1   Religious Beliefs about Health

Religion	Health Care Beliefs	Response to Health Crises
Hinduism	Accepts modern medical science.	Views illness as result of misuse of body. Considers therapy as transitory benefit.
Buddhism	Accepts modern medical science.	May ask for Buddhist priest for couseling. Family available for physical and emotional care.
Islam	Older, more conservative have fatalistic view and may resist compliance with medical science.	Uses faith healing and group prayer. Submits to will of God.
Judaism	Sanctity of life is overriding belief. Sabbath regulations may interfere with therapeutic procedures.	Obligated to seek medical care. Supported by family and friends.
Christianity	Seeks will of God in suffering but accepts modern medical science.	Uses prayer, faith healing, laying on of hands, sacraments.

cerned about bodily ills. The devotees of Buddhism have rich multireligious influences from Confucianism, Christianity, and Shintoism. Some branches and sects of Buddhism emphasize differing practices; for example, the Theravada branch uses an intellectual approach, the Mahayana branch emphasizes involvement with humanity, and the Zen sect practices austerity. Followers of Hinduism and Buddhism usually accept modern medical science.

In Islam, the believer is considered to be a unique individual with an eternal soul. Moslems (Muslims) pray five times daily, facing Mecca. Older or more conservative Moslems may have a fatalistic view and may resist compliance with medical treatment.

Jews believe in the sanctity of life. This basic principle overrides any conflicting beliefs and promotes acceptance of modern medical science. Observance of Sabbath regulations may interfere with scheduled therapeutic procedures.

Christians generally regard themselves as children of God, redeemed by Christ and destined for eternal life. They seek to discern the will of God in life and suffering, but their beliefs generally do not conflict with modern medical practice (Table 31-1).

Health Crises

Hindus may view illness as the result of misuse of the body or as a consequence of sins committed in a previous life. However, they generally do not oppose medical treatment but consider its benefits transitory. Buddhist clients or their families may ask to have a Buddhist priest for counseling during illness. A family member usually remains with the sick person to care for physical and emotional needs.

Moslems use faith healing to provide psychological support rather than to treat the pathological condition. Family members are a great comfort to a Moslem, and

Moslems consider group prayer strengthening, but there is no priest. The person submits to God's will in health and in illness.

In Judaism, the belief in the sanctity of life obligates the sick to seek medical care. Various laws apply to the donation or transplantation of organs. Visiting the sick is considered a religious obligation for Jews.

Christians may want to receive communion from their minister or priest during illness; Roman Catholics may wish to receive several sacraments: reconciliation, the Eucharist, and anointing of the sick. Jehovah's Witnesses are generally opposed to blood transfusions. Some religious sects believe in faith healing and some in laying on of hands (Table 31-1).

Birth

No special birth ritual is required by Hinduism. Buddhist rites such as infant presentation, affirmation, confirmation, or ordination are performed in late childhood. According to Islamic doctrine, if abortion occurs after 130 days gestation, the fetus is treated as a fully developed human being. Ritual circumcision is required by Orthodox and Conservative Jews on the eighth day after birth. Reform Jews favor ritual circumcision but do not consider it a religious imperative. Among Jews a fetus is buried, not discarded.

Various forms of baptism are practiced by Christians. Both Episcopalians and Roman Catholics require infant baptism; the former do not baptize aborted fetuses and stillborn infants but the latter do. Baptists, Seventh-Day Adventists, Baha'i followers, and Mennonites are some of the religious groups that do not practice infant baptism. The form of baptism differs from sect to sect. For example, sprinkling is sufficient for the Orthodox Presbyterians and Methodists, whereas the Pentacostals, Mormons, Baptists, and Church of Christ members require immersion (Table 31-2).

TABLE 31-2   Religious Practices Related to Life Events

Religion	Birth	Death
Hinduism	No special ritual.	Priest ties thread around neck or wrist, pours water into mouth. Only the family touches and washes body before its cremation.
Buddhism	Infant presentation, affirmation, confirmation, ordination.	Presence of Buddhist priest. Last rite chanting.
Islam	In case of abortion after 130 days gestation, fetus is treated as fully developed human being.	Before death, confession of sins and asking forgiveness of family. Only the family touches and washes body.
Judaism	Ritual circumcision. Fetal burial.	Oppose autopsy and cremation. Ritual cleansing of body by members of ritual burial society.
Christianity	Infant baptism required by Episcopalians and Roman Catholics. Baptism of aborted fetus and stillborn infants by Roman Catholics.	Last rites optional for Episcopalians and Lutherans, mandatory for Eastern Orthodox Christians and Roman Catholics.

Death

To Hindus, death and rebirth are nearly synonymous. After death, certain rites are prescribed. The priest may tie a thread around the neck or wrist to indicate a blessing; he may pour water into the mouth. The family washes the body, which is then cremated. The family of a Buddhist may wish to have a priest called in at the time of death; last rite chanting is often practiced at the bedside.

Before death the Islamic client confesses sins and asks for forgiveness of the family. After death the family washes the body, then turns toward Mecca. As with Hindus, only relatives and friends touch the body. No autopsy is performed unless required by law.

All Orthodox Jews and some Conservative Jews also oppose autopsy and cremation. Human remains sometimes must be cleansed by members of a ritual burial society, and burial is always carried out as soon as possible. Since customs vary, the nurse should always consult the deceased's family to determine their preference.

Among Christians, no rituals are required before or after death by Christian Scientists, Church of Christ members, and Jehovah's Witnesses. Last rites are optional for Episcopalians and Lutherans but mandatory for Eastern Orthodox Christians and Roman Catholics. Additional restrictions may apply to cremation, autopsy, and burial of amputated parts or burial in consecrated ground (Table 31-2).

Diet

Hindus have many dietary restrictions. Some sects are vegetarian, believing meat and intoxicants to be too stimulating to the senses. Some Buddhists also are vegetarians. Most members of the Buddhist religion practice moderation and do not use alcohol, tobacco, and drugs.

Eating pork is prohibited by Islam, and Ramadan, the ninth month of the Muhammedan or Muslim year (around June and July), is a period of daylight fasting. Many Orthodox, Conservative, and some Reform Jews strictly observe kosher dietary laws, which prohibit eating pork and shellfish and eating any meat with milk or

TABLE 31-3   Religious Dietary Regulations Affecting Health Care

Religion	Dietary Practices
Hinduism	Some sects are vegetarians, prohibiting meat and intoxicants.
Buddhism	Some are vegetarians; most do not use alcohol, tobacco, or drugs.
Islam	Eating pork is prohibited. Ramadan is period of daylight fasting.
Judaism	Some observe kosher dietary laws (prohibit eating pork and shellfish, eating meat with milk or milk products; regulate food preparation).
Christianity	Some groups (Seventh-Day Adventists, Baptists, and Mormons) prohibit use of alcohol, coffee, tea, and tobacco. Roman Catholics fast and abstain from meat on Ash Wednesday and Good Friday. They fast for 1 hour before Communion.

milk products. Jews also have regulations about food preparation.

Many Christian traditions have no dietary proscriptions. Some groups, such as Seventh-Day Adventists, Baptists, and Mormons, prohibit the use of alcohol, coffee, and tea; certain groups include tobacco with these prohibitions. Roman Catholics fast and abstain from meat on Ash Wednesday and Good Friday; some older Catholics continue to adhere to Friday abstinence. Armenian Catholics fast during Lent, and several branches of Christianity fast 1 to 6 hours before communion (Table 31-3).

■ ■ ■

The spiritual dimension of being is more than adherence to religious dogma or practices. Spirituality includes the belief in the influence of their beliefs, a Supreme Being, or a God as a direction and will in life. The nurse must address the client's spiritual needs in providing holistic health care.

SPIRITUAL HEALTH AND THE NURSING PROCESS

ASSESSMENT

Fish and Shelly (1978) define spiritual health as meaning and purpose in life and love and relatedness with other human beings. Brallier (1978) enumerates the progressive or cumulative characteristics of holistic health: realization of human potential, affirmation of the uniqueness and unlimited potential of each person, and achievement of a balanced dynamic integration of body, mind, and spirit.

Stoll (1979) suggests that when making a spiritual assessment, the nurse include specific questions in the nursing history about the client's concept of a Supreme Being, the client's source of strength and hope, the significance of religious practices and rituals to the client, and the client's perceived relationships between spiritual beliefs and health. According to Lafferty (1979), positive spiritual health choices for clients seeking to improve their quality of life include meditation and prayer, value-oriented spiritual or religious discussion, reading a spiritual book or attending a religious or spiritual meeting, and developing a highly valued personal characteristic or eliminating a weak personal trait. These needs should be a part of the spiritual assessment.

Spiritual needs may be intensified in certain life situations, such as birth, death, a major health crisis, anxiety, apprehension, fear, newly diagnosed serious or chronic disease, isolation, and psychiatric episodes. Spiritual assessment should be an extension of the psychosocial assessment and should be pursued to the extent that the nurse intends to use the information for planning client and family care.

Determining who or what sustains the client will help in planning for spiritual health. The answers to the following questions about spiritual health will influence nursing care:

1. Who is the client's God? a Supreme Being? a governing principle? money? power? another human being?
2. What is the client's relationship with a Supreme Being or God? one of fear or of love?
3. How does the client express this spiritual relationship? Are spiritual/religious practices part of this expression?
4. How does the client view himself? positively or negatively? worthy of God's love?
5. Does the client act authentically and relate openly?
6. Does the client assume responsibility for behavior and its consequences?
7. How effectively does the client relate to family and friends?
8. How effectively does the client relate to health care personnel? to other clients? to strangers?
9. Does the client see illness as a Supreme Being or God's punishment? or as an indication of love?
10. Does the client view illness as threatening?
11. How have the client's diagnosis and therapy affected self-concept? emotional state? will to live? cooperation with rehabilitation?

Spiritually healthy persons generally believe in a Supreme Being and view their ultimate welfare and peace in terms of their relationship to this being and the world at large. They are generally aware of their limitations as human beings but strive to act in accordance with their beliefs. They assume life's responsibilities with joy and cheerfulness.

As the nurse observes and analyzes the behaviors that demonstrate the client's level of spiritual health, it becomes obvious that the client's attitudes toward a Supreme Being, God, self, and others demonstrate the value the client places on spiritual health. Reactions to adversity, setbacks, delays in plans, aging, sickness, and suffering give clues to the client's spiritual values. As the nurse assesses the client's state of spiritual health, signs of unmet spiritual needs may emerge.

If the client is inconsistent with professed beliefs and actions, a nursing diagnosis of spiritual distress may be indicated. The client may express anger at the Supreme Being, God, a member of the pastoral care team, or the nurse. The client may question the meaning of life and suffering. Verbalizations about internal conflicts of be-

---

✁ *Research Highlight* ✍

Miller studied characteristics of loneliness and spiritual well-being in 64 chronically ill adults with rheumatoid arthritis and 64 randomly selected healthy adults to determine if a relationship existed between the variables. He also attempted to determine if a significant difference in loneliness and spiritual well-being existed between the ill and the healthy group. Two instruments were used for data collection: the Abbreviated Loneliness Scale (ABLS) and the Spiritual Well-Being Scale (SWB) with the subscales of Existential Well-Being (EWB) and Religious Well-Being (RWB). A negative relationship was found between loneliness and spiritual well-being in both the ill and the healthy groups with no significant difference in loneliness between the two groups.

Ill subjects had significantly higher SWB ($p < .01$) and RWB ($p < .001$) scores than healthy subjects. No differences in EWB were found. A canonical analysis of data from the ill subjects demonstrated that those with low ABLS scores were younger and had very low RWB and high EWB scores. High RWB scores were found in older female subjects.

Miller, JF: Assessment of loneliness and spiritual well-being in chronically ill and healthy adults, J Prof Nurs 1 (1):79, 1985.

---

liefs and required treatment may indicate a spiritual need. For example, if a client believes disease is a punishment for sinfulness, cooperation with therapy will aggravate guilt and prevent the restitution necessary through suffering. If clients believe that eternal life follows temporal life, they may repudiate any attempt at treatment and rehabilitation.

Observation of the client's affect and attitude, behaviors, verbalizations, interpersonal relationships, and environment might give clues to spiritual needs. Miller's study of loneliness and spiritual well-being (1985) showed a negative relationship between the two variables in both ill and healthy people (see research highlight).

Therefore, spiritual assessment continues throughout all interactions with the client. Do the client's words and actions reflect the respect and reverence as professed toward humanity? Are the client's spiritual values reflected in interaction with visitors? Do the client's get-well cards reflect appreciation of prayer and contain inspirational verse? Is the client openly questioning the reason for existence or suffering? Does the client seek spiritual assistance or admit an inability to continue usual religious practices? Request for prayers may in-

dicate a spiritual value or need. The client may ask the nurse about the moral implications of certain procedures in relation to beliefs about human life.

The conceptual model of human nature in physiological, psychosocial, and spiritual dimensions offers an additional approach to assessing spiritual needs. Questions such as the following can be derived from this model: To what extent have the client's physical disability and the therapeutic regimen altered ability to maintain relationships with the Supreme Being and others? Are there moral or ethical implications of the diagnosis and treatment that conflict with the client's religious or spiritual values? Do the etiology, diagnosis, and treatment of the disease conflict with the client's belief system?

NURSING DIAGNOSIS AND PLANNING

NANDA has defined spiritual distress and suggested etiologies and defining characteristics (see box). The client's answers to questions in the nursing history and the nurse's observations of the client's behaviors and interrelationships give clues to spiritual needs. However, clues must be validated and clarified before the nurse plans interventions. In the realm of spiritual care, the importance of the nurse's own spiritual aspirations, inspiration, and perception cannot be overemphasized. The nurse must remain aware of the responsibility to provide for clients' spiritual needs. To be attuned to spiritual aspects of care, a nurse should be aware of a personal spiritual dimension and be comfortable in discussing spiritual matters. In addition, the nurse's perception of clues to the client's spiritual needs requires sensitivity, active listening, and responding to what is heard. Less than one third of patients' spiritual problems were recognized by a majority of oncology nurses, according to Highfield and Cason (1983) (see research highlight, p. 799).

The nurse seeks validation from the client about a diagnosis of "spiritual distress." If the client concurs with the diagnosis, the nurse and the client together plan steps to meet this spiritual need. If the nurse has doubts about the client's ability to recognize spiritual needs, consultation with the family may provide clarification. If both the client and the family deny the existence of a spiritual need, the nurse should accept their decision. The nurse may need to find out if the client's minister, priest, or other spiritual adviser or a member of the pastoral care team has already recognized and ministered to the client's spiritual needs. Ideally the health

Spiritual Distress (Distress of the Human Spirit)

DEFINITION

Distress of the human spirit is a disruption in the life principle pervading a person's entire being and integrating and transcending one's biologic and psychosocial nature.

ETIOLOGIES

- Separation from religious and cultural ties
- Challenged belief and value system, e.g., result of moral or ethical implications of therapy or result of intense suffering

DEFINING CHARACTERISTICS

- Expresses concern with meaning of life and death and/or belief systems
- Shows anger toward God (as defined by the person)
- Questions meaning of suffering
- Verbalizes inner conflict about beliefs
- Verbalizes concern about relationship with deity
- Questions meaning for own existence
- Chooses not to participate or is unable to choose in usual religious practices
- Seeks spiritual assistance
- Questions moral and ethical implications of therapeutic regimen
- Displaces anger toward religious representatives
- Describes nightmares or sleep disturbances
- Alters behavior or mood evidenced by anger, crying, withdrawal, preoccupation, anxiety, hostility, apathy, etc.
- Regards illness as punishment
- Does not experience that God is forgiving
- Is unable to accept self
- Engages in self-blame
- Denies responsibilities for problems
- Describes somatic complaints

From Kim, MJ, et al.: Pocket-guide of nursing diagnosis, ed. 2, St. Louis, 1987, The C.V. Mosby Co.

⚕ Research Highlight ⚕

Highfield and Cason examined nurses' awareness of their clients' spiritual needs and problems, their ability to recognize signs of spiritual health and identify signs of spiritual problems. The authors devised a 49-item questionnaire based on Clinebell's "religious-existential" framework, identifying and defining four spiritual needs: (1) for meaning and purpose in life, (2) to give love, (3) to receive love, (4) for hope and creativity.

Thirty-five oncology nurses in a 1200-bed private hospital responded; 80% were registered nurses and 20% licensed vocational nurses. Their average age was 32 years and average length of practice was 10 years. The only items clearly identified with the spiritual dimension were those with direct reference to God or to a religous belief. Fifty-six percent of items indicating spiritual health were identified with the psychosocial dimension by more than half the sample. Twenty-four of the 31 behaviors and conditions were identified as psychosocial problems rather than spiritual. Less than one third (29%) of the client's spiritual problems were recognized as such by 74% of the sample.

Highfield, MF, and Cason, C: Spiritual needs of patients: are they recognized? Canc Nurs 6(3):187, 1983.

care team works together to identify and meet all the needs of a client, including spiritual needs (see sample nursing diagnosis box).

Dickenson (1975) suggests that ministry and spiritual care are inherent in nursing. She identifies the following factors in the nurse-client relationship that demonstrate the nurse's commitment to the client's spiritual health: support, self- and other-awareness, understanding, openness, and nonjudgmental acceptance. Several circumstances, however, may cause the nurse to be uncomfortable in providing spiritual care. One impediment may be the past role of spirituality or organized religion in the nurse's life.

An authoritarian upbringing may cause the nurse to rebel against the religious practices of childhood. The nurse may believe that religion or the spiritual dimension is a private matter for the client, although only 10% of critical-care nurses surveyed in Yancey's study (1987) indicated that spiritual concerns were too personal to discuss (see research highlight, p. 801). Some nurses may consider spiritual care as done only if and when time permits. The majority of the respondents in Yancey's study, however, disagreed that health care professionals are too busy to give spiritual care, contradicting the findings of Piles' research (1986). In Piles' study, 87.1% said lack of time was an obstacle to performing spiritual care (see research highlight, p. 801).

Some nurses feel unprepared to address the spiritual aspect of care with clients or have the misconception that spiritual needs should be left to the pastoral care department. Spirituality is interrelated with other dimensions of being human, and nurses should consider

Sample Nursing Diagnoses for Spiritual Distress		
Defining Characteristics	**Nursing Diagnoses**	**Related Factors**
Questioning meaning and purpose in life Ambivalent about belief system Expressing feelings of apathy, uselessness, withdrawal	Spiritual distress	• Lack of meaning and purpose in life • Permanent disability • Retirement age
Verbalizing belief in uncaring deity Demonstrating unresponsiveness to loved ones Suspicious of care of nurse	Spiritual distress	• Religious oppression • Rejection by family or significant others • Past negative experiences in the health care system • Lack of love and relatedness
Verbalizing belief in unforgiving deity Viewing illness as punishment or vindication Confessing past faults	Spiritual distress	• Unhealthy religious fear • Unresolved guilt • Difficulty in forgiving others or accepting forgiveness of others • Lack of forgiveness

spiritual health when planning care (see care plan box, p. 802). A concern for spirituality need not be confined to the pastoral care department, just as care directed toward psychosocial health is not a specialized matter for psychiatrists only. In the spiritual dimension, as in other dimensions, the nurse is assisting the client toward a state of well-being and a sense of fulfillment.

IMPLEMENTATION

When the nurse identifies the client's spiritual needs and arrives at a diagnosis of spiritual distress, plans should be made to meet this need. Resources included in the plan are nursing interventions, family involvement, and counseling by the clergy. Other possible sources for spiritual care are members of the pastoral care department and nurses' support groups.

NURSING INTERVENTIONS

After having determined what beliefs sustain the client's spirituality, the nurse's responsibility is to support and enhance this belief system or find someone able to do so. The nurse should not impose religious or spiritual beliefs on clients or their families nor should a nurse ever attempt to convert a patient. The nurse's sincerity, patience, and awareness of the client's spiritual distress will encourage the client to discuss spiritual values. The

nurse's own spirituality is a form of support in assisting the client to clarify beliefs about the Supreme Being, the spiritual dimension of life, and the meaning of suffering and pain. Soeken and Carson (1986) demonstrated that those baccalaureate and graduate nursing students who scored higher on a Spiritual Well-Being Scale expressed more positive attitudes toward providing spiritual care (see research highlight, p. 801).

How the client views self is another area for intervention. If the nurse consistently treats the client as a unique individual with significant value and unlimited potential, the client's self-concept will be enhanced. The nurse should consider the client's wishes when scheduling activities and should provide the client with privacy and personal time.

Individuals at any point on the health-illness continuum have a need to be alone. The nurse may help a hospitalized client gain from solitude through self-examination and redirection, a new perspective of a relationship with a belief system, a Supreme Being, or God, and a more positive self-concept.

If clients ask the nurse to pray for them or with them, it is appropriate to do so. If nurses are not comfortable in this situation, they should be honest with the client and offer to locate other sources of support. Prayer can be offered aloud or in silence according to the client's wishes. Prayer has various purposes in different religions: praise, petition, thanksgiving, and reparation for sin. The client may want to praise God and offer thanks for blessings or to request health or freedom from pain.

ϟ *Research Highlight* ϟ

Yancey assessed nurses' attitudes and practices on spiritual care. The sample population of 230 registered nurses, members of the American Association of Critical Care Nurses, responded to a previously validated, 2-part, mailed questionnaire, the Health Professional's Spiritual Role Scale (HPSR). The first part of the HPSR measured attitudes toward spiritual care and the second portion assessed frequency of performed spiritual practices.

A statistically significant relationship was found between attitudes and practices. Those nurses who had higher scores on the attitude scale demonstrated more frequent performance of spiritual care practices. Among the variables, years of experience, level of educational preparation, and exposure to nursing theory, only the last showed a statistically significant correlation with attitude and practice. Note the following findings: (1) 90% affirmed that spiritual care is a responsibility of the health care professional, (2) 87% agreed that health care professionals are uncomfortable discussing spiritual matters with patients, (3) only 10% indicated that spiritual concerns are too personal to discuss, (4) 25% strongly disagreed and 46% disagreed to a lesser extent that health care professionals are too busy to give spiritual care, and (5) 90% rejected the statement that spiritual well-being is not as important as physical well-being.

Yancey, V: Spiritual care: attitudes and practices of intensive care unit nurses, unpublished master's thesis, St. Louis, 1987, St. Louis University.

ϟ *Research Highlight* ϟ

Piles discovered the practicing professional registered nurse's role in providing spiritual care based on educational preparation for that role. With the use of a questionnaire, 300 randomly selected nurses were chosen, 75 from each of the four National League for Nursing regions of the continental United States.

Of the 300 respondents, 96.5% agreed that holistic care included spiritual care, 86.6% disagreed that only clergy and lay ministers can provide spiritual care, 65.9% felt inadequately prepared to perform such skills, and 89.2% recommended that spiritual care content be included in every basic nursing program. Respondents said lack of time (87.1%) and lack of knowledge (70.6%) were the only obstacles that hindered the performance of spiritual care skills.

Piles, C: Spiritual care: role of nursing education and practice: a needs survey for curriculum development, unpublished doctoral dissertation, St. Louis, 1986, St. Louis University.

ϟ *Research Highlight* ϟ

Soeken and Carson examined the relationship between the spiritual well-being of nurses and nursing students and their attitudes toward providing spiritual care for patients. A convenience sample of 29 senior-year baccalaureate nursing students and 24 graduate nursing students completed two research instruments, the Spiritual Well-Being Scale (SWB) and the Health Professional's Spiritual Role (HPSR). The majority of the respondents (77.3%) considered themselves to be members of religious groups. No differences were found between graduate and undergraduate students in this respect. Scores on both tools tended to be in the upper range, indicating positive religious and existential well-being, and an overall positive attitude toward providing spiritual care. Students with a higher level of spiritual well-being expressed more positive attitudes toward providing spiritual care. No correlation was found between age and spiritual well-being, attitudes toward roles, or appropriateness of behavior, nor did numbers of years of nursing experience among graduate students relate to other measures.

Soeken, KL and Carson VJ: Study measures nurses' attitudes about providing spiritual care, Health Progr 67(3):52, 1986.

The client should be allowed time to express a particular need.

INVOLVEMENT OF FAMILY AND FRIENDS

Relationships with others help sustain a person's belief system. The nurse should urge family and friends to visit the client and demonstrate their love and concern. In some cases, working with or through family or friends to provide the client's spiritual care is the most effective way to meet this need. Members of parish or church groups may visit, or they can be encouraged to send cards and assurance of prayers for recovery.

Including family members in a prayer service is a thoughtful gesture if this is appropriate to the client's religion and family members are comfortable participating. Reading favorite religious passages or prayerbooks may be requested and appreciated by the client and family. Encouraging clients to keep significant symbols nearby can be a source of consolation and spiritual

Sample Nursing Care Plan for Spiritual Distress

Nursing Diagnosis	Goal	Expected Outcomes	Nursing Interventions
Spiritual distress related to lack of forgiveness	Client is able to be forgiven.	Client will demonstrate self-acceptance. Client will indicate reconciliation with Supreme Being.	Suggest positive qualities of client. Illustrate ways behavior reflects values. Refer client to specific scriptures or sacred readings.

support. Because a visit to the hospital chapel or attendance at services can be important to the hospitalized client and family, a trip to the chapel or directions for finding the prayer room should be included when orienting the client and family to the medical facility. Arrangements may need to be made with personnel of the pastoral care department for the patient and family to receive the sacraments, especially communion (see care plan box).

ROLE OF THE CLERGY

Some hospitalized clients find a visit from their clergyman or spiritual adviser consoling. If the clergy has known the client and family prior to the current health problem, the support offered can provide continuity. The clergy or spiritual adviser understands the religious belief system of the client and can focus on the potential spiritual growth resulting from illness and suffering. The minister or pastor may pray with the client and family and perform religious rituals or administer sacraments.

The nurse should ask clients if they would like to have their minister, priest, or spiritual adviser notified of their hospitalization. All clergy should be made welcome in nursing units. Keeping them informed of physiological and psychosocial, as well as spiritual, concerns, when requested by the client or family, helps in providing holistic health care. The nurse shows respect for the client's spiritual values and needs by willingly cooperating and by making easier the administration of sacraments, rites, and rituals of the client's religion.

Providing privacy for the client and clergy or spiritual adviser is a thoughtful and sensitive gesture. If the nurse is unsure about the proper routine in a client's religion, asking the minister, the family, or the client is appropriate. The nurse can adapt spiritual care to the client's religious tenets without sacrificing personal beliefs.

OTHER RESOURCES

Other resources can assist in easing clients' spiritual health. Especially helpful are members of a hospital's pastoral care department, who can visit the client, ad-

minister sacraments or rites, and provide religious objects when requested. Taped meditations and televised religious services may also be available through the pastoral care department.

Pastoral care associates may serve also as counselors and consultants for nursing personnel. Discussion groups can help nurses recognize their own spiritual needs so they can respect the client's right to do the same. Such groups can also focus on the responsible and appropriate application of the nursing process to spiritual needs.

EVALUATION

Attainment of spiritual health can be considered a lifelong goal. However, to evaluate the effectiveness of nursing interventions in this dimension of health care, the nurse may compare the client's level of spiritual health with the behaviors and needs noted in the original assessment (see evaluation box). The following questions may be helpful:

1. Is the client's belief system stronger?
2. Do the client's professed beliefs support and direct actions and words?
3. Does the client gain peace and strength from spiritual resources (such as prayer and minister's visits) to face the rigors of treatment, rehabilitation, or impending death?
4. Does the client seem more in control and have a clearer self-concept?
5. Is the client at ease in being alone? in having life's plans changed?
6. Is the client's behavior appropriate to the occasion?
7. Has reconciliation of any differences taken place between the client and others?
8. Are mutual respect and love obvious in the client's relationships with others?

It is helpful to consider how the client looks and feels when spiritual needs are met. The client should be ex-

Sample Evaluation of Interventions for Spiritual Distress

Goals	Evaluative Measures	Expected Outcomes
Client discovers meaning and purpose in life.	Be alert for expression of belief that life has meaning. Question goals and plans for future.	Client states belief that pattern of life is directed by Supreme Being.
Relationships are significant and supportive.	Note manner of relating to significant others, nurses. Determine congruency of words and actions in relation to others.	Relatives and friends are loving and supportive. Client responds to affection in positive manner.
Forgiveness is given and received.	Listen for verbal evidence of self-acceptance and acceptance and understanding of others. Observe for peacefulness after reconciliation.	Spiritual distress from lack of self-acceptance and acceptance of others is reduced.

periencing emotions appropriate to the situation, developing a strong, realistic self-image and warm, open interpersonal relationships, and maintaining a sense of mission in life and confidence and trust in a Supreme Being. A client whose spiritual needs are met will be peaceful regardless of illness and suffering.

If the client is comfortable in expressing spiritual needs to the nurse or in sharing beliefs and religious resources, the nurse can assume that the psychological climate is encouraging verbalization of these needs. Does the nursing care plan schedule time for quiet, for prayer, for a visit to the chapel, and for attendance at services? Is provision for spiritual health considered as important as plans for medical and nursing care of a physiological or psychological illness?

Thus a nurse's evaluation of the attainment of spiritual health should include observation of the client's life situations and the nursing environment.

SUMMARY

Nursing care that neglects the client's belief system cannot be called holistic. To provide spiritual care, the nurse must understand what spiritual health is and be able to recognize the spiritually healthy person. As with other dimensions of care, the norm is identified first for comparison during assessment. If spiritual needs are identified in the assessment, plans are made to intervene appropriately. In implementing the plan for spiritual care, nursing interventions are individualized according to the client's specific needs. The family's involvement and the ministrations of spiritual advisers are sought when indicated. Resources for facilitating client's spiritual care and for providing support for nurses are used as necessary. The rewards of meeting clients' spiritual needs include personal and professional fulfillment and enrichment.

KEY CONCEPTS

✓ Spiritual health is when a person feels secure in a relationship with a Supreme Being or a system of beliefs, a presence with or in each person and in the world.

✓ To provide spiritual care in nursing, the nurse must understand spiritual health and be able to recognize the spiritually distressed person.

✓ Nurses should be aware of the client's general spiritual needs and facilitate the client's chosen practices.

✓ The spiritual dimension of care is not limited to the practices and dogma of organized religions.

✓ When making a spiritual assessment, the nurse includes questions about the client's concept of a Supreme Being, source of strength and hope, significance of religious practices and rituals, and perceived relationships between spiritual beliefs and health.

✓ The client's contradictory actions or attitudes may indicate spiritual distress.

✓ To be attuned to spiritual aspects of care, nurses should be aware of their own spiritual dimension and be comfortable in discussing spiritual matters.

✓ The nurse should use available resources such as family members, clergy, and other members of the health care team to help the client maintain or regain a state of spiritual health.

REFERENCES

Brallier, LW: The nurse as holistic health practitioner, Nurs Clin North Am 13(4):643, 1978.

Dickenson, SC: The search for spiritual meaning, Am J Nurs 75(10):1789, 1975.

Fish, S, and Shelly, JA: Spiritual care: the nurse's role, Downers Grove, Ill., 1978, InterVarsity Press.

Hanley, K: Fostering development in faith, Human Devel 6(2):21, 1985.

Lafferty, JA: Credo for wellness, Health Educ 10(5):10, 1979.

Meeks, LB: The role of spiritual health in achieving high level wellness, Health Values 1(5):222, 1977.

Peck, ML: The therapeutic effect of faith, Nurs Forum 22(2):153, 1981.

Sevensky, RL: Religion and illness: an outline of their relationship, South Med J 74(6):745, 1981.

Stoll, R: Guidelines for spiritual assessment, Am J Nurs 79(9):1574, 1979.

Studzinski, R: Adult faith is reward for long life, Envoy 15(2):4, 1986.

Research Articles

Highfield, MF, and Cason, C: Spiritual needs of patients: are they recognized? Canc Nurs 6(3):187, 1983.

Miller, JF: Assessment of loneliness and spiritual well-being in chronically ill and healthy adults, J Prof Nurs 1(1):79, 1985.

Piles, C: Spiritual care: role of nursing education and practice, A needs survey for curriculum development, unpublished doctoral dissertation, St. Louis, 1986, St. Louis University.

Soeken, KL, and Carson, VJ: Study measures nurses' attitudes about providing spiritual care, Health Progr 67(3):52, 1986.

Yancey, V: Spiritual care: attitudes and practices of intensive care unit nurses, unpublished master's thesis, St. Louis, 1987, St. Louis University.

ADDITIONAL READINGS

Buys, SAM: Discussion series sensitizes nurses to patient's spiritual needs, Hosp Progr 62(10):44, 1981.

Ellis, C: Course prepares nurses to meet patients' spiritual needs, Health Progr 67(3):76, 1986.

Hoyman, HS: Models of human nature and their impact on health education, Nurs Digest 3(5):37, 1975.

Kasanof, D, Levy, J, and Striffler, RC: When religious belief affects therapy, Patient Care 8(19):99, 1974.

Kim, MJ, and Moritz, DA, editors: Classification of nursing diagnoses, proceedings of the third and fourth conferences (NANDA), New York, 1986, McGraw-Hill Book Co.

Kim, MJ, et al.: Pocket-guide of nursing diagnoses, ed. 2, St. Louis, 1987, The C.V. Mosby Co.

Kraft, WF: Spiritual growth in adolescence and adulthood, Human Devel 4(4):14, 1983.

Miller, JF: Inspiring hope, Am J Nurs 85(1):22, 1985.

Newman, M: Theory development in nursing, Philadelphia, 1979, F.A. Davis Co.

Peterson, EA: The physical . . . the spiritual . . . can you meet all of your patient's needs? J Gerontol Nurs 11(10):23, 1985.

Pumphrey, JB: Recognizing your patient's spiritual needs, Nurs 77 7(12):64, 1977.

Ruffing-Rahal, MA: The spiritual dimension of well-being implications for the elderly, Home Healthc Nurse 2(2):12, 1984.

Shelly, JA: Spiritual care workbook: a companion to spiritual care; the nurse's role, Downers Grove, Ill., 1978, InterVarsity Press.

Stallwood, J, and Stoll, R: Spiritual dimensions of nursing practice. In Beland, I, and Passos, J, editors: Clinical nursing: pathophysiological and psychosocial approaches, ed. 3, New York, 1975, Macmillan Publishing Co.

Wheelock, RD: Unmet patient needs, Hosp Progr 55(7):60, 1974.

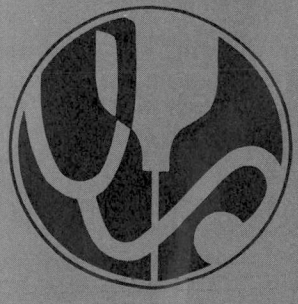

UNIT 7

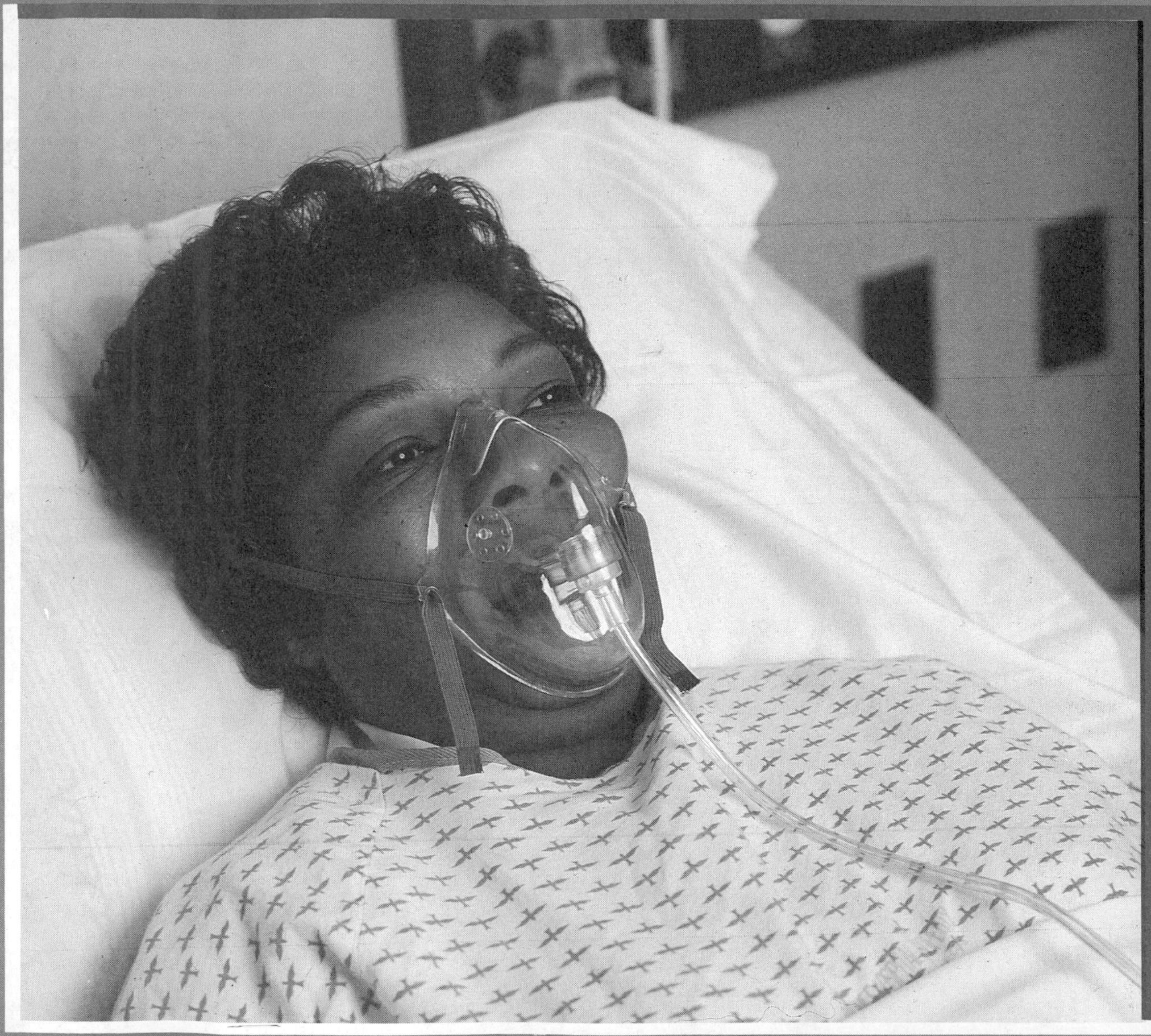

Basic Physiological Needs

Clients in both health and illness may need assistance in meeting basic physiological needs. These needs include good hygiene; nutrition; sleep and comfort; oxygenation; fluid, electrolyte, and acid-base balances; and unimpaired urinary and bowel elimination. Many health problems can disrupt the client's ability to meet such needs, and the unmet need may become the primary health problem. Thus the nurse must understand the processes related to the client's ability to meet these needs and the way to incorporate interventions addressing them into the nursing care plan. Although the needs discussed in this unit are principally physiological, the psychosocial dimension is often also involved, and care is planned holistically to restore, maintain, or promote total health.

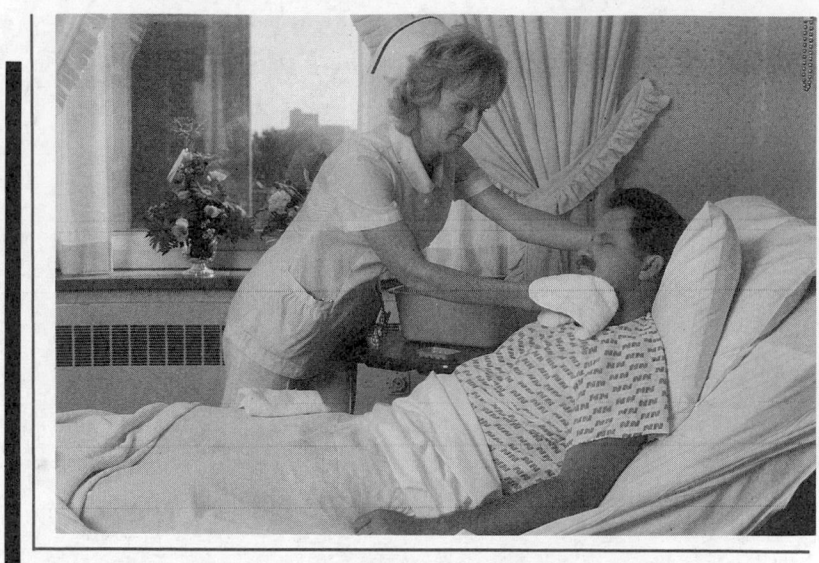

OBJECTIVES

Mastery of content in this chapter will enable the student to:

- Define the key terms listed.
- Identify common skin problems and related interventions.
- Describe factors that influence personal hygiene practices.
- Discuss conditions that may put a client at risk for impaired skin integrity.
- Describe the types of bathing techniques used depending on a client's physical condition.
- Successfully perform a complete bed bath and back rub.
- Discuss factors that influence the condition of the nails and feet.
- Explain the reason for the importance of a diabetic client to understand foot care.
- Describe the methods used for cleaning and cutting the nails.
- Describe clients at risk for poor oral hygiene.
- Discuss measures used to provide special oral hygiene and successfully provide oral hygiene.
- List common hair and scalp problems and their related interventions.
- Discuss how to assess the needs of clients requiring eye, ear, and nose care.
- Describe the steps followed in making an occupied, unoccupied, and a surgical hospital bed.

KEY TERMS

Acne
Apocrine Gland
Buccal
Cerumen
Dermatitis
Dermis
Dysphagia
Epidermis
Erythema
Gingiva
Halitosis
Hirsutism
Hygiene
Keratosis
Mastication

Nasal
Neuropathy
Oral Hygiene
Paronychia
Partial Bed Bath
Perineal Care
Periodontal Disease
Plantar Wart
Podiatrist
Pruritus
Sebum
Stomatitis
Trendelenburg Position
Vernix Caseosa

Hygiene

CHAPTER OUTLINE

A nurse works with a wide variety of clients who require assistance with personal hygiene or must learn proper hygiene techniques. Hygiene is the science of health. The self-care measures people use to maintain their health is personal hygiene.

Maintenance of personal hygiene is necessary for an individual's comfort, safety, and sense of well-being. Whereas well people are capable of meeting their own hygiene needs, ill people may require the nurse's assistance to carry out routine hygiene practices. In addition, several factors influence the client's hygiene practice. The nurse determines a client's ability to perform self-care and provides hygiene care according to the client's needs and preferred practices. While providing routine hygienic care, the nurse assesses the client's physical and emotional state. For example, complete assessment of the integument can be done during the client's bath. Because hygienic care often requires close contact with the client, the nurse can use communication skills to promote the therapeutic relationship and to learn about the client's emotional needs. During hygiene care the nurse can also teach clients health promotion practices. The nurse must also consider clients' specific physical limitations, beliefs, values, and habits. Individual hygienic preferences do not significantly affect health and can usually be incorporated into the nurse's plan of care. The nurse needs to preserve as much of the client's independence as possible, ensure privacy, and foster the client's physical well-being.

FACTORS INFLUENCING HYGIENE PRACTICE

The manner in which a person performs personal hygiene can be influenced by a number of factors. Generally people do not perform hygienic care in the same way, and the nurse can provide individualized care only after knowing the client's unique hygiene practices.

Body Image

A client's general appearance reflects the importance hygiene holds for him or her. Body image is a person's subjective concept of his or her physical appearance. This image can change frequently. A person's body image will affect the way in which hygiene is maintained. If the client is neatly groomed, the nurse considers all details of grooming when planning care and consults the client before making decisions about how hygienic care should be provided. In contrast, the client who appears unkempt or uninterested in hygiene requires education about the importance of hygiene. The nurse must not convey feelings of disapproval or revulsion when caring for a client whose hygiene is obviously poor.

When the client's body image changes as a result of surgery or a physical ailment, the nurse must make an extra effort to promote hygiene. For example, a young woman who has undergone a thyroidectomy may be concerned about the appearance of the scar in her neck. In addition to helping the client maintain good grooming practices, the nurse can discuss ways to cover the scar with ties or scarves until it becomes fainter.

Social Practices

The social groups to which a client relates can influence personal hygienic practices. During childhood, children acquire the hygiene practices of their parents. Family customs, the number of people in the house, and the availability of hot water are just a few of the factors influencing a child's hygienic care. Later in life, friends and work groups shape the expectations a person has about his or her personal appearance and the care taken to maintain adequate hygiene.

Socioeconomic Status

A person's economic resources influence the type and extent of hygienic practices used. The nurse should determine if the client can afford necessary hygienic supplies such as deodorant, shampoo, toothpaste, and cosmetics.

Knowledge

Knowledge about the importance of hygiene and its implications for well-being influences a person's hygiene practices. However, knowledge alone is not enough; the person must also be motivated to maintain self-care. Often learning about an illness or condition will encourage the client to improve hygiene practices. For example, when diabetic clients are aware of the effect of diabetes on the circulation to the feet, they are more likely to learn the proper techniques for foot care.

Cultural Variables

A client's cultural beliefs and personal values influence hygienic care. People from diverse cultural backgrounds follow different self-care practices. In North America, for example, many people take daily showers or tub baths. In the Far East, cleanliness is viewed as essential to a person's well-being. In European countries, however, it is not unusual to bathe completely only once a week. When caring for clients with different hygiene practices, the nurse avoids being judgmental or forcing the client to change practices.

Personal Preferences

Each client has individual desires and preferences on when to bathe, shave, or perform hair care. Likewise, clients select different hygiene products, for example, soap, shampoo, deodorant, or toothpaste, according to personal preferences. Clients also have preferences regarding how hygiene is performed. For example, one man may prefer to shave before a bath, whereas another shaves after taking a shower. Client preferences should help the nurse develop a more individualized plan of care. The nurse does not attempt to change a client's preferences unless the client's health is affected. For example, a male client with diabetes must carefully keep his feet clean to avoid the risk of infection. The nurse must explain and reinforce good foot care if the client is known to have repeated infections.

Physical Condition

People who suffer certain illnesses or who have undergone surgery often lack the physical energy or dexterity to perform personal hygiene. A client whose arm has been placed in a cast or who is in traction will require assistance in performing a complete bath. Serious cardiac, neurological, pulmonary, and metabolic conditions may exhaust or incapacitate clients and require the nurse to perform total hygienic care.

TYPES OF HYGIENE CARE

The nurse provides a variety of hygiene measures throughout the course of a day and can often schedule

Hygienic Care Schedule

EARLY MORNING CARE

- Nursing personnel on the night shift provide basic hygiene to clients getting ready for breakfast, scheduled tests, or early morning surgery. "AM care" includes offering a bedpan or urinal if the client is not ambulatory, washing the client's hands and face, and assisting with oral care.

MORNING OR AFTER BREAKFAST CARE

- In care performed after breakfast, the nurse assists by offering a bedpan or urinal to clients confined to bed; providing a bath or shower and oral, foot, nail, and hair care; giving a back massage; changing the client's gown or pajamas; and changing the bed linens and straightening the client's bedside unit and room.

AFTERNOON CARE

- Hospitalized clients often undergo many exhausting diagnostic tests or procedures in the morning. In rehabilitation centers, clients may participate in physical therapy during the morning. Afternoon hygiene care includes washing the hands and face, assisting with oral care, offering a bedpan or urinal, and straightening bed linen.

EVENING OR HOUR-OF-SLEEP-CARE

- Before bedtime the nurse offers personal hygiene care that helps a client relax to promote sleep. "PM care" may include changing soiled bed linens, gowns, or pajamas; assisting the client in washing the face and hands; providing oral hygiene; giving a back massage; and offering the bedpan or urinal to nonambulatory clients.

other care measures around the times hygiene is planned. The box describes the types of hygienic care commonly performed at certain times of day.

CARE OF THE SKIN

The skin is an active organ with the functions of protection, secretion, excretion, temperature regulation, and sensation (Table 32-1). The skin has three primary layers: epidermis (outer layer), dermis, and subcutaneous. The epidermis is composed of several thin layers of cells undergoing different stages of maturation. The innermost layer of the epidermis generates new cells that migrate slowly toward the epidermal surface. These cells replace the dead cells that are continuously shed from the skin's outer surface. The epidermis also contains melanocytes, special cells that produce the melanin or dark pigment of the skin. Exposure to sunlight causes the melanocytes to produce melanin, which gives some people a tan. Darker-skinned races have more active melanocytes, which produce more melanin. The distribution of pigmentation in dark-skinned people varies widely.

Bacteria commonly reside on the skin's outer surface. These resident bacteria (for example, *Corynebacterium*) are normal flora (see Chapter 43) that do not cause disease but instead inhibit the multiplication of disease-causing microorganisms.

The dermis is a thicker skin layer containing bundles of collagen and elastic fibers to support the epidermis. Nerve fibers, blood vessels, sweat glands, sebaceous glands, and hair follicles course through the dermal layer. Blood vessels in the dermis give skin its pink tint. Sebaceous glands secrete sebum, an oily, odorous fluid, into the hair follicles. Sebum lubricates the skin and hair to keep them supple and pliant. There are two types of sweat glands: eccrine and apocrine. The eccrine glands are distributed throughout the skin but are more abundant in the forehead, palms, and soles. Sweat excreted from the eccrine glands assists in temperature control through evaporation. The apocrine glands can be found in the axillary and genital areas. The bacterial decomposition of sweat from these glands is responsible for body odor. In the ears, ceruminous glands secrete cerumen into the external ear canal. This heavy, oily substance traps foreign material entering the ear.

The subcutaneous tissue layer contains blood vessels, nerves, lymph, and loose connective tissue filled with fat cells. The fatty tissue serves as a heat insulator of the body. Subcutaneous tissue also provides support for upper skin layers. Very little subcutaneous tissue can be found underlying the oral mucosa.

The skin exchanges oxygen, nutrients, and fluid with underlying blood vessels, synthesizes new cells, and eliminates dead nonfunctioning cells. The cells of the integument require adequate nutrition and hydration to resist injury and disease. Adequate circulation is essential to maintain cell life. When a person's physical condition changes, the skin often reflects this by alterations in color, thickness, texture turgor, temperature, and hydration (see Chapter 13). As long as the skin remains intact and healthy, its physiological function remains optimal.

ASSESSMENT

Nursing assessment is an ongoing process that occurs as the nurse gives hygiene care. The nurse does not assess all body regions before a bath or shampoo. However,

TABLE 32-1 Function of the Skin and Implications for Care

Function/Description	Implications for Care
PROTECTION	
The epidermis is a relatively impermeable layer that prevents entrance of microorganisms. Although microorganisms reside on the skin surface and in hair follicles, the relative dryness of the skin's surface inhibits bacterial growth. Sebum removes bacteria from hair follicles. The acidic pH of the skin further retards bacterial growth.	Weakening of the epidermis occurs by scraping or stripping its surface as by use of dry razors, tape removal, or improper turning or positioning techniques. Excessive dryness causes cracks and breaks in the skin and mucosa that allow bacteria to enter. Emollients soften skin and prevent moisture loss, soaking of the skin improves moisture retention, and hydration of the mucosa prevents dryness. However, constant exposure of the skin to moisture causes maceration or softening, which promotes bacterial growth. Bed linen and clothing should be kept dry. Misuse of soap, detergents, cosmetics, deodorant, and depilatories can cause chemical irritation. Alkaline soaps neutralize the protective acid condition of the skin. Cleansing of skin removes excess oil, sweat, dead skin cells, and dirt that can promote bacterial growth.
SENSATION	
The skin contains sensory organs for touch, pain, heat, cold, and pressure.	Friction should be used judiciously to avoid causing discomfort during bathing. Smoothing linen removes sources of mechanical irritation. Removing rings from nurse's fingers prevents the nurse from accidentally injuring the client's skin. Bath water should not be excessively hot or cold.
TEMPERATURE REGULATION	
Body temperature is controlled by radiation, evaporation, conduction, and convection.	Factors that interfere with heat loss can alter a person's temperature control. Wet bed linen or gowns interfere with convection and conduction. Excess blankets or bed coverings can interfere with heat loss through radiation and conduction. Coverings can promote heat conservation.
EXCRETION AND SECRETION	
Sweat acts to promote heat loss by evaporation. Sebum lubricates skin and hair.	Perspiration and oil can harbor microorganisms. Bathing removes excess body secretions, although excessive bathing can cause drying of skin.

the nurse must determine whether the client can tolerate hygiene procedures, which can often be exhausting. An assessment will guide the nurse in identifying the type of care required by the client.

Most assessment occurs as the nurse ministers to the client's hygienic needs. For example, during oral care, condition of the teeth and mucosa can be observed. Hygiene care allows the nurse to make assessment findings for a variety of health care problems and thus helps to set health care priorities.

PHYSICAL ASSESSMENT OF THE SKIN

While assisting a client with personal hygiene, the nurse assesses all external body surfaces. Using the skills of inspection and palpation (see Chapter 13), the nurse looks for alterations in the integument, determines the client's need for hygiene, and notes changes of the integument in response to nursing and medical therapies.

The nurse determines the condition of the skin by observing its color, texture, thickness, turgor, temperature, and hydration. Chapter 13 describes in detail the techniques for assessing each of these characteristics. The box on p. 814 describes normal skin characteristics.

The nurse also assesses for characteristics most influenced by hygiene measures (Table 32-2). Are there areas of dry skin as a result of too frequent baths, excessive use of soap, or use of harsh alkaline soaps? Have areas of skin maceration formed as a result of improper drying? Are there callused areas on the feet or hands that might benefit from soaking and the application of lotion?

While inspecting the skin the nurse notes the presence and condition of any lesions (see Chapter 13). Certain types have implications for hygiene measures. When the

TABLE 32-2   Common Skin Problems

Characteristics	Implications	Interventions
DRY SKIN		
Flaky, rough texture on exposed areas such as hands, arms, legs, or face	Skin may become infected if the epidermal layer is allowed to crack.	Bathe less frequently. Rinse body of all soap because residue left on skin can cause irritation and breakdown. Add moisture to air through use of humidifier. Increase fluid intake when skin is dry. Use moisturizing lotion to aid in healing process. The lotion forms a protective barrier and helps maintain fluid within the skin. Use creams to clean skin that is dry or allergic to soaps and detergents.
ACNE		
Inflammatory, papulopustular skin eruption, usually involving bacterial breakdown of sebum; appears on face, neck, shoulders, and back	Infected material within pustule can spread if area is squeezed or picked. Permanent scarring can result.	Wash hair and skin thoroughly each day with hot water and soap to remove oil. Cosmetics should be used sparingly, since oily cosmetics or creams accumulate in pores and tend to make the condition worse. Dietary restrictions may need to be implemented. Foods found to aggravate the condition should be eliminated from diet. Exposure to ultraviolet rays, either from sunshine or a heat lamp, may help control acne. Caution should be used to prevent burning of skin. Use prescribed topical antibiotics for severe forms of acne.
HIRSUTISM		
Excessive growth of body and facial hair, especially in women	Hirsutism may cause a negative body image by giving a female a male appearance.	The following may be used to remove unwanted hair: depilatories (can cause infection, rashes, or dermatitis); shaving (safest method); electrolysis (permanently removes hair by destroying hair follicles); tweezing (lasts only temporarily); bleaching of hair (lasts only temporarily).
SKIN RASHES		
Skin eruption that may result from overexposure to sun or moisture or from an allergic reaction; may be flat or raised, localized or systemic, pruritic or nonpruritic	If the skin is continually scratched, inflammation and infection may occur. Rashes can also cause discomfort.	Wash area thoroughly and apply antiseptic spray or lotion to prevent further itching and aid in healing process. Warm soaks may relieve inflammation.
CONTACT DERMATITIS		
Inflammation of skin characterized by abrupt onset with erythema, pruritus, pain, and appearance of scaly oozing lesions; seen on face, neck, hands, forearms, and genitalia	Dermatitis is often difficult to eliminate because the person is usually in continual contact with a substance causing the skin reaction. The substance may be hard to identify.	The condition usually disappears when exposure to causative agents (for example, cleansers and soaps) is avoided.
ABRASION		
Scraping or rubbing away of epidermis; may result in localized bleeding and later weeping of serous fluid	Infection occurs easily because of loss of protective skin layer.	Nurses should be careful not to scratch clients with jewelry or fingernails. Wash abrasions with mild soap and water. Use of a dressing or bandage could increase risk of infection owing to retained moisture.

Normal Skin Characteristics

- Intact, without abrasions
- Feels warm when palpated
- Localized changes in texture can be palpated across skin's surface
- Good turgor (elastic and firm) with skin generally smooth and soft
- Skin color varies from body part to body part

---

nurse observes skin problems, it helps to explain proper skin care to the client. For example, a rash on the skin often indicates an allergic reaction. The nurse teaches the client about the proper use of medications prescribed for the rash and cautions against use of over-the-counter drugs that may prove useless or even worsen the rash. Likewise, the nurse educates the client about avoiding use of irritants such as harsh soaps or cosmetics that can aggravate the condition.

DEVELOPMENTAL CHANGES

A client's age influences the normal condition of the skin and the type of hygiene measures required. The neonate's skin is relatively immature with the epidermis and dermis loosely bound together. The skin is extremely thin. Since any friction against the skin layers can cause bruising, the nurse must handle the neonate carefully during bathing. A break in the neonate's skin can easily lead to infection.

In a toddler the skin layers are more tightly bound together. The child thus has a greater resistance to infection and skin irritation. However, because of the child's more active play and the absence of established hygiene habits, greater attention is needed from parents and care givers to provide thorough hygiene.

During adolescence the growth and maturation of the integument are increased. In girls, estrogen secretion causes the skin to become soft, smooth, and thicker in texture with increased vascularity. In boys, male hormones produce an increased thickness of the skin with some darkening in color. Sebaceous glands become more active, predisposing adolescents to acne. Eccrine and apocrine sweat glands become fully functional during puberty. Adolescents usually begin to use antiperspirants. More frequent bathing and shampooing also become necessary to reduce body odors. Sweating is usually more pronounced in boys. The growth of body hair increases during adolescence as a result of hormonal changes. The body hair has a characteristic pattern of distribution, which the nurse can assess (see Chapter 13). Pubic and axillary hair develops in both sexes. Beard

⚔ Research Highlight ⚕

Frantz and Kinney studied whether sebum secretions and other external variables, for example, frequency of bathing, nutritional and fluid intake, and exposure to the sun, were associated with the occurrence of dry skin in the elderly. Participating were 76 elderly white individuals ranging from 65 to 97 years of age.

Actual samples of sebum were obtained and measured. The elderly subjects were asked about skin dryness, and the researchers looked for the presence of rough, scaly, flaking skin on skin surfaces.

Of the 76 subjects, 45 (59%) showed evidence of dry skin and 31 (41%) did not. Age and sex showed no statistical association with dry skin. The study also found no association between nutritional and fluid intake and frequency of bathing with dry skin. Most interesting, even though a decrease in sebum secretion in the elderly was identified, the researchers did not find an association between the presence of dry skin and reduced sebum secretion. The researchers suggest that a variety of factors may act together to cause dry skin in the elderly.

Frantz, RA, and Kinney, CK: Variables associated wih skin dryness in the elderly, Nurs Res 35(2):98, 1986.

---

and mustache hair grows in boys as a result of testicular androgens. Some girls and women have increased androgens levels causing hirsutism, or growth of facial hair.

The condition of an adult's skin depends on hygiene practices and exposure to environmental irritants. Normally the skin is elastic, well hydrated, firm, and smooth. With age the skin loses its resiliency and moisture, and sebaceous and sweat glands become less active (see research highlight). The epithelium thins and elastic collagen fibers shrink, making the skin fragile and subject to bruising and breaking. These changes warrant caution when turning and repositioning the elderly. Typically the elderly person's skin is dry and wrinkled, which can be aggravated by the sun. Daily bathing may cause the skin to become excessively dry.

SELF-CARE ABILITY

When a client becomes unable to bathe or perform personal skin care, the nurse provides the necessary assistance. To determine if a client requires a bed bath instead of a tub bath or shower, the nurse should assess the client's balance, activity tolerance, and muscle strength and coordination. The degree of assistance needed by a client during bathing may also depend on vision, the ability to sit without support, hand grasp, and range of motion of extremities. If a client's cognitive function is impaired the nurse's help probably will be needed.

RISKS FOR SKIN IMPAIRMENT

The nurse looks for certain conditions that place a client at risk for impaired skin integrity.

IMMOBILIZATION. A client who is unable to move freely as a result of illness or some external restraint is at risk for skin breakdown. The dependent body parts are exposed to pressure from underlying surfaces (for example, a mattress, a body cast, or a wrinkled layer of linen) reducing circulation to affected body parts. Chapter 42 describes how impairment of circulation to dependent body parts can result in decubitus ulcer formation. The nurse should be aware of clients who require assistance to turn and change position. Localized redness and tenderness are early signs of pressure on dependent body parts.

REDUCED SENSATION. Many clients are unable to sense an injury to the skin's surface. Clients with paralysis, circulatory insufficiency, or local nerve damage do not receive normal transmission of nerve impulses when excessive heat or cold, pressure, friction, or chemical irritants are applied to the skin. The nurse can easily assess the status of a client's sensory nerve function by checking for pain, tactile, or temperature sensation (see Chapter 13).

NUTRITIONAL ALTERATIONS. Adequate nutrients are essential for maintaining the normal integrity of the skin. Clients with limited caloric and protein intake have impaired tissue synthesis. The skin becomes thinner, less elastic, and smoother and a loss of subcutaneous tissue occurs. Poor digestion and absorption of nutrients (as caused by inflammatory conditions of the bowel or bowel surgery), excessive protein metabolism (as caused by fever, burns, or surgery), and excessive loss of protein (as caused by blood loss, wound exudate, or burns) place clients at risk for nutritional imbalances. Any hospitalized client who is not permitted to eat is a candidate for nutritional problems.

SECRETIONS AND EXCRETIONS ON THE SKIN. Moisture on the skin's surface is a medium for bacterial growth and can cause softening of epidermal cells. Perspiration, urine, watery fecal material, and wound drainage can accumulate on the skin's surface, resulting in skin breakdown and infection. The nurse gives particular attention to body areas, such as under the woman's breasts, the perineal area, or under the arms, where moisture may collect and skin surfaces may rub against each other and cause friction.

VASCULAR INSUFFICIENCY. In peripheral vascular disease either the arterial blood supply to tissues is inadequate or venous return is impaired, causing circulatory stasis in dependent extremities. Inadequate blood flow to the skin results in ischemia and breakdown. Clients with this disease have a high risk of infection because delivery of nutrients and white blood cells to injured tissues is inadequate.

EXTERNAL DEVICES. Often a client has some type of external device applied to or around the skin that has the potential for exerting pressure or friction against the skin's surface. A cast, cloth restraint, bandage, dressing, or orthopedic brace can rub against the skin and cause breakdown. The nurse assesses all skin surfaces exposed to any external device.

NURSING DIAGNOSIS

The nurse's assessment reveals the condition of the client's skin and the client's need for and ability to maintain personal hygiene needs. Defining characteristics direct the nurse to diagnose specifically the client's actual or potential health problems (see sample nursing diagnoses box on p. 816).

Examples of Nursing Diagnoses Related to Skin Integrity and the Need for Thorough Skin Care

NANDA-APPROVED NURSING DIAGNOSES

Impaired skin integrity related to:
- Pressure
- Physical immobilization
- Exposure to chemical irritants

Potential impaired skin integrity related to:
- Immobilization
- Vascular insufficiency
- Inadequate nutritional intake

Altered peripheral tissue perfusion related to:
- Impaired arterial blood flow
- Impaired venous return

Bathing/hygiene self-care deficit related to:
- Pain
- Forced immobilization
- Musculoskeletal weakness

Impaired tissue integrity related to:
- Altered circulation
- Nutritional deficit
- Mechanical irritation

Sample Nursing Diagnoses for Clients Needing Skin Care

Defining Characteristics	Nursing Diagnoses	Related Factors
Disrupted skin surface (for example, burn, abrasion) Destruction of skin layers	Impaired skin integrity	▪ Exposure to chemical substance ▪ Mechanical pressure ▪ Physical immobilization
Inability to wash body or body parts because of reduced strength, poor dexterity, reduced level of consciousness	Bathing/hygiene self-care deficit	▪ Presence of cast ▪ Musculoskeletal weakness ▪ Mental confusion
Cool skin temperature Diminished arterial pulsations Slow healing foot or leg lesions	Altered peripheral tissue perfusion	▪ Interrupted arterial blood flow

---

If the client has the potential for skin breakdown, the nurse plans preventive measures. The factors contributing to the problem determine the nurse's interventions.

If the client has skin breakdown, the nurse must provide care that promotes healing of injured skin surfaces and prevents infection. The nurse also eliminates factors that may lead to further tissue injury. Examples of nursing diagnoses are shown in the nursing diagnoses box.

PLANNING

Providing skin care has many purposes other than maintaining a client's cleanliness. A bath or shower helps the client relax, stimulates circulation to the skin, provides exercise through range-of-joint motion during bathing, improves self-image, and stimulates the rate and depth of respirations (see box at right). The interaction between nurse and client during bathing and skin care gives the nurse an opportunity to develop a meaningful relationship with the client.

Planning should focus on the types of methods of skin care the nurse will deliver and on the variety of nursing care measures the nurse can perform as a client bathes. Teaching, providing emotional support, and values clarification are just some of the types of interaction the nurse can include during hygiene.

Considering the client's hygiene preferences before planning care is also important. One client may prefer only a partial bath in the morning, and another may enjoy showering just before bed. The type of hygiene the client desires or requires will determine the supplies and equipment the nurse must prepare.

The client's condition influences the plan for delivering hygiene. A seriously ill client usually needs a daily bath because body secretions accumulate and the client is unable to maintain cleanliness (see care plan box). An elderly client at home may require a visit from the nurse to assist with a tub bath. If clients are normally inactive during the day and their skin tends to be dry, the nurse may need to bathe the client only twice a week. For clients who are weakened or possess poor muscle strength and coordination, the nurse must plan for necessary assistance. For example, an obese client who has had difficulty getting out of a tub should have a tub chair, hand rails, or extra personnel available for help.

Timing is also important in planning hygiene care.

Purposes of Bathing

▪ **Cleansing the skin.** Removes perspiration, some bacteria, sebum, and dead skin cells, which minimizes skin irritation and reduces chance of infection.

▪ **Stimulation of circulation.** Good circulation is promoted through the use of warm water and gentle stroking of the extremities.

▪ **Improved self-image.** Bathing promotes relaxation and a feeling of being refreshed and comfortable.

▪ **Reduction of body odors.** Excessive secretion of sweat from apocrine glands located in the axilla and pubic areas cause unpleasant body odors. Bathing and use of antiperspirants minimize odors.

▪ **Promotion of range of motion.** Movement of the extremities during bathing maintains joint function.

Sample Nursing Care Plan for Clients Needing Skin Care			
Nursing Diagnosis	**Goal**	**Expected Outcomes**	**Nursing Interventions**
Potential impaired skin integrity related to immobilization	Skin will remain intact and free of odors.	Skin is intact, warm, smooth, soft, and well hydrated. Odors are reduced or eliminated.	Provide daily total baths. Provide perineal care after each voiding and defecation. Apply skin lotion to areas of skin that become easily reddened: coccyx, heels, scapula, and greater trochanters. Change linen after client has been diaphoretic.

Being interrupted in the middle of a bath to go to an x-ray examination can frustrate and embarrass a client. The nurse should try to plan hygiene care around tests and procedures the client must undergo. This can be difficult in a hospital setting because tests may not be scheduled for specific times.

Goals for clients receiving skin care include:
1. Skin will remain intact and free of body odors
2. Joint range of motion is maintained
3. Client achieves a sense of comfort and well-being
4. Client participates in and understands methods of skin care

IMPLEMENTATION

BATHING

Bathing a client is a part of total hygienic care. Nurses provide categories of baths: cleaning and therapeutic (see box below). A physician's order is necessary for baths designed for therapeutic purposes. The order will designate bath temperature, the body part being treated (in the case of soaks), and any medicated solution used, for example, saline, sodium bicarbonate, or potassium permanganate.

Text continued on p. 823.

Types of Therapeutic Baths

HOT WATER TUB BATH

- Immersion in hot water helps relieve muscle soreness and spasm. However, a danger of causing burns exists. Water temperature should be 45°-46° C (113°-114.8° F) for adults.

WARM WATER TUB BATH

- Bathing in warm water relieves muscle tension. Water temperature should be 43° C (109.4° F).

COOL WATER BATH

- Bathing in cool water can relieve tension or lower body temperature. Precautions must be taken to avoid chilling. Water temperature should be tepid (37° C [98.6° F]) rather than cold. This type of bath is especially effective in reducing the body temperature of a small child with a fever.

SOAK

- Local application of water or medicated solution can remove dead tissue or soften crusted secretions. Aseptic technique is necessary when cleaning open or abraded areas of the skin. Soaks are also useful in reducing pain and swelling of inflamed or irritated skin surfaces.

SITZ BATH

- A sitz bath cleanses and reduces inflammation of the perineal and anal areas of a client who has undergone rectal or vaginal surgery or childbirth or who has local rectal irritation from hemorrhoids or fissures. Water temperature depends on the client's condition but should be 43°-45° C (109.4°-113° F).

PROCEDURE 32-1

Bathing a Client

STEPS	RATIONALE
1. Assess client's preferences for bathing practices: frequency of bathing, time of day bathing preferred, type of hygiene products used.	Promotes client's participation in care and sense of comfort.
2. Review orders for precautions concerning client's movement or positioning.	Prevents accidental injury to client during bathing activities.
3. Explain procedure and ask client for suggestions or ways to prepare supplies. If partial bath is to be performed, ask client how much of bath he or she wishes to complete.	Promotes client's cooperation and participation.
4. If shower or tub bath is to be done, schedule use of facilities if private bath unavailable.	Prevents unnecessary waiting that can cause fatigue.
5. Adjust room temperature and ventilation, and close room doors and windows.	Warm room, free of drafts, prevents rapid loss of body heat during bathing. Ensures privacy.
6. Prepare necessary equipment and supplies:	
a. Two bath towels	Separate towel and washcloth are used for client's face and body to enhance feeling of cleanliness.
b. Two washcloths	
c. Washbasin (for complete or partial bed bath)	
d. Soap and soap dish	
e. Bath blanket (for complete or partial bed bath)	Bath blanket maintains client's warmth during procedure.
f. Clean gown or pajamas	
g. Hygienic aids, such as skin lotion, deodorant, and/ or powder	
h. Bedpan or urinal and toilet paper	For client to use before bath.
i. Linen hamper or laundry bag	
j. Disposable gloves	Prevents contact with potentially infected body secretions.

COMPLETE OR PARTIAL BED BATH

1. Offer client bedpan or urinal. Provide towel and washcloth.	Client will feel more comfortable after voiding. Prevents interruption of bath.
2. Wash hands.	Reduces transmission of microorganisms.
3. Lower side rail and assist client in assuming comfortable position maintaining body alignment.	Aids nurse's access to client. Maintains client's comfort throughout procedure.
4. Bring client toward side closest to you. Place hospital bed in high position.	When nurse does not have to reach across bed, strain on back muscles is minimized.
5. Loosen top covers at foot of bed. Place bath blanket over top sheet. Fold and remove top sheet from under blanket. If possible, have client hold bath blanket while the nurse withdraws sheet.	Removal of top linens prevents their becoming soiled or moist during bath. Blanket provides warmth and privacy.

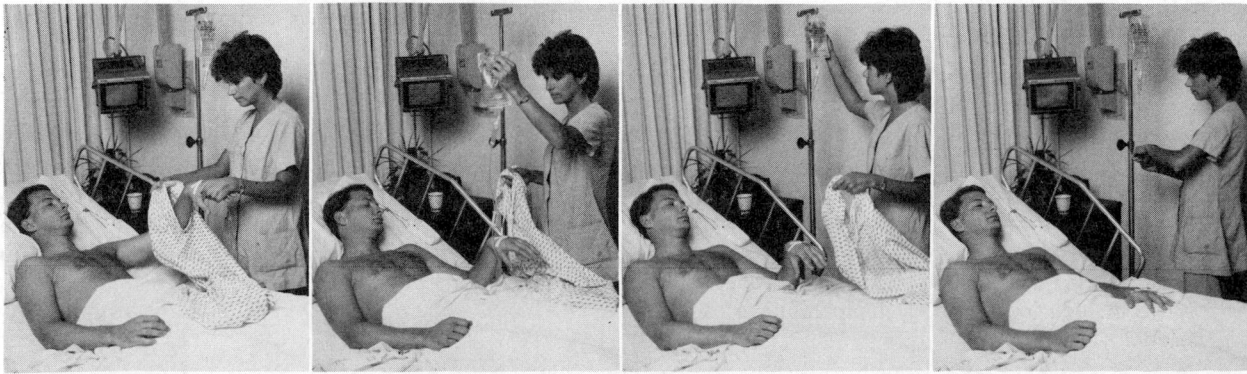

Step 7

STEPS	RATIONALE
6. If top sheet is to be reused, fold it for replacement later. If not, dispose in laundry bag, taking care not to allow linen to contact your uniform.	Proper disposal prevents transmission of microorganisms.
7. Remove client's gown or pajamas. If an extremity is injured or has reduced mobility, begin removal from *unaffected* side. If client has intravenous (IV) tube, remove gown from arm *without* IV first, then lower IV container and slide gown covering affected arm over tubing and container. Rehang IV container and check flow rate (see illustrations).	Provides full exposure of body parts during bathing. Undressing unaffected side first allows easier manipulation of gown over body part with reduced ROM.
8. Pull side rail up. Fill washbasin two-thirds full, with water between 43° and 46° C (110° and 115° F). Have client place fingers in water to test temperature tolerance. OPTION: Place plastic container of bath lotion in bath water.	Raising side rail maintains client's safety as nurse leaves bedside. Warm water promotes comfort and prevents unnecessary chilling. Testing temperature prevents accidental burning of client's skin. Keeps lotion warm for application to client's skin.
9. Remove pillow if allowed and raise head of bed 30-45 degrees. Place bath towel under client's head.	Removal of pillow makes it easier to wash client's ears and neck. Placement of towel prevents soiling of bed linen.
10. Place bath towel over client's chest.	Prevents soiling of bath blanket.
11. Fold washcloth around fingers of your hand to form a mitt (see illustration). Immerse mitt in water and wring thoroughly.	Mitt retains water and heat better than loosely held washcloth, keeps cold edges from brushing against client, and prevents splashing.
12. Wash client's eyes with plain warm water. Use different section of mitt for each eye. Move mitt from inner to outer canthus. Soak any crustations on eyelid for 2-3 minutes with damp cloth before attempting removal. Dry eye thoroughly but gently.	Soap irritates eyes. Use of separate sections of mitt reduces infection transmission. Bathing eye from inner to outer canthus prevents secretions from entering nasolacrimal duct. Pressure can cause internal injury.
13. Ask client about preference for using soap on the face. Wash, rinse, and dry well forehead, cheeks, nose, neck, and ears. (Men may wish to shave either at this point or after bath.)	Soap tends to dry face more quickly, since it is exposed to air more than other body parts.
14. Remove bath blanket from over client's arm that is farthest from you. Place bath towel lengthwise under arm. OPTION: Raise side rail and move to other side to wash arm.	Bathing far side first prevents reaching over clean area.
15. Lower side rail. Bathe arm with soap and water using long, firm strokes from distal to proximal areas (fingers to axilla). Raise and support arm above head (if possible) while thoroughly washing axilla.	Soap lowers surface tension and facilitates removal of debris and bacteria when friction is applied during washing. Long, firm strokes stimulate circulation. Movement of arm exposes axilla and exercises joint's normal ROM.
16. Rinse and dry arm and axilla thoroughly. If client uses deodorant or talcum powder, apply it.	Excess moisture causes skin maceration or softening. Deodorant controls body odor.

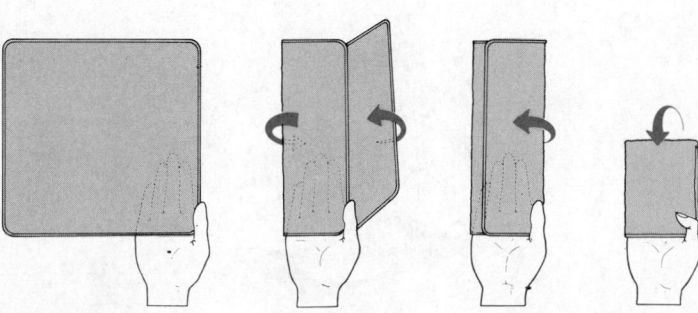

Step 11

Continued.

PROCEDURE 32-1, cont'd

Bathing a Client

STEPS	RATIONALE
17. Fold bath towel in half and lay it on bed beside client. Place basin on towel. Immerse client's hand in water. Allow hand to soak for 3-5 min before washing hand and fingernails (Procedure 32-5). Remove basin and dry hand well.	Soaking softens cuticles and calluses of hand and loosens debris beneath nails. Soaking also enhances feeling of cleanliness. Thorough drying removes moisture from between fingers.
18. Repeat Steps 14-17 for other arm.	
19. Check temperature of bath water and change water if necessary.	Use of warm water maintains client's comfort.
20. Cover client's chest with bath towel and fold bath blanket down to umbilicus.	This prevents unnecessary exposure of body parts.
21. With one hand, lift edge of towel away from chest. With mitted hand, bathe chest using long, firm strokes. Take special care to wash skinfolds under female client's breasts. It may be necessary to lift breast upward while bathing underneath it. Keep client's chest covered between wash and rinse periods. Dry well.	Towel maintains warmth and privacy. Secretions and dirt collect easily in areas of tight skinfolds.
22. Place bath towel lengthwise over chest and abdomen. (Two towels may be needed.) Fold blanket down to just above pubic region.	Prevents chilling and exposure of body parts.
23. With one hand, lift bath towel. With mitted hand, bath abdomen, giving special attention to bathing umbilicus and abdominal folds. Stroke from side to side. Keep abdomen covered between washing and rinsing. Dry well.	Moisture and sediment that collect in skinfolds predispose client to skin maceration and irritation.
24. Apply clean gown or pajama top. If one extremity is injured or immobilized, always dress affected side first. (This step may be omitted until completion of bath; gown should not become soiled during remainder of bath.)	Maintains client's warmth and comfort. Dressing affected side first allows easier manipulation of gown over body part with reduced ROM.
25. Cover chest and abdomen with top of bath blanket. Expose far leg by folding blanket over toward midline. Be sure perineum is draped.	Prevents unnecessary exposure.
26. Bend client's leg at knee by positioning your arm under leg. While grasping client's heel, elevate leg from mattress slightly and slide bath towel lengthwise under leg.	Towel prevents soiling of bed linen. Support of joint and extremity during lifting prevents strain on musculoskeletal structures.
27. Ask client to hold the foot still. Place bath basin on towel on bed and secure its position next to the foot to be washed.	Sudden movement by client could cause spillage of bathwater. (This step is omitted if client unable to hold leg in basin.)

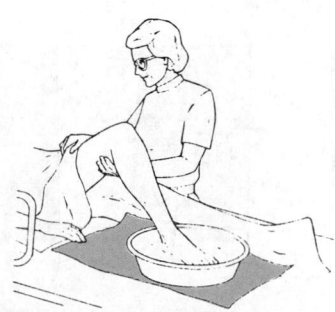

Step 28

STEPS	RATIONALE
28. With one hand supporting lower leg, raise it and slide basin under lifted foot. Make sure foot is firmly placed on bottom of basin. Allow foot to soak while you wash leg (see illustration).	Proper positioning of foot prevents pressure from being applied from edge of basin against calf. Soaking softens calluses and rough skin. (Note: if client is unable to hold leg, do not immerse; simply wash with washcloth.)
29. Use long, firm strokes in washing from ankle to knee and from knee to thigh. Dry well.	Promotes venous return.
30. Cleanse foot, making sure to bathe between toes. Clean and clip nails as needed (Procedure 32-5). Dry well. If skin is dry, apply lotion.	Secretions and moisture may be present between toes. Lotion helps to retain moisture and soften skin.
31. Repeat Steps 25-30 for other leg and foot.	
32. Cover client with bath blanket, raise side rail for client's safety, and change bathwater.	Drop in water temperature during bathing can cause chilling. Clean water reduces microorganism transmission.
33. Lower side rail. Assist client in assuming prone or side-lying position (as applicable). Place towel lengthwise along client's side.	Exposes back and buttocks for bathing.
34. Keep client draped by sliding bath blanket over shoulders and thighs.	Maintains warmth and prevents unnecessary exposure.
35. Apply disposable gloves	Prevents contact with microorganisms in body secretions.
36. Wash, rinse, and dry back from neck to buttocks using long, firm strokes. Pay special attention to folds of buttocks and anus. (Give a backrub.) (Procedure 32-4).	Skinfolds near buttocks and anus may contain fecal secretions that harbor microorganisms.
37. Change bathwater and washcloth.	Prevents transfer of microorganisms from anal area to genitalia.
38. Assist client in assuming sidelying or supine position. Cover chest and upper extremities with towel and lower extremities with bath blanket. Expose only genitalia. (If client can help, covering entire body with bath blanket may be preferable.) Wash, rinse, and dry perineum (Procedure 32-3). Give special attention to skinfolds.	Maintains client's privacy. Clients capable of performing partial bath usually prefer to wash their own genitalia. Skinfolds are a site for accumulation of secretions and/or moisture.
39. Dispose of gloves in receptacle.	Prevents transmission of microorganisms.
40. Apply any additional body lotion or oil as desired.	Moisturizing lotion prevents dry, chapped skin.
41. Assist client in dressing.	
42. Comb client's hair. Women may want to apply makeup.	Maintains client's body image.
43. Make client's bed (Procedures 32-11 and 32-12).	Provides clean surrounding environment.
44. Remove soiled linen and place in dirty linen bag. Clean and replace bathing equipment. Replace call light and personal possessions. Leave room as clean and comfortable as possible.	Prevents transmission of infection. Clean environment promotes client's comfort. Keeping call light and articles of care within reach promotes client's safety.
45. Wash hands.	Reduces transmission of microorganisms.

TUB BATH OR SHOWER

1. Check tub or shower for cleanliness. Use cleaning techniques according to agency policy. Place rubber mat on tub or shower bottom. Place disposable bathmat or towel on floor in front of tub or shower.	Cleaning prevents transmission of infection. Mats prevent slipping and falling.
2. Collect all hygienic aids, toiletry items, and linen requested by client. Place within easy reach of tub or shower.	Placing items close at hand prevents possible falls when client reaches for equipment.
3. Assist client to bathroom if necessary. Have client wear robe and slippers en route to bathroom.	Assistance prevents accidental falls. Wearing robe and slippers prevents chilling.

Continued.

PROCEDURE 32-1, cont'd

Bathing a Client

STEPS	RATIONALE
4. Demonstrate to client how to use call signal for assistance when in hospital or extended care facility.	Bathrooms are equipped with signaling devices in case client feels faint or weak or needs immediate assistance. Clients prefer privacy during bath if safety is not jeopardized.
5. Place "occupied" sign on bathroom door when in hospital or extended care facility.	Maintains client's privacy.
6. Fill bathtub halfway with warm water (43° C [109.4° F]). Ask client to test water, and adjust water temperature if it is too warm or too cold. Explain which faucet controls hot water. If client is taking shower, turn shower on and adjust water temperature before client enters shower stall.	Adjusting water temperature prevents accidental burns. The elderly and clients with neurological alterations (for example, spinal cord injury) are high risk for burns due to reduced sensation.
7. Instruct client to use safety bars when getting in and out of tub or shower.	Prevents slipping and falls.
8. Caution client against use of bath oil in tub water.	Oil causes tub surfaces to become slippery, predisposing client to accidental falls.
9. Instruct client not to remain in tub longer than 20 min. Check on client every 5 min.	Prolonged exposure to warm water may cause vasodilation and pooling of blood, leading to lightheadedness or dizziness.
10. Return to bathroom when client signals, and knock before entering.	Provides for client privacy.
11. For client who is unsteady, drain tub of water before client attempts to get out of it. Place bath towel over client's shoulders.	Prevents accidental falls. Client may become chilled as water drains.
12. Assist client in getting out of tub as needed and assist with drying.	Moisture may cause excessive softening of skin and promote spread of infection.
13. Assist client as needed in donning clean gown or pajamas, slippers, and robe. (In home setting client may don regular clothing.)	Maintains warmth to prevent chilling.
14. Assist client to the room and help him assume comfortable position in bed or chair.	Maintains relaxation gained from bathing.
15. Clean tub or shower according to agency policy. Remove soiled linen and place in dirty linen bag. Discard disposable equipment in proper receptable. Place "unoccupied" sign on bathroom door. Return supplies to storage area.	Prevents transmission of infection through soiled linen and moisture.
16. Wash hands.	Reduces transfer of microorganisms.

EVALUATION OF BATH TECHNIQUES

1. Observe client's behavior and ask if he feels fatigued or uncomfortable.	Determines client's tolerance to bathing activities.
2. Note areas on skin that were previously soiled, reddened, or showed early signs of breakdown.	Techniques used during bathing should leave skin clean and clear.
3. Record type of bath and client's tolerance of bathing. Also note condition of skin and any significant findings such as reddened skin areas or joint or muscle pain. Record level of assistance required by client.	Timely documentation maintains accuracy of client's record. Condition of skin documents response to therapy such as turning and positioning.

Illustrations from Sorrentino, SA: Mosby's textbook for nursing assistants, ed. 2, St. Louis, 1987, The C.V. Mosby Co.

PROCEDURE 32-2

Tepid Sponging

STEPS	RATIONALE
1. Assess client's body temperature and pulse.	Provides baseline for evaluating response to therapy. Sudden circulatory changes may alter pulse.
2. Explain to client that purpose of sponging with tepid water is to cool body slowly. Briefly describe steps of procedure.	Procedure can be uncomfortable because of cool applications. Anxiety over procedure can increase body temperature.
3. Prepare necessary equipment and supplies: a. Bath basin e. Waterproof pad b. Tepid water f. Bath blanket (37° C or 98.6° F) g. Thermometer c. Bath thermometer d. Washcloths	Tepid water prevents sudden heat loss and chilling.
4. Close room door or curtain.	Ensures privacy.
5. Wash hands.	Reduces transfer of microorganisms.
6. Place waterproof pads under the client and remove the gown.	Pads prevent soiling of the bed linen. Removing the gown provides access to all skin surfaces.
7. Keep the bath blanket over body parts not being sponged. Close the windows and door to prevent drafts in the room.	The bath blanket prevents chilling.
8. Check the water temperature.	Tepid water prevents chilling.
9. Immerse washcloths in water and apply wet cloths under each axilla and over the groin. If using tub, immerse client for 20-30 min.	The axilla and groin contain large superficial blood vessels. The application of washcloths promotes cooler temperature of the body's core by conduction. Immersion provides more effective heat loss.
10. Gently sponge an extremity for 5 min. Note the client's response. The opposite extremity may be covered by a cool washcloth. In tub, gently squeeze water over client's back and chest.	This prevents a sudden temperature fall and minimizes the risk of developing chills.
11. Dry the extremity and reassess the client's pulse and body temperature. Observe the client's response to therapy.	The client's response to therapy is monitored to prevent a sudden temperature change.
12. Continue sponging the other extremities, back, and buttocks for 3-5 min each. Reassess the temperature and pulse every 15 min.	This prevents a sudden temperature fall and minimizes the risk of developing chills.
13. Change the water and reapply sponges to the axilla and groin as needed.	The water temperature rises as a result of exposure to the client's warm body surface.
14. When the body temperature falls to slightly above normal, discontinue the procedure.	This prevents a temperature drift to a subnormal level. Follow institutional guidelines.
15. Dry the extremities and body parts thoroughly. Cover the client with a light bath blanket or sheet.	Drying and covering the client prevent chilling. An excessively heavy covering may increase body temperature.
16. Dispose of equipment and change the bed linen if soiled. Wash hands.	Controls the transmission of infection.
17. Measure the client's body temperature and pulse.	Temperature indicates the response to therapy. Dysrhythmias may be a complication of therapy.
18. Record the time the procedure was started and terminated, vital sign changes, and the client's response.	Recording communicates the care provided in an accurate and timely fashion.

The extent of the client's bath and the methods used for bathing depend on the client's physical capabilities and the degree of hygiene required. A complete bed bath is for clients who are totally dependent and require total hygienic care (Procedure 32-1).

A partial bed bath consists of bathing only body parts that would cause discomfort or odor if left unbathed (for example, hands, face, perineal area, and axillae). Dependent clients in need of only partial hygiene or self-sufficient bedridden clients who are unable to reach all body parts receive a partial bed bath.

The *tub bath* or *shower* can be used to give a more thorough bath than a bed bath. Washing and rinsing all body parts are easier. Safety is of primary concern because the surface of a tub or shower stall is slippery. Clients vary in how much help they will need. Some tubs are specially designed for dependent clients.

Tepid sponging is used when a client's temperature is very high. It can be soothing but can also be uncomfortable, depending on the client's skin temperature. Tepid water is used to avoid the chilling effect of cold water and to promote slow cooling, avoiding temperature fluctuations (Procedure 32-2).

Whatever type of bath the client receives, the nurse should follow these guidelines:

1. Provide privacy. Close the door or pull room curtains around the bathing area. While bathing the client, expose only the areas being bathed.
2. Maintain safety. Keep side rails up while you are away from the client's bedside. (Particularly important for dependent or unconscious clients.) Place the call light in the client's reach if you must leave the room temporarily.
3. Maintain warmth. The room should be kept warm, since the client is partially uncovered and may easily be chilled. Control drafts and keep windows closed.
4. Promote the client's independence as much as possible during bathing activities. Offer assistance as needed.

BATHING AN INFANT

An infant can be bathed in much the same way as an adult, either by a sponge bath or in a small tub. However, the nurse should take special precautions. Because an infant's temperature control mechanisms are still immature, prolonged exposure of body parts may cause rapid cooling. When giving a sponge bath, the nurse keeps the infant covered as much as possible. When giving a tub bath, the nurse should work quickly and be sure the water temperature is warm enough to prevent chilling. Henningson et al. (1981) note that bathing a newborn by immersion causes less heat loss and less crying.

The surface of an infant's skin has a pH of about 4.95 soon after birth (Whaley and Wong, 1987). This acid covering helps prevent the growth of bacteria on the skin's surface. Thus, plain water is preferred for bathing. Alkaline soaps such as Ivory, oils, powder, and lotion can alter the skin's pH and provide a medium for bacterial growth.

Care of the umbilical cord is a special consideration for the newborn. The umbilical stump is an excellent medium for bacterial growth. Triple dye is used by many institutions to prevent infection. The daily application of alcohol to the base of the cord aids drying. Normally the umbilical stump falls off in 14 to 17 days (Wilson et al., 1985) with proper care.

The nurse also gives special care to infants who have been circumcised. A small amount of bleeding normally occurs from the penis. The physician applies a sterile gauze dressing impregnated with petrolatum jelly around the circumcised area. The nurse may periodically clean the penis with moistened cotton balls until the dressing can be removed permanently (Whaley and Wong, 1987).

In hospitals where there is rooming-in of the infant and mother, the infant's bath is an excellent opportunity to involve the parents in the child's care. The parents can examine the infant's body parts and learn about normal variations in skin characteristics. A parent may worry about minor birth injuries unless the nurse explains how they occur and when they will disappear.

SPONGE BATH. Newborn infants are bathed after vital signs have stabilized. Nurses wear gloves when initially handling infants whose skin has become soiled from the blood of the mother. Initial washing only involves cleansing blood from the face and head. The vernix caseosa, a grayish-white, cheeselike substance covering the skin, may temporarily provide insulation and lubricating properties. The vernix caseosa dries and disappears within 24 to 48 hours.

Supplies for the bath include a shirt, a diaper (disposable or plain cloth), safety pins, a soft washcloth, cotton balls, a towel, and facial tissue. Plain water is used for bathing. A mild soap, for example, Ivory, should be used only for soiled areas such as around the anus. Optional supplies include alcohol for cleansing the umbilical cord and petrolatum jelly to prevent diaper rash.

The nurse prepares a basin with water at 38° to 40.5° C (100° to 105° F) so it feels comfortably warm when tested on the inside of the nurse's forearm. To prevent cooling, the nurse washes the infant's face, eyes, ears, and scalp before removing the shirt and diaper. The towel may also be kept over the infant for warming. The nurse cleans the infant's eyes and ears with clean, moistened cotton balls or a washcloth. The eyes are gently wiped from the inner to the outer canthus, using a clean cotton ball with each stroke or turning the cloth so only a clean part touches the eyes. While washing the face the nurse inspects the nares for crusted secretions. Cotton-tipped swabs should not be used to clean the nares or ears because an infant may move suddenly, causing the swab to break and damage the eardrum or mucous membranes. A rolled wisp of dampened cotton or the twisted end of the washcloth works well for cleaning the external ear canal and pinna. The infant's scalp can be cleaned by wiping off any secretions with a washcloth. However, if shampooing is necessary, the nurse secures the baby's head with one hand and positions it over the bath basin. A mild soap is best for shampooing. The nurse rinses the scalp by pouring water from a small cup or container over the infant's head into the basin.

Thorough drying is necessary to prevent evaporative heat loss.

The nurse then undresses the infant for the remainder of the bath. The towel is again used to drape areas not being washed. Keeping the infant covered may be difficult, since infants often kick and twist. Because of the infant's sensitive skin, little rubbing should be done when cleansing. However, the nurse gives special attention to the folds in the neck and axillae and creases at joints. For example, neck creases often collect regurgitated food, which may cause a rash. The umbilical cord should be cleansed with mild soap and water and dried thoroughly. Alcohol may be applied to the umbilicus to help dry it and to reduce chances of infection. Then the nurse dresses the infant in a shirt.

The nurse bathes the infant's buttocks and genitalia last. For a girl it is important to retract the labia fully in order to remove the vernix caseosa once it has dried. If the vernix caseosa is thick and adherent, the nurse may choose to remove it gradually during successive diaper changes to avoid causing unnecessary irritation during one bath. The vulva is cleaned from front to back to prevent spread of microorganisms from the anal area to the urethra. This technique for preventing urinary infection should be explained to the parents.

In male infants, the nurse washes carefully around the penis and scrotum. Noncircumcised infants should not have the foreskin retracted, since it is often too tight. Later, after the foreskin loosens, the nurse should teach the parents how to retract the foreskin, cleanse the area, and return the foreskin to its position. No special care is required around a circumcised penis. The nurse usually cleans off any blood with a clean cotton ball or washcloth. The original petrolatum jelly dressing remains in place for only a day.

The nurse bathes the buttocks last. Fecal material can be removed with facial tissue. Using mild soap helps ensure thorough cleansing of the anal area. After thorough drying, the application of a thin layer of petolatum jelly or ointment helps retain skin moisture and prevents diaper rash.

After the bath the nurse applies a clean diaper, which should fit snugly around the thighs and abdomen to prevent leakage of urine. If the child is circumcised, the diaper should fit loosely to prevent friction against the penis. The diaper should always be below the umbilical site until it is completely healed. The nurse fastens the diaper with the back overlapping the front to permit full flexion of the hips.

TUB BATH. Infants can be given a tub bath after the umbilicus has healed. Supplies for the tub bath are the same as those for a sponge bath. Supplies should be within easy reach. The face, neck, ears, eyes, and scalp are washed before the infant is undressed and immersed in the tub. The nurse lowers infants slowly into the tub to avoid startling them. The child must always be held firmly with one hand. A child is never left unattended in the bathinette. Often infants enjoy the sensation of being immersed in water, and older infants may enjoy playing during the bath. Body creases are much easier to clean and rinse in a tub bath. After the bath, the nurse wraps the infant completely in a towel and gently pats him dry, paying special attention to body creases. Application of body lotion to dry, cracked areas of the skin is soothing and provides important tactile stimulation.

PERINEAL CARE

Usually perineal care (pericare) is part of the complete bed bath (Procedure 32-3). Clients most in need of meticulous perineal care are those at greatest risk for acquiring an infection, for example, clients who have indwelling urinary catheters, are recovering from rectal or genital surgery, or have undergone childbirth. A client who is able to perform self-care should be allowed to do so. Many nurses are embarrassed about providing perineal care, particularly to clients of the opposite sex. Male nurses often seek out a female team member to provide hygiene to female clients, and vice versa. Embarrassment should not cause the nurse to overlook the client's hygiene needs. A professional, dignified attitude can reduce embarrassment and put the client at ease.

If a client performs self-care, various problems such as vaginal or urethral discharge, skin irritation, and unpleasant odors may go unnoticed. The nurse must be alert for complaints of burning during urination or localized soreness or pain in the perineum. The nurse also inspects bed linen for signs of discharge. Clients most at risk for skin breakdown in the perineal area are those with urinary or fecal incontinence, rectal and perineal surgical dressings, and indwelling urinary catheters.

BACKRUB

A backrub usually follows the client's bath. It promotes relaxation, relieves muscular tension, and stimulates skin circulation. During the backrub the nurse can assess the condition of the client's skin.

An effective backrub takes 3 to 5 minutes. The nurse should first inquire if the client would like a backrub because some clients dislike physical contact. The nurse should also consult the client's record for contraindications before offering a backrub (Procedure 32-4).

EVALUATION

During and at the completion of the client's bathing and skin care, the nurse evaluates success of the interventions. For each goal established in the plan of care,

Text continued on p. 830.

PROCEDURE 32-3

Perineal Care

STEPS	RATIONALE
1. Identify clients at risk for developing infection of genitalia, urinary tract, or reproductive tract (for example, presence of indwelling catheter, fecal incontinence, or surgical incision).	Secretions that accumulate on surface of skin surrounding female and male genitalia act as reservoir for infection. Traumatized tissues provide route for introduction of infectious organisms.
2. Explain procedure and its purpose to client.	Helps minimize anxiety during procedure that is often embarrassing to nurse and client.
3. Prepare necessary equipment and supplies:	Used when administering a bed bath.
a. Washbasin	
b. Soap dish with soap	
c. Two or three washcloths	
d. Bath towel	
e. Bath blanket	
f. Waterproof pad or bedpan	Prevents soiling of bed linen.
g. Toilet tissue	
h. Disposable gloves	Prevents contact with microorganisms in body secretions.
Additional supplies when pericare is given during times other than a bath:	
a. Cotton balls or swabs	Used for cleansing menstruating women or around indwelling catheters.
b. A solution bottle or container filled with warm water or prescribed rinsing solution	
c. Waterproof bag	For disposal of cotton balls.
4. Pull curtain around client's bed or close room door.	Maintains client's privacy.
5. Assemble supplies at bedside.	Ensures orderly procedure.
6. Raise bed to comfortable working position.	Facilitates good body mechanics.
7. Lower side rail and assist client in assuming dorsal recumbent (female) or supine (male) position.	Provides easy access to genitalia.
8. Female Perineal Care	
a. Position waterproof pad under client's buttocks or place bedpan under client.	Prevents bed linen from becoming wet.
b. Fold the top bed linen down toward foot of bed and raise the client's gown up above the genital area.	Exposes perineal area for easy accessibility.
c. Drape client by placing bath blanket with one corner between client's legs, one corner pointing toward each side of bed, and one corner over client's chest. Tuck side corners around client's legs and under hips (see illustrations).	Draping prevents unnecessary exposure of body part and maintains client's warmth and comfort during procedure.
d. Raise side rail. Fill washbasin with water that is approximately 41° to 43° C (105° to 109.4° F).	Prevents client from accidentally falling. Proper water temperature prevents burns to perineum.
e. Place washbasin and toilet tissue on overbed table. Place washcloths in basin.	Equipment placed within nurse's reach prevents accidental spills.

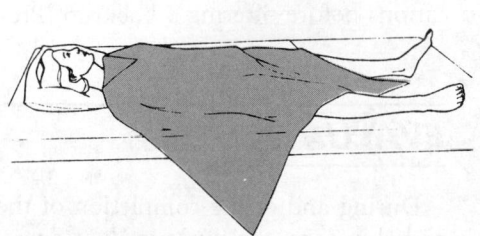 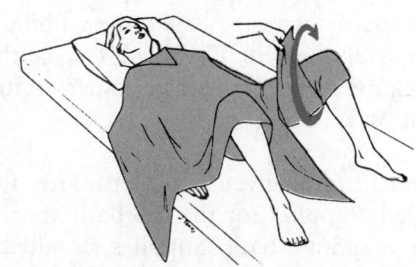

Step 8c

STEPS	RATIONALE
f. Lower side rail and help client flex her knees and spread her legs apart.	Provides full exposure of female genitalia.
g. Wash hand and apply disposable gloves. Fold lower corner of bath blanket up between client's legs onto her abdomen.	Minimizes transmission of microorganisms. Keeping client draped until procedure begins minimizes anxiety.
h. Wash and dry the client's upper thighs.	Buildup of perineal secretions can soil surrounding skin surfaces.
i. Wash the labia majora. Then use your nondominant hand to gently retract labia from thigh; with dominant hand, wash carefully in skinfolds. Wipe in direction from perineum to rectum. Repeat on opposite side using separate section of washcloth. Rinse and dry area thoroughly.	Skinfolds may contain body secretions that harbor microorganisms. Wiping from perineum to rectum reduces chance of transmitting fecal organisms to urinary meatus.
j. Separate labia with your nondominant hand to expose urethral meatus and vaginal orifice. With dominant hand, wash downward from pubic area toward rectum in one smooth stroke (see illustration). Use separate section of cloth for each stroke. Cleanse thoroughly around labia minora, clitoris, and vaginal orifice.	Cleansing method reduces transfer of microorganisms to urinary meatus. (For menstruating women or clients with indwelling urinary catheters, cleanse with cotton balls.)
k. If client is on bedpan, pour warm water over perineal area.	Rinsing removes soap and microorganisms more effectively than wiping.
l. Dry perineal area throughly.	Retained moisture harbors microorganisms.
m. Fold lower corner of bath blanket back between client's legs and over perineum. Ask client to lower legs and assume side-lying position.	Side-lying position provides access to anal area for cleansing.
n. Clean anal area by first wiping off fecal material with toilet tissue. Wash by wiping from vagina toward anus with one stroke. Discard washcloth. Repeat with clean cloth until skin is clear of fecal material (see illustration).	Fecal material contains large numbers of microorganisms that can cause vaginal or urinary tract infection.
o. Rinse area well and dry with bath towel.	Rinsing removes soap and microorganisms.
p. Remove disposable gloves and dispose in proper receptacle.	Moisture and body secretions on gloves can harbor microorganisms.
q. Assist client in assuming comfortable position and cover with sheet.	Client's comfort minimizes emotional stress of procedure.
r. Remove bath blanket and dispose of all soiled bed linen. Return unused equipment to storage area.	Reduces transmission of infection.

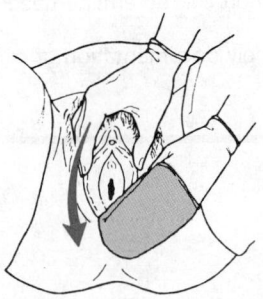

Step 8j

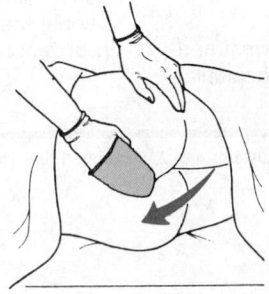

Step 8n

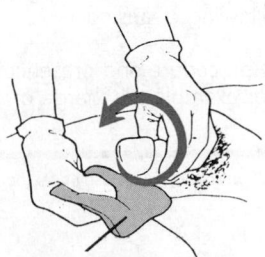

Disposable
washcloth

Step 9h

Continued.

PROCEDURE 32-3

Perineal Care

STEPS	RATIONALE
s. Raise side rail and lower bed to proper height. Return client's room to its condition before procedure.	Prevents client from accidentally falling. Clean environment enhances client's comfort.
t. Wash hands.	Reduces transmission of infection.
9. Male Perineal Care	
a. Position waterproof pad under client's buttocks.	Prevents bed linen from becoming wet.
b. Drape client by placing bath blanket with one corner between client's legs, one corner pointing toward each side of bed, and one corner over client's chest. Tuck side corners around client's legs and under hips.	Draping prevents unnecessary exposure of body parts and maintains client's warmth and comfort.
c. Raise side rail. Fill washbasin with water that is approximately 41° to 43° C (105° to 109.4° F).	Prevents client from accidentally falling. Proper water temperature prevents burns to perineum.
d. Place washbasin and toilet tissue on overbed table. Place washcloths in washbasin.	Easy access to supplies prevents accidental spills.
e. Lower side rail, wash hands, and apply disposable gloves.	Prevents nurse's exposure to and transmission of microorganisms.
f. Lower top corner of bath blanket below client's perineum. Gently raise penis and place bath towel underneath.	Towel prevents moisture from collecting in inguinal area.
g. Gently grasp shaft of penis. If client is uncircumcised, retract foreskin. If client has an erection, defer procedure until later.	Gentle handling reduces chance of client having an erection. Secretions capable of harboring microorganisms collect underneath foreskin.
h. Wash tip of penis at urethral meatus first. Using circular motion, cleanse from meatus outward. Discard washcloth and repeat with clean cloth until penis is clean. Rinse and dry gently (see illustration).	Direction of cleansing moves from area of least contamination to area of most contamination, preventing microorganisms from entering urethra.
i. Return foreskin to its natural position.	Tightening of foreskin around shaft of penis can cause local edema and discomfort.
j. Wash shaft of penis with gentle but firm downward strokes. Pay special attention to underlying surface of penis.	Vigorous massage of penis can lead to erection, which can cause embarrassment for client and nurse. Underlying surface of penis may have greater accumulation of secretions.
k. Rinse and dry penis thoroughly. Instruct client to spread his legs apart slightly.	Abduction of legs provides easier access to scrotal tissues.
l. Gently cleanse scrotum. Lift it carefully and wash underlying skinfolds. Rinse and dry.	Pressure on scrotal tissues can be very painful to client. Secretions collect between skinfolds.
m. Fold bath blanket back over client's perineum and assist client in turning to side-lying position.	Draping promotes comfort and minimizes client's anxiety. Side-lying position provides access to anal area.
n. Clean anal area following Steps n-t of female perineal care.	
10. Inspect surface of external genitalia and surrounding skin following cleansing.	Thick secretions may cover underlying skin lesions or areas of breakdown. Evaluation can determine need for additional therapy.
11. Record procedure and presence of any abnormal findings (for example, discharge or condition of genitalia).	Ensures accurate and timely documentation of care.

Illustrations from Sorrentino, SA: Mosby's textbook for nursing assistants, ed. 2, St. Louis, 1987, The C.V. Mosby Co.

PROCEDURE 32-4

Administering a Backrub

STEPS	RATIONALE
1. Identify factors or conditions such as rib or vertebral fractures, burns, or open wounds that contraindicate a backrub.	Massage of sensitive tissues might lead to further tissue injury.
2. For clients with history of hypertension or dysrhythmias, assess pulse and blood pressure.	Massage may cause autonomic nervous system stimulation that induces changes in heart rate and blood pressure. Research has not shown consistent relationships between human touch and the cardiac response of those being touched (Weiss, 1986).
3. Explain procedure and desired position to the client.	Helps promote relaxation.
4. Prepare necessary equipment and supplies: a. Bath blanket b. Bath towel c. Skin application (lotion, alcohol, or powder)	Lotion lubricates skin and prevents friction during massage. Alcohol cools skin but has drying effect. Powder reduces friction during massage.
5. Adjust bed to high, comfortable position.	Ensures proper body mechanics and prevents strain on nurse's back muscles.
6. Adjust light, temperature, and sound within room.	Environmental distractions can prevent client from relaxing.
7. Lower side rail and help client assume either prone or side-lying (Sims') position with back toward nurse. Close curtain around bed.	Position makes it easier to apply necessary pressure to back muscles. Privacy promotes client's relaxation.
8. Expose client's back, shoulders, upper arms, and buttocks. Cover remainder of body with bath blanket. Lay towel alongside client's back.	Prevents unnecessary exposure of body parts.
9. Wash your hands in warm water. Warm lotion either in your hands or by placing container under warm water. Place small amount of lotion in hands.	Cold causes muscle tension.
10. Explain to client that lotion will feel cool and wet.	Warning client reduces startle response.
11. Apply hands first to sacral area, massaging in circular motion. Stroke upward from buttocks to shoulders. Massage over scapulas with smooth, firm stroke. Continue in one smooth stroke to upper arms and laterally along sides of back down to iliac crests. Do not allow your hands to leave client's skin. Continue massage pattern for 3 min.	Gentle, firm pressure applied to all muscle groups promotes relaxation. Continuous contact with skin's surface is soothing and stimulates circulation to tissues.
12. Knead skin by grasping tissue between your thumb and fingers. Knead upward along one side of spine from buttocks to shoulders and around nape of neck. Knead or stroke downward toward sacrum. Repeat along other side of back.	Kneading increases circulation to muscles. Continuous motion is soothing and relieves muscle tension.
13. End massage with long stroking movements and tell client you are ending massage.	Long stroking is most soothing of massage movements.
14. If lying on side, ask client to turn to opposite side, and massage other hip.	
15. Wipe excess lubricant from client's back with bath towel. Retie gown or assist with pajamas. Help client to comfortable position. Open curtain and raise side rails as needed.	Excess lotion can be an irritant. Comfortable position enhances backrub's effects.
16. Dipose of soiled towel and wash your hands.	These measures promote infection control.
17. Ask client about comfort or note any areas of muscle pain or tension.	Degree of relief gained will depend on length of massage, client's ability to relax, and degree of discomfort before massage.
18. Reassess pulse and blood pressure.	Gentle back massage may increase heart rate and systolic blood pressure.
19. Record client's response to massage and condition of skin.	Accurate documentation describes client's response to therapy.

Sample Evaluation of Interventions for Clients Needing Skin Care

Goals	Evaluative Measures	Expected Outcomes
Skin will remain intact and free of odors.	Inspect surfaces of skin after cleansing. Inspect existing lesions for cleanliness and reduction in drainage. Take time to note presence of obvious body odors.	Skin is intact, warm, smooth, soft, and well hydrated. Areas of skin impairment show signs of healing (for example, reduced drainage or inflammation). Odors are reduced or eliminated.
Joint range of motion is maintained.	Exercise joint through range of motion during bathing of body part.	Joints move within same range of motion as client's baseline. Normal joints move freely without discomfort.
Client achieves sense of comfort and well-being.	Question client about sense of comfort. Observe client's body movements or gestures.	Client verbalizes less discomfort and sense of relaxation. Client is calm. Body movements are purposeful and relaxed. Client expresses positive statements about sense of well-being.
Client participates in and understands methods of skin care.	Observe client's initiation of and assistance with bathing activities. Observe if client asks questions regarding self-care measures. Ask client to explain proper technique to follow in bathing.	Client initiates hygiene measures or participates in bathing with nurse's assistance. Client describes proper hygienic methods to maintain skin integrity.

the nurse evaluates accomplishment of expected outcomes. Evaluation involves physical assessment measures, as well as questions directed toward the client (see evaluation box).

CARE OF THE FEET AND NAILS

The feet and nails often require special attention to prevent infection, odors, and injury to tissues. Often people are unaware of foot or nail problems until pain or discomfort occurs. Problems result from abuse or poor care of the feet and hands such as biting nails or trimming them improperly, exposure to harsh chemicals, and wearing ill-fitting shoes.

The feet are important to a person's physical and emotional health. Foot pain can cause a person to walk differently, causing strain on different muscle groups. Many people must walk or stand comfortably to perform their jobs effectively. Poor job performance can lead to emotional stress.

ASSESSMENT

PHYSICAL ASSESSMENT

Assessment of the feet involves a thorough examination of all skin surfaces, the shape, size, and number of toes, the shape of the foot, and the condition of the toenails. The nurse inspects for presence of lesions and notes whether areas of dryness, inflammation, or cracking are present. The areas between the toes should be carefully checked. The heels, soles, and sides of the feet are prone to irritation from ill-fitting shoes. The toes are normally straight and flat. The feet should be in straight alignment with the ankle and tibia. Table 32-3 reviews common types of foot and nail problems.

It is also important to assess the client's gait. Painful disorders of the feet can cause limping or an unnatural gait. The nurse asks if the client has discomfort of the feet and what factors aggravate the pain. Foot problems may result from bone or muscular alterations rather than skin disorders.

Clients with peripheral vascular disease, such as those with diabetes, should be assessed for adequacy of circulation to the feet. Chapter 13 describes the signs of

TABLE 32-3   Common Foot and Nail Problems

Condition	Characteristics	Implications	Interventions
Callus	Thickened portion of epidermis, consisting of a mass of horny, keratotic cells; usually flat, painless, and found on undersurface of foot or on palm of hand; caused by local friction or pressure	Condition may cause discomfort when wearing tight-fitting shoes.	Advise the client to wear gloves when using tools or objects that may create friction on palmar surfaces. Encourage the client to wear comfortable shoes. Soak callus in warm water and Epsom salts to soften cell layers. Use a pumice stone to remove callus after it softens. Applications of creams or lotions can reduce reformation.
Corns	Keratosis caused by friction and pressure from shoes; seen mainly on toes, over a bony prominence; usually cone shaped, round, and raised	Conical shape compresses underlying dermis, making it thin and tender. Pain is aggravated when tight-fitting shoes are worn. Tissue can become attached to bone if allowed to grow. Client may suffer alteration in gait owing to pain.	Surgical removal may be necessary depending on severity of pain and size of corn. Avoid use of oval corn pads, which increase pressure on toes and reduce circulation.
Plantar warts	Fungating lesion that appears on sole of foot; caused by papilloma virus	Warts may be contagious. They are painful and make walking difficult.	Treatment ordered by physician may include applications of salicylic acid, electrodesiccation (burning with an electrical spark), or freezing with solid carbon dioxide.
Athlete's foot (tinea pedis)	Fungal infection of the foot; scaliness and cracking of skin between toes and on soles of feet; small blister containing fluid may appear; apparently induced by wearing of constricting footwear, for example, sneakers	Athlete's foot can spread to other body parts, especially the hands. It is contagious and frequently recurs.	Feet should be well ventilated. Drying feet well after bathing and applying powder help prevent infection. Wearing of clean socks or stockings reduces incidence. Physician may order application of griseofulvin, miconazole, or tolnaftate.
Ingrown nails	Toenail or fingernail growing inward into soft tissue around nail; often results from improper nail trimming	Ingrown nails can cause localized pain when pressure is applied.	Treatment is frequent hot soaks in antiseptic solution and removal of portion of nail that has grown into the skin. Instruct the client on proper nail trimming techniques.
Ram's horn nails	Unusually long curved nails	Attempt by nurse to cut nails may result in damage to nail bed with risk of infection.	Refer the client to a podiatrist.
Paronychia	Inflammation of tissue surrounding nail after a hangnail or other injury; occurs in people who frequently have their hands in water; common in diabetic clients	Area can become infected.	Treatment is hot compresses or soaks and local application of antibiotic ointments. Paronychia can be prevented by careful manicuring.
Foot odors	Result of excess perspiration promoting microorganism growth	Condition may cause discomfort due to excess perspiration.	Frequent washing, use of foot deodorants and powders, and wearing clean footwear will prevent or reduce this problem.

arterial and venous insufficiency. Palpation of the dorsalis pedis and posterior tibial pulses indicates whether adequate blood flow is reaching peripheral tissues. Edema and changes in skin color, texture, and temperature can indicate that the client is in need of special hygienic care.

If a client is diabetic the nurse should also check for neuropathy, which is a degeneration of the peripheral nerves characterized by a loss in sensation. This is done by checking the client's sensation to light touch, pin prick, and temperature (see Chapter 13). The nails of the feet and hands are assessed using inspection and palpation.

A normal healthy nail is transparent, smooth, and convex with pink nail beds and translucent white tips. In black clients, a brown or black pigmentation is normally present between the nail and nail base. The nail is surrounded by a cuticle, which slowly grows over the nail and must be regularly pushed back. The skin around the nail beds and cuticles should be smooth and without inflammation. The nurse asks female clients if they frequently polish their nails and use polish remover, since chemicals in these products cause excessive nail dryness. Disease can change the shape and curvature of nails (see Chapter 13). Inflammatory lesions of the nail bed cause the formation of thickened, horny nails, which can separate from the nail bed.

DEVELOPMENTAL FACTORS

The nurse's assessment considers the special needs of the elderly, who often are unable to maintain proper foot and nail care. Noting the presence of poor vision, hand tremors, obesity, or the inability to bend over will reveal the level of assistance required by the elderly client. If foot or nail problems stay unresolved, an elderly person can easily become disabled. The nurse also assesses common problems of the aged. They often have dry feet because of a decrease in sebaceous gland secretion, dehydration of epidermal cells, and poor condition of footwear. Fissures that result in itching commonly develop. Fungal infections commonly occur under toenails, causing dirty yellow streaks or total discoloration. The nails also become opaque, scaly, and hypertrophied.

If an elderly client has chronic foot problems, the nurse should assess the type of home remedies used. Many over-the-counter preparations, such as those to treat corns, can damage normal skin layers. Burns or ulcerations resulting from these products increase the risk of infection.

FOOTWEAR

The types of footwear worn can predispose clients to foot and nail problems. Children or young adults who frequently fail to wear socks may have excess perspiration that promotes fungal growth. Tight or ill-fitting shoes or socks may cause certain skin lesions and interfere with circulation in the feet. The nurse also assesses whether clients wear clean footwear daily, since repeated use of soiled footwear can lead to infection. Shoes should fit snugly, not tightly, and provide support for the arch of the foot. When the person stands, shoes should be at least ½ inch longer than the largest toe, and wide enough to accommodate a weight-bearing foot. The widest part of the foot should match the widest part of the shoe (Graham and Morley, 1984).

KNOWLEDGE OF FOOT AND NAIL CARE PRACTICES

The nurse determines a client's knowledge about foot and nail care to assess educational needs. Does the client

Sample Nursing Diagnoses for Foot and Nail Problems

Defining Characteristics	Nursing Diagnoses	Related Factors
Inflammation of soft tissues surrounding nail Pull or tear in the skin Tenderness of tissues	Impaired skin integrity	• Injury to nail • Poor nail-care practices
Abnormal gait Inability to bear weight on foot Restricted movements	Impaired physical mobility	• Foot lesion • Ill-fitting shoes
Excess moisture around toes Foot odors Cracking of skin between toes Reduced arterial pulses	Potential impaired skin integrity	• Ill-fitting shoes • Poor hygiene practices • Impaired arterial perfusion

Examples of Nursing Diagnoses Related to Foot and Nail Problems

NANDA-APPROVED NURSING DIAGNOSES

Pain related to:
- Callus formation
- Ingrown toenails

Impaired physical mobility related to:
- Painful foot lesion

Bathing/hygiene self-care deficit related to:
- Visual disturbance
- Altered hand coordination

Impaired skin integrity related to:
- Impaired arterial perfusion
- Improper nail-cutting practices
- Friction of shoes
- Injury to nails

Potential impaired skin integrity related to:
- Impaired arterial perfusion
- Ill-fitting footwear

Potential for infection related to:
- Broken or traumatized skin

Knowledge deficit about foot/nail care related to:
- Information misinterpretation
- Lack of exposure to information

know how to cut nails? Does the client use over-the-counter products for nail care and grooming? It is especially important to assess the knowledge of diabetic clients because they must inspect their feet daily. Because of vascular insufficiency and neuropathy, a diabetic is at risk for injury to the feet. Any trauma to a diabetic's foot can easily lead to infection.

NURSING DIAGNOSIS

An assessment of the condition of a client's feet and nails will reveal the presence of any actual or potential health problems. The sample nursing diagnoses box lists the defining characteristics for select nursing diagnoses. As in the case with skin care, the nature of a client's foot or nail problems directs the nurse to perform supportive or preventive nursing care. Examples of nursing diagnoses are shown in the nursing diagnoses box.

PLANNING

The nurse may provide foot and nail care during the client's bed bath or at a separate time in the day according to the client's preference. Many community health nurses visit clients at home solely to provide foot and nail care. See the care plan box for an example.

If a client's nails are extremely hard or if a client is unable to perform personal nail care, a podiatrist can provide nail care. The podiatrist is trained in the treatment of nail and foot problems.

Goals for clients receiving nail and foot care include:
1. Skin and nail surfaces will remain intact and smooth.
2. Client achieves sense of comfort and cleanliness.
3. Client walks and bears weight normally.
4. Client understands and performs methods for foot and nail care correctly.

Sample Nursing Care Plan for Foot and Nail Problems

Nursing Diagnosis	Goals	Expected Outcomes	Nursing Interventions
Impaired physical mobility related to foot lesion	Client walks and bears weight normally.	Client wears shoes and walks in a normal gait. Client denies discomfort during walking or bearing weight.	Soak feet daily, cleanse thoroughly, and dry. Apply baby oil to dry areas. Trim client's nails weekly. Inspect client's existing shoes and make recommendations for a properly fitting pair.
	Client understands and performs regular foot care.	Client describes proper foot care practices.	Instruct client about method of inspecting condition of feet daily.
		Client selects proper footwear to minimize foot problems.	Instruct client about cleansing feet and nail trimming.

Nail and Foot Care

STEPS	RATIONALE
1. Identify clients at risk for foot or nail problems including:	
a. Elderly clients	Changes in sensory and motor function with aging impair self-care practices. Physiological changes of aging alter condition of foot and nails.
b. Clients with diabetes	Vascular changes associated with diabetes reduce blood flow to peripheral tissues.
c. Clients with heart failure or renal disease	These conditions can cause tissue edema and reduced blood flow to extremeties.
d. Clients who have had a cerebrovascular accident or stroke	Residual paralysis or reduced sensation can cause abnormal walking patterns resulting in friction and pressure on feet.
2. Obtain physician's order for cutting nails if agency policy requires it.	Client's skin may be accidentally cut. Certain clients are more at risk for infection depending on their medical condition.
3. Explain procedure to client, including fact that proper soaking requires several minutes.	Client must be willing to place fingers and feet in basins for 10-20 min. Client may become anxious or fatigued.
4. Prepare necessary equipment and supplies:	

4. Prepare necessary equipment and supplies:

a. Washbasin	g. Emery board
b. Emesis basin	h. Body lotion
c. Washcloth	i. Disposable bath mat
d. Bath or face towel	j. Paper towels
e. Nail clippers	k. Disposable gloves (optional)
f. Orange stick	

STEPS	RATIONALE
5. Wash hands. Arrange equipment on overbed table.	Easy access to equipment prevents delays. Reduces transmission of infection.
6. Pull curtain around bed or close room door (if desired).	Maintaining client's privacy reduces anxiety.
7. Assist client to bedside chair if possible. Place disposable bath mat on floor under client's feet. Place call light within client's reach.	Sitting in chair makes it easier to immerse feet in basin. Bath mat protects feet from exposure to soil or debris. Call light maintains safety of environment.
8. Fill wash basin with water at 43°-44° C (100°-110° F). Test temperature of water.	Warm water softens nails and thickened epidermal cells, reduces inflammation of skin, and promotes local circulation. Proper water temperature prevents burns of skin.
9. Place basin on bath mat and help client place the feet in basin.	Clients with muscular weakness or tremors may have difficulty positioning feet.
10. Adjust overbed table to low position and place it over client's lap.	Easy access prevents accidental spills.
11. Fill the emesis basin with water at 43°-44° C (100°-110° F) and place basin on paper towels on overbed table.	Warm water softens nails and thickened epidermal cells.
12. Instruct client to place fingers in emesis basin and place his or her arms in comfortable position.	Prolonged positioning can cause discomfort unless normal anatomical alignment is maintained.
13. Allow client's feet and fingernails to soak for 10-20 min. Rewarm water in 5 minutes if needed.	Softening of corns, calluses, and cuticles ensures easy removal of dead cells and easy manipulation of cuticle.
14. Clean gently under fingernails with orange stick while fingers are immersed. Then remove emesis basin and dry fingers thoroughly.	Orange stick removes debris under nails that harbors microorganisms. Thorough drying impedes fungal growth and prevents maceration of tissues.
15. With nail clippers, clip fingernails straight across and even with tops of fingers. Shape nails with emery board.	Cutting straight across prevents splitting of nail margins and formation of sharp nail spikes that can irritate lateral nail margins. Filing prevents cutting nail too close to nail bed.
16. Push cuticle back gently with orange stick.	Reduces incidence of inflamed cuticles.
17. Move overbed table away from client.	Provides easier access to feet.

STEPS	RATIONALE
18. Put on disposable gloves (optional) and scrub callused areas of feet with washcloth.	Gloves prevent transmission of fungal infection. Friction removes dead skin layers.
19. Clean gently under nails with orange stick. Remove feet from basin and dry them thoroughly.	Removal of debris and excess moisture reduces chances of infection.
20. Clean and trim toenails using procedures in Steps 15 and 16.	
21. Apply lotion to feet and hands and then assist client back to bed and into comfortable position.	Lotion lubricates dry skin by helping to retain moisture.
22. Remove disposable gloves and dispose in receptacle. Clean and return equipment and supplies to proper place. Dispose of soiled linen in hamper. Wash hands.	Prevents transmission of infection.
23. Inspect nails and surrounding skin after soaking and nail trimming.	Evaluates condition of skin. Allows nurse to note any rough nail edges remaining.
24. Record procedure and observations. Report any breaks in the skin.	Documents procedure and client's response. Abnormalities may pose risk of infection.

IMPLEMENTATION

Foot and nail care involves soaking to soften cuticles and layers of horny cells, thorough cleansing, drying, and proper trimming of nails. The nurse may provide the care in bed for an immobilized client or have the client sit in a chair (Procedure 32-5). The nurse must take time during the procedure to teach the client proper techniques for cleaning and nail trimming and tips on selecting proper footwear. By allowing the client to perform a part of foot and nail care, the nurse can stress principles related to preventing infection and tissue injury.

A diabetic client or one with peripheral vascular disease is at risk for foot and nail problems. A diabetic has a poor peripheral blood supply to the feet. In addition, sensation in the feet can become reduced. Any trauma to a diabetic's foot can often go unnoticed. With a break in the skin, infection can easily develop as a result of poor circulation. The nurse can advise these clients to use the following guidelines:

1. Wash and soak the feet daily using lukewarm water. Thoroughly pat the feet dry, and dry well between the toes.
2. Do not cut corns or calluses or use commercial removers. Consult a physician or podiatrist.
3. If the feet tend to perspire apply a bland foot powder.
4. If dryness is noted along the feet or between the toes, apply lanolin, baby oil, or even corn oil and rub gently into the skin.
5. File the toenails straight across and square; do not use scissors or clippers. Consult a podiatrist as needed.
6. Do not use over-the-counter preparations to treat athlete's foot or ingrown toenails. Consult a physician or podiatrist.
7. Teach the client to avoid wearing elastic stockings, knee-high hose, or constricting garters and not to cross the legs. Both impair circulation to the lower extremities.
8. Inspect the feet daily, including tops and soles of the feet, heels, and the area between the toes.
9. Wear clean socks or stockings daily. Socks should be free of holes or darns that might cause pressure.
10. Do not walk barefoot.
11. Wear properly fitting shoes. Soles of shoes should be flexible and nonslipping. Lamb's wool can be used between toes that rub or overlap. Shoes should be sturdy, closed in, and not restrictive to the feet.
12. Exercise regularly to improve circulation to the lower extremities: walk slowly, elevate, rotate, flex, and extend the feet at the ankle. Dangle the feet over the side of the bed 1 minute, then extend both legs and hold them parallel to the bed while lying supine for 1 minute, and finally rest 1 minute (Jordan and Nickerson, 1982).

Sample Evaluation of Interventions for Foot and Nail Problems

Goals	Evaluative Measures	Expected Outcomes
Skin and nail surfaces will remain intact and smooth.	Inspect integrity of skin surrounding nails and palpate the contour and smoothness of nail edges.	Skin will be smooth without cuts. Nails are short and straight without split ends.
	Inspect condition of cuticles.	Cuticles are intact. Previously inflamed tissues become less reddened and tender.
Client achieves sense of comfort and cleanliness.	Ask client about sense of comfort following nail and foot care.	Client verbalizes feeling clean and comfortable.
Client walks and bears weight normally.	Observe client's gait.	Wears shoes and walks normal gait.
	Note client's facial expression while walking or weight bearing.	Denies discomfort during walking or weight bearing.
	Ask client if pain is experienced while walking or standing.	
Client understands and performs methods of foot and nail care.	Observe client perform nail and foot care.	Client performs nail and foot care correctly.
	Ask client to describe techniques for cutting nails, cleansing feet, and to identify type of footwear to be worn.	Client describes proper nail and foot care practices. Client takes steps to prevent nail or foot problems.

13. Avoid applying hot-water bottles or heating pads to the feet. Use warm soaks or extra coverings instead.
14. Any minor cuts should be washed immediately and dried thoroughly. Only mild antiseptics, for example, neosporin ointment, should be applied to the skin. Avoid iodine or mercurochrome. Contact a physician for treatment of cuts or lacerations.

EVALUATION

A client's response to nail and foot care is best evaluated over several days. If the client has any existing problems, it may take time for the alterations to improve. The nurse also instructs the client on ways to evaluate personal nail and foot care practices. The evaluation box outlines the evaluation of nail and foot care.

ORAL HYGIENE

The oral cavity is lined with mucous membrane continuous with the skin. The membrane is an epithelial tissue that lines and protects organs, secretes mucous to keep passageways of the digestive system moist and lubricated, and absorbs nutrients.

The oral or buccal cavity consists of the lips surrounding the opening of the mouth, the cheeks running along the side walls of the cavity, the tongue and its muscles, and the hard and soft palate forming the roof of the cavity. The oral mucosa is normally light pink and moist. The teeth are the organs of chewing or mastication. A normal tooth consists of three parts: crown, neck, and root (Fig. 32-1). The crown, covered by a layer of enamel, is the exposed portion of a tooth. Enamel is the hardest tissue in the body and is suited to the cutting, tearing, and grinding movement of teeth. The neck of a tooth is the narrow portion surrounded by the gums or gingivae. The root of a tooth is the portion that fits into the jaw's socket. The periodontal membrane lies just below the gum margins and surrounds a tooth and holds it firmly in place. The dentin makes up the greatest part of a tooth's shell and contains the pulp cavity that houses connective tissue, blood and lymphatic vessels, and sensory nerves. Healthy teeth appear white, smooth, shiny, and properly aligned.

Oral hygiene helps maintain the healthy state of the mouth, teeth, gums, and lips. Brushing cleans the teeth of food particles, plaque, and bacteria, massages the gums, and relieves discomfort resulting from unpleasant odors and tastes. Flossing further helps to remove plaque

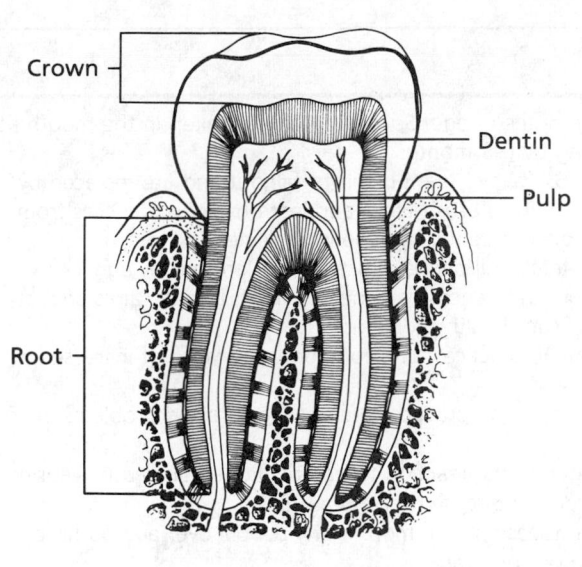

Fig. 32-1   A normal tooth.

and tartar between teeth to reduce gum inflammation and infection. Complete oral hygiene gives a sense of well-being and thus can stimulate appetite.

The nurse's responsibilities in oral hygiene are maintenance and prevention. The nurse can help clients maintain good oral hygiene by teaching them correct techniques or by actually performing hygiene for weakened or disabled clients. Often the nurse must make referrals to a dentist for problems requiring special care. Educating clients about common gum and tooth disorders and methods of prevention can motivate them to follow good oral hygiene practices.

ASSESSMENT

PHYSICAL ASSESSMENT

Chapter 13 describes in detail the assessment of the lips, teeth, buccal mucosa, gums, palate, and tongue. The nurse inspects all areas carefully for color, hydration, texture, and presence of lesions. Clients who do not follow regular oral hygiene practices may have receding gum tissue, inflamed gums, discolored teeth (particularly along gum margins), dental caries, missing teeth, and halitosis. Localized pain is a common symptom of gum disease and certain tooth disorders. Whenever palpating lesions in the mouth, the nurse must wear gloves and wash hands thoroughly before and after the examination. Infection of the mouth may involve organisms such as *Treponema pallidum, Neisseria gonorrhoeae,* and herpesvirus hominis.

DEVELOPMENTAL CHANGES

Throughout a person's life span, physiological changes affect the condition and appearance of structures in the oral cavity (Table 32-4). As a person grows older, oral hygiene practices change to further influence the teeth and mucosa. Assessment of a client's developmental level helps in determining the types of hygiene problems to expect.

HYGIENE PREFERENCES AND PRACTICES

The nurse assesses the client's oral hygiene practices to identify errors in technique, deficiencies in types of practices, and the client's knowledge level about dental care. Some helpful questions include the following:

1. How often does the client brush his or her teeth?
2. What type of toothpaste or dentifrice is used?
3. Does the client have dentures? When and how are they cleaned?
4. Does the client use mouthwash or lemon-glycerin preparations?
5. Does the client floss? If so, how often?
6. When was the client's last dental visit?
7. How often does the client visit a dentist?

Asking the client to demonstrate brushing and flossing techniques will be useful when developing a teaching plan.

RISK FACTORS FOR ORAL HYGIENE PROBLEMS

Certain clients are at risk for oral problems because of lack of knowledge about oral hygiene, an inability to perform oral care, or an alteration in the integrity of teeth and mucosa resulting from disease or treatments (Table 32-5).

COMMON ORAL PROBLEMS

It helps a nurse to be familiar with common oral problems. Each problem presents recognizable signs and symptoms and influences not only the type of hygiene but also the type of teaching the nurse must provide.

The two major types of real problems are dental caries (cavities) and periodontal disease (pyorrhea). *Dental caries* is the most common oral problem of younger people. The development of cavities is a pathological process that involves the eventual destruction of the tooth enamel through decalcification. Decalcification is a result of an accumulation of mucin, carbohydrates, and lactic acid bacilli in the saliva normally found in the mouth, which forms a coating on the teeth called *plaque.* Plaque is transparent and colorless and adheres to the teeth, particularly near the base of the crown at the gum margins. The plaque prevents normal acid dilution and neutralization and thus prevents the dissolution of bacteria in the oral cavity. The acid eventually destroys the tooth enamel and in severe cases the pulp or inner spongy tissue of the tooth. A cavity first begins as a chalky white

TABLE 32-4 Physiological Development of the Mouth

Developmental Level	Changes
Infant	Deciduous teeth begin to erupt at about 5 months of age. Solid food can be taken in the mouth at 5-6 months of age with chewing beginning by 6-8 months.
18 months-6 years	Twenty deciduous teeth are present. By age 6, "baby" teeth begin to fall out and are replaced by the permanent teeth. By age 2, child can begin to brush teeth and learn hygiene practices from parents. Dental caries may becomes a problem if dental hygiene is neglected.
6-12 years	Deciduous teeth are replaced by permanent teeth. All permanent teeth are present by age 12 except second and third molars. Definite food preferences become apparent. Dental caries and irregularity in the spacing of teeth are significant health problems.
12-18 years	All permanent teeth are present. Dental hygiene practices tend to improve because of increased awareness of body image.
18-40 years	Third molars appear. Good oral hygiene and nutrition practices are needed to avoid problems in later years.
Pregnancy	Changes in female sex hormones may exaggerate the reaction to irritants in dental plaque, causing gingivitis and increased risk of severe peridontal disease (Deliefde, 1984).
40-65 years	Loss of teeth, usually a result of periodontal disease, is common. Many people over age 55 have lost some or all of their teeth because of poor oral care.
65 years and over	Aging teeth become brittle, drier, and darker in color. Teeth become uneven, jagged, and fractured after years of crushing and grinding. Gums lose vascularity and tissue elasticity, causing dentures to fit poorly. Eating habits often change, and malnutrition may be a problem.

TABLE 32-5 Risk Factors for Oral Problems

Type of Client	Risk Factors
Clients who are paralyzed, seriously ill, or have physical restrictions to upper extremities (for example, cast or dressing).	Lacks upper extremity strength or dexterity needed to perform oral hygiene.
Unconscious, confused, combative, or depressed clients.	Unable or unwilling to attend to personal hygiene needs.
Diabetic clients.	Prone to dryness of mouth, gingivitis, periodontal disease, and loss of teeth.
Clients who are on fluid restrictions (see Chapter 37), have nasogastric tubes, receive continuous nasal oxygen, or are mouth-breathers.	Prone to dehydration and drying of mucous membranes. Thick secretions develop on the tongue and gums. Lips become cracked and reddened.
Clients undergoing radiation therapy.	Causes soreness, dysphagia, dryness, and taste changes.
Clients receiving chemotherapeutic drugs.	Cause ulcerations and inflammation of the mucosa.
Clients experiencing oral surgery, trauma to the mouth, placement of oral endotracheal tubes or airways.	Tissues in oral cavity become traumatized with swelling, ulcerations, inflammation, and possible bleeding.

discoloration of the tooth. As the cavity advances, the tooth takes on a brown or black discoloration.

For people more than 35 years of age, the most common oral problem is *periodontal disease* or pyorrhea. Periodontal disease is a long-term process involving infection and destruction of the supporting structures of the teeth: the gingivae (gums), cementum, ligaments, and alveolar bone. Periodontal disease progresses in four stages: (1) gingivitis or inflammation of the gums, (2) periodontitis, (3) acute necrotizing ulcerative gingivitis, and (4) destruction of the tooth-supporting structure (Levine, 1973). Symptoms of periodontal disease include bleeding gums, swollen inflamed tissues, receding gumlines with the formation of gaps or pockets between the teeth and gums, and the eventual loss of teeth. If proper oral care is not maintained, dead bacteria, called tartar, can collect at the gumline. The tartar attacks the gums and fibers attached to the teeth, resulting in lost teeth. The best preventive measures are regular flossing and brushing.

Other oral problems include *stomatitis,* an inflammatory condition of the mouth resulting from contact with irritants such as tobacco or from vitamin deficiency, infection by bacteria, viruses, or fungi, or use of chemotherapeutic drugs; *glossitis,* an inflammation of the tongue resulting from infectious disease or injury from a burn, bite, or other injury; and *gingivitis,* an inflammation of the gums usually resulting from poor oral hygiene or occurring as a sign of leukemia, vitamin deficiency, or diabetes mellitus.

Sample Nursing Diagnoses for Oral Hygiene Problems

Defining Characteristics	Nursing Diagnoses	Related Factors
Coated tongue Oral lesions Dry mouth Stomatitis Halitosis Tooth caries	Altered oral mucous membrane	• Radiation of oral cavity • Ineffective oral hygiene • Mouth breathing • Fluid restrictions
Unable to explain proper oral hygiene practices Brushes teeth incorrectly Requests information about oral hygiene	Knowledge deficit about oral hygiene	• Misunderstanding of hygiene practices • Lack of exposure to information on hygiene care
Oral lesions Dry mouth Buildup of plaque along gum margins Bleeding of gums or mucosa	Potential for infection	• Ineffective hygiene practices • Ill-fitting dentures • Oral mucosa trauma

Halitosis (bad breath) is a common problem of the oral cavity. It may be the result of poor oral hygiene, ingestion of certain foods, or an infection or disease process. Proper oral hygiene can eliminate the odors unless the cause is a systemic condition such as liver disease or diabetes.

The nurse frequently encounters *cheilosis* in clients. The disorder involves cracking of the lips, especially at the angle of the mouth. Riboflavin deficiency, mouth breathing, and excess salivation may cause cheilosis. Lubrication of the lips helps retain moisture, and antifungal or antibacterial ointments discourage microorganism growth.

A final problem the nurse should be able to recognize is *oral malignancy*. Malignancies appear as lumps or ulcers in or around the mouth. They are commonly found in clients with a history of pipe smoking or use of chewing tobacco. The most common site is at the base of the tongue. Early detection of oral cancers is vital to the success of treatment. Any sore in the mouth that does not heal should be brought to the attention of a dentist.

NURSING DIAGNOSIS

The nurse's assessment may reveal actual or potential alterations in the integrity of mouth structures (see sample nursing diagnoses box). Likewise, pertinent nursing diagnoses may reflect problems or complications result-

Examples of Nursing Diagnoses Related to Oral Hygiene Problems

NANDA-APPROVED NURSING DIAGNOSES

Altered oral mucous membrane related to:
• Oral trauma
• Restricted fluid intake
• Ineffective oral hygiene

Pain related to:
• Gingivitis
• Loose teeth

Altered nutrition: less than body requirements related to:
• Ill-fitting dentures
• Gingivitis

Bathing/hygiene self-care deficit related to:
• Altered level of consciousness
• Upper extremity weakness

Body-image disturbance related to:
• Halitosis
• Absence of teeth

Knowledge deficit about oral hygiene related to:
• Misunderstanding hygiene practices

Potential for infection related to:
• Oral mucosa trauma

ing from alterations of the oral cavity. The nurse's findings may also reveal a client's need for assistance with hygienic care. Examples of nursing diagnoses related to oral hygiene are shown in the nursing diagnoses box.

PLANNING

Developing a care plan for clients in need of oral hygiene involves considering the client's personal preferences, emotional status, and physical capabilities. The nurse must establish a good relationship with the client to assist with oral hygiene practices. Some clients are very sensitive about the condition of their mouths and are reluctant to let someone else care for them. In many cases clients are also unaware that they are at risk for serious dental and periodontal disease and thus require extensive education (see care plan box).

Goals for clients in need of oral hygiene include the following:
1. Oral mucosa is intact and well hydrated.
2. Teeth are without new dental caries.
3. Client is able independently to perform correct oral hygiene care.
4. Client achieves sense of comfort.
5. Client understands oral hygiene practices.

IMPLEMENTATION

ORAL HYGIENE

Good oral hygiene requires preventive and therapeutic measures. Proper care will prevent oral disease and tooth

destruction. Clients in hospitals or long-term care facilities often do not receive the aggressive care they need. Oral care must be provided on a regular daily basis, with frequency of hygiene measures dependent on the condition of the client's oral cavity.

Brushing, flossing, and irrigation are necessary for proper cleansing. Clients will also benefit from a proper diet, which excludes foods promoting plaque formation and tooth decay and promotes healthy periodontal structures. Clients of all ages should have a dental checkup at least every 6 months.

DIET

To prevent tooth decay, clients may have to change their eating habits reducing intake of carbohydrates, especially sweet snacks between meals. Sweet or starchy food adheres to tooth surfaces. If a client eats sweets, it is important to brush within 30 minutes to reduce the action of plaque. Eating acid-containing fruits, for example, apples and fibrous foods such as fresh vegetables also reduces plaque. The acidic quality of fruits eliminates bacteria that forms on teeth. A well-balanced diet ensures integrity of oral tissues.

For pregnant women, appropriate nutrients are essential for development of the fetus' primary teeth. The recommended amount of daily calcium intake is 1200 mg for the pregnant adult and 1600 mg for the pregnant adolescent (Neeson and May, 1986). Four to six cups of milk a day meet the calcium requirement.

BRUSHING

Thorough brushing of the teeth at least four times a day (after meals and at bedtime) is basic to an effective oral hygiene program. A toothbrush should have a

---

Sample Nursing Care Plan for Oral Hygiene Problems

Nursing Diagnosis	Goal	Expected Outcomes	Nursing Interventions
Knowledge deficit regarding oral hygiene related to misunderstanding of hygiene practices.	Client independently performs oral hygiene care correctly.	Client describes steps to follow in brushing and flossing.	Assist client two to three times in administering complete oral care (brushing and flossing). Explain risks of poor oral care. Provide client with booklet, *Protect Your Teeth.*
		Oral hygiene techniques are properly demonstrated.	Provide opportunity after instruction for client to perform oral care. Show client how to assess condition of teeth and gums.

PROCEDURE 32-6

Brushing and Flossing Teeth of Dependent Clients

STEPS	RATIONALE
1. Determine client's ability to grasp and manipulate toothbrush.	Elderly clients or those with changes in level of consciousness or musculoskeletal or nervous system alterations may be unable to hold toothbrush with firm grip or manipulate brush. Nurse can determine level of assistance required.
2. Explain procedure to client and discuss preferences regarding use of hygienic aids.	Some clients feel uncomfortable about having a nurse care for their basic needs. Client involvement with procedure minimizes anxiety.
3. Prepare necessary equipment and supplies: a. Toothbrush with straight handle and small, soft, rounded bristles	Soft, rounded bristles stimulate gums without causing bleeding.

b. Toothpaste or dentifrice
  c. Dental floss
  d. Water glass with cool water
  e. Mouthwash (optional)
	Only serves to provide aftertaste.

f. Straw
  g. Emesis basin
  h. Face towel and paper towels
  i. Disposable gloves
	Prevents contact with oral secretions.

4. Wash hands.	Reduces transmission of microorganisms.
5. Place paper towels on overbed table and arrange other equipment within easy reach.	Towels collect moisture and spills from emesis basin.
6. Pull curtain or close room door (optional if client only brushing teeth).	Provides for client's privacy. When brushing is part of bathing and total hygiene, privacy is essential.
7. Raise bed to comfortable working position. Raise head of bed (if allowed) and lower side rail. Move client or help client move toward you. Side-lying position can be used.	Raising bed and positioning client prevent nurse from experiencing muscle strain. Semi-Fowler's position helps to prevent client from choking or aspirating.
8. Place towel over client's chest.	Prevents soiling of gown and bed linen.
9. Position overbed table within easy reach and adjust height as needed.	Easy accessibility of supplies ensures smooth, safe procedure.
10. Apply gloves.	Prevents contact with microorganisms in saliva.
11. Apply toothpaste to brush, holding brush over emesis basin. Pour small amount of water over toothpaste.	Moisture aids in distribution of toothpaste over tooth surfaces.
12. Hold toothbrush bristles at 45-degree angle to gum line (see illustration). Be sure tips of the bristles rest against and penetrate under the gum line. Brush inner and outer surfaces of upper and lower teeth by brushing from gum to crown of each tooth. Use short vibrating strokes and brush each tooth separately. Clean biting surfaces of teeth by holding top of bristles parallel with teeth and brushing gently back and forth (see illustration). Brush sides of teeth by moving bristles back and forth (see illustration).	Angle allows for brush to reach all tooth surfaces and to clean under gum line where plaque and tartar accumulate. Back-and-forth motion dislodges food particles caught between teeth and along chewing surfaces.

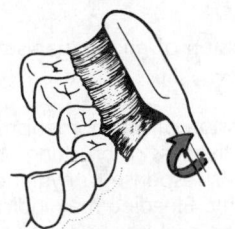 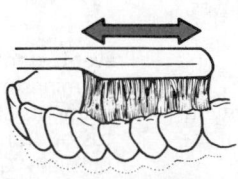 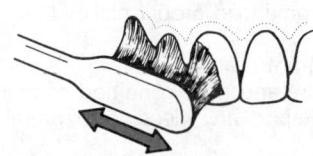

Step 12

Continued.

PROCEDURE 32-6, cont'd

Brushing and Flossing Teeth of Dependent Clients

STEPS	RATIONALE

13. Hold brush at 45-degree angle and lightly brush over surface and sides of tongue. Avoid initiating gag reflex.

Microorganisms collect and grow on tongue's surface. Gagging is uncomfortable and may cause aspiration of toothpaste.

14. Allow client to rinse mouth thoroughly by taking several sips of water, swishing it across all tooth surfaces, and spitting it into emesis basin.

Irrigation removes food particles.

15. Allow client to gargle or rinse mouth with mouthwash.

Mouthwash leaves pleasant taste in mouth.

16. Remove curved basin and assist in wiping client's mouth.

Promotes sense of comfort.

17. Prepare for flossing by having client wash hands, if client is to floss independently.

Reduces transmission of microorganisms.

18. Prepare two pieces of dental floss approximately 25 cm (10 inches) in length. Opinion differs over use of waxed versus unwaxed floss. Waxed floss frays less easily. Food particles adhere to unwaxed floss.

Adequate length needed to grasp floss firmly and insert over surfaces of teeth.

19. Wrap the ends of floss around the third finger of each hand. Using thumb and index finger, stretch floss and insert between two upper teeth. Move floss up and down in seesaw motion between teeth from under the gum lines up to top of each tooth's crown. Be sure to clean outer surface of back molar. Make a figure "C" around the edge of the tooth being flossed. Work systematically along each set of teeth.

Proper insertion and movement of floss along tooth surfaces mechanically removes plaque and tartar.

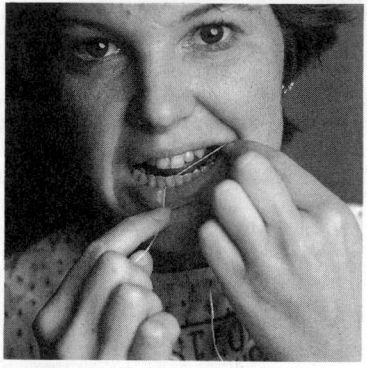

Step 20

20. Take a clean piece of floss and wrap around third finger of each hand. Using the two index fingers stretch floss and insert between two lower teeth (see illustration).

Frayed floss becomes caught between teeth and can be torn off. This can lead to gum inflammation and infection. Position of hands helps to reach lower tooth surfaces.

21. Move floss up and down, between gum lines and crown of lower teeth one at a time.

Upward motion of floss removes plaque and tartar.

22. Allow client to rinse mouth thoroughly with tepid water and spit into emesis basin. Assist in wiping client's mouth.

Irrigation removes plaque and tartar from oral cavity.

23. Assist client to comfortable position, remove bedside table, raise side rail, and lower bed to its original position.

Provides for client's comfort and safety.

24. Wipe off overbed table, discard soiled linen and paper towels in appropriate containers, remove soiled gloves, and return equipment to proper place.

Prevents transmission of microorganisms.

25. Wash hands.

Prevents transmission of microorganisms

26. Inspect condition of oral cavity.

Determines effectiveness of brushing and rinsing.

27. Record procedure and note condition of oral cavity in nurse's notes. Report any bleeding or presence of lesions.

Documents client's response to hygiene measures and status of oral cavity. Bleeding may indicate serious systemic problem. Certain oral lesions may be cancerous.

straight handle and a brush small enough to reach all areas of the mouth. Elderly clients with reduced dexterity and grip may require an enlarged toothbrush handle that provides an easier grip. This can be accomplished by piercing a soft rubber ball and pushing the brush handle through or by gluing a short piece of plastic tubing around the handle. An even, rounded brushing surface with soft, multitufted, nylon bristles is best. Rounded, soft bristles stimulate the gums without causing abrasion and bleeding. All tooth surfaces—inner, outer, and chewing—should be brushed thoroughly (Procedure 32-6). Electric toothbrushes may be used, but the nurse must check for any electrical hazards. Unflavored oral care sponges are used with clients unable to tolerate brushing because of oral trauma or bleeding tendencies.

A fluoride toothpaste is preferred for brushing teeth. Fluoride has been shown to reduce the incidence of tooth decay. Most toothpastes are pleasant tasting. The lemon-glycerin sponges still used in many institutions can have harmful effects on teeth and mucosa. Glycerin has an astringent effect, drying and shrinking gums and mucous membranes. The lemon, if used extensively, exhausts the salivary reflex through overstimulation and can erode teeth enamel (Macmillan, 1981). Since swabbing fails to clean teeth adequately, plaque accumulates around the base of the teeth. The glycerin provides nourishment for bacteria. A swabstick containing an aqueous solution of sorbitol, sodium, carboxymethylcellulose, and electrolytes has been shown effective in treating dry mouth. Moi-Stir is a salivary supplement that improves moisture and texture of the tongue and mucous membranes (Poland, 1987).

Whether a brush or sponge is used, thorough rinsing after brushing is important to remove dislodged food particles and excess toothpaste. Some people enjoy using mouthwash for its pleasant taste. Used over a long period of time, however, mouthwash dries mucosa.

When teaching clients about mouth care, the nurse reminds them not to share toothbrushes at home and not to drink directly from a bottle of mouthwash. Cross-contamination occurs easily. The use of disclosure tablets or drops to stain the plaque that collects at the gumline can be useful for showing clients how effectively they brush.

The amount of assistance needed by the client in brushing the teeth may vary. Many clients are able to perform their own oral care and should be encouraged to do so. The nurse observes the client to be sure proper techniques are used. Other clients need total assistance with hygiene. Procedure 32-6 reviews steps for assisting partially dependent clients with mouth care.

SPECIAL ORAL HYGIENE

Some clients require special oral hygiene methods either because of their level of dependence on the nurse or the presence of oral mucosa problems.

UNCONSCIOUS CLIENTS. These clients are susceptible to drying of mucosa-thickened salivary secretions, since they are unable to eat or drink, frequently breathe through the mouth, and often receive oxygen therapy. The unconscious client also cannot swallow salivary secretions that accumulate in the mouth. These secretions often contain gram-negative bacteria that can cause pneumonia if aspirated into the lungs. Procedure 32-7 describes mouth care for debilitated clients.

CLIENTS AT RISK FOR STOMATITIS. Chemotherapy, radiation, and nasogastric tube intubation can cause stomatitis. Clients should rinse their mouths before and after each meal using a solution containing ½ to 1 teaspoon of salt to 1 pint of water (Wilson, 1986). To remove thick mucus, use sodium bicarbonate solution, 1 teaspoon to 1 pint of water.

CLIENTS WITH DIABETES. Visits to the dentist are needed every 3 or 4 months. All tissues should be handled gently with a minimum of trauma. Clients should be taught to follow rigid cleansing schedules.

ORAL INFECTIONS. The nurse notifies a physician when signs of an infection such as coated ulcerations or a red, dry swollen tongue are seen. Yogurt (containing active cultures) with every meal is effective against yeast infections (Wilson, 1986). Liquid topical antibiotics can be applied to mucosal surfaces with a soft sponge or by having clients rinse the oral cavity with the medication. Clients who wear dentures must remove them before using topical antibiotics.

FLUORIDE USE

In many communities the water supply now contains fluoride. Even though fluoride has not been proved to eliminate tooth decay, it is known to prevent dental caries (Whaley and Wong, 1987). People who do not have fluoridated water available can obtain fluoride in the form of mouthwash, toothpaste, or supplements. Most toothpastes on the market today contain fluoride and can help prevent tooth decay. Fluoride supplements can be given to children beginning at the age of 2 weeks. Supplements are available without a prescription and can be taken with water, juice, or milk. The family dentist should be consulted concerning the amount of fluoride to be given.

Excessive fluoridation can result in a discoloration of tooth enamel. Clients should be advised to watch for this condition. Parents should keep fluoride supplements out of the reach of children.

FLOSSING

Dental flossing is necessary for effective removal of plaque and tartar between teeth. Flossing involves insertion of waxed or unwaxed dental floss between all

PROCEDURE 32-7

Performing Mouth Care for the Unconscious or Debilitated Client

STEPS	RATIONALE
1. Assess for presence of client's gag reflex.	Reveals client's risk for aspiration.
2. Position client in Sims' or side-lying position with head turned well toward dependent side (see illustration).	Allows secretions to drain from mouth instead of collecting in back of pharynx. Prevents aspiration.
3. Explain procedure to client.	Unconscious client may retain ability to hear.
4. Prepare necessary equipment and supplies:	
a. Anti-infective solution (for example, hydrogen peroxide diluted in equal parts of water)	Loosens crustations and acts as anti-infective.
b. Sponge toothbrush or tongue blade wrapped in single layer of gauze; small toothbrush	Brush cleans teeth most effectively. Sponge or swab stimulates and cleans gums and mucosa.
c. Padded tongue blade	Keeps mouth open and teeth separated during procedure without traumatizing oral structures
d. Face towel	
e. Emesis basin	
f. Paper towels	
g. Water glass with cool water	
h. Petroleum jelly	Lubricates lips.
i. Portable suction machine (optional) with rubber catheter	Removes retained oral secretions while oral cavity is cleansed.
j. Disposable gloves	Oral cavity contains highly infectious microorganisms.
5. Wash hands and apply disposable gloves.	Reduces transfer of miroorganisms.
6. Place paper towels on overbed table and arrange equipment. Turn on suction machine and connect tubing to suction catheter.	Prevents soiling of table top. Equipment prepared in advance ensures smooth, safe procedure.
7. Pull curtain around bed or close room door.	Provides privacy.
8. Raise bed to its highest horizontal level; lower side rail.	Use of good body mechanics with bed in high position prevents injury to nurse and client.
9. Bring client close to side of bed and near you; be sure client's head is turned toward mattress.	Proper positioning of head prevents aspiration.
10. Place towel under client's face and emesis basin under client's chin.	Prevents soiling of bed linen.
11. Carefully retract client's upper and lower teeth with padded tongue blade by inserting blade quickly but gently between the back molars. Insert when client is relaxed, if possible.	Prevents client from biting down on nurse's fingers and provides access to oral cavity.
12. Clean mouth using brush or tongue blade moistened with peroxide and water. Have second nurse suction as secretions accumulate during cleansing. Clean chewing and inner tooth surfaces first. Clean outer tooth surfaces. Swab roof of mouth and inside cheeks. Gently swab or brush tongue but avoid stimulating gag reflex (if present). Moisten clean swab or toothette with water to rinse. Repeat rinse several times. Suction any remaining secretions.	Brushing action removes food particles between teeth and along chewing surfaces. Swabbing helps remove secretions and crustations from mucosa and moistens mucosa. Suction removes secretions and fluid that can collect in posterior pharynx. Repeated rinsing removes peroxide that can be irritating to mucosa.

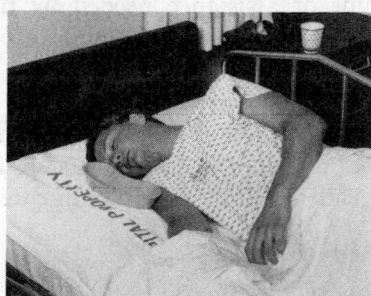

Step 2

STEPS	RATIONALE
13. Apply thin layer of petroleum jelly to lips.	Lubricates lips to prevent drying and cracking.
14. Explain to debilitated client that procedure is completed.	Provides meaningful stimulation to unconscious or less responsive client.
15. Remove gloves and dispose in proper receptacle.	Prevents transmission of microorganisms.
16. Reposition client comfortably, raise side rail, and return bed to original position.	Maintains client's comfort and safety.
17. Clean equipment and return to its proper place. Place soiled linen in proper receptacle.	Proper disposal of soiled equipment prevents spread of infection.
18. Wash hands.	Reduces transmission of microorganisms.
19. Inspect oral cavity.	Determines efficacy of cleansing. Once thick secretions are removed, underlying inflammation or lesions may be revealed.
20. Record procedure, including pertinent observation (for example, presence of bleeding gums, dry mucosa, ulcerations, or crusts on tongue) and report any unusual findings to nurse in charge or physician.	Documents response of client to nursing therapy. Bleeding may indicate more serious systemic problems. Lesions of oral cavity can be cancerous.

tooth surfaces, one at a time. The seesaw motion used to pull floss between teeth removes plaque and tartar from tooth enamel. If toothpaste is applied to the teeth before flossing, the fluoride can come in direct contact with tooth surfaces, aiding in cavity prevention. Flossing once a day is sufficient. Because it is important to clean all teeth surfaces thoroughly, the nurse should not rush to complete flossing. Placing a mirror in front of the client will help the nurse demonstrate the proper methods for holding the floss and cleaning between the teeth. Flossing is most easily done immediately after brushing (Procedure 32-6).

DENTURE CARE

Clients should be encouraged to clean their own dentures as frequently as natural teeth to prevent gingival infection and irritation (Procedure 32-8). The nurse must assist with denture care if clients become disabled, incapacitated, or confused. Dentures are the client's personal property and should be handled with care, since they can easily be broken. The nurse always stores dentures in an enclosed, labeled cup during soaking or when the dentures are not being worn. The client is discouraged from wrapping in facial or toilet tissue or placing dentures on meal trays, since the dentures may accidentally be thrown away.

EVALUATION

The beneficial outcomes of oral hygiene may not be seen for several days. Repeated cleansing is often needed to remove thick encrustations of the tongue and to restore the mucosa's hydration to normal. Likewise, it will take many weeks of rigorous hygiene to reduce incidence of dental caries. The evaluation box (p. 847) outlines the evaluation of oral hygiene care.

HAIR CARE

A person's appearance and feeling of well-being often depend on the way the hair looks and feels. Illness or disability may prevent a client from maintaining daily hair care. An immobilized client's hair soon becomes tangled. Dressings may leave sticky blood or antiseptic solutions on the hair. Proper hair care is important to the client's body image. Brushing, combing, and shampooing are basic hygiene measures for all clients. Clients should be permitted to shave when their condition allows.

Hair growth, distribution, and pattern can be indicators of a person's general health status (see Chapter 13). Hormonal changes, emotional and physical stress,

PROCEDURE 32-8

Cleaning Dentures

STEPS	RATIONALE

1. Ask client if dentures are loose fitting and if there is any gum or mucous membrane tenderness or irritation. After dentures are removed, nurse should inspect oral cavity and denture surfaces.

   Ill-fitting dentures rub against gums and mucous membranes. Area of irritation may require special care.

2. Explain procedure to client and assure that individual practice preferences will be used (when appropriate).

   Promotes client's understanding and cooperation.

3. Prepare necessary equipment and supplies:
   a. Soft-bristled toothbrush — Used to brush gums and tongue.
   b. Denture toothbrush
   c. Emesis basin or sink
   d. Denture dentifrice or toothpaste
   e. Water glasses (for warm and cool water)
   f. Single 4 × 4 gauze — Used to remove dentures.
   g. Washcloth
   h. Plastic denture cup
   i. Disposable gloves — Prevents contact with microorganisms in saliva.

4. Wash hands.

   Reduces transmission of microorganisms.

5. Arrange supplies on bedside table or near sink.

   Accessibility of supplies ensures smooth, organized procedure.

6. Pour emesis basin half full with tepid water or place washcloth in sink and run water until it is approximately 1 in deep.

   Water aids in distribution of dentifrice over denture surfaces. Cloth in bottom of sink protects dentures against breakage. Hot water can cause warping or softening of dentures.

7. Apply disposable gloves.

   Reduces transmission of infection.

8. Ask client to remove dentures and place them in emesis basin. If client is unable to remove dentures, grasp upper plate at front with thumb and index finger wrapped in gauze. Use steady downward pull. Gently lift lower denture from jaw and rotate one side downward to remove from client's mouth. Place dentures in emesis basin.

   Gauze prevents accidental slipping while handling dentures. Rotating denture at angle reduces pulling of lips during removal.

9. Apply dentifrice to denture and brush surfaces of dentures (see illustrations). Hold dentures close to water. Hold brush horizontally and use back-and-forth motion to cleanse biting surfaces. Hold brush horizontally and use short strokes from top of denture to biting surfaces of teeth to clean outer tooth surface. Hold brush vertically and use short strokes to clean inner tooth surfaces. Hold brush horizontally and use back-and-forth motion to clean undersurface of dentures.

   Cleansing prevents food and bacteria from collecting on denture surfaces and prevents odor and stain buildup. Holding dentures close to water reduces chance of breakage, because water will break fall if dentures slip.

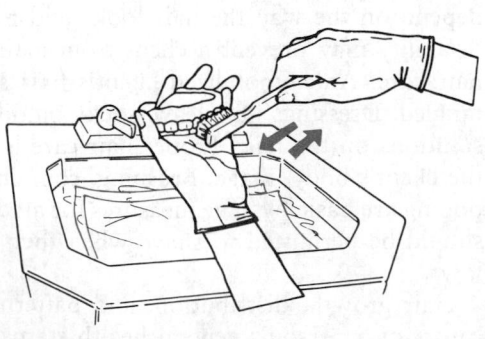
Step 9

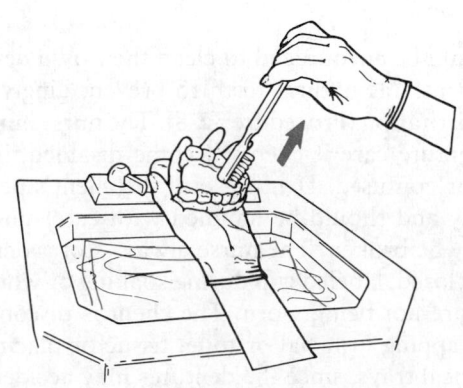

STEPS	RATIONALE
10. Rinse dentures thoroughly in tepid water.	Warm water dilutes and rinses dentifrice more effectively than cool water.
11. Return dentures to client or store in tepid water in denture cup.	Storage protects dentures from breakage. Tepid water keeps dentures well-moistened to make eventual insertion easier. Plastic dentures become brittle and warp if not kept moist.
12. Empty emesis basin and add fresh cool water. Apply toothpaste to soft toothbrush and gently brush client's gums, palate, and tongue.	Brushing helps stimulate circulation to gums and removes residual film of debris on gums and mucosa.
13. Have client rinse mouth thoroughly.	Rinsing removes all food particles and secretions.
14. Reinsert dentures if client desires or allow client to do so. Begin by gently inserting moistened upper denture. Have client use finger to press denture firmly in place, then insert moistened lower denture.	Bulkier upper denture easier to insert first when client has both upper and lower plates. Moistening lubricates denture for easier insertion. Applying gentle pressure to upper denture seals it against palate.
15. Dispose of gloves in proper receptacle. Clean and store supplies. Wash hands.	Controls spread of infection.
16. Ask client if dentures feel comfortable.	Cleansing removes sources of irritation.
17. Record procedure on flow sheet or nurses' notes.	Accurate and timely documentation maintains accuracy of client's record.

Illustrations from Sorrentino, SA: Mosby's textbook for nursing assistants, ed. 2, St. Louis, 1987, The C.V. Mosby Co.

Sample Evaluation of Interventions for Oral Hygiene Problems

Goals	Evaluative Measures	Expected Outcomes
Oral mucosa is intact and well hydrated.	Inspect condition of tongue, gums, and lining of cheeks. Observe condition of lips.	Mucosa is moist, intact, and has a uniform color. Tongue is well-hydrated. Lips are smooth, hydrated.
Teeth are without new dental caries.	Inspect teeth surfaces.	Teeth are white, smooth, and shiny. Teeth are free of food particles and plaque.
Client independently performs oral hygiene care correctly.	Observe client perform brushing, flossing, denture care. Ask client to describe oral hygiene techniques.	Oral hygiene techniques are properly demonstrated. Client describes steps to follow in brushing, flossing, or denture care.
Client achieves sense of comfort.	Question client if discomfort is noted in oral cavity. Observe facial expression for signs of discomfort.	Client denies oral pain or irritation.
Client understands oral hygiene practices.	Ask client to explain purpose of regular oral hygiene.	Client explains preventive measures against tooth decay and plaque.

TABLE 32-6   Hair and Scalp Problems

Problem	Characteristics	Implications	Interventions
Dandruff	Scaling of the scalp accompanied by itching; in severe cases, dandruff on eyebrows	Dandruff causes a person embarrassment. If dandruff enters the eyes, conjunctivitis may develop.	Shampoo regularly with a medicated shampoo. In severe cases a physician's advice may be needed.
Ticks	Small gray-brown parasites that burrow into the skin and suck blood	Ticks transmit several diseases to people. The most common are Rocky Mountain spotted fever and tularemia.	Do not pull ticks from skin because the sucking apparatus remains and may become infected. Placing a drop of oil or ether on the tick or covering it with petrolatum jelly eases removal. Oil suffocates the tick.
Pediculosis (lice)	Tiny grayish white parasite insects that infest mammals		
Pediculosis capitis (head lice)	Found on the scalp attached to hair strands; eggs look like oval particles, similar to dandruff; bites or pustules may be observed behind ears and at hairline	Head lice are difficult to remove and may spread to furniture and other people if not treated.	Shampoo with Kwell shampoo and repeat 12-24 hours later. Change bed linens.
Pediculosis corporis (body lice)	Tend to cling to clothing so may not be easily seen; body lice suck blood and lay eggs on the clothing and furniture	The client itches constantly. Scratches seen on skin may become infected. Hemorrhagic spots may appear on the skin where lice are sucking blood.	Client should bathe or shower thoroughly. After skin is dried, Kwell lotion should be applied. After 12-24 hours another bath or shower should be taken. Bag any infested clothing or linen until laundered.
Pediculosis pubis (crab lice)	Found in pubic hair; crab lice are grayish white with red legs	Lice may spread through bed linen, clothing, or furniture or between persons via sexual contact.	Shave hair off affected area. Cleanse as for body lice. If lice were sexually transmitted, partner must be notified.
Hair loss (alopecia)	Occurs in all races, mostly in women. Balding patches seen in periphery of hair line. Hair becomes brittle and broken. Causes from use of hair curlers, Afro picks, tight braiding, and use of hot comb.	Patches of uneven hair growth and loss alter client's appearance.	Stop hair-care practices that damage hair.

aging, infection, and certain diseases can affect characteristics of the hair. The hair shaft is an inert structure; any changes in its color or condition occur as a result of hormonal activity and nutrient supply to the hair follicle. Table 32-6 describes common hair and scalp problems and nursing interventions.

ASSESSMENT

PHYSICAL ASSESSMENT

Before performing hair care, the nurse assesses the condition of the hair and scalp (see Chapter 13). Normally the hair is clean, shiny, untangled, and the scalp is clear. The hair of black-skinned clients is usually thicker, drier, and curlier than lighter-skinned clients. Evenness of hair growth can be influenced by several factors. Baldness in men is usually a genetic condition. The loss of hair (alopecia) can result from improper hair care practices (Table 32-6) or use of chemotherapy medications.

DEVELOPMENTAL CHANGES

During a person's life span changes in the growth, distribution, and condition of body hair can influence the type of hygiene a person requires (Table 32-7).

TABLE 32-7 Physiological Development of Hair Growth

Age	Condition of Hair
Infant	Infants may have little or no scalp hair at birth. Scalp hair grows by the first year. Fine body hair (lanugo) is present on the forehead, cheeks, shoulders, and back.
Child	Scalp hair is lustrous, silky, strong, and elastic. Hair of black-skinned child is curlier and coarser.
Middle childhood to puberty	Androgenic hormones cause an increase in thickening and darkening of scalp hair, the growth of hair in the axilla and pubic areas in both sexes, and growth of facial hair in boys.
Adolescence	Boys may acquire additional amounts of distribution of body hair, such as on the chest. An increase in sebaceous gland activity causes hair to become oily.
Adulthood	Men with genetic tendency develop baldness.
Older adult	Axillary and pubic hair diminish in women. Scalp hair becomes thinner and depleted of melanin, causing gray coloring. Older women may develop chin and facial hair because of decreased estrogen production. Men experience balding or a receding hair line.

SELF-CARE ABILITY

The nurse assesses a client's physical ability to care for hair. Painful conditions of the upper extremities such as arthritis, a weakened hand grip, fatigue, and physical encumberances, for example, a cast or dressing, are just some of the conditions that will impair a client's ability to perform hair care.

HAIR-CARE PRACTICES

One way to assess a person's hair-care practices is by observing the appearance of the hair. Dull, tangled, dirty hair indicates improper care. Unkempt hair may be the result of lack of interest, depression, or physical inability to care for the hair.

By assessing a client's preferred hair style, the nurse can attempt to arrange the client's hair in the same manner. Asking the client to assist or teach the nurse how to style the hair correctly gives the client a greater sense of independence.

The nurse also assesses the type of hair care products

Examples of Nursing Diagnoses for Clients Requiring Hair and Scalp Care

NANDA-APPROVED NURSING DIAGNOSES

Dressing/grooming self-care deficit related to:
- Altered level of consciousness
- Physical immobility or weakness

Impaired skin integrity related to:
- Scalp laceration
- Insect bite

Pain related to:
- Scalp lesion
- Accumulated secretions in the hair

Body image disturbance related to:
- Unkempt physical appearance

Potential for infection related to:
- Scalp laceration
- Insect bites

---

a client prefers to use, as well as the time of day when hair care is usually performed. Assessment of shaving products is necessary with male clients.

NURSING DIAGNOSIS

The problems most likely to be identified by the nurse following assessment of the hair and scalp center on comfort and grooming. If actual lesions or abnormalities involving the scalp are identified, nursing diagnoses focus on the integrity of the scalp (see nursing diagnoses box). The sample nursing diagnoses box outlines defining characteristics for select nursing diagnoses.

PLANNING

Good hair care practices must be done routinely to meet the client's hygiene needs. It is important for the nurse to remember that the client remains aware of his or her appearance at all times. Therefore an effective plan (see care plan box) allows the client to initiate and participate in hygiene measures whenever possible.

Goals for clients in need of hair and scalp care include the following:

1. Hair and scalp will be clean and healthy
2. Client achieves a sense of comfort and self-esteem
3. Client will participate in hair-care practices

Sample Nursing Diagnoses for Clients Requiring Hair and Scalp Care

Defining Characteristics	Nursing Diagnoses	Related Factors
Client is unable to comb or brush hair. Client is unable to obtain hair care products. Client is unable to wash hair.	Dressing/grooming self-care deficit	• Physical immobility • Activity intolerance • Pain of upper extremities
Open laceration is along surface of scalp. There is bleeding with matting of hair. Bites or pustules are behind the ears and at hair line. Hemorrhageic spots are on skin. Abrasions or scratches are on skin.	Impaired skin integrity	• Scalp laceration • Insect bite • Exposure to chemicals
Client verbalizes concern about appearance of hair. Client avoids looking at self in mirror. Hair appears disheveled, tangled.	Body image disturbance	• Unkempt physical appearance • Inability to perform hair care independently

---

Sample Nursing Care Plan for Clients Requiring Hair and Scalp Care

Nursing Diagnosis	Goal	Expected Outcome	Nursing Interventions
Body image disturbance related to inability to perform hair care independently	Client achieves sense of comfort and self-esteem.	Client demonstrates positive self-esteem by looking in mirror and interacting with staff and family.	Brush hair at least three times daily. At night, braid hair. Provide a shampoo once every four days. Have client instruct about way to style hair.

IMPLEMENTATION

BRUSHING AND COMBING

Frequent brushing helps keep hair clean and distributes oil evenly along hair shafts. Combing merely styles the hair and prevents it from becoming tangled. Short-tooth combs are adequate for short hair, but large-tooth combs are preferred for curly hair. Combs with sharp, irregular teeth may scratch the scalp. The client able to perform self-care should be encouraged to maintain hair care daily. However, clients with limited mobility and poor coordination and those who are confused or seriously weakened by their illness require the nurse's help.

A client's long hair can easily become matted after he or she is confined to bed even for a short period. When lacerations or incisions involve the scalp, blood and topical medications can also cause tangling. Frequent brushing and combing keeps long hair neatly groomed. However, braiding of hair can help to avoid repeated tangles. The nurse asks the client's permission to braid hair. If braids are made too tightly, balding patches can develop.

To brush hair properly the nurse parts the hair into two sections and then separates each section into two more sections. Parting allows for ease in brushing smaller sections of hair. The nurse brushes from the scalp toward the hair ends. If tangles are present, the nurse uses the fingers to separate a small lock of hair, grasps it firmly near the scalp, and combs the loose end of the lock. Anchoring the tangled hair prevents painful pulling of the scalp during combing. If hair is excessively tangled, the nurse should comb out only a few sections at a time. Moistening hair with water or alcohol often frees tangles for easier combing. The nurse never cuts the client's hair without written consent.

The hair of black-skinned clients requires special attention. The thick, coarse, curly hair of black clients often becomes very dry and brittle. Clients who have an "Afro" hair style usually comb their hair with a special comb that has long teeth, spaced far apart. The open-toothed comb causes less pulling during combing. Wetting the client's hair with water before combing prevents trauma to the hair. To comb "Afro" hair styles, start at the client's neckline and slowly lift and fluff the hair outward until you reach the forehead. Comb one side of the client's head at a time, then repeat on the other side.

The nurse should caution black clients against hair-care practices that can damage hair. Daily braiding of hair is more damaging than corn rows. The tight braids may cause balding patches. The use of petroleum jelly and a hot comb for straightening hair may cause chronic inflammation and permanent scarring of the scalp. Application of hair straighteners with alkaline chemicals may cause hair to become brittle.

SHAMPOOING

Frequency of shampooing depends on a person's daily routine. The nurse should remind hospitalized clients that staying in bed, excess perspiration, or treatments that leave blood or solutions in the hair may require more frequent shampooing. For clients at home the nurse's greatest challenge may be to find ways the client can shampoo the hair without injury.

If the client is able to take a shower or bath, the hair can usually be shampooed without difficulty. A shower chair may be used for the client who is ambulatory but becomes tired or faint. Handheld shower nozzles allow clients to wash their hair during a tub bath or shower. Clients who are allowed to sit in a chair can usually be shampooed in front of a sink. If the client is forced to sit at the bedside, it is possible to shampoo the hair as the client leans forward over a washbasin.

If a client is unable to sit but can be moved, the nurse may transfer the client to a stretcher for transportation to a sink or shower equipped with a handheld nozzle. The nurse places a towel or small pillow under the client's head and neck, allowing the head to hang slightly over the stretcher's edge. Caution is needed with clients who have suffered neck injuries, because hyperextension of the neck could cause further injury.

If the client is unable to sit in a chair or be transferred to a stretcher, shampooing must be done with the client in bed. Many institutions require a physician's order for the procedure (Procedure 32-9). After shampooing, clients may like having their hair rolled on curlers or styled. Most health care centers have portable hair dryers. Dry shampoos that reduce the need to wet the client's hair are also available.

Black clients usually apply various types of oil preparations to the hair before or after shampooing. Oil prevents drying and subsequent breaking off of hair at the follicles or ends. Grier (1976) recommends a solution of alcohol and mineral oil to remove old oils that adhere to the hair shaft. The alcohol is an antiseptic and cleansing agent. The mineral oil cleans and lubricates the hair. The nurse confers with clients to determine the preferred type of oil preparation. Olive oil, baby oil, or Vasoline hair oil are commonly used. The application of an oil generally makes combing easier.

Normally, it is necessary for black clients to shampoo their hair only once or twice a week. Water shampoos tend to make their hair curlier and harder to comb. A mild shampoo is preferred if black clients have had their hair straightened.

SHAVING

Shaving of facial hair can be done after the bath or shampoo. Women may prefer to shave their legs or axillae during the bath. When assisting a client, the nurse should take care to avoid cutting the client with razor blades. Clients prone to bleeding, such as those receiving anticoagulant medications (heparin or coumadin) or high doses of aspirin, and those with bleeding disorders (hemophilia or leukemia) may prefer to use an electric razor. Before using an electric razor, check for any electrical hazards.

When a razor blade is used for shaving, the skin must be softened to prevent pulling, scraping, or cuts. For example, placing a warm washcloth over the male client's face for a few seconds, followed by the application of shaving cream or a lathering of mild soap, will effectively soften the skin. If the client is unable to shave his own face, the nurse may perform the shave. To avoid causing discomfort or razor cuts, the nurse holds the razor at a 45-degree angle to the skin and gently pulls the skin taut while using short, firm razor strokes in the direction the hair grows. Short downward strokes work best to remove hair over the upper lip. Often a client can explain the best way to move the razor. After the shave is completed, wash the client's face thoroughly to remove soap and hair. After drying the face assist in applying powder or an after-shave lotion to the client's face.

MUSTACHE AND BEARD CARE

Male clients with mustaches or beards require daily grooming. Keeping these clean is important because food

PROCEDURE 32-9

Shampooing Hair in Bed

STEPS	RATIONALE
1. Determine if any risks exist that might contraindicate shampooing or positioning. (Obtain physician's order as needed.)	Certain medical conditions (for example, cervical neck injuries, open incisions, a tracheostomy) may place client at risk of injury because of positioning, exposure to moisture, or manipulation of scalp.
2. Review physician's orders to determine if medicated shampoo is ordered.	For conditions such as lice or dandruff, special shampoos may be ordered.
3. Explain procedure to client.	Client may be anxious about positioning or risk of water entering eyes.
4. Prepare necessary equipment and supplies: a. Two bath towels b. Face towel or washcloth c. Shampoo (hair conditioner and cream rinse optional) d. Water pitcher e. Plastic shampoo trough f. Washbasin g. Bath blanket h. Waterproof pad i. Clean comb and brush j. Hair dryer k. Bottle of hydrogen peroxide (optional)	Conditioner reduces tangles. Used to pour water over hair. Diverts water to basin to prevent soiling bed linen. Cleans hair matted with blood.
5. Wash hands.	Reduces transmission of microorganisms.
6. Arrange equipment in convenient place and lower side rail.	Easy access to equipment and client prevents interruptions during procedure.
7. Place waterproof pad under client's shoulders, neck, and head. Position client supine with head and shoulders at top edge of bed. Place plastic trough under client's head and washbasin at end of trough, being sure trough spout extends beyond edge of mattress.	Prevents soiling of bed linen.
8. Place rolled towel under client's neck and bath towel across client's shoulders.	Slight hyperextension of neck minimizes problem of water draining down back of neck.
9. Brush and comb client's hair.	Removing tangles results in more thorough cleansing.
10. Obtain water at about 43°-44° C (110° F) and fill pitcher.	Proper water temperature prevents burns to face and scalp.
11. Ask client to hold face towel or washcloth over eyes.	Prevents shampoo or water from entering eyes.
12. With water pitcher slowly pour water over hair until it is completely wet. Apply small amount of shampoo.	Water aids in distribution of shampoo suds over hair.
13. Work up with both hands. Start at hairline and work toward back of neck. Lift head slightly with one hand to wash back of head. Shampoo sides of head. Massage scalp by applying pressure with fingertips.	Systematic progression over hair and scalp ensures thorough cleansing. Massage increases scalp circulation. Use of fingernails during massage can cause scratching of scalp.
14. Rinse hair with water. Make sure water drains into basin. Repeat rinsing until hair is free of shampoo. To speed drainage from trough, press down on its spout.	Retained shampoo leaves dull finish on hair. Dried shampoo may cause scalp irritation.
15. Repeat Steps 12-14.	Ensures thorough cleansing.
16. Apply conditioner or rinse if requested and rinse hair thoroughly.	Conditioner prevents excess drying. Cream rinse makes combing and brushing easier.
17. Wrap client's head in bath towel. Dry client's face with cloth used to protect the eyes. Dry off any moisture along neck or shoulders.	Retained moisture may cause cooling and chills.
18. Dry client's hair and scalp. Use second towel if first becomes saturated.	
19. Comb hair to remove tangles and dry with dryer or remaining towel as quickly as possible.	Drying prevents chilling.

STEPS	RATIONALE
20. Assist client to comfortable position and complete styling of hair.	Promotes client's sense of well-being.
21. Return equipment to its proper place. Discard soiled linen in linen hamper. Wash hands.	Maintains cleanliness of environment and controls transmission of infection.
22. Ask client how the hair feels.	Client will experience sense of cleanliness after shampooing.
23. Inspect condition of hair.	Shampooing should leave hair in clean condition.
24. Record procedure and any pertinent findings related to condition of hair or scalp.	Documents client's response to therapy and condition of hair or scalp should further treatment be necessary.

particles can easily collect in the hair. If the client is unable to care for himself, the nurse should trim, comb, or wash the beard or mustache when needed or at the client's request. The nurse never shaves off a mustache or beard without the client's consent.

EVALUATION

The nurse's evaluation of the outcomes of interventions are listed in the evaluation box.

CARE OF THE EYES, EARS, AND NOSE

Special attention is given to the cleansing of the eyes, ears, and nose during the client's bath. However, clients may also have special problems requiring cleansing of these organs throughout the day.

Eyes

The eyes are one of our most important organs. The partial or total loss of vision is devastating, not only because it leads to dependence on others, but also be-

Sample Evaluation of Interventions for Clients Requiring Hair and Scalp Care

Goals	Evaluative Measures	Expected Outcomes
Hair and scalp will be clean and healthy.	Inspect condition of hair and scalp.	Hair is clean, shiny, and untangled.
		The scalp is clean with fewer areas of infestations.
		Existing scalp lacerations or lesions are clean and without drainage or inflammation.
Client achieves a sense of comfort and self-esteem.	Question client if areas of tenderness exist along the scalp.	Client denies discomfort.
	Observe client's behaviors toward perceived image.	Client expresses positive statements about appearance.
		Client demonstrates positive self-esteem by looking in mirror, interacting with others, or discussing appearance.

cause the person's ability to view the world is lost. Normally no special care is required for the eyes, since they are continually cleansed by tears and the eyelids and lashes prevent entrance of foreign particles. A person needs only to remove any dried secretions that have collected on the inner canthus or the eyelashes. Unconscious clients are at risk for eye injury because the blink reflex may be absent. In these clients excessive drainage frequently collects along eyelid margins. Special attention is also needed for clients who have had eye surgery or an eye infection that can result in increased discharge or drainage. The nurse often has the responsibility of assisting clients in the care of eyeglasses, contact lenses, or artificial eyes.

Ears

Changes in hearing acuity can be frustrating and produce anxiety. A person with normal hearing also becomes frustrated when the hearing-impaired individual cannot understand what is being said. Hygiene of the ears has implications for hearing acuity only when wax or foreign substances collect in the external ear canal and interfere with sound conduction. The nurse should be sensitive to any behavioral cues that might indicate a hearing impairment (see Chapter 44). When caring for a client with a hearing aid, the nurse instructs the client on proper cleansing and maintenance techniques.

Nose

The nose provides for the sense of smell but also controls the temperature and humidity of inhaled air and prevents entrance of foreign particles into the respiratory system. The accumulation of crusted secretions within the nares can impair olfactory sensation and breathing. Irritation of nasal mucosa can cause swelling, leading to obstruction of the nares. Typically hygiene care of the nose is simple, but clients with nasogastric, enteral feeding, or endotracheal tubes that enter the nose may require special attention.

ASSESSMENT

PHYSICAL ASSESSMENT

Chapter 13 describes in detail the techniques used to assess the condition and function of the eyes, ears, and nose.

Normally the eyes are free of infection. The conjuctivae are clear, pink, and without inflammation. The eyelid margins are in close approximation with the eyeball, and the lashes are turned outward. The lid margins

are normally without inflammation, drainage, or the presence of lesions. The client's eyebrows should be symmetrical. Flaking of skin around the eyebrows may indicate dandruff.

Assessment of the external ear structures includes inspection of the auricle, external ear canal, and tympanic membrane. While performing hygiene measures, the nurse is most concerned with noting the presence of accumulated cerumen or drainage in the ear canal, local inflammation, or pain.

The nurse inspects the nares for signs of inflammation, discharge, lesions, edema, and deformity. The nasal mucosa is normally pink, clear, and without discharge. For clients with any form of tubing exiting the nose, the nurse should look at the nares surfaces that come in contact with the tubing. Friction from tubing can cause tissue sloughing, localized tenderness, inflammation, and even bleeding.

Assessing Client's Use of Sensory Aids

EYEGLASSES

- Purpose for wearing glasses (for example, reading, distance, or both)
- Methods used to clean glasses
- Presence of symptoms (for example, blurred vision, headaches, irritation)

CONTACT LENSES

- Type of lens worn
- Frequency and duration of time lenses are worn (include sleep time)
- Presence of symptoms (for example, burning, excess tearing, redness, irritation, swelling, or sensitivity to light)
- Techniques used by the client to cleanse, store, insert, and remove lenses
- Use of eye drops or ointments
- Use of an emergency identification bracelet or card that warns others to remove the client's lenses in case of an emergency

ARTIFICIAL EYE

- Method used to insert and remove the eye
- Method for cleansing the eye
- Presence of symptoms (for example, drainage, inflammation, or pain involving the orbit)

HEARING AID

- Type of aid worn
- Methods used to cleanse aid
- Client's ability to change battery and adjust hearing-aid volume

Sample Nursing Diagnoses for Eye, Ear, or Nose Problems

Defining Characteristics	Nursing Diagnoses	Related Factors
Abrasion of ear canal Ulceration in nasal mucosa Chronic irritation (for example, scratching ears, presence of nasal tube) Accumulated drainage	Potential for infection	• Broken skin or mucosa • Poor hygiene practices
Unable to explain methods for performing hygiene Client observed performing hygiene measures incorrectly Requests information about hygiene	Knowledge deficit about personal hygiene	• Lack of exposure to information • Information misinterpretation
Hearing acuity reduced Ear canal impacted with cerumen Ear canal swollen	Sensory/perceptual alterations (auditory)	• Obstruction in ear canal

USE OF SENSORY AIDS

For clients who wear eyeglasses, contact lenses, artificial eyes, or hearing aids, the nurse assesses the client's knowledge and methods used to care for the aids, as well as the presence of any problems caused by the aids. The box outlines factors to assess for clients using sensory aids. The nurse's findings have implications for client education.

SELF-CARE ABILITY

The nurse assesses a client's physical ability to perform eye, ear, and nose care, as well as care of any sensory aids. Clients who are unable to grasp small objects, have limited mobility in the upper extremities, have reduced vision, or who are seriously fatigued will require assistance from the nurse.

NURSING DIAGNOSIS

The nurse's assessment may reveal an actual alteration in the function of sensory organs, a problem in the client's ability to perform personal hygiene, or a deficit in the client's understanding of how to perform hygiene. Defining characteristics that include physical findings of client behaviors and knowledge lead to forming accurate nursing diagnoses (see sample nursing diagnoses box). The nursing diagnoses box lists common nursing diagnoses the nurse may identify.

Examples of Nursing Diagnoses Related to Eye, Ear, or Nose Problems

NANDA-APPROVED NURSING DIAGNOSES

Bathing/hygiene self-care deficit related to:
• Physical limitations
• Visual impairment
Knowledge deficit about personal hygiene related to:
• Lack of exposure to information
• Information misinterpretation
Pain related to:
• Physical irritation of eye
• Inflammation of ear canal
• Mechanical irritation of nares
Potential for infection related to:
    Poor hygiene practices
Sensory/perceptual alterations (visual, auditory, or olfactory) related to:
    Obstruction in ear canal
• Nasal obstruction

PLANNING

The client's personal preference and habits again are considered as the nurse plans hygienic care. The eyes, ears, and nose are sensitive to irritating or painful stimuli. Extra care must be taken to avoid injury to tissues. The care plan box describes basic guidelines for a client

Sample Nursing Care Plan for Clients Needing Ear Care

Nursing Diagnosis	Goal	Expected Outcomes	Nursing Interventions
Sensory/perceptual alteration: (auditory) related to obstruction in ear canal.	Normal sensory function is present.	Client is able to hear conversation in normal tone of voice. Client responds appropriately to questions.	Instruct client in proper method for regular ear care. Instruct client's wife about proper technique for weekly irrigation of ear canal. Caution client to call physician if hearing worsens.

requiring ear care. The goals of care for the client include the following:

1. Absence of infection
2. Normal sensory organ function
3. Understanding of methods used to care for the eyes, ears, and nose

IMPLEMENTATION

BASIC EYE CARE

Cleansing of the eyes is usually performed during the bath and involves washing with a clean washcloth moistened in water. The use of soap may cause burning and irritation and is usually omitted. The nurse wipes from the inner to the outer canthus of the eye to prevent secretions from draining into the lacrimal sac. A separate section of the washcloth is used each time to prevent spread of infection. If a client has dried secretions that are not removed easily with wiping, the nurse first may place a damp cloth or cotton ball on the lid margins to loosen the secretions. Direct pressure should never be applied over the eyeball, since this may cause serious injury.

The unconscious client may require more frequent eye care. Secretions may collect along the lid margins and inner canthus when the blink reflex is absent or when the eye does not close totally. It may be necessary to place an eye patch over the involved eye(s) to prevent corneal drying and irritation. Lubricating eye drops may be administered according to the physician's orders.

CLEANING GLASSES. Glasses are made of hardened glass or plastic that is impact resistant to prevent shattering. Nevertheless, because of the cost of glasses, the nurse uses care when cleaning glasses and should protect

them from breakage or other damage when not worn. Glasses should be put in their case and in a drawer of the bedside table when not in use.

Warm water is sufficient for cleaning glass lenses. A soft tissue is best for drying to prevent scratching of the lens. Plastic lenses may scratch easily, and require special cleansing solutions and drying tissues.

CONTACT LENS CARE. A contact lens is a small, round, sometimes colored disk that fits on the cornea of the eye over the pupil. The lens floats on the tear layer that lubricates the eye. A variety of contact lenses exist. Hard lenses are rigid, durable, and optically precise. The hard plastic lens can be uncomfortable and difficult to fit. The plastic is not oxygen permeable. The avascular cornea gets much of its oxygen from tears and the air, thus a hard lens must be removed after several hours of wear (12 to 14 hours). Hard lenses are relatively easy to clean and handle.

Soft contact lenses are less durable, more comfortable, and less likely to cause corneal epithelial damage because they are oxygen permeable. Certain soft lenses can be left in place for weeks or months, which is an advantage in the very young or old who have difficulty manipulating lenses. Disadvantages of the soft lenses are that they absorb topical medications, can be sites for infection, may stimulate superficial corneal vascularization, and can accumulate allergenic proteins (Gittinger, 1984). The lenses are often very thin and pliable and thus can easily tear. Extra precautions are needed to clean and manipulate soft lenses.

A third type of contact lens is the rigid gas-permeable lens. It allows oxygen to pass directly through the lens and can be worn either daily or for an extended period (up to 7 days).

A contact lens provides the following certain advantages over eye glasses:

Contact Lens Care

DO

- Wash and rinse hands thoroughly before handling a lens.
- Keep fingernails clean.
- Remove lenses from their storage case *one at a time* and place on the eyes.
- Start with the same lens (left or right) each time of insertion.
- Use lens placement technique learned from eye specialist.
- Use proper lens care products.
- Wear the lenses daily and follow the prescribed wearing schedule.
- Remove a lens if it becomes uncomfortable.
- Keep regular appointments with the eye specialist.
- Remove during sunbathing, showering, or swimming.

DO NOT

- Use soaps that contain cream or perfume for cleaning lenses.
- Let fingernails touch lenses.
- Mix up lenses.
- Exceed prescribed wearing time.
- Use saliva to wet lenses.
- Use homemade saline solution or tap water to wet or clean lenses.

TABLE 32-8   Common Problems for Contact Lens Wearers

Problem	Cause
Uncomfortable lens	Dirty or damaged lens
	Dust on eyelash enters eye
	Eye infection
Redness of the eye	Lens overwear
	Sensitivity to lens care solution
	Allergy
	Eye infection
Blurred vision	Dirty or damaged lens
	Mix up of left with right lens
	Corneal irritation
	Wearing a lens inside out (soft lenses only)
Excess tearing	Corneal irritation
	Lens overwear
	Eye infection

1. Improves clarity of vision
2. Safer than eye glasses during certain physical activities
3. Smoothes optically irregular surfaces of the eye
4. Provides a more attractive appearance for the wearer

Most clients will prefer caring for their contact lenses themselves. An eye specialist will instruct clients on the proper techniques to care for the lens. The box lists some common guidelines for all contact lens wearers that the nurse can reinforce during hygienic care. Clients should also be aware of the symptoms of problems that may be related directly or indirectly to contact lens use (Table 32-8).

The basic steps of contact lens care include cleaning to remove accumulation of deposits from tear film, rinsing to remove lens debris after cleaning, disinfecting to protect eyes from infection, and lubricating to replace water lost from lens and tears through evaporation. A variety of products are available for lens care, and each type of lens requires a different cleansing technique.

Some eye specialists also recommend periodic enzyme cleansing in addition to daily cleansing. The enzymes dissolve protein deposits on the lens surface. Some lenses can be cleaned with electrical heat disinfecting units.

Clients may require assistance from the nurse with contact lens care, insertion, and removal. It is important that a nurse protect those clients who are unable to care for their lenses properly. Prolonged wearing of contact lenses can cause serious corneal damage. Clients who become unconscious, restricted from moving their hands, or who lose clear judgment because of psychiatric illness, temporary mental confusion, or substance abuse should have their lenses removed immediately. Procedure 32-10 describes one technique for the care of contact lenses. Lenses need not be reinserted in these clients until they are more capable of caring for the lenses themselves.

ARTIFICIAL EYES. Clients with artificial eyes have had an enucleation of an entire eyeball as a result of tumor growth, severe infection, or eye trauma. Some artificial eyes are permanently implanted. Others should be removed for routine cleansing. Clients with artificial eyes usually prefer to care for their own eyes rather than having a nurse assist them. The nurse should respect the client's wishes and help by obtaining necessary equipment.

For clients who are scheduled for surgery, are unconscious, or are unable to move their arms, head, or neck, the nurse assists with removal and cleansing of artificial eyes.

To remove an artificial eye, the nurse retracts the lower eyelid and exerts slight pressure just below the eye. This

PROCEDURE 32-10

Taking Care of Contact Lenses

STEPS	RATIONALE
1. Assess client's ability to manipulate and hold contact lens.	Determines level of assistance required in care.
2. After lenses are removed, inspect eye for signs of corneal irritation.	Signs of corneal irritation may require client to refrain from contact use.
3. Discuss procedure with client.	Client can assist by explaining technique that may aid in removal and insertion.
4. Prepare necessary equipment and supplies for lens removal:	
a. Contact lens storage container (see illustration)	Separate cups labeled R for right lens and L for left lens. Protects lens breakage. (Certain lenses are stored dry, whereas others are stored in solution.)
b. Suction cup (optional)	Used to remove hard lens from unconscious or debilitated client.
c. Sterile saline	Used to moisten cornea before lens removal.
5. Prepare necessary equipment and supplies for cleaning and insertion:	
a. Lenses in storage container	
b. Wetting or lubricating solution	Keeps cornea moist and lens lubricated.

HARD LENSES

a. Sterile lens-cleaning solution	Cleans lens surface.
b. Sterile lens disinfectant and/or enzyme solution	Reduces microorganisms present. Enzyme reduces protein deposits.
c. Cotton ball or cotton-tipped applicator	Used to spread cleaner over surface of hard lens.
d. Bath towel	
e. Emesis basin	
f. Glass of warm tap water	

SOFT LENSES

a. Sterile lens-cleaning solution	Cleans lens surface.
b. Sterile lens disinfectant or enzyme solution	Reduces microorganisms and protein deposits.
c. Rinsing solution	Cleans lens of debris.
6. Have client assume supine or sitting position in bed or chair.	Provides easy access for nurse while retracting eyelids and manipulating lens.
7. Removing soft lenses	
a. Wash hands.	Prevents transmission of microorganisms.
b. Place towel just below client's face.	Catches lens if one should accidentally fall from the eye.
c. Add a few drops of sterile saline to client's eye.	Lubricates eye to facilitate lens removal.
d. Locate the position of the lens by gently retracting the client's upper and lower eyelids and asking client to look up, down, or to the side.	Lens may easily become displaced. Lens must be directly over cornea for proper removal.
e. Ask client to look forward	Eases tipping of lens during removal.
f. Using thumb of nondominant hand, retract client's lower eyelid.	Exposes lower edge of lens.
g. With pad of index finger of dominant hand, gently slide lens down off cornea onto the sclera or white of the eye.	Positions lens for easy grasping. Use of finger pad prevents injury to cornea and damage to lens.
h. Pull the upper eyelid down gently with the index finger of the nondominant hand and compress the lens slightly between the thumb and index finger.	Causes soft lens to double up. Air enters underneath lens to release suction.
i. Grasp lens between pads of fingertips of dominant hand, and lift out lens.	Prevents scratching of lens or cornea with the fingernails.
j. Hold lens in palm of cupped hand.	Protects lens from damage.
k. Place lens in proper cup of storage case. Be sure lens is centered properly.	Ensures proper lens will be reinserted into correct eye.

STEPS	RATIONALE

l. Repeat Steps c-k for other lens. Secure cover over storage case.

Proper storage prevents cracking or tearing.

m. Dispose of towel, and wash hands.

Reduces transmission of infection.

8. Removing hard lenses

   a. Wash hands.

Reduces transmission of microorganisms.

   b. Place towel just below client's face.

Catches lens if one should accidentally fall from the eye.

   c. Be sure lens is positioned directly over cornea. If it is not ask client to look forward and apply gentle pressure against lower eyelid with thumb or index finger and position lens properly.

Correct position of lens allows for easy removal from eye.

   d. Use both thumbs and gently retract the client's upper and lower eyelids of one eye until they are beyond the edges of the lens. Do not exert pressure directly on the eye.

Exposes lens fully.
Avoids pressure that can cause discomfort or injure cornea.

   e. Carefully move the margins of both eyelids toward the edges of the lens.

Eyelid margins trap the edges of the lens.

   f. While holding the top eyelid stationary, lift the bottom edge of the contact lens by pressing the lower lid under the lens.

Releases suction of lens on cornea. Lens tips forward.

   g. Bring the margins of both eyelids together to slide the lens off the eye (see illustration).

Minimizes any irritation of eye during lens removal.

   h. With thumb and forefinger grasp lens as it rises from eye.

   i. Cup lens in your hand.

Protects lens from breakage.

   j. Place lens in proper cup labeled L for left eye or R for right eye. Center lens in cup.

Both lenses may not have the same prescription.
Proper storage prevents cracking, tearing, or chipping.

   k. Repeat Steps c-j for other lens. Secure cover over storage case.

Proper storage prevents damage to lens.

   l. Dispose of towel and wash hands.

Controls spread of infection and keeps client's environment neat.

9. Cleansing contact lenses

   a. Wash hands.

Reduces transmission of microorganisms.

   b. Assemble supplies at bedside.

Provides easy access to supplies.

   c. Place towel over work area.

Towel helps to prevent lens breakage.

   d. Open lens container carefully, taking care not to flip lens caps open suddenly.

Prevents lenses from being accidentally spilled or flipped out of case.

   e. If lens has been soaking in disinfectant or enzyme solution, simply rinse with either saline (soft lenses) or tap water (hard lenses). Rinse thoroughly.

Special disinfecting solutions can effectively clean lenses soaked from 2-4 hr.

   f. If lenses have not been disinfected, pick up one lens at a time with your fingertips and place in palm of the hand or on knuckle.

Prevents scratching of lens surface.

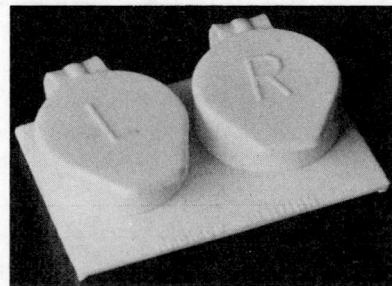

Step 4a

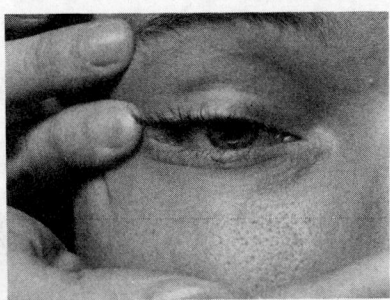

Step 8g

Continued.

PROCEDURE 32-10, cont'd

Taking Care of Contact Lenses

STEPS	RATIONALE
g. Apply 2-3 drops of cleansing solution and spread cleaner evenly over both sides of lens surface, using either fingertips, applicator, or cotton ball.	Spread evenly to cover all surfaces.
h. Gently stroke surface of lens using fingertips or applicator in a circular motion for at least 20 seconds. (Keep lens and finger wet.)	Removes tear film and debris. Moistened lens prevents scratching.
i. Hold lens over emesis basin. Rinse both sides of lens thoroughly with warm tap water (hard lens) or rinsing solution (soft lenses).	Use of basin prevents loss of lens. Rinsing removes sediment and debris.
j. Reinsert lens immediately after cleaning unless storing overnight or disinfecting.	Prevents contamination if lens is replaced in storage container.
k. Repeat steps e-j for other lens.	
l. If lenses are to be disinfected, place each in correct slot of storage container and add disinfecting solution. Close storage container tightly (see illustration).	Ensures all surfaces of lens are exposed to disinfectant.
m. Allow lenses to remain in disinfectant for the correct time indicated on product instructions.	Some solutions need only be applied for 10 minutes. Others may be used for several hours.
n. Open storage case, discard solution, and clean and rinse each lens thoroughly before insertion.	Removes disinfectant that may irritate eye.
o. Clean storage container using hot water and rinsing solution. Keep open to air while drying.	Prevents build up of microorganisms.
p. Wash hands.	Prevents transmission of microorganisms.
10. Inserting hard lenses	
a. Wash hands.	
b. Place towel over client's chest.	Towel will catch dropped lens and avoid breakage.
c. Apply drop of wetting solution to both sides of lens surface. Spread solution over lens.	Lubricates lens so that it slides easily over and adheres to cornea.
d. Place right lens concave side up on top of index finger of dominant hand.	Proper manipulation of lens ensures easy insertion. Inner surface of lens should face up so that it is applied against cornea.
e. Instruct client to bend the head gently backward or look straight ahead, while retracting both upper and lower eyelids (see illustration); place lens gently over center of cornea.	Hard lens is rigid and can be placed as client looks straight ahead. Retraction of lids promotes easy insertion between lid margins.
f. Ask client to close the eyes briefly and avoid blinking.	Helps to secure position of lens.
g. Be sure lens is centered properly by asking client if vision is blurred.	If lens slips to side of cornea or into conjunctival sac, vision will blur.
h. Repeat Steps c-g for left eye.	
i. Assist client to comfortable position.	Promotes client's comfort.

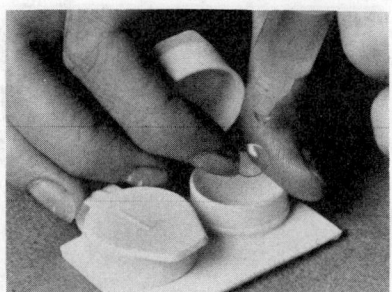

Step 9l

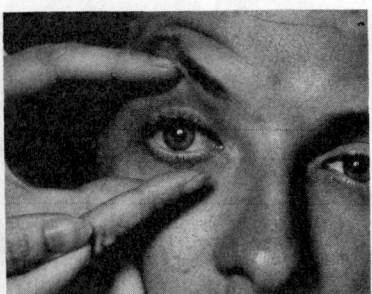

Step 10e

STEPS	RATIONALE
j. Wash hands and discard soiled supplies.	Prevents infection and maintains a neat environment.
k. Store lens container and wetting and cleansing solutions in client's bedside drawer.	
11. Inserting soft lenses	
a. Wash hands.	Prevents transmission of microorganisms
b. Place towel over client's chest.	Towel will catch lens to avoid scratching or tearing.
c. Hold a regular soft lens at its edges between thumb and index finger of your dominant hand. Flex the lens slightly and note if edges point inward. Reverse position if edges point out.	Ensures that correct side of lens is applied over cornea. A lens applied inside out causes blurred vision and minor discomfort.
d. Hold an ultrathin lens on the tip of the index finger of your dominant hand. Note if edges turn inward.	Flexing of an ultrathin lens can cause it to fold and stick together.
e. Wet the right lens with saline, and place it right side up on the tip of your index finger. Be sure the finger is dry.	The wet lens will adhere readily to the moist cornea instead of the dry finger during placement.
f. Have client look up or to the side. Retract both eyelids.	Client's position eases application to surface of eye. Lens should fit easily between eyelid margins.
g. Place soft lens directly over sclera; it may be necessary to press lightly to make lens adhere to eye. Be sure to insert proper lens in each eye.	Placement will allow lens to move over cornea. Prescriptions may differ.
h. Have client close the eye and roll it toward lens.	Maneuver centers soft lens over cornea.
i. Be sure lens is centered properly by asking client if vision is blurred.	If lens slips to side of cornea or into conjuctival sac, vision will blur.
j. If client's vision is blurred:	
(1) Retract eyelids.	
(2) Locate position of lens.	
(3) Ask client to look in direction opposite of lens and with your index finger, apply pressure to lower eyelid margin and position lens over cornea.	
(4) Have client look slowly toward lens.	Technique repositions lens over center of cornea as client looks toward lens.
k. Repeat Steps c-j for left eye.	
l. Assist client to comfortable position.	Promotes client's comfort.
m. Wash hands and discard soiled supplies. Store lens container and wetting and cleansing solutions in client's bedside drawer.	Prevents infection and maintains a neat environment.
12. Ask client if lenses feel comfortable after reinsertion.	Determines if any debris may be caught between lens and cornea.
13. Record or report any signs or symptoms of visual alterations noted during procedure.	May indicate presence of eye injury or disease.
14. Record on nursing care plan or Kardex times of lens insertion and removal.	Determines safe period of time for insertion.

action causes the artificial eye to rise from the socket because the suction holding the eye in place has been broken. The nurse may also use a small, rubber-bulb syringe or medicine dropper bulb to create a suction effect. The suction created by placing the bulb tip directly over the eye and squeezing lifts the artificial eye from the socket.

The artificial eye is usually made of glass or plastic.

Warm normal saline will clean the prosthesis effectively. The nurse also cleans the edges of the eye socket and surrounding tissues with soft gauze moistened in saline or clean tap water. Any signs of infection should be reported immediately, since bacteria can spread to the neighboring eye, underlying sinuses, or underlying brain tissue. To reinsert the eye, the nurse retracts the upper and lower lids and gently slips the eye into the socket, fitting it neatly under the upper eyelid. An artificial eye may be stored in a labeled container filled with tap water or saline.

PRESERVING VISION. All clients will benefit from learning a few simple guidelines for their visual health:

1. Clients under the age of 40 should have an eye examination regularly every 3 to 5 years. Routine testing for glaucoma is advised for all adults over age 40 every 2 years.
2. Common symptoms of eye disorders include pain, photophobia, blurred vision, burning, itching, excess tearing, halos around lights, and floaters.
3. Avoid home remedies for eye problems or injuries. Treatment for chemicals or dust that enters the eye includes flushing the eye continuously with tepid water for at least 10 minutes.
4. Never try to remove a foreign object from the eye. Seek medical attention immediately.

CLEANING THE EARS

The nurse cleans the client's ears as a routine part of a bed bath. The clean end of a moistened washcloth, rotated gently into the ear canal, works best for cleaning. When cerumen is visible, gentle downward retraction at the entrance of the ear canal may cause the wax to loosen and slip out. The nurse instructs clients never to use bobby pins or toothpicks to remove ear wax. The use of such objects can cause trauma to the ear canal and rupture of the tympanic membrane. Use of cotton-tipped applicators should also be avoided, since they can cause wax to become impacted within the canal.

Children are the most common age group to have impacted cerumen. Excessive or impacted cerumen can usually be removed only by irrigation. The procedure first involves instilling one to two drops of mineral oil in the impacted ear(s) twice daily for 4 to 5 days (Watkins, 1984). Then the instillation of approximately 250 ml of warm water (37° C or 98.6° F) into the external ear canal will mechanically wash away loosened wax. Cold or hot water will cause nausea or vomiting. The child may sit or lie on his or her side with the affected ear up. The nurse places a small curved basin under the affected ear to catch the irrigating solution. A Water Pik (set on no. 2 setting) or a bulb irrigating syringe can be used to irrigate the ear canal. The tip of the syringe or pik should not occlude the ear canal to avoid exerting pressure against the tympanic membrane. Gentle irrigation directed toward the top of the canal will loosen the cerumen from the sides of the ear canal. Once the canal is clear, the nurse wipes off any moisture from the client's ear and inspects the canal for remaining cerumen.

HEARING AIDS. Chapter 44 discusses the need for and use of hearing aids. Hearing loss is a common health

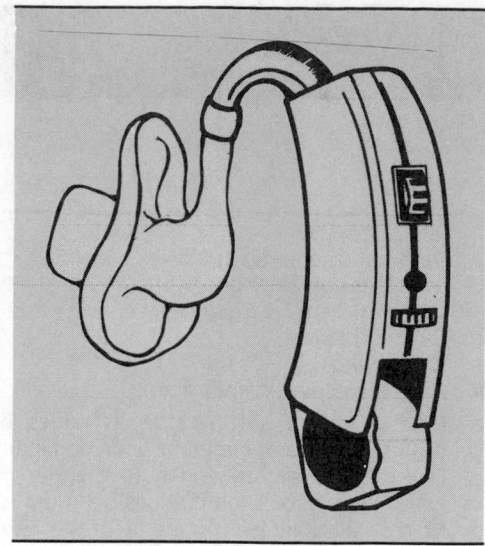

Fig. 32-2   Behind-the-ear hearing aid.

problem. The ability to hear is vital for persons to be able to communicate normally and react appropriately within their environment. Four types of hearing aids are available to clients. One is the behind-the-ear hearing aid, shaped like a shrimp that fits around and behind the ear. It is the most common type of hearing aid used (Fig. 32-2). Another is the body-aid, which is a bulky instrument used for severe hearing loss. A fitted ear mold connects to a receiver and transmitter the size of a cigarette case. The in-the-ear hearing aid is a small device that fits in the ear canal. An eyeglass aid fits into the ear canal and attaches to a battery located on the arm of the eyeglass frame. The care of a hearing aid involves routine cleansing, battery care, and proper insertion technique (Proc. 32-11).

NOSE CARE

The client can usually remove secretions from the nose by gently blowing into a soft tissue. This may be all the daily hygiene that is needed. The nurse cautions the client against harsh blowing that creates pressure capable of injuring the eardrum, nasal mucosa, and even sensitive eye structures. Bleeding from the nares is a key sign of harsh blowing or mucosal irritation.

If the client is unable to remove nasal secretions, the nurse assists by using a wet washcloth or a cotton-tipped applicator moistened in water or saline. The applicator should never be inserted beyond the length of the cotton tip. Excessive nasal secretions can also be removed by suctioning. Nasal suctioning is contraindicated in clients who have had nasal or brain surgery.

When clients have tubes inserted through the nose, the nurse should change the tape anchoring the tube at least once a day (see Chapter 46). When tape becomes

PROCEDURE 32-11

Care of a Behind-the-Ear Hearing Aid

Steps	Rationale
1. Assess client's knowledge of and routines for cleansing and caring for hearing aid.	Determines client's understanding and need for health education. Nurse will adapt method of care to client's procedure.
2. Determine whether client can hear clearly with use of aid by talking slowly and clearly in normal voice tone.	Inability to hear may indicate faulty function of hearing aid.
3. Have client suggest any additional tips for care; explain that you are going to clean and replace hearing aid.	Client becomes uncomfortable when unable to hear clearly. Explain all steps before removing aid to minimize confusion and anxiety.
4. Assess whether hearing aid is working by removing from client's ear. Close battery case and turn volume slowly to high. Cup hand over earmold. If aid emits no sound, replace batteries and assess again.	Determines need for new battery. Feedback squeal will cause harsh whistling sound.
5. Check to be sure plastic connecting tube is not twisted or cracked.	Cracked or twisted tube prevents transmission of sound.
6. Check to see if earmold is cracked or has rough edges.	Can cause irritation to external ear canal.
7. Check for accumulation of cerumen around earmold and plugging of opening in mold.	Prevents clear sound reception and transmission.
8. Prepare necessary equipment and supplies:	
a. Emesis basin	Used to soak ear mold.
b. Mild soap and warm water	
c. Pipe cleaner (optional)	Used to clean plastic connecting tube.
d. Syringe needle (optional)	Used to clean opening in ear mold.
e. Soft towel	
f. Washcloth	
g. Storage case	
9. Cleaning hearing aid	
a. Wash hands.	Reduces transmission of microorganisms.
b. Assemble supplies at bedside table or sink area.	Procedure can be performed without delays.
c. Detach earmold from battery device.	Moisture entering battery and transmitter will cause permanent damage to aid.
d. Add warm water and soap to emesis basin. Soak ear mold for several minutes.	Soaking removes cerumen that can accumulate on mold.
e. Wash ear canal with washcloth moistened in soap and water. Rinse and dry.	Removes cerumen and debris.
f. If cerumen has built up in hole of earmold, carefully clean hole with tip of syringe needle.	Wax will prevent normal sound transmission.
g. Rinse earmold thoroughly with clear water.	Soap may form residue that blocks opening in mold.
h. Allow mold to dry thoroughly after wiping with soft towel.	Water droplets left in connecting tube could enter hearing aid and damage parts.
i. Clean connecting tube with pipe cleaner (optional).	Removes moisture and debris that can interfere with sound transmission and hearing aid function.
j. Reconnect ear mold to hearing aid device before inserting or storing hearing aid.	Reassembly allows nurse to check functioning.
k. Store hearing aid in storage case if client is about to bathe, walk in the rain, use a hair dryer, sit under sun lamp or heat, go to surgery or major procedure or sleep or if client is diaphoretic.	Protects hearing aid against damage and breakage.
10. Inserting hearing aid	
a. To reinsert hearing aid first check batteries (Step 4); replace batteries as needed.	Necessary for proper sound amplification. Always change batteries over soft surface (for example, towel or bed) to avoid breakage.
b. Turn aid off and turn volume control down.	Will protect client from sudden exposure to sound.
c. Place earmold in external ear canal. Be sure ear bore (hole) in mold is placed into canal first. Shape of mold indicates correct ear. Gently press and twist until mold feels snug.	Proper fit ensures optimum sound transmission.

Continued.

PROCEDURE 32-11, cont'd

Care of a Behind-the-Ear Hearing Aid

STEPS	RATIONALE
d. Gently bring connecting tube up and over toward back of ear, avoiding kinking. Battery device fits around upper ear (see illustration).	Ensures correct function of hearing aid device and maintains client's comfort.
e. Adjust volume gradually to comfortable level for talking to client in regular voice at a 1-1.25 m (3-4 feet) distance.	Gradual adjustment prevents exposing client to harsh squeal or feedback. Client should hear nurse comfortably.
f. Remove soiled equipment from bedside. Dispose of used supplies. Wash hands.	Maintains clean environment and reduces risk of infection.

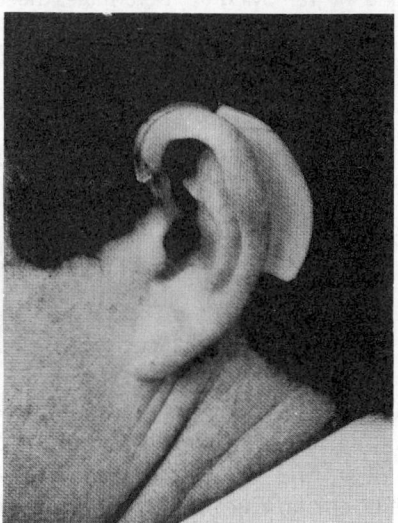

Step 10d

11. Return to client to assess whether hearing is clear or hearing aid is producing inappropriate feedback sound.	If earmold is not securely in place, it will squeal or not function.
12. Document that aid is removed and stored if client is going to surgery or special procedure.	Protects nurse from liability of loss of hearing aid.
13. Report to nursing staff difficulties client has in communicating.	Improves continuity of care in communication techniques for client.
14. Note on nursing kardex that client uses hearing aid.	

Illustration from Long, BC, and Phipps, WJ: *Essentials of medical-surgical nursing,* ed. 2, St. Louis, 1989, The C.V. Mosby Co.

moist from nasal secretions, the skin and mucosa can easily become macerated. The up and down movement of tubing causes tissue sloughing. The nurse should know how to tape tubing correctly to minimize tension or friction on the nares. When sloughing occurs, it may be necessary to remove the tube and insert one through the other naris. The nurse should always clean the nares thoroughly around the tubing because secretions accumulate.

EVALUATION

Evaluation of eye, ear, and nose care must be individualized on the basis of the client's existing sensory function. Hygienic care alone will not improve sensory function beyond a client's baseline level. The evaluation box outlines the nurse's evaluation measures.

Evaluation of Interventions for Eye, Ear, and Nose Problems

Goals	Evaluative Measures	Expected Outcomes
Infection is absent.	Inspect condition of the conjunctiva and lid margins of the eye.	Conjunctiva will remain clear and pink. Eyelid margins are without drainage or crustations.
	Question client about symptoms of eye problems.	Client denies symptoms of burning, itching, excess tearing.
	Inspect condition of external ear canal. Gently palpate tragus of ear. Question client about ear discomfort.	Canal is clear without redness, areas of excoriation, or purulent discharge. Client denies discomfort as ear is palpated.
	Inspect condition of nares.	Nares are clear without inflammation or purulent drainage.
Normal sensory organ function is present.	Evaluate client's visual acuity and ability to hear normal conversation (allow client to use own aids during testing).	Client is able to visually identify objects with the same accuracy as prior to hygiene (for example, read newsprint, recognize faces). Client is able to hear conversation in normal tone of voice and respond appropriately to questions.
Client understands method used to care for the eyes, ears, and nose.	Ask client to explain hygiene methods to use.	Client describes techniques for basic eye, ear, and nose care.
	Observe client perform personal hygiene.	Client performs hygiene measures correctly, including care of any sensory aids.
	Ask client to discuss ways to maintain visual health.	Client describes precautions to take for visual health.

CLIENT'S ROOM ENVIRONMENT

Attempting to make client's rooms as comfortable as their home environments is one of the nurse's priorities. Clients with severe illness may be restricted to bed for many days. Likewise, clients immobilized by traction apparatus, casts, or monitoring equipment do not always enjoy the luxury of leaving their rooms as they wish. Clients hospitalized in semiprivate rooms must share the environment with another person. Chronically disabled persons living in nursing homes or skilled care facilities are often confined to rooms for long periods. The client's room should be comfortable, safe, and large enough to allow the client and visitors to move about freely. The nurse is able to control factors such as room temperature, ventilation, noise, and odors to creat a more comfortable environment. Keeping the room neat and orderly also contributes to the sense of well-being.

Maintaining Comfort

Providing a comfortable environment depends on age, severity of illness, and level of normal daily activity. Depending on the client's age and physical condition, room temperature should be between 20° and 23° C (68° and 74° F). Infants, the elderly, and the acutely ill may need a warmer temperature. However, some critically ill clients benefit from cooler temperatures to lower the body's metabolic demands. A client physically active will usually be more comfortable in a cool room.

A good ventilation system keeps stale air and odors from lingering in the room. Because drafts may occur as the air moves about the room, the nurse must protect the acutely ill, infants, and the elderly by ensuring that they are adequately dressed and covered with a lightweight blanket. Clients who complain of excess drafts, despite the nurse's interventions, may need to be moved to a different room.

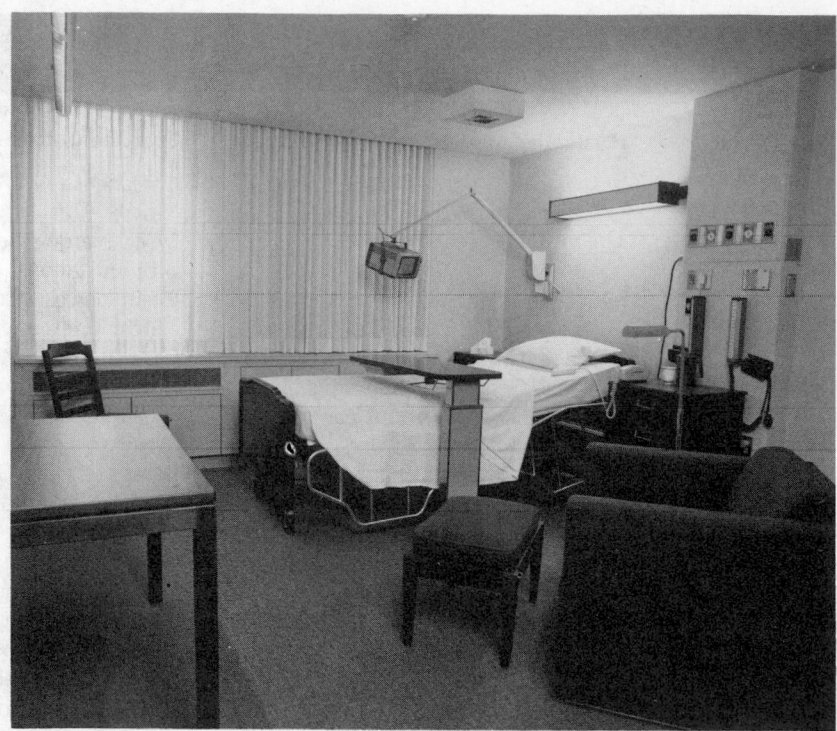

Fig. 32-3   A typical hospital room.

Good ventilation also reduces lingering odors caused by draining wounds, vomitus, bowel movements, and the failure to empty bedpans and urinals promptly. Body, breath, or smoking odors may also be offensive to some people. Room deodorizers help in eliminating many unpleasant odors. Nurses should always empty and rinse bedpans or urinals promptly after use. Thorough hygiene measures are the best way to control body or breath odors. Hospitalized clients can generally choose to stay in a room where smoking is not permitted. The nurse should monitor visitors who attempt to smoke in client's rooms and explain that smoke can be irritating to the clients breathing. Many health care institutions prohibit smoking in nursing care areas.

Ill clients seem to be more sensitive to the noises commonly heard within a hospital environment: the clanging of metal equipment, wheelchairs or stretchers moving down halls, or loud talking and laughter at the nurse's station. Until the client is familiar with the hospital noise, the nurse should try to control the noise level by handling equipment properly, making sure equipment is in proper working order, and controlling voice volume. The nurse also explains the source of any unfamiliar noises.

Proper lighting is necessary for the safety and comfort of the client and health care workers. A brightly lit room is usually stimulating. When clients attempt to fall asleep, the nurse reduces lighting levels. Room lighting can be adjusted by closing or opening drapes, regulating overbed and floor lights, and closing or opening room doors.

Controlling stimuli within the room environment helps to promote the client's feeling of security. A comfortable environment enhances the client's ability to gain needed rest and sleep so all energy can be direct to recovery.

Room Equipment

A typical hospital room (Fig. 32-3) contains certain basic pieces of furniture: overbed table, bedside stand,

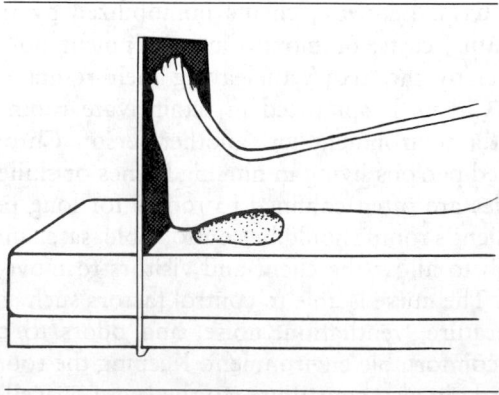

Fig. 32-4   Footboard.

chairs, lights, and beds. Special equipment designed for comfort or positioning of clients includes footboards (Fig. 32-4), special mattresses, bed boards, and bed cradles (see box).

OVERBED TABLE

The overbed table rolls on wheels and can be adjusted to various heights over the bed or a chair. Usually two storage areas are under the tabletop. The table provides ideal working space for the nurse performing procedures and also serves as a surface to place meal trays, toiletry items, and objects frequently used by the client.

BEDSIDE STAND

The bedside stand is used to store the client's personal articles as well as hygiene equipment such as the bath basin, extra towels, or an emesis basin. The telephone, water pitcher, and drinking cup are commonly found on a bedside table.

CHAIRS

Most hospital rooms contain two types of chairs: an armless straight-backed chair and an upholstered lounge chair with arms. The lounge chair is used by the client and visitors and is usually placed at the foot of the bed or alongside it. Straight-backed chairs are convenient when temporarily transferring the client from the bed, as during bedmaking. A straight-backed chair is also more maneuverable than the larger lounge chair. Nurses frequently place clean linen on the chair or hang linen bags over the chair back.

LIGHTS

Each room usually has an overbed light in addition to a floor or table lamp. Movable lights that extend over the bed from the wall should be positioned for easy reach but moved aside when not in use to prevent clients or staff from bumping their heads. Gooseneck or special examination lights are portable standing lights used to provide extra illumination during bedside procedures.

A call light is at each client's bedside. When a client presses a button located on the side rail of the bed or at the end of an extension cord, a light goes on at the nurses' station or just outside the client's room. The call-light signal indicates a client needs assistance. It is important for the nurse to respond to a call light as soon as possible. In addition to call lights, most hospitals have intercoms that allow clients to talk to a staff person at the nurses' station. Many hospital units also have emergency signal lights that nurses use to call for assistance when clients are in trouble.

BEDS

Because a bed is the piece of equipment used most by a client, it should be designed for comfort, safety, and adaptability for changing positions.

The typical hospital bed consists of a firm mattress on a metal frame that can be raised and lowered horizontally. The frame is divided into three sections so the operator can raise and lower the head and foot of the bed, in addition to inclining the entire bed with the headboard up or down. Table 32-9 lists common bed positions. Most beds are powered by electrical motors, but some beds are run manually or by hydraulic power.

The position of a bed is usually changed by electrical controls on the side of the bed, at the foot of the bed, or in a bedside cable. Clients can thus raise or lower sections of the bed without expending much energy. It is important for nurses to instruct clients on the proper use of controls and to caution them against raising the bed to a position that might cause harm. A hospital bed is usually 65 to 70 cm (26 to 28 inches) above the floor at its lowest level. In the home most beds are 50 to 55 cm (20 to 22 inches) high. The greater height of a hospital bed prevents undue musculoskeletal strain on the

TABLE 32-9 Common Bed Positions

Position	Description	Uses
Fowler's	Head of bed raised to angle of 45 degrees or more; semisitting position.	Preferred while client eats; used during nasogastric tube insertion and nasotracheal suction; promotes lung expansion.
Semi-Fowler's	Head of bed raised approximately 30 degrees; incline less than Fowler's position.	Promotes lung expansion.
Trendelenburg	Entire bed frame tilted with head of bed down.	For postural drainage; facilitates venous return in clients with poor peripheral perfusion.
Reverse Trendelenburg	Entire bed frame tilted with foot of bed down.	Used infrequently; promotes gastric emptying and prevents esophageal reflux.
Flat	Entire bed frame horizontally parallel with floor.	For clients with vertebral injuries and in cervical traction. Position used for clients who are hypotensive. Position generally preferred by clients for sleeping.

nurse and the client. It is unnecessary for the nurse to reach across or bend down while caring for clients, and clients can move from the bed to a chair with minimal stress on their hips and knees.

Beds contain a number of safety features. Locks located on the wheels or casters should be used whenever the bed is stationary to prevent accidental movement during performance of a procedure (for example, transferring the client from the bed to a stretcher). Side rails, located on both sides of a bed, protect clients from accidental falls, help clients position themselves, and provide upper extremity support as a client gets out of bed. Side rails are adjustable, metal frames that raise and lower by pushing or pulling a knob. The nurse never leaves the bedside when a side rail is lowered with the client still in bed. Each bed also has a special removable headboard. This feature is important in emergency situations when the medical team must have easy access

to the client's head during cardiopulmonary resuscitation (see Chapter 36).

Most beds have firm, water-repellent mattresses. A mattress should have an even surface for the client's comfort. Most mattresses have handles on the sides to be used when the mattresses are removed or turned over.

Special beds, frames, and mattresses have been designed to help nurses care for bedridden clients and their special needs. Some beds and frames help to turn immobilized clients or maintain correct body alignment at all times (see box). They make it easier for nurses to lift or position clients. Some beds also have specially designed mattresses or surfaces that reduce risk or pressure sore formation.

BEDMAKING. Making a bed is an important responsibility of the nurse. It is essential for the nurse to keep the bed as clean and comfortable as possible. This re-

Special Beds and Mattresses

- **CircOlectric bed**—consists of bed frame–turning mechanism that rotates vertically in a circular fashion up to 210 degrees. Used for clients with spinal cord injuries and severe burns.
- **Rotokinetic treatment table**—rotates a client up to 270 degrees continuously from the extreme left lateral to the extreme right lateral position. Used for severely immobilized clients and clients with multiple trauma or spinal cord injuries.
- **Clinitron bed**—distributes clients' weight evenly over its support surface. Works through fluidization. Air is forced upward through the mattress that contains tiny ceramic microspheres. Used for immobilized clients and clients in severe pain.
- **Flotation pads**—mattress-like pad contructed of silicone or polyvinyl chloride gel encased in a vinyl-covered square. Serves as an artificial layer of fat to pad bony prominences. Fits in center of larger foam mattress.
- **Egg crate mattress**—foam mattress with foam rubber peak designed to disperse and evenly distribute a client's weight.
- **Air mattress (pressure cycling)**—rubberized mattress that fits over regular bed mattress. Connected with a pressure cycling device that intermittently inflates and deflates to create a cycling effect that minimizes pressure on bony prominences.

quires frequent inspections to be sure linen is clean, dry, and wrinkle free.

The nurse usually makes a bed in the morning after the client's bath, as the client is bathing and showering, or when the client is out of the room for tests or procedures. Throughout the day the nurse straightens linen that becomes loose or wrinkled. The bed linen should also be checked for food particles after meals and for wetness or soiling. Any linen that becomes wet or soiled should be changed.

When changing the bed linen, the nurse follows basic principles of asepsis by keeping soiled linen away from the uniform. It is best to place soiled linen in special linen bags before discarding it in the linen hamper. The nurse never fans linen so as to avoid air currents, which can spread microorganisms. Dirty linen should never be placed on the floor to avoid transmitting infection. If clean linen touches the floor, it is immediately discarded.

During bedmaking the nurse must use proper body mechanics. The bed should always be raised to its highest position before changing linen so the nurse does not have

to bend or stretch over the mattress. When making an occupied bed, the nurse should also use the principles of body mechanics while turning and repositioning the client (see Chapter 41).

The client's privacy, comfort, and safety are all important when making a bed. Using side rails, keeping call lights within the client's reach, and maintaining the proper bed position help promote a client's comfort and safety. After making a bed, the nurse always returns it to the lowest horizontal position to prevent accidental falls.

Whenever possible, the nurse should make the bed while it is unoccupied (Procedure 32-12). If the client is confined to bed, the nurse organizes bedmaking activities to conserve time and energy (Procedure 32-13). When making an unoccupied bed, the nurse follows the same basic principles for bedmaking. However, the nurse loosens the bed linen on both sides, removes all soiled linen simultaneously, and places the clean base and top linen on one side before going to the other side.

An unoccupied bed can be either open or closed. In an open bed the top covers are folded back so a client can easily get into bed. In a closed bed the top sheet, blanket, and bedspread are drawn up to the head of the mattress and under the pillows. A closed bed is prepared in a hospital room before a new client is admitted to that room.

A surgical, recovery, or postoperative bed is an open version of the unoccupied bed. The top bed linen is arranged in a way that allows a surgical client to transfer easily from a stretcher to the bed (Fig. 32-5). The top sheets and spread are not tucked or mitered at the corners. Instead, the top sheets are folded lengthwise or crosswise at the foot of the bed. If a client is returning from surgery, the nurse always makes a complete linen change. Once a client is discharged, all bed linen is sent

Text continued on p. 878.

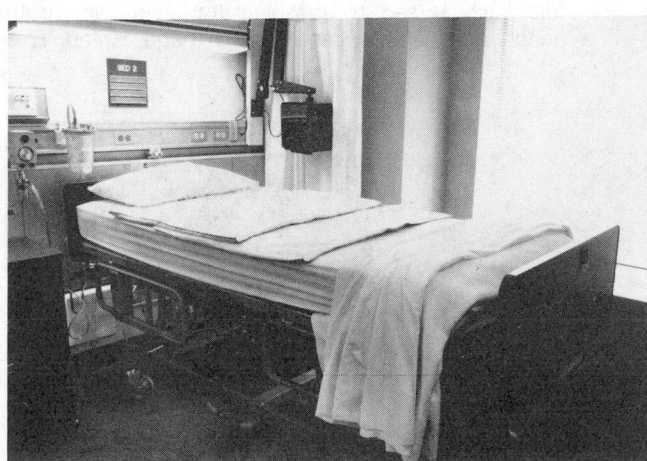

Fig. 32-5 Surgical or recovery bed.

PROCEDURE 32-12

Making an Unoccupied Bed

STEPS	RATIONALE
1. Assess potential for client being incontinent or having excess drainage on bed linen.	Determines need for protective waterproof pads or bath blankets on bed.
2. Assess client's activity orders and physical mobility.	Determines level of activity allowed, including whether client should be out of bed.
3. If client is in bed, explain that you wish to change bed while he or she is sitting up. Ask if he feels able to sit in chair and assist as necessary.	Client should not feel inconvenienced by procedure. Client may feel anxious if uncomfortable or fatigued.
4. Prepare needed quipment and supplies:	
a. Linen bags	Used to collect linens.
b. Mattress pad (need only be changed when soiled)	
c. Bottom sheet (flat or fitted)	
d. Draw sheet	Used to help lift or move client and to protect bottom sheet from soiling.
e. Top sheet (flat)	
f. Blanket	
g. Bedspread	
h. Waterproof pads or bath blankets (optional)	To lay under client at points where drainage is expected. Reduces soiling of bed linen.
i. Pillow cases	Used to place linen on in order of use.
j. Bedside chair or table	
5. Wash hands.	Reduces transmission of microorganisms.
6. Assemble equipment and arrange it on bedside chair or table. Remove all unnecessary equipment, such as overbed table.	Assembling all equipment provides for smooth flow of procedure and ensures client's comfort. Placing linen on clean surface minimizes spread of infection.
7. Lower side rail on your side of bed and remove call light.	Provides easy access to bed.
8. Adjust bed height to comfortable working position.	Raising bed minimizes strain on nurse's back and muscles.
9. On your side, loosen linen, starting at top of bed. Move along sides and then down toward foot. Move to other side of bed, lower side rail, and loosen all linen.	Loosening linen makes it easier to remove.
10. Remove bedspread and blanket separately by folding each into ball or folded square and discarding into linen bag if they are not to be reused. Do not allow uniform to come in contact with soiled linen (see illustration). Avoid fanning or shaking linen.	Reduces transmission of microoogranisms.
11. If spread or blanket is to be reused, fold as follows: fold each spread by grasping top edge with both hands, one hand at center; other hand at end. Fold	Folding method facilitates replacement and prevents wrinkling.

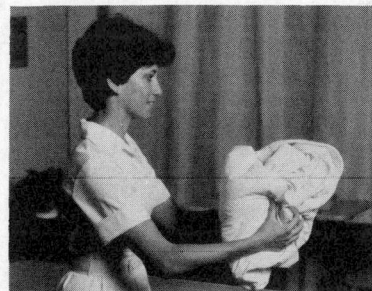

Step 10

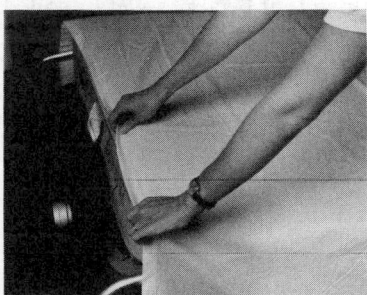

Step 18

STEPS	RATIONALE
top edge down, even with the bottom edge. Pick up spread at center and fold so that farthest side comes even with nearest side. Bring top and bottom edges together again. Place folded spread or blanket over back of chair.	
12. Remove soiled pillow cases by grasping closed end with one hand and slipping pillow out with other. Discard pillow cases in linen bag and place pillows on table.	Pillows slide out easily, minimizing chance of contact with soiled linen.
13. Fold each piece of remaining bed linen separately into ball or folded square and discard into linen bag.	Attempting to fold all soiled linen at once creates bulky bundle that is difficult to discard and may easily come in contact with the nurse's uniform.
14. Slide mattress toward head of bed.	If mattress slides toward foot of bed when head of bed is raised, it is difficult to tuck in linen.
15. Wipe off any moisture on mattress with washcloth moistened in antiseptic solution; dry thoroughly.	Reduces transmission of microorganisms.
16. Stand at side of bed where linen is placed. Spread mattress pad over mattress.	Time is saved by making half of bed first and then moving to opposite side.
17. Smooth out all wrinkles in pad.	Wrinkles or folds of linen are source of chronic irritation against client's skin.
18. Unfold bottom sheet lengthwise and place the vertical center crease of the sheet lengthwise along center of the bed. Fold sheet's top layer over toward opposite side of bed. Smooth bottom layer of sheet across mattress on your side; bring edge over side of mattress. Allow it to hang 25 cm (10 in) over mattress edge. Hem of bottom edge of sheet should lie seam down, even with bottom edge of mattress (see illustration). Pull remaining top portion of sheet over top edge of mattress.	Method of unfolding linen saves nurse's time and energy. Making one side of bed at a time avoids excess movement. Proper placement of linen ensures adequate length will be available to cover opposite side of bed. Keeping seam edge down eliminates source of irritation to client's skin. If bottom edge of sheet is not tucked in, it can later be changed without removing top linen.
19. While standing at head of the bed, miter top corner of bottom sheet.	Mitered corner is not loosened easily.

19.
a. Face head of bed diagonally. Place hand that is away from head of bed under top corner of mattress near mattress edge and lift.
b. With other hand, tuck top edge of bottom sheet smoothly under mattress so side edges of sheet above and below mattress would meet if brought together.
c. Face side of bed and pick up top edge of sheet approximately 45 cm (18 in) down from top of mattress (see illustration).
d. Lift sheet and lay it on top of mattress to form neat, triangular fold, with lower base of triangle even with mattress side edge (see illustration).
e. Tuck lower edge of sheet, hanging free below mattress, under mattress. Tuck with your palms down. Do this without pulling triangular fold (see illustration).
f. Hold portion of sheet covering side edge of mattress in place with one hand. With other hand, pick up top of triangular linen fold and bring it down over side of mattress. Tuck this portion of sheet under mattress (see illustration).

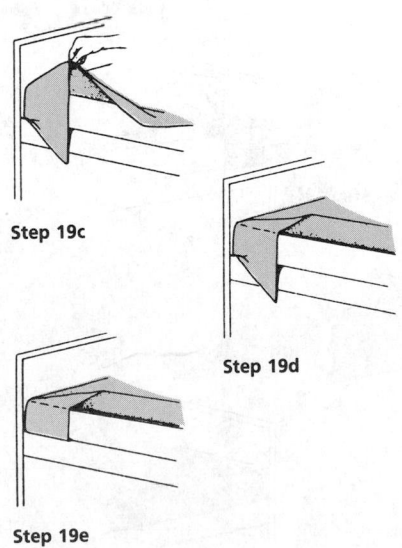

Step 19c

Step 19d

Step 19e

Continued.

PROCEDURE 32-12, cont'd

Making an Unoccupied Bed

STEPS	RATIONALE
20. Tuck remaining portion of sheet under mattress. Keep linen smooth (see illustration).	Folds of linen can irritate client's skin.
21. Open drawsheet so it unfolds in half. Lay center fold along middle of the bed lengthwise. Fanfold top layer at center of bed. Smooth bottom layer of drawsheet out over mattress.	Drawsheet is used to lift and reposition client. Placement under client's torso distributes most of body weight over sheet.
22. Tuck excess edge under mattress, keeping palms down.	Anchors sheet in place to prevent sliding and wrinkling.
23. Move to opposite side of bed.	One side of bed is completed before nurse moves to other side.
24. Spread fanfolded bottom sheet smoothly over edge of mattress from head to foot of bed.	Wrinkles can cause irritation.
25. Miter top corner of bottom sheet (Step 19). When tucking corner be sure sheet is taut.	Taut sheet eliminates wrinkles and folds that can rub client's skin.
26. Facing side of bed, grasp remaining edge of bottom sheet, lean back, keeping your back straight, and pull as you tuck excess linen tightly under mattress. Proceed from head to foot of bed. (Avoid lifting mattress during tucking to ensure tight fit.)	Proper use of body mechanics while tucking linen prevents injury to nurse.
27. Smooth folded drawsheet over bottom sheet. Grasp edge of drawsheet with palms down, lean back, and tuck sheet tightly under mattress. Tuck first at middle, then at top, and then at bottom (see illustration).	Tucking first at top or bottom may pull sheet sideways, causing poor fit.
28. If needed, apply waterproof pad or bath blanket over drawsheet.	Pad collects body secretions and drainage, protecting linen from becoming soiled.
29. Move to side of bed where linen is located. Place top sheet over bed with vertical center fold lengthwise down middle of bed. Open sheet out from head to foot, being sure top edge of sheet is seam up and even with top edge of mattress. Spread excess sheet over bottom edge of mattress. (Do not fan top sheet over the bed.)	Placement ensures equal distribution of sheet over bed. Positioning sheet with seam up prevents irritation of client's skin. Avoid fanning because it creates air currents, which can spread microorganisms throughout room.

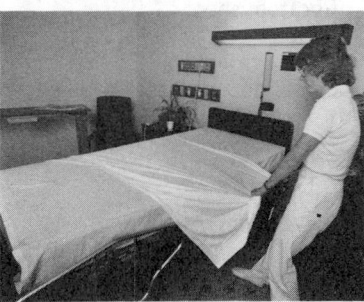

Step 27

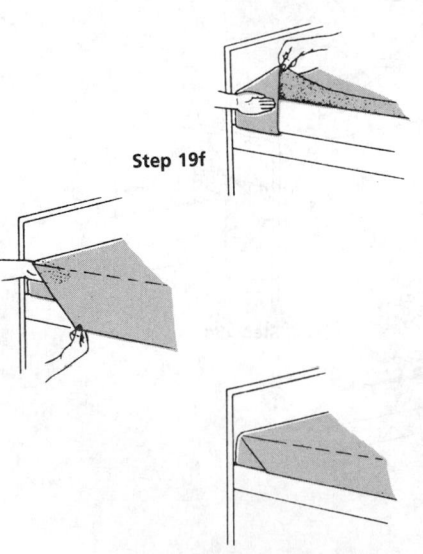

Step 19f

Step 20

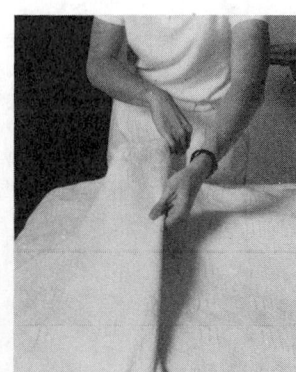

Step 30

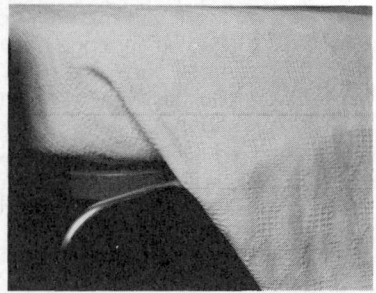

Step 36

STEPS	RATIONALE
30. Make horizontal toe pleat: stand at foot of bed and form fold in sheet 5-10 cm (2-4 in) across bed. Pull sheet up from bottom to make fold. Fold should be approximately 15 cm (6 in) from bottom edge of mattress (see illustration).	Allows for free movement of client's feet and prevents friction against surface of toes.
31. Tuck in remaining portion of sheet on one side of foot of mattress (optional).	Anchors top sheet so that client can move freely.
32. Place blanket on bed, unfolding it so that crease runs lengthwise along middle of bed. Top edge should be parallel with edge of top sheet and 15-20 cm (6-8 in) down from top mattress edge. Bottom edge should hang over mattress. Spread blanket evenly over bed.	Blanket provides adequate warmth. Cuff will be formed with sheet folded over top edge of blanket and spread.
33. Place spread over bed according to Step 30. Be sure top edge of spread extends about 2.5 cm (1 in) above blanket's edge. Then tuck top edge of spread over and under top edge of blanket.	Spread gives bed a neat appearance and provides extra warmth.
34. Make a cuff by running edge of top sheet down over top edge of blanket and spread.	Smooth cuff protects client's face from irritation.
35. Standing on one side at foot of bed, lift mattress corner slightly with one hand and with other hand tuck top sheet, blanket, and spread together under mattress. Be sure you have not pulled out toe pleat of sheet so linens are loose enough for client to move.	Pressure sores can develop on client's toes and heels if feet rub between tight-fitting bed sheets. Lifting mattress too high can loosen bottom linen.
36. Make modified mitered corner with top sheet, blanket, and spread: pick up side edge of top sheet, blanket, and spread approximately 45 cm (18 in) up from foot of mattress. Lift linens to form triangular fold and lay it on bed. Tuck loose edge hanging down under side of mattress. Pick up triangular fold and bring it down over mattress, holding linen in place along side of mattress. Do not tuck tip of triangle (see illustration).	Modified mitered corner secures top linen but keeps even edge of top sheet, blanket, and spread draped over mattress.
37. Go to other side: spread sheet, blanket, and spread evenly. Fold top edge of spread over blanket and make cuff with top sheet (as in Step 34). Make modified mitered corner at foot of bed (as in Step 36).	Nurse saves time and energy by completing one side of bed at time.
38. Apply clean pillowcase. With one hand, grasp pillowcase at center of closed end. Gather case, turning it inside out over hand holding it. With same hand, pick up middle of one end of pillow. Pull pillowcase down over pillow with other hand. Be sure corners of case fit evenly over pillow.	This method makes it easy to slide case smoothly over pillow.
39. Position pillow(s) at center of head of bed.	Maintains neat appearance.
40. Place call light within client's reach and return bed to comfortable height.	Provides for client's safety.
41. If client is to return to bed, fold back top covers to one side or fanfold them to bottom third of bed.	Folding back covers makes it easy for client to return to bed.
42. Rearrange furniture and place any personal items within easy reach.	Neat environment promotes sense of well-being.
43. Discard dirty linen in linen hamper or chute. Wash hands.	Prevents transmission of microorganisms.
44. Evaluate client's tolerance to sitting up in chair: compare heart rate to previous resting rate. Ask if client feels weak, dizzy, or fatigued; assess blood pressure if client complains of dizziness or weakness.	Client's inability to tolerate exertion, even low levels of exercise, may be reflected in changes in vital signs or subjective report of symptoms.
45. Assist client in returning to bed.	

Illustrations from Sorrentino, SA: Mosby's textbook for nursing assistants, ed. 2, St. Louis, 1987, The C.V. Mosby Co.

Making an Occupied Bed

STEPS	RATIONALE
1. Determine potential for client being incontinent or having excess drainage on bed linen.	Determines need for protective waterproof pads or extra bath blankets on bed.
2. Check client's chart for orders or specific precautions for movement and positioning.	Ensures client's safety as well as use of proper body mechanics for nurse and client.
3. Explain procedure to client, noting that client will be asked to turn on side to roll over linen.	Minimizes anxiety and promotes client's cooperation.
4. Prepare needed equipment and supplies:	
a. Linen bags	Used to collect linen.
b. Bath blanket	Provides warmth.
c. Mattress pad (need only be changed when soiled)	
d. Bottom sheet (flat or fitted)	
e. Draw sheet	Used to help lift or move client at points where drainage is expected. Reduces soiling of bed linen.
f. Top sheet (flat)	
g. Blanket	
h. Bedspread	
i. Waterproof pads (optional)	Lay under client at points where drainage is expected. Reduces soiling of bed linen.
j. Pillow case(s)	
k. Bedside chair or table	
5. Wash hands.	Reduces transmission of microorganisms.
6. Assemble equipment and arrange it on bedside chair or table. Remove all unnecessary equipment.	Assembling all equipment provides for smooth procedure and ensures client's comfort. Placing linen on clean surface minimizes spread of infection.
7. Draw room curtain around bed or close door.	Maintains client's privacy, thus promoting emotional and physical comfort.
8. Adjust bed height to comfortable working position.	Raising bed horizontally minimizes strain on nurse's back. It is easier to remove and apply linen evenly to bed in flat position.
9. Lower side rail on your side of bed. Remove call light.	Provides easy access to bed and linen.
10. Loosen top linen sheet at foot of bed.	Loosening linen makes it easier to remove.
11. Remove bedspread and blanket separately by folding them into squares and placing them in linen bag (if not to be reused). Do not allow linen to contact uniform. Do not fan or shake linen.	Reduces transmission of microorganisms.
12. If blanket and spread are to be reused, fold by bringing top and bottom edges together. Fold side farthest from your working side over onto nearer bottom edges together again. Place folded linen over back of chair.	Folding method facilitates replacement and prevents wrinkling.
13. Cover client with bath blanket in following manner: unfold bath blanket over top sheet. Ask client to hold top edge of bath blanket. If client is unable to help, tuck top of bath blanket under his or her shoulder. Grasp top sheet under bath blanket at client's shoulders and bring sheet down to foot of bed. Remove sheet and discard it in linen bag.	Bath blanket provides warmth and keeps body parts covered during linen removal.
14. With assistance from another nurse slide mattress toward head of bed.	If mattress slides toward foot of bed when head of bed is raised, it is difficult to tuck linen and is uncomfortable for client.
15. Position client on his or her side on far side of bed, facing away from you. Adjust pillow under client's head. Be sure side rail is up.	Moving client to side provides space for placement of clean linen. Side rail ensures client's safety.
16. Loosen bottom linens, moving from head to foot of bed.	Prepares for removal of all bottom linen simultaneously.

STEPS	RATIONALE

17. Fanfold bottom sheet and draw sheet toward client: first drawsheet, then bottom sheet. Tuck edges of linen just under client's buttocks, back, and shoulders. Do not fanfold mattress pad if it is to be reused (see illustration).

Provides maximum work space for placing clean linen. Later, when client turns to other side, soiled linen can be easily removed.

18. Wipe off any moisture on mattress with towel and appropriate disinfectant.

Reduces transmission of microorganisms.

19. Apply clean linen to exposed half of bed.
    a. Place clean mattress pad on bed by folding it lengthwise with center crease in middle of bed. Fanfold top layer over mattress. (If pad is reused, simply smooth out any wrinkles.)

Applying linen over bed in successive layers minimizes energy and time nurse uses in bed making.

    b. Unfold bottom sheet lengthwise so center crease is situated lengthwise along center of bed. Fanfold sheet's top layer toward center of bed alongside client. Smooth bottom layer of sheet over mattress and bring edge over your side of mattress. Allow sheet's edge to hang about 25 cm (10 in) over mattress edge. Hem of bottom sheet should lie seam down and even with bottom edge of mattress (see illustration).

Proper positioning of linen on one side ensures that adequate linen will be available to cover opposite side of bed. Keeping seam edges down eliminates irritation to client's skin.

20. Miter bottom sheet at head of bed:
    a. Face head of bed diagonally. Place hand that is away from head of bed under top corner of mattress, near mattress edge, and lift.

Mitered corner cannot be loosened easily even if client moves about frequently in bed.

    b. With other hand, tuck top edge of bottom sheet smoothly under mattress so side edges of sheet above and below mattress would meet if brought together.
    c. Face side of bed and pick up top edge of sheet at approximately 45 cm (18 in) down from top of mattress.
    d. Lift sheet and lay it on top of mattress to from neat triangular fold, with lower base of triangle even with mattress side edge.
    e. Tuck lower edge of sheet, which is hanging free below mattress, under mattress. Tuck with palms down. Do this without pulling triangular fold.
    f. Hold portion of sheet covering side edge of mattress in place with one hand. With other hand, pick up top of triangular linen fold and bring it down over side of mattress. Tuck this portion of sheet under mattress.

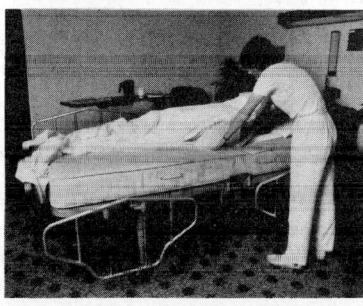

Step 17

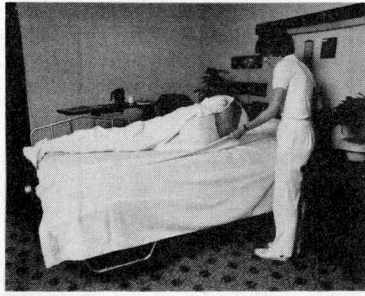

Step 19b

21. Tuck remaining portion of sheet under mattress, moving toward foot of bed. Keep linen smooth.

Folds of linen are source of irritation.

22. Open draw sheet so it unfolds in half. Lay center fold along middle of bed lengthwise and position sheet so it will be under client's buttocks and torso. Fanfold top layer toward client with edge alongside client's back. Smooth bottom layer out over mattress and tuck excess edge under mattress (keep palms down).

Draw sheet is used to lift and reposition client. Placement under client's torso distributes most of client's body weight over sheet.

Continued.

PROCEDURE 32-13, cont'd

Making an Occupied Bed

STEPS	RATIONALE
23. Place waterproof pad over draw sheet with center fold against client's side. Fanfold far half toward client.	Used to protect bed linen from soiling.
24. Raise side rail on working side and go to other side.	This maintains client's safety during turning.
25. Lower side rail. Assist client to roll slowly onto his other side, over folds of linen.	This exposes opposite side of bed for removal of soiled linen and placement of clean linen.
26. Loosen edges of soiled linen from underneath mattress.	Loosening linen makes it easier to remove.
27. Remove soiled linen by folding it into a bundle or square, with soiled side turned in. Discard it in linen bag.	Reduces transmission of microorganisms.
28. Spread clean fanfolded linen smoothly over edge of mattress from head to foot of bed.	Smooth linen will not irritate client's skin.
29. Assist client in rolling back into supine position. Reposition pillow.	Client's comfort is maintained.
30. Miter top corner of bottom sheet (Step 20). When tucking corner be sure sheet is taut.	Taut sheet eliminates irritating wrinkles and folds.
31. Facing side of bed, grasp remaining edge of bottom sheet. Lean back, keeping your back straight, and pull as you tuck excess linen tightly under mattress. Proceed from head to foot of bed. (Avoid lifting mattress during tucking to ensure tight fit.)	Proper use of body mechanics while tucking linen prevents injury to nurse.
32. Smooth fanfolded draw sheet out over bottom sheet. Grasp edge of sheet with palms down, lean back, and tuck sheet tightly under mattress. Tuck from middle to top and then to bottom.	Tucking first at top or bottom may pull sheet sideways, causing poor fit.
33. Place top sheet over client with center fold lengthwise down middle of bed. Open sheet from head to foot and unfold it over client.	Sheet should be equally distributed over bed by correctly positioning center fold.
34. Ask client to hold clean top sheet, or tuck sheet around client's shoulders. Remove bath blanket and discard it in linen bag (see illustration).	Sheet prevents exposure of body parts. Having client hold sheet encourages client participation in care.
35. Place blanket on bed, unfolding it so that crease runs lengthwise along middle of bed. Unfold blanket to cover client. Top edge should be parallel with edge of top sheet and 15-20 cm (6-8 in) down from top sheet's edge.	Blanket should be placed to cover client completely and provide adequate warmth.
36. Place spread over bed according to Step 31. Be sure top edge of spread extends about 2.5 cm (1 in) above blanket's edge. Tuck top edge of spread over and under top edge of blanket.	Spread gives bed neat appearance and provides extra warmth.

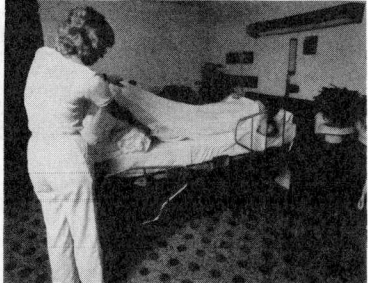

Step 34

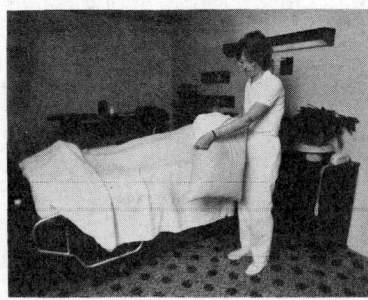

Step 41c

STEPS	RATIONALE
37. Make cuff by turning edge of top sheet down over top edge of blanket and spread.	Smooth cuff protects client's face from rubbing against blanket or spread.
38. Standing on one side at foot of bed, lift mattress corner slightly with one hand and tuck top linens under mattress. The top sheet and blanket are tucked under together. Be sure linens are loose enough to allow for movement of client's feet. (You may make horizontal toe pleat [Procedure 24-11, Step 30]).	Tucking all top linens together makes neat-appearing bed. Pressure sores can develop on client's toes and heels from feet rubbing between tight fitting bed sheets.
39. Make modified mitered corner with top sheet, blanket, and spread:	
a. Pick up side edge of top sheet, blanket, and spread approximately 45 cm (18 in) up from foot of mattress. Lift linens to form triangular fold and lay it on bed.	Modified mitered corner secures top linen but keeps an even edge of blanket and top sheet draped over mattress.
b. Tuck lower edge of sheet, which is hanging free below mattress, under mattress. Do not pull triangular fold.	
c. Pick up triangular fold and bring it down over mattress while holding linen in place along side of mattress. Do not tuck tip of triangle.	
40. Raise side rail. Make other side of bed; spread sheet, blanket, and bedspread out evenly; fold top edge of spread over blanket and make cuff with top sheet (Step 37); make modified mitered corner at foot of bed (Step 39).	Side rail protects client from accidental falls.
41. Change pillowcase	
a. Have client raise head. While supporting his or her neck with one hand, remove pillow. Allow client to lower head.	Support of neck muscles prevents injury during flexion and extension of neck.
b. Remove soiled case by grasping pillow at open end with one hand and pulling case over pillow with other hand. Discard case in linen bag.	Pillows slide out easily, thus minimizing contact with soiled linen.
c. Grasp clean pillowcase at center of closed end. Gather case, turning it inside out over hand holding it. With same hand pick up middle of one end of pillow. Pull pillowcase down over pillow with other hand (see illustration).	Method makes it easy to slide pillowcase over pillow.
d. Be sure pillow corners fit evenly in corners of pillowcase.	Poorly fitting case constricts fluffing and expansion of pillow.
43. Place call light within client's reach and return bed to comfortable position.	Ensures client's safety and comfort.
44. Open room curtains. Rearrange furniture. Place personal items within easy reach on overbed table or bedside stand. Return bed to comfortable height.	Neat environment promotes sense of well-being.
45. Discard dirty linen in linen hamper or chute and wash hands.	Prevents transmission of microorganisms.

to the laundry, the mattress and bed are cleaned by housekeeping personnel, and new bed linen is applied.

LINENS. The nurse collects linens in order of their use. This makes it easier for the nurse to make the bed without having to stop and search for specific linen pieces. It is important to collect not only bed linens but also the client's personal linens such as bath towels and washcloths. The nurse should avoid bringing excess linen to the client's room, since it can easily become contaminated. Linen should be collected in the following order: linen bag for soiled linen, mattress pad (optional), bottom sheet (flat or fitted), cotton or plastic-backed drawsheet, top sheet (flat), blanket, bedspread, pillowcases, bath towels, hand towel, washcloths, hospital gown, and blanket.

Linens are pressed and folded in a manner to prevent the spread of microorganisms and to make bedmaking easier. Bed linens have a center crease that the nurse places in the center of the bed from the head to the foot. The linens unfold easily to the sides, with creases often fitting over the mattress edge.

When removing soiled linen, the nurse rolls up the linen with the side on which the client was lying rolled inside. Soiled linen should never come in contact with the nurse's uniform.

A complete linen change is not always necessary. The nurse may reuse the mattress pad, sheet, blanket, and bedspread for the same client if they are not wet or soiled. All linen should be removed from the client's room at the time of discharge.

SUMMARY

Hygiene measures cover a variety of basic physical needs that clients are often unable to meet themselves. The nurse's responsibility includes assessing a client's physical condition, personal hygiene habits, ability to perform self-care, and body image. Promoting a client's independence and participation in personal hygiene is a part of the nurse's role.

A nurse should be resourceful when delivering hygiene measures. Take time for therapeutic communication, client teaching, and providing emotional support. Likewise, whenever the client needs assistance, the nurse can conduct portions of a physical examination.

The nurse uses considerable judgment and planning to anticipate certain clients' hygiene needs. Debilitated and seriously ill clients are significant challenges to the nurse.

KEY CONCEPTS

✓ Hygiene is a personal matter, and the nurse considers all factors influencing a client's personal hygiene routine.

✓ The nurse assumes responsibility for providing clients' daily hygiene needs if they are unable to care for themselves adequately.

✓ Providing hygienic care gives the nurse the opportunity to assess all external body surfaces, as well as the client's emotional state.

✓ Assisting the client with or providing daily hygiene needs allows the nurse to use teaching and communication skills to develop a meaningful relationship with the client.

✓ The client's personal preferences must always be considered as the nurse plans the client's daily hygiene care.

✓ The nurse must maintain the client's privacy and comfort when providing the client's daily care.

✓ During assessment of the skin and oral mucosa, the nurse observes characteristics most influenced by hygiene measures.

✓ Clients who are immobilized and poorly nourished and who have reduced sensation or peripheral circulation are at risk for altered skin integrity.

✓ Gloves should be worn by nurses during hygienic care when the risk of contacting body fluids is high.

✓ Techniques used during tepid sponging are designed to minimize the risk of a client chilling.

✓ Clients with diabetes require special consideration when a nurse provides nail and foot care.

✓ When administering oral care to unconscious clients, the nurse takes measures to prevent them from aspirating fluid into their lungs.

✓ Clients who wear contact lenses must learn proper self-care techniques to avoid corneal injury.

✓ The evaluation of hygiene care is based on the client's expression of a sense of comfort, relaxation, well-being, and an understanding of personal hygiene techniques.

REFERENCES

Deliefde, B: The dental care of pregnant women, NZ Dent J 80:41, 1984.

Grier, ME: Hair care for the black patient, Am J Nurs 76:1781, 1976.

Henningson A, et al.: Bathing or washing babies after birth? Lancet 2:1401, 1981.

Jordan, J, and Nickerson, D: Hygiene. In Guthrie, D, and Guthrie, R, editors: Nursing management of diabetes mellitus, ed. 2, St. Louis, 1982, The C.V. Mosby Co.

Macmillan, K: New goals for oral hygiene, Can Nurse 77(3):40, 1981.

Neeson, JD, and May, KA: Comprehensive maternity nursing: nursing process and the childbearing family, New York, 1986, J.B. Lippincott Co.

Watkins, S: Clearing impacted ears, Am J Nurs 84:1107, 1984.

Whaley, LF, and Wong, DL: Nursing care of infants and children, ed. 3, St. Louis, 1987, The C.V. Mosby Co.

Wilson, CB, et al.: When is umbilical cord separation delayed? J Pediatr 107:292, 1985.

Research Article

Poland, JM: Comparing Moi-Stir to lemon glycerine swabs, Am J Nurs 87:422, 1987.

ADDITIONAL READINGS

Carden, RC: The ins and outs of contact lenses, RN 48:48, 1985.

Centers for Disease Control: Recommendations for prevention of HIV transmission in health care settings, MMWRR 36 (suppl. 25):3s, 1987.

Chenger, P, and Kovacik, A: Dental hygiene during pregnancy: a review, MCN 23:342, 1987.

Davis, M: Getting to the root of the problem: hair grooming techniques for black patients, Nurs 77 7:60, 1977.

Dyer, E, et al.: Dental health in adults, Am J Nurs 76:1156, 1976.

Ebersole, P, and Hess, P: Toward healthy aging: human needs and nursing response, ed. 2, St. Louis, 1986, The C.V. Mosby Co.

Forbes, K, and Stokes, SA: Saving the diabetic foot, Am J Nurs 84:884, 1984.

Frantz, RA, and Kinney, CK: Variables associated with skin dryness in the elderly, Nurs Res 35(2):98, 1986.

Gannon, EP, and Kadezabeck, E: Giving your patients meticulous mouth care, Nurs 80 10:14, 1980.

Levine, P: Safeguarding your patients against periodontal disease, RN 36:38, 1973.

Maurer, J: Providing optimal oral health, Nurs Clin North Am 12:4, 1977.

Michelson, D: How to give a good back rub, Am J Nurs 78:1197, 1978.

Nurses' drug alert: Nicotine gum and dental work protection, Am J Nurs 85:171, 1985.

Osguthorpe, NC: If your patient has contact lenses, Am J Nurs 84:1255, 1984.

Petton, S: Your role in radiation therapy, RN 48:32, 1985.

Roach, LB: Assessing skin changes: the subtle and the obvious, Nurs 74 4:64, 1974.

Schweiger, JL, Lang, JW, and Schweiger, JW: Oral assessment: how to do it, Am J Nurs 80:654, 1980.

Sorrentino, SA: Mosby's textbook for nursing assistants, ed. 2, St. Louis, 1987, The C.V. Mosby Co.

Sykes, J: Black skin problems, Am J Nurs 79:1092, 1979.

Thibodeau, GA: Textbook of anatomy and physiology, ed. 12, St. Louis, 1987, The C.V. Mosby Co.

Wilson, D: Make mouth care a must for your patients, RN 49:39, 1986.

Winslow, EH: Oxygen uptake and cardiovascular responses in control adults and acute myocardial infarction patients during bathing, Nurs Res 34:164, 1985.

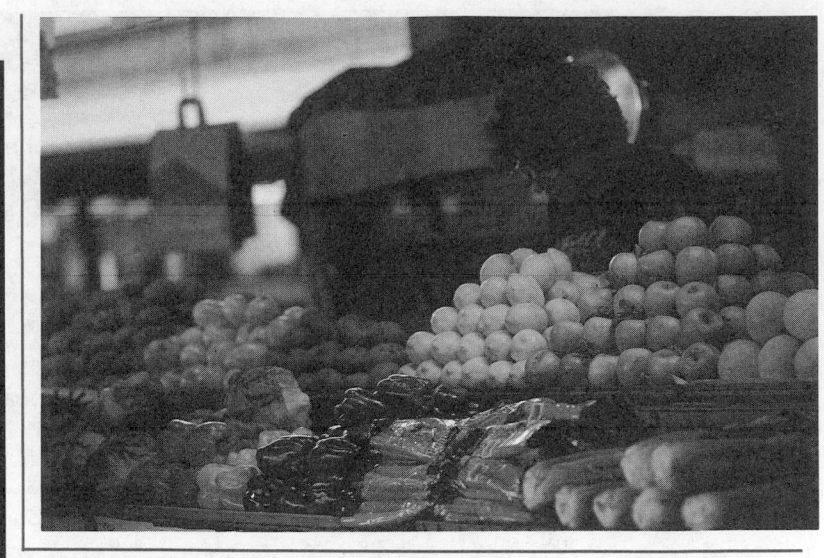

OBJECTIVES

Mastery of content in this chapter will enable the student to:

- Define the key terms listed.
- List the six categories of nutrients and explain why each is necessary for nutrition.
- Explain the importance of a balance between energy intake in foods and energy output.
- List the end products of carbohydrate, protein, and lipid metabolism.
- Explain the significance of saturated, unsaturated, and polyunsaturated lipids in nutrition.
- Describe the basic four food groups, and discuss their values in planning meals for good nutrition.
- Explain recommended daily allowances (RDAs).
- List seven dietary guidelines for health promotion.
- Discuss the major areas of nutritional assessment.
- Identify three major nutritional problems and describe clients at risk for these problems.
- State the goals for enteral nutrition.
- Describe the procedure for initiating and maintaining tube feedings.
- Describe methods to avoid the complications associated with tube feedings.
- State the goals of total parenteral nutrition.
- Describe the procedure for initiating and maintaining total parenteral nutrition.
- Discuss the importance of diet counseling in evaluation and client teaching before discharge.

KEY TERMS

Anabolism	Glycolysis
Anorexia	Hemosiderosis
Ariboflavinosis	Hypermetabolism
Atherosclerosis	Intrinsic Factor
Beriberi	Ketoacidosis
BMR	Legume
Cachexia	Malnutrition
Catabolism	Megadose
Catalyst	Metabolism
Collagen	Organic Foods
Cretinism	Oxidation
Emaciation	Pellagra
Enzyme	Peristalsis
Gluconeogenesis	RDAs
Glycerol	Satiety
Glycogen	Tryptophan

Nutrition

The science of nutrition is relatively young, although nutritional support has always been a factor in the care of the sick. Because most other forms of treatments were lacking, early client care relied heavily on the preparation and administration of food to maintain the body's strength and fight disease.

Before World War II, nursing schools provided instruction in nutrition and diet therapy, laboratory courses in food preparation, and clinical experiences in the preparation and serving of therapeutic diets. The battlefield hospitals provided the surgical, pharmacological, and medical technologies necessary to save the lives of the casualty victims. In addition, implementation of diets adequate in carbohydrates, fats, and proteins promoted wound healing and reduced the rate of complications in the soldiers recovering from the war-related injuries.

After the war, knowledge about illness and trauma increased, changing the attitudes of people about hospitals. Hospitals were regarded as facilities for the restoration of health rather than placement facilities for the terminally ill.

Nursing curricula began to place greater emphasis on the impact of nutrition on health maintenance and health restoration. Nursing students were not only taught normal and therapeutic nutrition but were also taught the role of the clinical dietitian in clinical facilities.

During the late 1960s and early 1970s nursing curricula began to integrate nutrition content rather than having a single course. This resulted in nurses delegating too much of the nutritional therapy to the dietician, assuming that the total burden is on the shoulders of the dietician. Therefore, nurses lost some of their interest in nutritional therapy and did not appropriately consult with the clinical nutritionist regarding therapeutic diet plans.

Today, interest in health promotion and prevention of disease is increasing. This interest has also led to a greater awareness of the link between nutrition and the onset of acute and chronic illnesses. Research documented the link between food high in saturated fats, animal fats, and cholesterol with coronary artery disease. Foods high in grains and fiber are associated with reduced risk of colorectal cancers. High caffeine intake has been positively correlated with fibrocystic breast disease and certain cardiovascular symptoms. Finally, the specialty of critical care nursing and medicine has ongoing research on the impact of proteins on wound healing or the impact of excessive carbohydrates on weaning a person from a mechanical ventilator.

At present, diet therapy is recognized as an important adjunct to treatment. In some illnesses, such as non-insulin-dependent diabetes mellitus or mild hypertension, diet therapy may be the only therapy initiated. Other conditions, such as severe ulcerative colitis, require stronger treatments, for example, total parenteral nutrition. Other conditions such as prolonged infections, trauma, or head and neck surgeries require enteral feedings by way of a nasogastric tube feeding.

PRINCIPLES OF NUTRITION

The body requires food to (1) provide energy for organ function, body movement, and work, (2) maintain body temperature, and (3) provide raw materials for enzyme function, growth, replacement of cells, and repair.

Metabolism refers to all the biochemical reactions within the body. It consists of anabolic reactions that build substances and body tissue and catabolic reactions that break down substances. Food is ingested, digested, and absorbed to produce the energy needed for these reactions.

People's energy requirements vary and are influenced by many factors. The energy requirement of an awake person at rest is called the basal metabolic rate (BMR). The BMR is the energy needed at a person's lowest level of cellular function. Such things as age, body size, body temperature, activity, environmental temperature, growth, sex, nutritional state, emotional state, and food intake affect individual energy requirements beyond the BMR.

When energy requirements are completely met by calorie intake in food, people maintain their activity level without weight change. When the number of calories ingested exceeds the energy needs, the person gains weight; when the number of calories ingested fails to meet energy requirements, the person will lose weight. Energy requirements vary from day to day, reflecting changes in the factors that influence them.

Nutrients are foods that contain the elements necessary for body function. The six categories of nutrients are water, carbohydrates, proteins, lipids, vitamins, and minerals. Energy needs are met by the metabolism of carbohydrates, proteins, and lipids. Water is needed because nutrients must be in solution for absorption and transportation. Although vitamins and minerals do not provide energy, they are involved in the reactions that produce energy.

Foods are sometimes described according to the density of their nutrients. Nutrient density is the proportion of essential nutrients to the number of calories. Foods with the most nutrients in proportion to their total calories are said to have high density. Foods with low nutrient density provide an energy source but lack essential nutrients (for example, alcohol and refined sugar).

Water

Water is the most important nutrient because the function of cells depends on a fluid environment. Water composes 60% to 70% of total body weight. A lean person's body contains more water than an obese person's body. Infants have the greatest percentage of total body weight as water; elderly people have the least. The proportion of water in total body weight decreases with age. Infants and elderly people are most vulnerable to water deprivation or water loss. Yet no one, when deprived of water, can survive for more than a few hours in a desert or a few days in the most protective environment.

A person's fluid needs are met by drinking liquids, by eating solid foods such as fresh fruits and vegetables, and by water produced when food is oxidized during the digestive processes. In a healthy individual the fluid intake from all sources equals the fluid output through elimination, respiration, and sweating. An ill person can have an increased need for fluid, as is the case with an increased body temperature or hypermetabolic state. In addition, an ill person can have a decreased need for fluid intake, as in cardiopulmonary or renal diseases.

Thirst is a protective mechanism that alerts the conscious person to the need for fluids. Thirst is a less reliable guide to the need for fluids in the confused client. Infants experience thirst, although they may not be able to communicate this need.

Carbohydrates

Carbohydrates are composed of carbon, hydrogen, and oxygen. The ratio of hydrogen to oxygen is the same as in water: two hydrogen ions for every oxygen ion.

Carbohydrates are obtained primarily from plant foods; the only important source of animal carbohydrate is the lactose in milk (milk sugar). The carbohydrate content of the diet tends to be greater in families with limited resources for food expenditure. Carbohydrates may contribute as much as 90% of the total caloric intake in other parts of the world where grains, such as rice and corn, are a major ingredient of every meal.

Carbohydrates are classified according to their sugar units or saccharides. Monosaccharides such as glucose (dextrose) or fructose cannot be broken down into a more basic sugar unit. Disaccharides such as sucrose, lactose, and maltose are composed of two monosaccharides and water. Polysaccharides such as glycogen are composed of many sugar units. They are insoluble in water and are digested with varying degrees of completeness. Glycogen is the form in which the body stores carbohydrates. It is synthesized from glucose and stored in the liver and muscles.

Plants store carbohydrate as starch. Starch is made up of granules enclosed by cellulose walls. When starch is cooked, the granules swell and burst their cellulose wall. Raw starch foods are more difficult to digest than the same foods after cooking, since the freeing of the granules from the cellulose permits greater contact with digestive enzymes and more complete digestion.

Starch digestion consists of several steps (Fig. 33-1). Dextrin is also produced commercially and is used to increase the digestibility of foods such as baby foods, cereals, and toasted breads.

Some polysaccharides cannot be digested because humans do not have enzymes capable of breaking them down. Nevertheless, these polysaccharides have a role in human nutrition because they add fiber to the diet. Fiber is receiving increasing attention as a dietary factor in disease prevention and treatment. Examples of fiber are agar and pectin, which are used to form gels and as thickening agents, carrageen (Irish moss), which is used to increase the smoothness of ice creams and sauces, and lignin, a woody substance added to breads.

The metabolism of 1 g of carbohydrate produces 4 calories (17 joules). Carbohydrate metabolism may produce three different results: catabolism into energy, carbon dioxide, and water; anabolism into glycogen for storage; and conversion into fat (adipose tissue) for storage. Carbohydrates contribute to the total caloric requirements, but no specific daily allowances for carbohydrates are required. Carbohydrates are the body's preferred energy source and are needed for the metabolism of lipids and for protein sparing (replacing protein in meeting energy needs). In order to keep the body in acid-base balance, at least 50 to 100 g of carbohydrate is needed daily. A majority of carbohydrates should be derived from natural sugars and polysaccharides.

Proteins

Proteins are composed of hydrogen, oxygen, carbon, and nitrogen. Most proteins also contain sulfur and phosphorus. Because of their high molecular weight and tendency to form colloidal solutions, proteins do not readily pass through body membranes. Amino acids are the most important components of proteins; they are essential for synthesis of body tissue in growth, maintenance, and repair. Protein can also be used as a source of energy.

Protein foods tend to be expensive, and their contribution to total caloric intake is usually higher in affluent families and developed countries. Protein intake is of particular importance during periods of rapid growth and after disease and injury.

Proteins are classified as simple, conjugated, or derived. Simple proteins are hydrolyzed into amino acids or their derivatives. Albumin and globulin are simple proteins. The combination of a simple protein with a nonprotein substance will produce a conjugated protein. Examples of conjugated proteins are mucoprotein, which is formed by the combination of a carbohydrate group and a simple protein, and lipoprotein, formed by a combination of a lipid and a simple protein. Derived proteins are formed during the hydrolysis of protein. For example, peptides and proteases occur during stages in the digestion of protein.

Another method of classifying protein is based on its nutritional value. This classification identifies proteins as either complete or incomplete. A complete protein contains all the essential amino acids in sufficient quantity to support growth and maintain nitrogen balance. Complete proteins are also referred to as high–biological value proteins. Examples of complete or high–biological value proteins are meat, fish, poultry, milk, and eggs.

An incomplete protein does not contain all the essential amino acids or does not have them in sufficient

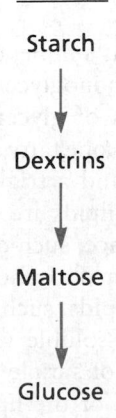

Starch

↓

Dextrins

↓

Maltose

↓

Glucose

Fig. 33-1 Digestion of starch.

Essential and Nonessential Amino Acids

ESSENTIAL	NONESSENTIAL
▪ Histidine	▪ Alanine
▪ Isoleucine	▪ Arginine
▪ Leucine	▪ Asparagine
▪ Lysine	▪ Aspartic acid
▪ Methionine	▪ Citrulline
▪ Phenylalanine	▪ Cysteine
▪ Threonine	▪ Cystine
▪ Tryptophan	▪ Glutamic acid
▪ Valine	▪ Glycine
	▪ Hydroxyglutamic acid
	▪ Hydroxyproline*
	▪ Norleucine*
	▪ Proline
	▪ Serine
	▪ Thyroxine*
	▪ Tyrosine

*Whether these are true amino acids is questionable.

quantity to support growth and maintain nitrogen balance. Examples of incomplete proteins are cereals, legumes, and vegetables. The combination of one incomplete protein with another incomplete protein (which contains the missing amino acids or increases the amount of amino acids) in the same dish or meal will supply the essential amino acids (see box) to support growth and maintain nitrogen balance.

Because the body cannot synthesize essential amino acids, the diet must provide them. Nonessential amino acids need not be present in the diet because the body can manufacture them from the breakdown of other amino acids. Incomplete proteins that combine to act as complete proteins are called complementary proteins. Grains and legumes are complementary proteins. Incomplete proteins can also be made complete by the supplementation of synthetic amino acids. The addition of synthetic lysine to wheat is an example of amino acid supplementation.

Protein is the body's only source of nitrogen, and 16% of protein is nitrogen. Nitrogen balance is an important concept. The body is in nitrogen balance when the intake and output of nitrogen are equal. When the intake of nitrogen exceeds the output, the body is in positive nitrogen balance, as in growth, normal pregnancy, and wound healing. The nitrogen retained by the body is used for building, repair, or replacement of body tissues.

Negative nitrogen balance occurs when the body is losing more nitrogen than it is taking in. The increased nitrogen loss is the result of body tissue destruction. Negative nitrogen balance is associated with infection, fever, starvation, injury, and prolonged immobilization.

Protein can be used to provide energy, but because of protein's essential role in growth, maintenance, and repair, it is important that protein be spared to carry out its own unique functions. Protein sparing is the provision of sufficient carbohydrate in the diet to meet the energy needs of the body to spare protein for its role in nitrogen balance and tissue building.

Protein is metabolized to yield amino acids, nitrogen, and 4 kcal (17 joules) per gram. Amino acids are anabolized into tissues, hormones, and enzymes. Amino acids can also be converted to fat and stored as adipose tissue or catabolized into energy via gluconeogenesis, carbon dioxide, and water.

The required daily allowance for protein ranges from 2.2 g/kg body weight for infants under 6 months to 56 g for males 15 years or older (Table 38-8). Pregnant women require an additional 30 g and lactating women an additional 20 g above their usual daily need of 44 to 46 g.

Nutrition experts believe that the intake of protein in America is generally greater than required. Protein foods are expensive to buy and to produce in terms of the economic use of land and fodder. In addition, meats, whole milk, cheese, and eggs are not pure protein. They also contain significant amounts of saturated fatty acids and cholesterol. Nutritional guidelines recommend the reduction of saturated fats and cholesterol.

Lipids

Lipid is a comprehensive term applied to compounds that are insoluble in water but soluble in organic solvents, such as ethanol, ether, benzene, and acetone. Lipids include fats that are solid at room temperature and oils that are liquid at room temperature. Lipids are composed of carbon, hydrogen, and oxygen, but the proportion of each element differs from that of carbohydrate.

Lipids are classified as simple, compound, or derived. Simple lipids, such as monoglycerides, diglycerides, and triglycerides, are esters of glycerol and fatty acids. A monoglyceride contains one fatty acid, a diglyceride contains two fatty acids, and a triglyceride contains three fatty acids. Compound lipids are simple lipids combined with a nonlipid substance, such as carbohydrate in glycolipids, phosphorus in phospholipids, and protein in lipoproteins. Derived lipids, such as cholesterol, steroid hormones, and the fat-soluble vitamins, are produced during the breakdown of simple or compound lipids.

Approximately 98% of the lipid in foods and 90% of the lipid in the human body are in the form of triglycerides. Triglycerides are termed simple when the three fatty acids that comprise them are the same. A mixed triglyceride is composed of two or three different fatty acids. High blood levels of triglycerides have been linked to atherosclerosis.

Health care workers are also interested in the relationship between dietary intake of fatty acids and blood cholesterol levels. Increased blood cholesterol levels are associated with atherosclerosis and resulting cerebrovascular accidents (stroke) and coronary occlusion.

A saturated fatty acid contains as much hydrogen as it can hold. An unsaturated fatty acid can take up another hydrogen atom, and a polyunsaturated fatty acid can take up many more hydrogen atoms. Unsaturated and polyunsaturated fatty acids are oils. They have a low melting point and are liquid at room temperature. Hydrogenation is a process by which these oils are made more solid by the addition of hydrogen. The addition of hydrogen also makes them more saturated. Ingestion of saturated fatty acids appears to increase blood cholesterol levels. Ingestion of unsaturated fatty acids has a minimal effect on blood cholesterol, and polyunsaturated fatty acids appear to lower blood cholesterol levels.

Fatty acids are usually not purely saturated, unsaturated, or polyunsaturated. Most animal fats have high proportions of saturated fatty acids; most vegetable fats have higher amounts of unsaturated and polyunsaturated fatty acids.

Linoleic acid is the only essential fatty acid. Since the body is unable to synthesize linoleic acid, it is dependent on an adequate dietary intake. Linoleic acid is a polyunsaturated fatty acid found in safflower, soybean, corn, cottonseed, and peanut oils.

Fat is the body's form of stored energy. The glycerol portion of lipids can be converted to glucose by gluconeogenesis. All body cells except the red blood cells and the central nervous system cells can oxidize fatty acids for energy. After a period of starvation, even the central nervous system can adapt to the use of amino acids and ketones as energy sources.

The metabolism of 1 g of lipid yields 9 kcal (38 joules), more than twice the energy provided by carbohydrates or proteins. Lipids account for 35% to 45% of the American diet, with the percentage usually increasing with affluence. Nutritional guidelines recommend a reduction of lipid intake to 20% of the total caloric intake, with some authorities suggesting even lower intakes.

Vitamins

Vitamins are organic substances, present in minute amounts in foods, that are essential to normal metabolism. The body is unable to synthesize vitamins in the required amounts and depends on dietary intake. Research is constantly improving the understanding of the role of vitamins in human physiology. New vitamins have been identified and recommended allowances established or revised.

Although they are contained in many foods, vitamins are affected by processing, storage, and preparation. Vitamin content is usually highest in fresh foods that are used quickly after minimal exposure to heat, air, or water. Vitamins are classified as water soluble and fat soluble.

WATER-SOLUBLE VITAMINS

The water-soluble vitamins are vitamin C and vitamin B complex, which consists of eight different vitamins. Water-soluble vitamins cannot be stored in the body and must be provided in the daily food intake. It was once assumed that, because water-soluble vitamins are not stored in the body, hypervitaminosis of these vitamins does not occur. However, recent studies of people who took megadoses of vitamin C and vitamin B_6 indicate that toxicity can occur. Vitamins are chemicals used as catalysts in biochemical reactions. When there is enough of any specific vitamin to meet the catalytic demands, the rest of the vitamin supply acts as a free chemical and may be toxic to the body. Table 33-1 lists the characteristics of water-soluble vitamins.

FAT-SOLUBLE VITAMINS

The fat-soluble vitamins—A, D, E, and K—can be stored in the body, and therefore daily intake is not needed. However, with the exception of vitamin D, these vitamins should be provided by dietary intake. Toxicity to some fat-soluble vitamins has been recognized for years. Toxicity is usually the result of megadoses of synthetic vitamins, but it has also been reported in people whose diet includes a large intake of fish liver.

Processing, storage, and preparation of foods have less effect on fat-soluble vitamin content, and many foods are fortified by the addition of vitamins A and D. The characteristics of the fat-soluble vitamins are listed in Table 33-2 (p. 888).

Minerals

Minerals are inorganic elements that are essential to the body because of their role as catalysts in biochemical reactions. Minerals are classified as macrominerals when the daily requirement is 100 mg or more and microminerals when less than 100 mg is needed daily. Because the required amount of microminerals is usually very small or a trace, microminerals are also referred to as trace elements. The characteristics of macrominerals are summarized in Table 33-3 (p. 889). Those of microminerals are summarized in Table 33-4 (p. 890).

In addition to the microminerals in Table 33-4, arsenic, nickel, silicon, tin, vanadium, and possibly cad-

TABLE 33-1 Water-Soluble Vitamins

Vitamin	Functions	Effects of Deficiency	Effects of Excess	Sources	RDA Range (Adults)
C (ascorbic acid)	Production of collagen, integrity of capillary walls, formation of red blood cells, metabolism of amino acids, reduction of iron salts, protection of other vitamins from oxidation	Scurvy, poor wound healing, bleeding gums, loose teeth, bruising	Kidney stones, scurvy on withdrawal, urinary tract infection	Citrus fruits, potatoes, cabbage, tomatoes, broccoli, strawberries, cantaloupe, green peppers	60 mg/day
VITAMIN B COMPLEX					
B$_1$ (thiamine)	Component of enzymes, carbohydrate oxidation, important component in oxidative conversion of pyruvic acid and hence the citric acid cycle	Beriberi (rare), polyneuritis, mental confusion, muscular weakness, ataxia, tachycardia, cardiac enlargement	None known	Pork, fish, eggs, poultry, dried beans, whole grains, wheat germ, oatmeal, bread, pasta	1.5 mg/day
B$_2$ (riboflavin)	Metabolism of nutrients, essential for growth, coenzymes function in the oxidation and reduction of fat, carbohydrates, and proteins	Ariboflavinosis: cracks at mouth corners, scaly desquamation of skin around mouth, eye irritation, glossitis, photophobia	Ulcer, elevated blood glucose level, increased uric acid levels in blood	Milk, whole grains, green vegetables, liver	1.7 mg/day
Niacin	Essential for protein utilization, glycolysis, fat synthesis, tissue repair	Pellagra: weakness, anorexia, lassitude, indigestion; severe pellagra: dermatitis, diarrhea, dementia	Ulcer, liver dysfunction, elevated blood glucose level, increased blood uric acid levels	Meats, dairy products, whole grains, cereals, tuna	20 mg/day
B$_6$ (complex of pyridoxine, pyridoxal, pyridoxamine)	Metabolism of nutrients, synthesis of nonessential amino acids, conversion of tryptophan to niacin, proper function of blood and central nervous system cells	Anemia, irritability, skin lesions, cracks at corners of mouth	None reported	Whole grains, liver, fish, poultry, green beans, nuts, meats, potatoes	2.0 mg/day

From Grant, JA, and Kennedy-Caldwell, C: Nutritional support in nursing, New York, 1988, Grune & Stratton.
†From Estimated safe and adequate daily dietary intakes, Committee on Dietary Allowances, Food and Nutrition Board, National Academy of Sciences—National Research Council, Washington, D.C., amended, July 1, 1985.

TABLE 33-1—cont'd

Vitamin	Functions	Effects of Deficiency	Effects of Excess	Sources	RDA Range (Adults)
Folacin, folic acid	Metabolism of some amino acids, maturation of red blood cells, synthesis of purines and pyrimidines, which are necessary for RNA and DNA	Macrocytic anemia	None reported	Liver, green leafy vegetables, meat, fish, poultry, whole grains	400 μg/day
B_{12} (cobalamin)	Manufacture of enzymes essential to the metabolism of nutrients, nucleic acid, and folic acid; proper function of the cells of the bone marrow, gastrointestinal tract, and nervous system, formation of purines, therefore RNA and DNA	Pernicious anemia and neurological disorders	None reported	Milk, eggs, cheese, meat, fish, poultry, foods of animal origin (plant foods contain no vitamin B_{12})	6 μg/day
Pantothenic acid	Metabolism of nutrients, synthesis of cholesterol and steroid hormones, activity of adrenal cortex	None known	Increased need for thiamin	Meats, whole grain cereals, legumes	10 mg/day[†]
Biotin	Synthesis of fatty acids, utilization of glucose, metabolism of protein, utilization of vitamin B_{12} and folic acid	None known	None known	Liver, kidneys, dark green vegetables, egg yolk, green beans	300 μg/day[†]

mium are known to play as yet unidentified roles in human nutrition. The field of minerals is currently a major area of nutrition research.

DIGESTION

The only nutrients the body can use in their ingested form are monosaccharides, water, vitamins, some minerals, and alcohol. All other foods must be broken down into simpler form for absorption.

Digestion consists of mechanical breakdown by chewing, churning, mixing with fluid, and chemical reactions by which food is reduced to its simplest form. The flow of digestive juice is under hormonal control. Enzymes are an essential component of the chemistry of digestion. They are proteinlike substances that act as catalysts to speed up biochemical reactions. As catalysts, enzymes are not part of the end product of the reaction. Most enzymes have one specific function, although some enzymes are able to enter into several closely related reactions. Enzyme activity is regulated by the pH of the intestinal contents. Each enzyme functions best at a specific pH and will be inactivated by major variations from that level. The secretions of the gastrointestinal tract have vastly different pH levels; saliva is relatively neutral, gastric juice is highly acid, and the secretions of the small intestine are alkaline.

TABLE 33-2   Fat-Soluble Vitamins

Vitamin	Functions	Effects of Deficiency	Effects of Excess	Sources	RDA Range (Adults)
A (retinol, retinal, and retinoic acid)	Growth and maintenance of epithelial tissue, maintenance of visual acuity in dim light, necessary for proper immune functions, especially antigen recognition	Night blindness, rough scaly skin, dry mucous membranes, decreased resistance to infection, faulty tooth and bone development	Nausea, vomiting, abdominal pain, and growth failure in children; weight loss in adults; megadoses: hair loss, bone swelling and tenderness, joint pain, hepatomegaly, splenomegaly	Whole milk, whole milk products, eggs, green leafy vegetables, yellow fruits and vegetables, fish liver oil, liver	5000 IU/day
D (cholecalciferol, ergosterol)	Absorption and utilization of calcium in bone and tooth development	Rickets and delayed dentition in children, osteomalacia in adults	Megadoses: loss of appetite, vomiting, growth failure, weight loss	Sunlight, fortified milk, fortified margarines, fish liver oils	400 IU/day
E (tocopherol)	Protection of vitamins A and C and polyunsaturated fatty acids from oxidation, synthesis of heme	Increased hemolysis of red blood cells and macrocytic anemia in premature infants	Interference with the utilization of vitamins A and K, prolonged prothrombin time, intestinal irritability	Vegetable oils, green leafy vegetables, milk, eggs, meats, cereals	30 IU/day
K	Essential to prothrombin formation and blood clotting	Hemorrhagic disease of the newborn, prolonged clotting time in adults	Hyperbilirubinemia in infants, vomiting in adults	Green leafy vegetables	10-140 μg/day†

From Grant, JA, and Kennedy-Caldwell, C: Nutritional support in nursing, New York, 1988, Grune & Stratton.
†From Estimated safe and adequate daily dietary intakes, Committee on Dietary Allowances, Food and Nutrition Board, National Academy of Sciences—National Research Council, Washington, D.C., amended July 1, 1985.

The mechanical, chemical, and hormonal activities of digestion are interdependent. Enzyme activity is dependent on the mechanical breakdown of food to increase its surface area for chemical action. Hormones regulate the flow of digestive secretions needed for enzyme supply, and digestion may also be slowed down or speeded up by strong emotional states. The secretion of digestive juice and motility of the gastrointestinal tract are regulated by physical, chemical, and hormonal factors, and they are intricately bound to psychological, emotional, and nervous system alterations.

Digestion begins in the mouth where food is mechanically broken down by chewing. The food is mixed with saliva, which contains ptyalin (salivary amylase), an en-zyme that acts on cooked starch to begin its conversion to maltose. The longer food is chewed, the more starch digestion occurs in the mouth. Proteins and fats are broken down physically but remain unchanged chemically because no enzymes are in the mouth to act on them. Chewing reduces food particles to a size suitable for swallowing, and saliva provides lubrication to further ease swallowing.

Swallowed food enters the esophagus and is moved along by peristaltic waves. At the cardiac sphincter, the upper opening of the stomach, the presence of the food mass causes the sphincter to relax and allow the food to enter the stomach.

The stomach acts as a reservoir for food. Food remains

TABLE 33-3 Macrominerals

Mineral	Functions	Effects of Deficiency	Effects of Excess	Sources	RDA Range (Adults)
Calcium	Formation of teeth and bones, contraction of muscle fibers, transmission of nerve impulses, activation of enzymes, permeability of cell membranes, coagulation of blood, cardiac function	Tingling of fingers and around mouth, muscle cramps, carpopedal spasm, tetany, convulsions, pathological fractures	Relaxed skeletal muscles, cardiac irregularities	Milk, milk products, leafy vegetables, fish and small edible bones	1000 mg/day
Magnesium	Supports function of B vitamins; utilization of calcium, potassium, and protein; maintenance of electrical activity in nerves and muscles	Neuromuscular irritability, confusion, hallucinations, growth failure	Lethargy, diarrhea	Whole grains, nuts, legumes, green vegetables	400 mg/day
Phosphorus	Formation of bone and teeth, activation of B vitamins, transfer of energy within cells, promotion of normal muscle and nerve activity, metabolism of carbohydrate, regulation of acid-base balance, transmission of hereditary traits	Hemolytic anemia, defective white blood cell function, delayed clotting, bone pain, pathological fractures	Erosion of jaw	Pork, beef, dried peas and beans, milk and milk products	1000 mg/day

From Grant, JA, and Kennedy-Caldwell, C: Nutritional support in nursing, New York, 1988, Grune & Stratton.

in the stomach for varying periods depending on the type of meal, gastric motility, and psychological influences. In general, carbohydrate meals spend the least amount of time in the stomach, lipid meals the longest, and protein meals an intermediate period. Large food intake decreases gastric motility and increases the length of time food remains in the stomach. Food remains in the stomach for an average period of 3 hours, with a range of 1 to 7 hours.

The activity of ptyalin continues in the stomach until the presence of hydrochloric acid decreases the pH sufficiently to inactivate it. The stomach churns the food mass, mixing it with gastric secretions and causing further breakdown in the size of the food particles. The acid environment favors the action of pepsin. Pepsin is an enzyme that splits proteins into proteases and peptones. Lipase, an enzyme that functions best in an alkaline medium, is able to act on emulsified fats such as butter, egg yolk, milk, and cream at near-neutral pH levels. Lipase splits emulsified fats into fatty acids and glycerol.

Food leaves the stomach at the pyloric sphincter as an acid, liquefied mass called chyme. Chyme flows into the duodenum and is quickly mixed with bile, intestinal juices, and pancreatic secretions. Bile emulsifies fat to permit enzyme action, and it holds fatty acids in solution.

Intestinal secretions contain seven enzymes: lipase for fat digestion, aminopolypeptidase and dipeptidase for

TABLE 33-4 Microminerals

Mineral	Functions	Effects of Deficiency	Effects of Excess	Sources	RDA Range (Adults)
Copper	Essential to hemoglobin formation, cofactor in synthesis of phospholipids, formation and activity of some enzymes, synthesis of prostaglandin	Abnormal blood cell development in infants, bone demineralization	Headache, dizziness, heartburn, weakness, nausea, vomiting, diarrhea, Wilson's disease	Liver, kidney, shellfish, nuts, raisins	2 mg/day
Fluoride	Formation of teeth, prevention of dental caries	Poor dental health	Mottling, pitting, and discoloration of tooth enamel	Fluoridated water, seafood, toothpaste, mouthwash	4 mg/day[†]
Iodine	Basic component of thyroid hormones	Cretinism in infants, depressed thyroid activity	Toxic goiter	Iodized salt, seafood, food additives, dough oxidizers, dairy disinfectants, coloring agents	150 μg/day
Iron	Essential to the formation of hemoglobin, synthesis of vitamins, purines, and antibodies	Anemia, fatigue, weakness, lethargy	Hemosiderosis, acute iron poisoning from accidental ingestion in infants and children: cramps, abdominal pain, nausea, vomiting, black stools, cirrhosis of the liver	Liver, lean meats, whole grains, enriched breads and cereals, green leafy vegetables	18 mg/day; pregnant women need 30-60 mg/day of supplemental iron over required RDA
Zinc	Connective tissue integrity, involvement in immune response, formation of enzymes and insulin	Impaired wound healing, decreased sensations of taste and smell, skin lesions	Fever, nausea, vomiting, diarrhea	Oysters, liver, meats, poultry, legumes, nuts	15 mg/day

From Grant, JA, and Kennedy-Caldwell, C: Nutritional support in nursing, New York, 1988, Grune & Stratton.
[†]From Estimated safe and adequate daily dietary intakes, Committee on Dietary Allowance, Food and Nutrition Board, National Academy of Sciences—National Research Council, Washington, D.C., amended July 1, 1985.

protein digestion, and amylase, sucrase, lactase, and maltase for carbohydrate digestion.

Pancreatic juice contains five enzymes: amylase, which digests starch; lipase, which breaks down emulsified fats; and trypsin, chymotrypsin, and carboxypolypeptide, which enter into reactions with proteins.

Peristalsis continues in the small intestine, mixing the secretions with the chyme. The mixture becomes increasingly alkaline, inhibiting the action of the gastric enzymes and promoting the action of the duodenal secretions. The major portion of digestion occurs in the small intestine, producing glucose, fructose, and galactose from carbohydrates; amino acids from proteins; and fatty acids and glycerol from lipids.

ABSORPTION

The small intestine is also the site of absorption of simple nutrients. The small intestine is lined with numerous villi that project into the lumen and greatly increase the surface area available for absorption. Table 33-5 describes the means and route of absorption of major nutrients.

The intestinal contents continue to move by peristaltic action into the large intestine. Water is the only nutrient absorbed from the large intestine. Other nutrients remaining in the intestinal contents when they reach the large intestine are lost to the body and will be excreted as waste products. When intestinal motility is increased,

TABLE 33-5   Intestinal Absorption of Some Major Nutrients

Nutrient	Form	Means of Absorption	Control Agent or Required Cofactor	Route
Carbohydrate	Monosaccharides (glucose and galactose)	Competitive	—	Blood
		Selective	—	
		Active transport via sodium pump	Sodium	
Protein	Amino acids	Selective	—	Blood
	Some dipeptides	Carrier transport systems	Pyridoxine (pyridoxal phosphate)	Blood
	Whole protein (rare)	Pinocytosis	—	Blood
Fat	Fatty acids	Fatty acid-bile complex (micelles)	Bile	Lymph
	Glycerides (mono-, di-)		—	Lymph
	Few triglycerides (neutral fat)	Pinocytosis	—	Lymph
Vitamins	B_{12}	Carrier transport	Intrinsic factor (IF)	Blood
	A	Bile complex	Bile	Blood
	K	Bile complex	Bile	From large intestine to blood
Minerals	Sodium	Active transport via sodium pump	—	Blood
	Calcium	Active transport	Vitamin D	Blood
	Iron	Active transport	Ferritin mechanism	Blood (as transferritin)
Water	Water	Osmosis	—	Blood, lymph, interstitial fluid

From Williams, SR: Nutrition and diet therapy, ed. 6, St. Louis, 1989, The C.V. Mosby Co.

as in diarrhea, the body loses nutrients that move through the small intestine too quickly for complete absorption.

Metabolism

Nutrients absorbed in the intestines, including water, are transported through the circulatory system to body tissues. Through metabolism, nutrients are converted by chemical changes into a number of substances the body requires. Carbohydrates, protein, and fat undergo metabolism to produce chemical energy and to maintain a dynamic balance of tissue buildup and breakdown. To carry out the body's work, the chemical energy produced by metabolism is converted to other types of energy by different tissues. Muscle contracture involves mechanical energy, the nervous system involves electrical energy, the mechanisms of heat production involve thermal energy, and so on, and these forms of energy all originate in metabolism. The interrelationships of protein, carbohydrate, and fat metabolism are depicted in Fig. 33-2.

The two basic types of metabolism are anabolism and catabolism. Anabolism is the production of more complex chemical substances by synthesis of nutrients. Catabolism is the breakdown of chemical substances into simpler substances. Although catabolism produces some energy, both processes require energy, which must be provided from either food or stored energy sources.

Storage

Some but not all of the nutrients required by the body are stored in body tissues. The body's major form of stored energy is fat stored in the adipose tissue, which has an almost unlimited capacity. Glycogen is stored in small reserves in liver and muscle tissue, and protein is stored in muscle mass. When the body's energy requirements exceed the energy supplied by ingested nutrients, stored energy is used; conversely, unused energy is stored, principally in fat.

Fat-soluble vitamins are also stored in limited reserves and are released to meet the body's needs when not provided sufficiently by dietary intake. Water-soluble vitamins are not stored and therefore must be provided by daily dietary intake.

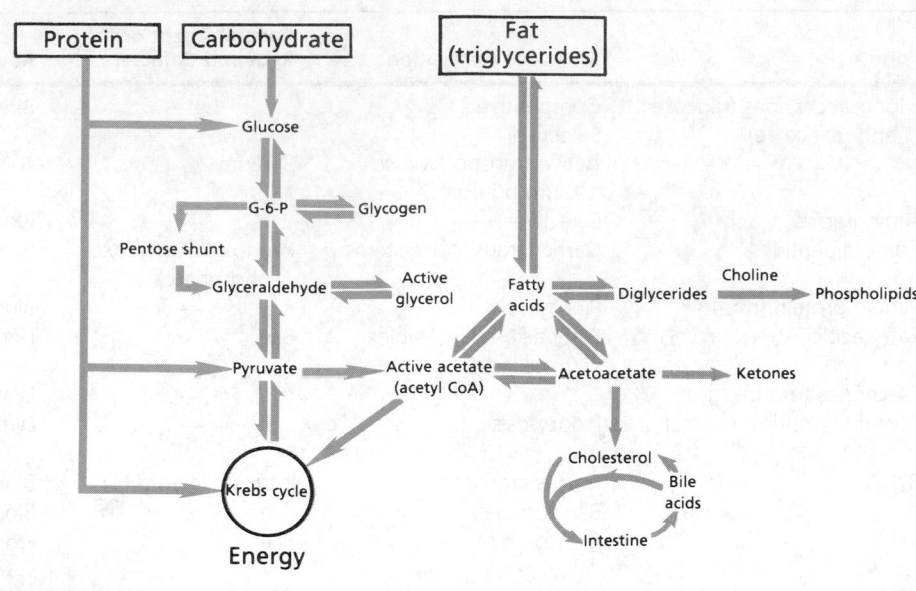

Fig. 33-2 Summary of metabolism of the nutrients. Note metabolic interrelationships of carbohydrate, protein, and fat.

From Williams, SR: Nutrition and diet therapy, ed. 6, St. Louis, 1989, The C.V. Mosby Co.

ELIMINATION

The intestinal contents move through the various segments of the large intestine by peristalsis. As the material moves toward the rectum, water is absorbed into the mucosa. The longer the material stays in the large intestine, the more water is absorbed and the firmer the remaining solid material becomes.

The end products of digestion include cellulose and similar fibrous substances that the body is unable to digest, sloughed cells from the intestinal walls, mucus, digestive secretions, water, and microorganisms.

FOUNDATIONS OF AN ADEQUATE DIET

Basic Four Food Groups

The basic four food groups were introduced in 1956 as one of the earliest recommendations by the U.S. Department of Agriculture (USDA). It was suggested that selecting foods from a wide variety of milk, meat, bread and cereal products, and fruits and vegetables would ensure the required amounts of needed nutrients. The four food groups are used as a guide for meal planning. In addition, this classification has the specific variations for the different developmental ages (Table 33-6). The basic dietary plan provides an average of 1200 calories

per day. Additional foods to round out meals and meet energy requirements can be selected from enriched cereals, complex carbohydrates, and additional grains.

The basic four food groups is not a problem-free solution to dietary management, and there are four weaknesses of the plan. First, no provision is made for the portions of fast or prepackaged food items, which are popular in today's dietary regimen. Second, the grouping does not include any recommendations for daily fluid intake, which should equal 6 to 8 glasses of fluid per day. Third, no recommendation is made for fiber intake, which is grossly lacking in today's dietary patterns. Fourth, the plan does not identify those foods that may be high in calories but low in nutritional value.

While the basic four food group plan does not ensure that the client will ingest the recommended daily allowances for carbohydrates, proteins, fats, vitamins, and minerals, it has one major advantage. It is easily remembered and can be used as a buying and food-preparation guide for clients who are on regular diets and seek a balanced diet.

Recommended Daily Allowances

The Committee on Dietary Allowances of the Food and Nutrition Board of the National Academy of Sciences has published a list of recommended daily allowances (RDAs) since 1943. The RDAs are the level of intake of essential nutrients considered, in the judgment of the committee on the basis of scientific knowledge,

TABLE 33-6 Daily Dietary Guide: The Basic Four Food Groups

Food Group and Nutrients	Daily Amounts*
Milk Milk, cheese, ice cream, or other products made with whole or skimmed milk Nutrients: calcium, protein, riboflavin	Children under 9: 2-3 cups Children 9-12: 3 or more cups Teenagers: 4 or more cups Adults: 2 or more cups Pregnant women: 3 or more cups Nursing mothers: 4 or more cups (1 cup = 8 ounces fluid milk or designated milk equivalent†)

Meats
Beef, veal, lamb, pork, poultry, fish, eggs
Nutrients: protein, iron, thiamine
Alternates: dry beans, dry peas, nuts, peanut butter
	2 or more servings
	Count as 1 serving:
	  2-3 ounces of lean, boneless, cooked meat, poultry, or fish
	  2 eggs
	  1 cup cooked dry beans or peas
	  4 tbsp peanut butter

Vegetables and fruits
Nutrients: niacin, riboflavin, vitamin A, vitamin C, smaller amounts of other vitamins and minerals
	4 or more servings
	Count as 1 serving:
	  ½ cup of vegetable or fruit or a portion such as 1 medium apple, banana, orange, potato, or ½ a medium grapefruit, melon
	Include:
	  A dark-green or deep-yellow vegetable or fruit rich in vitamin A at least every other day
	  A citrus fruit or other fruit or vegetable rich in vitamin C daily
	  Other vegetables and fruits including potatoes

Bread and cereals
Nutrients: thiamine, niacin, riboflavin, iron, protein
	4 or more servings of whole grain, enriched or restored
	Counts as 1 serving:
	  1 slice of bread
	  1 ounce (1 cup) ready-to-eat cereal, flake or puff varieties
	  ½-¾ cup cooked cereal
	  ½-¾ cup cooked pastas (macaroni, spagetti, noodles)
	  Crackers: 5 saltines, 2 square graham crackers, etc.

From Williams, S: Nutrition and diet therapy, ed. 5, St. Louis, 1985, The C.V. Mosby Co.
*Use additional amounts of these foods or added butter, margarine, oils, sugars, etc., as desired or needed.
†Milk equivalents: 1 ounce cheddar cheese, 3 servings cottage cheese, 1 cup fluid skimmed milk, 1 cup buttermilk, ½ cup dry skimmed milk powder, 1 cup ice milk, 1⅔ cups ice cream, ½ cup evaporated milk.

to be adequate to meet the nutritional needs of practically all healthy people. The RDAs were originally designed as a guide for planning and securing food supplies for national defense during World War II. Now they are revised every 5 years to incorporate changes and new knowledge based on research. The 1985 RDAs are contained in Tables 33-1 through 33-4. The RDAs are designed for population groups, not for individuals, and they exceed the requirements for most healthy individuals.

In 1941 the Food and Drug Administration established minimum daily requirements, standards that represented minimum intake for each nutrient. These standards were replaced in 1968 by the U.S. recommended daily allowances (U.S. RDAs), which are used only in food labeling. Unless a food has added nutrients or the manufacturer makes nutritional claims for it, nutritional labeling is voluntary. In most cases the single value used is the highest amount listed in the RDA (excluding recommendations for infants or pregnant or lactating women). In labeling, amounts present are expressed as a percentage of the U.S. RDAs. The U.S. RDA for iron is 18 mg, for example, and if a serving of oatmeal contains 0.72 mg of iron, the container would be labeled to indicate that one serving contains 4% of the U.S. RDA for iron.

The Canadian recommended daily nutrient allowance is published by the Committee for Revision of the Canadian Dietary Standard, Bureau of Nutritional Sciences, Health, and Welfare (Table 33-7). The Canadian standards for 1982 list 15 age categories and requirements for pregnant and lactating women.

TABLE 33-7 Recommended Nutrient Intakes for Canadians: Average Energy Requirements and Summary Examples

Age	Sex	Average Height (cm)[c]	Average Weight (kg)[c]	Requirements[a,b]					
				kcal/kg[c,d]	MJ/kg[d]	kcal/day[e]	MJ/day[f]	kcal/cm[g]	MJ/cm[f]
MONTHS									
0-2	Both	55	4.5	120-100	0.50-0.42	500	3.0	9	0.04
3-5	Both	63	7.0	100-95	0.42-0.40	700	2.8	11	0.05
6-8	Both	69	8.5	95-97	0.40-0.41	800	3.4	11.5	0.05
9-11	Both	73	9.5	97-99	0.41	950	3.8	12.5	0.05
YEARS									
1	Both	82	11	101	0.42	1100	4.8	13.5	0.06
2-3	Both	95	14	94	0.39	1300	5.6	13.5	0.06
4-6	Both	107	18	100	0.42	1800	7.6	17	0.07
7-9	M	126	25	88	0.37	2200	9.2	17.5	0.07
	F	125	25	76	0.32	1900	8.0	15	0.06
10-12	M	141	34	73	0.30	2500	10.4	17.5	0.07
	F	143	36	61	0.25	2200	9.2	15.5	0.06
13-15	M	159	50	57	0.24	2800	12.0	17.5	0.07
	F	157	48	46	0.19	2200	9.2	14	0.06
16-18	M	172	62	51	0.21	3200	13.2	18.5	0.08
	F	160	53	40	0.17	2100	8.8	13	0.05
19-24	M	175	71	42	0.18	3000	12.4		
	F	160	58	36	0.15	2100	8.8		
25-49	M	172	74	36	0.15	2700	11.2		
	F	160	59	32	0.13	1900	8.0		
50-74	M	170	73	31	0.13	2300	9.6		
	F	158	63	29	0.12	1800	7.6		
75+	M	168	69	29	0.12	2000	8.4		
	F	155	64	23	0.10	1500	6.0		
Pregnancy (additional)[h]									
Lactation (additional)[h]									

From Bureau of Nutritional Sciences, Department of National Health and Welfare, Ottawa, Canada, 1982.

[a]Recommended nutrient intakes for Canadians, 1982—Committee for the revision of the Dietary Standard for Canada, Bureau of Nutritional Sciences, Department of National Health and Welfare. Recommended intakes of energy and of certain nutrients are not listed in this table because of the nature of the variables upon which they are based. The figures for energy are estimates of average requirements for expected patterns of activity. For nutrients not shown, the following amounts are recommended: thiamin, 0.4 mg/100 kcal (0.48 mg/5000 kJ); riboflavin, 0.5 mg/1000 kcal (0.6 mg/5000 kJ); niacin, 6.6 NE/1000 kcal (7.9 NE/5000 kJ); vitamin B_6, 15 µg, as pyridoxine, per gram of protein intake; phosphorus, same as calcium.

Recommended intakes during periods of growth are taken as appropriate for individual representative of the midpoint in each age group. All recommended intakes are designed to cover individual variations in essentially all of a healthy population subsisting upon a variety of common foods available in Canada. It is emphasized that these are examples of the application of the RNI to particular classes of individuals and/or particular situations.

[b]Requirements can be expected to vary within a range of ±30%.

[c]Figures rounded to the closest whole number when ≥10 and to the closest 0.5 when <10.

[d]First and last figures are averages of the beginning and at the end of the 3-month period.

[e]Figures rounded to the nearest 50 when <1000 and to the nearest 100 when ≥1000.

[f]Figures include 2 decimals if value is <1 and 1 decimal if ≥1.

Other Dietary Guidelines

Before 1977, most public advice on dietary planning was based on the Basic Four Food Groups. In 1977 the Senate Select Committee on Nutrition and Human Needs formulated guidelines for Americans, designed to help them avoid some of the nutrition-related problems identified by research studies. These guidelines, which are directed to the problems of obesity, excessive intake of fat, cholesterol, sugar, salt, and inadequate intake of fiber, relate to heart disease, cancer, gastrointestinal disorders, diabetes mellitus, and other health problems. These guidelines were controversial because specific recommendations about a number of nutrients were made (Ranhotra, 1985).

The USDA and the Department of Health and Human Services issued dietary guidelines in 1980. These guidelines consisted of seven categories and were revised in 1985, with recommendations that they be evaluated in

of Recommended Nutrient Intakes

	Fat-Soluble Vitamins			Water-Soluble Vitamins			Minerals				
Protein (g/day)[i]	Vit A (RE/day)[j]	Vit D (μg/day)[k]	Vit E (mg/day)[l]	Vit C (mg/day)	Folacin (μg/day)[m]	Vit B$_{12}$ (μg/day)	Ca (mg/day)	Mg (mg/day)	Fe (mg/day)	I (μg/day)	Zn (mg/day)
11[n]	400	10	3	20	50	0.3	350	30	0.4[o]	25	2[p]
14[n]	400	10	3	20	50	0.3	350	40	5	35	3
16[n]	400	10	3	20	50	0.3	400	45	7	40	3
18	400	10	3	20	55	0.3	400	50	7	45	3
18	400	10	3	20	65	0.3	500	55	6	55	4
20	400	5	4	20	80	0.4	500	65	6	65	4
25	500	5	5	25	90	0.5	600	90	6	85	5
31	700	2.5	7	35	125	0.8	700	110	7	110	6
29	700	2.5	6	30	125	0.8	700	110	7	95	7
38	800	2.5	8	40	170	1.0	900	150	10	125	6
39	800	2.5	7	40	170	1.0	1000	160	10	110	7
49	900	2.5	9	50	160	1.5	1100	220	12	160	9
43	800	2.5	7	45	160	1.5	800	190	13	160	8
54	1000	2.5	10	55	190	1.9	900	240	10	160	9
47	800	2.5	7	45	160	1.9	700	220	14	160	8
57	1000	2.5	10	60	210	2.0	800	240	8	160	9
41	800	2.5	7	45	165	2.0	700	190	14	160	8
57	1000	2.5	9	60	210	2.0	800	240	8	160	9
41	800	2.5	6	45	165	2.0	700	190	14[q]	160	8
57	1000	2.5	7	60	210	2.0	800	240	8	160	9
41	800	2.5	6	45	165	2.0	800	190	7	160	8
57	1000	2.5	6	60	210	2.0	800	240	8	160	9
41	800	2.5	5	45	165	2.0	800	190	7	160	8
15	100	2.5	2	0	305	1.0	500	15	6	25	0
20	100	2.5	2	20	305	1.0	500	20	6	25	1
25	100	2.5	2	20	305	1.0	500	25	6	25	2
20	400	2.5	3	30	120	0.5	500	80	0	50	6

[q]Figures rounded to the nearest 0.5
[h]Pregnancy: Add 100 kcal during the first trimester and 300 for the second and third trimesters. Lactation: Add 450 kcal/day.
[i]The primary units are grams per kilogram of body weight. The figures shown here are only examples.
[j]One retinol equivalent (RE) corresponds to the biological activity of 1 μg of retinol, 6 μg of β-carotene or 12 μg of other carotenes.
[k]Expressed as cholecalciferol or ergocalciferol.
[l]Expressed as d-α-tocopherol equivalents, relative to which β and γ-tocopherol and α-tocotrienol have activities of 0.5, 0.1, and 0.3 respectively.
[m]Expressed as total folate.
[n]Assumption that the protein is from breast milk or is of the same biological value as that of breast milk and that between 3 and 9 months adjustment for the quality of the protein is made.
[o]For the infant it is assumed that breast milk is the source of iron up to 2 months of age.
[p]Based on the assumption that breast milk is the source of zinc up to 2 months of age.
[q]After the menopause the recommended intake is 7 mg/day.

1990 and every 5 years thereafter (see box on p. 896).

Pennington (1981) attempts to incorporate limitation of problem nutrients, available food supplies, and health promotion into the basic recommendations. This plan consists of four food groups and four levels of consumption. The four food groups are group I: vegetables and fruit; group II: grains; group III: vegetable, dairy, and meat sources of protein; and group IV: luxury foods such as desserts, sweets, fats, and alcohol.

The four levels of consumption are level I: liberal; level II: moderate; level III: very moderate; and level IV: sparse. Food groups I and II should be taken at the first level of consumption. Food group III contains foods to be taken at three different levels. Legumes in group III are to be consumed liberally or at level I and skim and low-fat milk dairy products, lean meat, and poultry at level II or moderate intake. Luncheon meats, whole milk dairy products, sausage, nuts, seeds, peanuts, eggs, and

1985 Dietary Guidelines

Eat a Variety of Foods

- Fruits and vegetables
- Whole grain and enriched breads, cereals, and other grain products
- Milk, cheese, yogurt, and other milk products
- Meat, poultry, fish, eggs, and dry peas and beans

Maintain Reasonable Body Weight

Avoid Too Much Fat, Saturated Fat, and Cholesterol

- Choose lean meat, fish, and poultry
- Use dry peas and beans as protein sources
- Use low-fat milk and milk products
- Use of egg yolk and organ meats moderately
- Limit consumption of butter, cream, heavily hydrogenated fats and oils and foods high in palm and coconut oil
- Trim off excess fat on meats
- Broil, bake, or boil rather than fry

Eat Foods With Adequate Starch and Fiber

- Substitute starches for fat and sugars
- Use whole grain breads and cereal, fruits, vegetables, nuts

Avoid Too Much Sugar

- Use less sugar and high-sugar foods
- Avoid between-meal sweets
- Avoid foods whose labels contain sucrose, glucose, and lactose
- Select foods canned without syrup or with light syrup

Avoid Too Much Sodium

- Learn to enjoy unsalted food
- Cook with only a small amount of added salt
- Add little or no salt at the table
- Limit intake of salty foods
- Read food labels
- Use new, lower sodium products

Drink Alcoholic Beverages in Moderation

Data from Ranhotra, G: Dietary recommendations, 1977-1985.

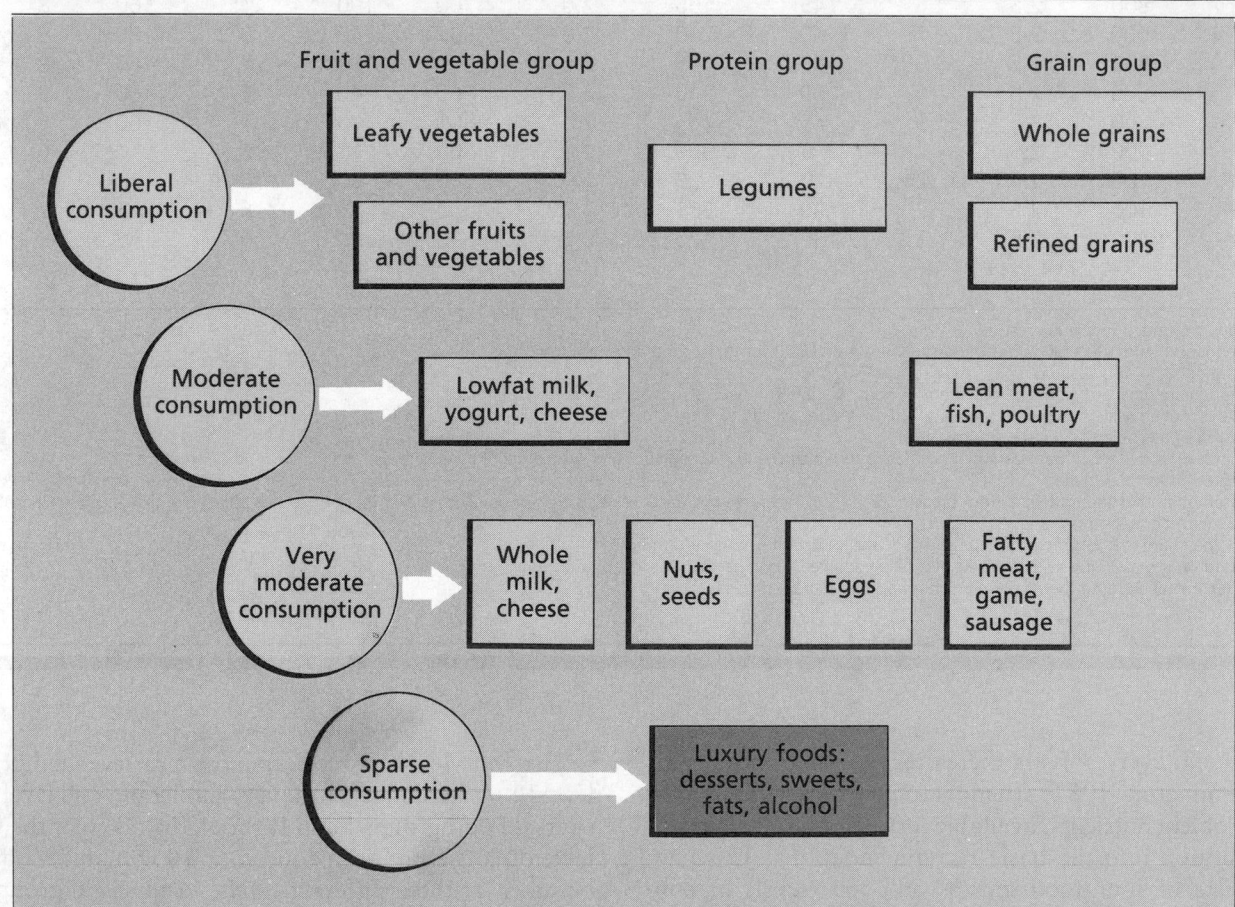

Fig. 33-3 A suggested food guide, shown as an inverse pyramid.
Modified from Pennington, J: J Nutr Educ 13:53, 1981.

TABLE 33-8   Portion Sizes and Suggested Servings Per Day from the Inverse Pyramid Food Guide

Food Group	Example of Portion Sizes	Suggested Servings Per Day	
		Teens and Adults	**Children**
Vegetables and fruits	¼-1 c raw, ½ c cooked leafy greens ¼-½ c dried fruit ½ c fruit or vegetable juice ¼ c other fruits and vegetables	6 or more with at least 1 from leafy greens	4 or more with at least 1 from leafy greens
Grains and grain products	1 slice bread, 1 waffle, 1 tortilla ½ c cooked cereal ½ c rice, noodles, grits ¾-1 c ready-to-eat cereal	6 or more with at least 3 from whole grains	4 or more with at least 2 from whole grains
Protein foods*	1 c milk, yogurt 1 oz cheese, meat, fish, poultry 1 egg ½ cooked legumes 2 tbsp peanut butter 2 oz seeds, nuts	6 to 15 with at least 2 from dairy foods and at least 4 from others	6 to 15 with at least 3 from dairy foods and at least 3 from others
Luxury foods	Desserts 　½ c pudding, ice cream 　2 cookies 　Small slice cake Fats 　1 tbsp butter, oil Sweets 　1 tbsp sugar, honey Alcohol 1 oz liquor 4 oz wine 12 oz beer	**Children, teens, and adults** Desserts 　1 or less Fats 　4 or less Sweets 　4 or less **Adults only** Alcohol—1 or less	

From Pennington, J: J Nutr Education 13:54, 1981.
*Small portion sizes are specified in order to encourage a wide variety.

fatty meats or game should be consumed at level III or very moderately. Sparse consumption of foods in the luxury group IV is recommended. Fig. 33-3 shows the food guide as a inverse pyramid. Table 33-8 lists the recommended intake and serving sizes.

Alternative Food Patterns

Long before recommended allowances and guidelines were issued, many people followed special patterns of food intake based on religion, cultural background, ethics, health beliefs, personal preference, or concern for the efficient use of land to produce food. Such special diets are not necessarily more or less nutritional than diets based on the basic four food groups or other nutritional guidelines, since good nutrition depends on a balanced intake of all required nutrients. A common dietary pattern is the vegetarian diet.

VEGETARIAN DIETS

Vegetarianism is the consumption of a diet consisting predominantly of plant foods. Vegetarians may be ovo-lactovegetarians, who avoid meat, fish, and poultry but include eggs and milk in their diet, or lactovegetarians, who include milk in the diet but avoid eggs. Vegans, or pure vegetarians, consume only plant foods, avoiding meat, poultry, or fish.

DEVELOPMENTAL VARIABLES IN NUTRITION

Infants

Infancy is marked by rapid growth and high energy requirements. The average birth weight of an American baby is 3.2 to 3.4 kg (7 to 7½ pounds). The infant usually doubles birth weight at 4 to 5 months and triples it at 1 year of age. An energy intake of approximately 117 kcal/kg body weight is needed in the first half of infancy and 108 kcal/kg in the second half. A full-term newborn infant is able to digest and absorb simple carbohydrates, proteins, and a moderate amount of fat. Amylase, the starch-splitting enzyme, is not present at birth. Infants need a high amount of fluid, because a large portion of the infant's total body weight is water.

BREAST-FED INFANTS

Breast milk is the ideal food for infants. The current recommendation is that breast milk be the major source of nutrients in the first 6 months. Breast milk contains antibodies to protect against antigens in infant formulas and foods. As the infant grows, the gastrointestinal tract can fight against antigenic proteins.

Breast milk also provides protective maternal antibodies and promotes bonding between mother and child. The lipid content of breast milk is better absorbed than that of other infant foods. Breast-feeding may prevent infant obesity and protect against hypercholesterolemia in later life. At the end of the nursing period, breast milk has a higher fat content that is thought to provide satiety and stop the infant from sucking. The high cholesterol level of breast milk is thought to foster the development of more efficient cholesterol metabolism.

Breast-fed infants need a source of vitamin C, fluoride, vitamin D, and iron. Diluted orange juice can be introduced at 1 to 2 months of age, gradually decreasing the amount of diluent until the infant is receiving full-strength juice. Fluoride should be given as a supplement in areas where the water supply is not fluoridated or if the infant does not drink enough fluoridated water to meet needs. Vitamin D is also given as a vitamin supplement. After 4 months, when the fetal store of red blood cells is exhausted, the infant needs a dietary source of iron. Premature infants need iron earlier and appear to absorb it better than full-term infants.

BOTTLE-FED INFANTS

Bottle-fed infants are usually given 5% to 10% glucose 4 hours after birth. But ingesting refined sugar at an early age may produce a desire later for sweet foods. The infant who handles the glucose feeding well progresses to diluted formula and then to full-strength formula. Infant formulas can also be fortified with vitamins and minerals to resemble human milk.

Neither undiluted whole milk nor skim milk should be used as a basis for infant formulas. Whole milk has excess protein and requires dilution, and skim milk lacks linoleic acid. In addition, bottle-fed babies need a fluoride supplement if the water supply is not fluoridated. They also should be given diluted orange juice or a vitamin C supplement at 1 to 2 months of age.

INTRODUCTION TO SOLID FOOD

The ability to swallow voluntarily is not fully developed until 10 to 12 weeks of age. Before that time swallowing must be stimulated by sucking. The amount of saliva needed to ease swallowing solid food is not secreted until about 3 months of age. The extrusion reflex (pushing food out of the mouth with the tongue) lasts until the infant is 4 months old. Taste sensation is not present until 3 to 4 months of age. Spoon feeding is thus not a good idea until 4 to 6 months of age.

Enriched rice cereal, the first solid food for both breast-fed and bottle-fed infants, may be given at 4 to 6 months of age. Other grain cereals will follow later. They provide iron, calcium, phosphorus, thiamine, riboflavin, and niacin. Meat is an alternative first food for breast-fed babies. Some pediatricians prefer it because of its iron and protein content. Vegetables are usually given at 7 months, fruits at 8 months, and meat and cottage cheese at 9 months. Earlier ingestion of meat by bottle-fed infants results in excess protein intake.

Infants should be given new foods in small servings, one new food at a time, to identify allergies. They should be exposed to a wide variety of foods to ensure intake of essential nutrients. The texture of solid food progresses from strained to mashed to minced to chopped to cut table foods.

Toddlers and Preschoolers

The growth rate slows during the toddler period (1 to 3 years of age). The toddler needs fewer calories but an increased amount of protein in relation to body weight. Toddlers are more interested in their environment and increasing motor skills than in food.

The toddler needs two servings (16 ounces) daily from the milk group to supply protein, calcium, riboflavin, and vitamins A and B_{12}. Fortified milk provides vitamin D and additional vitamin A. Whole milk should be used until the toddler reaches 2 years of age because of the linoleic acid in the milk fat. One half of the toddler's protein intake should consist of high-biological–value proteins. Toddlers who consume more than 24 ounces of milk daily instead of other foods may develop a milk anemia. Lean red meats, as a part of the 1 to 3 ounces of meat group foods, are a good source of iron, as are whole grains, enriched cereals, and breads. When giving meats to a toddler, the portion should be cut small to avoid the possibility of choking. Hot dogs are are dangerous for children at this age.

The toddler should receive four servings daily from the fruit and vegetable group. One serving daily should be a good source of vitamin C. Green leafy vegetables and deep yellow fruits and vegetables should be served frequently. Toddlers like bite-sized raw vegetables but should not be given raw carrots because they could choke on them.

The toddler's four servings from the bread and cereal group should include whole grain or enriched breads, cereals, and pastas. Infant cereals may continue to be used because of their higher iron content. Sugar-coated cereals and sugar on cereals should be avoided. Toddlers often prefer dry cereal. In addition to the basic four food groups, the toddler should have 1 to 2 teaspoons of margarine or butter for vitamin A.

Good nutritional habits should be started early, with fruit desserts, custards, puddings, and ice cream emphasized instead of cakes, pies, and cookies.

During the preschool years, from ages 3 to 6, children gain an average of 2 kg (4½ pounds) of body weight and 5 to 8 cm (2 to 3 inches) in height a year. At the end of the preschool period, the child's weight is double that at 1 year of age and height is 1½ times that at 1 year. The average 6-year-old weighs 19 kg (42 pounds) and stands 105 cm (42 inches) high. Growth slows during the preschool period, but energy requirements are increased.

Daily protein needs are increased to 40 g, half of which should be high-biological–value proteins. Calcium and iron remain important. Fruits and vegetables should be encouraged to provide vitamins A and C. Interest in food continues to be overshadowed by interest in the enlarging environment and motor skills. Several small meals may be preferable to the traditional three.

Preschoolers need 16 ounces of milk daily, 1 to 3 ounces from the meat group, four servings from the fruit and vegetable group (including a daily source of vitamin C and frequent servings of leafy green and deep yellow vegetables and fruits), four servings of whole grain or enriched foods from the bread and cereal group, and 1 to 2 teaspoons of margarine or butter.

School-Age Children

School-age children, 6 to 12 years old, grow at a slower and steadier rate, with a gradual decline in energy requirements per unit of body weight. The school-age child gains 3 to 5 kg (6½ to 11 pounds) in weight and 6 cm (2½ inches) in height a year until puberty.

The appetites of school-age children are greater than those of younger children, and food intake is more varied. Recommended intake includes two servings from the milk group, 2 to 3 ounces of meat group foods, three to four servings from the fruit and vegetable group (with a daily source of vitamin C and a source of vitamin A every other day), three to four servings from whole grain and enriched breads and cereals, and 1 to 2 teaspoons of margarine or butter.

Despite better appetites and more varied food intake, the diets of school-age children should be carefully assessed for adequate protein and vitamin A and C. Milk intake usually exceeds recommendations, but failure to eat a proper breakfast and unsupervised intake at school may result in an improper or inadequate diet.

Adolescents

During adolescence, physiological age is a better guide to nutritional needs than chronological age. Adolescence begins with the growth spurt of puberty at the end of childhood and ends with the completion of physical growth. Caloric needs are greatly increased to meet increased metabolic demands. Girls need approximately 2000 to 2500 kcal a day; boys need 2500 to 3000 kcal a day. Protein needs increase to a daily requirement of 50 to 60 g. Calcium is essential for the rapid bone growth of adolescence, and girls need a continuous source of iron to replace menstrual losses. Iodine supports increased thyroid activity, and B complex vitamins support the heightened metabolic activity.

Adolescents' requirements from the basic four groups include three or more servings from the milk group; two or more from the meat group; four or more from the vegetable-fruit group (with a daily source of vitamin C and a source of vitamin A every other day); two to six or more from the bread and cereal group, with emphasis on whole grains; and 1 to 2 tablespoons of margarine or butter.

The adolescent's diet is influenced by many factors other than nutritional needs, including concern about body image and appearance, desire for independence, and fad diets. Nutritional deficiencies may occur in adolescent girls as a result of dieting and using oral contraceptives. The nutrients involved are folic acid, vitamin B_6, vitamin C, thiamine, riboflavin, and iron. The adolescent boy's diet may be inadequate in total calories, protein, iron, folic acid, B vitamins, and iodine.

Pregnant teenage girls must meet their own nutritional needs and the additional demands of the fetus. Pregnancy occurring within 4 years after menarche (which usually occurs at 10½ to 13 years in America) places mother and fetus at risk because of anatomical and physiological immaturity. The fetus has an increased risk of low birth weight, malformation, and mortality.

The caloric intake of the pregnant adolescent should permit an 11 to 13 kg (24- to 29-pound) total weight gain, usually achieved by increasing the caloric intake by 300 kcal daily.

Most teenage girls do not want to gain weight. Counseling related to the nutritional needs of pregnancy may be very difficult, and suggestions are better than rigid directions. The diet of a pregnant adolescent is most apt to be deficient in calcium, iron, and vitamins A and C.

Young and Middle Adults

The demands for most nutrients are reduced as the growth period ends. Mature adults need nutrients for energy, maintenance, and repair. Energy needs usually decline over the years. Obesity may become a problem because of decreased physical exercise, increased dining out, or the ability to afford more luxury foods.

Adult women who use oral contraceptives need extra folic acid, vitamin C, riboflavin, vitamin B_6, and vitamin B_{12}. Those who use intrauterine devices need additional vitamin C and iron to compensate for increased menstrual flow.

Young and middle-aged adults are subject to the same recommendations from the basic four food groups: two or more servings from the milk group, four or more from the vegetable-fruit group (with a daily source of vitamin C and three to four weekly servings of sources of vitamin A continuing), four or more from the whole grain or enriched bread and cereal group, and 1 to 2 tablespoons of margarine or butter.

PREGNANCY

Poor nutrition during pregnancy can cause low birth weight in infants and decreased chances of survival. Generally, the fetus' needs are met at the expense of the mother's needs. However, if nutrient sources are not available, both mother and fetus will suffer. The nutritional status of the mother at the time of conception is important in terms of nutritional reserves and basic eating habits. Often significant aspects of fetal growth and development occur before pregnancy is even suspected.

The energy requirements of pregnancy are related to body weight and activity. A total weight gain of 10 to 15 kg (22 to 33 pounds) is recommended.

Caloric intake should be sufficient to meet energy needs and to spare protein for anabolism. Inadequate weight gain and weight gain above 15 kg (33 pounds) are not desirable. In the event of undesirable gains or losses, the food intake should be evaluated. Pregnant women should be cautioned against fasting as a method of weight control, because fasting leads to ketoacidosis, which can be dangerous to the fetus.

Food intake in the first trimester should include balanced portions of essential nutrients with emphasis on quality. Protein intake throughout pregnancy is increased by 30 g or a 65% to 68% increase over prepregnancy. High-risk mothers are advised to double their normal protein intake. High-biological–value protein should supply two thirds of the protein intake.

Calcium intake should be increased by 50% per day. Calcium is needed for fetal tooth and bone development and blood clotting. Calcium intake is especially critical in the third trimester when fetal bones are mineralized.

Pregnant women need more iron than can be supplied by even the most ideal diet. Iron needs are increased by 30 to 60 mg a day. Iron is needed to correct preexisting deficiencies and to provide for increased maternal blood volume, for fetal blood storage, and for blood loss during delivery.

Iodine needs are increased by 25 mg (15% to 17%) because of increased activity of the thyroid gland.

Because vitamin A is needed for cell development, epithelial tissue maintenance, and tooth and bone development, requirements are increased by 200 retinol equivalents (20% to 25%).

Pregnancy also increases requirements for B vitamins, which are needed for enzyme production necessitated by increased metabolic activity. Folic acid intake is particularly important for DNA synthesis and the growth of red blood cells. Inadequate intake of folic acid may lead to megaloblastic anemia, a type of anemia seen in women who have had many pregnancies.

Vitamin C requirements are increased by 20 mg (30%) to provide the intercellular cement in connective and vascular tissue and to enhance the absorption of iron. Vitamin D needs are increased by 5 µg (100%), because this vitamin promotes the absorption of calcium and phosphorus needed for tooth and bone development.

The pregnant woman should have four or more servings from the milk group; four or more from the meat group; five to seven from the vegetable-fruit group (including a citrus fruit and a potato daily, and leafy green or dark yellow vegetables and fruits three to four times a week); two to four or more from the enriched or whole grain bread and cereal group; and at least 1 to 2 tablespoons of margarine or butter daily.

Pregnant women should increase their fluid intake by drinking 6 to 8 glasses of water daily. They should avoid saccharin, alcohol, excessive caffeine, and all drugs not specifically ordered.

LACTATION

Lactation requires further increases in nutrition. The production of breast milk increases energy requirements. The lactating woman needs 500 kcal above her prepregnancy requirement.

Protein requirements are reduced to 20 g per day, 10 g less than during pregnancy. The need for calcium remains the same as during pregnancy. Although the lactating woman requires less protein, folacin, and iron as compared to the pregnancy requirements, there is an increased need for vitamin A, niacin, riboflavin, iodine, and zinc over pregnancy needs. The need for vitamins C, D, E, B_6, B_{12}, and thiamine and for the minerals calcium, phosphorus, and magnesium are the same for the pregnant and the lactating woman, but the lactating woman requires more fluid.

The increased calories from the basic food groups should be provided by leafy green vegetables, citrus fruits, whole grains, milk, meats, and poultry to provide vitamins A and C, niacin, riboflavin, and zinc. She should continue to drink a quart of milk daily or its equivalent from the milk group. Fluid intake should total at least 3 quarts a day. Caffeine, alcohol, and drugs are excreted in breast milk and should be used only under a physician's supervision.

Older Adults

Adults 65 years and older have decreased needs for niacin, thiamine, riboflavin, and B vitamins associated with energy production. Decreased activity of the thyroid gland reduces the need for iodine. There seems to be no need for an increase in any nutrient.

Numerous factors influence the nutritional status of the older adult. Income is probably the most important, because a fixed income may reduce the amount of money used to buy food. Health is another important influence; the older adult may be on a therapeutic diet or have difficulty eating because of physical symptoms, lack of teeth, or dentures. Food shopping and preparation may be difficult because of physical disability or lack of transportation. Living alone decreases the interest and pleasure of preparing and eating meals.

Taste acuity normally declines with age. The taste buds that recognize sweet and salt are the first to deteriorate, leaving bitter and sour as the dominant taste sensations. Dentures also increase bitter and sour taste sensations. A normal decline in gastric secretions results in less efficient digestion.

The basic four food group selections for older adults are the same as for younger adults, although the way foods are prepared or the types of foods selected may need to be changed. Diets of older adults are typically low in protein foods and high in breads, cakes, and cereals. Meats may be avoided because of cost or because they are difficult to chew. Cheese, eggs, and peanut butter are used to provide protein. Milk continues to be an important food, particularly for the older woman who needs adequate calcium to protect against osteoporosis. Whole grain cereals and breads should be encouraged. Cream soups and meat-based vegetable soups are good for the older adult with chewing problems. The diet of the older adult should contain choices from all food groups and may require vitamin supplements.

NUTRITION AND THE NURSING PROCESS

Nurses are in an excellent position to recognize signs of poor nutrition and to take steps to initiate change. Close daily contact with clients and their families enable nurses to make observations about a client's physical status, food intake, weight gain or loss, and response to therapy. By using the four techniques of assessment, the nurse is able to identify actual or potential problems in nutritional status and implement appropriate nursing, medical, and nutritional therapies to reduce or reverse the client's nutritional alterations.

Nurses should investigate the reasons for decreased or excessive food intake and provide clients with alternatives. An equally important nursing responsibility is an awareness of indications that parenteral feeding can be replaced with oral feedings or that a nasogastric, gastric, or jejunostomy feeding tube is no longer necessary. In addition, the nurse is responsible for indicating when intravenous fluids should be supplemented with enteral or parenteral feedings.

Nurses in all settings should be alert to clients at risk because of nutritional problems. Both overweight and underweight clients are at risk for nutritional deficits because a 20% deviation from the client's ideal body weight is considered a high-risk factor. Both gross increases or decreases in body weight may reduce the body's protein reserve.

In the assessment component of the nursing process, the nurse gathers data to make a diagnosis of the client's nutritional problem or the potential for nutritional complications. Once the nutritional needs of the client are identified, the nurse designs specific interventions to meet those needs.

ASSESSMENT

Nurses make nutritional assessment part of daily nurse-client relationships. Because food and fluid are basic biological needs of all human beings, a nutritional assessment is essential. Nutritional assessment is particularly important for clients at risk for nutritional problems related to hospitalization, life-style habits, and other factors.

The following nutritional assessment goals as outlined by the American Society of Parenteral and Enteral Nutrition (ASPEN) are to:

1. Identify nutritional deficiencies adversely affecting health.
2. Obtain specific information to assist in planning and delivering nutritional care.
3. Evaluate the efficacy of nutritional care, modifying the nutritional care plan as needed to obtain the desired result (Forlaw and Grant, 1983).

The nutritional assessment consists of nursing history, observation, anthropometry, and laboratory data. In addition, the assessment is individualized to assess adequately each client to determine those clients at risk for nutritional alterations.

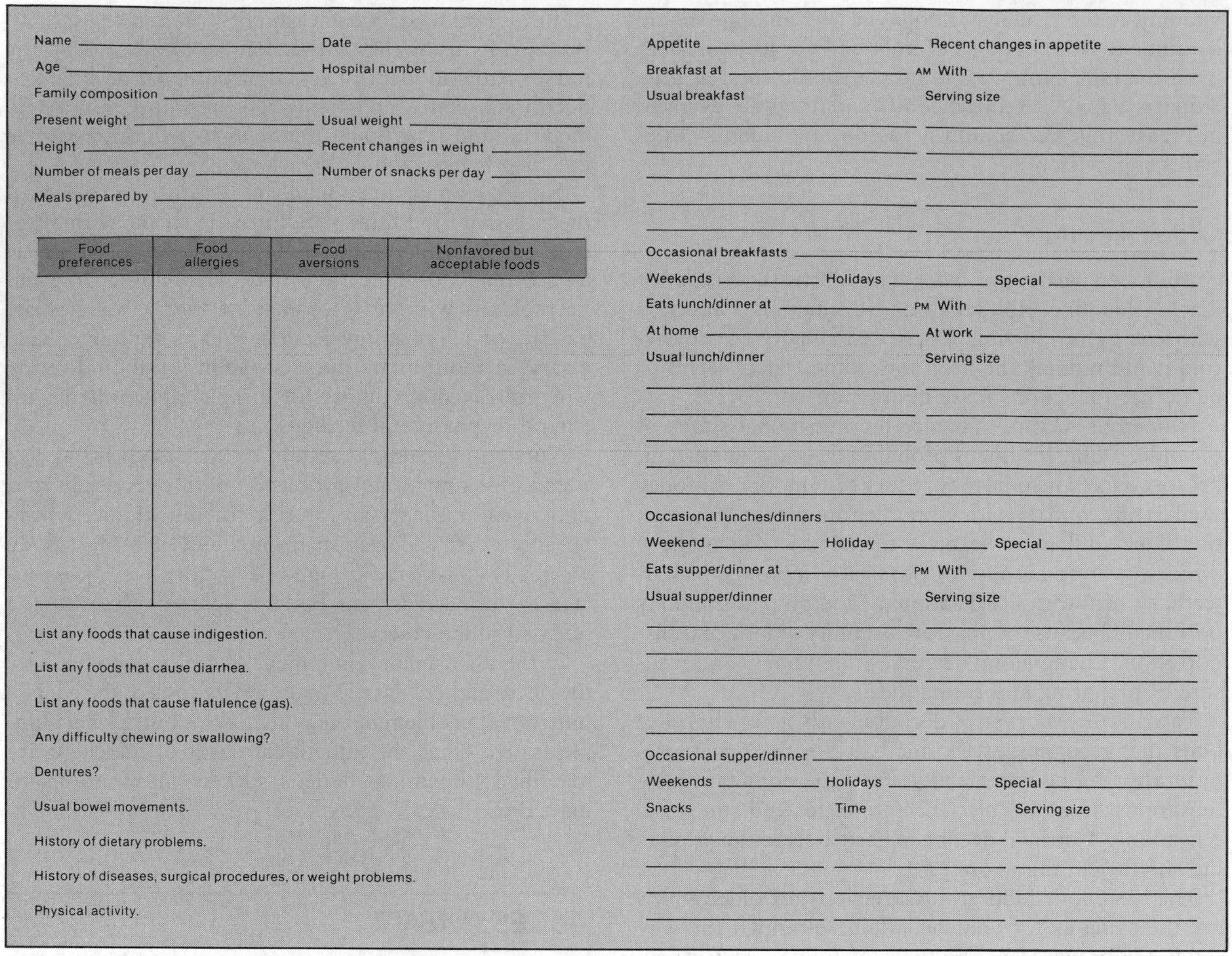

Name _____ Date _____

Age _____ Hospital number _____

Family composition _____

Present weight _____ Usual weight _____

Height _____ Recent changes in weight _____

Number of meals per day _____ Number of snacks per day _____

Meals prepared by _____

Food preferences	Food allergies	Food aversions	Nonfavored but acceptable foods

List any foods that cause indigestion. _____

List any foods that cause diarrhea. _____

List any foods that cause flatulence (gas). _____

Any difficulty chewing or swallowing? _____

Dentures? _____

Usual bowel movements. _____

History of dietary problems. _____

History of diseases, surgical procedures, or weight problems. _____

Physical activity. _____

Appetite _____ Recent changes in appetite _____

Breakfast at _____ AM With _____

Usual breakfast — Serving size

Occasional breakfasts _____

Weekends _____ Holidays _____ Special _____

Eats lunch/dinner at _____ PM With _____

At home _____ At work _____

Usual lunch/dinner — Serving size

Occasional lunches/dinners _____

Weekend _____ Holiday _____ Special _____

Eats supper/dinner at _____ PM With _____

Usual supper/dinner — Serving size

Occasional supper/dinner _____

Weekends _____ Holidays _____ Special _____

Snacks — Time — Serving size

Fig. 33-4 Diet history.

From Bodinski, LH: The nurse's guide to diet therapy, New York, 1982, John Wiley & Sons, Inc.

NURSING HISTORY

In addition to the general nursing history (see Chapter 6), the nurse can obtain a more specific diet history to assess the client's actual or potential nutritional needs. The diet history focuses on the client's habitual intake of food and liquids, as well as information about preferences, allergies, problems, and other relevant areas. Fig. 33-4 provides an example of a diet history.

In addition, a detailed record can be kept of the client's food intake over a 3-day period, including a weekend day. This record allows the nurse to calculate the client's nutritional intake and to compare this with recommended daily allowances to determine whether the client's usual dietary habits are providing all nutrients in required amounts.

In the nursing history the nurse also gathers information about the client's activity level to determine the energy need and compare it with the client's food intake.

FACTORS INFLUENCING DIETARY PATTERNS. A final area for the nurse to assess is a set of factors that influence the client's dietary pattern and nutritional status (see box). These factors include the client's health status, cultural background, religion, socioeconomic status, personal preference, psychological factors, use of alcohol or drugs, and misinformation of beliefs about food values.

Health Status. A good appetite is generally accepted as a sign of health, while anorexia is an almost universal symptom of disease. Anorexia also occurs as a side effect of drug therapy and as a response to treatment. Yet medical personnel tend to be unconcerned about anorexia and believe that a client's appetite will return when the condition is corrected. It is important, however, to recognize that nutritional support is an essential part of recovery.

Factors Influencing Dietary Patterns

HEALTH STATUS

- A good appetite is a sign of health.
- Anorexia is usually a symptom of disease or can be a side effect of drugs.
- Nutritional support is an essential part of recovery from any medical treatment.

CULTURE AND RELIGION

- Cultural and religious patterns and restrictions concerning food must be taken into account.
- Special foods and diets should be given when appropriate.
- Older clients are more apt to cling to ethnic food habits; this tendency may be increased during illness.

SOCIOECONOMIC STATUS

- Food expenses are not fixed, and spending varies according to the amount of money available.
- Whether someone is around to prepare food determines the amount of convenience foods used.

PERSONAL PREFERENCE

- Individual likes and dislikes are perhaps the strongest influence on diet.
- Foods associated with pleasant memories tend to become favorite foods; those associated with unpleasant memories tend to be avoided.
- Luxury foods may be used as status symbols.
- Individual preferences must be considered when planning a therapeutic diet.

PSYCHOLOGICAL FACTORS

- Individual motivations to eat balanced meals and individual perceptions about diet are strong influences.
- Food has strong symbolic value for many people (for example, milk may symbolize helplessness; meat may symbolize strength).

ALCOHOL AND DRUGS

- Excess alcohol use contributes to nutritional deficiencies because money may be spent on alcohol instead of food, and alcohol may replace part of the diet and depress appetite.
- Excess alcohol can also affect gastrointestinal organs.
- Drugs that depress appetite can lower intake of essential nutrients.
- Drugs can also deplete nutrient stores and lessen their absorption in the intestines.

MISINFORMATION AND FOOD FADS

- Food myths can be the result of cultural background, peer pressure, and a desire to control one's own diet choices.
- Food fads often involve erroneous beliefs that certain foods are especially healthy (for example, yogurt is more nutritional than milk, oysters increase sexual potency, or honey is healthier than sugar).
- Nurses must be careful not to be condescending when teaching a client that foods may not have the qualities attributed to them.

Culture and Religion. The influence of religion and culture on a client's attitude toward food is often overlooked. Health care workers often attribute a client's refusal to eat or to comply with a dietary regimen to anorexia or lack of understanding.

It is not possible to be familiar with all the dietary practices of all religions and cultures, but nurses should be familiar with the food practices of the predominant religions and cultures in their area of practice. If they ask questions about individual practices, clients are usually happy to explain their practices and grateful for the interest and concern expressed.

Cultural patterns should be considered in planning therapeutic diets; ethnic dishes should be included whenever appropriate. Nurses need to familiarize themselves with the ingredients in ethnic foods to recognize their contribution to the diet.

Socioeconomic Status. The amount of family income available for buying food varies. Food expenses are not always a fixed amount as are rent and mortgage payments. When money is tight, therefore, many people spend less on food.

It is generally assumed that people with higher incomes purchase more proteins and fats and fewer complex carbohydrates, while people with lower incomes do the opposite. This is not always true because some people with an interest in nutrition are convinced of the soundness of dietary guidelines and plan their meals accordingly. Some people with limited income also follow dietary guidelines and purchase adequate amounts of protein foods despite a limited budget.

In addition to food purchases, a family must consider food preparations. When no one is at home to prepare meals, more convenience foods must be used. When someone has the time to convert inexpensive foods into appealing meals, more of the food budget can be used to ensure that all necessary nutrients are included.

The impact of advertising and the lack of knowledge about the contents of processed foods also influence food purchases. It cannot be assumed that the person with enough money will purchase foods containing the essential nutrients.

Personal Preference. Individual food likes and dislikes are perhaps the strongest influence on food intake. A given food preference may have a tie to the past; the reason for the preference may no longer be remembered although the food remains a favorite. Certain foods, usually those associated with childhood, make people feel safe and protected and are often desired during periods of stress. Children tend to adopt the food preferences and habits of their parents, and these preferences may persist throughout life.

Clients who follow a therapeutic diet need help to understand the reasons for the diet. The client's food preferences should be considered in planning the diet. When a client does not like a particular food in the diet, an appropriate substitute should be found, to increase the palatability of the diet.

Psychological Factors. Closely related to matters of personal preference are psychological factors, which also influence clients' dietary patterns. Eating patterns vary widely among individuals as a result of differences in education, family influences, values, attitudes, behavioral patterns, and other factors. One person may be highly motivated to eat balanced meals every day, for example, whereas another may be less interested in nutrition and may eat whatever is most convenient most of the time. Perceptions about diet also vary: one person may perceive that vitamins are important and daily supplements necessary, whereas another may believe that vitamin needs are satisfied by eating an occasional fresh fruit or vegetable. The nurse assesses such psychological factors in planning and implementing dietary teaching or counseling.

Another psychological factor is the symbolic value of food. For some people, milk symbolizes maternal security, whereas to others it may symbolize helplessness. Therefore some clients may drink a great deal of milk whereas others reject it because of symbolic associations. Similarly, to some clients meat symbolizes strength and masculinity, and vegetables and fruits symbolize femininity, significantly affecting dietary patterns.

ALCOHOL AND DRUGS. The client's ingestion of alcohol and use of prescription, over-the-counter, or illegal drugs may also affect nutritional status either directly or indirectly by influencing dietary patterns.

The excessive ingestion of alcohol contributes to nutritional deficiencies in several ways. Money used to buy alcoholic beverages might otherwise have been spent on more nutritional foods. Alcohol may replace part of the diet, thus reducing the intake of nutrients from other foods. Alcohol can also depress the appetite. Furthermore, excessive ingestion of alcohol can affect gastrointestinal organs, reducing the efficiency of digestion and absorption of nutrients.

The effects of drugs on nutrition vary widely, depending on the type and actions of the drugs. Drugs that depress the appetite, including nonprescription drugs sold to dieters, can lower the intake of essential nutrients. Other drugs can deplete stores of nutrients or lessen their absorption in the intestines. The nurse should therefore take note of any drugs in the nursing and medical histories in order to minimize or counteract their effects on the client's nutritional status.

MISINFORMATION AND FOOD FADS. For many people dietary patterns are influenced by misinformation or myths about the values of certain foods. A food fad is a shared perception that a particular food is especially healthy, can cure an illness, can increase sexual potency, should be avoided because of negative health effects, and so on. Some food myths are rooted in cultural background, some arise because of the popular interest in natural foods, some involve peer pressure, and some persist because of the desire to exert greater control over health status through diet. Although it is true that good nutritional practices improve health, many food fads and myths have no scientific basis. Often the foods do not have the properties claimed by those believing in the fad or myth. If such beliefs have the potential to disrupt a client's dietary pattern, the nurse may use teaching or counseling techniques to ensure that the client's diet provides adequate nutrition. Because people's food beliefs are often closely related to their philosophy of life or other life-style factors, the nurse must be careful not to seem condescending or put the client on the defensive when discussing food values and correcting misinformation. This is particularly true when the client is from a culture different from the nurse's. Table 33-9 presents a few examples of food fads and myths and the truth about these foods.

PHYSICAL ASSESSMENT

As in other kinds of nursing assessment, the nurse observes the client for signs of actual or potential nutritional needs. Because improper nutrition affects all body systems, clues to malnutrition may be observed during physical assessment (see Chapter 30). When the general physical assessment of body systems is complete, the nurse can recheck pertinent areas to evaluate the client's nutritional status. The clinical signs of nutritional status (Table 33-10, p. 906) provide guidelines for observation during the physical assessment.

ANTHROPOMETRY. Anthropometry is a system of measurement of the size and makeup of the body and specific body parts. Anthropometric measurements that aid in identifying nutritional problems include weight,

TABLE 33-9   Examples of Food Fads and Myths

Food	Common Misinformation	Nutritional Facts
Honey	Thought healthier than sugar, a curative for coughs or colds, better than sugar for digestion	No special curative powers, no significant differences in digestion
Yogurt	Thought to ensure good health, more nutritious than milk	Essentially equivalent to milk in nutritional qualities
Citrus fruits	Thought to cause acid indigestion	Stomach acid production unaffected by citrus fruits
Cabbage, onions	Thought to taint breast milk	Lactation requires specific nutrients, and breast milk is not tainted by any food
Gelatin	Thought in large amounts to build strong nails	Not necessary for nail formation, which depends on general nutrition, nail care, and other factors
Oysters, raw egg, rare lean beef	Thought to increase fertility or sexual potency	No food affects sexual potency
Raw milk	Thought more nutritious than pasteurized milk	Pasteurized milk may contain slightly less vitamin C but also includes vitamin D; raw milk carries a greater risk of contamination

height, wrist circumference, mid-upper arm circumference (MAC), and triceps skinfold (TSF).

Unless contraindicated, a client's height and weight should be obtained on hospital admission or entry into an outpatient care setting. A client should always be weighed at the same time each day, on the same scale, and with the same clothing or linen. The client's height and weight can be compared to the usual measurements and to standards for normal height-weight relationships.

Wrist circumference is used to estimate the client's body frame. A tape measure is used to measure the smallest portion of the client's wrist, distal to the styloid process (Fig. 33-5). Body frame normal values include 9 to 11 cm (small), 11 to 12 cm (medium), and 12 to 14 cm (large).

The MAC determines muscle wasting. The client should be sitting because measurements while the client is supine may decrease accuracy. If the client is bedridden, the measurement can be obtained with the client's arm placed across the chest. The client's nondominant arm is relaxed, and the nurse measures the circumference at the midpoint of the arm, between the tip of the acromial process of the scapula and the olecron process of the ulna (Fig. 33-6). Measurement of the nondomi-

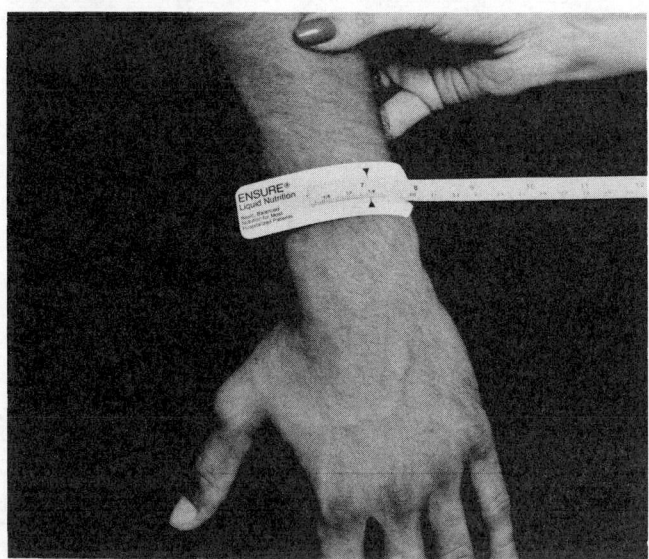

Fig. 33-5   Wrist circumference.

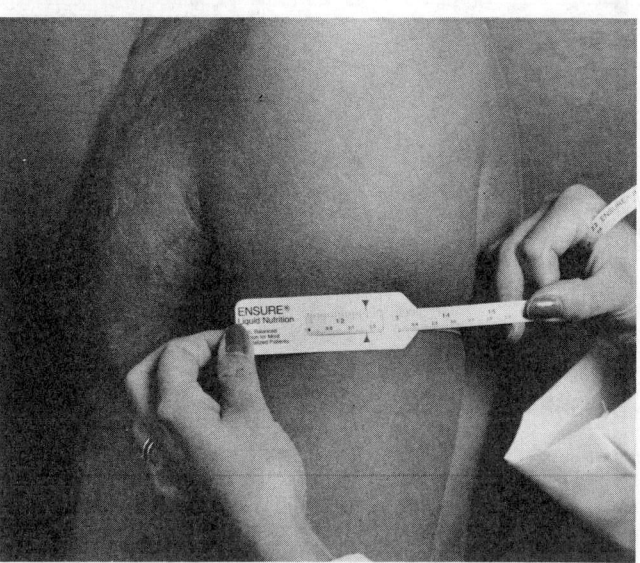

Fig. 33-6   Mid-upper arm circumference.

TABLE 33-10 Clinical Signs of Nutritional Status

Body Area	Signs of Good Nutrition	Signs of Poor Nutrition
General appearance	Alert, responsive	Listless, apathetic, cachectic
Weight	Normal for height, age, body build	Overweight or underweight (special concern for underweight)
Posture	Erect, arms and legs straight	Sagging shoulders, sunken chest, humped back
Muscles	Well-developed, firm, good tone, some fat under skin	Flaccid, poor tone, underdeveloped, tender, edema, wasted appearance, cannot walk properly
Nervous control	Good attention span, not irritable or restless, normal reflexes, psychological stability	Inattentive, irritable, confused, burning and tingling of hands and feet (paresthesia), loss of position and vibratory sense, weakness and tenderness of muscles (may result in inability to walk), decrease or loss of ankle and knee reflexes, absent vibratory sense
Gastrointestinal function	Good appetite and digestion, normal regular elimination, no palpable organs or masses	Anorexia, indigestion, constipation or diarrhea, liver or spleen enlargement
Cardiovascular function	Normal heart rate and rhythm, no murmurs, normal blood pressure for age	Rapid heart rate (above 100 beats per minute), enlarged heart, abnormal rhythm, elevated blood pressure
General vitality	Endurance, energetic, sleeps well, vigorous	Easily fatigued, no energy, falls asleep easily, looks tired, apathetic
Hair	Shiny, lustrous, firm, not easily plucked, healthy scalp	Stringy, dull, brittle, dry, thin, and sparse, depigmented, can be easily plucked
Skin (general)	Smooth, slightly moist, good color	Rough, dry, scaly, pale, pigmented, irritated, bruises, petechiae, subcutaneous fat loss
Face and neck	Skin color uniform, smooth, pink, healthy appearance, not swollen	Greasy, discolored, scaly, swollen, skin dark over cheeks and under eyes, lumpiness or flakiness of skin around nose and mouth
Lips	Smooth, good color, moist, not chapped or swollen	Dry, scaly, swollen, redness and swelling (cheilosis), or angular lesions at corners of the mouth or fissures or scars (stomatitis)
Mouth, oral membranes	Reddish pink mucous membranes in oral cavity	Swollen, boggy oral mucous membranes
Gums	Good pink color, healthy, red, no swelling or bleeding	Spongy, bleed easily, marginal redness, inflamed, gums receding
Tongue	Good pink color or deep reddish in appearance, not swollen or smooth, surface papillae present, no lesions	Swelling, scarlet and raw, magenta color, beefy (glossitis), hyperemic and hypertrophic papillae, atrophic papillae
Teeth	No cavities, no pain, bright, straight, no crowding, well-shaped jaw, clean, no discoloration	Unfilled caries, absent teeth, worn surfaces, mottled (fluorosis), malpositioned
Eyes	Bright, clear, shiny, no sores at corner of eyelids, membranes moist and healthy pink color, no prominent blood vessels or mound of tissue or sclera, no fatigue circles beneath	Eye membranes pale (pale conjunctivas), redness of membrane (conjunctival injection), dryness, signs of infection, Bitot's spots, redness and fissuring of eyelid corners (angular palpebritis), dryness of eye membrane (conjunctival xerosis), dull appearance of cornea (corneal xerosis), soft cornea (keratomalacia)
Neck (glands)	No enlargement	Thyroid enlargement
Nails	Firm, pink	Spoon shape (koilonychia), brittle, ridged
Legs, feet	No tenderness, weakness, or swelling; good color	Edema, tender calf, tingling, weakness
Skeleton	No malformations	Bowlegs, knock-knees, chest deformity at diaphragm, beaded ribs, prominent scapulas

From Williams, SR: Nutritional guidance in prenatal care. In Worthington-Roberts, BS, Vermeersch, JA, and Williams, SR: Nutrition in pregnancy and lactation, ed. 3, St. Louis, 1985, The C.V. Mosby Co; Grant, JA, and Kennedy-Caldwell C: Nutritional support in nursing, New York, 1988, Grune-Stratton.

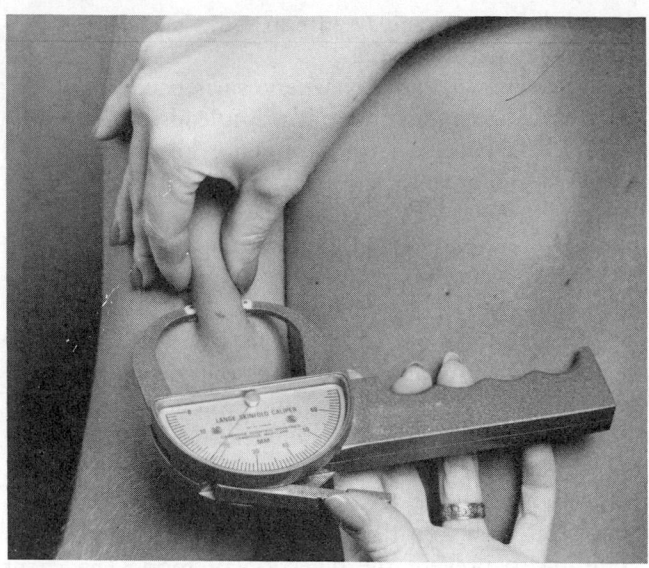

Fig. 33-7 Triceps skin fold.

nant arm prevents false recordings secondary to increased muscle mass from activities of daily living or employment. Normal values are 28.3 cm (male) and 28.5 cm (female).

Skinfold measurements are used to determine fat content of subcutaneous tissue. TSF is the most common and easiest to measure. With the thumb and forefinger, pinch lengthwise a double fold of fat about 1 cm above midpoint of the MAC. With the other hand, place teeth of calipers on either side of the fat fold (Fig. 33-7). The nurse averages the measurements from three readings. Normal values include 12.5 cm (males) and 16.5 cm (females). Other anatomical areas for skinfold measurements include the biceps, scapula, and abdominal muscles.

The mid-arm muscle circumference (MAMC) is an estimation of skeletal mass. It is calculated from the MAC and TSF anthropometric measures. The formula is $MAMC = MAC - (TSF \times 3.14)$. The normal values include 25.3 cm (males) and 23.2 cm (females).

LABORATORY DATA

Laboratory values useful in nutritional assessment include the complete blood counts, serum albumin level, transferrin level, and urinary concentrations of urea nitrogen and creatinine (Table 33-11). A low red blood cell count and depressed hemoglobin value indicate anemia. The hemoglobin and hematocrit values can also reflect the state of hydration. Serum levels of albumin and transferrin are used to identify protein-calorie malnutrition (PCM). Reduced levels of albumin and transferrin in adults also indicate a visceral protein deficit.

Urine specimens collected every 24 or 48 hours are

TABLE 33-11 Common Laboratory Tests to Evaluate Nutritional Status

Test	Purpose	Abnormal Findings
Serum album normal: 4-5.5 mg/dl	Maintain serum protein levels Maintain fluid and electrolyte balance Useful in determining prolonged protein wasting	Abnormal values may take up to 2 weeks before they are reflected in blood studies. Abnormalities in liver and kidney diseases, stress, dehydration, infection. <2.5 mg/dl indicates severe protein depletion.
Transferrin normal: 170-250 mg/dl	More specific indicator of protein/calorie malnutrition than albumin Blood protein binds with iron	Abnormal values respond quickly to changes in protein intake. Decreased in liver disease and chronic renal failure.
Total lymphocyte count (TLC) normal: >1800	Impaired nutritional intake depresses immune system, which is reflected in TLC	Depleted in all immunosuppressed clients.
Hemoblobin normal: 12-15 g/dl	Measures oxygen and iron carrying capacity of the blood	Decrease may indicate some form of anemia or can be lowered with blood loss.
Blood urea nitrogen (BUN) normal: 10-20 mg/dl	Measures breakdown of dietary protein Measures urea production in the liver and excretion in the kidneys	Elevated with excessive protein intake. Depressed with low protein intake. Elevated in liver and renal disease. Falsely elevated in hypovolemic dehydration.
Creatinine excretion in 24-hour urine	Creatinine formation and excretion reflects total muscle mass Indirect measure of skeletal muscle mass depletion	Abnormally low in renal disease. Abnormally low in severe malnutrition and starvation.

helpful in assessing nutritional status. The urea nitrogen level is related to the use of exogenous protein and to nitrogen balance. Creatinine is used with height to indicate changes in lean tissue mass.

CLIENTS AT RISK FOR NUTRITIONAL PROBLEMS

Any client with a condition that interferes with the ability to ingest, digest, or absorb adequate nutrients should be considered at risk. Congenital anomalies and surgical revisions of the gastrointestinal tract interfere with normal function. Clients fed solely by the intravenous route for more than 10 days are at risk for nutritional deficiencies.

Increased demand for nutrients to meet heightened metabolic needs is a factor in caring for infants and pregnant women. Clients who are otherwise healthy may have a potential for actual or potential nutritional deficiencies related to poor dietary habits. Also at risk are clients who are obese, who have anorexia nervosa or bulimia, who have undergone surgery or are immobilized, or those with cancer who may or may not be receiving radiotherapy.

OBESITY. Obesity is a condition in which there is a 20% increase above ideal body weight. Obesity cuts across all socioeconomic levels and is a risk factor in most of the leading causes of death. Our culture stresses slenderness, so excessive weight causes psychological problems, inconvenience, and unhappiness in addition to its impact on health.

To lose weight, a person must burn some of the body's store of fat. When insufficient calories are ingested to meet the daily energy needs, the body is forced to burn its reserve stores for energy. A person may lose weight either by reducing food intake or increasing energy needs through increased activity. The best plan for weight loss combines reduced food intake with increased exercise. The best diet plan is to adopt a well-balanced diet for life. The basic four food groups in the recommended serving sizes supply approximately 1200 kcal a day and provide a safe basis for weight reduction. Once the ideal body weight is reached, the intake can be adjusted upward to maintain this weight. This prevents the tendency to regain weight after the dieting stops. Following the guidelines and reducing intake of fats and refined sugars should also reduce weight.

ANOREXIA NERVOSA. Anorexia nervosa is a biopsychosocial disorder in which self-imposed starvation is used to establish identity and control, marked by denial of being underweight, hunger, and fatigue. It may be metabolic and possibly hereditary. Usually a problem in family dynamics is present; early feeding patterns and attitudes toward food have also been implicated. The desirability of a slender figure in today's society is considered a potent factor.

The client with anorexia nervosa is usually an adolescent girl. Extreme undernutrition leads to secondary endocrine disorders such as amenorrhea and delayed sexual development. The client may also go on food binges followed by self-induced vomiting or cathartic purges. The treatment of anorexia nervosa is a combination of psychotherapy, behavior modification, and dietary therapy.

BULIMIA. Bulimia or the binge-purge syndrome occurs in half of the clients with anorexia nervosa, but not all bulimic clients have anorexia nervosa. The syndrome appears to develop with an abnormal craving for food accompanied by the desire to remain slender. The client gorges on food to satisfy the craving and then induces vomiting to prevent the digestion of food. The client may also use laxatives or enemas to increase gastric motility so nutrients are not absorbed. The practice of secretly vomiting after eating usually starts with occasional binges and gradually becomes a daily activity and the preferred way of controlling weight. Frequent vomiting, laxative abuse, and overuse of enemas lead to electrolyte imbalances (hypokalemia being the most serious), esophageal lesions, dental caries, endocrine disturbances, and metabolic changes. Treatment includes dietary education, hospitalization, psychotherapy, drug therapy with phenytoin (Dilantin), group therapy, and behavioral modification.

POSTOPERATIVE CLIENTS. Surgery interferes with food intake. Preoperative preparation usually involves at least an 8-hour period of fasting. The resumption of food intake postoperatively varies with the client, the surgical procedure, complications, and the surgeon's protocol (see Chapter 46).

Unless the surgical procedure dictates an alternative feeding method, clients who have had mouth and throat surgery must chew and swallow food in the presence of excision sites, sutures, or otherwise manipulated tissue. The ingestion of food causes discomfort, and clients are usually reluctant to eat or drink. Fluids are usually offered first. The use of a straw may be helpful in some cases, such as dental surgery, but is specifically contraindicated in others, such as cleft palate repairs. Soft foods are sometimes easier to swallow than liquids. Hot fluids, tart juices, and fiber should be avoided after throat and mouth surgery. Milk, yogurt, sherbet, ice cream, ginger ale, and diluted fruit juices are usually allowed.

When surgery is performed on the stomach and intestines, an alternative method of food intake is usually prescribed to allow the suture line to heal and edema to subside. Nasogastric suction may also be used to prevent gastric and intestinal secretions from irritating the re-sected areas. When oral intake is restricted for a short period, fluids are usually given intravenously. Gastric surgery may limit the amount of food that can be ingested at any one time. Intestinal surgery may interfere with absorption of nutrients, depending on the length of intestine involved and the location.

The diversion of intestinal wastes through the creation of artificial openings in the abdomen (ileostomy, colostomy) affects fluid loss and electrolyte balance. Clients with ileostomies also lose some of their ability to absorb vitamin B_{12}. Clients with ileostomies and colostomies have dietary concerns related to the consistency of the ostomy waste and control of odor.

IMMOBILIZED CLIENTS. Extended immobilization can result in deossification and osteoporosis of bones and in hypercalcemia. Hypercalcemia predisposes clients to kidney and bladder stones; it is a particular problem in children and adolescents because of their rapid bone growth. Early ambulation is the best way to prevent immobilization problems. When ambulation is not possible, adequate quantities of high-biological–value protein help prevent skin breakdown and infections, and high phosphorus intake in the early weeks of immobilization reduces blood calcium levels. Generous fluid intake also protects against kidney stones. Range-of-motion exercises for noninvolved joints provide some activity.

CANCER AND RADIOTHERAPY. Malignant cancer cells compete with normal cells for nutrients, increasing the metabolic needs of the client. Clients with cancer typically complain of anorexia and taste distortions. Nutritional support and the correction of nutritional deficits can enable clients to benefit from therapies previously denied them. Optimal nutrition improves cancer survival rates, as well as the quality of life.

Although radiotherapy destroys the rapidly dividing neoplastic cells, it also destroys normal cells. Clients in good nutritional states can tolerate larger doses of radiation. Radiotherapy usually causes anorexia, nausea, and vomiting. Irradiation of the head and neck can lead to taste and smell distortions, decreased salivation, and dysphagia. Irradiation of the abdomen and pelvis can result in malabsorption and diarrhea.

NURSING DIAGNOSIS

The nursing assessment ends with the nurse clustering relevant data to determine if actual or potential nutritional problems exist (see nursing diagnoses box). A

Examples of Nursing Diagnoses Related to Altered Nutritional Status

NANDA-APPROVED NURSING DIAGNOSES

Altered nutrition: less than body requirements related to:
- NPO status
- Excessive dieting
- Anorexia
- Self-induced vomiting
- Alcoholism
- Excessive use of enemas or laxatives
- Food fads
- Alternative diet forms

Altered nutrition: more than body requirements related to:
- Excessive caloric intake

Altered nutrition: potential for more than body requirements related to:
- Dysfunctional eating patterns
- Closely spaced pregnancies

Feeding self-care deficit related to:
- Impaired mobility of both arms

Impaired swallowing related to:
- Surgical trauma
- Muscular weakness

Body-image disturbance related to:
- Obesity

Impaired social interaction related to:
- Poor body image from obesity

Fluid volume excess related to:
- Hypoalbuminemia

Fluid volume deficit: actual related to:
- Inadequate fluid intake

Potential for infection related to:
- Intravenous nutritional therapy
- Inadequate food intake

---

deficit may occur when any one or multiple nutrients are not ingested, poorly digested, or incompletely absorbed. Specific diagnoses are related to the actual nutritional deficiency. The nursing diagnosis may also involve a general nutritional deficiency or problems that place the client at risk for nutritional deficiencies.

The nursing diagnostic statement is based on supporting diagnostic characteristics present in the assessment data base (see sample nursing diagnoses box). In addition, the suspected cause or etiology of the diagnosis is stated. Identification of causes further individualizes the nursing diagnostic statement and subsequent plan of care.

Sample Nursing Diagnoses for Altered Nutritional Status

Defining Characteristics	Nursing Diagnoses	Related Factors
Unplanned weight loss Weight less than 20% of ideal body weight Aversion to food Impaired taste Inflamed buccal mucosa Abdominal pain Diarrhea	Altered nutrition: less than body requirements	▪ Inability to ingest, digest, or absorb nutrients due to physiological, psychosocial, or economical factors
Weight 20% over ideal body weight Sedentary activity High fat and carbohydrate intake High food intake at the end of the day	Altered nutrition: more than body requirements	▪ Excessive intake in relation to metabolic need
Familial obesity Observed use of food as a reward Dysfunctional eating patterns	Altered nutrition: potential for more than body requirements	▪ Hereditary predisposition ▪ Excessive intake ▪ Psychological conditioning related to food

PLANNING

Planning to maintain a proper nutritional status is better than having to correct deficits (see care plan box). The identification of those clients at risk for nutritional problems should result in a care plan that will prevent nutritional problems or minimize them if they should occur. Nutritional education and counseling are important for the client on a regular diet to prevent disease and to promote health. The clients on a therapeutic diet who understand the rationale for the diet are more likely

Sample Nursing Care Plan for Altered Nutritional Status

Nursing Diagnosis	Goal	Expected Outcomes	Nursing Interventions
Altered nutrition: less than body requirements related to inability to swallow nutrients	Client returns to within 10% of ideal body weight.	Client will gain 0.5 to 1 lb/week. Client will retain all nutrients. Diarrhea or vomiting is absent. Serum electrolytes and other blood chemistry levels indicate improving nutritional status. There is no edema. There are no skin or mouth lesions.	Weigh client daily. Take a daily colorie count. Institute nasogastric tube feedings: gradually increase rate and strength to tolerance and need. Do a daily stool count. Perform daily serum electrolyte levels until stable, then 3 days/week. Perform serum chemistry levels weekly, monitor skin and mouth for lesions every 8 hours. Record intake and output. Observe for fluid and electrolyte imbalances as needed.

to comply with it. For this group of clients the plan is based on one or more of the following goals:

1. Clients return to within 10% of ideal body weight.
2. Clients maintain fluid and electrolyte balance within normal limits.
3. No complications result from therapies designed to assist clients to return to within 10% of ideal body weight.

In the health care and home care settings, some clients with physiological conditions that cause more severe cases of malnutrition require total parenteral nutrition (TPN) to meet fluid, electrolyte, and nutritional needs. TPN is a nutritionally adequate hypertonic solution consisting of glucose, amino acids, lipids, minerals, and vitamins given through an indwelling peripheral or central intravenous catheter. Clients most at risk for requiring TPN are those suffering from severe trauma, febrile states, cancer, or severe malnutrition. The nursing care plan for clients receiving TPN is based on one or more of the following additional goals:

1. Clients maintain a positive nitrogen balance when illness prevents them from absorbing sufficient amounts of nutrients.
2. The delivery of essential nutrients for wound healing and restoration of body tissues is increased.
3. Clients with severe physiological conditions affecting nutritional status receive nutrients.
4. The clients' gastrointestinal tracts heal.

IMPLEMENTATION

Ill or debilitated clients usually have poor appetites despite the efforts of dietitians, nurses, families, friends, and other support people. Nurses can help by displaying interest in the client's intake, by understanding the influences that reduce appetite, and by a willingness to do everything possible to improve intake.

One of the most disruptive influences on intake is diagnostic testing. Some blood and radiographic studies require the client to fast. Therefore the client's breakfast is usually withheld until the client returns from the test or the testing is completed. Although microwave ovens make it possible for the client to have a hot meal after the test, clients may be too fatigued to eat properly.

Stress is another influence on client intake. Clients who are worried about their families, finances, employment, or their illness itself are unable to eat or to eat enough to compensate for the effect of stress on their metabolism.

Medications also affect the client's intake and, in some cases, the utilization of nutrients. Medications can affect the client's sensations of taste or smell, and as a result, food is not as appetizing. Second, medications can cause nausea or vomiting. The client is anorexic because of the nausea or the nutrients are vomited before the client has properly digested them. Also, medications such as insulin and thyroid hormones can affect the client's metabolism.

Nurses are able to design implementation measures around three general areas to promote their clients' nutrition. These areas include measures to stimulate the client's appetite, enteral nutritional therapies, and parenteral nutritional therapies.

STIMULATING APPETITE

A nurse can help to stimulate the client's appetite through environmental adaptations, consultation with a diet therapist, special diets and food preferences, and client and family counseling.

ENVIRONMENT. Nurses are responsible for providing an environment conducive to eating. The client's room should be free of reminders of treatments completed or yet to come. The environment should be free of odors. Mouth care should be provided when necessary to remove any unpleasant tastes. The client needs to be positioned comfortably, so the meal can be more enjoyable. If the client has visitors or needs any hygiene requirements before eating, sufficient time is given to permit anticipation and preparation for the meal.

In addition, when a client refuses a portion of the meal, every effort should be made to replace it with a suitable alternative.

DIET THERAPIST. After a meal the client's intake is evaluated and charted; nurses should recognize that they share responsibility with the dietitian for food intake and should work cooperatively with the diet therapist. Sharing information about a client's concerns and response to diet therapy will benefit the nurse, the diet therapist, and the client. The client's education about the therapeutic diet should be a shared responsibility. The dietitian is the expert in diet therapy, but the nurse can relate the dietary modification to the client's condition and explain how the diet contributes to the overall plan of care.

SPECIAL DIETS. Nurses should be familiar with the special diets used in client care, so they can select appropriate between-meal liquids and snacks, monitor food brought in by visitors, and offer acceptable food supplements (Fig. 33-8).

A regular hospital diet contains approximately 2500 kcal and consists of appropriate servings from a variety of food groups. In some hospitals the regular diet has been changed to reflect the dietary guidelines by de-

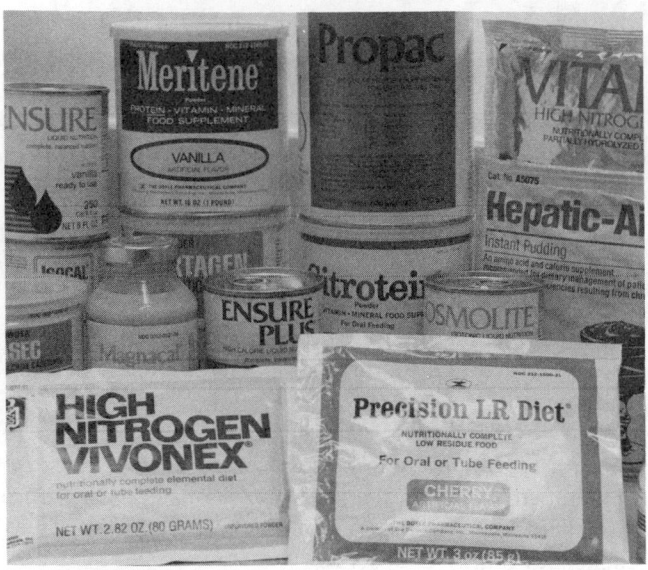

Fig. 33-8   Various diet supplements.

creasing lipids and increasing complex carbohydrates. No particular food restrictions are in the regular diet, but foods that are difficult to digest and fried foods are usually kept to a minimum.

A *light diet* is composed of foods that are easily digested and quickly emptied from the stomach. Rich, heavy foods such as fatty foods, pastries, concentrated sweets, and fibrous fruits and vegetables are eliminated from the light diet. Foods are usually prepared simply.

The major modification in the *soft diet* is texture. The soft diet usually contains sufficient calories in the same percentages of protein, carbohydrate, and lipid as in the regular diet. The soft diet is designed to include foods that are easily chewed and digested. Harsh, fibrous foods, rich foods, and strongly flavored foods are omitted.

DIET THERAPY IN DISEASE MANAGEMENT

Good nutrition is important in both health and illness, but the specific dietary intake pattern that results in good nutrition must often be modified for clients with particular diseases. Diet modifications are necessary to correspond with the body's ability to metabolize certain nutrients, to correct nutritional deficiencies related to the disease, and to eliminate certain foods from the diet that may be harmful to persons with the disease.

GASTROINTESTINAL DISEASES. The treatment of *ulcerative colitis* may include a liquid diet in the acute stage, a low-residue diet during recovery, and thereafter a bland diet high in protein, calories, vitamins, and minerals and low in fat. Vitamins and iron supplements are generally required because absorption is decreased.

The treatment of *diarrhea* may include a diet high in vitamins to counteract decreased absorption, low in residue, and high in calories if the client is emaciated.

The treatment of *malabsorption syndrome,* including sprue and celiac disease, includes a gluten-free diet. Gluten is present in wheat, rye, and oats.

The treatment of *acute enteritis* generally involves fasting initially, followed by a liquid diet, and thereafter a bland diet.

Acute gastritis is generally treated by a liquid diet initially, with a gradual transition to a low-residue diet and thereafter a bland diet. The treatment for *chronic gastritis* involves eliminating from the diet the foods or liquids that cause inflammation and thereafter permitting only easily digested foods.

The treatment of *diverticulitis* in which perforation has not occurred includes a liquid diet or low-residue diet until the infection subsides, after which a high-fiber diet is generally prescribed.

Peptic ulcers are better controlled with medications such as cimetidine. This classification of drugs is antihistamine—H_2 receptor and blocks secretion of hydrochloric acid (HCl) Clients are also encouraged to avoid foods that increase stomach acidity.

CARDIOVASCULAR DISEASES. The general goals of dietary treatment of cardiovascular diseases include preventing stomach distention to avoid pressure against the heart, reducing the client's weight if needed, and lowering blood lipids to lessen the risk of atherosclerosis.

The treatment of *myocardial infarction* includes a liquid diet for several days, progressing to a low-fat, low-sodium, high-carbohydrate soft diet during recovery, followed by a diet moderately low in fat and protein and high in carbohydrates.

The exact role of cholesterol and saturated fat intake in *atherosclerosis* remains debatable, but dietary therapy for treatment and prevention generally includes maintaining a recommended weight and a diet low in saturated fats and cholesterol.

The treatment of *hypertension* includes weight reduction to normal if the client is overweight and a diet low in sodium and moderately low in fats.

DIABETES. Adult-onset diabetes (non-insulin-dependent diabetes mellitus [NIDDM]) can usually be controlled by diet therapy alone. Juvenile-onset diabetes (insulin-dependent diabetes mellitus [IDDM]) requires both insulin and dietary restrictions. In both cases the diet is individualized according to the client's age, build, weight, and activity level. Fats are moderately controlled, and complex carbohydrates make up a higher percentage of the diet than simple carbohydrates. Foods for dietary planning are classified in six exchange groups, in which each item has about the same value as other foods in the same group. Meals are planned around balanced numbers of food exchanges.

RENAL DISEASES. The dietary treatment of *acute glomerulonephritis* depends on individual tolerances but may begin with a limited liquid diet for a few days, gradually returning to a normal diet limited in protein. The diet for *chronic glomerulonephritis* is generally high in carbohydrates and fat, with protein amounts equal to normal plus the amount lost in urine.

The treatment of renal failure may begin with a diet of selected fruit juices only or beverages containing carbohydrates and fats. A diet of essential carbohydrates and amino acid protein, but one that is also low in whole protein foodstuffs, follows.

Dietary treatment for *renal stones* depends on the type of stones. For calcium phosphate stones the diet is low in calcium and high in acid ash. For uric acid stones the diet is low in purines. For calcium oxalate stones the diet avoids all foods high in calcium and oxalates.

PSYCHOSOCIAL EFFECTS OF SPECIAL DIETS. Because foods have symbolic meanings for clients and are closely related to life-style, habits, cultural background, and other aspects of the individual, many clients have difficulty adjusting to special diets. Many clients had previously considered mealtime something to look forward to, a pleasurable period distinct from routines or an interlude from work activities. The special diet, especially a bland diet, makes eating a dull affair. In addition, eating with others may have been a primary form of social interaction for the client, but now the client eats alone in a hospital room or at home and cannot eat the same foods as other family members. In such situations the nurse and other health care professionals should recognize the actual or potential psychosocial factors and make plans to counteract negative effects. For example, the nurse can find substitutes for dietary foods to match the client's preference or can make meals more appealing with spices or condiments. Family members or others can also be involved, both to maintain the social value of mealtimes and to provide support when practical by joining in the client's diet. Counseling techniques may be employed to help family members support the client through conversation and other means. A little imagination can go a long way to make a restricted diet more satisfactory.

HANDICAPPED CLIENTS. Clients with disabilities that interfere with independent food intake should be allowed to do as much as possible for themselves. The nurse should prepare the tray, cutting food into bite-sized pieces, buttering bread, and pouring liquids. Special eating utensils should be used if they will contribute to the client's independence. Some disabled clients may become tired from their efforts to feed themselves. The nurse should determine if the client who stops eating is still hungry and needs assistance to finish the meal. The results of self-feeding should be evaluated on the basis of food intake and not neatness. The client's success should be recognized and commended. The nurse who finds a way to aid the disabled client to eat more independently should share this information by incorporating it in the care plan.

CLIENT AND FAMILY COUNSELING

Clients discharged from a hospital with a diet prescription often need dietary counseling to plan meals that meet specific diet requirements or general nutrition needs. Similarly, in other health care settings, clients with nutrition deficits or specific problems such as overweight may require assistance in menu planning and compliance with recommended diet therapies. The nurse's counseling role often includes the family and community resources as well.

Meal planning must take into account the family's budget and differences in the preferences of family members. Specific foods are chosen on the basis of the dietary prescriptions or standard dietary guidelines such as the basic four food groups. But meals should also provide a variety of foods and contrasting colors and consistencies. For families on limited budgets, substitutes can be used. For example, beans or cheese dishes can often replace meat in a meal, and evaporated or dry skim milk can be used for many cooking purposes. The method of preparation may also be modified when it is necessary to minimize certain substances; for example, baking rather than frying reduces fat intake, and lemon juice or spices can be used to replace salt in a low-sodium diet.

Planning menus a week in advance has several benefits. In addition to helping ensure good nutrition or compliance with a specific diet, such planning based on three balanced meals a day helps family members avoid impulse eating of less nutritional foods. Fruit and other nutritional items can be included in the plan for between-meal snacks. Careful advance planning can also help the family stay within the allotted budget because planned food buying is generally more economical than last-minute shopping, which may include more expensive processed and packaged foods. Often a simple tip can be of value in meal planning, such as advice to avoid grocery shopping when hungry, which can lead to spontaneous purchases of more expensive or less nutritional foods not included in meal plans.

Finally, the nurse can assist the client with referral to community resources for assistance with dietary problems. Assistance in obtaining food is provided by several government programs such as food commodities, food stamps, and school lunch programs. Private organizations such as Meals on Wheels programs also provide assistance. Volunteer health agencies, such as the American Heart Association and the American Diabetes Association, provide nutrition consultation, diet counseling, and educational materials. Other community groups also offer planned menus and other nutritional guidelines.

ENTERAL FEEDINGS

Enteral feedings are the ingestion or the instillation of nutrients by way of the gastrointestinal tract. The ingestion of whole food, semisolid food, or liquids by the enteral route is preferable because these feedings offer a safe, selective, economical alternative to parenteral nutrition (Grant and Kennedy-Caldwell, 1988). Enteral feedings can be approached in two ways, oral and tube feedings. Tube feedings also offer a variety of approaches and are detailed in the tube-feeding section of this chapter.

ORAL FEEDINGS

Assisting Clients with Feeding. Being fed deprives clients of the independence they gained over their food intake as toddlers. At best, being fed is an unpleasant experience. Nurses can improve client feeding by carefully protecting clients' dignity and actively involving them in the process. Any material used to protect a client's clothing should be referred to as a napkin, not a bib. The nurse should allow the client time to empty the mouth after every spoonful, attempting to match the speed of feeding to the client's readiness and asking frequently if it is too fast or slow. The nurse should also allow clients to direct the order in which they wish to eat food items, and conversation about topics other than food should be an integral part of the process. The nurse who has several clients to feed should use ingenuity to prevent an assembly line approach that is devastating to the client's self-esteem.

TUBE FEEDINGS.
When the client is unable to ingest, chew, or swallow food but is still able to digest and absorb nutrients, a feeding tube is ordered. Feeding tubes can be inserted nasally into either the stomach or small intestine or surgically into the stomach (gastrostomy). A newer method involves the percutaneous gastrostomy (PEG) tube placement.

Nursing research has investigated the problems associated with feeding tube placement, type of feeding instilled, rate of feeding, and the complications associated with the tube feeding itself. Chapter 11 offers a brief synopsis of these problems as they are reported in nursing research literature.

Liquid diets may be clear liquid (transparent fluids) or include full liquids (foods that are liquid at room or body temperature). A clear liquid diet does not provide sufficient calories and usually is given for only 1 to 2 days. Clear liquids, which do not provide lipid, contain only about 480 kcal of carbohydrate and 40 kcal of protein. Caloric and protein intake can be increased by the inclusion of egg white and gelatin to clear liquid diets. Although full liquid diets provide adequate calories, they usually are low in iron and lack fiber.

A *bland diet* is designed to eliminate any food that is chemically, mechanically, or thermally irritating. Stimulating liquids and spicy foods are eliminated, and foods are served warm or cool rather than hot or cold.

A *low-residue diet* is designed to reduce the contents of the intestinal tract. This diet limits fiber and other foods that leave a high level of residue in the intestines. Milk and milk products leave a high intestinal residue and are limited to 8 ounces a day in a low-residue diet. Clear fluids, meats, fats, and eggs are permitted. Cheese, fried foods, and highly seasoned foods are avoided. Only refined cereals and white bread are permitted, and all vegetables except peeled white potatoes are excluded. Although fruits are not permitted, fruit juices are allowed. A low-residue diet usually provides insufficient calcium, iron, and vitamins. It is not designed to be used for more than 3 or 4 days.

Until recently, large-bore rubber or plastic feeding tubes were used for nasogastric tube feedings. However the problems associated with these tubes—local irritation, pharyngitis, otitis, sinusitis, and esophageal sphincter incompetence—led to the development of the more pliable and flexible small-bore feeding tubes (Fig. 33-9) (Metheny, Spies, and Eisenberg, 1988). For the adult,

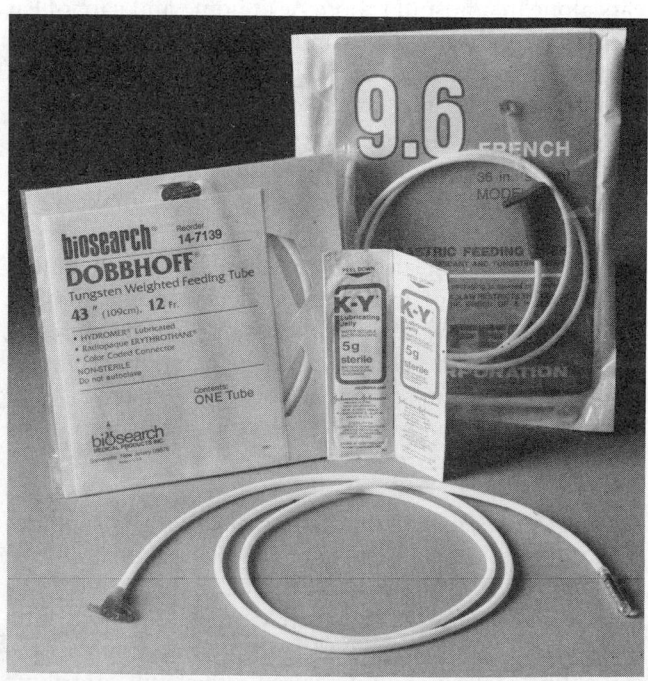

Fig. 33-9 Small-bore feeding tubes.

PROCEDURE 33-1

Initiating Enteral Tube Feedings

STEPS	RATIONALE
1. Assess client for enteral tube feedings: impaired swallowing, head or neck surgery, decreased level of consciousness.	Identify clients who need tube feedings before they become nutritionally depleted.
2. Verify physician's order.	Tube feedings must be ordered by a physician. Order should include formula, route, amount, and frequency.
3. Place client in a high-Fowler's position.	Reduces the risk of pulmonary aspiration in the event the client should vomit or regurgitate the feeding.
4. Assemble the following equipment:	Ensures prompt, efficient completion of the feeding.
a. Disposable gavage bag and tubing	Provides container for feeding.
b. Asepto syringe (60 ml size)	Formula can be administered via syringe for bolus feedings. Syringe can also be used to verify placement of large-bore feeding tubes.
c. Prescribed formula and amount	
d. Infusion pump designed for feeding tubes	Pump is necessary to regulate continuous tube feedings.
e. Disposable gloves	Prevents transmission of microorganisms.
5. Wash hands. Apply gloves.	Protects nurse from transmission of blood-borne infection from gastric contents.
6. Determine placement of gastric tube.	Measures verify placement of tube in the client's stomach. These measures have proven effective and safe for large-bore feeding tubes. Review section on tube feedings and Chapter 46.
a. Aspirate gastric secretions and check gastric residual.	Presence of gastric secretions indicates that the distal end of the tube is in the stomach. Residual volume indicates if gastric emptying is delayed. Delayed gastric emptying means that 150 ml or more remains in the stomach.
b. Inject 20-30 ml of air into the end of the tube. Auscultate over the epigastrum for a gurgling bubbling sound.	Documents the presence of air entering the client's stomach. Auscultation of air is not a reliable indicator to verify placement of small-bore feeding tubes.
7. Auscultate for bowel sounds.	Indicates presence of peristalsis and ability of gastrointestinal tract to digest nutrients.
8. Administer tube feeding.	
a. BOLUS OR INTERMITTENT FEEDING	
(1) Pinch proximal end of the feeding tube.	Prevents air from entering the client's stomach.
(2) Attach syringe to end of tube and elevate 18 inches above the client's head.	
(3) Fill syringe with formula. Allow syringe to empty gradually, refilling until prescribed amount has been delivered to the client.	
(4) If gavage bag is used, attach bag to the end of the feeding tube and raise bag 18 inches above client's head. Fill bag with prescribed amount of formula, allow bag to empty gradually.	Gradual emptying of tube feeding by gravity from a syringe or gavage bag reduces the risk of diarrhea induced by bolus tube feedings.
b. CONTINUOUS DRIP METHOD	
(1) Hang gavage bag to IV pole.	Method is designed to deliver a prescribed hourly rate of feeding that reduces the risk of diarrhea. Clients who receive these feedings should have their gastric residuals checked every 6-8 hours.
(2) Connect end of bag to the proximal end of the feeding tube.	
(3) Connect infusion pump and set rate.	
9. Remove and dispose of gloves in the proper receptacle. Wash hands.	Prevents transmission of microorganisms.
10. When tube feedings are not being administered, clamp the proximal end of the feeding tube.	Prevents air from entering the stomach between feedings.
11. Administer water via feeding tube as ordered with or between feedings.	Provides client with source of water to help maintain fluid and electrolyte balance.
12. Record amount and type of feeding in nurses' notes.	Documents the administration of feeding.

most of these tubes are 8 to 12 Fr tubes and 36 to 43 inches in length and are manufactured with attached weights to assist both introducing the catheter into the gastrointestinal tract and maintaining the desired location (Grant and Kennedy-Caldwell, 1988).

Chapter 46 discusses the placement of the large-bore nasogastric tube, which is frequently placed during abdominal surgery for the purposes of gastric decompression and irrigation. This section and the procedures described focus solely on the small-bore feeding tube and gastrostomy tube feedings. Procedure 33-1 details the complete procedure for administering a tube feeding and the feeding process itself. Before actual placement of the tube, the nurse must determine the appropriate tube length by measuring the total distance from the client's nose to ear to xiphoid (Fig. 33-10). This length provides the distance from the nose to the stomach in 98% of clients. For tubes that are placed into the duodenum or jejunum, add an additional 20 to 30 cm (Grant and Kennedy-Caldwell, 1988).

The alert client should be in a high-Fowler's position. The comatose client should be placed in a semi-Fowler's position. The tip of the nares is lubricated with a water-soluble lubricant. The tube is gently inserted along the floor of the nostril. The tube should not be forced, since this can cause kinking and discomfort (Grant and Kennedy-Caldwell, 1988). Small sips of water can help the client swallow the tube when its tip reaches the back of the client's throat. Continue instructing client to swallow until the desired length of the tubing is swallowed. If the client is unable to assist, pass the tube along the floor of the nostril. Check the back of the client's throat to

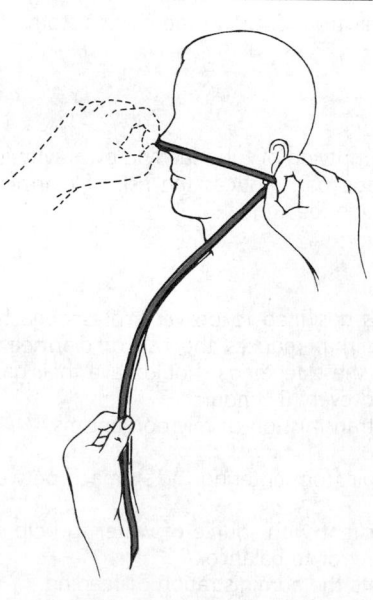

Fig. 33-10 Measurement for length of a feeding tube.

determine that the tube has not coiled in the posterior pharynx. Flex the client's head toward the chest, closing off the glottis so that the risk of the tube entering the trachea is reduced (Grant and Kennedy-Caldwell, 1988). Continue advancing the tube until the desired length has been passed.

Verification of the placement of these small-bore feeding tubes is difficult and different from the large-bore tubes. Historically, large-bore feedings tube placement has been verified by withdrawing gastric contents from the tube, injecting air through the nasogastric tube while auscultating the stomach for a gurgling or bubbling sound, or asking the client to speak (Perry and Potter, 1986; Metheny and Snively, 1983; Metheny, Spies, and Eisenberg, al., 1988). Unfortunately, these methods do not apply as readily to small-bore nasogastric tubes. A clinical study reported that over 50% of the attempts to aspirate even small volumes of fluid through small-bore feeding tubes were unsuccessful (Metheny, Spies, and Eisenberg, 1988). Fortunately, it is easier to aspirate fluid from some types of small-bore tubes. A laboratory study examining various small-bore feeding tube properties (for example, material and tube diameter) found that the polyurethane tubes were better than those made of silicone and that 10 and 12 Fr tubes were superior to 8 Fr tubes in terms of volume of fluid aspirated (Metheny, Eisenberg, and McSweeney, 1988). However, physical properties of feeding tubes also need to be studied in a clinical setting because a number of variables were not addressed in this study.

Inability to satisfactorily measure gastric contents by gastric aspiration into a syringe interferes with the nurse's ability to measure gastric retention of tube feeding solution. Thus, it becomes even more important to assess the client for abdominal distention, nausea, and vomiting. Failure to note a markedly distended abdomen predisposes the client to regurgitation and possible aspiration of gastric contents. The need to keep the head of the bed elevated is essential to prevent pulmonary aspiration.

Because of the difficulty in withdrawing fluid from small-bore feeding tubes, nurses frequently rely on the auscultatory method to confirm nasogastric feeding tube placement. This method consists of insufflating 10 to 30 ml of air through the tube while auscultating the epigastrum or left upper quadrant for a gurgling or bubbling sound. Yet, many sources in the literature report that "pseudoconfirmatory gurgling" can occur when the tube is elsewhere such as in the esophagus or lung (Miller, Tomlinson, and Sahn, 1985; Muthuswamy et al., 1982). Metheny, Spies, and Eisenberg (1988) reported that nurses were unable to discern gastric tube location by the auscultatory method. For example, nurses reported hearing air when the tube was in the esophagus, duodenum, jejunum, and stomach.

It is generally accepted that the ability to speak is hindered by the inadvertent respiratory placement of a firm, large-bore feeding tube. However, a number of clients reported being able to speak when small-bore tubes accidentally entered the respiratory tract (Rombeau and Barot, 1981; McDanal, Wheeler, and Ebert, 1983). Thus, this method is not a reliable means to test for inadvertent respiratory placement of small-bore pliable tubes.

Little has been written on how the nurse should check for placement of small-bore nasointestinal feeding tubes. Nurses in practice frequently report using the auscultatory method, even though its reliability is in serious question.

Another study by Metheny, Spies, and Eisenberg (1986) examines nasoenteral feeding-tube displacement. In this study, 92% of the subjects were fed with the small-bore feeding tubes, and a sizable number of these tubes were found by radiological examination to be spontaneously displaced. That is, the distal tips of the tubes dislocated upwardly in the gastrointestinal tract while the proximal external portion of the feeding tube remained taped in place. Displacement was associated with risk factors such as coughing, vomiting, suctioning, and decreased level of consciousness.

Currently used bedside methods to test placement of small-bore feeding tubes are frequently ineffective. At present, the most reliable method is radiographic verification. This method is costly and not without risk. Therfore, new methods to test placement need to be explored. In the meantime, the nurse must have a high index of suspicion for tube displacement in clients at risk and employ meticulous assessment skills.

The solutions used for tube feedings must be nutritionally adequate, tolerated by the client, and appropriate to the area of the gastrointestinal tract to which they are delivered. The wide variety of commercial products available have become popular for tube feedings. They are easy to prepare and offer standard nutritional content. The commercial preparations differ in osmolarity, digestibility, caloric density, lactose content, viscosity, and lipid content. Ensure is an example of a commercial food for clients who can digest protein and fat. Like similar products from other manufacturers, it provides 1 kcal/ml. Flexical is an example of a food for tube feeding that is ready to be absorbed. It (and similar products) provides 1 kcal/ml. A high-density product for tube feeding is available for clients with fluid restrictions. It is concentrated and provides 2 kcal/ml.

Clients may be maintained indefinitely on tube feedings, which can provide all the essential nutrients except fiber. Although cramping and diarrhea are commonly associated with tube feedings, these symptoms usually subside when the flow rate or the concentration of the solution is reduced.

TOTAL PARENTERAL NUTRITION

Parenteral nutrition is a complex form of therapy designed to provide daily nutritional requirements by the intravenous route. The success of this form of nutrition depends on the dietary prescription, management of the intravenous catheter, dressing care, and complications resulting from the therapy itself (Grant and Kennedy-Caldwell, 1988).

Clients who are unable to ingest or digest enteral nutrition are candidates for TPN. TPN is contraindicated in clients whose gastrointestinal tract is functional within 7 to 10 days, when the client is well nourished and when minimal stress and trauma are present. It is also of limited value for the client in an untreatable disease state such as widely advanced metastatic malignancy. Last, it should not be used when the risks outweigh the benefits (Grant and Kennedy-Caldwell, 1988).

TPN solutions are hyperosmolar, that is, highly concentrated, and as a result are infused through central lines. The solution itself is tailored to the client's specific nutritional needs, with some common elements for all clients (see box). A typical solution consists of approximately 25% dextrose and 3% to 4% protein, supplying close to 1000 calories per liter (Grant and Kennedy-Caldwell, 1988). Electrolyte needs vary with the client's general status.

FAT EMULSIONS. Clients may also require nutritional supplements through fat emulsions. Fat emulsions provide supplemental calories to prevent essential fatty acid deficiencies (Atkins and Oakley, 1986). These nutrients can be administered through a separate peripheral line, through the central line by Y connector tubing (see Chapter 37), or as an additive to the TPN solution. The last option is based on research findings that fats (also called lipids) can be added to TPN solutions without causing incompatibility problems or compromising the solution's stability (Atkins and Oakley, 1986). Fat emulsions should be administered sterilely into a patent intravenous line. The emulsion should not be used if it appears oily or appears to have separated.

The recommended initial infusion rate for fat emulsions is 1 ml per minute. Reactions to this emulsion can include dyspnea, cyanosis, allergy, nausea, vomiting, headache, chest pain, back pain, pressure over the eyes, or dizziness. The appearance of any of these symptoms warrants stopping the infusion and immediately notifying the physician. If the client tolerates the fat emulsion, the rate can gradually be increased as ordered by the physician.

INITIATING TPN. TPN requires a large-gauge intracatheter threaded into a central vein such as the jugular or subclavian or large peripheral vein. Nurses do not insert central catheters but assist in the procedure.

The procedure is sterile and requires the following equipment:

1. Sterile drapes
2. Sterile gloves
3. Sterile Betadine swabs
4. Alcohol
5. Topical anesthetic (lidocaine)
6. Betadine ointment
7. Sterile 4 × 4 and 2 × 2 gauze pads, or transparent dressing
8. Tape
9. Parenteral solution
10. Parenteral infusion tubing
11. Intracatheter needle
12. Sutures
13. In-line filter
14. Infusion pump

The nurse explains the procedure to the client and witnesses informed consent. The client is taught to perform the Valsalva maneuver, bearing down with mouth closed and holding a breath. This increases venous filling of the vein and reduces the risk of an air embolism during needle insertion. Once the client has learned the technique satisfactorily, the catheter can be inserted.

The client is placed in the Trendelenburg position to dilate the central veins in the neck and shoulder. The physician drapes the venipuncture site with sterile barriers and cleanses the site with Betadine swabs followed by alcohol wipes. Lidocaine is injected for local anesthesia. The physician punctures the vein and looks for a nonpulsatile blood return. A pulsating blood return indicates that an artery, not the vein, was punctured. When the physician begins to thread the intracatheter through the needle, the nurse instructs the client to do the Valsalva maneuver.

After placement of the catheter the needle is removed and an intravenous infusion is connected to the hub of the catheter. The physician sutures the catheter in place and covers the site with a sterile dressing. A chest x-ray film is used to identify any complications such as accidental puncture of the lung or the parietal pleura.

Clients receiving TPN should have their vital signs measured and their blood glucose monitored every 4 hours or as ordered by the physician. The nurse should be alert for changes and report any to the physician.

Medications or blood should not be given through the TPN line because this increases the risk of bacterial contamination. In a life-or-death situation the TPN line may be the only intravenous line available and will need to be used for emergency treatment.

Beginning an Infusion. Before beginning an infusion the nurse compares the physician's order with the solution prepared by the pharmacy. The nurse connects the TPN infusion tubing to a filter and places the inser-

tion spike in the solution. The tubing is filled with the solution and hung at the bedside. The nurse attaches the tubing to the infusion pump.

Infusion Flow Rate. Clients initially receive low doses of TPN solution, such as 1 liter per 24 hours, typically gradually increasing to 3 liters per 24 hours. The solution should be delivered over a 24-hour period; the rate is included in the physician's orders.

Too rapid administration of this hypertonic infusion can result in osmotic diuresis, dehydration, and death (see Chapter 37). Infusion pumps help to regulate the flow. If an infusion falls behind schedule, the nurse should not attempt to catch up because a hyperosmotic reaction could result (Metheny and Snively, 1983).

MAINTAINING THE TPN SYSTEM. The infusion flow should be assessed every hour. All clients receiving TPN should be connected to an infusion pump. The nurse should also evaluate the catheter and infusion line for patency.

Preventing Complications. After the catheter is inserted, a chest x-ray film is used to document correct placement of the catheter in the superior vena cava, proximal to the right atrium (Munro-Black, 1984). The film can also show a pneumothorax, which may occur if the needle punctures the pleura during insertion. Pneumothorax assessment findings include chest pain, dyspnea, and coughing; the rapidity of onset and the degree of symptoms depend on the severity of the pneumothorax.

A second complication is the development of an air embolus during insertion of the catheter or changing of the tubing. This can be prevented by having the client do the Valsalva maneuver and placing the client in the Trendelenburg position.

Hyperglycemia is caused by a high concentration of dextrose in the TPN solution. Risk factors for hyperglycemia include increased secretion of adrenal hormones, increased age, and renal disease (Metheny and Snively, 1983). Hyperglycemia, which can cause dehydration, nausea, headache, and weakness, can also occur when the rate of infusion is too rapid. The risk of hyperglycemia can be reduced by giving the solution at the prescribed rate. If the solution falls behind schedule, the nurse should not increase the rate of flow unless ordered by the physician. Checking the urine for glucose and acetone every 4 to 6 hours can identify signs of glucose intolerance. Clients receiving TPN may be given insulin injections to increase the body's ability to metabolize the increased glucose. Once the TPN has been discontinued, the insulin injections are discontinued.

Hypoglycemia can occur if TPN is abruptly discontinued. The high glucose concentration of the TPN so-

TABLE 33-12 Interventions for Preventing Metabolic Complications of TPN

Intervention	Rationale
Weigh client daily.	Documents that the client is maintaining or gaining weight and has a proper fluid balance
Record intake and output.	Provides data base for ongoing fluid-balance assessment
If client is allowed oral intake, maintain calorie count of foods eaten.	Provides data needed to calculate TPN caloric requirement
Obtain urine to measure glucose and acetone every 4 to 6 hours.	Determines if client is excreting glucose in the urine and if an insulin supplement is needed
Obtain blood samples for measurement of iron, transferrin, and white blood cells.	Evaluates cellular nutritional status
Continually assess the client's fluid and electrolyte status.	Prevents circulatory overload, dehydration, and electrolyte imbalances
Maintain infusion rate as ordered. Do not speed up or slow down infusion unless instructed by the physician or a severe complication occurs.	Prevents hyperglycemia, osmotic diuresis, hypoglycemia, and fluid overload

lution has stimulated the client's pancreas to secrete more insulin. The client may also be receiving supplemental insulin injections. If the TPN infusion is too slow or abruptly discontinued, there is too little blood glucose and too much insulin, and hypoglycemia occurs. Symptoms of hypoglycemia include occipital headaches, cold clammy skin, dizziness, tachycardia, and tingling of the extremities and circumoral regions (Metheny, 1987). Hypoglycemia can be prevented by maintaining an accurate infusion rate and a gradual reduction of the TPN solution. The gradual reduction allows the pancreas time to adapt to the decreased glucose load. If the TPN solution must be discontinued abruptly, a 5% or 10% glucose in water solution usually provides enough glu-

Sample Evaluation of Interventions for Altered Nutritional Status

Goals	Evaluative Measures	Expected Outcomes
Client returns to within 10% of ideal body weight.	Weigh client.	Weight shows appropriate gain or loss.
	Observe client for signs of nutritional deficits.	Physical and laboratory indications of nutritional deficits are absent.
Client's fluid and electrolyte status remains within normal limits.	Observe client for signs of dehydration or overhydration.	Signs of dehydration or overhydration are absent.
	Palpate skin for loss of turgor.	Skin turgor remains normal.
	Palpate skin for signs of edema.	Edema is absent.
	Weigh client daily.	There is no excessive weight loss or gain.
	Monitor electrolyte levels.	Electrolyte levels remain within normal limits.
Complications are prevented.	Observe for electrolyte imbalance.	Electrolyte levels remain within normal limits.
	Observe for signs of infection.*	Erythema, pain, swelling are absent at venipuncture site.
	Obtain blood glucose levels.*	Blood glucose levels remain within normal range.

*Evaluative measures associated with total parenteral nutrition

cose to prevent rebound hypoglycemia until the client's pancreatic insulin rate decreases in about 12 to 24 hours (Grant, 1980; Grant and Kennedy-Caldwell, 1988).

Fluid overload causes an increase in extracellular fluid volume. If severe, fluid overload can result in pulmonary edema and congestive heart failure. Signs and symptoms include shortness of breath, tachycardia, weak pulse, hypertension or hypotension, confusion, decreased urine output, rales, or pitting edema. Fluid overload can be prevented by maintaining an accurate rate of infusion and monitoring the client's central venous pressure. If signs of fluid overload occur, the nurse *slows* the infusion rate, notifies the physician, and remains with the client continually assessing the client's status.

The major metabolic complications of TPN can be prevented by continually implementing seven nursing interventions (Table 33-12). These interventions are designed for early identification and treatment of these complications.

EVALUATION

The value of the nurse's activities in meeting the client's nutritional needs is unknown until they are evaluated. Nutritional assessment must be ongoing to evaluate the results of nursing interventions. Care plans must be constantly updated to avoid continuing ineffective actions and to strengthen support of effective interventions. Adequate time should be allowed to test a nursing approach to a problem. Behavior change in a client is as valid an indicator of success as weight gain or laboratory results.

Nurses should establish outcomes for nursing actions and be alert for signs that goals are being met (see evaluation box). Whenever possible the client should be an active participant in the planning and evaluation of care.

SUMMARY

Nurses must understand the functions of the basic nutrients and how they are metabolized to produce energy. An understanding of the guidelines for the selection of an adequate diet is essential so nurses can teach clients about diet and answer questions related to diet. Nurses should also be alert to current research findings and their impact on dietary recommendations. They should be familiar with alternative food patterns followed by some clients and have a knowledge of the influence of age on dietary needs.

Nurses must be able to assess the nutritional status of clients. They must also recognize that many divergent factors influence a client's food intake and that these factors must be considered in attempting to modify food intake.

Nurses must be able to identify clients at risk for nutritional problems and be aware of common nutritional conditions. They should be aware of the importance of their interaction with others in the area of food intake, be familiar with common hospital diets, and be able to assist clients at mealtime.

Finally, nurses must evaluate their activities in the area of nutritional support to revise those that prove ineffective and continue those that are effective.

KEY CONCEPTS

✓ The nutrients needed by the body to carry out vital functions are water, carbohydrates, proteins, lipids, vitamins, and minerals.

✓ Body weight is maintained when food intake equals energy output.

✓ Carbohydrates are anabolized into glycogen and adipose tissue or catabolized into energy.

✓ Proteins are anabolized into tissue, hormones, or enzymes or catabolized into energy.

✓ Lipids may be anabolized into adipose tissue or catabolized into energy.

✓ Proteins are essential for growth, maintenance, and repair.

✓ The essential amino acids and the essential fatty acids must be supplied by dietary intake because the body is unable to synthesize them from other ingested substances.

✓ Digestion is the mechanical and chemical process by which food is broken down into its simplest form for absorption. Digestion and absorption occur mainly in the small intestine.

✓ Recommended daily allowances (RDAs), another basis for diet selection, were formulated for population groups, not individuals.

✓ Guidelines for dietary change advocate reduced intake of fat, saturated fat, salt, refined sugar, and cholesterol and increased intake of complex carbohyrates and fiber.

✓ Age affects the requirements for essential nutrients. Periods of rapid growth increase the need for protein, vitamins, and minerals.

✓ Because improper nutrition can affect all body systems, nutritional assessment includes a review of the total physical assessment.

✓ Nurses can improve food intake of clients by thoughtful attention to the preparation of both client and environment before meals are served.

✓ Disabled clients should be supported in their efforts to eat as independently as possible.

✓ Proper feeding techniques can protect the dependent client from loss of dignity and self-esteem.

✓ Special hospital diets alter the composition, texture, digestibility, and residue of foods to suit client's particular needs.

✓ Tube feedings can be used for clients who are unable to ingest food but are able to digest and absorb foods.

✓ Total parenteral nutrition (TPN) supplies essential nutrients in appropriate amounts to support life through the introduction of a concentrated nutrient solution into a large central vein or the right atrium of the heart.

✓ Evaluation of the outcomes of nursing intervention in the area of nutritional support is essential to revise, update, or continue nursing activities.

REFERENCES

Atkins, JM, and Oakley, CW: A nurse's guide to TPN, RN 6:20, 1986.

Forlaw, B, and Grant, P: Introduction to nutritional and physical assessment of the adult patient for the nurse, Aspen, Colo., 1983, American Society for Parental and Enteral Nutrition (ASPEN).

Grant, J: Handbook of total parenteral nutrition, Philadelphia, 1980, W.B. Saunders Co.

Grant, JA, and Kennedy-Caldwell, C: Nutritional support in nursing, New York, 1988, Grune and Stratton.

Metheny, NM: Fluid and electrolyte balance, Nursing considerations, Philadelphia, 1987, J.B. Lippincott Co.

Metheny, NM, and Snively, WD, Jr.: Nurse's handbook of fluid balance, ed. 4, Philadelphia, 1983, J.B. Lippincott Co.

Munro-Black, J: The ABC's of total parenteral nutrition, Nurs 84 14:50, 1984.

Pennington, J: Considerations for a new food guide, J Nutr Educ 13:2, 1981.

Perry, AG, and Potter, PA: Clinical nursing skills and techniques, St. Louis, 1986, The C.V. Mosby Co.

Rohantra, G: Dietary recommendations: 1977-1985, Research Department Technical Bulletin 7(8), 1985.

Rombeau, J, and Barot, L: Enteral nutritional therapy, Surg Clin North Am 61:605, 1981.

Research Articles

McDanal, J, Wheeler, D, and Ebert, J: A complication of nasogastric intubation: pulmonary hemorrhage, Anesthesiology 59:356, 1983.

Metheny, NA, Eisenberg, P, and McSweeney, M: Effect of feeding tube properties and three irrigants on clogging rates, Nurs Res 37(1):165, 1988.

Metheny, NA, Spies, M, and Eisenberg, P: Frequency of nasoenteral tube displacement and associated risk factors, Res Nurs Health, 9(3):241, 1986.

Metheny, NA, Spies, M, and Eisenberg, P: Measures to test placement of nasoenteral feeding tubes, West J Nur Res, Aug. 1988.

Miller, K, Tomlinson, J, and Sahn, S: Pleuropulmonary compliations of enteral tube feeding, Chest 88:203, 1985.

Muthuswamy, P, Patel, K, and Rajendran, R: Isocal pneumonia with respiratory failure, Chest 81:390, 1982.

ADDITIONAL READINGS

Baker, DJ: 10 years of TPN at home, Am J Nurs 84:1248, 1984.

Birdsall, C: When is TPN safe? Am J Nurs 85:73, 1985.

Bodinski, L: A nurse's guide to diet therapy, New York, 1982, John Wiley & Sons, Inc.

Buergel, N: Monitoring nutritional status in the clinical setting, Nurs Clin North Am 14:2, 1979.

Bureau of Nutritional Sciences, Department of National Health and Welfare: Recommended nutrient intakes for Canadians, 1982, Ottawa, Canada, 1982, The Department of National Health and Welfare.

Butterworth, C: The skeleton in the hospital closet, Nutr Today 9:4, 1974.

Butterworth, C, and Blackburn, G: Hospital malnutrition and how to assess the nutritional status of the patient, Nurs Digest 4:6, 1976.

Caly, J: Assessing adults' nutrition, Am J Nurs 77:10, 1977.

Carr, P: When the patient needs TPN at home, RN 6:25, 1986.

Cerrato, P: Will IV feeding endanger your patient? RN 12:59, 1986.

Ciseaux, A: A view from the mirror, Am J Nurs 80:8, 1980.

Claggett M: Anorexia nervosa: a behavioral approach, Am J Nurs 80:8, 1980.

Committee on Dietary Allowances, Food and Nutrition Board, National Academy of Sciences—National Research Council: Estimated safe and adequte daily dietary intakes, Washington, D.C., 1980, The Academy.

Copeland, E, Van Elys, J, and Shils, M: Nutrition and cancer, 1978, American Cancer Society.

Department of Agriculture and Department of Health and Human Services: Nutrition and your health: dietary guidelines for Americans, Washington, D.C., 1980, U.S. Government Printing Office.

Dwyer, J: Vegetarianism, Contemp Nutr 4:6, 1979.

Goodhart, R, and Shils, M, editors: Modern nutrition in health and disease, ed. 6, Philadelphia, 1980, Lea & Febiger.

Greenburg, J: Why your hospitalized patient won't eat, Consultant 19:9, 1979

Howard, R, and Herbold, N: Nutrition in clinical care, ed. 2, New York, 1982, McGraw-Hill Book Co.

Hui, Y: Human nutrition and diet therapy, Belmont, Calif., 1983, Wadsworth Publishing Co.

Johnson, S: A safer gastrostomy for the high-risk patient, RN 3:29, 1986.

Keithley, J: Proper nutritional assessment can prevent hospital malnutrition, Nurs 79 9:2, 1979.

Lucas, A: Anorexia nervosa, Contemp Nutr 3:8, 1978.

Lucas, A: Bulimia and vomiting syndrome, Contemp Nutr 6:4, 1981.

Maxwell, M, and Klienan, C, editors: Clinical disorders of fluid and electrolyte metabolism, ed. 3, New York, 1980, McGraw-Hill Book Co.

McDaniel, J: Diet therapy in the nursing school curriculum, J Am Diet Assoc 70:3, 1977.

Mertz, W: Trace elements, Contemp Nutr 3:2, 1978.

Moore, MC: Do you still believe these myths about tube feeding? RN 5:51, 1987.

National Academy of Sciences: Recommended daily allowances, ed. 9, Washington, D.C., 1985, The Academy.

Pennington, J: J Nutr Educ 13:54, 1981.

Richardson, T: Anorexia nervosa: an overview, Am J Nurs 80:8, 1980.

Robinson, C, and Weigley, E: Basic nutrition and diet therapy, New York, 1984, Macmillan Publishing Co.

Rose, J: Nutritional problems in radiotherapy patients, Am J Nurs 78:6, 1978.

Rose, J, editor: Nutrition and killer diseases, Park Ridge, N.J., 1982, Noyes Publications.

Rudman, D, and Williams, P: Megavitamins: use and misuse, N Engl J Med 309:8, 1983.

Schaumburg, H, et al.: Sensory neuropathy from pyridoxine abuse: a new megavitamin syndrome, N Engl J Med 309:8, 1983.

Senate Select Committee on Human Needs: Dietary goals for the United States, Washington, D.C., 1977, US Government Printing Office.

Shapcott, D: Essential trace mineral deficiencies and cardiovascular disease. In Rose, J, editor: Nutrition and killer diseases, Park Ridge, N.J., 1982, Noyes Publications.

Suitor, C, and Crowley, M: Nutrition: principles and application in health promotion, ed. 2, Philadelphia, 1984, JB Lippincott Co.

Thiele, VF: Clinical nutrition, ed. 2, St. Louis, 1980, The C.V. Mosby Co.

Williams, SR: Nutritional guidance in prenatal care. In Worthington-Roberts, BS, Williams, SR, and Vermeersch, JA: Nutrition in pregnancy and lactation, ed. 4, St. Louis, 1989, The C.V. Mosby Co.

Williams, SR: Nutritional and diet therapy, ed. 6, St. Louis, 1989, The C.V. Mosby Co.

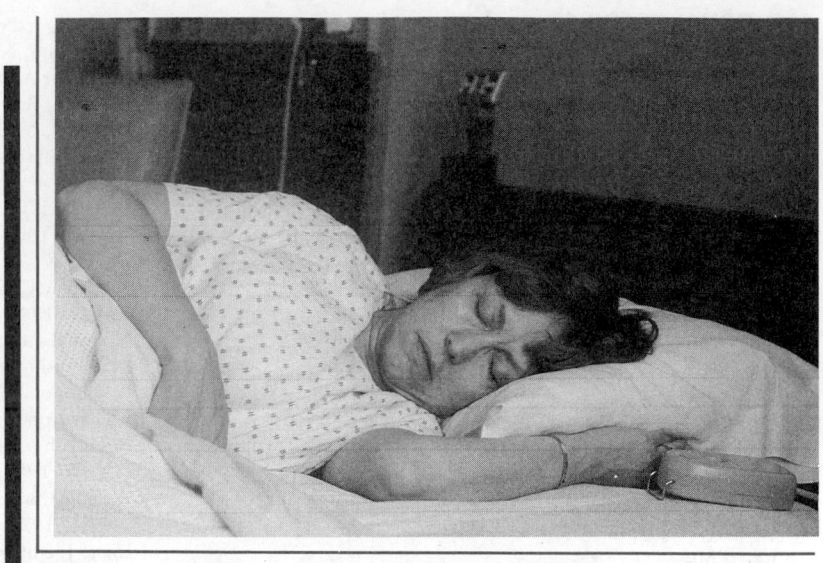

OBJECTIVES

Mastery of content in this chapter will enable the student to:

- Define the key terms listed.
- Describe the differences and similarities between rest and sleep.
- Explain the effect the 24-hour sleep-wake cycle has on biological function.
- Discuss mechanisms that regulate sleep.
- Describe the stages of a normal sleep cycle.
- Explain the functions of sleep.
- Compare and contrast the sleep requirements of different age groups.
- Identify factors that normally promote and disrupt sleep.
- Describe common sleep disorders.
- Conduct a sleep history for a client.
- Identify relevant nursing diagnoses related to sleep problems.
- Identify nursing interventions designed to promote a normal sleep cycle for an adult and child.
- Describe ways to evaluate sleep therapies.

KEY TERMS

Angina
Apnea
Biological Clock
BSR
Cataplexy
Central Sleep Apnea
Circadian Rhythm
Delusions
Enuresis
Fatigue
Hypnotic
Infradian Rhythm
Insomnia
Narcolepsy

Nocturia
Nocturnal Enuresis
NonREM or NREM Sleep
Obstructive Sleep Apnea
Paranoia
Polysomnogram
Reflux
REM Sleep
Reticular Activating System
Sedative
Sleep Deprivation
Somnolence
Tranquilizer
Ultradian Rhythm

Sleep

The need for sleep and rest is important in the quality of life for all persons. All individuals need and receive different amounts and qualities of sleep and rest. Physical and emotional health depend on the ability to fulfill these basic human needs.

Nurses work with clients who often have preexisting sleep disturbances, as well as clients who develop sleep problems as a result of illness or the effects of hospitalization. A sleep problem may cause a client to seek health care, or it may be a problem to which the client has adjusted. When a person becomes ill, rest and sleep are important for normal recovery. During illness, a client often requires more sleep and rest than normal. However, the nature of an illness may prevent the client from gaining adequate rest and sleep. The environment of a hospital or long-term care facility and the activities of health care personnel may also make it difficult for the client to sleep, as in the following hypothetical situation.

Carol, a 28-year-old woman, is hospitalized for acute inflammation of the gallbladder. Pain has caused additional symptoms of nausea and vomiting. She has two young children at home, and her husband is out of town on business. Carol is concerned that it will be difficult for her parents to watch the children. The nurses are ordered to monitor Carol's condition by checking vital signs every 4 hours. An intravenous (IV) line is inserted into Carol's left arm, adding to her discomfort. Her anxiety seems to grow as the pain worsens. Carol continually watches the slow drip of the IV. When she lies flat on her back, the pain increases, but this is her normal sleeping position. Despite having received an analgesic late the preceding evening, Carol reports in the morning that she was unable to sleep.

Nurses work with clients like Carol every day. To help a client gain needed rest and sleep, a nurse must understand the nature of sleep, the factors influencing it, and the client's sleep habits. Each client requires an individualized approach. The nurse's interventions can be effective for both short-term and long-term sleep disturbances.

COMPARING SLEEP AND REST

A person at rest feels mentally relaxed, free from worry, and physically calm. Rest does not imply inactivity, although we often think of it as settling down in a comfortable chair or lying in bed. A person at rest is free from physical or mental exertion. All persons have their own habits for obtaining rest and are usually able to adjust to new environments or conditions that affect the ability to rest. Rest may be gained from reading a book, practicing a relaxation exercise (see Chapter 35), or taking a long walk.

Nurses frequently care for clients on bedrest. This treatment confines clients to bed to reduce physical and psychological demands on the body. A person on bedrest is not necessarily rested. A client on bedrest still may have emotional worries that prevent complete relaxation. Depending on others for care may cause a client on bedrest to feel stressed.

Sleep is a state of rest that occurs for sustained periods. The reduced consciousness during sleep provides time for the repair and recovery of body systems for the next period of wakefulness. A sleeping person interacts less with the environment. Sleep restores a person's energy and feeling of well-being.

When persons enter a hospital or other health care facility, their rest and sleep habits can easily be changed by hospital routines. The extent of change depends on the physiological and psychological state of the client, as well as the environmental surroundings in which the client is placed. The nurse must always be aware of a client's need for rest. Inadequate rest causes fatigue, irritability, and the inability to make sound decisions, and to cope with stressors. The lack of rest for long periods of time can cause illness or worsening of existing illness. The nurse can help clients learn the importance of rest and ways to promote it.

Promoting Rest

Many factors determine a person's ability to gain adequate rest. In the home the nurse helps clients develop behaviors conducive to rest and relaxation. This may include control of factors in the environment or changing certain life-style habits. In a health care setting nurses

---

Conditions for Proper Rest

PHYSICAL COMFORT
- Eliminate sources of physical irritation.
- Control sources of pain
- Provide warmth
- Maintain hygiene
- Maintain proper anatomical alignment or positioning
- Remove environmental distractions

FREEDOM FROM WORRY
- Able to make own decisions
- Participate in personal health care
- Have knowledge needed to understand health problems and implications
- Practice restful activities regularly

SUFFICIENT SLEEP
- Obtain average hours of sleep needed to avoid fatigue
- Follow good sleep hygiene habits

---

must be able to promote rest in an environment that is often stressful. Loud or unfamiliar noises, irritating lighting, loss of privacy, frequency of therapeutic procedures, and a variety of health care personnel can all interfere with a client's rest. The box lists basic conditions needed to ensure proper rest.

PHYSIOLOGY OF SLEEP

Sleep is a set of complete physiological processes involving a sequence of states within the central nervous system (Hoch and Reynolds, 1986). Each sequence can be identified by specific behaviors and patterns of brain activity. Instruments such as the electroencephalogram (EEG), which measures electrical activity in the cerebral cortex, the electromyogram (EMG), which measures muscle tone, and the electrooculogram (EOG), which measures eye movements, provide information about the physiology of sleep.

Circadian Rhythms

Each person's life is a series of rhythms that influence and regulate physiological function and behavioral responses. The most familiar rhythm is the 24-hour, day-night cycle known as the diurnal or circadian rhythm (derived from Latin: *circa* means about and *dies* means day). Another rhythm is the woman's menstrual cycle, an infradian (longer than 24 hours) rhythm. The stage of sleep known as REM (rapid eye movement) is an ultradian (less than 24 hours) rhythm lasting from 10 to 60 minutes. Circadian rhythms influence the pattern of major biological functions. The fluctuation and predictability of body temperature, heart rate, blood pressure, hormone and electrolyte secretions, and sensory acuity depend on the 24-hour circadian cycle.

The 24-hour sleep-wake cycle continues to operate even when external factors that influence behavior such as clocks and social and work routines are removed. However, each person has an individualized free-running sleep-wake cycle. Some people are able to fall asleep at 8 PM, while others go to bed at midnight or early in the morning. People also tend to differ as to the time of day they function best. Horne and Ostberg (1976) described two groups of people, *morning* and *evening* types. The morning person prefers to go to bed early and get up early, performing best in the morning. The evening person prefers later nights and getting up later, functioning best in the evenings. In hospitals or extended care facilities all clients tend to be treated the same. Little attention is given to adapt care to an individual's preference for sleep. If a person's sleep-wake cycle is altered significantly, desynchronization occurs. This results in a poorer quality of sleep. Reversals in the sleep-wake cycle such as sleeping during the day instead of the night (or vice versa for people who work nights) can signal serious illness. Anxiety, restlessness, irritability, and an impairment in judgment are common symptoms of desynchronization.

The biological rhythm of sleep frequently becomes synchronized with other body functions. Changes in body temperature, for example, correlate with sleep patterns. Normally, body temperature peaks in the afternoon, decreases gradually, and then drops sharply after a person falls asleep (see Chapter 12). When a person's sleep-wake cycle becomes disrupted—for example, by rotating job shifts or frequent environmental disturbances—other physiological functions change as well. The integrity of a client's sleep-wake cycle can influence the client's overall state of health.

Sleep Regulation

The control and regulation of sleep is believed to depend on the interrelationship between two antagonistic cerebral mechanisms. Both intermittently activate and suppress the brain's higher centers to control sleep and wakefulness. One mechanism causes wakefulness, while the other causes sleep. The reticular activating system (RAS) is located in the upper brainstem region. It is believed to contain special cells that maintain a person's alertness and wakefulness. The RAS receives sensory input visually and in the form of auditory pain and tactile stimuli. Activity from the cerebral cortex (for example, emotions or thought processes) also stimulate the RAS. Recent studies reported by Canavan (1984) and Chuman

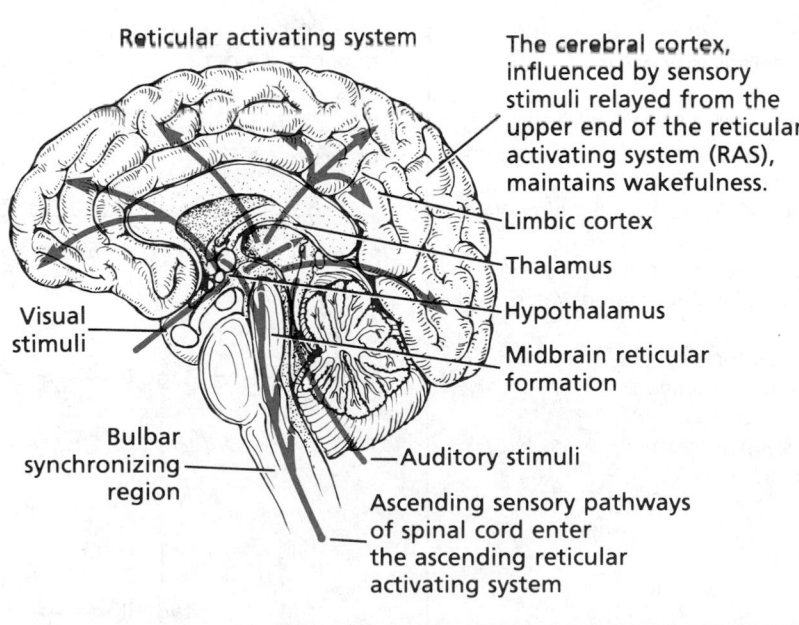

Fig. 34-1   RAS and BSR control sensory input, intermittently activating and suppressing the brain's higher centers to control sleep and wakefulness.

Stages of Sleep

STAGE 1: NONREM

- Lightest level of sleep
- Lasts a few minutes
- Decreased physiologic activity begins with gradual fall in vital signs and metabolism
- Person easily aroused by sensory stimuli such as noise
- If person awakes, feels as though daydreaming

STAGE 2: NONREM

- Period of sound sleep
- Relaxation progresses
- Arousal is still easy
- Lasts 10 to 20 minutes
- Body functions continue to slow

STAGE 3: NONREM

- Initial stages of deep sleep
- Sleeper is difficult to arouse and rarely moves
- Muscles completely relaxed
- Vital signs decline but remain regular
- Lasts 15 to 30 minutes

STAGE 4: NONREM

- Deepest stage of sleep
- Very difficult to arouse sleeper
- If sleep loss has occurred, sleeper will spend considerable portion of night in this stage
- Stage responsible for restoring and resting the body
- Vital signs significantly lower than during waking hours
- Lasts approximately 15 to 30 minutes
- Sleepwalking and enuresis may occur

REM SLEEP

- Stage of vivid, full-color dreaming (less vivid dreaming may occur in other stages)
- Usually begins every 50 to 90 minutes after sleep has begun
- Typified by autonomic response of rapidly moving eyes, fluctuating heart and respiratory rates, and blood pressure.
- Loss of skeletal muscle tone
- Responsible for mental restoration
- Sleeper most difficult to arouse
- Duration of REM sleep increases with each cycle and averages 20 minutes

(1983) suggest that wakefulness is the result of neurons releasing catecholamines like norephinephrine.

Sleep is believed to be produced by the release of serotonin from specialized cells in the raphe sleep system of the pons and medial forebrain area. This area of the brain has also been called the bulbar synchronizing region (BSR). Whether a person remains awake or falls asleep depends on a balance of impulses received from higher centers (for example, thoughts), peripheral sensory receptors (for example, sound or light stimuli), and the limbic system (emotions) (Fig. 34-1).

As people try to fall asleep, they close their eyes and assume a relaxed position. Stimuli to the RAS decline. If the room is dark and quiet, activation of the RAS further declines. At some point the BSR takes over, causing a person to fall asleep.

Sleep Cycle

Studies with the EEG, EMG, and EOG show different levels of brain activity indicating different stages of sleep. Sleep involves two phases: rapid eye movement (REM) sleep and nonREM sleep (see box). NonREM sleep is further divided into four stages, through which a sleeper progresses during a typical sleeping cycle. The sleeping stages are highly individualized.

Normally, in an adult the routine sleep pattern begins with a presleep period during which the person is aware only of a gradually developing drowsiness. This period normally lasts 10 to 30 minutes, but if a person has difficulty falling asleep, it may last an hour or more.

As adults fall asleep, they progress through the four stages of nonREM sleep. At the end of the fourth stage they come out of deep sleep, go back to stage two, and then enter a period of REM. It usually averages 90 minutes for a person to reach REM sleep. Each person varies, but a typical night's sleep consists of four to six such cycles.

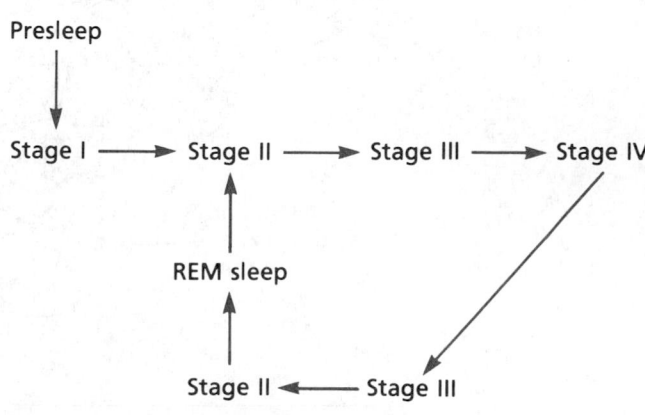

Fig. 34-2 The adult sleep cycle.

As the period of sleep progresses, stages III and IV shorten and the period of REM lengthens. REM sleep may last 30 to 60 minutes during the last sleep cycle. People on the average awaken five times during the night and are twice as likely to awaken from REM sleep as any other stage (Langford et al., 1972).

Not all people progress consistently through the stages of sleep. For example, a sleeper may fluctuate for short intervals between stages II, III, and IV before entering REM stage. The amount of time spent in each stage varies throughout the night (Fig. 34-2). The number of sleep cycles depends on the total amount of time spent sleeping.

FUNCTIONS OF SLEEP

Theories on the function of sleep fall into two categories: restorative-synthetic and behavioral.

Traditionally, sleep is viewed as a time of restoration and preparation for the next period of wakefulness. During nonREM sleep a person's biological functions slow. A healthy adult's normal heart rate throughout the day averages 70 to 80 beats per minute or less if the individual is in excellent physical condition. However, during sleep the heart rate falls to 60 beats per minute or less. This means the heart beats 10 to 20 fewer times in each minute during sleep or 60 to 120 fewer times in each hour. Clearly, then, restful sleep is beneficial in preserving cardiac function.

During nonREM sleep the body repairs and renews epithelial and specialized cells, such as brain tissue. Stage IV sleep may trigger production of growth hormone for bone growth, protein synthesis, and tissue repair. This is especially true in children, who experience more stage IV sleep.

The body conserves energy during sleep. The skeletal muscles relax progressively, and the absence of muscular contraction preserves chemical energy for more vital cellular processes. The lowering of the basal metabolic rate further conserves the body's energy supply.

REM sleep appears to be a cycle of brain activity important for learning, memory, and behavioral adaptation. The brain filters stored information of the day's activities. The person who is asleep may be able to solve problems and gain new insights. Dreaming allows a person to clarify emotions and prepare the mind for events of the next day.

The benefits of sleep for behavior become more obvious when a person is deprived of sleep. A loss of REM sleep leads to feelings of confusion and suspicion. If people are deprived of stage 3 and 4 sleep, they feel withdrawn and physically uncomfortable (Williams et al., 1967). No clear cause-and-effect relationship exists between sleep deprivation and a specific body dysfunc-tion (Webster and Thompson, 1986). However, various body functions can be altered when prolonged sleep deprivation occurs.

Dreams

Dreams occur during both nonREM and REM sleep. The dreams of REM sleep are more vivid and elaborate. REM dreams progress in content throughout the night from dreams about current events to emotional dreams of childhood or the past. Personality can influence the quality of dreams; for example, a creative person usually has creative dreams and a depressed person usually dreams of helplessness.

Most people dream about immediate concerns such as an argument with a spouse, plans for a wedding, or worries over work. Sometimes a person is unaware of fears that are represented in bizarre dreams. Psychologists attempt to analyze the symbolic nature of dreams. For example, an apple may represent a forbidden object, the sense of rushing to an unknown destination may represent an unresolved conflict, or a lion may symbolize rage. A person's ability to describe a dream and interpret its significance may help resolve personal concerns or fears.

The dreams of REM sleep are believed to be functionally important. Sigmund Freud believed dreams were a product of a person's unconscious desires and served to release psychological tensions. Thus the nature and occurrence of dreams became a basis for psychotherapy.

Another theory suggests that dreams erase certain fantasies or nonsensical memories. Most dreams are forgotten. In fact, during REM sleep, consolidation of short-term memory is impaired. To remember a dream, a person must consciously think about the dream on awakening. People who recall dreams vividly usually awake just after a period of REM sleep. Some theorists therefore believe that people dream in order to forget. They discourage clients from attempting to remember dreams so that undesirable thought patterns are effectively forgotten.

Other theorists believe that dreams serve to consolidate memories for emotional and mental equilibrium.

Normal Sleep Requirements

No specific number of hours of sleep are needed to ensure adequate rest. One person may function well with 4 hours of sleep while another requires 10 hours. Each person has a unique biological clock for determining the duration of sleep.

NEONATES

A neonate averages 16 hours of sleep daily, with a range of 10 to 23 hours. The child enters the world in a state of wakefulness, with eyes open wide and sucking behavior vigorous. After about an hour the newborn becomes quiet and less responsive to internal and external stimuli. A period of sleep lasting up to 4 hours follows. The child will then awaken again and often become overly responsive to stimuli. Hunger, pain, cold, or other stimuli frequently cause crying. For the first week the neonate sleeps almost constantly to recover from the birth process. Approximately 50% of the sleep of a newborn is REM sleep, which stimulates the higher brain centers. This is essential for development, since the neonate is not awake long enough for significant external stimulation.

INFANTS

Infants usually develop a nighttime pattern of sleep by age 3 months. The infant may take several naps during the day but usually sleeps an average of 10 to 12 hours a night. The infant commonly awakens early in the morning, although it is not unusual for an infant to awaken during the night. If awakening during the night continues, the problem may be with diet because hunger frequently awakens the child. Large infants sleep longer than smaller ones because of their greater stomach capacity. Infants between 1 month and 1 year of age sleep an average of 14 hours a day. REM sleep predominates in the infant's sleep cycle.

TODDLERS

By the age of 2 years children sleep through the night and take one or two daily naps. At 3 years the second nap is usually eliminated. The percentage of REM sleep begins to fall because the toddler has access to a variety of meaningful external stimuli. As the brain matures there is less need for internal stimulation. Parents often face the problem of a toddler's unwillingness to go to bed at night, an expression of the child's need for autonomy. The child prefers to stay awake and spend time with parents and siblings to satisfy the need to explore and be curious.

PRESCHOOLERS

The preschooler's main problem in getting enough sleep is difficulty in relaxing or quieting down after a long, active day. Many preschoolers also have problems with bedtime fears, waking during the night, or nightmares. Parents are most successful in getting preschoolers to bed by establishing a consistent bedtime ritual. Children should not be allowed to become manipulative by sleeping with parents or by staying up past a reasonable hour. When nightmares occur, the parent should comfort the child in the child's own bed. The total daily sleep needs for a preschooler average 10 to 11 hours.

SCHOOL-AGE CHILDREN

The amount of sleep needed during the school years is highly individualized because of childrens' varying states of activity and levels of health. The school-age child usually does not require a nap. Throughout the school years a child is in need of 10 to 12 hours of sleep. The 6- or 7-year-old child can usually be persuaded to go to bed by encouraging quiet activities beforehand. The older child becomes resistant out of a need to be independent. Many older children seek a later bedtime as a symbol of dominance over younger children. Parents are usually successful in getting the older child to bed by using a firm, consistent approach.

ADOLESCENTS

An adolescent usually spends an active day that is both mentally and physically exhausting. Often the desire to spend time with peers prevents adolescents from realizing their need for sleep. Once bedtime approaches, however, the adolescent offers little resistance to sleep. An adolescent averages 8 to 9 hours of sleep nightly.

ADULTS

The average daily amount of sleep varies considerably among adults. Most adults in the 20- to 50-year-old age group average 6 to 8½ hours of sleep. However, 5% to 10% of this age group sleep more than 9 hours, and 2% to 5% sleep less than 6 hours without difficulty. Approximately 20% of the time is spent in REM sleep, 50% to 60% in a light stage I or II sleep, and 20% in the deeper stage III or IV sleep. One of the more inconsistent sleep habits among adults is the time they go to sleep. Most healthy adults do not require regular naps.

OLDER ADULTS

The amount of sleep a person gets as age increases does not change, although the quality of sleep deteriorates (Kales and Kales, 1974). REM sleep continues to occur cyclically at intervals of 90 minutes in all age groups. Throughout life there is a progressive decrease in stages 3 and 4 nonREM, and the elderly have almost no stage 4 sleep (Clapin-French, 1986). An elderly person awakens more often during the night and has an increase in total wake time. It may also take more time for an elderly person to fall asleep (Ross et al. 1986).

Hayter (1983) studied the sleep habits of older persons and found that the majority of elderly nap during the day. Some may nap more than once a day, but some elderly nap only occasionally during a week's time. Hayter's work showed that napping is not an attempt to compensate for sleep lost at night. However, nappers were found to get more total sleep time than those who did not nap.

The changes in an elderly person's sleep pattern are

due to changes in the central nervous system that affect the regulation of sleep. Sensory impairment, common with aging, may reduce a person's sensitivity to time cues that maintain circadian rhythms. The elderly also often suffer a variety of chronic illnesses that can impair the quality of sleep.

FACTORS AFFECTING SLEEP

Factors that promote sleep in one person may hinder sleep in another. A single factor may not be the only cause for a person's sleep problem. Physiological, psychological, and environmental factors can alter the quality and quantity of sleep.

Physical Illness

Any illness that causes pain, physical discomfort (such as difficulty swallowing), anxiety, or depression can result in sleep difficulties. Persons with such alterations may have trouble falling or staying asleep. Illnesses also force clients to sleep in positions to which they are unaccustomed. Assuming an awkward position while in traction can interfere with falling and staying asleep.

Respiratory disease often interferes with sleep. Clients with chronic lung disease (such as emphysema) are short of breath and frequently cannot sleep without two or three pillows to raise their heads. Asthma, bronchitis, and allergic rhinitis alter the rhythm of a person's breathing and disturb sleep. A person with a common cold has nasal congestion, sinus drainage, and an inflamed throat, all of which impair breathing and the ability to relax.

Coronary heart disease is characterized by episodes of sudden chest pain and irregular heart rates. Clients with this disease are often afraid to go to sleep because of a possible attack at night. The attacks have been found to occur more often during REM sleep (Ross et al., 1986). Death from heart disorders most frequently occurs at night, especially between 5:00 and 6:00 AM when REM sleep lasts longer.

Hypertension often causes early morning awakening and fatigue. Hypothyroidism decreases stage 4 sleep, while hyperthyroidism causes persons to take more time to fall asleep.

Nocturia, or urination during the night, disrupts sleep and the sleep cycle. This condition is most common in elderly people with reduced bladder tone or in persons with cardiac disease, diabetes, urethritis, or prostatic disease. Once a person awakens to urinate, returning to sleep may be difficult.

The elderly often experience "restless leg syndrome," which occurs during the presleep stage. The person experiences recurrent, rhythmical movements of the feet and legs. An itching sensation is felt deep in the muscles. Relief comes only from moving the legs, which prevents the person from relaxing long enough to fall asleep. The restless leg syndrome is a benign condition. In contrast, a person who has severe leg cramps during the night may have a problem with arterial circulation.

Persons with peptic ulcer disease often awaken in the middle of the night. Gastric acid levels reach a peak in the stomach around 1:00 and 3:00 AM (McNeil et al., 1986), causing stomach pain.

Drugs and Substances

Various types of drugs affect the pattern and quality of sleep a person enjoys (see box). Medications prescribed for sleep often cause more problems than benefits. The elderly often take a variety of drugs to control or treat chronic illness and the combined effects of several drugs can seriously disrupt sleep. One substance that may help a person to sleep is L-tryptophan, a protein found in foods such as milk, cheese, and meats.

Life-Style

The routine a person follows during the course of a day may influence sleep patterns. An individual working

---

Drugs and Their Effects on Sleep

HYPNOTICS
- Provide only temporary (1 week) increase in quantity of sleep
- Eventually cause "hangover" during daytime: excess drowsiness, confusion, decreased energy
- May worsen sleep apnea in the elderly

DIURETICS
- Cause nocturia

ANTIDEPRESSANTS AND STIMULANTS
- Suppress REM sleep

ALCOHOL
- Speeds onset of sleep
- Disrupts REM sleep
- Awakens person during night and causes difficulty returning to sleep

CAFFEINE
- Prevents person from falling asleep
- May cause a person to awaken during night

a rotating shift—for example, 2 weeks of days followed by a week of nights—has difficulty adjusting to the altered sleep schedule. The body's internal clock might be set for the person to fall asleep at 11 PM but the work schedule forces him to go to sleep at 9 AM instead. The individual often can sleep only 3 or 4 hours because the body's clock perceives that it is time to be awake and active. Only after several weeks of working a nightshift does a person's biological clock adjust. Other alterations in routine that are capable of disrupting sleeping patterns include performing unaccustomed heavy work, engaging in late night social activities, and changing evening mealtime.

Sleep Patterns

The duration of sleep and the time sleep begins influence succeeding attempts to fall asleep. For example, when a person awakens earlier than usual, the circadian rhythm is reset. The next night the person will be able to fall asleep earlier than the previous night. If a person follows the natural sleep rhythm and sleeps an extra hour, the rhythm will be delayed an hour the first night, 2 hours the second night, and so on (Hauri, 1982). A person who experiences temporary sleep deprivation as a result of an active social evening, lengthened work schedule, or late-night television watching usually feels sleepy the next day. Sleep deprivation may result in difficulty performing tasks and remaining attentive. Chronic lack of sleep is much more serious than temporary sleep deprivation and can cause serious alterations in a person's ability to perform daily functions.

Emotional Stress

Worry over personal problems or situations can disrupt sleep. Emotional stress causes a person to be tense and often leads to frustration when sleep does not come. Stress may also cause a person to try too hard to fall asleep, to awaken frequently during the sleep cycle, or to oversleep. Continued stress causes poor sleep habits.

Elderly clients frequently experience losses that lead to emotional stress. Retirement, physical impairment, death of a loved one, or loss of economic security are examples of situations that predispose the elderly to anxiety and depression. With emotional stress the elderly experience delays in falling asleep, earlier appearance of REM sleep, frequent awakening, increased total bed time, feelings of sleeping poorly, and early awakening (Colling, 1983).

Environment

The environment in which a person sleeps has a significant influence on the ability to fall and remain asleep.

Good ventilation is essential for restful sleep. The size, firmness, and position of the bed can affect the quality of sleep. Harder surfaces cause more body movement (Schmidt-Kessen and Kendel, 1973). Hospital beds are often harder than those at home. If a person usually sleeps with another individual, sleeping alone can cause wakefulness.

Sound also influences sleep. The level of noise needed to awaken a person depends on the stage of sleep (Webster, 1986). Low-level noise is more likely to arouse a person from stage 1 sleep, while louder noise awakens people in stage 3 or 4 sleep. Some persons require silence to fall asleep while others prefer background noise such as soft music. In hospital settings, noise creates a problem for clients. Noise in hospitals is usually new or strange, thus clients are prone to awaken. The level of noise in hospitals can be very loud. Normal conversation measures approximately 50 decibels. Seidlitz (1981) found that a wall suction machine measured 67 decibels, a client coughing was 70 decibels, and a nurse opening a package of rubber gloves registered 86 decibels. People-induced noises, related to nursing staff talking, is also a major source of increased sound levels. Intensive care units are sources for very loud noise levels. Close proximity of clients, noise from confused and very ill clients, and disturbances caused by emergencies all make the environment unpleasant.

Light levels may affect a person's ability to fall asleep. Clients may prefer a room to be dark while others keep a soft light on at all times. Clients also may have trouble sleeping, depending on the temperature of a room. A room that is too warm or too cold causes a client to become restless. Sleeping at temperatures higher than 24° C has been found to cause poorer quality sleep (Schmidt-Kessen and Kendel, 1973).

Exercise and Fatigue

A person who is moderately fatigued usually achieves restful sleep, especially if the fatigue is the result of enjoyable work or exercise. Exercising 2 hours before bedtime allows the body to cool down and maintains a state of fatigue that promotes relaxation. However, excess fatigue resulting from exhausting or stressful work can make falling asleep difficult.

Caloric Intake

Weight loss or gain influences a person's sleep pattern. When a person gains weight, sleep periods become longer with fewer interruptions. Weight loss can cause short and fragmented sleep. Certain sleep disorders may be the result of the semistarvation diets popular in our weight-conscious society.

SLEEP DISORDERS

Sleep problems are common among clients. The problem may bring a client to seek health care or the effects of illness or hospitalization may create the sleep disorder. The best way to diagnose sleep disorders is through the use of a nighttime polysomnogram. This involves use of the EEG, EMG, and EOG to monitor the client's stages of sleep and wakefulness.

Insomnia

Insomnia is a symptom of clients with chronic difficulty falling asleep (initial insomnia), difficulty remaining asleep (intermittent insomnia), or inability to go back to sleep after awakening (terminal insomnia). The insomniac complains of insufficient quantity and quality of sleep. Frequently, however, the client gets more sleep than is realized. Insomnia may signal an underlying physical or psychological disorder.

Persons may experience insomnia only temporarily, usually a result of situational stresses such as family or work problems, jet lag, illness, or loss of a loved one. The insomnia may recur, but between episodes the client is able to sleep well.

Insomnia is most commonly associated with poor sleep habits. If the condition continues, the fear of not being able to sleep can be enough to cause wakefulness. During the day, a person with chronic insomnia may feel sleepy, fatigued, depressed, and anxious.

Insomnia may become a condition that continues for years. Treatment is usually symptomatic, including improved sleep hygiene measures, biofeedback, and relaxation techniques. The exact cause of insomnia is unknown. In drug-dependence insomnia the client is unable to fall asleep because of excessive use of hypnotic medications. Such a client benefits from a gradual withdrawal of hypnotics.

Sleep Apnea

The easiest description of sleep apnea is the cessation of breathing for a time during sleep. There are two types: central and obstructive.

Apnea is the cessation of airflow through the nose and mouth for at least 10 seconds (Block, 1980). In obstructive apnea the upper airway becomes blocked and nasal airflow stops for as long as 30 seconds (Feierman, 1985). The person still attempts to breathe as chest and abdominal movement continue. During the apneic period, each successive diaphragmatic movement becomes stronger until the obstruction is relieved. Central apnea involves defects in the brain's respiratory center. The impulse to breathe temporarily fails, and nasal airflow and chest wall movement cease. The oxygen saturation

of a person's blood falls slightly. No treatment exists for central sleep apnea.

Obstructive apnea causes a serious decline in a client's arterial oxygen level (see Chapter 36). Serious hypoxemia may cause cardiac dysrhythmias, right heart failure, pulmonary hypertension, and anginal attacks. Men tend to be more frequently affected, particularly those who have recently gained weight. The most frequent time of naturally occurring death is 6 AM, and some researchers believe that sleep apneas are a cause.

A person with sleep apnea typically snores at night and complains of excessive daytime sleepiness. Three types of treatment are helpful: weight reduction, surgical removal of the tonsils and uvula in the posterior pharynx, and the use of continuous positive airway pressure (CPAP). CPAP requires a client to wear a mask over the nose with room air delivered through the mask pressure. The air pressure keeps the airway open and prevents its collapse. The CPAP device is 100% effective.

Narcolepsy

Narcolepsy is a condition associated with the complaint of daytime sleepiness with abnormality of REM sleep. During the day a person may suddenly feel an overwhelming wave of sleepiness and fall asleep. REM sleep can occur within 15 minutes after sleep. Cataplexy or sudden muscle weakness with intense emotions such as anger, sadness, or laughter may occur in the day. A person with narcolepsy may also have hallucinations that are almost real dreams occurring just as the person falls asleep. The person may not know the difference between a dream and reality. Finally, sleep paralysis, or the feeling of being unable to move or talk just before waking or falling asleep, is another symptom.

The greatest problem with narcolepsy is that individuals fall asleep at inappropriate times. Unless a person understands the disorder, a sleep attack can easily be mistaken for laziness, lack of interest in activities, or drunkenness. Clients are treated with stimulants that increase wakefulness and medications that suppress REM sleep. Brief daytime naps further help to reduce narcoleptic attacks. Factors that increase a narcoleptic's drowsiness, for example, liquor or exhausting activities, should be avoided.

Sleep Deprivation

Although not a true sleep disorder, sleep deprivation is a problem many clients experience as a result of hospitalization. Sleep deprivation involves decreases in the amount, quality, and consistency of sleep. When sleep becomes interrupted or fragmented, changes in the normal sequence of sleep stages occur, and cycles cannot

---

Sleep Deprivation Symptoms

PHYSIOLOGICAL SYMPTOMS

- Hand tremors
- Decreased reflexes
- Slowed response time
- Reduction in word memory
- Decreased reasoning, judgment
- Cardiac dysrhythmias

PSYCHOLOGICAL SYMPTOMS

- Moods
- Disorientation
- Irritability
- Decreased motivation
- Fatigue
- Sleepiness
- Hyperactivity

Components of a Sleep History

- Description of client's sleeping problem
- Severity of sleep problem
- Daytime symptoms
- Normal sleep pattern
- Medical history
- Current life events
- Emotional and mental status
- Bedtime rituals and environment
- Report from bed partner
- Sleep/wake log
- Behaviors of sleep deprivation

---

be completed (Fisher, 1984). Gradually a cumulative sleep deprivation develops.

Clients may experience a variety of physiological and psychological symptoms (see box). The severity of symptoms often is related to the duration of sleep deprivation. Causes of sleep deprivation may include illness (such as fever, difficulty breathing, pain), sleep disorders, emotional stress, environmental disturbances, and changes in sleep patterns (such as shift work).

The most effective treatment for sleep deprivation is elimination or correction of factors that disrupt a person's normal sleep pattern. Nurses play an important role in treating sleep deprivation problems.

Other Sleep Disorders

Sleep problems common in children include sleep walking (somnambulism), night terrors, nightmares, noctural enuresis (bedwetting), and tooth grinding. When adults have these problems, it may indicate more serious disorders. Specific treatment for each of these disorders varies. However, in all cases, it is important to support the client and maintain his or her safety. For example, a sleepwalker is unaware of surroundings and is slow to react. Thus, the risk of falls are great. A nurse should not startle a sleepwalker but instead gently awakens the sleeper and leads him or her back to bed.

ASSESSMENT

In an effort to promote a normal restful sleep for a client, the nurse should assess a client's sleep history (see

box). The choice of sleep therapies will depend on the factors and conditions that typically promote the client's sleep and those impacting on the current problem. Fig. 34-3 is a sleep questionnaire developed by McNeil et al. (1986) that can be used to assess a hospitalized client's sleep patterns. Clapin-French (1986) strongly recommends the use of a sleep history, particularly in the care of the elderly client (see research highlight).

Description of Sleeping Problems

The nurse asks the client to describe any sleep problems. Open-ended questions may help the client describe

---

✄ Research Highlight ✄

The elderly frequently experience sleep disturbances associated with age-related changes in sleep physiology. Clapin-French (1986) assessed the factors involved in changes in sleep patterns of elderly clients in long-term care facilities and evaluated the extent of the use of a nursing sleep history by the nursing staff. Of the 102 elderly adults studied, 71% received some type of sleep medication regularly. Significant shifts in sleep patterns after admission occurred in the clients taking medication. However, only 54% had a nursing sleep history conducted by the nursing staff. Clients may receive inappropriately large amounts of sleep medications without adequate assessment of factors promoting the sleep problems. A detailed assessment of a client's sleep pattern should be a routine part of a nursing history.

Clapin-French, E: Sleep patterns of aged persons in long-term care facilities, J Adv Nurs 11:57 Jan. 1986.

THE SLEEP QUESTIONNAIRE

At home, what do you do at bedtime to help you sleep? _____

_____

Some of the statements may *appear* to be the same, but each is different and should be rated as such.*

A. I think I have difficulty with sleep
   a. in the hospital
   b. at home
B. I sleep more at home than in the hospital.
C. When I awaken in the hospital, I feel fatigued and groggy.
D. It takes me longer than 30 minutes to fall asleep in the hospital.
E. Since I've been in the hospital, I awaken frequently at night.
F. In the hospital, if I wake up in the middle of the night it takes me longer than 30 minutes to fall back to sleep.
G. It bothers me that I now go to bed at a different time than I would like.
H. It bothers me that I get up at a different time each morning.
I. Hospital staff awaken me while I'm sleeping.
J. I am awakened at night for treatments.
K. During the day, there is little time for rest.
L. At night I am awakened by noises.
M. At night I am awakened by light.
N. The mattress in the hospital bothers my sleep.
O. The pillow in the hospital bothers my sleep.
P. Having a roommate in the hospital affects my sleep.
Q. I sleep in a very warm room.
R. I have pain at night.
S. The medicines I take keep me awake.
T. My illness keeps me awake at night.

1. I drink coffee, tea, cola, or cocoa during the day.
2. I drink coffee, tea, cola, or cocoa around sleeping time.
3. I exercise during the day.
4. I exercise around sleeping time.
5. I smoke during the day.
6. I smoke around sleeping time.
7. I have unpleasant conversation during the day.
8. I have unpleasant conversation around sleeping time.
9. I have negative thoughts during the day.
10. I have negative thoughts around sleeping time.
11. I think about what happened during the day and at sleeping time plan for tomorrow.
12. I read during the day.
13. I read around sleeping time.
14. I eat around sleeping time.
15. I watch TV during the day.
16. I watch TV around sleeping time.
17. I have pleasant conversation during the day.
18. I have pleasant conversation around sleeping time.
19. I have positive thoughts during the day.
20. I have positive thoughts around sleeping time.
21. I drink alcohol around sleeping time.

*Response choices were: *Never, Rarely, Sometimes, Often, Very Often.*

Fig. 34-3 A sleep questionnaire can be used to assess sleep patterns.

From McNeil, BJ, et al.: Sleep questionnaire, AJN 86(1):261, 1986. © 1986. Reproduced with permission from American Journal of Nursing Company.

problems more fully. For example, "Tell me what type of problem you have falling asleep," or "Describe what a normal night of sleep is like," encourages clients to describe the nature of any disturbances.

The nurse learns the type of sleep disturbances the client has, when it started, its duration, and its frequency. Clients often can recall the situations leading to their sleep problem. Questions such as "When you awaken in the middle of the night, what is the reason for it?" help to clarify the problem. It is important to know if the client has trouble falling asleep, staying asleep, awakening early, or if a combination of problems exist.

Parents are usually successful in learning why their children have trouble sleeping. Children often are able to relate fears or worries that inhibit their ability to fall asleep. If a child frequently awakens in the middle of a bad dream, the parent can identify the problem but perhaps does not understand the meaning of the dream. Parents can also describe the typical behavior patterns that foster or impair sleep. For example, excessive stimulation from active play or having several friends over to visit may predictably impair a child's sleep.

Severity of Sleeping Problems

How severe is the client's sleeping problem, and what are the effects on the client? The nurse will assess the number of nights a week the client has difficulty sleeping, the length of time it takes to fall asleep, the frequency of awakening, and the length of time it takes to fall asleep after awakening. In the hospital setting the nurse may monitor the actual number of hours of sleep a client receives. If the nurse cannot remain in the client's room to observe sleep, however, it is possible to note the number of times the client awakens as care is delivered during the night.

A chronic sleep disturbance will influence a client's ability to perform daily activities. If the problem is more recent, clients are better able to recall factors leading to the problems. Parents are able to tell the nurse how long the problem has existed, how it has progressed, and the child's response to the disturbance. The nurse can then assess the severity of the condition based on information about the frequency of episodes of night terrors, bad dreams, enuresis, or difficulty falling asleep at night.

Daytime Symptoms

It is important to learn if the client's sleep problem interferes with daily functioning. Does the client feel tired, irritable, or have difficulty concentrating? Is it necessary for the client to nap during the day? Has the client noticed a problem in meeting work responsibilities or

maintaining interpersonal relationships since the sleep disturbance began?

During the history the nurse observes the client's behaviors. If the client moves slowly and without energy or appears apathetic and unenthusiastic, inadequate sleep may be the problem. Failure to remain alert and failure to concentrate during questioning are other relevant observations.

Young children often display symptoms of sleep problems during play or in school. A child may easily become irritable or angry. Some children fall asleep in school at inappropriate times. A nurse can often sense a young child's overall lack of energy and enthusiasm during play or during interactions with other children.

Normal Sleep Pattern

The client or the parent should be asked to describe the normal sleep pattern that existed before the sleep disturbance. Questions might concern the typical hour the person went to sleep, the average length of sleep, and the number of times the person awakened during the night. The client's problem may be drastically different from his normal pattern or may prove to be relatively minor. Hospitalized clients may need or want more sleep as a result of illness, or they may require less sleep since they are less active. A client may think it is necessary to try to sleep longer than normal. These changes can disrupt a person's sleep pattern and eventually make sleeping difficult.

Medical History

The nurse determines if the client has any preexisting health problems that might interfere with sleep. Does the client have a history of psychiatric problems? A manic depressive sleeps more when depressed than when manic. A schizophrenic may have fragmented sleep. Does the client have a history of psychiatric problems? Does the client suffer from any chronic diseases or painful disorders that interfere with sleep? The nurse also assesses the client's medication history, including a description of over-the-counter and prescribed drugs. The nurse may also assess a client's daily caffeine intake at this time.

Current Life Events

The nurse learns if the client is experiencing any changes in life-style. A person's occupation may offer a clue to the nature of a sleep problem, particularly if the person works rotating shifts. Questions about social activities, recent traveling, or mealtime schedules will help to clarify the sleep assessment.

Emotional and Mental Status

Is the client experiencing any emotional stress related to illness or situational crises such as loss of job or loved one? How do the client's emotions affect the ability to sleep? If a client is anxious, excitable, angry, or normal, mental preoccupations can seriously disrupt sleep.

Bedtime Rituals

Assessing the client's bedtime ritual is helpful. What does the client do before going to bed? Does the client drink a glass of milk, take a sleeping pill, eat a snack, watch television, or exercise? The nurse assesses habits that are beneficial compared with those that disturb a person's sleep. Not all clients are alike. Watching television may bore one person to sleep while another individual may stay awake during a suspenseful movie.

Hospitalization often interferes with bedtime rituals. Restrictions caused by a person's illness may prevent the client from eating or drinking. Exercise may also be a contraindication to sleep. A nurse learns how hospital routines affect the person's ability to fall asleep.

The nurse should pay special attention to a child's bedtime rituals. The parents can report whether it is necessary, for example, to read the child a bedtime story, rock the child to sleep, or engage in quiet play.

Bedtime Environment

The nurse asks the client to describe normal bedroom conditions. Is the bedroom dark, or are there any sources of light? Is the door to the room usually open or closed? Does the client listen to the radio or watch television in the bedroom? On what type of bed and mattress does the client sleep? Does any type of noise prevent the client from falling asleep? Does a child require the company of a parent to fall asleep? The nurse may learn that changes in the home environment are necessary to promote a client's sleep.

In a hospital setting the nurse needs to know the client's normal environment compared to what exists in the hospital room. There may be environmental distractions such as a roommate's television, an electronic monitor in the hallway, a noisy nurses' station, or another client who cries out at night. The nurse identifies factors in the hospital environment that can be reduced or controlled.

Bed Partner

Information from a client's bed partner may reveal the nature of certain sleep disorders. A bed partner, for example, can report the pattern of the client's falling asleep or awakening. Partners of clients with apnea often complain that their sleep is disturbed by the clients snoring and restless movement. Often a partner must sleep in a different bed or room. The nurse should ask the client's bed partner whether the client has pauses or interruptions of breathing or snoring during sleep. Some partners mention becoming fearful when the client apparently stops breathing and then struggles before airflow returns. The partner may also be the best source to describe the frequency of narcoleptic attacks in a client.

Sleep-Wake Log

If the cause of a sleep problem is unclear, the nurse may ask the client and bed partner to keep a sleep-wake log for 2 weeks. The nurse should not rely only on the client's casual description of the problem. Descriptions of the worst sleeping nights may distort the real problem. Entries into the log include physical activities, mealtimes, type of intake (alcohol and caffeine), time and length of daytime naps, evening and bedtime rituals, and the hour the client tries to fall asleep. A partner can be helpful in recording the estimated hour the client falls asleep, the frequency of middle-of-the-night awakenings, and the time the client awakens in the morning. The log is helpful, but sometimes its completion can distract persons from sleeping.

Behaviors of Sleep Deprivation

Some clients are unaware of their sleep problems. The nurse observes for behaviors such as irritability, disorientation (similar to a drunken state), or slurred speech. If sleep deprivation has lasted a long time, psychotic behavior such as delusions and feelings of paranoia may develop. For example, a client may report seeing strange objects or colors in the room. The client may act afraid when the nurse enters the room.

Clients with chronic sleep disorders usually have mild symptoms of sleep deprivation. Clients hospitalized in intensive care units for an extended time may show the "ICU syndrome" of sleep deprivation. Constant environmental stimuli within the ICU, such as strange noises from equipment or the frequent monitoring and care given by nurses, and ever-present lights, confuse clients. Soon a client cannot tell the difference between night and day. Repeated environmental stimuli coupled with the client's poor physical status, lead to sleep deprivation.

NURSING DIAGNOSIS

The nurse's assessment will reveal clusters of data that indicate whether a sleep problem exists or if the nature of a person's sleep creates other nursing diagnoses (see nursing diagnoses box). For example, a 36-year-old female is a busy lawyer whose work keeps her up until 1 or 2 AM when her normal bedtime is 11 PM. She complains of awakening at least once every night and still feeling tired in the morning. She also admits to losing her temper more often at work. The defining characteristics of changes in normal sleep pattern and verbal complaints of not feeling rested point to the nursing diagnosis "sleep pattern disturbance."

The nurse's diagnosis should identify the probable cause for the problem such as psychological stress involving work so appropriate interventions can be planned. If the probable cause or related factors are incorrectly defined, the client may not benefit from care.

Sleep problems may affect clients in other ways. For example, a nurse may find that a client with sleep apnea has problems with a spouse. The spouse is tired and frustrated over the client's continued snoring at night. Plus the spouse is concerned that the client is breathing improperly and thus is in physical danger. The nursing diagnosis of "ineffective family coping" indicates that the nurse must provide support to the client and spouse so that they can understand sleep apnea and obtain the medical treatment needed.

When choosing a nursing diagnosis following assess-

Examples of Nursing Diagnoses Related to Sleep Disturbances

NANDA-APPROVED NURSING DIAGNOSES

Sleep pattern disturbance related to:
- Environmental disturbances
- Chronic illness
- Emotional/situational stress

Potential for injury related to:
- Attacks of sleepwalking/narcolepsy

Ineffective family coping: compromised related to:
- Spouse's poor understanding of sleep problem

Self-esteem disturbance related to:
- Incidents of bed-wetting

Altered thought processes related to:
- Sleep deprivation

Sample Nursing Diagnoses for Sleep Disturbances

Defining Characteristics	Nursing Diagnoses	Related Factors
Client verbalizes inability to fall asleep.	Sleep pattern disturbance	• Chronic illness
Client has interrupted sleep.		
Client awakens earlier or later than desired.		• Situational stress: loss of job or loved one
Client verbalizes feeling tired, irritable.		• Environmental disturbances
Changes in behavior (restless, disorientation) present.		• Alcohol ingestion
Client has frequent attacks of sleep walking, narcolepsy.	Potential for trauma	• Sleepwalking
Client has history of injury from falls.		• Narcoleptic attack
Hospital environment is unfamiliar.		
Spouse complains about client's snoring and disruptive sleep pattern.	Ineffective family coping: compromised	• Spouse's and client's poor understanding of sleep apnea
Client expresses concern over spouse's lack of understanding.		
Sleep log indicates frequent sleep interruptions. Spouse moves to different bedroom.		

ment, the nurse must be sure appropriate defining characteristics are identified. This ensures an accurate, individualized diagnosis suited to the client's needs. The sample nursing diagnoses box lists examples of nursing diagnoses for clients with sleep problems.

disorder. The goals of any care plan for a client needing sleep or rest include:

1. Obtaining a sense of restfulness following sleep
2. Experiencing fewer symptoms of sleep deprivation
3. Identifying factors that promote or disrupt sleep
4. Establishing an adequate sleep pattern

PLANNING

After identifying each nursing diagnosis, the nurse develops a plan of care (see care plan box). An individualized plan of care can be developed only after understanding the client's perception of a normal sleep pattern and the various factors that disrupt the client's sleep. Together the nurse and client develop realistic interventions that will promote rest and sleep. Even the client's bed partner may have useful suggestions for the plan of care.

In a hospital setting it is important for the nurse to plan treatments or routines so that the client will be able to rest. Other staff members should be aware of the plan of care so they can cluster activities at certain times to reduce awakenings.

The success of sleep therapy depends on an approach that fits the client's life-style and the nature of any sleep

IMPLEMENTATION

Clients need adequate sleep and rest to recover from physical illness. Nursing care in an acute care setting will differ from that provided in a client's home. The primary differences are in the environment and the nurse's ability to support the client's normal sleep habits. The client's age will also influence the type of therapies that are most effective. Whatever the cause or related factor for a sleep problem, the nurse performs specific interventions that promote normal sleep patterns.

Environmental Controls

All clients require a sleeping environment with a comfortable room temperature, minimal sources of noise, a comfortable bed, and proper lighting. Infants sleep best

---

Sample Nursing Care Plan for Sleep Disturbances

Nursing Diagnosis	Goals	Expected Outcomes	Nursing Interventions
Sleep pattern disturbance related to environmental disturbances	Client will obtain a sense of restfulness after sleep within 48 hours. Client will establish an adequate sleep pattern.	Client will fall asleep within 30 minutes of going to bed. Client will have no more than one period of awakening during sleep. Client will sleep at least 7 hours. Client will describe a feeling of restfulness after awakening.	Encourage client to ambulate in hallway for 10 minutes, 1 to 2 hours before bedtime Provide client with glass of milk 30 minutes before bedtime (9 PM) Measure vital signs between 9 and 9:30 PM Offer analgesic for leg pain (as needed) at 9 PM Assist client with positioning in bed and offer backrub at 9:30 PM Keep room door closed and light on in bathroom only. Control sources of environmental noise.

Control of Noise in the Hospital

- Close doors to a client's room.
- Reduce volume of nearby telephone and paging equipment.
- Wear rubber-soled shoes; avoid wearing clogs.
- Turn off bedside equipment not in use such as oxygen or suction equipment.
- Avoid abrupt loud noise such as toilet flushing or moving a bed.
- Keep necessary conversations at low levels, particularly at night.
- Conduct discussions or nursing report in a private, separate area away from client rooms.
- Turn off television or radio unless client prefers soft music.

---

when the room temperature is 18° to 21° C (65° to 69.8° F) at night. Cribs should be positioned away from open windows or drafts. The infant is covered with a light, warm blanket. Children and adults vary more in regards to comfortable room temperature. Some prefer to sleep without covers. The elderly often require extra blankets or covers. Many older clients sleep wearing socks.

It helps to eliminate sources of distracting noise so that a bedroom is as quiet as possible. In a hospital setting the nurse can control noise in several ways (see box). At home, it may require the cooperation of people living with the client to reduce noise. For example, the volume of a television watched by family members in another room can be reduced. Some clients are used to sleeping with familiar inside noises, such as the hum of a fan.

A bed and mattress should provide support and comfortable firmness. Bed boards can be placed underneath mattresses to add support. The position of the bed in the room may make a difference for some clients. An infant's bed must be a safe environment. To reduce the chance of suffocation, pillows or the ends of loose blankets should not be placed in the crib. A loose-fitting plastic mattress cover should not be used, since an infant might pull it over the face and cause suffocation. Infants are positioned in bed usually on their stomach or side to prevent suffocation or aspiration of stomach contents. The nurse places infants on their stomach or side until they are able to turn their heads side-to-side. For any client prone to confusion or falls, the bed's side rails should be positioned up. A call light should also be placed within the client's reach, so the client may ask for help when needed.

Clients vary in regard to the amount of light preferred at night. Infants sleep best in softly lit rooms. Light should not shine directly on the infant's eyes. A small table lamp in the infant's room prevents leaving the infant in total darkness. An elderly client may sleep best with a dim light. This reduces the chance of confusion and prevents falls enroute to the bathroom. If street lights shine through windows or if a client sleeps during the day, heavy shades, drapes, or slatted blinds are helpful. Nurses should close curtains between clients in semi-private rooms. Lights on a hospital nursing unit can be dimmed at night.

Promoting Bedtime Rituals

Bedtime rituals relax a client in preparation for sleep. It is always important for persons to go to sleep when they feel fatigued or sleepy. Going to bed while one is fully awake and thinking about other things can cause insomnia and interfere with the bed as a stimulus for sleep.

Newborns and infants sleep through so much of the day that a specific ritual is hardly necessary. However, quieting activities, such as holding the infant snugly in a blanket, singing or talking softly, and gently rocking, will help infants fall asleep.

A bedtime ritual used consistently helps young children avoid attempts to delay sleeping. Toddlers and pre-schoolers may be too excited and full of energy to go to bed. Reading children stories, allowing them to sit in the parent's or nurse's lap while listening to music, or listening to a child's prayer are routines that can be associated with preparing for bed. Quiet activities such as coloring and reading work well with school-age children.

Adults should learn to avoid excessive physical or mental stimulation just before bedtime. Physical exercise can promote sleep if performed at least 2 hours before bedtime. Reading a light novel, watching a relaxing television program, or listening to music helps a person relax. Clients should not try to finish office work or resolve family problems before bedtime. The bedroom should not be used as a place to work. The bedroom should always be associated with sleep.

Working towards a consistent time for sleep helps most clients gain a healthy sleep pattern and strengthens the rhythm of the sleep-wake cycle. Persons should also void before retiring, so they are not kept awake by a full bladder.

Relaxation exercises are a useful bedtime ritual. Slow, deep breathing for a minute or two induces calm. Rhythmic contraction and relaxation of muscles (see Chapter 35) alleviates tension and prepares the body for rest (Hoch and Reynolds, 1986). Guided imagery, praying, meditation, and yoga may also promote sleep.

Read + Know

Comfort Measures For Promoting Sleep

- Administer analgesics and/or sedatives about 30 minutes before bedtime.
- Encourage clients to wear loose-fitting nightwear.
- Remove any irritants against the client's skin such as moist or wrinkled sheets or drainage tubing.
- Position and support body parts to protect pressure points and aid muscle relaxation.
- Offer a massage just before bedtime.
- Administer necessary hygiene measures.
- Keep bed linen clean and dry.
- Provide a comfortable mattress.
- Encourage client to void before hour of sleep.

Promoting Comfort

A person falls asleep only after feeling comfortable and relaxed. The nurse can use several measures to promote a client's comfort (see box). Minor irritants can keep clients awake. Diapers should be changed before placing infants in bed. Soft cotton nightclothes keep an infant or small child warm and comfortable.

Hospital beds tend to be harder than ones at home. A hard surface can cause more body movement (Schmidt-Kessen and Kendel, 1973). Compared with bed at home, hospital beds also are often of a different height, length, or width. Keeping beds clean and dry and in a comfortable position may help clients relax.

Some clients suffer painful illnesses requiring special comfort measures such as application of dry or moist heat, use of supportive dressings or splints, and proper positioning.

Providing for personal hygiene improves a client's sense of comfort. A warm bath or shower before bedtime can be relaxing. Clients restricted to bed should be offered the opportunity to wash the face and hands. Toothbrushing and care of dentures also help to prepare the client for sleep.

Establishing Periods of Rest and Sleep

In a hospital or extended care setting it is difficult to provide clients with the time needed to rest and sleep. The nurse can help by scheduling treatments, procedures, and routines for times when clients are awake. For example, if a client's physical condition has been stable, the nurse should avoid awakening the client to check vital signs. Unless maintaining a drug's therapeutic blood level is essential, medications should be given during waking hours. The nurse should work with the ra-

diology department and other support services to plan therapies at intervals that allow clients time for rest.

When the client's condition demands more frequent monitoring, the nurse can plan activities to allow for extended rest periods. For example, if a client needs frequent dressing changes, is receiving intravenous therapy, and has drainage tubes from several sites, the nurse should not make a separate trip into the room to check each individual problem. Instead the nurse should use a single visit to change the dressing, regulate the intravenous system, and empty the drainage tubes. In the home setting, it may help to encourage clients to stay physically active during the day so they are more likely to sleep at night. Increasing daytime activity lessens problems with falling asleep.

It is common for the elderly to nap for short intervals during the day. Hayter (1985) suggests that older clients take afternoon naps to restore the body physically. Hoch and Reynolds (1986) recommend naps to be taken at the same time each day to maintain a consistent schedule.

Controlling Physiological Disturbances

For clients with physical illness, the nurse can help control symptoms that disrupt sleep. For example, a client with respiratory abnormalities should sleep with two pillows or in a semisitting position to ease the effort to breathe. The client may benefit from taking prescribed bronchodilators before sleep to prevent airway obstruction. A client with a hiatal hernia also needs special care. After meals the client may experience a burning sensation as a result of gastric reflux. To prevent sleep disturbances, the client should eat a small meal several hours before bedtime and sleep in a semisitting position.

Stress Reduction

Sources of emotional stress can interfere with sleep. Likewise the inability to sleep can make a person feel irritable and tense. When clients feel emotionally upset, they should be encouraged not to force sleep. Otherwise, insomnia frequently develops, and soon bedtime is associated with the inability to relax.

A client who has difficulty falling asleep may find it helpful to get up and pursue a relaxing activity, such as reading or sewing rather than staying in bed and thinking about sleep.

In a health care setting a nurse on the nightshift should take time to sit and talk with clients who are unable to sleep. This will help the nurse determine the factors that are keeping the client awake. Explaining procedures or answering questions may give the client the peace of mind needed to fall asleep.

Children often have bedtime fears, awaken during the night, or have nightmares. The fears are usually normal for the child's age, for example, fear of the dark, strange noises or intruders. After a nightmare, parents should talk to the child about fears to provide a cooling-down period. The child is comforted but left in his own bed. The child's fears should not be used as an excuse to delay bedtime.

Bedtime Snacks

Some persons enjoy a bedtime snack while others cannot sleep after eating. A perfect snack includes a dairy product such as warm milk or cocoa that contains L-tryptophan. A full meal before bedtime can often cause gastrointestinal upset and interfere with a person's ability to fall asleep.

Nurses should discourage clients from drinking caffeine before bedtime. The stimulant can cause a person to stay awake or awaken throughout the night. Alcohol is capable of interrupting sleep cycles and reducing the amount of deep sleep. Coffee, tea, colas, and alcohol act as diuretics and may cause persons to awaken in the night to void.

Administering Sleep Medications

Several hypnotic drugs are considered safe in promoting sleep: flurazepam (Dalmane), chlordiazepoxide (Librium), chloral hydrate, methaqualone (Quaalude), and diazepam (Valium). These hypnotics cause the least disruption to the sleep cycle. Nurses should caution clients against taking hypnotics with alcoholic beverages. Clients should also avoid activities requiring motor coordination while under the influence of hypnotics.

The use of nonprescription sleeping medications is not advisable. Clients should learn the risks of such drugs, especially the long-term effects of sleep disruption. The nurse can help clients to use behavioral measures instead of drugs to cure sleep problems.

Client Teaching

To develop good sleep habits at home, clients and their bed partners should learn techniques that promote sleep and conditions that interfere with sleep. Parents of young children can also learn good sleep hygiene habits.

Sample Evaluation of Interventions for Sleep Disturbances

Goals	Evaluative Measures	Expected Outcomes
Client obtains sense of restfulness after sleep.	Note client's verbal expression of sense of restfulness. Note client's report of number of awakenings and sleep duration. Ask spouse or partner to describe client's daytime behaviors and behavior before falling asleep.	Client expresses a feeling of being rested. Client falls asleep within 20 to 30 minutes. Client reports fewer awakenings during sleep than before therapy. Client is able to return to sleep within minutes after awakening. Client is able to sleep the desired length of time. Client recalls episodes of dreaming. Client describes bedtime rituals conducive to relaxation
Client experiences fewer symptoms of sleep deprivation.	Note client's verbal description of feelings after sleep. Note client's description of behaviors at work or at home during the day. Observe nonverbal expressions and behaviors.	Client expresses a feeling of being rested. Client describes fewer episodes of feeling irritable, depressed, or anxious. Client reports being able to complete work related responsibilities successfully. Client appears relaxed and demonstrates clear memory, judgment, and reasoning.
Client understands factors that promote or disrupt sleep.	Note client's or partner's description of good sleep habits. Note client's or partner's description of factors that disrupt sleep.	Client describes use of good sleep habits in the home setting. Client and partner can discuss factors or behaviors that disrupt sleep.

Clients will benefit more from instructions based on information about their home setting and the client's life-style. For example, a suggestion for the client to control noise at night has little use if the client lives near a busy airport. Any suggestions for relaxing bedtime activities should include activities the client enjoys.

Clients should also learn how disease states can affect sleep. For example, a client with a hiatal hernia should learn to avoid eating large meals before bedtime. This prevents an irritating regurgitation of food into the esophagus that causes burning and keeps the person from being able to fall or stay asleep. Another important topic for client education is proper use of sleep medications. Clients should learn about alternative measures for promoting sleep (for example, relaxation and warm baths). A client should also be taught the hazards of sleeping medications to avoid side effects or drug-dependence insomnia.

EVALUATION

Each client has a different need for sleep and rest. For this reason the evaluation of therapies designed to promote sleep and rest must be individualized. Clients in relatively good health may not need as much sleep or require as many adjustments to their sleep patterns as clients whose physical conditions are poor.

The nurse is effective in promoting rest and sleep if the goals of care are met. The nurse uses evaluative criteria in determining the outcome of all sleep therapies (see evaluation box).

SUMMARY

Each day a person needs sleep to protect and restore body functions. Normally the sleep-wake cycle follows a 24-hour rhythm that is coordinated with other physiological functions such as body temperature and hormonal secretions. Sleep is a rhythm within a rhythm. After falling asleep, a person passes through a series of stages that help the body to rest and recover.

All age groups have different sleep requirements and sleep habits. A person's age affects the type of sleep therapies used by the nurse. The nurse's care may differ in the home setting compared to measures used to promote sleep in a hospital or extended care setting.

Many factors can promote or disrupt sleep, and a number of sleep disorders can cause specific problems for clients. The nurse is responsible for assessing the nature of any sleep pattern. The client's participation in the plan of care will ensure an individualized approach to sleep therapy.

KEY CONCEPTS

✓ Rest is not inactivity but a feeling of physical calm and freedom from worry.

✓ Sleep is a sustained period of rest during which a person experiences a reduced level of consciousness.

✓ The 24-hour sleep-wake cycle is a circadian rhythm that influences physiological function and behavior.

✓ The control and regulation of sleep depends on a balance between central nervous system regulators.

✓ During a typical night's sleep a person passes through several sleep cycles, each of which contain five separate stages of sleep.

✓ REM sleep is the stage of vivid dreaming that helps restore mental function.

✓ No specific number of hours of sleep is needed by each person to rest.

✓ Neonates, infants, and young children require more sleep than older children and adults.

✓ The elderly awaken more often during the night, and stage 4 sleep declines.

✓ Symptoms of various disease processes may disrupt sleep.

✓ Long-term use of sleeping pills may lead to difficulty in initiating and maintaining sleep.

✓ The hectic pace of a person's life-style, emotional and psychological stress, and alcohol ingestion all disrupt the sleep pattern.

✓ An environment with a darkened room, reduced noise, a comfortable bed, and good ventilation promotes sleep.

✓ The most common type of sleep disorder is insomnia, which is characterized by the inability to fall asleep or remain asleep during the night.

✓ Assessment of a client's sleep history involves an analysis of the client's normal sleep pattern, the nature of the sleep disturbance, and the identification of factors that impair the client's sleep.

✓ Diagnosing a client's sleep problem depends on identifying factors that impair sleep.

✓ In using environmental controls to promote sleep, the nurse should consider the client's home environment and normal life-style.

✓ A bedtime ritual of relaxing activities prepares a person physically and mentally for sleep.

✓ Pain control is essential to promote a client's ability to sleep.

✓ One of the most important nursing interventions for promoting sleep is establishing periods for sleep and rest.

REFERENCES

Block, AJ: Respiratory disorders during sleep. I. Heart Lung 9:1011, 1980.

Canavan, T: The psychobiology of sleep. Nurs 84, 2:682, 1984.

Chuman, MA: The neurological basis of sleep, Heart Lung 12:177, 1983.

Colling, J: Sleep disturbances in aging: a theoretical and empiric analysis, ANS 6:36, 1983.

Feierman, JR: Disordered sleep, Emerg Med 17:160, 1985.

Fisher, ME: ICU syndrome, Crit Care Nurs 4:39, 1984.

Hauri, P: Current concepts: the sleep disorders, ed. 2, Kalamazoo, Mich., 1982, The Upjohn Co.

Hoch, C, and Reynolds, C III: Sleep disturbances and what to do about them, Geriatr Nurs 7:24, 1986.

Kales, A, and Kales, J: Sleep disorders: recent findings in the diagnostic and treatment of disturbed sleep, N Engl J Med 290:487, 1974.

Langford, GW, et al.: Spontaneous arousals from sleep in human subjects, Psychonomic Science 28:228, 1972.

McNeil, BJ, et al.: Sleep quetionnaire, AJN 86(1):261, 1986.

Ross, MS, et al.: When sleep won't come: helping our elderly clients, Can Nurs 82:14, 1986.

Seidlitz, P: Excessive noise levels determintal to patients, staff, Hosp Prog 62:54, 1981.

Research Articles

Clapin-French, E: Sleep patterns of aged persons in long-term care facilities, J Adv Nurs 11:57, 1986.

Hayter, J: Sleep behavior of older persons, Nurs Res 32:242, 1983.

Hayter, J: To nap or not to nap? Geriatr Nurs 6:104, 1985.

Horne, JA, and Ostberg, O: A self-assessment questionnaire to determine morningness-eveningness in human circadian rhythms, Int J Chronobiology 4:97, 1976.

Schmidt-Kessen, W, and Kendel, K: Einfluss der Raumtemperatur auf den Nachtschlaf, Res Exp Med 160:220, 1973.

Webster, RA, and Thompson, DR: Sleep in hospital, J Adv Nurs 11:447, 1986.

Williams, RL, et al.: Effects of prolonged stage four and 1-REM sleep deprivation, EEG, task performance and psychologic responses, SAM-TR-67-59, United States Air Force School of Aerospace Medicine, Florida University, Gainesville, 1967.

ADDITIONAL READINGS

Brewer, MJ: To sleep or not to sleep: the consequences of sleep deprivation, Crit Care Nurs 5:35, 1985.

Ebersole, P, and Hess, P: Toward healthy aging: human needs and nursing response, ed. 3, St. Louis, 1989, The C.V. Mosby Co.

Fernsebner, B: Sleep deprivation in patients, AORN J 37:35, 1983.

Fosnot, H: When the patterns of sleep go askew, Patient Care 14:122, 1980.

Hayter, J: The rhythm of sleep, Am J Nurs 80:457, 1980.

Helton, MC, et al.: The correlation between sleep deprivation and the intensive care unit syndrome, Heart Lung 9:464, 1980.

Melnechuk, T: The dream machine, Psychology Today, 17:22, 1983.

Orem, J, and Barnes, CD, editors: Physiology in sleep, New York, 1980, Academic Press.

Potempa, K, et al.: Chronic fatigue, Image: J Nurs Sch, 18:165, 1986.

Reynolds, CF III et al.: Sleeping pills for the elderly: are they ever justified? J Clin Psychiatry 46:9, Feb. 1985.

Schirmer, MS: When sleep won't come, J Gerontol Nurs 9:16, 1983.

Simmons, FB, et al.: The palatopharyngoplasty operation for snoring and sleep apnea: an interim report, Otolaryngol Head Neck Surg 92:375, 1984.

Synder-Halpern, R: The effect of critical care unit noise on patient sleep cycles. CQ, 7:41-51, 1985.

Taub, JM: Acute shifts in sleep-wakefulness: effects on performance and moods, Psychosom Med, 36:164, 1974.

Walseben, J: Sleep disorders, Am J Nurs 82:936, 1982.

Weaver, TE, and Millman, RP: Broken sleep, Am J Nurs 86:146, 1986.

Whaley, LF, and Wong, DL: Nursing care of infants and children, ed 3, St. Louis, 1987, The C.V. Mosby Co.

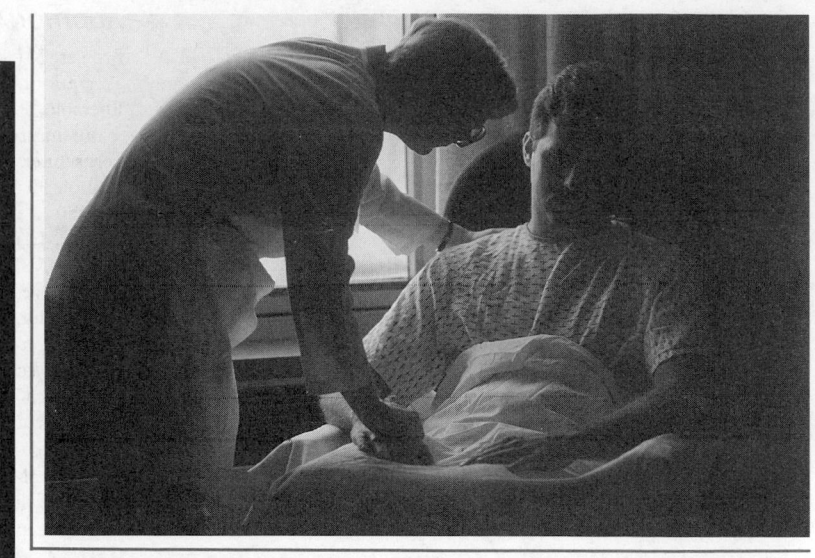

OBJECTIVES

Mastery of content in this chapter will enable the student to:

- Define the key terms listed.
- Discuss common misconceptions about pain.
- Identify components of the pain experience.
- Discuss the three phases of behavioral responses experienced with pain.
- Explain the relationship of the gate control theory to select nursing therapies for pain relief.
- Perform an assessment of a client experiencing pain.
- Describe guidelines for individualizing pain therapies.
- Identify the techniques and rationale for selecting pain therapies.
- Explain common causes for undertreatment of pain with analgesics.
- Discuss the purpose and services of a hospice program.
- Provide nursing therapies that prevent or reduce a client's pain.

KEY TERMS

Afferent
Analgesic
Anesthesia
Chordotomy
Concomitant Symptoms
Cutaneous Stimulation
Efferent
Endorphin
Epidural
Exacerbation
Intractable Pain
Localized Pain
Narcotic
Neurotransmitter
Noxious
Pain
Perception
Placebo
Radiating Pain
Reaction
Reception
Referred Pain
Remission
Threshold
Tolerance
Transcutaneous Electrical Nerve Stimulation (TENS)

Comfort

Everyone experiences some type or degree of pain. Pain that results from a cut finger or decayed tooth is self-limiting, predictable, and tolerated well by most people. Pain from a terminal illness, an unknown or undiagnosed source, or a serious injury is indeterminate in length, unpredictable in its course, and less tolerated. The person in pain feels distress or suffering and seeks relief.

A client values the nurse's ability to bring relief from suffering. However, the nurse cannot see or feel the client's pain. No two persons experience pain in the same way, and no two painful events create identical responses or feelings in a person. Total relief never comes for many individuals in pain, and the nurse can only use interventions that minimize it.

Nurses care for clients in many settings and situations that provide the opportunity to promote comfort. The nurse has a responsibility to discover what the experience of pain is like and to initiate measures that either provide relief or help the client learn to cope.

NATURE OF PAIN

Pain is much more than a single sensation caused by a specific stimulus. Pain is subjective and highly individualized, and the interpretation and meaning of pain involve psychosocial and cultural factors. The person experiencing pain is the only authority about his or her pain. According to McCaffery (1980), "Pain is whatever the experiencing person says it is, existing whenever he says it does." Pain cannot be objectively measured, such as with an x-ray or blood test. Although certain types of pain create predictable signs and symptoms, often the nurse can only assess pain by relying on the client's words and behavior. Only the client knows whether pain is present and what the experience is like. To help a client gain relief, the nurse must believe that the pain exists.

Pain is a protective physiological mechanism. A person with a sprained ankle avoids bearing full weight on the foot to prevent further injury. Pain is a warning that tissue damage has occurred. The client who is unable to feel sensations, such as one with a spinal cord tumor will be unaware of pain-inducing injuries.

Pain is a leading cause of disability and one of the most common reasons for seeking health care. As the average life span increases, more people have chronic disease in which pain is a common symptom. In addition, medical advances have resulted in diagnostic and therapeutic measures that are often uncomfortable. Pain is one of the most common problems faced by nurses, yet it is a source of frustration and is often one of the most misunderstood problems the nurse confronts.

PREJUDICES AND MISCONCEPTIONS

Health care personnel often hold prejudices toward clients in pain. When there is a lack of objective evidence pointing to the source of pain, nurses may find it hard to believe it exists. The attitudes many nurses have about clients in pain are partly due to the traditional medical model of illness. This model supports the belief that disordered body states result from physical causes. Thus pain is viewed as a physical response to organic dysfunction. Under these assumptions pain for which there is no organic basis may be labeled "psychogenic" or "unreal" (Taylor et al., 1984). When no obvious source of pain can be found nurses often negatively stereotype the pain sufferer as a complainer or difficult client.

Taylor et al. (1984) studied 268 registered nurses who worked in a variety of specialty and general medical-surgical units. Each nurse was asked to read a one paragraph description of a hypothetical client, described as either an acute or chronic pain sufferer. After reading the paragraph each nurse estimated the suffering of the hypothetical client and rated the client on a series of personality and behavioral traits. The study showed the majority of nurses attributing significantly less suffering to the hypothetical clients in chronic, long-term pain than those with acute pain of short duration. The nurses also felt that the hypothetical clients who had no signs of pathology suffered less than those with pathological signs. The study also showed nurses to have negative attitudes toward clients having low back pain.

Common Biases and Misconceptions about Pain

- Drug abusers and alcoholics overact to discomforts.
- Clients with minor illnesses have less pain than those with severe physical alterations.
- Administering analgesics regularly will lead to the client's drug dependence.
- The amount of tissue damage in an injury can accurately indicate pain intensity.
- Health care personnel are the best authorities on the nature of the client's pain.
- Psychogenic pain is not real.

The extent to which nurses make assumptions about clients in pain seriously limits the nurse's ability to offer pain relief. Unfortunately, all people are influenced by prejudices based on their culture, education, and experience. Too often nurses allow misconceptions about pain (see box) to affect their willingness to intervene. Many nurses even avoid acknowledging a client's pain because of their own fear and denial.

To help a client gain comfort or relief, the nurse must view the experience through the client's eyes. Acknowledging personal prejudices or misconceptions will also help the nurse address the client's problem more professionally. The nurse who becomes an active, knowledgeable observer of a client in pain will make a more objective analysis of the pain experience. The client makes the diagnosis that pain is present, and the nurse works to apply techniques and skills that ultimately give relief.

COMPONENTS OF THE PAIN EXPERIENCE

Pain is a complex interplay of physical, emotional, and behavioral reactions. To best understand the pain experience it helps to describe the three components of pain: reception, perception, and reaction. A client in pain cannot discriminate between the components. However, understanding each stage will help the nurse recognize factors that can cause pain, symptoms that accompany pain, and actions of therapies.

Reception

Reception is the neurophysiological component of the pain experience. Pain results from actual or potential tissue damage and is caused by a physical stimulus. Nox-

TABLE 35-1   Physical Sources of Pain

Source	Type of Stimulus	Pathophysiological Processes
Trauma	Mechanical, chemical	Tissue damage, inflammation, direct irritation of nerve endings
Ischemia	Chemical	Decreased blood flow to body part (for example, blocked coronary artery)
Alteration in body fluids	Mechanical	Edema distending body tissues
Duct distention	Mechanical	Overstretching of duct's narrow lumen (for example, passage of kidney stone through ureter)
Perforated visceral organ	Chemical	Chemical irritation by secretions on sensitive nerve endings (for example, ruptured appendix or duodenal ulcer)
Space-occupying lesion (tumor)	Mechanical	Irritation of peripheral nerves by growth of lesion within a confined space
Burn (heat or extreme cold)	Thermal	Inflammation or loss of superficial layers of epidermis causing increased sensitivity of nerve endings.

ious (pain) stimuli may result from thermal, mechanical, chemical, or electrical stimuli.

Thermal stimuli result from skin contact with hot or cold substances. Pressure, friction, tension, and stretching are mechanical stimuli. Chemical stimuli originate from substances within the body, such as gastric enzymes and histamines, or from substances outside the body such as caustic chemicals. An electrical current causes an electrical stimulus. Table 35-1 summarizes physical alterations that elicit pain-producing stimuli. The nurse's awareness of factors that cause pain can aid in prevention and use of pain relief therapies.

Once tissue damage occurs, free nerve endings found in skin, muscle, bone, and mucous membranes convert pain stimuli into electrical nerve impulses. Not all tissues contain receptors that transmit pain signals. The brain and alveoli of the lung are examples of tissues insensitive to pain. Some receptors respond only to one type of pain stimulus while others are also sensitive to temperature and pressure. The pain threshold is reached when a stimulus is intense enough to creat a nerve impulse. Normally the physiological pain threshold does not differ among individuals even of different racial or cultural backgrounds (Guyton, 1985).

Nerve impulses resulting from the painful stimulus travel along afferent peripheral nerve fibers to the spinal cord where it synapses with spinal nerves. Two types of peripheral nerve fibers conduct painful stimuli. Unmyelinated C fibers are small and conduct impulses slowly, and myelinated A fibers are larger and conduct impulses rapidly. The A fibers send impulses that localize the source of pain and detect pain intensity. C fibers relay impulses of a more diffuse nature. For example, after stepping on a nail, a person initially feels a sharp localized pain, which is the result of A-fiber transmission. Within a few seconds pain becomes more diffuse and widespread until the whole foot aches because of C-fiber innervation. Both A and C fibers enter the spinal cord through the dorsal roots of spinal nerves and travel up and down segments of the spinal cord before crossing over to the opposite side. After synapsing with longer nerve fibers in the dorsal and spinothalamic nerve tracts, pain impulses travel up the spinal cord. Fig 35-1 shows the normal pain reception pathway. Once the pain impulse ascends the spinal cord, information is transmitted quickly to higher centers in the brain, including the reticular formation, limbic system, thalamus, and sensory cortex.

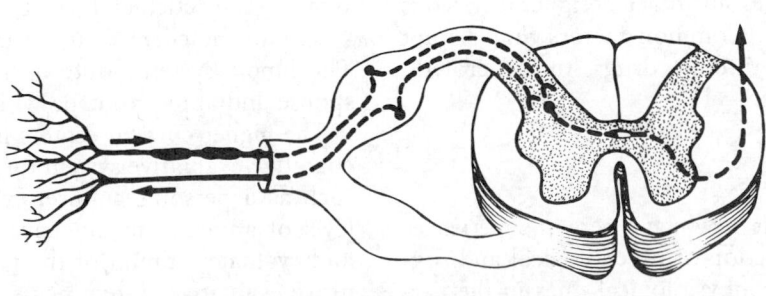

Fig. 35-1   Pain reception pathway.

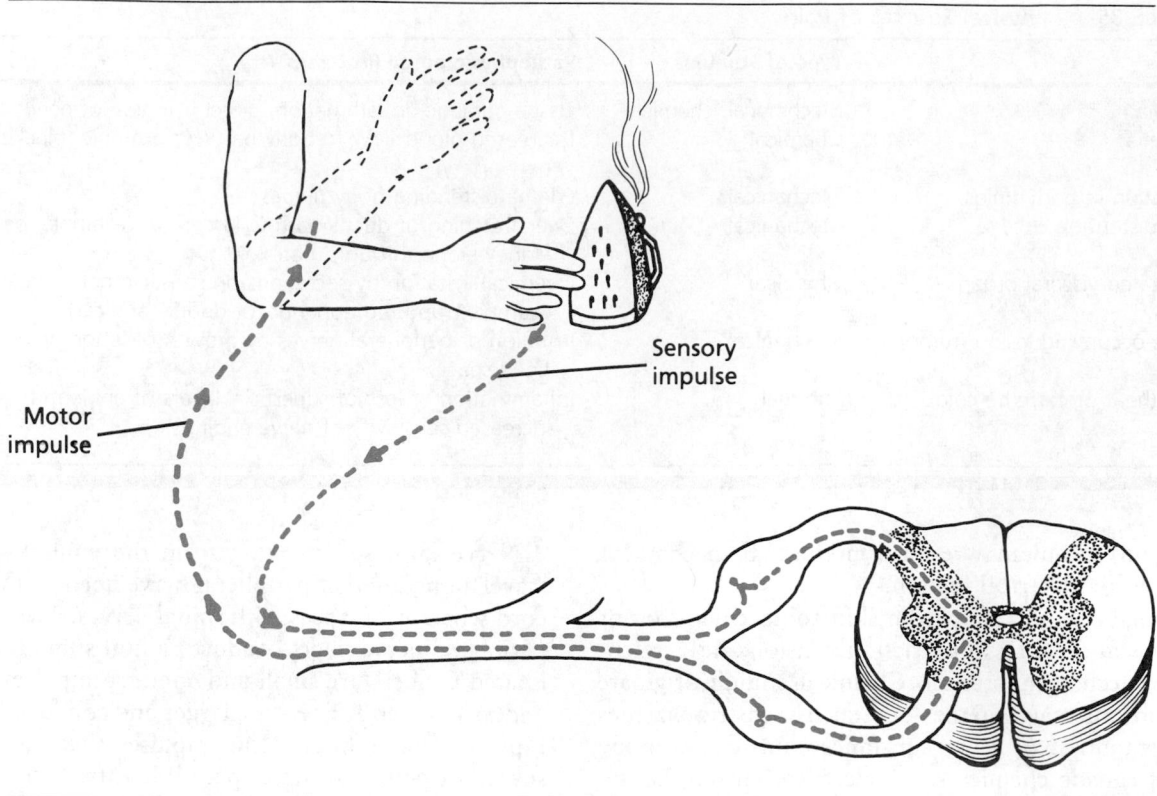

Fig. 35-2 Protective reflex to pain stimulus.

There is also a protective reflex response that occurs with pain reception (Fig. 35-2). A fibers send sensory impulses to the spinal cord, where they synapse with spinal motor neurons. The motor impulses travel via a reflex arc along efferent nerve fibers back to a peripheral muscle near the site of pain stimulation. Contraction of the muscle leads to a protective withdrawal from the source of pain. For example, when a person accidentally touches a hot iron, a burning sensation is felt but the hand also reflexively withdraws from the iron's surface. When superficial fibers in the skin are stimulated, a person moves away from the pain source. If internal tissues such as muscle or mucous membranes become stimulated, tightening and guarding of muscles occur.

Pain reception requires an intact peripheral nervous system and spinal cord. Common factors that disrupt pain reception include trauma, drugs, tumor growth, and metabolic disorders.

Perception

Perception is the point at which a person experiences pain. There is an interaction of psychological and cognitive factors with neurophysiological ones in the perception of pain. Meinhart and McCaffery (1983) describe three interactional systems of pain perception as sensory-discriminative, motivational-effective, and cognitive-evaluative. The sensory-discriminative system involves an interaction of nerve transmission between the thalamus and sensory cortex. As a result a person perceives the location, severity, and character of pain. A functional nervous system is required for pain perception. Any factor that lowers a client's level of consciousness such as analgesics, anesthetics, or cerebral disease impairs pain perception. In contrast, conditions that heighten a person's awareness or sensitivity to stimuli increase pain perception. Sensory restriction and sleep deprivation increase pain perception.

The reticular formation and limbic system in the brainstem are important to the motivational-affective system. The reticular formation creates a defensive response in the client to interrupt or avoid pain stimuli. The limbic system controls the client's emotional response and ability to cope with pain.

The higher cortical centers in the brain influence the cognitive-evaluative system for pain perception. Factors such as a person's culture, experience with pain, and level of anxiety can influence how a person processes and evaluates stimuli of the pain experience. The cognitive-evaluative system helps a person interpret intensity and quality of pain so action can be taken.

Each person learns from painful experiences in an

individual way. Previous experience does not necessarily mean a person will accept pain more easily in the future. If a person has had frequent episodes of pain without relief or bouts of severe pain, personal perceptions are those of anxiety or even fear. In contrast, if a person has had repeated experiences with the same type of pain but the pain has successfully been relieved, it becomes easier to interpret the pain sensation. As a result, the client is better prepared to take necessary actions in relieving the pain.

When a client has had no experience with pain, the first perception of pain can impair the ability to cope with it. For example, after abdominal surgery it is common for a client to experience severe incisional pain for several days. Unless the client is aware of this, the onset of pain may be viewed as a serious complication. Rather than participate actively in postoperative breathing exercises (see Chapter 46), the client may lie immobile in bed and breathe shallowly in fear that something has gone wrong. The nurse should prepare the client with a clear explanation of the type of pain that will be experienced and what can be done to reduce it.

Values about pain and the manner in which it should be expressed are also a part of pain perception. If the client views pain as a personal weakness or a deserved punishment, he or she may not express discomfort. If the client perceives pain as unwarranted or as a threat to comfort and existence, the individual is less hesitant to express pain. A person who values the support of significant others, is likely to feel the need to express pain openly.

Anxiety often increases perception of pain. An emotionally healthy person is usually able to tolerate moderate or even severe pain better than one whose emotions are less stable.

ENDORPHINS

The body contains a natural supply of morphine-like substances called endorphins. Stress and pain activate endorphins. Located within the brain, spinal cord, and gastrointestinal tract, they regulate and modify painful stimuli by affecting neurotransmitters. Analgesia results when certain endorphins attach to opiate receptors in the brain. People who have less pain than others from a similar injury generally have higher endorphin levels. Pain relief measures such as transcutaneous electrical nerve stimulation and acupuncture are believed to cause release of endorphins. The effects of placebos may also be related to endorphin levels. But, it is not known how some persons are able to activate their endorphins.

Endorphins may cause differences in sensitivity to pain. In some persons, anxiety over pain may release endorphins. In chronic pain, endorphins often cease to function (Meinhart and McCaffery, 1983).

Reaction

The reaction to pain is the physiological and behavioral responses that occur once pain is perceived.

PHYSIOLOGICAL RESPONSES

As pain impulses ascend the spinal cord toward the brainstem and thalamus, the autonomic nervous system becomes stimulated as part of the stress response. Pain of low to moderate intensity and superficial pain elicit the "flight-or-fight" reaction of the general adaptation syndrome (see Chapter 28). Stimulation of the sympathetic branch of the autonomic nervous system results in physiological responses summarized in Table 35-2. If the pain is unrelenting, severe, or deep, typically originating from involvement of the visceral organs (such as with a myocardial infarction and colic from gallbladder

TABLE 35-2   Physiological Responses to Pain

Response	Cause or Effect
SYMPATHETIC STIMULATION*	
Dilation of bronchial tubes and increased respiratory rate.	Provides greater O_2 intake
Increased heart rate	Provides greater O_2 transport
Peripheral vasoconstriction (pallor, elevation in blood pressure)	Elevates blood pressure with shift of blood supply from periphery and viscera to skeletal muscles and brain
Increased blood glucose	Provides additional energy
Diaphoresis	Controls body temperature during stress
Increased muscle tension	Prepares muscles for action
Dilation of pupils	Affords better vision
Decreased gastrointestinal motility	Frees energy for more immediate activity
PARASYMPATHETIC STIMULATION†	
Pallor	Blood supply shifts away from periphery
Muscle tension	Result of fatigue
Decreased heart rate and blood pressure	Vagal stimulation
Rapid, irregular breathing	Body defenses begin to fail under prolonged stress of pain
Nausea and vomiting	Return of gastrointestinal function
Weakness or exhaustion	Expenditure of physical energy

*Pain of low to moderate intensity and superficial pain
†Severe or deep pain

or renal stones), the parasympathetic nervous system goes into action. Sustained physiological responses to pain could cause serious harm to an individual. Except in cases of severe traumatic pain, which may send a person into shock, most people reach a level of adaptation in which physical signs return to normal. Thus a client in pain will not always exhibit physical signs throughout its duration.

BEHAVIORAL RESPONSES

Meinhart and McCaffery (1983) describe three phases of a pain experience: anticipation, sensation, and aftermath. The anticipation phase occurs before onset of perceived pain. A person knows that pain will occur. In situations of traumatic injury or unforeseen painful procedures a person will not anticipate pain. The anticipation phase is perhaps most important, since it can affect the other two.

Anticipation of pain often allows a person to learn about pain and its relief. With adequate instruction and support, clients learn to understand pain and control anxiety before it occurs. Nurses play an important role in helping clients during the anticipatory phase. With proper guidance, clients become aware of the unknown and thus cope with their discomfort. In situations where clients are too fearful or anxious, anticipation of pain can heighten the perception of pain severity.

Sensation of pain occurs when pain is felt. How people choose to react to discomfort varies widely. A person's tolerance to pain is the point at which there is an unwillingness to accept pain of greater severity or duration. How well a person tolerates pain depends on attitudes, motivation, and values.

Pain threatens physical and psychological well-being. A client may be reluctant to express pain, considering it a sign of weakness. Often clients believe that being a "good patient" means not expressing pain to avoid bothering people around them. Another reason clients may not express pain is that maintaining self-control is important in their culture. The client with high pain tolerance is able to endure periods of severe pain without assistance. Often a nurse must encourage such a client to accept pain-relieving measures so activity or nutritional intake is not seriously curtailed.

In contrast, a client with low pain tolerance may seek relief before pain occurs. For example, a client may request an aspirin in anticipation of a headache. The client's ability to tolerate pain significantly influences the nurse's perceptions of degree of the discomfort. Often the nurse is willing to attend to the client whose pain tolerance is high. Yet it is unfair to ignore the needs of the client who cannot tolerate even minor pain.

Typical body movements and facial expressions that indicate pain include holding the painful part, bent posture and facial grimacing. A client may be more ex-

TABLE 35-3 Disorders that Cause Pain

Disorder	Pain Characteristics
Kidney disease	Abdominal aching
	Tenderness and pain in the back area of the costovertebral angle
Angina pectoris	Crushing sensation in chest, often radiating down left shoulder and arm
Ruptured intravertebral disc	Low back pain accompanied by pain radiating down the leg
Gastric ulcer	Burning pain around umbilicus; referred pain in shoulder
Trigeminal neuralgia	Lightning-like or stabbing pain along distribution of trigeminal nerve, involving gums, lips, mouth, nose, and chin

pressive by crying or moaning. Often a client expresses discomfort through frequent requests to the nurse. The nurse soon learns to recognize patterns of behavior that reflect pain. However, lack of pain expression does not necessarily mean that the client is not experiencing pain. Unless a client openly reacts to pain, it is difficult to determine the nature and extent of discomfort. A role of the nurse is helping the client communicate the pain response effectively. A nurse's knowledge of the disease or illness helps anticipate the client's pain. For example, a ruptured intravertebral disc in a lower lumbar vertebra typically causes severe low back pain in addition to pain that radiates or extends down the leg. Table 35-3 summarizes common disorders that cause pain.

The aftermath phase of pain occurs when it is reduced or stopped. Even though the source of discomfort is controlled, a client may still require the nurse's attention. Pain is a crisis. After a painful experience clients may experience physical symptoms such as chills, nausea, vomiting, anger, or depression. If there are repeated episodes of pain, aftermath responses can become serious health problems in themselves. The nurse helps clients gain control and self-esteem to minimize fear over potential pain experiences.

GATE CONTROL THEORY OF PAIN

There have been several attempts to explain the complexity of pain in terms of the relationship of physiological, psychological, and cognitive variables. The gate control theory, proposed by Melzack and Wall (1965) is the most comprehensive. The theory suggests that pain impulses can be regulated or even blocked by gating

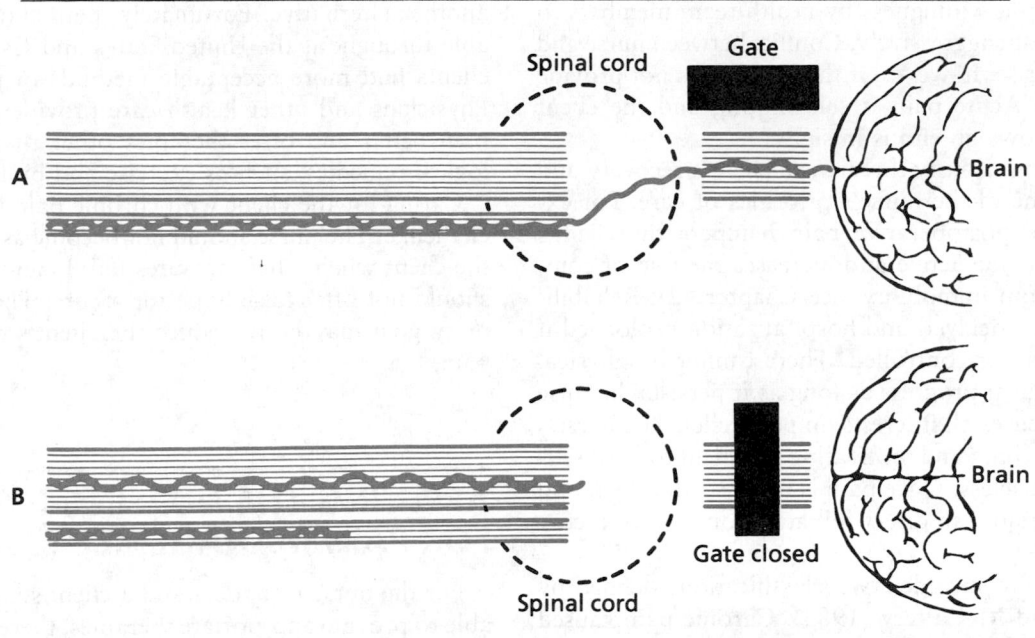

Fig. 35-3 Diagrammatic sketch of gate control theory. **A,** Small type C nerve fibers conduct pain impulses to the brain. **B,** Synapses are stimulated by impulses traveling across large nerve fibers acting as gates to block pain impulses.

mechanisms located along the central nervous system. The proposed location of the gates is in the dorsal horn of the spinal cord. When gates are open, pain impulses flow freely. When gates are closed, pain impulses become blocked. Partial opening of the gates may also occur.

Small C fibers carry most potentially painful impulses. Excitation of C fibers inhibits gating mechanisms so that pain stimuli flow easily to cortical centers of the brain. Large A fibers pass through the same gating mechanisms (Fig. 35-3). Whether the gates remain open or closed depends on whether competing messages from larger nerve fibers stimulate the gating mechanism. A bombardment of large-fiber sensory impulses such as those from the pressure of a backrub or the heat of a warm compress will close the gates to pain stimuli. Transmission of pain impulses from the spinal cord to the cerebral cortex can be inhibited or facilitated, thus altering pain perception.

It is also believed that the reticular formation in the brainstem can send inhibitory signals to gating mechanisms. When there is excess sensory input, as in the case of pain, the reticular formation can close gates. Some clients can be distracted from pain by removing the sensation of pain from their center of attention. Auditory or visual stimuli can distract clients and help make pain more tolerable.

Gating mechanisms can also be altered by thoughts, feelings, and memories. The cerebral cortex and thala-

mus can influence whether pain impulses reach a person's conscious awareness. The realization that, in a sense, there is conscious control over how pain is perceived helps explain the different ways people react and adjust to pain. The gate control theory gives the nurse a conceptual basis for pain relief measures.

ACUTE AND CHRONIC PAIN

Everyone experiences some level of pain throughout the day. Common examples include the ache of over-exercised muscles, the burning discomfort from eye strain, or pressure felt from sitting in one position for too long. These minor discomforts rarely cause one to seek health care.

The pain that nurses most often observe in clients includes acute and chronic pain, classified by the duration for which pain lasts. Acute pain is defined by Meinhart and McCaffery (1983) as pain that has a rapid onset, varies in intensity, and lasts for a brief time or up to 6 months. The function of acute pain is to warn persons of impending injury or disease. Acute pain eventually resolves with or without treatment once a damaged area heals.

Clients in acute pain are frightened, anxious, and expect relief quickly. The time sequence of acute pain usually results in a willingness by health team members to treat acute pain aggressively. Conflict between nurse and client may arise, however, if the nurse does not provide quick relief. Acute pain is self-limiting and the client therefore knows an end is in sight.

Acute pain seriously threatens a client's recovery and should be one of the nurse's priorities of care. For example, acute postoperative pain hampers the client's ability to become active and increases the risk of complications from immobility (see Chapter 42). Rehabilitation may be delayed and hospitalization prolonged if acute pain is not controlled. There cannot be physical or psychological progress as long as it persists, because the client focuses all interests on pain relief. The nurse's efforts at teaching and motivating the client toward self-care will be useless. Once pain is relieved, the client and health care team can direct full attention toward recovery.

Chronic pain includes two classifications defined by Meinhart and McCaffery (1983). Chronic pain caused by uncontrolled cancer is often called intractable pain. It can last a prolonged time until a client's death. Health care workers usually are willing to treat cancer pain as aggressively as acute pain. Often, however, family members are unwilling to administer needed narcotics for fear of causing side effects such as lethargy or drug dependence.

The other form of chronic pain is benign or persistent and lasts for more than 6 months. The problem with benign, chronic pain is that there may not be a known disease or injury causing the pain. An injured area may have healed long ago, yet pain persists. The client with chronic pain often has periods of remissions (partial or complete disappearance of symptoms) and exacerbations (increase in severity). The unpredictabilty of chronic pain frustrates the client, frequently leading to psychological depression. The pain becomes part of every aspect of the individual's life. Chronic pain is a major cause of psychological and physical disability leading to problems such as loss of job, inability to perform simple daily activities, sexual dysfunction, and social isolation from family and friends.

The person with chronic pain often does not show overt symptoms. The individual does not adapt to the pain but seems to suffer more with time as physical and mental exhaustion occur. Symptoms of chronic pain include fatigue, insomnia, anorexia, weight loss, depression, hopelessness, and anger.

The life of a person with chronic pain can be tragic. Often the person consults many physicians and therefore accumulates various medications and therapies. However, taking several medications may result in undesirable side effects. Clients desperate for pain relief may fall prey to quackery, for example, special liniments, diets, or pain-relief devices. Alcohol abuse may become

another alternative. Fortunately, pain clinics are available throughout the United States and Canada to help clients find more acceptable methods of pain control. Physicians and other health care providers understand pain better and offer therapies other than pharmacological remedies, such as exercise and biofeedback.

Caring for the client with chronic pain is an unusual challenge. The nurse should not become as frustrated as the client when relief measures fail. Likewise, the nurse should not offer false hope for a cure. The nurse's primary goal may be to reduce the client's perception of pain.

APPLYING THE NURSING PROCESS FOR PAIN MANAGEMENT

For the nurse to understand a client's pain and to be able to provide appropriate therapies, there is a need for a systematic approach to pain management. The nursing process is the best model to ensure accurate analysis and management of pain.

ASSESSMENT

The key to assessing pain is not ignoring the client. The nurse should explore the pain experience thoroughly. Nurses cannot allow personal biases to prejudice assessment of pain. Viewing the pain from the client's perspective will enable a more accurate assessment.

When assessing pain, the nurse must be sensitive to the client's level of discomfort. If pain is acute or severe, it is unlikely that the client can provide a detailed description of the entire pain experience. During an episode of acute pain the nurse primarily assesses the client's physiological responses as well as the location, severity, and quality of the pain. A more thorough pain assessment takes time and should be conducted when the client becomes more alert and attentive.

CLIENT'S EXPRESSION OF PAIN

A problem in pain assessment is that many clients fail to report or discuss discomfort. In a study by Jacox and Stewart (1973), two thirds of the 72 clients studied were reluctant to discuss pain and tried instead to remain calm and silent. To complicate pain assessment more, many nurses believe that if clients have pain they will report it. This is not always true.

A client must trust a nurse and perceive the nurse's willingness to help before discussing the pain experience openly. If a client senses that the nurse doubts that pain exists, little information will be shared. The nurse must develop a positive therapeutic relationship and encourage clients to discuss pain. The nurse avoids aggravating pain with a lengthy assessment.

The nurse should learn how the client communicates discomfort. Can the client communicate verbally? Will nonverbal behaviors be the best source of information? If the client speaks a different language, pain assessment will be difficult. A family member or interpreter may be necessary to describe the client's feelings and sensations. Often clients in pain will confide in only one person.

CLASSIFICATION OF THE PAIN EXPERIENCE

The nurse should identify the phase of pain the client is undergoing. Whether the client is in the anticipatory, sensation, or aftermath phase influences not only the client's symptoms but the types of therapies most likely to relieve pain. Clients likely to be in the anticipatory phase include those scheduled to undergo invasive diagnostic or therapeutic procedures, surgery, and those with a history of recurring pain such as the anginal pain of myocardial ischemia. These clients may be anxious, fearful, or they may ask questions about upcoming pain. Clients in the sensation phase generally demonstrate signs and symptoms of discomfort. Clients with traumatic injuries and post-operative clients are in a condition that discourages the nurse from asking several detailed questions. The client who is sensing pain, especially if severe, wants relief fast. When a person is in the aftermath of discomfort the nurse must assess carefully for physical or psychological aftereffects. The client may express apologies to the nurse for acting "improperly" during the pain experience.

It is important for the nurse to assess if the client's pain is acute or chronic. If the pain is acute a detailed assessment is needed of pain characteristics. With chronic pain the nurse determines if it is intermittent, persistent, or of limited duration. Once the phase or type of pain is assessed, findings direct the nurse to conduct further assessment or begin specific interventions.

CHARACTERISTICS OF PAIN

The nature of the pain experience provides more detailed information for the nurse. Assessment data help establish medical and nursing diagnoses, as well as determine pain relief therapies.

ONSET AND DURATION. The nurse asks questions to determine the onset, duration, and time sequence of pain. When did the pain begin? How long has it lasted? Does it occur at the same time each day? How frequently does it recur?

It may be easier to diagnose the nature of pain by identifying time factors. The onset of sudden and severe pain is easier to assess than gradual, mild discomfort.

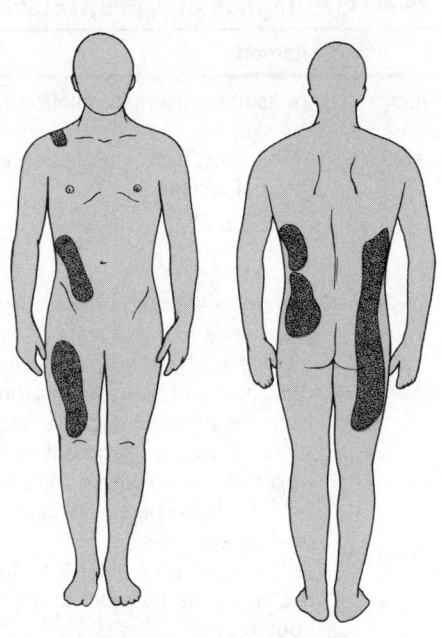

Fig. 35-4   Diagrammatic figures used to locate a client's pain.

An understanding of the time cycle of a client's pain helps the nurse know when to intervene and anticipate discomfort.

LOCATION. To assess pain location the nurse asks the client to point to the area of discomfort. To localize the pain more specifically, the nurse then has the client trace the area from the most severe point outward. This will be difficult to do if pain is diffuse, or involves large segments of the body. Some assessment tools have figures of the body (Fig. 35-4) on which the nurse can draw the location of the pain. This can be useful as a baseline if the pain should change.

When recording pain location the nurse uses anatomical landmarks and descriptive terminology. The statement, "The pain is localized in the upper right abdominal quadrant" is more specific than "The client states the pain is in his abdomen." Knowing a client's disease or illness can help the nurse locate pain more easily.

Pain, classified by location, may be superficial or cutaneous, deep or visceral, referred or radiating (Table 35-4).

SEVERITY. The severity or intensity of pain reaches a maximal intensity that a client perceives. Any increase in pain stimuli beyond that point will not cause greater pain. The cause of pain may be a clue to the intensity of discomfort, but this is not a reliable predictor (Meinhart and McCaffery, 1983).

TABLE 35-4 Classification of Pain by Location

Type	Definition	Characteristics	Examples
Superficial or cutaneous	Pain resulting from stimulation of the skin	Short duration, localized; usually a sharp sensation	Needle stick; small cut or laceration
Deep visceral	Pain resulting from stimulation of internal organs	Diffuse, may radiate in several directions; duration varies but usually lasts longer than superficial pain; pain may be sharp, dull, or unique to organ involved	Crushing sensation (for example, angina pectoris); burning sensation (for example, gastric ulcer)
Referred	Common phenomenon in visceral pain, since many of the organs themselves have no pain receptors; however, sensory neurons from the affected organ enter the same spinal cord segment as neurons from areas where the pain is felt; the brain perceives pain in unaffected areas	Pain is felt in a part of the body separate from the source of pain and may assume any characteristic	A myocardial infarction may cause referred pain to the jaw, left arm, and left shoulder; kidney stones may refer pain to the groin area
Radiating	A sensation of pain extending from the initial site of injury to another body part	Pain feels as though it travels down or along a body part; may be intermittent or constant	Low back pain from a ruptured intravertebral disc accompanied by pain radiating down the leg from sciatic nerve irritation

Intensity is one of the most subjective characteristics of pain. Clients are usually asked to describe pain severity by using terms such as mild, moderate, severe, or unbearable. The meaning of these terms can differ between nurse and client.

Descriptive scales are an objective means of measuring pain severity (Fig. 35-5). A numerical scale consists of a line divided by numbered points, which indicate pain intensities. A descriptive scale follows the same principle except that the points are described by increasing levels of severity. A visual analog scale does not have labeled subdivisions. Only the ends of the scale are labeled, giving the client total freedom in identifying severity. A pain scale should be designed so that it is easy for the nurse to administer and is not time consuming for the client to complete. If the client can easily understand the scale, the description should be more accurate.

Descriptive scales are useful not only in assessing the severity of pain but also in evaluating changes in the client's condition. The nurse can use the scales after therapy or when symptoms become aggravated to judge whether the pain has decreased or increased.

The nurse does not use pain scales to compare one client with another. Although the scales lend relative objectivity to measurement, the severity of pain is too subjective to permit comparisons between individuals.

QUALITY. Another subjective characteristic of pain is its quality. Because there is no common or specific pain vocabulary in general use, the words a client may choose to describe pain can apply to any number of things. Often, a client describes pain as "crushing," "throbbing," "sharp," "dull," or "burning." A client's pain is often indescribable.

Assessment is more accurate if a client can describe the sensation after open-ended questions. For example, the nurse might ask, "Tell me what your pain feels like." If a client cannot find words to describe the sensation the nurse may assist by giving examples of words to choose. Meinhart and McCaffery (1983) report that the qualities of pricking, burning, and aching are useful to first describe pain. Later the client may choose more descriptive terms.

There is some consistency in the way people describe certain types of pain. The pain associated with a myocardial infarction is often described as crushing or viselike, whereas the pain of a surgical incision is often described as sharp and stabbing. When the client's descriptions fit the pattern forming in the nurse's assessment, a clearer analysis can be made of the nature and type of pain.

PAIN PATTERN. There are many factors that can affect the character of pain. It can be helpful to assess specific events or conditions that precipitate or aggravate pain (Table 35-5). Body functions or movements may cause variation in pain (Adams, 1980). For example, a change in posture that causes pain usually indicates

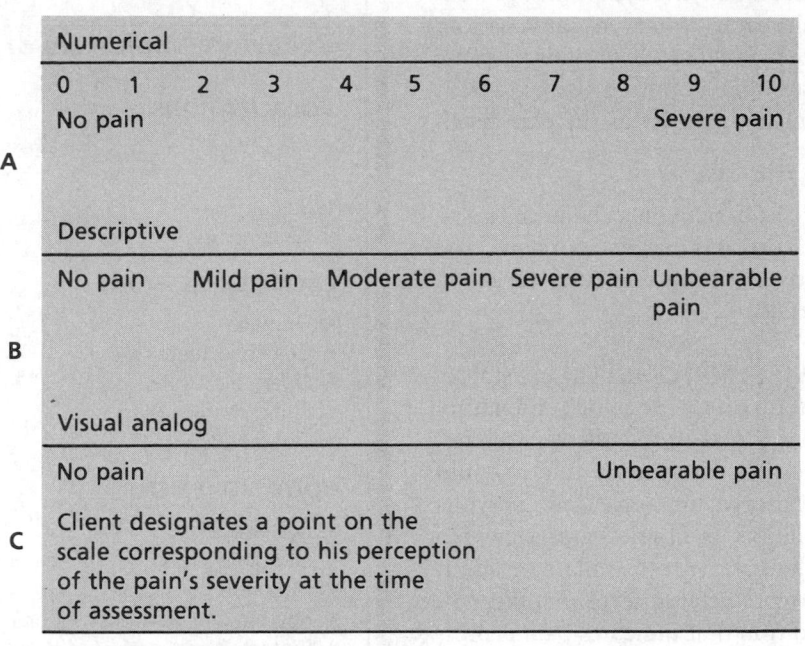

Fig. 35-5   Sample pain scales. A, Numerical. B, Descriptive. C, Visual analog.

bone, muscle, or ligament alterations. Once the nurse identifies precipitating or aggravating factors it is easier to plan interventions to avoid worsening the pain.

Relief Measures.   It is also useful to know if a client has an effective way for relieving pain (see box). What works best for the client will often work best for the nurse. Clients gain comfort from knowing the nurse is willing to try their relief measures. In the home setting the nurse must be sure that relief measures are safely being used. The nurse's assessment of relieving factors should also include identification of practitioners, for example, internist, orthopedist, chiropractor, or dentist whose services the client has sought. Clients with chronic pain are more likely to try alternative health care methods.

CONCOMITANT SYMPTOMS. Symptoms that often accompany pain include nausea, headache, dizziness, urination, constipation, or restlessness. Certain types of

---

Potential Pain Relief Measures

- Postion Change
- Analgesics
- Ice bag
- Massage

- Heating Pad
- Eating
- Rest

TABLE 35-5   Examples of Precipitating and Aggravating Factors Related to Pain Sources

Source of Pain	Precipitating/Aggravating Factors
Angina pectoris (insufficient blood flow through coronary arteries)	Physical exertion; emotional stress; exposure to cold temperature; eating large meal
Ruptured intravertebral disk	Bending over or stretching; lifting objects
Gastric ulcer	Tension; going to work; coffee or liquor ingestion
Urinary tract infection	Micturition (urinating)
Gallbladder inflammation	Eating foods high in fat content
Appendicitis	Sudden jarring or vibration of bed while lying down
Pharyngitis (sore throat)	Swallowing, talking
Peripheral vascular disease (insufficient blood flow to extremities)	Exercise (walking or running)
External otitis (inflammation of outer ear canal)	Rubbing or scratching ear canal; excessive drying of skin
Pleuritis	Inhaling deeply and coughing

pain have predictable accompanying symptoms. For example, severe rectal pain often results in constipation. The pain of an inflamed gallbladder or kidney stone frequently causes nausea and vomiting. Concomitant symptoms may be as much a priority as the pain itself.

EFFECTS OF PAIN ON THE CLIENT

By recognizing the effects of pain on a client, the nurse is able to identify the nature and existence of pain. The nurse becomes a detective, sorting out clues revealing the client's pain experience.

PHYSICAL SIGNS AND SYMPTOMS. The physiological response to pain can reveal the existence and nature of pain and the potential threat to the client's welfare. When a client experiences discomfort the nurse should assess vital signs and observe for autonomic nervous system involvement (Table 35-2). Physiological signs can reveal pain in clients who try not to complain or admit discomfort. There is no predictable level or extent of change in a client's condition that indicates pain is present.

The nurse should not confuse signs and symptoms of pain with other behavioral or pathological changes. For example, a client who is highly anxious will also exhibit an elevated heart and respiratory rate; one who is seriously dehydrated has an increased pulse because of volume depletion. The nurse considers all signs and symptoms before determining that pain is the cause.

It is helpful to determine which clients are at greater risk for having pain. The client's health status indicates whether pain is an expected symptom. The postoperative client and the victim of serious trauma are just two examples of those who will probably experience acute pain.

If pain continues unrelieved, the nurse looks for signs of physical exhaustion. Decreasing vital sign values indicate parasympathetic nerve response. The client becomes less responsive to stimuli within the environment. The nurse should measure vital signs more often if the client's condition deteriorates.

BEHAVIORAL EFFECTS. When a client experiences pain the nurse assesses verbalization, vocal response, facial and body movements, and physical contact with other persons. The client's verbal report of pain is a vital part of the total assessment. How well a client communicates pain may depend on the nurse's willingness to listen or understand, the client's assumptions about the cause or source of pain, and the client's cognitive level. Many clients cannot verbalize discomfort because of the inability to communicate. An infant, an unconscious client, a disoriented or confused person, an aphasic person and a client who speaks a foreign language are unable to explain their pain experience. The

---

Behavioral Indicators of Effects of Pain

VOCALIZATIONS
- Moaning
- Crying
- Screaming
- Gasping

FACIAL EXPRESSIONS
- Grimace
- Clenched teeth
- Open, alert eyes
- Biting the lips
- Tightened jaw

BODY MOVEMENT
- Restlessness
- Immobilization
- Muscle tension
- Rhythmic or rubbing motions
- Protective movement of body parts

SOCIAL INTERACTION
- Avoidance of conversation
- Focus only on activities for pain relief
- Avoidance of social contacts
- Reduced attention span

---

nurse must use therapeutic communication skills (see Chapter 19) and understand personal biases about pain to communicate effectively with client or family members.

Groaning, grunting, or crying are examples of vocalizations used to express pain (see box). Certain vocalizations may be involuntary and without warning when an acute attack of pain occurs. For some clients vocalizations are culturally acceptable ways to communicate.

Subtle facial expressions or body movements often reveal more about the character of pain than precise questioning. Does the client grimace or begin to toss or turn at regular intervals? Does the amount of restlessness or protective movement increase as the assessment progresses? Does the client react more uncomfortably while assuming different positions?

Some nonverbal expressions characterize sources of pain. The client with chest pain often grabs or holds the chest. A child or adult with severe abdominal pain often assumes a fetal position. A client with a severe headache may squint or rub the temples. The nonverbal expression of pain may support or contradict other information about pain. If a woman in labor reports that her labor pains are occurring more frequently and if she begins to massage her abdomen more frequently, the client's report is confirmed. If a client complains of severe abdominal pain but continues to grasp his chest, a more detailed assessment may be necessary.

The nature of pain either causes a person to attend to the discomfort and fight it or give in to the discomfort and withdraw socially. The extent to which a client interacts with the environment can clue the nurse as to the intensity or nature of pain. The more severe the pain, generally the greater its effect on the client's life-style (Timmermans and Sternbach, 1976).

INFLUENCE ON ACTIVITIES OF DAILY LIVING.
Clients who live with daily pain experience changes in their ability to participate in routine activities. Assessment of these changes reveals the extent of the client's disability and adjustments necessary to help the client participate in self-care.

The nurse asks the client if pain interferes with sleep. Is there difficulty falling asleep? Are sleeping pills or other medications needed to induce sleep? Does the pain awaken the client during the night? The client may have insomnia as a result of the pain.

Depending on the location of pain the client may have difficulty performing normal hygiene measures. Can the client dress independently or shampoo hair? Does the pain restrict mobility to the point that the client is no longer able to bathe in a bathtub? A client with severe arthritis, for example, may find it painful to grasp eating utensils. The nurse determines from the assessment the client's need for assistance with self-care activities. The nurse also considers the need for family members or friends to assist the client with basic hygiene.

Pain can seriously impair the ability to maintain normal sexual relations. Conditions such as arthritis, degenerative diseases of the hip, and chronic back pain make it difficult for a person to assume usual positions during intercourse. When assessing the extent to which pain has affected sexual activity, the nurse determines the frequency of sexual relations before and after the onset of pain. It also helps to learn if a client is physically unable to participate or if the desire for sexual intercourse has been diminished by the pain.

The ability of a person to work can be seriously threatened by pain. The more physical activity required in a job, the greater the risk of discomfort when the pain is associated with musculoskeletal and certain visceral alterations. Pain related to emotional stress will likely be increased in the individual whose job involves tension-laden decision making. The nurse assesses the work the client does and the ability to function in a regular job. The daily chores of the homemaker are assessed in the same manner as a job outside the home. The nurse assesses if it is necessary for the client to stop activity

occasionally because of the pain. Often the nurse can help clients select ways of minimizing or controlling the pain so they remain productive.

It is also important to include an assessment of how pain affects social activities. The pain may be so debilitating that the client becomes too exhausted to socialize. The nurse identifies the client's normal social activities, the extent to which they have been disrupted, and whether the client wishes to participate.

CLIENT'S COPING RESOURCES.
The experience of pain can be lonely. The pain may cause partial or total disability. Clients often find various ways to cope with the physical and psychological effects of pain. The nurse's assessment includes identification of the client's coping resources. These can be used in the nurse's plan of care to support the client and offer a degree of pain relief.

Coping resources are more than just methods or techniques. A client may depend on the emotional support of a spouse, children, other family members, or friends. Although pain still exists, the presence of a loved one can minimize loneliness and fear. A client's religious beliefs can also provide comfort. Reading scriptures or saying a prayer gives many individuals an inner strength to cope more effectively with discomfort. Being actively involved in household chores or other work can be another mechanism for coping.

The nurse asks the client what factors help in accepting or adjusting to the pain experience. Having the client describe what he typically does during an episode of pain may reveal coping resources.

SOCIOCULTURAL INFLUENCES ON THE PAIN EXPERIENCE

Throughout life we learn to respond to situations by observing others in our environment. Each person's culture influences how one learns to react to and express pain. People respond to pain in different ways. The nurse must never assume to know how each client will respond. However, an understanding of cultural background, socioeconomic status, and personal attributes will help the nurse assess pain and its meaning for a client more accurately.

Many studies describe the influence of culture on the pain experience. Miller and Shuter (1982) found that whites used more pain disclosure statements than blacks. The same was true for clients over 40 years of age compared with younger clients. Several studies have shown that the more educated and affluent respond quicker to symptoms and seek medical care for conditions that persons in lower social classes ignore. Nurses must learn there are ways to respond to pain other than their own. An assessment of cultural influences on the way clients respond or react to pain will assist a nurse in determining

TABLE 35-6 Situational Factors in the Pain Experience

Situational Factor	Nursing Assessment	Questions to Consider
Meaning of pain	Meaning and value of pain perceived by the client	Is pain associated with dying or disability? Does the client perceive a need to change his life-style? Does pain threaten the client's body image?
Knowledge and under-standing	Level and extent of information the client has received about pain	What has the client been told to expect? What does the client expect the pain to feel like? Does the client believe the pain can be relieved? When does the client believe he will feel pain and for how long?
Level of consciousness	Client's ability to respond appropriately to the environment and perceive pain	Does the client respond to pain or other stimuli? What medications is the client receiving? What are the dosages and expected effects of the medications? How is a disease process affecting the level of consciousness?
Presence and attitudes of others	The individuals whom the client uses as a source of support during the pain experience	In whom does the client confide about the pain experience? How does this person provide support? What is the person's understanding and acceptance of the client's pain?

the significance of pain to the client and what measures will be more effective in providing pain relief.

SITUATIONAL FACTORS

There are situational factors surrounding any pain experience that influence the client's reaction to pain (Table 35-6). The nurse's assessment should include all of these factors since many of them can be altered to help a client adjust more easily to pain. The meaning of pain to a client is very important. When pain threatens a client's life situation the client experiences greater pain intensity (Craig, 1986). When pain is merely temporary and poses little threat to clients, pain perception is less.

The client must have access to information about the pain experience. An understanding of pain will influence the client's response and perceptions. If the client is uninformed about factors such as intensity, duration, or nature of pain, the experience will be more unpleasant.

A client's level of consciousness influences pain perception and response. Analgesics, sedatives, and anesthetics depress functions of the central nervous system. Disease processes may also alter level of consciousness and response to pain.

Another situational variable that can significantly affect pain response is the presence and attitudes of significant others. Persons of different sociocultural groups have different expectations of people to whom they complain about pain (Meinhart and McCaffery, 1983). A person in pain often depends on a significant other to help support, assist, or provide protection. An absence

of family or friends can often make the pain experience more stressful.

NURSING DIAGNOSIS

The development of an accurate nursing diagnosis for a client in pain ensures the nurse's accountability and responsibility for pain management. The nurse analyzes data collected on the client and begins to interpret patterns of pain. For example, an assessment reveals that a 56-year-old male client has complained of an aching back pain during repeated visits to a clinic for 8 months. During that time the client has avoided physical activity and has become withdrawn from friends. He complains of an inability to sleep and loss of appetite. He walks awkwardly and frequently supports the small of his back with his hand. The defining characteristics of pain greater than 6 months, a change in life-style and activities, an impairment in physical activity, and social withdrawal all point to a diagnosis of "comfort, altered: chronic pain."

The nurse's diagnosis should focus on the specific nature of the pain (see sample nursing diagnoses box). This ensures that the most appropriate pain relief measures will be chosen.

The nurse may make diagnoses other than "comfort, altered." The extent to which pain affects a client's life-

Sample Nursing Diagnoses For Pain

Defining Characteristics	Nursing Diagnoses	Related Factors
Verbalization of pain less than 6 months Vocalization of discomfort Vital sign changes Restlessness and protective behavior: Facial grimacing	Acute pain	• Traumatic laceration • Surgical incision • Burn • Pathological process
Verbalization of pain longer than 6 months Use of several practitioners to seek pain relief Avoidance of physical activity Sleep disturbance Vital sign changes	Chronic pain	• Chronic physical disability (for example, arthritis, ruptured intravertebral disk, or cancer)
Immobilized or reduced movement of body part Localized pain involving body part Reluctance to attempt movement	Impaired physical mobility	• Pain (for example, surgical wound, injury, or chronic physical disability)

Examples of Nursing Diagnoses for Pain

NANDA-APPROVED NURSING DIAGNOSES

Anxiety related to:
• Unrelieved pain.
Acute pain related to:
• Physical injury/trauma
• Chemical injury
• Biological disturbances
Chronic pain related to:
• Chronic physical disability
• Chronic psychosocial disability
Ineffective individual coping related to:
• Chronic pain
Impaired physical mobility related to:
• Musculoskeletal pain
• Incisional pain
Self-care deficit related to:
• Musculoskeletal pain
Disturbance in self-concept related to:
• Chronic pain
Sexual dysfunction related to:
• Pain

style and general state of health determines if other nursing diagnoses are relevant. For example, the nurse's assessment may reveal that a client suffers pain of the hands and shoulders. As a result, the client is unable to remove or fasten necessary items of clothing. The client has the pain of crippling arthritis. The nursing diagnosis would be "self-care deficit: grooming related to arthritic pain." The client would have a nursing diagnosis of "altered comfort" to direct the nurse's interventions toward pain relief. The additional diagnosis of "self-care deficit" would lead the nurse to assist the client with alternative measures for performing self-care.

In choosing a nursing diagnosis the nurse must be sure that appropriate defining characteristics are identified. This ensures an accurate, individualized diagnosis suited to the client's needs. The nursing diagnoses box lists examples of nursing diagnoses appropriate to clients with pain.

PLANNING

For each nursing diagnosis identified the nurse develops a plan of care individualized to the client's needs (see care plan box). Together the nurse and client set realistic expectations for pain relief measures and the degree of pain relief to expect. A therapy that works for one client will not work for all. In the home setting, the nurse will likely use some of the remedies the client has

Sample Nursing Care Plan for Pain

Nursing Diagnosis	Goal	Expected Outcomes	Nursing Interventions
Pain related to movement of abdominal incision and skin irritation	Client achieves a sense of well-being and comfort within 2 hours of therapy.	Client will remain mobile and verbalize less pulling of incision with movement. Client will verbalize minimal discomfort during dressing change and show no nonverbal signs of discomfort. Client will state that he remains pain free 1 to 2 hours after dressing change. Client will deny irritation around incision.	Instruct client to splint incisional area with flat of hands, while turning or raising from bed. Provide music therapy (client prefers classical music) 30 minutes before each dressing change. Administer prescribed morphine 8 mg IM and Tylenol 10 gr, 30 minutes before dressing change. Cleanse skin around abdominal wound with mild soap and water to remove antibiotic solution.

adopted. The nurse cannot, however, use therapies that are unsafe. It is important for the client to understand that complete pain relief cannot be guaranteed, but that it will be attempted.

It may be important to include the client's family in the plan of care. The family may need to administer care in the home setting. In an acute care setting the family must understand the nature and extent of the client's pain and the forms of therapy to be used. Family members who show a disinterest or prejudicial view toward the client's pain can slow the client's recovery.

1. Obtaining a sense of well-being and comfort
2. Maintaining the ability to perform self-care
3. Maintaining existing physical and psychosocial function
4. Understanding the pain experience

To establish an effective plan of care, the nurse includes two important elements of care: establishing a therapeutic relationship with the client and educating the client about pain.

THERAPEUTIC RELATIONSHIP

The client in pain is highly vulnerable and is at the mercy of anyone who may attempt halfheartedly to "make him feel better." The client is not always convinced that someone is concerned with his or her welfare. The client in pain needs someone to trust. If the nurse is unable to establish a therapeutic relationship with the client, any resultant mistrust can heighten the client's awareness of pain. Unless the client has a means to ex-

press concerns or fears about pain, the reaction to the pain experience may become inappropriate. Often a client will become angry, or complain about the nurse's care when needs for pain relief are ignored.

The nurse can best help by seeing the client as a total person and conveying a sense of caring. Giving careful attention to the client's concerns during the assessment is one way of building the client's confidence in the nurse. Promptness in attending to the client's needs further establishes a strong therapeutic relationship. Making judgments about the validity of pain, bartering pain relief in return for "good" client behavior, and controlling sources of pain relief will destroy the client's trust in the nurse.

A successful nurse-client relationship depends in part on the nurse's ability to respect the client's response to pain. Many nurses value firm self-control. However, a client may need to cry, moan, or even become angry. Whatever the client's response, he or she should not feel ashamed or fearful that the nurse will not be accepting.

EDUCATION

A client is better prepared to handle almost any situation when he or she understands it. The experience of pain is no exception. Teaching a client about the pain experience reduces anxiety and helps the client achieve a sense of control. For example, a client may be entering a clinic or hospital the first time for diagnostic tests. If the client knows there are to be tests but does not understand them, the client might fantasize about the experience. Fears are enhanced if friends have had unpleasant experiences in similar circumstances. Fear increases perception of painful stimuli.

During the anticipatory phase of the pain experience the nurse plans to teach the client about the procedures and associated discomfort. Price et al. (1980) found that when clients received instruction about an upcoming painful experience, they perceived the actual experience as less unpleasant. Clients changed the way they evaluated the pain sensation and thus tolerated pain more effectively.

For some clients early forewarning of pain can be a problem. The highly anxious or fearful client is often irrational and unable to learn from the nurse's explanations. Such clients tend to fantasize horrible events if they receive information too early about painful procedures. If a client seems unlikely to benefit from advance preparation, it is best to explain invasive procedures a short time before they occur. It is not alwasy easy to know whether a client can accept an impending unpleasant experience. If a client is typically anxious or if previous teaching has not relieved anxiety, the nurse must use judgment in knowing when to tell the client.

Relevant play is a type of teaching that works well with children. Play reduces anxiety that might otherwise be created if the nurse tries to explain complicated procedures. For example, if a child is to have a laceration of the arm sutured, it helps to let the child put sutures into a doll's arm. Almost any procedure or situation can be acted out with dolls or other appropriate toys.

IMPLEMENTATION

The nature of pain and the extent to which it affects physical and psychosocial well-being determines the choice of pain relief therapies. Acute pain, for example, often requires use of analgesics to quickly deliver relief to the client. There are surgical remedies available for chronic pain disorders. Nurses can, however, independently use pain relief measures that complement those prescribed by a physician. Witt (1984) describes characteristics of ideal nursing interventions for chronic pain management. These interventions should be within the scope of the average nurse's qualifications to use them effectively, not require special equipment likely to be unavailable in many health care settings, not interfere with the client's medical treatments, not be subject to a physician's approval or supervision, and not require the client's informed consent. The nurse can play an important role in helping clients use techniques for acute and chronic pain relief. If there is doubt about a nursing therapy, the nurse must consult the client's physician. The least invasive or safest therapy should be tried first.

GUIDELINES FOR INDIVIDUALIZING PAIN THERAPY

In providing pain relief measures it is important for the nurse to choose therapies suited to the client's unique pain experience. McCaffery (1979) suggests nine useful guidelines for individualizing pain therapy:

1. *Use different types of pain relief measures*—Using more than one therapy has an additive effect in reducing pain. In addition, the character of pain may change throughout the day, requiring several different therapies. Combining physical and psychological approaches, for example, analgesics and relaxation, controls all components of the pain experience.

2. *Provide pain relief measures before pain becomes severe*—An ounce of prevention is worth a pound of cure. It is easier to prevent severe pain than to relieve it once it exists. Giving an analgesic half an hour before a client must walk or perform an activity is an example of controlling pain early.

3. *Use measures the client believes are effective*—The client is the expert on his or her own pain. The client may have ideas about what measures to use (for example, rubbing lotion on a swollen finger) and when to use them that will make pain therapy successful.

4. *Consider the client's ability or willingness to participate in pain relief measures*—Some clients cannot actively assist with pain therapy because of fatigue, sedation, or altered levels of consciousness. However, there are variations of pain relief measures that require little effort, such as relaxation exercises in bed or listening to music as a distraction. The nurse will not relieve pain by forcing an unwilling client to participate in therapy. The depressed client with chronic pain has little motivation to participate.

5. *Choose pain relief measures on the basis of the client's behavior reflecting the severity of pain*—It would be poor judgment to administer a potent narcotic if a client has only mild pain. The nurse carefully assesses what the client says and how he or she behaves before choosing pain therapy. Some clients acquire relief from severe pain after using only mild analgesics. Only the client can determine the potency of an effective therapy.

6. *If a therapy is ineffective at first, encourage the client to try it again before abandoning it*—Often anxiety or doubt prevents a therapy from relieving pain. Some approaches, such as distraction, require practice. Some measures that seem ineffective may merely require adjustment to become effective. For example, the dosage of an analgesic may be increased if severe pain is initially unrelieved. The nurse should be patient and understanding in helping the client learn to use measures that do not afford immediate relief.

7. *Keep an open mind about what may relieve pain*—New ways are often found to control pain. There is still much to be learned about the pain experience.

Rejecting a client's nonconventional therapies will lead to mistrust. It is, however, the nurse's responsibility to monitor therapies to ensure the client's safety and well-being.

8. *Keep trying*—The nurse can easily become frustrated when efforts at pain relief fail. It is important not to abandon the client when pain persists. The client in severe chronic pain who is ignored may choose suicide as an alternative. If the client gains no relief, the nurse should reassess the situation and consider whether alternative therapies are needed.

9. *Protect the client*—A pain therapy should not cause more distress than the pain itself. The nurse always observes response to therapy. Any pain relief measure may cause side effects, such as fatigue, anxiety, or additional pain. The nurse's aim is to relieve pain without disabling the client mentally, emotionally, or physically.

PREVENTING PAIN RECEPTION

A basic nursing responsibility is protecting the client from harm. One simple way to promote comfort is by removing or preventing painful stimuli (see box). This is especially important for clients who are immobilized or disabled.

Often, pain can be avoided by maintaining normal body function. For example, a client who is allowed to become constipated may suffer from distention and abdominal cramping. The nurse actively intervenes to ensure that the normal elimination process continues.

The nurse anticipates stimuli that may cause pain. Before performing procedures, the nurse considers the client's condition, aspects of the procedure that may be uncomfortable, and techniques to avoid causing pain. For example, consider a client with knee pain caused by arthritis. The nurse knows that any extreme flexion of the knee causes much pain. Before walking the client to the bathroom the nurse makes sure an elevated toilet seat is available. The client can then be seated and raise up with minimal discomfort.

It takes only simple consideration of the client's comfort and a little extra time to avoid pain-producing situations. Knowledge of factors that precipitate or aggravate pain helps the nurse prevent discomfort. The client with coronary artery disease is taught to avoid stressful exercise and large meals that normally cause painful attacks. Learning proper lifting techniques and avoiding sudden turning movements helps a client with a history of back pain avoid discomfort on the job.

The nurse also reduces the extent to which pain receptors are stimulated. Covering an open wound with bandages reduces irritation to sensitive nerve endings. Turning a client stops transmission of impulses from pressure sites on bony prominences.

CUTANEOUS STIMULATION

One way to prevent or reduce pain perception is through cutaneous stimulation. This is stimulation of a person's skin to relieve pain. A massage, warm bath, application of liniment, hot and cold therapies, and transcutaneous electric nerve stimulation (TENS) are simple ways to reduce pain perception. The specific way in which cutaneous stimulation works is unclear. One suggestion is that it causes release of endorphins. Based on the gate-control theory, it is suggested that cutaneous stimulation activates large diameter sensory nerve fibers. Thus when a heating pad is applied to the skin, impulses fail to travel along the smaller nerve fibers. Synaptic gates close to transmission of pain impulses.

Cutaneous stimulation requires the nurse to touch the client. Work by Krieger (1975) suggests that therapeutic touch alone may result in a client's improved sense of well-being. Touch can communicate caring and thus help clients relax.

A massage or backrub (see Chapter 32) are low-cost, safe ways to use cutaneous stimulation. A massage may lessen pain and promote muscular relaxation. The nurse can use massage on one body part or several. It takes about 10 minutes to correctly massage a single body part. Procedure 35-1 describes the techniques of massage.

Cold and heat applications (see Chapter 47) are routine measures that can be used in the home. Ice bags, ice massage, heating pads, and hot or cold compresses relieve pain and promote healing of injured tissues. Ice massage and application of cold packs are two types of cold therapy that are particularly effective for pain relief. Ice massage involves use of a large ice cube or a small

---

Controlling Painful Stimuli in the Client's Environment

- Tighten wrinkled bed linen.
- Remove tubing on which client is lying.
- Loosen constricting bandages.
- Change wet dressings.
- Position client in anatomical alignment.
- Check temperature of hot or cold applications, including bath water.
- Lift client up in bed, do not pull.
- Position client correctly on bed pan.
- Avoid exposing skin or mucous membranes to irritants (for example, diarrheal stool, wound drainage).
- Prevent urinary retention by keeping Foley catheters patent and free-flowing.
- Prevent constipation with fluids, diet, and exercise.

PROCEDURE 35-1

Massage Techniques

STEPS	RATIONALE
1. Assess the following: a. Condition of body part to be massaged b. Character of client's pain c. Contraindications to positioning (for example, neck injury)	Massaging overly sensitive or damaged skin can cause further tissue injury. Provides a baseline to determine effectiveness of massage in relieving pain. Massage of some body parts cannot be achieved without proper positioning and thus may be contraindicated.
2. Prepare the following supplies: a. Skin lubricant (oil or lotion) b. Pillow (optional)	Eases movement of hands over client's skin.
3. Explain procedure: positioning, duration of massage, body parts to be massaged, purpose of massage.	Anticipation and understanding of the procedure helps client to relax and cooperate.
4. Instruct client to tell you if the massage becomes painful or feels especially good.	Avoids injury to client. Client is best judge of what therapy is effective in reducing pain or muscle tension.
5. Close door or pull curtains.	Ensures privacy.
6. Wash hands.	Reduces transmission of microorganisms.
7. Position height of bed to comfortable working level and lower side rail.	Promotes proper use of body mechanics by the nurse. Makes access to client easy.
8. After determining area to be massaged, position body part appropriately: a. Hands: place arms on pillow with client sitting or supine. b. Arms: same as step a. c. Neck: Position client prone.	Promotes venous return and supports arms comfortably. Provides easy access to neck muscles.
9. Drape client to expose only the body parts to be massaged.	Promotes client's comfort, warmth, and privacy.
10. Apply lotion to your hands and warm while rubbing hands together.	Prevents startling client and promotes comfort.
11. Massage each body part at least 10 minutes: a. Hands—make contact first with one hand and then the other. Using both hands, slowly open the client's palm, gliding your fingers over the palmar surface. While supporting the hand use both thumbs to apply friction to the palm. Use your thumbs in a circular motion to stretch the palm outward. Massage each finger outward. Massage each finger separately, using a corkscrew-like motion from base of finger to the tip. With your thumb and finger knead each small muscle in the client's fingers. Glide your hands smoothly from fingertips to wrists. Repeat for other hand.	Improves likelihood that muscular relaxation and reduced perception of pain will occur. Relaxes clenched muscles of the fingers and palm.
b. Arms—Use a gliding stroke to massage from client's wrist to forearm. With thumb and forefinger of both hands, knead muscles from client's forearm to shoulder. Continue kneading biceps, deltoid, and triceps muscles. Finish with gliding strokes from the wrist to the shoulder.	Thicker muscles require more kneading to cause relaxation.
c. Neck—Support the neck at the hairline with one hand and massage up the neck with a gliding stroke. Knead muscles on one side of neck. Switch hands to support neck and knead other side of neck. Stretch the neck slightly with one hand at the top and the other at the bottom.	Movement of neck may interfere with ability to massage muscles fully. Relieves tension felt in deeper neck muscles.
12. During the massages, note any nonverbal cues indicating the client's level of comfort.	Excess pressure to muscle groups or stretching of sensitive tissues may cause discomfort.
13. During the massage, note which muscles are relaxed versus tight.	Tense muscles require more massage to achieve relaxation.

Continued.

PROCEDURE 35-1, cont'd

Massage Techniques

STEPS	RATIONALE
14. Once the massage is complete, allow client to relax in the assumed position. Give client time to relax or fall asleep.	Benefit of massage is increased by client remaining inactive. Stimulation of muscles reduces pain perception and promotes full relaxation.
15. Wash hands and store supplies.	Reduces transmission of microorganisms.
16. Record in nurses' notes: Body part massaged, client's response to massage, and change in level of comfort.	Documents therapy and client's response. Provides information for choosing massage in the future for pain relief.
17. Return to room 30 min later to evaluate client's level of comfort.	Determines degree of pain relief obtained.

paper cup filled with water and frozen (ice rises out of the cup to create a smooth surface for massage). The massage is simple. A nurse or the client can apply the ice with firm pressure to the skin, followed by a slow steady circular massage over the area. Cold may be applied near the pain site, on the opposite side of the body corresponding to the pain site, or on a site located between the brain and pain site. It takes about 5 to 10 minutes to use cold application. Each client will respond differently to the site of application that is most effective. However, application near the actual site of pain tends to work best. Clients will feel four types of sensation: cold, burning, aching, and numbness. When numbness occurs the ice should be removed. Melzack et al. (1980) found ice massage to be effective for tooth or mouth pain when ice was placed on the web of the hand between the thumb and index finger. This point on the hand is an acupuncture point that apparently influences nerve pathways to the face and head. Cold applications are also effective before invasive needle punctures such as intramuscular injections, bone marrow punctures, or lumbar punctures. When using any form of cold or hot application, the nurse must instruct the client to avoid injury to the skin. Clients can easily be burned by their incorrect use.

Transcutaneous electric nerve stimulation (TENS) involves stimulation of the skin with a mild electrical current passed through external electrodes. The therapy requires a physician's order. The TENS unit consists of three parts (Figure 35-6): a battery-powered transmitter, lead wires, and electrodes. The electrodes are placed directly over or near the site of pain. Hair or skin preparations should be removed before attaching the electrodes. When a client feels pain the transmitter is turned on. The TENS unit creates a buzzing or tingling sensation. The client may adjust the intensity and quality of skin stimulation. The tingling sensation can be applied as long as pain relief lasts. In a study conducted by Taylor et al. (1983) clients who received TENS reported greater pain relief than clients who received narcotic analgesics.

Cutaneous stimulation can provide effective, tempo-

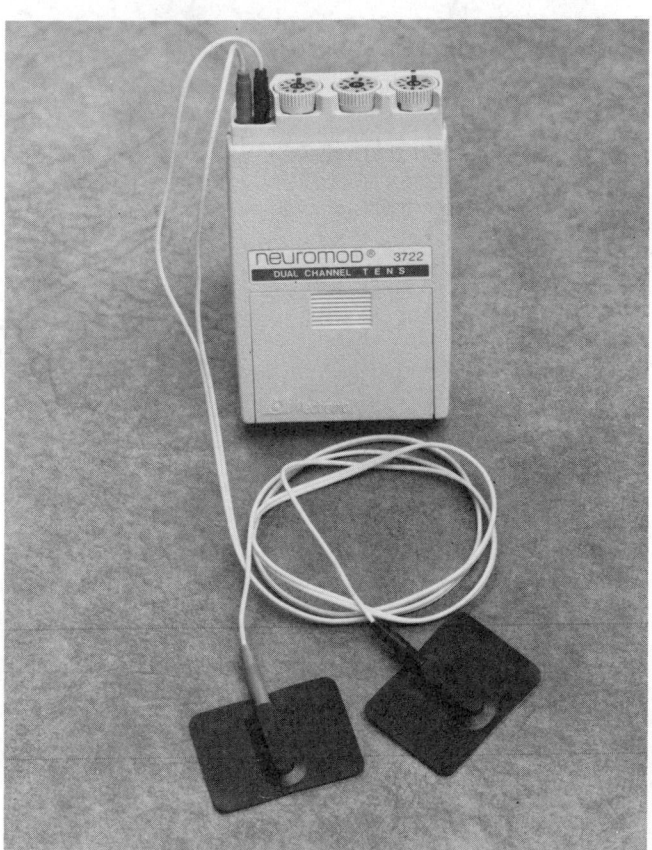

Fig. 35-6 TENS.

rary pain relief. To enhance its effects, the nurse helps the client assume a comfortable position, eliminates environmental irritants such as noise or bright lights, and explains the purpose of therapy. Cutaneous stimulation should not be used on sensitive skin areas (such as burns, rashes, or bruises), incisions, inflamed areas, or underlying fractures.

DISTRACTION

The reticular activating system (RAS) inhibits painful stimuli if a person receives sufficient or excessive sensory input. With meaningful sensory stimuli, a person can ignore or become unaware of pain. Pleasurable stimuli also cause the release of endorphins to relieve pain. Persons who are bored or in isolation only have their pain to think about and thus perceive it more acutely. Distraction helps direct attention to something else. As a result, there is not a full awareness of pain. Distraction often can increase pain tolerance, but there is one disadvantage. If it works, health care personnel or family may question the existence or severity of a person's pain. Distraction may work best for short, intense pain lasting a few minutes such as during a procedure or while waiting for an analgesic to work (Mayer, 1985).

The nurse assesses types of activities the client enjoys that may act as distractions. These might include singing, describing photos or pictures aloud, listening to music, playing games, or other rhythmic activities. Most distractions can be used in a hospital, home, or long-term care facility.

One effective distraction is music. There are some institutions that have music therapists. However, the nurse can use music creatively in many clinical situations. Clients generally either prefer to perform (play an instrument or sing a song) or listen to music. Music

that initially matches a person's mood is usually best (Bailey, 1985). For example, a lonely person might initially enjoy a solo instrument or vocalist. Selections might progress to musical groups or even symphonic works. The box suggests ways to use music effectively.

RELAXATION AND GUIDED IMAGERY

Clients can alter affective-motivational and cognitive pain perception through relaxation and guided imagery. Relaxation is mental and physical freedom from tensions or stress. The ability to relax physically promotes mental relaxation as well. Relaxation techniques provide clients with self-control when pain occurs. These techniques reverse the physical and emotional stress that occurs with pain. Clients who use relaxation techniques successfully experience several physiologic and behavioral changes (see box, below). The nurse obtains a physician's order for relaxation therapy if there is any legal uncertainty of the nurse's action or if the client's physical condition is unstable. Relaxation techniques include meditation, yoga, Zen, guided imagery, and progressive relaxation exercises.

Relaxation with or without guided imagery relieves tension headaches, labor pain, acute anticipated episodes of pain (for example, a needle stick), and chronic pain disorders. It may take five to ten training sessions before clients can effectively minimize pain (Carney, 1983). Relaxation training can be practiced indefinitely and is usually without side effects. Carney (1983) notes studies that show 60% to 70% of clients with tension headache can reduce activity by at least 50% with relaxation.

For effective relaxation, the client's participation and cooperation are needed. The nurse explains the technique in detail to help establish realistic goals for pain relief. Considerable practice is needed to achieve consistent pain reduction. The nurse describes common sensations the client may experience such as a decrease in temperature or numbness of a body part. These sensory changes are the feedback to which the client attends as the exercises progress. The nurse is a coach, guiding the

---

Using Music to Control Pain

- Match musical selections to a client's taste. Consider age and background.
- Earphones avoid annoying other clients or staff and help client to concentrate on music
- If pain is acute, it often helps to increase the volume of music. As pain decreases, the volume should be reduced.
- If background music is provided, select general types suited to the client's preferences.
- Have the client concentrate on the music and emphasize rhythm by tapping fingers or patting the thigh.
- Encourage clients to use music, particularly when it is enjoyed in the home.

Effects of Relaxation

- Decreased pulse, blood pressure, and respirations.
- Decreased oxygen consumption.
- Decreased muscle tension.
- Decreased metabolic rate.
- Heightened concentration on single idea.
- Lack of attention to environmental stimuli.
- No voluntary change of position.

Adapted from Dimotto, JW: Relaxation, Am J Nurs 84:754, 1984

Body Positions for Relaxation

SITTING

- Sit with back resting against entire back of chair.
- Place feet flat on the floor.
- Keep legs separated.
- Hang arms at the side or rest on chair arms.
- Keep head aligned straight with spine.

LYING

- Keep legs separated with toes pointed slightly outward.
- Rest arms at sides without touching sides of body.
- Keep head aligned straight with spine.
- Use thin, small pillow under the head.

---

client slowly through steps of the exercise. The nurse does not teach relaxation techniques when the client is in acute discomfort because an inability to concentrate will make the exercises ineffective.

The client may use guided imagery and relaxation exercises together or separately. In either case the nurse makes the environment as quiet as possible. Closing curtains or turning off room lights decreases irritating stimuli. Every effort is made to minimize distractions. The client may sit in a comfortable chair or lie in bed (see box). A light sheet or blanket for warmth often helps the client feel more comfortable.

In guided imagery the client creates an image in the mind, concentrates on that image, and gradually becomes less aware of pain. The nurse coaches the client in forming the image and helping concentrate on the sensory experience. Initially the nurse asks the client to think of a pleasant scene or experience that enables use of all the senses. The client describes the image and the nurse records it so it can be used during later exercises. The nurse uses specific information given by the client and does not make changes in the client's image. For example, if the client imagines a scene of relaxing on a cool bed of grass, the nurse does not add a dog. If the client is fearful of dogs, the nurse's description may create tension and anxiety. The following is an example of a portion of a guided imagery exercise:

Imagine yourself lying on a cool bed of grass with the sounds of rushing water from a nearby stream. It's a warm, balmy day. You turn to see a patch of blue wildflowers in bloom and can smell their fragrance.

Guided imagery works best when the client is able to use all senses. The nurse sits close enough to the client to be heard but is not intrusive. A calm, soft voice helps the client focus more completely on the suggested image.

As the client relaxes it is unnecessary for the nurse to speak continuously. If the client shows signs of agitation, restlessness, or discomfort, the nurse should stop the exercise and begin later.

Progressive relaxation of the entire body takes about 15 minutes. The client pays attention to the body, noting areas of tension. Tense areas are replaced with warmth and relaxation. Some clients relax better with eyes closed. Soft background music can be helpful.

The relaxation exercise involves a combination of controlled breathing exercises and a series of contractions and relaxation of muscle groups. The client begins by breathing slowly and diaphragmatically, allowing the abdomen to rise slowly and the chest to expand fully. The nurse coaches the client in breathing slowly and gradually while relaxing the entire body. While the client establishes a regular breathing pattern, the nurse begins to coach the client to pay attention to tense muscle groups. The nurse directs the client to locate the area of muscular tension, think about how it feels, tense the muscles fully, and then completely relax them. This creates the sensation of removing all discomfort and stress. Gradually the client can relax the muscles without first tensing them. When full relaxation is achieved, pain perception is lowered and anxiety toward the pain experience becomes minimal. The following is an example of how a nurse coaches a client:

Let's begin by finding as comfortable a position as possible. Arms at your side . . . legs uncrossed. . . . Move until you feel at ease. . . . Take a deep breath. Feel your stomach and chest slowly rise. . . . Relax. . . . Now breathe out slowly . . . slowly . . . and relax.

Count to 4, inhaling on 1 and 2, exhaling on 3 and 4. . . . Continue to breathe slowly. . . . Your body is beginning to relax. . . . Think relax. . . . Feel the parts of your body. . . . Notice any tension in your muscles. . . . Continue to breathe slowly . . . . and relax.

Concentrate on your face . . . . your jaws . . . . your neck. . . . Notice any tightness. . . . Breathe in warmth and relaxation. . . . Concentrate on any tension in your hands. . . . Notice how it feels. . . . Now make a fist. A tight fist! As you begin to exhale, relax your fist. . . . Good! Notice how your hand feels. . . . Think relax. . . . Your hand feels warm . . . . heavy or light. . . . Just relax more . . . . and more. Now focus on your forearms. . . . Notice any tension. . . . Relax your arms. . . . Feel your body relaxing. . . . Let the feelings of relaxation spread from your fingers and hands through the muscles of your arms.

As with guided imagery, if the client becomes agitated or uncomfortable, the nurse stops the exercise. If the client seems to have difficulty relaxing only part of his body, the nurse can slow the progression of the exercise and concentrate on the tensed body part. The client must also know from the beginning that the exercise can be stopped at any time. With practice the client can perform relaxation exercises independently.

ANTICIPATORY GUIDANCE

Modifying anxiety associated with pain directly relieves pain and also adds to the effects of other pain relief measures. Moderate anxiety may be useful when a client anticipates a painful experience. Clients can learn what is to be expected during a painful procedure or event. Knowledge about pain helps a client control anxiety and cognitively gain a level of pain relief.

The nurse gives clients information that prevents misinterpretation of the painful event and promotes understanding of what to expect. Information given to clients includes explanation of:

1. Occurrence, onset, and expected duration of pain
2. Quality, severity, and location of pain
3. Information on how the client's safety is assured
4. Cause of the pain
5. Methods nurse and client take for pain relief.
6. Expectations of the client during a procedure

An example of anticipatory guidance is preoperative teaching (see Chapter 46). Explanation of the incisional pain the client will feel and methods used to control it helps the client adapt postoperatively.

The nurse cannot say that the client will experience no pain. Anticipatory guidance gives an honest explanation of the pain experience. The nurse also gives instruction on pain relief techniques so the client will be prepared to cope with discomfort.

PHARMACOLOGICAL PAIN THERAPY

Several pharmacological agents provide pain management. All require a physician's order. The nurse's judgment in the use of medications and management of clients receiving pharmacological therapies helps ensure the best pain relief possible.

ADMINISTERING ANALGESICS

Analgesics can provide clients effective pain relief. However, nurses and physicians often have misconceptions about the dangers and effects of analgesics. In a study by Marks and Sachar (1973), hospitalized medical clients were found to be undertreated with the narcotic meperidine (Demerol). Nurses and physicians undertreated clients because of incorrect pharmacologic information, concerns about addiction, anxiety over errors in judgment while using a narcotic analgesic, and administering less medication than was ordered. In a study by Rankin and Snider (1984), a group of nurses completed a questionnaire measuring their perceptions of pain suffered by cancer clients. The study showed that 89% believed clients had adequate pain control. However, 67% assessed that the clients suffered moderate pain. Often nurses' uncertainty with correct administration of analgesics leads only to a reduction in pain, not relief.

Nurses must understand the drugs available for pain relief and their pharmacological effects. Pharmacological agents act at different levels of the nervous system to create pain relief. A drug may act at the peripheral receptor level or at the central nervous system level. The most common peripheral analgesics include acetylsalicylic acid (aspirin), acetaminophen (Tylenol), and the nonsteroidal antiinflammatory drugs, ibuprofen (Motrin) and naproxen (Naprosyn). These drugs act primarily on peripheral receptors to diminish reception of pain stimuli.

Narcotic analgesics such as morphine, meperidine (Demerol), and codeine act on higher centers of the brain to modify perception of and reaction to pain. Morphine is a derivative of opium and has three characteristic analgesic effects: (1) raising the pain threshold and thereby reducing pain perception; (2) reducing anxiety and fear, which are components of the reaction to pain; and (3) inducing sleep even in the presence of severe pain. The danger of morphine and other narcotic analgesics is the potential for depression of vital nervous system functions. Opiates cause respiratory depression by depressing the respiratory center within the brainstem. Clients also experience an alteration in mental processes. The following are characteristics of an ideal analgesic:

1. Rapid onset
2. Effective over a prolonged time
3. Effective for all ages
4. Used orally and parenterally
5. Free of severe side effects
6. Nonaddicting
7. Inexpensive

Sedatives, antianxiety agents, and muscle relaxants are often prescribed to clients in chronic pain or clients who have other symptoms associated with pain. However, these are often of little benefit. Sedatives are the drugs most often prescribed to chronic pain sufferers (Brena, 1983). These can cause drowsiness and impairment of coordination, judgment, and mental alertness. Misuse of sedatives and antianxiety agents is a serious health problem that can cause disabling illness behaviors.

Analgesics require careful assessment, application of pharmacological principles (see Chapter 15), and common sense. A person's response to an analgesic is highly individual. A relatively mild nonnarcotic may prove as effective as a potent narcotic for some clients, or an orally administered analgesic may bring the same relief as an injectable form of analgesic. It is the nurse's responsibility to follow a few basic principles:

1. Know the client's previous response to analgesics.
2. Select the proper medication when more than one is ordered.
3. Know the accurate dosage.
4. Assess the right time and interval for administration.

It is helpful to know whether the client has previously gained relief from analgesics. The client can usually provide this information. If possible the nurse notes if a nonnarcotic was as successful as a narcotic. Previous dosages and routes of administration should be assessed to help prevent undertreatment. A client who has remained comfortable receiving an oral dose of codeine every 6 hours will look skeptically at the nurse who enters the room with a syringe. If a client has not recently received any form of analgesic, the nurse must obtain a history of allergies.

Selecting the proper medication can often be difficult. Frequently a physician will order several analgesics from which to choose. Generally a more potent medication is ordered for severe pain, whereas a milder analgesic is prescribed for less acute pain. For pain that is mild to moderate, it is safer to start with a nonnarcotic or milder form of narcotic. Nonnarcotics can also be alternated with narcotics. Pain may be aggravated by physical distress and fatigue and require a more potent medication. A nonnarcotic may be adequate later in the day when pain has subsided.

Choosing oral medication over an injection is not always simple. An injection acts quicker. A narcotic can achieve its maximum effect one hour after an injection. An oral medication may take as long as two hours. Therefore, a client waits for pain relief, but it worsens instead and the oral medication is less effective by the time peak action occurs. For acute and intermittent pain, injections quickly bring relief. If pain is chronic and persistent, an oral drug often gives longer, more sustained relief. The nurse should also know the comparative potencies of analgesics in oral and injectable form. For example, a physician may order: Demerol 50-100 mg, IM or PO every 3-4 hours prn. This order leaves much to the judgment of the nurse and would require clarification. Consider the confusion created by such an order. The nurse must select the best dosage, route, and time interval. The maximum dose of Demerol (100 mg) has about the same analgesic strength as 13 mg morphine intramuscular (IM) (Heidrich and Perry, 1982). The lowest dose of 50 mg by mouth (PO) is equal to the strength of two aspirin. If nurses on succeeding shifts choose different routes for the same dosages the client will not receive the same level of analgesia and pain control will be poor. Nurses must provide controlled, sustained pain relief.

Since nurses often fear overtreating clients in pain, a helpful rule to follow is that severe pain requires a greater amount of analgesic to relieve it. Doses at the upper end of normal prescribed ranges are usually safe. If a well-meaning nurse administers a low dose that proves ineffective, the client may suffer until a drug can again be given.

The nurse has the primary role in determining the time and interval for analgesic administration. Narcotic analgesics are usually ordered on a prn (as needed) basis. For example, the medication order is oral codeine 30 mg every 3 to 4 hours prn. If a client receives a dose at 7 AM, the nurse may not administer the drug again until 10 AM at the earliest. However, the client may not need it until late afternoon. It is important to administer analgesia as soon as pain occurs and before it increases in severity. The client should be an active participant in telling the nurse when pain perception occurs. The nurse also assesses the client frequently for nonverbal expressions of pain. If any pain-producing procedure, such as walking, sitting up, or a dressing change, is scheduled the nurse should give an analgesic before the activity. The drug should be administered so that its peak effect is reached during the client's most active time.

There are benefits in giving clients more control over their pain therapy. When clients depend on nurses for analgesia, an erractic cycle of alternating pain and analgesia often occurs. The client feels pain and asks for a medication. The nurse may be unable to deliver the medication promptly. Within an hour after drug administration, analgesia finally occurs. Pain relief may last only a half hour. The client may be sedated as long as an hour. Then, gradually, the client again feels discomfort. A drug delivery system called patient-controlled analgesia (PCA) allows clients to administer pain medications when they want them. The PCA is a portable computerized pump with a chamber for a syringe. The pump intravenously delivers a small preset dose of medication, usually morphine. To receive a dose the client pushes a button on a cord attached to the pump (Fig. 35-7). A timer allows the system to deliver no more than a specified number of doses every hour to avoid overdoses. Each dose may be as small as 1 cc or 1 mg of morphine sulfate every 6 minutes. The pump has a locked safety system that prevents tampering. Even

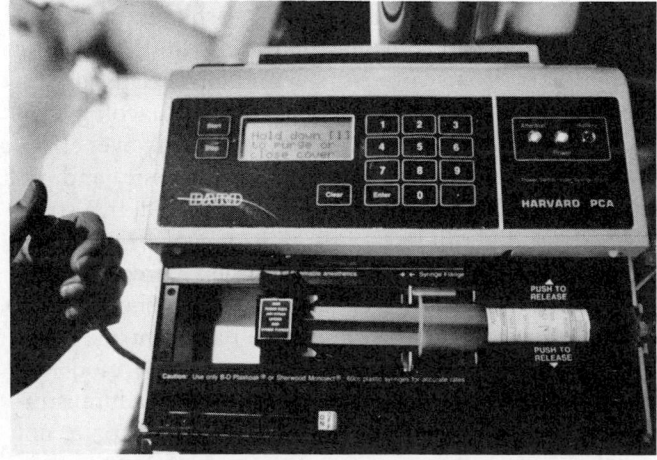

Fig. 35-7 Patient-controlled analgesic device.

though a dose can only be released every 6 minutes, each time the client pushes the button a small bell alarms. The bell acts as a placebo. The client believes a dose is delivered with each ring of the bell. Benefits of the PCA include the following:

1. Clients have control over their pain.
2. Pain relief does not depend on nurse availability.
3. Clients tend to take less medication.
4. Small doses of analgesics delivered at short intervals stabilize serum drug concentrations for more sustained pain relief.

Success of the PCA depends on the client's ability to use it. The nurse should provide a thorough explanation and demonstration to the client.

LOCAL ANESTHETICS. Local anesthesia is the loss of sensation to a localized body part. Physicians use local anesthesia while suturing a wound, moving a painful body part, delivering an infant, and performing some surgery. Local anesthesia has fewer risks than general anesthesia, which causes loss of consciousness and depression of vital functions.

Local anesthetics can be applied topically on skin and mucous membranes or injected to anesthetize a part of the body. Local anesthetics block the function of sensory, motor, and autonomic neurons supplying the affected area. Thus, when the client temporarily loses sensation of a body part, motor and autonomic function is also lost. Smaller sensory nerve fibers are more sensitive to local anesthetics than large motor fibers. As a result, the client loses sensation before losing motor function, and, conversely, motor activity returns before sensation.

Local anesthetics can cause side effects depending on their absorption into the circulation. Itching or burning of the skin or a localized rash are common after topical applications. Application to vascular mucous membranes increases the chance of systemic effects such as a change in heart rate. Injection of anesthetics increase the risk of systemic side effects, depending on the amount of drug used and the area injected.

Table 35-7 summarizes the types of local anesthesia by injection. Each produces a different level of anesthesia as a result of the amount of anesthetic used and location of the spinal nerve affected (Fig. 35-8).

The nurse assists the physician during use of local anesthesia by providing emotional support to the client, watching for systemic side effects, and protecting the client from injury. Many clients are apprehensive about whether an anesthetic will prevent pain. The nurse explains how the local anesthetic will be applied and the sensations the client will experience. Injection of an anesthetic can be painful if the physician does not first numb the injection site. The nurse prepares the client for such discomfort.

It is common for clients to fear paralysis, since epidural and spinal injections come close to the spinal cord. The nurse explains where the needles are inserted and warns clients that they will temporarily lose motor and autonomic function (for example, bowel and bladder function).

Before the client receives an anesthetic, the nurse determines the history of allergies. To monitor systemic effects of local anesthetics, the nurse assesses blood pressure and pulse. Spinal anesthesia may also cause variations in respiratory rate.

After administration of a local anesthetic the nurse protects the client from injury until full sensory and motor function returns. Pain is a normal protective

TABLE 35-7   Local Anesthesia Techniques

Type	Area Injured	Area Anesthetized	Indications for Use
Infiltration	Superficially under skin or mucous membranes	Small peripheral nerves to area infiltrated	Small incisions of the skin; insertion of sutures to close cuts or wounds; minor dental repairs
Peripheral nerve block	Area surrounding large peripheral nerve at point above bifurcation of nerve	Wider area than with infiltration; numbs entire body part (for example, hand, upper gums, foot)	Major dental repairs; manipulation or reduction of extremity fractures; minor hand and foot surgery
Epidural or peridural nerve block	In lumbosacral region of spinal cord; anesthetic injected around major nerve roots exiting base of spinal cord at site outside dura mater	Lower trunk and extremities	Delivery of newborn; major surgery to lower trunk and extremities (for example, hemorrhoidectomy, appendectomy, vascular repair)
Spinal nerve block	Anesthetic injected around major nerve root within subarachnoid space of spinal cord	Lower trunk and extremities	Major surgery to lower trunk and extremities; clients who would be at risk with general anesthesia

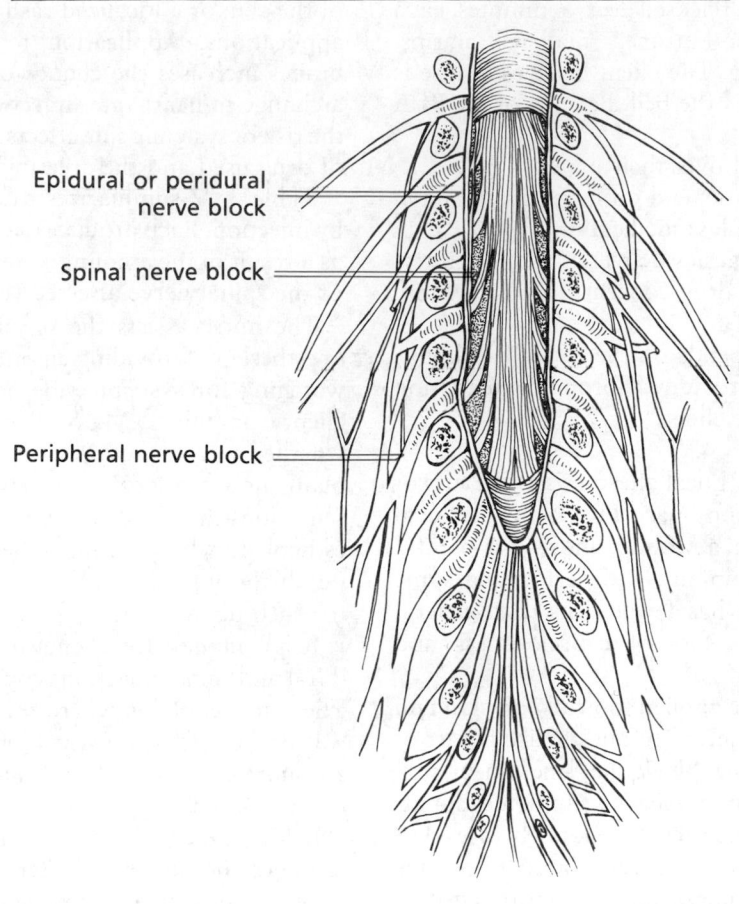

Epidural or peridural nerve block

Spinal nerve block

Peripheral nerve block

Fig. 35-8 Injection sites for peripheral, spinal, and epidural or peridural nerve blocks.

mechanism. Until a local anesthetic is absorbed and metabolized, the client must be careful in using an anesthetized body part. For example, after an injection into a joint, the nurse warns the client to avoid using the joint until function returns. For clients with topical anesthesia the nurse avoids applying heat or cold to numb areas. After spinal anesthesia the client stays in bed until sensory and motor function returns. The nurse assists the client during the first attempt at getting out of bed.

PLACEBOS Often a nurse's reassuring words will seem to bring about pain relief even though there are no direct physiological or chemical effects on a client. A placebo is any treatment that produces an effect because of its intent and not its physical or chemical properties (McCaffery, 1982). An inactive substance such as injectable normal saline or oral preparations of sugar are often prescribed as if they were medication. The pharmacy can prepare placebos in the form of capsules or tablets to make them look the same as medications.

Considerable argument exists over how placebos relieve pain. Some researchers believe that placebos in-

crease endorphin levels. Others believe that they create a psychological sense of pain relief, lowering a person's pain perception. Whatever the mode of action, when the placebo is administered correctly, the client is convinced that it will provide pain relief. The client's belief that a placebo is a real form of therapy may be the necessary factor in relieving pain.

The nurse requires a physician's order before administering a placebo. The placebo is not to be used as a form of punishment or as a test to prove whether the client is really in pain. The nurse may choose to give the placebo by telling the client it is a medication, or explain its purpose and desired effect. The nurse may also choose not to give the placebo. It is important for nurses to consider their values related to the ethics of administering placebos.

The nurse enhances the chances of a placebo working by explaining that its intent is to relieve pain. It is also helpful to provide a quiet, comfortable environment that enables the client to relax. Trust in the nurse relieves doubt the client might have about the therapy's benefit. The nurse administers the placebo as though it were an actual pain medication, assesses the client's pain carefully, and evaluates and records the placebo's effects.

PROMOTING WELLNESS

Pain can seriously disable and immobilize an individual. The effect of pain on physical mobility can alter self-care activities. Pain can also change a person's sexuality and desire to socialize with others. The nurse helps the client and appropriate family members find ways to cope with pain and maintain a functional life-style.

The nurse acts to minimize potential effects of immobilization (see Chapter 42) by practicing good positioning techniques. Regular turning, range of motion exercise, and anatomical alignment of body parts reduce painful contractures from forming. When a client is mobile the nurse makes sure painful body parts are protected. Elastic bandages, braces, splints, or even pillows can support injured parts during movement. If crutches or other assistive devices are required, the nurse makes sure they are used properly. Otherwise, the client may be at risk for further injury or pain.

Painful disorders of the upper extremities create difficulty in eating, bathing, grooming, and dressing. The nurse may refer a client to an occupational therapist who can devise ways to maintain function even when finger movement or grasp is impaired. Eating utensils, comb and brush, and a toothbrush can be attached to extension devices. They have enlarged handles or splints that allow clients to pick up the items. Clothing fasteners made from velcro tape make it easier for clients to remove or apply clothing. Shirts or blouses can be sewn so garments can simply be pulled on over the head.

A warm bath can be relaxing therapy. Personal cleanliness also promotes comfort. If chronic pain exists the nurse should encourage family members to help clients maintain hygiene practices in the home.

With fatigue, pain perception can increase. Procedures within a health care setting should be planned around rest periods. Clients with chronic discomfort should be encouraged to rest before social activities in the home.

A person with pain may avoid sexual activity for fear that it will cause or aggravate discomfort. The need for sexual warmth is not, however, negated by pain (Cash, 1984). Clients can learn to sexually express themselves regardless of pain. A client whose movement is restricted by pain may not be able to assume the most common male on top position used for intercourse. Alternative side-lying or rear-entry positions may be less uncomfortable and strenuous. Nurses should also caution clients about the fact that tranquilizers, muscle relaxants, and narcotics decrease libido and potency.

SURGICAL MEASURES FOR PAIN RELIEF

When a client's pain persists despite medical treatment and it is clear that the pain is physical and not psycho-logical, surgical therapies may give relief. A posterior rhizotomy involves surgically cutting the dorsal roots of a spinal nerve. The resection involves the posterior root of the spinal cord. It is effective for relieving both localized acute pain in the area supplied by the nerve root and deep visceral pain. The client loses sensation of pain but retains full motor function.

A chordotomy is more extensive involving resection of the thoracic or cervical spinal cord at various levels. The procedure is used to treat intractable or unrelieved pain. The higher the focus of pain, the higher the site selected for a chordotomy. For example, pain in the thorax, upper extremities, and shoulders requires a high cervical chordotomy. The risks of the procedure are great, since permanent paralysis may result from edema of the cord or accidental resection of motor nerves. After the procedure the client has a permanent loss of both pain and temperature sensation in the affected areas. If the surgery is uncomplicated, the senses of touch and position are retained.

A dorsal column stimulator is a battery-powered device that blocks pain impulses from reaching the spinal cord. A small electrode is surgically implanted near a sensory nerve believed to be transmitting the pain impulses. The device works like transcutaneous nerve stimulation. The client wears a battery-powered transmitter that sends electrical signals to block pain stimuli. When pain is felt, the client turns on the transmitter, which creates a mild buzzing or tingling sensation. The buzzing may last as long as pain relief occurs. The transmitter stimulates large sensory fibers entering the spinal cord and inhibits small pain fibers.

CLIENTS WITH INTRACTABLE PAIN

Intractable pain cannot be permanently relieved. The pain can become so debilitating that a client assumes a dependent role on others. Chronic intractable pain encompasses a person's total existence. The client will try anything to gain relief. Worldwide it is estimated that 25% of all persons with cancer die without relief from severe pain (Daut and Cleeland, 1982). Cleeland (1984) further notes that one in three people with metastatic cancer reports pain that interferes with the quality of life. One of the greatest nursing challenges is to care for the client with intractable pain.

When therapy to control the spread of cancer fails, analgesic medications may be the only way to alleviate suffering. Administration of analgesics in treatment of cancer-related pain requires application of principles different from those used to treat acute pain. When a client with cancer first experiences pain, it is best to begin with a higher medication dosage than will be needed for relief. The physician slowly decreases the dosage to the amount needed, thus providing the client with immediate pain relief.

Too often opiates are underprescribed since physicians fear depression of the central nervous system. For example, most opiates such as codeine and morphine have an average duration of action ranging between 2 and 4 hours. However, standard prescriptions are for opiates to be given every 4 hours. The client is needlessly exposed to unnecessary discomfort as the blood level of the drug is at its lowest point at the end of the fourth hour, before the next dose (Brena, 1983).

Studies show that drug dependence is low among clients with cancer-related pain. Administering the right drug and the required dose at the proper interval alleviates the fear of pain, protects the client from drug-seeking behavior, and reduces the incidence of tolerance and dependence. For clients with cancer the aim of drug therapy is to anticipate and minimize pain rather than cure it. It is therefore necessary to give required doses on a regular basis. Prescribing analgesics on a prn basis for cancer clients is ineffective and causes more suffering. The cancer client must take an analgesic regularly, even when the pain, nausea, and other symptoms subside.

Despite the problems many chronic pain sufferers have, there are medications that can provide some pain relief. Methadone and oral morphine are useful. Methadone has several advantages: (1) a high oral potency, (2) long duration of action, (3) a cumulative effect that maintains a steady analgesic level to prevent pain, and (4) a relative lack of interference with a client's mood (Maxwell, 1980). Once a client's methadone dosage becomes regulated, only two daily doses may be required. Opiate cocktails also achieve a significant level of pain relief for cancer clients. Brompton's mixture, Val-Streck elixir, and modified Brompton's mixtures do not interfere with mental alertness. Bromptom's mixture includes a combination of drugs: morphine or methadone (narcotic analgesic), cocaine or an amphetamine (central nervous system stimulant that reduces sedation and respiratory depression caused by the narcotic), a phenothiazine (antipsychotic and antiemetic), and ethyl alcohol. The mixture often contains a fruit-flavored syrup to improve its taste. Brompton's mixture is easier to take than repeated injections. The client learns to adjust the dosage to ensure adequate pain relief. There is argument that Brompton's mixture is not as effective as morphine alone. However, the limited sedative effect of the cocktail offers an advantage.

A popular measure for treatment of severe intractable cancer pain is morphine administered by continuous intravenous (IV) drip. Continuous IV drip provides more uniform and better pain control because lower doses of the drug are used and thus there are fewer side effects. Although a client receives a continuous infusion of morphine, the total daily dose may be less than with regular conventional intramuscular injections. Candidates for continuous drip therapy include clients with severe pain for which oral and intermittent parenteral narcotics provide minimal relief, clients with severe vomiting who are unable to take medications orally, clients with clotting disorders who cannot tolerate injections without bruising, and clients unable to swallow orally administered medications.

Continuous drip morphine is given in the acute care setting as well as the home. In the hospital the drug is mixed in an intravenous solution of either dextrose in water (D5W) or lactated Ringer's solution. The morphine is delivered by an infusion control pump (see Chapter 37) to ensure a safe, accurate, and steady rate of infusion. The prescribed dosage of morphine depends on the severity of the client's pain, tolerance to the medication, and previous history of drug use. Dosages may range from 4 mg per hour, with 100 mg morphine added to 500 ml IV fluid, to higher doses with 200 mg morphine added to 500 ml IV fluid. The higher the concentration of morphine, the smaller the amount of fluid the client receives. Each agency has guidelines for morphine dosage and infusion rates.

When a client is first placed on continuous drip morphine the nurse must make careful ongoing assessments. To prevent overdosage and central nervous system depression, the nurse records a baseline blood pressure and respiratory rate before the infusion begins. Once the infusion starts, the nurse monitors vital signs as often as every 15 to 30 minutes for the first few hours until the client gains pain relief at a constant dosage. If blood pressure or respirations decrease, the infusion rate is reduced according to the physician's order or agency policy. If the client continues to show signs of severe respiratory depression, the physician will order the infusion discontinued. The narcotic antagonist naloxone (Narcan) should be available to reverse respiratory depression.

In the home setting, clients may use ambulatory infusion pumps. The pumps are lightweight, compact (about the size of a transistor radio), and allow free movement. The pump is battery powered and worn in a pouch attached to a belt or harness. The bag of medication and intravenous fluid fits inside the pump. A dosage of morphine, delivered continuously over 24 hours, is slowly infused into a central venous catheter. The pumps differ from a PCA device, which only delivers small, preset doses of medication. These large catheters inserted into the client's subclavian vein in the hospital, are relatively easy to maintain. The client and family learn to manage the pump, observe for drug side effects, and maintain function of the central venous catheter (see box). Since the client is initially managed on morphine in the hospital before going home, the risk of side effects is not as great unless the client or family member increases drug doses. A home health nurse makes routine visits to be sure the client manages the pump correctly.

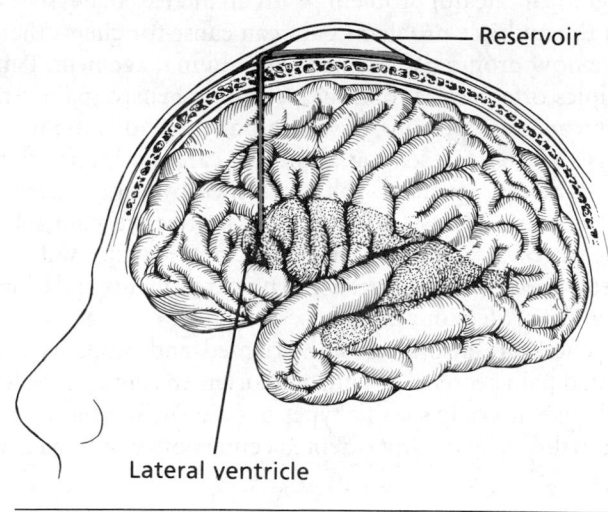

Tips in Managing Morphine Administered via Ambulatory Infusion Pumps

- Observe for side effects:
  - Sedation
  - Hypotension
  - Dizziness or fainting
  - Nausea
  - Vomiting
  - Respiratory depression
  - Constipation
- Be prepared to administer naloxone (Narcan) IM to reverse respiratory depression.
- Keep the central venous catheter patent. Maintain minimum pump flow rate. Irrigate catheter routinely with heparin flush.
- Prevent air from entering central venous catheter. Clamp catheter when infusion has stopped.
- Prevent infection at catheter site. Keep site clean with soap and water.

Fig. 35-9   Ommaya reservoir.

The intravenous fluid bag and tubing are usually changed about once a week by the nurse. This maintains the sterility of the system.

Chronic pain can become so intolerable that opiates or other analgesics given by conventional routes become ineffective. Giving opioids directly into the spinal column can produce effective analgesia with fewer systemic side effects. Small volumes of a local anesthetic (bupivacaine) or morphine are infused either into the epidural or subarachnoid (intrathecal) space in one of three ways. A small catheter is inserted through the skin and between two lumbar vertebrae to rest in the epidural space. The physician may also surgically implant an epidural catheter with a subcutaneous refillable reservoir. The final option is to surgically implant an Ommaya reservoir just underneath the scalp. The reservoir has a small thin catheter that is threaded by the surgeon through a small hole in the skull into the lateral ventricle (Fig. 35-9).

Clients receive medications intraspinally by continuous infusion or by intermittent bolus. The local anesthetic blocks conduction of nerve fibers peripherally around the area of the spinal cord injected. The bupivacaine also blocks the sympathetic nervous system locally. This can cause problems (such as hypotension, reduced intestinal peristalsis or bladder dysfunction). In contrast, intraspinal morphine stimulates opiate receptor sites in the central nervous system, as if a large dose of endorphins were administered (Alberico, 1984). Physicians usually administer intrathecal drugs. However, more nurse specialists and home care nurses are becoming responsible for the procedure. Table 35-8 lists nursing implications for clients with intraspinal catheter infusions.

The nurse uses all available pain relief measures for the client with cancer. The nurse-client relationship can help the client adapt to chronic pain. The client must feel that those responsible for managing the pain are competent and dependable.

PAIN CLINICS AND HOSPICES

During the last decade, health professionals from the United States and Canada have recognized pain as a

TABLE 35-8   Nursing Care of Clients with Intraspinal Infusions

Goal	Actions
Prevent catheter displacement	Limit client's activity.
	Secure catheter (if not connected to implanted reservoir) carefully to outside skin.
Maintain catheter function	Check external dressing around catheter site for dampness or discharge (CSF leak may develop).
Prevent infection	Use strict aseptic technique when caring for catheter.
	Change IV tubing every 24 hours.
Prevent undesirable complications	Monitor vital signs (hypotension, respiratory depression, and bradycardia indicate systemic absorption).
	Assess for blurred vision, ringing in the ears, or a metallic taste (toxicity).
Maintain urinary and bowel function	Monitor intake and output.
	Assess for bladder and bowel distention.

significant health problem. With an increased awareness of the multiple problems pain can cause for clients there are now programs designed for pain management. Pain clinics offer several options. A comprehensive pain center can treat persons on an in-patient and out-patient basis. Staff representing all health care disciplines such as nursing, medicine, physical therapy, and dietetics work with clients to find the most effective pain relief measures. A comprehensive clinic provides not only diverse therapy but research into new treatments and training for professionals.

There are also syndrome-oriented and modality-oriented pain centers. A syndrome-oriented center cares for clients with only specific types of pain such as back pain or arthritis. Modality-oriented centers offer only specific types of treatment, such as biofeedback, acupuncture, or TENS.

Hospices are programs for care of the terminally ill. Hospice comes from the Latin word "hospes", which means a place to rest. Often hospice programs are affiliated with hospitals. The programs help terminally-ill clients continue to live at home in comfort and privacy with the help of a hospice health care team. Pain control is a priority for hospices. Clients receive the proper dosage and forms of analgesics that provide pain relief. Under the guidance of hospice nurses, families learn how to monitor the client's symptoms and become the primary care givers. A hospice client may become hospitalized in the event of a brief acute care crisis or family problem.

Sample Evaluation of Interventions for Pain

Goals	Evaluative Measures	Expected Outcomes
Client obtains sense of well-being and comfort.	Note client's verbal expression of level of comfort. Note nonverbal behaviors. Use descriptive pain scales after each therapy.	Client expresses a reduced intensity of pain. There are fewer non-verbal expressions of discomfort. Client selects a lower number or point on the pain scale compared to the rating before therapy.
Client maintains ability to perform self-care.	Observe client during dressing, eating, bathing, grooming.	Client is able to independently perform self-care activities with or without self-care devices.
Client maintains existing physical and psychosocial function.	Evaluate physical function previously impaired by client's pain (such as range of motion, strength, posture, ambulation).	Client will show an improved level of physical function. Clients with acute pain may show an improvement equal to level of physical function before pain occurred. Clients with chronic pain are more debilitated. They will be able to function better during pain relief than when pain reoccurs.
	Evaluate client's willingness to socialize or interact with others.	Client will initiate more conversations, and participate in more social activities.
Client understands the pain experience.	Assess client's knowledge of the nature and the cause of pain, choice of therapy, and expected benefits of therapy. Assess client's ability to avoid worsening pain. Assess client's knowledge of medications related to dosage, action, time of administration, and side effects.	Client will correctly describe type and nature of pain and factors that aggravate discomfort. Client will describe ways to avoid worsening the pain. Client will administer analgesics or other medications correctly.

EVALUATION

The client is the best resource for evaluating the effectiveness of pain relief measures. The nurse must continually determine whether the character of the client's pain has changed and whether individual therapies are effective. The nurse is successful in treating pain if the goals of care are met. The nurse uses evaluative criteria in determining the outcome of pain relief therapies (see evaluation box).

If the nurse determines that a client continues to have discomfort after therapy, it may be necessary to try additional therapies. For example, if an analgesic provides only partial relief, the nurse may add relaxation exercises or guided imagery exercises.

The nurse also evaluates the client's perceptions of the effectiveness of therapy. The client may be able to help decide the best times to attempt a treatment. For example, the client is the best judge of whether a therapy works when anxiety and irritability are absent or when the pain is most severe.

The nurse also determines tolerance to therapy, as well as the overall relief obtained. For example, if a nurse administers an analgesic, side effects from the medication must be assessed in addition to the client's reported pain relief. Similarly, after turning a client the nurse should return to determine if the client is tolerating the new position and if pain has subsided. If a therapy aggravates discomfort, the nurse stops it immediately and seeks an alternative.

The nurse and client should not become frustrated if a given therapy does not act quickly. Time and patience are necessary to maximize the chances of a therapy working. The nurse considers what factors may be influencing the client's perceptions or reactions to pain. For example, a backrub may prove ineffective if the client has just learned the results of diagnostic tests and has had no opportunity to express concerns. The nurse evaluates the entire pain experience to determine what therapies are most effective and when they should be administered.

SUMMARY

The experience of pain is different for each person. The meaning pain conveys, the threat to comfort, and the potential implications of serious illness make the experience highly subjective but very real. Pain is a problem faced in every health care setting. The nurse is most effective in providing comfort by understanding the nature of pain and the client's perceptions, eliminating personal prejudices about pain, and working closely with the client to find the best pain relief measures.

KEY CONCEPTS

✓ Pain is largely a subjective experience.

✓ Pain is a protective mechanism that warns of tissue injury.

✓ A nurse's misconceptions about pain often result in doubt as to the degree of the client's suffering and an unwillingness to provide relief.

✓ Knowledge of the three components of the pain experience—reception, perception, and reaction—provides the nurse with guidelines for determining pain relief measures.

✓ An interaction of psychologic and cognitive factors affect a person's pain perception.

✓ Sensory messages from large nerve fibers can theoretically close synaptic gates to block transmission of pain stimuli.

✓ A number of therapies that provide pain relief may act by causing an increase in endorphin levels.

✓ The nature of a person's past experience with pain will affect the ability and willingness to cope with future discomfort.

✓ A client's pain tolerance influences the nurse's perceptions of the seriousness of discomfort.

✓ The difference between acute and chronic pain involves duration of discomfort, physical signs and symptoms, and the client's perceptions regarding pain relief.

✓ Chronic pain can affect every aspect of a person's life and lead to serious behavioral problems.

✓ The nurse does not attempt to assess the pain history while the client is experiencing severe discomfort.

✓ Pain scales lend objectivity to the measurement of pain and serve as tools to evaluate effectiveness of pain therapies.

✓ Clients who live with daily pain experience changes in their routine living activities.

✓ Pain can cause physical signs and symptoms similar to the signs and symptoms of certain disease processes.

✓ A nurse's assessment of a client in pain may lead to a nursing diagnosis of an alteration in comfort to diagnoses related to the physical and behavioral problems resulting from pain.

✓ Clients waiting to undergo invasive tests may gain some relief from pain by anticipatory guidance.

✓ Central to a nurse's plan for pain relief is developing a therapeutic relationship with the client and educating the client about pain.

✓ The nurse individualizes pain therapy by collaborating closely with the client, using assessment findings, and trying a variety of therapies.

✓ Eliminating sources of painful stimuli is a basic nursing measure for promoting a client's comfort.

✓ Progressive relaxation exercises and guided imagery promote a sense of relaxation and lessen awareness of pain.

✓ Proper administration of analgesics require the nurse to know the client's response to the drugs, select the proper medication, and administer an accurate dose in a timely manner.

✓ Using a regular schedule for analgesic administration helps prevent pain.

✓ Respiratory depression is a side effect of opiates.

✓ When pain interferes with a person's ability to perform self-care, the nurse may provide assistive devices for clients.

✓ The nurse's primary role in caring for a client who receives local anesthesia is protecting the client from injury.

✓ The client with intractable cancer-related pain requires dosages of analgesics that give immediate relief so that drug-seeking behaviors leading to drug dependence are avoided.

✓ The aim of therapy for cancer clients is to anticipate and prevent pain rather than treat it.

✓ Evaluation of the client's pain therapy requires consideration of the changing character of pain, response to therapy, and the client's perceptions of a therapy's effectiveness.

REFERENCES

Adams, RD: Pain: general considerations. In Isselbacher, KJ, et al., editors: Harrison's principles of internal medicine, ed. 9, New York, 1980, McGraw-Hill Book Co.

Alberico, JG: Breaking the chronic pain cycle, Am J Nurs 84:1222, 1984.

Baily, LM: Music's soothing charms, Am J Nurs 85:1280, 1985.

Brena, SF: In Brena, SF, and Chapman, SL, editors: Management of patients with chronic pain, New York, 1983, SP Medical and Scientific Books.

Carney, RM: Clinical applications of relaxation training, Hosp Prac 18(7):83, 1983.

Cash, JT: Sexuality and chronic pain, Am J Nurs 84:1417, 1984.

Cleeland, CS: The impact of pain on the patient with cancer, Cancer 54 (suppl):2635, 1984.

Craig, KD: Social modelling influences in pain. In Sternbach, RA, editor: The psychology of pain, ed. 2, New York, 1986, Raven Press.

Daut, RL, and Cleeland, CS: The prevalence and severity of pain in cancer, Cancer 50:1913, 1982.

Guyton, AC: Anatomy and physiology, New York, 1985, Saunders College Publishing.

Heidrich, G, and Perry, S: Helping the patient in pain, Am J Nurs 82:1828, 1982.

Krieger, D: Therapeutic touch: the imprimatur of nursing, Am J Nurs 75:784, 1975.

Maxwell, MB: How to use methadone for the cancer patient's pain, Am J Nurs 80:1606, 1980.

Mayer, DK: Non-pharmacologic management of pain in the person with cancer, Adv Nurs 10:325, 1985.

Mayer, DK, and Coyle, N: Spinal relief of cancer pain, Am J Nurs 86:1050, 1986.

McCaffrey, M: Nursing management of the patient with pain, ed. 2, Phildelphia, 1979, J.B. Lippincott Co.

McCaffrey, M: Understanding your client's pain, Nurs 80 10:26, 1980.

McCaffery, M: Would you administer placebos for pain? These facts can help you decide, Nurs 82 12:22, 1982.

Meinhart, NT, and McCaffery, M: Pain: a nursing approach to assessment and analysis, Norwalk, Conn., 1983, Appleton-Century-Crofts.

Miller, JF, and Shuter, R: An exploratory study of pain expression styles among blacks and whites, Int J Intercult Rel 6:281, 1982.

Price, DD, et al: Psychophysical analysis of experimental factors that selectively influence the affective dimension of pain, Pain 8(2):137, April 1980.

Rankin, MA, and Snider, B: Nurse's perceptions of cancer patient's pain, Canc Nurs 7:149, 1984.

Taylor, AG, et al.: How effective is TENS for acute pain? Am J Nurs 83:1171, 1983.

Taylor, AG, et al.: Duration of pain, condition, and physical pathology as determinants of nurses assessment of patients in pain, Nurs Res 33:4, 1984.

Timmermans, G, and Sternback, RA: Human chronic pain and personality: a canonical correlation analysis. In Bonica, JJ, and Albe-Fessard, D, editors: Advances in pain research and therapy, vol. 1, New York, 1976, Raven Press.

Witt, J: Relieving chronic pain, Nurs Pract 9:36, 1984.

Research Articles

Jacox, AK, and Stewart, M: Psychosocial contingencies of the pain experience, Iowa City, 1973, University of Iowa College of Nursing.

Marks, RM, and Sachar, EJ: Undertreatment of medical inpatients with narcotic analgesics, Ann Intern Med 78:173, 1973.

Melzack, R, and Wall, PD: Pain mechanisms: a new theory, Science 150:971, 1965.

Melzack, R, et al.: Relief of dental pain by ice massage of the hand, Can Med Assoc J 122:189, 1980.

ADDITIONAL READINGS

Barnett, DC, and Hair, B: Use and effectiveness of transcutaneous electrical nerve stimulation in pain management, J Neurosurg Nurs, 13:323, 1981.

Bast, C, and Hayes, P: Patient-controlled analgesia, Nurs 86 16(1):25, 1986.

Bast, C, and Hayes, P: PCA: a new way to spell pain relief, RN 49(8):18, 1986.

Boyer, MW: Continuous drip morphine, Am J Nurs 82:603, 1982.

Bonica, JJ, and Albe-Fessard, D, editors: Advances in pain research and therapy, vol. 1, New York, 1976, Raven Press.

Cook, JD: The therapeutic use of music: a literature review, Nurs Forum 20:253, 1981.

Cook, JD: Music as an intervention in the oncology setting, Canc Nurs, 9:23, 1986.

Dimotto, JW: Relaxation, Am J Nurs 84:754, 1984.

Gramse, CA: For control of severe pain: dorsal column stimulation, Am J Nurs 78:1022, 1978.

Hannon, D, et al.: Pain: portable relief for terminal patients, RN 48:37, 1985.

Haslam, DR: Age and the perception of pain, Psychonomic Sci 15:86, 1969.

Hauck, SL: Pain: problem for the person with cancer, Canc Nurs 9:66, 1986.

Kaido, RF: Age and morphine analgesia in cancer patients with postoperative pain, Clin Pharmacol Rev 28:823, 1980.

Kanner, RM, and Portenoy, RK: Are the people who need analgesics getting them? Am J Nurs 86:589, 1986.

Keller, E, and Bzdek, VM: Effects of therapeutic touch on tension headache pain, Nurs Res 35:101, 1986.

Locsin, R: The effect of music on the pain of selected postoperative patients, J Adv Nurs 6:19, 1981.

McCaffery, M: How to relieve your patients' pain fast and effectively with oral analgesics, Nurs 80 10:58, 1980.

McCaffery, M: Relieving pain with noninvasive techniques, Nurs 80 10:55, 1980.

Melzack, R: The McGill pain questionnaire: major properties and scoring methods, Pain 1:277, 1975.

Moertel, CG: Relief of pain with oral medications, Aust NZ J Med 6(suppl 1):1, 1976.

Moore, DE, and Blacker, HM: How effective is TENS for chronic pain? Am J Nurs 83:1175, 1983.

Moulin, DE, and Coyle, N: Spinal relief of cancer pain, Am J Nurs 86:1050, 1986.

Proctor, MR, and Warfield, CA: Biofeedback pain control, Hosp Pract 104, 1984.

Rahr, V: Giving intrathecal drugs, Am J Nurs 86:829, 1986.

Wells, N.: The effect of relaxation on postoperative muscle tension and pain, Nurs Res 31:236, 1982.

Williams, DJ: Pushbutton pain relief puts the patient in control, 85:1458, 1985.

Zahourek, RP: Hypnosis in nursing practice. I. Emphasis on the "problem patient" who has pain, J Psychosoc Nurs 20:13, 1982.

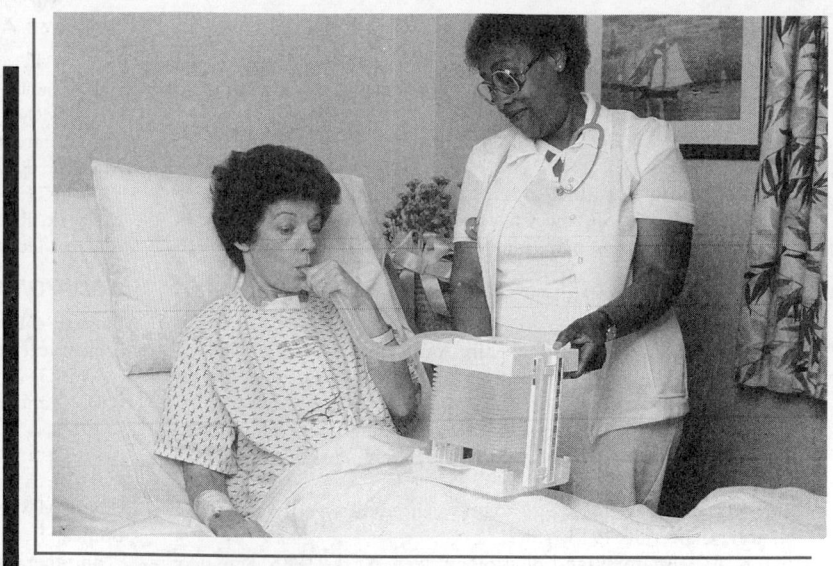

OBJECTIVES

Mastery of content in this chapter will enable the student to:

- Define the key terms listed.
- Describe the gross structure and function of the respiratory system.
- Identify processes involved in ventilation, perfusion, and exchange of respiratory gases.
- Describe neural and chemical regulation of respiration.
- Explain how a client's level of health, age, life-style, and environment can affect tissue oxygenation.
- Identify causes and effects of hyperventilation, hypoventilation, and hypoxemia.
- Perform a nursing assessment of the respiratory system.
- Develop nursing diagnoses for altered oxygenation.
- Describe nursing interventions to increase activity tolerance, maintain or promote lung expansion, promote mobilization of pulmonary secretions, maintain a patent airway, promote oxygenation, and restore cardiopulmonary function.
- Develop evaluation criteria for the nursing care plan for the client with altered oxygenation.

KEY TERMS

Alveolar Hyperventilation
Alveolar Hypoventilation
Atelectasis
Bronchoscopy
Cardiac Arrest
Chest Percussion
Chest Physiotherapy
Coccidioidomycosis
Cough
Diffusion
Ear Oximeter
Erythrocyte
Flail Chest
Hemoptysis

Hypovolemia
Hypoxia
Incentive Spirometry
Nebulization
Orthopnea
Oxygen Therapy
Passive Smoking
Pneumothorax
Polycythemia
Postural Drainage
Pulmonary Function Tests
Pursed-Lip Breathing
Thoracentesis
Ventilation
Vibration

Oxygenation

Oxygen is a basic human need and is required for life. The nurse often encounters clients who are unable to meet oxygen needs independently. To help clients meet their oxygen needs the nurse must understand respiratory physiology.

Respiratory physiology involves oxygenation of the body through the mechanisms of ventilation, perfusion, and transport of respiratory gases. In addition, neural and chemical regulators control fluctuations in respiratory rate and depth to meet tissue oxygen demands.

Level of health, age, life-style, and environment also affect the ability to meet tissue oxygen needs. When a client is unable to meet oxygen requirements, hyperventilation, hypoventilation, or hypoxemia may result.

This chapter discusses respiratory physiology, factors affecting oxygenation, hyperventilation, hypoventilation, hypoxia, and care of the client unable to meet oxygen needs. Through the nursing process the nurse assesses and diagnoses oxygenation needs, plans and implements nursing interventions to meet them, and evaluates the client's response to nursing care.

RESPIRATORY PHYSIOLOGY

Most cells in the body obtain much of their energy from chemical reactions involving oxygen. Cells must also eliminate carbon dioxide (Vander, Sherman, and Luciano, 1980). For this exchange of respiratory gases to occur, the organs, nerves, and muscles of respiration must be intact. In addition, the central nervous system

Major Anatomic Structures of the Thorax and Their Functions

INSPIRATORY MUSCLES
Diaphragm

Contraction causes the diaphragm to descend, creating a negative pleural pressure and increasing the vertical dimension of the lungs, which contributes to inflation of the lungs, (Fig. 36-2, *A*). The increase in vertical dimension and the decrease in intrapulmonary pressure (negative with respect to atmospheric pressure) causes air to enter the lungs.

External Intercostal

- Contraction elevates the anterior ends of the ribs, causing them to move upward and outward. This increases the anteroposterior dimension of the thorax.

Accessory Muscles

- Accessory muscles include the scalene, sternocleidomastoid, and trapezius muscles. Contraction elevates the first two ribs and elevates the sternum.

EXPIRATORY MUSCLES
Internal Intercostal

- Contracture pulls ribs down and in, thereby decreasing the anteroposterior diameter of the thorax.

Abdominal Respiratory

- Abdominal respiratory muscles include the rectus, transverse abdominis internal oblique, and external oblique muscles. Contraction depresses lower ribs, forces the diaphragm up, and decreases the vertical dimension of the thoracic cavity (Fig. 36-2, *B*).

PLEURAL SPACE

- A potential space, which is only a thin film of liquid lying between the outer layer of the lung (visceral pleura) and the inner layer of the chest cavity (parietal pleura). It permits a smooth, gliding movement of lungs along the chest wall. Normally air is not present in the pleural space.

LUNGS
Left (Two Lobes) and Right (Three Lobes)

- Transfers oxygen from the atmosphere into the alveoli and transfers carbon dioxide from the alveoli to the lungs and excreted as a waste product. Filters toxic material from circulation; metabolizes compounds, such as angiotensin I, bradykinin, and prostaglandins; and is a reservoir for blood.

Alveoli

- Transfers oxygen and carbon dioxide to and from the blood through the alveolar membrane. These tiny air sacs expand during inspiration, greatly increasing the surface area over which exchange of gases occurs (Fig. 36-1).

---

must be able to regulate the cycle of inspiration and expiration.

Structure and Function

Respiration can be altered by conditions or diseases that occur in the pulmonary system, resulting in changes of structure and function. The respiratory muscles, pleural space, lungs, and alveoli (Fig. 36-1) are essential to the three major purposes of the respiratory system: ventilation, perfusion, and exchange of respiratory gases (see box).

Ventilation

Ventilation is the process by which gases are moved into and out of the lungs. Adequate ventilation requires coordination of the muscular and elastic properties of the lung and thorax, as well as intact innervation. The major inspiratory muscle is the diaphragm, which is innervated by the phrenic nerve. This nerve exits the spinal cord at the fourth vertebra. Spinal cord disruption at the fourth cervical level can sever the phrenic cervical nerve and impair the diaphragm's function. The cervical vertebrae are commonly injured in diving and automobile accidents. These clients may be dependent on a ventilator for the rest of their lives because the diaphragm does not descend for inspiration. For adequate ventilation, the lungs must be able to do the work of breathing and move respiratory gases into and out of the lungs.

WORK OF BREATHING

The work of breathing is effort required to expand and contract the lungs. It is determined by the degree of compliance of lung tissue, resistance of the airway, presence of active expiration, and use of accessory muscles of respiration (Groër and Shekleton, 1983).

Compliance is the ability of the lungs and thorax to

expand in response to increased intraalveolar pressure (Groër and Shekleton, 1983). Simply stated, compliance is the ability of the lungs to expand. Compliance is decreased in diseases such as pulmonary edema, interstitial fibrosis, or pleural fibrosis. In addition, congenital or traumatic structural abnormalities, such as kyphosis or fractured ribs, decrease compliance.

Airway resistance is the pressure difference between the mouth and the alveoli in relation to the rate of flow of inspired gas. Airway resistance can be increased by an airway obstruction, such as foreign body, or small airway disease, such as asthma, or tracheal edema. When resistance is increased, the amount of air traveling through the anatomical airways is decreased.

Active expiration is the use of muscle groups to contract the lungs. Expiration is a passive process that depends on elastic recoil properties of the lungs and requires little or no muscle work. Elastic recoil is produced by elastic fibers in lung tissue and by surface tension in the fluid film lining the alveoli (Bushnell, 1981).

Accessory muscles of respiration, the sternocleidomastoid muscle groups, can increase lung volume during inspiration. Clients with chronic obstructive pulmonary disease, especially emphysema, frequently use these muscles to increase lung volume. During assessment the nurse may observe the client's clavicles being elevated in the inspiratory phase of respiration.

Decreased compliance, increased airway resistance, active expiration, or use of accessory muscles increases the work of breathing, resulting in an increased energy expenditure. To meet this expenditure the body increases its metabolic rate. Consequently the need for oxygen is increased. This sequence is a vicious circle for a client with impaired ventilation and causes further deterioration of respiratory status.

VOLUMES

Normal volumes within the lung are measured through pulmonary function testing. Some of these measurements are taken with a spirometer, which measures the volume of air entering or leaving the lungs. Variations in lung volumes may be associated with health states such as pregnancy, exercise, obesity, or obstructive and restrictive pathological conditions of the lung. The amount of surfactant, degree of compliance, and strength of respiratory muscles can affect pressures and volumes within the lungs as well.

PRESSURES

Gases are moved into and out of the lungs, through a process involving pressures (Fig. 36-2). Intrapleural pressure is negative to (less than) atmospheric pressure, which is 760 mm Hg at sea level. For air to flow into the lungs, intrapleural pressure must become more negative, setting up a pressure gradient between the at-

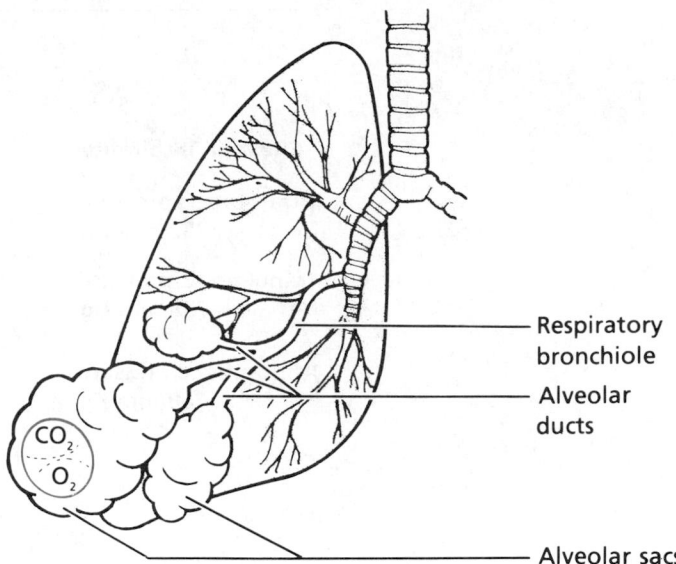

Fig. 36-1   Alveoli at the terminal end of the lower airway. From Groer, MW, and Shekleton, ME: Basic pathophysiology: a conceptual approach, ed. 2, St. Louis, 1983, The C.V. Mosby Co.

mosphere and alveoli, which moves air into the lungs. In addition, intra-alveolar pressures become slightly negative with respect to atmospheric pressure, increasing airflow into the air sacs. When atmospheric air is introduced into the intrapleural space, the negative pull is equalized, resulting in contraction of the lung (Fig. 36-2).

Perfusion

The primary function of pulmonary circulation is to move blood to and from the blood-gas barrier so gas exchange can occur. Pulmonary circulation is also a reservoir for blood so the lung can increase its blood volume without large increases in pulmonary artery or venous pressures. Finally, this circulatory system filters blood to remove small thrombi before they reach the brain or other vital organs (West, 1979).

PULMONARY CIRCULATION

Pulmonary circulation begins at the pulmonary artery, which receives mixed venous blood from the right ventricle. Blood flow through this system depends on the pumping ability of the right ventricle, which has an output of about 5 to 6 liters per minute. The flow continues from the pulmonary artery through the pulmonary arterioles, pulmonary capillaries (where the exchange of gases takes place), pulmonary venules, and pulmonary veins. It returns oxygenated blood to the left atrium.

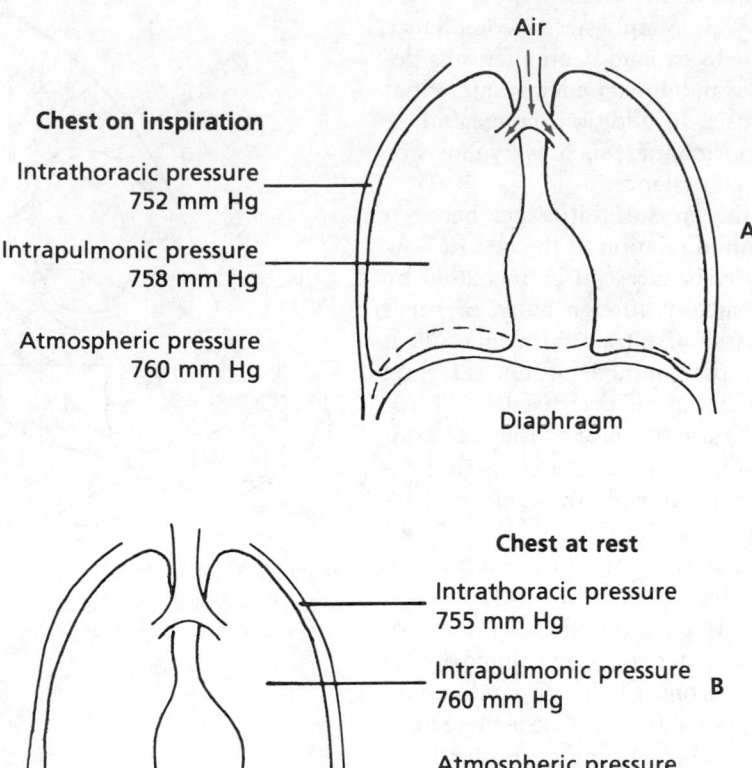

Fig. 36-2 **A,** Contraction of the diaphragm to increase vertical dimensions of the lungs. **B,** Relaxation of the diaphragm decreasing vertical dimensions of the lungs.
From Wade, JF: Comprehensive respiratory care, ed. 3, St. Louis, 1982, The C.V. Mosby Co.

DISTRIBUTION

Pressures within the pulmonary circulatory system are low in comparison to those in the systemic circulatory system. The normal pulmonary systolic arterial pressure is between 20 and 30 mm Hg, the diastolic pressure is less than 12 mm Hg, and the mean pressure is less than 20 mm Hg (Daily and Schroeder, 1985). Because of low pressure and low resistance the walls of the pulmonary vessels are thinner than those in the systemic circulation and contain less smooth muscle. The lung accepts the total cardiac output from the right ventricle and, except in cases of alveolar hypoxia, does not direct blood flow from one region to another.

Exchange of Respiratory Gases

Respiratory gases are exchanged in the alveoli and body tissues. Oxygen is transferred from the lungs to the blood, and carbon dioxide is transferred from the blood to the alveoli to be exhaled as a waste product.

At the tissue level, oxygen is transferred from the blood to tissues, and carbon dioxide is transferred from tissues to the blood to return to the alveoli and be exhaled. This transfer depends on the process of diffusion.

DIFFUSION

Diffusion is movement of molecules from an area of high concentration to an area of lower concentration. Diffusion of respiratory gases can be affected by thickness of the membrane across which gases diffuse and by the membrane's surface area.

Increased thickness of the membrane decreases the rate of diffusion because respiratory gases take longer to diffuse. In clients with pulmonary edema, pulmonary infiltrate, or a pulmonary effusion, thickness of the respiratory membrane is increased. As a result, diffusion is slowed and delivery of oxygen to tissues is impaired.

The surface area of the membrane can be altered as a result of a chronic disease (such as emphysema), an acute disease (such as a pneumothorax), or a surgical process (such as a lobectomy). The surface area is decreased when fewer alveoli are functioning.

OXYGEN TRANSPORT

The oxygen transport system consists of the lungs and cardiovascular system. Adequate oxygen delivery depends on the amount of oxygen entering the lungs (ventilation), blood flow to the lungs and tissues (perfusion), adequacy of diffusion, and the capacity of blood to carry oxygen. The capacity to carry oxygen is influenced by the amount of dissolved oxygen in the plasma, the amount of hemoglobin, and the affinity of hemoglobin for oxygen.

Only a relatively small amount of required oxygen, about 3%, is dissolved in the plasma. Most oxygen is transported by hemoglobin. The hemoglobin molecule serves as a carrier for oxygen and carbon dioxide. The hemoglobin molecule combines with oxygen to form oxyhemoglobin. The maximal amount of oxygen that can be combined with hemoglobin is called the oxygen capacity. Each gram of hemoglobin can combine with 1.39 ml of oxygen (West, 1979). When total hemoglobin is multiplied by this figure, the product is the total oxygen-carrying capacity of hemoglobin. The oxyhemoglobin molecule is easily reversible, allowing hemoglobin and oxygen to dissociate, which frees oxygen to enter tissues.

CARBON DIOXIDE TRANSPORT

The transport of respiratory gases includes movement of carbon dioxide. Carbon dioxide diffuses into red blood cells and is rapidly hydrated into carbonic acid because of the presence of carbonic anhydrase. The carbonic acid then dissociates into hydrogen (H^+) and bicarbonate (HCO_3^-) ions. The hydrogen ion is buffered by hemoglobin, and the HCO_3^- diffuses into the plasma (Ganong, 1983) (see also Chapter 37). In addition, some of the carbon dioxide in red blood cells reacts with amino acid groups, forming carbamino compounds. This reaction can occur rapidly without the presence of an enzyme. Reduced hemoglobin (deoxyhemoglobin) can combine with carbon dioxide more easily than oxyhemoglobin, and therefore the majority of carbon dioxide is transported by venous blood.

Regulation of Respiration

The main purpose of respiratory regulation is to supply sufficient oxygen to meet the body's demands, such as exercise, infection, or pregnancy. In addition, respiratory regulation promotes exhalation of metabolically produced carbon dioxide, which is a determinant of acid-base status. Adequacy of respiratory regulation is measured by arterial blood gases (see Chapter 37).

There are two respiratory regulators: neural regula-

Neural and Chemical Regulation of Respiration

NEURAL REGULATION

- Maintains rhythm and depth of respiration, as well as the balance between inspiration and expiration.

Cerebral Cortex

- Voluntary control of respiration, delivers impulses to the respiratory motor neurons by way of the spinal cord. Voluntary control of respiration accommodates speaking, eating, and swimming.

Medulla Oblongata

- Automatic control of respiration, which occurs continuously.

CHEMICAL REGULATION

- Maintains appropriate rate and depth of respirations based on changes in the blood's carbon dioxide (CO_2), oxygen (O_2), and hydrogen ion (H^+) concentration.

Chemoreceptors

- Located in the medulla and aortic and carotid bodies. Changes in chemical content of O_2, CO_2, and H^+ stimulate chemoreceptors, which, in turn, stimulate neural regulators to adjust the rate of depth of ventilation to maintain normal arterial blood gases. Chemical regulation can occur during routine physical exercise or in some illnesses. Chemical regulation is a short-term adaptive mechanism.

---

tors and chemical regulators. Neural regulation includes the central nervous system control of respiratory rate, depth, and rhythm. Chemical regulation involves the influence of chemicals, such as carbon dioxide and hydrogen ions, on the rate and depth of respiration (see box).

FACTORS AFFECTING OXYGENATION

Adequacy of ventilation, perfusion and transport of respiratory gases from the lungs to tissues is influenced by four factors: (1) physiological, (2) developmental, (3) life-style, and (4) environmental.

Physiological Factors

Any condition that affects respiratory system functioning directly affects the ability to meet the body's oxygen demands. The general classifications of respiratory disorders include hyperventilation, hypoventilation, hypoxia, and hypercapnia. These are described in detail later in the chapter.

Other physiological processes also affect oxygenation (Table 36-1). These include alterations that affect the oxygen-carrying capacity of blood, such as the anemias; alterations in the ability of the myocardial pump to perfuse ventilated regions of the lung and to deliver oxygenated blood to tissues; and increases in the body's metabolic demands. The increased demand may be normal, such as during pregnancy, or result from an abnormal process, such as fever and infection. Alterations that affect chest wall movement or the central nervous system also affect oxygenation.

DECREASED OXYGEN-CARRYING CAPACITY

As noted earlier, hemoglobin carries 97% of the diffused oxygen to tissues. Thus any process that decreases or alters hemoglobin decreases the oxygen-carrying capacity of blood. Anemia and inhalation of toxic substances are two disorders that decrease carrying capacity.

Anemia is characterized by below normal levels of hemoglobin in the blood. Anemia reflects one or more of three basic processes: decreased hemoglobin production, increased red cell destruction, or blood loss. Assessment findings in clients with anemia include fatigue, decreased activity tolerance, increased breathlessness, pallor, and increased heart rate. Severe anemia in the elderly can cause cardiac failure.

Carbon monoxide is the most common toxic inhalant decreasing the oxygen-carrying capacity of blood. A bond of the carbon monoxide molecule with the hemoglobin molecule is stronger than the bond between hemoglobin and oxygen. Because of the bond's strength, carbon monoxide is not easily dissociated from hemoglobin. Elevated carbon monoxide blood levels are found in clients who have attempted suicide by sitting in a car with the motor running in a closed garage, who have survived dwelling fires, and who have inhaled "side stream" smoke from cigarettes at home or work.

Assessment findings for clients with carbon monoxide poisoning depend on the percentage of hemoglobin saturated with carbon monoxide. An outstanding clinical feature is the absence of cyanosis. The skin of carbon monoxide victims can appear normal or cherry red. When 10% or less of the hemoglobin is saturated with carbon dioxide, there are usually no symptoms. If 10% to 20% is saturated, the client complains of a headache resulting from cerebral vasodilation. A 20% to 30% saturation causes chest pain as a result of myocardial hypoxia. When 30% to 40% is saturated, the client

TABLE 36-1 Physiological Processes Affecting Oxygenation

Process	Effect on Oxygenation
Anemia	Decreases oxygen-carrying capacity of blood.
Toxic inhalant (for example, carbon monoxide)	Decreases oxygen-carrying capacity of blood. Carbon monoxide displaces oxygen from hemoglobin and decreases the capacity of blood to carry oxygen.
Airway obstruction	Limits inspired oxygen delivered to the alveoli.
High altitudes	Decreases inspiratory oxygen concentration because atmospheric oxygen concentration is lower.
Hypovolemia and left-sided heart failure	Reduces cardiac output and perfusion to ventilated regions of the lung.
Fever	Increases metabolic rate and tissue oxygen demand.
Decreases chest wall motion (for example, musculoskeletal impairments)	Prevents descent of the diaphragm and reduces anterior-posterior diameter of the thorax on inspiration, thereby reducing the volume of inspired air.

experiences a severe headache, chest pain, weakness, nausea, and vomiting. As the amount of hemoglobin saturated with carbon monoxide increases, the client's heart rate and respiratory rate increase. When the hemoglobin is more than 50% saturated, Cheyne-Stokes respiration, coma, and death may result (Luce, Tyler, and Pierson, 1984).

DECREASED INSPIRED OXYGEN CONCENTRATION

When the concentration of inspired oxygen declines, the oxygen-carrying capacity of the blood is decreased. Decreases in the fraction of inspired oxygen concentration (FI_{O_2}) can be caused by an upper or lower airway obstruction (which limits delivery of inspired oxygen to alveoli), decreased environmental oxygen (as occurs at high altitudes), or decreased inspiration as the result of an incorrect oxygen concentration setting on respiratory therapy equipment.

An incorrect oxygen flow rate setting on oxygen therapy equipment can cause decreases in the FI_{O_2}. In addition, increased flow rates on oxygen therapy equipment can suppress the client's normal respiratory drive, resulting in slow, shallow respirations and hypoxemia. To avoid this, the nurse should determine that oxygen therapy is at the correct rate, by the correct route, for the correct client. Oxygen should be treated as a drug, and the "five rights" of drug administration should be followed (see Chapter 15).

DECREASED CARDIAC OUTPUT

Decreases in cardiac output reduce perfusion of the ventilated regions of the lung. As a result, there is a decrease in oxygen circulating to peripheral tissues. Common factors that decrease cardiac output are hypovolemia and left-sided heart failure.

HYPOVOLEMIA. Hypovolemia is a reduced circulating blood volume resulting from extracellular fluid losses such as shock or severe dehydration. If the loss is significant, fluid available for circulation is diminished. The body tries to adapt by increasing the heart rate and peripheral vasoconstriction in an effort to raise cardiac output.

LEFT-SIDED HEART FAILURE. Left-sided heart failure is an abnormal condition characterized by impaired function of the heart's left side and by elevated pressure and congestion in pulmonary veins and capillaries. If failure of the left ventricle is significant, the amount of blood ejected from the left ventricle drops greatly. As a result, cardiac output also falls.

Delivery of oxygen-rich hemoglobin to tissues depends on cardiac output. Decreases in cardiac output can cause tissue hypoxia, which may result in lower activity tolerance, breathlessness, dizziness, and confusion.

INCREASED METABOLIC RATE

Increases in metabolic activity of the body result in an increased oxygen demand. If the body systems are unable to meet this demand, the level of oxygenation declines. An increased metabolic rate is a normal response of the body to pregnancy, wound healing, and exercise, because the body in these situations is building tissue. Most people are able to meet the greater need for oxygen and do not display signs of oxygen deprivation.

The increased metabolism of the body during fever or infection is an adaptive response. The body attempts to meet the increased need for energy. If the infection or febrile state persists, the metabolic rate remains high and the body begins to break down protein stores. As the body continues to break down protein, muscle wasting occurs and the client has decreased muscle mass. Respiratory muscles, for example, diaphragm and intercostals, are also wasted and the client may not be able to do the work of breathing and eventually display signs and symptoms of hypoxemia.

CONDITIONS AFFECTING CHEST WALL MOVEMENT

Anything that reduces chest wall movement can result in decreased ventilation. If the diaphragm cannot fully descend with breathing, the volume of inspired air decreases and less oxygen is delivered to the alveoli and subsequently to tissues.

PREGNANCY. As the fetus grows during pregnancy, the greater size of the uterus pushes abdominal contents upward against the diaphragm. Thus, during the last trimester of pregnancy the inspiratory capacity of a pregnant woman declines. She may then experience shortness of breath on exertion and be easily fatigued.

OBESITY. Obese clients often have a heavy lower thorax and abdomen, which severely reduces lung volumes, particularly in the recumbent and supine positions. In some clients an obesity-hypoventilation syndrome develops in which oxygenation is decreased and carbon dioxide is retained, resulting in daytime sleepiness. The body tries to compensate by increasing red blood cell production. This results in polycythemia, an abnormally high number of red blood cells.

The obese client is also susceptible to pneumonia after an upper respiratory tract infection because the lungs cannot be fully expanded and pulmonary secretions are not mobilized in the lower lobes. The postoperative or immobilized client is at high risk for hypostatic bronchopneumonia. Pulmonary hygiene measures should be included in the nursing care plan to reduce the risks of hypostatic bronchopneumonia.

MUSCULOSKELETAL ABNORMALITIES. Musculoskeletal impairments in the thoracic region reduce oxygenation. Such impairments may result from abnormal structural configurations, trauma, muscular diseases, or diseases of the central nervous system.

Abnormal Structural Configurations. Abnormal structural configurations affecting oxygenation include those that affect the rib cage, such as pectus excavatum, and those that affect the vertebral column such as scoliosis. Pectus excavatum is a depression of the sternum that interferes with lung expansion. Kyphosis is an abnormal condition of the vertebral column characterized by increased convexity of the thoracic spine as viewed from the side. This abnormality produces a structural barrier to lung expansion. The angle of curvature can progress with time, resulting in severe hypoventilation and hypoxemia.

Trauma. Trauma to the chest wall may also impede inspiration. The person with multiple rib fractures develops a flail chest, in which fractures cause instability in part of the chest wall and paradoxical breathing, with the lung underlying the inspired area contracting on inspiration and bulging on expiration. This asynchronous chest wall movement can result in hypoxia.

Chest wall or upper abdomen incisions may also decrease chest wall movement and oxygenation. The client may breathe shallowly to minimize chest wall movement in order to avoid pain, thereby increasing the risk for hypostatic bronchopneumonia. Certain analgesics may also depress the respiratory center, thus decreasing respiratory rate. Therefore, with clients who have had surgery of the chest or upper abdomen, the nurse must use analgesics along with the techniques of coughing and deep breathing (see Chapter 35).

Muscle Diseases. Muscle diseases such as muscular dystrophy affect oxygenation of tissues. If muscular disease decreases the client's ability to expand and contract the chest, ventilation is impaired and atelectasis can occur.

Nervous System Diseases. Myasthenia gravis, Guillain-Barré syndrome, and poliomyelitis are examples of nervous system diseases that can affect respiratory functioning. Myasthenia gravis interferes with normal transmission of impulses from nerves to muscles. The disease involves the whole body, including muscles of respiration.

Guillain-Barré syndrome and poliomyelitis cause inflammation and paralysis of muscle groups. Guillain-Barré syndrome usually results in an ascending type of paralysis. If paralysis ascends to the thoracic region, respiratory muscles become paralyzed. This respiratory paralysis may later reverse, leaving the client with little or no residual paralysis. Poliomyelitis may lead to general or local paralysis. As with Guillain-Barré syndrome it may reverse, but poliomyelitis usually results in more residual paralysis.

Central Nervous System Alterations. Diseases or trauma involving the central nervous system, specifically the medulla oblongata and spinal cord, may result in impaired respiration. When the medulla oblongata is affected, neural regulation of respiration is damaged and abnormal breathing patterns may develop. Damage to the spinal cord can affect respiration in two ways. If the phrenic nerve is damaged, the diaphragm may not descend, thus reducing inspiratory lung volumes and causing hypoxemia. Spinal cord trauma below the fifth cervical vertebra usually leaves the phrenic nerve intact but damages nerves that innervate the intercostal muscles. This prevents the chest from expanding in the anterior-posterior diameter.

INFLUENCES OF CHRONIC DISEASE. The level of oxygenation can be decreased as a direct consequence of chronic disease, as with cardiopulmonary disease. It can also be decreased as a secondary effect, as with anemia in a client with osteoarthritis.

Chronic illness may also affect oxygenation as an indirect result of depression. A depressed client may not be interested in preparing meals or eating. When dietary intake declines, production of hemoglobin is diminished, and the oxygen-carrying capacity of blood declines.

Developmental Stage

The developmental stage of the client and the normal aging process can affect tissue oxygenation.

PREMATURE INFANT

A premature infant is at risk for hyaline membrane disease, which is thought to be caused by a surfactant deficiency. The surfactant-synthesizing ability of the lungs develops late in pregnancy and therefore may be lacking in premature infants (Groër and Shekleton, 1983).

INFANT AND TODDLER

Infants and toddlers are at risk for upper respiratory tract infections as a result of frequent exposure to other children. In addition, during the teething process some infants develop nasal congestion, which encourages bacterial growth and increases the potential for respiratory tract infection.

Upper respiratory tract infections are usually not dangerous, and the infant or toddler recovers with little difficulty. However, airway obstructions can develop. The two most common airway infections are bronchiolitis and acute epiglottitis. In addition obstruction can occur with aspirated foreign objects, such as food, buttons, or candy.

SCHOOL-AGE CHILD AND ADOLESCENT

School-age children and adolescents are exposed to respiratory infections and respiratory risk factors such as smoking. A healthy child usually does not have adverse pulmonary effects from respiratory infections. A person who starts smoking in adolescence and continues to smoke into middle age, however, has an increased risk for cardiopulmonary disease.

Research demonstrates that passive smoking or secondary smoking has harmful effects on the fetus, as well as on young children. Passive smoking is the smoke and toxic fumes inhaled by a nonsmoker from a smoker's cigarette. Continued exposure to passive smoke can result in chronic respiratory infections such as bronchitis.

OLDER ADULT

The respiratory system undergoes changes throughout the aging process. The connective tissue and bronchial tree undergo structural changes as the lungs lose elasticity. The alveoli are often enlarged and the bronchial ducts are dilated (Groër and Shekleton, 1983).

Ventilation and transfer of respiratory gases decline with age. Osteoporotic changes of the thoracic cage and kyphosis of the vertebrae occur normally with aging. With these changes the lungs are unable to expand fully, leading to lower oxygenation levels.

Normal changes in the lungs during aging increase the older adult's susceptibility to severe complications of infections, stress, and cardiac problems. Minor pulmonary infections can set off a series of responses leading to cardiopulmonary dysfunction.

Life-Style

A person's life-style may directly or indirectly affect the body's ability to meet oxygen requirements. Lifestyle factors that influence respiratory functioning include nutrition, exercise, cigarette smoking, substance abuse, and stress.

NUTRITION

Nutrition can affect respiratory function in three ways. First, severe obesity can decrease lung expansion because of the pressure of abdominal contents against the diaphragm and an increased O_2 demand on the body. Second, the malnourished client may experience respiratory muscle wasting, which results in decreased muscle strength and decreased respiratory excursion. The client may have a low activity tolerance demonstrated by dyspnea on exertion. Muscle weakness may also decrease the ability to cough productively, putting the client at risk for the accumulation of pulmonary secretions. Finally, both obese and malnourished clients are at risk for anemia.

EXERCISE

Exercise increases the body's metabolic activity and thus oxygen demands. The respiratory rate and depth of respirations increase, enabling the person to inhale more oxygen and expire excess carbon dioxide.

A physical exercise program has many benefits (see Chapter 42). People who exercise regularly have a lower pulse rate and blood pressure, increased blood flow, and greater oxygen extraction by working muscles. Fully conditioned people can increase oxygen consumption by 10% to 20% because of increased cardiac output. Regular exercise also benefits the client psychologically by enhancing the ability to perform activities of daily living and increasing sense of well-being (Luce, Tyler, and Pierson, 1984).

CIGARETTE SMOKING

Cigarette smoking is associated with a number of diseases, including lung cancer. The risk of lung cancer is 60 times greater for a person who smokes two packs of cigarettes a day than for someone who has never smoked. The mortality with lung cancer is about 90%, and is frequently diagnosed only when it has reached an advanced stage (Groër and Shekleton, 1983).

Cigarette smoking may lead to cardiovascular disease. The inhaled nicotine causes vasoconstriction of peripheral and coronary blood vessels. Thus cigarette smoking can worsen peripheral vascular and coronary artery diseases.

Smoking is also associated with recurrent respiratory tract infections, especially emphysema and chronic bronchitis. Smoking itself damages the ciliary clearance mechanism within the lungs and paralyzes cilia. As a result, cilia are unable to clear mucus from the airway, which leads to development of chronic bronchitis.

SUBSTANCE ABUSE

Excessive use of alcohol and other drugs can impair tissue oxygenation in two ways. First, the person who chronically abuses substances often has a poor nutritional intake. With the resultant decrease in iron-rich foods, hemoglobin production declines. Second, excessive use of alcohol and certain other drugs can depress the respiratory center in the central nervous system. The rate and depth of inspiration are reduced, decreasing the amount of oxygen inhaled. Thus less oxygen is available to tissues.

ANXIETY

A continuous state of severe anxiety increases the body's oxygen demand. The body responds to anxiety and other stresses by an increased rate and depth of respiration. Most people can adapt, but some, particularly those with chronic illnesses or acute life-threatening illnesses such as a myocardial infarction, cannot tolerate the oxygen demands associated with anxiety.

Environment

The environment can also influence the level of oxygenation. The incidence of pulmonary disease is higher in smoggy, urban areas than in rural areas. In addition, family members of smokers have a greater risk for respiratory tract infections or chronic illnesses because they passively inhale smoke.

The client's workplace similarly may increase the risk for pulmonary disease. Occupational pollutants include asbestos, talcum powder, dust, and airborne fibers. For example, farm workers in dry regions of the southwestern United States are at risk for coccidioidomycosis, a fungal disease caused by inhalation of spores of the windborne bacterium *Coccidioides immitis*.

Finally, altitude of the environment can affect oxygenation. In high altitudes the atmospheric oxygen pressure is lower, resulting in a lower percentage of inspired oxygen and decreased concentration of arterial oxygen.

ALTERATIONS IN RESPIRATORY FUNCTIONING

Alterations in respiratory function are caused by illnesses and conditions that affect ventilation or oxygen transport. The three primary alterations are hyperventilation, hypoventilation, and hypoxia.

Hyperventilation

The term "hyperventilation" is often used to refer to alveolar hyperventilation. It is a state of ventilation in excess of that required to maintain normal carbon dioxide levels in body tissues, thus excreting excess CO_2 (Groër and Shekleton, 1983).

Hyperventilation causes below normal carbon dioxide tension. Therefore the nurse must remember that hyperventilation is not associated with respiratory rate because an individual with tachypnea can still have an elevated carbon dioxide level and would therefore be hypoventilating.

Hyperventilation can be induced by anxiety, infections, drugs, or an acid-base imbalance. Acute anxiety can lead to hyperventilation resulting in loss of consciousness. Fever can result in hyperventilation as a result of compensatory mechanisms within the body. For each degree Fahrenheit increase in body temperature, there is a 7% increase in the metabolic rate (Groër and Shekleton, 1983). Higher metabolic rates increase carbon production. This, in turn, leads to increased respiration in clients without chronic obstructive pulmonary disease.

Hyerperventilation may also be chemically induced. Salicylate poisoning causes excessive stimulation of the respiratory center because of the body's attempt to compensate for carbon dioxide excess. Amphetamines also increase ventilation, primarily by raising carbon dioxide production.

Last, hyperventilation can occur as the body tries to compensate for metabolic acidosis. Ventilation increases to reduce the amount of carbon dioxide available to form carbonic acid (see Chapter 37).

Alveolar hyperventilation produces many signs and symptoms that can be identified by assessment (see box at left). Blood flow to major organs is diminished as a result of the vasoconstrictor effect of low carbon dioxide and reduced cardiac output. Hemoglobin does not release oxygen to tissues as readily, and tissue hypoxia results. As symptoms worsen, the client may become more agitated, which further increases the respiratory rate and can result in respiratory alkalosis.

Hypoventilation

Hypoventilation refers to alveolar hypoventilation, not the client's respiratory rate. It is a state such as hypercapnia, in which the carbon dioxide tension is elevated. Because too much carbon dioxide is in the blood, carbonic acid production increases and respiratory acidosis occurs (see Chapter 37).

Hypoventilation is caused by a pathophysiological mechanism. The central nervous system may be affected, as with a drug overdose or trauma to the brainstem, or the lungs may be affected. Severe atelectasis can produce hypoventilation. Atelectasis is a collapse of the alveoli that prevents normal respiratory exchange of oxygen and carbon dioxide. As alveoli collapse, less of the lung is capable of being ventilated and hypoventilation occurs.

The inappropriate administration of oxygen can also result in hypoventilation. Clients with chronic obstructive pulmonary disease have adapted to a high carbon dioxide level, and their only breathing stimulus is the hypoxic drive. High concentrations of oxygen, greater than 24% to 28% (1 to 3 L/minute), will obliterate the hypoxic drive. Thus elimination of the stimulus to breathe depresses or in some cases suppresses respiratory function and hypoventilation occurs.

Hypoventilation may cause many signs and symptoms revealed through physical assessment (see box at right). If untreated, the client's status can rapidly decline. Convulsions, unconsciousness, and death can result.

The goals of treatment for hypoventilation are first to restore or maintain optimal ventilatory function, second to improve tissue oxygenation, and third to restore or maintain acid-base balance (Groër and Shekleton, 1983).

Signs and Symptoms of Alveolar Hyperventilation

- Tachycardia
- Shortness of breath
- Chest pain
- Dizziness
- Light-headedness
- Decreased concentration
- Paresthesia
- Numbness (extremities, circumoral)
- Tinnitus
- Blurred vision
- Disorientation
- Tetany (carpopedal spasm)

Hypoxia

Hypoxia is inadequate cellular oxygenation that results from a deficiency in the delivery or use of oxygen at the cellular level (Groër and Shekleton, 1983). Hypoxia can be caused by (1) a decreased hemoglobin level and lowered oxygen-carrying capacity of the blood; (2) a diminished concentration of inspired oxygen as may occur at high altitudes; (3) inability of the tissues to extract oxygen from the blood as with cyanide poisoning; (4) decreased diffusion of oxygen from the alveoli to the blood as with pneumonia; and (5) poor tissue perfusion as with shock.

The clinical signs and symptoms of hypoxia include apprehension, restlessness, inability to concentrate, declining level of consciousness, dizziness, and behavioral changes (see box at right). The hypoxic client is unable to lie down and appears fatigued and agitated. Changes in vital signs include an increased pulse rate and increased rate and depth of respiration. However, as the hypoxia worsens, the respiratory rate may decline as a result of fatigue. During early stages of hypoxia the blood pressure is elevated, unless hypoxia is caused by shock. Cyanosis, a blue discoloration of the skin and mucous membranes caused by the presence of desaturated hemoglobin in capillaries, is a late sign of hypoxia. Cyanosis observed in the tongue and soft palate, where blood flow is high, indicates hypoxemia. Cyanosis elsewhere, as in the fingernail beds, may merely reflect stagnant blood flow (Luce, Tyler, and Pierson, 1984). Cyanosis is apparent when 5 g of hemoglobin per 100 ml of blood has been reduced to deoxyhemoglobin and has reached superficial capillaries (Groër and Shekleton, 1983). The nurse should observe other areas of the body besides skin for signs of cyanosis, such as the conjunctivae, mouth, nail beds, and peripheral circulation. The presence or absence of cyanosis, however, is not an absolute indicator of oxygenation status.

Dyspnea is another clinical sign of hypoxia. Dyspnea is shortness of breath or difficulty in breathing. Pathological dyspnea must be differentiated from physiological dyspnea, which is shortness of breath after exercise or excitement. Pathological breathlessness is a distressing sensation of not being able to catch one's breath (Groër and Shekleton, 1983).

Hypoxia is a life-threatening condition. Untreated, it can produce cardiac dysrhythmias that result in death. Hypoxia is treated by administration of oxygen, or by treatment of the underlying cause, such as shock or pneumonia.

ASSESSMENT

The nursing assessment of a client's respiratory functioning and determination of impairment should include data collected from the following areas:

1. Nursing history of the client's normal and present respiratory function, past impairments in respiratory functioning, and measures the client may use to optimize oxygenation.
2. Physical examination
3. Review of laboratory and diagnostic test results including sputum

Nursing History

The nursing history described here focuses on the client's ability to meet oxygen needs. The nursing history

---

Signs and Symptoms of Alveolar Hypoventilation

- Dizziness
- Headache (may be occipital only on awakening)
- Lethargy
- Disorientation
- Decreased ability to follow instructions
- Cardiac dysrhythmias
- Electrolyte imbalances
- Convulsions
- Coma
- Cardiac arrest

Signs and Symptoms of Hypoxia

- Restlessness
- Apprehension, anxiety
- Decreased ability to concentrate
- Decreased level of consciousness
- Increased fatigue
- Dizziness
- Behavioral changes
- Increased pulse rate
- Increased rate and depth of respiration
- Elevated blood pressure
- Cardiac dysrhythmias
- Pallor
- Cyanosis
- Clubbing
- Dyspnea

for respiratory function includes cough, shortness of breath, wheezing, pain, environmental exposures, frequency of respiratory tract infections, pulmonary risk factors, past respiratory problems, and medications.

COUGH

Cough is a sudden, audible expulsion of air from the lungs. The person breathes in, the glottis is partially closed, and the accessory muscles of expiration contract to expel the air forcibly. Coughing is a protective reflex to clear the trachea, bronchi, and lungs of irritants and secretions. In addition, the cough reflex prevents aspiration of foreign bodies into the lungs.

A cough is difficult to evaluate. Almost everyone has periods of coughing. Furthermore, clients with a chronic cough tend to deny, underestimate, or minimize their coughing, often because they are so accustomed to it that they are unaware of how frequently it occurs. A family member or significant other may be more objective about the client's frequency of coughing.

Once the nurse determines that the client has a cough, it must be identified as productive or nonproductive and its frequency assessed. A *productive cough* is one that results in sputum. Sputum is material coughed up from the lungs that may be expectorated through the mouth. It contains mucus, cellular debris, and microorganisms, and it may contain pus or blood. If a client is producing sputum, the nurse must obtain information regarding its color, taste, consistency, odor, and the presence of blood (see box). The nurse should also inquire if the sputum is produced at all times, just on rising from bed, or only when the client has a cold. If the sputum is discolored,

the nurse should inquire if it clears with coughing. Occasionally yellow sputum produced in the morning may clear with the second or third cough. The nurse inquires whether the amount has recently increased or decreased. The client should try to produce some sputum so the nurse can inspect it for color, consistency, and odor.

If hemoptysis (bloody sputum) is reported the nurse should be certain that it is associated with coughing. Hematemesis and bleeding from the upper respiratory tract are not usually associated with coughing (Smith, 1982). In addition the hemoptysis should be described according to amount, color, duration, and if mixed with sputum. Bright red sputum may indicate *Aspergillus* infection, lung abscess, tuberculosis, bronchogenic carcinoma, congestive heart failure, or pulmonary emboli. When a client reports bloody or blood-tinged sputum, diagnostic tests, such as examination of sputum specimens, chest x-ray examinations, bronchoscopy, or other x-ray studies, should be performed.

Coughing is classified as to the time when the client most frequently coughs. Clients with chronic sinusitis may cough only in the early morning or immediately after rising from a sleep. This clears the airway of mucus resulting from sinus drainage. Clients with chronic bronchitis generally produce sputum all day, although greater amounts are produced after rising from a semirecumbent or flat position. This is the result of the dependent accumulation of sputum in the airways and is associated with reduced mobility (see Chapter 42).

DYSPNEA

Dyspnea, or shortness of breath, can be a subjective finding (the client states that he feels short of breath) or an objective finding (exaggerated respiratory effort, use of the accessory muscles of respiration, flaring of the nares, and an extreme increase in the rate and depth of respirations) (Groër and Shekleton, 1983). Dyspnea is not always a direct reflection of the state of tissue oxygenation but may be a symptom of a discrepancy between the need for respiration and the body's ability to meet that need. The perception and occurrence of dyspnea depend on the client's state of mind, concentrations of carbon dioxide and oxygen in the blood, and adequacy of ventilation, perfusion, and transport of respiratory gases (Groër and Shekleton, 1983).

Jansen-Bjerklie, Carrieri, and Hudes (1986) studied the sensation of dyspnea across four classifications of pulmonary diseases: emphysema-bronchitis, restrictive, asthma, and vascular. They noted that while sensations of dyspnea were similar across all disease categories, the frequency, intensity, and periodicity of the dyspnea had the greatest effect on the quality and frequency of sensations reported (see research highlight). A second nursing study found a significant relationship between anxiety and reports of dyspnea and that dyspnea in clients

---

Range of Sputum Characteristics

COLOR
- Clear
- White
- Yellow
- Green
- Brown
- Red
- Streaked with blood

CONSISTENCY
- Frothy
- Watery
- Tenacious, thick

TASTE
- None

ODOR
- None
- Foul

PRESENCE OF BLOOD
- Occasionally
- Early morning
- Bright or dark red
- Tinged

with chronic obstructive pulmonary disease also resulted in distress on the somatic system and poor appetite (Gift, Plant, and Jacox, 1986).

The nursing history of dyspnea includes circumstances of its occurrence, such as with exertion, stress, or respiratory tract infection. The nurse also determines whether the client's perception of dyspnea affects the ability to lie flat. The client with true dyspnea is unable to lie flat. Orthopnea is an abnormal condition in which the person must use multiple pillows when lying down or sit to breathe. The presence of orthopnea is usually quantified, such as two- or three-pillow orthopnea. This means that the client perceives shortness of breath unless two or three pillows are used for sleeping.

WHEEZING

Wheezing is a form of rhonchus and is characterized by a high-pitched musical quality that does not clear with coughing. It is caused by high-velocity movement of air through a narrowed airway. Wheezing may be associated with asthma and acute bronchitis. Clients can usually describe when they wheeze and if it is present on inspiration or expiration.

The nurse should also obtain information about any precipitating factors such as a respiratory infection, allergens, exercise, or stress. Likewise, the nurse should

determine what the client uses for relief, such as rest or sitting upright. If the client uses a medication for relief, the nurse should determine what it is.

PAIN

Pain associated with respiration must be evaluated with regard to location, duration, radiation, and effect on respiration. Pleuritic chest pain is peripheral in location and may radiate to the scapular regions. It is worsened by inspiratory maneuvers, such as coughing, yawning, or sighing. Clients often describe pleuritic pain as knifelike. It lasts from a minute to hours and is always associated with inspiration. In addition, inspiratory pain is also typical of pericarditis.

Musculoskeletal pain may be present following exercise, rib trauma, or prolonged coughing episodes. This pain is also aggravated by inspiratory movements and may easily be confused with pleuritic chest pain (Smith, 1982).

ENVIRONMENTAL EXPOSURE

Environmental exposure to many inhaled substances is closely linked with respiratory disease. The nurse should investigate exposures in the client's home and workplace.

The most common environmental exposure in the home is cigarette smoke. The nurse should determine whether a client who is a nonsmoker is passively exposed to smoke. Passive smoke exposure occurs when the client breathes air containing smoke from another person's cigarette, cigar, or pipe.

An employment history should be obtained to assess exposure to substances such as fibers, fumes, or chemical inhalants. Dopico et al. (1984) noted that the respiratory effects of workers exposed to grain dust was similar to those of smokers and that the effects of smoking and grain dust were additive but not synergistic. In addition, exposure to minimal dust resulted in an increased incidence of symptoms associated with chronic obstructive pulmonary disease (Churg, et al., 1985). Last, respiratory symptoms such as coughing and wheezing were more prevalent in cotton textile workers than in the general population (Beck, Schachter, and Marinder, 1984).

Exposure to substances may occur during travel. Schistosomiasis infection can be acquired in Asia, Africa, the Caribbean, and South America. Coccidioidomycosis (valley fever) can be acquired, for example, in southwestern desert regions, from exposure to chicken farms, and river valleys, such as the Ohio and Mississippi valleys (Smith, 1982).

RESPIRATORY INFECTIONS

A nursing history should contain information about the client's frequency and duration of respiratory tract

---

✄ *Research Highlight* ✄

The purpose of this research was to compare recalled physical and emotional sensations during episodes of acute dyspnea across four types of pulmonary disease groups: emphysema-bronchitis, asthmatic, restrictive, and vascular. The study population consisted of 68 subjects. Measurements of temporal patterns of physical and emotional sensations before and after a dyspneic episode were identified. Researchers noted that the frequency of sensations were similar across all disease categories, but few signficant differences were identified. However, the frequency, intensity, and periodicity of the symptom of dyspnea had the greatest effect on the quality and the frequency of the symptoms reported. Asthmatics reported the lowest mean score and females reported the highest scores. Variables of pulmonary disease group, gender, fatigue, and support network were signficantly related to usual dyspnea. Pulmonary group, gender, and attendance at Better Breathers classes were significantly related to worst dyspnea.

Janson-Bjerklie, S, Carrieri, VK, and Hudes, M: The sensations of pulmonary dyspnea. Nurs Res 35(3):154.

infections. Although everyone occasionally experiences a common cold, with some people it frequently results in bronchitis or pneumonia. The nurse also asks about any known exposure to tuberculosis and about the results of the tuberculin skin test.

Because the acquired immunodeficiency syndrome (AIDS) may initially be diagnosed after *Pneumocystis carinii* or Mycobacterium pneumonia, the nurse should determine the client's exposure to illicit intravenous drug use and multiple heterosexual and homosexual contacts. These factors assist in identifying clients at risk for exposure to the AIDS virus. (Bennett, 1986).

RISK FACTORS

The nurse must also investigate familial and environmental risk factors. A family history of cancer, particularly lung cancer, or cardiovascular diseases should be noted. If the client's family has such a history, it is necessary to document which blood relatives have had the disease and their present level of health or age at time of death.

Other family risk factors include the presence of infectious diseases, particularly tuberculosis. The nurse should determine who in the client's household has been infected and the status of treatment.

Last, a complete employment history is necessary to identify exposure to substances such as asbestos, coal, or dust. This is particularly important with middle-aged and elderly adults who may have worked in places not regulated to protect workers from carcinogens.

MEDICATIONS

The last component of the nursing history should be medications the client is using. These include prescribed, over-the-counter, and illicit drugs and substances. Such medications may have adverse effects themselves or by interaction with other drugs. A person using a prescribed bronchodilator drug, for example, may decide that using an over-the-counter inhalant as well will be beneficial. This product may react with the prescribed medication by potentiating or decreasing its effect.

Illicit drugs, particularly parenterally administered narcotics, are often diluted with talcum powder. Their injection can cause pulmonary disorders resulting from the irritant effect of talcum powder on lung tissues.

The nursing health history of the respiratory system provides the nurse with a data base for the later physical examination. As with the total nursing history, this history helps identify factors that may affect the client's level of health.

TABLE 36-2 Inspection of Cardiopulmonary Status

Assessment	Abnormality	Cause
Eyes	Xanthelasma—yellow lipid lesions on eyelids	Associated with hyperlipidemia
	Corneal arcus—whitish opaque ring around junction of cornea and sclera	Abnormal finding in young to middle adults associated with hyperlipidemia (normal finding in elderly is arcus senilius)
	Pale conjuntivae	Associated with anemia
	Cyanotic conjunctivae	Associated with hypoxemia
	Petechiae on conjunctivae	Associated with fat embolus or bacterial endocarditis
Skin	Cyanosis—peripheral	Vasoconstriction and diminished blood flow
	Cyanosis—central	Hypoxemia
	Decreased skin turgor	Dehydration—may be a normal finding in the elderly as a result of decreased skin elasticity
	Edema—dependent	Associated with right- and left-sided heart failure
	Edema—periorbital	Associated with kidney disease
Fingertips and nailbeds	Cyanosis	Decreased cardiac output or hypoxia
	Splinter hemorrhages	Bacterial endocarditis
	Clubbing	Chronic hypoxemia
Mouth and lips	Cyanotic mucous membranes	Decreased oxygenation (hypoxia)
	Pursed-lip breathing	Associated with chronic lung disease
Neck veins	Distention	Associated with right-sided heart failure
Nose	Flaring nares	Air hunger, dyspnea
Chest	Retractions	Increased work of breathing, dyspnea
	Asymmetrical	Chest wall injury

Data from Dennison, R: Cardiopulmonary assessment: how to do it better in 15 easy steps, Nurs 86 16(4):34, 1986.

Physical Examination

The physical examination performed to assess the client's level of tissue oxygenation includes evaluation of the entire cardiopulmonary system. Skills of assessment, inspection, and percussion are used. The examination described here focuses on the client's cardiopulmonary status more specifically than the general physical assessment described in Chapter 13.

INSPECTION

Using inspection techniques the nurse does a head-to-toe observation of the client for skin and mucous membrane color, general appearance, level of consciousness, adequacy of systemic circulation, breathing patterns, and chest wall movement. (Table 36-2 through Table 36-4). Abnormalities detected result in detailed investigation of these areas during palpation, percussion, or auscultation.

Breathing patterns include respiratory rate, depth, and rhythm (Table 36-3). Breathing patterns can be altered by exercise, obesity, and an increased metabolic rate. Certain breathing patterns may indicate a change in the client's level of tissue oxygenation or a change in the acid-base balance.

Chest wall movements are observed to determine if the chest expands symmetrically or if abnormal paradoxical breathing is present. Abnormal chest wall movements can occur with a disease process or as a result of chest wall trauma (Table 36-4).

PALPATION

Palpation of the chest provides assessment data in several areas. Palpation documents the type and amount of thoracic excursion, elicits any areas of tenderness on light and deep palpation, and can identify tactile fremitus, thrills and heaves. With palpation the nurse can locate the cardiac point of maximal impulse (PMI). Pal-

TABLE 36-3   Assessment of Breathing Patterns

Pattern	Causes
Eupnea—normal respiratory rate; an adult range of 12-22 breaths/minute; normal tidal volume is 5-7 ml/kg body weight*	
Tachypnea—increased respiratory rate above the client's normal rate; characterized by quick, shallow respirations	Exercise, pregnancy, fever, pulmonary diseases, anxiety, neurological conditions, airway obstruction
Bradypnea—decreased respiratory rate below the client's normal rate	Drug overdose, central nervous system dysfunction, airway obstruction
Kussmaul respiration—abnormally deep, very rapid sighing type of respiration; tidal volume is increased as well as rate	Diabetic ketoacidosis
Ataxic respirations—uncoordinated respiratory patterns; no coordinated rate or depth of respiration	Central nervous system disorders
Cheyne-Stokes respiration—breathing pattern characterized by alternating periods of apnea and deep rapid breathing; cycle begins with slow, shallow breaths that gradually increase to abnormal depth and rate; respiration gradually subsides as breathing slows and becomes shallow	Congestive heart failure, bronchopneumonia, drug overdose, sleep, central nervous system damage

*Data from Luce, JM, Tyler, ML, and Pierson, DJ: Intensive respiratory care, Philadelphia, 1984, W.B. Saunders Co.

TABLE 36-4   Assessment of Abnormal Chest Wall Movement

Abnormality	Cause
Retraction—visible sinking in soft tissues of chest between and around firmer tissue of cartilaginous and bony ribs; retractions have a specific beginning point and worsen and there is a need for increased inspiratory effort; retractions may be observed at intercostal space, intraclavicular space, trachea, and substernally*	Any condition that causes increased inspiratory effort (for example, airway obstruction, asthma, tracheobronchitis)
Paradoxical breathing—asynchronous breathing; chest contracts during inspiration and expands during expiration	Flail chest
Increased anterior-posterior diameter	Senile emphysema or COPD

*Infants can experience sternal and substernal retractions with only slight inspiratory effort because of their chest pliability.

pation also allows the nurse to feel for abnormal masses or lumps in the axilla and breast tissue (see Chapter 13).

PERCUSSION

With percussion the nurse can detect abnormal fluid, air in the lungs, or diaphragmatic excursions. There are five percussion tones: resonance, hyperresonance, dullness, flatness, and tympany. Resonance is the sound produced by a healthy, non-smoker's lungs on normal inspiration. Hyperresonance is produced in healthy clients upon forced, deep inspiration and in children. Hyperresonance during regular inspiration indicates air-trapping, as with asthma, emphysema, or pneumothorax. Dullness is produced when there is fluid or consolidation within the lungs. Flatness, when produced at the bases of the lungs, may indicate a pleural effusion. When tympany is produced, the examiner is most likely percussing the gastric region and not lung tissue.

Percussion indicates the degree of diaphragmatic excursion (see Chapter 13), which results from obesity, pregnancy, organomegaly, ascites, and chronic obstructive pulmonary disease (COPD).

AUSCULTATION

Auscultation indentifies normal and abnormal heart and lung sounds, (see Chapter 13). Adventitious breath sounds occur with collapse of a lung region, fluid in lung field, or airway obstruction. Auscultation also evaluates response of the client to nursing interventions for improving respiratory status.

Auscultation of the cardiovascular system should assess for normal S_1 and S_2 sounds, the presence of abnormal S_3 and S_4, and murmurs and rubs (see Chapter 13). The examiner must identify location, radiation, intensity, pitch, and quality of a murmur. Last, auscultation is used to identify a bruit over the carotid arteries, abdominal aorta, and femoral arteries.

Physical examination enables the nurse to document abnormalities described in the nursing history, as well as identify abnormalities it does not include. In addition, repeated physical examination provides objective criteria for evaluating nursing care. Diagnostic tests to gather further information completes the assessment data base.

Diagnostic Tests

Many diagnostic tests can be performed to obtain data for respiratory assessment. They can determine adequacy of ventilation and oxygenation, allow inspection of structures of the respiratory system, and determine presence of abnormal cells or infection in the respiratory tract.

TESTS TO MEASURE ADEQUACY OF VENTILATION AND OXYGENATION

PULMONARY FUNCTION TESTS. Pulmonary function tests determine the ability of the lungs to efficiently exchange oxygen and carbon dioxide. Basic ventilation studies are performed with a spirometer and recording device as the client breathes through a mouthpiece into a connecting tube. Measurements include tidal volume, inspiratory reserve volume, residual volume, and forced expiratory volume.

Pulmonary function tests are usually performed in a pulmonary function laboratory. The nurse prepares the client by explaining the procedure. A nose clip prevents air from being inhaled or exhaled through the nose. The client breathes through a mouthpiece attached to a spirometer for measuring lung volume. The client is asked at appropriate times in the test to inhale or exhale as much air as possible. The nurse seeks the client's cooperation to ensure accurate results.

Providing information about the procedure decreases anxiety and encourages cooperative participation. Usually no other preparation is needed, although it may be beneficial if the client does not eat a large meal immediately before the test. A full stomach diminishes the ability to inhale deeply, resulting in inaccuracies.

ARTERIAL BLOOD GASES. Arterial blood gas measurement is performed in conjunction with pulmonary function tests to determine the hydrogen ion concentration, partial pressure of carbon dioxide and oxygen concentration, and oxyhemoglobin saturation. Arterial blood gas tests provide information about diffusion of gas across the alveolar capillary membrane and adequacy of tissue oxygenation (see Chapter 37).

OXIMETRY. Continuous measurements of capillary oxygen saturation is available by cutaneous oximeter devices. One of the most common is a finger oximeter. The nurse attaches a non-invasive sensor to the client's finger. The sensor monitors capillary blood oxygen saturation. Continuous monitoring of O_2 saturation is useful in assessing sleep disorders, exercise tolerance, and transient decreases in O_2 saturation.

However, cutaneous oximeter measurements are not completely accurate. They are most useful in detecting falls in O_2 saturation below 80 mm Hg. Elevated serum bilirubin or poor cutaneous perfusion leads to inaccurate oximeter results.

COMPLETE BLOOD COUNT. A complete blood count determines the number and type of red and white blood cells per cubic millimeter of blood. The nurse obtains a venous blood sample by using the venipuncture technique (see Chapter 37).

The complete blood count (CBC) also measures the hemoglobin. Hemoglobin is contained within the red blood cells (RBCs), also called erythrocytes. Each RBC contains 200 to 300 molecules of hemoglobin. Each molecule of hemoglobin contains several molecules of heme. It is the heme component that carries oxygen to the tissues. Each molecule of heme can carry one molecule of hemoglobin.

A deficiency in RBCs decreases the blood's oxygen carrying capacity. This is because there are fewer hemoglobin molecules available to carry oxygen to tissues. Conditions that result in decreased RBCs include anemias, whole blood loss, nutritional disorders, and others.

When RBCs are increased such as is the case with polycythemia in chronic lung conditions and cyanotic heart conditions the oxygen-carrying capacity of the blood is increased. But in these conditions the disease process causes the body to adapt through production of more RBCs. Increased RBCs increase blood viscosity and the client's risk for thrombus formation.

Normal values for a complete blood count vary with age and sex. The newborn's hemoglobin level is quite high, from 14 to 20 g/100 ml of blood. This value declines during the first year to 11 to 14 g/100 ml. From age 1 year through puberty, the normal hemoglobin value ranges between 11 and 13 g/100 ml of blood. The normal value for adult men is 14 to 18 g/100 ml, and for adult women 12 to 16 g/100 ml. The older adult is more likely to have deficiencies in hemoglobin as a result of chronic illness, decreased appetite, and poor nutrition.

TESTS TO VISUALIZE STRUCTURES OF THE RESPIRATORY SYSTEM

CHEST X-RAY EXAMINATION. A chest x-ray examination consists of a roentgenogram of the thorax that allows the physician and nurse to observe the lung fields for fluid (such as occurs with pneumonia), for masses (as with lung cancer), fractures (as with rib and clavicular fractures), and other abnormal processes (such as tuberculosis).

A chest x-ray examination is painless, requiring only that the client hold breath briefly during inspiration. Occasionally an expiratory film is taken.

BRONCHOSCOPY. Bronchoscopy is visual examination of the trachea and bronchial tree. The standard rigid, tubular metal bronchoscope or the narrower, flexible fiberoptic bronchoscope may be used. Bronchoscopy is performed to obtain biopsy and fluid or sputum samples for examination. It can also remove mucus plugs or foreign bodies that have become lodged in the airways.

The client is maintained in a fasting state before bronchoscopy. As with many invasive procedures, there is a risk that the client may gag and vomit. Maintaining the client in a fasting state reduces the risk.

The nurse also administers medications before the procedure. A sedative is usually administered, and atropine may be used occasionally to reduce oral secretions. The nurse continues to observe the client after the procedure for signs and symptoms of respiratory distress or hypoxia. Assessment of the client's gag/swallow reflex is obtained prior to initiating oral fluids.

LUNG SCAN. The most common lung scan is the computed tomogram (CT scan). CT scanning combines x-ray and computer technology. X-ray beams pass through a section or plane of the thorax from different angles, and the computer calculates tissue absorption and displays a printout and scan picture of the tissues showing densities of various intrathoracic structures. A CT scan can identify abnormal masses by size and location but cannot identify tissue types, which requires a biopsy.

CT scans are noninvasive and painless. The client usually requires no preparation. Occasionally a contrast medium may be injected during the procedure to assist with visualization of structures. If ordered, venipuncture is used to gain access to the client's circulatory system.

TESTS TO DETERMINE ABNORMAL CELLS OR INFECTION IN THE RESPIRATORY TRACT

THROAT CULTURES. A throat culture sample is obtained by swabbing the oropharynx and tonsillar regions with a culture swab. The throat culture determines presence of pathogenic microorganisms and the antibiotics to which they are most sensitive.

When obtaining a throat culture sample, the nurse inserts the swab into the pharyngeal region and passes it along reddened areas and areas of exudate. Some clients have an active gag reflex, making it difficult to obtain the specimen. The reflex may be less active if the client is sitting straight and leaning slightly forward. In addition, the client may be able to control gagging if informed that the procedure will take only a few seconds.

SPUTUM SPECIMENS. Sputum specimens identify a specific microorganism and its drug resistance and sensitivities. This specimen is referred to as "sputum for culture and sensitivity" (C and S). A sputum specimen may also be obtained to identify the presence of the tubercle bacillus (TB). This sputum specimen is called "sputum for acid-fast bacillus" (AFB). The AFB specimen is obtained serially in the early morning, usually for 3 consecutive days. Finally, sputum specimens are obtained to identify abnormal cells. This is called "sputum for cytology" and involves a serial collection of three early morning sputum specimens. Cytological sputum examination is performed to identify lung cancers by cell type.

If a client is unable to cough or produce sputum, the nurse may have to suction the airway to obtain the specimen. A sputum trap is attached to the suction catheter, which traps mucus. The nurse must avoid suctioning large amounts of sterile saline into the sputum trap. This dilutes the sputum and can make analysis difficult or impossible.

When sputum specimens are obtained, the nurse should record the color, consistency, amount, and odor of the sputum and that the specimen was sent to a specific laboratory for analysis on a specific date and time.

THORACENTESIS. Thoracentesis is surgical perforation of the chest wall and pleural space with a needle to aspirate fluid for diagnostic or therapeutic purposes or to remove a specimen for biopsy. The procedure is performed with aseptic technique, using a local anesthetic. The client usually sits upright with the anterior thorax supported by pillows or an over-the-bed table.

Whether this procedure is painful depends on the client's tolerance to pain (see Chapter 35). The nurse can reduce the client's anxiety by explaining the procedure and telling the client what to expect. The client must understand the importance of holding the breath as requested and of not coughing during the procedure. Sudden movements of the thorax may result in the lung being punctured by the thoracentesis needle. The client is instructed to notify the physician before coughing or sneezing so the needle can be withdrawn.

NURSING DIAGNOSIS

Clients with altered level of oxygenation can have nursing diagnoses that are primarily from a cardiovascular or pulmonary origin (see nursing diagnosis box). Each nursing diagnosis should be based on specific defining characteristics and should include the related etiol-

---

Examples of Nursing Diagnoses Related to Respiratory Dysfunction

NANDA-APPROVED NURSING DIAGNOSES

Ineffective airway clearance related to:
- Impaired cough
- Incisional pain
- Immobility
- Decreased level of consciousness

Impaired gas exchange related to:
- Decreased lung expansion
- Decreased level of consciousness
- Presence of pulmonary secretions
- Inadequate oxygen intake

Ineffective breathing pattern related to:
- Chest wall abnormality
- Immobility
- Use of analgesics
- Neuromuscular damage
- Airway obstruction

Decreased cardiac output related to:
- Acid-base disturbances
- Electrolyte imbalance

Potential for infection related to:
- Stasis of pulmonary secretions

Potential altered body temperature related to:
- Stasis of pulmonary secretions

Sample Nursing Diagnoses for Respiratory Dysfunction

Defining Characteristics	Nursing Diagnoses	Related Factors
Cough Adventitious lung sounds Tachypnea Dyspnea Cyanosis	Ineffective airway clearance	• Impaired cough reflex • Thick pulmonary secretions • Incisional pain • Immobility • Decreased level of consciousness
Altered chest wall motion Dyspnea Use of accessory muscles Nasal flaring Pursed-lip breathing Abnormal arterial blood gases Tachypnea Cough	Ineffective breathing pattern	• Chest wall abnormality • Immobility • Use of analgesics • Neuromuscular damage • Airway obstruction • Anxiety • Pain
Restlessness Change in vital signs Abnormal arterial blood gases Pulmonary secretions Decreased level of consciousness Acid base imbalance	Impaired gas exchange	• Decreased lung expansion • Decreased level of consciousness • Pulmonary secretions • Inadequate oxygen intake

ogy (see Chapter 7). The diagnostic label is validated by the defining characteristics or signs and symptoms.

Two recent nursing studies have validated nursing diagnoses as a result of pulmonary causes (McDonald, 1985; York, 1985). McDonald (1985) researched three diagnostic categories: (1) ineffective airway clearance, (2) ineffective breathing patterns, and (3) impaired gas exchange. The study validated a partial list of defining characteristics and identified 20 nursing interventions appropriate for the diagnostic categories. The second study attempted to validate defining characteristics associated with ineffective breathing patterns and ineffective airway clearance (York, 1985). In addition to identifying the most common defining characteristics for both categories, the researcher developed a model for validating other diagnostic classifications (York, 1985; York and Martin, 1986).

There are three major classifications of nursing diagnoses for clients with an altered level of oxygenation (see sample nursing diagnoses box). Through assessment the nurse identifies defining characteristics.

PLANNING

Clients with impaired respiration require a nursing care plan directed toward meeting the actual or potential oxygenation needs of the client (see care plan box). The plan includes one or more of the following client-centered goals:

1. Improved activity tolerance
2. Maintenance and promotion of lung expansion
3. Mobilization of pulmonary secretions
4. Maintenance of a patent airway

5. Maintenance or promotion of tissue oxygenation
6. Restoration of cardiopulmonary function

The client's level of health, age, life-style, and environmental risks affect the level of tissue oxygenation. Clients with severe impairments in oxygenation frequently require nursing interventions directed toward all six goals.

IMPLEMENTATION

Nursing interventions for promoting and maintaining adequate oxygenation include independent nursing actions (such as positioning, coughing techniques, and preventive health behaviors) and interdependent or dependent interventions (such as oxygen therapy, lung inflation techniques, hydration, medications, and; in some agencies, the use of chest physical therapy). These are the basic categories of nursing interventions.

Improved Activity Tolerance

Nursing interventions for improving activity tolerance primarily include noninvasive measures and health maintenance behaviors such as cardiopulmonary reconditioning and respiratory muscle training.

CARDIOPULMONARY RECONDITIONING

The major method of cardiopulmonary reconditioning is a structured rehabilitation program. Cardiopulmonary rehabilitation is defined as actively assisting the client to achieve and maintain an optimal level of health through controlled physical exercise, nutrition counseling, relaxation and stress management techniques, prescribed medications and oxygen, and adherence to the

---

Sample Nursing Care Plan for Respiratory Dysfunction

Nursing Diagnosis	Goal	Expected Outcomes	Nursing Interventions
Ineffective airway clearance related to thickened pulmonary secretions	Pulmonary secretions are removed.	Adventitious lung sounds are absent on auscultation.	Turn, cough, and deep breathe every 2 hours.
		Client has forceful, productive cough.	Suction if client unable to expectorate sputum.
		Sputum is clear, white, frothy.	Increase fluid intake to 1000 ml every 8 hours.
		Dyspnea is absent.	Perform postural drainage with percussion every 3 hours.
			Add high humidity to oxygen supply (if oxygen is ordered).

program. Goals of rehabilitation are defined by the client and the rehabilitation team.

As physical reconditioning occurs, the client's complaints of dyspnea, chest pain, fatigue, and activity intolerance should decrease. Researchers noted the amount of anxiety, depression, and somatic concerns decreased as clients participated in cardiopulmonary rehabilitation. This occurred whether or not there was clinical improvement in the cardiopulmonary disease itself (Shenkman, 1985; Agle et al., 1973).

In addition, those clients who adhered more strictly to their program realized more consistent benefits. However, adherence to a cardiopulmonary reconditioning program or other medical regimen requires motivation and behavioral changes by the client. A combination of client education, joint goal setting, client self-monitoring, and continuous support from care givers promotes adherence to prescribed programs (Kert, 1985; Steckel and Swain, 1977; Swain and Steckel, 1981).

RESPIRATORY MUSCLE TRAINING

Respiratory muscle training improves muscle strength and endurance, resulting in improved activity tolerance. It is believed that respiratory muscle training may prevent respiratory failure in clients with COPD (Kim, 1984).

One method for respiratory muscle training is the incentive spirometer resistive breathing device (ISRBD). Resistive breathing is achieved by placing a resistive breathing device into a volume-dependent incentive spirometer. Muscle training is achieved when the client uses the ISRBD on a scheduled routine, for example, twice a day for 15 minutes and or four times a day for 15 minutes. Larson and Kim (1984) studied nine clients with COPD and measured muscle training following use of the IRSBD. Subjects demonstrated a significant increase in respiratory muscle strength and sputum expectoration and a clinical improvement in exercise tolerance and performance of activities of daily living.

Maintenance or Promotion of Lung Expansion

Nursing interventions to maintain or promote lung expansion include noninvasive techniques such as positioning and breathing exercises. Lung expansion is also promoted by procedures using equipment such as incentive spirometers and intermittent positive-pressure breathing machines. Expansion can also be achieved by invasive procedures such as insertion of a chest tube.

POSITIONING

In the healthy, completely mobile person, adequate ventilation and oxygenation are maintained by frequent changes of position during the activities of daily living. However, when a person's mobility is restricted as a result of illness or injury, he or she is at risk for respiratory impairment. The most common types of impairments are stasis of pulmonary secretions and decreased chest wall expansion (see Chapter 42).

Frequent changes of position of partially or completely immobilized clients are simple and cost-effective methods for reducing the risks of pulmonary complications. Postoperative clients whose incisional pain limits chest wall expansion require frequent changes of position. Because chest wall expansion is limited, these clients are at risk for pooling of respiratory secretions and subsequent hypostatic bronchopneumonia. The care plan for the immediate postoperative period should include changing a client's position at least every 2 hours, and, unless contraindicated, the client's ambulation schedule should gradually increase the time spent out of bed. These two interventions in the postoperative nursing care plan promote full lung expansion and help reduce the risk of postoperative pulmonary complications (see Chapter 46).

BREATHING EXERCISES

Breathing exercises include techniques to improve ventilation and oxygenation. The three basic techniques are deep breathing and coughing exercises, pursed-lip breathing, and abdominal-diaphragmatic breathing. Deep breathing and coughing exercise is routine intervention for postoperative clients. The procedure is detailed in Chapter 46.

Pursed-lip breathing involves deep inspiration and prolonged expiration through pursed lips. Originally this breathing exercise was thought to decrease airway collapse by increasing intraluminal airway pressure near the mouth. However, recent research indicates that this technique benefits clients primarily by slowing the ventilatory rate, thereby increasing tidal volume and decreasing dead space ventilation. Alveolar ventilation remains the same, but the work of breathing decreases (Luce, Tyler, and Pierson, 1984).

Pursed-lip breathing exercises are useful in promoting adequate oxygenation and ventilation in anxious clients, as well as those with chronic obstructive pulmonary diseases. The client is instructed to take a deep breath and to exhale slowly through pursed lips while silently counting to four. Since this exercise affects exhalation, the client should be encouraged to increase the exhalation time. The client is usually able to perfect this technique by increasing the count during exhalation from four to eight. This exercise is best performed with the client sitting upright.

Abdominal-diaphragmatic breathing requires the client to relax intercostal and accessory respiratory muscles while taking deep inspirations and watching the abdomen move outward as the diaphragm descends. During expiration the client slowly and forcefully contracts abdominal muscles and observes the abdomen for inward movement as the diaphragm ascends. These exercises are initially taught with the client in the supine position and then are practiced while sitting and standing. The exercise is often used with the pursed-lip breathing technique. The pulmonary results of this exercise pattern include decreased air trapping and reduced work of breathing (Luce, Tyler, and Pierson, 1984). This exercise is also useful for clients with pulmonary disease, for postoperative clients, and women in labor to promote relaxation and provide pain control.

INCENTIVE SPIROMETRY

Incentive spirometry is a method of encouraging voluntary deep breathing by providing visual feedback to clients about their inspiratory volume. Incentive spirometry is used to prevent or treat atelectasis and is particularly useful for postoperative clients (Luce, Tyler, and Pierson, 1984).

Postoperative complications are prevented by reinflating collapsed alveoli and evacuating mucous. This is achieved through sustained maximal inspiration (SMI), which is defined as alveolar inflation to total lung capacity produced by high negative transpulmonary pressures. Incentive spirometry uses SMI and generates high negative transpulmonary pressures and increased lung volume with adequate alveolar inflation time (Weaver, 1981).

Flow-oriented incentive spirometers consist of one or more plastic chambers that contain free moving colored balls. The client inhales briskly to elevate the balls and to keep them floating as long as possible. The goal is to keep the balls elevated for as long as possible in order to ensure a maximal sustained inhalation. The goal is *not* to snap the balls to the top of the chamber with a rapid, very brief, low-volume breath. Even if a very slow inspiration does not elevate the balls, this pattern may achieve greater lung expansion (Luce, Tyler, and Pierson, 1984). The advantage of flow-oriented inspiratory spirometry is its low cost, but it does not determine the volume of inspiration.

Volume-oriented incentive spirometry devices have a bellows that is raised to a predetermined volume by an inhaled breath (Fig. 36-3, *A*). An achievement light or counter is used instead in some devices. (Fig. 36-3, *B*). Some devices are constructed so the light will not turn on unless the bellows is held at a minimal desired volume for a specified period to enhance lung expansion. The advantage of volume-oriented incentive spirometry is that a known volume of inspiration can be maintained.

Incentive spirometry encourages clients to breathe to their normal inspiratory capacity. When this method is used with a postoperative client, it helps to know the client's preoperative inspiratory capacity. Because of postoperative pain, a postoperative inspiratory capacity one half to three fourths of the preoperative volume is acceptable (Luce, Tyler, and Pierson, 1984).

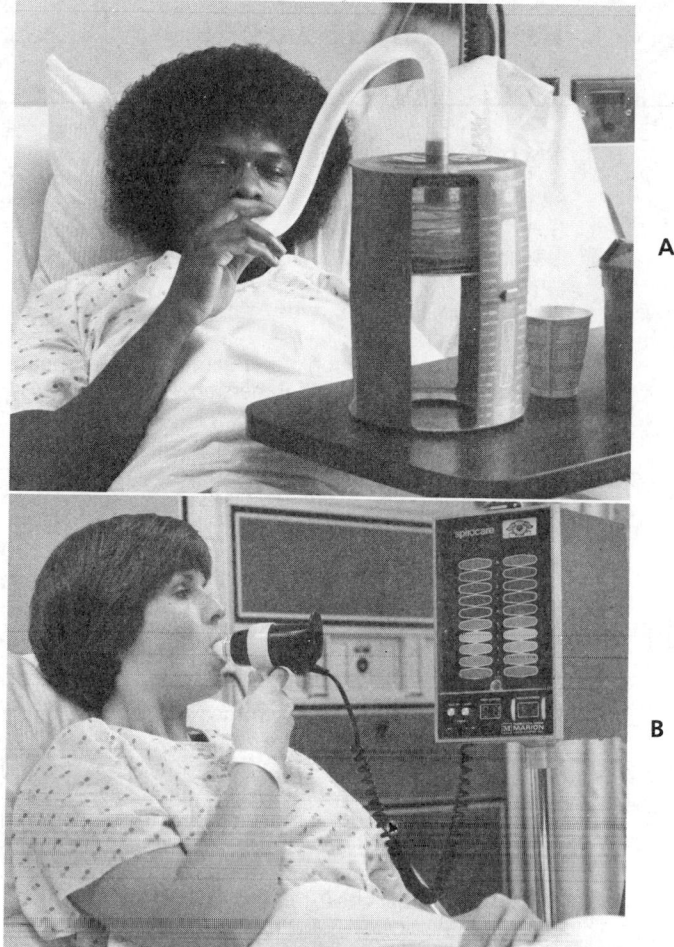

Fig. 36-3 Volume-oriented spirometer. **A,** Bellows visible to client. **B,** Achievement light indicator.

BLOW BOTTLES

Blow bottles are devices in which fluid is moved from one container to another by air pressure. The disadvantage of blow bottles is that they provide feedback only about exhalation. Hyperinflation of the lungs and the presumed benefit occur *only if a deep breath is taken before blowing into the bottle.*

A client instructed in proper use of the blow bottle may use frequent small breaths and the Valsalva maneuver to move the liquid. Therefore the nurse should teach the client to inhale deeply and then seal the lips tightly around the mouthpiece and exhale. Unless deep inhalation is achieved, expansion of lung alveoli does not occur.

INTERMITTENT POSITIVE-PRESSURE BREATHING

Intermittent positive-pressure breathing (IPPB) devices assist lung hyperinflation by applying positive pressure to the airways. Hyperinflation depends on the amount of pressure applied and on compliance of the

Care of Chest Tubes

STEPS	RATIONALE
1. Assess client to determine:	
a. Ease of respirations, anxiety, chest discomfort, breath sounds, respiratory rate, and regularity.	Ineffective chest tube drainage will impede the client's respiratory functioning.
b. Puncture dressing intact, drainage, and presence of subcutaneous emphysema.	A poorly secured puncture dressing can result in increased entry of air into the pleural space and subcutaneous emphysema.
c. Drainage: volume, type, rate, and bottle below chest level.	Provides continuous data to the amount and rate of chest tube drainage.
d. Drainage unit: bubbling, fluctuation appropriate, and water-seal straw submersion.	Determines accurate functioning of unit.
e. Suction: set at ordered level.	Determines correct suction setting.
2. Explain to client what you are observing and the frequency of observations.	Decreases client anxiety about the tubes.
3. Maintain client in a semi-Fowler's position and turn every 1 hour toward the lung in which the tube is positioned.	Promotes drainage of fluid (as with a hemothorax or postoperative thoractomy).
4. Have client cough and deep breathe every 2 hours. (Contraindicated in clients after a lobectomy.)	Promotes drainage of fluid and reexpansion of affected lung. The pressure from forceful coughing after lobectomy can increase risk of suture rupture at the stump of lung removal.
5. Wash hands.	Reduces transmission of infection.
6. Coil tubing flat on bed, which then falls into a straight line into the collection bottle.	Dependent drainage loops impede flow of fluid from the pleural space.
7. If ordered and hospital policy, strip tubing by: placing one hand securely on tube next to puncture site, and using second hand, compress tube sliding toward drainage unit. Release first hand and repeat procedure along the entire length of tubing. Some institutions may use a special chest-tube roller.	Stripping mechanically dislodges or pushes forward clots, fibrin, or debris. Increases suction effect and may cause client temporary discomfort. *Only used when clients have drainage from the chest tube, which, if left stagnant, may cause occlusion of the tube.*
8. Place two hemostats with rubber tubing over the tips at client's bedside.	Used for emergency measures if the chest-tube drainage bottles should accidentally break or become disconnected. Clamping the chest tubes is only an emergency measure. It protects the client against a large air leak from disconnection or breakage of the system. Excessive air leaks can lead to tension pneumothorax.
9. Wash hands.	Reduces transmission of infection.
10. Record in nurses' notes patency of chest tubes, presence of drainage, presence of fluctuations, client's vital signs, and level of comfort.	Documents accurate functioning of chest tubes and client's physical status.

chest wall. Clients with low compliance require higher IPPB pressures to achieve hyperinflation. Following inspiration, the machine automatically shuts off and passive exhalation occurs. The client's next inspiratory cycle triggers the machine to deliver the preset pressure.

More cost effective and portable incentive spirometers have all but replaced IPPB devices. However, in some institutions, IPPB is used to deliver aerosol bronchodilators or mucolytics to the client with pulmonary disease.

CHEST TUBES

A chest tube is a catheter inserted through the thorax to remove fluid or air and thus promote lung reexpansion. Chest tubes are used after chest surgery, chest trauma, and for pneumothorax or hemothorax (Procedure 36-1).

A *pneumothorax* is collection of air or other gas in the pleural space. The gas causes the lung to collapse because it obliterates the negative intrapleural pressure and a counterpressure is exerted against the lung, which is then unable to expand. A pneumothorax may occur spontaneously, result from an open chest wound or the rupture of an emphysematous vesicle on the surface of the lung, or follow severe coughing or an invasive procedure such as a thoracentesis or insertion of a subclavian intravenous line.

A client with a pneumothorax usually feels pain as atmospheric air irritates the parietal pleura. The pain may be sharp and pleuritic. Dyspnea is common and worsens as the size of the pneumothorax increases.

Hemothorax is an accumulation of blood and fluid in the pleural cavity between the parietal and visceral pleurae, usually as the result of trauma. The hemothorax produces a counterpressure and prevents the lung from full expansion. A hemothorax can also be caused by rupture of small blood vessels from inflammatory processes, such as pneumonia or tuberculosis. In addition to pain and dyspnea, signs and symptoms of shock can develop if blood loss is severe.

There are four types of chest tube drainage systems. The *one-bottle system* is the simplest closed drainage system because the single bottle serves as a collector and a water seal (Fig. 36-4, *A*). During normal respiration, fluctuations in the water-seal straw are expected. The fluid should descend with inspiration. A *two-bottle system* permits the liquid to flow into the collection bottle and air flows into the water-seal bottle (Fig. 36-4, *B*). Fluctuations in the water-seal straw are still anticipated. The advantage of the two-bottle system is that it permits more accurate measurement and observation of chest drainage (Erikson, 1981).

A *suction-three-bottle system* permits a pressure difference between the pleural space and the drainage bottles by pulling air from the bottles, causing the pressure to drop inside (Fig. 36-4, *C*). Usually -15 to -20 cm water is used for adults and a lesser amount for children

(Erikson, 1981). A *pleur-evac* system is a one-piece disposable molded plastic unit that duplicates the three-bottle system.

Chest tubes can cause nurses unnecessary worry. Knowing the basics of chest-tube management and troubleshooting maneuvers reduces side effects (Table 36-5).

Nursing research has investigated the effect of chest tube stripping in patients after cardiac surgery. The findings indicate that there was no effect in the reduction of bleeding from the surgical site. While the study population included only 30 subjects, the researchers noted that stripping resulted in little difference in chest-tube management and recommended further investigation (Duncan, Erickson, and Weigel, 1987).

SPECIAL CONSIDERATIONS. Clamping chest tubes is not necessary when walking the client. Simply handle the bottles carefully and maintain the drainage device below the client's chest. If the tubing disconnects from the bottles, cleanse the tips and reconnect. Instruct client to exhale as much as possible and to cough. These maneuvers rid the pleural space of as much air as possible.

Mobilization of Pulmonary Secretions

The ability of a client to mobilize pulmonary secretions may make the difference between a short, smooth postoperative recovery period and a long period involving complications with greater difficulty in achieving a maximal level of health. Nursing interventions that promote mobilization of pulmonary secretions include hydration, humidification, nebulization, and chest physiotherapy.

HYDRATION

Maintenance of an adequate systemic hydration keeps mucociliary clearance normal. In clients with adequate hydration, pulmonary secretions are thin, white, watery, and easily removed with minimal coughing. Excessive coughing required to clear thick, tenacious secretions is fatiguing and leaves the client with little energy (Feldman, 1982). Unless contraindicated, most clinicians recommend a fluid intake of 1500 to 2000 ml per day (Luce, Tyler, and Pierson, 1984). Adequacy of hydration can be determined by the color consistency, and ease of secretion expectoration.

HUMIDIFICATION

Humidification is the process of adding water to gas. Temperature is the most important factor affecting how much water vapor a gas can hold. The percent of water in the gas in relation to the gas's capacity for water is the relative humidity. Air or oxygen with a high relative humidity keeps the airways moist and loosens and mobilizes pulmonary secretions.

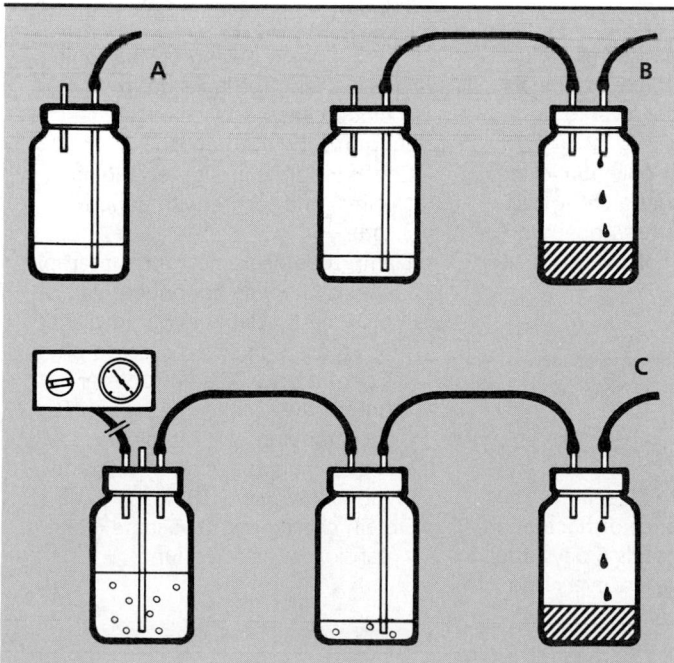

Fig. 36-4 Chest tube drainage. **A,** One-bottle system. **B,** Two-bottle system. **C,** Three-bottle system with suction.

Humidification is necessary for clients receiving oxygen therapy. Oxygen delivered to the upper airways, as with a nasal catheter, nasal cannula, or face mask, is humidified by bubbling it through water. Heating of these humidifiers is impractical because condensed moisture fills the narrow tubing. Therefore the relative humidity of oxygen delivered to the upper airways is only 30% (Luce, Tyler, and Pierson, 1984).

Another method is the humidity tent. This is used for infants and children with illnesses such as croup or tracheitis. Children with these disorders require high humidity to liquefy secretions and help reduce fever. The nebulizer at the top of the humidity tent must remain filled with water to prevent unhumidified air or oxygen from entering the tent. Air in the humidity tent can become cool and fall below 20° C (68° F), causing the child to become chilled. Therefore the nurse monitors the child's body temperature as well as respiratory status. Children in humidity tents require frequent changes of clothing and bed linen to remain warm and dry.

NEBULIZATION

Nebulization is a process of adding moisture or medications to inspired air by mixing particles of varying sizes with the air. A nebulizer uses the aerosol principle to suspend a maximal number of water drops or particles of the desired size in inspired air. Nebulization improves clearance of pulmonary secretions by altering the tracheobronchial mucosa. Therefore, nebulization is often used for administration of bronchodilators or mucolytic agents.

The major types of nebulizers are the jet-aerosol nebulizer and the ultrasonic nebulizer. A jet-aerosol nebulizer uses gas under pressure, and the ultrasonic nebulizer uses high-frequency vibrations to break up the water or medication into fine drops or particles. The drops of particles, when inspired with air or administered oxygen, are then deposited throughout the tracheobronchial tree.

CHEST PHYSIOTHERAPY

Chest physiotherapy (CPT) is a group of therapies used in combination to mobilize pulmonary secretions (see box on p. 1005). These therapies include postural drainage, chest percussion, and vibration. Chest physiotherapy should be accompanied by productive coughing. Suctioning is used if the client's ability to cough is inadequate.

Chest percussion involves striking the chest wall over the area being drained. The hand is positioned so the fingers and thumb touch and the hand is cupped (Fig. 36-5). Percussion on the surface of the chest wall sends waves of varying amplitude and frequency through the chest. The force of these waves can change the consistency of the sputum or dislodge it from airway walls (Luce, Tyler, and Pierson, 1984). Chest percussion is performed by alternating hand motion against the chest

TABLE 36-5 Troubleshooting Chest Tubes

Problem	Explanation	Solution
No fluctuation of the water level in the water-seal chambers	Water in the water-seal chamber fluctuates as the client breathes. Inhalation causes the water level to descend.	Check if client is lying on the tubing. Check tubing for kinks, loops or blood clots. Lung may be reexpanded.
Continuous bubbling in the water-seal chamber.	Bubbling should occur only during the first few minutes after a chest tube has been inserted after a pneumothorax or 24 hours following a lobectomy.	Check for air leak, tighten tubing joints, and secure with adhesive tape. Clamp tube near chest tube insertion site. If bubbling continues, leak is proximal to clamp either in client or at insertion site. Report to physician at once. Clamp tube for only a few seconds to prevent further trapping of air in pleural space and worsening of pneumothorax (Erickson, 1981).
Drainage from hemothorax has gone from bloody to scant serous drainage. No fluctuations in water seal is present.	Serous drainage, absence of fluctuation, and normal lung sounds 6 days after hemothorax indicates recovery and reexpansion of the lung.	Obtain chest x-ray to validate reexpansion of affected lung.

Data from Paulaw, D, and Jones, S: Test your skill at troubleshooting chest tubes, RN October, 1986; Erickson, R: Solving chest-tube problems, Nurs 81 81:62, 1981.

wall (Fig. 36-6).

Percussion is contraindicated in clients with bleeding disorders, osteoporosis, or fractured ribs. Caution should be taken to percuss the lung fields and not the scapular regions, or trauma may occur to the skin and underlying musculoskeletal structures.

Vibration is a fine, shaking pressure applied to the chest wall only during exhalation (Luce, Tyler, and Pierson, 1984). Vibration increases the exhalation of trapped air and may shake mucus loose and induce a cough. Vibration is not recommended in infants and young children.

Postural drainage is the use of positioning techniques that draw secretions from specific segments of the lungs and bronchi into the trachea. Coughing or suctioning normally removes secretions from the trachea. The procedure for postural drainage can include most lung segments (Table 36-6). Because clients may not require postural drainage of all lung segments, the procedure is based on clinical assessment findings. For example, clients with left lower lobe atelectasis may require postural drainage of only the affected region, whereas a child with cystic fibrosis may require postural drainage of all lung segments.

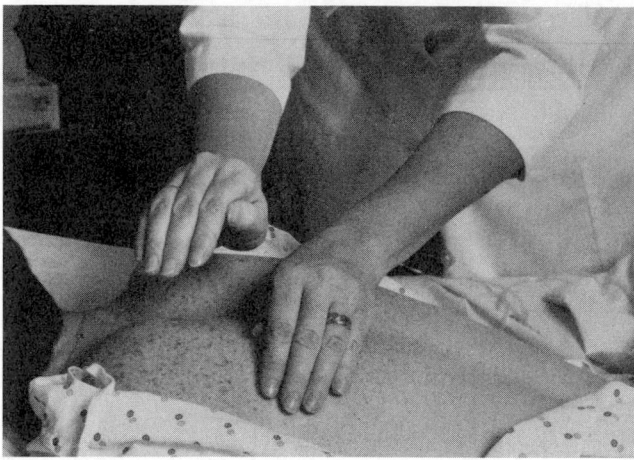

Fig. 36-6 Chest-wall percussion, alternating hand motion against the client's chest wall.

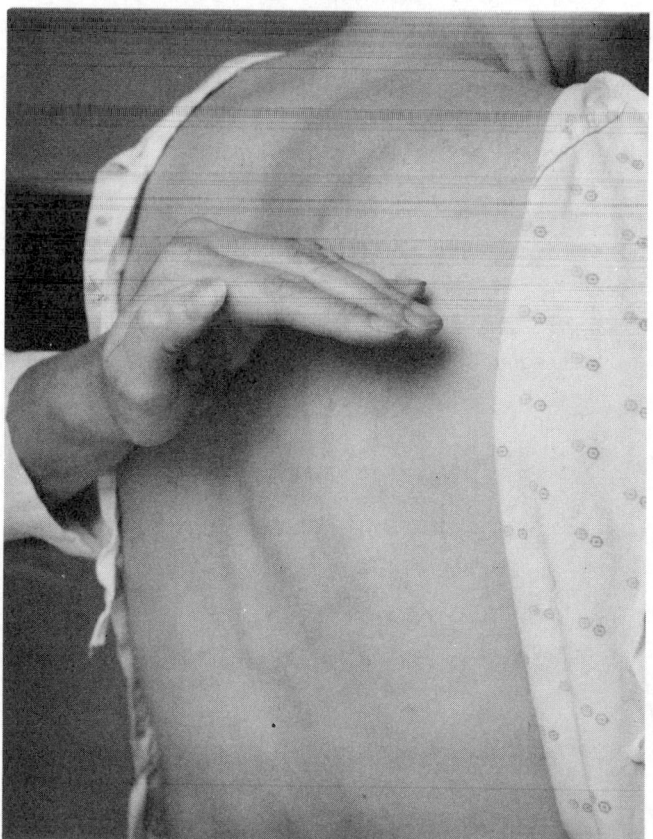

Fig. 36-5 Hand position for chest-wall percussion during physiotherapy.

Guidelines for Chest Physiotherapy

Nursing care and selection of CPT skills are based on specific assessment findings. The following guidelines help the nurse in physical assessment and subsequent decision making:

1. Know the client's normal range of vital signs. Conditions such as atelectasis and pneumonia requiring CPT can affect vital signs. The degree of change is related to the level of hypoxia, overall cardiopulmonary status, and tolerance to activity.
2. Know the client's medications. Certain medications, particularly diuretics and antihypertensives, cause fluid and hemodynamic changes. These may decrease the client's tolerance to the positional changes of postural drainage. Steroid medications increase the client's risk of pathological rib fractures and often contraindicate rib shaking.
3. Know the client's medical history. Certain conditions such as increased intracranial pressure, spinal cord injuries, or abdominal aneurysm resection contraindicate the positional changes of postural drainage. Thoracic trauma or surgery also may contraindicate percussion, vibration, and rib shaking.
4. Know the client's level of cognitive function. Participation in controlled cough techniques requires the client to follow instructions. Congenital or acquired cognitive limitations may alter the ability to learn and participate in these techniques.
5. Be aware of the client's exercise tolerance. CPT maneuvers are fatiguing. When the client is not used to physical activity, initial tolerance to the manuevers may be decreased. However, with gradual increases in activity and planned CPT, tolerance to the procedure improves.

TABLE 36-6 Positions for Postural Drainage

Lung Segment	Position of Client	Lung Segment	Position of Client
ADULT		Right middle lobe—posterior segment	Prone with thorax and abdomen elevated
Bilateral	High Fowler's	Both lower lobes—anterior segments	Supine in Trendelenburg position
Apical segments Right upper lobe—anterior segment	Sitting on side of bed Supine with head elevated	Left lower lobe—lateral segment	Right side lying in Trendelenburg position
Left upper lobe—anterior segment	Supine with head elevated	Right lower lobe—lateral segment	Left side lying in Trendelenburg position
Right upper lobe—posterior segment	Side lying with right side of chest elevated on pillows	Right lower lobe—posterior segment	Prone with right side of chest elevated in Trendelenburg position
Left upper lobe—posterior segment	Side lying with left side of chest elevated on pillows	Both lower lobes—posterior segments	Prone in Trendelenburg position
Right middle lobe—anterior segment	Three-fourths supine position with dependent lung in Trendelenburg position		

TABLE 36-6—cont'd

Lung Segment	Position of Client
CHILD	
Bilateral—apical segments	Sitting on nurse's lap, leaning slightly forward flexed over pillow
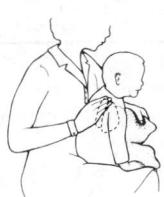	
Bilateral—middle anterior segments	Sitting on nurse's lap, leaning against nurse
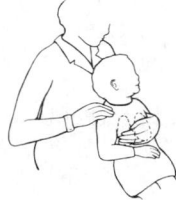	
Bilateral lobes—anterior segments	Lying supine on nurse's lap, back supported with pillow
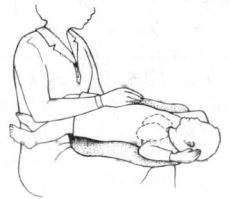	

Maintenance of a Patent Airway

The airway is patent when the trachea, bronchi, and large airways are free from obstructions. Three types of interventions are used to maintain a patent airway: coughing techniques, suctioning, and artificial airway.

COUGHING TECHNIQUES

Coughing is effective for maintaining a patent airway. Coughing permits the client to remove secretions from both the upper and lower airways. The normal series of events in the cough mechanisms are (1) deep inhalation, (2) closure of the glottis, (3) active contraction of the expiratory muscles, and (4) glottis opening. Deep inhalation increases lung volume and airway diameter. Thus air can pass to partially obstructing mucus plugs or other foreign matter. Contraction of the expiratory muscles against the closed glottis allows a high intrathoracic pressure to develop. As a result, when the glottis is opened, large flow of air is expelled at a high speed, providing momentum for mucus to move to the upper airway. After the cough the mucus can be expectorated or swallowed (Traver, 1982).

Various coughing techniques can be taught to different clients. Chapter 46 details the technique of deep breathing and coughing. Other cough techniques are cascade, huff, and quad coughing.

With the *cascade cough* the client takes a slow, deep breath and holds it for 2 seconds, while contracting expiratory muscles. Then the client opens his mouth and performs a series of coughs throughout the breath, thereby coughing at progressively lowered lung volumes. This technique promotes airway clearance and a patent airway in clients with large volumes of sputum.

With the *huff cough* the client, while exhaling, opens the glottis by saying the word "huff." The huff cough stimulates a natural cough reflex. This is generally effective only for clearing central airways, but with practice the client inhales more air and may be able to progress to the cascade cough.

The *quad cough* technique is used for clients without abdominal muscle control, such as those with spinal cord injuries. The client or nurse pushes inward and upward on the abdominal muscles toward the diaphragm while the client breathes with maximal expiratory effort, causing the cough (Luce, Tyler, and Pierson, 1984).

The effectiveness of coughing is evaluated by sputum expectoration, the client's report of swallowed sputum, or clearing of adventitious sounds on auscultation. Clients with chronic pulmonary diseases, upper respiratory tract infections, and lower respiratory tract infections should be encouraged to cough at least every 2 hours when awake. Clients with a large amount of sputum should be encouraged to cough every hour while awake and every 2 to 3 hours while asleep until the acute phase of mucus production has ended.

SUCTIONING TECHNIQUES

When a client is unable to clear respiratory tract secretions with coughing, the nurse must use suctioning to clear the airways. The three primary suctioning techniques are oropharyngeal and nasopharyngeal suctioning, orotracheal and nasotracheal suctioning, and suctioning an artificial airway.

These techniques are based on common principles. Because the oropharynx and trachea are considered sterile, sterile technique is required for suctioning. The mouth is considered clean, and therefore the suctioning of oral secretions should be performed after suctioning of the oropharynx and trachea. Each type of suctioning requires the use of a beaded-tip catheter with a ring of holes along the side of the catheter at the distal end.

OROPHARYNGEAL AND NASOPHARYNGEAL SUCTIONING. The oropharynx extends behind the mouth from the soft palate above the level of the hyoid

PROCEDURE 36-2

Oropharyngeal and Nasal Suctioning

STEPS	RATIONALE
1. Assess for signs and symptoms indicating presence of upper airway secretions: gurgling respirations, restlessness, vomitus in mouth, drooling.	Physical signs and symptoms result from decreased oxygen to tissues as well as pooling of secretions in upper airway.
2. Explain to the client how the procedure will help to clear the airway and relieve some of the breathing problems. Explain that coughing, sneezing, or gagging is normal.	Explanation of the procedure relieves the client's anxiety.
3. Prepare necessary equipment and supplies:	Ensures that procedure is completed quickly and efficiently.
a. Portable or wall suction unit with connecting tubing with Y connector if needed	
b. Sterile catheter	
c. Sterile water or normal saline, sterile basin	Used to clean catheter.
d. Sterile gloves	
e. Drape or towel	To protect linen and client's bedclothes.
f. Nasal or oral airway if indicated	Ensures access to airway.
4. Close door or pull curtain.	Ensures privacy.
5. Properly position the client.	
a. Place a conscious client with a functional gag reflex for oral suctioning in the semi-Fowler's position with head turned to one side. Place such a client for nasal suctioning in the semi-Fowler's position with neck hyperextended.	The gag reflex helps prevent aspiration of gastrointestinal contents. Positioning of the head to one side or hyperextending the neck promotes smooth insertion of the catheter into the oropharynx or nasopharynx, respectively.
b. Place an unconscious client in the side-lying position facing the nurse.	This position prevents the client's tongue from obstructing the client's airway, promotes drainage of pulmonary secretions, and prevents aspiration of gastrointestinal contents.
6. Place a towel on the pillow or under the client's chin.	Soiling of the bed linen or the client's bed clothes from secretions is prevented. Secretions on the towel can be discarded, thus reducing spread of bacteria.
7. Select the proper suction pressure for the client and the type of suction unit. For wall suction units this is 110-150 mm Hg in adults, 95-110 mm Hg in children, or 50-95 mm Hg in infants.	Proper suction pressure provides safe but effective negative pressure according to the client's age. Proper suction pressure decreases possibility of damage to mucous membranes and hypoxemia.
8. Wash hands.	Reduces transmission of microorganisms.
9. Pour sterile water or saline into sterile container.	Sterile solution is needed to lubricate the catheter to decrease friction and promote smooth passage of the catheter.
10. Apply a sterile glove to your dominant hand. Apply nonsterile glove to nondominant hand (suction kits may contain two sterile gloves).	Sterile glove maintains asepsis as catheter is passed into client's mouth or nose and reduces transmission of microorganisms. Nonsterile glove reduces transmission of microorganisms.
11. Using gloved hand, with catheter coiled, attach catheter to connecting tubing of suction machine.	Sterility is maintained.
12. Approximate the distance between the client's ear lobe and tip of the nose and place the thumb and forefinger of gloved hand at that point.	This distance ensures that the suction catheter remains in the pharyngeal region. Insertion of the catheter past this point places the catheter into the trachea.
13. Moisten distal 6-8 cm (3-4 in) catheter tip with sterile solution. Apply suction with catheter tip in the solution.	Moistening the catheter tip reduces friction and eases insertion of catheter. Applying suction while the catheter is in the sterile solution ensures that suction equipment is functioning before catheter is inserted.
14. Suction.	
a. For oropharyngeal suctioning, gently insert the catheter into one side of the mouth, and glide the catheter to the oropharynx. Do not apply suction during insertion.	Stimulation of the gag reflex is reduced. Application of suction pressure while introducing catheter into pharynx increases risk of damage to pharyngeal mucosa.

STEPS	RATIONALE
b. For nasopharyngeal suctioning, gently insert catheter into one nostril. Guide the catheter medially along the floor of the nasal cavity. Do not force the catheter. If one nostril is not patent, try the other. Do not apply suction during insertion.	The catheter avoids the nasal turbinates and enters more easily into nasopharynx. The risk of trauma to the oral and nasal mucosa during catheter insertion is reduced.
14. With nondominant hand, apply intermittent suction by occluding suction port with your thumb. Gently rotate the catheter as you withdraw it. The procedure should not take longer than 15 seconds.	Occlusion of suction port activates suction pressure. Suctioning is intermittently done as the catheter is withdrawn. Rotation removes secretions from all surfaces of the airway and prevents trauma from suction pressure on one area of the airway. Suctioning also removes air. The client's oxygen supply could be severely reduced if the procedure lasts longer than 15 seconds.
15. Flush the catheter with sterile solution by placing it in the solution and applying suction.	Flushing the catheter with sterile solution removes secretions from the catheter and lubricates the catheter for the next suctioning.
16. Allow the client to rest for 20-30 seconds before reinserting the catheter. Replace oxygen cannula if applicable.	Time between suctionings allows the client to increase oxygen intake.
17. Ask client to deep breathe and cough between suctions.	Deep breathing and coughing promote mobilization of secretions to the upper airway where they can be removed with the catheter. If the client is able to cough productively, further suctioning may not be needed if the airways are clear on auscultation.
If resuctioning is needed, repeat steps 13 through 15.	
18. Suction secretions in mouth or under tongue after suctioning the oropharynx or nasopharynx.	Sterile asepsis is maintained. The mouth should be suctioned only after sterile areas are thoroughly suctioned.
19. Discard catheter by wrapping it around gloved hand and pulling glove off around catheter.	Reduces the spread of bacteria from suction equipment.
20. Wash hands.	Reduces transmission of microorganisms.
21. Prepare equipment for next suctioning.	Ready access to suction equipment is provided, especially if the client is experiencing respiratory distress.
22. Observe client for absence of airway secretions, restlessness, oral secretions.	Indicates that secretions have been removed from oral and pharyngeal areas.
23. Record the amount, consistency, color, and odor of secretions and the client's reponse to the procedure; document client's presuctioning and postsuctioning respiratory status.	Recording this information documents that the procedure was completed and the client's status before and after.

bone and contains the tonsils. The nasopharynx is located behind the nose and extends to the level of the soft palate. Oropharyngeal or nasopharyngeal suctioning is used when the client is able to cough effectively but is unable to clear secretions by expectorating or swallowing. The suction procedure (Procedure 36-2) is used after the client has coughed. As the amount of pulmonary secretions is reduced and the client is less fatigued, he or she may be able to expectorate or swallow the mucus. This type of suctioning is then no longer required.

OROTRACHEAL AND NASOTRACHEAL SUCTIONING

Orotracheal or nasotracheal suctioning is necessary when the client with pulmonary secretions is unable to cough and does not have an artificial airway present. A catheter is passed through the mouth or nose into the trachea. The nose is the preferred route because stimulation of the gag reflex is minimal. The procedure is similar to nasopharyngeal suctioning, but the catheter tip is moved farther into the client to suction the trachea.

The entire procedure from catheter passage to its removal cannot take more than 15 seconds because oxygen does not reach the lungs during suctioning. Unless the client is in respiratory distress, he or she should be allowed to rest between passes of the catheter. If the client is using supplemental oxygen, the oxygen cannulae or mask should be replaced during rest periods.

ARTIFICIAL AIRWAY

An artificial airway is an oral airway or an endotracheal, nasotracheal, or tracheostomy tube. Indications for an artificial airway include decreased level of consciousness, airway obstruction, mechanical ventilation, and removal of tracheal secretions.

ORAL AIRWAY. The oral airway, the simplest type of artificial airway, prevents obstruction of the trachea by displacement of the tongue into the oropharynx in the unconscious client (Fig. 36-7). The oral airway extends from the teeth to the oropharynx, maintaining the tongue in the normal position. The correct size airway must be used. If the airway is too small, the tongue is not held in the anterior portion of the mouth. If it is too large, it may force the tongue toward the epiglottis and obstruct the airway.

The artificial oral airway is inserted by turning the curve of the airway toward the cheek and placing it over the tongue into the oropharynx. When the airway is in the oropharynx, the nurse turns it so the opening points downward. The correctly placed airway moves the tongue forward away from the oropharynx. The flange, the flat portion of the airway, should rest against the client's teeth.

If the nurse attempts to insert the oral airway with a curve toward the tongue, the client's natural airway can be further obstructed. Incorrect insertion merely forces the tongue back into the oropharynx.

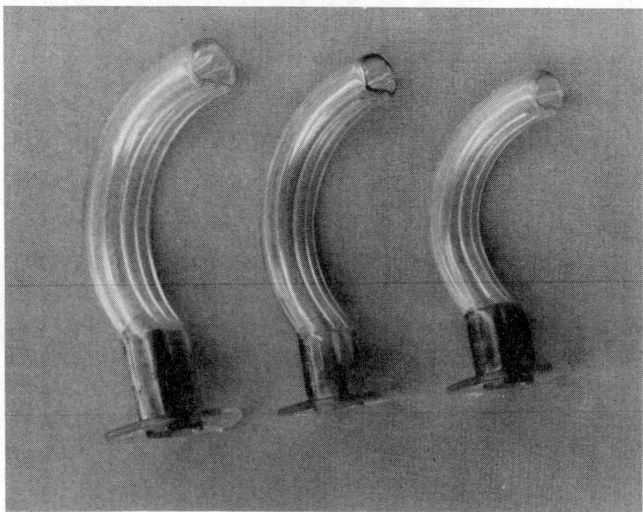

Fig. 36-7 Artificial oral airways.

The oral airway is commonly used for postoperative clients under general anesthesia. The client generally dislodges it by coughing it out on regaining consciousness.

The oral airway also promotes orotracheal suctioning in the unconscious client. The suction catheter can be passed through the center of the airway or along its side to gain access to the trachea.

TRACHEAL AIRWAY. Artificial tracheal airways include endotracheal, nasotracheal, and tracheal tubes. These allow easy access to the client's trachea for deep tracheal suctioning. Removal of tracheal secretions must be aseptic, atraumatic, and effective.

Asepsis involves using a freshly opened sterile suction catheter that is handled with a sterile glove. Secretion removal should be as atraumatic as possible. To avoid trauma, suction should never be applied during insertion of the catheter, but only during its withdrawal. The catheter is rotated and suction is applied intermittently during withdrawal.

Effective suctioning removes secretions from the right and left mainstem bronchi. Unless the catheter is unusually long, this procedure is almost impossible to accomplish with a nasotracheal tube (Wade, 1982). To suction each bronchus, the nurse turns the client's head away from the direction of the bronchus to be suctioned. For example, before the left bronchus is suctioned, the head is turned to the right.

■ ■ ■

Frequency of suctioning is determined by continued client assessment. If secretions are identified by inspection or auscultation techniques, suctioning is required. Sputum is not produced continuously or every 1 or 2 hours but occurs as a response to a pathological condition. Therefore there is no rationale for routine suctioning of all clients every 1 to 2 hours.

Maintenance and Promotion of Oxygenation

Promotion of lung expansion, mobilization of secretions, and maintenance of a patent airway assist the client in meeting oxygenation needs. However, some clients also require oxygen therapy to keep a healthy level of tissue oxygenation.

GOALS OF OXYGEN THERAPY

The goal of oxygen therapy is to prevent or relieve hypoxia. Any client with impaired tissue oxygenation can benefit from controlled oxygen administration. Oxygen is not a substitute for other treatment, however, and should be used only when indicated. Oxygen should be treated as a drug. It is expensive and has dangerous side effects. As with any drug, the dosage or concentration of oxygen should be continuously monitored. The nurse should routinely check the physician's orders to verify that the client is receiving the prescribed oxygen concentration. The "five rights" of medication administration also pertain to oxygen (see Chapter 15).

SAFETY PRECAUTIONS WITH OXYGEN THERAPY

Oxygen is a highly combustible gas. Although it will not spontaneously burn or cause an explosion, it can easily cause a fire to ignite in a client's room if it contacts a spark, as from a cigarette. Oxygen in high concentrations has a great combustion potential and fuels fire readily.

With increasing use of home oxygen therapy, clients and health care professionals must be aware of the dangerous combustible effects. Reports in the literature include information about incidents in the hospital settings, especially associated with oxygen tents in the pediatric setting and cigarette smoking (Gjerde and Kraemer, 1980). A recent article noted a case in which there was a hazard with home oxygen therapy. A client using a portable oxygen source attempted to sharpen lawn mower blades on a home grinder. As soon as the blades touched the grindstone and created sparks, the client felt a burning sensation around and within his nasal passages. Although he quickly removed the oxygen cannula, he received first-degree burns to the face and cheeks from the "blow torch" effect produced by the cannula (McCauley and Boller, 1987).

The nurse should promote safety by using the following measures. First, "no smoking" signs should be placed on the client's room door and over the bed. The client, visitors and roommates, and all personnel should be informed that smoking is not permitted in areas where oxygen is in use. The nurse should determine that all electrical equipment in the room is functioning correctly and is properly grounded (see Chapter 40). An electrical spark in the presence of oxygen can result in a severe fire. Finally, the nurse should know the hospital's fire procedures and the location of the closest fire extinguisher.

SUPPLY OF OXYGEN

Oxygen is supplied to the client's bedside either by oxygen tanks or through a permanent wall-piped system. Oxygen tanks are transported on wide-based carriers that allow the tank to be placed upright at the client's bedside. Regulators are used to control the amount of oxygen delivered. One common type is an upright flowmeter with a flow-adjustment valve at the top. A second type is a cylinder indicator with a flow-adjustment handle.

In the hospital or home, oxygen tanks are delivered with the regulator in place. In the hospital, connecting the regulator is usually done by the respiratory therapy department. Vendors are generally responsible for connecting the oxygen tank to the regulator for home use.

METHODS OF OXYGEN DELIVERY

Oxygen can be delivered to the client by nasal cannula, nasal catheter, face mask, or mechanical ventilator.

NASAL CANNULA. A nasal cannula is a simple, comfortable device (Procedure 36-3). The two cannulae, about 1.5 cm (½ inch) long, protrude from the center of a disposable tube and are inserted into the nostrils. Oxygen is delivered via the cannulae with a flow rate of up to 5 to 6 liters per minute. Higher flow rates dry airway mucosa and do not further increase inspired oxygen concentrations (Luce, Tyler, and Pierson, 1984). The nurse must know what flow rate produces a given percentage of inspired oxygen concentration (FIO_2).

NASAL CATHETER. Nasal catheters are used less frequently than nasal cannulae, but they are not obsolete. The procedure involves inserting an oxygen catheter into the nose to the nasopharynx. Because securing the catheter can cause pressure on the nostril, the catheter must be changed at least every 8 hours and inserted into the other nostril. For this reason the nasal catheter is often a less desirable method because the client may have pain when the catheter is passed into the nasopharynx and because trauma can occur to the nasal mucosa. In addition, even when the catheter is properly placed, gas flow can be misdirected into the stomach, causing serious and painful gastric distention. The relationship of oxygen flow rate in liters per minute and inspired oxygen concentration is the same as with nasal cannula.

TRANSTRACHEAL OXYGEN. Transtracheal oxygen is a method of oxygen delivery in which a small intravenous-size catheter is inserted directly into the trachea through a surgical tract in the lower neck. Oxygen is delivered directly into the trachea.

The transtracheal oxygen delivery system is more advantageous in clients needing continuous oxygen for several reasons. First, there is no oxygen lost to the atmosphere, which is the case with nasal cannula. Therefore the cost of oxygen delivery is less expensive. Second, because oxygen travels directly into the trachea as opposed to through the nose to the posterior pharynx and into the trachea, clients achieve adequate oxygenation at lower less costly flow rates. Third, clients are more likely to use oxygen as prescribed because of the mobility, comfort, and cosmetic improvement. Last, additional humidification is unnecessary because the nasopharynx, the area in most need of supplemental humidity, is bypassed (Am J Nurs, 1987).

Transtracheal oxygen is a potential source of danger to clients with chronic pulmonary disease who have a

PROCEDURE 36-3

Applying a Nasal Cannula

STEPS	RATIONALE
1. Inspect client for signs and symptoms associated with hypoxia and presence of airway secretions.	Left untreated, hypoxia can produce cardiac dysrhythmias and death. The presence of airway secretions decreases the effectiveness of oxygen delivery.
2. Explain to client and family what the procedure entails and the purpose of oxygen therapy.	Decreases client's anxiety, which reduces oxygen consumption and increases client cooperation.

3. Assemble needed supplies and equipment:
  a. Nasal cannula
  b. Oxygen tubing
  c. Humidifier
  d. Sterile distilled water
  e. Oxygen source with flowmeter
  f. "No smoking" signs
	Ensures that procedure is completed quickly and efficiently.

4. Wash hands.	Reduces transmission of infection.
5. Attach nasal cannula to oxygen tubing and attach to a humidified oxygen source adjusted to the prescribed flow rate.	Humidification prevents drying of nasal and oral mucous membranes and airway secretions.
6. Place tips of cannula into client's nares.	Directs flow of oxygen into client's upper respiratory tract.
7. Adjust elastic headband or plastic slide until cannula fits snugly and comfortably.	Client is more likely to keep cannula in place if it fits comfortably.
8. Maintain sufficient slack on oxygen tubing and secure to client's clothes.	Allows client to turn head without dislodging cannula and reduces pressure on tips of nares.
9. Check the cannula every 8 hours.	Patency of cannula and oxygen flow are ensured.
10. Keep the humidification jar filled at all times.	Inhalation of dehumidified oxygen is prevented.
11. Assess the client's nares and external nose for skin breakdown every 6-8 hours.	Because of the drying effects, prolonged use of nasal oxygen can increase the risk of skin breakdown in the client's nares and external nose.
12. Check the oxygen flow rate and the physician's orders every 8 hours.	Delivery of the prescribed oxygen flow rate is ensured.
13. Wash hands.	Reduces transmission of microorganisms.
14. Inspect client for relief of symptoms associated with hypoxia.	Indicates that hypoxia is corrected or reduced.
15. Observe client's nares and superior surface of both ears for skin breakdown.	Oxygen therapy can cause drying of nasal mucosa. Pressure on ears from cannula tubing or elastic can cause skin irritation.
16. Record in nurses' notes method of oxygen delivery, flow rate, patency of oxygen cannula, client response, and respiratory assessment.	Documents correct use of oxygen therapy and client's response.

---

history of carbon dioxide retention. This therapy must be carefully monitored. These clients may require lower oxygen flow rates than predicted.

Use of transtracheal oxygenation occurs in four steps. First is client orientation, evaluation, and selection. Not all clients requiring oxygen therapy can use this method of delivery. Some do not wish to have the surgical procedure, which is done under local anesthesia. Second is surgical insertion of the stent. The stent is a stoma-type access route directly into the trachea. Third is initiation of oxygen through a number 9 French catheter in an immature tract. Last, the final oxygen flow rate is delivered through a number 8 French catheter through the mature tract.

There is a 7-day waiting period before administration of oxygen into the transtracheal system. During this period clients have reported subcutaneous emphysema. This is an accumulation of air in subcutaneous tissues, in this case caused by coughing, which is common in these clients. It can also be caused by premature delivery of oxygen into the transtracheal catheter. Subcutaneous emphysema resolves when oxygen is removed from the catheter. A common practice is continued oxygen delivery by way of nasal cannula for one week before using the catheter.

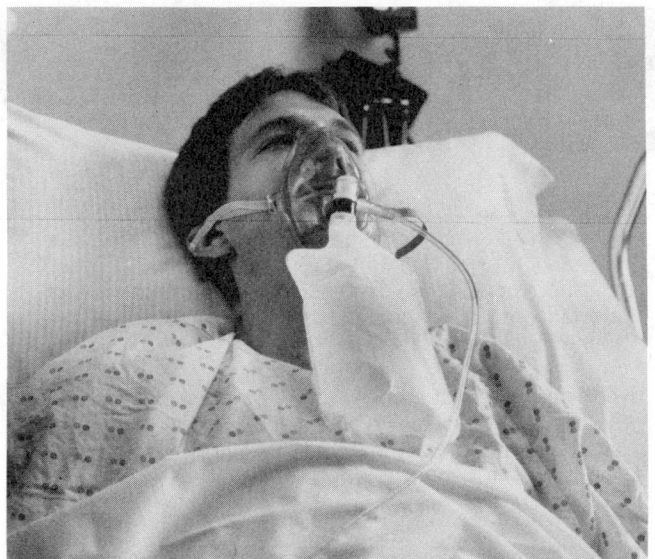

Fig. 36-8 Plastic face mask with reservoir bag.

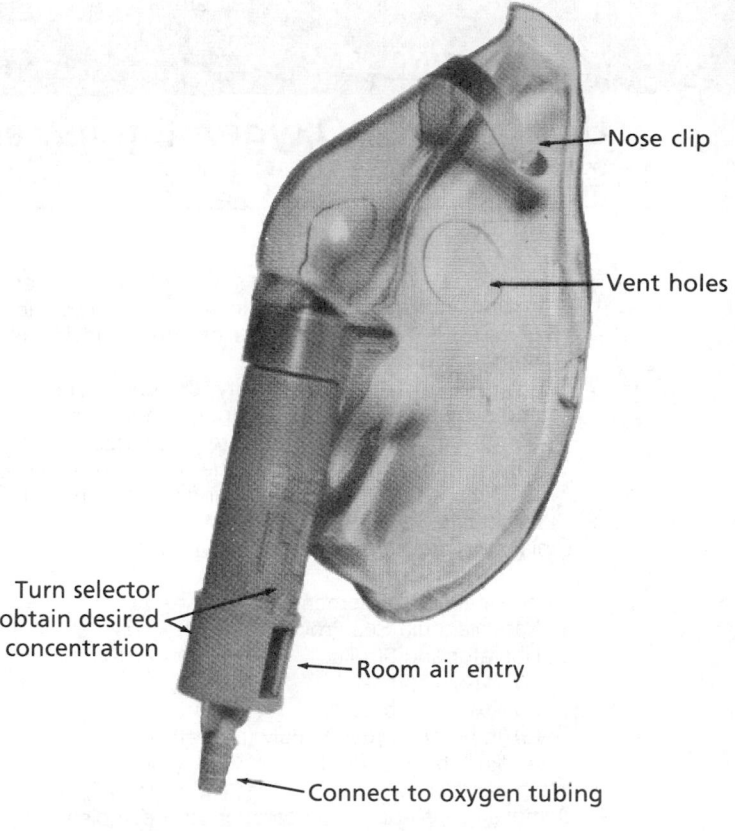

Nose clip

Vent holes

Turn selector
to obtain desired
O_2 concentration

Room air entry

Connect to oxygen tubing

Fig. 36-9 Venturi mask.
Courtesy Puritan-Bennett Corp., Overland Park, Kan.

OXYGEN MASKS. An oxygen mask is a device used to administer oxygen, humidity, or heated humidity. It is shaped to fit snugly over the mouth and nose and is secured in place with a strap. There are two primary types of oxygen masks: high and low concentration.

A plastic face mask with a reservoir bag (Fig. 36-8) and a Venturi mask (Fig. 36-9) are capable of delivering higher concentrations of oxygen. The plastic face mask with a reservoir bag can deliver 70% oxygen with a flow rate of 10 liters per minute. This oxygen mask maintains a high-concentration oxygen supply in the reservoir bag. The nurse should frequently inspect the bag to make sure it is inflated. If it is deflated, the client may be breathing large amounts of exhaled carbon dioxide.

The Venturi mask can be used to deliver oxygen concentrations of 24%, 28%, 35%, and 40% with oxygen flow rates of 4, 6, 8, and 10 liters per minute, respectively, depending on which flow control meter is selected (Wade, 1982).

The simple face mask (Fig. 36-10) is used for short-term oxygen therapy. It fits loosely and delivers oxygen concentrations from 30% to 60%. The mask is contraindicated for clients with carbon dioxide retention because retention can be worsened.

HOME OXYGEN. When home oxygen is required, it is usually delivered by nasal cannula. When a client has a permanent tracheostomy, however, a T-tube or tracheostomy collar is necessary. Three types of oxygen are used: compressed oxygen, liquid oxygen, and oxygen

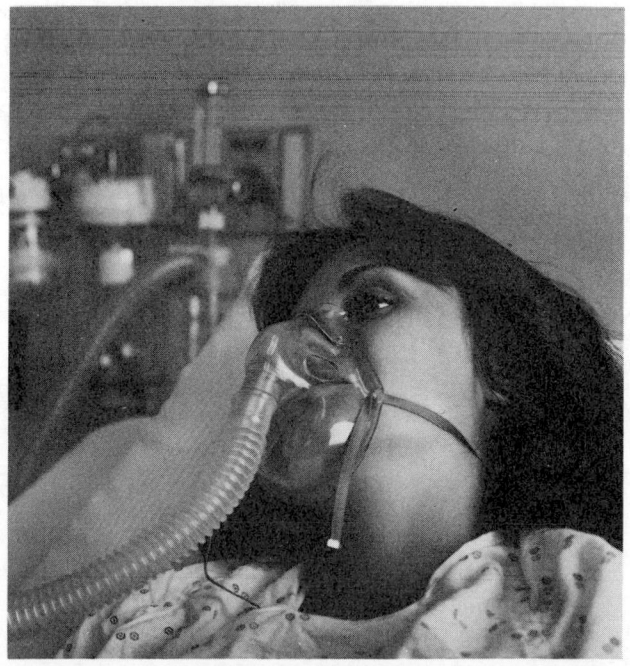

Fig. 36-10 Simple face mask.

PROCEDURE 36-4

Using Home Oxygen Equipment

STEPS	RATIONALE
1. Assess the following:	
a. Determine client's or family's ability to use oxygen equipment correctly, while in hospital, if possible, or assess for appropriate use of equipment in the home setting.	Physical or cognitive impairments may necessitate instructing family member or significant other how to operate home oxygen equipment.
b. Assess client's or family's ability to observe for signs and symptoms of hypoxia: apprehension, anxiety, decreased ability to concentrate, decreased level of consciousness, increased fatigue, dizziness, behavioral changes, increased pulse, increased respiratory rate, pallor, and cyanosis.	Hypoxia can occur at home when client uses oxygen. It can be caused by worsening of client's physical problem or another underlying condition, for example, change in respiratory status.
2. Explain the procedure to client and family.	Reinforces education received in the hospital. Enables client and family to ask questions.
3. Prepare needed equipment:	Ensures that procedure is completed quickly and efficiently.
a. Nasal cannula (see Procedure 36-3).	
b. Liberator and Stroller	
(1) Nasal cannula	
(2) Oxygen tubing	
(3) In-home oxygen supply (Liberator)	
(4) Portable system (Stroller)	
4. Wash hands.	Reduces transmission of infection.
5. Demonstrate steps for preparation and completion of oxygen therapy.	Demonstration is reliable technique for teaching psychomotor skill and enables client to ask questions.
6. Prepare the Liberator and Stroller for use:	
a. Place Liberator in a clutter-free environment (see illustration).	30 L Liberator replaces 3½ compressed oxygen cylinders but requires sufficient space.
b. Check oxygen levels of both Liberator and Stroller by depressing button at lower right corner and reading dial (see illustration).	Ensures timely and effective use of remaining oxygen supply and allows time for refill.
c. When necessary, refill Stroller by turning bayonet coupling lock on Stroller 45 degrees. Insert female adapter (Stroller) to male adaptor (Liberator) (see illustration).	Allows for secure connection between Liberator and Stroller to prevent leakage of oxygen into room air.
d. Select prescribe rate (see illustration).	Ensures delivery of prescribed amount of oxygen.
e. Lock flowmeter.	Prevents client from changing oxygen flow rate.

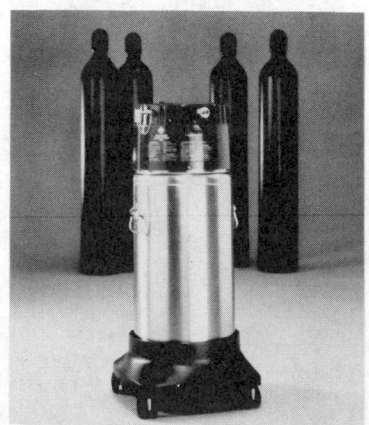

Step 6a

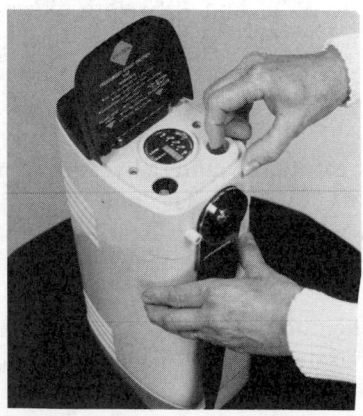

Step 6b

STEPS	RATIONALE
f. Connect nasal cannula and oxygen tubing to Stroller.	Connects oxygen source to delivery method.
g. Place Stroller on cart.	Allows client to ambulate freely without expending energy to carry Stroller.
7. Have client or family perform each step with guidance from nurse.	Allows nurse to correct errors in technique and discuss their implications.
8. Discuss signs and symptoms of respiratory tract infection: fever, increased sputum, change in color in sputum, foul sputum odor.	Respiratory tract infections increase oxygen demand and may affect oxygen transfer from lungs to blood.
9. Instruct client or family to notify physician if signs or symptoms of hypoxia or respiratory tract infections occur.	Can prevent severe exacerbation of client's pulmonary disease.
10. Wash hands.	Reduces transmission of infection.
11. Record teaching plan, information given to client, and validation of learning.	Provides written documentation for teaching plan for client and family. Documents client learning.

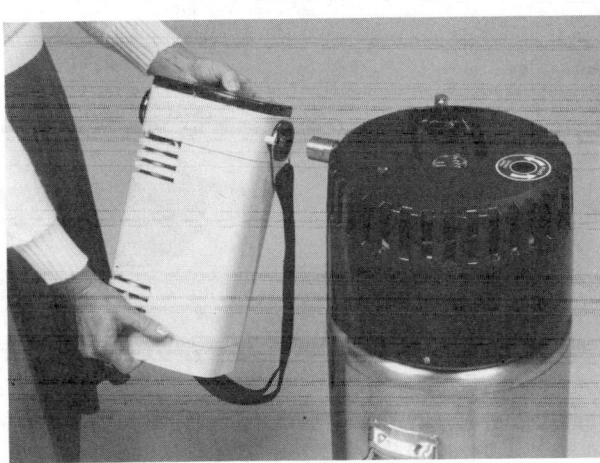

Step 6c

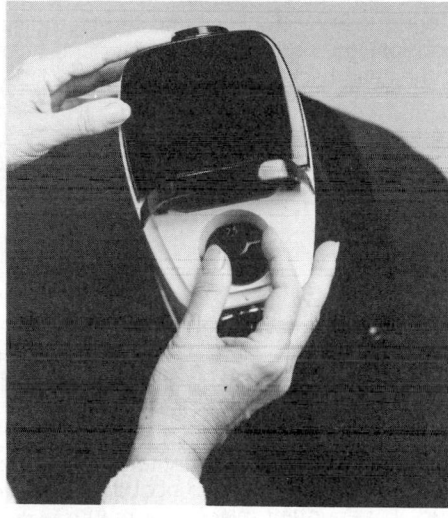

Step 6d

concentrators. In the home the major consideration is the oxygen delivery source.

Compressed oxygen requires several large oxygen tanks. Each tank lasts about 50 hours at 2 L/min. Liquid systems use a small portable tank filled from a reservoir in the home. Oxygen concentrators extract oxygen from the air and supply it to the client at prescribed flow rates (Traver, 1982).

Clients requiring home oxygen need extensive teaching so they are able to continue oxygen therapy efficiently and safely (Procedure 36-4). In preparation, the nurse must coordinate efforts of the client, primary nurse, visiting nurse, and home oxygen equipment ven-

dor. Second, the nurse must allow sufficient time for teaching so that the client is confident in maintaining the oxygen delivery system (Perry and Potter, 1986).

Special Considerations. The equipment vendor and nurse should instruct the client how frequently Liberator and Stroller must be filled. Small Liberator (4 pound) (Sprint) has a 4-hour capacity, whereas 9½ pound Stroller has an 8-hour capacity. Refilling occurs automatically and usually takes less than a minute. Also client must be cautioned against use of over-the-counter medications unless prescribed by a physician.

PROCEDURE 36-5

Cardiopulmonary Resuscitation

STEPS	RATIONALE

ONE NURSE

1. Assess for unresponsiveness: observe for spontaneous respirations: palpate carotid pulse; ask victim "Are you OK?"

   Prevents injury from attempted resuscitation of a person who has not suffered a cardiac or respiratory arrest.

2. Call for help: in a hospital setting, call a "code"; in a community setting, call an emergency phone number.

   Activates mechanism for additional personnel.

3. Place the victim supine on a hard surface or use a backboard.

   External compression of the heart is facilitated. The heart is compressed between the sternum and the hard surface.

4. Kneel at the level of the victim's shoulders.

   This position allows performance of rescue breathing and chest compressions without moving knees.

5. Open victim's airway:
   a. Head-tilt/chin-lift maneuver (adults and children): place one hand on victim's forehead and apply firm, backward pressure with the palm to tilt the head back. Place the fingers of the other hand under the bony part of the jaw near the chin and lift to bring the chin forward and the teeth almost to occlusion, thus supporting the jaw and helping to tilt the head back (see illustration).

   This maneuver is more effective in opening the airway than the previously recommended *head-tilt/neck-lift*.
   This maneuver removes the tongue or epiglottis as an airway obstruction.

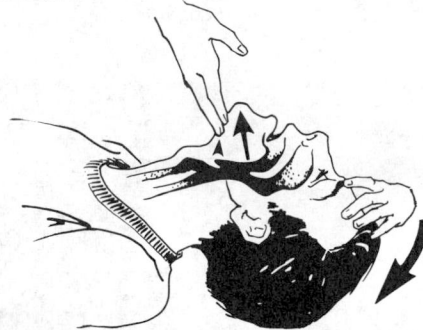

Step 5a

   b. Jaw thrust maneuver (adults and children): grasp angles of the victim's lower jaw and lift with both hands, thus displacing the mandible forward while tilting the head backward.

   This technique without head-tilt is the safest first approach to opening the airway of the victim with suspected neck injury because it can usually be accomplished without extending the neck.

6. Prepare for artificial respiration.
   a. For mouth-to-mouth resuscitation of an adult, pinch the victim's nose and occlude his mouth with yours. For an infant, place your mouth over the infant's nose and mouth.

   An airtight seal is formed and air is prevented from escaping from the nose.

   b. For Ambu bag resuscitation, use the proper size face mask and apply it over the victim's mouth and nose.

   An airtight seal is formed as the bag is compressed and oxygen enters the client.

7. Administer artificial respiration.
   a. For mouth-to-mouth resuscitation of an adult, blow two quick breaths into the victim's mouth. Adequate time for the two breaths (1-1½ seconds per breath) should be allowed to provide good chest expansion and decrease the possibility of gastric distention.

   In most adults this volume is 800 ml and is sufficient volume to make the chest rise. An excess of air volume and fast inspiratory flow rates are likely to cause pharyngeal pressures that exceed esophageal opening pressures, allowing air to enter the stomach and result in gastric distention, thereby increasing the risk of vomiting.

   b. For mouth-to-mouth resuscitation of an infant or child, administer two slow breaths, 1-1½ seconds per breath with a pause between for rescuer to take a breath.

   Since an infant's air passages are smaller with resistance to flow quite high, it is difficult to make recommendations about the force or volume of the rescue breaths. However, three factors should be remembered: (1) rescue breaths are the single most important maneuver in assisting a nonbreathing child, (2) an appropriate volume is one that makes the chest rise and fall, and (3) slow breaths provide an adequate volume at the lowest possible pressure, thereby reducing the risk of gastric distention.

STEPS	RATIONALE

c. For artificial respiration with an Ambu bag in an adult, compress the bag fully for two breaths.

d. For Ambu bag resuscitation in a child, use two small compressions of the bag.

Overinflation of the child's lungs is prevented.

8. Observe for rise and fall of the chest wall with each respiration. If lungs do not inflate, reposition the head and neck and check for visible airway obstruction, such as vomitus.

Observing chest wall movement ensures that artificial respirations are entering the lungs.

9. Suction any secretions from the airway. If suction is unavailable, turn the victim's head to one side.

Suctioning prevents airway obstruction. Turning the client's head to one side allows gravity to drain secretions.

10. Assess for presence of the carotid pulse; pulse check should take 5-10 seconds.

a. Carotid pulse is most central and accessible artery in children over 1 year. However, in an infant the short, chubby neck makes carotid difficult to palpate; brachial artery is recommended instead.

Carotid artery pulse will persist when the more peripheral pulses are no longer palpable. Performing external cardiac compressions on a victim who has a pulse may result in serious medical complications.

11. If victim is pulseless, begin external cardiac compressions:

Adult

a. Proper hand position (see illustration):

(1) Using middle index finger of the hand nearest the victim's legs, locate lower margin of rib cage on the side next to rescuer.

(2) Move fingers up the rib cage to the notch where the ribs meet the sternum. Place middle finger on notch and index finger next to it on the lower end of the sternum.

(3) Place long axis of the heel of the hand nearest victim's head on the long axis of the sternum next to the index finger.

(4) Remove first hand from notch, place on top of the hand on the sternum so that the hands are parallel to each other.

(5) Either extend or interlace fingers, but keep fingers off the chest.

Properly performed external chest compressions can produce systolic blood pressure peaks of more than 100 mm Hg, but the diastolic pressure is low, with the mean blood pressure in the carotid arteries seldom exceeding 40 mm Hg. Blood flow through the carotid artery is only one fourth to one third of normal.

Proper hand position results in maximal compression of the heart between the sternum and the vertebrae. If compressions occur over the xiphoid process, the victim's liver can be lacerated.

Reduces risk of rib fracture during compression.

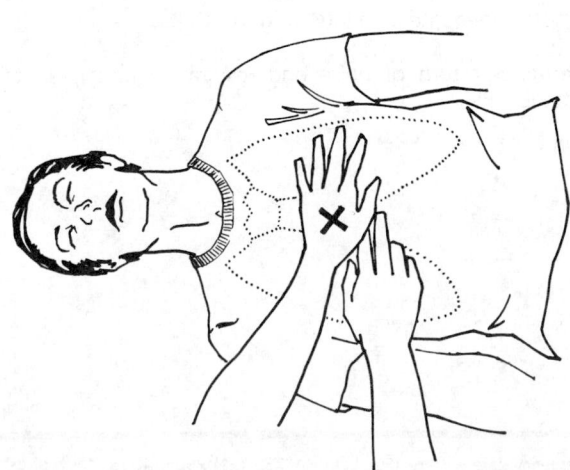

Step 11a (adult)

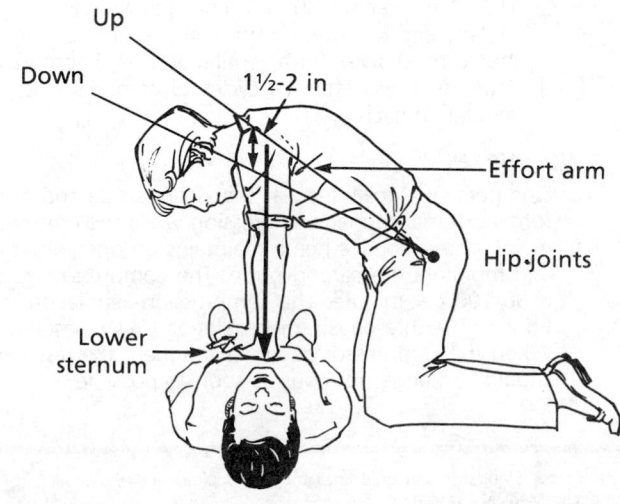

Step 11b (adult)

Continued.

PROCEDURE 36-5, cont'd

Cardiopulmonary Resuscitation

STEPS	RATIONALE
b. Lock elbows, maintain arms straight and shoulders directly over the hands on victim's sternum (see illustration):	In this manner the thrust for each compression is straight down on the sternum.
(1) Compress chest 3.8-5.0 cm (1½-2 in).	
(2) Compress chest 80-100 times per minute. Perform 15 external compressions with the mnemonic "one and, two and, three and . . ." to 15.	Faster rate increases blood flow with an increased flow to the brain and heart. Faster rate also allows a pause for ventilation in two-rescuer CPR.
c. Ventilate lungs with two ventilations as in step 7a.	
d. Reassess victim after four cycles (15 compressions: 2 ventilations each cycle).	Determines return of pulse and respiration and the need to continue CPR.
Infant (1-12 months)	
a. Proper hand position:	Proper hand position results in maximal compression.
(1) Draw an imaginary line between the nipples over the breast bone (sternum).	
(2) Place the index finger of the hand farthest from the infant's head just under the intermammary line where it intersects the sternum.	The area of compression is one finger's width below this intersection at the location of the middle and ring fingers.
b. Using two fingers compress 1.3-2.5 cm (½-1 in) at least 100 times per minute.	Promotes adequate cardiac output.
c. At the end of every fifth compression a pause should be allowed for a ventilation (1½ seconds).	Promotes adequate ventilation during CPR.
d. Reassess victim after ten cycles (5 compressions: 1 ventilation each cycle).	Determines return of pulse and respiration and the need to continue CPR.
Child (1-7 years)	
a. Proper hand position:	Proper position results in maximal compressions.
(1) Locate lower margin of the victim's rib cage on the side next to the rescuer with the middle and index fingers.	
(2) Follow the margin of the rib cage with the middle finger to the notch where the ribs and breast bone meet.	
(3) Place index finger next to middle finger.	
(4) Place heel of other hand next to the index finger with long axis of the heel parallel to sternum.	
b. Compress sternum with one hand 2.5-3.8 cm (1-1½ in) at a rate of 80-100 times per minute.	Promotes adequate cardiac output.
c. At the end of every fifth compression a pause should be allowed for a ventilation (1-1½ seconds).	Promotes adequate ventilation during CPR.
d. Reassess victim after 10 cycles (5 compressions: 1 ventilation each cycle).	Determines return of pulse and respiration and need to continue CPR.

TWO NURSES

12. One person is positioned at the victim's side and performs external cardiac compression while the other remains at the victim's head, maintains an open airway, and monitors the carotid pulse. The compression rate is 80-100 per minute. The compression-ventilation ratio is 5:1 with a pause for ventilation (1-1½ seconds). When the compressor becomes fatigued, the rescuers should exchange positions as soon as possible.

Data from Standards and guidelines for cardiopulmonary resuscitation (CPR) and emergency cardiac care (ECC), JAMA 255 (21):2905, 1986, copyright 1986, American Medical Association.

Restoration of Cardiopulmonary Functioning

If a client's hypoxia is severe and prolonged, cardiac arrest may result. A cardiac arrest is a sudden cessation of cardiac output and circulation. When this occurs, oxygen is not delivered to tissues, carbon dioxide is not transported from tissues, tissue metabolism becomes anaerobic, and metabolic and respiratory acidoses occur. Permanent heart, brain, and other tissue damage occurs within 5 minutes.

CARDIOPULMONARY RESUSCITATION

Cardiac arrest is characterized by an absence of pulse and respiration and by dilated pupils. If the nurse determines that the client has cardiac arrest, cardiopulmonary resuscitation (CPR) must be initiated. CPR is a basic emergency procedure of artificial respiration and manual external cardiac massage (Procedure 36-5). CPR has three main goals, called the ABCs of cardiopulmonary resuscitation: to establish an *a*irway, initiate *b*reathing, and maintain *c*irculation.

EVALUATION

Nursing interventions are evaluated by comparing the client's progress as a result of nursing therapies to the goals and desired outcomes of the nursing care plan. Each goal and category of interventions has objective evaluation criteria. These (see evaluation box) are examples of evaluation criteria for clients with altered oxygen; other criteria are based on the specific nursing diagnoses and goals of care.

When nursing measures directed to improve oxygenation are unsuccessful, the nurse must immediately modify the nursing care plan. New interventions are then developed. The nurse should not hesitate to notify the physician about a client's deteriorating oxygenation status. Prompt notification can avoid an emergency situation or even the need for cardiopulmonary resuscitation.

SUMMARY

Clients with impaired oxygenation require planned nursing care that focuses on returning the client to a maximal level of wellness. Many nursing interventions can be used to promote lung expansion, mobilize secretions, maintain a patent airway, promote oxygenation or to restore cardiopulmonary functioning.

Nursing interventions are individualized to the client's level of health, age, life-style, and needs. Many nursing skills are used to help the client achieve a maximal level of oxygenation.

Sample Evaluation of Interventions for Respiratory Dysfunction

Goals	Evaluative Measures	Expected Outcomes
Activity tolerance is improved.	Palpate client's radial pulse.	Pulse remains below 120 bpm.
	Observe and ask client about perception of dyspnea or breathlessness.	Client reports decreased dyspnea on exertion.
	Palpate client's radial pulse 10 minutes after exercise.	Baseline pulse rate returns 10 minutes after exercise.
	Instruct client to keep an activity record.	Client has gradual increase in activities of daily living.
Pulmonary secretions mobilized.	Auscultate all lung fields after 2 hours and after coughing and deep breathing or suctioning.	Adventitious lung sounds are absent.
	Inspect sputum produced by cough and/or suctioning.	Client has forceful productive cough. Sputum is clear, white, and frothy.
	Observe and ask client about perception of dyspnea or breathlessness.	Dyspnea is absent. Chest x-ray studies are clear.
Lung expansion improved.	Auscultate all lung fields every 2 hours and after coughing or suctioning.	Breath sounds are improved and adventitious lung sounds are absent.
	Observe chest wall motion when client is walking or sitting up.	Chest expansion is improved.
	Observe for signs of dyspnea.	Nasal flaring or reports of dyspnea are absent.

KEY CONCEPTS

✓ Metabolic activity of cells require oxygen.

✓ The primary function of the lungs is to transfer oxygen from the atmosphere into the alveoli and to transfer carbon dioxide out of the body as a waste product.

✓ Ventilation is the process of providing adequate oxygenation from the alveoli to the blood.

✓ Breathing requires the body to generate energy to expand the lungs; this is called the work of breathing.

✓ Compliance, or the ability of the lungs to expand and contract, depends on the function of musculoskeletal and neurological systems and on other physiological factors.

✓ Inspiration is an active process, and expiration is a passive process.

✓ The process of moving air in and out of the lungs is achieved with lung changes in pressures and lung volumes.

✓ Adequate oxygenation requires the heart to perfuse the ventilated regions of the lung.

✓ Respiratory gases are primarily transported by hemoglobin.

✓ Respiration is controlled by the central nervous system and by chemicals within the blood.

✓ Decreased hemoglobin levels alter the client's ability to transport oxygen.

✓ An increased metabolic rate increases tissue oxygen demand.

✓ Impaired chest wall movement reduces the level of tissue oxygenation.

✓ The normal aging process decreases elasticity of the lungs.

✓ Hyperventilation is a respiratory rate greater than that required to maintain normal levels of carbon dioxide.

✓ Hypoventilation causes carbon dioxide retention.

✓ Hypoxia occurs if the amount of oxygen delivered to tissues is too low.

✓ The nursing history includes information about the client's cough, dyspnea, wheezing, pain, environmental exposures, respiratory infection, risk factors, and use of medications.

✓ The nurse uses all assessment techniques when evaluating a client's level of oxygenation.

✓ Diagnostic and laboratory tests may be needed to complete the data base for a client with decreased oxygenation.

✓ The nursing process is used to restore or maintain the client's maximal level of wellness.

✓ Improper positioning can decrease ventilation and oxygenation.

✓ Breathing exercises improve ventilation and oxygenation.

✓ Incentive spirometry increases inhalation volumes.

✓ Hydration and humidification help liquefy and mobilize pulmonary secretions.

✓ Nebulization delivers small drops of water or particles of medication to the airways.

✓ Chest physiotherapy includes postural drainage, percussion, and vibration to mobilize pulmonary secretions.

✓ Coughing and suctioning techniques are used to maintain a patent airway.

✓ Oxygen therapy is used to improve levels of tissue oxygenation and is delivered by nasal cannula, nasal catheter, or oxygen mask.

✓ Cardiac arrest requires the use of cardiopulmonary resuscitation.

REFERENCES

Agle, DP, et al.: Multidiscipline treatment of chronic pulmonary insufficiency, Psychosom Med 35:41, 1973.

Beck, GJ, Schachter, EN, and Marinder, LR: The relationship of respiratory symptoms and lung function loss in cotton textile workers, Am Rev Resp Dis 130:6, 1984.

Bennett, JA: What we know about AIDS, Am J Nurs 86:1016, 1986.

Bushnell, SS: Respiratory intensive care nursing, ed. 2, 1981, Boston, Little, Brown & Co.

Churg, A, et al.: Small airways disease and mineral dust response, Am Rev Resp Dis 131:139, 1985.

Clinical News: Transtracheal oxygen: the nose knows the difference, Am J Nurs 87:421, 1987.

Daily, EK, and Schroeder, JS: Techniques in bedside hemodynamic monitoring ed. 3, St. Louis, 1985, The C.V. Mosby Co.

Dopico, GA, et al.: Epidemiologic study of clinical and physiologic parameters in grain handlers of Northern United States, Am Rev Resp Dis 130:759, 1984.

Duncan, CR, Erickson, RS, and Weigel, RM: Effect of chest tube management on drainage after cardiac surgery, Heart Lung, 16(1):1, 1987.

Erikson, R: Chest tubes: they're really not that complicated, Nurs 81 11(5):34, 1981.

Feldman, J: Chronic obstructive pulmonary disease. In Traver, GA, editor: Respiratory nursing: the science and the art, New York, 1982, John Wiley & Sons.

Ganong, WF: Review of medical physiology, ed. 13, Los Altos, Calif., 1983, Lange Medical Publications.

Gift, AG, Plant, SM, and Jacox, A: Psychologic and physiologic factors related to dyspnea in subjects with chronic obstructive pulmonary disease, Heart Lung 15(6):595, 1986.

Gjerde, GE, and Kraemer, R: An oxygen therapy fire, Resp Care 25:363, 1980.

Groër, MW, and Shekleton, MS: Basic pathophysiology: a conceptual approach, ed. 2, St. Louis, 1983, The C.V. Mosby Co.

Kerr, JAC: Adherence and self-care, Heart Lung 14(1):24, 1985.

Kim, MJ: Respiratory muscle training, Heart Lung 13:333, 1984.

Larson, M, and Kim, MJ: Respiratory muscle training with incentive spirometer resistive breathing device, Heart Lung 13:341, 1984.

Luce, JM, Tyler, ML, and Pierson, DJ: Intensive respiratory care, Philadelphia, 1984, W.B. Saunders Co.

McCauley, CS, and Boller, LR: The hazards of home oxygen therapy, N Engl J Med 316(2):107, 1987.

McDonald, BR: Validation of three respiratory nursing diagnoses, Nurs Clin North Am 20(4):697, 1985.

Paulaw, D, and Jones, S: Test your skill at trouble shooting chest tubes RN October 1986

Perry, AG, and Potter, PA: Clinical nursing skills and techniques: basic, intermediate, and advanced, St. Louis, 1986, The C.V. Mosby Co.

Shenkman, B: Factors contributing to attrition rates in a pulmonary rehabilitation program, Heart Lung 14(1):53, 1985.

Smith, SJ: Clinical assessment of the pulmonary patient. In Traver, GA, editor: Respiratory nursing: the science and the art, New York, 1982, John Wiley & Sons.

Steckel, S, and Swain, MA: Contracting with patients to improve compliance, Hospitals 15:81, 1977.

Swain, MA, and Steckel, S: Influencing adherence among hypertensives, Res Nur Health 4:213, 1981.

Traver, GA: Respiratory nursing: the science and the art, New York, 1982, John Wiley & Sons.

Vander, AJ, Sherman, JAH, and Luciane, DS: Human physiology: the mechanism of body function, ed. 3, New York, 1980, McGraw-Hill Book Co.

Wade, JF: Respiratory nursing care, ed. 3, St. Louis, 1982, The C.V. Mosby Co.

Weaver, TE: New life for lungs . . . through incentive spirometers, Nurs 81 11(2):53, 1981.

West, JB: Respiratory physiology, the essentials, ed. 2, Baltimore, 1979, The Williams & Wilkins Co.

York, K: Clinical validation of two respiratory nursing diagnoses and their defining characteristics, Nurs Clin North Am 20(4):657, 1985.

York, K, and Martin, PA: Clinical validation of respiratory nursing diagnoses: a model. In Hurley, MH, editor: Classification of nursing diagnoses: proceedings of the sixth conference (NANDA), St. Louis, 1986, The C.V. Mosby Co.

Research Article

Jansen-Bjerklie, S, Carrieri, VK, and Hudes, M: The sensation of pulmonary dyspnea, Nur Res 35(3):154, 1986.

ADDITIONAL READINGS

Dennison, R: Cardiopulmonary assessment: how to do it better in 15 easy steps Nurs 86 16(4):34, 1986.

Perry, AG, and Potter, PA: Shock: comprehensive nursing management, St. Louis, 1983, The C.V. Mosby Company.

Standards and guidelines for cardiopulmonary resuscitation (CPR) and emergency cardiac care, JAMA 255(21):2903, 1986.

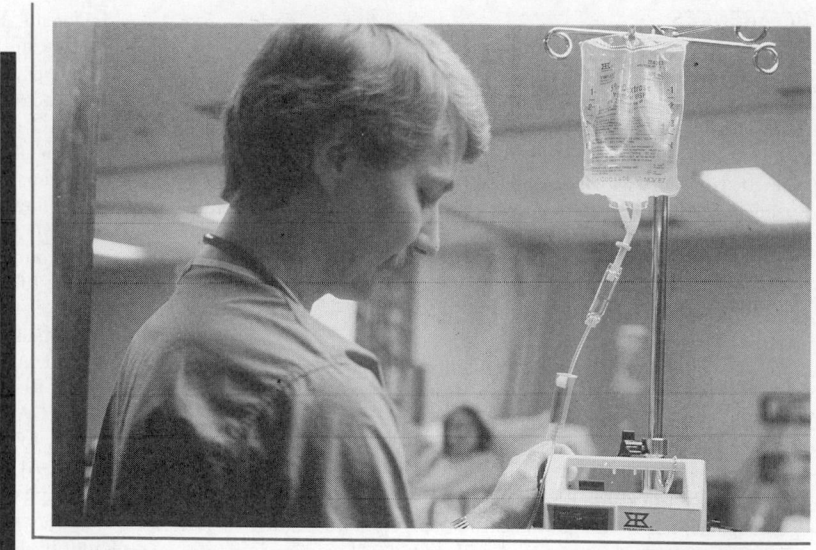

OBJECTIVES

Mastery of content in this chapter will enable the student to:

- Define the key terms listed.
- Describe the regulation and imbalances of sodium, potassium, calcium, magnesium, chloride, bicarbonate, phosphate, and acid base.
- Describe the volume disturbances of dehydration and overhydration.
- Discuss the variables affecting fluid, electrolyte, and acid-base balances.
- Compile a nursing history and complete a physical examination for fluid, electrolyte, and acid-base balance.
- Describe laboratory studies associated with fluid, electrolyte, and acid-base imbalances.
- Develop a nursing care plan for clients with fluid, electrolyte, and acid-base disturbance.
- Discuss the purpose of intravenous (IV) therapy.
- Distinguish between peripheral and central venous lines.
- Describe the procedure for initiating and maintaining an IV line and calculating IV flow rate.
- Demonstrate how to change IV solutions, tubing, and dressing and to discontinue an infusion.
- Discuss the complications of IV therapy.
- Discuss the procedure for administering a blood transfusion and nursing actions for a transfusion reaction.

KEY TERMS

Acidemia	Hydrostatic Pressure
Active Transport	Hypervolemia
ADH	Interstitial Fluid
Aldosterone	Intracellular Fluid
Alkalemia	Milliequivalent (mEq)
Anions	Osmosis
Arterial Blood Gases	Osmotic Pressure
Autotransfusion	Overhydration
Buffer	Plasma
Cations	Plasma Proteins
Compensation	Sodium Pump
Dehydration	Specific Gravity
Electrolyte	Urinometer
Extracellular Fluid	Vascular Access Devices
Hemolysis	Venipuncture
Hemosiderin	

Fluid, Electrolyte, and Acid-Base Balances

Fluid, electrolyte, and acid-base balances within the body are necessary to maintain health and function in all systems. These balances are maintained by the intake and output of water and electrolytes, their distribution in the body, and the regulation of renal and pulmonary function. Imbalances may result from many factors and are associated with illnesses. Therefore nursing care for many different kinds of clients includes assessment and correction of imbalances or maintenance of balance. Acid-base balance is necessary for many physiological processes, and imbalances resulting from many causes can alter respiration, metabolism, and central nervous system function.

A healthy, mobile, well-oriented adult is usually capable of maintaining normal fluid, electrolyte, and acid-base balances because of the body's adaptive mechanisms. However, the infant, the severely ill adult, the disoriented or immobile client, and the elderly are frequently unable to respond independently, and after a period of time the body's adaptive capacities are no longer capable of maintaining balance.

This chapter focuses on the distribution and composition of body water, the movement of body water from one compartment to another, the factors that regulate fluid and electrolyte balances, specific electrolyte and volume disturbances, and normal and abnormal acid-base relationships. Through the nursing process the nurse is able to assess, interpret, and restore fluid, electrolyte, and acid-base imbalances.

FLUID AND ELECTROLYTE BALANCES

Distribution of Body Fluids

Body fluids are distributed in two distinct compartments, one containing extracellular fluids and the other containing intracellular fluids.

Extracellular fluids are the portion of the body fluids comprising the interstitial fluid and blood plasma. Interstitial fluid fills the spaces between most cells of the body and provides a substantial portion of the body's liquid environment. About 16% of body weight consists of interstitial fluids. Another extracellular fluid is plasma, the watery, colorless, fluid portion of the lymph and blood in which the leukocytes, erythrocytes, and platelets are suspended. Plasma comprises 4% of body weight.

Intracellular fluids are liquids within cell membranes containing dissolved solutes essential to fluid and electrolyte balance and metabolism. Intracellular fluids constitute 80% of body weight. Many of the materials in the intracellular fluid compartment are the same as those located in the extracellular fluid space. However, the proportion of the substances is different. For example, a larger proportion of potassium exists in intracellular fluids than in extracellular fluids.

Composition of Body Fluids

The fluids circulating throughout the body in extracellular and intracellular fluid spaces are composed of electrolytes, minerals, and cells.

An *electrolyte* is an element or compound that, when melted or dissolved in water or another solvent, dissociates into ions and is able to carry an electric current. Positively charged electrolytes are *cations*. (Students may find it helpful to associate the "t" in cation [which has a positive charge] with a plus [+] sign.) Negatively charged electrolytes are called *anions*. The concentration of each electrolyte differs in extracellular and intracellular fluids. However, the total weight of anions and cations in each fluid compartment should be the same.

Electrolytes are commonly measured in milliequivalents per liter (mEq/L). This value represents the number of grams of the specific electrolyte (solute) dissolved in 1 liter of plasma (solution). Electrolytes are vital to neuromuscular function and acid-base balance.

Minerals, which are ingested as compounds, are usually referred to by the name of a metal, nonmetal, radical, or phosphate rather than by the name of the compound of which they are a part. Minerals play a vital role in regulating many body functions. They are consituents of all body tissues and fluids and are important in maintaining physiological processes. Minerals also act as catalysts in nerve response, muscle contraction, and metabolism of nutrients in foods. In addition, they regulate electrolyte balance and hormone production and strengthen skeletal structures.

Cells, which are also located in body fluids, are the functional fundamental units of all living tissue. Examples of cells within body fluids are the red blood cell (RBC) and the white blood cell (WBC).

Body fluids composed of electrolytes, minerals, and cells comprise a major portion of the total body weight. For body fluids to remain in appropriate intracellular or extracellular compartments, their movement must follow specific patterns.

Movement of Body Fluids

Body fluids are not static. Fluids and electrolytes shift from compartment to compartment to meet metabolic needs such as tissue oxygenation, response to illness, acid-base disturbances, or response to drug therapies. Body fluid and electrolyte movement is affected through diffusion, osmosis, active transport, or fluid pressures. In addition, movement of fluid components depends on cellular permeability.

DIFFUSION

Diffusion is a process in which solid, particulate matter in a fluid moves from an area of higher concentration to an area of lower concentration, resulting in an even distribution of the particles in the fluid. Substances that are diffusing therefore move down their concentration gradients or, more simply, move in a downhill direction (Groër, 1981). Fluids and electrolytes also diffuse across cellular membranes. For a substance to cross a membrane, the membrane must be permeable to that substance.

OSMOSIS

Osmosis is the movement of a pure solvent, such as water, through a semipermeable membrane from a solution that has a lower solute concentration to one that has a higher solute concentration. The membrane is permeable to the solvent but it is impermeable to the solute, the particulate matter. The rate of osmosis depends on the following factors: (1) the concentrations of the solutes in the solutions, (2) the temperature of the solutions, (3) the electrical charges of the solutes, and (4) the differences between the osmotic pressures exerted by the solutions.

The concentration of a solution is measured in osmols. An osmol is the amount of a substance in solution in the form of molecules, ions, or both, that has the same osmotic pressure as one mole of an ideal nonelectrolyte. The osmotic pressure of a solution is expressed as osmolarity, which is expressed in osmols or milliosmols per kilogram of the solution.

If the concentration of the solute is greater on one side of the permeable membrane, the rate of osmosis is quicker and a more rapid transfer of solvent across the membrane occurs. This continues until an equilibrium is reached.

ACTIVE TRANSPORT

Active transport is the movement of materials across the cell membrane by chemical activity that allows the cell to admit larger molecules than it would otherwise be able to admit. Unlike diffusion and osmosis, active transport requires metabolic activity and energy expenditure.

Active transport is enhanced by carrier molecules, such as insulin, within a cell that bind themselves to incoming molecules. For example, insulin binds itself to glucose and serves as a transport vehicle to permit entry of glucose into the cell. Active transport is the mechanism by which the cell absorbs glucose and other substances to carry out metabolic activities.

The criteria for active transport include movement against a concentration gradient, saturation motion, and metabolic work by the cell. Active transport can be inhibited by cooling the cell, starving it, by withholding glucose, and poisoning the cell (Groër, 1981). Examples of active transport in the body are found in sodium and potassium pumps. Sodium is pumped out of the cell. Potassium is pumped in, against a concentration gradient.

FLUID PRESSURES

The pressures exerted by different types of fluids also direct the movement of fluid between extracellular and intracellular fluid compartments. The basic pressures exerted on fluids are osmotic and hydrostatic pressures.

Osmotic pressure refers to the drawing power for water and depends on the number of molecules in the solution (Metheny and Snively, 1983). Osmotic pressure is exerted through a semipermeable membrane and is dependent on the activity of the solutes separated by the membrane. A solution with the same osmotic pressure or osmolarity as blood plasma is called *isotonic*. The intravenous (IV) administration of an isotonic solution prevents shifting of fluid and electrolytes from intracellular compartments. One substance affecting osmotic pressure is albumin, a serum protein naturally produced by the body. Albumin exerts colloid osmotic pressure, which assists in maintaining fluids in their proper fluid compartments.

A hypotonic solution that has a lesser concentration of solutes than is normal in body fluids may be administered to a client to help maintain fluid and electrolyte balance. For example, half normal saline (½ NS) may

be ordered for clients recovering from ketoacidosis. This hypotonic solution is ordered with other electrolyte solutions.

Hydrostatic pressure is the pressure exerted by a liquid. Blood and fluid entering the capillaries do so at a certain pressure. Like osmotic pressures, hydrostatic pressures assist in maintaining body fluids in their appropriate compartments. The shift in fluids from one compartment to another usually results from an adaptive regulatory mechanism the body institutes to maintain fluid and electrolyte balance.

Regulation of Body Fluids

FLUID INTAKE

Fluid intake is regulated primarily through the thirst mechanism. The thirst control center is located within the hypothalamus in the brain. Psychological factors and a "dry throat" create a sensation of thirst (Groër, 1981) (Fig. 37-1). Major physiological stimuli to the thirst center are increased plasma osmolarity and decreased blood volume.

Receptor cells called *osmoreceptors* continually monitor osmotic pressure. When too much fluid is lost, the osmoreceptors detect the loss and activate the thirst center. As a result the person feels thirsty and seeks water.

Water is also acquired from food intake, such as fruits, vegetables, and meat, and from the oxidation of food substances during digestion. As discussed in Chapter 33, water is one of the end products of the metabolism of

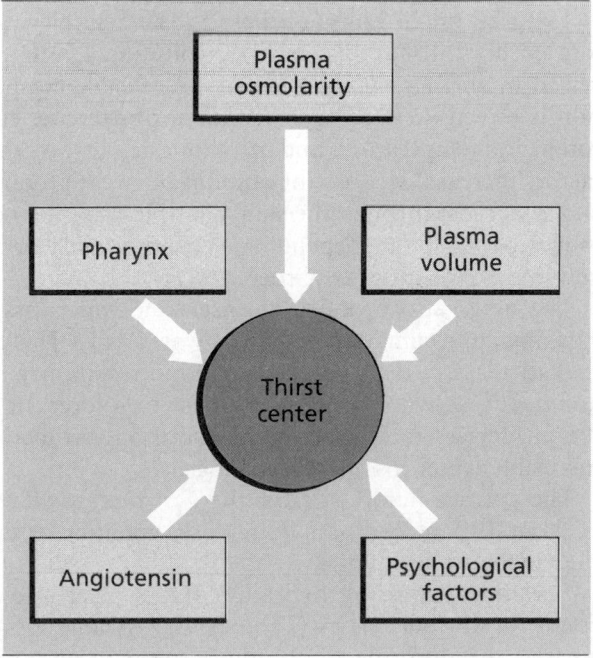

Fig. 37-1 Stimuli affecting the thirst mechanism.

carbohydrates, proteins, and fats. For each 100 calories of food metabolized, about 14 ml is acquired (Guyton, 1982). Fluid intake requires an alert state. Infants, clients with neurological or psychological impairments, and some of the elderly are unable to perceive or respond to thirst mechanisms. As a result, they are at risk for dehydration.

FLUID OUTPUT

Fluid output occurs through the following organs of water loss: the kidneys, the skin, the lungs, and the gastrointestinal tract.

The *kidneys* are the major regulatory organs of fluid balance. They receive about 170 liters of plasma to filter each day and in the adult produce 1.5 liters (1500 ml) of urine to be excreted. Approximately 1 ml of urine per kilogram of body weight per hour (1 ml/kg/hr) is produced by all age groups (Metheny, 1987). The amount of urine produced by the kidneys can be influenced by two hormones, antidiuretic hormone (ADH) and aldosterone. These hormones affect water and sodium excretion and can be stimulated by changes in blood volume. The regulatory effects of these hormones on the kidneys and total fluid balance are described in the following section.

Water loss from the *skin* is regulated primarily by the sympathetic nervous system, which activates the sweat glands. Stimulation of the sweat glands can result from muscular exercise, elevated environmental temperature, and increased metabolic activity as with a fever.

Water loss from the skin can be a sensible or insensible loss. Insensible water loss is continuous and is not perceived by the person. The average insensible water loss is 15 to 20 ml/24 hours (Groër, 1981). Sensible water loss occurs through excessive perspiration and is perceived by the person. The amount of sensible perspiration is directly related to the amount of exercise, environmental temperature, and metabolic activity. As these factors increase, so does the amount of sweat produced and water lost through the skin. Sensible water loss can range up to 5000 ml, depending on exercise and external and body temperatures (Groër, 1981).

The *lungs* also produce an insensible water loss by expiring approximately 400 ml of water daily. This loss may increase in response to changes in respiratory rate and depth, as with increased exercise or a fever. In addition, devices for oxygen administration can increase insensible water loss from the lungs.

The average fluid loss from the *gastrointestinal tract* is about 100 ml/24 hours. Obviously vomiting or diarrhea increases fluid loss.

The nurse assessing hydration status must also account for all fluid losses (Table 37-1). As fluid loss increases, the nurse needs to adjust the plan of care to increase fluid intake orally or parenterally to maintain

TABLE 37-1 Average Daily Fluid Output in a 70 Kg (187 lb) Adult

Organ or System	Amount (ml)
Kidneys	1500
Skin	
Insensible loss	600-900
Sensible loss	0-5000
Lungs	400
Gastrointestinal tract	100
TOTAL*	2600-2900

*Excludes sensible loss.

fluid balance. In addition, the nurse must be aware of the hormonal controls on fluid and electrolyte balance.

HORMONES

The major hormones affecting fluid and electrolyte balance are ADH and aldosterone. *ADH* decreases the production of urine by increasing the reabsorption of water by the kidney tubules. During transient periods of fluid volume deficit, as with vomiting and diarrhea or hemorrhage, the amount of ADH in the blood increases. As a result the water reabsorbed by the kidney tubules increases and is returned to the circulating blood volume. Urinary output declines in response to the hormone's action.

The stimulus for ADH secretion is an increase in blood osmolarity, which indicates a state of water deficit. The hormone itself is released by the posterior pituitary gland.

Aldosterone is a mineral corticoid, produced by the adrenal cortex, that regulates sodium and potassium balance. The presence of aldosterone causes the kidney tubules to excrete potassium and reabsorb sodium and, as a result, water is also reabsorbed and returned to the blood volume. Fluid deficits such as those produced by hemorrhage or gastrointestinal losses can stimulate the secretion of aldosterone into the blood.

A third class of hormones, *glucocorticoids,* also affects water and electrolyte balance. Whereas normal glucocorticoid hormone secretion does not result in major fluid imbalances, excesses of the hormone in the circulation alter fluid and electrolyte balance. For example, a client with Cushing's syndrome retains sodium and water because of the action of excess glucocorticoids. Likewise, a client receiving steroid medications, such as cortisone or prednisone, retains sodium and water.

The regulatory mechanisms for fluid and electrolyte balance are short-term methods of maintaining fluid balance during transient states such as exercise, viral and bacterial illness, vomiting, or diarrhea. However, when these conditions are prolonged, the body's regulatory mechanisms are insufficient, and fluid and electrolyte imbalances can occur.

Regulation of Electrolytes

The major cations—sodium, potassium, calcium, and magnesium—are located in the extracellular and intracellular fluid. Their actions affect neurochemical and neuromuscular transmissions, which influence muscular function, cardiac rhythm and contractility, mood and behavior, and gastrointestinal functioning.

CATIONS

Major cations within the body fluids include sodium (Na^+), potassium (K^+), calcium (Ca^{++}), and magnesium (Mg^{++}). Cations may be interchanged when one cation exits the cell and is replaced by another. This occurs because cells tend to maintain electrical neutrality. Therefore one positively charged ion must be exchanged with another positively charged ion.

SODIUM REGULATION. Sodium is the most abundant cation in the extracellular fluid. Sodium ions are involved in maintaining water balance, transmitting nerve impulses, and contracting muscles. The normal extracellular concentration of sodium is 136 to 144 mEq/L.

Water goes where sodium goes in fluid and electrolyte balances. For example, if the kidneys retain sodium, they retain water also. Conversely, if the kidneys excrete sodium, they excrete water. The action of many drugs (for example, diuretics) is based on this principle.

Sodium is regulated by salt intake, aldosterone, and urinary output. The major sources of sodium are table salt, processed meats, snack foods, and canned vegetables. In individuals with normal renal function the excretion of urine sodium can be increased to keep the serum sodium level within normal limits. When sodium intake decreases or a person loses body fluids (for example, through burns or trauma), the body attempts to conserve sodium through the secretion of aldosterone. Aldosterone exerts its action on the kidney tubules to reabsorb sodium, thus returning sodium to the extracellular fluid.

POTASSIUM REGULATION. Potassium is the predominant intracellular cation regulating neuromuscular excitability and muscle contraction. The sources of potassium include whole grains, meat, legumes, fruits, and vegetables. Potassium is needed for glycogen formation, protein synthesis, and correction of acid-base imbalances.

Potassium assists in regulating the acid-base balance because the potassium ion (K^+) can be exchanged with the hydrogen ion ($H+$). Therefore, in an acidotic state, a potassium ion is conserved and a hydrogen ion is excreted. The opposite occurs in alkalosis.

Potassium is regulated primarily by the kidneys. With increased aldosterone secretion, more potassium is excreted through the urine and the serum potassium level can fall. Another mechanism of regulation is the exchange with the sodium ion in the kidney tubule. When sodium is retained, potassium is excreted. The normal range for serum potassium is 3.5 to 5.0 mEq/L.

CALCIUM REGULATION. Calcium is the most abundant element in the body (Metheny and Snirely, 1983). The body requires calcium for cell membrane integrity and structure, adequate cardiac conduction, blood coagulation, bone growth and formation, and muscle relaxation. Calcium is in the following forms in body fluids: (1) ionized (4.5 mg/100 ml), (2) nondiffusible, which is calcium complexed to protein anions (5 mg/100 ml), and (3) calcium salts such as calcium citrate and calcium phosphate (1 mg/100 ml). Some clinical laboratories also report normal calcium values as mEq/L. Calcium in body fluid is a small percentage of the total body calcium. The major portion of calcium is in bones and teeth.

Calcium in extracellular fluid is regulated through the actions of the parathyroid and thyroid glands. Parathyroid hormone (PTH) controls the balance among bone calcium, gastrointestinal absorption of calcium, and kidney excretion of calcium. Thyrocalcitonin from the thyroid gland also has a minor role in determining serum calcium levels by inhibiting bone resorption of calcium.

MAGNESIUM REGULATION. Magnesium is the second most important cation of the intracellular fluids and is essential for enzyme activities, neurochemical activities, and muscular excitability. Plasma concentrations of magnesium range from 1.5 to 2.5 mEq/L.

Magnesium is indirectly regulated through renal excretion and some actions of parathyroid hormone. Altered magnesium levels, hypomagnesemia and hypermagnesemia are often associated with serious disease and produce symptoms reflecting altered neuromuscular function (Groër, 1981).

ANIONS

CHLORIDE REGULATION. Chloride is found in extracellular and intracellular fluid. The chloride ion balances cations within the extracellular fluid. If a negatively charged ion leaves the extracellular fluid and enters the intracellular fluid, a chloride ion will be exchanged and enter the extracellular fluid. The ion exchange maintains electrical neutrality.

Chloride is regulated through the kidneys. The amount of chloride excreted is related to dietary intake. A person with normal kidneys who has a high chloride intake will excrete a higher amount of urine chloride. Normal serum chloride levels range from 95 to 105 mEq/L.

BICARBONATE REGULATION. Bicarbonate (HCO_3^-) is the major chemical base buffer within the body. The bicarbonate ion is found in extracellular and intracellular fluid. The kidneys regulate bicarbonates. When the body needs to retain more base, the kidneys reabsorb greater quantities of bicarbonate and return it to the extracellular fluid. Normal arterial bicarbonate levels range between 22 and 26 mEq/L. The bicarbonate ion is an essential component of the carbonic acid–bicarbonate buffering system essential to acid-base balance.

PHOSPHATE REGULATION. Phosphate (PO_4^-) is a buffer anion in intracellular and extracellular fluid. Phosphate and calcium help develop and maintain bones and teeth. Phosphate also promotes normal neuromuscular action, participates in carbohydrate metabolism, and assists in acid-base regulation.

Serum phosphate concentration is regulated by the parathyroid hormone and by activated vitamin D (Groër, 1981). Phosphate is normally absorbed through the gastrointestinal tract in a range of 3 to 12 mg/100 ml. Calcium and phosphate are inversely proportional. If one rises, the other falls.

ACID-BASE BALANCE

Acid-base balance exists when the net rate at which the body produces acids or bases equals the rate at which acids or bases are excreted. This balance results in a stable concentration of hydrogen ions (H^+) in body fluids. The concentration of hydrogen ions in a body fluid is expressed as the pH value. The pH is a scale for measuring the acidity or alkalinity of a fluid. A pH value of 7 is neutral. Below 7 is acid, and above 7 is alkaline. An increase in the number of hydrogen ions in the bloodstream increases the acid component, thereby lowering the pH. Normal pH values range from 7.36 to 7.44.

The human body has regulatory mechanisms for maintaining the acid-base balance and for adapting to short-term changes in hydrogen ion concentration. Such changes occur during physical exercise, moderate anxiety states, and minor gastrointestinal upsets. The body can make adjustments for transient changes in pH (compensation). However, with severe trauma, uncontrolled diabetes mellitus, or shock, the body's normal compensatory mechanisms are unable to maintain the pH within a physiological range. In such cases, medical intervention is required.

The types of acid-base regulators within the body are chemical, biological, and physiological buffering systems. A *buffer* is a substance or group of substances that can absorb or release hydrogen ions to correct an acid-base imbalance.

Chemical Regulation

The largest chemical buffer in extracellular fluid is the carbonic and bicarbonate buffer system. This system can be expressed as the following equation:

$$CO_2 + H_2O \leftrightarrows H_2CO_3 \leftrightarrows H^+ + HCO_3^-$$
carbon dioxide · water · carbonic acid · hydrogen · bicarbonate

The carbonic acid–bicarbonate buffer system is the first buffering system to react to change in the pH of extracellular fluid, and it reacts within seconds. The excretion of carbon dioxide resulting from metabolism is controlled primarily by the lungs. The excretion of hydrogen and bicarbonate ions is controlled by the kidneys. The reaction of these substances buffers a strong acid or base to maintain a relatively constant pH (Fig. 37-2).

The carbonic acid–bicarbonate buffering system is the only strictly chemical buffering reaction combining excess ions of either charge. It can accept or donate hydrogen ions to correct an acid state (acidemia) or strongly alkaline state (alkalemia) (Stroot, Lee, and Barrett, 1984).

The carbonic acid–bicarbonte buffer responds immediately to acid-base imbalance, is an adaptive system, and has a relatively brief effect.

A second chemical buffering system involves the plasma proteins albumin, fibrinogen, prothrombin, and the gamma globulins, which constitute about 6% to 7% of blood plasma. These proteins can bind with or release hydrogen ions to correct acidosis or alkalosis. However, their capacity to maintain the acid-base balance of extracellular fluid is limited, and they cannot correct long-term imbalances.

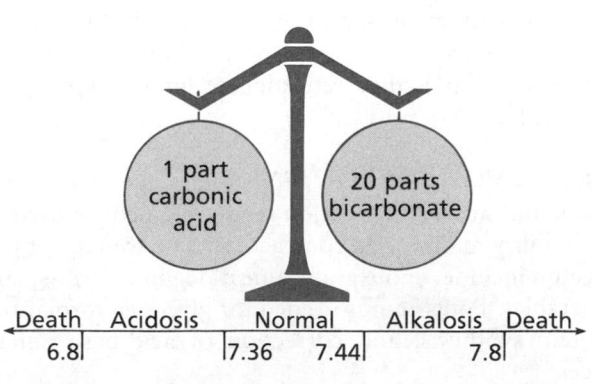

Fig. 37-2 Carbonic acid/bicarbonate ratio and pH.

Biological Regulation

Biological buffering occurs when hydrogen ions are absorbed or released by body cells. The hydrogen ion has a positive charge and must be exchanged with another positively charged ion, frequently potassium (K^+). In conditions with excessive acid, a hydrogen ion enters the cell and a potassium ion leaves the cell and enters the extracellular fluid. The extracellular fluid is thus less acidic because fewer hydrogen ions are present. As a result of this exchange, however, people with acidosis are also hyperkalemic. After the acidosis is corrected, potassium reenters the cells, and potassium levels return to normal.

Biological buffering occurs after chemical buffering and takes 2 to 4 hours. A second type of biological buffer is the hemoglobin-oxyhemoglobin system. When blood is oxygenated, chloride travels from the hemolgobin to the plasma. As chloride leaves the cell, bicarbonate enters. This process is part of the chloride shift and is a reciprocal exchange between these anions (Stroot, Lee, and Barrett, 1984).

Physiological Regulation

LUNGS

The physiological buffers in the body are the lungs and the kidneys. The lungs can provide a rapid adaptation to an acid-base imbalance. In fact, they can act to return the pH to normal before the biological buffers can.

Ordinarily, hydrogen ions and carbon dioxide provide the stimulus for respiration. When the concentration of hydrogen ions is altered, the lungs react to correct the imbalance by alternating the rate and depth of respiration. In alkalosis, the rate of respiration is reduced and the person retains carbon dioxide. The carbon dioxide combines with water in the blood to form carbonic acid, which helps to increase the acid component and balance the alkaline excess. If an excess in acid occurs, respiratory rate is increased and the lungs excrete larger amounts of carbon dioxide (Stroot, Lee, and Barrett, 1984). Therefore, less carbon dioxide is available to combine with water and create carbonic acid.

KIDNEYS

The kidneys can take from a few hours to several days to regulate acid-base abnormalities. They use three mechanisms to regulate hydrogen ion concentration. They can reabsorb bicarbonate during acid excess and excrete it during acid deficit. The kidneys use a phosphate ion ($PO_4^=$) to carry hydrogen ions by excreting phosphoric acid (H_3PO_4) and forming an acid base, and they can convert ammonia (NH_3) to ammonium (NH_4) by attaching a hydrogen ion to ammonia.

DISTURBANCES IN FLUID, ELECTROLYTE, AND ACID-BASE BALANCES

Disturbances in fluid, electrolyte, or acid-base balances can disrupt normal body processes. A client who loses body fluids through burns, illnesses, or trauma is at risk for electrolyte imbalances. In addition, untreated electrolyte imbalances (for example, potassium loss) result in acid-base disturbances.

Volume Disturbances

The basic types of volume disturbances are fluid volume deficits and fluid volume excesses. Fluid volume deficit (dehydration) is a state of water loss beyond the normal regulatory system's ability to repair (Groër), 1981). Fluid volume excess (overhydration) is an excess in the extracellular fluid.

DEHYDRATION

Water balance is maintained by fluid and output and hormonal regulation. When fluid output exceeds intake, dehydration occurs. Likewise, decreased reabsorption of water by the kidney from decreased ADH or aldosterone secretion can result in dehydration.

Dehydration is an excessive loss of water from body tissues. Dehydration also disturbs the balance of the essential electrolytes: sodium, potassium, and chloride. With water loss, the regulatory mechanisms within the body attempt to maintain cardiovascular function and perfusion to the vital organs. The hormonal controls also assist in conserving the remaining body water.

These mechanisms activate the sympathetic nervous system and cause vasoconstriction of the arterioles to maintain blood pressure and perfusion of the heart, lungs, and brain. The renal blood flow and glomerular filtration rate decrease, and urine output falls to maintain fluid in the extracellular fluid. Clinically dehydration can be observed in the following forms: isotonic, hypernatremic, and hyponatremic (Table 37-2).

Isotonic dehydration is a loss of fluid from the extracellular space but with no important effect on the solutes within the plasma (Table 37-2). With a loss of extracellular fluid, the major response of the body is to activate the sympathetic nervous system. The degree of sympathetic response is proportionate to the degree of extracellular fluid deficit. For example, when a person is in shock, activation of the sympathetic nervous system raises blood pressure, causes vasoconstriction, increases heart rate, and maintains blood supply to the vital organs and the kidney.

Hypernatremic dehydration is a loss of fluid with sodium excess. It is not marked by the cardiovascular signs and ultimate circulatory collapse of isotonic dehydra-

TABLE 37-2 Dehydration

Causes	Signs and Symptoms
ISOTONIC	
Losses from the gastrointestinal system, such as diarrhea, vomiting, or drainage from fistulas or tubes Third-space fluid shifts Loss of plasma or whole blood, as with burns or hemorrhage Excessive perspiration	*Physical examination:* initial hypotension, tachycardia, cardiac dysrhythmias, dry skin, poor skin turgor, dry mucous membranes, pallor, lethargy, weakness, oliguria *Laboratory findings:* urine specific gravity >1.025
HYPERNATREMIC	
Diabetes insipidus Interruption of the neurologically driven thirst mechanisms Diabetes mellitus (occasionally) Head trauma, tumors, or central nervous system lesions Infantile gastroenteritis	*Physical examination:* weight loss, poor skin turgor, thirst, muscle tremors, hypotension, tachycardia, fever, nuchal rigidity
HYPONATREMIC	
Chronic illness Malnutrition Underlying renal disease	Physical examination: Usually presents as a symptom of an underlying illness. Weight loss related to chronic illness or malnutrition

tion. Rather, it results from the loss of excess water from the extracellular fluid, which then becomes hyperosmolar, causing cellular dehydration with relative maintenance of the extracellular fluid volume. Hypernatremic dehydration (serum Na^+ 150 mEq/L) is associated with increased insensible water loss (Table 37-2). With increased insensible water loss, as with hyperventilation, the body normally responds with thirst and increased water intake and a decrease in urinary output. Elderly, young, immobile, confused, or neurologically impaired clients may be unable to perceive or respond to increased thirst.

Hyponatremic dehydration results from a loss of sodium from the extracellular fluid in excess of water loss. Hyponatremic dehydration is often associated with chronic illness and malnutrition (Table 37-2). When accompanying a chronic process, hyponatremic dehydration usually develops without symptoms. Clients with renal disease are very susceptible.

OVERHYDRATION

Overhydration is marked by an excess of water in the extracellular fluid and is a symptom of liver, renal, or cardiovascular disease. It can be caused iatrogenically by large amounts of isotonic saline solution or may occur because of shifts of interstitial fluid into the plasma. It can also follow humoral alterations and is marked by water intoxication.

Water intoxication is a condition in which the total body water volume is increased because of excess water ingestion or excess ADH secretion. The overall effect is dilution of the extracellular fluid volume with osmosis of water into the cells (Groër, 1981). It can be easily confused with hyponatremic dehydration because hyponatremia is present. However, in water intoxication, hyponatremia results from water excess rather than sodium loss.

When clients are overhydrated, excess fluid is often stored in interstitial spaces, with edema in the dependent body regions. However, during water intoxication, increases occur in the extracellular or circulating blood volume, as well as in the cells. Thus all body systems can be affected.

EXTRACELLULAR FLUID EXCESS. Extracellular fluid excess occurs when sodium and water are retained in the circulating blood volume. Because sodium and water are retained in equal proportions the condition may be referred to as *isotonic excess* or *circulatory overload.* Signs of the increased circulating blood volume are hypervolemia, edema, and weight gain.

Hypervolemia is an increase in the amount of fluid in the circulating blood volume. To compensate for the increase, the urinary output may increase in relation to fluid intake. An increase in blood pressure may occur. However, if the kidneys are able to excrete the excess sodium and water, the rise in blood pressure is transient. If the kidneys are unable to excrete the excess volume, neck vein distention, liver enlargement, increased venous pressure, and signs of pulmonary edema may occur.

Edema is the abnormal accumulation of fluid in interstitial spaces of tissues—in the pericardial sac, intra-

TABLE 37-3   Sodium Imbalances

Net Sodium Loss*	Net Water Excess*	Signs and Symptoms
Hyponatremia		
Kidney disease	Syndrome of inappropriate ADH secretion (SIADH)	*Physical examination:* apprehension, anxiety, personality change, postural hypotension, postural dizziness, abdominal cramping, nausea and vomiting, diarrhea, tachycardia, convulsions and coma, cold, clammy skin
Addison's disease		
Gastrointestinal losses	Increase of water over solute intake, when renal mechanisms are not functioning properly	
Increased sweating		
Diuretics		
Interruption of Na^+, K^+ pump with decreased cell K^+ and decreased serum Na^+	Hyperaldosteronism	
	Diabetic ketoacidosis	
	Oliguria caused by renal failure	
Use of diuretics combined with low-sodium diet	Psychogenic polydipsia	*Laboratory findings:* serum sodium < 136 mEq/L, urine specific gravity < 1.010
Metabolic acidosis		

Net Water Deficit*	Net Sodium Excess*	Signs and Symptoms
Hypernatremia		
Water deprivation	Ingestion of large amounts of concentrated salt solutions	*Physical examination:* thirst, dry and flushed skin, dry tongue and mucous membranes, pyrexia, agitation, convulsions, restlessness, excitability, oliguria or anuria
Urea diuresis		
Greatly increased insensible water loss	Iatrogenic administration of hypertonic saline solution parenterally	
Disorders in which thirst is either absent or not perceived		*Laboratory findings:* serum sodium > 144 mEq/L, urine specific gravity > 1.030 (if water loss is not caused by renal dysfunction)
Nephrogenic diabetes insipidus		

*Data from Groër, MW: Physiology and pathophysiology of the body fluids, St. Louis, 1981, The C.V. Mosby Co.

pleural space, peritoneal cavity, or joint capsules. When edema occurs, body weight increases. Edema is a symptom of conditions such as increased blood volume with decreased cardiac output, fluid overload, sodium retention, increased aldosterone, increased steroid production or administration, liver disease, loss of serum proteins, malnutrition, allergic reaction, neoplastic disease, and blocked lymphatic drainage.

Electrolyte Imbalances

SODIUM IMBALANCES

Hyponatremia is a less-than-normal concentration of sodium in the blood, which can take place when a net sodium loss or net water excess occurs (Table 37-3). Usually hyponatremia includes a decrease in the osmolarity of plasma and extracellular fluid (Groër, 1981).

When a sodium loss occurs, the body initially adapts by reducing water excretion to maintain serum osmolarity at near-normal levels. As sodium loss continues, the body continues to preserve the blood and interstitial (tissue) volume. As a result, the proportion of sodium in the extracellular fluid lessens. Hyponatremia caused by sodium loss can result in vascular collapse and shock. When a pure sodium deficit occurs, there is a distinct loss of extracellular fluid volume, a condition different from hyponatremia resulting from water excess.

Hyponatremia can develop when there are large excesses of extracellular fluid volume, which is also called *water excess*. With water excess, dilutional effects on all blood components (dilutional hyponatremia) occur.

Hypernatremia is a greater-than-normal concentration of sodium in the extracellular fluid, which can be caused by extreme water loss or an overall sodium excess (Table 37-3). When hypernatremia occurs, the body attempts to conserve as much water as possible through renal reabsorption. Interstitial osmotic pressure increases, and fluid shifts from the cells into the extracellular fluid, causing the cells to shrink and interrupting most of the physiological cellular processes.

Potassium is closely aligned to the regulation of sodium balance and imbalance. Frequently when sodium is retained, potassium is excreted, as when aldosterone is secreted.

TABLE 37-4 Additional Electrolyte Imbalances

Causes	Signs and Symptoms
HYPOKALEMIA	
Use of potassium-wasting diuretics	*Physical examination:* weakness and fatigue, muscle fatigue,
Diarrhea, vomiting, or other gastrointestinal losses	decreased muscle tone, intestinal distention, decreased
Alkalosis	bowel sounds, heart block (severe hypokalemia), pares-
	thesia, and weak, irregular pulse
Cushing's syndrome or adrenal hormone-producing tumors	*Laboratory findings:* serum potassium < 4 mEq/L,* ECG ab-
Renal disease	normalities: likely when potassium is < 3.0 mEq/L*
Extreme diaphoresis	
Excessive use of potassium-free intravenous solutions	
HYPERKALEMIA	
Renal failure	*Physical examination:* anxiety, irritability, cardiac dysrhythmias,
Hypertonic dehydration	hypotension, paresthesia, weakness
Massive cellular damage such as burns and trauma	*Laboratory findings:* serum potassium > 5 mEq/L, ECG find-
Iatrogenic administration of large amounts of potassium	ings. Usually appear with serum potassium > 7 mEq/L.[‡]
intravenously	These findings include bradycardia, heart block, dysrhyth-
Addison's disease (hypoadrenalism)	mias[†]
Acidosis	
Rapid infusion of stored blood	
Potassium-retaining diuretics	

*Data from Groër, MW: Physiology and pathophysiology of the body fluids, St. Louis, 1981, The C.V. Mosby Co.
[†]Levels > 8.5 mEq/L are frequently fatal as a result of cardiac arrest (Metheny, 1987).
[‡]Data from Metheny, NM, Overview of fluid and electrolyte problems: nursing considerations, Philadelphia, 1987, J.B. Lippincott Co.

POTASSIUM IMBALANCES

Hypokalemia is a condition in which an inadequate amount of potassium circulates in the extracellular fluid. When severe, hypokalemia can affect cardiac conduction by causing dangerous irregularities. Because the normal amount of potassium is so small, there is little tolerance for fluctuations in serum potassium levels.

Hypokalemia can result from several conditions (Table 37-4) and is often observed in clients recovering from massive cellular injuries such as burns, crushing injuries, or massive trauma. Initially the extracellular fluid becomes hyperkalemic because of the release of potassium from the damaged cells, but if renal function is normal, the excess potassium is excreted by the kidneys (Groër, 1981).

Hyperkalemia is a greater than normal amount of potassium in the blood. Severe hyperkalemia produces marked cardiac conduction abnormalities such as ventricular dysrhythmia and cardiac arrest (Metheny, 1987). The primary cause of hyperkalemia is renal failure, but other illnesses also result in increased potassium (Table 37-4). Any decrease in renal function diminishes the amount of potassium the kidney can excrete.

CALCIUM IMBALANCES

Hypocalcemia represents a drop in serum and ionized calcium and can result from several illnesses, some of which directly affect the thyroid and parathyroid glands (Table 37-4). The signs and symptoms of hypocalcemia correlate directly to the physiological role of serum calcium.

Hypercalcemia is an increase in the total serum concentration of calcium and ionized calcium. Frequently, hypercalcemia is a symptom of an underlying disease resulting in excess bone resorption with release of calcium (Table 37-4).

MAGNESIUM IMBALANCES

Hypomagnesemia occurs when the serum concentration level drops below 1.5 mEq/L. The causes of hypomagnesemia (Table 37-4) produce symptoms similar to hypocalcemia. Magnesium acts directly on the neuromuscular junction. Decreases in the serum magnesium concentration increases neuromuscular irritability (Metheny, 1987). *Hypermagnesemia* occurs when the serum concentration of magnesium rises above 2.5 mEq/L (Table 37-4). Hypermagnesemia diminishes the excitability of muscle cells.

TABLE 37-4—cont'd

Causes	Signs and Symptoms
HYPOCALCEMIA	
Rapid administration of blood transfusions containing citrate Hypoalbuminemia Parathyroid disease Vitamin D deficiency Neoplastic diseases Pancreatitis Rapid administration of citrated blood	*Physical examination:* numbness and tingling of fingers and circumoral region, hyperactive reflexes, positive Trousseau's sign, positive Chvostek's sign, tetany, muscle cramps, pathological fractures (chronic hypocalcemia) *Laboratory findings:* serum calcium < 4.5 mEq/L or 10 mg/100 ml, ECG changes
HYPERCALCEMIA[†]	
Hyperparathyroidism Metastatic tumors of bone Paget's disease Osteoporosis Prolonged immobilization	*Physical examination:* decreased muscle tone, anorexia, nausea and vomiting, weakness and lethargy, low back pain (retrorenal region from kidney stones), decreased level of consciousness, cardiac arrest *Laboratory findings:* serum calcium > 5.8 mEq/L or 10 mg/100 ml; roentgenographic examination shows generalized osteoporosis, widespread bone cavitation, radiopaque urinary stones; elevated BUN caused by fluid volume deficit or renal damage
HYPOMAGNESEMIA*	

Inadequate intake
  Malnutrition
  Alcoholism
Inadequate absorption
  Diarrhea, vomiting, nasogastric drainage, fistulas
  Excessive dietary calcium—competes with magnesium for transport sites
  Diseases of the small intestine
Hypoparathyroidism
Excessive loss
  Thiazide diuretics
Aldosterone excess
Polyuria
	Physical examination: muscular tremors, hyperactive deep tendon reflexes, confusion and disorientation, hallucinations, convulsions, tachycardia, hypertension, dysrhythmias, positive Chvostek's and Trousseau's signs
	Laboratory findings: serum magnesium level < 1.5 mEq/L or 1.8 mg/dl.[‡] Also associated with hypocalcemia and hypokalemia[‡]

HYPERMAGNESEMIA	
Renal failure Excess parenteral administration of magnesium	*Physical examination:* physician findings more frequent in acute elevations in magnesium levels. Depressed functioning, depressed deep tendon reflexes, depressed respirations, hypotension, flushing *Laboratory findings:* serum magnesium levels > 2.5 mEq/L

CHLORIDE IMBALANCES

Hypochloremia occurs when the serum chloride level falls below 95 mEq/L. Vomiting or prolonged and excessive nasogastric or fistula drainage can result in hypochloremia. A newborn can quickly develop hypochloremia as a result of diarrhea. Some diuretic medications also result in increased chloride excretion. When serum chloride levels fall, the body adapts by increased reabsorption of the bicarbonate ion, affecting acid-base balance, and metabolic alkalosis results.

Hyperchloremia occurs when the serum chloride level rises above 105 mEq/L and when the serum bicarbonate value falls. Hypochloremia and hyperchloremia rarely occur as single disease processes but are commonly associated with acid-base imbalance. No single set of symptoms is associated with these alterations.

Acid-Base Imbalances

The primary types of acid-base imbalance are respiratory acidosis, respiratory alkalosis, metabolic acidosis, and metabolic alkalosis.

Causes of Acid-Base Imbalances

RESPIRATORY ACIDOSIS

- Pneumonia
- Respiratory failure
- Atelectasis
- Drug overdose
- Paralysis of respiratory muscles (Guillain-Barré syndrome, poliomyelitis, myasthenia gravis)
- Traumatic injuries to the thorax (flail chest)
- Obesity
- Airway obstruction
- Head injuries
- Cerebrovascular accident (stroke)
- Drowning
- Cystic fibrosis

RESPIRATORY ALKALOSIS

- Anxiety
- Fear
- Anemia
- Hypermetabolic states
- Disorders of the central nervous system (head injuries, infections)
- Drugs (aspirin overdose)
- Asthma
- Pneumonia
- Inappropriate mechanical ventilator settings

METABOLIC ACIDOSIS

- Starvation
- Dehydration
- Diabetic ketoacidosis
- Renal failure
- Shock
- Diarrhea
- Drugs (methanol, ethanol, formic acid, paraldehyde, aspirin)
- Renal tubular acidosis (RTA)

METABOLIC ALKALOSIS

- Excessive vomiting
- Prolonged gastric suctioning
- Electrolyte disturbance
- Cushing's disease
- Drugs (steroids, sodium bicarbonate, diuretics)
- Hyperaldosteronism

RESPIRATORY ACIDOSIS

Respiratory acidosis is marked by an increased arterial carbon dioxide concentration ($Paco_2$), excess carbonic acid (H_2CO_3), and an increased hydrogen ion concentration (decreased pH). Respiratory acidosis is caused by hypoventilation or any condition that depresses ventilation (see box). Decreased ventilation may begin in the respiratory system (respiratory failure) or outside the respiratory system (drug overdose). In clients with respiratory acidosis the cerebrospinal fluid and brain cells become acidic, causing neurological changes. Hypoxemia occurs because of the respiratory depression, resulting in further neurological impairments. Electrolyte changes may accompany the acidosis.

RESPIRATORY ALKALOSIS

Respiratory alkalosis is marked by decreased $Paco_2$ and decreased hydrogen ion concentration (increased pH). Respiratory alkalosis results from excessive exhalation of CO_2, or hyperventilation (see box). Like respiratory acidosis, respiratory alkalosis can begin outside the respiratory system (anxiety) or within the respiratory system, such as in the initial phases of an asthmatic attack.

METABOLIC ACIDOSIS

Metabolic acidosis results from a rise in hydrogen ion concentration (decreased pH) in the extracellular fluid, caused by either a primary increase in hydrogen ion or a decrease in bicarbonate (Groër, 1981). Metabolic acidosis is caused by many conditions (see box). The types of metabolic acidosis, normochloremic and hyperchloremic, are classified according to the client's plasma chloride concentration.

METABOLIC ALKALOSIS

Metabolic alkalosis is marked by heavy loss of acid from the body or by increased levels of bicarbonate. The most common cause is vomiting. Metabolic alkalosis may also result when a client with a gastric acid disturbance ingests large amounts of sodium bicarbonate. Other causes are listed in the box.

VARIABLES AFFECTING FLUID AND ELECTROLYTE BALANCES

Fluid and electrolyte status is neither a static nor single physiological entity. Many variables can change the distribution of body fluid and electrolytes. In some instances, as with normal changes during pregnancy and exercise, fluid and electrolyte imbalance is a normal and expected response. However, some disease conditions, such as nausea and vomiting, have a more severe consequence, particularly with infants and the elderly.

During assessment the nurse identifies altered fluid states. To assess clients effectively, the nurse considers variables influencing fluid status, the way normal balance changes, and whether the change is a normal anticipated change or a consequence of a pathological process. The major factors that can affect fluid and electrolyte status include age, body size, environmental temperature, life-style, and level of health.

Age

Age affects distribution of body fluids and electrolytes. The major differences are observed in infants, the elderly, and pregnant clients.

INFANTS

The infant's proportion of total body water is greater than that of the school-age child, adolescent, or adult. However, although infants have a greater proportion of body water, they are not protected from fluid loss, such as that which occurs with diarrhea. In fact, infants are at greater risk for dehydration because their body water loss is proportionately greater per kilogram of body weight.

CHILDREN

In childhood illnesses, the regulatory and compensatory responses to imbalances are less stable and tend to operate within a more narrow range with less tolerance for large changes in balance. Children frequently respond to illness with a fever of higher temperature or longer duration than that of adults. Fever in childhood can profoundly affect water and electrolyte balance (Groër, 1981).

ADOLESCENTS

In adolescence, rapid and major changes occur in both anatomy and physiology. The increased growth rate increases metabolic processes and, as a result, the amount of water produced as an end product of metabolism. Changes in fluid balance are greater in adolescent girls because of hormonal changes associated with the menstrual cycle.

PREGNANT WOMEN

The pregnant woman experiences several changes in fluid and electrolyte balance. At about the fifteenth week of pregnancy, aldosterone secretion and excretion begin to rise, and in some cases the elevation can be 10 times normal (Metheny and Snively, 1983). Some physicians believe that this can cause fluid retention.

As the fetus and uterus grow, reaching their preterm size, they exert pressure on the inferior vena cava. This pressure, and the pressure of vascular congestion of the pelvis further increase venal caval pressure. As a result,

filtration of fluid from the vascular bed to the tissues increases, and hydrostatic edema results (Metheny and Snively, 1983). However, when the woman lies down, pressure on the vena cava is relieved, and after a period of time the edema disappears.

At the end of pregnancy, before delivery of the infant, the average woman's body has 6.5 liters of extra fluid. Of this amount, 3.5 liters is from the fetus, placenta, and amniotic fluid. The other 3 liters results from increases in blood volume, breast size, and uterus mass (Metheny and Snively, 1983).

The increase of 40% to 45% in circulating blood volume, which is reached about 2 to 6 weeks before delivery, includes increases in serum plasma and red blood cells. After delivery, the excess circulating blood volume declines rapidly, returning to near-normal ranges by the end of the first postpartum week (Metheny and Snively, 1983).

OLDER ADULTS

The elderly client's risk of fluid and electrolyte imbalance may be closely associated with decreased renal function and a consequent lack of urine concentration. The elderly may also have chronic illness, such as diabetes mellitus, cardiovascular disorders, or cancer, that can impair fluid balance. In addition, the total amount of body water decreases with age. For example, water comprises approximately 60% of the total body weight in young men, 52% in elderly men, and 52% in young women, and 46% in elderly women (Metheny and Snively, 1983).

■ ■ ■

Fluid and electrolyte changes occur normally with developmental changes. However, when an illness is also present, the client may be unable to adapt adequately to these changes. Therefore the nurse needs to include the fluid changes associated with aging and development in nursing assessment.

Body Size

Body size has an effect on the total body water. Because fat contains no water, the obese client has proportionately less body water. Women have more fat deposits, such as in the breasts and hips, than men. As a result, the total body water in women is less than in men of the same age.

Environmental Temperature

Fluid and electrolyte imbalances are associated with extremes in environmental temperature and relative humidity. The overall body response to environmental temperatures exceeding 28° to 30° C (82.4° to 86° F) is to increase sensible water loss by sweating, which cools the peripheral blood and helps to reduce body temperature.

The healthy adult can sweat about 1 liter per hour for 2 hours, losing about 5% of body weight without straining the cooling mechanism. However, after a body weight loss of 7% is exceeded, the cooling mechanism declines to conserve body water (Metheny and Snively, 1983).

The relative humidity of the environmental temperature also affects body water loss and body temperature regulation. The evaporation of sweat decreases at 60% humidity and ceases at 75% (Burch, Knochil, and Murphy, 1979).

The body responds with fluid changes to excessive environmental temperature. It increases peripheral vasodilation, which allows more blood to come to the surface for cooling. Sweating increases body fluid loss, which results in loss of sodium and chloride ions. The body also increases cardiac output and pulse rate. Finally, increased aldosterone secretion occurs, resulting in sodium retention and potassium excretion by the kidneys (Metheny and Snively, 1983). Each of these responses can affect overall fluid and electrolyte balance, and the nurse needs to assess the environment to determine actual or potential alterations in fluid and electrolyte balance.

Life-Style

Life-style can have an indirect effect on fluid and electrolyte balance. Habits that can affect fluid balance include diet, stress, and exercise.

DIET

Dietary intake of fluids, salt, potassium, calcium, and necessary carbohydrates, fats, and proteins helps to maintain normal fluid and electrolyte status. When nutritional intake is inadequate, the body tries to preserve its protein stores by breaking down glycogen and fat stores. However, after those resources are depleted, the body begins to destroy protein sources. Serum protein levels drop below normal, and hypoalbuminemia results. In hypoalbuminemia the serum colloid osmotic pressure is decreased and fluid shifts from the circulating blood volume and enters the interstitial fluid spaces, resulting in edema.

STRESS

The impact of stress on fluid and electrolyte balance can be understood in terms of the general adaptation syndrome (see Chapter 28). Stress increases aldosterone and glucocorticoid levels, leading to sodium and water retention. In addition, increased ADH secretion decreases urine output. The effect of the stress response is

to increase fluid volume. As a result, cardiac output, blood pressure, and perfusion to the major organs are increased.

EXERCISE

Exercise results in increased sensible water loss through sweat. The client who exercises can respond to the thirst mechanism and help to maintain fluid and electrolyte balance by increasing fluid intake. Athletes undergoing sustained vigorous exercise must have fluid loss replaced by a liquid that contains electrolytes. One such substance is Gatorade, which contains glucose, sodium, chloride, and potassium.

Level of Health

Generally, the better the client's health, the easier it will be to tolerate fluid and electrolyte changes.

SURGERY

Surgical procedures result in changes in fluid balance because of the body's stress response to surgical trauma during the second to fifth days after surgery. The more extensive the surgery, the greater the response of the body. Postoperative fluid imbalances result from increased secretion of aldosterone, glucocorticoids, and ADH. Increases in aldosterone and glucocortocoid result in sodium and chloride retention and potassium excretion. An increase in ADH results in decreased urinary output. These hormonal increases and the activity of the sympathetic nervous system help to maintain circulating blood volume and blood pressure after surgery.

After the immediate postoperative period, hormone secretion returns to normal levels, and excess sodium and water are excreted from the body. Postoperative fluid and electrolyte changes are normal and should be anticipated in surgical clients.

BURNS

In clients with severe second- or third-degree burns, body fluids are lost. The greater the body surface burned, the greater the fluid loss. The burned client loses body fluids by one of five routes. Plasma leaves the intravascular space and becomes trapped as edema. This is also called the plasma–to–interstitial fluid shift. Along with the shifting of fluid, serum proteins are lost from extracellular fluids. Plasma and interstitial fluids are lost as burn exudate, a visible fluid loss on the burned surface and common with second-degree burns. Water vapor and heat are lost because burned skin can no longer serve as a barrier against such losses. This loss increases in proportion to the amount of skin burned. Blood leaks from damaged capillaries, contributing to an already decreased extracellular fluid volume. Finally, sodium and water shift into the cells, again depleting extracellular fluid volume (Metheny and Snively, 1983).

CARDIOVASCULAR DISORDERS

The failing heart has a diminished cardiac output. As a result, perfusion to the kidneys is decreased and urinary output drops. The client retains sodium and water, and edema, circulatory overload, and pulmonary edema may result.

Fluid and electrolyte imbalances associated with heart failure can be controlled for a time with diuretic and cardiotonic medications and fluid and sodium restrictions. The goal of this treatment is to reduce the work of the left ventricle by relieving the excess extracellular fluid volume.

RENAL DISORDERS

Failing kidneys alter fluid and electrolyte balance. There is an abnormal buildup of sodium, chloride, and potassium, with an excess of toxic extracellular fluid. The fluid becomes toxic because the kidneys are unable to filter and excrete the waste products of cellular metabolism.

The severity of fluid and electrolyte imbalance is proportional to the degree of renal failure. Occasionally, acute renal failure, induced by shock or a decrease in extracellular fluid, may be reversible. Although chronic renal failure is progressive, the client may be treated successfully with dietary control of protein and salt intake, diuretic medications, and fluid restrictions.

CANCER

The types of fluid and electrolyte imbalances observed in a cancer client depend on the type and progression of the cancer. All the electrolyte imbalances discussed can occur in the client with cancer. In addition, cancer clients can develop third-space fluid accumulations that increase total body water, and there is actually a decrease in extracellular fluid volume (Metheny and Snively, 1983).

■ ■ ■

In addition to these categories of illness, fluid and electrolyte imbalances also occur with gastrointestinal disturbances and disease of the endocrine system. The changes are predictable, and therefore the nurse should anticipate fluid and electrolyte imbalances in postoperative or cancer clients.

In addition to these specific illnesses, the client's overall level of health influences fluid and electrolyte status. Clients with chronic illness and concomitant depression of the immune system and decreases in nutritional intake are at a greater risk for fluid and electrolyte imbalance than healthier persons who have gastroenteritis for 24 to 36 hours. In all cases the nurse must assess the actual or potential risk factors for fluid and electrolyte balances.

NURSING PROCESS IN ALTERATIONS IN FLUID AND ELECTROLYTE BALANCES

ASSESSMENT

During assessment of fluid and electrolyte balance the nurse identifies fluid volume overload and deficits. In addition, assessment helps the nurse to determine the effectiveness of therapy. For example, if a diuretic medication is prescribed for a client with congestive heart failure, the nurse assessing the client after therapy expects to note a decrease in weight, an increase in 24-hour urine output, and a decrease in or absence of dependent edema. The nurse also assesses fluid and electrolyte balance to detect adverse reactions to therapy. For example, if fluids are ordered for a client with progressive renal failure, the nurse may find, on the third day, that the 24-hour fluid intake exceeds renal output by four to one, that the client's weight is increased, and that dependent edema and abnormal lung sounds are present. Finally, fluid and electrolyte assessment helps the nurse anticipate needs for nursing care. For example, a client with edema who is placed on diuretic therapy should have a care plan to anticipate needs such as an increased use of the bathroom, bedpan, or urinal or instruction for a salt-restricted diet.

Assessment of fluid and electrolyte balance includes the following areas: nursing history, physical examination, measurement and recording of intake and output, and laboratory studies.

NURSING HISTORY

To collect data about fluid and electrolyte status the nurse must understand fluid regulation, electrolyte imbalances, and volume disturbances. In addition, the nurse needs to know why and how some diseases, treatments, drug therapies, and diet changes will alter fluid balance.

Clients with cardiovascular and renal diseases, severe burns or trauma, and endocrine disorders are at high risk for fluid and electrolyte disturbances. In addition, prolonged gastrointestinal upsets, particularly in the very young and the very old, can result in fluid or electrolyte imbalance.

Certain treatments such as IV therapy and total parenteral nutrition alter fluid balance. Prescribed drugs also increase the risk for fluid and electrolyte distur-

---

Risk Factors for Fluid, Electrolyte, and Acid-Base Imbalances

- Chronic diseases
  - Cancer
  - Cardiovascular disease such as congestive heart failure
  - Endocrine disease such as Cushing's disease and diabetes mellitus
  - Malnutrition
  - Chronic pulmonary disease
  - Renal disease such as progressive renal failure
- Trauma
  - Crush injuries
  - Head injuries
- Burns
- Drug therapy
  - Diuretics
  - Steroids
  - Spironolactone (Aldactone) or other aldosterone inhibitor agents
- Gastroenteritis
- Nasogastric suctioning
- Fistulas
- Intravenous therapy
- Total parenteral nutrition

---

bances. For example, diuretic medications usually increase the risk for sodium loss, which results in hypotonic dehydration. Conversely, administration of steroid preparations results in sodium retention and can cause fluid overload.

The nurse also collects the nursing history to identify potential or actual risk factors increasing the chances of fluid and electrolyte imbalances (see box, above). Eventually all types of chronic diseases have the potential to cause fluid or electrolyte imbalances. Because the progression of these diseases is usually slow, imbalances can be controlled. When nurses care for clients with chronic illnesses, however, they often find that the disease processes are no longer stabilized and fluid and electrolyte imbalances are present.

Head injuries can result in cerebral edema. Occasionally, this edema creates pressure on the pituitary gland, and as a result ADH secretion is changed. Two alterations can occur. Diabetes insipidus occurs when too little ADH is secreted and the client excretes large volumes of dilute urine with a low specific gravity. The second alteration is SIADH, in which there is continued secretion of ADH, which is seen clinically as water intoxication (Kubo and Grant, 1978). There are six indicators

of SIADH, including the following*:

1. Hyponatremia with hypoosmolarity of serum and extracellular fluids
2. Continued renal excretion of sodium
3. No other signs of volume depletion
4. Urine osmolarity above normal range
5. Normal renal function
6. Normal adrenal function

In addition, physical assessment and laboratory findings are consistent with fluid volume overload.

Burns can result in the loss of plasma through the burned skin surface. Thus a loss of both fluid and electrolytes occurs.

Drug therapies increase the risk for fluid and electrolyte disturbances. Although diuretic medications cause excretion of water, they can be potassium sparing such as spironolactone (Aldactone) or potassium wasting such as furosemide (Lasix).

Gastroenteritis and nasogastric suctioning result in loss of potassium and chloride ions. Hydrogen ions are also lost, causing a disturbance in acid-base balance.

Fistulas can also result in a loss of potassium. As a result, clients with fistulas are at risk for hypokalemia. The loss of potassium increases the risk for acid-base disturbances (see box at left).

PHYSICAL EXAMINATION

Because fluid, electrolyte, and acid-base disturbances can affect all systems, the nurse must systematically identify any abnormalities during the physical examination (Table 37-5 on p. 1040 and box at right).

MEASURING FLUID INTAKE AND OUTPUT

Measuring and recording all liquid intake and output during a 24-hour period helps to complete the assessment data base for fluid and electrolyte balance. Intake includes all liquids taken orally, by feeding tube, and parenterally. Liquid output includes urine, diarrhea, vomitus, gastric suction, and drainage from postsurgical tubes. Frequently the recording of such data is referred to as the I & O.

Generally, intake and output are routinely measured for clients after surgery and clients whose condition is unstable, who have fever, whose fluids are restricted, or who are receiving diuretic or IV therapy. The nurse neither needs nor should wait for a physician's order to begin intake and output measurements. Clients with chronic cardiopulmonary or renal illnesses and those whose health status has declined also receive such measurements.

Oral intake includes all liquids, such as gelatin, ice cream, soup, juice, and water, taken by mouth. Liquid

---

*From Lane, G, and Pierce, AG: When persistence pays off, Nurs 82 12:44, 1982.

Clinical Symptoms of Fluid, Electrolyte, and Acid-Base Imbalances

FLUID AND ELECTROLYTE BALANCES

Integumentary System
- Edema (circulatory overload)
- Dry skin (dehydration)

Cardiopulmonary System
- Cardiac dysrhythmias (hypokalemia)
- Jugular venous distention (circulatory overload)

Gastrointestinal System
- Increased viscosity of saliva (hyponatremia)
- Longitudinal furrows on tongue (hyponatremia)
- Chvostek's sign (hypocalcemia, hypomagnesemia)

Musculoskeletal System
- Hypotonicity (hyponatremia)
- Hypertonicity (hypernatremia)
- Muscle cramps, tetany (hypocalcemia)
- Deep tendon reflexes decreased or absent (hypercalcemia, hypermagnesemia)
- Increased or hyperactive reflexes (hypocalcemia, hypomagnesemia)
- Cold, clammy skin (hyponatremia)
- Velvety sheen of skin (hypernatremia)

ACID-BASE BALANCE

Central Nervous System
- Headache (metabolic alkalosis and acidosis, respiratory acidosis)
- Irritability (metabolic alkalosis, respiratory alkalosis)
- Lethargy (metabolic alkalosis and acidosis, respiratory acidosis)
- Decreases in level of consciousness (metabolic alkalosis and acidosis, respiratory acidosis)
- Dizziness (respiratory alkalosis and acidosis)

Cardiopulmonary System
- Tachycardia (metabolic alkalosis, respiratory acidosis)
- Bradycardia (metabolic alkalosis)
- Kussmaul respirations (metabolic acidosis)
- Cardiac dysrhythmias (metabolic acidosis, respiratory acidosis and alkalosis)
- Tachypnea (respiratory alkalosis)

Gastrointestinal System
- Nausea and vomiting (metabolic alkalosis and acidosis)
- Anorexia (metabolic acidosis)
- Diarrhea (metabolic acidosis)

Musculoskeletal System
- Numbness and tingling of extremities (metabolic alkalosis)
- Hypertonicity (metabolic alkalosis)
- Tetany (metabolic alkalosis, respiratory alkalosis)
- Muscle weakness (metabolic acidosis, respiratory alkalosis and acidosis)
- Tremors (respiratory acidosis)

intake also includes fluids given through nasogastric or jejunostomy feeding tubes, liquids given as IV fluids, and blood or its components.

Ambulatory clients' urinary output is recorded after each trip to the bathroom. These clients are instructed to save their urine in a container for the nurse to record the amount, or clients may be instructed to measure and record their own output. The output of a client who has an indwelling Foley catheter, drainage tube, or suction is recorded at the end of each nursing shift or more frequently (for example, every 2 hours) as the client's condition requires.

In the hospital, 8-hour intake and output records are attached to the bedside chart or room door. The records include all types of fluid intake and output and includes physicians' orders (Fig. 37-3, p. 1043).

The 24-hour totals are included in the client's chart. These 24-hour totals are usually recorded at midnight or 6 AM, depending on policy. The records note the type of intake and output and are broken down into 8-hour segments (Fig. 37-4. p. 1044).

Taking intake and output measurements is a procedure requiring help from the client and family and instructions from the nurse. The nurse explains the reasons the measurements are needed and provides the client with a copy of the hospital's metric conversions. The nurse instructs the client not to empty any container with voided fluids but to ask the nurse to do so. A client using a toilet should be instructed to use a calibrated insert, which attaches to the rim of the toilet bowl. After each urination the client notifies the nurse, who measures, records, and empties the urine and rinses the insert.

Clients occasionally receive a specific amount of a liquid medication every 1 to 2 hours. For example, antacids are commonly ordered in 30 ml doses every hour for clients who have or who are at risk for gastrointestinal bleeding. Over 24 hours this hourly antacid can

Text continued on p. 1045.

TABLE 37-5 Physical and Behavioral Nursing Assessment for Fluid, Electrolyte, and Acid-Base Balances

Assessment	Imbalance	Frequency
FLUID LOSS (MEASURED BY WEIGHT)		
2%-5% loss	Mild dehydration	On admission and daily
6%-9% loss	Moderate dehydration	
10%-14% loss	Severe dehydration	
20% loss	Death	
2% gain	Mild volume overload	
5% gain	Moderate volume overload	
8% gain	Severe volume overload	
HEAD (HEENT)		
Headache		
History	Metabolic or respiratory acidosis	Every hour
Irritability		
Observation	Metabolic or respiratory alkalosis	Every hour
Lethargy		
Observation	Metabolic acidosis or alkalosis, respiratory acidosis	Every hour
Dizziness		
History	Respiratory alkalosis or acidosis	Every hour
Fontanels (infant)		
Inspection:		Every hour
Depressed	Fluid volume deficit	
Bulging	Fluid volume overload	
Eyes		
Inspection:		Every 4 hours
Sunken		
Dry conjunctivae	Fluid volume deficit	
Decreased or absence of tearing		
Inspection:		Every 4 hours
Periorbital edema	Fluid volume overload	
Blurred vision		
Papilledema		
Ears		
None		
Bridge of nose		
Palpation: pinched skin remains raised	Fluid volume deficit	Every 2 hours

TABLE 37-5—cont'd

Assessment	Imbalance	Frequency
Throat and mouth		
Inspection:		
Sticky dry mucous membranes		
Dry cracked lips	Fluid volume deficit	Every 4 hours
Decreased saliva		
Increased viscosity of saliva	Hyponatremia	Every 2 hours
Longitudinal furrows on tongue	Hyponatremia	
Palpation: Chvostek's sign	Hypocalcemia, hypomagnesemia	
CARDIOVASCULAR SYSTEM		
Inspection:		Every hour
Flat neck veins	Fluid volume deficit	
Distended neck veins	Fluid volume overload	
Palpation:		
Dysrhythmias	Metabolic acidosis, respiratory alkalosis and acidosis	
Increased pulse rate	Metabolic alkalosis, respiratory acidosis	
Decreased pulse rate	Metabolic alkalosis	
Weak pulse	Fluid volume deficit	
Decreased capillary filling		
Bounding pulse rate	Fluid volume overload	
Auscultation:		
Blood pressure low with or without orthostatic changes	Fluid volume deficit	
Third heart sound	Fluid volume excess	
ECG: cardiac dysrhythmias	Hypokalemia	
RESPIRATORY SYSTEM		
Inspection:		Every hour
Increased rate	Fluid volume overload or deficit, respiratory alkalosis	
Dyspnea	Fluid volume overload, metabolic acidosis	
Auscultation:		
Rales		
Rhonchi	Fluid volume overload	
GASTROINTESTINAL SYSTEM		
Inspection:		Every 2 hours
Anorexia	Metabolic acidosis	
Sunken abdomen		
Vomiting	Fluid volume deficit	
Diarrhea		
Abdominal cramps	Metabolic acidosis or alkalosis	
Palpation: poor skin turgor	Fluid volume deficit	
Auscultation: hyperperistalsis with diarrhea or hypoperistalsis	Fluid volume deficit	

Continued.

TABLE 37-5 Physical and Behavioral Nursing Assessment for Fluid, Electrolyte, and Acid-Base Balances—cont'd

Assessment	Imbalance	Frequency
RENAL SYSTEM		
Inspection:		Every 2 hours
Oliguria or anuria	Fluid volume deficit or fluid volume overload	
Diuresis (if kidneys normal)	Fluid volume overload	
Specific gravity increased	Fluid volume deficit	
NEUROMUSCULAR SYSTEM		
Inspection:		Every hour
Numbness, tingling	Metabolic alkalosis	
Muscle cramps, tetany	Hypocalcemia, metabolic or respiratory alkalosis	
Irritability, lethargy, coma	Fluid volume deficit	
Tremors	Respiratory acidosis	
Disorientation	Fluid volume overload	
Palpation:		
Hypotonicity	Fluid volume deficit and hyponatremia	
Hypertonicity	Hypernatremia, metabolic alkalosis	
Percussion:		
Deep tendon reflexes decreased or absent	Hypercalcemia, hypermagnesemia	
Increased or hyperactive	Hypocalcemia, hypomagnesemia	
SKIN		
Body temperature		
		Every 1-2 hours
Increased	Hypernatremia	
Decreased	Fluid volume deficit	
Body surface		
Inspection:		
Velvety sheen	Hypernatremia	
Dry, scaly skin	Fluid volume deficit	
Palpation:		
Poor skin turgor	Fluid volume deficit	
Cold, clammy	Hyponatremia	
Warm, normal, "doughy" quality	Hypernatremia	
Extremities (dependent body parts: sacrum, back, legs)		
Inspection:		
Slow venous filling	Fluid volume deficit or fluid volume overload	
Palpation: edema (1+ to 4+)	Fluid volume overload or slow venous return (for example, pregnancy)	

Data from Groër, MW: Physiology and pathophysiology of the body fluids, St. Louis, 1981, The C.V. Mosby Co.; Keithley, JK, and Frauline, KE: Nurs 82 12:44, 1982; and Metheny, NM: Natl Intravenous Ther Assoc 4:38, 1981.

Barnes Hospital   **B-8**

DAILY INTAKE AND OUTPUT RECORD

17-4 Rev. 2/83

FROM 0700   /   /   TO 0700   /   /   Addressograph Plate

INTAKE

Coffee mug	- 180cc
Ice tea container to clear line (without ice)	- 250cc
Ice cream container (melted)	- 30cc
Sherbet container (melted)	- 50cc
Juice container	- 120cc
Milk carton	- 240cc
Paper cup (1/4 from brim)	- 240cc
Soup bowl (broth)	- 180cc
Gelatin container (melted)	- 100cc

ORDERS: (CIRCLE)

NPO
WATER
CLEAR FLUIDS
FULL FLUIDS

AMT. DESIRED
CC

RATE   GTTS/MIN.   CC/HR.

OUTPUT

SOURCE KEY:
V = VOIDED
C = CATHETER
INC = INCONTINENT

SOURCE KEY:
VOM. = VOMITUS
LIQ. S. = LIQUID STOOL
HV. = HEMOVAC
L.T. = LEVIN TUBE
T.T. = T. TUBE
OTHER

TIME	PARENTERAL SOLUTION IN BOTTLE KIND	AMT.(CC)	AMT.(CC) ABSORBED	ORAL KIND	AMT. (CC)	URINE SOURCE	AMT. (CC)	OTHER SOURCE	AMT. (CC)
0700 0800									
0800 0900									
0900 1000									
1000 1100									
1100 1200									
1200 1300									
1300 1400									
1400 1500									
8 HR. TOT.				8 HR. TOT.		8 HR. TOT.		8 HR. TOT.	
1500 1600									
1600 1700									
1700 1800									
1800 1900									
1900 2000									
2000 2100									
2100 2200									
2200 2300									
8 HR. TOT.				8 HR. TOT.		8 HR. TOT.		8 HR. TOT.	
2300 2400									
2400 0100									
0100 0200									
0200 0300									
0300 0400									
0400 0500									
0500 0600									
0600 0700									
8 HR. TOT.				8 HR. TOT.		8 HR. TOT.		8 HR. TOT.	
24 HR. TOT.				24HR. TOT.		24 HR. TOT.		24 HR. TOT.	

Fig. 37-3 Eight-hour fluid intake and output record.
Courtesy Barnes Hospital, St. Louis.

B-17

BARNES HOSPITAL
24 HOUR
INTAKE AND OUTPUT SUMMARY
(Retain in Patient's Record)

STAMP ADDRESSOGRAPH PLATE HERE

DATE	SHIFT	INTAKE: ORAL and/or TUBE FEEDING	INTAKE: IV (Incl. Blood and Plasma)	OUTPUT: URINE	OUTPUT: GASTRIC	OUTPUT: OTHER (specify)
	07000 1500					
	1500 2300					
	2300 0700					
	TOTAL					
	07000 1500					
	1500 2300					
	2300 0700					
	TOTAL					
	07000 1500					
	1500 2300					
	2300 0700					
	TOTAL					
	07000 1500					
	1500 2300					
	2300 0700					
	TOTAL					
	07000 1500					
	1500 2300					
	2300 0700					
	TOTAL					
	07000 1500					
	1500 2300					
	2300 0700					
	TOTAL					
	07000 1500					
	1500 2300					
	2300 0700					
	TOTAL					

Fig. 37-4 Twenty-four hour intake and output record.
Courtesy Barnes Hospital, St. Louis.

Laboratory Data for Fluid, Electrolyte, and Acid-Base Imbalances

FLUID AND ELECTROLYTE IMBALANCES

- Altered concentrations of sodium, chloride, and bicarbonate ions
- False elevation of red or white blood cell count because of hemoconcentration caused by dehydration
- False lowering of CBC values with overhydration
- False elevation of the BUN when client is dehydrated and extracellular fluid is hemoconcentrated
- False lowering of BUN because of overhydration and hemodilution
- Concentrated urine causes higher specific gravity of urine
- Overhydration causes a fall in specific gravity of urine

ACID-BASE IMBALANCES
Metabolic Alkalosis

- pH greater than 7.44
- $Paco_2$ normal or greater than 44 mm Hg if lungs are compensating
- Pao_2 normal
- O_2 saturation normal
- HCO_3^- above 26 mEq/L
- K^+ less than 3.5 mEq/L

Metabolic Acidosis

- pH less than 7.36
- $Paco_2$ normal, or less than 36 mm Hg if lungs are compensating
- Pao_2 normal, or less than 36 mm Hg if lungs are compensating
- O_2 saturation normal
- HCO_3^- below 22 mEq/L
- K^+ above 5.5 mEq/L

Respiratory Alkalosis

- pH 7.44 or greater
- $Paco_2$ less than 36 mm Hg
- Pao_2 normal
- O_2 saturation normal
- HCO_3^- normal
- K^+ below 3.5 mEq/L

Respiratory Acidosis

- pH less than 7.36
- $Paco_2$ greater than 44 mm Hg (unless the client has chronic obstructive pulmonary disease)
- Pao_2 normal or below 80 mm Hg depending on severity of acidosis
- O_2 saturation normal or below 95% depending on severity of acidosis
- HCO_3^- normal in early respiratory acidosis
- K^+ above 5.5 mEq/L

amount to a significant intake and should always be recorded on the intake record.

The amounts of fluid intake and output are essential for obtaining an accurate data base. This information helps to maintain an ongoing evaluation of hydration status and to prevent severe imbalances.

LABORATORY STUDIES

Laboratory tests are performed to obtain further objective data about fluid, electrolyte, and acid-base balance (see box). These tests include serum electrolyte levels, complete blood count, blood urea nitrogen (BUN), blood creatinine, urine specific gravity, and arterial blood gases.

Serum electrolytes are measured to determine the hydration status, the electrolyte concentration of the blood plasma, and acid-base balance. Electrolytes frequently measured include sodium, potassium, chloride, and bicarbonate ions. The severity of the illness determines the frequency of the electrolyte measurements. Serum electrolytes are routinely collected from any client entering a hospital setting as a screening test for alterations.

The complete blood count (CBC) is a determination of the number and type of red and white blood cells per cubic millimeter of blood. Changes in the CBC occur in response to dehydration or overhydration. Serious alterations in the CBC, such as anemia, can also affect oxygenation status.

Blood creatinine levels are useful in measuring kidney function. Creatinine is a normal byproduct of muscle metabolism and is excreted at fairly constant levels, regardless of factors such as fluid intake, diet, or exercise.

The urine specific gravity test measures the urine's degree of concentration. The specific gravity can be measured at the bedside using a urinometer (see Chapter 38). Normally the urine specific gravity ranges between 1.010 and 1.025. Because water has a specific gravity of 1.000, urine with a lower specific gravity (1.010) is more dilute than urine with a higher specific gravity (1.025).

NURSING DIAGNOSIS

Assessment reveals clusters of data indicating problems with fluid, electrolyte, acid-base balance, or other related problems (see nursing diagnoses box). Nursing diagnoses resulting from the assessment have supporting defining characteristics, which are contained within the data base, and expected causes or etiologies. Identification of expected causes further individualizes the nursing diagnostic statement and subsequent plan of care (see sample nursing diagnoses box).

Examples of Nursing Diagnoses Related To Fluid, Electrolyte, and Acid-Base Disturbances

NANDA-APPROVED NURSING DIAGNOSES

Actual or *potential fluid volume deficit* related to:
- Loss of plasma associated with burns
- Chronic malnutrition
- Inappropriate use of medications

Fluid volume excess related to:
- Sodium retention
- Excessive water ingestion

Impaired tissue integrity related to:
- Edema

Impaired gas exchange related to:
- Hypoventilation
- Acid-base disturbance

Ineffective breathing pattern related to:
- Acid-base disturbance

PLANNING

After identifying nursing diagnoses, the nurse develops a plan of care (see care plan box). The care plan is individualized according to the client's acute or chronic fluid, electrolyte, or acid-base imbalance. Clients with altered fluid, electrolyte, and acid-base imbalances require a nursing care plan directed toward meeting actual or potential fluid needs. The plan is based on one or more of the following goals:

1. Fluid, electrolyte, and acid-base balance are restored and maintained.
2. Causes of imbalance are identified and corrected.
3. Client has no complications from therapies needed to restore balance.

IMPLEMENTATION

When a client's volume is depleted, fluids and electrolytes can be replaced orally, with IV administration of fluids and blood components, or through total parenteral nutrition if the fluid deficit is caused by malnutrition. For clients with fluid volume excess the nurse implements measures to reduce fluids, such as fluid intake restrictions, reduced sodium intake, and administration of diuretics.

CORRECTING FLUID AND ELECTROLYTE IMBALANCES

DAILY WEIGHING. All clients with fluid and electrolyte disturbances should be weighed daily. Otherwise, a client can gain 2.7 to 3.6 kg (6 to 8 pounds) before edema is observed (Folk-Lightly, 1984). Weight should be determined at the same time each day, and the same scale should be used. The client should also wear the same clothes, or if a bed scale is used, the same number of sheets should be on the scale with each daily weighing.

Sample Nursing Diagnoses for Fluid, Electrolyte, and Acid-Base Disturbances

Defining Characteristics	Nursing Diagnoses	Related Factors
Hypotension Thirst Decreased urine output Weight loss Decreased skin turgor Dry skin Dry mucous membranes Weakness	Actual or potential fluid volume deficit	- Altered regulatory mechanisms - Active fluid loss (for example, bleeding) - Excessive losses through normal routes (for example, diarrhea) - Medication use
Edema Weight gain, pulmonary congestion, crackles, jugular vein distention, restlessness, anxiety	Fluid volume excess	- Altered regulatory mechanisms - Excess fluid intake - Excess sodium intake
Confusion Restlessness Hypercapnia Increased secretions	Impaired gas exchange	- Hypoventilation - Medication - Increased pulmonary secretions

Sample Nursing Care Plan for Fluid, Electrolyte, and Acid-Base Disturbances

Nursing Diagnosis	Goal	Expected Outcomes	Nursing Interventions
Fluid volume deficit related to excessive diarrhea	Fluid and electrolytes return to normal values.	Serum electrolytes are within normal limits. Hypotension or orthostatic changes are absent. Skin turgor is normal. Mucous membranes are moist. Urine output increases (>70 ml per hour). Diarrhea is not present.	Infuse IV fluids at 125 ml/hr. Keep NPO until 24 hours after last diarrheal stool. Start oral fluids with 30 ml clear liquids. Advance to full liquid diet when client tolerates a liquid diet for 24 hours with no further diarrhea.

INTAKE AND OUTPUT MEASUREMENTS. In addition to providing assessment data, intake and output records provide current information about fluid balance. Intake and output measurements can indicate if excess fluid volume is excreted in the urine. Likewise, they can show whether the excretion of fluids through the kidneys has diminished.

The nurse should measure, not estimate, intake and output. Both the client and family should be aware that *all* intake and output must be measured.

ENTERAL REPLACEMENT OF FLUIDS

Oral. Unless contraindicated, oral replacement of fluids and electrolytes is appropriate as long as the client is not vomiting, is not experiencing a profound fluid loss, or does not have a mechanical obstruction in the gastrointestinal tract. Clients unable to tolerate solid foods may still be able to ingest fluids.

Oral fluid replacement is easily implemented in the home and hospital. Mild illness such as viral diarrhea, respiratory tract infections, and fevers may cause fluid and electrolyte disturbances. In addition, clients recovering from anesthesia or gastrointestinal surgery usually receive clear liquids first and then advance to a regular diet if they tolerate the liquids.

Tube Feedings. Fluids need not be replaced by mouth. They can also be replaced internally through nasogastric, gastrostomy, or jejunostomy feeding tubes.

When replacing fluids by mouth in a client with fluid

TABLE 37-6 Oral Fluids

Solution	Calories (Kcal/30ml)	HCO₃⁻ (mEq/L)	Na⁺ (mEq/L)	Ca⁺⁺ (mEq/L)	K⁺ (mEq/L)	Mg⁺⁺ (mEq/L)	Cl⁻ (mEq/L)	Predominant Carbohydrate
Water								
Pedialyte (oral electrolyte solution)	6.0		30.0	4.0	20.0	4.0	30.0	Dextrose
Lytren (oral electrolyte solution)	9.0 (isotonic)		30.0	4.0	25.0	4.0	25.0	Glucose
5% glucose in water	6.0							Glucose
10% glucose in water	12.0							Glucose
Pepsi-Cola	13.2	7.3	6.5		0.8			Sucrose
Coca-Cola	14.4	13.4	0.4		12.0			Sucrose
Ginger ale	10.0	3.6	3.5					Sucrose
Gatorade	5.5		23.0		3.0		17.0	Glucose, sucrose
Lemon-lime soda	9.6		7.5	0.3	0.2			
Broth, beef (canned)	6.0		55.0					
Tea, unsweetened	0.25				Trace			

From Groër, MW: Physiology and pathophysiology of the body fluids, St. Louis, 1981, The C.V. Mosby Co.

deficit, the nurse should choose fluids with adequate calories and electrolyte content (Table 37-6), but if fluids are replaced through a feeding tube, the physician usually prescribes a nutritional supplement (see Chapter 33).

RESTRICTION OF FLUIDS. Clients who retain fluids and have a fluid volume overload require restricted fluid intake. These clients have renal failure, congestive heart failure, cor pulmonale, or SIADH.

Fluid restriction is often difficult for clients, particularly if they are taking medications that dry the oral mucous membranes. The nurse should explain the reason fluids are restricted. In addition, the client should know how much fluid is permitted orally and that ice chips, gelatin, and ice cream are considered fluid.

Given this information, the client should help to decide the amount of fluid with each meal, between meals, before bed, and with medications. Frequently clients on fluid restriction can swallow a number of pills with as little as 1 ounce (30 ml) of liquid.

A good rule of thumb for fluid restrictions is to allow half the allotted total oral fluids between 8 AM and 4 PM, the period when clients usually are more active and receive two meals and most of their oral medications. Then an additional two fifths of the allotted total fluid is permitted between 4 PM and 11 PM, permitting fluids with meals and evening visitors. Between the hours of 11 PM and 8 AM the remainder of the total fluid allotment is permitted. Because the client is usually asleep during this period, fluid needs decrease.

The nurse should also ensure that clients receive their favorite fluids (unless contraindicated). For example, if a client can have only 200 ml of fluid with breakfast and hates cranberry juice but likes apple or grape juice, the nurse should be sure the diet kitchen has this information.

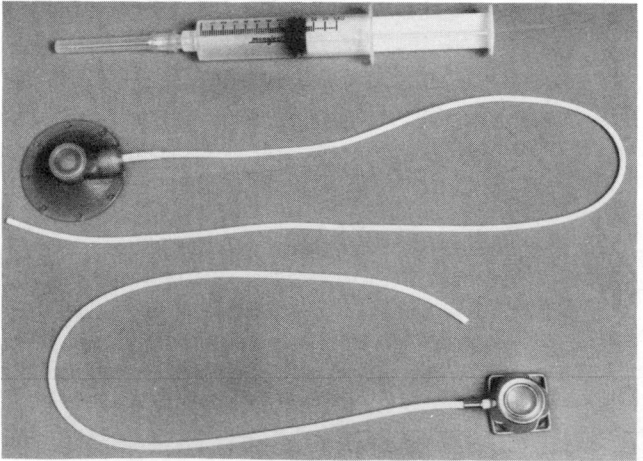

Fig. 37-5 Examples of implantable silicone venous catheters.

PARENTERAL REPLACEMENT OF FLUID AND ELECTROLYTES. Fluid and electrolytes may be replaced through infusion directly into the blood rather than intake through the digestive system. Parenteral replacement includes total parenteral nutrition, IV fluid and electrolyte therapy, and blood replacement.

Vascular Access Devices. Vascular access devices are catheters, cannulas, or infusion ports designed for long-term repeated access to the vascular system (Fig. 37-5). These devices are safer and have improved mechanisms for delivering long-term IV therapy. Increased use of central venous catheters and implanted infusion ports require nurses to be educated in the care of these devices.

With increasing risk to health care workers for transmission of the human immunodeficiency virus (HIV), the causative agent presently identified for AIDS, and other infectious diseases, the principles of body fluid substance isolation must be practiced when administering parenteral fluids. The CDC has issued guidelines pertaining to exposure to body substances (see box).

Health care workers must consider all clients as potentially infected with HIV and other blood-borne pathogens and adhere rigorously to risk of exposure to blood and body fluids. (CDC, 1987). Universal precautions should be used with all clients, especially those in obstetric, operating room, critical care, and emergency care settings in which the risk of blood exposure is increased and infection status may be unknown (see box). In addition, precautions for invasive procedures are followed when surgical entry into tissues, cavities, or organs or repair of major traumatic injuries occurs (CDC, 1987).

Total Parenteral Nutrition. Total parenteral nutrition (TPN) is a nutritionally adequate hypertonic solution consisting of glucose and other nutrients and electrolytes given through an indwelling peripheral or central IV catheter. TPN is used as an intervention in severe cases of malnutrition. Chapter 33 fully describes its administration.

IV Therapy. The goal of IV fluid administration is to correct or prevent fluid and electrolyte disturbances in clients who are or may become acutely ill. For example, a client with third-degree burns over 40% of the body is critically ill and has severe fluid and electrolyte imbalances. Fluid therapy must be continuously regulated in these clients because of continual changes in fluid and electrolyte balance. A client allowed to ingest nothing by mouth for 2 days after an appendectomy receives IV fluid replacement to prevent fluid and electrolyte imbalances. The infusion is discontinued with resumption of normal intake.

When IV fluid administration is required, the nurse must know the correct solution, equipment needed, and the procedures required to initiate an infusion, regulate the fluid infusion rate, maintain the system, identify and correct problems, and discontinue the infusion.

TYPES OF SOLUTIONS. Many prepared electrolyte solutions are available for use. Electrolyte solutions fall into the following categories: isotonic, hypotonic, and hypertonic. A solution is *isotonic* if the total electrolyte content approximates 310 mEq/L. A *hypotonic* solution is one in which the total electrolyte is below 250 mEq/L. A *hypertonic* solution has a total electrolyte content of 375 mEq/L or greater (Metheny and Snively, 1983).

Universal Precautions to Prevent Transmission of HIV as They Pertain to IV Therapy

- Gloves should be worn for touching blood and body fluids, mucous membranes, or nonintact skin of all clients, for handling items or surfaces soiled with blood or body fluids, and for performing venipuncture and other vascular access procedures.
- Gloves should be changed after contact with each client.
- Hands and other skin surfaces should be washed immediately and thoroughly if contaminated with blood or other body fluids. Hands should be washed immediately after gloves are removed.
- To prevent needlestick injuries, needles should not be recapped, purposely bent or broken by hand, removed from disposable syringes, or otherwise manipulated by hand.
- Used needles, syringes, and IV fluid equipment should be placed in puncture-resistant containers for disposal. The puncture-resistant containers should be located as close as practical to the use area.
- Health care workers who have exudative lesions or weeping dermatitis should refrain from all direct care and from handling invasive equipment until the condition resolves.
- Pregnant health care workers are not known to be at greater risk of contracting HIV infections than health care workers who are not pregnant. However, if a health care worker develops HIV infection during pregnancy, the infant is at risk of infection resulting from perinatal transmission. Because of this risk, pregnant health care workers should strictly adhere to precautions to minimize the risk of HIV transmission.

From Centers for Disease Control: Recommendations for prevention of HIV transmission in health care settings, MMWR 36 (Suppl. 25):3s, 1987.

In general, isotonic fluids are used for extracellular volume replacement, as for fluid deficit after prolonged vomiting. The decision to use a hypotonic or hypertonic solution is based on the specific electrolyte imbalance.

Certain additives are frequently instilled into IV solutions, most commonly vitamins and potassium chloride (KCl). The physician's order includes required additives, for example:

Bottle #1: 1000 ml—D5W with 20 mEq KCl and 1 ampule of multivitamins

Clients with normal kidneys who are receiving nothing by mouth should have potassium added to IV solutions. If the physician's order for such a client does not include potassium, the nurse should double-check the order. Kidneys routinely excrete potassium, and if there is no potassium intake orally or parenterally, hypokalemia can quickly develop.

The nurse collects and, if necessary, prepares the solution using the "five rights" of medication administration described in Chapter 15.

EQUIPMENT. Correct selection and preparation of equipment assists in safe and quick placement of an IV line. Because fluids are instilled into the bloodstream, sterile technique is necessary, and therefore the nurse must have all needed equipment organized and at the bedside. The nurse who must leave the bedside to obtain another piece of equipment must start the procedure again. Standard equipment includes IV solution and tubing, needles (Fig. 37-6), antiseptic, tourniquet, gloves, dressing, and armboard.

The arm board is used to reduce movement of the extremity with the IV infusion in place and to maintain the extremity in a flat position. Arm boards may be used when inserting an IV line on the dorsal surface of the hand.

Other IV equipment includes solution containers, various types of tubing, and volume control devices. An injectable antibiotic medication such as ampicillin may be added to a small IV solution bag containing 50 ml and "piggybacked" into the main line to be administered over a 30- to 40-minute period (see Chapter 15). The type and amount of solution depend on the medication added and the client's physiological status. For example, when ampicillin is administered parenterally, it must be infused within 1 hour after the drug was prepared. Otherwise the medication loses its potency. Different tubing types are used to administer a medication. A drug given rapidly needs to be infused with macrodrip tubing. In addition, clients may require IV extension tubing to increase mobility or to facilitate changes in position. Volume control devices are used with children, with clients with renal or cardiac failure, or with critically ill clients to prevent sudden uncontrolled rapid infusion of large

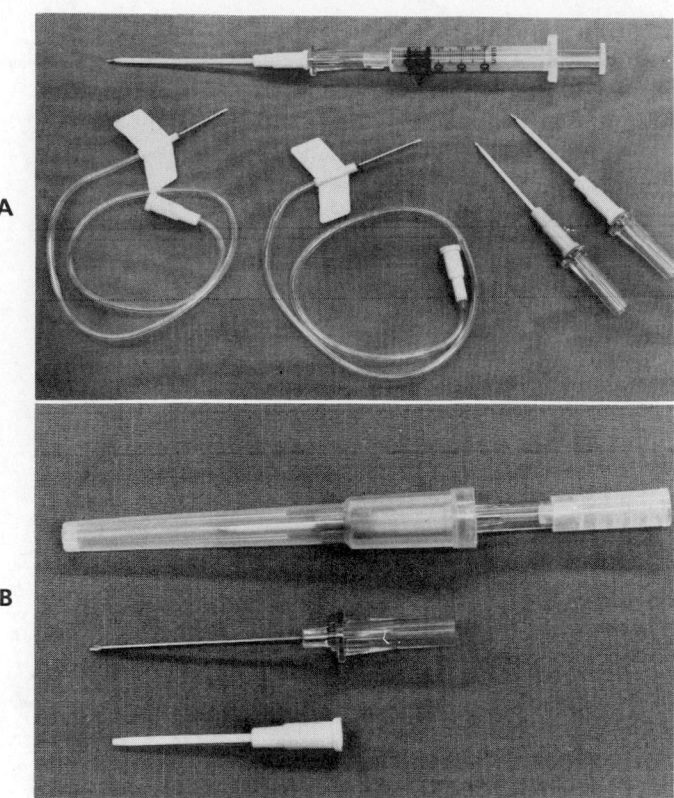

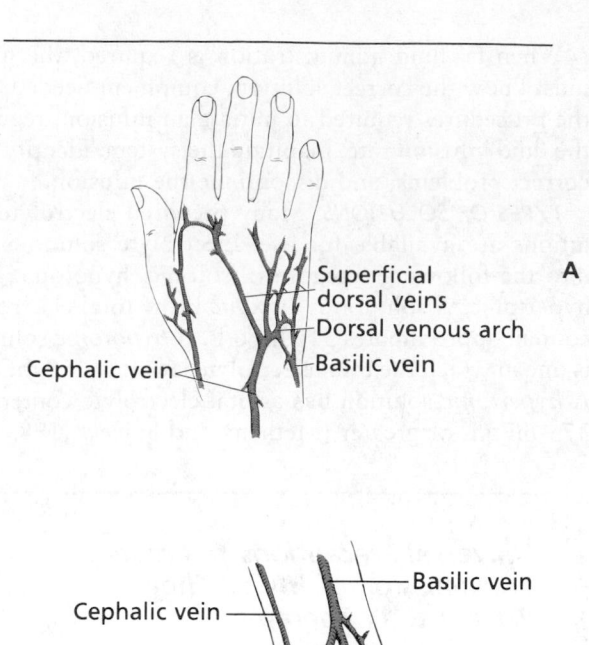

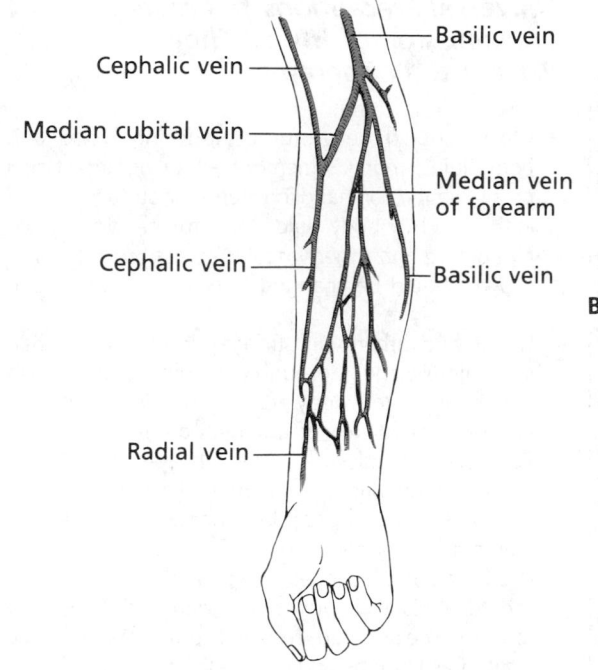

Fig. 37-6 **A,** *Beginning at top and moving clockwise:* Angiocatheter attached to syringe, two angiocatheters of different gauges, two butterfly needles. **B,** Components of an angiocatheter. *Top to bottom:* Angiocatheter in sterile container, metal stylet to pierce the skin, plastic catheter to remain in the vein.

volumes. (Additional information on volume control devices is presented in the section on regulating the infusion flow rate.)

INITIATING THE THE INTRAVENOUS LINE. After the equipment is collected at the bedside, the nurse prepares to place the IV line by assessing the client for the venipuncture site (Procedure 37-1). A venipuncture is a technique in which a vein is punctured transcutaneously by a sharp rigid stylet (for example, a butterfly needle or cannula such as an angiocatheter containing a flexible plastic catheter) or by a needle attached to a syringe. The general purposes of venipuncture are to collect a blood specimen, to instill a medication, to start an IV infusion, or to inject a radiopaque or radioactive tracer for special examinations. Procedure 37-1 describe venipuncture for IV infusion.

The nurse assessing the client for potential venipuncture sites should consider conditions, cautions, and contraindications that exclude certain sites. Because very young and elderly clients have fragile veins, the nurse should avoid sites that are easily moved or bumped such as the dorsal surface of the hand. It is often difficult to

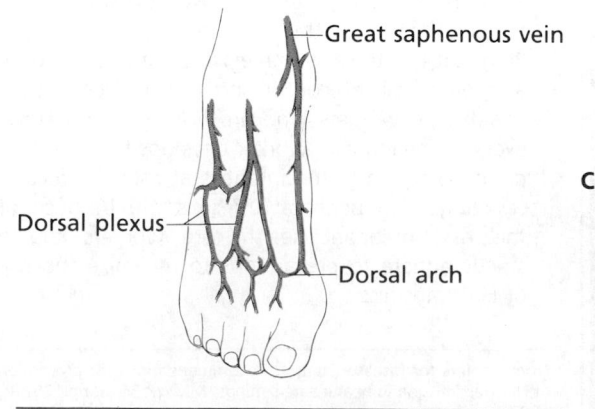

Fig. 37-7 Common IV sites. **A,** Dorsal surface of the hand. **B,** Inner arm. **C,** Dorsal surface of the foot.

Text continued on p. 1055.

PROCEDURE 37-1

Venipuncture with an Angiocatheter

STEPS	RATIONALE

1. Observe for signs and symptoms indicating fluid or electrolyte imbalances:
  a. Sunken eyes
  b. Periorbital edema
  c. Greater than 2% increase or decrease in body weight
  d. Dry mucous membranes
  e. Flattened or distended neck veins
  f. Change from baseline vital signs
  g. Irregular pulse rhythm
  h. Auscultation of rales or rhonchi in lungs
  i. Poor skin turgor
  j. Increased or decreased bowel sounds
  k. Decreased urine output
  l. Behavioral changes
  m. Confusion
	Because fluid and electrolyte disturbances can affect every system in the body, nurse must systematically assess client to identify abnormalities related to fluid or electrolyte imbalance. Daily weights document fluid retention or loss. Change in body weight of 1 kg corresponds to 1 L of fluid retention or loss.

2. Identify client and explain procedure.	Reduces anxiety and promotes cooperation.

3. Assemble necessary equipment for initiating IV line:
 	
  a. Correct solution
  b. Proper needle for venipuncture (Fig. 37-6)
  c. Infusion set (infants and children require a 60 gtt/ml drip and often a volume control device)
  d. IV tubing
  e. Alcohol and povidone-iodine cleansing swabs
  f. Tourniquet
  g. Arm board
  h. Gauze and providone-iodine ointment
  i. Tape
  j. Towel to place under client's hand
  k. IV pole
  l. Gloves
	Correct selection and preparation of equipment assist in safe and quick placement of IV line.

4. Identify accessible vein for placement of IV needle or catheter.
  a. Avoid bony prominences.
  b. Use most distal portion of vein first.
  c. Avoid placing IV over client's wrist.
  d. Avoid placing IV in client's dominant hand.
	Selection of appropriate vein promotes ease and placement of IV catheter and needle.

5. Wash hands.	Reduces transmission of microorganisms.
6. Organize equipment on clutterfree bedside stand or overbed table (see illustration).	Reduces risk of contamination and accidents.

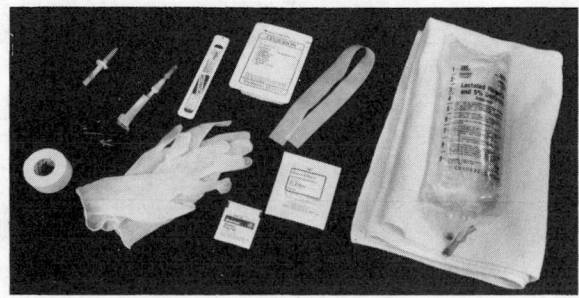

Step 6

Continued.

PROCEDURE 37-1, cont'd

Venipuncture with an Angiocatheter

STEPS	RATIONALE
7. Open sterile packages using aseptic technique (see Chapter 43).	Maintains sterility of equipment and reduces spread of microorganisms.
8. Check solution, using "five rights" of drug administration. Make sure any prescribed additives, such as potassium and vitamins, have been added. NOTE: When using bottled IV solution, remove metal cap and metal and rubber disks beneath cap.	IV solutions are medications and should be double-checked to reduce risk of error. Permits entry of infusion tubing into solution.
9. Open infusion set, maintaining sterility of both ends.	Prevents bacteria from entering infusion equipment and thus bloodstream.
10. Place roller clamp (see illustration) about 2 to 4 cm (1 to 2 in) below drip chamber.	Close proximity of roller clamp to drip chamber allows more accurate regulation of flow rate.
11. Move roller clamp to "off" position.	Prevents accidental spillage of fluid on client, nurse, bed, or floor.
12. Insert infusion set into fluid bag. a. Remove protective cover from IV bag without touching opening (see illustration). b. Remove protector cap from tubing insertion spike, not touching spike, and insert spike into opening of IV bag (see illustration). Or insert spike into black rubber stopper of IV bottle.	Maintains sterility of solution. Prevents contamination of solution from contaminated insertion spike.
13. Fill infusion tubing. a. Compress drip chamber and release. b. Remove needle protector and release roller clamp to allow fluid to travel from drip chamber through tubing to needle adapter. Return roller clamp to off position after tube is filled. c. Be certain tubing is clear of air and air bubbles. d. Replace needle protector.	Creates suction effect; fluid enters drip chamber. Removes air from tubing and permits it to fill with solution. Large air bubbles can act as emboli. Maintains system sterility.
14. Select appropriate IV needle or angiocatheter.	Needle or angiocatheter is necessary to puncture the vein and instill IV fluid.
15. Select distal site of vein to be used.	If sclerosing or damage to vein occurs, proximal site of same vein is still usable.
16. If large amount of body hair is present at needle insertion site, shave it.	Reduces risk of contamination from bacteria on hair. Also assists in maintaining intactness of IV dressing and makes removal of adhesive tape less painful.
17. If possible, place extremity in dependent position.	Permits venous dilation and visibility.
18. Place tourniquet 10 to 12 cm (5 to 6 in) above insertion site. Tourniquet should obstruct venous, not arterial, flow (see illustration). Check presence of distal pulse.	Diminished arterial flow prevents venous filling.

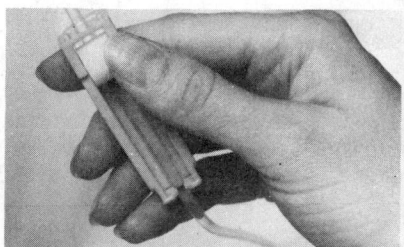

Step 10

Step 12a

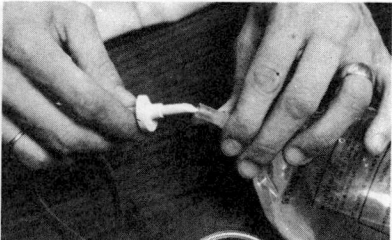

Step 12b

STEPS	RATIONALE

19. Select well-dilated vein (see illustration). Client may have to make a fist if vein in hand or arm is selected.
    NOTE: Be sure needle adapter end of infusion set is nearby and on sterile gauze or towel.
20. Apply disposable gloves.

21. Cleanse insertion site with povidone-iodine solution, followed by alcohol (see illustration).
22. Perform venipuncture.
    Butterfly needle: place needle at 30-degree angle with bevel up about 1 cm (1½ in) distal to actual site of venipuncture (see illustration).
    Angiocather: insert bevel up at 30-degee angle distal to actual site of venipuncture.

Muscle contraction increases venous distention.

Permits smooth, quick connection of infusion to needle after vein is punctured.
Decreases exposure to HIV, hepatitis, and other blood borne organisms.
Povidone-iodine is topical antiinfective; alcohol is topical antiseptic. Together, they reduce skin surface bacteria.
Allows nurse to place needle parallel with vein. Thus, when vein is punctured, risk of puncturing both sides is reduced.

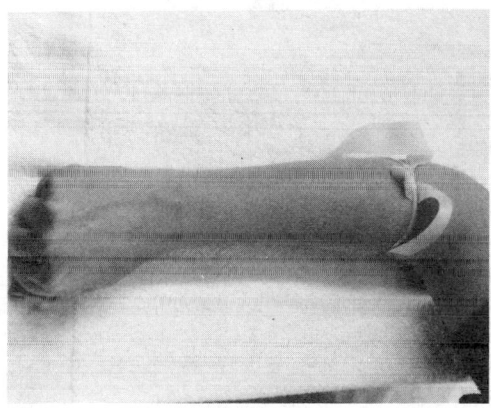

Step 18

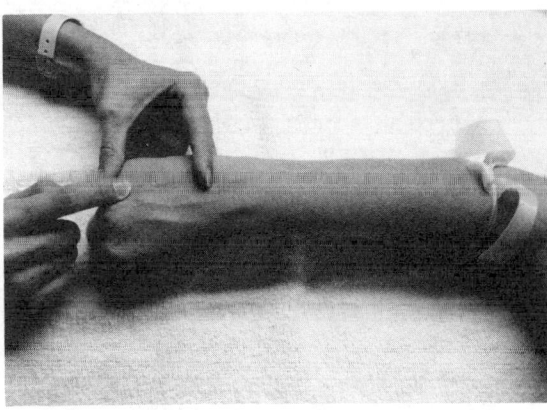

Step 19

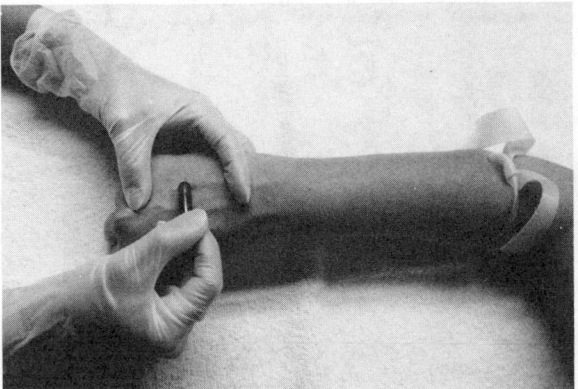

Step 21

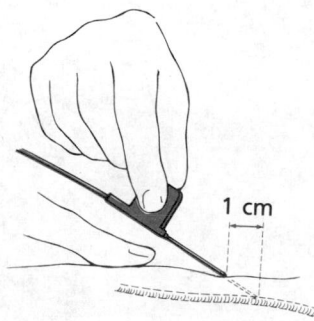

1 cm

Step 22

Continued.

Venipuncture with an Angiocatheter

STEPS	RATIONALE
23. Look for blood return through tubing of butterfly needle or angiocatheter, indicating that needle has entered vein. Advance catheter approximately ¼ into vein and then remove stylet (see illustration). Continue advancing flexible catheter or butterfly needle until hub rests at venipuncture site.	Increased venous pressure from tourniquet increases backflow of blood into catheter or tubing. Stylet helps to puncture skin and advance catheter but must be removed to avoid puncture of vein.
24. Connect needle adapter of infusion to hub of angiocatheter or needle. To maintain sterility, do not touch point of entry of either needle adapter or inside hub of angiocatheter (see illustration).	Prompt connection of infusion set maintains patency of vein.
25. Stabilizing catheter with one hand, release tourniquet. Release roller clamp to begin infusion at a rate to maintain patency of IV line.	Permits venous flow and prevents clotting of vein and obstruction of flow of IV solution.
26. Secure IV catheter or needle. a. Place narrow piece (½ in) of tape under catheter, and cross tape over catheter.	Prevents accidental removal of catheter from vein.

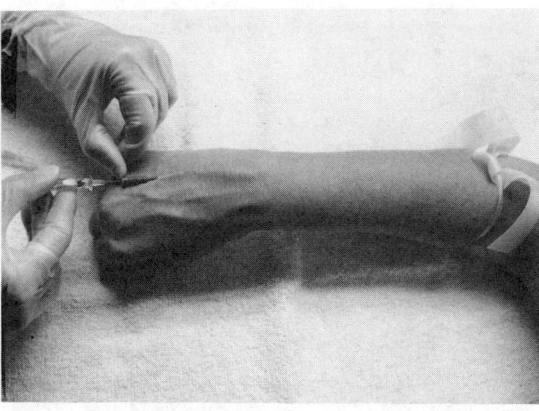

Step 23

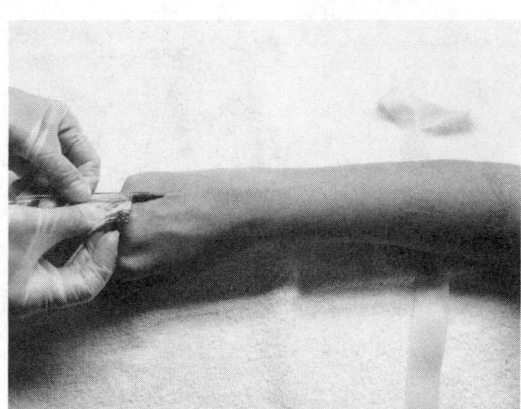

Step 24

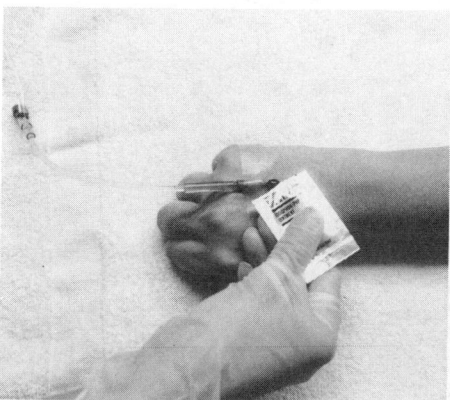

Step 26b

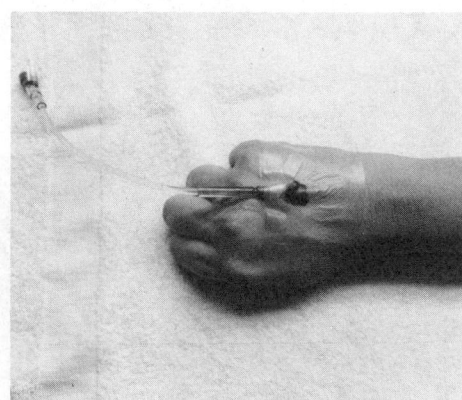

Step 26d

STEPS	RATIONALE
b. Place povidone-iodine solution at venipuncture site (see illustration).	Solution ointment is topical antiseptic germicide that reduces bacteria on skin and decreases risk of local or systemic infection. When transparent dressing is used, povidone-iodine solution is recommended; ointment interferes with adherence of dressing to skin.
c. Place second piece of narrow tape directly across catheter.	
d. Place transparent dressing over venipuncture sites, following manufacturer's directions (see illustration). (Alternatively, place third piece of narrow tape under IV insertion needle adapter, and cross tape over infusion tubing. Place 2 × 2 gauze over catheter and secure it with 1 in piece of tape.)	Prevents accidental disconnection of IV infusion.
e. Secure infusion tubing to catheter with piece of 1 in tape.	Further stabilizes connection of infusion to catheter.
27. Write date and time of placement of IV line on IV dressing.	Provides immediate data as to when IV was inserted and subsequent dressing changes.
28. Adjust flow rate to correct drops per minute	Maintains correct rate of flow for IV solution.
29. Discard gloves and supplies and wash hands.	Reduces transmission of microorganisms.

30. Observe client to determine the response to IV fluid therapy every hour.
  a. Correct amount of solution infused as prescribed
  b. Proper flow rate gtt/minutes
  c. Patency of IV catheter or needle
  d. Absence of infiltration, phlebitis, or inflammation
	Provides continuous evaluation of type and amount of fluid delivered to client. Hourly inspection prevents accidental fluid overload or inadequate infusion rate.

31. Record in nurses' notes type of fluid, insertion site, flow rate, size and type of IV catheter or needle, when infusion was begun. Note client's response to IV fluid, amount infused, and integrity and patency of IV system according to agency policy.	Documents initiation of IV fluid therapy as ordered by physicians. Follow-up documentation provides data about the response to therapy.

insert an IV line in clients who have had many venipunctures because their veins may be sclerosed with scar tissue. An obese client presents problems for venipuncture because of the difficulty in locating superficial veins. The thin and emaciated client's veins are also difficult to puncture. Although they may be visible, the veins are quite fragile, and as a result the nurse may puncture through the entire vein instead of placing the needle or catheter within it. When a client is severely dehydrated or has decreased extracellular fluid, as with shock, the veins may collapse. The collapse results from decreased circulating blood volume. When veins collapse, venipuncture becomes extremely difficult, but it is also a lifesaving measure. For these difficult clients, venipuncture should be performed by someone with the necessary expertise.

Venipuncture is contraindicated in a site that has signs of infection, infiltration, or thrombosis. An infected site is red, tender, swollen, and possibly warm to the touch.

Exudate may be present. An infected site is not used because of the danger of introducing bacteria from the skin surface into the bloodstream.

Common IV puncture sites include the hand and the arm (Fig. 37-7, *A* and *B*, p. 1050). However, the superficial veins of the foot can be used if the client is nonambulatory (Fig. 37-7, *C*, p. 1050). The use of the foot for an IV site is more common with pediatric clients and is generally avoided in the adult.

After completing the assessment for venipuncture sites, the nurse carefully explains the procedure to the client. The nurse should explain the reason the infusion was ordered, its expected results, and the nurse's expectations of the client.

The venipuncture and IV infusion procedure has many steps. Procedure 37-1 describes the steps for using an angiocatheter, but the procedure is the same with a butterfly needle.

Large catheters placed into a central vein such as the

Regulating Intravenous Flow Rates

STEPS	RATIONALE
1. Observe patency of IV line and needle.	For fluid to infuse at proper rate, IV line and needle must be free of kinks, knots, or clots.
a. Open drip regulator and observe for a rapid flow of fluid from IV solution into drip chamber, then close drip chamber to prescribed rate.	Rapid flow of fluid into drip chamber denotes patency of IV line. Closing drip chamber to prescribed rate prevents fluid overload.
b. If fluid does not flow, lower IV fluid bottle/bag below level of infusion site and observe for blood return.	Indicates needle is patent and in vein. Venous pressure is greater than pressure in IV tubing.
2. Check client's medical record for correct solution and additives. Usual order includes: solution for 24 hr, usually divided into 2 or 3 L. Occasionally, IV order contains only 1 L to keep vein open (KVO). Record also shows time over which each liter is to infuse.	IV fluids are medications. "Five rights" are followed to decrease chance of medication error.
3. Know calibration in drop per milliliter (gtt/ml) of infusion set:	Microdroppers, also called minidrip, universally deliver 60 gtt/ml. However, commercial parenteral administration sets for macrodrip exist. Nurse should know which company's infusion set hospital uses.

Microdrip: 60 gtt/ml
Macrodrip (Metheny and Snively, 1983):
Abbott Lab   15 gtt/ml
Tranvenol Lab   10 gtt/ml
McGaw Lab   15 gtt/ml

4. Select one of the following formulas to calculate flow (Metheny and Snively, 1983):

   After hourly rate has been determined, formula will give correct flow rate.

   a. $\text{ml/hr} = \dfrac{\text{total volume}}{\text{hours of infusion}}$

   b. drop factor $\times$ ml/min = drops/minute

      or

   c. $\dfrac{\text{Total volume} \times \text{drop factor}}{\text{Infusion time in minutes}} = \text{drops/minute}$

STEPS	RATIONALE
5. Place infusion pump or volume control device at bedside if ordered or available.	Reduces risk of infusion of incorrect fluid.
6. Read physician's orders and follow "five rights" to be sure you have correct solution and proper additives.	IV fluids are medications; following "five rights" decreases chance of medication error.
a. IV fluids are usually ordered for 24 hr period, indicating how long each liter of fluid should run; for example, an IV order for a client is:	Determines volume of fluid that should infuse hourly.

     (1) Bottle 1: 1000 ml D5W
              with 20 mEq KCl
              8 AM to 4 PM
        Bottle 2: 1000 ml D5W
              with 20 mEg KCl
              4 PM to 12 midnight
        Bottle 3 1000 ml D5W
              with 20 mEq KCl
              12 midnight to 8 AM
       Total 24 hr IV intake: 3000

STEPS	RATIONALE
7. Determine hourly rate by dividing volume by hours, for example.	Provides even infusion of fluid over prescribed hourly rate.

$$\frac{1000 \text{ ml}}{8} = 125 \text{ ml/hr}$$

or if 4 liters are ordered for 24 hr:

$$\frac{4000}{24} = 166.7 \text{ ml} = 167 \text{ ml/hr}$$

STEPS	RATIONALE
8. Place adhesive tape vertically on IV bottle or bag next to volume markings. Mark adhesive tape based on hourly flow rate. For example, if entire volume of fluid is to be infused over an 8-, 10-, or 12-hour period, respective designations will be marked on the tape.	Time taping IV bag gives nurse visual cue as to whether fluids are being administered over correct time period.
9. After hourly rate has been determined, calculate minute rate based on drop factor of infusion set. Minidrip or microdrip infusion set has drop factor of 60 drops (gtt) per milliliter. Regular drip or macrodrip infusion set used here has drop factor of 15 gtt/ml. Using formula, calculate minute flow rates:	This allows nurse to calculate minute flow rate based on this formula:

Bottle 1: 1000 ml with 20 KCl

$$\frac{\text{total volume} \times \text{drop factor}}{\text{infusion time in minutes}}$$

Volume is divided by time.

Microdrip:
$$\frac{125 \text{ ml} \times 60 \text{ gtt/ml}}{60 \text{ min}} =$$

$$\frac{7500 \text{ gtt}}{60} = 125 \text{ gtt/min}$$

Macrodrip:
$$\frac{125 \text{ ml} \times 15 \text{ gtt/ml}}{60 \text{ min}} = 31 \text{ to } 32 \text{ gtt/min}$$

STEPS	RATIONALE
10. Time flow rate by counting drops in drip chamber for 1 min by watch, then adjust roller clamp to increase or decrease rate of infusion (see Illustration).	Determines if fluids are being administered too slowly or fast.
11. Follow this procedure for infusion pump:	
a. Place electronic eye on drip chamber below origin of drop and above fluid level in chamber (see Illustration).	IV infusion pumps monitor IV fluids based on flow rate or drops per minute. Infusion pumps have electronic eye that counts number of drops flowing from administration set.
b. IV infusion tubing is placed with ridges of control box in direction of flow; that is, portion of tubing nearest IV bag at top and portion of tubing nearest client at bottom. Required drops per minute are selected, door to control tubing is shut, power button is turned on, and start button is pressed.	Infusion pumps move fluid by compressing and milking tubing, thus propelling fluid through tubing.
c. IV tube drip regulator must be in open position while infusion pump is in use.	

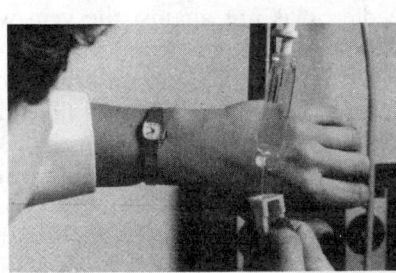

Step 10

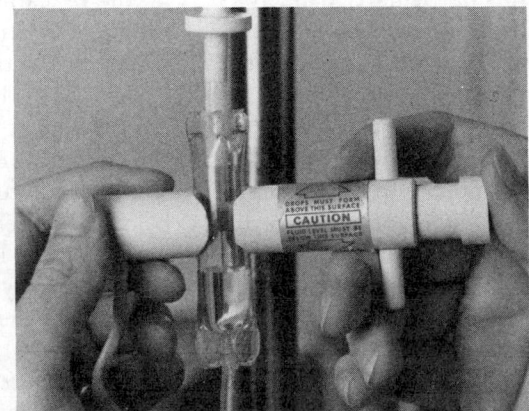

Step 11a

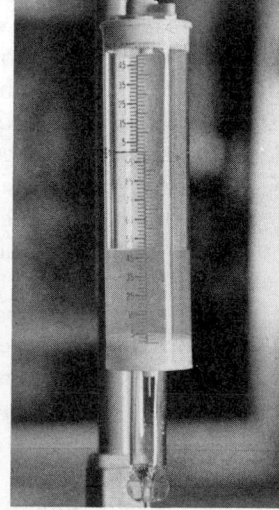

Step 12a

Continued.

Regulating Intravenous Flow Rates

STEPS	RATIONALE
d. Monitor infusion rates at least hourly	Infusion pumps are not infallible and do not replace frequent, accurate assessments.
e. Assess patency of IV system when alarm sounds.	Alarm indicates that electronic eye has not noted precise number of drops from drip chamber.
12. Follow this procedure for volume control device.	
a. Place volume control device between IV bag and insertion spike of infusion set (see illustration).	Reduces risk of sudden increases in fluid volume.
b. Place 2 hr of fluid into device.	Prevents IV line from running dry if nurse does not return in exactly 60 min. In addition, if accidental increase in flow rate occurs, client receives at most only 2 hr fluid allotment.
c. Assess IV system at least hourly and add fluid to volume control device. Regulate flow rate.	Maintains patency of IV system.
13. Observe client to determine response to IV therapy and restoration of fluid and electrolyte balance. Signs of infiltration include: inflammation at site; clot in IV catheter, kink or knot in infusion tubing.	Signs and symptoms of dehydration or overhydration warrant changing rate of fluid infused.
14. Record rate of infusion, gtt/min and ml/hr, in nurses' notes every 4 hr.	Documents that prescribed IV flow is being delivered to client.

subclavian vein are used to monitor central venous pressure (CVP) and to deliver large volumes of fluids and total parenteral nutrition. Although these catheters are inserted by physicians, nurses are responsible for maintaining them.

REGULATING THE INFUSION FLOW RATE. After the IV infusion is secured and the IV line is patent, the nurse must regulate the rate of infusion according to physician's orders (Procedure 37-2). An infusion rate that is too slow can lead to further cardiovascular and circulatory collapse in a client who is dehydrated, in shock, or critically ill. An infusion rate that is too rapid can result in fluid overload, which is particularly dangerous in some cardiovascular, kidney, and neurological disorders. The nurse calculates the infusion rate to prevent too slow or too rapid administration.

Infusion pumps regulate the flow of IV fluids. They are designed to deliver a measured amount of fluid over a period of time, and IV infusion pumps monitor IV fluids based on the flow rate or drops per minute. Infusion pumps have an electronic eye that counts the number of drops flowing from an IV administration set. The electronic eye must be placed on the drip chamber below the origin of the drop and above the fluid level in the chamber.

The IV infusion tubing is placed within the ridges of the control box in the direction of flow (that is, the portion of the tubing nearest the IV bag is at the top and the portion of tubing nearest the client is at the bottom). The required drops per minute are selected, the door to the control chamber is shut, the power button is turned on, and the start button is pressed.

The infusion pump's electronic eye monitors the drip rate. If the required number of drips per minute is not achieved, an alarm will sound. The alarm can be sounded if the IV bag is empty, the infusion tubing is kinked, or the vein is clotted. If the alarm sounds, the nurse investigates and corrects the cause of the drip rate problem.

IV flow rates can be affected by the patency of the IV needle or catheter, infiltration, a knot or kink in the tubing, the height of the solution, and the position of the client's extremity.

Patency of the IV needle or catheter means that there are no clots at the tip of the needle or catheter and that the catheter or needle tip is not against the vein wall. The nurse can assess patency by lowering the IV bag below the level of IV insertion site and observing for a blood return. If no blood return occurs and fluid does not flow easily from the drip chamber when the roller clamp is opened, a clot may be present at the catheter tip.

An *infiltration* may be present when the IV insertion site is cool, clammy, swollen, and in some cases painful. An infiltration occurs when the IV needle or catheter has become dislodged from the vein and is in the subcutaneous space. When an infiltration occurs, the IV line must be discontinued and a new line inserted.

A *knot or kink* in the tubing can decrease the flow rate. Occasionally the tubing is kinked underneath IV dressing, which requires the nurse to open the dressing to locate the problem. Frequently the flow rate will resume after the tubing is straight. The client may also occlude the tubing by lying or sitting on it.

The *height* of the IV bag can affect flow rates. Raising the bag may increase the flow rate because of gravity.

The *extremity* position can decrease flow rates, particularly with IV sites at the wrist. Occasionally the use of an arm board helps to keep the wrist flat. Sometimes, it is more comfortable for the client to have an infusion started in a new location rather than dealing with a site that causes problems. However, before discontinuing the infusion that is hampered by an extremity position, the nurse must be sure the client has other accessible veins.

These influences on IV flow rates can occur with any client at any time. When caring for a client with an infusion, the nurse should assess the site and the infusion rate at least every hour.

Children, the elderly, clients with severe head trauma, and clients susceptible to volume overload must be protected from sudden increases in infusion volumes. Sudden increases can occur accidentally. For example, a restless client may with a sudden movement loosen the roller clamp and increase the flow rate, or the flow rate may be accidentally increased if the client ambulates. A sudden increase in IV volume can kill the client or make him critically ill. Volume control devices, such as a Volutrol or buret, can prevent sudden increases in volume (see Chapter 15).

The volume control device is placed between the IV bag and insertion spike of the infusion set. Most control devices can hold 150 ml. Nurses usually put 2 hours' worth of fluid in the buret. Therefore, if the client is to have only 30 ml per hour, the nurse places 60 ml in the volume control device. If the nurse does not return to the client in exactly 1 hour, the IV line does not run dry. In addition, if an accidental increase in flow rate occurs, the client receives at most only 2 hours' allotment of fluid instead of 500 or 1000 ml.

MAINTAINING THE SYSTEM. After the IV line is in place and the flow rate regulated, the nurse must maintain the system. The nurse provides comfort and hygiene measures, assistance with meals, and assistance with ambulation. IV catheters and drugs, especially those with potassium, can cause discomfort and burning sensations. Clients must be reassured that occasional discomfort is normal. Sometimes, discomfort is relieved by repositioning the extremity, but occasionally it is necessary to start a new IV line in a larger vein.

Because a client with an infusion in the arm finds it difficult to meet hygiene needs, the nurse should help with bathing and changing gowns. Gowns are changed by following six steps for maximum arm mobility and speed:

1. Remove the sleeve of the gown from the uninvolved arm
2. Remove the sleeve of the gown from the involved arm
3. Remove the IV bottle or bag from its stand and pass it and the tubing through the sleeve
4. Place the IV bottle or bag and tubing through the sleeve of the clean gown
5. Place the involved arm through the gown sleeve
6. Place the uninvolved arm through the gown sleeve

The client with an arm or a hand infusion is able to walk, unless contraindicated. A walking IV pole, a standard V pole with wheels, is needed. The nurse helps the client out of bed and places the pole next to the involved arm. The client is instructed to hold onto the pole with the involved hand and to push it while walking. The nurse should assess the equipment to make sure that the IV bag is at the proper height, that there is no tension on the tubing, and that the flow rate is correct. The nurse should instruct the client to report any blood in the tubing, a stoppage in the flow, or increased discomfort.

Because clients receiving IV therapy to restore a fluid volume deficit may require frequent changing of solutions, the nurse should allow adequate time for this.

Occasionally, clients require an IV infusion to deliver a drug every 4, 6, or 8 hours. An hourly infusion flow of about 10 to 15 ml per hours is used to keep the vein open (KVO) using a microdrip infusion set. Generally these clients do not use an entire IV solution bag. However, they should have a new solution bag or bottle at least once every 24 hours because the sterility of the solution cannot be guaranteed for longer than a day. When an IV solution container is changed, the nurse uses sterile technique and follows an organized procedure (Procedure 37-3).

Technically, IV tubing can remain sterile for 48 hours. However, most institutions recommend that new sterile tubing be used every 24 hours. The procedure is much simpler and more efficient if the nurse changes the infusion tubing when preparing to hang a new IV bag or bottle (Procedure 37-4). To prevent entry of bacteria into the bloodstream, sterility must be maintained.

The dressing over the IV insertion site is changed according to hospital policy to enable the nurse to inspect the site for possible signs of infection or early signs of infiltration (Procedure 37-4). The recent use of transparent dressings enables the nurse to continually assess venipuncture sites. The more common practice of daily dressing changes has been reduced to every 48 to 72 hours with the transparent dressings.

PROCEDURE 37-3

Changing IV Solutions and Tubing

CHANGING IV SOLUTION

1. Identify client. Assess physician's orders and client and have the next solution prepared at least 1 hr before needed. If the solution is prepared in the pharmacy, be sure it has been delivered to the floor. Check that the solution is correct and properly labeled.

Ensures correct client undergoes procedure. Prevents finding an empty IV bag without having a replacement bag. Checking prevents medication error.

2. Prepare to change the solution when it only remains in the neck of the bottle or bag.
3. Be sure the drip chamber is half full.
4. Wash hands.
5. Prepare new solution for changing. If using plastic bag, remove protective cover from entry site. If using glass bottle: remove metal cap, metal disk, and rubber disk.

Prevents air from entering the IV tubing and the vein from clotting from lack of IV flow.
Provides IV fluid to the vein while bag is being changed.
Reduces transmission of microorganisms.
Permits quick, smooth, and organized change from old to new solution.

6. Move roller clamp to reduce flow rate.

Prevents solution remaining in drip chamber from emptying while changing solutions.

7. Remove old solution from IV pole.
8. Quickly remove spike from old IV solution, and without touching tip, spike new solution bottle.
9. Hang new bag or bottle of solution.

Brings work to nurse's eye level.
Reduces risk of solution in drip chamber (Step 3) running dry and maintains sterility.
Allows gravity to assist with delivery of IV fluid into drip chamber.

10. Check for air in tubing.
11. Make sure drip chamber contains solution.
12. Regulate flow rate to prescribed rate.

Reduces risk of air embolus.
Reduces risk of air entering IV tubing.
Maintains measures to restore fluid balance and deliver IV fluid as ordered.

13. Observe IV system for patency, absence of infiltration, phlebitis, or inflammation. Observe response to IV therapy.

Provides ongoing evaluation of response to IV fluid therapy.

CHANGING INTRAVENOUS TUBING

14. Determine when a new infusion set is warranted:
    a. Hanging first solution of day
    b. Puncture of infusion tubing
    c. Contamination of tubing

    d. Occlusions in IV tubing can occur after infusion of packed red blood cells, whole blood, or albumin.

IV tubing should be changed daily and procedure is simplified when changing tubing with new solution.
Punctured tubing results in leakage of fluid.
Contamination of tubing can allow entry of bacteria into bloodstream.
Whole blood or blood component products have potential to occlude or partially occlude IV tubing.

15. Assemble the following:
    a Infusion tubing
    b. Sterile 2 × 2 or 4 × 4 gauze
    c. If a new IV dressing must be applied:
       (1) Sterile 2 × 2 gauze or sterile 4 × 4 gauze
       (2) Povidone-iodine ointment
       (3) Adhesive remover
       (4) Povidone-iodine solution
       (5) Alcohol swabs
       (6) Strips of tape or polyurethane film dressing
       (7) Disposable gloves

Enables nurse to efficiently and safely complete procedure.

NOTE: Follow hospital guidelines for dressing changes. Some agencies use transparent dressings without ointment.

STEPS	RATIONALE
16. Explain procedure to client.	Promotes cooperation and prevents sudden movement of extremity, which could dislodge needle or catheter.
17. Wash hands.	Reduces transmission of microorganisms.
18. Open new infusion set, keeping protective coverings over infusion spike and insertion site for butterfly needle or IV catheter.	Provides nurse with ready access to new infusion set and maintains sterility of infusion set.
19. Apply nonsterile disposable gloves.	Decreases risk of exposure to HIV, hepatitis, and other blood-borne bacteria.
20. Place sterile 2 × 2 or 4 × 4 gauze on bed near IV puncture site.	Provides sterile field for new sterile needle adapter before connection to IV needle or catheter.
21. If needle or catheter hub is not visible, remove IV dressing. Do not remove tape that secures needle or catheter to skin.	Needle hub must be accessible to provide smooth transition when removing old tubing and inserting new tubing.
22. Take new IV tubing and move roller clamp to "off" position.	Prevents spillage of solution after new bag or bottle is spiked.
23. Slow rate of infusion by regulating drip rate on old tubing.	Prevents complete infusion of solution remaining in tubing.
24. With old tubing in place, compress drip chamber and fill chamber.	Provides surplus of fluid in drip chamber so there is sufficient fluid to maintain IV patency while changing to new tubing.
25. Discontinue old tubing from solution and hang drip chamber over IV pole.	Allows fluid to continue to flow through IV catheter while nurse prepares new tubing.
26. Place insertion spike of new tubing into old IV solution opening and hang solution on pole.	Permits flow of fluid from solution into new infusion tubing.
27. Compress and release drip chamber on new tubing.	Allows drip chamber to fill and promote rapid, smooth flow of solution through new tubing.
28. Open roller clamp, remove protective cap from needle adapter, and flush tubing with solution.	Removes air from tubing and replaces it with fluid.
29. Place needle adapter of new IV tubing, with protective cap off, between sterile 2 × 2 or 4 × 4 gauze near IV site.	Provides smooth, quick insertion of new tubing into needle hub, while maintaining sterility of infusion tubing.
30. Turn roller clamp on old tubing to "off" position.	Prevents spillage of fluid as tubing is removed from needle hub.
31. Stabilize hub of IV catheter or needle and gently pull out old tubing. Maintain stability of hub and insert needle adapter of new tubing into hub.	Prevents accidental displacement of catheter or needle.
32. Open roller clamp on new tubing.	Permits solution to enter catheter or tubing.
33. Regulate IV drip according to physician's orders and monitor rate hourly.	Maintains infusion flow at prescribed rate.
34. If necessary, apply new dressing (Procedure 37-4).	Reduces risk of bacterial infection from skin.
35. Discard old tubing and gloves in container for contaminated materials.	Prevents transmission of microorganisms.
36. Wash hands.	Reduces transmission of microorganisms.
37. Evaluate flow rate and observe connection site for leakage.	Maintains prescribed rate of flow of IV therapy and determines if fit is secure.
38. Record changing of tubing and solution on client's record and place piece of tape with date and time below level of drip chamber. Record fluid infused on I & O form.	Documents procedure and records that measures to maintain sterility were carried out. Provides visual cue to all care providers of when IV tubing was changed.

Changing an IV Dressing

STEPS	RATIONALE
1. Assess need to change dressing. a. Determine when IV dressing was last changed. Many institutions require nurse to write date and time on dressing itself.	Provides information regarding length of time that present dressing has been in place. In addition, nurse is able to plan for dressing change.
b. Observe present dressing for moisture.	Moisture is medium for bacterial growth. Moisture on sterile dressing renders dressing contaminated.
c. Observe present dressing for intactness.	Nonadhering dressing increases risk of bacterial contamination to venipuncture site or displacement of IV catheter.
d. Observe IV system for proper functioning or complications: kinks in infusion tubing or IV catheter; infiltration; inflammation.	Unexplained decrease in flow rate or pain and swelling at venipuncture site require nurse to investigate placement and patency of IV catheter.

2. Assemble necessary equipment:
  a. Sterile 2 × 2 gauze or transparent dressing
  b. Sterile 4 × 4 gauze or transparent dressing
  c. Povidone-iodine ointment
  d. Adhesive remover
  e. Povidone-iodine solution
  f. Alcohol swabs
  g. Strips of tape or polyurethane film dressing
  h. Disposable gloves
	Enables nurse to efficiently and safely complete procedure.

3. Explain procedure to client. Explain that affected extremity must remain still and length of procedure.	Assists in obtaining client cooperation and gives time frame around which client can plan personal activities.
4. Wash hands.	Reduces transmission of microorganisms.
5. Apply disposable gloves.	Reduces risk to HIV, hepatitis, and other blood-borne bacteria.
6. Remove tape and gauze from old dressing one layer at a time, leaving tape that secures IV needle or catheter in place.	Prevents accidental displacement of catheter or needle, which can occur if catheter tubing becomes tangled between two layers of dressing.

7. If infiltration, phlebitis, or clot occur or if ordered to do so by physician, discontinue IV infusion.
  a. Turn roller clamp to off position.
  b. Place gauze or alcohol pad over venipuncture site and remove catheter or needle by pulling straight away from site.
	Prevents spillage of IV fluid on bed, client, nurse, or floor.
	Prevents damage to vein.

c. Apply pressure to site for 1 to 2 min.	Controls bleeding or hematoma formation.
8. If IV is infusing properly, gently remove tape securing needle or catheter. Stabilize needle or catheter with one hand.	Exposes venipuncture site; prevents accidental displacement of catheter or needle.
9. Use adhesive remover to cleanse skin and remove adhesive residue.	Adhesive residue decreases ability of new tape to adhere tightly to skin.
10. Using circular motion, cleanse insertion site with povidone-iodine solution followed by alcohol.	Circular motion prevents cross-contamination from skin bacteria near venipuncture site. Povidone-iodine is a topical antiinfective; alcohol is a topical antiseptic. Together, they reduce skin surface bacteria.
11. Replace single strip adhesive tape to anchor IV catheter or needle.	Prevents accidental displacement of catheter or needle.
12. Place povidone-iodine ointment on venipuncture site.	Ointment is a topical antiseptic germicide that reduces skin bacteria and reduces risk of local or systemic infection. If a transparent dressing is used, povidone-iodine solution rather than ointment is recommended because an ointment interferes with adherence of dressing to the skin. In addition, the solution must be completely dry before application of transparent dressing.
13. Place 2 × 2, 4 × 4, or a clear dressing over venipuncture site. If a transparent dressing is selected, apply it in the direction of hair growth.	Provides barrier against bacteria. Reduces discomfort when dressing is removed.

STEPS	RATIONALE
14. Anchor IV tubing with additional pieces of tape.	Prevents accidental displacement of IV needle or catheter or separation of IV tubing from needle adapter.
15. Place date and time of dressing change directly on dressing (following agency policy).	Documents dressing change.
16. Discard equipment in appropriate container, remove and dispose of gloves, and wash hands.	Reduces transmission of microorganisms.
17. Reassess functioning and patency of IV system in response to changing IV dressing.	Validates that IV is patent and functioning correctly.
18. Record in nurses' notes time IV dressing was changed. Include patency of IV system and observation of venipuncture site.	Documents that dressing was changed, how IV system is functioning, and that venipuncture site is free of infection.

COMPLICATIONS OF IV THERAPY. The major complications of IV therapy are infiltration, phlebitis, fluid overload, bleeding, and infection.

An *infiltration* occurs when IV fluids enter the subcutaneous space around the venipuncture site. This is manifested as swelling (from increased tissue fluid) and pallor (caused by decreased circulation) around the venipuncture site. Fluid may be flowing through the IV line at a decreased rate or may have stopped flowing. Pain may also occur with an infiltration. Pain usually results from edema and increases proportionately as the infiltration worsens.

When infiltration occurs, infusion must be discontinued and, if necessary, reinserted into another extremity. To reduce discomfort caused by infiltration, the nurse should raise the extremity, which promotes venous drainage and helps decrease edema, and wrap the extremity in a warm towel for 20 minutes, which increases circulation and reduces pain and edema.

Phlebitis is an inflammation of the vein caused by the catheter or by the chemical irritation of additives and drugs given intravenously. Signs and symptoms of phlebitis include pain, increased skin temperature over the vein, and in some instances a red line traveling along the path of the vein. The IV line must be discontinued and a new line inserted in another vein. Warm, moist heat on the site of phlebitis can offer some relief to the client. Phlebitis is potentially dangerous because blood clots (thrombophlebitis) can occur and in some cases may result in emboli.

Fluid overload occurs when the client has received too rapid administration of solutions. Assessment findings are similar to those of fluid volume overload. The nurse should *slow* the rate of infusion, notify the physician, and be prepared to give diuretic medications. Prompt action is necessary to prevent worsening of the condition or even death.

Bleeding can occur around the venipuncture site while the infusion is taking place. Bleeding is common in clients who have received heparin or who have a bleeding disorder. If bleeding occurs around the venipuncture site and the catheter is within the vein, a pressure dressing may be applied over the site to control it. Bleeding from a vein is usually a slow, continuous seepage and is not fatal.

Infusion-related *infections* are caused by contamination of the IV system, venipuncture site, or the solution itself (Messner and Gorse, 1987). Clinical manifestations of these infections include purulent thrombophlebitis, cellulitis, and site infections, as evidenced by erythema, swelling, and pain at the venipuncture site.

Infusion-related infections can be reduced by four interventions. The nurse uses vigorous hand-washing techniques to remove gram-negative organisms before applying gloves for the venipuncture procedure (Tomford, Hershey, and McLakin, 1984). The nurse also changes "keep open" IV solutions at least every 24 hours. The nurse should also replace all peripheral venous catheters, including heparin locks, at least every 72 hours and preferably every 49 hours (CDC, 1987). In addition, the nurse maintains sterility of the IV system when changing tubing, solutions, and dressings (Axnick and Yarbrough, 1984).

DISCONTINUING IV INFUSIONS. Discontinuing an infusion is necessary after the prescribed amount of fluids has been infused, when an infiltration occurs, if phlebitis is present, or if the infusion catheter or needle develops a clot at its tip. The nurse discontinuing an infusion first

PROCEDURE 37-5

Administering a Blood Transfusion

STEPS	RATIONALE
1. Explain the procedure to the client. Determine if there have been prior transfusions and note reactions, if any.	Clients who have had blood transfusion in the past may have greater fear of transfusion.
2. Ask the client to report chills, headache, itching, or rash immediately.	These are signs of a transfusion reaction. Prompt reporting and discontinuation of transfusion can help to minimize a reaction.
3. Be sure client has signed any necessary consent forms.	Some agencies require clients to sign consent forms before receiving any blood component transfusions.
4. Wash hands. Apply disposable gloves.	Reduces risk for transmission of HIV, hepatitis, and other blood-borne bacteria.
5. Establish IV line with large-gauge (#18 or #19) catheter. Refer to Procedure 37-1 for venipuncture technique.	Large-gauge catheters permit infusion of whole blood and prevent hemolysis.
6. Use infusion tubing that has an in-line filter. Tubing should also be a **Y**-type administration set (see illustration).	Filter removes any debris and tiny clots from the blood. Y-type set permits administration of additional products or volume expanders easily and immediate infusion of 0.9% sodium chloride solution after completion of the infusion.
7. Hang a solution container of 0.9% normal saline to be administered after blood infusion.	Prevents hemolysis of red blood cells.
8. Follow agency protocol in obtaining blood products from the blood bank. Request blood when you are ready to use it.	Whole blood or packed red blood cells must remain in a cold (1° to 6° C) environment.
9. With another registered nurse, correctly identify blood product and client.	One nurse reads out loud while the other nurse listens and double-checks the information.
a. Check the compatibility tag attached to the blood bag and the information on the bag itself.	Verifies that the ABO group, Rh type, and unit number match.
b. For whole blood, check ABO group and Rh type, which is on client's chart.	Verifies that they match those on the compatibility tag and blood tag.

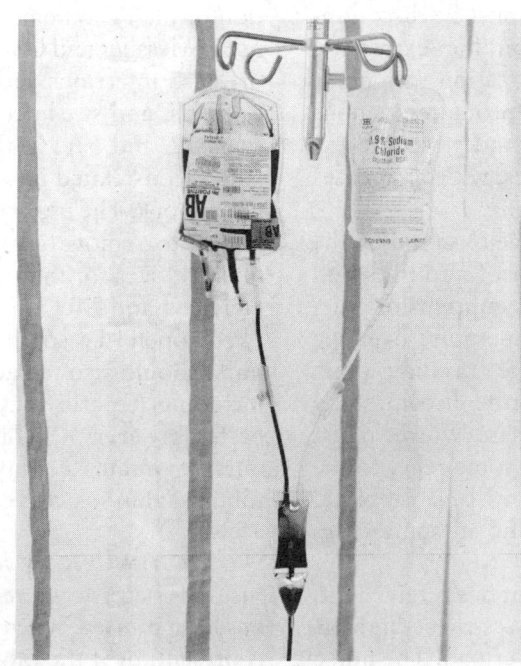

Step 6

STEPS	RATIONALE
c. Double-check the blood product with the physician's order.	Verifies correct blood component.
d. Check expiration date on the bag.	After 21 days, blood has only 70% to 80% of the original number of cells and 23 mEq/L of potassium.*
e. Inspect the blood for clots.	An anticoagulant, citrate-phosphate-dextrose (CPD), is added to blood and permits preserved blood to be stored for 21 days. Another anticoagulant, citrate-phosphate-dextrose-adenine (CPD-A), allows storage for 35 days.* If clots are present, return blood to the blood bank.
f. Ask client's name, and check armband.	Verifies correct client. Do not administer blood to a client without an arm band. The identification name and number on the wristband must be identical to those on the blood compatibility tag.
10. Obtain baseline vital signs.	Verifies pretransfusion temperature, pulse rate, blood pressure, and respirations.
11. Begin transfusion a. Prime the infusion line with 0.9% normal saline. b. Begin transfusion slowly by first filling the in-line filter. c. Adjust the rate to 2 ml per minute for the first 15 minutes, and remain with client. If you suspect a reaction, *stop* the transfusion and notify the blood bank and the physician.	Prevents hemolysis. If the filter is not filled, the transfusion will not infuse properly.
12. Monitor vital signs. a. Take vital signs every 5 min for the first 15 min of the transfusion and every hour thereafter. b. Observe for flushing, itching, dyspnea, hives, or rash.	Documents any change in vital sign status that could indicate early warning of a transfusion reaction. May indicate an early sign of a tranfusion reaction.
13. Maintain the prescribed infusion rate using infusion pumps, if necessary.	Infusion pumps maintain the prescribed rate.
14. Remove and dispose of gloves. Wash hands.	Reduces transmission of microorganisms.
15. Continually observe for adverse reactions.	Adverse reactions can occur at any point during the transfusion (Table 37-7).
16. Record the administration of the blood or blood product.	Documents administration of the blood component.

*Data from Metheny, NM, and Snively, WD, Jr.: Nurse's handbook of fluid balance, ed. 4, Philadelphia, 1983, J.B. Lippincott Co.

applies disposable gloves and removes the tape and dressing in the same manner as for the daily infusion dressing changes. The nurse then moves the roller clamp to the off position to prevent spillage of IV fluid. The nurse places a gauze or alcohol pad over the venipuncture site and, using the other hand, withdraws the catheter needle by pulling straight back away from the puncture site. The nurse applies pressure to the site for 1 to 2 minutes to control bleeding and prevent hematoma formation. Clients who have received heparin require longer pressure because of the action of heparin on blood-clotting mechanisms. If needed, the nurse applies a sterile dressing over the venipuncture site. The nurse records the amount of fluid infused and the time of the discontinuation.

Blood Replacement. Blood replacement or transfusion is the IV administration of whole blood or a component such as plasma, packed red blood cells, or platelets. The following list includes objectives for blood transfusion:

1. To increase circulating blood volume after surgery, trauma, or hemorrhage
2. To increase the number of red blood cells and to maintain hemoglobin levels in clients with severe anemia

3. To provide plasma-clotting factors to help to control bleeding in clients with hemophilia

BLOOD GROUPS AND TYPES. The most important grouping for transfusion purposes is the ABO system, which includes the following groups: A, B, O, and AB. The determination of blood groups is based on the presence or absence of A and B red cell antigens. Individuals with A antigens, B antigens, or no antigens belong to groups A, B, and O. Respectively, the person with A and B antigens have AB blood (Porth, 1986).

Agglutinins, or antibodies that work against the A and B antigens, are called *anti-A* and *anti-B agglutinins.* These agglutinins occur naturally (Patrick, et al., 1986). Individuals with type A blood naturally produce anti-B agglutinins in their plasma. Similarly, type B individuals naturally produce anti-A agglutinins in their plasma. A type O individual naturally produces both agglutinins, which is why a person with type O blood is considered a universal donor. An AB type individual produces neither antibody, which is why type AB individuals can be universal recipients. If blood that is mismatched with the client's blood is transfused, a transfusion reaction occurs. The transfusion reaction is an antigen-antibody reaction and can range from a mild response to severe anaphylactic shock.

Another consideration when matching for blood transfusions is the *Rh factor,* an antigenic substance in the erythrocytes of most people. A person with the factor is Rh positive, whereas a person without it is Rh negative. If the blood given to an Rh-positive person is Rh negative, *hemolysis,* or red blood cell destruction, and anemia occurs. If an Rh-negative mother gives birth to an Rh-positive baby, the infant may be exposed to antibodies to the mother's Rh-negative factor, and red blood cell destruction and erythroblastosis fetalis result.

AUTOTRANSFUSION. Autotransfusion is the collection, anticoagulation, filtration, and reinfusion of blood from an active bleeding site. Because the reinfused blood is the client's own, there are many advantages to autotransfusion. The risk of technical errors of blood typing and crossmatching is eliminated. Possible adverse effects associated with homologous blood transfusion are also eliminated. In addition, dependence on homologus blood banks is reduced, and possible exposure to serum hepatitis, HIV, and other blood-borne infections is eliminated.

When an elective surgical procedure is anticipated and transfusions are required, some individuals choose to give one or more units of their own blood in advance. This blood is stored and is available intraoperatively and postoperatively. This, too, is a type of autotransfusion.

BLOOD TRANSFUSIONS. Transfusing blood or blood components is a nursing procedure. The nurse is responsible for assessment before and during the tranfusion and regulation of the transfusion (Procedure 37-5, p. 1064).

If the client has an IV line in place, the nurse should assess the venipuncture site for signs of infection or infiltration. The nurse should also determine if the IV venipuncture was performed with an 18- or 19-gauge angiocatheter. The large catheter promotes flow because the molecules of blood and its components are larger than the molecules of IV fluids. A large catheter also prevents hemolysis. The nurse should determine that the catheter is patent and functioning properly. The nurse should have the proper in-line filter and tubing for blood transfusion. The tubing should be primed with 0.9% normal saline to prevent hemolysis of red blood cells. Other solutions such as D5W (dextrose 5%) cause the red blood cells to swell and rupture because of the hypotonicity of the solution compared with whole blood or packed red blood cells.

Pretransfusion assessment also includes obtaining information from the client. The nurse asks whether the client knows the reason for the blood transfusion and whether the client has ever had a transfusion or a transfusion reaction. A client who has had a transfusion reaction is usually at no greater risk for a reaction with a subsequent transfusion. However, the client may be anxious about the transfusion, necessitating nursing intervention.

Pretransfusion assessment must include a baseline measurement of vital signs. These values must be recorded before the nurse gives any blood products because a change in vital signs can indicate a transfusion reaction.

When giving a transfusion, the nurse explains the procedure, asks the client to report any side effects, and makes sure the client has signed an informed consent. The nurse establishes the line, hangs a solution container of 0.9% normal saline for after the transfusion, and follows established procedures for obtaining blood products. The nurse, with another registered nurse, then checks the identity of the blood products, the client, and the compatibility of the blood and the client. Just before the transfusion the nurse monitors vital signs. The transfusion begins with a prime of the line with 0.9% normal saline, and the rate of infusion is begun slowly. The infusion is maintained, side effects monitored, and the transfusion recorded.

Clients with severe blood loss such as with a hemorrhage may receive rapid transfusions through a central venous pressure catheter. A blood warming device is often necessary because the tip of the central venous pressure catheter lies in the superior vena cava, above the right atrium. Rapid administration of cold blood can result in cardiac dysrhythmias (Querin and Stahl, 1983).

During blood infusion the client is at risk for a reaction, particularly during the first 15 minutes. Therefore the nurse should remain with the client and assess color and vital signs. The rate of a transfusion is usually specified in the physician's orders. Ideally a unit of whole blood or packed red blood cells is transfused in 2 hours. However, a client with a low fluid tolerance can have a transfusion over 4 hours (Querin and Stahl, 1983).

TRANSFUSION REACTIONS. A transfusion reaction is a systemic response by the body to blood incompatible with that of the recipient. It is caused by red cell incompatibility or allergic sensitivity to the leukocytes, the platelets, or the plasma protein components of the transfused blood or to the potassium or citrate preservative in the blood. Blood transfusion can also result in disease transmission.

Several types of reactions can result from blood transfusions. General adverse reactions (Table 37-7) range from immediate onset of fever, chills, and skin rash to hypotension, shock, and a delayed reaction that may not occur until several days or weeks after the transfusion.

A second category of reactions includes diseases transmitted by blood donors who are asymptomatic. Certain diseases transmitted through transfusions are malaria, hepatitis, and AIDS. Because all units of blood collected must undergo serological testing and AIDS screening, the risk of acquiring blood-borne infections from transfusions is reduced.

Correct administration of blood and blood products reduces the risk of transfusion reactions. The nurse, although not actually a participant in the blood labeling process, is responsible for determining that the blood delivered to the nursing unit corresponds to the client's blood type listed in the medical record. Two nurses should check the blood against the client's identification number, blood group, and complete name. If even a minor discrepancy exists, the blood should not be given and the blood bank laboratory should be notified.

In addition to allergic reactions and the transmission of illnesses, certain risks (hyperkalemia, hypocalcemia, and circulatory overload) are associated with blood transfusions.

Stored blood may cause hyperkalemia. Blood that is 1 day old has a plasma potassium content of approximately 7 mEq/L, and blood stored for 21 days has a plasma potassium content of 23 mEq/L (Metheny and Snively, 1983). The increase in potassium is related to the destruction of red blood cells. At the end of 21 days, about 20% to 30% of the cells are destroyed. Because the major intracellular cation is potassium, potassium enters the plasma as cells are destroyed. The potassium level of a client receiving several units of blood should be measured frequently. If the potassium level is elevated, the client should be given an ion exchange resin such as sodium polystyrene sulfonate (Kayexalate).

In some clients, blood infusion can result in hypocalcemia because of the action of the citrated blood as it combines with ionized calcium (Metheny and Snively, 1983). Two preservatives often added to blood, citrate-phosphate-dextrose and citrate-phosphate-dextrose-adenine, contain more citrate than is needed to combine with calcium in the blood collected for the transfusion. Therefore, when tranfused blood is infused into the bloodstream, the preservative combines with the ionized calcium, and tetany can result. The risk of hypocalcemia increases with the number of blood transfusions the client receives.

Iron overload (hemosiderosis) can occur in clients who receive frequent transfusions. One milliliter of blood contains 1 mg of iron (Mountcastle, 1979). Hemosiderosis is an abnormal desposit of iron in a variety of tissues, usually in the form of hemosiderin, an iron-rich pigment that is a product of red blood cell hemolysis. Clients at risk for hemosiderosis are those with illnesses involving chronic, extensive destruction of red blood cells, such as anemias, thalassemia major, or splenic dysfunction.

Circulatory overload is a risk when a client receives massive whole blood or packed red blood cell transfusions for hemorrhagic shock or when a client with normal blood volume receives blood. Clients particularly at risk for circulatory overload are the elderly and those with cardiopulmonary diseases.

Blood reactions are life-threatening but with a suspected reaction, some nursing actions can maintain the client's physiological stability. In the event of a suspected reaction, the nurse should do the following:
1. Stop the transfusion immediately.
2. "Piggyback" 0.9% normal saline into the IV line. The nurse should not turn off the blood and turn on the 0.9% normal saline on the Y-tubing infusion set, which will merely infuse the blood in the tubing into the client. Even a small amount of mismatched blood can cause a major reaction.
3. Notify the physician.
4. Remain with the client, observe signs and symptoms, and monitor vital signs every 5 minutes.
5. Prepare to administer emergency drugs, such as antihistamines, vasopressors, fluids, and steroids.
6. Prepare for CPR.
7. Obtain a urine specimen and send it to the laboratory.
8. Save the blood container and tubing for return to the laboratory.
9. Complete and necessary paperwork, such as reports about transfusion reaction and nurses' notes.

Although anaphylactic transfusion reactions are relatively rare, they can occur with any client. Correct administration of blood and blood products prevents reactions. When a client has a transfusion reaction, prompt nursing actions can decrease the severity of the response.

TABLE 37-7   Adverse Reactions to Blood Transfusions

Type	Cause	Onset	Signs or Symptoms	Nursing Actions
Febrile nonhemolytic (most common reaction; usually occurs in previous transfusion recipients or multiparous clients)	Antigen-antibody reaction to white blood cells or platelets contained in blood product	Immediately or within 6 hours after transfusion	Fever (with or without chills), headache, nausea and vomiting, nonproductive cough, hypotension, chest pain, dyspnea	Stop transfusion. Keep vein open. Notify physician and blood bank. Take vital signs p.r.n.
Allergic urticarial (generally innocuous)	Allergic reaction to plasma-soluble antigen contained in blood product	Anytime during transfusion or within 1 hour after transfusion	Skin rash	Slow transfusion to keep-vein-open rate. Notify physician and blood bank. Take vital signs p.r.n.
Delayed hemolytic (more common than acute hemolytic; frequently missed; occurs in previous transfusion recipients or multiparous clients)	Incompatibility of RBC antigens other than ABO group	Days to weeks after transfusion	Decreasing hemoglobin level, possible persistent lowgrade fever	Notify physician and blood bank.
Acute hemolytic (potentially life threatening)	ABO group incompatibility	Usually during first 5 to 15 minutes, but may occur any time during transfusion	*Mild form:* fever, chills, back pain, hypotension, nausea, vomiting, flushing, hematuria, oliguria *Severe form (in addition to above):* dyspnea, chest pain, anuria, shock, disseminated intravascular coagulation	Stop transfusion. Keep vein open. Notify physician and blood bank. Take vital signs p.r.n. Assess for signs and symptoms of shock. Monitor intake and output; check for decreased urinary output. Start resuscitative measures p.r.n.
Anaphylactic (extremely rare: potentially life threatening)	Idiosyncratic reaction in patients with immunoglobulin A (IgA) deficiency, sensitized to IgA through previous transfusion or pregnancy	Immediately (after transfusion of only few milliliters of blood)	Severe respiratory and cardiovascular collapse (with dyspnea and tachypnea, tachycardia, hypotension, and cyanosis), severe gastrointestinal disturbances (with nausea, vomiting, diarrhea, and cramping)	Stop transfusion. Keep vein open. Notify physician and blood bank. Take vital signs every 15 minutes (or p.r.n.) Start resuscitative measures p.r.n.

CORRECTING ACID-BASE IMBALANCES

Nursing interventions to promote acid-base balance are performed to support prescribed medical therapies. The nurse's knowledge of respiratory physiology also allows for dependent nursing activities to be performed. Because physicians often order a variety of drug therapies to correct acid-base imbalances, the nurse must maintain a functional IV line.

PROCEDURE 37-6

Arterial Puncture

STEPS	RATIONALE
1. Collect the following equipment and bring it to the bedside:	Permits quick and efficient performance.
a. Heparinized 5 ml syringe	Prevents coagulation of the arterial sample.
b. ⅝ in 20-gauge needle	Promotes atraumatic cannulization of artery.
c. Crushed ice for arterial blood sample	Decreases oxygen metabolism of the sample.
d. Local anesthetic	Reduces local pain when more than one attempt is necessary and reduces likelihood of arterial spasm.
e. Topical skin antibacterial scrub and alcohol wipes	Reduces the entry of surface bacteria into puncture site.
f. Air lock or cap for syringe	Prevents air from entering blood after sample has been obtained, thus altering the results of the blood gas analysis.
g. 2 × 2 gauze	Allows application of pressure after arterial puncture.
h. Disposable gloves	Reduces risk of exposure to HIV, hepatitis, and other blood-borne bacteria.
2. Check client's identity. Explain the procedure and the client's responsibility.	Ensures correct client undergoes procedure. Prevents hyperventilation due to anxiety and a resulting temporary change in blood gases.
3. Palpate the radial artery.	The radial artery is selected because it is superficially located, has collateral circulation, and is not adjacent to a large vein.
4. Hyperextend the client's wrist over a rolled towel.	Maintains the radial artery in a superficial position.
5. Wash hands. Apply disposable gloves.	Reduces risk of exposure to HIV, hepatitis, and other blood-borne bacteria.
6. **Cleanse the site** with a circular motion using providone-iodine followed by an alcohol wipe.	**Reduces the risk of skin bacteria entering puncture site.**
7. Apply local anesthetic. Xylocaine 2% is usually injected subcutaneously.	Anesthetic reduces pain and subsequent hyperventilation in some clients and decreases the likelihood of arterial spasm.
8. Flush a 5 ml syringe with 0.5 ml of 1:1000 heparin solution and then empty the syringe, leaving heparin in the needle (Metheny and Snively, 1983).	Heparin in the needle prevents clotting of blood sample. Excess heparin in the syringe affects the pH value of the sample blood.
9. Insert the needle at an angle while stabilizing the client's artery with your free hand (see illustration).	Minimizes formation of a hematoma at the puncture site.
10. Observe for a pulsating flow of blood into the syringe.	Indicates the puncture of an artery.
11. Withdraw 3 to 5 ml of blood.	Provides a sufficient amount for analysis.
12. Remove the needle and syringe from the artery. Cork the syringe with air lock. Be sure to expel any air in the syringe.	Prevents entry of air into syringe. If air enters the syringe, the blood must be discarded to avoid inaccurate blood gas results.
13. Rotate the syringe so blood mixes with heparin.	Prevents clotting of the sample.

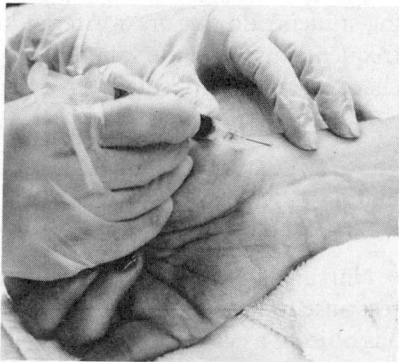

Step 9

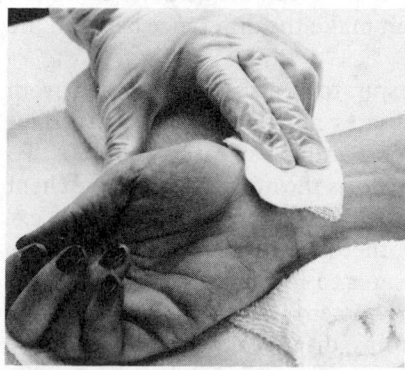

Step 16

Continued.

PROCEDURE 37-6, cont'd

Arterial Puncture

STEPS	RATIONALE
14. Submerge the syringe in crushed ice.	Reduces the rate of oxygen metabolism of the sampled blood.
15. Label the specimen with client's name, body temperature, and (for clients on oxygen therapy) inspired oxygen concentration.	Normally a 6% change in arterial Pao_2 occurs with each degree of centigrade of body temperature (Metheny and Snively, 1983). Measurement of oxygen concentration is important in evaluating the effectiveness of oxygen therapy.
16. Apply pressure to the puncture site by applying 2 × 2 gauze over the site and holding for 5 minutes. Length of time may be increased for clients receiving anticoagulants (see illustration).	Reduces the risk of hematoma formation and damage to the artery.
17. Discard equipment in appropriate container, remove and dispose of gloves, and wash hands.	Reduces transmission of microorganisms.
18. Record in nurses' notes time of arterial blood gas and from which extremity the specimen was drawn.	Documents arterial blood gas specimen was obtained.

The nurse should frequently check the physician's orders for new medications or fluids. The metabolic requirements for clients with acute acid-base disturbances continually change. Prescribed drugs, such as insulin or sodium bicarbonate, and fluid and electrolyte replacement should be given promptly. The physician usually gives written and oral orders to the nurse during the acute phase. To ensure communication, however, the nurse checks the client's chart hourly for new written orders. The nurse should evaluate the patency and functioning of the IV line at frequent intervals.

The nurse implements appropriate nursing measures to promote ventilation and oxygenation (see Chapter 36). This is particularly important for the client with respiratory acidosis. Stasis of pulmonary secretions and decreased lung expansion worsen the acidotic condition and in some clients can make the difference between life and death.

For clients with respiratory alkalosis resulting from anxiety, the nurse initiates nursing measures to reduce the anxiety after first correcting respiratory alkalosis. To correct respiratory alkalosis the nurse instructs the client to breathe into a paper bag so the client rebreathes exhaled carbon dioxide, thereby providing carbon dioxide that combines with water to form carbonic acid, which increases blood acidity. After the respiratory alkalosis is corrected, the symptoms disappear. At this point the nurse may be able to assist the client in determining the cause of anxiety and methods to control it. Some clients

with repeated anxiety attacks need professional counseling, and the nurse should make an appropriate and prompt referral.

The nurse develops interventions to protect the client from complications. Clients with acid-base disturbances usually require repeated arterial blood gas analysis. This procedure provides arterial blood samples for analysis of hydrogen ion concentration.

ARTERIAL BLOOD GASES. Arterial blood gas determinations require the removal of blood from an artery to determine acid-base status and adequacy of ventilation and oxygenation. Arterial blood gas samples are drawn from a peripheral artery, such as the radial artery, or from an arterial line. In some agencies, nurses are responsible for radial artery punctures. Beginning nursing students do not draw arterial blood gas samples but frequently assist in the sampling process and care for the client after the procedure (Procedure 37-6).

EVALUATION

Nursing interventions are evaluated by comparing the response to nursing therapies with each goal. Each goal has objective evaluation criteria. The criteria in the evaluation box are examples of expected outcomes based on the specific goals of care.

Sample Evaluation of Interventions for Fluid, Electrolyte, and Acid-Base Disturbances

Goals	Evaluative Measures	Expected Outcomes
Fluid and electrolyte balance are restored and maintained.	Inspect the skin for edema or dry, scaly skin. Palpate for poor skin turgor, absence of edema, or weak pulse. Inspect the oral cavity for dry, sticky mucous membranes, decreased saliva, or longitudinal furrows on tongue. Inspect for electrolyte imbalance such as weight loss or gain, Chvostek's sign, cardiac dysrhythmias, anuria, or oliguria. Auscultate for adventitious lung sounds or third heart sound. Obtain vital signs for tachycardia, bradycardia, hypotension, hypertension, or orthostatic hypotension. Obtain and observe for electrolyte imbalance, as evidenced by laboratory findings.	Vital signs return to baseline normals. Normal skin turgor returns. Edema is absent. Excessive weight loss or gain is absent. Lungs are clear. Serum electrolytes, arterial blood gases, and blood chemistry are normal.
Causes of imbalance are identified and corrected.	Observe for vomiting, diarrhea, or wound drainage. Observe for complications associated with fluid replacement. Obtain blood samples, and observe for electrolyte imbalances, as evidenced by laboratory findings.	Client experiences no vomiting or diarrhea. Client experiences no fluid losses. Serum electrolyte levels are normal.
Client has no complications from therapies needed to restore fluid, electrolyte, and acid-base balances.	Observe that correct type and amount of fluid has been given. Observe for patent intravenous catheter or needle as indicated by adequate blood return or absence of infiltration or inflammation. Palpate the venipuncture site for pain, swelling, erythema, or exudate. Inspect the IV infusion system for break in aseptic technique. Obtain vital signs and observe for signs of fluid overload or fluid deficit. Obtain and observe for electrolyte imbalance or abnormal glucose levels, as evidenced by laboratory findings.	Vital signs are normal (baseline). Serum electrolytes, arterial blood gases, and blood chemistry are normal. Signs of infection or infiltration at venipuncture site are absent. Signs of thrombus or phlebitis along access vein are absent. Correct fluid and rate are administered.

SUMMARY

Clients with altered fluid and electrolyte status require nursing care plans designed to assist in restoring normal fluid volume and electrolyte concentrations. The nurse restores fluid balance through oral fluid replacement, administration of IV fluids, or maintenance of fluid restrictions. Electrolytes can be given orally or parenterally. The nurse also treats underlying illness that may cause fluid and electrolyte imbalances.

Acid-base imbalances may result from a number of underlying illnesses. With minor imbalances, the body compensates by chemical, biological, and physiological regulatory mechanisms. With more severe imbalances, however, medical and nursing interventions are required because acid-base imbalances are life threatening. Each type of imbalance involves clinical signs and symptoms assessed by the nurse.

When providing care to clients with altered fluid, electrolyte, or acid-base balances, the nurse uses all components of the nursing process to maintain and restore balance. In so doing, the nurse continually monitors for changes in the client's status.

KEY CONCEPTS

✓ Body fluids are distributed in extracellular and intracellular fluid compartments.

✓ Body fluids are composed of electrolytes, minerals, cells, and water.

✓ Body fluids are regulated through fluid intake, output, and hormonal regulation.

✓ Intracellular fluid is the largest fluid compartment in the body.

✓ Acid-base balance depends on the hydrogen ion concentration in the blood.

✓ The body's chemical buffering system is the first system to respond to acid-base abnormalities.

✓ Biological buffering occurs when hydrogen ions are absorbed or released by the cells to compensate for acid-base imbalances.

✓ Physiological buffering involves compensatory responses in the lung or kidneys. Volume disturbances include fluid volume deficits and excesses.

✓ Chronic and severe, acute illnesses increase the risk for fluid, electrolyte, and acid-base imbalances.

✓ Very young or old clients are at greater risk for fluid, electrolyte, and acid-base imbalances.

✓ Assessment for fluid, electrolyte, and acid-base includes the nursing history, physical and behavioral assessment, measurements of intake and output, daily weighing, specific laboratory data such as CBCs and measurement of serum electrolytes, BUN, specific gravity, and arterial blood gases.

✓ Fluid deficits can be corrected by oral or parenteral administration of fluid.

✓ Complications of IV therapy include infiltration, phlebitis, fluid overload, and bleeding at the infusion site.

✓ Blood transfusions replace fluid volume loss resulting from hemorrhage, anemia, or coagulation disorders.

✓ Administration of blood or blood products requires the nurse to follow specific guidelines to prevent transfusion reactions.

✓ Careful monitoring of the client receiving a transfusion identifies potential transfusion reactions early.

✓ The risks of transfusion include transfusion reactions, hyperkalemia, hypocalcemia, circulatory overload, and blood-borne infections.

✓ Acid-base balance depends on the hydrogen ion concentration in the blood.

✓ Respiratory acidosis is characterized by increased carbon dioxide concentration, excess carbonic acid, and increased hydrogen ion concentration.

✓ Respiratory alkalosis is characterized by decreased carbon dioxide, and hydrogen ion concentrations.

✓ Metabolic acidosis is characterized by a rise in hydrogen ion concentration.

✓ Metabolic alkalosis is characterized by a decrease in hydrogen ion concentration.

✓ The goals of therapy for acid-base imbalances are treatment of the underlying illness and restoration of the arterial pH to normal.

REFERENCES

Axnick, KR, and Yarbrough, M: Infection control: an integrated approach, St. Louis, 1984, The C.V. Mosby Co.

Burch, G, Knochil, J, and Murphy, R: Stay on guard against heat syndromes, Patient Care 13:1, 1979.

Centers for Disease Control: Recommendations for prevention of HIV transmission in health care settings, MMWR 36(suppl. 25):3s, 1987.

Folk-Lightly, M: Solving the puzzles of patient's fluid imbalances, Nurs 84 14:34, 1984.

Groër, MW: Physiology and pathophysiology of the body fluids, St. Louis, 1981, The C.V. Mosby Co.

Guyton, AC: Textbook of medical physiology, ed. 6, Philadelphia, 1982, W.B. Saunders Co.

Kubo, WM, and Grant, MM: The syndrome of inappropriate secretion of antidiuretic hormone, Heart Lung 7:465, 1978.

Lane, G, and Pierce, AG: When persistence pays off, Nurs 82 12:44, 1982.

Messner, RL, and Gorse, GJ: Nursing management of peripheral intravenous sites, Focus Crit Care 14(2):25, 1987.

Metheny, NM: Overview of fluid and electrolyte balance: nursing considerations, Philadelphia, 1987, J.B. Lippincott Co.

Metheny, NM, and Snively, WD, Jr.: Nurse's handbook of fluid balance, ed. 4, Philadelphia, 1983, J.B. Lippincott Co.

Mountcastle, VC: Medical physiology, ed. 14, St. Louis, 1979, The C.V. Mosby Co.

Patrick, ML, et al.: Medical-surgical nursing: pathophysiological concepts, Philadelphia, 1986, J.B. Lippincott Co.

Querin, J, and Stahl, L: Twelve simple sensible steps for successful blood transfusions, Nurs 83 13:34, 1983.

Stroot, VR, Lee, CA, and Barrett, C: Fluid and electrolytes, ed. 3, Philadelphia, 1984, F.A. Davis Co.

Tomford, JW, Hershey, CO, McLakin, CE: Intravenous therapy team peripheral venous catheter-associated complications: a prospective controlled study, Arch Intern Med 144:1191, 1984.

ADDITIONAL READINGS

Centers for Disease Control: Guidelines for the prevention and control of nosocomial infections, MMWR 30, 1981.

Dennis, EMP: An ambulatory infusion pump for pain control: a nursing approach for home care. Canc Nurs 7:309, 1984.

Emminizer, S, Klopp, EH, and Haven, JM: Autotransfusion: current status, Heart Lung 10:83, 1981.

Feldstein, A: Detect phlebitis and infiltration, Nurs 86 16:44, 1986.

Goodman, MS, and Weekham, R: Venous access devices: an overview, Oncol Nurs Forum 11:16, 1984.

Groër, MW, and Shekleton, ME: Basic pathophysiology: a conceptual appraoch, ed. 2, St. Louis, 1983, The C.V. Mosby Co.

Harper, RA: A guide to respiratory care: physiology and clinical applications, Philadelphia, 1981, J.B. Lippincott Co.

Howard, M, Puri, V, and Paidiputy, B: The effects of fluid resuscitation in the critically ill patient, Heart Lung 13:649, 1984.

Jones, S: New IV catheters that can do it all, RN 48:20, 1985.

Kaye, W: Catheter- and infusion-related sepsis: the nature of the problem and its solution, Heart Lung, 11:221, 1982.

Keithley, JK, and Frauline, KE: What's behind that IV line? Nurs 82 12:33, 1982.

Keyes, JL: Fluid, electrolyte, and acid-base regulation, Belmont, Calif., 1985, Wadsworth Inc.

Klass, K: Troubleshooting central line complications, Nurs 87 87:58, 1987.

Lee, CA, Stroot, VR, and Schaper, CA: What to do when acid-base problems hang in the balance, Nurs 75 5:32, 1975.

Luce, JM, Tyler, ML, and Pierson, DJ: Intensive respiratory care, Philadelphia, 1984, W.B. Saunders Co.

Masoorli, ST, and Piercy, S: A life-saving guide to blood products, RN, 32, 1984.

Maxwell, M, and Klienan, C, editors: Clinical disorders of fluid and electrolyte metabolism, ed. 3, New York, 1980, McGraw-Hill Book Co.

Metheny, NM: Overview of fluid and electrolyte imbalances, NITA 4:38, 1981.

Metheny, NM: Nursing care of patients with syndrome of inappropriate antidiuretic hormone secretion, NITA 5:240, 1982.

Miller, D: Tips on drawing blood through a heparin lock, RN 49:22, 1986.

Pauley, SY: Transfusing therapy for nurses, II. NITA 8:51, 1985.

Popovsky, MA, and Taswell, HF: Role of IV and transfusion nurses in autologous transfusion, NITA 7:385, 1984.

Runquist, B, Aspina, J, and Hibbard, L: A new approach for problem IV dressings, RN 47:49, 1984.

Smith, LG: Reactions to blood transfusions, Am J Nurs 84:1096, 1984.

Whaley, LF, and Wong, DL: Nursing care of infants and children, ed 3, St. Louis, 1987, The C.V. Mosby Co.

Wiseman, M: Setting standards for home IV therapy, Am J Nurs 85:421, 1985.

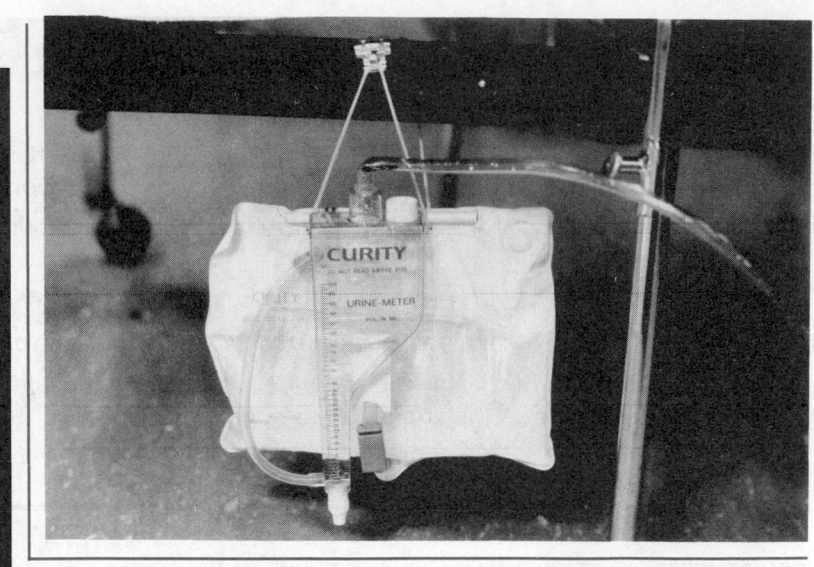

OBJECTIVES

Mastery of content in this chapter will enable the student to:

- Define the key terms listed.
- Explain the function of each organ in the urinary system.
- Describe the process of urination.
- Identify factors that commonly influence urinary elimination.
- Compare and contrast common alterations in urinary elimination.
- Obtain a nursing history for a client with urinary elimination problems.
- Identify nursing diagnoses appropriate for clients with alterations in urinary elimination.
- Obtain urine specimens.
- Describe characteristics of normal and abnormal urine.
- Describe the nursing implications of common diagnostic tests of the urinary system.
- Discuss nursing measures to promote normal micturition.
- Describe nursing measures to reduce episodes of incontinence.
- Insert a urinary catheter.
- Discuss nursing measures to reduce urinary tract infection.
- Irrigate a urinary catheter.

KEY TERMS

Anuria	Nephron
Bacteriuria	Neurogenic Bladder
Cystitis	Neuropathy
Diuresis	Nocturia
Dysuria	Oliguria
Endocrine	Polyuria
Enuresis	Reflux
Fistula	Renal
Glomerulus	Residual Urine
Glycosuria	Retroperitoneal
Hematuria	Ureterostomy
Ketonuria	Urgency
Meatus	Urinary Frequency
Micturition	Urinary Incontinence

Urinary Elimination

Normal elimination of urinary wastes is a basic function most people take for granted. When the urinary system fails to function properly, the cardiovascular, endocrine, and nervous systems can be affected. Clients with alterations in urinary elimination may also suffer emotionally from resulting body image changes. The nurse provides understanding and a sensitivity to clients' needs. With elderly clients in particular, the nurse must know the reasons for problems and find acceptable solutions.

PHYSIOLOGY OF URINE ELIMINATION

Urinary elimination depends on the function of four organs: kidneys, ureters, bladder, and urethra. Kidneys remove wastes from the blood and from urine. Ureters transport urine from the kidneys to the bladder. The bladder holds urine until the urge to urinate develops. Urine leaves the body through the urethra. All organs of the urinary system must be intact and functional for successful removal of urinary wastes (Fig. 38-1).

Kidneys

Kidneys are reddish brown, bean-shaped organs that lie on either side of the vertebral column behind the abdominal peritoneum and against deep muscles of the back. The kidneys rest at a level with the twelfth thoracic and third lumbar vertebrae. Normally the left kidney is

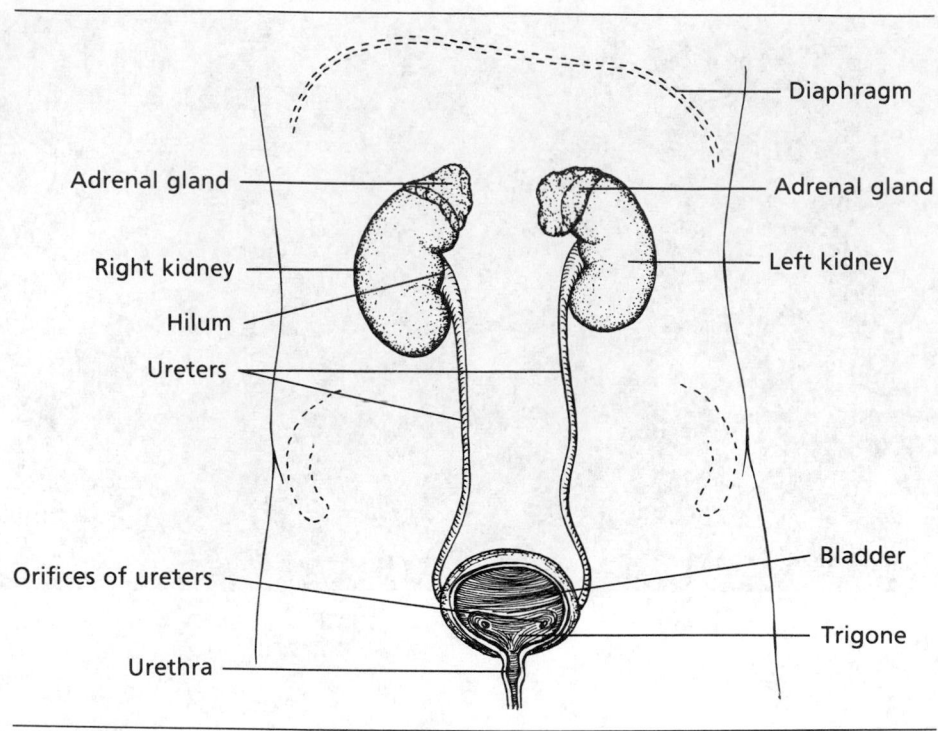

Fig. 38-1   Organs of the urinary system

1.5 to 2 cm (⁶/₁₀ to ⁸/₁₀ inch) higher than the right. Each measures about 12 cm by 7 cm and weighs 120 to 170 g. An adrenal gland lies on the superior pole of each kidney. Each kidney is covered by a tough capsule, surrounded by a cushion of fat.

The kidneys filter wastes that collect in the blood. Blood reaches each kidney by the renal artery that branches from the abdominal aorta. The renal artery enters the kidney at the hilum. Almost 20% to 25% of the body's cardiac output circulates daily through the kidneys. The kidney contains almost 1 million cells called nephrons. Each nephron, the functional unit of the kidney, is capable of forming urine. The nephron is composed of the glomerulus, Bowman's capsule, proximal convoluted tubule, loop of Henle, distal tubule, and collecting duct (Fig. 38-2).

Blood reaches nephrons by tiny arterioles. A cluster of blood vessels forms the glomerulus, which is the initial site of urine formation. The glomerular capillaries are porous and permit filtration of water and substances such as glucose, amino acids, urea, creatine, and major electrolytes into Bowman's capsule. Protein does not normally filter through the glomerulus. Protein in the urine (proteinuria) is a sign of glomerular injury. The glomerulus filters about 125 ml of filtrate per minute.

Not all of the glomerular filtrate is excreted as urine. Once the filtrate leaves the glomerulus, it passes through a system of tubules and collecting ducts where water

and substances such as glucose, amino acids, uric acid, and sodium and potassium ions are selectively reabsorbed back into the plasma. Other substances such as hydrogen ions, potassium ions, and ammonia are secreted back into the tubules. About 99% of the filtrate is reabsorbed into the plasma, with the remaining 1% comprising urine. Thus the kidneys play a key role in fluid and electrolyte balance. The normal adult 24-hour output of urine is about 1500 to 1600 ml. An output of 60 ml of urine per hour is generally normal. An output of less than 30 ml per hour may indicate renal alterations. This amount varies with food and fluid intake. The volume of urine formed at night is about half that formed during daytime, since intake and metabolism decline. Nocturia, or excessive urination at night, can be a sign of renal alteration. In a healthy person, the intake of water in food and fluids balances the output of water in urine, feces, and insensible losses in perspiration and respiration.

Ureters

Urine leaves the tubules and enters collecting ducts that transport it to the renal pelvis. A ureter joins each kidney pelvis for the initial exit route for urinary wastes. Ureters are long tubular structures, 25 to 30 cm (10 to 12 inches) long and 1.25 cm (½ inch) in diameter in the adult, extending down behind the peritoneum to join at

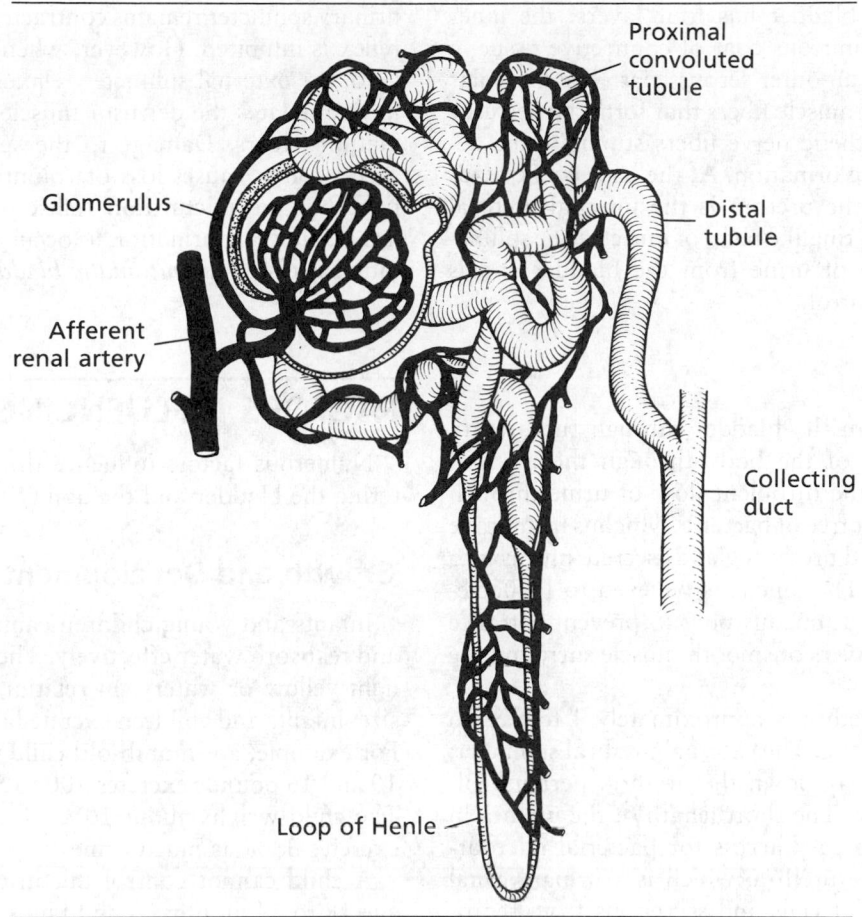

Glomerulus

Afferent
renal artery

Proximal
convoluted
tubule

Distal
tubule

Collecting
duct

Loop of Henle

Fig. 38-2   Renal nephron.

the floor of the bladder in the pelvic cavity. Urine drain-ing from the ureters to the bladder is sterile.

Three layers of tissue form the wall of the ureter. The inner layer is a mucous membrane continuous with the lining of the renal tubules and urinary bladder. The mu-cous lining is an excellent medium for growth and spread of microorganisms. The middle layer consists of smooth muscle fibers; it helps transport urine through the ureters by peristaltic waves stimulated by urine in the renal pelvis. An outer layer of fibrous connective tissue sup-ports the ureters.

Peristaltic waves cause the urine to enter the bladder in spurts rather than steadily. To prevent the reflux of urine from the bladder into the ureters, a small flaplike fold of mucous membrane acts as a valve and covers the juncture of the ureters with the bladder.

An obstruction within the ureters, such as a kidney stone (renal calculus), results in strong peristaltic waves that attempt to move the obstruction into the bladder. Simultaneously a reflex response causes the renal arte-rioles to constrict to reduce urine production in the kid-ney on the affected side.

Bladder

The urinary bladder is a hollow, distensible, muscular organ that is a reservoir for urine and the organ of excretion. When empty, the bladder lies in the pelvic cavity behind the symphysis pubis. In the male the blad-der lies against the rectum posteriorly, and in the female it rests against the anterior wall of the uterus and vagina.

The bladder's shape changes as it becomes filled with urine. The walls of the bladder can expand. Normally it holds approximately 600 ml of urine. Pressure within the bladder is usually low, a factor that protects against infection.

When the bladder is full, the superior surface expands up into a dome and pushes above the symphysis pubis. A greatly distended bladder may reach the umbilicus. In a pregnant women the fetus pushes against the bladder, causing a feeling of fullness and reducing the bladder's capacity.

At the base of the bladder is the trigone. An opening exists at each of the trigone's three angles: two at the base of the trigone for the ureters and one at the apex for the urethra.

The wall of the bladder has four layers: the inner mucous coat, a submucous coat of connective tissue, a muscular coat, and an outer serous coat. The muscular layer has bundles of muscle fibers that form the detrusor muscle. Parasympathetic nerve fibers stimulate the detrusor muscle during urination. At the base of the bladder where it joins the urethra is the internal urethral sphincter, made of a ringlike band of muscle. The sphincter prevents escape of urine from the bladder and is under voluntary control.

Urethra

Urine travels from the bladder through the urethra and passes outside of the body through the urethral meatus. Normally the turbulent flow of urine through the urethra washes it free of bacteria. Mucous membrane lines the urethra, and urethral glands secrete mucus into the urethral canal. The mucus is believed to be bacteriostatic and forms a mucous plug to prevent entrance of bacteria. Thick layers of smooth muscle surround the urethra.

In women the urethra is approximately 4 to 6.5 cm (1½ to 2½ inches) long. The external urethral sphincter, located about halfway down the urethra, permits voluntary flow of urine. The short length of the urethra in females provides an easy access for bacterial microorganisms. In men the urethra, which is a urinary canal and a passageway for cells and secretions from reproductive organs, is 20 cm (8 inches) long. It has three sections: the *prostatic urethra,* the *membranous urethra,* and the *penile urethra.*

In a female the urinary meatus is located between the labia minora, above the vagina and below the clitoris. In a male the meatus is located at the distal end of the penis.

Act of Urination

Urination, micturition, and voiding are all terms for the process by which urine is expelled from the urinary bladder. The bladder normally holds as much as 600 ml of urine. However, the desire to urinate can be sensed when the bladder contains only a small amount of urine (150 to 200 ml in an adult, 50 to 200 ml in a child). As the volume of urine increases, the bladder walls stretch, sending sensory impulses to the micturition center in the sacral spinal cord. Parasympathetic impulses from the micturition center stimulate the detrusor muscle to contract rhythmically. The internal urethral sphincter also relaxes so urine may enter the urethra, although voiding does not yet occur. As the bladder contracts, nerve impulses travel up the spinal cord to the midbrain and cerebral cortex. A person is thus conscious of the need to urinate. If the person chooses not to void, the external urinary sphincter remains contracted and the micturition reflex is inhibited. However, when a person is ready to void, the external sphincter relaxes, the micturition reflex stimulates the detrusor muscle to contract, and urination occurs. Damage to the spinal cord above the sacral region causes loss of voluntary control of urination, but the micturition reflex pathway may remain intact, allowing urination to occur reflexively. This condition is called an *automatic bladder.*

FACTORS INFLUENCING URINATION

Numerous factors influence the volume of urine entering the bladder and the ability to urinate.

Growth and Development

Infants and young children cannot concentrate urine and reabsorb water effectively. Their urine thus appears light yellow or watery. In relation to their small body size, infants and children excrete large volumes of urine. For example, a 6-month-old child who weighs between 10 and 16 pounds excretes 400 to 500 ml of urine daily. The child weighs about 10% of an adult's weight but excretes 33% as much urine.

A child cannot control micturition voluntarily until age 18 to 24 months. A child must be able to recognize the feeling of bladder fullness, to hold urine for 1 to 2 hours, and to communicate the sense of urgency to a parent. As in the case of toilet training for defecation, the young child needs a parent's understanding, patience, and consistency. A child may not gain full control of micturition until the age of 4 or 5. Boys are generally slower than girls. Daytime control of micturition is easier to accomplish than nighttime control and occurs earlier in the child's development, usually by 2 years of age.

The adult normally voids 1500 to 1600 ml of urine daily. The kidney is able to concentrate urine effectively, producing a normal amber-colored urine. A person does not void excessively during the night because of a reduction of renal blood flow during rest and because of the kidney's ability to concentrate urine.

The process of aging impairs micturition. Problems of mobility sometimes make it difficult for the elderly to reach a toilet in time. Elderly people may be too weak to rise from a toilet seat without assistance. Chronic neurological disease such as parkinsonism or cerebrovascular accident (stroke) impairs the sense of balance and makes it difficult for men to stand while voiding. If an elderly person loses control of thought processes, the ability to control micturition is unpredictable. The person may lose the ability to sense a full bladder or be unable to recall the procedure for voiding.

Changes in kidney and bladder function also occur with aging. The kidney's ability to concentrate urine declines. Thus the elderly often experience nocturia, excessive urination at night. The bladder loses its muscle tone and capacity to hold urine, resulting in increased frequency of urination. Because the bladder cannot contract as effectively, an elderly person often retains urine in the bladder after voiding. Residual urine increases the risk for bacterial growth and development of urinary infection.

Sociocultural Factors

Cultural and gender norms vary on the privacy of urination. North Americans expect toilet facilities to be private, whereas some European cultures accept communal toilet facilities. Social expectations (for example, school recesses) influence the time of urination.

The nurse's approach to a client's elimination needs must consider cultural and social habits. If a client prefers privacy, the nurse tries to prevent interruptions as the client voids. A client who is less sensitive to the need for privacy should be treated with understanding and acceptance.

Psychological Factors

Anxiety and emotional stress do not change the characteristics of urine, but may cause a sense of urgency and increase frequency of urination. An anxious person may have the urge to void even after voiding only a few minutes earlier.

Anxiety may also prevent a person from being able to urinate completely. Emotional tension makes it difficult to relax abdominal and perineal muscles. If the external urethral sphincter is not completely relaxed, voiding may be incomplete and urine retained in the bladder.

Personal Habits

Privacy and adequate time to urinate are usually important to most people. Some people need distractions (for example, reading) to relax.

Muscle Tone

Weak abdominal and pelvic floor muscles impair bladder contraction and control of the external urethral sphincter. Poor control of micturition can result from muscle wasting caused by prolonged immobility, stretching of muscles during childbirth, menopausal muscle atrophy, and damage to muscles from trauma.

Continuous drainage of urine through an indwelling catheter causes loss of bladder tone. The bladder remains relatively empty and thus is never stretched to capacity. When a muscle is not stretched regularly, atrophy develops. When a catheter is removed, the client may have difficulty regaining urinary control.

Fluid Intake

The kidneys maintain a sensitive balance between retention and excretion of fluids. If fluids and the concentration of electrolytes and solutes are in equilibrium, an increase in fluid intake causes an increase in urine production. Ingested fluids increase the body's circulating plasma and thus increase the volume of glomerular filtrate and urine excreted.

Ingestion of certain fluids has a direct influence on urine production and excretion. Alcohol inhibits the release of antidiuretic hormone (ADH) and thus promotes urine formation. Coffee, tea, cocoa, and cola drinks that contain caffeine increase diuresis and the frequency of micturition. Foods that contain a high fluid content, such as fruits and vegetables, may also increase urine production.

Disease Conditions

Several diseases affect the ability to micturate. Any lesion of peripheral nerves leading to the bladder causes loss of bladder tone, reduced sensation of bladder fullness, and difficulty in controlling urination. For example, diabetes mellitus and multiple sclerosis cause neuropathies that alter bladder function.

Diseases that slow or hinder physical activity interfere with the person's ability to void. Rheumatoid arthritis, degenerative joint disease, and parkinsonism are examples of conditions that make it difficult to reach and use toilet facilities. A client with rheumatoid arthritis often cannot sit on or rise from a toilet without an elevated seat.

Renal and bladder disease obviously affects micturition. Acute and chronic renal failure are caused by a variety of factors that alter function of the nephrons. Eventually reduced glomerular filtration and oliguria develop.

Irritation or inflammation of the bladder caused by infection or obstruction results in incomplete bladder emptying during micturition. Benign prostatic hypertrophy or enlargement of the prostate gland, a common condition in older men, results in obstruction to urine outflow and impairment of bladder tone.

Febrile conditions influence urine production. The client who becomes diaphoretic loses a large amount of fluids through insensible water loss, which decreases urine production. However, the increased body metabolism associated with fever increases accumulation of body wastes. Although urine volume may be reduced, it is highly concentrated.

Surgical Procedures

The stress of surgery initially triggers the general adaptation syndrome (see Chapter 28). The posterior pituitary gland releases an increased amount of ADH, which increases water reabsorption and reduces urine output. The surgical client is often in an altered state of fluid balance before surgery, which aggravates the reduction in urine output. The stress response also elevates the level of aldosterone, resulting in reduction in urine output in an effort to increase circulatory fluid volume.

Anesthetic agents and narcotic analgesics slow the glomerular filtration rate, reducing urine output. These pharmacological agents also impair sensory and motor impulses traveling between the bladder, spinal cord, and brain. Clients recovering from anesthesia and deep analgesia are often unable to sense bladder fullness and are unable to initiate or inhibit micturition. Spinal anesthetics, in particular, create the risk of urinary retention because of an inability to sense the need to void.

Surgery of lower abdominal and pelvic structures can impair urination because of local trauma to surrounding tissues. The edema and inflammation associated with healing may obstruct the flow of urine from the bladder or urethra, interfere with relaxation of pelvic and sphincter muscles, or cause discomfort during voiding. After surgery involving the bladder and urethra, clients routinely need urinary catheters.

The surgical formation of a ureterostomy (urinary diversion) either temporarily or permanently bypasses the bladder and urethra as the exit routes for urine. The client with a ureterostomy has a stoma on the abdomen to drain urine.

Medications

Diuretics prevent reabsorption of water and certain electrolytes to increase urine output. Urinary retention may be caused by use of anticholinergics (for example, atropine), antihistamines (for example, Sudafed), antihypertensives, (for example, Aldomet), and beta-adrenergic blockers (for example, Inderal). There are medications that change the color of urine (for example, amitriptyline turns it blue-green, cascara turns it yellow to red, indomethacin turns it green, and warfarin sodium [Coumadin] turns it orange).

Diagnostic Examinations

Examinations of the urinary system can influence micturition. Procedures such as an intravenous pyelogram or urogram require that the client not take fluids orally before the test. A restriction in fluid intake commonly lowers urine output. Diagnostic examinations (for example, cystoscopy) that involve direct visualization of urinary structures may cause localized edema of the urethral passageway and spasm of the bladder sphincter.

The client often has urinary retention following such a procedure and may pass red- or pink-tinged urine because of bleeding resulting from trauma to the urethral or bladder mucosa.

ALTERATIONS IN URINARY ELIMINATION

The most common urinary problems encountered by the nurse involve disturbances in the act of micturition. These disturbances result from impaired bladder function, obstruction to urine outflow, or inability to voluntarily control micturition. Some clients may have permanent or temporary changes in the normal pathway of urinary excretion. The ureterostomy client has special problems, since urine drains to the outside through an artificial opening (stoma) on the abdominal wall.

Urinary Retention

Urinary retention is accumulation of urine in the bladder with inability of the bladder to empty fully. Urine collects in the bladder, stretching its walls and causing feelings of pressure, discomfort, tenderness over the symphysis pubis, restlessness, and diaphoresis.

Urine production slowly fills the bladder and prevents activation of stretch receptors. After distending beyond a certain point the bladder becomes unable to contract.

A key sign is absence of urine output over several hours and formation of bladder distention. The client under the influence of anesthetics or analgesics may feel only pressure, but the alert client has severe pain as the bladder distends beyond its normal capacity. In severe urinary retention the bladder may hold as much as 2000 to 3000 ml of urine.

As retention progesses, *retention with overflow* may develop. Pressure in the bladder builds to a point that the external urethral sphincter is unable to hold back urine. The sphincter temporarily opens to allow a small volume of urine (25 to 60 ml) to escape. As urine exits, the bladder pressure falls enough to allow the sphincter to regain control and close. With retention overflow the client voids small amounts of urine two or three times an hour with no real relief of distention or discomfort. Bladder spasms may occur with voiding.

Retention occurs as a result of urethral obstruction, surgical trauma, alterations in motor and sensory innervation of the bladder, medication side effects, and anxiety.

Lower Urinary Tract Infections

Urinary tract infections account for 40% of hospital-acquired (nosocomial) infections in the United States (Burgener, 1987). Bacteria in the urine (bacteriuria) may lead to the spread of organisms into the bloodstream and kidneys.

Microorganisms can enter the urinary tract through the urethral meatus or through the bloodstream. The ascending route through the urethra is more common. Bacteria inhabit the distal urethra, external genitalia, and vagina in women. Organisms enter the urethral meatus easily and travel up the inner mucosal lining to the bladder. Women are more susceptible to infection because of the proximity of the anus to the urethral meatus and because of the female's short urethra. In the male, prostatic secretions contain an antibacterial substance that reduces urinary tract infection. Th elderly and clients with progressive underlying disease are also at risk.

In a healthy person with good bladder function, organisms are flushed out during voiding. However, bladder distention reduces blood flow to the mucosal and submucosal layer, and tissues become more susceptible to bacteria. Residual urine in the bladder is an ideal site for microorganism growth. The pH and chemical makeup of urine also affect the spread of organisms.

The most common cause of infection is urinary tract instrumentation. For example, the introduction of a catheter or diagnostic instrument through the urethra provides a direct route for microorganisms. With an indwelling bladder catheter, bacteria ascend along the outside of the catheter on the urethral wall or travel up the catheter's lumen. The catheter interferes with the normal voiding mechanism that acts as a defense against organisms entering the urethra. Local irritation to the urethra or bladder further predisposes tissues to bacterial invasion.

Urinary tract infections acquired in health institutions also result from contaminated hands of personnel, irrigation fluids, and rectal thermometers.

Poor perineal hygiene is a common cause of urinary tract infection in females. Inadequate handwashing, failure to wipe from front to back after voiding or defecating, and frequent sexual intercourse predispose females to urinary tract infection. In some young girls cystitis develops due to exposure to ingredients in bubble baths or shampoo used in the bathtub (Rogers, 1986). Any interference with the free flow of urine can cause infection. A kinked or obstructed catheter and any condition resulting in urinary retention can cause infection of the bladder.

Clients with urinary tract infections have pain or burning during urination (dysuria) as urine flows past inflamed tissues. Fever, chills, nausea and vomiting, and malaise develop as the infection worsens. An irritated bladder causes a frequent and urgent sensation of the need to void. Irritation to bladder and urethral mucosa results in blood-tinged urine (hematuria). The urine appears concentrated and cloudy because of the presence of bacteria. If infection spreads to the kidneys, flank pain, tenderness, low-grade fever, and chills are common symptoms.

Urinary Incontinence

Urinary incontinence is the loss of control over micturition. It may be temporary or permanent. The client cannot control the external urethral sphincter. Leakage of urine may be continuous or intermittent. The five types of incontinence are total, functional, stress, reflex, and urge (Table 38-1).

Incontinence should not be associated only with the elderly and senile. It may develop in people of every age, although it is more common in adults. Incontinence causes a person to feel like a social outcast. Clothing becomes wet with urine, and the accompanying odor adds to embarrassment. Clients with this problem often avoid social activities for fear of an episode occurring.

The elderly have special problems with incontinence because of physical limitations and the environment in which they live. An elderly person with restricted mobility has a greater chance of being incontinent because of inability to reach toilet facilities in time. Low-set chairs and beds raised well above the floor may be obstacles for the elderly who must get up to reach a toilet. An elderly client who has difficulty undoing buttons or manipulating zippers faces another obstacle. The elderly client often lacks the energy to walk very far at one time, and if there is only one toilet in the home, the distance may be too far for the client with urge incontinence.

Continued episodes of incontinence create the potential for skin breakdown. The acidic character of urine is irritating to skin. The immobilized client who has frequent incontinence is especially at risk for decubitus ulcers.

Enuresis

Enuresis is repeated involuntary urination in children who have reached the age when voluntary control is possible. Usually this is around age 5 (Whaley and Wong, 1987).

Episodes occur more commonly at night (nocturnal enuresis), usually during deep sleep (see Chapter 34). Enuresis may occur during the day (diurnal enuresis) when the child is engaged in play and unaware of a full bladder. Some children are enuretic during a temper tantrum or dispute with a sibling or playmate.

Primary enuresis means that the child has never had a long dry or symptom-free period. *Secondary* or *acquired enuresis* occurs after a dry period of at least a year.

Theories explaining the cause of enuresis include heredity, delayed development, sibling rivalry, emotional trauma during toilet training, food allergies, and behavior problems.

TABLE 38-1 Types of Urinary Incontinence

Type	Description	Causes	Symptoms
Total	Total uncontrollable and continuous loss of urine	Neuropathy of sensory nerves, trauma or disease of spinal nerves or urethral sphincter, fistula between bladder and vagina	Constant flow of urine at unpredictable times, nocturia, unawareness of bladder filling or incontinence
Functional	Involuntary unpredictable passage of urine in client with intact urinary and nervous systems	Change in environment, and sensory, cognitive, or mobility deficits	Strong urge to void causes loss of urine before reaching appropriate receptacle
Stress	Increased intraabdominal pressure causes leakage of small amount of urine	Coughing, laughing, vomiting, or lifting with full bladder, obesity, third trimester uterus, incompetent bladder outlet, weak pelvic musculature	Dribbling of urine with increased intraabdominal pressure, urinary urgency and frequency
Urge	Involuntary passage of urine following a strong sense of urgency to void	Decreased bladder capacity, irritation of bladder stretch receptors, alcohol or caffeine ingestion, increased fluid intake	Urinary urgency, abnormal frequency (more often than every 2 hours), bladder contracture or spasm, nocturia, voiding in small (less than 100 cc) or in large (more than 550 cc) amounts
Reflex	Involuntary loss of urine occurs at somewhat predictable intervals when a specific bladder volume is reached	Upper spinal cord injury or disease involving area above reflex arc, blocking cerebral awareness. Lower spinal cord injury blocks impulses to the reflex arc	Unawareness of bladder filling, no urge to void, uninhibited bladder contraction/spasm at regular intervals

The condition tends to be more common in boys and in children of lower socioeconomic families. Bed wetting is more often seen in children who live in homes with poor cleanliness habits.

Urinary Diversions

A urinary stoma to divert the flow of urine from the kidneys directly to the abdominal surface is done for several reasons (see box). A urinary diversion may be temporary or permanent. Fig. 38-3 illustrates several urinary diversions.

The ileal loop or conduit involves separating a loop of intestinal ileum with its blood supply intact. The surgeon implants the ureters into the ileum, which is an outlet for urine drainage. The ileum is not a reservoir. The remaining ileum is reconnected to the rest of the digestive tract. The disadvantage is that, if urine outflow becomes obstructed, the ileal conduit absorbs fluids and electrolytes and can cause metabolic alterations.

A ureterostomy involves bringing the end of one or both ureters to the abdominal surface. To avoid the need for two collecting devices, a transureteroureterostomy

---

Possible Indications for Urinary Diversions

- Cancer of the bladder, prostate, urethra, vagina, uterus, or cervix
- Trauma
- Radiation injury to the bladder
- Vesicovaginal fistula
- Urethrovaginal fistula
- Neurogenic bladder
- Chronic cystitis
- Chronic urinary incontinence that is unmanageable by conservative means

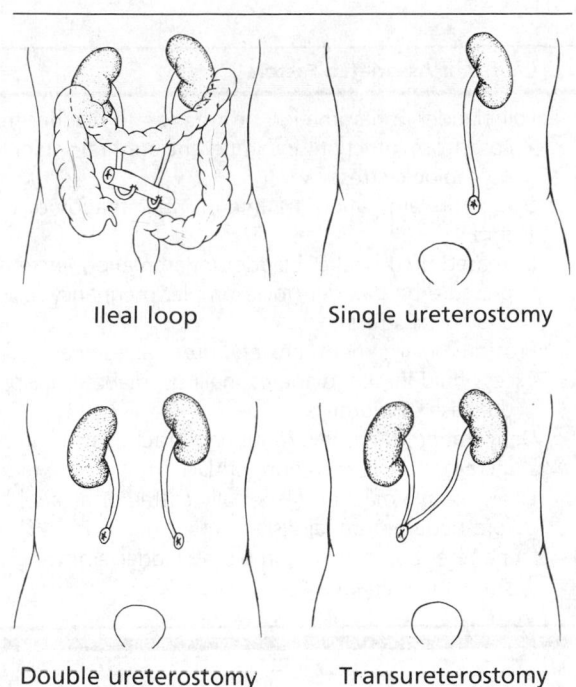

Fig. 38-3 Types of urinary diversions.

Ileal loop   Single ureterostomy

Double ureterostomy   Transureterostomy

connects the ureters and brings one out through the abdominal wall.

The client with a urinary diversion must wear a stomal pouch continuously because there is no sphincter control for regulation of urine flow. Local irritation and skin breakdown occur when urine comes in contact with the skin for long periods.

A urinary diversion poses threats to a client's body image. The client must wear an artificial device to collect urine, and must learn to manage it. However, the client can wear normal clothing, engage in physical activity, travel, and have sexual relations.

ASSESSMENT

To identify a client's urinary elimination problem and gather data for a care plan, the nurse obtains a nursing history, performs a physical assessment, assesses the client's urine, and reviews information from diagnostic tests and examinations.

Nursing History

The nursing history includes a review of the client's elimination patterns and symptoms of urinary altera-

tions, as well as an assessment of factors that may be affecting the ability to urinate normally.

1. Pattern of urination—Ask the client about daily voiding patterns including frequency and times of day, normal volume at each voiding, and history of recent changes. Frequency varies among individuals. The common times for urination are on awakening, following meals, and before bedtime. Most people void an average of 5 or more times a day. The client who voids frequently during the night may have renal disease. Information about the pattern of urination is necessary to establish a baseline of comparison.

2. Symptoms of urinary alterations—Certain symptoms specific to urinary alterations may occur in more than one type of disorder. During an assessment the nurse asks the client about the symptoms listed in Table 38-2. The nurse also assesses if the client is aware of conditions or factors that precipitate or aggravate symptoms.

3. Factors affecting urination—The nurse summarizes factors in the client's history that normally affect urination such as:

   a. Medication history, including over-the-counter drugs.

   b. Environmental barriers at home or health care setting. Client may need elevated toilet seat, grab bars, portable commode.

   c. Sensory restrictions such as clients with visual problems who may have trouble reaching toilet facilities. If the client has difficulty with hand coordination, the nurse assesses the type of clothing and ease in using clothing fasteners.

   d. Past illness such as urinary tract infection or surgery increases the risk for recurrent problems. Chronic diseases (for example, multiple sclerosis) that impair bladder function require the nurse to consider preventive care measures. Clients returning from surgery often have difficulty voiding the first few hours until the effects of anesthesia disappear.

   e. Presence of urinary diversion. If the client has a urinary diversion, the nurse assesses its location, function, condition of surrounding skin, and usual methods for management (type of appliance or pouch, type of skin barriers or applications, methods used to reduce skin irritation, frequency of appliance changes, and the type of nighttime drainage system).

   f. Personal habits. If a client becomes hospitalized the nurse assesses the extent to which personal habits are altered. Privacy is often difficult to accomplish in a health care setting, particularly if a client must use a bedpan.

   g. Presence of indwelling catheter. Clients recovering from major surgery and those suffering critical

TABLE 38-2 Common Symptoms of Urinary Alterations

Symptoms	Description	Causes or Associated Factors
Urgency	The feeling that a person needs to void immediately	Full bladder, inflammation or irritation to bladder mucosa from infection, incompetent urethral sphincter, psychologic stress
Dysuria	Painful or difficult urination	Bladder inflammation, trauma or inflammation of urethra
Frequency	Voiding at frequent intervals	Increased fluid intake, bladder inflammation, increased pressure on bladder (for example, pregnancy, psychological stress)
Hesitancy	Difficulty initiating urination	Prostate enlargement, anxiety, urethral edema
Polyuria	Voiding a large amount of urine	Excess fluid intake, diabetes mellitus, diabetes insipidus, use of diuretics
Oliguria	Diminished urinary output in relation to fluid intake	Dehydration, renal failure, urinary tract obstruction, increased ADH secretion (SIADH)
Nocturia	Urination, particularly excessive, at night	Excess intake of fluids (especially coffee or alcohol before bedtime), renal disease
Dribbling	Leakage of urine despite presence of voluntary control of micturition	Urine retention from incomplete bladder emptying, stress incontinence

illness or disability often have an indwelling catheter to aid urinary drainage and provide a measurement of urine output. Presence of a catheter places a client at risk for infection.

h. Fluid intake. A client's physical condition will affect the frequency with which the nurse monitors fluid intake (see Chapter 37). Regular intake and output measurements help assess a client's overall fluid balance.

Physical Assessment

It is important for the nurse to assess skin integrity. Often problems with urinary elimination are associated with fluid and electrolyte disturbances. The nurse assesses the skin's hydration status by noting texture and turgor. Assessment of the oral mucosa also reveals whether the client's hydration is adequate (see Chapter 37). To assess urinary function the nurse examines the kidneys, bladder, and urethral meatus (see Chapter 13).

KIDNEYS

The only way to assess the position, shape, and size of kidneys is by deep palpation of the abdomen. Much practice is needed to become adept at kidney palpation.

If the kidneys become infected or inflamed, flank pain typically develops. The nurse can assess for flank tenderness early in the disease by percussing the costovertebral angle (the angle formed by the spine and twelfth rib). Inflammation of the kidney results in pain during percussion.

BLADDER

Normally the bladder rests below the symphysis pubis and cannot be examined by the nurse. When distended, the bladder rises above the symphysis pubis at the midline of the abdomen and just below the umbilicus. During physical assessment the nurse may note a swelling or convex curvature of the lower abdomen. When distention is not visible, the nurse lightly palpates the lower abdomen. The bladder normally feels smooth and rounded. As the nurse applies light pressure to the bladder, the client may feel tenderness or even pain. Palpation may also cause the urge to urinate. Percussion of a full bladder yields a dull percussion note.

URETHRAL MEATUS

The female client assumes a dorsal recumbent position to provide full exposure of the genitalia. The nurse uses the nondominant hand to retract the labial folds to see the urethral meatus. Normally the meatus is pink and appears as a small slitlike opening below the clitoris and above the vaginal orifice. There is normally no discharge from the meatus. Drainage may indicate infection. The nurse notes its color and consistency. A clear watery drainage is likely to be urine.

Women with vaginal infections are susceptible to urinary tract infections because the vaginal discharge may travel easily to the urethral meatus. Elderly women commonly have vaginitis as a result of hormonal deficiencies. The nurse inspects the vaginal orifice carefully and describes any drainage. Infection is indicated by reddened, inflamed vaginal mucosa.

The male's urethral meatus is normally a small opening at the tip of the penis. A hypospadias is a congenitally formed opening of the urethra on the undersurface of the penis. The nurse inspects the meatus for discharge and inflammation. It may be necessary to retract the foreskin in uncircumcised males to see the meatus.

Assessment of Urine

Assessment of urine involves measuring the client's fluid intake and urine output and observing characteristics of the client's urine.

INTAKE AND OUTPUT

The nurse assesses the client's average daily fluid intake. If a precise measurement of fluid intake is needed from the client who is at home, the nurse may ask the client to show a commonly used glass or cup on which the intake estimate is based.

In a health care setting the nurse measures a client's fluid intake when the physician orders intake and output measurements (see Chapter 37). The nurse includes all sources, including oral intake, intravenous fluid infusions, tube feedings, and fluid instilled into nasogastric tubes.

Because it is often difficult for the client to estimate volumes of urine voided, the nurse must obtain measurements. A change in urine volume is a significant indicator of fluid imbalance or kidney disease. While caring for the client, the nurse assesses volume by measuring (with plastic receptacles, bedpans or urinals, or a catheter bag) urinary output with each voiding. Special urimeters attach between indwelling catheters and drainage bags and are a convenient means of measuring urine volume on a regular basis (Fig. 38-4). A urimeter holds 100 to 200 ml of urine. After measuring urine from a urimeter, the nurse can drain the cylinder into the urinary drainage bag or into a receptacle for disposal.

When urine from a drainage bag is measured, it is best to use a separate plastic graduate receptacle. Scales on the bags offer only an approximate volume.

With the normal daily urinary output being about 1500 to 1600 ml, the nurse reports any extreme increase or decrease in volume. A repeated hourly output of less than 30 ml is cause for concern. Similarly, high volumes of urine, over 2000 ml daily, should be reported to a physician.

CHARACTERISTICS OF URINE

The nurse inspects the client's urine for color, clarity, and odor.

COLOR. Normal urine ranges from a pale, straw color to amber, depending on its concentration. Urine is usually more concentrated in the morning. As the person drinks more fluids, urine becomes less concentrated.

Bleeding from the kidneys or ureters causes urine to become dark red; bleeding from the bladder or urethra causes a bright red urine. Various drugs also change urine color (see box). Beets, rhubarb, and blackberries may cause red urine. Special dyes used in intravenous diagnostic studies eventually discolor urine. Dark amber urine may be the result of high concentrations of bilirubin caused by jaundice of the liver. Urine containing bilirubin can be detected by the appearance of yellow

---

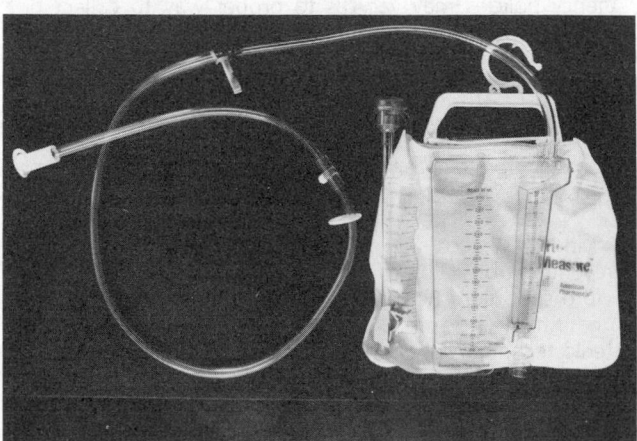

Fig. 38-4 Urimeter.

Examples of Drugs that Discolor Urine

YELLOW URINE

- Cascara
- Vitamin B_2
- Phenacetin

ORANGE URINE

- Azo Gantrisin
- Sulfonamides

PINK OR RED URINE

- Thorazine
- Ex-Lax
- Phenytoin (Dilantin)

GREEN OR BLUE-GREEN URINE

- Amitriptyline (Elavil)
- Vitamin B complex

BROWN OR BLACK URINE

- Injectable iron compounds
- Levodopa (L-dopa)
- Nitrofurantoin

Collecting a Midstream (Clean-Voided) Specimen

STEPS	RATIONALE

1. Assess client's mobility and balance in being able to use toilet facilities independently.

   Determines level of assistance required by client.

2. Refer to medical record for indications of urinary infection.

   Helps nurse understand purpose of specimen procedure for client.

3. Assess client's understanding of purpose of test and method of collection.

   Information allows nurse to clarify misunderstandings and promotes client's cooperation.

4. Prepare following equipment and supplies:

   Agency policy may determine type of equipment to use.

   a. Commercial kit for clean-voided urine (see illustration), sterile cotton balls, or 2 × 2 inch gauze pads

   Used to clean, rinse, and dry perineum.

   b. Antiseptic solution such as povidone-iodine

   c. Sterile water

   Rinses antiseptic solution. Antiseptic solution can alter test results if allowed to enter specimen.

   d. Sterile gloves
   e. Sterile specimen container
   f. Soap, towel, washcloth

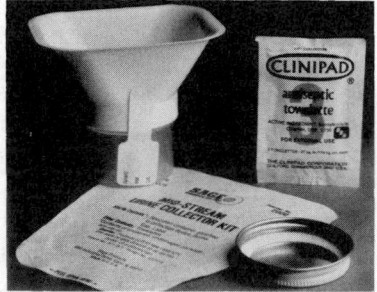

Step 4a

   g. Bedpan (for nonambulating clients), specimen hat, bedside commode, or potty chair

   Allows women to void in toilet seat in usual fashion. Children more likely to use familiar facilities.

   h. Completed specimen identification label
   i. Completed laboratory requisition form

   Completion of label and requisition before collecting specimen prevents confusing it with other specimens and ensures more rapid transport to laboratory.

5. Explain procedure to client:
   a. Reason midstream specimen is needed

   Helps client provide specimen independently.

   b. How client/family member can assist
   c. How to obtain specimen free of feces

   Feces change characteristics of urine and may cause abnormal values.

6. Provide client fluids to drink ½ hr before collecting specimen.

   Improves likelihood of client being able to void.

7. Refer to agency procedures for specimen collection methods.

   Agency policies may vary as to proper way to collect or handle specimens.

8. Wash hands.

   Reduces transfer of infection.

9. Provide privacy for client who will give specimen in bed by closing curtain around bed or closing room door.

   Privacy allows client to relax and produce a specimen more quickly.

10. Give client or family member towel, washcloth, and soap to cleanse perineal area or assist client as needed to cleanse perineum.

    Clients prefer to wash their own perineal area whenever possible.

11. Assist bedridden client onto bedpan.

    Provides easy access to perineal areas to collect specimen.

12. Put on sterile gloves (see Chapter 43).

    Prevents introduction of microorganisms on nurse's hands into specimen. Reduces risk of transmission of microorganisms to nurse.

13. Using surgical asepsis, open sterile kit or prepare sterile tray.

    Sterile technique is essential to maintain sterility of equipment and specimen.

14. Pour antiseptic solution over cotton balls unless kit contains prepared gauze pads in antiseptic solution.

    Cotton ball or gauze is used to cleanse perineum.

15. Open specimen container and place cap with sterile inside surface up and do not touch inside of container.

    Contaminated specimen is most frequent reason for inaccurate reporting of urinary cultures and sensitivities.

STEPS	RATIONALE

16. Assist or allow client to independently cleanse perineum and collect specimen:
  a. For a male:
    (1) Hold penis with one hand and using circular motion and antiseptic swab, cleanse end of penis, moving from center to outside.
	Cleanse from area of least contamination to area of greatest contamination to decrease bacterial levels.

(2) If agency procedure indicates, rinse area with sterile water and dry with cotton balls or gauze pad.	Prevents contamination of specimen with antiseptic solution.
(3) After client has initiated urine stream, pass specimen container into stream and collect 30-60 ml.	Initial urine flushes out microoogranisms that normally accumulate at urinary meatus and prevents their collection in specimen.
b. For a female: (1) Spread labia minora with thumb and forefinger of nondominant hand.	Provides access to urethral meatus.
(2) Cleanse area with cotton ball or gauze, moving from front (above urethral orifice) to back (toward anus). Repeat this movement 3 times (left side, right side, and center), using separate cotton balls.	Prevents contamination of urinary meatus with fecal material.
(3) If agency procedure indicates, rinse area with sterile water, and dry with cotton.	Prevents contamination of specimen with antiseptic solution.
(4) While continuing to hold labia apart, client should initiate stream and after stream achieved, pass specimen container into stream and collect 30-60 ml.	Initial stream flushes out microorganisms that accumulate at urethral meatus.
17. Remove specimen container before flow of urine stops and before releasing labia or penis. Client finishes voiding into bedpan or toilet.	Prevents contamination of specimen with skin flora.
18. Replace cap securely on specimen container (touch only outside).	Retains sterility of inside of container and prevents spillage of urine.
19. Cleanse any urine from exterior surface of container.	Prevents transfer of microorganisms to others.
20. Remove gloves, dispose in proper receptacle.	Prevents transfer of microoogranisms.
21. Remove bedpan (if applicable) and assist client to comfortable position.	Promotes relaxing environment.
22. Wash hands.	Reduces transmission of infection.
23. Label specimen and attach laboratory requisition.	Prevents inaccurate identification that could lead to errors in diagnosis or therapy.
24. Take specimen to laboratory within 15 minutes or immediately refrigerate.	Bacteria grow quickly in urine and the specimen should be analyzed immediately to obtain correct results.
25. Record date and time urine specimen was obtained in nurse's notes.	Documents implementation of physician's order.

foam when a specimen is shaken. The nurse reports any abnormal color to the physician, especially if the cause is unknown.

CLARITY . Normal urine appears transparent at the time of voiding. Urine that stands several minutes in a container becomes cloudy. Freshly voided urine in clients with renal disease may appear cloudy because of protein concentration. Urine also appears thick and cloudy as a result of bacteria.

ODOR. Urine has a characteristic odor. The more concentrated the urine, the stronger the odor. Bacteria in the urine causes an ammonia odor which is common in clients who are repeatedly incontinent. A sweet or fruity odor occurs from acetone or acetoacetic acid, by-products of incomplete fat metabolism, seen with diabetes mellitus or starvation.

URINE TESTING

The nurse is frequently responsible for collecting urine specimens for laboratory testing. The type of test determines the method of collection. All specimens are labeled with the client's name, date, and time of collection.

SPECIMEN COLLECTION

Random Specimen. A random routine urine specimen can be collected with a client voiding naturally or through a Foley catheter or urinary diversion collection bag. The specimen should be clean but need not be sterile. Random specimens are used for urinalysis testing or measurements of specific gravity, pH, or glucose.

The client voids into a clean urine cup, urinal, or bedpan. Many clients are able to do this independently. However, mobility restrictions or poor vision may require the nurse to assist. It is easier to collect a specimen if the client drinks a glass of fluid 30 minutes before the procedure. A client should void before defecating so that feces do not contaminate the specimen. Female clients are also instructed not to place toilet tissue in the bedpan. Only 120 ml (4 oz) of urine is needed for accurate testing.

Once the specimen is collected the nurse places the lid tightly on the specimen container, washes off any urine that splashed on the outside of the container, places the container in a paper or plastic bag, and sends the labeled specimen promptly to the laboratory.

Clean-Voided or Midstream Specimen. To obtain a specimen relatively free of the microorganisms growing in the lower urethra, the nurse instructs the client on the method for obtaining a clean-voided specimen (Procedure 38-1). This type of specimen is needed to test urine for culture and sensitivity. A client begins the urinary stream and then during the middle portion of voiding collects the specimen. The initial stream of urine cleans or flushes the urethral orifice and meatus of resident bacteria. It is easiest for clients to obtain clean-voided specimens while using toilet facilities.

Sterile Specimen. Another method for collecting a urine specimen for culture is by obtaining it from an indwelling catheter. It is no longer recommended to catheterize a client just to obtain a specimen, since the risk of causing an infection is high. A urine specimen is also not collected for culture from urine drainage bags unless it is the first urine drained into a new sterile bag. Bacteria grow rapidly in drainage bags and would give a false measurement of bacteria.

For an indwelling retention catheter, the nurse uses a sterile syringe to withdraw urine. The nurse washes hands and applies nonsterile gloves to prevent transmission of microorganisms. A 3 ml syringe with a small-gauge needle (23- or 25-gauge) is best to prevent creation of a hole in the catheter port. However, if blood is suspected in the urine, a large-bore needle prevents breakdown of red blood cells. It is safe to insert a needle directly into the end of a self-sealing rubber catheter. Silastic, plastic, or silicone catheters are not self-sealing. Most urinary catheters have special ports to withdraw specimens. First the nurse clamps the tubing just below the site chosen for withdrawal, allowing fresh, uncontaminated urine to collect in the tube. The nurse then wipes the catheter or port with a disinfectant swab. Inserting the needle at a 30-degree angle ensures entrance into the catheter lumen. While aspirating 3 to 5 ml of urine the nurse must be careful not to raise the tubing, which would cause urine to flow back into the bladder.

After obtaining the specimen the nurse transfers the urine into a sterile container using sterile aseptic technique. The nurse removes the gloves, properly disposes of equipment, and washes hands to reduce the transfer of microorgansims to other clients and health care workers. The laboratory requisition should indicate how the specimen was collected.

Timed Urine Specimens. Some tests of renal function and urine composition, such as measuring levels of adrenocortical steroids and hormones and creatinine clearance tests, require collection of urine over 2, 12, or 24 hour intervals.

The timed collection period begins after the client urinates. The nurse indicates the starting time on the gallon container and on the laboratory requisition, and discards the first sample (check agency policy). The client then collects all urine voided in the timed period.

Each voiding is collected in a clean container and immediately emptied into the larger gallon container. Some tests require the client to void at specific times. Each specimen must be free of feces or toilet tissue.

Any missed specimens will make test results inaccurate. The nurse should remind the client to void before defecating so that urine is not contaminated by feces. The collection jar usually contains a preservative or requires refrigeration. The laboratory should be consulted for instructions. The client should void the last specimen as close as possible to the end of the timed period.

Double-Voided Specimen. For accurate measurement of glucose and ketones in the urine the specimen must be "fresh." Urine that has been in the bladder for several hours does not reveal the amount of glucose and ketones in the urine at the time of testing. Ideally the client voids 30 to 45 minutes before the time a test specimen is required. The nurse discards the first specimen and then has the client drink at least 8 ounces of fluid. The client then voids a second or double-voided specimen for testing. The second specimen accurately reflects composition of urine recently filtered by the kidneys.

Urine Collection in Children. Specimen collection from infants and children is often difficult. Adolescents and school-age children are usually able to cooperate, although they may be embarrassed. Preschool children and toddlers have difficulty voiding on request. Offering a young child fluids 30 minutes before requesting a specimen may help. The nurse must use terms for urination that the child can understand. A young child may be reluctant to void in unfamiliar receptacles. A potty chair or bedpan placed under the toilet is usually effective. The nurse must use special collection devices for infants or toddlers who are not toilet trained. Clear, plastic, single-use bags with self-adhering material can be attached over the child's urethral meatus.

The nurse prepares an infant by first washing the genitalia, perineum, and surrounding skin with soap and water or an antiseptic. Thorough drying is necessary, because the bag's adhesive does not stick to a moist, powdered, or oily surface. The nurse attaches the bag from back to front, first to the perineum and then toward the symphysis pubis. In girls the perineum should be gently stretched to ensure that the bag has a leak-proof fit. In boys the scrotum and penis fit inside the collection bag. A diaper is placed over the bag. The nurse checks the bag often and removes it as soon as urine is available. An active child can easily loosen the bag and cause a leak. For a clean-voided specimen the nurse uses a sterile collection bag.

COMMON URINE TESTS

Urinalysis. The laboratory performs a urinalysis on a specimen obtained by any of the previously described methods. Table 38-3 lists normal values for a urinalysis. The specimen should be examined as soon as possible, preferably within 2 hours. It should be the first voided specimen in the morning to ensure a uniform concentration of constituents. For a quick screening the nurse can perform certain portions of the urinalysis with special reagent strips or tablets. The nurse dips the strips into urine or applies droplets to tablets and then watches for a color change.

Specific Gravity. The specific gravity is the weight or degree of concentration of a substance compared with an equal volume of water. To measure specific gravity the nurse uses a urinometer and cylinder (Fig. 38-5). The urinometer has a specific gravity scale at the top and a weighted mercury bulb at the bottom. The nurse pours a urine specimen into a clean, dry cylinder. Next the nurse suspends and lightly twirls the weighted urinometer into the cylinder of urine. The concentration of dissolved substances in the urine determines the depth at which the urinometer will float.

With the urinometer at eye level the nurse reads the measurement at the base of the meniscus at the level of the urine. The specific gravity of a morning urine specimen voided by a fasting client reflects the kidney's max-

TABLE 38-3 Routine Urinalysis Values

Measurement (Normal Value)	Interpretation
pH (4.6 to 8.0)	Helps indicate acid-base balance. Urine that stands for several hours becomes alkaline from bacterial invasion.
	Selected antibiotics (for example, neomycin and streptomycin) are more effective against urinary tract infections if the pH is alkaline.
Protein (up to 8 mg/100 ml)	Normally not present in urine. Seen in renal disease because damage to glomerular membrane allows protein to enter urine. However, a temporary presence of protein in the urine can occur after strenuous exercise, exposure to cold, or psychological stress.
Glucose (not normally present)	Diabetic clients have glucose in urine as a result of inability of tubules to reabsorb high glucose concentrations (over 180 mg/100 ml). Ingestion of high concentrations of glucose may cause some to appear in urine of healthy persons.
Ketones (not normally present)	Poorly controlled diabetic clients experience a breakdown of fatty acids. The end product of fatty acid metabolism is ketones. Clients with dehydration, starvation, or excessive aspirin ingestion also have ketonuria.
Blood (up to two red blood cells)	Damage to glomerulus or tubules may cause blood cells to enter urine. Trauma or disease of lower urinary tract also causes hematuria.
Specific gravity (1.01 to 1.03)	Measures concentration of particles in the urine. A high specific gravity reflects concentrated urine, and a low specific gravity reflects diluted urine. Dehydration, reduced renal blood flow, and an increase in ADH secretion elevate specific gravity. Overhydration and inadequate ADH secretion reduce specific gravity.

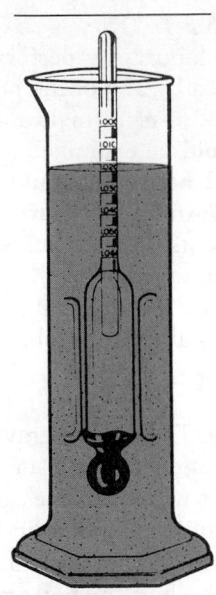

Fig. 38-5   Measurement of urine specific gravity using a uri-nometer.

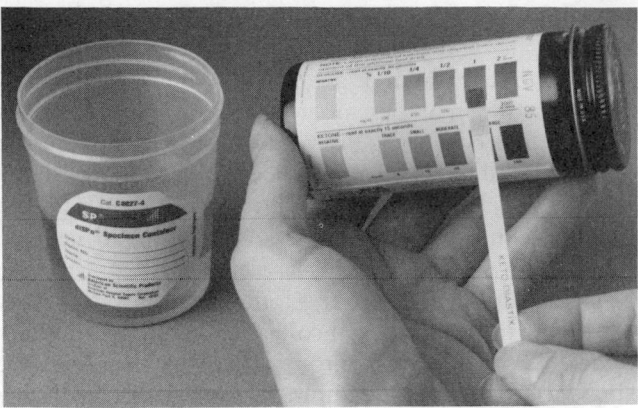

Fig. 38-6   Checking results on a glucose reagent strip.

imum concentrating ability. A specific gravity below 1.01 reflects an inability of the kidneys to concentrate urine or an insufficient secretion of ADH. An elevated specific gravity can indicate dehydration. Radiopaque substances given for x-ray procedures may cause a falsely high specific gravity.

Urine Culture. A urine culture simply requires a sterile sample of urine. It takes about 72 hours before the laboratory can report findings of bacterial growth. If bacteria are present, an additional test for sensitivity determines which antibiotics are effective.

Glucose and Ketones. An accurate measurement of glucose and ketones always requires a double-voided specimen. Several products, including Keto-Diastix, Multistix, and Tes-Tape reagent strips, are used to detect glucose and ketone. The strips contain chemicals that change color when exposed to glucose and ketone. The nurse dips a strip in a urine specimen and pulls it out. After a selected time period (10 to 15 seconds), the nurse compares the strip's color with that of the chart on the bottle. The color scale measures the quantity of glucose or ketone in urine (Fig. 38-6). The range on the color scale extends from negative, trace, 1+, 2+, to 3+. Urine glucose levels are no longer considered a reliable indicator for assessing a diabetic's level of control. Blood glucose monitoring is a more accurate test and can be done by the client after performing a simple fingerstick.

DIAGNOSTIC EXAMINATIONS. The two approaches for visualizing urinary structures are direct and indirect. The nursing implications for urinary diagnostic examinations are similar to those for gastrointestinal examinations.

Indirect Visualization. To view the entire urinary system the physician orders indirect visualization tests. The clients receives an intravenous injection of either a contrast dye or radioisotope. Normally the injected medium takes only a few minutes to circulate and be excreted. Because the kidneys and ureters lie behind the intestines, it is necessary with tests such as the intravenous pyelogram (IVP) to give the client cathartics to promote adequate emptying of the bowel. An upper gastrointestinal examination and small bowel series (see Chapter 39) cannot be done for 2 to 3 days before an IVP because remaining barium in the intestines will obscure the view.

The IVP requires that x-ray studies be taken at specific intervals over a 30- to 60-minute period as the dye concentrates. The client may also be asked to void during the procedure to measure bladder emptying.

An IVP allows indirect visualization of kidneys, renal pelvis, ureters, and bladder following injection of an intravenous radiopaque dye. The physician observes for the presence of renal artery blockage, urinary tumors, vascular abnormalities, and trauma. Nursing implications before the test include:

1. Observe client sign informed consent.
2. Nurse assesses the client for history of iodine allergy, which predicts allergies to the IVP dye.
3. Client receives cathartic on evening before test.
4. Client takes nothing by mouth after midnight.
5. Nurse explains that facial flushing is normal during dye injection and that client may feel dizzy or warm.

6. Nurse explains that physician starts an intravenous infusion for dye injection.
7. Nurse explains that test involves x-ray studies taken at several intervals, with client to void near the end of the test.

Nursing implications during the test include:

1. Nurse assesses intravenous site for signs of infiltration of dye into tissues (for example, swelling, redness, pain).
2. Nurse observes for signs of allergic reaction to dye (for example, respiratory distress, fall in blood pressure).
3. Nurse reminds the client of normal sensations caused by dye injection.

Nursing implications after the test include:

1. Client may receive normal diet afterward.
2. Nurse encourages fluid intake to minimize dehydration caused by fasting.

Renal scanning uses radioactive isotopes to outline urinary structures. The isotope can be detected without the need of a bowel preparation. A renal scan measures radioactive concentrations while the client assumes a supine, prone, or sitting position. A very low dosage of radioisotope is used, so no precautions against radioactive exposure are needed.

A renal scan allows indirect visualization of the urinary tract following intravenous injection of a radioisotope. The physician observes for renal artery blockage and primary renal disease indicated by a delay in isotope excretion. The test is indicated for clients unable to receive IVP drugs. Nursing implications before the test include:

1. Observe client sign informed consent.
2. Nurse explains that radioisotope is injected intravenously through an existing IV line or needle.
3. Nurse explains that client will feel no discomfort but must lie still.
4. Nurse explains there is no risk of radioactive exposure.

Nursing implications during the test include:

1. Nurse assists the client to change positions during the test.
2. Nurse explains that the machine measuring the isotope uptake is similar to a Geiger counter.

A nursing implication after the test:

1. Nurse instructs the client to resume normal activities.

The indirect urinary examinations are relatively painless, except for the intravenous injection of dye or isotope. The nurse does not routinely give a sedative before the test unless the physician views the client as highly anxious.

Direct Visualization. To view the interior of the bladder and urethra the physician performs a cystos-

copy. The cystoscope looks much like a urinary catheter although it is not as flexible. It is inserted through the client's urethra. The instrument has an outer plastic or rubber sheath, an obturator that keeps the scope rigid during insertion, a telescope for viewing the bladder and urethra, and a channel for inserting catheters or special surgical instruments.

The procedure is painful during instrument insertion. Unless the client lies still, there is risk of bladder perforation. The client may have the test with local or general anesthesia. Because the test requires insertion of a foreign object into a sterile cavity, the client receives large amounts of fluids (intravenously or orally) before and during the procedure to maintain a continuous urine flow and to flush out any bacteria. During the test urine and tissue specimens may be collected.

The physician usually performs the cystoscopy in a hospital cystoscopy room. Special cystoscopy tables minimize stress and fatigue clients may experience from maintaining one position for a prolonged time. Nursing implications before the test include:

1. Observe client sign informed consent.
2. Client receives cathartics on evening before the test.
3. If local anesthetic is to be used, the nurse encourages oral fluids.
4. If general anesthetic is to be used, the client takes nothing by mouth after midnight.
5. Nurse explains that insertion of cystoscope is similar to insertion of urethral catheter.
6. Nurse explains the importance of lying still during the test.
7. Nurse explains that an intravenous line will be started to give fluids during the test.
8. Nurse gives the client a sedative and/or analgesic.

Nursing implications during the test include:

1. Nurse assists the client to assume a lithotomy position.
2. Nurse prepares the perineal area with antiseptic solution.
3. Nurse explains (if client is awake) that insertion of cystoscope causes an urge to void.
4. Nurse reminds client to be still.

Nursing implications after the test include:

1. Nurse instructs the client to remain in bed as ordered.
2. Nurse assesses for signs of urinary retention and first voiding.
3. Nurse observes characteristics of urine, noting bloody or cloudy urine.
4. Nurse encourages increased fluid intake.
5. Nurse observes for fever, dysuria, or drop in blood pressure.

NURSING DIAGNOSIS

A thorough assessment of the client's urinary elimination function ensures the nurse's ability to make relevant and accurate nursing diagnoses. The diagnosis may be potential or actual, depending on risks or health alterations (see nursing diagnoses box). The diagnosis may focus on a urinary elimination alteration or associated problems.

Identification of defining characteristics leads the nurse to select an appropriate diagnosis (see sample nursing diagnoses box). Specifying related factors for each diagnosis allows selection of individualized nursing interventions.

PLANNING

The nurse plans therapeutic interventions for clients with urinary elimination problems, and preventive interventions may be required for clients with potential urinary problems (see care plan box). The nurse plans therapies according to severity of risks to the client.

It is important to consider the client's home environment and normal elimination routines when planning therapies. Reinforcement of good health habits that are already followed will improve compliance with the plan of care.

The client with actual or potential alterations in urinary elimination learns to recognize signs of change and to prevent serious problems. Alterations in urinary elimination pose a high risk to a client's overall state of health.

Planning care also involves an understanding of the client's need to control body function. Alterations in urinary elimination can be embarrassing, uncomfortable, and often frustrating. The nurse and client work together to establish ways of maintaining client involvement in nursing care and to maintain normal elimination patterns when possible.

In an effort to promote normal urinary elimination, goals for the client include:

1. Understanding normal urinary elimination
2. Achieving normal micturition
3. Achieving complete bladder emptying
4. Freedom from infection
5. Skin integrity maintained
6. Gaining a sense of comfort

Associated problems require interventions that often have no direct effect on urinary elmination. Unless the nurse intervenes, however, associated problems are likely to continue. Problems involved with urinary elim-

---

Examples of Nursing Diagnoses Related to Urinary Elimination

NANDA-APPROVED NURSING DIAGNOSES

Pain related to:
- Urethral inflammation
- Urinary retention

Toileting self-care deficit related to:
- Limited lower extremity mobility

Impaired skin integrity or potential impaired skin integrity related to:
- Incontinence of urine

Altered patterns of urinary elimination related to:
- Sensory motor impairment
- Traumatized urethral tissue

Body-image disturbance related to:
- Feelings about ureterostomy
- Feelings about frequent incontinence

Functional incontinence related to:
- Mobility restrictions
- Unfamiliar toileting facilities

Potential for infection related to:
- Urethral catheter insertion
- Poor personal hygiene

Reflex incontinence related to:
- Loss of voluntary control of micturition

Stress incontinence related to:
- Increased intraabdominal pressure
- Weak pelvic musculature

Total incontinence related to:
- Loss of voluntary control of micturition
- Presence of anatomic fistula

Urge incontinence related to:
- Alcohol ingestion
- Irritation of bladder mucosa

Urinary retention related to:
- Weakened detrusor muscle

---

ination alterations are often interrelated and complex. The nurse must also anticipate problems that may develop as a result of therapy. For example, diagnosis of potential for infection is appropriate whenever a client has an indwelling catheter.

IMPLEMENTATION

Client Education

Success of therapies aimed at eliminating or minimizing urinary elimination problems depends in part on

Sample Nursing Diagnoses for Urinary Elimination

Defining Characteristics	Nursing Diagnoses	Related Factors
Dysuria Frequency Hesitancy Urgency	Altered patterns of urinary elimination	• Sensory-motor impairment • Infection
Bladder distention Small, frequent dribbling Overflow incontinence	Urinary retention	• Inhibition of voiding reflex • Weakened detrusor muscles
Urgency Frequency Bladder spasm Nocturia	Urge incontinence	• Increased fluid intake • Alcohol intake • Overdistended bladder • Enlarged prostate

successful client education. The nurse instructs clients on their specific elimination problem. For example, a client who practices poor hygiene will benefit from learning about normal sterility of the urinary tract and ways to prevent infection. It may also be useful to discuss the basic mechanism for urine production and voiding for clients with an elimination alteration. Knowledge of factors that promote normal urine production and voiding can also be helpful. Clients learn the significance of symptoms of urinary alterations so early preventive

Sample Nursing Care Plan for Urinary Elimination

Nursing Diagnosis	Goals	Expected Outcomes	Nursing Interventions
Urinary retention related to weakened detrusor muscle	Client will achieve complete bladder emptying.	Bladder will be nondistended after voiding.	Instruct client on use of pelvic floor (Kegel) exercises during nonvoiding times.
		Client will deny feeling of bladder fullness after voiding.	Administer Bethanechol 2.5 mg subcutaneously 3 hours after last voiding (maximum four times daily).
		Residual urine will be less than 50 ml.	Catheterize client immediately after voiding for residual urine.
	Client will be free of infection.	Urine remains clear amber.	Maintain fluid intake of 2000 to 2500 ml fluids daily. (Client prefers cranberry juice and iced tea.)
		Client is free of symptoms of urinary tract infections.	Offer client mild soap and water for perineal hygiene after each voiding.

health care can be initiated.

The nurse can easily incorporate teaching during nursing care delivery. For example, if the nurse is attempting to increase the client's fluid intake, a good time to discuss benefits is while giving fluids with medications or meals. The nurse may be more successful in teaching about perineal hygiene during a bath or while giving catheter care. Much of the information the nurse offers is practical in nature. The nurse can easily include family members in informal discussions.

Promoting Normal Micturition

Many nursing measures have been designed to promote normal voiding in clients at risk for urination difficulties and in clients with established urination problems. The nurse can initiate many of them independently.

STIMULATING MICTURITION REFLEX

The client's ability to void depends on feeling the urge to urinate, being able to control the urethral sphincter, and being able to relax during voiding. The nurse can help foster relaxation and stimulate the reflex to void by helping clients assume the normal position for voiding. Females are better able to void in a squatting position. This position promotes contraction of the pelvic and intraabdominal muscles that assist in sphincter control and bladder contraction. If the client is unable to use toilet facilities, the nurse positions the client in a squatting position on a bedpan (see Chapter 39) or bedside commode. The male client voids more easily in the standing position. At times it may be necessary for one or more nurses to assist the male client to stand. If the male client cannot reach toilet facilities, he may stand at the bedside and void into a urinal, a metal or plastic receptacle for urine (Fig. 38-7).

Other measures that promote relaxation and ability to void include sensory stimuli. The sound of running water helps many clients void through the power of suggestion. Stroking the inner aspect of the client's thigh may stimulate sensory nerves and promote the micturition reflex. Placing the client's hand in a pan of warm water often promotes voiding. It is easier for a person to relax and void when sitting on a bedpan that has been warmed. The nurse can also pour warm water over the client's perineum and create the sensation to urinate. If the client's urine output is to be measured, the nurse must first measure the volume of water to be poured over the perineal area. Offering clients a drink may also promote voiding.

MAINTAINING ELIMINATION HABITS

Many clients follow routines to promote normal voiding. In a hospital or long-term care facility the nurse's

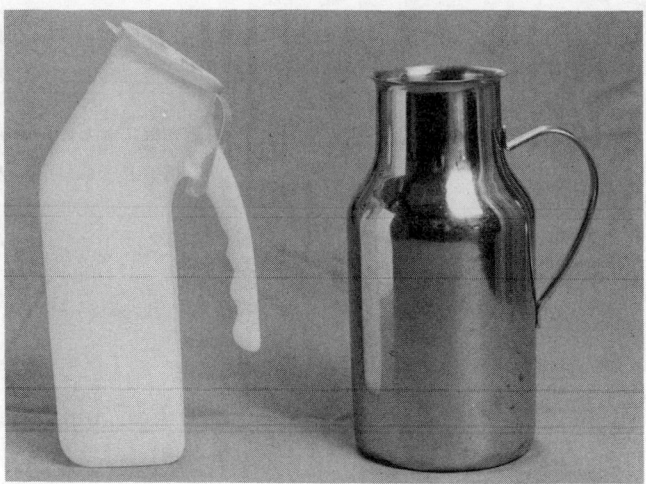

Fig. 38-7 Types of male urinals.

routines may conflict with those of the client. Integrating the client's habits into the plan of nursing care fosters a normal voiding.

The client usually requires time to void. Asking a client to void quickly so he or she can be transported to x-ray testing, or requesting a urine specimen as soon as possible, does not contribute to normal voiding habits. The client should be given at least 30 minutes to provide a specimen. The nurse learns the times when a client normally voids, such as on awakening or before meals, and offers the opportunity to use toilet facilities then. Also important is the need to respond to the client's urge to urinate. Delay in assisting the client to the bathroom may interfere with normal micturition.

Privacy is essential for normal voiding. If the client cannot reach the bathroom, the nurse makes sure the bedside area is enclosed by a curtain. In the home the debilitated client may prefer using a bedside commode enclosed behind a partition or room divider. Some clients are embarrassed by the sound of voiding. Running water or flushing the toilet masks the sound. Often young children are unable to void in the presence of persons other than their parents.

If the client typically uses special measures to void, the nurse should encourage their continued use at home and, when possible, in the institution. The client may be able to relax and void more easily while reading or listening to music. A drink of coffee or a sip of beer may also promote urination.

MAINTAINING ADEQUATE FLUID INTAKE

A simple method of promoting normal micturition is maintaining good fluid intake. A client with normal renal function who does not have heart disease or alterations requiring fluid restriction should drink 2000 to 2500 ml of fluid daily. However, an average daily intake of 1200 to 1500 ml of fluids is usually adequate.

When fluid intake is increased, the excreted urine flushes out solutes or particles that may collect in the urinary system. Because a client is unlikely to be willing to drink 2500 ml of water daily, the nurse should offer fluids the client prefers. Vegetables and fruits contain a high fluid content.

At home it may be helpful to set a schedule for drinking fluids (for example, with meals or medications). To prevent nocturia, fluids should not be taken just before bedtime.

Promoting Complete Bladder Emptying

Under normal conditions some urine remains in the bladder because urinary sphincters close. The sphincters provide more pressure than the pressure of urine in the bladder. Thus, persons normally remain continent and dry. Urinary incontinence, however, occurs either from pressure in the bladder being too great or the sphincters being too weak. Urinary retention occurs from a strong or contracted sphincter that prevents normal bladder emptying.

Measures that promote micturition may help clients with incontinence or retention. There are additional measures used to promote and control bladder emptying so that clients gain a sense of elimination control (Table 38-4).

STRENGTHENING PELVIC FLOOR MUSCLES

Clients who have difficulty starting or stopping the urine stream may benefit from pelvic floor (Kegel) exercises (Table 38-5). These exercises improve the strength of pelvic floor muscles and consist of repetitive contractions of muscle groups (Kane et al., 1984). A client begins these exercises during voiding to learn the technique. They are then practiced at nonvoiding times. Improvement is usually gradual. Clients should be alert and motivated to perform the exercises.

MEDICATIONS

Drug therapy given alone or along with other therapies can help treat problems of incontinence and retention. There are two types of medications. One relaxes a spastic bladder to thereby increase bladder capacity. The other stimulates the bladder.

The bladder is innervated by the parasympathetic nervous system. When urine is present in the bladder, stress or urge incontinence may result from hyperactivity of the bladder muscle that suddenly increases intravesicular pressure. Uncontrolled bladder contractions may be caused by local irritants to the bladder such as stones or infection. Drugs that depress the neurotransmitter acetylcholine, which stimulates the bladder, reduce in-

continence caused by bladder irritation. Examples of these anticholinergic drugs include propantheline (Pro-Banthine) and oxybutynin chloride (Ditropan). The anticholinergics can cause cardiac dysrhythmias and should be used with caution in clients with heart disease.

TABLE 38-4 Treatment Options for Incontinence

Primary Treatment	Other Treatments
ACUTE	
Management of the acute illness	Catheter
Appropriate toileting schedule	
Alteration of the environment	
Modification of drug regimen	
Adequate bowel care	Protective undergarments
Treatment of UTI	
Treatment of atrophic urethritis and vaginitis	
General supportive measures	
URGE	
Anticholinergic drug therapy	
Bladder retraining	
Treatment of associated UTI	
Treatment of associated vaginitis	Biofeedback
	Intravaginal electrical stimulation
STRESS	
Conditioning (Kegel) exercises	Estrogen
	Alpha-adrenergic agonists
Surgery	Intravaginal electrical stimulation
Bladder neck suspension	Artificial sphincter
OVERFLOW	
Surgery	
Intermittent catheterization	Indwelling catheter
FUNCTIONAL	
Habit training	Scheduled toileting
	Incontinence undergarments
	Environmental alterations
	Supportive measures
	Catheters
	Indwelling
	External
	Skin care

From Orzeck, S, and Ouslander, JG: Urinary incontinence: an overview of causes and treatment, J Entero Ther 14:24, 1987.

TABLE 38-5 Pelvic Floor Exercises

Exercise Steps	Rationale
EXERCISE I	
Instruct client to learn to feel the pelvic muscles.	Assists client in feeling anterior muscles of pelvic floor.
Have client try to stop the flow of urine during urination and then to restart it.	Control technique is learned.
Practice with each voiding.	
EXERCISE II	
Have client assume a sitting or standing position.	Assists client in feeling posterior muscles of pelvic floor.
Instruct client to tighten muscles around anus without tensing leg, buttock, or abdominal muscles.	
EXERCISE III	
Have client tighten the posterior muscles and then slowly contract anterior muscles while counting slowly to four.	Improves pelvic muscle control, and aids relaxation of sphincters during voiding.
Then relax muscles completely.	
Repeat exercise 4 times per hour while awake, for 3 months.	
EXERCISE IV	
Situps.	Strengthens abdominal muscles for bladder control.

Anticholinergics may also cause constipation and a dry mouth.

When the bladder empties, the detrusor muscle contracts in response to parasympathetic stimulation. Incomplete bladder emptying results from impaired innervation or weakness of the detrusor muscle. The client experiences retention and overflow incontinence. Cholinergic drugs increase contraction of the bladder and improve emptying. Bethanechol (Urecholine) stimulates parasympathetic nerves to increase bladder wall contraction and relax the sphincter. Bethanechol can be given by subcutaneous or oral routes. The nurse should administer the first dose 3 to 4 hours after the last voiding to be sure the bladder contains urine. To gain the drug's peak effect, the nurse administers it shortly before micturition is attempted (15 to 30 minutes subcutaneously, 30 to 60 minutes orally). Cholinergic drugs may cause diarrhea as a side effect.

BLADDER RETRAINING

The goal of bladder retraining is to restore a normal pattern of voiding by inhibiting or stimulating voiding (Orzeck and Ouslander, 1987). This is useful in clients with a cerebrovascular accident, overdistention, a bladder injury, an indwelling urinary catheter, or an acute illness that caused incontinence. For bladder retraining to be successful, clients must be alert and physically able to follow a training program.

The nurse first assesses the client's pattern of urination (for example, frequency, time, habits, volume). This information allows the nurse to plan a program that often takes 2 weeks or more to learn. The actual time for training depends on a client's condition. If an indwelling catheter has been inserted 6 to 12 months, bladder capacity is greatly reduced and permanent bladder wall changes may occur (Kristiansen et al., 1983). If the client has an underlying urinary tract infection, this should be treated at the same time.

The following measures will help the incontinent client gain control over urination:

1. Learning exercises to strengthen the pelvic floor
2. Initiating a toileting schedule
    a. Upon awakening
    b. Every 2 hours during the day and evening
    c. Before getting into bed
    d. Every 4 hours at night
3. Using methods to initiate voiding (for example, running water, stroking the inner thigh)
4. Using methods to relax to aid complete bladder emptying (for example, reading, deep breathing)
5. Never ignoring the urge to void
6. Taking fluids approximately 30 minutes before planned voiding times
7. Limiting fluids after supper to no more than 150 to 200 ml (5 to 7 ounces); avoiding tea, coffee, alcohol, and other caffeine drinks.
8. Taking prescribed diuretic medication or fluids that increase diuresis (such as tea or coffee) early in the morning
9. Progressively lengthening or shortening periods between voiding
10. Offering protective undergarments to contain urine and reduce the client's embarrassment (do not use diapers)
11. Following a weight control program if obesity is a problem

These guidelines help the client to establish a routine for voiding and to control factors that might increase the number of incontinent episodes.

HABIT TRAINING

A client with functional incontinence may benefit from habit training, which simply helps clients improve voluntary control over urination. A flexible toileting schedule based on the client's pattern is established.

The nurse helps the client to the bathroom before incontinent episodes occur. Fluids and medications are timed to prevent interference with the toileting schedule. Clients with moderate or severe mental and/or physical function can benefit. Positive reinforcement to reward successful voiding and neutral interaction when accidental incontinence occurs helps reinforce success.

CATHETERIZATION

Catheterization of the bladder involves introducing a rubber or plastic tube through the urethra and into the bladder. The catheter provides a continuous flow of urine in clients unable to control micturition or those with obstructions. Because bladder catheterization carries the risk of urinary tract infection, it is preferable to rely on other measures. Catheterization is no longer used routinely.

TYPES OF CATHETERIZATION. Intermittent and indwelling retention catheterization are the two forms of catheter insertion. With the *intermittent* technique a straight single-use catheter is introduced for a period long enough to drain the bladder (5 to 10 minutes). When the bladder is empty, the nurse immediately withdraws the catheter. Intermittent catheterization can be repeated as necessary. An *indwelling* or Foley catheter remains in place for an extended period until a client is able to void completely and voluntarily. It may be necessary to change indwelling catheters periodically.

The straight single-use catheter (Fig. 38-8) has a single lumen with a small opening about 1.3 cm (½ inch) from the tip. Urine drains from the tip, through the lumen, to a receptacle. An indwelling Foley catheter has a small inflatable balloon that encircles the catheter just below the tip. When inflated, the balloon rests against the bladder outlet to anchor the catheter in place (Fig. 38-9). The indwelling retention catheter also has as many as two or three separate lumens within the body of the catheter (Fig. 38-8). One lumen drains urine through the catheter to a collecting tube. A second lumen carries sterile water to and from the balloon when it is inflated or deflated. A third (optional) lumen may be used to instill fluids or medications into the bladder. It is easy to determine the number of lumens by the number of drainage and injection ports at the catheter's end.

A third type of catheter has a curved tip. A Coudé catheter (Fig. 38-8) is used on male clients who may have enlarged prostates with obstructions along the urethra. The Coudé is less traumatic during insertion because it is stiffer and easier to control than the Foley catheter.

Catheters come in many diameters to fit the size of a client's urethral canal. The CDC suggests nurses use as small a catheter as possible consistent with good drainage to minimize urethral trauma (Wong, 1982). Paraurethral glands that bathe the urethra in its natural lubrication become blocked if a catheter lumen is too large.

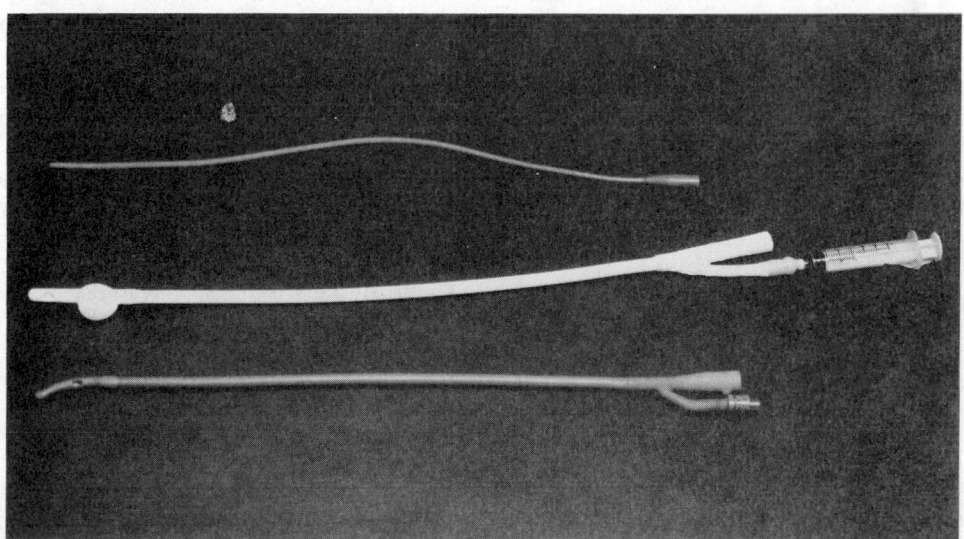

Fig. 38-8 Type of catheters. *Top,* Straight catheter; *middle,* indwelling double-lumen catheter with inflated balloon; *bottom,* Coudé catheter.

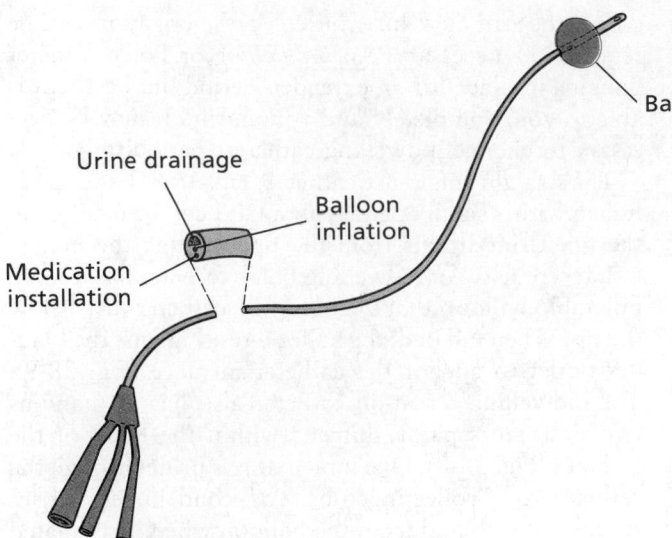

Fig. 38-9 Foley catheter with balloon inflated.

The French system is used for catheter gauge sizing. The larger the gauge number, the larger the catheter. Children usually require a no. 8 or no. 10 French. Women require a no. 14 to no. 16, while men need a no. 16 to no. 18.

Balloons on retention catheters also come in many sizes, depending on the volume of fluid or air needed to inflate them. The 5 ml and 30 ml sizes are most common.

INDICATIONS FOR CATHETERIZATION. Catheterization may be indicated for many reasons. When the need for catheterization is short term and minimizing infection is a priority, the intermittent method is best. Intermittent catheterization is also preferred for persons with spinal cord injuries who have no bladder control. By intermittently draining the bladder on a routine basis,

these clients have fewer infections. Indwelling catherization is used when long-term bladder emptying is necessary. Table 38-6 outlines specific indications for catheterization.

CATHETER INSERTION. Urethral catheterization requires a physician's order. The nurse must use strict aseptic technique (see Chapter 43). Organizing equipment before the procedure prevents interruptions. The steps for inserting an indwelling and a single-use straight catheter are basically the same. The difference lies in the procedure taken to inflate the indwelling catheter balloon and secure the catheter. While inserting an indwelling catheter the nurse has the opportunity to collect needed specimens. Procedure 38-2 lists steps for performing female and male urethral catheterization.

SELF-CATHETERIZATION. Some clients with chronic disorders such as spinal cord injury learn to perform self-catheterization. The client must be able to physically manipulate equipment and assume a position for successful catheterization. The nurse teaches the client anatomy of the urinary tract, knowledge of clean versus sterile technique, the importance of a limited fluid intake regimen, and the frequency of self-catheterization. Generally, a goal is to have clients perform self-catheterizations every 6 to 8 hours.

Text continued on p. 1104.

TABLE 38-6 Indications for Catheterization

| Intermittent Catheterization | Indwelling Catheterization | |
	Short-Term	Long-Term
Relieve discomfort of bladder distention and provide decompression	Obstruction to urine outflow (for example, prostate enlargement)	Cases of severe urinary retention with recurrent episodes of urinary tract infection
Obtain a sterile urine specimen	Clients undergoing surgical repair of the urethra and surrounding structures	Clients with skin rashes, ulcers, or wounds irritated by contact with urine
Assess presence of residual urine when bladder empties incompletely	Prevent urethral obstruction from blood clots	Terminally ill clients for whom bed linen changes are painful
Long-term management of clients with spinal cord injuries, neuromuscular degeneration, incompetent bladders	Provides means to measure output in critically ill or comatose clients	
	Provides continuous or intermittent bladder irrigations	

less infection than foley, less stone formation

PROCEDURE 38-2

Inserting a Straight or Indwelling Catheter

STEPS	RATIONALE
1. Assess status of client:	
a. When client last voided	May indicate likelihood of bladder fullness.
b. Level of awareness or developmental stage	Reveals client's ability to cooperate during procedure.
c. Mobility and physical limitations of client (nurse can request additional nursing personnel to assist with this procedure if necessary)	Affects way that nurse will position client.
d. Client's age	Determines catheter size to use. No. 8-10 French gauge is generally used for children and 14-16 for women. No. 12 may be considered for young females. No. 16-18 is used for male clients unless larger size is ordered by physician.
e. Distended bladder	Can indicate need to insert catheter if client is unable to void independently. Clients at risk for distension include postpartum women, postoperative clients, and men with prostatic hypertrophy.
f. Presence of pathological condition that may impair passage of catheter (for example, enlarged prostate gland)	Obstruction prevents passage of catheter through urethra into bladder.
g. Allergies	Determines allergy to antiseptic, tape, or rubber.
2. Prepare necessary equipment and supplies:	Promotes organization of nurse's activities, thereby increasing efficiency
a. Sterile gloves*	Procedure is considered sterile.
b. Sterile drapes, one fenestrated	
c. Lubricant*	Minimizes urethral trauma during insertion.
d. Antiseptic cleansing solution*	
e. Cotton balls or gauze squares	
f. Forceps	
g. Prefilled syringe with sterile water	Used to inflate balloon of indwelling catheter.
h. Catheters of correct size and type for procedure (intermittent or indwelling)	
i. Flashlight or gooseneck lamp	Helps in seeing urinary meatus of female client.
j. Bath blanket	Promotes privacy by draping client.
k. Waterproof absorbent pad	Positioning under client prevents soiling of bed linens.
l. Trash receptacle	
m. Disposable gloves; basin with warm water; soap; face cloth; towel	Providing perineal care prior to introducing catheter helps reduce risk of urinary tract infection. Provides opportunity to examine female's urethral meatus or to retract foreskin of uncircumcised male.
n. Sterile drainage tubing and collection bag (may be preattached to catheter); tape; safety pin; elastic band	If indwelling catheter is to be inserted, tape, elastic band, and pin help secure position of catheter, thus preventing trauma to external urethral sphincter.
o. Receptacle or basin (usually bottom of tray)	Provides area for urine to drain when straight or indwelling catheter is used.
p. Specimen container	For sterile urine specimen to determine presence of bacteria.
3. Explain procedure to client. Also describe pressure sensation that will be felt during catheter insertion.	Reduces client's anxiety and promotes cooperation throughout procedure.
4. Arrange for extra nursing personnel to assist, if appropriate.	May be necessary to assist with positioning dependent client. Promotes use of correct body mechanics and client's safety.
5. Wash hands.	Reduces transmission of infection.
6. Raise bed to appropriate working height.	Promotes use of proper body mechanics.

Continued.

Inserting a Straight or Indwelling Catheter

STEPS	RATIONALE
7. Facing client, stand on left side of bed if right-handed (on right side if left-handed). Clear bedside table and arrange equipment.	Successful catheter insertion requires nurse to assume comfortable position with all equipment easily accessible.
8. Raise side rail on opposite side of bed.	Promotes client safety.
9. Close cubicle or room curtains.	Reduces client's embarrassment and aids in relaxation during procedure.
10. Place waterproof pad under client	Prevents soiling of bed linen.
11. Position client.	
a. For female client, assist to dorsal recumbent position (supine with knees flexed). Ask client to relax thighs so as to externally rotate them. (Legs may be supported with pillows.)	Provides good view of perineal structures.
b. Postion female client in side-lying (Sims') position with upper leg flexed at knee and hip if unable to be supine (optional).	Alternate position if client cannot abduct leg at hip joint (for example, arthritic joints). Also, this position may be more comfortable for client. Support client with pillows, if necessary, to maintain position.
c. For male client, assist to assume supine position with thighs slightly abducted.	Supine position prevents tensing of abdominal and pelvic muscles.
12. Drape client.	Avoids unnecessary exposure of body parts and maintains client's comfort.
a. For female client, drape with bath blanket. Place blanket diamond fashion over client; one corner at client's neck, side corners over each arm and side, and last corner over perineum. Raise gown above hips.	
b. For male client, drape upper trunk with bath blanket and cover lower extremities with bed sheets, exposing only genitalia.	
13. Wash perineal area with soap and water as needed; dry. Disposable gloves should be worn.	Presence of microorganisms near urethral meatus is reduced.
14. Position lamp to illuminate perineal area. (When using flashlight, assistant holds it.)	Permits accurate identification and good view of urethral meatus.
15. Remove and dispose of gloves	Prevents transmission of microorganisms.
16. Open catheterization kit and catheter (if packaged separately) according to directions, keeping bottom of container sterile.	Prevents transmission of microorganisms from table or work area to sterile supplies.
17. Put on sterile gloves (see Chapter 43).	Allows nurse to handle sterile supplies without contamination.
18. Organize supplies on sterile field; open inner sterile package containing catheter; pour sterile package of antiseptic solution in correct compartment containing sterile cotton balls; open packet containing lubricant; remove specimen container (lip should be loosely placed on top) and prefilled syringe from collection compartment of tray and set them aside on sterile field.	Maintains principles of surgical asepsis and organizes work area. All activities requiring the nurse to use both hands are to be completed before cleansing the urethral meatus.
19. When inserting a retention catheter, test the catheter balloon by injecting fluid from the prefilled syringe into balloon valve. Balloon should inflate fully without leakage. Withdraw fluid and leave syringe on port of catheter.	Checks integrity of balloon. A balloon that leaks or inflates improperly is replaced.
20. Appiy sterile drape.	
a. For female client, allow top edge of drape to form cuff over both hands. Place drape down on bed between client's thighs. Slip cuffed edge just under client's buttocks, taking care not to touch contaminated surface with gloves.	Outer surface of drape covering nurse's hands remains sterile until touched by buttocks. Sterile drape against sterile gloves is sterile.

STEPS	RATIONALE
b. Pick up fenestrated sterile drape and allow it to unfold without touching an unsterile object. Apply drape over client's perineum exposing labia and being sure not to touch contaminated surface.	Maintains sterility of work surface.
c. For male client, apply drape over his thighs just below penis. Pick up fenestrated sterile drape, allow it to unfold, and drape it over penis with fenestrated slit resting over penis.	Maintains sterility of work surface.
21. Place sterile kit and its contents on sterile drape between client's thighs.	Provides easy access to supplies during catheter insertion.
22. Open urine specimen container, keeping top sterile.	Prepares container for transfer of urine.
23. Apply lubricant along sides of catheter tip. Females: 2.5-5 cm (1-2 in) Males: 7.5-12.5 cm (3-5 in)	Allows easy insertion of catheter tip through urethral meatus.
24. Cleanse urethral meatus.	
a. Female client: With nondominant hand carefully retract labia to fully expose urethral meatus. Maintain position of nondominant hand throughout remainder of procedure.	Full visualization of meatus is provided. Full retraction prevents contamination of meatus during cleansing. Closure of labia during cleansing requires that procedure be repeated because area has become contaminated.
b. With dominant hand pick up cotton ball with forceps and clean perineal area, wiping front to back from clitoris toward anus. Use new clean cotton ball for each wipe: along near labial fold, along far labial fold, directly over meatus.	Cleansing reduces number of microorganisms at urethral meatus. Use of single cotton ball for each wipe prevents transfer of microorganisms. Preparation moves from area of least contamination to that of most contamination. Dominant hand remains sterile.
c. Male client: If client is not circumcised, retract foreskin with nondominant hand. Grasp penis at shaft just below glans. Retract urethral meatus between thumb and forefinger. Maintain nondominant hand in this position throughout catheter insertion.	Minimizes chance of erection occurring (if an erection develops, discontinue procedure). Accidental release of foreskin or dropping of penis during cleansing requires process to be repeated because area has become contaminated.
d. With dominant hand pick up cotton ball with forceps and clean penis. Cleanse using cotton once around penis, starting at meatus and working toward base.	Reduces number of microorganisms at meatus and moves from area of least contamination to most contamination. Dominant hand remains sterile.
25. Pick up catheter with gloved dominant hand approximately 5 cm (2 in) from catheter tip. Hold end of catheter loosely coiled in palm of dominant hand (optional: may grasp catheter with forceps). Place distal end of catheter in urine tray receptacle unless already attached to drainage bag.	Collection of urine prevents soiling of client's bed linen and allows accurate measurement of urinary output.
26. Insert catheter:	
a. Female client (see illustration): with nondominant hand continuing to retract labia	
(1) Ask client to take a deep breath and slowly insert catheter through meatus. (If no urine appears, catheter may be in vagina. If catheter is in vagina, leave catheter in place; obtain and insert another catheter and then remove the first catheter.)	Relaxation of external sphincter aids in insertion of catheter. (Catheter in vagina is no longer sterile. Leaving first catheter in place helps prevent inserting second catheter in vagina.)
(2) Advance catheter approximately 5-7.5 cm (3 in) in adult, 2.5 cm (1 in) in child, or until urine flows out catheter's end. If inserting a retention catheter, advance another 5 cm (2 in) after urine appears. Do not force catheter against resistance.	Female urethra is short. Appearance of urine indicates that catheter tip is in bladder or lower urethra. Further advancement of catheter ensures bladder placement. Balloon of retention catheter must be advanced into bladder. Forceful insertion may traumatize urethra.
(3) Release labia and hold catheter securely with nondominant hand.	Bladder or sphincter contraction may cause accidental expulsion of catheter.

Continued.

PROCEDURE 38-2, cont'd

Inserting a Straight or Indwelling Catheter

STEPS	RATIONALE
b. Male client (see illustration): lift penis to position perpendicular to client's body and apply light traction upward.	Straightens urethral canal to ease catheter insertion.
(1) Ask client to bear down as if to void and slowly insert catheter through meatus.	Relaxation of external sphincter aids in insertion of catheter.
(2) Advance catheter 17.5-22.5 cm (7-9 in) in adult and 5-7.5 cm (2-3 in) in young child, or until urine flows out catheter's end. If resistance is felt, withdraw catheter; do not force it through urethra.	Adult male urethra is long. Appearance of urine indicates catheter tip is in bladder or urethra. Resistance to catheter passage may be caused by urethral strictures or enlarged prostate. Further advancement of catheter ensures proper placement.
If inserting a retention catheter, advance another 5 cm (2 in) after urine appears.	Ensures balloon is advanced into bladder.
(3) Release penis and hold catheter securely with dominant hand.	Bladder or sphincter contraction may cause accidental expulsion of catheter.
27. Collect urine specimen as needed: Fill specimen cup or jar to desired level (20-30 ml) by holding end of catheter in dominant hand over cup (or collect specimen from sterile drainage bag). With dominant hand pinch catheter to stop urine flow temporarily, then release catheter to allow remaining urine in bladder to drain into collection tray. Cover specimen cup and set it aside for labeling.	Allows sterile specimen to be obtained for culture analysis.
28. Allow bladder to empty fully about, 750-1000 ml (unless institution policy restricts maximal volume of urine to drain with each catheterization).	Retained urine may serve as reservoir for growth of microorganisms. Rapid emptying of large volume of urine may cause engorgement of pelvic blood vessels and hypovolemic shock.
29. Remove straight single-use catheter.	
a. Withdraw catheter slowly but smoothly until removed.	Discomfort to client is minimized.
30. Inflate balloon of indwelling catheter.	
a. While holding catheter with thumb and little finger of dominant hand at meatus, take end of catheter and place it between first two fingers of nondominant hand.	Catheter should be anchored while syringe is manipulated.
b. With free dominant hand attach syringe to injection port at end of catheter. (In some sets syringe is already connected.)	Port connects to lumen leading to inflatable balloon.

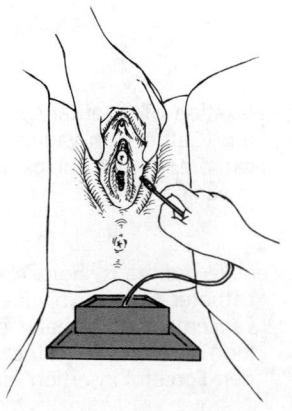

Step 26a

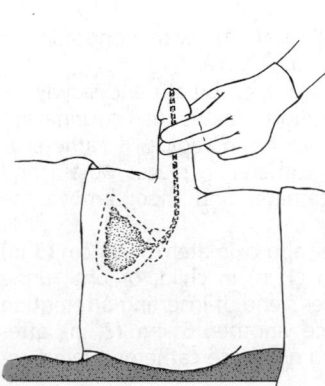

Step 26b

STEPS	RATIONALE
c. Slowly inject total amount of solution. If client complains of sudden pain, aspirate back solution and advance catheter farther. Inject no more fluid than balloon size indicates.	Balloon within bladder is inflated. If balloon is malpositioned in urethra, pain will occur during inflation.
d. After inflating balloon fully, release catheter with nondominant hand and pull gently to feel resistance (see illustration). Then move catheter slightly back into bladder. Disconnect syringe.	Inflation of balloon anchors catheter tip in place above bladder outlet to prevent removal of catheter. Gentle pulling ensures proper placement and anchoring. Advancing catheter upward minimizes pressure on bladder neck.

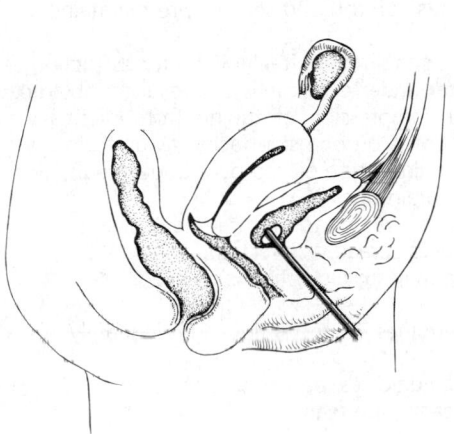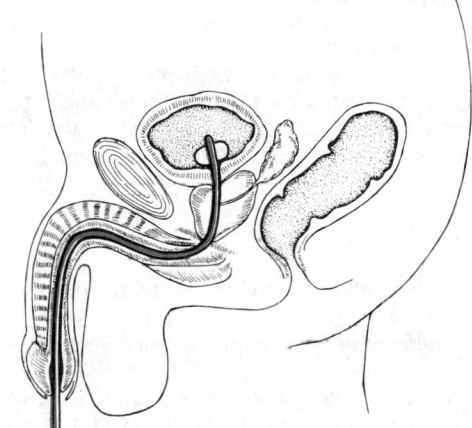

Step 28d

STEPS	RATIONALE
31. Attach end of catheter to collecting tube of drainage system, unless already connected to bag. Place drainage bag in a dependent position (see illustration).	Closed system for urine drainage is established. Dependent position of drainage bag promotes flow of urine away from bladder.
32. Tape catheter.	
a. For female client, tape catheter to the inside of the thigh with strip of nonallergenic tape. Allow for slack so that movement of thigh does not create tension on catheter.	Anchoring of catheter minimizes trauma to urethra and meatus during client's movement. Catheter positioned over the thigh prevents kinking. Nonallergenic tape prevents skin breakdown.

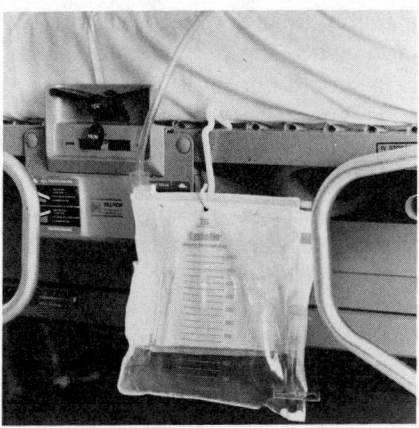

Step 31

Continued.

PROCEDURE 38-2, cont'd

Inserting a Straight or Indwelling Catheter

STEPS	RATIONALE
b. For male client, tape catheter to top of his thigh or lower abdomen (with penis directed toward abdomen). Allow for some slack in catheter, so that movement does not create tension on catheter.	Anchoring catheter to lower abdomen is thought to reduce pressure on urethra at junction of penis and scrotum, thus reducing possibility of tissue necrosis in this area.
32. Be sure there are no obstructions or kinks in tubing. Place excess coil of tubing on bed and fasten it to bottom sheet with clip from drainage set or with rubber band and safety pin.	Patent tubing allows free drainage of urine by gravity and prevents backflow of urine into bladder.
33. Remove gloves and dispose of equipment, drapes, and urine in proper receptacles.	Prevents transmission of infection.
34. Assist client to comfortable position. Wash and dry perineal area as needed.	Client's comfort and security are maintained.
35. Instruct client on ways to lie in bed with catheter: side-lying facing drainage system with catheter and tubing draped over lower thigh; side-lying facing away from system, catheter and tubing extending between legs.	Urine should drain freely without obstruction. Placing catheter under extremities can result in obstruction as result of compression of tubing from client's weight. When client is on one side facing away from system, catheter should not be placed over upper thigh; this forces urine to drain uphill.
36. Caution client against pulling on catheter.	Reduces trauma to urethral meatus.
37. Wash hands.	Reduces spread of infection.
38. Palpate bladder and ask if client remains uncomfortable.	Determines if distention is relieved.
39. Observe character and amount of urine in drainage system.	Determines if urine is flowing adequately.
40. Report and record: type and size of catheter inserted; amount of fluid used to inflate balloon; characteristics of urine; amount of urine.	Communicates pertinent information to all members of health care team.

*These items may be contained on the catheterization tray or they may have to be added after the sterile field is established. May depend upon whether disposable or nondisposable trays are used by the institution.

CLOSED DRAINAGE SYSTEMS. After inserting an indwelling catheter it is necessary to maintain a closed urinary drainage system to minimize the risk of infection. Urinary drainage bags are plastic and capable of holding about 1000 to 1500 ml of urine. The bag should hang on the bed frame without touching the floor when the bed is in its lowest position. A drainage bag should not be placed over or on the bed's side rails. The bag also fits on the frames of most wheelchairs. When the client ambulates, the nurse or client carries the bag below the client's waist. *The nurse should never raise a drainage bag and tubing above the level of the client's bladder.* Urine in the bag and tubing can become a medium for bacteria, and infection is likely to develop if urine flows back into the bladder.

Most drainage bags contain an antireflux valve to prevent urine from reentering the drainage tubing and contaminating the client's bladder. A spigot at the base of the bag provides a means for the nurse to empty the bag. The spigot should always be clamped, except during emptying, and tucked into the protective pouch at the bag's side.

To keep the drainage system patent the nurse: (1) checks for kinks or bends in the tubing; (2) avoids positioning the client on the drainage tubing; and (3) observes for clots or sediment that may occlude the collecting tubing.

ROUTINE CATHETER CARE. Clients with indwelling catheters in place have a number of special care needs. Nursing measures are directed at preventing infection and maintaining unobstructed flow of urine through the catheter drainage system.

Fluid Intake. All clients with catheters should have a daily intake of 3000 ml if permitted. This can be met through oral ingestion or intravenous infusion. A high fluid intake produces a large volume of urine that flushes the bladder and keeps catheter tubing free of sediment.

PROCEDURE 38-3

Indwelling Catheter Care

STEPS	RATIONALE
1. Assess for episode of bowel incontinence or client's report of discomfort at catheter insertion site.	Accumulation of secretions or fecal material causes irritation to perineal tissues and acts as site for bacterial growth.
2. Prepare necessary equipment and supplies:	Ensures an orderly procedure.
a. Sterile catheter care kit	
(1) Sterile gloves	
(2) Cotton balls or application swabs	
(3) Sterile drape	
(4) Antiseptic cleansing solution (for example, povidone-iodine)	
(5) Antibiotic ointment (for example, neomycin)	
(6) Sterile forceps	
(7) Kit container for discarded cotton or swabs	
b. Bath blanket or towels	Used to drape client.
c. Waterproof absorbent pad	Prevents soiling of bed linen.
3. Explain procedure to client. Offer client opportunity to perform self-care if able.	Reduces anxiety and promotes cooperation. Embarrassment during procedure may motivate client to perform own hygiene.
4. Provide privacy by closing room door or bedside curtain.	Maintains client's self-esteem.
5. Wash hands.	Reduces transmission of infection.
6. Position client:	
a. Female in dorsal recumbent position	Ensures easy access to perineal tissues.
b. Male in supine position	
7. Place waterproof pad under client.	Protects bed linen from soiling.
8. Drape bath blanket on bed clothes so that only perineal area is exposed.	Prevents unnecessary exposure of body parts.
9. Open sterile catheter care kit using sterile aseptic technique.	Maintains organized, sterile work area.
10. Put on sterile gloves (see Chapter 43).	Allows nurse to handle sterile supplies without contamination.
11. Apply sterile drapes over client's perineum.	Outer surface of drape provides a sterile work area.
12. Pour antiseptic solution on cotton balls or swabs. Apply antiseptic ointment to cotton ball (check client for allergies to antiseptic).	Prepares solutions for easy application, minimizing risk of contamination.
13. With nondominant hand:	
a. Gently retract labia of female client to fully exposure urethral meatus and catheter insertion site, maintaining position of hand throughout procedure	Provides full visualization of urethral meatus. Full retraction of tissues prevents contamination of meatus during cleansing. Accidental closure of labia or dropping of penis during cleansing requires process to be repeated.
b. Retract foreskin if client not circumcized, and hold penis at shaft just below the glans, maintaining position of hand throughout procedure	
14. Assess urethral meatus and surrounding tissues for inflammation, swelling, and discharge. Note amount, color, odor, and consistency of discharge. Ask client if burning or discomfort is felt.	Determines presence of local infection and status of hygiene.
15. Cleanse perineal tissues:	
a. Female client—use a separate cotton ball and forceps to cleanse each labum majus, moving down toward the anus. Repeat process to cleanse the labia minora, then cleanse around the urethral meatus moving down the catheter, and be sure to cleanse each side	Cleansing reduces the number of microorganisms at the urethral meatus. Use of single cotton ball for each wipe prevents transfer of microorganisms. Cleansing moves from area of least contamination to most. Dominant hand remains sterile.

Continued.

PROCEDURE 38-3, cont'd

Indwelling Catheter Care

STEPS	RATIONALE
b. Male client—while spreading the urethral meatus, cleanse around the catheter first, then use a clean cotton ball with forceps and wipe in a circular motion around the meatus and glans	
16. Reassess urethral meatus for discharge.	Determines if cleansing is complete.
17. Take a new cotton ball with forceps and wipe in a circular motion along the length of the catheter for about 10 cm (4 in).	Reduces presence of secretions or drainage on outside catheter surface.
18. Apply antiseptic ointment at urethral meatus and along 2.5 cm (1 in) of the catheter.	Further reduces growth of microorganisms at insertion site.
19. Place client in safe, comfortable position.	Promotes client's comfort.
20. Remove gloves. Dispose of contaminated supplies and wash hands.	Prevents spread of infection.
21. Record and report condition of perineal tissues, the procedure, client's response, and any abnormalities noted.	Provides data to document procedure and informs staff of client's condition.

Perineal Hygiene. Buildup of secretions or encrustations at the catheter insertion site is a source of infection. Nurses provide perineal hygiene (see Chapter 32) at least twice daily or as needed for any client with a retention catheter. Soap and water are effective in reducing the number of organisms present around the urethra. It is very important for the nurse not to accidentally advance the catheter up into the bladder during cleansing. Otherwise, bacteria may be introduced.

Catheter Care. In addition to routine perineal hygiene, many institutions recommend clients with catheters receive special care twice daily and after defecation or bowel incontinence to help minimize discomfort and infection (Procedure 38-3).

REMOVAL OF INDWELLING CATHETER. Two important principles to follow when removing an indwelling catheter are to (1) promote normal bladder function and (2) prevent trauma to the urethra. Loss of muscle tone in the bladder is a common problem after prolonged catheterization. Bladder reconditioning, which can reduce the loss of bladder tone, requires a physician's order and is begun at least 10 hours before catheter removal (Williamson, 1982). The nurse clamps the indwelling catheter to allow urine to accumulate. The volume of urine stretches the bladder's walls to stimulate muscle tone. Three hours later the nurse unclamps the catheter and allows urine to drain for 5 minutes. The process is repeated two more times. After the conditioning procedure the nurse removes the catheter. Clients who receive bladder conditioning are believed to be able to feel the urge to avoid sooner than those with no conditioning.

To remove a catheter the nurse requires a clean disposable towel, a trash receptacle, and a sterile syringe the same size as the volume of solution within the catheter's inflated balloon. Disposable gloves are optional. The end of each catheter contains a label that denotes the volume of solution (5 to 30 ml) within a balloon.

The nurse positions the client in the same position as during catheterization. Some institutions recommend collecting a sterile urine specimen at this time. After removing the tape, the nurse places the towel between the female's thighs or over the male's thighs. The nurse inserts the syringe into the injection port. Most ports are self-sealing and require only the tip of the syringe to be inserted. The nurse slowly withdraws all of the solution to deflate the balloon totally. If a portion of the solution remains, the partially inflated balloon will traumatize the urethral canal as the catheter is removed. Following deflation the nurse explains that the client will feel a burning sensation as the catheter is withdrawn. The nurse then pulls the catheter out smoothly and slowly.

It is normal for the client to experience dysuria, especially if the catheter has been in place several days or weeks. The catheter causes inflammation of the urethral canal. Until the bladder regains full tone, the client may also have an increased frequency of urination.

The nurse notes when the client first voids after cath-

PROCEDURE 38-4

Applying a Condom Catheter

STEPS	RATIONALE
1. Assess status of client to determine need for condom catheter.	Client continuously incontinent of urine is at risk for skin breakdown.
2. Prepare necessary equipment and supplies:	
a. Rubber condom sheath (proper size)	
b. Strip of elastic tape and skin prep	
c. Urinary collection bag with drainage tubing or leg bag and straps	Urinary leg bag allows client to remain mobile.
d. Basin with warm water and soap	
e. Towels and wash cloths	
f. Disposable gloves	Protects nurse's hands; reduces client's risk of infection.
g. Bath blanket	
h. Razor (optional)	
3. Explain procedure to client.	Reduces anxiety and promotes cooperation.
4. Wash hands.	Reduces transmission of infection.
5. Provide privacy by closing room door or bedside curtain.	Maintains client's self-esteem.
6. Assist client into supine position. Place bath blanket over his upper torso. Fold sheets so that client's lower extremities are covered; only genitalia should be exposed.	Promotes client comfort; draping prevents unnecessary exposure of body parts.
7. Assess condition of penis.	Baseline to compare changes in condition of skin after condom application.
8. Put on disposable gloves. Provide perineal care (see Chapter 32) and dry thoroughly. Shave hair at base of penis.	Removes irritating secretions. Rubber sheath rolls onto dry skin more easily. Hair adheres to condom, and pulls during condom removal.
9. Prepare urinary drainage collection bag and tubing or prepare leg bag for connection to condom, if necessary. Clamp off drainage exit ports. Secure collection bag to bed frame; bring drainage tubing up through siderails onto bed.	Provides easy access to drainage equipment once condom is in place.
10. Apply skin prep to penis and allow to dry.	
11. With nondominant hand, grasp penis along shaft. With dominant hand, hold condom sheath at the tip of penis and smoothly roll sheath onto penis.	Prepares penis for easy condom placement.
12. Allow 2.5-5 cm (1-2 in) of space between tip of glans penis and end of condom catheter.	Space at end allows free passage of urine into collecting tubing when client passes urine.
13. Encircle penile shaft with strip of elastic adhesive. Strip should touch only condom sheath. Apply snugly, but not tightly.	Condom must be secured so it is snug and will stay on but not too tight to cause constriction of blood flow.
14. Connect drainage tubing to end of condom catheter. Be sure condom is not twisted.	Allows urine to be collected and measured. Keeps client dry. Twisted condom obstructs urine flow.
15. Place excess coiling of tubing on bed and secure to bottom sheet.	Prevents looping of tubing and promotes free drainage of urine.
16. Place client in safe, comfortable position.	Promote's client's comfort.
17. Remove gloves. Dispose of contaminated supplies and wash hands.	Prevents spread of infection.
18. Observe urinary drainage.	Determines if normal voiding is occurring.
19. Regularly inspect skin on penile shaft for signs of breakdown or irritation.	Indicates if condom or urine is causing irritation or if adhesive is too restrictive.
20. Record and report time of catheter application, condition of skin, and voiding pattern.	Provides data to determine change in elimination status.

eter removal and assesses for bladder distention. If over 8 hours elapses before the client voids, it may become necessary to catheterize again. If the volume voided is small, residual urine may be in the bladder.

ALTERNATIVES TO CATHETERIZATION

To avoid the risks associated with catheters inserted through the urethra, there are two alternatives for urinary drainage. Suprapubic catheterization involves surgical placement of a catheter through the abdominal wall above the symphysis pubis and into the urinary bladder. The physician performs the procedure under local or general anesthesia. The catheter is anchored in place with sutures, a commercially prepared body seal, or both. Urine drains into a urinary drainage bag. The suprapubic catheter is relatively painless and reduces the incidence of infection commonly seen with retention catheters. Clients with chronic incontinence or loss of bladder control benefit most from a suprapubic catheter. Women who have undergone a hysterectomy may also benefit temporarily from the insertion of a suprapubic catheter during the postoperative course.

The suprapubic catheter can become blocked by sediment, clots, or the abdominal wall itself. Nurses must monitor the client's intake and output carefully, observe for signs of kidney infection (for example, flank tenderness, chills, fever), and monitor the appearance of urine. Spread of infection to the kidneys may indicate removal of the catheter. A suprapubic catheter must remain patent at all times. The nurse also administers skin care around the insertion site.

The second is the *condom* catheter. It is suitable for incontinent or comatose male clients who still have complete and spontaneous bladder emptying. The condom is a soft, pliable, rubber sheath that slips over the penis. It may be worn at night only or continuously, depending on the client's needs. A strip of elastic tape fits around the top of the condom to secure it in place (Fig. 38-10). Some types of condoms are applied with skin paste. Care must be taken not to contract the band tightly, or blood supply to the penis will be impaired. Standard adhesive tape should never be used to secure a condom catheter because it does not expand with change in penis size, and blood supply to the penis is impaired.

The end of the condom fits into a plastic drainage tubing. A drainage bag can be attached to the side of the bed or strapped to the client's leg. The condom catheter itself poses little risk of infection. Infections with condom catheters usually result from buildup of secretions around the urethra, trauma to the urethral meatus, or buildup of pressure in the outflow tubing. Procedure 38-4 reviews application of the condom catheter.

The nurse should change a condom catheter daily to

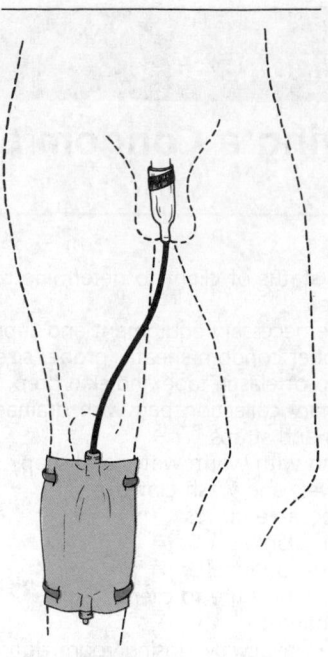

Fig. 38-10   Condom catheter with leg drainage bag.

check for skin irritation. With each catheter change the nurse cleans the urethral meatus and penis thoroughly. Twisting of the condom at the drainage tube attachment irritates the skin and obstructs urine outflow. The drainage tubing must be checked often for patency.

Prevention of Infection

One of the most important considerations for a client with urinary alterations is the need to prevent infection. Good perineal hygiene involving cleansing the urethral meatus after each voiding is essential. A daily intake of 2000 to 2500 ml of fluids dilutes urine and promotes regular micturition, which flushes the urethra of microorganisms.

Infection can develop in a catheterized client in a number of ways. Maintaining a closed urinary drainage system is important in infection control. A break in the system can lead to introduction of microorganisms. Sites at risk are at place of catheter insertion, the drainage bag, the spigot, tube junction, and junction of tube and bag (Fig. 38-11). In addition, the nurse monitors the patency of the system to prevent pooling of urine within tubing. Urine in the drainage bag is an excellent medium for microorganism growth. Bacteria can travel up drainage tubing to grow in pools of urine. If this urine flows back into the client's bladder, an infection will likely develop. The box gives suggestions for ways to prevent infections in catheterized clients.

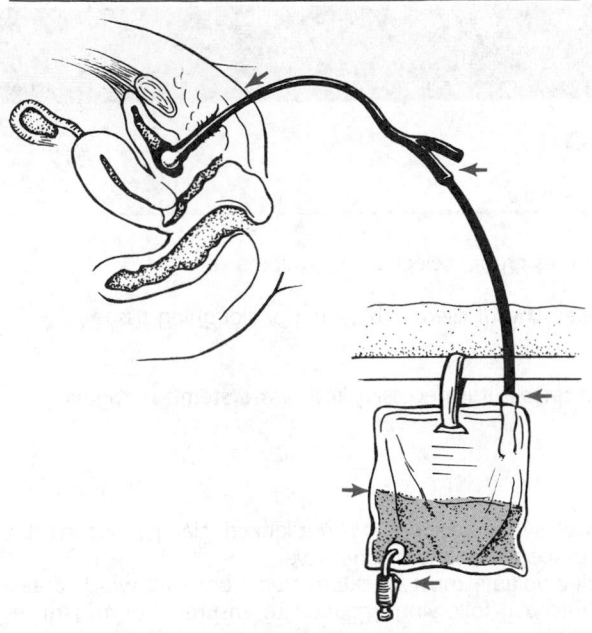

Fig. 38-11   Potential sites for introduction of infectious organisms into a urinary drainage system.

HANDWASHING

Good handwashing practices are basic to infection control. Handwashing is necessary before the nurse handles a catheter or the drainage system. When the nurse goes from a client with a catheter to one without, handwashing can prevent cross-contamination. The nurse also cautions clients against handling a catheter with unclean hands.

ACIDIFYING URINE

An acid urine tends to inhibit growth of microorganisms. Meats, eggs, whole-grain breads, cranberries, prunes, and plums increase urine acidity. The foods metabolize into acid end products that eventually enter the urine. Cranberry juice increases urine acidity, whereas fruit juices such as orange or grapefruit juice produce alkaline urine. However, large volumes of juice must be taken to actually change urine pH. High doses of ascorbic acid may lower urine pH.

CATHETER IRRIGATIONS AND INSTILLATIONS

To maintain the patency of indwelling urinary catheters, it sometimes becomes necessary to irrigate or flush a catheter. Blood, pus, or sediment can collect within tubing and result in bladder distention and the build-up of stagnant urine. Instillation of a sterile solution ordered by the physician will clear the tubing of accumulated material. For clients with bladder infections, a physician

---

Tips for Preventing Infection in Catheterized Clients

- Follow good handwashing techniques.
- Do not allow the spigot on the drainage bag to touch a contaminated surface.
- Do not open the drainage system at connection points to obtain specimens or measure urine.
- If the drainage tubing becomes disconnected, do not touch the ends of the catheter or tubing. Wipe the ends of the tube with antiseptic solution before reconnecting.
- Each client should have a separate receptacle for measuring urine to prevent cross-contamination.
- Prevent pooling of urine and reflux of urine into the bladder.
  - Avoid raising the drainage bag above the level of the client's bladder.
  - If it becomes necessary to raise the bag during transfer of the client to a bed or stretcher, clamp the tubing.
  - Avoid allowing large loops of tubing to dangle from bedside.
  - Before client exercises or ambulates, drain all urine from tubing into bag.
- Avoid prolonged clamping or kinking of the tubing (except during conditioning).
- Empty the drainage bag at least every 8 hours.
- Remove the catheter as soon as possible after confering with physician.

---

may order a bladder irrigation to include instillation of an antiseptic solution to wash out the bladder or treat a local infection. In both types of irrigations sterile aseptic technique is followed.

Before performing an irrigation, the nurse assesses the catheter for blockage. If the amount of urine in the drainage bag is less than the client's intake or less than the output during the previous shift, blockage can be expected. If urine does not drain freely, the nurse milks the tubing. Milking is done by gently squeezing then releasing the drainage tube in an alternating fashion. The nurse should always milk from the client to the drainage bag so a clot or sediment will not be forced back into the catheter.

There is disagreement in the nursing literature about the most effective procedure for irrigations. Studies have shown higher or equal infection rates in clients receiving irrigation than those with nonirrigated catheters (Dudley and Barriere, 1981; Gelmon, 1980). This was the case even with closed irrigation systems. Contamination of

Closed and Open Catheter Irrigation

STEPS	RATIONALE
1. Assess physician's order for type of irrigation and irrigating solution to use.	Ensures proper selection of equipment.
2. Assess color of urine and presence of mucus or sediment.	Determines if client is bleeding or sloughing tissue.
3. Determine type of catheter in place:	
a. Triple lumen (one lumen to inflate balloon, one to instill irrigation solution, and one to allow outflow of urine)	Indicates if it is necessary to break system for irrigation.
b. Double lumen (one lumen to inflate balloon, one to allow outflow of urine)	
4. Determine patency of drainage tubing.	Ensures drainage tubing is not kinked, clamped incorrectly, or looped below bladder level.
5. Assess amount of urine in drainage bag.	Urine volume must be subtracted from that which drains into bag following irrigation to ensure all of irrigant returns.
6. Collect necessary equipment and supplies.	
a. Closed intermittent method:	
(1) Sterile irrigating solution	
(2) Sterile graduated cup	
(3) Sterile 30 to 50 ml syringe	Used to instill irrigant into catheter.
(4) Sterile 19- to 22-gauge, 1 inch needle	
(5) Antiseptic swab	
(6) Screw clamp	Temporarily occludes catheter as irrigant is instilled.
(7) Bath blanket	
b. Closed continuous method:	
(1) Sterile irrigating solution, correct bag or solution	
(2) Irrigation tubing with clamp (with or without Y connector)	Clamp regulates irrigation flow rate. Y-connector allows IV bags to be connected to tubing.
(3) Metric container	For measuring urine output in drainage bag.
(4) IV pole	
(5) Antiseptic swab	
(6) Y connector (optional)	Connects irrigation tubing to double-lumen catheter.
(7) Bath blanket	
c. Open method:	
(1) Disposable, sterile irrigation tray and set	
(2) Bulb syringe or 60 ml, piston-type syringe	Provides necessary force to dislodge clot.
(3) Sterile collection basin	
(4) Waterproof drape	
(5) Sterile solution container	
(6) Antiseptic swabs	
(7) Sterile gloves	
(8) Ordered irrigating solution at room temperature, cold solution may cause bladder spasm.	
(9) Tape	
(10) Bath blanket	
7. Explain procedure and purpose to client.	Helps client to relax and cooperate during procedure.
8. Wash hands.	Reduces transmission of infection.
9. Provide privacy, pull curtains around bed, fold back covers so that catheter is exposed at junction where it connects to drainage tubing. Cover client's chest with bath blanket.	Promotes client comfort; shows respect for client while exposing area nurse must see.
10. Assess lower abdomen for bladder distention.	Detects if catheter is malfunctioning, blocking urinary drainage.

STEPS	RATIONALE
11. Position client in dorsal, recumbent, or supine position.	Promotes client comfort and provides easy access to catheter. Promotes flow of irrigating solution into bladder.

12. Closed intermittent irrigation:
  a. Prepare the prescribed sterile irrigating solution in the sterile graduated cup
  b. Draw the sterile solution into the syringe using aseptic technique
  c. Clamp the indwelling retention catheter below the soft injection port
  d. Cleanse the catheter injection port with an antiseptic swab (same port used for specimen collections)
  e. Insert needle or syringe through port at a 30-degree angle
  f. Slowly inject fluid into the catheter and bladder
 	
  g. Withdraw syringe and remove clamp, allow solution to drain into urinary drainage bag (it is optional to keep tubing clamped to allow instilled fluid to remain in bladder)
	Ensures irrigating fluid remains sterile.
	
	Occlusion of catheter will provide resistance against which irrigant can be forcefully instilled into catheter.
	Reduces transmission of infection.
	
	Ensures needle tip enters lumen of catheter.
	
	Slow, continuous pressure will dislodge clots and sediment without traumatizing bladder wall.
	Allows drainage to flow by gravity.

13. Closed continuous irrigation:
  a. Using aseptic technique insert tip of sterile irrigation tubing into bag containing irrigation solution
  b. Close clamp on tubing and hang bag of solution on IV pole
  c. Open clamp and allow solution to flow through tubing, keeping end of tubing sterile, close clamp
  d. Wipe off irrigation port of 3-lumen catheter or attach a sterile Y connector to double-lumen catheter, then connect to irrigation tubing
  e. Be sure drainage bag and tubing are securely connected to either drainage port of 3-lumen catheter or other arm of Y connector
	Prevents entrance of microorganisms.
	
	Prevents loss of irrigating solution.
	
	Removes air from tubing.
	
	The third catheter lumen or Y connector provides means for irrigating solution to enter bladder. System must remain sterile.
	Ensures that urine and irrigating solution will drain from bladder.

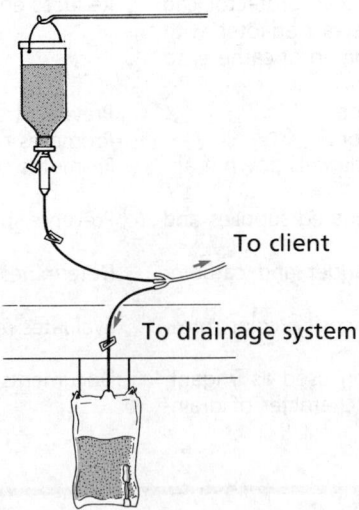

To client

To drainage system

Step 13g

Continued.

Closed and Open Catheter Irrigation

STEPS	RATIONALE
f. For an intermittent flow, clamp tubing on drainage system, open clamp on irrigation tubing and allow prescribed amount of fluid to enter bladder (100 ml is normal for an adult), close irrigation tubing clamp, then open drainage tubing clamp	Fluid instills through catheter into bladder, flushing system. Fluid drains out after irrigation is completed.
g. For a continuous irrigation (see illustration), calculate drip rate and adjust clamp on irrigation tubing accordingly, be sure clamp on drainage tubing is open, check volume of drainage in drainage bag	Ensures continuous even irrigation of catheter system. Prevents accumulation of solution in bladder, which may cause bladder distention and possible injury.
14. Open irrigation:	
a. Open sterile irrigation tray, establish sterile field, pour amount required of sterile solution into sterile solution container, replace cap on large container of solution	Adheres to principles of surgical asepsis.
b. Don sterile gloves (see Chapter 43).	Reduces transmission of infection.
c. Position waterproof drape under catheter	Prevents soiling bed linen.
d. Aspirate 30 ml of solution into irrigating syringe	Prepares irrigant for instillation into catheter.
e. Move sterile collection basin close to client's thigh	Prevents soiling of bed linen and prohibits reaching over sterile area.
f. Disconnect catheter from drainage tubing, allowing urine to flow into sterile collection basin; cover open end of drainage tubing with sterile protective cap. Position this tubing so that it stays coiled on top of bed.	Maintains sterility of inner aspect of catheter lumen and drainage tubing, reduces potential of inducing pathogens into bladder.
g. Insert tip of syringe into lumen of catheter and gently instill solution	Gentle instillation reduces incidence of bladder spasm but clears catheter of obstruction.
h. Withdraw syringe, lower catheter, allow solution to drain into basin; repeat instilling solution and draining several times until drainage is clear	Allows drainage to flow by gravity. Provides for adequate flushing of catheter.
i. If solution does not return, have client turn onto side facing nurse; if changing position does not help, reinsert syringe and gently aspirate the solution	Change in position may move tip of catheter in bladder, increasing likelihood that fluid instilled will flow out.
j. Once irrigation is completed, remove protector cap from drainage tubing adapter, swab adapter with alcohol swab, and reinsert into lumen of catheter to reestablish closed drainage system	Reduces entrance of microorganisms into system.
15. Reanchor catheter to client with tape.	Prevents trauma to urethral tissue.
16. Assist client into comfortable position.	Promotes relaxation and rest.
17. Lower bed to its lowest position, side rails down if appropriate.	Promotes client safety.
18. Remove gloves. Dispose of contaminated supplies and wash hands.	Prevents spread of infection to other clients.
19. Calculate fluid used to irrigate bladder and catheter and subtract from volume drained.	Determines accurate urinary output.
20. Assess characteristics of output: viscosity, color, presence of clots.	Evaluates response to therapy.
21. Record type and amount of solution used as irrigant, amount returned as drainage, and character of drainage.	Documents procedure and client's tolerance.

irrigating fluids and equipment and disconnection of the catheter system may be factors in causing infection.

Burgener (1987) recommends that a closed system be maintained during intermittent irrigations or instillations. The nurse uses a sterile 30 to 50 ml syringe with a 19 to 22- gauge, 1-inch needle to inject a prescribed solution into the catheter. This technique is effective for irrigating a partially blocked catheter or for bladder instillations. Steps for using this closed system are outlined in Procedure 38-5.

When a single intermittent irrigation is required, this procedure is safer and less likely to introduce infections into the urinary tract. There are two additional methods for catheter irrigation. One is a closed bladder irrigation system (Procedure 38-5). This system provides for frequent intermittent or continuous irrigation of a catheter without disrupting the sterile catheter system. It is used most often in clients who have had genitourinary surgery and are at risk for blood clots and mucous fragments occluding a catheter. The other system involves opening the closed drainage system to instill bladder irrigations (Procedure 38-5). This technique poses greater risk for causing infection. However, it may be needed when cath-eters become blocked and it is undesirable to change the catheter.

Maintenance of Skin Integrity

The normal acidity of urine is irritating to skin. When urine becomes alkaline, encrustations or precipitate collects on the skin, fostering breakdown. Continuous exposure to urine of the perineal area or the skin surrounding an ostomy leads to gradual maceration and excoriation. Washing with mild soap and warm water is the best way to remove urine from skin. Body lotion keeps skin moisturized and provides a barrier to the urine. Clients who wet their clothing should receive a partial bath and a clean set of clothes after each voiding.

When the skin becomes irritated or inflamed, the physician may prescribe a cream or spray containing steroids to reduce inflammation (for example, Kenalog). If fungal growth develops, the antifungal drug nystatin (Mycostatin), available in cream or powder form, is effective.

The client with an ostomy has a special hygiene problem because urine drains from the ostomy site continuously. Often the drainage pouch or appliance becomes

---

Sample Evaluation of Interventions for Urinary Elimination

Goals	Evaluative Measures	Expected Outcomes
Client will understand normal urinary elimination.	Ask client to explain normal voiding process. Ask client to describe factors that promote or impair urinary elimination. Observe client's self-care habits related to toileting.	Client will verbalize understanding of urinary elimination and follow appropriate health care practices promoting elimination.
Client will achieve normal micturition.	Measure urinary output and compare with intake. Observe client's ability to void.	Client will void at least 1500-1600 ml urine daily. Client is able to void without use of medications or catheterization.
Client will achieve complete bladder emptying.	Palpate bladder for distention after voiding. Catheterize, using straight catheter, for residual urine after voiding.	Bladder will be nondistended. Residual urine will be less than 50 ml after voiding.
Client will be free of infection.	Obtain urine culture. Assess client for signs of dysuria, burning, itching at urethral meatus, urgency or frequency. Observe characteristics of urine.	No bacterial growth. Client will remain symptom free. Urine will be clear, amber, without sediment.
Skin integrity will be maintained.	Observe condition of urethra and surrounding skin. Observe skin around urinary stoma.	Skin will remain dry, intact, without inflammation or excoriation.
Client will gain a sense of comfort.	Evaluate if client feels burning or pain during urination. Palpate bladder for distention.	Client voids without dysuria. Bladder is nondistended.

moist and slips from the skin. Continual oozing of urine around the stoma causes skin breakdown. Skin barriers provide a layer of protection between the client's skin and the ostomy pouch. When urine leaks, it frequently covers the outer skin barrier. It is also helpful for the client with an ostomy to select an appliance that fits snugly against the skin's surface around the stoma.

Promotion of Comfort

Clients with urinary alterations become uncomfortable as a result of the symptoms of urinary problems. Frequent or unpredictable voiding, dysuria, and painful distention are all sources of discomfort.

The incontinent client gains comfort from having clean, dry clothing. When stress incontinence is the problem, a protective pad or sanitary belt offers protection against soiling. Wet clothing adheres to the skin and can cause rubbing and irritation.

Dysuria may be relieved by giving urinary analgesics that act on the urethral and bladder mucosa. Phenazopyridine helps relieve dysuria, burning, and itching. It comes combined with sulfonamide antibiotics in preparations such as Azo Gantanol and Azo Gantrisin. The sulfonamide provides additional antibacterial action. Clients taking drugs with phenazopyridine should be aware that their urine may appear orange. They must drink large amounts of fluids to prevent toxicity from the sulfonamides and to maintain optimal flow through the urinary system.

If the client has local discomfort from an inflamed urethra, a warm sitz bath may provide pain relief (see Chapter 32). The warm water soothes inflamed tissues near the urethral meatus by improving blood supply. The client is often relaxed after a sitz bath so voiding occurs easily.

Pain of distention cannot be relieved unless the client is able to empty the bladder. Methods for stimulating micturition may be the only sources of pain relief.

EVALUATION

To evaluate outcomes and response to nursing care the nurse measures the effectiveness of all interventions. The optimal outcome is the client's ability to urinate voluntarily without symptoms (for example, urgency, dysuria, or frequency). The urine should be an amber color, clear, without abnormal constituents and within the normal range of pH and specific gravity. The client should be able to identify factors that may influence the ability of void normally.

The nurse also evaluates specific interventions designed to promote normal urinary function and prevent complications of urinary alterations (see evaluation box).

Using the nursing process, the nurse collects data related to the client's voiding pattern, exposure to risks for urinary tract alteration, and physical condition. Laboratory analysis of urine specimens and diagnostic review of urinary structures provide further information for nurse's data base. Nursing diagnoses are the basis for the plan of care.

Nursing interventions promote normal urination and provide support to clients unable to maintain continence. Because of the urinary tract's vulnerability to infection, one of the nurse's primary concerns is infection control. The client with urinary alterations may also suffer embarrassment, social isolation, and depression. Whether the client's alteration is temporary (as with catheterization) or long term (as with ureterostomy), the nurse must maintain the client's privacy and dignity.

SUMMARY

Normal elimination of urinary wastes requires maintenance of urinary function. The nurses' therapies either promote or minimize the factors that influence proper urinary function. Each client has a different pattern of elimination and follows different personal toileting habits.

KEY CONCEPTS

- ✓ The act of micturition or voiding is influenced by voluntary control from higher brain centers, as well as involuntary control from the spinal cord.
- ✓ Symptoms common to urinary disturbances include urgency, dysuria, polyuria, oliguria, and difficulty in starting the urinary stream.
- ✓ When collected properly, a clean-voiding urine specimen does not contain bacteria picked up from the urethral meatus.

✓ A client can better understand the importance of perineal hygiene by knowing that the urinary tract is normally sterile.

✓ Methods of promoting the micturition reflex assist clients in sensing the urge to urinate and controlling urethral sphincter relaxation.

✓ An increased fluid intake results in increased urine formation that flushes particles and solutes from the urinary system.

✓ An indwelling urinary catheter remains in the bladder for an extended period, making the risk of infection greater than with intermittent catheterization.

✓ Since urine drains almost continuously from a ureterostomy, there is a risk of skin breakdown around a stoma site.

✓ A primary function of the elimination process is fluid balance.

✓ Catheter irrigation becomes necessary when the catheter becomes occluded with sediment or blood clots.

✓ A catheter drainage system should be positioned to allow free drainage of urine by gravity.

✓ Condom catheters are applied snugly but not so tightly as to constrict blood flow.

✓ Since urine drains almost continuously from a ureterostomy, there is a risk of skin breakdown around a stoma site.

REFERENCES

Dudley, MN, and Barriere, SL: Antimicrobial irrigations in the prevention and treatment of catheter-related urinary tract infections Am J Hosp Pharm 38(1):59, 1981.

Kane, RL, et al.: Essentials of clinical geriatrics, New York, 1984, McGraw-Hill Book Co.

Kristiansen, P, et al.: Long-term urethral catheter drainage and bladder capacity, Neurol Urodyn 2:134, 1983.

Orzeck, S, and Ouslander JG: Urinary incontinence: an overview of causes and treatment, J Entero Ther 14:20, 1987.

Rogers, W: Shampoo urethritis (letter). Am J Dis Childh 139:748, 1985.

Whaley, LF, and Wong, DL: Nursing care of infants and children, ed. 3, St. Louis, 1987, The C.V. Mosby Co.

Williamson, ML: Reducing post-catheterization bladder dysfunction by reconditioning, Nurs Res 31:28, 1982.

Wong, ES: Guidelines for the prevention of catheter-associated urinary tract infections. In Guidelines for the prevention and control of nosocomial infections, p. 1, Atlanta, 1982, US Centers for Disease Control.

Research Articles

Burgener, S: Justification of closed intermittent urinary catheter irrigation/installation: a review of current research and practice, J Adv Nurs 12:229, 1987.

Gelmon, ML: Antibiotic irrigation and catheter-associated urinary tract infections, Nephron 25:259, 1980.

ADDITIONAL READINGS

Alteresco, V: Theoretical foundations for an approach to urinary incontinence, J Entero Ther 13:105, 1986.

Bates, P: A troubleshooter's guide to indwelling catheters, RN 44:63, 1981.

Bello-Reuss, E, and Reuss, L: Homeostatic and excretory functions of the kidney. In Klahr, S, editor: The kidney and body fluids in health and disease, New York, 1983, Plenum Medical Book Co.

Bielski, M: Preventing infection in the catheterized patient, Nurs Clin North Am 15:703, 1980.

Brundage, DJ: Nursing management of renal problems, ed. 2, St. Louis, 1980, The C.V. Mosby Co.

Demmerle, B, and Bantol, MA: Nursing care of the incontinent person, Geriatric Nurs 1:246, 1980.

De sautels, RE: Managing the urinary catheter, Nurs Digest 3:30, 1975.

Erickson, PJ: Ostomies: the art of pouching, Nurs Clin North Am 22:311, 1987.

Greengold, BA, and Ouslander, JG: Bladder retraining, J Gerontol Nurs 12:31, 1986.

Harty, JI, and Catalona, WJ: Management aspects of the genitourinary system. In Etheredge, E, editor: Management techniques in surgery, New York, 1986, John S. Wiley Co.

Mandelstam, D: Strengthening pelvic floor muscles, Geriatric Nurs 1:251, 1980.

Nurses' drug alert: Urinary tract irritation from shampoo, Am J Nurs 86:66, 1986.

Pagana, KD, and Pagana, TJ: Diagnostic testing and nursing implications: a case study approach, ed. 2, St. Louis, 1986, The C.V. Mosby Co.

Petillo, MH: The patient with a urinary stoma, Nurs Clin North Am 22:263, 1987.

Robb, SS: Urinary incontinence verification in elderly men, Nurs Res 34:278, 1985.

Wilde, MH: Living with a Foley, Am J Nurs 86:1121, 1986.

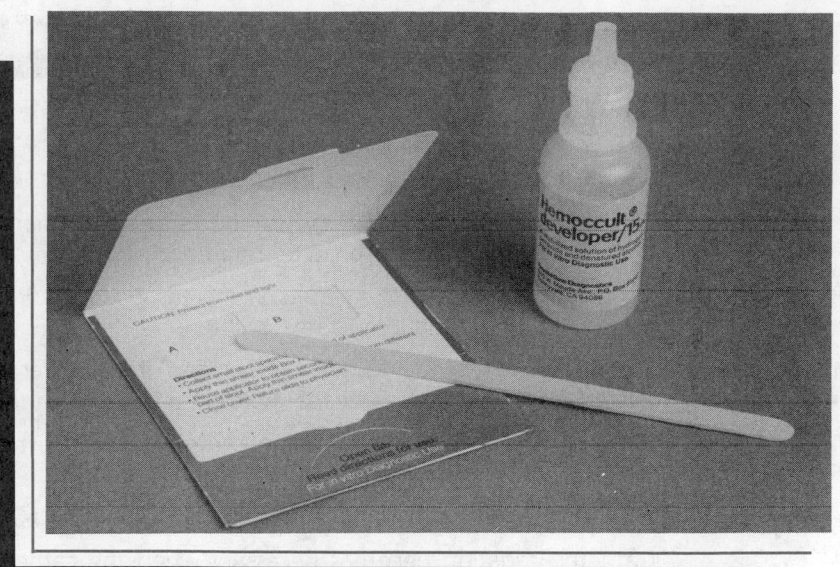

OBJECTIVES

Mastery of content in this chapter will enable the student to:

- Define the key terms listed.
- Discuss the role of gastrointestinal organs in digestion and elimination.
- Describe four functions of the large intestine.
- Explain the physiology of normal defecation.
- List and discuss psychological and physiological factors that influence the elimination process.
- Describe common physiological alterations in elimination.
- Assess a client's elimination pattern.
- Perform a guaiac test for occult blood.
- List nursing diagnoses related to alterations in elimination.
- Describe nursing implications for common diagnostic examinations of the gastrointestinal tract.
- Administer an enema.
- List nursing measures aimed at promoting normal elimination.
- Discuss the relationship between the structure and function of a colostomy and nursing care required.

KEY TERMS

Amylase	Excoriation
Biopsy	Feces
Bolus	Flatulence
Cathartic	Guaiac Test
Chyme	Haustral Contraction
Colitis	Hemorrhoids
Colon	Laxative
Constipation	Masticate
Contrast Medium	Melena
Crohn's Disease	Ostomate
Defecation	Ostomy
Diarrhea	Paralytic Ileus
Diverticula	Regurgitation
Endoscopy	Stoma
Enema	Tarry
Enterostomal Therapist	

Bowel Elimination

Regular elimination of bowel waste products is essential for normal body functioning. Elimination alterations may cause problems with the gastrointestinal and other body systems. These alterations can be embarrassing and frustrating. Because bowel function depends on the balance of several factors, each client has a unique elimination pattern.

Clients often need assistance from the nurse to maintain normal elimination habits. Illness may prevent them from following their bowel management program. Clients may become physically unable to use normal toilet facilities. The home environment may present obstacles for clients with altered mobility, requiring changes in bathroom fixtures.

To manage a client's elimination problems, the nurse must understand normal elimination and factors that create alterations. Supportive nursing care respects the client's privacy and emotional needs. Measures designed to promote normal elimination should also minimize discomfort.

NORMAL DIGESTION AND ELIMINATION PROCESS

The gastrointestinal (GI) tract is a series of hollow mucous membrane–lined muscular organs whose primary purposes are to (1) absorb fluid and nutrients and (2) prepare food for absorption and use by the body's cells (Fig. 39-1). The volume of fluids absorbed by the GI tract is high, making fluid balance a key function of

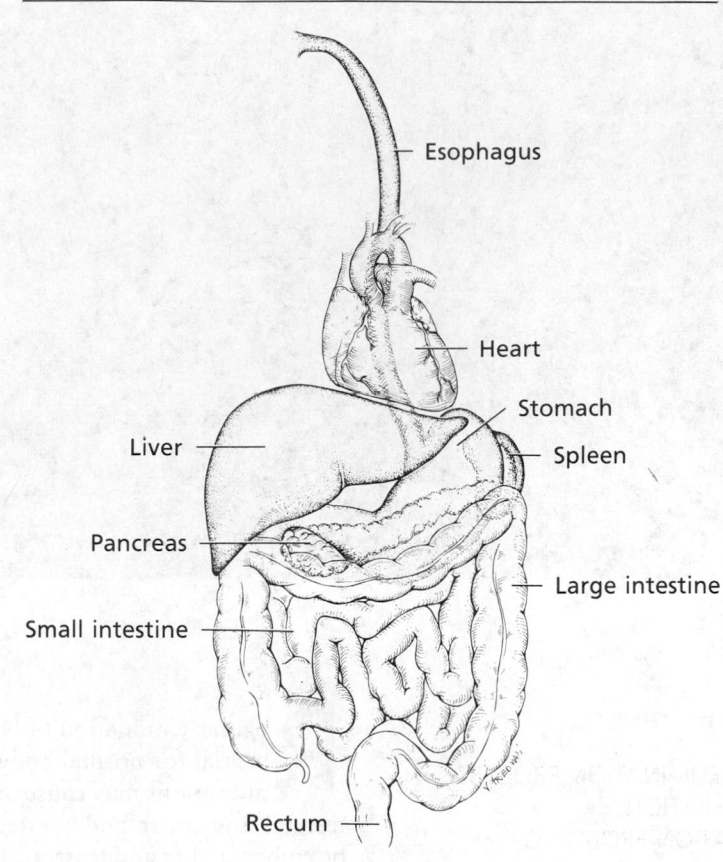

Fig. 39-1 Organs of the gastrointestinal system (with the heart as a reference point).

elimination. In addition to ingested fluids and foods, the GI tract also receives many secretions from organs such as the gallbladder and pancreas (Table 39-1). Any disorder that seriously impairs normal absorption or secretion of GI fluids will cause fluid imbalance.

The GI tract mechanically and chemically breaks down nutrients into a suitable size and form. All digestive organs work together to ensure that the mass or

TABLE 39-1 Gastrointestinal Tract Fluid Balance

	Ingested and Secreted (ml)	Absorbed (ml)
Food and drink	1500	
Saliva	1500	
Gastric juice	3000	
Pancreatic juice	2000	
Bile	500	
Small intestine		5850
Colon		2500
Feces		150
TOTAL	8500	8500

bolus of food reaches the areas of nutrient absorption safely and effectively. The teeth masticate (chew) food, breaking it down to a suitable size for swallowing. Salivary secretions contain enzymes that initiate digestion of certain food elements. Saliva dilutes and softens the bolus of food in the mouth for easier swallowing.

Esophagus

As food enters the upper esophagus, it passes through the upper esophageal sphincter, which is a circular muscle that prevents air from entering the esophagus and food from refluxing (moving backward) into the throat. The bolus of food travels approximately 25 cm (10 inches) down the esophagus. Food is pushed along by slow peristaltic waves produced by alternating contractions of smooth muscle. As a portion of the esophagus contracts behind the food bolus, the circular muscle in front of the bolus relaxes. A peristaltic wave propels food toward the next wave (Fig. 39-2). Peristalsis moves food throughout the length of the GI tract.

In 15 seconds the bolus of food moves down the esophagus and reaches the lower esophageal sphincter.

Although no muscular sphincter lies between the esophagus and the stomach, a pressure difference exists at the lower end of the esophagus. The lower esophageal pressure is 10 to 40 mm Hg, whereas pressure within the stomach is 5 to 10 mm Hg. The pressure gradient normally prevents reflux of stomach contents back into the esophagus. Factors influencing lower sphincter pressure include antacids, which minimize reflux, and fatty foods and nicotine, which increase reflux.

Stomach

In the stomach, food is temporarily stored and mechanically broken down for digestion and absorption. The stomach secretes hydrochloric acid (HCl), mucus, the enzyme pepsin, and intrinsic factor. The concentration of HCl influences stomach acidity and the body's acid-base balance (see Chapter 37). For every HCl molecule secreted into the stomach, a bicarbonate (HCO_3^-) molecule enters the blood plasma. HCl helps mix and break down food in the stomach. Mucus protects the stomach mucosa from acidity and enzyme activity. Pepsin digests proteins, although not much digestion occurs in the stomach. Intrinsic factor is the essential component needed for vitamin B_{12} absorption in the intestine. Lack of intrinsic factor results in pernicious anemia.

Before food leaves the stomach, it is changed into a semifluid material called **chyme.** Chyme is more easily digested and absorbed than solid food. Clients who have portions of their stomach removed or who have rapid stomach emptying (as with colitis) have serious digestive problems because food is not broken down into chyme. Food enters the small intestine before being adequately broken down to a semifluid form. Absorption is less efficient, and nutritional alterations can develop.

Small Intestine

During normal digestion chyme leaves the stomach and enters the small intestine. The small intestine is a tube about 2.5 cm (1 inch) in diameter and 6 m (20 feet) in length. It contains three divisions: duodenum, jejunum, and ileum. Chyme mixes with digestive enzymes (such as bile and amylase) while traveling through the small intestine. Segmentation (alternating contraction and relaxation of smooth muscle) churns the chyme, further breaking down food for digestion (Fig. 39-2). As chyme mixes, forward peristaltic movement temporarily ceases to permit absorption. Chyme travels slowly down the small intestine to allow absorption.

Most nutrients and electrolytes are absorbed in the small intestine. Enzymes from the pancreas (such as amylase) and bile from the gallbladder are released into the duodenum. The intestine breaks down fats, proteins, and carbohydrates into basic elements (see Chapter 33). Nu-

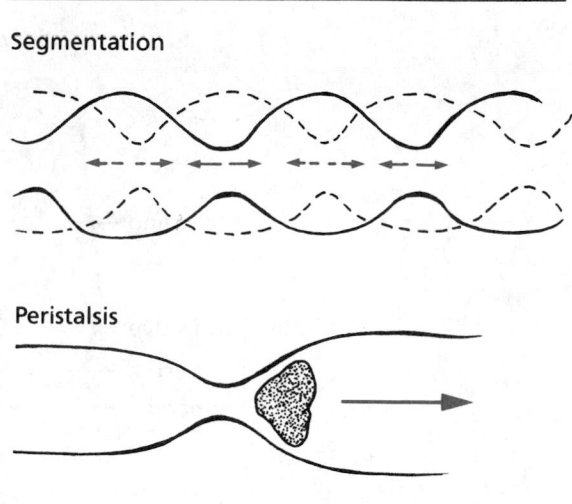

Fig. 39-2 Segmented and peristaltic waves.

trients are almost entirely absorbed by the duodenum and jejunum. The ileum absorbs certain vitamins, iron, and bile salts. If small intestine function is impaired, the digestive process is greatly altered (for example, inflammation, surgical resection, or obstruction can disrupt peristalsis, reduce the area of absorption, or block passage of chyme). Electrolyte and nutrient deficiencies then develop.

Large Intestine

The lower gastrointestinal tract is named the large intestine (colon) because its diameter is larger than the small intestine. However, its length of 1.5 to 1.8 m (5 to 6 feet) is much shorter. The large intestine is divided into the cecum, colon, and rectum (Fig. 39-3). It is the primary organ of bowel elimination.

CECUM

Unabsorbed chyme enters the large intestine at the cecum through the ileocecal valve, which is a circular muscle layer that prevents colon contents from regurgitating (returning to the small intestine).

COLON

Although watery chyme enters the colon, the volume of water lessens as chyme moves along it. The colon is divided into four sections: ascending, transverse, descending, and sigmoid. The colon is made of muscular tissue, which allows it to eliminate large quantities of waste.

The colon has four interrelated functions: absorption, protection, secretion, and elimination. A large volume of water and a significant amount of sodium and chloride are absorbed by the colon daily. As food passes through

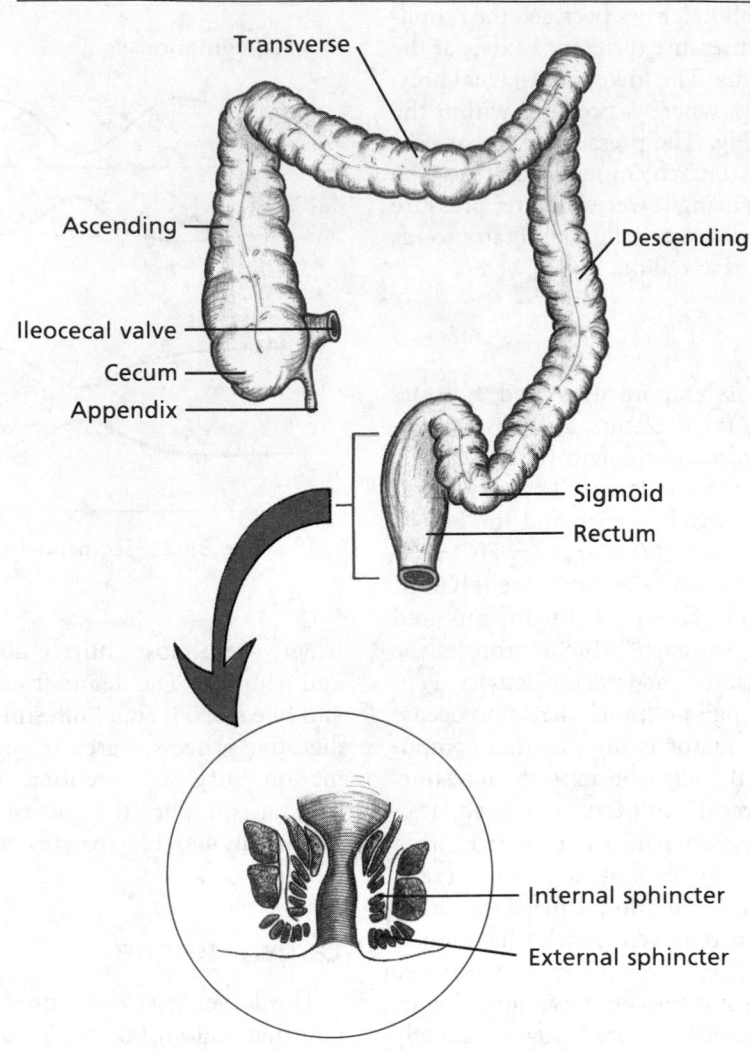

Ascending

Ileocecal valve

Cecum

Appendix

Transverse

Descending

Sigmoid

Rectum

Internal sphincter

External sphincter

Fig. 39-3 Divisions of the large intestine.

the colon, haustral contractions occur. These are similar to segmental contractions of the small intestine but last longer—up to 5 minutes. The contractions produce large sacs in the colon's wall, providing a large surface area for absorption.

As much as 2.5 liters of water may be absorbed by the colon in 24 hours. On the average, 55 milliequivalents (mEq) of sodium and 23 mEq of chloride are absorbed daily. The amount of water absorbed from chyme depends on the speed at which colonic contents move. Chyme is normally a soft, formed mass. If the speed of peristaltic contractions is abnormally fast, there is less time for water to be absorbed and the stool will be watery. If peristaltic contractions slow down, a hard mass of stool forms, resulting in constipation.

The colon protects itself by releasing a supply of mucus. Mucus is normally clear to opaque with a stringy consistency. Mucus lubricates the colon, preventing trauma to its inner walls. Lubrication is especially important near the distal end of the colon where contents become drier and harder.

The secretory function of the colon aids in electrolyte balance. Bicarbonate is secreted in exchange for chloride. About 4 to 9 mEq of potassium is released each day by the large intestine. Serious alterations in colon function can cause electrolyte imbalance.

Finally, the colon removes waste products and gas (flatus). Flatus results from air swallowing, diffusion of gas from the bloodstream into the intestine, and bacterial action on nonabsorbable carbohydrates. Fermentation of carbohydrates (such as in cabbage and onions) produces intestinal gas, which can stimulate peristalsis. An adult normally forms 7 to 10 liters of flatus daily.

Slow peristaltic contractions move contents through

the colon. Intestinal contents are the main stimulus for contraction. Waste products and gas exert pressure against the walls of the colon. The muscle layer stretches, stimulating the reflex that initiates contraction.

Mass peristaltic movements push undigested food toward the rectum. These movements are unlike the frequent peristaltic waves in the small intestine (usually heard during auscultation) in that they occur only three or four times daily.

When these mass peristaltic movements occur, large segments of the colon contract as a result of gastrocolic and duodenocolic reflex responses. These occur when the stomach or duodenum is filled with food. Filling initiates nerve impulses that stimulate the colon's muscular walls. Mass peristalsis is strongest during the hour after mealtime.

RECTUM

Waste products that reach the sigmoid portion of the colon are called feces. The sigmoid stores feces until just before defecation.

The rectum is the final division of the gastrointestinal tract. Its length varies according to age:

Infant	2.5 to 3.8 cm (1 to 1.5 inches)
Toddler	5 cm (2 inches)
Preschooler	7.5 cm (3 inches)
School age	10 cm (4 inches)
Adult	15 to 20 cm (6 to 8 inches)

Normally the rectum is empty of feces until defecation. It contains vertical and transverse folds of tissue. Each vertical fold contains an artery and veins. If the veins become repeatedly distended from pressure during the straining of defecation, permanent dilations called hemorrhoids form. Hemorrhoids can make defecation painful.

When the fecal mass or gas moves into the rectum to distend its walls, defecation begins. The process involves involuntary and voluntary control. The internal sphincter is a smooth muscle innervated by the autonomic nervous system. As the rectum distends, sensory nerves are stimulated and carry impulses that cause the internal sphincter to relax, allowing more feces to enter the rectum. At the same time impulses travel to the brain to create awareness of the need to defecate.

As the internal sphincter relaxes, so does the external sphincter. The person who is toilet trained can voluntarily control the external sphincter. If the time for defecation is not right, constriction of the levator ani muscles closes the anus and defecation is delayed. At the time of defecation, the external sphincter relaxes. Pressure can be exerted to expel feces through an increase in intraabdominal pressure or a Valsalva maneuver. A Valsalva maneuver is voluntary contraction of abdominal muscles during forced expiration with a closed glottis (holding one's breath while straining). Relaxation of the levator ani muscle allows feces to be expelled. If the act of defecation is voluntarily stopped, feces remain in the rectum until the defecation reflex is restimulated. The act of defecation can be promoted by flexing the thigh muscles (which puts pressure on the abdomen) and sitting (which increases pressure down on the rectum).

TABLE 39-2 Factors Affecting Elimination

Factors Promoting Elimination	Factors Impairing Elimination
Stress-free environment	Emotional stress (anxiety or depression)
Ability to follow personal bowel habits, privacy	Failure to heed the defecation reflex, lack of time or privacy
High-fiber diet	High-carbohydrate and high-fat diet
Normal fluid intake (fruit juices, warm liquids)	Reduced fluid intake
Exercise (walking)	Immobility or inactivity
Ability to assume a squatting position	Inability to squat because of immobility, advanced age, musculoskeletal deformities, pain, or advanced pregnancy; pain during defecation
Properly administered laxatives and cathartics	Use of narcotic analgesics, antibiotics, or general anesthetics and overuse of cathartics

FACTORS AFFECTING ELIMINATION

Knowledge of the factors affecting elimination lets the nurse anticipate measures required to maintain a normal elimination pattern (Table 39-2). An understanding of how these factors alter normal elimination provides guidelines for reversing their effects.

Age

Developmental changes that affect elimination occur throughout life. An infant has a small stomach capacity and less secretion of digestive enzymes. Some foods such as complex starches are tolerated poorly. Food passes quickly through an infant's intestinal tract because of rapid peristalsis. The infant is unable to control defecation because of a lack of neuromuscular development. This development usually does not take place until 2 to 3 years of age.

During adolescence there is rapid growth of the large intestine. The secretion of hydrochloric acid increases, particularly in males. Adolescents typically eat more during this growth period.

The elderly often experience changes in the gastrointestinal system that impair digestion and elimination. Many lose their teeth and thus the ability to chew food thoroughly. Food enters the digestive tract only partially chewed and cannot be digested, since the amount of digestive enzymes in saliva and the volume of gastric acids fall with aging. The inability to digest fat-containing foods reflects a loss of the enzyme lipase.

With age, peristaltic action declines and esophageal emptying is slowed. Sluggish emptying of the esophagus can cause discomfort in the epigastric section of the abdomen. Absorptive properties of the intestinal mucosa change, causing protein, vitamin, and mineral deficiencies. The elderly also lose muscle tone in the perineal floor and anal sphincter. Although the integrity of the external sphincter may remain intact, the elderly may have difficulty controlling bowel evacuation. Because of slowing of nerve impulses, some are less aware of the need to defecate.

Diet

Regular daily food intake helps maintain a regular pattern of peristalsis in the colon. The food a person eats influences the process of elimination. Fiber, the undigestible residue in the diet, provides the bulk in fecal material. Bulk-forming foods stretch the bowel walls, creating peristalsis and initiating the defecation reflex. An infant's immature bowel cannot usually tolerate fiber-containing foods until several months of age. By stimulating peristalsis, bulk foods pass quickly through the intestines, keeping the stool soft. The following foods contain a higher amount of fiber than others:

1. Raw fruits (apples, oranges)
2. Cooked fruits (prunes, apricots)
3. Greens (spinach, kale, cabbage)
4. Raw vegetables (celery, zucchini)
5. Whole grains (cereal, breads)

Convenience foods such as pizza, pot pies, and sugar-coated cereals tend to be low in fiber. They are popular for people with active life-styles or who live alone (such as the elderly).

Ingestion of a high-fiber diet improves the likelihood of a normal elimination pattern if other factors are normal. Gas-producing foods such as onions, cauliflower, and beans also stimulate peristalsis. The gas that is formed distends intestinal walls, increasing colon motility. Some spicy foods may increase peristalsis but also cause indigestion and watery stools.

Some foods, such as milk and milk products, are difficult or impossible for some people to digest. This is caused by a lactose intolerance. Lactose, a simple form of sugar found in milk, is normally broken down by the enzyme lactase. The inability to digest lactose results from a failure to produce lactase. Intolerance to specific foods may result in diarrhea, gaseous distention, and cramping.

Fluid Intake

An inadequate intake of fluids or disturbances causing loss of fluid (such as vomiting) affect the character of feces. The colon continues to reabsorb fluid from chyme and thus feces become dry and hardened. Fluid liquefies intestinal contents, easing their passage through the colon. Reduced fluid intake slows passage of food through the intestine. An adult should drink 6 to 8 glasses (1400 to 2000 ml) of fluid daily. Hot beverages and fruit juices soften stool and increases peristalsis. A large ingestion of milk may slow peristalsis in some persons and cause constipation.

Physical Activity

Physical activity promotes peristalsis, whereas immobilization depresses colonic motility. Early ambulation after illness is encouraged to ensure maintenance of normal elimination.

Maintaining tone of skeletal muscles used during defecation is important. Weakened abdominal and pelvic floor muscles impair the ability to increase intraabdominal pressure and to control the external sphincter. Muscle tone may be weakened or lost as a result of long-term illness or of neurological disease that impairs nerve transmission.

Psychological Factors

The function of almost all body systems can be impaired by prolonged emotional stress (see Chapter 28). If an individual becomes anxious, afraid, or angry, the stress response initiates impulses from the parasympathetic division of the autonomic nervous system. This response allows the body to restore defenses. The digestive process is accelerated and peristalsis is increased to provide nutrients needed for defense. Side effects of increased peristalsis are diarrhea and gaseous distention. If a person becomes depressed, the autonomic nervous system slows impulses and peristalsis can decrease. A number of diseases of the gastrointestinal tract are believed to be worsened by stress, including ulcerative colitis, gastric ulcers, and Crohn's disease.

A child's elimination pattern may be upset by the method of toilet training. Forcing a child to learn toilet training before nervous and muscular systems are developed is a waste of time. Punishing children for accidents will make toilet training stressful. A child needs understanding and patience to avoid problems such as chronic constipation.

Personal Habits

Personal elimination habits influence bowel function. The act of defecation is a private matter. Most people benefit from being able to use their own toilet facilities at a time that is most effective and convenient for them. A busy work schedule is one factor that may disrupt a person's normal habits and result in alterations such as constipation. A person should learn the best time for regular elimination (for example, after meals or on awakening).

Hospitalized clients can rarely maintain privacy during defecation. Bathroom facilities are often shared with a roommate whose hygienic habits may be quite different. The client's illness often limits physical activity and requires use of a bedpan or bedside commode. The sights, sounds, and odors associated with sharing toilet facilities or using bedpans are often embarrassing. Embarrassment prompts clients to ignore the urge to defecate, which may begin a vicious cycle of discomfort. Therapies may be needed if alterations such as constipation develop, making the problem even more significant and anxiety producing.

Position During Defecation

Squatting is the normal position during defecation. Modern toilets are designed to facilitate this posture, allowing the person to lean forward, exert intraabdominal pressure, and contract the thigh muscles. However, an elderly client or one with joint disease such as arthritis may be unable to rise from a low toilet seat. Attachments that raise the seat enable the client to get off the toilet without assistance. Clients who use such attachments, as well as short people, may require a footstool for proper hip flexion.

For the client immobilized in bed, defecation is often difficult. In a supine position it is impossible to contract the muscles used during defecation. Assisting the client to a more normal sitting position on a bedpan enhances the ability to defecate.

Pain

Normally the act of defecation is painless. However, a number of conditions, including hemorrhoids, rectal surgery, and abdominal surgery, may result in discomfort. In these instances the client often suppresses the urge to defecate in order to avoid pain. Constipation is a common problem for clients with pain during defecation.

Pregnancy

As pregnancy advances and the size of the fetus increases, pressure is exerted on the rectum. A temporary obstruction created by the fetus impairs passage of feces. Constipation is a common problem during the last trimester. A pregnant woman's frequent straining during defecation may result in formation of permanent hemorrhoids.

Surgery and Anesthesia

General anesthetic agents used during surgery cause temporary cessation of peristalsis (see Chapter 46). Inhaled anesthetic agents block parasympathetic impulses to the intestinal musculature. The anesthetic's action slows or stops peristaltic waves. The client who receives local or regional anesthesia is less at risk for elimination alterations, since bowel activity is affected minimally or not at all.

Surgery that involves direct manipulation of the bowel temporarily stops peristalsis. This condition, called paralytic ileus, usually lasts about 24 to 48 hours. If the client remains inactive or is unable to eat after surgery, return of normal bowel function may be further delayed.

Medications

Medications are available for promoting defecation. Laxatives and cathartics soften the stool and promote peristalsis. When used correctly laxatives and cathartics safely maintain normal elimination patterns. However, chronic use of cathartics causes the large intestine to lose muscle tone and become less responsive to stimulation by laxatives. Laxative overuse can also cause serious diarrhea that may lead to dehydration and electrolyte depletion. Mineral oil, a common laxative, decreases fat-soluble vitamin absorption.

Medications such as dicyclomine hydrochloride (Bentyl) suppress peristalsis and treat diarrhea. Several medications have side effects that may impair elimination. Narcotic analgesics depress peristalsis in the gastrointestinal tract. Opiates commonly cause constipation. Anticholinergic drugs, such as atropine or glycopyrrolate (Robinul), inhibit gastric acid secretion and depress gastrointestinal motility. Although useful in treating hyperactive bowel disorders, anticholinergics can cause constipation in a client with normal bowel function. Many antibiotics produce diarrhea as a result of irritation and inflammation of the gastrointestinal mucosa. If the diarrhea and associated abdominal cramping become severe, the client may need to change medications.

Diagnostic Tests

Diagnostic examinations involving visualization of gastrointestinal structures often require that portions of the bowel be empty of contents. A client is not allowed to eat or drink after midnight of the day preceding such examinations as a barium enema, endoscopy of the lower gastrointestinal tract, or an upper gastrointestinal (UGI) series. In the case of a barium enema or endoscopy, the client usually receives cathartics and an enema. Emptying the bowel interferes with elimination until normal eating is resumed.

Barium examination procedures pose an additional problem. Barium hardens if allowed to stay in the gastrointestinal tract. This can lead to constipation or bowel impaction. A client should receive a cathartic to promote elimination of barium. Failure to evacuate all barium may require that the client receive a cleansing enema.

COMMON BOWEL ELIMINATION PROBLEMS

The nurse may care for clients who have or are at risk for having elimination problems due to physiological changes in the gastrointestinal tract, surgical alteration of intestinal structures, or disorders impairing defecation.

Constipation

Constipation is a symptom, not a disease. It is a decrease in frequency of bowel movements, accompanied by prolonged or difficult passage of hard, dry stools. Straining during defecation is an associated sign. When intestinal motility slows, the fecal mass becomes exposed over time to the intestinal walls and most of the fecal water content is absorbed. Little water is left to soften and lubricate stool. Passage of a dry stool may cause rectal pain.

There is no correct number of daily or weekly bowel movements. Each person has a normal pattern that the nurse must assess. If a person often has fewer than two bowel movements each week, there is cause for concern. The elderly tend to report more problems with constipation if they are unable to have daily bowel movements. In this case their concern is unwarranted.

The causes of constipation are:

1. *Irregular bowel habits*—When normal defecation reflexes are ignored, they tend to become weakened. Children at play, professionals, and hospitalized clients unwilling to use a bedpan are examples of people that may suppress the defecation urge. Change in routine can quickly disrupt normal defecation patterns.
2. *Inadequate diet*—A low-fiber diet that is high in animal fats (meats, dairy products, eggs) and refined sugars (rich desserts) can cause constipation. Loss

of teeth may cause the elderly to eat soft, processed foods that contain little fiber. Low fluid intake further impairs peristalsis and fecal lubrication.

3. *Lack of exercise*—Lengthy bedrest after an illness and lack of regular exercise cause constipation.
4. *Medications*—Heavy use of laxatives causes loss of intestinal muscle tone with resultant loss of normal defecation reflexes. Laxatives promote complete emptying of the lower colon, and time is needed to refill it with bulk. An anxious client may repeat a laxative dosage to have another bowel movement. The colon eventually loses muscle tone and responds only to laxatives or enemas. Tranquilizers, opiates such as codeine and morphine, anticholinergics, and iron cause constipation.
5. *Age*—Slowed peristalsis and loss of abdominal muscle elasticity place the elderly at risk for constipation. Decreased intestinal secretion of mucus reduces lubrication and adds to the problem. Many elderly live alone and eat improper diets that are low in fiber.
6. *Disease*—Abnormalities of the gastrointestinal tract such as bowel obstruction, diverticulitis, and paralytic ileus cause constipation. Clients with spinal cord injury or tumor may also have elimination alterations caused by blockage of nerve impulses to the colon.

Constipation is a significant hazard to health. Straining during defecation causes problems to the client with recent abdominal or rectal surgery. The effort to pass a stool can cause sutures to separate, reopening the wound. In addition, clients with a history of cardiovascular disease or diseases causing elevated intraocular pressure (glaucoma) and intracranial pressure should prevent constipation and avoid using the Valsalva maneuver. Straining during defecation is usually accompanied by holding the breath. As a result, the intrathoracic pressure and the heart rate drop. This sudden change in heart rate can be easily withstood by a person with a healthy heart, but the client with cardiac instability should avoid a Valsalva maneuver. Exhaling through the mouth during straining avoids a Valsalva maneuver.

Impaction

Fecal impaction results from unrelieved constipation. It is a collection of hardened feces, wedged in the rectum, that cannot be expelled. In cases of severe impaction the mass may extend up into the sigmoid colon. Clients who are debilitated, confused, or unconscious are most at risk for impaction. They are too weak or unaware of the need to defecate. Frequent repetition of practices that promote constipation can also cause impaction, as can failure to pass barium contrast medium after a gastrointestinal examination.

An obvious sign of impaction is the inability to pass a stool for several days despite a repeated urge to defecate. When a continuous oozing of diarrheal stool suddenly develops, impaction should be suspected. The liquid portion of feces located higher in the colon seeps around the impacted mass. Loss of appetite (anorexia), abdominal distention and cramping, and rectal pain may accompany the condition. The nurse who suspects an impaction can gently perform a digital examination of the rectum and palpate the impacted mass. Some institutions require a physician's order for a nurse to perform a rectal examination because of the risk of causing vagal stimulation that slows a client's heart rate. Another danger with digital examination is bowel perforation, especially with the older adult and those with neoplastic colon diseases.

Diarrhea

Diarrhea is an increase in the number of stools and the passage of liquid, unformed feces. It is a symptom of disorders affecting digestion, absorption, and secre-

TABLE 39-3   Conditions That Cause Diarrhea

Condition	Physiological Effects
Emotional stress (anxiety)	Increased intestinal motility
Intestinal infection (streptococcal or staphylococcal enteritis)	Inflammation of intestinal mucosa, increased mucus secretion in colon
Food allergies	Reduced digestion of food elements
Food intolerance (greasy foods, coffee, alcohol, spicy foods)	Increased intestinal motility, increased mucus secretion in colon
Medications	
Iron	Irritation of intestinal mucosa
Antibiotics	Suprainfection allowing overgrowth of normal flora, inflammation and irritation of mucosa
Laxatives (short term)	Increased intestinal motility
Colon disease (colitis, Crohn's disease)	Inflammation and ulceration of intestinal walls, reduced absorption of fluids, increased intestinal motility
Surgical alterations	
Gastrectomy	Loss of reservoir function of stomach, food dumped into duodenum too quickly for proper absorption
Colon resection	Reduced size of colon, reduced amount of absorptive surface

tion in the gastrointestinal tract. Intestinal contents pass through the small intestine and colon too quickly to allow the usual absorption of fluid. Irritation within the colon may be an added factor that results in an increased mucus secretion. As a result, feces become watery so the client may be unable to control the urge to defecate. It is often difficult to assess diarrhea in infants because of their wide variation in bowel habits. An infant who is bottle fed may have one firm stool every second day, while a breast-fed baby may pass five to eight small, soft stools daily. It is important for the mother or nurse to note (1) any sudden increase in number of stools, (2) any reduction in fecal consistency with an increase in fluid content, and (3) a tendency for feces to be greenish.

Excess loss of colonic fluid can result in serious fluid and electrolyte imbalance. Infants and the elderly are particularly susceptible (see Chapter 37) to associated complications. Since repeated passage of diarrheal stools also exposes the skin of the perineum and buttocks to irritating intestinal contents, meticulous skin care is needed to prevent skin breakdown. The client may experience abdominal cramping, nausea, and vomiting, depending on the severity of the diarrhea.

Many conditions cause diarrhea (Table 39-3). The aim of treatment is first to remove precipitating conditions and then slow peristalsis. Any irritation to the intestinal mucosa must be eliminated.

Incontinence

Fecal incontinence is the inability to control passage of feces and gas from the anus. Physical conditions that impair anal sphincter function or control can cause incontinence. Conditions that create frequent, loose, large-volume, watery stools also predispose to incontinence.

Mental disorders such as schizophrenia, severe depression, or anxiety and dementia may prevent the client from being aware of the need to defecate.

Incontinence can harm a client's body image. In many situations the client is mentally alert but physically unable to avoid defecation. The embarrassment of soiling one's clothes can lead to social isolation. The client must depend on the nurse for a basic need. Clients with mental or sensory alterations often are unaware that they have passed a stool. The nurse must understand and support the client even though repeated cleaning of an incontinent client can become frustrating.

Like diarrhea, incontinence predisposes the skin to breakdown. The nurse must check often to be sure anal and perineal regions are clean and dry.

Flatulence

As gas accumulates in the lumen of the intestines, the bowel wall stretches and distends (flatulence). It is a common cause of abdominal fullness, pain, and cramping. Normally intestinal gas escapes through the mouth (belching) or the anus (passing of flatus). However, if there is a reduction in intestinal motility resulting from opiates, general anesthetics, abdominal surgery, or immobilization, flatulence may become severe enough to cause distention with shortness of breath. Accumulation of gas forces the diaphragm up and reduces lung expansion.

A person normally produces several liters of intestinal gas daily. Swallowed air makes up over 75% of intestinal gas. Bacterial decomposition of food in the colon releases methane gas. Carbon dioxide is a product of fermentation in the bowel. Any factor that causes gas will increase intestinal flatulence (for example, ingestion of onions, beans, and cauliflower).

Hemorrhoids

Hemorrhoids are dilated, engorged veins in the lining of the rectum. They are either external or internal. External hemorrhoids are clearly visible as protrusions of skin. If the underlying vein is hardened, there may be a purplish discoloration. Internal hemorrhoids have an outer mucous membrane. Increased venous pressure from straining at defecation, pregnancy, congestive heart failure, and chronic liver disease can cause hemorrhoids.

Hemorrhoids bleed easily when stretched. Passage of a hard stool commonly causes bleeding. The hemorrhoids become inflamed and tender, and clients may complain of itching and burning. Because pain worsens during defecation, the urge to defecate may be ignored, resulting in constipation.

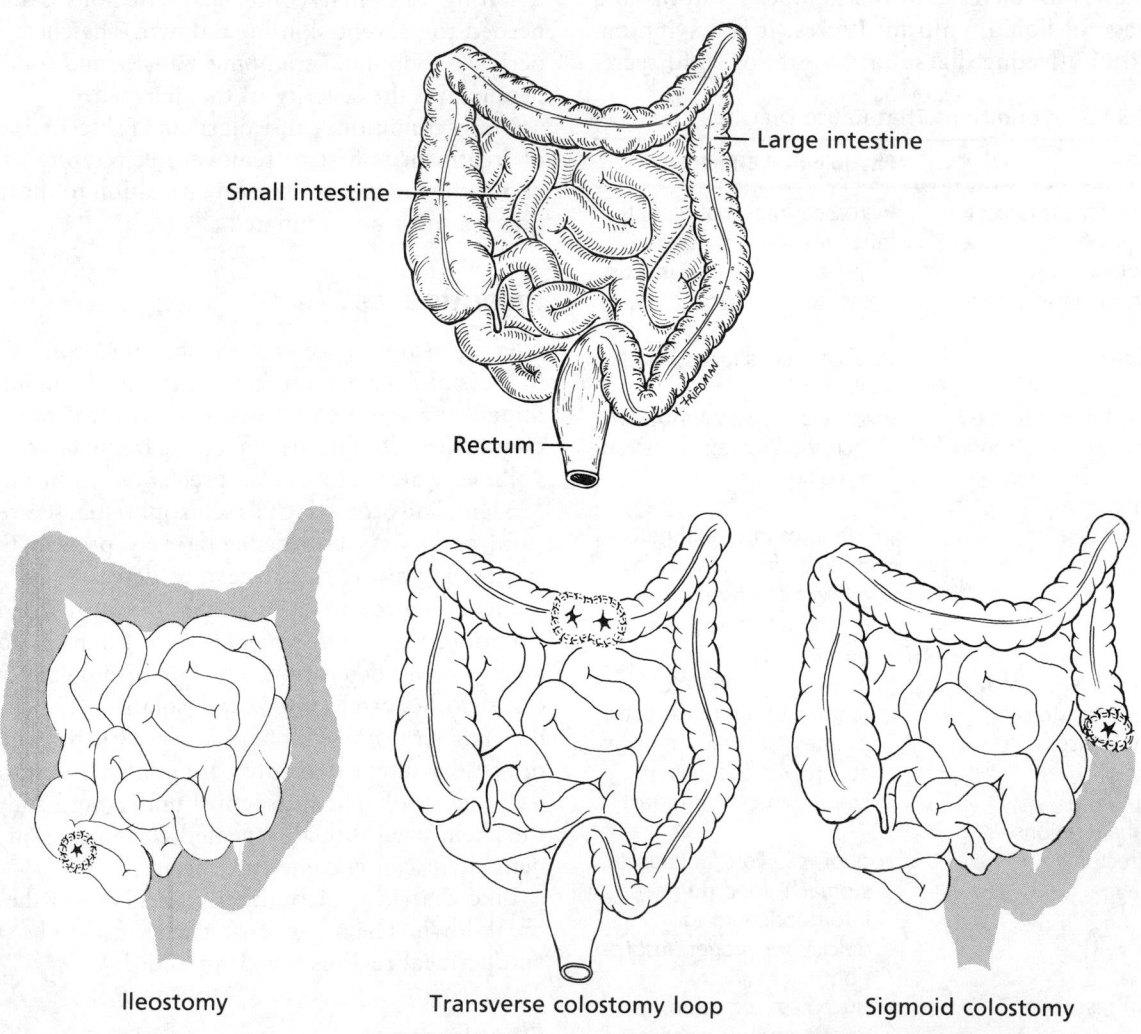

Large intestine

Small intestine

Rectum

Ileostomy   Transverse colostomy loop   Sigmoid colostomy

Fig. 39-4 Normal intestines and three types of ostomies (shaded areas indicate excised tissue).

BOWEL DIVERSIONS

Certain diseases cause conditions that prevent normal passage of feces through the rectum. This creates the need for a temporary or permanent artificial opening (stoma) in the abdominal wall. Surgical openings are formed in the ileum (ileostomy) or colon (colostomy) (Fig. 39-4). Ends of the intestines are then brought through the opening to create the stoma. The stoma is covered with a plastic pouch or bag to collect fecal material.

The location of the ostomy determines the consistency of stool. An ileostomy bypasses the entire large intestine. As a result, stools are frequent and liquid. The same is true for a colostomy of the ascending colon. A colostomy of the transverse colon generally results in a more solid, formed stool. The sigmoid colostomy emits almost normal stool. The location of a colostomy is determined by the client's medical problem and general condition.

The following lists the three types of colostomy construction:

1. Loop colostomy
2. End colostomy
3. Double-barrel colostomy

A loop colostomy is usually performed in a medical emergency when closure of the colostomy is anticipated in the near future. The surgeon pulls a loop of bowel onto the abdomen. A communicating wall remains between the proximal and distal bowel. A plastic rod or rubber catheter is temporarily placed underneath the bowel loop to keep it from slipping back (Fig. 39-5, *A*). The surgeon then opens the bowel and sutures it to the skin of the abdomen. The loop ostomy has two openings through the stoma. The proximal end drains stool while the distal portion drains mucous. Within 7 to 10 days the plastic rod is removed.

The end colostomy consists of one stoma formed from the proximal end of the bowel with the distal portion of the gastrointestinal tract removed. Most clients with end colostomies suffer cancer of the bowel. In some cases the rectum is also removed.

The double-barrel colostomy consists of two distinct stomas: the proximal functioning stoma and the distal nonfunctioning stoma. Unlike the loop colostomy, a double-barrel colostomy has the bowel severed (Fig. 39-5, *B*).

Ostomies such as the ileostomy that emit frequent liquids stools create a management challenge. A bag or pouch must always be worn. Regular defecation cannot be achieved, because of a continuous oozing of stool. The bag must be emptied, washed, and replaced throughout the day. Skin care is vital to prevent exposure to fecal irritants.

A colostomy in the transverse or sigmoid colon is simpler to manage. The client may continue to wear a pouch at all times even though bowel movements may occur only once or twice daily. Selected foods can be eaten at prescribed intervals so that bowel movements occur at a convenient time. Therefore the client may not need to wear a pouch. A physician may order routine irrigations of the ostomy, similar to giving an enema. This allows the person to empty the bowel regularly and eliminate a pouch. Irrigations are not performed as routinely as in the past.

An ostomy causes serious body image changes, particularly if it is permanent. Clients often perceive a stoma as a form of mutilation. Even though clothing conceals the ostomy, the client feels different. Many clients have difficulty maintaining or initiating normal sexual relations. An important factor in the client's reactions is the character of fecal secretions and the ability to control them. Foul odors, spillage, or leakage of liquid stools and inability to regulate bowel movements give the client a loss of self-esteem.

ASSESSMENT

To assess bowel elimination pattern and determine abnormalities, the nurse collects a nursing history, physical assessment of the abdomen, inspection of fecal characteristics, and a review of pertinent test results.

Nursing History

The nursing history provides a review of the client's normal bowel pattern and habits. What a client describes as "normal" may be different from factors and conditions that tend to promote normal elimination. Identifying normal and abnormal patterns and habits allows the nurse to determine the client's problems. Much of the nursing history can be organized around the factors that affect elimination. The nurse then applies this knowledge through questions to determine the presence and extent of GI alterations. A typical nursing history of a client's elimination status includes:

1. *Determination of the usual elimination pattern*—frequency and time of day are included.
2. *Identification of routines followed to promote normal elimination*—examples are drinking hot liquids, using a laxative, eating specific foods, or taking time to defecate during a certain part of the day.
3. *Description of any recent change in elimination pattern*—this information is perhaps the most significant, since elimination patterns are variable and the client can best detect change. Determine the client's last bowel movement. If there were changes, ask the client to suggest a cause.

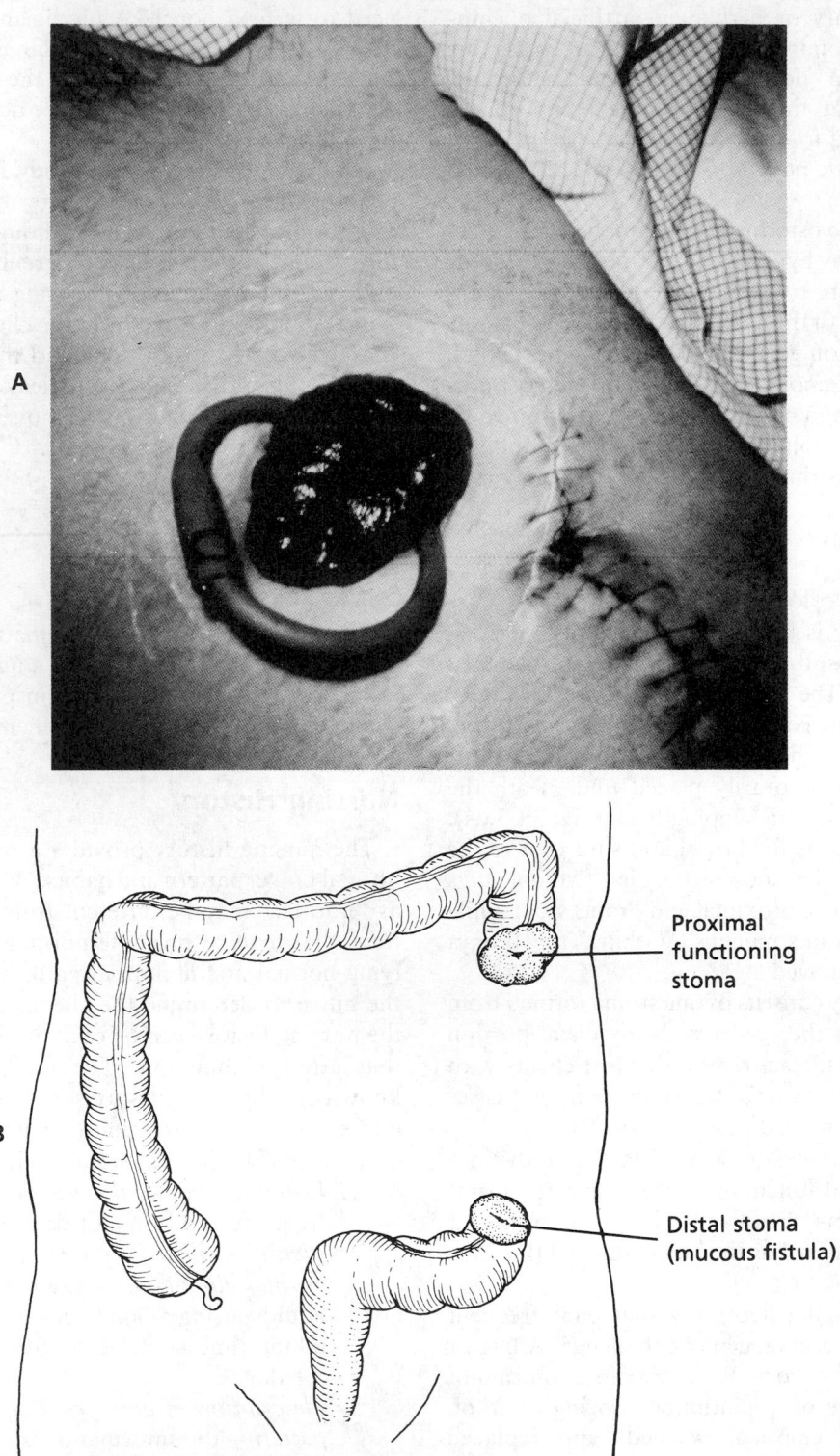

Fig. 39-5 A, A transverse loop colostomy supported with a flexible red rubber catheter. B, Double-barrel colostomy in the descending colon.

From Broadwell, DC, and Jackson, BS: Principles of ostomy care, St. Louis, 1982, The C.V. Mosby Co.

4. *Client's description of usual characteristics of the stool*—the nurse determines if the stool is normally watery or formed, soft or hard, and the typical color. The client also describes a normal stool's shape.

5. *Diet history*—determine the client's dietary preferences for a day. The nurse measures servings of fruits, vegetables, cereals, and breads. Is mealtime regular or irregular and are certain foods eaten infrequently?

6. *Description of daily fluid intake*—this includes the type and amount of fluid. The client may have to estimate the amount using common household measurements.

7. *History of exercise*—ask the client to describe the type and amount of daily exercise. Simply asking the client if the client exercises is not adequate because it leaves the judgment solely to the client. For example, a client who walks back and forth in an office may perceive this as adequate exercise. Therefore, the nurse asks for a specific description of exercise patterns.

8. *Assessment of the use of artificial aids at home*—the nurse assesses if the client requires the use of enemas, laxatives, or special foods before having a bowel movement. If so, the nurse asks how often the client uses them.

9. *History of surgery or illnesses affecting the gastrointestinal tract*—this information can often help to explain symptoms. In addition, it provides the nurse with an idea of the potential for maintaining or restoring a normal elimination pattern.

10. *Presence and status of artificial orifices*—if the client has an ostomy the nurse assesses frequency of fecal drainage, character of feces, appearance and condition of the stoma (color, swelling, irritation), type of appliance used, and methods used to maintain the ostomy's function.

11. *Medication history*—does the client take medications (such as laxatives, antacids, iron supplements, and analgesics) that might alter defecation or fecal characteristics?

12. *Emotional state*—the client's emotions can significantly alter frequency of defecation. During assessment, observation of the client's emotions, tone of voice, and mannerisms can reveal significant behaviors indicating stress.

13. *Social history*—if the client is not independent in bowel management, who assists and how?

Physical Assessment

The nurse assesses the status of GI function (see Chapter 13).

MOUTH

An assessment includes inspection of the client's teeth and gums. Poor dentition or poorly fitting dentures will influence the ability to chew.

ABDOMEN

The nurse inspects all four abdominal quadrants for contour, shape, symmetry, and skin color. Inspection also includes noting masses, peristaltic waves, scars, venous patterns, stomas, or lesions. Normally peristaltic waves are not visible. However, observable peristalsis may be a sign of intestinal obstruction.

Abdominal distention appears as an overall outward protuberance of the abdomen. Intestinal gas, large tumors, or fluid in the peritoneal cavity may cause distention. A distended abdomen feels tight and the skin appears taut as if stretched. Daily measurement of the abdomen's girth using a tape measure will reveal whether distention is increasing. Measurements should be taken over the same anatomical landmarks (for example, umbilicus) to provide an accurate chronological measurement. If masses are present, they appear as localized bulges or protuberances.

The nurse auscultates the abdomen before palpation to avoid changing the frequency of bowel sounds. The diaphragm of the stethoscope is used to assess bowel sounds in each of the quadrants (see Chapter 13). While auscultating, the nurse notes the character and frequency of bowel sounds. The nurse assesses bowel sounds as normal or too loud, absent, hyperactive, or hypoactive. An increase in pitch or "tinkling" sound may be heard with abdominal distention. Absent or hypoactive sounds occur with paralytic ileus after abdominal surgery. High-pitched and hyperactive bowel sounds occur with small intestine obstruction and inflammatory disorders.

During palpation and percussion it is important for the client to relax. Tensing abdominal muscles interferes with palpating underlying organs or masses. The nurse palpates with a light, gentle touch. Palpation of a tender or sensitive area causes a guarding or voluntary tightening of abdominal muscles. If the nurse locates an unusual mass, deep palpation may be necessary for further examination. A mass may indicate presence of a tumor. The nurse should not apply deep palpation unless trained in the skill.

Percussion detects lesions, fluid, or gas within the abdomen. Familiarity with the five percussion notes (see Chapter 13) also permits identification of underlying abdominal structures. Gas or flatulence will create a tympanic note. Masses, tumors, and fluid are dull to percussion.

RECTUM

The nurse inspects the area around the anus for lesions, discolorations, inflammation, and hemorrhoids.

TABLE 39-4 Fecal Characteristics

Characteristic	Normal	Abnormal	Cause
Color	Infant: yellow; adult: brown	White or clay	Absence of bile
		Black or tarry	Iron ingestion or upper gastrointestinal (GI) bleeding
		Red (melena)	Lower GI bleeding, hemorrhoids
		Pale with fat	Malabsorption of fat
Odor	Pungent; affected by food type	Noxious change	Blood in feces or infection
Consistency	Soft, formed	Liquid	Diarrhea, reduced absorption
		Hard	Constipation
Frequency	Varies: infant four to six times daily (breast fed) or one to three times daily (bottle fed); adult daily or two to three times a week	Infant more than six times daily or less than once every 1 to 2 days; adult more than three times a day or less than once a week	Hypomotility or hypermotility
Amount	150 g per day (adult)		
Shape	Resembles diameter of rectum	Narrow, pencil-shaped	Obstruction, rapid peristalsis
Constituents	Undigested food, dead bacteria, fat, bile pigment, cells lining intestinal mucosa, water	Blood, pus, foreign bodies, mucus, worms	Internal bleeding, infection, swallowed objects, irritation, inflammation

Abnormalities should be carefully recorded. To examine the rectum the nurse uses gentle palpation. After donning a clean disposable glove, the nurse lubricates the index finger with petrolatum jelly. The nurse then asks the client to bear down and, as the client does so, the nurse passes the index finger through the relaxed anal sphincter toward the client's umbilicus. The sphincter usually constricts around the nurse's finger. The nurse should methodically palpate all sides of the rectal wall for nodules or irregularities in texture. The rectal mucosa is normally smooth and soft. Pushing the index finger forcefully against the rectal wall or extending the finger too far may cause discomfort. Vigorous stimulation should be avoided to prevent triggering a vagal nerve reflex that can lower the heart rate.

The findings of an abdominal assessment may give clues as to the nature of gastrointestinal alterations. For example, abdominal distention coupled with auscultation of hyperactive bowel sounds suggests gaseous formation, presence of obstruction, or inflammation of the bowel. The nurse's assessment will then focus on other factors or conditions.

Fecal Characteristics

Inspection of fecal characteristics (Table 39-4) reveals information about the nature of elimination alterations. Several factors can influence each characteristic. A key to assessment is knowing if there have been any recent changes. The client can best provide this information.

Laboratory and Diagnostic Tests

Laboratory and diagnostic examinations yield useful information concerning elimination problems. Laboratory analysis of fecal contents can detect pathological conditions such as tumors, hemorrhage, and infection. Diagnostic studies allow the physician to visualize all segments of the gastrointestinal tract. Diagnostic tests such as endoscopy permit direct visualization of structures. Tests such as the barium enema or an upper gastrointestinal (UGI) series require ingestion of a contrast medium that outlines structures on x-ray examination.

FECAL SPECIMENS

The nurse is directly responsible for ensuring that specimens are accurately obtained, properly labeled in appropriate containers, and transported to the laboratory on time. Institutions provide special containers for fecal specimens. Some tests require specimens to be placed in chemical preservatives.

Medical aseptic technique should be used during collection of stool specimens (see Chapter 13). Because about 25% of the solid portion of a stool is bacteria from the colon, the nurse should wear disposable gloves when handling specimens.

Handwashing is necessary for anyone who might come in contact with the specimen. Often the client is capable of obtaining the specimen if properly instructed. Explain that feces cannot be mixed with urine or water. For this reason the client must defecate into a clean, dry bedpan or special container than can be placed under the toilet seat.

TABLE 39-5 Screening for Colon Cancer

Risk Factors	Warning Signs	Screening Tests
Age: over 50 Family history: colon polyps History of inflammatory bowel disease (colitis, Crohn's disease) Living in urban area Diet: high intake of fats, low fiber intake	Change in bowel habits Rectal bleeding	Digital rectal examination every year after age 40 Guaiac test for occult blood every year after 50 Proctoscopy every 3 to 5 years after age 50, following two annual negative examinations

Tests performed by the laboratory for occult (microscopic) blood in the stool and stool cultures require only a small sample. The nurse collects about an inch of formed stool or 15 to 30 ml of liquid diarrheal stool. To avoid contact with feces while transferring solid specimens to a container, the nurse should wear gloves and use a wooden tongue depressor. The nurse must pour liquid specimens carefully into the proper container. Tests for measuring the output of fecal fat require 3- to 5-day collection of stool. All fecal material must be saved throughout the test period.

After obtaining a specimen the nurse tightly seals the container and completes laboratory requisition forms. The nurse then records specimen collections in the client's medical record. It is important to avoid delays in sending specimens to the laboratory. Some tests such as measurement for ova and parasites require the stool to be warm. When stool specimens are allowed to stand at room temperature, bacteriological changes that alter test results can occur.

GUAIAC TEST. A common laboratory test that can be done at home or at the client's bedside is the guaiac test, which measures microscopic amounts of blood in the feces. Small amounts of blood are normally lost daily in the feces from minor abrasions of nasopharyngeal and oral surfaces. Quantities of blood greater than 50 ml arising from the upper gastrointestinal tract can be seen as melena. Guaiac tests help reveal visually undetectable blood. It is a useful diagnostic screening test for colon cancer (Table 39-5).

Clients who are receiving anticoagulants or who have a bleeding disorder or a GI disorder known to cause bleeding (for example, intestinal tumors, bowel inflammation, ulcerations) should be guaiac tested. The most common guaiac test is the Hemoccult slide test (Procedure 39-1).

DIAGNOSTIC EXAMINATIONS

A client may have a diagnostic test as an outpatient or inpatient. Visualization of GI structures may be by a direct or an indirect approach.

DIRECT VISUALIZATION. Instruments introduced either through the mouth (upper GI viewing) or the rectum (lower GI viewing) allow the physician to inspect the integrity of mucosa, blood vessels, and organ parts. A fiberoptic endoscope is an optical instrument with a lens viewer, a long flexible tube, and a light source at the end. It allows viewing of structures at the tip of the tube and insertion of special instruments for biopsy. The tube is flexible to minimize trauma and discomfort to the client.

Proctoscopes and sigmoidoscopes are rigid tube-shaped instruments with attached light sources. The proctoscope looks like a speculum with a light. These instruments are less flexible than fiberoptic scopes and more capable of causing the client discomfort.

Upper gastrointestinal (UGI) endoscopy or gastroscopy allows visualization of the esophagus, stomach, and duodenum. The physician inspects for tumors, vascular changes, mucosal inflammation, ulcers, hernias, and obstructions. A gastroscope enables the physician to remove tissue specimens for biopsy, remove abnormal tissue growth (polyps), and coagulate sources of bleeding. Nursing implications before the test include:
1. Client signs informed consent.
2. Client takes nothing by mouth after midnight.
3. Client removes dentures.
4. Nurse explains that the client may feel fullness in the throat and a sense of gagging during the test.
5. Nurse explains that the client will be unable to speak as the endoscope enters the esophagus.
6. Nurse positions the client in the left Sims' or left lateral position.
7. Nurse gives a sedative and an anticholinergic.

Nursing implications during the test include:
1. Nurse describes steps of the test to the client.
2. Nurse places tissue specimens in a properly labeled container that is sealed tightly.
3. Nurse has emergency equipment available in case of respiratory complications.

Nursing implications after the test include:
1. Because the client's throat is anesthetized, the nurse instructs the client to avoid eating or drinking until

Measuring Occult Blood in Stool

STEPS	RATIONALE

1. Assess client's medical history for bleeding or gastrointestinal disorder.

Routine screening can be instituted by nurse.

2. Assess type of medications client receives. Note those drugs that have potential for causing gastrointestinal mucosal bleeding.

Anticoagulants will increase risk of bleeding in gastrointestinal tract, even from minor trauma to mucosa. Long-term use of steroids and acetylsalicylic acid can irritate mucosa.

3. Refer to physician's order for medication or dietary modifications/restrictions before test.

Medications such as iron supplement and bismuth compounds can cause stools to resemble melena. Rare meats can cause same results.

4. Prepare necessary equipment and supplies:
   a. Paper towel
   b. Hemoccult test supplies (see illustration):
      (1) Cardboard hemoccult slide
      (2) Wooden applicator
      (3) Hemoccult developing solution
   c. Disposable gloves

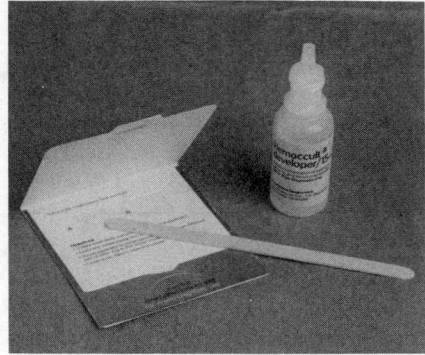

Step 4b

5. Explain purpose of test and how client can assist.

Client's understanding of test's purpose provides cooperation and minimizes anxiety.

6. Be sure dietary or medication restrictions were followed.

Ensures accurate test results.

7. Wash hands.

Reduces transmission of infection.

8. Apply clean disposable gloves.

Reduces transmission of microorganisms from fecal specimen to nurse's hands.

9. Obtain uncontaminated stool specimen.

Specimen is obtained in clean, dry container and not contaminated with urine, water, or toilet tissue.

10. Use tip of wooden applicator to obtain small portion of feces.

Small specimen is sufficient for measuring blood content in feces.

11. Perform Hemoccult slide test.
    a. Open flap of slide and apply thin smear of stool on paper in first box (see illustration).

Guaiac paper inside box is sensitive to fecal blood content.

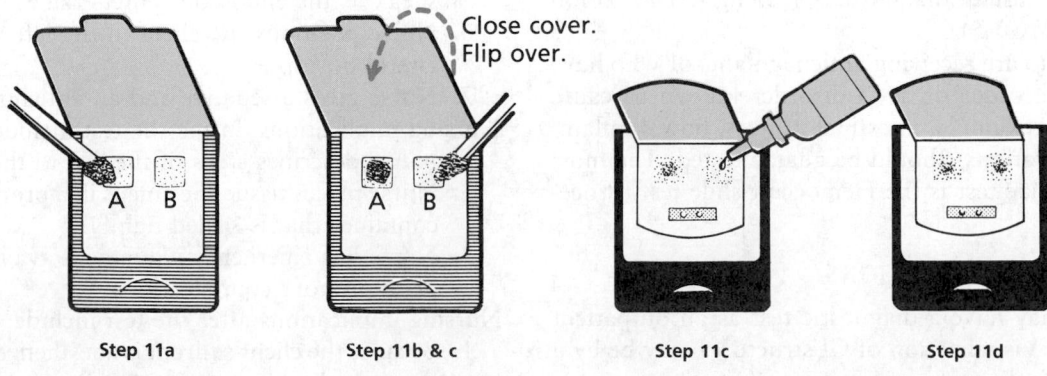

Close cover.
Flip over.

Step 11a	Step 11b & c	Step 11c	Step 11d

STEPS	RATIONALE
b. Obtain second fecal specimen from different portion of stool and apply thinly to slide's second box (see illustration).	Findings of occult blood are more conclusive for gastrointestinal bleeding when entire specimen is found to contain blood.
c. Close slide cover and turn slide over to reverse side (see illustration). Open cardboard flap and apply 2 drops of Hemoccult developing solution on each box of guaiac paper (see illustration).	Developing solution penetrates underlying fecal specimen. Presence of blood is indicated by change in color of guaiac paper.
d. Read results of test after 30-60 sec (see illustration). Note color changes.	Bluish discoloration indicates presence of occult blood (guaiac positive). No change in color of guaiac paper indicates negative results.
e. Dispose of test slide in proper receptacle.	Reduces transfer of microorganisms.
12. Wrap wooden applicator in paper towel, remove gloves, and dispose in proper receptacle.	Feces contain large numbers of microorganisms.
13. Wash hands.	Reduces spread of infection.
14. Record results of test in nurses' notes and note unusual fecal characteristics.	All test results should be documented promptly. Findings may indicate need for further diagnosis.

the gag reflex returns (2 to 4 hours). To check for the gag reflex the nurse places a tongue blade at the back of the client's tongue.

2. Nurse explains that hoarseness and a sore throat are normal for several days; cool fluids and normal saline gargling relieve soreness.
3. Nurse observes for bleeding, fever, abdominal pain, difficulty swallowing, and difficulty breathing.

Sigmoidoscopy allows visualization of the anus, rectum, and sigmoid colon. Proctoscopy allows visualization of the anus and rectum. Both tests enable the physician to collect tissue specimens and coagulate sources of bleeding. Nursing implications before the test include:

1. Client signs an informed consent.
2. Client receives an enema the night before and the morning of the test; laxatives are optional.
3. Client may be allowed a light breakfast.
4. Nurse explains that the client will feel discomfort and the urge to defecate as the instruments are inserted.
5. During the test the physician uses air to distend the bowel for better visualization; nurse explains that the client will feel "gas pains."
6. Nurse positions the client in a knee-chest position face down; Sims' position on the left side is acceptable.
7. Nurse drapes the client to avoid unnecessary exposure and minimize embarrassment.

Nursing implications during the test include:

1. Nurse keeps the client draped and observes for respiratory distress (especially in clients with lung disease who cannot tolerate a head-down position).
2. Nurse provides the physician with long cotton swabs for removing mucus.
3. Nurse places tissue specimens in a properly labeled container that is sealed tightly.

Nursing implications after the test include:

1. Nurse observes for rectal bleeding, rectal or abdominal pain, and fever.
2. Nurse cautions the client to observe for blood in stools and to report bleeding to a physician.

INDIRECT VISUALIZATION. When direct visualization is impossible (as with deeper GI structures), the physician relies on indirect x-ray examination. The client either ingests a contrast medium or has the medium given as an enema. One of the most common media is barium, a white, chalky, radiopaque substance that the client drinks like a milkshake. It is used in UGI studies and barium enemas. Contrast media usually contain a flavoring agent for better taste.

An upper gastrointestinal (UGI) study is an x-ray study of an ingested contrast medium that allows the physician to visualize the lower esophagus, stomach, and duodenum. The physician notes ulcerations, inflammation, tumors, and anatomical malposition of organs. The patency of organs and the pyloric valve are also observed. Nursing implications before the test include:

1. Client signs an informed consent.
2. Client takes nothing by mouth after midnight.
3. Nurse explains that the test may take several hours and requires frequent position changes; nurse explains that discomfort is minimal except for lying on a hard examination table.
4. Nurse explains that barium has a chalky taste (some preparations contain artificial flavoring).

A nursing implication during the test is:

1. The test is done in the radiology department; a technician explains the steps of the test.

Nursing implications after the test include:

1. Client may resume eating after the test.
2. Client must expel the barium to avoid bowel impaction; nurse instructs the client to increase fluid intake (at least 2 liters after the test); the physician may order a mild laxative or enema; stools are lightly colored until the barium is expelled.

Small bowel follow-through (continuation of UGI) allows the physician to examine the small intestine. The flow of barium through the intestine may suggest motility problems. A barium enema allows indirect visualization of the lower colon to reveal location of tumors, polyps, and diverticula. The physician can also detect positional abnormalities. Nursing implications before the test include:

1. Client signs informed consent.
2. Bowel preparation varies; client may receive any of the following the evening before the test:
   a. Clear liquids for lunch and supper
   b. One glass of water 8 to 10 hours before the test
   c. Stimulant cathartics
   d. An enema
3. On the day of the test the client receives additional cathartic by suppository.
4. Nurse explains the purpose of extensive bowel preparation.
5. Nurse explains that a lengthy procedure may cause fatigue.
6. Nurse observes the results of enemas and cathartics to ensure the bowel is empty before the test.
7. Nurse explains that the client may feel cramping and fullness once the barium is instilled.
8. Nurse explains that the client will be instructed to change positions often (supine, prone, and sidelying).

A nursing implication during the test is:

1. Client expels barium after first set of x-ray films (30 minutes); a repeat film is taken to check for barium retention.

Nursing implications after the test include:

1. Client may resume eating after the test.
2. Nurse instructs the client to increase intake of oral

fluids to promote barium evacuation and to counteract dehydrating effects of the cathartics.

3. Nurse instructs the client to observe stools for barium; the physician may order a mild cathartic.
4. Nurse offers the hospitalized client a warm bath for comfort.

NURSING DIAGNOSIS

The nurse's assessment of the client's bowel function reveals data that may indicate an actual or potential elimination problem or a problem resulting from elimination alterations (see nursing diagnosis box). Associated problems such as body image changes or skin breakdown require interventions unrelated to bowel function impairment. However, in some instances the nurse must direct as much attention to the elimination problem as to the associated problem.

The nurse's ability to identify the correct diagnosis depends not only on the thoroughness of assessment but also on recognition of defining characteristics and factors that can impair elimination. The nurse's responsibility is to determine the client's risk and institute measures to ensure maintenance of normal bowel function.

Examples of Nursing Diagnoses Related to Bowel Elimination Problems

NANDA-APPROVED NURSING DIAGNOSES

Constipation related to:
- Immobility
- Improper dietary habits
- Insufficient fluid intake

Diarrhea related to:
- Emotional stress
- Food intolerance

Bowel incontinence related to:
- Spinal cord injury
- Inability to attend to defecation

Pain related to:
- Hemorrhoidal inflammation

Toileting self-care deficit related to:
- Musculoskeletal weakness
- Fatigue

Actual or potential impaired skin integrity related to:
- Fecal incontinence

Body image disturbance related to:
- Presence of ostomy
- Fecal incontinence

Sample Nursing Diagnoses for Bowel Elimination Problems

Defining Characteristics	Nursing Diagnoses	Related Factors
Frequency less than usual pattern Hard formed stool Straining at stool Decreased bowel sounds	Constipation	• Immobility • Improper dietary habits • Pain on defecation • Medications
Abdominal pain Increased frequency of stools Loose, liquid stool Cramping	Diarrhea	• Dietary intake • Stress • Medications
Disruption of skin surface Redness, excoriation, weeping of skin	Impaired skin integrity	• Exposure to diarrheal stool

The sample nursing diagnoses box gives examples of nursing diagnoses with defining characteristics and related causes.

PLANNING

With nursing diagnoses defined, the nurse's plan of care should incorporate the client's elimination habits or routines as much as possible. If the habits caused the elimination problem, the nurse will help the client learn new ones. Each person's defecation pattern is unique.

For this reason, the nurse and client must work together closely to plan effective interventions. The care plan box includes a sample care plan.

When clients are disabled or debilitated by illness, it will be necessary to include the family in the plan of care. Often family members have the same ineffective elimination habits as the client. Thus, client-family teaching is an important part of the nurse's plan. Other health team members such as dietitians and enterostomal therapists can be a valuable resource in the plan of care.

The goals of care for clients with elimination problems include:

1. Understanding normal elimination

Sample Nursing Care Plan for Bowel Elimination Problems

Nursing Diagnosis	Goals	Expected Outcomes	Nursing Interventions
Constipation related to improper dietary habits	Client will understand food and fluid intake required to promote soft, formed stools.	Client will describe dietary sources high in fiber. Client will explain the normal fluid intake to promote defecation. Client will prepare a 24-hour menu including high-fiber foods and fluids.	Instruct client on foods he prefers that stimulate peristalsis (wheat, bread, apples, lettuce, celery, apricots). Administer 8 glasses of fluids (prefers orange and grape juice) daily.
	Client will attain regular defecation habits.	Client defecates routinely following meals. Stool will be soft and formed.	Encourage client to take time to defecate 30 to 60 min after breakfast. Discuss with client physical effects of ignoring the defecation reflex.

2. Attaining regular defecation habits
3. Understanding and maintaining proper fluid and food intake
4. Achieving a regular exercise program
5. Achieving comfort
6. Maintaining skin integrity
7. Maintaining self-concept

IMPLEMENTATION

Success of the nurse's interventions depends on improving the client's and family members understanding of bowel elimination. In the home, hospital, or long-term care facility, clients capable of learning can be taught effective bowel habits.

The nurse should teach the client and family about proper diet, adequate fluid intake, and fluids that stimulate or slow peristalsis. This often can best be done during the client's meal time. The client should also learn the importance of establishing regular bowel routines, regular exercise, and taking appropriate measures when elimination problems develop. When complications develop from elimination problems, the nurse can teach the client and family members how to give proper skin care, administer enemas, and monitor drug effects.

The special needs of ostomy clients often require extensive education. Clients learn the skills needed to apply stomal appliances, irrigate colostomies (when appropriate), and administer skin care.

Promotion of Regular Bowel Habits

One of the most important habits a nurse can teach a client regarding bowel habits is to take time for defecation. Ignoring the urge to defecate and not taking time to defecate completely are common causes of constipation. To establish regular bowel habits, a client must know when the urge to defecate normally occurs.

The nurse advises the client to begin establishing a routine during a time when defecation is most likely to occur, usually an hour after meals. If attempts are made to defecate during the time when mass colonic peristalsis occurs, the chances of success are great. If a client is restricted to bed or requires assistance in ambulating, the nurse should offer a bedpan or help the client reach the bathroom. The nurse must be prompt in assisting before the urge disappears.

Many clients have established rituals for defecation. In a hospital or long-term care facility, the nurse should make certain that treatment routines do not interfere with the client's schedule. It is also important to provide privacy. When a client forced to use a bedpan shares a room with another person, the nurse should curtain off the client's area so the client can relax, knowing that interruptions will not occur. The call light should always be placed within the client's reach. Bathroom doors should be closed, although the nurse may stand close by in case the client needs assistance.

Promotion of Normal Defecation

To help clients evacuate bowel contents normally and without discomfort, a number of interventions may be helpful. These interventions act by stimulating the defecation reflex, affecting the character of feces, or increasing peristalsis.

SQUATTING POSITION

The nurse may need to assist clients who have difficulty squatting because of muscular weakness and mobility problems. Regular toilets are too low for clients unable to lower themselves to a squatting position because of joint- or muscle-wasting diseases. Clients can purchase elevated toilet seats for the home. With such a seat, less effort is needed to sit or stand. In orthopedic and rehabilitation units in a health care center, toilet seats are elevated.

POSITIONING ON BEDPAN

A client restricted to bed must use a bedpan for defecation. Women use bedpans to pass both urine and feces, whereas men use bedpans only for defecation. Sitting on a bedpan can be extremely uncomfortable. The nurse should help position the client comfortably.

Two types of bedpans are available (Fig. 39-6). The regular bedpan, made of metal or hard plastic, has a curved smooth upper end and a sharp-edged lower end, and is about 5 cm (2 inches) deep. A fracture pan, designed for client with body or leg casts, has a shallow upper end about 1.3 cm (1/2 inch) deep. The upper end of either pan fits under the buttocks toward the sacrum, with the lower end just under the upper thighs. The pan should be high enough so feces enter the pan. A metal bedpan should be warmed with water first.

The most important element for the nurse to consider in positioning the client is preventing muscle strain and discomfort. A client should never be placed on a bedpan and then left with the bed flat unless activity restrictions demand it. If the bed is flat, the hips remain hyperextended. Sometimes it may be necessary to have the bed flat when placing the client on the bedpan. After the client is on it, the nurse raises the head of the bed 30 degrees. Raising the client to a 90-degree angle can make positioning difficult. In a sitting position, the client must rise straight up while using the strength of the arms as the nurse positions the pan. Most clients are too weak to accomplish this. Clients who have had abdominal

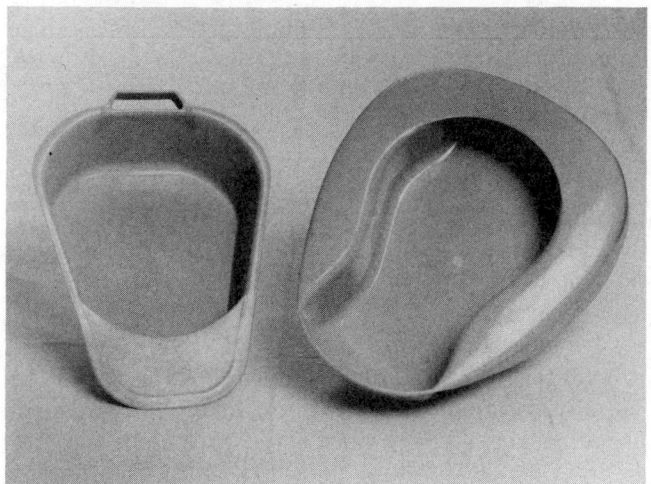

Fig. 39-6 Types of bedpans: *From left,* fracture bedpan and regular bedpan.

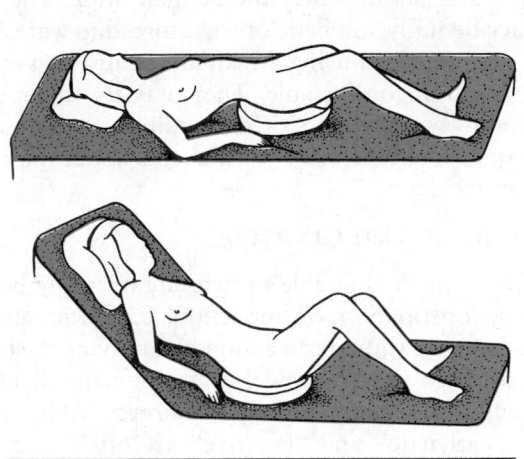

Fig. 39-7 Positions on a bedpan. *Top,* improper positioning of client. *Bottom,* proper position reduces client's back strain.

surgery are hesitant to exert strain on suture lines. Furthermore, the nurse risks injury in trying to lift the client onto the bedpan.

Fig. 39-7 demonstrates proper and improper positions of clients on bedpans. The best method is to be sure the client is positioned high in the bed. The nurse raises the client's head about 30 degrees, which prevents hyperextension of the back and provides support to the upper torso as the client raises the hips by bending the knees and lifting the hips upward. The nurse places a hand palm up under the client's sacrum, resting the elbow on the mattress and using it as a lever to help in lifting, while slipping the pan under the client. Clients who have overhead trapeze frames can easily lift themselves by grasping the trapeze bar.

If the client is immobile or it is unsafe to allow the client to exert such effort, the client can roll onto the bedpan by using the following steps:

1. Lower the head of the bed flat and assist the client to roll over onto one side, backside toward you.
2. Apply powder lightly to back and buttocks to prevent skin from sticking to the pan.
3. Place the bedpan firmly against the buttocks, down into the mattress with the open rim toward the client's feet (Fig. 39-8).
4. Keeping the hand against the bedpan, place the other around the client's far hip. Ask the client to roll back onto the pan, flat in bed. *Do not shove the pan under the client.*
5. With the client positioned comfortably, raise the head of the bed 30 degrees.
6. Place a rolled towel or small pillow under the lumbar curve of the client's back for added comfort.
7. Raise the knee gatch or ask the client to bend the

knees to assume a squatting position. Do not raise the knee gatch if contraindicated.

The nurse should maintain the privacy of a client using a bedpan. The call light and a supply of toilet paper should be within easy reach. When the client finishes, the nurse responds to the call signal immediately and removes the pan. The client may require assistance with wiping. To remove the pan the nurse asks the client to roll off to the side or raise the hips. The nurse holds the pan steady to avoid spilling. The nurse should avoid pulling or shoving the pan from under the client's hips, because this can pull the client's skin and cause tissue injury. Once the pan is removed, the nurse, while wearing gloves, cleans the anal and perineal areas.

The nurse should immediately empty the bedpan's contents either into the toilet or in a special receptacle in the utility room. A spray faucet attached to most toilets allows the nurse to rinse the bedpan thoroughly. The client uses the same bedpan each time.

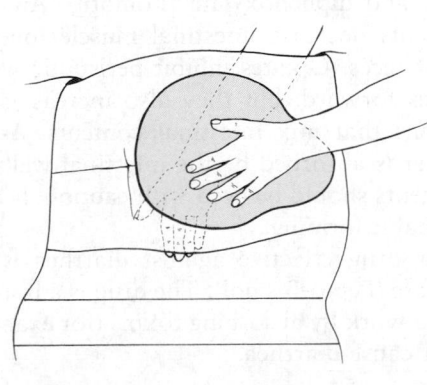

Fig. 39-8 Positioning an immobilized client on a bedpan.

The nurse should offer the bedpan often. The client may accidentally soil bedclothes if forced to wait. Many clients try to avoid using a bedpan because it is embarrassing and uncomfortable. They may try to get to the bathroom even though their conditions prohibit ambulation. The nurse must warn clients about the risk of falls or accidents.

CATHARTICS AND LAXATIVES

Often a client is unable to defecate normally because of pain, constipation, or impaction. Cathartics and laxatives have the short-term action of emptying the bowel. They are also used in bowel evacuation for clients undergoing GI tests and abdominal surgery. Although the terms "cathartic" and "laxative" are often used interchangeably, cathartics have a stronger effect on the intestines.

Cathartics and laxatives are available in oral, tablet, and powder suppository dosage forms (see Chapter 15). The same medication can sometimes be classified as a cathartic or a laxative, depending on the amount used. Although the oral route is more commonly used, cathartics that come prepared as suppositories are more effective because of their stimulant effect on the rectal mucosa. Cathartic suppositories such as bisacodyl (Dulcolax) may act within 30 minutes. The nurse should give the suppository shortly before the client's usual time to defecate or immediately after a meal.

The nurse teaches clients about the potential harmful effects of repeated use of laxatives. The client should understand that laxatives and cathartics are not meant for long-term maintenance of bowel function.

Five types of cathartics are available. The drug classes are based on the method by which the agent promotes defecation (Table 39-6).

ANTIDIARRHEAL AGENTS

For clients with diarrhea, frequent passage of liquid stools becomes a problem. The most effective antidiarrheal agents are opiates such as codeine phosphate, paregoric, and diphenoxylate (Lomotil). Antidiarrheal opiate agents decrease intestinal muscle tone to slow passage of feces. Opiates inhibit peristaltic waves that move feces forward, but they also increase segmental contractions that mix intestinal contents. As a result more water is absorbed by the intestinal walls. Antidiarrheal agents should be used with caution, because opiates are habit forming.

Another drug effective against diarrhea is bismuth subsalicylate (Pepto-Bismol). The drug is a bismuth salt, believed to work by absorbing toxins (for example, bacteria) that cause diarrhea.

ENEMAS

An enema is instillation of a solution into the rectum and sigmoid colon. The primary reason for an enema is to promote defecation by stimulating peristalsis. The volume of fluid instilled breaks up the fecal mass, stretches the rectal wall, and initiates the defecation reflex. Enemas are also given as a vehicle for drugs that exert a local effect on rectal mucosa.

The most common use for an enema is temporary relief of constipation. Other indications include removing impacted feces; emptying the bowel before diagnostic tests, surgery, or childbirth; and beginning a program of bowel training.

Clients should be discouraged from relying on enemas to maintain bowel regularity. Enemas do not treat the cause of constipation. As with laxative abuse, frequent use of enemas destroys normal defecation reflexes.

TYPES OF ENEMAS. There are several types of enemas. *Cleansing enemas* promote the complete evacuation of feces from the colon. They act by stimulating peristalsis through the infusion of a large volume of solution or through local irritation of the colon's mucosa. Suggested maximum volumes are:

Infant	150-250 ml
Toddler	250-350 ml
School-age child	300-500 ml
Adolescent	500-750 ml
Adult	750-1000 ml

Cleansing enemas include tap water, normal saline, hypertonic saline, and soapsuds solution. Each solution exerts a different osmotic effect (see Chapter 37), influencing the movement of fluids between the colon and interstitial spaces beyond the intestinal wall. Infants and children can tolerate only normal saline because they are at risk for fluid imbalance.

Tap water is hypotonic and exerts a lower osmotic pressure than fluid in interstitial spaces. After infusion into the colon, tap water escapes from the bowel lumen into interstitial spaces. The net movement of water is low; the infused volume stimulates defecation before large amounts of water leave the bowel. Tap water enemas should not be repeated because water toxicity or circulatory overload can develop if large amounts of water are absorbed.

Physiologically normal saline is the safest solution to use because it exerts the same osmotic pressure as fluids in interstitial spaces surrounding the bowel. The volume of infused saline stimulates peristalsis. Giving saline enemas does not create the danger of excess fluid absorption. If prepared saline is not available at home, 500 ml (1 pint) of tap water mixed with 1 teaspoon of table salt can be substituted.

Hypertonic solutions infused into the bowel exert osmotic pressure that pulls fluids out of interstitial spaces. The colon fills with fluid, and the resultant distention promotes defecation. Clients unable to tolerate large volumes of fluid benefit most from this type of enema.

TABLE 39-6   Common Types of Laxatives and Cathartics

Classification	Agent/Brand Name	Action	Indications	Risks
Bulk-forming	Methylcellulose/Colo-gel, Hydrolose Plantago seed/Meta-mucil Naturacil	High fiber content absorbs water and increases solid intestinal bulk. Stretches intestinal wall to stimulate peristalsis.	Least irritating and safest cathartic. Drug of choice for chronic constipation (pregnancy, low-residue diet). May also be used to relieve a mild watery diarrhea.	Can cause an obstruction if not mixed with at least 240 ml of water or juice and swallowed quickly. Caution in using bulk-forming laxatives that also contain stimulants.
Emollient or wetting	Docusate sodium/Coloctyl Disonate Colace Docusate calcium/Surfak Docusate potassium/Dialose	Stool softeners are detergents that lower surface tension of feces, allowing water and fat to penetrate. May increase secretion of water by intestine.	Useful for short-term therapy to relieve straining on defecation (hemorrhoids, perianal surgery, pregnancy, recovery from myocardial infarction).	Little value for treatment of chronic constipation.
Saline	Magnesium Citrate/Citrate of Magnesium Citroma Magnesium hydroxide/Milk of Magnesia Sodium phosphate/Phospho-Soda Fleet Enema	Contains salt preparation not absorbed by intestines. Osmotic effect increases pressure in bowel to act as stimulant for peristalsis. May also lubricate feces.	Used only for acute emptying of bowel (for example, endoscopic examination, suspected poisoning, acute constipation).	Do not use in long-term management of constipation. Avoid using in clients with kidney dysfunction (toxic buildup of magnesium). Avoid phosphate salts for clients on fluid restriction.
Stimulant cathartics	Bisacodyl/Dulcolax castor oil/Neoloid, Purge Casanthranol/Dialose Plus, Peri-Colace Danthron/Modane Bulk Doxidan Phenolphthalein/Correctol Ex-Lax	Irritates intestinal mucosa to increase motility. Decreases absorption in small bowel and colon. Phenolphthalein and danthron may cause pink or red color to urine.	May be used to prepare bowel for diagnostic procedures.	May cause severe cramping. Not to be used long term. Chronic use may cause fluid and electrolyte imbalances. Avoid during pregnancy and lactation.
Lubricants	Mineral oil/Haley's MO Petrogalar Plain	Coats fecal contents, allowing for easier passage of stool. Reduces water absorption in colon.	Used to prevent straining on defecation (hemorrhoids, perianal surgery).	Decreases absorption of fat soluble vitamins (A, D, E, and K). Can cause dangerous form of pneumonia if aspirated into lungs.

Contraindications for this type of enema are clients who are dehydrated and young infants. A hypertonic solution of 120 to 180 ml (4 to 6 ounces) is usually effective. The commercially prepared Fleet's enema is the most commonly used.

Soapsuds may be added to tap water or saline to create the additional effect of intestinal irritation. Only pure castile soap is safe. Harsh soaps or detergents can cause serious bowel inflammation. The recommended ratio of soap to solution is 5 ml (1 teaspoon) of castile soap to 1000 ml of warm water or saline.

A physician may order a high or low cleansing enema. High enemas are given to cleanse the entire colon. Fluid is delivered at a high pressure by raising the enema container to a high level. During administration of a regular enema, the enema can or bag is held 12 to 18 inches (4.8 to 7.2 cm) above the client's hips. Thus with a high enema the can will be raised to 18 inches or slightly higher. The client is asked to turn from the left lateral to the dorsal recumbent, over to the right lateral position. The position change ensures that fluid reaches the large intestine. With a low enema the nurse holds the can 12 inches or less above the client's hips. A low enema cleans only the rectum and sigmoid colon.

Oil retention enemas lubricate the rectum and colon. The feces absorb the oil and become softer and easier to pass. To enhance action of the oil, the client retains the enema for several hours if possible.

Carminative enemas provide relief from gaseous distention. They improve the ability to pass flatus. An example of a carminative enema is MGW solution, which contains 30 ml of magnesium, 60 ml of glycerin, and 90 ml of water.

A *return flow enema,* or Harris flush, is a mild colonic irrigation that helps to expel flatus. The nurse first administers a small amount (100 to 200 ml) of mild enema solution into the client's rectum and colon. Then the nurse lowers the enema container to allow the solution to flow back through the rectal tube and into the container. Repeating this process several times aids in reducing flatus and promoting peristalsis.

Medicated enemas contain drugs. An example is polystyrene sodium sulfonate (Kayexalate), used to treat clients with dangerously high serum potassium levels. This drug contains a resin that exchanges sodium ions for potassium ions in the large intestine. Another medicated enema is neomycin solution, an antibiotic used to reduce bacteria in the colon before bowel surgery.

ENEMA ADMINISTRATION. The nurse administers enemas in commercially packaged disposable units or with reusable equipment prepared before use. Sterile technique is unnecessary, because the colon normally contains bacteria. However, the nurse needs to wear gloves to prevent the transmission of fecal microorganisms.

The nurse should explain the procedure, including the position to assume, precautions to take to avoid discomfort, and the length of time necessary to retain the solution before defecation. If the client is to receive the enema at home, the nurse explains the procedure to a family member.

Often the physician orders "enemas till clear." This means that the enema is repeated until the client passes fluid that is clear and contains no fecal material. It may be necessary to give as many as three enemas, but the nurse should caution the client against using more than three. Excess enema use seriously depletes fluids and electrolytes. If the enema fails to return a clear solution after three times (check agency policy), the physician should be notified.

When an enema is given to a child, it is helpful to have a parent assist. The child should understand each step of the procedure and be able to see the equipment beforehand.

Giving an enema to a client unable to contract the external sphincter can pose difficulties. The nurse gives the enema with the client positioned on the bedpan. Giving the enema with the client sitting on the toilet is unsafe because the curved rectal tubing can abrade the rectal wall. Procedure 39-2 outlines the steps for enema administration.

DIGITAL REMOVAL OF STOOL

For clients with an impaction, the fecal mass may be too large to be passed voluntarily. If enemas fail, the nurse must break up the fecal mass with the fingers and remove it in sections. The procedure can be very uncomfortable for the client. Excess rectal manipulation may cause irritation to the mucosa, bleeding, and stimulation of the vagus nerve, which results in a reflex slowing of the heart rate. Because of the procedure's potential complications, a physician's order is necessary for the nurse to remove a fecal impaction.

The steps for removing stool digitally include the following:

1. Explain the procedure and help the client lie on the side with knees flexed and back toward you.
2. Drape the trunk and lower extremities wih a bath blanket and place a waterproof pad under the buttocks. Keep a bedpan next to the client.
3. Apply disposable gloves and lubricate the index finger of your dominant hand with lubricating jelly.
4. Gently insert the index finger into the rectum and advance the finger slowly along the rectal wall toward the umbilicus.
5. Gently loosen the fecal mass by massaging around it. Work the finger into the hardened mass.
6. Work the feces downward toward the end of the rectum. Remove small pieces at a time and discard into bedpan.
7. Reassess the client's heart rate and look for signs of fatigue. Stop the procedure if the heart rate drops significantly or the rhythm changes.
8. Continue to clean feces and allow the client to rest at intervals.
9. Once completed, offer a washcloth and towel to wash and dry the buttocks and anal area. Assist as needed.
10. Remove bedpan and dispose of feces. Remove gloves by turning them inside out, then discard.
11. Assist client to toilet or clean bedpan if urge to defecate develops.
12. Wash your hands. Record results of disimpaction by describing fecal characteristics.
13. The procedure may be followed by enemas or cathartics.

PROCEDURE 39-2

Administering a Cleansing Enema

STEPS	RATIONALE
1. Assess status of client; last bowel movement; normal bowel patterns; presence of hemorrhoids; mobility; external sphincter control.	Determines presence of factors that indicate need for enema and that influence method of administration.
2. Review physician's order for enema.	To determine how many enemas client will require; to determine type of enema to be given (oil retention, carminative, medicated). Nurse must know this to organize equipment and prepare client.
3. Collect appropriate equipment:	Organizes nurse's activities, thereby increasing efficiency.

Enema bag administration:

STEPS	RATIONALE
a. Enema container	Depends on type of enema to be administered. For example, a commercially prepared Fleet's enema is already packaged.
b. Tubing and clamp, if not already attached to container, as in disposable set.	

c. Appropriately sized rectal tube
   Adult - #22 to #30 French
   Child - #12 to #18 French
	Rectal tubing should be small enough to fit diameter of client's anus and large enough to prevent leakage of solution from around tube.

d. Ordered correct volume of solution warmed to: 40.5°-43° C (105°-109° F) for an adult and 37° C (98.6° F) for a child	Nurse must be aware of how much fluid a client can safely tolerate; hot water can burn intestinal mucosa; cold water can cause abdominal cramping and is difficult to retain.
e. Bath thermometer	Used to measure temperature of solution.
f. Lubricating jelly	Reduces friction and irritation to rectal mucosa.
g. Waterproof pad	Prevents soiling bed linens.
h. Bath blanket	Covers client's trunk and lower extremities and reduces exposure of body parts.
i. Toilet tissue	For cleansing perineal area after defecation.
j. Bedpan, plus either a commode chair or access to toilet	Depends on client's level of mobility.
k. Disposable gloves	To protect nurses hands and reduce spread of microorganisms.
l. Wash cloth, towel, and basin	To cleanse client after procedure. This will depend on client's level of mobility.
m. IV pole	To hang solution container on.

Prepackaged enema:

STEPS	RATIONALE
a. Prepackaged disposable bottle with rectal tip	Contains solution and smooth tip for insertion.
b. Disposable gloves	
c. Lubricating jelly	
d. Waterproof pad	
e. Bath blanket	
f. Toilet tissue	
g. Bedpan or commode	
h. Washcloth, towel, and basin	
4. Correctly identify client and explain procedure.	Reduces client's anxiety and promotes cooperation throughout procedure.
5. Assemble enema bag with appropriate solution and rectal tube.	
6. Wash hands.	Reduces transmission of infection.
7. Provide privacy by closing curtains around bed or closing door to room.	Reduces embarrassment for the client.
8. Raise bed to appropriate working height for nurse, and raise side rail on opposite side.	Promotes use of good body mechanics and client safety.

Continued.

Administering a Cleansing Enema

STEPS	RATIONALE
9. Assist client into left side-lying (Sims') position with right knee flexed. Children may also be placed in dorsal recumbent position. Position clients with poor sphincter control on bedpan in comfortable dorsal recumbent position.	Sims' position allows enema solution to flow downward by gravity along natural curve of sigmoid colon and rectum, thus improving retention of solution. (Clients with poor sphincter control cannot retain all of enema solution.)
10. Place waterproof pad under client's hips and buttocks.	Prevents soiling linen.
11. Cover client with bath blanket, exposing only rectal area.	Provides warmth, reduces exposure of body parts, and allows client to feel more relaxed and comfortable.
12. Place bedpan or commode in easily accessible position. If client will be expelling contents in toilet, ensure that toilet is free.	In case client is unable to retain enema solution.
13. Put on disposable gloves.	Prevents transmission of microorganisms from feces.
14. Administer enema using prepackaged disposable container.	
a. Remove plastic cap from rectal tip. Tip is already lubricated, but more jelly can be applied as needed.	Lubrication provides for smooth insertion of rectal tube without causing rectal irritation or trauma.
b. Gently separate buttocks and locate rectum. Instruct client to relax by breathing out slowly through the mouth.	Breathing out promotes relaxation of external anal sphincter.
c. Insert tip of bottle gently into rectum. Advance tip 7.5-10 cm (3-4 in) in adult, 5.-7.5 cm (2-3 in) in child, or 2.5-3.75 cm (1-1.5 in) in infants.	Gentle insertion prevents trauma to rectal mucosa.
d. Squeeze bottle until all solution has entered rectum and colon. (Most bottles contain about 250 ml of solution.)	Hypertonic solutions require only small volumes to stimulate defecation.
15. Administer enema using enema bag.	
a. Add warmed solution to enema bag. (Warm tap water as it flows from the faucet. Place saline container in basin of hot water before adding saline to enema bag.) Check temperature of solution with bath thermometer or by pouring small amount of solution over inner wrist.	Hot water can burn intestinal mucosa. Cold water can cause abdominal cramping and is difficult to retain.
b. Raise container, release clamp, and allow solution to flow long enough to fill tubing.	Removes air from tubing.
c. Reclamp tubing.	Clamping prevents further loss of solution.
d. Lubricate 3-4 in of tip of rectal tube with lubricating jelly.	Lubricant allows smooth insertion of rectal tube without risk of irritation or trauma to the mucosa.
e. Gently separate buttocks and locate rectum. Instruct client to relax by breathing out slowly through mouth.	Breathing out promotes relaxation of external anal sphincter.
f. Insert tip of rectal tube slowly by pointing tip in direction of client's umbilicus. Length of insertion is 7.5-10 cm (3-4 in) for adult, 5-7.5 cm (2-3 in) for child, and 2.5-3.75 cm (1-1.5 in) for infant.	Careful insertion prevents trauma to rectal mucosa from accidental lodging of tube against rectal wall. Insertion beyond proper limit can cause bowel perforation.
g. Hold tubing in rectum constantly until end of fluid instillation.	Bowel contraction can cause expulsion of rectal tube.
h. Open regulating clamp and allow solution to enter slowly with container at client's hip level.	Rapid infusion can stimulate evacuation of rectal tube.
i. Raise height of enema container slowly to appropriate level above anus: 30-45 cm or 12-18 in for high enema, 30 cm or 12 in for low enema, 7.5 cm or 3 in for infant. Infusion time varies with volume of solution administered (for example, 1 liter in 10 min).	This allows for continuous slow infusion of solution. Raising container too high causes rapid infusion and possible painful distention of colon. High pressure can cause rupture of the bowel in infants.

STEPS	RATIONALE
j. Lower container or clamp tubing if client complains of cramping or if fluid escapes around rectal tube.	Temporary cessation of infusion prevents cramping. Cramping may prevent client from retaining all fluid, altering effectiveness of enema.
k. Clamp tubing after all solution is infused.	Clamping prevents entrance of air into rectum.
16. Place layers of toilet tissue around tube at anus and gently withdraw rectal tube.	Provides for client's comfort and cleanliness.
17. Explain to client that feeling of distention is normal. Ask client to retain solution for 5-10 minutes or as long as possible while lying quietly in bed. (For infant or young child gently hold buttocks together for a few minutes.)	Solution distends the bowel. Length of retention varies with type of enema and client's ability to contract anal sphincter. Longer retention promotes more effective stimulation of peristalsis and defecation.
18. Discard enema container and tubing in proper receptacle or rinse out thoroughly with warm soap and water if container is to be reused.	Controls transmission and growth of microorganisms.
19 Remove gloves by pulling them inside out and discard in trash can.	Prevents transmission of microorganisms.
20. Assist client to bathroom or help position client on bedpan.	Normal squatting position promotes defecation.
21. Observe character of feces and solution (caution client against flushing toilet before inspection).	When enemas are ordered "until clear," is is essential to observe contents of solution passed.
22. Assist client as needed to wash anal area with warm soap and water.	Fecal content can irritate skin. Hygiene promotes client's comfort.
23. Wash hands.	Reduces transmission of infection.
24. Inspect character of stool and fluid passed.	Determines if stool is evacuated or fluid is retained.
25. Record pertinent information: a. Type and volume of enema given b. Color, amount, and consistency of fecal return	Communicates pertinent information to all members of health care team. Prompt recording improves documentation of treatment results.

BOWEL TRAINING

The client with incontinence is unable to maintain bowel control. A bowel training program can help some clients achieve normal defecation, especially those who still have some neuromuscular control. The training program involves setting up a daily routine. By attempting to defecate at the same time each day and using measures that promote defecation, the client gains control of bowel reflexes. The program requires time, patience, and consistency. The physician determines the client's physical readiness and ability to benefit from bowel training. A successful program includes:

1. Assessing the normal elimination pattern and recording times when the client is incontinent
2. Choosing a time in the client's pattern to initiate defecation control measures
3. Giving stool softeners orally every day or a cathartic suppository at least half an hour before the selected defecation time. (Lower colon must be free of stool so suppository contacts intestinal mucosa.)
4. Offering a hot drink or fruit juice (or whatever fluids normally stimulate peristalsis for the client) before the defecation time
5. Assisting the client to the toilet at the designated time
6. Providing privacy and setting a time limit for defecation (15 to 20 minutes)
7. Instructing the client to lean forward at the hips while sitting on the toilet, to apply manual pressure with the hands over the abdomen, and to bear down but not strain to stimulate colon emptying
8. Not criticizing or conveying frustration if the client is unable to defecate
9. Providing regular meals with adequate fluids and fiber
10. Maintaining normal exercise within the client's physical ability

The client will require positive reinforcement and encouragement. It often takes several days to weeks before training is successful.

PROCEDURE 39-3

Pouching a Colostomy or Ileostomy

STEPS	RATIONALE
1. Assess condition of existing bag for leakage and note appearance of underlying stoma and surgical incision. Question client about presence of discomfort at or around stoma.	Determines need to change bag. Leakage of contents causes skin irritation. Stoma and peristomal sutures should be inspected daily to note early signs of complications.
2. Note amount of drainage from stoma.	Pouches should be emptied when half full to avoid premature leakage. Liquid output, common in postoperative phase, will cause appliance to melt down and wear out sooner. Copious output will also increase deterioration of appliance. Ileostomy output is more corrosive to appliance and skin and requires more durable equipment.
3. Assess skin around stoma, noting presence of scars, folds, or protuberance of skin.	Determine site for pouch placement and size of underlying skin barrier. Allow 1½ to 2 in of skin barrier on all sides of stoma to ensure secure seal.
4. Determine client's knowledge and understanding of ostomy.	Reveals client's level of acceptance of ostomy and assists nurse in determining extent to which client should be allowed to participate in care.
5. Collect appropriate equipment:	
a. Skin barriers (Stomahesive, Hollihesive, karaya paste or powder)	Maintains skin integrity.
b. Ostomy bag (see illustration)	Contains stool; allows emptying from bottom without removal; is odor proof; can be cut to fit changing stoma sizes.
c. Clamp	Pouch should be drainable to avoid frequent changes; therefore, needs clamp.
d. Hypoallergenic tape	Reinforces pouch to skin barrier.
	Prevents skin irritation.

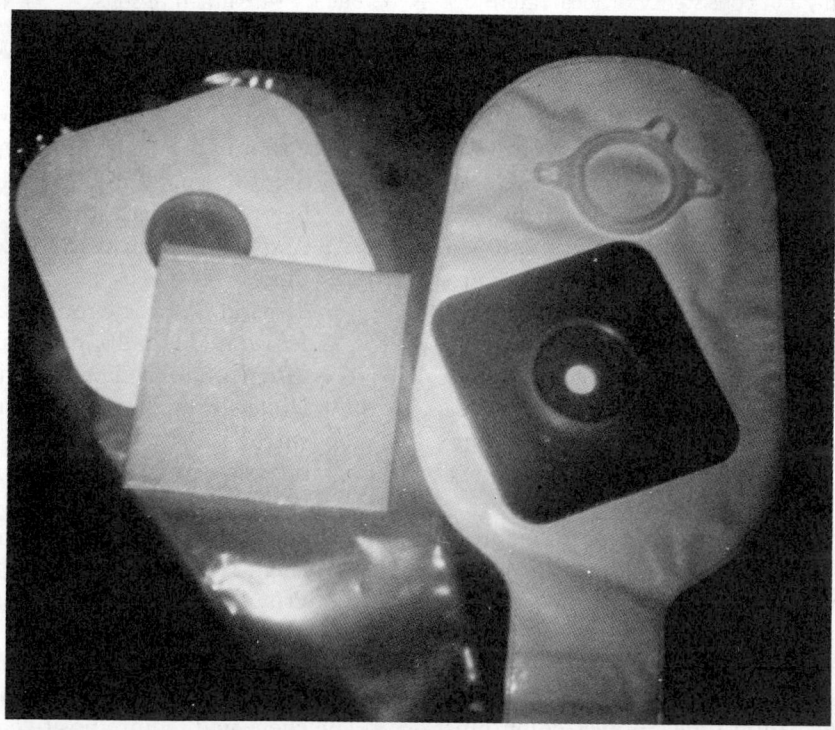

Step 5b

STEPS	RATIONALE
e. Washcloth, towel, wash basin with warm water	Cleansing of skin around stoma.
f. Skin cleanser (Sween or Bard) or mild soap	Removes irritating drainage from skin.
g. Disposable gloves	Prevents contact with microorganisms in feces.
6. Select optimal time to change pouch (when client is comfortable, between meals, or before administration of medications that may affect bowel function).	Teaching is ineffective if client is in pain. Signs and smells of ostomy may reduce appetite. Changing pouch goes smoother whan ostomy is least likely to function.
7. Explain procedure (if client is unfamiliar with technique), otherwise allow client to organize steps for pouch change. Be sure client observes procedure.	Encourage client's participation in care. Ultimately client must assume self-care.
8. Position client supine or sitting for pouch application; if client is able to stand, help him assume standing position.	When client is lying or standing, there are fewer wrinkles in skin and pouch.
9. Wash hands and apply gloves.	Reduces transmission of infection.
10. Close room curtains or door.	Provides privacy.
11. If pouch is full, remove clamp and empty contents through bottom into bedpan.	Prevents spillage on client's skin.
12. Remove old appliance as one piece.	Reduces trauma; jerking can cause skin tears.
13. Wash skin gently with skin cleanser or with regular soap and water. Remove secretions from skin.	Secretions act as irritant to skin. Bacteria in fecal secretions can enter incisional area (new colostomy) and cause infection.
14. Rinse soap off thoroughly. Blot dry.	Use of any soap could result in film or residue being left behind. These residues can result in chemical reactions or burns and can cause premature leakage because of interference with pouch adhesion. Blot dry gently to avoid trauma to stoma, which normally bleeds easily.
15. If blood appears after washing, reassure client that small amount is normal. Clarify what is abnormal.	Minimizes client's anxiety, since bowel has rich vascular supply. Client must be able to recognize complications.
16. Observe condition of skin and stoma. Encourage client to make these observations daily.	Allows for early monitoring of complications. Stoma is at risk for necrosis during first postoperative week; necrosis is evidenced by dark color, dry appearance, failure to bleed, and actual sloughing. Client observation aids in acceptance and adjustment; client also develops habit of observing for skin-stomal problems, which are more easily correctable if detected and reported early.
17. If abdominal crease is present or if contour is irregular, fill in with paste-type barrier.	Provides smooth surface for application of skin barrier and pouch's faceplace.
18. Allow paste to dry for 1-2 min.	Prevents alcohol burns to skin.
19. If abdominal contour is flat or after paste has dried, prepare skin barrier using skin sealant or karaya paste. Cut hole in barrier slightly larger than stoma, up to 1/16 in (see illustration). Cut radial slits from center of hole. Cut rounded corners on edges of skin barrier.	Close fit of barrier around stoma prevents contact of skin with effluent. Barrier cut too tight will loosen from peristalsis of stoma. Slits allow barrier opening to expand if stoma becomes edematous. Rounded corners adhere better to skin.
20. Prepare ostomy pouch; cut hole in center of faceplate 1/8 in larger than hole in barrier.	Avoids risk of paper cut of stoma and ensures better seal with barrier.
21. Remove paper backing from pouch faceplate and apply to shiny, noncovered side of barrier (see illustration).	Reduces risk of wrinkling that can occur if wafer is applied to skin before pouch is attached; gives better leakproof seal.
22. Remove backing from barrier and apply it and pouch as unit to skin (see illustration). Smooth out from center. Hold in place for 1-3 min. Apply in position that facilitates emptying.	Creates wrinkle-free, secure seal onto skin.
23. Apply hypoallergenic tape as needed to edges of faceplate over skin barrier.	Adds extra reinforcement.

Continued.

PROCEDURE 39-3, cont'd

Pouching a Colostomy or Ileostomy

STEPS	RATIONALE
24. Fold bottom edges of pouch over to fit clamp. Secure clamp.	Prevents leakage of pouch contents.
25. Dispose of old appliance in pastic bag and dispose in trash chute. (Be sure this is not a reusable appliance, since they should be washed and reused several times.)	Avoids odors lingering in room, which is unpleasant to client and staff.
26. Remove soiled gloves and dispose in proper receptacle.	Reduces transmission of infection.
27. Wash hands.	Reduces transmission of infection.
28. Assist client to comfortable position if necessary.	Ensures client comfort.
29. Record pertinent information: type of pouch and skin barrier, amount and appearance of feces, condition of stoma and surrounding skin.	Documents care and provides data for later determining change in client's condition.

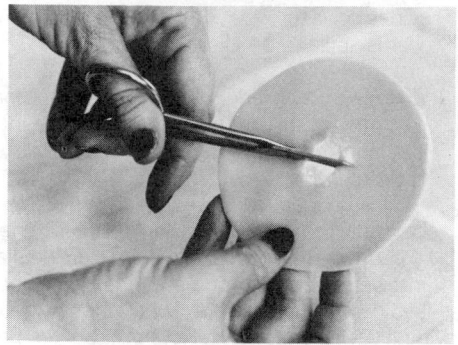

Step 19

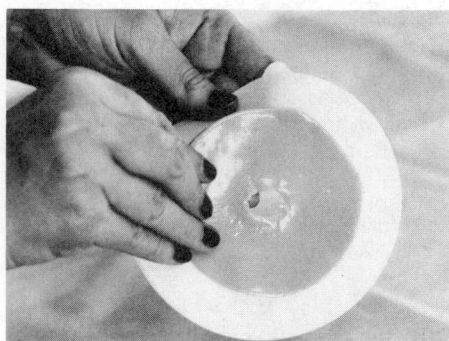

Step 21

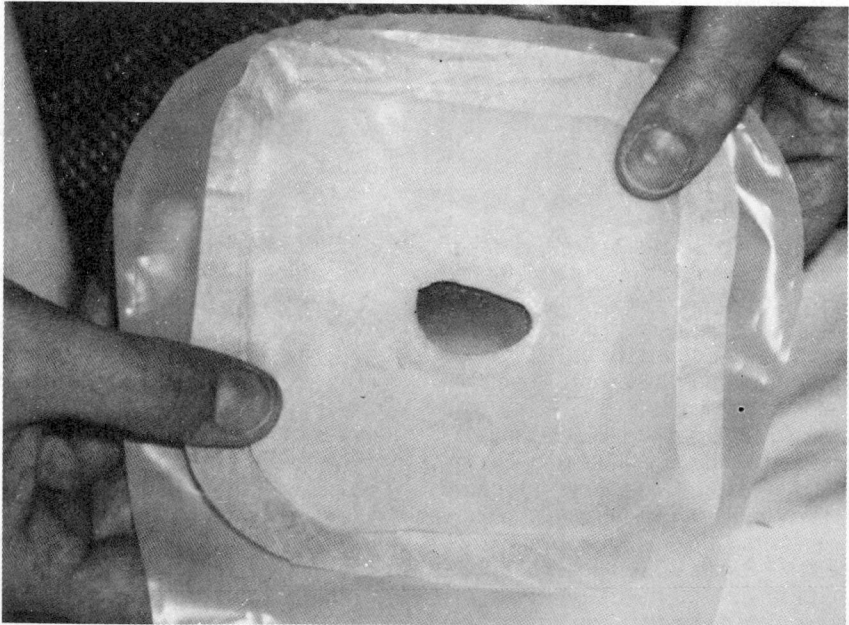

Step 22

Care of Ostomies

Clients who have temporary or permanent bowel diversions face unique health care problems. Their pattern of bowel elimination differs from those with an intact colon. They must wear a pouch or appliance to collect stool emitted from the stoma. Some clients learn to irrigate their ostomy to establish a regular bowel elimination routine. Clients with ostomies must also follow good health practices such as maintaining proper dietary habits and exercising regularly to maintain a normal elimination pattern.

POUCHING OSTOMIES

Ostomies require a pouch to collect fecal material. An effective pouching system protects the skin, contains fecal material, remains odor free, and is comfortable and inconspicuous. A person wearing a pouch should feel secure in particpating in any activity.

There are many pouching systems available. To ensure that a pouch fits well and meets the client's needs, the nurse considers the (1) type of ostomy, (2) size and contour of the abdomen, (3) condition of the skin around the stoma, (4) physical activities of the client, (5) client's personal preference, and (6) cost of equipment. An enterostomal therapist (ET) is a nurse trained to care for ostomy clients. The staff nurse collaborates with the ET nurse to be sure the correct pouching system is used.

A pouching system consists of a pouch and skin barrier. Pouches come in one and two piece systems that are disposable or reusable. Skin barriers include wafers, pastes, powders, and liquid film that is applied to the skin around the stoma. A good skin barrier protects the skin and prevents irritation from repeated removal of the pouch. Procedure 39-3 describes steps for applying one type of pouch system.

IRRIGATING A COLOSTOMY

To establish a pattern of regular defecation, clients with descending and sigmoid colostomies often irrigate their ostomy. The muscular quality of the colon allows it to be safely irrigated with a relatively large volume of water. The irrigation acts like an enema, distending the bowel and stimulating peristalsis. Fluid is instilled into the colon via the stoma. Elimination thus occurs at a time chosen by the client. The irrigation also cleans the colon of gas and odor. Gentle lavage is performed to reduce the risk of bowel perforation.

Surgical creation of a colostomy can seriously change a person's body image due to the appearance of the stoma and loss of bowel control. Regaining control of fecal elimination through irrigation helps emotional adjustment. The client can also gain greater freedom without the need to wear a stomal pouch continuously.

The physician will recommend when to begin irriga-

Contraindications to Colostomy Irrigation

- Ascending colostomies
- Temporary colostomies
- Disease in remaining colon (diverticulosis, inflammatory disease)
- Infant or child
- Physical limitations (arthritis, paralysis)
- Mental limitations (confusion, dementia, retardation)
- Inadequate sanitary facilities
- Stomal abnormalities (prolapse, hernia)
- Client's lack of interest and motivation to learn

---

tions and their frequency. Eventually clients develop their own schedule for irrigations. However, it is usually necessary to perform the procedure the same way every day or every other day. Some clients have physical or mental limitations that make colostomy irrigations unwise (see box). Young children and infants should not receive colostomy irrigations. Infants are at risk for bowel perforation. Young children often cannot sit still for the procedure.

Clients may find irrigation to be a problem. The procedure is time consuming (45 to 60 minutes) and they may be unwilling to interrupt their life-style. For many irrigation is unpleasant. The nurse's emotional support can help clients make a choice. Alternate methods of ostomy management are available, such as dietary control or laxative use. If a client initially decides against irrigations, the decision can be changed later. Procedure 39-4 outlines the steps for an ostomy irrigation.

Maintenance of Proper Fluid and Food Intake

In choosing a diet for promoting normal elimination, the nurse should consider the frequency of defecation, characteristics of feces, and types of foods that either impair or promote defecation. The client with frequent constipation or impaction requires an increased intake of high-fiber foods and more fluids. However, the client should realize that diet therapy provides only long-term relief of elimination problems and may not give immediate relief from problems such as constipation.

When diarrhea is a problem, the nurse can recommend foods of low fiber content and discourage foods that typically cause gastric upset or abdominal cramping. The client with diarrhea is susceptible to potassium loss from heavy loss of GI contents. Fruits and vegetables contain

PROCEDURE 39-4

Irrigating a Colostomy

STEPS	RATIONALE

1. Assess frequency of defecation and character of stool.

Unrelieved constipation characterized by hardened feces can indicate need to irrigate colon.

2. Assess time when client normally irrigates ostomy. With a new ostomy, confer with physician for order.

Maintains an established routine for bowel emptying.

3. Assess client's understanding of procedure and ability to perform techniques.

Determines level of client participation.

4. Collect appropriate equipment:
   a. Graduated container
   b. Tubing with regulatory clamp
   c. Catheter with cone (see illustration)

Organizes your activities, thereby increasing efficiency.

Provides control of fluid instillation into colon.

Because stoma has no sphincters there is no way for client to willfully retain solution. Therefore it is given via a cone, or tube with a backflow device, to prevent premature loss of solution.

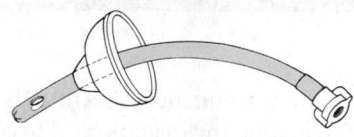

Step 4c

   d. Irrigation sleeve, with or without belt
   e. Water-soluble lubricant

   f. Clamps

   g. New appliance
   h. Disposable gloves
   i. Bedpan (optional)
   j. Washcloth, towel, wash basin
   k. IV pole
   l. Liquid cleanser

Directs flow of irrigating fluid from stoma into toilet.
Makes insertion of cone into stoma easier. Water-soluble lubricants will not harm plastic equipment.
May use to close both top and bottom of sleeve allowing ambulation after solution has returned and while awaiting final results.
Will need new pouch when irrigation completed.
Prevents contact with microorganisms in fecal fluids.
Used if client is confined to bed.

5. Prepare client by explaining procedure.

Allays fears by explaining stoma is not painful. Ensures cooperation.

6. Choose proper time for irrigation, about 1 hr after meal.

Coordinates irrigation during normal time of duodenocolic reflex.

7. Assist client with positioning.
   a. If ambulatory, have client sit on chair in front of toilet
   b. If confined to bed rest, have client lie on side.

Allows for directing sleeve into toilet for drainage of fecal contents and irrigant.

8. Wash hands and apply gloves
9. Close bathroom door or room curtains.

Reduces transmission of infection.
Provides privacy.
Allows access to stoma.

10. Remove appliance and cleanse skin as normally done in changing enterostomy pouch.

11. Apply irrigation sleeve. Roll up so that bottom just touches water in toilet. (For client confined to bed, clip bottom of drain sleeve.)

Directs flow of stool into toilet. Rolling up sleeve prevents it from stopping up plumbing when commode is flushed. Also keeps end of sleeve clean.

12. Fill graduated container with required solution (usually 500-1000 ml tepid water). Hang on IV pole so bottom of container is level with client's shoulder.

500-1000 ml is sufficient to distend colon and trigger effective emptying. Cold water results in syncope and hot water could damage stoma or intestine. Height of bag creates pressure gradient for fluid to enter colon.

13. Attach cone to irrigating tube. Allow enough fluid to run through entire length of tube.

Flushes air out of tube. Air is expelled from tubing because it causes an air lock and will not let solution flow.

14. Apply lubricant to cone.

Prevents trauma to stoma.

15. Insert cone through top of irrigation sleeve.

Ensures containment of stool within sleeve.

16. Insert cone gently but firmly into stoma (see illustration). Stoma should be dilated before first irrigation with gloved, lubricated finger to determine direction of bowel lumen.

Stoma easily injured. Inserting tube toward direction of bowel facilitates introduction of solution.

STEPS	RATIONALE
17. Begin flow of solution and readjust position of cone as necessary (see illustration).	In order to get sufficient distention solution must not leak around cone. Client or nurse may need to redirect direction of cone and slowly increase firmness against stoma until solution flows in easily and leakage around cone ceases.
18. Adjust flow of solution by raising or lowering irrigating container. To aid in this, bottom of irrigator bag should be hung 18 in above stoma.	Administration too rapidly results in cramping and inability to hold sufficient volume for adequate results.
19. Administer 500-1000 ml of solution slowly over 15 min, pausing when client cramps but not removing cone until above amount is given.	Usually 500-1000 ml is required to empty colon. Pauses prevent premature leakage of solution because cone replaces sphincter.
20. When solution runs in, clamp tubing and remove cone making sure sleeve fits around hand. Should obtain small gush of fluid, then returns in spurts.	Clamping tubing prevents return of results into irrigator. Sleeve should be placed properly to avoid gush of solution over top of sleeve. If colon was distended sufficiently, contracting of bowel musculature results in return of solution in intermittent spurts.
21. Clamp top of sleeve.	Prevents leakage at top.
22. When most of solution has returned (15 to 20 min), rinse sleeve with water, fold end up, fasten it to the top, and have client ambulate (unless restricted to bed).	Allows ambulation. Prevents leakage. Entire procedure takes about 1 hr and client may become tired of sitting.
23. When all of feces have returned, rinse sleeve out with water and special liquid cleanser and remove. Then you may wash sleeve out with soap and water rinse and air dry.	Prevents sleeve from deteriorating permitting reuse. Controls odor.

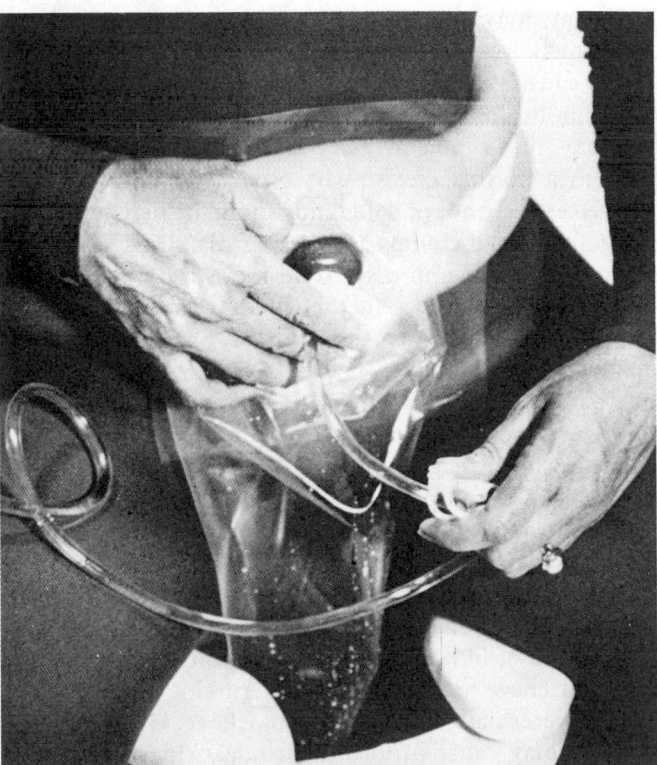

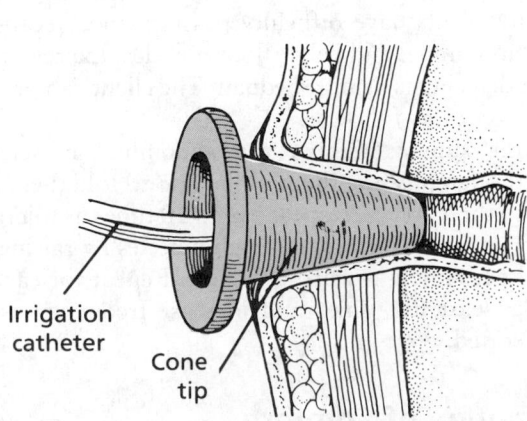

Irrigation
catheter
Cone
tip

Step 16

Step 17

Continued.

Irrigating a Colostomy

STEPS	RATIONALE
24. Apply new pouch according to procedure (Procedure 39-3).	Avoids leakage and skin problems.
25. Dispose of equipment no longer needed. Remove gloves by turning them inside out and dispose in receptacle.	Reduces transmission of microorganisms.
26. Wash hands.	Prevents cross contamination.
27. Inspect volume and character of fecal material and fluid that returns following irrigation.	Determines if irrigant is retained (serious fluid imbalances can occur if retained). Character and amount of stool reveals success at cleaning bowel.
28. Note client's response during irrigant infusion. Ask if he or she feels cramping or abdominal pain.	Reveals client's tolerance of irrigation.
29. Palpate and auscultate abdomen after return of irrigant.	Evaluates for potential complication of bowel perforation.
30. Assist client to comfortable position.	Ensures client comfort.
31. Record pertinent information: a. Character of feces b. Tolerance to procedure	Communicates pertinent information to members of health care team.

Step 16 illustration from Broadwell, DC, and Jackson, BS: Principles of ostomy care, St. Louis, 1982, The C.V. Mosby Co.; © 1978 CIBA-GEIGY. Reproduced and adapted with permission from Clinical Symposia—by John Craig, MD. All rights reserved. Step 17 illustration from Broadwell, DC, and Jackson, BS: Principles of ostomy care, St. Louis, 1982, The C.V. Mosby Co.

potassium but are not ideal because they have a high fiber content. Better foods are baked chicken, seafood, pork, veal, and evaporated and dry nonfat instant milk. Supplements may be ordered by the physician, but they are extremely irritating to gastric mucosa.

Illness-causing diarrhea can be debilitating. If the client cannot tolerate foods or liquids orally, IV therapy (with potassium supplements) are necessary. The client returns to a normal diet slowly, often beginning with fluids. Excessively hot or cold fluids stimulate peristalsis, causing abdominal cramps and further diarrhea. As the tolerance to liquids improves, solid foods are ordered.

Diet therapy is important for clients with ostomies. During the first weeks after surgery, many physicians recommend low-fiber diets, particularly for ileostomy clients because the small bowel requires time to adapt to the diversion. Low-fiber foods include bread, noodles, rice, cream cheese, eggs (not fried), strained fruit juices, lean meats, fish, and poultry. As ostomies heal, clients can eat almost any food. High-fiber foods such as fresh fruits and vegetables help to ensure a more solid stool needed to achieve success at irrigation. Blockage must be avoided. The stoma's surgical construction can affect the likelihood of blockage. Ileostomy clients should eat slowly and chew food completely. Drinking 10 to 12 glasses of water daily also prevents blockage. High-fiber foods that may cause problems include stringy meats, mushrooms, popcorn, wild fruits such as cherries, and some seafoods such as shrimp or crab. Ostomy clients may benefit from avoiding foods that cause gas and odor, including broccoli, cauliflower, dried beans, and brussels sprouts.

Promotion of Regular Exercise

A daily exercise program helps prevent elimination problems. Walking, riding a stationary bicycle, or a swim stimulates normal peristalsis. Clients who are sedentary at work are most in need of regular exercise.

For a client temporarily immobilized, the nurse should attempt ambulation as soon as possible. If the condition permits, the nurse will assist a postoperative client to walk to a chair on the evening of the day of surgery. The postsurgical client should walk farther each day.

Some clients have difficulty passing stool because of weak abdominal and pelvic floor muscles. Exercises help bedridden clients using a bedpan. The client can practice the exercises as follows:

1. Lie supine; tighten the abdominal muscles as though pushing them to the floor. Hold them tight to three; relax. Repeat five to 10 times as tolerated.
2. Flex and contract the thigh muscles by raising one knee slowly toward the chest. Repeat for each leg at least five times and increase frequency as tolerated.

Promotion of Comfort

Many clients have discomfort from alterations in elimination. Pain results when hemorrhoidal tissues are directly irritated. Flatulence can also create discomfort, particularly if abdominal distention develops.

The primary goal for the client with hemorrhoids is to have soft-formed stools. Proper diet, fluids, and regular exercise improve the likelihood of stools being soft. If the client becomes constipated, passage of hard stools will cause bleeding and irritation.

Local heat provides temporary relief to swollen hemorrhoids. A sitz bath is the most effective means of heat application (see Chapter 47).

Often hemorrhoids become so enlarged that they cover the rectum. To prevent trauma to tissues the nurse must use caution when inserting rectal thermometers, suppositories, or rectal tubes. A generous amount of lubricating jelly will reduce friction when inserting an object past a hemorrhoid. Often the client is better able to insert an object safely into the rectum. The nurse should never attempt to force an object into the rectum without full view of the anus. When hemorrhoids cause chronic pain, surgical removal is the best treatment.

To relieve the discomfort of flatulence, the nurse should use measures that either reduce flatus or promote its escape. Air swallowing increases flatus. The client can reduce the amount of air swallowed by not drinking carbonated beverages, not using straws for drinking, and not chewing gum or hard candies. When flatulence becomes severe as a result of reduced peristalsis, a nasogastric tube is often used.

When flatulence results in abdominal cramping, ambulation promotes passage of flatus. Having the client walk down the hall may be enough to stimulate peristalsis and relieve gas.

When conservative measures fail, flatulence can be relieved by insertion of a rectal tube. The client assumes a side-lying position while the nurse inserts the tube in the same manner as for an enema (Procedure 39-2). Because fluid is not instilled into the bowel, the nurse can advance the tube deeper to reach areas where flatus has accumulated (15 cm or 6 inches in an adult, 5 to 10 cm or 2 to 4 inches in a child).

After inserting the tube the nurse instructs the client to lie quietly in bed. To prevent the tube from being dislodged, the nurse may tape it to one of the buttocks. A gauze dressing or waterproof pad placed around the open end of the rectal tube will catch liquid fecal material.

Continual use of rectal tubes can cause irritation and eventual excoriation of the anus and rectal mucosa. A rectal tube should not remain in place longer than 30 minutes. The physician will determine the frequency with which the tube can be inserted. If flatulence persists, the nurse should notify the physician.

The return-flow enema is another means to expel flatus. The alternating instillation and drainage of fluid into and out of the colon and rectum stimulates passage of flatus.

The client with diarrhea or fecal incontinence is at risk for skin breakdown when fecal contents remain on the skin. The same problem exists for the client with an ostomy that drains liquid stool. Liquid stool is usually acidic and contains digestive enzymes. Irritation from repeated wiping with toilet tissue aggravates skin breakdown. Bathing the skin after soiling is helpful but may result in more breakdown unless the skin is thoroughly dried.

The nurse should instruct the client on cleansing the anal area with mild soap and water after each passage of stool. When a client with an ostomy removes the pouch covering the stoma, the surrounding skin should be thoroughly cleaned.

When caring for a debilitated, incontinent client who is unable to ask for assistance, the nurse should check often for defecation. The anal areas can be protected with petrolatum jelly, zinc oxide, or another ointment that holds moisture in the skin, preventing drying and cracking. Yeast infections of the skin can develop easily. Several powdered antifungal agents are effective against yeast. Baby powder or cornstarch should not be used because they have no medical properties and they frequently cake on the skin and become difficult to remove.

Promotion of Self-Concept

When a client has a bowel elimination problem, there is a risk that a threat to self-concept will be experienced. Frequent incontinence, foul odorous stools, or an ostomy appliance are just a few factors that may cause clients to perceive a change in body image. The result may be a client who avoids socializing with others or is unwilling to assume responsibility for self-care. The client with an ostomy often sees a stoma as a form of mutilation. This client may thus have difficulty maintaining or initiating sexual relations with a partner.

The nurse can play an important role in restoring a client's self-concept through the following interventions:

1. Give clients an opportunity to discuss concerns or fears about elimination problems.
2. Provide clients and families with information to understand and manage the elimination problem.
3. Give positive feedback when the client attempts self-care measures.
4. Help clients with ostomies to manage their condition but do not expect them to like it.
5. Provide clients privacy during care.
6. Show clients acceptance and understanding.

Often, clients with an elimination problem go through a process similar to grieving (see Chapter 26). The nurse's support is essential to help them return to a more normal life-style.

Sample Evaluation of Interventions for Bowel Elimination Problems

Goals	Evaluative Measures	Expected Outcomes
Client understands normal elimination.	Ask client to describe factors that affect elimination.	Client will explain effects of diet, fluids, exercise, stress, medications, and personal habits on elimination.
	Ask client to discuss factors in history that places him or her at risk for elimination problems.	
Regular defecation is attained.	Observe character of stools. Record frequency of defecation. Observe client's ability to defecate (if using bedpan).	Client will attain a regular schedule of defecation, passing soft-formed stools without excess straining.
Client understands and maintains proper fluid and food intake.	Ask client or family member to create a meal plan.	Meal plan will include foods suited to client's elimination needs and which promote normal defecation.
	Measure client's fluid intake.	Client will have a minimum intake of 1400 to 2000 ml daily.
Client achieves regular exercise program.	Observe client initiate active exercises daily.	Client will ambulate down halls or report activities (daily walking, swimming).
	Ask client to describe benefits of regular exercise.	Client will explain that regular exercise stimulates intestinal peristalsis.
Client achieves comfort.	Ask client if any discomfort is experienced, such as during defecation.	Client will not have burning or pain during defecation.
	Inspect anal area.	Tissue is intact, without evidence of bleeding or inflammation.
	Palpate abdomen.	Abdomen is flat, soft, without distention.
Skin integrity is maintained.	Inspect perianal or peristomal skin.	Skin is clean, intact, without excoriation or inflammation.
	Ask client to explain methods for keeping skin intact.	Client will be able to explain that fecal contents irritate skin. Client will explain steps used to pouch ostomy.
Client attains a positive self-concept.	Observe client's level of participation in self-care.	Client initiates good elimination hygiene practices (for example, skin care).
		Client with ostomy changes pouch and cleans skin around stoma.
	Ask client about feelings related to elimination problems.	Client will verbalize acceptance of any alteration in elimination.

EVALUATION

The effectiveness of the nurse's care depends on success in meeting the expected outcomes of care (see evaluation box). Optimally, the client will be able to defecate soft-formed stools regularly. The client will also gain information needed to establish a normal elimination pattern.

SUMMARY

Normal elimination of fecal wastes requires maintenance of gastrointestinal function. Each client has a different defecation pattern and presents risks for alterations in elimination. The nurse provides therapies that promote or minimize factors that affect peristalsis or the absorption and secretion of intestinal contents. Much of the nurse's care involves educating clients about daily activities or habits that affect defecation.

Clients become dependent on the nurse when the ability to control body functions is lost. The nurse's approach with clients who have elimination problems must be sensitive and understanding.

✓ A primary function of the elimination process is fluid balance.

✓ Mechanical breakdown of food elements, gastrointestinal motility, and selective absorption and secretion of substances by the large intestine influence the character of feces.

✓ Mass peristalsis in the large intestine is strongest an hour after mealtime.

✓ Food high in fiber content and an increased fluid intake keep feces soft.

✓ Regular use of laxatives can lead to constipation.

✓ Vagal stimulation, which slows the heart rate, may occur during straining while defecating, taking rectal temperatures, and enemas.

✓ The greatest danger from diarrhea is development of fluid and electrolyte imbalance.

✓ The location of an ostomy influences consistency of the stool.

✓ Assessment of a person's elimination pattern should focus on bowel habits, an analysis of factors that normally influence defecation, a review of recent changes in elimination, and a physical examination.

✓ A guaiac test is recommended for clients who take anticoagulants, who have a bleeding disorder or gastrointestinal disorder causing bleeding, or who are at risk for colon cancer.

✓ Indirect and direct visualization of the lower gastrointestinal tract requires cleansing of the bowel before the procedure.

✓ The nurse should consider frequency of defecation, fecal characteristics, and effect of foods on gastrointestinal function when selecting a diet promoting normal elimination.

✓ Proper positioning on a bedpan allows the client to assume a position similar to squatting without experiencing muscle strain.

✓ Cathartics or laxatives should be administered shortly before the usual time of defecation.

✓ Proper administration of an enema is the slow instillation of a warm solution in the proper volume.

✓ Irrigation of an ostomy follows the same principles as an enema administration except a special irrigating tube is needed and the client cannot control passage of feces.

✓ Dangers during digital removal of stool include traumatizing the rectal mucosa and promoting vagal stimulation.

✓ Skin breakdown can occur after repeated exposure to liquid stool.

ADDITIONAL READINGS

Alterescu, V: The ostomy, Am J Nurs 85:1241, 1985.

Alterescu, V: The ostomy, what do you teach the patient? Am J Nurs 85:1250, 1985.

Alterescu, V: Theoretical foundations for an approach to fecal incontinence, J Entero Ther 13:44, 1986.

Alterescu, KB: Colostomy, Nurs Clin North Am 22:281, 1987.

Aman, RA: Treating the patient, not the constipation, Am J Nurs 80:1634, 1980.

American Cancer Society: Guidelines for the cancer-related check-up: recommendations and rationale, 30:18, 1980.

Bitterman, RA: Getting the bowels under control, Emerg Med 19:69, March 15, 1987.

Broadwell, DC, and Jackson, BS: Principles of ostomy care, St. Louis, 1982, The C.V. Mosby Co.

Burggraf, V, and Donlan, B: Assessing the elderly, Am J Nurse 85:872, 1985.

Davis, A, et al.: Bowel management, a quality assurance approach to upgrading programs, J Gerontol Nurs 12:13, 1986.

Dolinger, R: How radiation complicates stoma care, RN 49:32, 1986.

Erickson, PJ: Ostomies: the art of pouching, Nurs Clin North Am 22:311, 1987.

Gershenson, DM, and Smith, DB: Enteric diversions in ostomy care and the cancer patient, Orlando, Fla., 1986, Grune & Stratton, Inc.

Guyton, AC: Human physiology and mechanisms of disease, ed. 3, Philadelphia, 1982, WB Saunders Co.

Pagana, K, and Pagana TJ: Diagnostic testing and nursing implications, ed. 2, St. Louis, 1986, The C.V. Mosby Co.

Smith, DB: The ostomy, how is it managed? Am J Nurs 85:1246, 1985.

Tedesco, FJ: Laxative use in constipation, Am J Gastroenterol 80:303, 1985.

Thibodeau, GA: Anatomy and physiology, St. Louis, 1987, The C.V. Mosby Co.

Whaley, LF, and Wong, DL: Nursing care of infants and children, ed. 3, St. Louis, 1987, The C.V. Mosby Co.

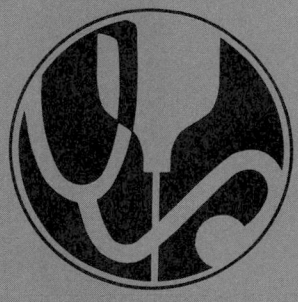

UNIT 8

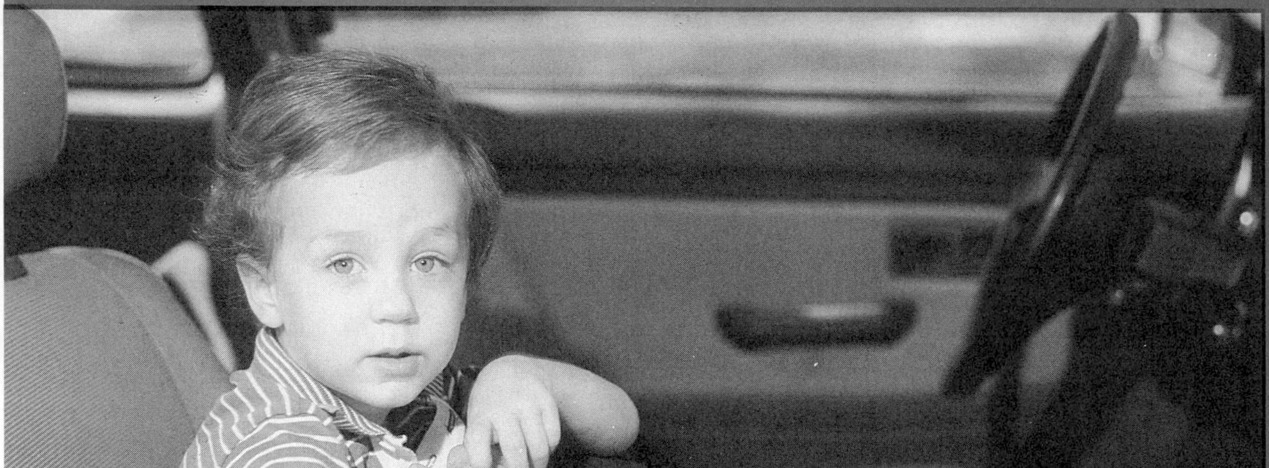

Providing a Safe Environment

An important aspect of nursing care is a safe environment. Health problems often threaten the need for physiological and psychosocial safety, which, if unmet, may further have an impact on overall health. The first four chapters in this unit emphasize protection of the client through promoting safety and effective body mechanics, minimizing the hazards of immobility, and using aseptic techniques and controlling infection. The last two chapters involve clients with sensory alterations or at risk for substance abuse, whom the nurse may address with special nursing interventions.

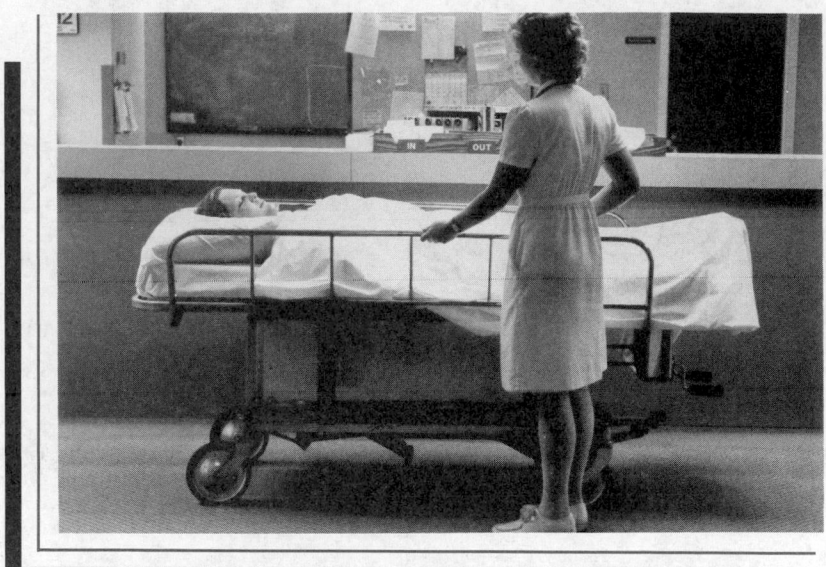

OBJECTIVES

Mastery of content in this chapter will enable the student to:

- Define the key terms listed.
- Describe how unmet basic physiological needs of oxygen, fluids, nutrition, and temperature can threaten a client's safety.
- Discuss methods to reduce physical hazards.
- Describe current methods to reduce the transmission of pathogens and parasites.
- Describe present methods of pollution control.
- Discuss the specific risks to safety as they pertain to the client's developmental age.
- Describe the four categories of risks in a health care agency.
- State nursing diagnoses associated with risk to a client's safety.
- Develop a nursing care plan for clients whose safety is threatened.
- Describe nursing interventions specific to the client's age for reducing risk of falls, fires, poisonings, and electrical hazards.
- Describe methods to evaluate interventions designed to maintain or promote a client's safety.

KEY TERMS

Air Pollution

Carbon Monoxide

Decibel

Food and Drug Administration (FDA)

Food Poisoning

Incident Report

Noise Pollution

Poison

Poison Control Center

Pollutant

Relative Humidity

Restraint

Water Pollution

Safety

Nursing care directed toward health maintenance and illness prevention involves promoting the client's safety in the community or within the health care environment, which is just as essential as meeting hygiene and nutrition needs. Protection and safety are basic to survival, and these needs continue throughout the life span.

Defined broadly, an environment is all of the many factors, physical and psychosocial, that influence or affect the life and survival of the client. A safe environment in the client's home, workplace or school, neighborhood, or a health care agency is comfortable, maintains the client's privacy, and reduces to a minimum the risks of injury, infection, and untoward effects from treatments or medications.

A safe health care environment reduces the length of treatment or hospitalization, the frequency of treatment-related accidents, the potential for lawsuits, the number of work-related injuries to personnel, and the overall cost of health services. In addition, a safe health care environment allows the professional and paraprofessional staff to function at its optimal level.

Safety in the home reduces the risk of accidents and illnesses and the subsequent need for health care service. Safety is positively correlated to health promotion: the greater the safety in a home, the greater the level of health promotion in that home.

ENVIRONMENTAL SAFETY

A safe environment is one in which (1) basic needs are achievable, (2) physical hazards are reduced, (3) transmission of pathogens and parasites is reduced, (4) sanitation is maintained, and (5) pollution is controlled.

Basic Needs

Meeting basic human needs is necessary for achieving safety and security needs (see Chapter 27). Frequently certain physiological needs, including oxygen, optimal humidity, nutrition, and optimal temperature, influence a person's safety.

OXYGEN

The nurse must be aware of factors in a client's environment that decrease the amount of available oxygen. One of the most common environmental hazards in the home is an improperly functioning furnace. A furnace that is not operating properly or is not properly vented introduces carbon monoxide into the environment. *Carbon monoxide* is a colorless, odorless, poisonous gas produced by the combustion of carbon or organic fuels. Carbon monoxide binds strongly with hemoglobin, preventing the formation of oxyhemoglobin and thus reducing the supply of oxygen delivered to the tissues (see Chapter 36). A client who moves to a new residence or who has an older furnace should be encouraged to have the furnace inspected. This inspection is usually performed free of charge or for a nominal fee. Public buildings such as schools, hospitals, and businesses are required by municipal codes to have periodic furnace inspections to reduce the risk of carbon monoxide poisoning.

Carbon monoxide poisoning can be caused in other ways, such as the inadvertent inhalation of automobile or truck exhaust fumes in a poorly ventilated area or a closed garage. The risk of carbon monoxide poisoning can increase in blizzard conditions because people stranded in their vehicles in a snowstorm may attempt to keep warm by running the engine. The poisoning can also occur if the exhaust system is faulty or blocked and gas leaks into a vehicle with tightly sealed windows.

HUMIDITY

The relative humidity of the air in the environment may affect the client's health and safety. *Relative humidity* is the amount of water vapor in the air as compared with the maximum amount of water vapor that the air could contain at the same temperature. The comfort zone for humidity varies from person to person, but most people are comfortable when the humidity is between 60% and 70%.

When the relative humidity is high, the skin's moisture evaporates slowly. Thus during hot, humid weather people feel uncomfortably hot and sticky. If the relative humidity is low, the skin's moisture evaporates quickly. This is why people feel less hot and uncomfortable when the temperature is 32.2° C (90° F) with a relative humidity of 30% than when the temperature is 32.2° C with a relative humidity of 85%.

Modern air conditioners and forced air furnaces enable people to control the temperature of the home and work environments, but they also remove humidity. As a result, people in these environments may have dry mucous membranes of the nose and throat, increasing their risk of respiratory tract infections. Thus many people have attached humidifiers to their furnaces to raise the humidity of the environment when the furnace is operating.

Increasing the environmental humidity has therapeutic benefits. Children and adults with upper respiratory tract infections usually experience improvement in their symptoms when a humidifier is placed in the room while they sleep. The humidifier increases the relative humidity of the inhaled air, which helps to liquefy secretions and improve breathing.

NUTRITION

Meeting nutritional needs adequately and safely requires environmental controls and knowledge. In the home the client needs a refrigerator and a freezer compartment to keep perishable foods fresh. An adequate water supply is needed to clean fresh produce and dishes. Some provision for garbage collection is necessary to maintain sanitary conditions.

Clients and other food preparers need basic information regarding safety in food handling and preparation. Fresh vegetables and fruits should be washed before storing or use to remove insecticides, dirt, and pathogens. Fresh meat, poultry, and fish stored in a refrigerator should be used within 24 to 36 hours unless they are kept in a refrigerated meat keeper that guarantees freshness. The safest approach is to freeze fresh meat immediately after purchase and to thaw it just before use. Poultry should always be defrosted in the refrigerator rather than at room temperature because organisms can grow quickly. Food products should not be used after their expiration dates. Finally, people who do their own canning of vegetables should take care to perform the canning procedure correctly to prevent growth of botulism-causing organisms and other pathogens.

TEMPERATURE

The comfort zone for environmental temperature varies among individuals, but the usual comfort range is between 18.3° and 23.9° C (65° and 75° F). Temperature extremes that frequently occur during the winter and summer affect not only comfort and productivity but safety as well.

Exposure to severe cold for prolonged periods causes frostbite and hypothermia. Hypothermia occurs when the core body temperature is 35° C (95° F) or below.

The person experiences increased confusion and a declining level of consciousness that can result in coma. Shivering is present in the early stages, and trembling may occur on one side of the body or in one extremity. Ultimately the client's vital signs, pulse, and blood pressure decline, and death ensues.

The elderly, children, and clients with spinal cord injuries (for example, paraplegia and quadriplegia) are at a higher risk for hypothermia, which is believed to be a result of autonomic nervous system response. Chronic or acute illness increases a person's susceptibility to hypothermia. Similarly, the ingestion of alcohol interferes with the client's temperature regulation and increases the risk for hypothermia.

Exposure to extreme heat can result in heatstroke or heat exhaustion. In either case the body's electrolyte balance is changed, the core body temperature rises, and brain damage results when the core body temperature reaches 41.1° C (106° F). The client becomes confused, the level of consciousness declines, and coma can result. The chronically ill, the elderly, the young, and the poor are at greatest risk for injury from extreme heat (see Chapter 12).

Reduction of Physical Hazards

Physical hazards in an environment may threaten safety. These hazards can result in a physical injury, such as a sprained ankle from slipping on an unsecured rug, or a psychological injury, such as that which occurs when a person's home has been burglarized. Many physical hazards can be minimized by adequate lighting, reduction in clutter, and security measures.

ENSURING ADEQUATE LIGHTING

Adequate lighting reduces physical hazards by illuminating areas in which the client moves and works. Outside the home, lighting brightens walkways from the street to the house, from the garage to the house, and on the stairs up to the front or back door. Inside the house the halls, staircases, and individual rooms need adequate lighting so residents can safely carry out activities of daily living. Night lights in dark halls, bathrooms, and rooms of children and the elderly help to maintain safety by reducing the risk of falls. A night light in a guest room can help to orient an overnight guest who needs to get up in the middle of the night. Adequate lighting also helps to protect the home and its inhabitants from crime. Well-lighted garages, walkways, and doorways discourage intruders from entering the premises or hiding in shadows.

DECREASING CLUTTER

Injuries in the home frequently result from objects on the stairs and floor, wet spots on the floor, and clutter on bedside tables, closet shelves, the top of the refrigerator, or bookshelves. The risk of injury from clutter is greatest for the elderly and those with impaired vision.

To reduce the risk of injury, all clutter should be removed. Halls and traffic areas should remain free of equipment and furniture. Necessary objects such as clocks, glasses, tissues, or medications should remain on bedside tables within reach of an ill client, but nonessential materials such as books, needlework, or newspapers should be placed elsewhere.

SECURING THE HOME

People need to take precautions to secure their homes from intruders, who constitute a threat to both physical and mental safety. When assessing the client's home for safety, the nurse should evaluate the presence and quality of locks on doors and windows. Adequate exterior lighting can also reduce the risk of home break-ins.

For the client who is relocating, it might be helpful to inquire about the crime rate in the proposed location. Statistics about crimes rates can be obtained from the local police department and home insurance companies.

Reduction of Transmission of Pathogens and Parasites

A pathogen is any microorganism capable of producing an illness. A parasite is an organism living in or on another organism and obtaining nourishment from it. Pathogens and parasites can be found in water, food, people, and insects and other animals.

In a health care agency effective and efficient methods are used for the control of pathogen transmission, including techniques of medical and surgical asepsis and infection control (see Chapter 43).

The transmission of pathogens from person to person can be reduced and in some cases prevented by immunizations. *Immunization* is the process by which resistance to an infectious disease is produced or augmented. Immunity is acquired following the oral administration or injection of an antigen, which causes production of an antibody within the body. The body is then immune to the effects of the harmful pathogens. The discovery of the immunization process for smallpox led the way for the biomedical advances of immunizations for other communicable diseases. As a result the incidence of many highly communicable diseases has been greatly reduced.

The rising rate of AIDS and other sexually transmitted diseases (STDs) is increasing the public's awareness of pathogenic transmission. Safe sexual practices through the correct use of condoms and decreases in casual sexual activities reduce an individual's risk for STDs.

The human immunodeficiency virus (HIV), the causative pathogen of AIDS, is also transmitted through intravenous substance abuse. Drug abusers frequently share syringes and needles, and it is this sharing that increases the risk of acquiring AIDS. The HIV pathogen is blood-borne: thus it is transmitted via contaminated syringes and needles (CDC, 1987).

FOOD SANITATION

Improperly processed or contaminated food can cause illness and death by transmission of pathogens and parasites. Commercially processed and packaged foods are subject to Food and Drug Administration (FDA) regulations and usually contain a minimal amount of contaminants. The FDA is a federal agency responsible for the enforcement of federal regulations regarding the manufacture, processing, and distribution of food, drugs, and cosmetics to protect consumers against the sale of impure or dangerous substances.

The risk of contamination is greatest when food is processed incorrectly. *Food poisoning* is the toxic processes resulting from the ingestion of a food contaminated by toxic substances or by bacteria containing toxins. Kinds of food poisoning include (1) bacterial food poisoning such as botulism, which originates from improper food canning, (2) toadstool poisoning from the mistaken ingestion of toadstools instead of mushrooms, (3) shellfish poisoning from eating contaminated shellfish such as lobster or crab, (4) parasitic infestation from contaminated meat, poultry, or fish, such as *Salmonella* from contaminated poultry, and (5) chemical poisoning from ingesting insecticide sprays on unwashed fruits and vegetables.

INSECT AND RODENT CONTROL

Adequate control of fleas and ticks on domestic animals and in the environment reduces the incidence of bites, skin irritations, and disease transmission. Tick bites are the mode of transmission for Rocky Mountain spotted fever.

Rodents also transmit pathogens. A rat or mouse can transmit rat-bite fever, which in the United States is caused by the *Streptobacillus moniliformis* organism and in the Far East by the *Spirillum minus* organism. Although both of these organisms are sensitive to penicillin, the best approach to rat-bite fever is prevention, which is achieved by reducing the rodent population through proper disposal of garbage.

DISPOSAL OF HUMAN WASTES

The transmission of pathogens and parasites is also controlled by adequate disposal of human waste through proper construction and repair of sewers and drains. Without a satisfactory sewer and waste system, the population is at risk for illnesses transmitted through human feces. Examples of these diseases are typhoid fever and hepatitis.

Pollution Control

A healthy environment is free of pollution. People commonly think of pollution in terms of air or water pollution, but noise can also be a form of pollution presenting health risks.

Air pollution is the contamination of the environmental atmosphere by substances known as pollutants. A pollutant is a harmful chemical or waste material discharged into the water or atmosphere. Prolonged exposure to air pollution increases the risk for pulmonary disease. In urban regions, industrial wastes and vehicle exhausts are common contributors to air pollution. In the home, school, or workplace, cigarette smoke is the primary cause of air pollution. Environmental pollutants can also occur from improper disposal of radioactive and bioactive waste products such as dioxin.

Water pollution is the contamination of lakes, rivers, and streams, usually by industrial pollutants. Industries found guilty of polluting the water are often required by the courts to pay for the clean-up.

Water treatment facilities filter harmful contaminants from the water, but there are often flaws within water systems. If water exiting the treatment facility becomes contaminated, the public is notified to boil their water. Flooding frequently causes damage to water treatment stations, requiring the boiling of drinking water.

Noise pollution occurs when the noise level in an environment becomes uncomfortable to its inhabitants. Noise levels are measured in units of sound intensity called decibels. Noise level tolerances vary from individual to individual and are influenced by the person's health status. A high noise level over a period of time can produce hearing loss. If the noise level is maintained or the person does not use protective earplugs, complete deafness can result.

The health care agency can also be noise polluted. Even when the noise level is not high enough to affect clients' hearing acuity, it may produce a syndrome called sensory overload. *Sensory overload* is a marked increase in the intensity of auditory and visual stimuli. It disrupts cerebral processing of information and problem solving and increases anxiety, paranoia, hallucinations, depression, and unrealistic feelings (Lindenmuth, Breu, and Malooley, 1981).

Pollution—air, water, and noise—can impair the level of health of all those exposed to the pollutants. A nurse assessing a client's environment may be the first to recognize the potential threat to the client from pollution.

ASSESSMENT

Nurses provide care to clients and their families in their homes or communities. Clients who are ill, illiterate, poor, or elderly often require the nurse's help to achieve a safe environment. To do this the nurse needs to understand what contributes to a safe environment in the home or health care agency and then thoroughly assess the environment for threats to safety.

Community

RISKS AT DEVELOPMENTAL STAGES

Threats to a client's safety within the community are influenced by the client's developmental stage, as well as life-style habits, mobility status, sensory impairments, and safety awareness (see Unit 5). In the United States and Canada, accidents are the leading cause of death in people between 1 and 44 years of age.

INFANT, TODDLER, AND PRESCHOOLER. Home accidents kill, disfigure, and permanently disable thousands of children each year, with children under age 5 being at greatest risk for death. Two conclusions can be drawn about the underlying causes or precipitating factors in childhood accidents (Roy, 1982). First, accidents

TABLE 40-1   Expected Motor Development Changes that Increase Risk of Injury in Infants and Toddlers

Age	Motor Development	Hazard
1 mo	Can hold head midline and parallel to body; unable to hold head erect.	If not supported, infant's head flops forward or backward.
2 mo	Grasp reflex present; grasps and holds object for few moments or longer.	Able to grasp electrical cords and other dangerous items on floor.
3 mo	May begin to roll from back to abdomen; bears weight on forearms.	Increased risk of falling off bed, changing table, and counter.
4 mo	Increased grasping ability and explores new objects with mouth.	Able to pick up small objects, which usually go immediately into the mouth.
	Increased ability to roll from abdomen and from side to side and to move in rocking motion.	Increased risk of falling from surfaces.
5 mo	Ability of locomotion increases by rocking, rolling, twisting.	Able to purposefully move toward objects that may be dangerous.
	Able to grasp bottle, but should not be left unattended.	Risk of choking on contents; drinking from bottle in supine position can increase risk of ear infections and dental caries in baby and permanent teeth.
	Ability to grasp small objects increases.	Increased risk of choking on small objects.
6 mo	Creeps by propelling on abdomen, steering with arms and legs.	Able to move to potential dangers, such as electrical outlets and household cleaners.
7 mo	May be crawling; able to sit alone for short periods of time.	Able to move rapidly from one spot to another.
8 mo	May be able to pull to standing position; able to sit unsupported.	Can easily fall unless helped back to sitting or lying position.
9 mo	Begins to crawl up stairs; can stand and move by using furniture for support (walking may occur any time after age 8 mo).	Can lose balance and fall down stairs; can lose balance with wobbly furniture; can bruise self on sharp corners of tables and bookcases.
10 mo	Climbs up and tries to climb down from chairs; able to change from prone to sitting position.	May fall from chair; unable to judge distances or limits.
11 mo	Interested in feeding self.	Unless foods are cut into small pieces, choking may result.
12 mo	May climb out of crib (although rare at this age, it can occur).	Increased risk of falling out of crib or playpen.
	Takes covers off plastic screwtop containers.	Able to open and possibly taste harmful substances.
15 mo	Walks with help; cannot walk around corners or stop suddenly without losing balance.	Loses sense of balance and easily falls.
18 mo	Runs clumsily and falls often.	May injure head from severe falls.
	Moves furniture and climbs on furniture.	May pull furniture over on self; falls off furniture.
24 mo	Able to turn door knobs.	Can independently open closed door and may ingest harmful products stored in cabinet, closet, or bathroom.

Information adapted from Whaley, LF, and Wong, DL: Nursing care of infants and children, ed. 3, St. Louis, 1987, The C.V. Mosby Co.; Potter, PA, and Perry, AG: Basic nursing, St. Louis, 1987, The C.V. Mosby Co.

involving children are largely preventable, but frequently parents need to be shown the specific dangers by nurses and other health care professionals. Second, as the infant grows, accident potential increases. The newborn's accident potential is influenced by people or external agents, but growth and the acquisition of new motor skills place the active child at risk for injuries (Table 40-1). Accident prevention thus requires health education for parents and removal of dangers where possible.

SCHOOL-AGE CHILD. When children enter school, their environment expands to include the school, transportation to and from school, school friends, and after-school activities. Each of these is a potential threat to the child's safety. Injuries can be minor such as falling and bruising the child's knee or major such as being hit in the head by a baseball.

Through discussions and examples, parents, teachers, and nurses instruct children how to safely cross the street, how to choose the proper foods to eat, how to brush their teeth, and how to do other hygiene measures.

Since school-age children are participating in more activities outside their immediate home and neighborhood environments, they are at greater risk of injury from strangers. Therefore the child should be warned repeatedly not to accept candy, food, gifts, or rides from strangers. In addition, children need to know what to do if a stranger approaches them. Frequently neighborhoods have a "block home" or "safe house." In these homes the owner ensures that an adult is home during the times when children are walking to and from school. If a stranger approaches a child, the child can run to that home and the adult will protect the child and call the proper authorities. Nurses can work with school systems or neighborhoods to initiate such a system to protect their children.

Sports safety is stressed in school sports, but parents and health professionals can reinforce these safety tips by insisting that children wear protective gear while participating in sports in the home. For example, schools provide hard batting helmets for baseball games, and parents should also provide this equipment when children are playing baseball in their own backyards. Nurses can also work with neighborhood sports programs to provide education on safe sports and proper use of protective equipment. Participation in sports programs may include instruction on proper nourishment provided during breaks from the actual physical activity.

ADOLESCENT. As children enter adolescence, they begin to develop a sense of identity and their own values, which may conflict with parental values. In addition, the adolescent begins to separate emotionally from the family, and the peer group begins to have a stronger influence.

TABLE 40-2 Changes That May Indicate Substance Abuse

Change	Cause
Bloodshot eyes	Alcohol
Slurred speech	Alcohol, depressants
Restlessness	Alcohol withdrawal, stimulants
Sleepiness	Alcohol, depressants
Erratic appetite	Alcohol, depressants, stimulants
Clumsiness	Alcohol, stimulants, depressants
Urinary frequency	Alcohol
Blackouts	Alcohol
Susceptibility to illness	Alcohol, stimulants, depressants
Dilated pupils	Stimulants

Modified from Rice, MA, and Kibbee, PE: Matern Child Nurs J 8:134, 1983.

The struggle toward identity may cause the teenager to experience shyness, fear, and anxiety, with resulting dysfunction at home, at school, or within the peer group. Psychoactive substances, such as drugs and alcohol, may make the world more bearable for the troubled teenager. Unfortunately, substances used for this purpose put the adolescent at a high risk for continued alcohol or drug abuse (Rice and Kibbee, 1983).

Long-term habitual use of drugs or alcohol results in subtle but recognizable behavioral changes (Table 40-2). The nurse should be aware, however, that medical and emotional problems can produce similar behavioral changes. Moodiness and confusion are typical adolescent behavior patterns (Rice and Kibbee, 1983).

When assessing the adolescent for possible substance abuse, the nurse must look for environmental and psychosocial clues. Environmental clues include drug-oriented magazines, beer and liquor bottles, drug paraphernalia, blood spots on clothing, burns on clothing, or the continual wearing of long-sleeved shirts in hot weather and dark glasses indoors. Psychosocial clues include failing grades, change in dress, increased absenteeism from school, increased aggressiveness, changes in interpersonal relationships, isolation, erratic behavior, avoidance of eye contact, bragging about drug abuse, and increased time spent in the bathroom.

When adolescents learn to drive, their environment expands and so does their potential for injury. The young driver must be taught and expected to comply with rules and regulations regarding driving and use of a car. In addition to municipal regulations, each family places regulations on the teenage driver. Common rules include proper use of seat belts, use of alcohol, riding in a car when someone is under the influence of alcohol or drugs, and curfews setting a time to be home with the car.

Because this is a period when adolescents develop mature sexual physical characteristics, they also begin to have physical relationships with other adolescents. This age group requires prompt and correct instruction regarding safe sexual practices and birth control. In addition, information needs to be provided about the risks of early sexual activity. For example, early intercourse and multiple sexual partners are correlated with cervical cancer. This age group also needs counseling on peer pressure. Specifically, how does the teenager handle constant pressure to participate in sex or drug activities? Many school health programs have instituted the "Just Say No" program. But for many of these teens, just saying "no" is difficult, and in some cases insufficient, particularly for teens who view themselves as not fitting in. Frequently they think by joining in with these activities, acceptance is immediate.

ADULT. The threats to an adult client's safety are frequently related to life-style habits, which are presented in a later section of this chapter. The client who uses alcohol excessively, for example, is at greater risk for motor-vehicle accidents. The long-term smoker has a greater risk of cardiovascular or pulmonary disease as a result of the inhalation of smoke into the lungs and the effect of nicotine on the circulatory system (vasoconstriction). Likewise, the adult experiencing a high level of stress is more likely to have an accident or illnesses such as headaches, gastrointestinal disorders, and infections (see Chapter 28).

OLDER ADULT. Accidental injury from falls, automobile collisions, and burns is a leading cause of death among the elderly (Cooper, 1981). Of all fatal home falls, 82% are experienced by adults over 65 years of age. The elderly are more likely to fall as a result of the physiological changes that occur during the aging process (see box).

Some of these changes, such as slowed response time and sensory impairments, can increase the elderly client's risk for automobile accidents and burns.

OTHER RISK FACTORS

LIFE-STYLE. A client's life-style can increase safety risks. At greater risk of injury are people who drive or operate machinery while under the influence of chemical substances, who work at jobs inherently more dangerous, and who are risk-takers or daredevils. In addition, people experiencing stress, anxiety, fatigue, alcohol or drug withdrawal, or who are taking prescribed medications may be more accident prone. Because of these factors, these clients may be too preoccupied to notice the source of potential accidents such as a cluttered stair or a stop sign.

MOBILITY. A client with impaired mobility has many kinds of safety risks. First, immobilization itself can pre-

---

Physiological Changes Common to the Aging Process that Increase the Risk of Falls

- Decreased circulation in the brain causing dizziness and fainting
- Mechanical obstruction of vertebral arteries to the brain caused by crushed osteoporotic vertebrae
- Decreased auditory acuity
- Decreased night vision, color vision, visual acuity
- Arteriosclerosis
- Orthostatic hypotension
- Loss of sense of position
- Diminished space perception
- Decreased muscle mass, strength, coordination
- Decreased ability to balance
- Osteoporosis and increased stress on weight-bearing areas resulting in an unsteady gait and susceptibility to fractures
- Decreased muscle activity necessary for adequate venous return
- Decreased capacity of blood vessels
- Slowed nervous system response

Modified from Witte, NS: Am J Nurs 79:1950, 1979.

---

dispose the person to other physiological and emotional hazards, which in turn can further restrict mobility and independence (see Chapter 42). A client with impaired mobility is at risk for injury when entering motor vehicles and buildings that are not equipped for the handicapped.

SENSORY IMPAIRMENTS. Clients with visual, hearing, or communication impairments, such as aphasia, illiteracy, or language barriers, are at greater risk for injury in the community. Such clients may not be able to perceive a potential danger or express needs for assistance.

SAFETY AWARENESS. Some clients are unaware of safety precautions, such as keeping medicine away from children or reading the expiration date on food products. A complete nursing assessment should help the nurse identify the client's level of knowledge regarding home safety so that deficiencies can be corrected with an individualized nursing care plan.

Health Care Agency

The basic types of risks to a client's safety within the health care environment are (1) falls, (2) client-inherent

High-Risk and Risk-Prone Conditions Leading to Falls in Hospital

HIGH-RISK CONDITIONS

- Neurological disorders
  □ Parkinsonism
  □ Brain tumor
  □ Seizure disorder
  □ Cerebrovascular accident
  □ Head injury
  □ Spinal cord injury
  □ Multiple sclerosis
- Debilitating disease
  □ Anemia
  □ Pulmonary disease
  □ Coronary artery disease
  □ Cushing's disease
  □ Diabetes mellitus
  □ Cancer (especially metastatic)

RISK-PRONE CONDITIONS

- Difficulties with gait or locomotion
  □ Use of walker, cane, crutches, or wheelchairs
  □ Prosthesis
  □ Dizziness
- Debilitation
  □ Nosocomial—bowel preparation, invasive procedures, postoperative status
  □ Natural—restrictive pain, diminished caloric intake, prolonged bed rest
- Mental status deterioration
  □ Confusion
  □ Disorientation
  □ Depression
  □ Mental retardation
  □ Organic brain syndrome
- Central nervous system alterations
  □ Tranquilizers
  □ Sedatives
  □ Substance abuse
  □ Anesthesia
- Sensory deficits
  □ Blindness
  □ Eye patches
  □ Hearing loss
  □ Hemiplegia
  □ Paraplegia
  □ Quadriplegia
  □ Proprioceptive loss
- Language barrier

Modified from Lynn, FH: Am J Nurs 80:1098, 1980.

⚯ Research Highlight ⚯

Jankin, Reynolds, and Swiech made a retrospective chart review on two groups of patients. Patients 60 years of age and older who fell during hospitalization (N = 331) were compared with a random sample of patients 60 years of age and older who were hospitalized during the same time period but did not fall (N = 300). For both groups, 2 days of hospital record review were sampled. In the fall group, record review included admission day and the day preceding the fall. In the group who did not fall, their admission day and a random hospital day was reviewed.

The study identified seven statistically significant variables that increased the patient's risk of injury. The significant variables included general weakness, decreased mobility of lower extremities, sleeplessness, incontinence, confusion, depression, and substance abuse. Many of these variables have also been supported by other nursing research studies (Innes and Thurman, 1983; Nickens, 1985; and Perry, 1982).

Jankin, JK, Reynolds, BA, and Swiech, K: Patient falls in the acute care setting: identifying risk factors, Nurs Res 35:214, 1986.

accidents, (3) procedure-related accidents, and (4) equipment-related accidents. The nurse learns to recognize factors associated with these four potential problem areas and to take steps to prevent or minimize accidents in the institution.

An accident necessitates the filing of an incident report, a confidential document that completely describes any client accident occurring on the premises of a health care agency. It documents how the accident occurred, any reactions by or effects on the client, and what was done for the client. The incident report is for internal use and is filed with the agency's insurance and legal departments and quality assurance office. In the event of a lawsuit, the incident report is available to the hospital attorneys. Incident reports are also collected by risk managers, who monitor trends and frequencies of incidents in the workplace. Repeated occurrences of incidents in an area will lead managers to take preventive actions.

In addition to completing the incident report, the nurse must document the accident in the client's medical record and describe its effects on the client's health status. The nurse does not write "incident report completed" in the medical record because the incident report is for internal use only (Lynn, 1980).

FALLS. Of all clients admitted to a hospital, extended care facility, or nursing home, 2% experience a fall, and

---

Home Assessment for Falls

HOME EXTERIOR

* Are sidewalks uneven?
* Are steps in good repair?
* Do steps have handrails?
* Are handrails securely fastened?
* Is there adequate lighting?
* Can client sit down and get up from outdoor furniture easily?

HOME INTERIOR

* Are lights bright enough to compensate for limited vision?
* Are stairways adequately lit?
* Are there enough night lights to improve vision during darkness?
* Do throw rugs have secure rubber backings?
* Are rooms uncluttered to permit easy mobility?
* Do chairs and stools provide sufficient support for sitting down and getting up?
* Is temperature within a comfortable range (65° to 75° F)?
* Do door thresholds impair mobility?

STAIRS

* Are stairways well-illuminated?
* Are steps in good repair?
* Are step edges clearly marked with colored tape?
* Are handrails available on both sides of stairways?
* Are handrails securely fastened to walls?

KITCHEN

* Is the gas stove pilot light in good repair?
* Are chairs of proper height for ease in sitting down and getting up?
* Are storage areas easily reached?
* Are floors slippery?
* Is there adequate light?
* Are mats nonskid?

BATHROOM

* Is there a mat or skidproof strips in the tub or shower?
* Does the tub/toilet have grab bars nearby?
* Will the client need an elevated toilet seat to get on and off easily?
* Is the medication cabinet well-illuminated?

BEDROOM

* Are the bed and chairs of adequate height to allow for getting on and off easily?
* Are rugs/carpets nonskid or well anchored to the floor?
* Are night lights available?
* Are light switches accessible?
* Is there adequate lighting?

From Tideiksaar, R: Geriatric falls in the home, Home Health Nurse, 4(2):21, 1986.

2% of those who fall have a fracture (Lynn, 1980). Falls result from slipping or sliding, knees buckling under, fainting, or tripping over tubes, equipment, or furniture. A client can fall from the bed, wheelchair, toilet, or commode or while walking. The occurrence of falls increases during the evening and nighttime hours. Risk factors include age, degree of physical or mental debility, psychomotor status, and use of medications (see box).

Nurse researchers have investigated client falls in acute, long-term, and home settings (see research highlight). Reduction in the risks and frequency of falls reduce complications, length of stay, and the client's ultimate limits of independence.

When delivering nursing care in the home, the nurse must also assess this environment for the potential of falls (see box). Assessment and subsequent prevention of falls reduces the chance for further physical impairments to the client. In addition, family members and friends are also protected from injury. The prevention of injury to the primary care giver of a client in need of nursing care in the home in turn reduces future hospitalization of the client.

CLIENT-INHERENT ACCIDENTS. Client-inherent accidents are accidents other than falls in which the client is the primary factor. Examples of client-inherent accidents are self-inflicted cuts, injuries, and burns; ingestion or injection of foreign substances; self-mutilation or setting fires; and pinching fingers in drawers or doors.

The nurse must file a complete and accurate incident report for client-inherent injuries. A thorough report describing the client's physical and behavioral status as well as the incident is necessary for studying risk factors within the agency that require preventive action and for protecting the institution and health care professionals from any subsequent lawsuits (see Chapter 18).

Checklist for Electrical Hazards

- Ungrounded equipment
- Frayed cords
- Circuits overloaded by too many appliances in one area
- Improperly functioning equipment
- Use of extension cords
- Tangled or cluttered cords
- Use of electrical appliances near sink, bathtub, shower, or damp areas
- Electrical cords or appliances within reach of young children
- Noninsulated wiring in basement or crawlspace

Examples of Nursing Diagnoses for Safety Risks

NANDA-APPROVED NURSING DIAGNOSES

Potential for poisoning related to:
- Improperly prepared or stored foods
- Accessibility to medications, household cleaners, or poisonous plants
- Impaired vision

Potential for suffocating related to:
- Use of outdated or broken infant cribs or playpens
- Improperly vented furnace

Potential for trauma related to:
- Cluttered home environment
- High crime area
- Improper or inadequate lighting

Altered thought processes related to:
- Substance abuse
- Side effects of prescribed medications
- Sensory overload

Impaired home maintenance management related to:
- Limited financial resources
- Physical inability to maintain surroundings

Knowledge deficit related to:
- Unfamiliarity with child-care safety
- Environmental safety

Potential altered body temperature related to:
- Exposure to temperature extremes

PROCEDURE-RELATED ACCIDENTS. Procedure-related accidents are those that occur during therapy. They include medication and fluid administration errors, improper application of external devices, and accidents related to improper performance of procedures, such as dressing changes.

The nurse can prevent many procedure-related accidents. For example, correct administration of medications, using the "five rights" described in Chapter 15, helps to prevent medication errors. In addition, proper administration of intravenous fluids prevents fluid overload or deficit (see Chapter 37). Also, injury from the introduction of pathogens is reduced when surgical asepsis is used for sterile dressing changes (see Chapter 43) or invasive procedures, such as insertion of a Foley catheter (see Chapter 38). Finally, correct use of body mechanics and transfer techniques reduces the risk of injuries from transfer procedures (see Chapter 41).

EQUIPMENT-RELATED ACCIDENTS. Equipment-related accidents are those that result from the malfunction, disrepair, or misuse of equipment or from an electrical hazard. To avoid injury, personnel should not operate monitoring or therapy equipment without instruction.

A checklist should be used to assess potential electrical hazards to reduce the risk of electrical fires, electrocution, or injury from improperly wired equipment (see box).

NURSING DIAGNOSIS

The nursing diagnoses identify risks to the client's safety based on the data provided by the nursing as-

sessment. The assessment reveals clusters of data that indicate when a client has an actual or potential risk to his or her safety (see nursing diagnoses box). General categories involve threats related to poisoning, inhalants, pollutants, or trauma.

The nursing diagnostic statement identifies the expected cause such as impaired vision, substance abuse, or side effects of prescribed medications. The expected causes are individualized so that appropriate interventions can be planned. As the nurse develops the nursing diagnostic statement, the nurse must be sure that the appropriate defining characteristics are present in the assessment database. The sample nursing diagnoses box lists examples of nursing diagnoses for clients with threats to their safety.

PLANNING

The care plan for maintaining the client's safety has a primary goal of prevention of illness or injury (see care plan box). The client's developmental stage, life-style, and level of health impact on the individualized care plan for the client's safety.

Sample Nursing Diagnoses for Safety Risks

Defining Characteristics	Nursing Diagnoses	Related Factors
Lack of interest in learning Inaccurate follow through of instruction Inaccurate ability to state or perform safety measure	Knowledge deficit	• Unfamiliarity with child-care safety • Unfamiliarity with environmental safety
Weakness Poor visual acuity Lack of safety precautions Increased crime statistics	Potential for trauma	• Cluttered home environment • High crime area • Improper or inadequate lighting

Clients with actual or potential risks to their safety require a nursing care plan directed toward meeting their safety needs. The plan is based on one or more of the following client-centered goals:

1. Maintaining an environment that is adapted to motor, sensory, and cognitive developmental needs
2. Acquiring knowledge related to potential threats to safety
3. Reducing the potential for injury
4. Reducing the risk of accidental poisonings

IMPLEMENTATION

Nursing interventions are directed at maintaining the client's safety in the home environment as well as in the health care agency. Because most nursing measures are applicable in both environments, the interventions are presented in two sections: developmental considerations and environmental protections. The first category of interventions includes those specific to each developmental age for reducing risks for that particular age group. En-

Sample Nursing Care Plan for Safety Risks

Nursing Diagnosis	Goal	Expected Outcomes	Nursing Interventions
Knowledge deficit related to unfamiliarity with child-care safety.	Parents will gain knowledge about potential threats to child's safety.	Parents identify hazards in the child's home and community. Modifiable hazards in the home and community are reduced 100%.	Through three 20-minute teaching sessions, the nurse teaches parents potential hazards in child's environment. Through home assessment, the nurse identifies potential safety threats. Parents remove potential hazards from child's reach. Instruct parents how to use Mr. Yuk label on potentially hazardous substances. Instruct parents on appropriate use of syrup of ipecac, that is, this emetic is not used for caustic poisonings nor for the ingestion of gasoline (Procedure 40-1.)

TABLE 40-3 Nursing Interventions to Promote Safety of Infants, Toddlers, and Preschoolers

Intervention	Rationale
Use large soft toys without plastic eyes, nose, or mouth.	The small parts can be dislodged by baby and accidental aspiration can occur.
If a playpen with mesh sides is used, do not leave one side down.	The baby's head can become wedged between the playpen pad and the lowered mesh side, and asphyxiation can occur.
Never leave the sides of the crib down or turn away from a baby on a changing table.	The child can suddenly roll and fall from the crib or changing table.
Hold baby at feeding time; do not prop the bottle.	This increases bonding with the parent and reduces the risk of choking.
If formula is used, be sure to read the instructions. Most formulas must be diluted with water.	Using undiluted formula can cause fluid and electrolyte imbalances in the newborn.
Discontinue the use of the infant seat at 3 months or earlier if the infant is very mobile.	At 3 months, active infants may be able to propel themselves out of the seat and fall.
Baby proof the house for small objects, sharp objects, and toxic and poisonous substances.	Babies explore their world with their hands and mouth, and small objects can result in choking. Toxic and poisonous substances require prompt action (see later section on poison).
Cover electrical outlets with protective covers (Fig. 40-1).	Electrical wall outlets are at babies' eye level and stimulate their curiosity. A crawling baby will frequently attempt to play with electrical wall plates regardless of the number of toys available.
Use guardrails at the top and bottom of stairs and at the doorway of rooms considered off-limits to a crawling or walking toddler.	This prevents the child from falling down the stairs or being exposed to rooms with unguarded dangers.
Never leave a baby unattended in infant seat, walker, stroller, or high chair.	An active child can easily slide out of these devices and fall.
Never leave a baby or child unattended in a bath or wading pool.	Accidental drowning may occur.
Never attach a pacifier to a child with a string around the neck.	The string may become easily tangled, and stangulation can result.
Restrain a child in the back seat of an automobile. Children under 4 should be in an approved car seat (Fig. 40-2). Older children should be restrained with a seat belt.	In the event of a sudden stop or an auto accident, an unrestrained child is bounced against hard, sharp surfaces of the vehicles interior and injuries result.
Plastic bags, such as those for storing fruit or dry cleaning, should be removed from home.	If the child places these over the head, the air supply decreases and the child suffocates.
Install strong dead-bolt locks on doors well beyond the toddler's reach, even when the child is standing on a chair.	This prevents the child from leaving the home without the parent's knowledge, reducing danger of child getting lost, freezing to death, or being abducted.
Use the words "no" and "don't" to convey that an object or action increases the child's risk of injury, such as playing with matches (Fig. 40-3).	Improperly using these words renders them meaningless to the child.
Teach the child to swim at an early age, but always provide supervision.	The child will be able to enjoy the water safely. A child who knows how to swim can still get in difficulty in the water and needs supervision.
Teach the child how to cross the street and how to walk in parking lots.	This provides the child with self-protection against dangers from automobiles.
Teach the child not to talk to or accept anything from a stranger and to notify parents or a responsible adult if approached by a stranger.	This reduces the risk of injury or abduction by a stranger. Reporting the stranger's presence helps law enforcement personnel investigate and remove a threat.
Do not allow the child to run with a sucker or popsicle in the mouth.	The child may fall, and the stick from the sucker or popsicle can cause a puncture injury or a foreign body in the child's airway.
Impress on the child not to eat anything found on the street or in the grass.	The substance may be poisonous and can cause severe illness.
Use back burners on stoves and get into the habit of turning pot handles toward the wall.	This reduces the risk of the child pulling down a pot of hot liquid and being burned.
Remove doors from unused refrigerators and freezers, and instruct the child not to hide in these items.	The door may latch and on older models cannot be released from the inside; as a result aphyxiation can occur.

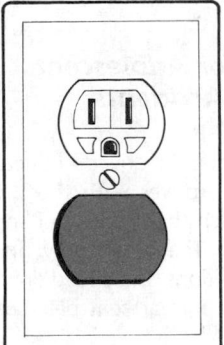

Fig. 40-1 Safety covers for electrical outlets.

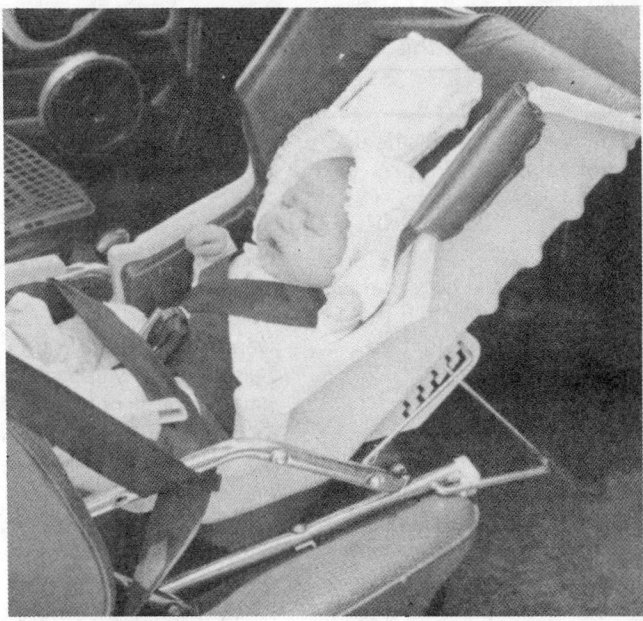

Fig. 40-2 Infant car seat.
From Whaley, LF, and Wong, DL: Nursing care of infants and children, ed. 3, St. Louis, 1987, The C.V. Mosby Co.

vironmental interventions are developed to modify the environment so that present or potential hazards are eliminated or minimized.

Developmental Considerations

INFANT, TODDLER, AND PRESCHOOLER

Infants and preschoolers depend on adults to protect them from injury. Growing children are curious and completely trusting of their environment and do not perceive themselves to be in danger.

Nurses are frequently in a position to educate parents or guardians about reducing risks of injuries for young children. Nurses working in prenatal clinics can easily incorporate safety into the care plan of the childbearing family. Community health nurses can assess the home environment and show parents how to promote safety in their homes. The nurse can teach both the child and the parent or guardian about safety (Table 40-3 and Figs. 40-1 to 40-2).

SCHOOL-AGE CHILD

School-age children increasingly explore their environment. They have friends outside their immediate neighborhood; they may walk to school, and they become more active in school, church, and community activities. All of these activities help the child to develop social skill and independence, but they also increase the risk of injury, such as falls from playground equipment, sports injuries, etc. The school-age child begins to align some activities with those of the adult, learning from parents, teachers, and often television heroes. This patterning of behavior and activities is not necessarily a threat to the child, except when the child imitates an adult behavior that presents safety risks, such as operating an electric saw. Some nursing interventions help to guide the parent to provide for the safety of the school-age child (Table 40-4).

Approximately 20% of school-age children are also at risk for depression (Rhyne et al., 1986). Loss and impaired parent-child relationships are primary causative factors. The school-age child commonly exhibits depression through changes in appetite, sleeping, activity levels, and apathy. Prompt recognition results in prompt intervention in the form of family or individual counseling or support groups.

ADOLESCENT

When children approach their adolescent years, much of their time is spent away from home and with their peer group. During adolescence young people learn to drive. Risks to the adolescent's safety therefore involve many factors outside the home environment. Adults serve as role models for adolescents, and through example and education, can help adolescents minimize risks to their safety. The box lists measures by which nurses and parents can help the adolescent prevent accidents.

Adolescent adjustment to responsibilities and changes in their bodies may result in mood swings, withdrawal, or even depression. In addition, this age population has a high incidence of suicide because of depression, poor body image, or feelings of decreased self-worth. Suicide has devastating effects upon the family because they are left with feelings of loss, anger, inadequacy, and pain. Nurses can provide emotional support to these families

TABLE 40-4 Nursing Interventions to Promote Safety of the School-Age Child

Intervention*	Rationale
Teach the child the safe use of equipment for play and work activities.	The child needs to learn that some equipment is for play and other is for work and that improper use can result in injury.
Teach the child how to ride a bicycle safely and the responsibilities that go with bicycling.	If bicycling is prohibited on sidewalks, the child must learn to obey traffic signals and ride with traffic patterns or identify safe locations for bicycle riding.
Teach the child, when roller skating, to wear a protective helmet and knee and elbow pads.	When children roller skate, they fall; protective devices reduce the risk of serious injury.
Never allow the child to operate appliances while alone in the house.	If an electrical mishap were to occur, no one would be available to help the child.
If a parent chooses to have firearms in the house, teach the parent to keep them unloaded, locked up, and out of reach.	This prevents injury from accidental discharge or improper use.

*In addition to those in Table 40-3 appropriate for the school-age child.

Measures for Adolescents to Prevent Accidents

- Enroll teenagers in driver's education courses and make practice drives with them in good and bad weather. Teach them how to handle a motor vehicle in a skid. Teach the new driver to adhere to driving regulations and speed limits.
- Teach them to wear seat belts while driving or as passengers.
- Instruct them not to drive after using a psychoactive substance or enter an automobile when the driver has been using such substances.
- Form a contract with teenagers that, if they drink at a party, they call home for a ride with no questions asked.
- Teach adolescents not to drive with others who are drinking or under the influence of drugs.
- Help them develop safe eating, sleeping, and relaxation habits.
- Inform them of the dangers of psychoactive substances.
- Inform them of the dangers of unsafe sexual practices. Teach adolescents safe-sex decisions and practices.
- Recognize changes in adolescents' behavior and mood.
- Listen to them.
- Do not try to be a buddy; remain a parent.

---

along with referrals to counselors and support groups such as Survivors of Suicide (Hoffman, 1987).

ADULT

Risks to young and middle adults frequently result from life-style factors, such as child rearing, high-stress states, inadequate nutrition, excessive alcohol intake, and substance abuse. Adults need to be taught that their safety is in fact threatened, and as a result their life-style needs to be modified.

Stress management centers (see Chapter 28) and health promotion activities (see Chapter 2) have been incorporated into many community service programs as well as hospitals. In addition, neighborhood centers, community clinics, and outpatient clinics are equipped to assist the adult in modifying life-style habits that present risks to health, such as smoking, overeating, lack of exercise, and alcoholism.

OLDER ADULT

As noted earlier, most injuries to the elderly involve falls, auto accidents, and burns (Cooper, 1981). The

advancing age and the concurrent physiological changes in vision, hearing, mobility, circulation, and the ability to make quick judgments may predispose some elderly to falls and other accidents. In addition, many of the medications given to the elderly make falls more likely (Cooper, 1981). Nursing interventions designed to reduce the risk of falls compensate for the physiological changes of aging (Table 40-5 and box on p. 1172).

Automobile accidents are more likely to occur with the elderly because of three specific physiological changes. First, changes in visual acuity and depth perception prevent the client from quickly observing situations in which an accident is likely to occur. Second, decreased hearing acuity alters the elderly client's ability to hear emergency vehicle sirens or car and truck horns. Last, because of decreased nervous system response, the elderly may be unable to react as quickly as they once could to avoid an accident (Ebersole and Hess, 1989) (see box on p. 1173).

Pedestrian accidents among the elderly can also be reduced by persuading the elderly to take five precautions: (1) wear reflectorized garments when walking at

TABLE 40-5   Measures to Prevent Falls in the Home of the Elderly

Measure	Rationale
STAIRS	
Install treads with a uniform depth of 9 inches and 9-inch risers (vertical face of the steps).	If stairs are of uniform size, the elderly need not continually adjust their vision.
Install uniform-textured or plain-colored surfaces on each tread, and mark the edge of the tread with a contrasting color.	Uniform textures or color help to decrease vertigo. Marking the edge of the tread provides the client with an obvious visual clue to the end of the stair.
Ensure proper lighting of each tread. Block sun or lightbulb glare with translucent shades or screen or use lower wattage bulbs.	An elderly client's vision is unable to accommodate quickly to changes in lighting.
Ensure adequate head room so users need not duck to negotiate stairs.	Sudden changes in a client's head position may result in dizziness.
Remove protruding objects from staircase walls.	Decreased peripheral vision may prevent the client from seeing the object.
Maintain outdoor walkways and stairs in good condition, free of holes, cracks, and splinters.	Decreased visual acuity can prevent the elderly from seeing any structural defect.
HANDRAILS	
Install smooth but slip-resistant handrails at least 2 inches from the wall.	The 2-inch distance allows the client to grasp the handrail firmly for support.
Secure handrail firmly so that user's weight is supported, especially at the bottom and top of the stairway.	The elderly have the greatest risk of falling at the top and bottom of stairs because their center of gravity is being shifted and their balance is unstable.
Install guard rails in the bathroom near the toilet or tub.	This enables the elderly to have support while rising from a sitting to standing position.
FLOOR COVERINGS	
Secure all carpeting, mats, and tile; place nonskid backing under small rugs.	A sudden slip may cause dizziness and inability of an elderly person to regain balance. A decrease in muscle strength may decrease their ability to adjust to a slip and prevent a fall.

night, (2) stand on the sidewalk, not in the street, when waiting to cross a street, (3) always cross at corners, not in the middle of the block, particularly if the street is a major one, (4) whenever possible, cross with the traffic light, not against it, and (5) look left, right, and left again before entering the street or crosswalk.

Burns and scalds are also more apt to occur with the elderly who are at greater risk for several reasons. They may forget and leave hot water running or become confused when turning the dials on a stove. Impaired visual acuity and sense of smell increase the danger that the elderly may not detect smoke or gas fumes (Cooper, 1981). The nursing measures developed for preventing burns are designed to minimize the risk from impaired vision and hearing (see box).

Environmental Considerations

Nursing interventions directed toward eliminating environmental threats include general preventive measures, such as meeting basic needs, reducing physical hazards, reducing pathogen and parasite transmission, and controlling pollution effects, as well as specific measures to reduce the risk of accidental injuries from falls, fires, poisoning, and electrical hazards.

GENERAL PREVENTIVE MEASURES

Nursing interventions can contribute to a safer environment by helping the client meet the basic physiological needs of oxygen, humidity, nutrition, and temperature.

Nurses use effective and efficient methods to control pathogen transmission. These include techniques of *medical asepsis*, the removal or destruction of disease-causing organisms or infected material, and *surgical asepsis*, protection against infection by the use of sterile techniques (see Chapter 43). Pathogen transmission from person to person can be reduced or prevented by *immunization*, the process by which resistance to an infectious disease is acquired through the administration

---

Risk and Fall Assessment

Diagnosis: _____
Primary: _____
Secondary: _____

PLEASE CHECK ONLY THOSE DATA THAT PERTAIN

General Data

___ Age over 60
___ History of falls prior to admission
___ Post op: 24-48 hours
___ Falls during this admission or previous admission (within 1 year)

Physical Status

___ Dizziness/unbalanced
___ Unsteady gait
___ Joint difficulties
___ Fatigue
___ Paresis/paralysis
___ Seizure disorder
___ Impaired vision
___ Impaired hearing
___ Nocturia

Mental Status

___ Confused or disoriented
___ Impaired judgment
___ Impaired memory
___ Unable to understand instruction

Medications

___ Diuretics
___ Narcotics, sedatives, psychotropics, hypnotics, tranquilizers, antidepressants
___ Antihypertensives, beta-blockers, calcium channel blockers
___ Laxatives, cathartics

Ambulatory Devices

___ Walker ___ Geri-chair
___ Crutches ___ Wheelchair
___ Cane

Restraining Devices

___ Posey jacket ___ Posey belt
___ Soft restraints ___ Other
___ Side rails

Language Status

___ Aphasia
___ Primary language other than English

Adapted with permission from Fife, DD, et al.: A risk/falls program: code orange for success, Nurse Manage 15(911):50, 1984.

---

of an antigen and the body's consequent production of an antibody. In the home environment, awareness of safe methods of food handling helps reduce the risk of pathogen and parasite transmission through contaminated food.

SPECIFIC SAFETY CONCERNS

FALLS. Modifications in the client's home or health care environment can easily reduce the risk of falls. A heavy or debilitated client in a bed or wheelchair or on a toilet should be properly secured or supported. Excess furniture and equipment should be removed, and a weakened client should wear rubber-soled shoes or slippers for walking or transferring. Clients need to be instructed to inspect canes, walkers, and crutches to be sure the rubber tip is intact.

With clients in the home or hospital setting, certain safeguards can be implemented or taught to the family to minimize the risk of falls (see box and Figs. 40-3 and

40-4). In addition, confused, disoriented, very young, or very old clients may require the use of restraints and side rails to protect them from falling out of bed.

Restraints. A restraint is any one of numerous devices used to immobilize a client or an extremity. The use of restraints involves a psychological adjustment for the client and family, and the nurse should assist them in adapting to this necessary change (Table 40-6, p. 1175). As with other procedures, the nurse must follow specific guidelines when using restraints (Procedure 40-1). The overall objectives for restraints are:

1. To reduce the risk of the client falling out of bed or from chair or wheelchair
2. To prevent interruption of therapy such as traction, intravenous infusions, nasogastric tube feeding, or Foley catheter
3. To prevent the confused or combative client from removing life-support equipment
4. To reduce the risk of injury to others by the client

Steps the Elderly Can Take to Prevent Automobile Accidents

- See your physician if you suspect you have a hearing problem.
- Leave your car window partially open to let you hear warning signals.
- Set the air conditioner or heater and the radio low so that their noise does not mask outside sounds.
- Place mirrors on both sides of the car, and use them and a wide rear-view mirror when you change lanes or pass other vehicles.
- Stop frequently to stretch your muscles and rest your eyes.
- Schedule regular eye examinations to check for vision changes or health problems that may affect your vision.
- Follow the physician's recommendations, if any, about limiting when and where you drive.
- Before driving, give yourself time to adjust to new lenses, especially bifocals or trifocals.
- Wear good quality sunglasses to reduce glare. Wear them only during the day.
- Keep windshield and all windows clean inside and out. Replace worn wiper blades. Keep headlights, tail lights, and turn signals clean to maintain maximum lighting.
- If you take medication, know its long- and short-term effects on your driving ability.
- Do not smoke while driving at night. Smoking impairs vision.
- Do not drive when you have been drinking.
- Enroll in a driver training course through your state motor vehicle department.
- Take circuitous routes to avoid freeways.

From Cooper, S: Accidents and older adults. Copyright 1981, American Journal of Nursing Company. Reprinted with permission from Geriatric Nursing, July/August, vol. 2.

Steps the Elderly Can Take to Prevent Burns

- Do not smoke in bed or when sleepy.
- When cooking, do not wear loose-fitting clothing (bathrobes, nightgowns, pajamas).
- Learn to use a microwave oven.
- Set thermostats for water heater or faucets so water does not become too hot.
- Install a portable hand fire extinguisher and smoke detectors in the kitchen.
- Keep access to outside door(s) unobstructed.
- Identify emergency exits in public buildings.
- If you consider entering a boarding or foster home, check to see that it has smoke detectors, a sprinkler system, and fire extinguishers.
- Wear clothing that is nonflammable or treated with a permanent flame-retardant finish. Fabrics of animal hair, wool, or silk are less flammable.
- Use several electrical outlets to avoid overloading.

From Cooper, S: Accidents and older adults. Copyright 1981, American Journal of Nursing Company. Reprinted with permission from Geriatric Nursing, July/August, vol. 2.

Measures to Prevent Falls in the Health Care Setting

- Identify clients at risk for falling (see box on p. 1172).
- Assign clients at risk rooms near the nurse's station.
- Alert all nursing/health care personnel to client's increased risk of falling, for example, Kardex notation or sign on client's room or over his bed.
- Use nightlight in room.
- Reinforce to client/family the need for assistance when ambulating or getting up.
- Side rails up.
- Call lights easily accessible, prompt answering of call light.
- Client's personal and diversional items within easy reach.
- Scheduled toileting routine.
- Reassessment of client's risk of falling each shift.
- Frequent observation of client.
- Proper use of restraints or sitters.

When used correctly, restraints benefit the client. For legal purposes it is important that the nurse be familiar with agency policy and procedures for the appropriate use of restraints. Most institutions require a physician's order. When the nurse makes an independent judgment to apply restraints, it is important to document the assessment of the client's activity and behavior, the conclusions about the client's status, the nursing action, and the fact that the action was explained to both the client and family. In addition, the nurse notes specifically the type of restraint selected and where the restraints were applied.

Side Rails. Chapter 41 discusses side rails as a device for increasing the client's mobility and stability in bed or when moving from bed to chair. Side rails also help prevent the unconscious client from falling out of bed or from a stretcher (Fig. 40-5). However, the use of side rails alone for a disoriented client may cause only more confusion and further injury. Frequently a confused client who is determined to get out of bed attempts to climb over the side rail or climbs out at the foot of the bed. Either attempt usually results in a fall. Therefore for the confused client, a jacket restraint is often used with the side rails elevated.

FIRES. Both the home and the hospital environment are always at risk for fires. Accidental home fires typically result from smoking in bed, careless extinguishing of cigarette butts in trash cans, grease fires, or electrical fires resulting from faulty wiring or appliances. Institutional fires typically result from a client smoking in bed or from an electrical or anesthetic-related fire.

The interventions described here are directed toward fires occurring in health care agencies, but the same principles apply for fires in the home. It is important to have a plan of action in the event of fire (see box, p. 1175).

If a fire occurs in a health care agency, the nurse has three major priorities: (1) to protect clients from injury, (2) to report the location of the fire, and (3) to contain the fire. Upon observing a fire, the nurse should immediately report its exact location. The nurse may then attempt to extinguish the fire if there is no immediate threat to clients.

When hospital or institutional fires occur, all personnel are mobilized to evacuate clients. Clients who are close to the fire, regardless of its size, are at risk of injury and should be moved to another area. If a client requires oxygen but not life support, the nurse discontinues the oxygen, which is combustible and can fuel an existing fire. If the client is on life support, the nurse may need to maintain the client's respiratory status manually with an Ambu bag (see Chapter 36) until the client is moved away from the threat of fire. Ambulatory clients can be directed to walk by themselves to a safe area and in some cases may be able to assist in moving clients in wheelchairs. Bedridden clients are generally moved from the scene of a fire by a stretcher, their bed, or a wheelchair. If none of these methods is appropriate, clients must be carried from the area. If a client must be carried, the nurse should be careful not to overextend physical limits for lifting, since injury to the nurse can result in further injury to the client. If fire department personnel are on the scene, they can help evacuate the clients.

Once a fire has been reported and clients are out of danger, nurses and other personnel must take measures to contain or put out the fire, such as closing doors and

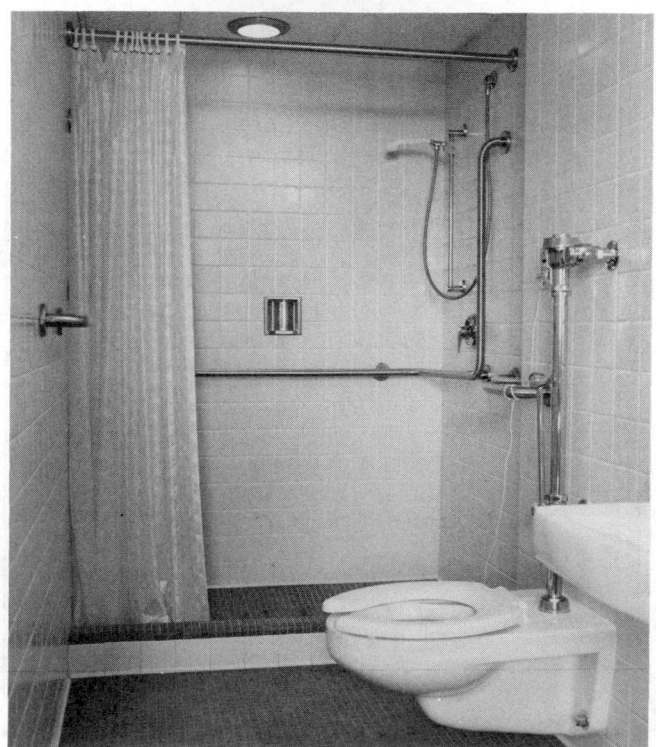

Fig. 40-3 Safety bars around toilets and showers.

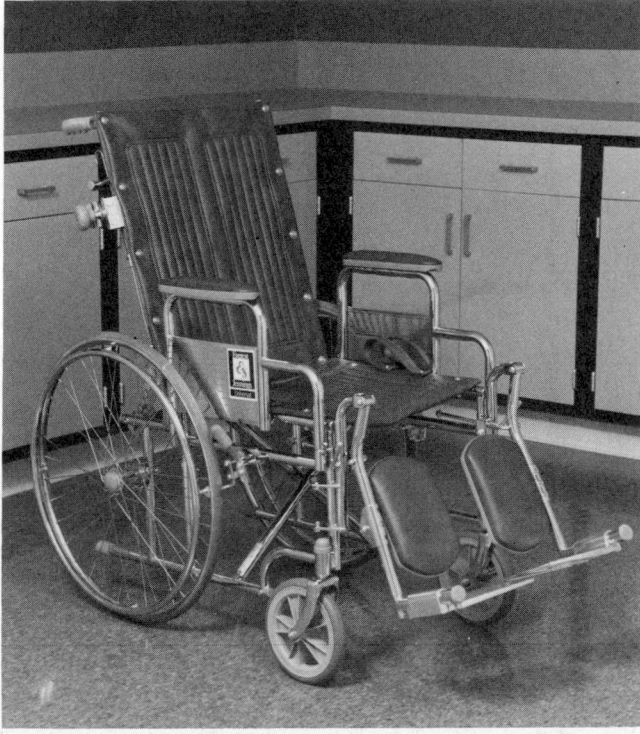

Fig. 40-4 Safety lock on wheelchairs.

TABLE 40-6 Guidelines for the Use of Restraints

Guideline	Rationale
The restraint should be selected to reduce the client's movement only as much as necessary.	Overrestraining a client so activities are unduly restricted can exacerbate the hazards of immobility.
If a restraint is necessary, the nurse should carefully explain to the client and family the type of restraint and why the restraint is needed.	Restraint can increase confusion or hostility in both the client and family. Explanation of the restraint can reduce or even prevent some of these negative perceptions.
Restraint should not exacerbate the client's health problem.	Restraints that are too tight can impair circulation to the distal extremities.
Restraint should not interfere with treatment.	Restraints placed over intravenous sites can impede the flow of fluid into the client's circulation. Restraints attached to fractured or dislocated extremities can impair healing.
Bony prominences should be padded before applying a restraint.	Padding reduces the risk of injury to the skin from pressure.
Restraints should be changed whenever they become soiled or damp.	Soiled or damp restraints increase the risk of skin breakdown.
Restraints should be secured in such a manner that they cannot be undone by the client.	When a client is able to undo restraints, the whole purpose of the restraint is negated.
Any restraint applied to a client in bed should be attached to the bed frame (see step 10 illustration in Procedure 40-1), not the side rails.	Release of the side rails while the restraint remains attached can result in injury to the client's musculoskeletal system.
Restraints should be removed every 4 hours. The client should not be left unattended.	Removal provides an opportunity to assess skin integrity and to provide skin care, often by massaging the areas on which the restraints were applied. A previously restrained client who is left unattended can cause self-injury or can injure others.
Frequent (up to every 1 hour) circulation checks when extremity restraints are used.	Checks reduce the risk of vascular extremity injury from poor distal circulation due to tightening of the restraint.

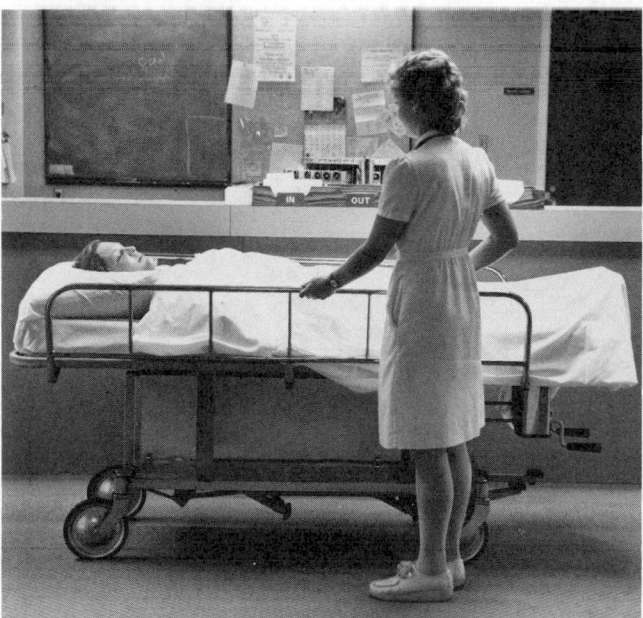

Fig. 40-5 Side rails in the up position on a stretcher.

Fire Containment Guidelines

- Know the telephone number for reporting a fire, and be sure the number is attached to all telephones.
- Know the agency's or unit's fire drill or fire evacuation routine.
- Post accurate, easy-to-follow routes to fire exits.
- Know the location of fire extinguishers, how to use them, and which type of extinguisher to use for a specific fire (Table 40-7).
- Report a fire before attempting to extinguish it, regardless of its size.
- Keep hallways free of unnecessary equipment or furniture.
- Keep fire hoses clear at all times.
- Periodically check the efficiency of fire extinguishers.
- Post signs on the outside of elevators warning people to take the stairs in the event of a fire.

PROCEDURE 40-1

Applying Restraints

STEPS	RATIONALE

1. Identify clients whose safety is maintained by use of restraints: confused or disoriented clients; clients requiring immobilization of extremity; children requiring immobilization of elbow joint to prevent dislodgment of therapeutic equipment.

Restraints are used to reduce risk of client falling out of bed, chair, or wheelchair; prevent interruption of therapy such as traction, IV infusions, or nasogastric tube feedings; prevent confused or combative client from injuring himself by removing Foley catheters, surgical drains, or life support equipment; reduce risk of injury to others by client.

2. Check physician's order and assess type of restraint needed.

Nursing assessment aids in determining what type of restraint to use. Physician's order protects nurse from liability.

3. Explain carefully to client and/or family why restraint is necessary, type of restraint selected, and anticipated duration of restraint.

Restraints can increase confusion or combativeness in client. In addition, family may express anger about restraint. Explanation and reinforcement can reduce or even prevent some of these negative perceptions.

4. Prepare the following equipment for application of selected restraint:
   a. Proper restraint
   b. Padding to protect bony prominences

Nurse is able to complete restraining procedure without having to leave client partially restrained.

Padding protects circulation to distal portion of extremity if wrist or ankle restraints are selected.

5. Wash hands.

Reduces transmission of microorganisms.

6. Apply selected restraint:
   a. Jacket restraint: vestlike garment that usually crosses in back of client but may also cross in front (Fig. 41-27 in Chapter 41).

Restrains client while lying or reclining in bed and while sitting in chair or wheelchair. Are useful in home care settings but should not be used unless other methods to maintain client safety have failed.

   b. Belt restraint: Device that secures client on stretcher (see illustration). Avoid placing belt too tightly across client's chest or abdomen.

Restrains center of gravity and prevents client from rolling off stretcher or sitting up while on stretcher.

   c. Extremity restraints (ankle or wrist restraint): Designed to immobilize one or all extremities. Commercially available limb restraints are composed of sheepskin and foam pad that comes in contact with skin. *Modification* of commercial restraint can be devised by making clove hitch restraint, a strip of cloth that does not tighten if client pulls against it. Clove hitch is made in two steps. Make figure eight with strip of cloth, and then pick up loops (see illustrations). Before attaching restraint to client's limbs, place gauze or padding around extremity to be restrained and then place loops of clove hitch directly over padded surface (see illustration).

Maintains immobilization of extremity to protect client from injury from fall or accidental removal of therapeutic device such as an IV tube or Foley catheter.

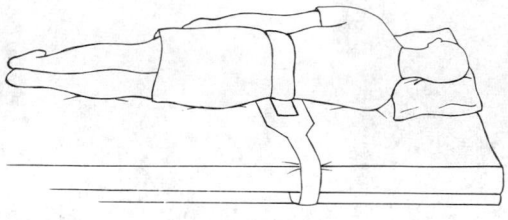

Step 6b

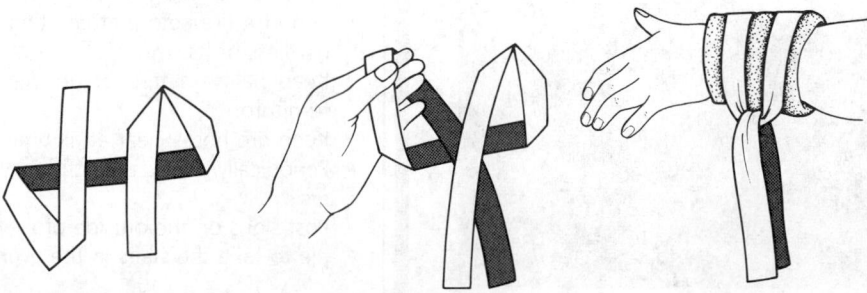

Step 6c

STEPS	RATIONALE
d. Mitten restraint: thumbless mitten devices (see illustration) to restrain client's hands.	Prevents clients from dislodging invasive equipment, removing dressings, or from scratching.
e. Elbow restraint: Piece of fabric with slots in which tongue blades are placed so that elbow joint remains rigid (see illustration).	Used with infants and children to prevent elbow flexion.
f. Mummy restraint: Blanket or sheet is opened on bed or crib with one corner folded toward center. Child is placed on blanket with shoulders at fold with feet toward opposite corner. With child's right arm straight down against the body, right side of blanket is pulled firmly across right shoulder and chest and secured beneath left side of body. Left arm is placed straight against side, and left side of blanket is brought across shoulder and chest and locked beneath child's body on right side. Lower corner is folded and brought over body and tucked or fastened securely with safety pins (Whaley and Wong, 1987).	Maintains short-term restraint of small child or infant for examination or treatment involving head and neck. Mummy device effectively controls movement of child's torso and extremities.
7. Pad bony prominences before applying restraint.	Padding decreases injury to underlying skin.
8. Secure restraints so they cannot be undone by client.	When client is able to undo restraints, purpose of restraint is negated.
9. Attach restraints applied to client in bed or on stretcher to bed frame (see illustration), not side rails.	Release of side rails while restraint remains attached can result in injury to client's musculoskeletal system.
10. Wash hands.	Reduces transmission of microorganisms.
11. Completely remove restraints at least every 4 hrs for 30 min. Client should not be left unattended.	Provides opportunity to assess skin integrity and provide skin care. Areas on which restraints were applied are often massaged.
12. Assess adequacy of restraint and presence of any potential injury to musculoskeletal system every 4 hrs. Observe color of extremity and palpate pulses below extremity.	Timely assessment enables nurse to routinely observe musculoskeletal system and prevent any complications from restraint device.
13. Observe for correct application of restraint every 4 hrs.	Incorrect application of restraints can result in injury to client's musculoskeletal system from falls or muscle strains.
14. Record in nurse's notes nursing assessment both before and after restraints were used, focusing on client's safety, client's level of orientation, type of restraint selected, client's response to restraint.	Documents that client's physical safety was at risk and that specific restraint was warranted.

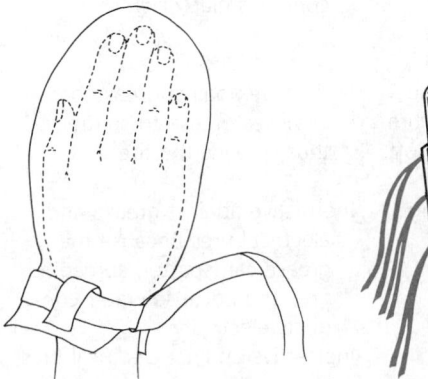

Step 6d

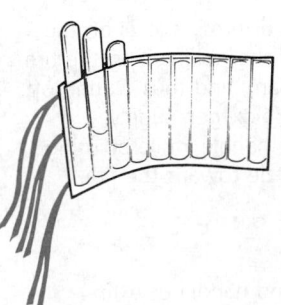

Step 6e

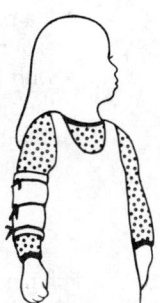

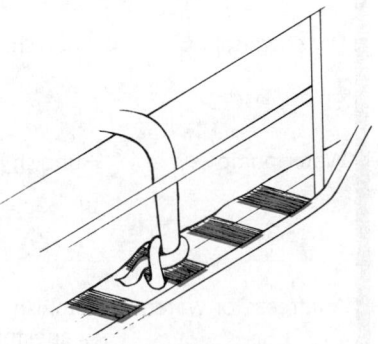

Step 9

windows, turning off oxygen and electrical equipment, and using a fire extinguisher.

The three basic types of fires for which extinguishers are used are paper and rubbish (type A), grease and anesthetic gas (type B), and electrical (type C). The appropriate extinguisher must be used for each type (Table 40-7).

POISONING. A poison is any substance that impairs health or destroys life when ingested, inhaled, or absorbed by the body. Specific antidotes or treatments are available for only some types of poisons. The capacity of body tissue to recover from the poison determines the reversibility of the effect. Poisons can impair the respiratory, circulatory, central nervous, hepatic, gastrointestinal, and renal systems of the body. Accidental poisonings are a greater risk for the toddler, the preschooler, and the young school-age child.

The nurse can help parents reduce the risk of accidental poisoning by placing poison labels on hazardous substances (Fig. 40-6). With adolescents and young or middle adults, poisonings are often caused by insect or snake bites. Drug and other substance poisonings in this age group are commonly related to suicide attempts or drug experimentation. The elderly client is also at risk for poisoning because diminished eyesight may cause an accidental ingestion of a toxic substance. The impaired memory of some elderly clients may result in accidental overdosage of prescribed medications.

In the home the two major sources of poisons are plants (see box, below) and household cleaners (see box, p. 1180). Experts recommend that when poisoning is suspected, the nurse or family member call a poison control center, a facility that provides information regarding all aspects of intoxication, treatment, and referrals. The nurse should teach parents that calling such a center for information before attempting home remedies can save their child's life.

Procedure 40-2 lists accepted interventions for accidental poisonings that the nurse may teach to a parent or guardian.

ELECTRICAL HAZARDS. Much of the equipment used in health care settings is electrical and must be well-maintained in a safe condition to prevent electrical hazards.

The electrical plug of grounded equipment has three prongs. The rounded, longer prong is the ground. Theoretically the ground prong carries any stray electrical current back to the ground, hence its name. The other two prongs carry the power to the piece of electrical equipment (Cooper, 1983).

Improperly grounded or malfunctioning electrical equipment increases the risk of electrical injury and fire. The use of a prevention checklist when assessing the client's environment can reduce injuries from electrical sources in both the health care agency and the home (see box).

TABLE 40-7 Types of Fire Extinguishers and Their Uses

Type	Class of Fire	How to Use	Precautions
Carbon dioxide (CO_2)	Grease, electrical	Direct CO_2 into the flame, thus cutting off the fire's oxygen supply.	
Soda and acid (water extinguisher)	Paper and rubbish, wood	Turn canister upside down, thereby mixing the soda and acid. CO_2 is then produced, releasing the water extinguisher under pressure. To stop the flow, turn canister right side up.	Ineffective against grease and electrical fires because it causes grease to spatter, thereby spreading the fire, and water conducts electricity.
Dry chemical	Rubbish, electrical	Pull a pin or press a level on the extinguisher, blanketing the fire with foam, and thus cutting off the fire's oxygen supply.	Ineffective against grease because it causes grease to spatter and thus spreads the fire
Water pump	Rubbish, wood	Pump the handle while pointing the nozzle toward the fire.	Ineffective against grease and electrical fires because the grease can spatter, spreading fire, and because water conducts electricity
Antifreeze or water	Rubbish, wood, grease, anesthetics	Pull pin and handle of extinguisher, and direct extinguisher toward fire.	Ineffective against electrical fires because water conducts electricity

If a client receives an electrical shock, the nurse should immediately determine if the client has a pulse. If the client is without a pulse, cardiopulmonary resuscitation (CPR) should be initiated and emergency personnel notified (see Chapter 36). If the client has a pulse, is alert, and oriented, the nurse should quickly obtain vital signs and assess the skin for signs of thermal injury. The client's physician is notified. If an electrical shock occurs in the client's home, the nurse follows the same proce-

dure but should have the client go to the emergency room and then notify the personal physician.

RADIATION. Radiation is a health hazard in the hospital environment and the community. In the hospital setting, particularly in large medical centers, radiation hazards can arise from the nuclear medicine diagnostic centers and the research laboratories as well. Clients also have radiation implants for the treatment of certain types

---

Poisonous Plants

These plants contain a wide variety of poisons, and symptoms may vary from a mild stomach ache, skin rash, and swelling of the mouth and throat to involvement of the heart, kidneys, or other organs. The poison center can give you more specific information of these plants or others that may be poisonous and are not on this list. Many plants do not cause toxicity unless ingested in very large amounts.

- Acorn (oak)
- Akee fruit
- Anemone
- Angel trumpet tree
- Apricot (kernels, leaves)
- Arrowhead
- Autumn crocus
- Avocado (leaves)
- Azalea
- Baneberry
- Belladonna
- Betel nut palm
- Bird of paradise
- Bittersweet
- Black locust
- Bleeding heart
- Buckeye
- Buttercup
- Caladium
- Calla lily
- Castor bean
- Century plant
- Cherries (pits)
- Chinaberry
- Choke cherry
- Christmas rose
- Climbing nightshade
- Cowbane
- Daffodil
- Daphne
- Deadly nightshade
- Delphinium
- Desert potato
- Devil's ivy
- Dieffenbachia
- Dumbcane
- Dutchman's breeches

- Elderberry
- Elephant ear
- English ivy
- Euonymus
- Fava bean
- Flags (iris)
- Four o'clock
- Foxglove
- Goldenchain
- Holly berries
- Horsetail reed
- Hyacinth
- Hydrangea
- Indian turnip
- Inkberry
- Iris
- Jack-in-the-pulpit
- Japanese yew
- Jasmine
- Jequirty bean
- Jerusalem cherry
- Jimson weed seeds
- Jonquil
- Lantana
- Larkspur
- Lingustrum
- Lily of the valley
- Lobelia
- Locoweed
- Lucky nut
- Marsh marigold
- Mayapple
- Mistletoe berries
- Monkshood
- Moonseed
- Morning glory
- Mother-in-law plant

- Mountain laurel
- Mulberries (green)
- Narcissus
- Nightshade
- Oleander
- Peach (seeds)
- Pencil tree
- Peony
- Periwinkle
- Peyote
- Philodendron
- Pigeonberry
- Poinsettia
- Poison hemlock
- Poison ivy
- Pokeweed/pokeberries
- Potato (all green parts)
- Primrose
- Privet
- Ranunculus
- Rhododendron
- Rhubarb leaves
- Rosary pea
- Snow drop
- Sorrel
- Star of Bethelem
- Swiss cheese plant
- Thornapple
- Threadleaf
- Tobacco
- Tomato (all green parts)
- Tulip bulb
- Virginia creeper
- Water hemlock
- Wisteria
- Yellow jessamine
- Yew berries

From Missouri Poison System: Poisonous plants, St. Louis, 1987, Cardinal Glennon Memorial Hospital for Children.

Common Poisonous Household Chemicals

- Alcoholic beverages
- Ammonia
- Antifreeze
- Ant syrup or paste
- Automotive products
- Bathroom bowl cleaner
- Bleach
- Boric acid
- Camphophenique
- Charcoal lighter
- Cleaning fluid
- Clinitest tablets
- Cologne
- Copper and brass cleaners
- Corn and wart remover
- Detergents
- Dishwasher detergents
- Disinfectants
- Drain cleaners
- Epoxy glue kit

- Furniture polish
- Garden sprays
- Gasoline
- Gun cleaners
- Hair dyes
- Insecticides
- Iodine
- Iron medications
- Kerosene
- Lighter fluid
- Model cement
- Muriatic acid
- Mushrooms
- Nail polish
- Nail polish remover
- Oven cleaner
- Paint
- Paint remover
- Paint thinner
- Perfume

- Permanent wave solutions
- Pesticides
- Pine oil
- Plants
- Prescription and nonprescription medicines
- Rat poisons
- Rubbing alcohol
- Shaving lotion
- Silver polish
- Snail bait
- Spot removers
- Strychnine
- Sulfuric acid
- Super glue
- Turpentine
- Veterinary products
- Weed killers
- Window wash solvent

From St. Louis Regional Poison Center Network: Poisonous household chemicals, St. Louis, 1983, Cardinal Glennon Memorial Hospital for Children.

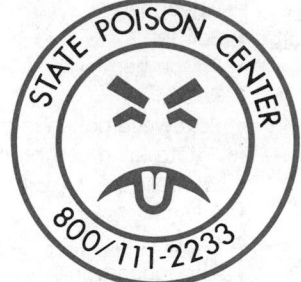

Fig. 40-6 ''Mr. Yuk'' label.

From Billings, DM, and Stokes, LG: Medical-surgical nursing: common health problems of adults and children across the life span, ed. 2, St. Louis, 1986, The C.V. Mosby Co.

of cancers, (for example, advanced prostate cancer).

Hospitals and medical centers have guidelines on the care of clients who require radiation implants. These clients are isolated to one room, and nursing and medical personnel follow procedures to reduce their risk and other client's risk to exposure.

Hospital laboratories require personnel to attend a course on radiation hazards and to pass a specific test regarding these hazards. In addition, researchers and laboratory workers must follow strict policies when using radioactive substances. Failure to follow these guidelines can result in loss of research funds, loss of research space, and loss of employment.

Prevention of Electrical Hazards

- Use only grounded equipment.
- Check electrical equipment for frayed cords or visible signs of damage before use.
- Avoid overloading outlets.
- If extension cords must be used, make sure they are taped to the ground with *electrical tape* to prevent others from tripping over the cord and pulling out the plug.
- Never pull a plug using the cord. Pull a plug by gripping it firmly and pulling it straight out of the wall socket.
- Send equipment that has been dropped to the biomedical department before reuse.
- Report any shocks experienced while using equipment.
- Believe a client who reports a tingling sensation or shocks from the equipment, and have the equipment evaluated for stray current. If possible, unplug equipment until evaluation takes place.
- If you do not understand how to operate a piece of equipment, ask for assistance.

Modified from Cooper, KC: Focus 10:17, 1983.

PROCEDURE 40-2

Intervening in Accidental Poisonings

STEPS	RATIONALE
1. Identify the type and amount of substance ingested.	This information will help to determine the correct type and amount of antidote needed for the victim.
2. Call the poison control center before attempting any intervention.	Poison control centers have all the information needed to treat the poisoned client or to offer referral to treatment centers.

3. If instructed to induce vomiting:
  a. Infants 0-12 months—ipecac is only administered under direction of a physician
  b. Children (1 year-12 years)—1 tablespoon (15 ml) of ipecac
  c. Adults—2 tablespoons (30 ml) of ipecac
	Households should keep syrup of ipecac in an easily accessible place. Ipecac causes vomiting and emptying of the stomach, rather than gagging or retching. Poison control experts recommend these dosages and do not advise inducing vomiting with substances other than ipecac (Aronow et al., 1985). Vomiting should only be induced under physician's instruction and is not induced with ingestion of gasoline or other caustic poisons.

4. Give oral fluids to assist vomiting:
  a. Children (1 year to 12 years)—5 to 15 ml/kg up to 8 oz of water
  b. Adults—16 oz of water
	Assists in emptying of the stomach and further avoids gagging and retching.

5. If requested to do so, save vomitus and deliver to poison control center.	Laboratory analysis can determine what further treatment is necessary.
6. Place victim with the head turned to side.	This reduces the risk of aspiration.
7. Vomiting is *never* induced for the following substances: lye, household cleaners, grease or petroleum products, furniture polish.	Vomiting can increase the area of internal burns (in case of lye) and the risk of aspiration.
8. Vomiting is *never* induced in an unconscious victim.	Vomiting increases the risk of aspiration.
9. If instructed by the poison control center to bring the person to the emergency room, call an ambulance.	Ambulance personnel will be able to provide emergency measures if needed. In addition, the parent or guardian may be too upset to drive safely.

The community is at risk for radiation exposure because of incorrect disposal and transportation of radioactive waste products. Community health agencies and the Environmental Protection Agency (EPA) follow specific, strict guidelines for the disposal of radioactive waste. If radioactive leak occurs, these community agencies institute measures to contain the leak to prevent exposure to surrounding neighborhoods, to clean up radioactive leaks as quickly as possible, and to ensure that injured parties receive prompt medical care.

EVALUATION

The interventions for reducing the threat to a client's safety are evaluated by comparing the client's response to each of the nursing therapies for each goal. The nurse uses the objective evaluative outcome criteria established during the planning phase (see evaluation box).

SUMMARY

A safe environment is essential to maintaining and restoring a client's health. Nurses working in a structured health care setting or in a community-based agency are the client's first line of defense against falls, environmental hazards, medication errors, poisoning, and other injuries.

The client's risk for injury increases with declining health status, decreases in mobility, and reduced functioning of special senses. In addition, clients at opposite ends of the life span, the very young and the elderly, have greater risks to their safety.

The nursing process is used to reduce the risk of injury through specific nursing interventions and client education. The nurse promotes a safe environment by removing threats to safety and by teaching clients and their families about hazards in their homes.

Sample Evaluation of Interventions for Safety Risks

Goals	Evaluative Measures	Expected Outcomes
An environment adapted to the motor, sensory, and cognitive developmental needs of the client is maintained.	Observe client's environment for absence of actual or potential threats to safety.	Environment is free of threats to safety.
	Evaluate through inspection or percussion the client's motor, sensory, or cognitive status for appropriate environmental modifications.	Client makes environmental changes consistent with motor, sensory, or cognitive status.
The client acquires knowledge related to potential threats to personal safety.	Inspect client's environment for removal of hazards.	Environment is free of hazards.
	Observe client's safe use of home appliances, medications, health care equipment.	Client correctly uses medication, equipment, or treatments.
Potential for injury is reduced.	Observe client for side effects or adverse reactions to medications.	Side effects or adverse effects are absent.
	Inspect client's skin and musculoskeletal system for injury.	Skin and tissues are intact. Musculoskeletal system has no injury.
	Inspect equipment.	Electrical grounding and functioning are correct.
Risk of accidental poisoning is reduced.	Observe the client's self-medication administration.	Client follows "five rights" for medication administration.
	Inspect environment for potential poisonings.	Poisonous substances are absent. "Mr. Yuk" labels are correctly used.
		Syrup of ipecac is in the home.
		Client knows appropriate use of ipecac.
		Client posts phone number of local poison control center.

KEY CONCEPTS

✓ A safe health care environment reduces the length of treatment or hospitalization, the frequency of treatment-related accidents, the potential for lawsuits, the number of work-related injuries to personnel, and the overall cost of health service.

✓ In the community a safe environment is one in which basic needs are achievable, physical hazards are reduced, transmission of pathogens and parasites is reduced, pollution is controlled, and sanitation is maintained.

✓ Factors that reduce the amount of available atmospheric oxygen include an improperly functioning furnace and high carbon monoxide levels from automobile exhaust and cigarette smoke.

✓ Prolonged exposure to extremely hot or cold environmental temperatures can reduce the client's level of health or even cause death.

✓ Reduction of physical hazards in a client's environment includes providing adequate lighting, decreasing clutter, and securing the home.

✓ The transmission of pathogens and parasites is reduced through medical and surgical asepsis, immunization, food sanitation, insect and rodent control, and disposal of human wastes.

✓ Children under 5 years of age are at greatest risk for home accidents that may result in severe injury and death.

✓ The school-age child is at risk for injury at home, at school, and traveling to and from school.

✓ Adolescents are at risk for auto accidents and substance abuse.

✓ Threats to an adult's safety are frequently associated with poor life-style habits.

✓ Risks of injury for the elderly are directly related to the physiological changes of the aging process.

✓ Risks to client safety within a health care agency include falls and client-inherent, procedure-related, and equipment-related accidents.

✓ Nursing interventions for promoting a client's safety are individualized for the client's developmental stage, life-style, and environment.

✓ Nursing interventions are developed to modify the client's environment for protection from falls, fires, poisonings, and electrical hazards.

✓ The nursing care plan to promote safety is continually evaluated to identify new or continued risks to the client.

REFERENCES

Aronow, R, et al.: Comments from AAPCC to U.S. Food and Drug Administration on poison treatment drug products, Vet Hum Toxicol 28:343, 1985.

Centers for Disease Control: Recommendations for prevention of HIV transmission in health care settings, MMWR, Aug. 1987.

Cooper, KL: Electrical safety: the electrically sensitive ICU patient, Focus 10:17, 1983.

Cooper, S: Common concern—accidents and older adults, Geriatr Nurs 2:287, 1981.

Ebersole, P and Hess, P: Toward healthy aging: human needs and nursing process, ed. 3, St. Louis, 1989, The C.V. Mosby Co.

Hoffman, Y: Surviving a child's suicide, Am J Nurs 87:955, 1987.

Lindenmuth, JE, Breu, CS, and Malooley, JA: Sensory overload, Am J Nurs 80:1465, 1981.

Lynn, FH: Incidents—need they be accidents? Am J Nurs 80:1098, 1980.

Rhyne, MC, et al.: Children at risk for depression, Am J Nurs 86:1374, 1986.

Rice, MA, and Kibbee, PE: Review: identifying the adolescent substance abuser, Matern Child Nurs 8:139, 1983.

Roy, G: Home accidents: developmental risks, Community Outlook, August 11, 1982.

Whaley, LF, and Wong, DL: Nursing care of infants and children, ed. 3, St. Louis, 1987, The C.V. Mosby Co.

Research Articles

Innes, EM, and Thurman, WG: Evaluation of patient falls, QRB 9(2):30, 1983.

Nickens, H: Intrinsic factors in falling among the elderly, Intern Med 145:1089, 1985.

Perry, BC: Falls among the elderly—a review of the methods and conclusions of epidemiologic studies, Geriatr Soc 30:367, 1982.

ADDITIONAL READINGS

Baptiste, MS, and Feck, G: Preventing tap water burns, Am J Public Health 70:727, 1980.

Davidson, M, and Grant, E: Accidental hypothermia: a community hospital perspective, Postgrad Med 70:42, 1981.

Doyle, JT: You swallowed your what? RN 48:40, 1985.

Ferguson, D, and Beck, C: H.A.L.F.—a tool to assess elderly abuse within the family, Geriatr Nurs 4:30, 1983.

Fife, DD, et al.: A risk/falls program: code orange for success, Nurse Manag 15(11):50, 1984.

Ford, AH: Use of automobile restraining devices for infants, Nurs Res 29:281, 1980.

Gray-Victrey, M: Education to prevent falls, Geriatr Nurs 5:179, 1984.

Hernandez, M, and Miller, J: How to reduce falls, Geriatr Nurs 7(2):97, 1986.

Innes, EM: Maintaining fall prevention, QRB July, 217.

Janken, JK, Reynolds, BA, and Swiech, K: Patient falls in the acute care setting: identifying risk factors, Nurs Res 35:215, 1986.

Jones, MK: Fire, Am J Nurs 84(11):1368, 1984.

Tideiksaar, R: Geriatric falls in the home, Home Healthc Nurse 4(2):21, 1986.

Riffle, KL: Falls: kinds, causes and prevention, Geriatr Nurs 3:165, 1982.

Rivara, FP, and Berger, LR: Consumer product hazards: setting priorities for research and regulatory action, Am J Public Health 70:701, 1980.

Roy, G: Home accidents—can they be prevented? Community Outlook, August 11, 1982.

Witte, NS: Why the elderly fall, Am J Nurs 75:1950, 1979.

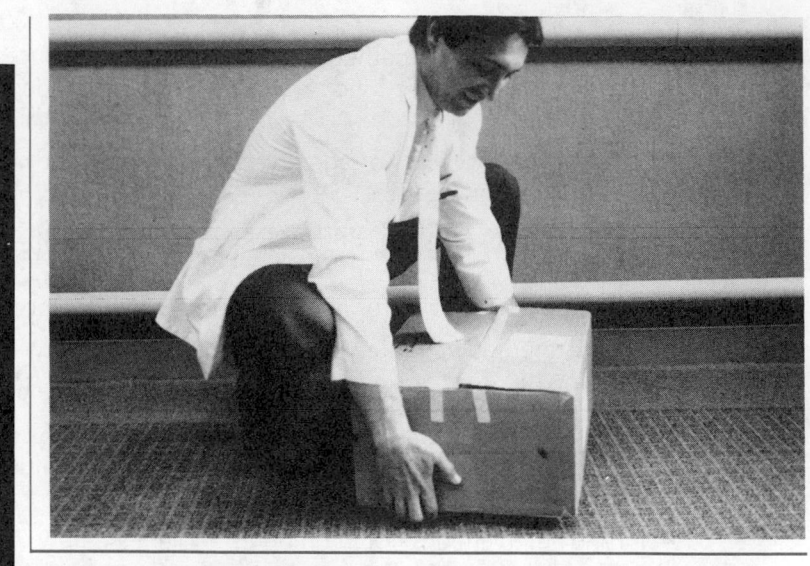

OBJECTIVES

Mastery of content in this chapter will enable the student to:

- Define the key terms listed.
- Describe the roles of the skeleton, skeletal muscles, and nervous system in regulation of movement.
- Discuss physiological and pathological influences on body alignment and joint mobility.
- Assess for alterations in body alignment and joint mobility.
- State the correct nursing diagnoses for impaired body alignment and joint mobility.
- Write nursing care plans for impaired body alignment and joint mobility.
- Describe the procedure for assisting a client to move up in bed and moving a helpless client up in bed.
- Describe the procedure for repositioning a helpless client.
- Describe the procedures for assisting clients to a sitting position.
- Describe the procedure for transferring a client from bed to chair.
- Describe the procedure for a three-person carry.
- Describe complete range of joint motion exercises.
- Describe crutch safety.
- Describe the five crutch gaits.
- Evaluate the nursing plan for maintaining body alignment and joint mobility.

KEY TERMS

Achilles Tendon
Activity Tolerance
Antagonistic Muscles
Antigravity Muscles
Body Mechanics
Cartilage
Cartilaginous Joint
Cerebellum
Crutch Gait
Exercise
Fibrous Joint
Flat Bones
Footboard
Fracture
Friction
Gravity

Hand Rolls
Hand-Wrist Splints
Irregular Bones
Isometric Contraction
Isotonic Contraction
Joints
Ligaments
Long Bones
Muscle Tone
Myoneural Junction
Neurotransmitter
Pathological Fractures
Posture
Proprioception
Proprioceptors
Restraints

Body Mechanics

Clinical nursing requires the nurse to incorporate knowledge and skills into practice. One component of knowledge and skill is body mechanics, a broad term used to describe coordinated efforts of the musculoskeletal and nervous systems.

Many nursing activities such as lifting a client, transferring a client from bed to chair, or positioning an immobilized client require muscle exertion by the nurse. To reduce the risk of injury to both the client and nurse, the nurse must practice proper body mechanics.

Body mechanics includes knowing how and why certain muscle groups are used. The nurse also needs to understand the regulation of movement, including how coordinated body motion involves integrated functioning of the skeletal system, skeletal muscle, and nervous system. In addition, certain muscle groups are used primarily for movement and others primarily for posture.

This chapter describes how and why movement is regulated; the basics of integrated functions of the skeleton, skeletal muscles, and nervous systems; posture and body alignment; and joint mobility. The focus is on body alignment and joint mobility. Immobility and its impact on the client are detailed in Chapter 42.

OVERVIEW OF BODY MECHANICS

Body mechanics is the coordinated effort of the musculoskeletal and nervous systems to maintain balance, posture, and body alignment during lifting, bending, moving, and performing activities of daily living. Use of proper body mechanics reduces risk of injury to the

1185

musculoskeletal system. Proper mechanics also facilitates body movement, which allows physical activity without muscle strain and excessive use of muscle energy.

In clinical situations nurses assist clients to turn, walk, and increase their activities. A nurse may also need to move an immobilized client. The best protection for the nurse while administering care is to practice principles of body mechanics. This will reduce the risk of injury.

Body mechanics is concerned with the three areas of alignment, balance, and coordinated movement.

Body Alignment

Body alignment refers to the condition of the joints, tendons, ligaments, and muscles in various body positions. There are correct and incorrect body alignments for standing, sitting, and lying down. Correct body alignment reduces strain on musculoskeletal structures and is associated with adequate muscle tone. Proper body alignment contributes to balance.

Body Balance

Body balance is achieved when there is a wide base of support, the center of gravity is within the base of support, and a vertical line falls from the center of gravity through the base of support. When the body is improperly balanced, the center of gravity is displaced, increasing the force of gravity and the possibility of falling.

Body balance is also enhanced by posture. The better the posture, the greater the balance. The nurse can maintain proper body alignment by using two simple techniques. First, the base of support can easily be widened by separating the feet to a comfortable distance. Second, balance is increased by bringing the center of gravity closer to the base of support. This is achieved by bending the knees and flexing the hips until the person is squatting and still maintaining proper back alignment.

Coordinated Body Movement

Weight is the force exerted on a body by gravity. When an object is lifted, the lifter must overcome the object's weight and know its center of gravity. In symmetrical objects the center of gravity is located at the exact center of the object. Because people are not geometrically perfect, their centers of gravity are usually at 55% to 57% of standing height and are located in the midline. The force of weight is always directed downward, which is why an unbalanced object falls. Clients who are unsteady fall because, as their centers of gravity become unbalanced, the gravitational force of their weight eventually causes them to fall. Therefore the nurse needs to

design nursing interventions that protect such clients from falling and ensure their safety (see Chapter 40).

Friction is a force that occurs in a direction to oppose movement. As the nurse turns, transfers, or moves a client up in bed, friction must be overcome. A nurse can reduce friction by following some basic principles.

First, the greater the surface area of the object to be moved, the greater the friction. If a client is unable to assist in moving up in bed, the client's arms should be placed across the chest. This decreases surface area and reduces friction.

Second, a passive or immobilized client produces greater friction to movement. Thus, whenever possible, the nurse should use some of the client's strength and mobility when lifting, transferring, or moving the client up in bed. This can be done by explaining the procedure and telling the client when to move. The client then knows what is being done, what to do, and when.

Third, friction can be reduced by lifting rather than pushing a client. Lifting has an upward component and decreases the pressure between the client and the bed or the chair. The use of a pull sheet reduces friction because the client is more easily moved along the bed's surface.

REGULATION OF MOVEMENT

Coordinated body movement involves integrated functioning of the skeletal system, skeletal muscle, and nervous system. Because these three systems cooperate so closely in mechanical support of the body, they can be considered almost a single functional unit. The skeleton and skeletal muscles contribute to the shape of the body in both its length and width, and to distribution of fat that determines body construction (Strand, 1978). In addition, the skeletal system provides body support structures for movement, and muscles provide necessary strength. The nervous system permits initiation and voluntary control of movement.

Skeletal System

The skeleton is the body's supporting framework and is comprised of 206 bones. There are four types of bones in the skeleton: long, short, flat, and irregular. *Long bones* contribute to height (such as the femur, fibula, and tibia in the leg) and length (such as the phalanges of the fingers and the toes). *Short bones* occur in clusters and, when combined with ligaments and cartilage, usually permit movement of the extremities. Two examples of short bones are carpal bones in the foot and the patella in the knee. *Flat bones* provide structural contour, such as bones in the skull and the ribs in the thorax. *Irregular bones* make up the vertebral column and some bones of the skull, such as the mandible.

In addition to providing supporting structure of the body, the skeleton has four other functions. First, the skeleton provides attachments for muscles and ligaments. These attachments allow movement of parts of the skeleton, such as opening and closing the mouth or extending an arm or a leg. Second, the skeleton protects vital organs; for example, the skull protects the brain, and the ribs protect the heart and lungs. Third, bones assist in regulation of calcium balance. Bones are able to store calcium and release it to the circulation as needed. The regulation of calcium balance is controlled by the parathyroid hormone. Fourth, the internal structure of bones contains bone marrow, participates in red blood cell production, and acts as a reservoir for blood. Although the last two functions are indirectly related to movement, they should not be overlooked when assessing a client's strength and mobility.

Clients with altered calcium regulation and metabolism are at risk for developing pathological fractures, which can occur in all bones but are most common in the ribs and weight-bearing bones. These fractures result from weakened bone tissue and are frequently caused by osteoporosis or neoplasms. Osteoporosis, which results from increased bone resorption of calcium and decreased bone formation, is frequently observed in postmenopausal women, immobilized clients, and clients receiving long-term steroid therapy. Neoplasms result from primary bone tumors and metastases from primary cancers, such as those of the lung, breast, or prostate. Osteoporosis and bone neoplasms weaken the bone's structure so that fractures may result from simple weight bearing activities of daily living.

Clients with altered bone marrow function or diminished red blood cell production are usually weakened and fatigue easily. Weakness and fatigue not only decrease mobility of these clients but place them at risk of falling. Both falling and immobilization result in trauma to the musculoskeletal system, and the nurse must identify these risks early in assessment of the client's mobility and body alignment.

CHARACTERISTICS OF BONE

The characteristics of bone include firmness, rigidity, and elasticity. Firmness results from inorganic salts such as calcium and phosphate that are laid down in the bone matrix. Firmness is related to the bone's rigidity, which is necessary to keep long bones straight and enables them to withstand weight bearing. In addition, bones have a degree of elasticity and skeletal flexibility that changes with age.

Composition of the skeleton changes throughout the life span. The newborn has a large amount of cartilage and is highly flexible but is unable to support weight. The toddler's bones are more pliable than those of an elderly person and are better able to withstand falls.

Discussion of the skeletal system's role in regulation of movement would be incomplete without a brief summary of the role of joints, ligaments, tendons, and cartilage.

JOINTS

Joints are connections between bones. Each joint is classified according to its structure and degree of mobility. There are four classifications of joints: synostotic, cartilaginous, fibrous, and synovial.

The *synostotic joint* occurs when bones are jointed by bones. No movement is associated with this type of joint, and the bony tissue that forms between the bones provides strength and stability. The classic example of this type of joint is the sacrum, in which vertebrae are joined together (Fig. 41-1, *A*).

The *cartilaginous or synchondrodial joint* has little movement but is elastic and uses cartilage to unite body surfaces. Cartilaginous joints are found when bones are exposed to a constant pressure, such as the costosternal joints between the sternum and ribs (Fig. 41-1, *B*).

The *fibrous or syndesmodial joint* has a tough layer of fibrous connective tissue that binds bones firmly together. Because of the flexibility of connective tissue, some movement of the joint is permitted. For example, the connective tissue between the tibia and fibula joins the bones in a fibrous joint at their distal ends, where they provide a socket for the upper part of the talar bones of the foot (Strand, 1978). Together these bones and connective tissues form the ankle joint, which permits plantar and dorsal flexion of the foot (Fig. 41-1, *C*).

The *synovial or true joint* is a freely movable joint in which contiguous bony surfaces are covered by articular cartilage and connected by ligaments lined with a synovial membrane. Joining of the humeral radius and ulna by cartilage and ligaments forms a pivotal joint (Fig. 41-1, *D*). Other types of synovial joints are ball-and-socket joint, such as the hip joint, and hinge joints, such as interphalangeal joints of fingers.

LIGAMENTS

Ligaments are white, shiny, flexible bands of fibrous tissue binding joints together and connecting bones and cartilages. Ligaments are elastic and aid joint flexibility and support (Fig. 41-2). In addition, some ligaments have a protective function. For example, ligaments between the vertebral bodies, nonelastic ligaments and the ligamentum flavum, prevent damage to the spinal cord during movement of the back.

TENDONS

Tendons are white, glistening, fibrous bands of tissue that connect muscle to bone. Tendons are strong, flexible, and inelastic and occur in various lengths and thick-

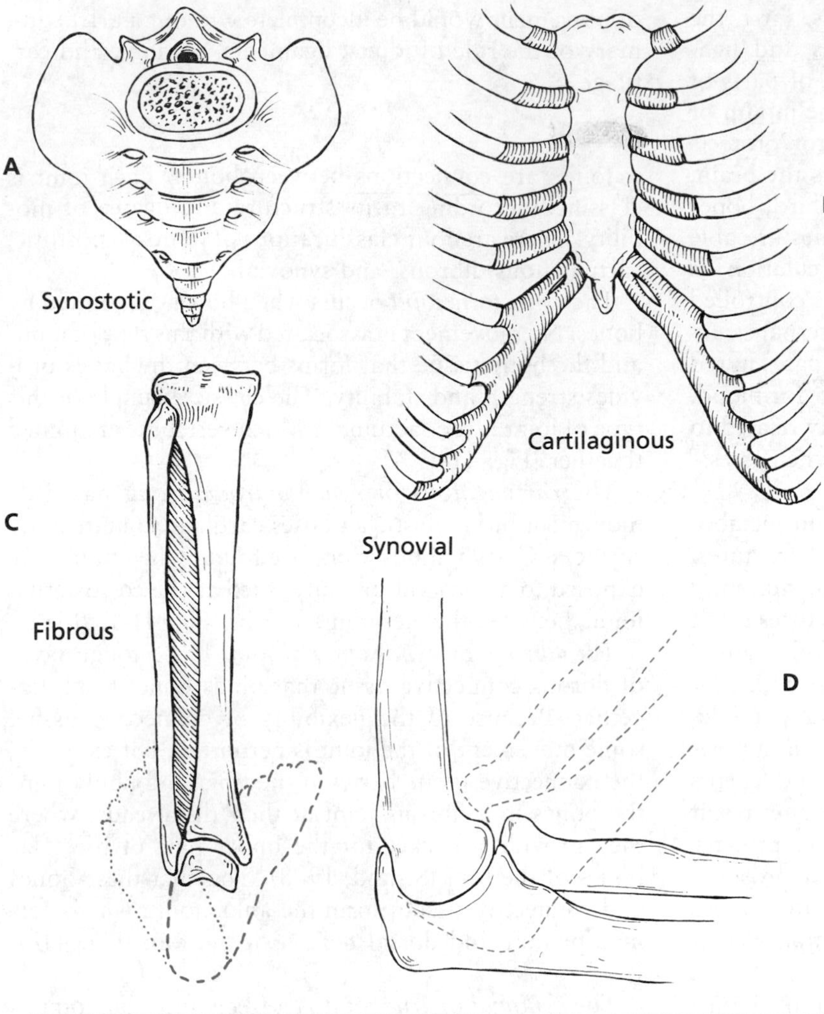

A

Synostotic

B

Cartilaginous

C

Synovial

Fibrous

D

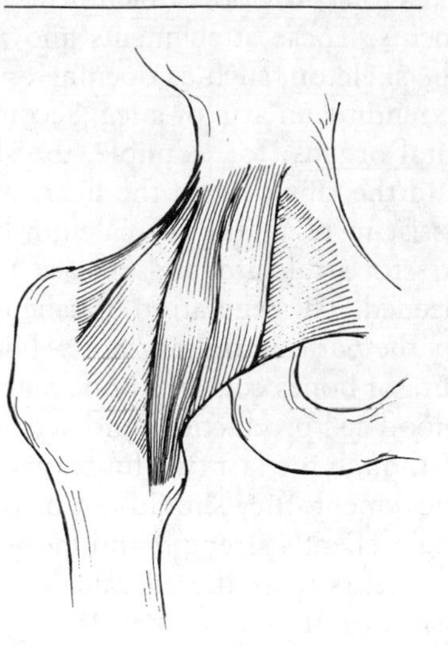

Fig. 41-2 Ligaments of the hip joint.

Fig. 41-1 Joint types.

nesses. The Achilles tendon (tendo calcaneus) is the thickest and strongest tendon in the body. It begins near the middle of the posterior of the leg and attaches the gastrocnemius and soleus muscles in the calf to the calcaneal bone in the back of the foot (Fig. 41-3).

CARTILAGE

Cartilage is nonvascular, supporting connective tissue located chiefly in the joints and in the thorax, trachea, larynx, nose, and ear. The fetus has a large amount of temporary cartilage, which is replaced by bone during infancy. Permanent cartilage is unossified except in advanced age and diseases such as osteoarthritis.

Joints, ligaments, tendons, and cartilage permit strength and flexibility of the skeleton. Strength enables the skeletal system to support the body. Flexibility is demonstrated through range of joint motion, which is discussed in a later section of this chapter. However,

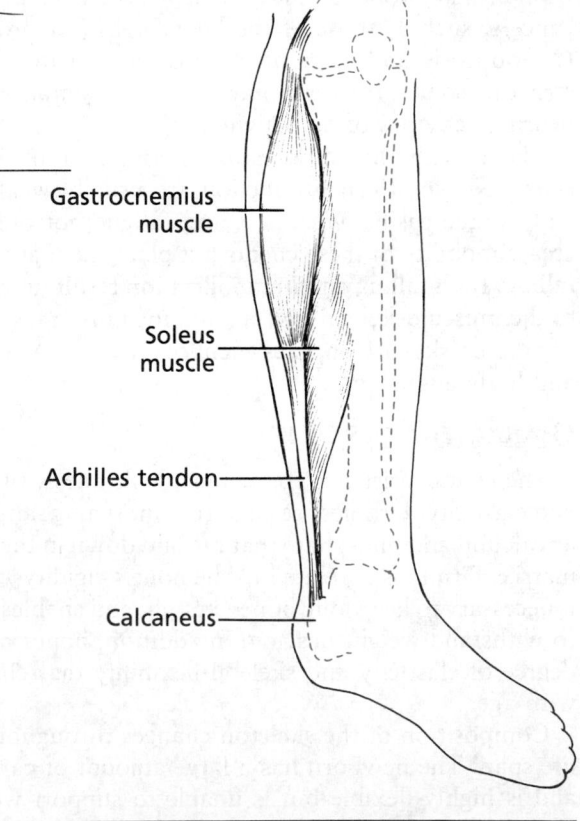

Gastrocnemius muscle

Soleus muscle

Achilles tendon

Calcaneus

Fig. 41-3 Achilles tendon.

strength and flexibility of the skeleton do not result entirely from these four structures; adequate skeletal muscle is also necessary.

Skeletal Muscle

Movement of bones and joints involve active processes that must be carefully integrated to achieve coordination. Skeletal muscles, because of their ability to contract and relax alternatively, are the working elements of movement. Contractile elements of the skeletal muscle are enhanced by its anatomical structure and attachment to the skeleton.

Muscle contraction is stimulated by an electrochemical impulse that travels from the nerve to the muscle across the myoneural junction. The electrochemical impulse causes the thin actin-containing filaments to shorten, thus contracting the muscle. Removal of the stimulus results in muscle relaxation.

There are two types of muscle contractions: isotonic and isometric. In *isotonic* contraction, increased muscle tension results in muscle shortening. *Isometric* contraction causes an increase in muscle tension or muscle work but no shortening of the muscle. Voluntary movement is a combination of isotonic and isometric contractions—for example, what occurs when the nurse lifts a client up in bed. Initially, the client's weight causes increased tension in the muscles of the nurse's arms until the tension (isometric) is equal to the weight to be lifted and the weight of the lower arm. When this equilibrium is reached, continued stimulation to the muscles results in muscle shortening (isotonic), bending the elbow, and the client is lifted off the bed.

Although isometric contractions do not result in muscle shortening, energy expenditure is increased. This type of muscle work is comparable to having a car in neutral with the driver continually depressing the accelerator and racing the engine. The driver is not going anywhere but is certainly expending a large amount of energy. It is important for the nurse to recognize the energy expenditure associated with isometric exercises because they are contraindicated in some illnesses such as cardiopulmonary disease.

Each skeletal muscle is capable of isometric and isotonic contractions. Some skeletal muscles are concerned primarily with movement, while others are concerned primarily with posture.

MUSCLES CONCERNED WITH MOVEMENT

Muscles concerned primarily with movement are located near the skeletal region where movement is caused by leverage. Leverage occurs when specific bones, such as the humerus, ulna, and radius, and the associated joints, such as the elbow joint, act together as a lever. Thus the force applied to one end of the bone to lift a weight at another point tends to rotate the bone in the direction opposite that of the applied force. Muscles that attach to bones of leverage provide necessary strength to move the object.

Leverage is characteristic of movements of the upper extremities. Arm muscles are parallel to one another and extend the full length of the bones. The long parallel muscles provide strength and work together with the bones and joints to enable lifting an object with the arms.

MUSCLES CONCERNED WITH POSTURE

Muscles associated primarily with maintaining posture are short and featherlike in appearance because they converge obliquely at a common tendon. Muscles of the lower extremities, trunk, neck, and back are concerned primarily with posture. These muscle groups work together to stabilize and support body weight standing or sitting. It is these muscles that allow an individual to maintain a sitting or standing posture for a period of time.

MUSCLE REGULATION OF POSTURE AND MOVEMENT

Posture and movement can be reflections of personality and mood. For example, an individual with a dramatic personality gestures with the hands to illustrate an idea, and a person who is fatigued or depressed may slouch.

Posture and movement are also dependent on the skeleton and the shape and development of skeletal muscles. Coordination and regulation of different muscle groups depend on muscle tone and activity of antagonistic, synergistic, and antigravity muscles.

MUSCLE TONE. Muscle tone or tonus is the normal state of balanced muscle tension. Tension is achieved by alternate contraction and relaxation of neighboring fibers of a specific muscle group. Muscle tone enables a body part to be maintained in a functioning position without muscle fatigue. In addition, muscle tone promotes venous return to the heart, as is the case with leg muscles. Continuous contraction and relaxation of the muscle fibers pumps venous blood toward the heart.

Muscle tone is achieved through continual use of muscles. Activities of daily living require muscle action and help to maintain muscle tone. As a result of immobility or prolonged bed rest, a client's activity level and muscle tone decrease (see Chapter 42).

MUSCLE GROUPS. The antagonistic, synergistic, and antigravity muscle groups are coordinated by the nervous system and work together to maintain posture and initiate movement.

Antagonistic muscles work together to bring about movement at the joint. During movement the active mover muscle contracts while its antagonist relaxes. For example, when flexing the arm, the active biceps brachii contracts and its antagonist, the triceps brachii, relaxes. During extension of the arm the active triceps brachii contracts and the new antagonist, the biceps brachii, relaxes.

Synergistic muscles contract together to accomplish the same movement. When the arm is flexed, the strength of contraction of the biceps brachii is increased by contraction of the synergistic muscle, the brachialis. Thus with synergistic muscle activity there are now two active movers, the biceps brachii and the brachialis, that contract while the antagonistic muscle, the triceps brachii, relaxes.

Antigravity muscles are specifically involved with stabilization of joints. These muscles continuously oppose the effect of gravity on the body and permit the person to maintain an upright or sitting posture (Strand, 1978). In an adult the antigravity muscles are the extensors of the leg, gluteus maximus, quadriceps femoris, soleus muscles, and muscles of the back.

Skeletal muscles support posture and carry out voluntary movement. Muscles are attached to the skeleton by tendons, which provide strength and permit motion. Movement of the extremities is voluntary and requires coordination from the nervous system.

Nervous System

Movement and posture are regulated by the nervous system. The major voluntary motor area, located in the cerebral cortex, is the precentral gyrus or motor strip. A majority of motor fibers descend from the motor strip and cross at the level of the medulla. Thus the motor fibers from the right motor strip initiate voluntary movement for the left side of the body, and the opposite is true for movement on the right side of the body.

During voluntary movement, impulses descend from the motor strip to the spinal cord. An impulse exits the spinal cord through efferent motor nerves and travels through nerves to muscles, where movement occurs. This impulse is propelled by synapses, which keeps the impulse traveling in one direction. Most motor fibers are encased in a myelin sheath and are called myelinated fibers. Along the myelinated fibers is a series of indentations known as nodes of Ranvier. These nodes increase impulse transmission because the impulse is able to jump from node to node.

Transmission of the impulse from the nervous system to the musculoskeletal system is an electrochemical event and requires a neurotransmitter. Basically, neurotransmitters are chemicals such as acetylcholine that transfer the electric impulse from the nerve across the myoneural junction to muscle. The neurotransmitter reaches a muscle and stimulates it, causing movement.

Movement can be impaired by disorders that alter neurotransmitter production, transfer across the synaptic cleft, or activation of muscle activity. Posture, or the position of the body in relation to the surrounding space, is also regulated by the nervous system. Posture requires coordination of proprioception and balance.

PROPRIOCEPTION

Proprioception is achieved through stimuli originating from within the body regarding spatial position and muscular activity. Proprioception in the body is monitored by proprioceptors, which are any nerve endings located in muscles, tendons, and joints.

As a person carries out activities of daily living, proprioceptors are continuously monitoring muscle activity and body position. For example, the proprioceptors on the soles of the foot contribute to correct posture while standing or walking. In standing there is continuous pressure on the bottom of the feet. The proprioceptors monitor the pressure, communicating this information through the nervous system to the antigravity muscles. The standing person remains upright until deciding to change position. As a person walks, the proprioceptors on the bottom of the feet monitor pressure changes. Thus when the bottom of the moving foot comes in contact with the walking surface, the individual automatically moves the stationary foot forward. The proprioceptors allow people to walk without having to watch their feet.

BALANCE

When standing, running, lifting, or performing activities of daily living, a person must have adequate balance. Balance is assisted through control by the nervous system, specifically by the cerebellum and the inner ear. The major function of the cerebellum is to coordinate voluntary movement, particularly highly skilled movements such as those required in golf and skiing (Strand, 1978). In addition, the cerebellum assists in balance, such as permitting a person to stand on one foot with eyes closed (Romberg test of cerebellar function; see Chapter 13).

Within the inner ear are semicircular canals, three fluid-filled structures that assist in maintaining balance. Fluid within the canals has a certain inertia, and when the head is suddenly rotated in one direction, the fluid within the canal in the same direction remains stationary for a moment while the canal turns with the head. This allows a person to change position suddenly without losing balance.

Impairment of Movement

Smooth, coordinated, and purposeful movement results from integration of structure and function of the skeleton, skeletal muscle, and nervous system. When any of these are damaged or destroyed, movement is impaired. The skeleton can be damaged by fractured bones or joints and torn ligaments, tendons, and cartilage. Disease affecting the composition of bone, such as osteoporosis or neoplasms, restricts movement. Muscle abnormalities, such as muscular dystrophy, decrease muscle strength and mobility. Diseases of the nervous system, such as multiple sclerosis, or damage to the nervous system, such as a spinal cord injury, restricts voluntary motor activity. Each of these diseases or injuries increases the risk for actual or potential impairment of body alignment or joint mobility. Assessment of these impairments is presented in a later section.

PRINCIPLES OF BODY MECHANICS

Proper body mechanics is as important to the nurse and client as proper nutrition. It affects both of their levels of wellness. Correct body mechanics is necessary to health promotion, and prevention of disability.

The nurse uses a variety of muscle groups for each nursing activity, such as walking during nursing rounds, administering medications, lifting and transferring clients, and moving objects. The physical forces of weight and friction can influence body movement. Correctly used, these forces increase the nurse's efficiency. Incorrect use can impair the nurse's ability to lift, transfer, and position clients. The nurse also incorporates knowledge of physiological and pathological influences on body alignment. The box lists principles that are useful in a variety of settings.

DEVELOPMENTAL CHANGES

Throughout life the body's appearance and functioning undergo change. The greatest impact is observed in childhood and old age.

Infant

The newborn infant's spine is flexed and lacks the anteroposterior curves of the adult. The first spinal curve occurs when the infant extends the neck from the prone position. As growth and stability increase, the thoracic spine straightens and the lumbar spinal curve appears, which allows sitting and standing. The infant's musculoskeletal system is flexible. The extremities are flexed and joints have complete range of joint motion. As the newborn matures, the musculoskeletal system becomes stronger and the infant is able to resist movement and reach out and grasp objects (see Chapter 22). As the baby grows, musculoskeletal development permits support of weight for standing and walking. Posture is awkward because the head and upper trunk are carried forward. Since body weight is not evenly distributed along a line of gravity, the child is off balance and falls easily.

Principles of Body Mechanics

- The wider the base of support and the lower the center of gravity, the greater the stability.
- The equilibrium of an object is maintained as long as the line of gravity passes through its base of support.
- When the line of gravity shifts outside the base of support, the amount of energy required to maintain equilibrium is increased.
- Equilibrium is maintained with least effort when the base of support is broadened in the direction in which movement occurs.
- Stooping with hips and knees flexed and the trunk in good alignment distributes the work load among the largest and strongest muscle groups and helps to prevent back strain.
- The stronger the muscle group, the greater the work it can perform safely.
- Use of a larger number of muscle groups for an activity distributes the work load.
- Facing the direction of movement prevents abnormal twisting of the spine.
- Pushing, pulling, or sliding an object on a surface requires less force than lifting it, since lifting involves moving the object's weight against the pull of gravity.
- Moving an object by rolling, turning, or pivoting requires less effort than lifting it, since momentum and leverage are used to advantage.
- Use of a lever when lifting an object reduces the amount of weight lifted.
- The less the friction between the object moved and surface on which it is moved, the less the force required to move it.
- Moving an object on a level surface requires less effort than moving on an inclined surface, because the pull of gravity is less on a level surface.
- Working with materials that rest on a surface at a good working level requires less effort than lifting them above the working surface.
- Contraction of stabilizing muscles preparatory to activity helps to prevent ligaments and joints from strain and injury.
- Dividing balanced activity between arms and legs protects the back from strain.
- Variety of position and activity helps to maintain good muscle tone and prevent fatigue.
- Alternating periods of rest and activity help prevent fatigue.

From Winters, M: Protective body mechanics in daily life and nursing, Philadelphia, 1952, W.B. Saunders Co.

Toddler

The toddler's posture—slightly swaybacked with a protruding abdomen—is awkward. As the child walks, the legs and feet are usually far apart and the feet are slightly everted. Toward the end of the toddler stage posture appears less awkward, curves in the cervical and lumbar vertebrae are accentuated, and foot eversion disappears (Daniels and Worthingham, 1977).

School-Age Child

By the third year the body is slimmer, taller, and better balanced. Abdominal protrusion is decreased, the feet are not as far apart, and arms and legs have increased in length. The child also appears more coordinated. From the third year through beginning adolescence the musculoskeletal system continues to develop. Long bones in the arms and legs grow. Muscles, ligaments, and tendons become stronger, resulting in improved posture and increased muscle strength. Greater coordination enables the child to perform tasks that require fine motor skills (see Chapter 23).

Adolescent

The adolescent stage is usually initiated by a tremendous growth spurt (see Chapter 23). Growth is frequently uneven. As a result, the adolescent may appear awkward and uncoordinated. Adolescent girls usually grow and develop earlier than boys. Hips widen, and fat is deposited in the upper arms, thighs, and buttocks. The boy's changes in shape are usually the result of long bone growth and increased muscle mass. Legs become longer and hips narrower. Muscular development increases in the chest, arms, shoulders, and upper legs.

Adult

An adult who has correct posture and body alignment feels good, looks good, and generally appears self-confident. The healthy adult also has the necessary musculoskeletal development and coordination to carry out activities of daily living (see Chapter 24). Normal changes in posture and body alignment in adulthood occur mainly in pregnant women. These changes result from the body's adaptive response to weight gain and the growing fetus. The center of gravity shifts toward the anterior. The pregnant woman leans back and is slightly swaybacked and may complain of backache.

Older Adult

The aging process results in musculoskeletal changes (see Chapter 25). Degenerative joint changes may decrease range of joint motion. Skeletal muscle mass and strength may be reduced. Changes in the structure of the bone matrix may result in fragile, brittle bones (Hudson, 1983).

The elderly walk more slowly and appear less coordinated. They may also take smaller steps, keeping the feet closer together, which decreases the base of support. Thus body balance is unstable, and they are at greater risk for falls and injuries.

PATHOLOGICAL INFLUENCES ON BODY ALIGNMENT AND MOBILITY

A variety of pathological conditions affect body alignment and joint mobility. Although a complete description of each condition is beyond the scope of the chapter, the student needs knowledge about musculoskeletal disorders. Through tables and summaries this section provides baseline information about these pathological influences, which are broken down into six categories: postural abnormalities, pathophysiological mechanisms affecting bone formation, altered joint mobility, impaired muscle development, damage to the central nervous system, and direct trauma to the musculoskeletal system. A subsequent section describes in detail nursing procedures used to maintain or restore body alignment and joint mobility.

Postural Abnormalities

Congenital or acquired postural abnormalities affect the efficiency of the musculoskeletal system, as well as body alignment, balance, and appearance. During physical assessment the nurse observes body alignment and range of joint motion (see Chapter 13). Postural abnormalities impair alignment, mobility, or both.

The nurse requires some knowledge about characteristics, causes, and treatment of common postural abnormalities (Table 41-1). The nurse uses this baseline knowledge first to improve the client's body alignment during lifting, transfer, and positioning. Second, because some postural abnormalities affect range of joint motion, the nurse maintains range of joint motion in affected joints and uses the client's range in remaining joints. Last, the nurse is able to design nursing interventions to strengthen affected muscle and joint groups, improve the client's posture, and adequately use affected and unaffected muscle groups.

Pathophysiological Mechanisms Affecting Bone Formation

The skeleton provides structural support for the body, protects soft tissues and organs, and is the anchoring

TABLE 41-1 Postural Abnormalities

Abnormality	Description	Cause	Treatment
Torticollis	The head is inclined to the affected side, in which the sternocleidomastoid muscle is contracted	Congenital or acquired	Surgery, heat, support, or immobilization depending on the cause and severity
Lordosis	Exaggeration of the anterior convex curve of the lumbar spine	Congenital; temporary as with pregnancy	Based on cause; frequently treated with spine-stretching exercises
Kyphosis	Increased convexity in the curvature of the thoracic spine	Congenital; rickets; tuberculosis of the spine	Based on cause and severity; includes spine-stretching exercises, sleeping without pillows, using a bed board, bracing, and spinal fusion
Kypholordosis	Combination of kyphosis and lordosis	Congenital	Based on cause; similar to methods used in kyphosis or lordosis
Scoliosis	Lateral curvature of the spine, unequal heights of hips and shoulders	Congenital; poliomyelitis; spastic paralysis; unequal leg length	Based on cause and severity; immobilization and surgery
Kyphoscoliosis	Abnormal anteroposterior and lateral curvature of the spine	Congenital; poliomyelitis; cor pulmonale	Based on cause and severity; immobilization and surgery
Congenital hip dysplasia	Hip instability with limited abduction of the hips and, occasionally, adduction contractures; head of the femur does not articulate with the acetabulum because of abnormal shallowness of the acetabulum	Congenital; more common with breech deliveries	Maintaining continuous abduction of the thigh so that the head of the femur presses into the center of the acetabulum; abduction splints, casting, or surgery
Knock-knee (genu valgum)	Legs curved inward so that the knees knock together as the person walks	Congenital; rickets	Knee braces and surgery if not corrected by growth
Bowlegs (genu varum)	One or both legs bent outward at the knee; normal until 2-3 years of age	Congenital; rickets	Slowing the rate of curving if not corrected by growth; in the case of rickets, vitamin D, calcium, and phosphorus intake increased to normal ranges
Clubfoot	95%: medial deviation and plantar flexion of the foot (equinovarus); the remaining 5%: lateral deviation and dorsiflexion (calcaneovalgus)	Congenital	Based on the degree and ridigity of the deformity; casts, splints such as the Denis Browne splint, and surgery
Foot-drop	Characterized by plantar flexion, inability to invert the foot because of peroneal nerve damage	Congenital; trauma; improper position of the immobilized client	Cannot be corrected; may be prevented through physical therapy
Pigeon-toes	Internal rotation of the forefoot or the entire foot, common in infants	Congenital; habitual	Corrected by growth or by wearing reversed shoes

site for the origin and insertion of muscles. In addition, the bone affects calcium metabolism and blood formation in the body. The functional activities of bone cells include modeling, remodeling, and repairing. Modeling involves the growth processes that allow bones of the newborn to develop into the large, identically shaped bones of the adult. Modeling is dependent on dietary and physiological factors. Remodeling occurs in the growing and the fullgrown skeleton and involves coupling of the constantly occurring processes of bone resorption and formation. Repair is the cellular process that occurs in response to a fracture (Groër and Shekleton, 1983).

Nurses care for clients who have actual or potential alterations in modeling, remodeling, or repair of bone. A later section on direct trauma to the musculoskeletal system describes bone repair.

Altered Joint Mobility

Joint mobility can be altered by inflammation, degeneration, or articular disruption. Arthritis is an inflammation of the joints characterized by swelling and pain. It can result from a direct inflammatory reaction in the joint tissue such as gouty arthritis, an infectious process such as septic arthritis, or an immune-mediated inflammatory process such as rheumatoid arthritis.

Joint degeneration is demonstrated by changes in articular cartilage combined with hypertrophic changes at the articular bone ends (Groër and Shekleton, 1983). Synovial and cartilaginous joints are equally affected, and degenerative changes commonly affect weight-bearing joints. Although degenerative joint disease is not caused by inflammation, it is frequently termed osteoarthritis.

Articular disruption may be as mild as a sprain or as severe as dislocation. In articular disruption there is trauma to the articular capsules, such as a tear in a sprain, or a separation in a dislocation. Articular disruption is usually the result of trauma, but it can also be congenital, as with congenital hip dysplasia.

Inflammation, degeneration, or articular disruption alters the degree of joint mobility of affected joints. Nurses must know the cause of limited joint mobility, how to assess it, and design nursing interventions directed toward maintaining and improving a client's range of joint motion. Chapter 13 describes the assessment of range of joint motion. The section on intervention in this chapter provides a step-by-step procedure for maintaining range of joint motion.

Impaired Muscle Development

Inadequate development of skeletal muscles affects body alignment, balance, and mobility. Muscular dys-

trophies are the most common developmental impairments of skeletal muscles. These are a group of genetically transmitted diseases characterized by progressive pathological changes in the skeletal muscles, resulting in muscle wasting and weakness (Groër and Shekleton, 1983).

Damage to the Central Nervous System

Damage to any component of the central nervous system that regulates voluntary movement results in impaired body alignment and mobility. The motor strip in the cerebrum can be damaged by trauma from a head injury, ischemia from a cerebrovascular accident (stroke), or bacterial infection from meningitis. Motor impairment is directly related to the amount of destruction of the motor strip. For example, in the case of a person with a right-sided cerebral hemorrhage with complete necrosis, destruction of the right motor strip and left-sided hemiplegia are consequences. However, a person with a right-sided head injury will have cerebral edema and damage (but not destruction) of the motor strip, and with extensive physical therapy, voluntary movement may gradually return to the left side.

Because voluntary motor fibers descend from the motor strip in the cerebrum down the spinal cord, trauma to the spinal cord also impairs mobility. The most common trauma is transection of the spinal cord in which motor fibers are cut. This can cause a complete bilateral loss of voluntary motor control below the level of the trauma. Spinal cord trauma frequently results from diving or automobile accidents or gunshot or knife wounds to the neck and back.

Direct Trauma to the Musculoskeletal System

Direct trauma to the musculoskeletal system can result in bruises, contusions, sprains, and fractures. The more severe fractures are the focus of discussion in this section. A fracture is a disruption of bone tissue continuity. Fractures most commonly result from direct external trauma, but they can also occur as a consequence of some deformity of the bone, as with pathological fractures of osteoporosis, Paget's disease, and osteogenesis imperfecta.

As the fracture heals, bone begins to repair. During repair the fractured bone initiates a cellular process that results in bone formation. Young children are able to form new bone more easily than adults and, as a result, have few complications after a bone fracture. Treatment includes positioning the fractured bone in proper alignment and immobilizing it to promote normal healing and restore function. Immobilization results in some muscle atrophy, loss of tone, and joint stiffness.

Any acquired or congenital condition that affects the structure of the musculoskeletal or nervous system impairs body alignment or joint mobility. Impairment can be temporary or permanent. Regardless of duration of the impairment, the nursing care plan includes interventions that maintain the present level of alignment and joint mobility, as well as interventions designed to increase the client's level of motor function.

NURSING PROCESS FOR IMPAIRED BODY ALIGNMENT AND MOBILITY

Based on data collected during assessment, the nurse determines the client's care plan. When assessing a client's body alignment and joint mobility, the nurse also evaluates the client's ability to perform activities of daily living.

ASSESSMENT

Nursing assessment of body alignment and joint mobility is usually conducted during the complete physical assessment. In this section on assessment and subsequent sections on the components of the nursing care plan, the content is divided into two categories: body alignment and joint mobility. This division is intended to help the student assess the client, diagnose problems, and plan, deliver, and evaluate nursing care. However, remember that body alignment and joint mobility are closely related.

BODY ALIGNMENT

The assessment of body alignment can be carried out with the client standing, sitting, or lying down. This assessment has six objectives:
1. Determining normal physiological changes in body alignment resulting from growth and development
2. Identifying deviations in body alignment caused by poor posture
3. Providing an opportunity for the client to observe his or her posture
4. Identifying learning needs of the client for maintaining correct body alignment
5. Identifying the presence of trauma, muscle damage, or nerve dysfunction
6. Obtaining information concerning other factors that contribute to poor alignment, such as fatigue, malnutrition, and psychological problems

The first step in assessing body alignment is to put the client at ease so that an unnatural or rigid position is not assumed. When assessing body alignment of an immobilized or unconscious client, pillows and positioning supports should be removed from the bed and the client placed in the supine position.

STANDING. The nurse should focus assessment of body alignment for the standing client on the following points:
1. The head is erect and midline.
2. When observed posteriorly, the shoulders and hips are straight and parallel.
3. When observed posteriorly, the vertebral column is straight.
4. When the client is observed laterally, the head is erect and the spinal curves are aligned in a reversed S pattern. The cervical vertebrae are anteriorly convex, the thoracic vertebrae are posteriorly convex, and the lumbar vertebrae are anteriorly convex.
5. When observed laterally, the abdomen is comfortably tucked in and the knees and ankles are slightly flexed. The person appears comfortable and does not seem conscious of the flexion of knees or ankles.
6. The client's arms are comfortably at the sides.
7. Feet are placed slightly apart to achieve a base of support, and the toes are pointed forward.
8. When the client is viewed anteriorly, the center of gravity is in the midline, and the line of gravity is from the middle of the forehead to a midpoint between the feet. Laterally the line of gravity runs vertically from the middle of the skull to the posterior third of the foot (Fig. 41-4).

SITTING. The nurse assesses alignment of the sitting client by the following observations:
1. The head is erect, and the neck and vertebral column are in straight alignment.
2. The body weight is evenly distributed on the buttocks and thighs.
3. The thighs are parallel and in a horizontal plane.
4. Both feet are supported on the floor. With clients of short stature, a footstool is used and the ankles are comfortably flexed (Fig. 41-5).
5. A 2 to 4 cm (1- to 2-inch) space is maintained between the edge of the seat and the popliteal space on the posterior surface of the knee. This space ensures that there is no pressure on the popliteal artery or nerve to decrease circulation or impair nerve function.
6. The client's forearms are supported on the armrest, in the lap, or on a table in front of the chair.

It is particularly important to assess alignment when sitting if the client has muscle weakness, muscle paral-

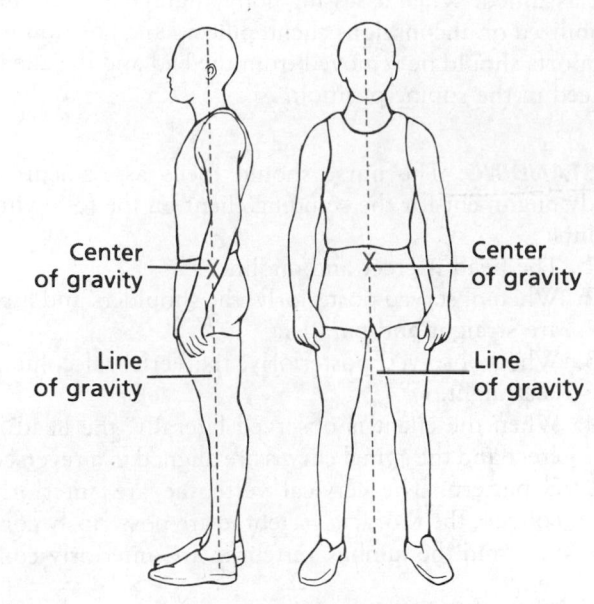

Fig. 41-4 Correct body alignment when standing.

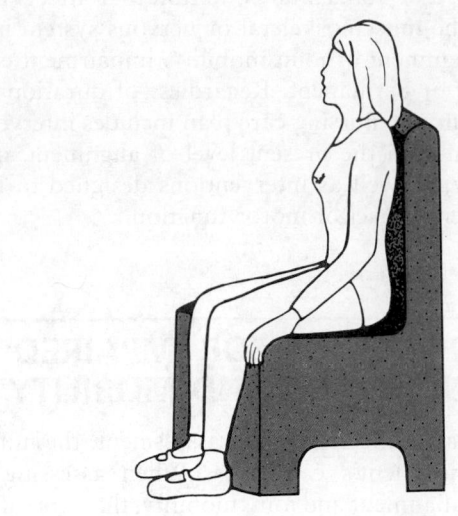

Fig. 41-5 Correct body alignment when sitting.

ysis, or nerve damage. Because of these alterations, the client has diminished sensation in the affected area and is unable to perceive pressure or decreased circulation. Proper alignment while sitting reduces the risk of musculoskeletal system damage in such a client.

LYING DOWN. People who are conscious have voluntary muscle control and normal perception of pressure. As a result they usually assume the position of comfort when lying down. Because their range of motion, sensation, and circulation are within normal limits, they change positions when they perceive muscle strain and decreased circulation.

Assessment of body alignment while lying down requires that the client be placed in the lateral position with all but one pillow and all positioning supports removed from the bed (Fig. 41-6). The body should be supported by an adequate mattress. The vertebrae should be in straight alignment without observable curves. This assessment provides baseline data concerning the client's body alignment.

Conditions that create a risk of damage to the musculoskeletal system when lying down include clients with impaired mobility, such as those in traction or with arthritis; clients with decreased sensation, such as those with hemiparesis resulting from a stroke; clients with impaired circulation, such as those with diabetes; and clients with lack of voluntary muscle control, such as those with spinal cord injuries.

When a nursing assessment indicates that a client is at risk for damage to the musculoskeletal system while

lying down, nursing interventions are directed toward maintaining proper body alignment while rotating the client. Detailed procedures for the semi-Fowler's, supine, prone, lateral, and Sims' positions are presented in the intervention section of this chapter.

MOBILITY

Assessment of a client's mobility enables the nurse to determine coordination and balance while walking, ability to carry out activities of daily living, and ability to participate in an exercise program. Assessment of mobility has three components: range of joint motion, gait, and exercise.

RANGE OF JOINT MOTION. Range of joint motion is the maximal amount of movement possible at a joint in one of the three planes of the body: sagittal, frontal, and transverse. The *sagittal plane* is a line that passes through the body from front to back, dividing the body into a left and a right side. The *frontal plane* passes through the body from side to side and divides the body into front and back. The *transverse plane* is a horizontal line that divides the body into upper and lower portions (Bilger and Greene, 1973).

Joint mobility in each of the planes is limited by ligaments, muscles, and construction of the joint. However, there are joint movements specific to each plane. In the sagittal plane, movements are flexion and extension (fingers and elbows) and hyperextension (hip). In the frontal plane, movements are abduction and adduction (arms and legs) and eversion and inversion (feet). In the transverse plane, movements are pronation and supination (hands), internal and external rotation (knees), and dor-

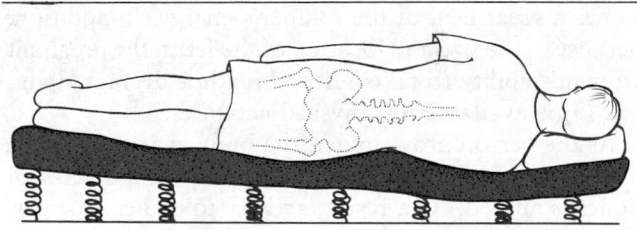

Fig. 41-6   Correct body alignment when lying down.

siflexion and plantar flexion (feet).

When assessing range of joint motion the nurse asks questions and makes observations to collect data about joint stiffness, swelling, pain, limited movement, and unequal movement. Clients whose joint mobility is restricted because of illness, disability, or trauma require exercise of joints to reduce the hazards of immobility. These exercises, performed by the nurse, are called passive range of joint motion exercises. The nurse takes each affected joint through its complete range of motion.

GAIT. Gait is the manner or style of walking, including rhythm, cadence, and speed. Assessing a client's gait allows the nurse to draw conclusions about balance, posture, and ability to walk without assistance.

Initially the nurse observes the overall appearance of the walking client. Normally, the adult posture is well aligned. The actual activity of walking takes place in a four-phase sequence: heel strike, stance, push-off, and swing (Daniels and Worthingham, 1977). During *heel strike* the foot is about at a right angle to the leg. The knee is extended but not locked, in a readiness for slight flexion as the body weight is shifted forward into the stance phase. During *stance* the trunk is maintained in a vertical position with the head and neck properly aligned. At *push-off* there is plantar flexion of the foot and hyperextension of the metatarsophalangeal joints of the toes. During swing the foot easily clears the floor with good alignment. Rhythm of movement is unchanged and remains coordinated.

EXERCISE

Exercise is physical activity for conditioning the body, improving health, and maintaining fitness. It can also be used as therapy for correcting a deformity or restoring the overall body to a maximal state of health. When a person exercises, physiological changes occur in body systems (see box at right).

ACTIVITY TOLERANCE. The nurse's assessment of the client's energy level includes the physiological effects of exercise and activity tolerance. Activity tolerance is the kind and amount of exercise or work that a person

is able to perform. Assessment is necessary when planning any activity such as walking, range of joint motion, or activities of daily living for clients with acute or chronic illness. In addition, knowledge of the client's activity tolerance is needed to plan other nursing therapies.

Activity tolerance assessment includes data from physiological, emotional, and developmental domains (see box, p. 1198). This provides the nurse with baseline data about the client's activity patterns and tolerance (Gordon, 1976). In addition, this assessment is applicable in all clinical settings and is quickly completed.

The client who experiences changes in physiological function on exercise such as dyspnea or chest pain will not tolerate activity as well as the client who does not. Likewise, the weak or debilitated client is unable to sustain activity because the greater energy needed to complete the activity creates fatigue and generalized weakness.

People who are depressed, worried, or anxious are frequently unable to tolerate exercise. Depressed clients are usually not motivated to participate. Clients who are worried or anxious fatigue easily because they expend a great deal of energy in worry and anxiety. Thus they may experience physical and emotional exhaustion.

Physiological Effects of Exercise on Major Body Systems

- **Cardiovascular.** Increased cardiac output from a resting value of 5 liters/minute to a maximum of 35 liters/minute in trained athlete*; strengthening of the cardiac muscle; increased heart rate; increased venous return; dilation of skeletal muscle arterioles (localized hyperemia)
- **Respiratory.** Increased respiratory rate and depth; increased alveolar ventilation reaching as high as 120 liters/minute[†]
- **Metabolic.** Increased use of circulatory glucose and fatty acids; increased breakdown of muscle and liver glycogen stores into glucose; increased triglyceride breakdown; increased use of fatty acids for body fuel; increased metabolic rate; increased production of body heat
- **Musculoskeletal.** Increased muscle tone; increased muscle size; increased strength; maintenance of joint mobility

---

*Data from Vander, RJ, Sherman JH, and Luccano, DS: Human physiology: the mechanisms of body function, New York, 1979, McGraw-Hill Book Co.
[†]Data from Guyton, AC: Function of the human body, ed. 4, Philadelphia, 1974, W.B. Saunders Co.

Developmental changes also affect activity tolerance. As the infant enters the toddler stage, the activity level increases and the need for sleep declines. The child entering nursery school, preschool, or primary grades expends mental energy in learning and may require more rest after school before strenuous play. The adolescent going through puberty may require more rest because much of the body's energy is expended for growth and hormone changes.

A pregnant woman has fluctuations in her energy tolerance. During the first trimester she may have increased fatigue. Hormonal changes and fetal development use body energy, and the woman may be unable or unmotivated to carry out physical activities. The second trimester of pregnancy usually results in a return of activity tolerance to the prepregnancy state. In fact some women feel their activity tolerance is greater during this period. During the last trimester fetal development consumes a great deal of the mother's energy. In addition, because of the size and location of the fetus, the pregnant woman's ability to take a deep breath is decreased and less O_2 is available for physical activities.

As the person grows older, the body changes, muscle mass is reduced, posture changes, and composition of bones is altered. As a result, activity tolerance changes. The individual may still exercise, but will do it at a reduced intensity.

CARDIOVASCULAR SYSTEM. To sustain the increased skeletal muscle activity during exercise, the blood supply delivered to muscles must increase, which is achieved by an increased cardiac output. Initially the heart rate increases during exercise. Contractile force of the cardiac muscle of the left ventricle increases, as does the volume of blood ejected (stroke volume). Increases in heart rate and stroke volume increase cardiac output.

In addition, dilation of arterioles within skeletal muscles increases delivery of blood and oxygen to muscle tissue. The body surface becomes warm and red as a result of localized hyperemia from arteriolar dilation.

RESPIRATORY SYSTEM. The increased physiological activity during exercise requires an increased supply of oxygen (O_2) to body tissues. To increase O_2 available for tissue, the person must increase O_2 inhaled. First, the body can increase depth of respiration, which results in increased tidal volume. Tidal volume is the amount of air inhaled and exhaled. Increased tidal volume results in more O_2 inhaled. Second, the respiratory rate quickens during exercise. Third, increased tidal volumes and respiratory rate cause increased alveolar ventilation. Measurement of alveolar ventilation is determined by multiplying the respiratory rate by the tidal volume. Thus, increasing both rate and tidal volume increases alveolar ventilation. Last, the increased respiratory rate increases excretion of carbon dioxide (CO_2). During exercise the body's metabolic activity increases, and CO_2 is formed as a waste product. The increased respiratory rate allows a person to "blow off" excess CO_2, which helps maintain the body's acid-base balance.

METABOLIC SYSTEM. Exercise requires the body to mobilize fuel to provide energy required for muscle contraction. Three major fuels are used by exercising muscle: circulatory glucose, circulatory fatty acids, and stored glycogen. To make these available, overall metabolic activity of the body increases, producing more body heat and waste products, such as CO_2.

MUSCULOSKELETAL SYSTEM. Exercise affects functioning and strength of the musculoskeletal system. During exercise muscle tone, size, and strength increase. The person is then able to exercise longer with each strengthening of muscles. Joint mobility is also maintained because exercise requires movement of body parts.

There is an overall improvement of physiological functioning as a result of exercise. All systems become stronger and function more efficiently. In nursing, certain interventions are directed toward exercise. However, nurses often care for clients whose mobility is restricted and, as a result, develop nursing therapies designed to reduce the hazards of immobility (see Chapter 42).

NURSING DIAGNOSIS

Nursing diagnoses identifying actual or potential alterations in body alignment and joint mobility are based on data collected during the nursing assessment. Analysis reveals clusters of data that indicate the presence or potential for a problem (see nursing diagnoses box).

Body alignment and joint mobility are intertwined. A person with poor body alignment may have reduced mobility. In identifying nursing diagnoses, the nurse is able to design nursing strategies that reduce or prevent hazards associated with poor body alignment or reduced joint mobility.

Alterations in body alignment can result from developmental changes, postural abnormalities, abnormalities in bone formation, impaired muscle development, damage to the central nervous system, and direct trauma to the musculoskeletal system.

The nursing diagnostic statement identifies expected causes, such as pressure or restricted mobility. Expected causes are individualized so that interventions can be planned.

As the diagnostic statement is developed, the nurse makes sure that appropriate defining characteristics are present in the assessment data base. The sample nursing diagnoses box lists examples for clients with poor body alignment or impaired joint mobility.

PLANNING

Improper body alignment and impaired joint mobility affects joint groups, and impairments can be localized

---

Examples of Nursing Diagnoses Related to Improper Body Mechanics and Impaired Joint Mobility

NANDA-APPROVED NURSING DIAGNOSES

Activity intolerance related to:
- Poor body alignment
- Decreased mobility

Potential for injury related to:
- Improper body mechanics
- Improper positioning
- Improper transfer techniques

Actual or potential impaired skin integrity related to:
- Restricted mobility
- Improper positioning
- Pressure

Impaired physical mobility related to:
- Reduced range of joint motion

Sample Nursing Diagnoses for Improper Body Mechanics and Impaired Joint Mobility

Defining Characteristics	Nursing Diagnoses	Related Factors
Broken skin Altered mobility Malnutrition Unsteady gait History of falls Disorientation	Potential for injury	• Improper positioning • Improper body mechanics
Limited range of motion Decreased muscle strength Inability to move, transfer, ambulate Impaired coordination	Impaired physical mobility	• Activity intolerance • Depression • Pain • Cognitive impairment • Musculoskeletal impairment

Sample Nursing Care Plan for Improper Body Mechanics and Impaired Joint Mobility

Nursing Diagnosis	Goals	Expected Outcomes	Nursing Interventions
Impaired physical mobility related to pain	Client improves mobility. Verbal and nonverbal complaints of pain are reduced.	Client ambulates two times per day and evening shift. Client positions self. Client does not express a lack of willingness to move.	Instruct client on the use of Patient Controlled Analgesia (PCA). Teach client relaxation techniques two times per shift. Observe return demonstration of relaxation techniques. Teach client proper position techniques. Encourage regular periods of ambulation. Inspect skin for signs of injury.

or generalized to include all joints. In addition they can be short-term, progressive, or permanent.

Clients at risk for hazards associated with improper body alignment and impaired joint mobility require a nursing care plan directed toward meeting these special needs (see care plan box).

The plan is based on one or more of these goals:
1. Maintain proper body alignment
2. Regain proper body alignment or optimal level of body alignment
3. Reduce injuries to the skin and musculoskeletal systems resulting from improper body mechanics or alignment
4. Achieve full or optimal range of joint motion
5. Prevent contractures

The primary nursing goal is to maintain proper body alignment. Frequently this is included in the nursing care plan before impairments are observed. Maintaining body alignment is especially important in clients with actual or potential limitations in mobility. For example, a comatose client should be positioned with pillows and the position changed at least every 2 hours to reduce the risk of poor alignment and future injury to the skin and musculoskeletal system.

IMPLEMENTATION

BODY ALIGNMENT

To maintain proper body alignment the nurse correctly lifts the client, uses proper positioning techniques,

and safely transfers clients from bed to chair or bed to stretcher. Procedures described in this section incorporate principles of body mechanics that are needed to maintain or restore body alignment.

LIFTING TECHNIQUES. The rate of injuries in occupational settings has increased in recent years, and more than half are back injuries that are the direct result of improper lifting and bending techniques (Owens, 1980). The most common back injury is strain on the lumbar muscle group, which includes the muscles around the lumbar vertebrae. Muscle injury to these areas affects the ability to bend forward, backward, and side to side. In addition, the ability to rotate the hips and lower back is decreased.

The nurse is at risk for injury to lumbar muscles in lifting, transferring, or positioning the immobilized client. Before lifting, the nurse should assess ability to lift the client or object by determining these basic lifting criteria:
1. *Position of weight*—The weight to be lifted should be as close to the lifter as possible. Positioning the object in such a manner uses the lifting force of the nurse because the object is in the same plane.
2. *Height of the object*—The best height for lifting vertically is slightly above the level of the middle finger of a person with the arm hanging at the side (Owens, 1980). This is about 2 feet off the ground and is closer to the lifter's center of gravity.
3. *Body position*—When the lifter's body position varies with different lifting tasks, a general rule is applicable to most lifting situations: the body is

PROCEDURE 41-1

Proper Lifting

STEPS	RATIONALE
1. Assess the four basic lifting measures: position of weight, height of object, body position, and maximum weight.	Determine if you are able to do it yourself or require help.

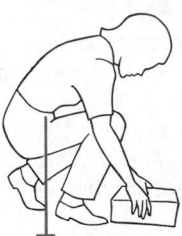

STEPS	RATIONALE
2. Lift object correctly from below center of gravity (see illustration):	
a. Come close to the object to be moved.	Increases body balance during the lift.
b. Enlarge your base of support by placing feet slightly apart.	Maintains better body balance, thus reducing risk of falling.
c. Lower your center of gravity to the object to be lifted.	Increases body balance and enables muscle groups to work together in a synchronized manner.
d. Maintain proper alignment of the head and neck with the vertebrae.	Reduces risk of injury to the lumbar vertebrae and muscle groups.
3. Lift object correctly from shelf above center of gravity:	
a. Use safe, stable step stool.	Raises center of gravity closer to object.
b. Stand as close to shelf as possible.	Moves center of gravity closer to object.
c. Quickly transfer weight of object from shelf to arms and over base of support.	Reduces danger of falling by moving lifted object close to center of gravity over base of support.

positioned so that multiple muscle groups work together in a synchronized manner.

4. *Maximum weight*—Each nurse should know the maximum weight that is safe to carry—safe for the nurse as well as the client. An object is too heavy if its weight is 35% or more of a person's body weight. Therefore a nurse who weighs 130 pounds should not try to lift an immobilized 100-pound person. Although the nurse may be able to do it, there is a risk of dropping the client or causing injury to the nurse's back.

In lifting, the nurse should follow a procedure designed to protect the musculoskeletal system (Procedure 41-1). First the nurse's body is brought close to the object to be lifted. Second, the feet are slightly apart. Third, with the head erect and the neck and vertebrae in proper alignment, the nurse's center of gravity is lowered toward the object to be lifted.

Lifting an object from a high shelf increases risks because it is more difficult to maintain body balance. To reach an object overhead, people often stand on tiptoe with their feet together, thereby decreasing their base of support, elevating their center of gravity, and ultimately decreasing their balance.

The nurse who must lift an object from a high shelf should (1) use a safe, stable step stool or ladder for elevation; (2) stand as close to the shelf as possible; and (3) quickly transfer the weight of the object from the shelf to the arms and over his or her base of support. These principles maintain the lifter's base of support and align the object's weight close to the lifter's center of gravity.

POSITIONING TECHNIQUES. Clients with impaired nervous, skeletal, or muscular system functioning and increased weakness and fatigability often require help from the nurse to attain proper body alignment while in bed or sitting. Several devices are available for the nurse to maintain good body alignment for clients while they are being positioned (Table 41-2).

Pillows are readily available in hospitals or extended care facilities. However, when the client is at home, the supply is limited. Before using a pillow, the nurse should determine if it is the proper size. A thick pillow under the client's head increases cervical flexion. A thin pillow under body prominences may be inadequate to protect skin and tissue from damage caused by pressure. When additional pillows are unavailable or if they are an im-

TABLE 41-2 Devices Used for Proper Positioning

Device	Uses
Pillow	Provides support of body or extremity; elevates a body part; splints incisional area to reduce postoperative pain during activity or coughing and deep breathing
Footboard or Posey footguard	Maintains feet in dorsal flexion
Trochanter roll (Fig. 41-8)	Prevents external rotation of legs when the client is in the supine position
Sandbag	Provides support and shape to the body contours; immobilizes an extremity; maintains specific body alignment
Hand roll	Maintains the thumb slightly adducted and in opposition to the fingers; maintains fingers in a slightly flexed position
Hand-wrist splint	Individually molded for the client to maintain proper alignment of the thumb; slightly adducted in apposition to the fingers; maintains the wrist in slight dorsal flexion
Trapeze bar	Enables the client to raise trunk from the bed; enables the client to transfer from bed to wheelchair; allows the client to perform exercises that strengthen upper arms
Side rail	Allows the weak client to roll from side to side or to sit up in bed
Bed board	Provides additional support to the mattress and improves vertebral alignment

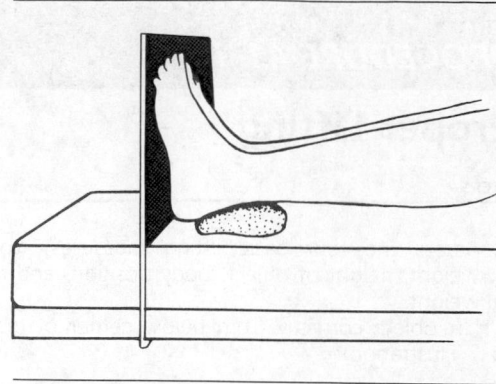

Fig. 41-7 Footboard.

is in the neutral position or in inward rotation. When correct alignment of the hip is achieved, the patella faces directly upward.

Sandbags are sand-filled plastic tubes that can be shaped to body contours. Sandbags can be used in place of or in addition to trochanter rolls. They immobilize an extremity or maintain body alignment.

Hand rolls maintain the thumb in slight adduction and in opposition to the fingers. A hand roll maintains the hand, thumb, and fingers in a functional position. Hand rolls can be made by folding a washcloth in half, rolling it lengthwise, and securing it with tape. The roll is placed against the palmar surface of the client's hand. The nurse evaluates the hand roll to make sure the hand is indeed in a functional position. If washcloths are in short supply, a roll of Kerlix can be used.

Hand-wrist splints are individually molded for the client to maintain proper alignment of the thumb (slight adduction) and the wrist (slight dorsiflexion). These splints should be used only by the client for whom the splint was made.

The *trapeze bar* descends from a securely fastened overhead bar that is attached to the bed frame. It allows the client to pull with upper extremities to raise the trunk off the bed, to assist in transfer from bed to wheelchair, or to perform upper arm exercises (Fig. 41-9).

Restraints are devices used for immobilization, especially of confused or disoriented clients. A common jacket restraint is the Posey jacket (Fig. 41-10). When placing the jacket on the client, the nurse laps one side over the other on the client's back. The ties are placed under the loop on the jacket and secured to the bed, chair, or wheelchair frame. Restraints should *never* be tied to bedside rails because the client may be injured if a side rail is lowered with the restraint in place. (See Chapter 40 for safety principles in using restraints.)

Side rails, bars positioned along the sides of the bed, ensure client safety (see Chapter 40) and are also useful for increasing mobility. In addition, they allow the weak

proper size, the nurse can fold sheets, blankets, or towels.

A *footboard* is placed perpendicular to the mattress, parallel to and touching the plantar surfaces of the client's feet (Fig. 41-7). The footboard prevents footdrop by maintaining the feet in dorsiflexion. After placing it on the bed, the nurse needs to determine if it is correctly placed, since a small client's feet may not reach the board. A Posey footguard is a manufactured device that uses foam structures to maintain the client's feet in the dorsiflexed position.

The *trochanter roll* prevents external rotation of the legs when the client is in a supine position. To form a trochanter roll, a cotton bath blanket is folded lengthwise to a width that will extend from the greater trochanter of the femur to the lower border of the popliteal space (Fig. 41-8). The blanket is placed under the buttocks and then rolled counterclockwise until the thigh

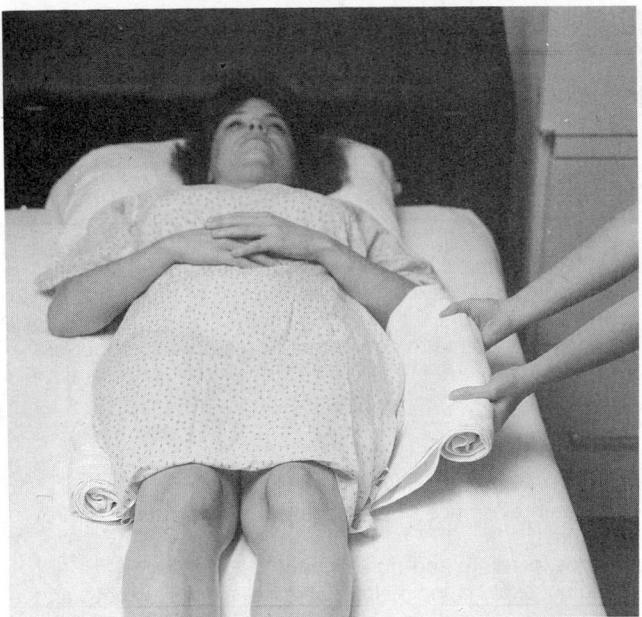

Fig. 41-8 Trochanter roll.

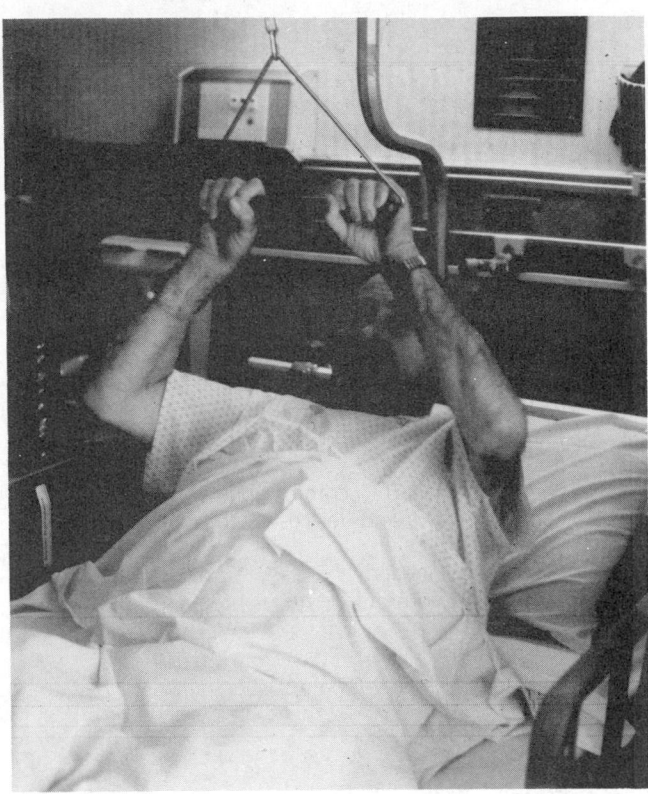

Fig. 41-9 Client using a trapeze bar.

client to roll from side to side or sit up in bed.

Bed boards are plywood boards placed under the entire mattress. They are useful for increasing back support and alignment, especially with a soft mattress.

All of these devices, except hand and wrist splints, are readily available in a hospital or community setting. Hand-wrist splints are designed to mold to the contour of the hand, and they are most commonly used to increase function in a client with limited mobility related to nervous system dysfunction such as hemiplegia after a cerebrovascular accident (stroke).

Although each procedure for positioning has specific guidelines, there are some general ones the nurse should follow for clients who require positioning assistance (Procedure 41-2).

Various positions are described in the following paragraphs and include guidelines for each.

These guidelines reduce the risk of injury to the musculoskeletal system when the client is in a sitting position or lying in bed. When joints are unsupported, their alignment is impaired. Likewise, if joints are not positioned in a slightly flexed position, their mobility is decreased. During positioning the nurse also assesses for pressure points. When actual or potential pressure areas exist, nursing interventions involve removal of the pressure, decreasing risk for development of pressure sores, and further trauma to the musculoskeletal system.

Supported Fowler's Position. In the supported Fowler's position, the head of the bed is elevated 45 to 60 degrees and the client's knees are slightly elevated without pressure to restrict circulation in the lower legs.

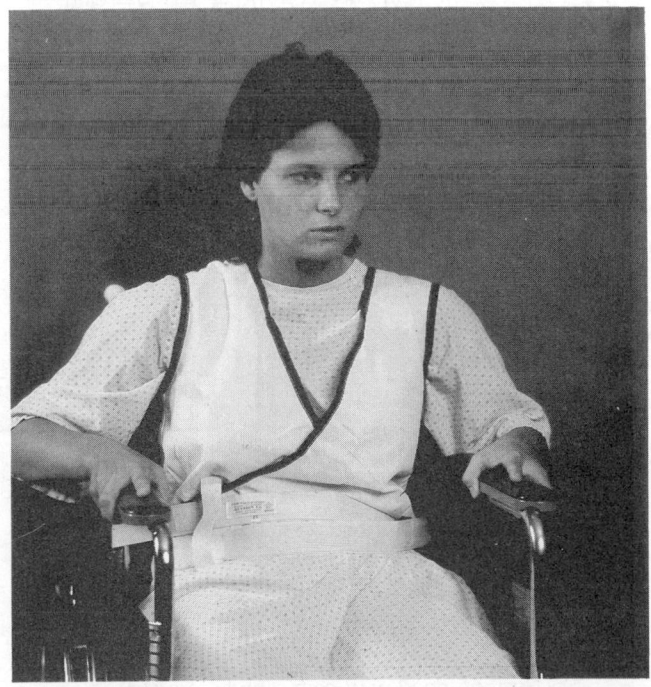

Fig. 41-10 Client restrained with Posey jacket looped through wheelchair arms.

PROCEDURE 41-2

Positioning Clients in Bed

STEPS	RATIONALE
1. Assess client's body alignment and comfort level while client is lying down.	Provides baseline data concerning client's body alignment and comfort level. Determines ways to improve position and alignment.

2. Prepare the following equipment and supplies:
  a. Pillows   e. Hand rolls
  b. Footboard f. Restraints
  c. Trochanter g. Side rails
  d. Sandbags
	Provides easy access to equipment necessary for proper positioning.

3. Raise level of bed to comfortable working height.	Raises level of work toward nurse's center of gravity.
4. Remove pillows and devices used in previous position.	Reduces interference from bedding during positioning procedure.
5. Get help as needed.	Provides for client and nurse safety.
6. Explain procedure to client.	Providing explanation helps decrease client's anxiety and increase cooperation.
7. Wash hands.	Reduces transmission of infection.
8. Provide for client privacy.	Ensuring client's mental comfort is as important as ensuring physical comfort.
9. Put bed in flat position.	Provides easy access to client and allows nursing personnel to reposition client without working against gravity.
10. Move client to head of bed.	Maintains client's comfort. Allows room for proper positioning. Helps maintain proper body alignment.
11. Positioning client in supported Fowler's position a. Elevate head of bed 45°-60°.	Increases comfort, improves ventilation, and increases client's opportunity to socialize or relax.
b. Rest head against mattress or on small pillow.	Prevents flexion contractures of cervical vertebrae.
c. Use pillows to support arms and hand if client does not have voluntary control or use of hands and arms.	Prevents shoulder dislocation from effect of downward gravitational pull of unsupported arms, promotes circulation by preventing venous pooling, prevents flexion contractures of arms and wrists.
d. Position pillow at lower back.	Supports lumbar vertebrae and decreases flexion of vertebrae.
e. Place small pillow or roll under thigh.	Prevents hyperextension of knee and occlusion of popliteal artery from pressure from body weight.
f. Place small pillow or roll under ankles.	Prevents prolonged pressure on heels from mattress.
g. Place footboard at bottom of client's feet (see illustration).	Maintains dorsal flexion and prevents foot drop.

Step 11g

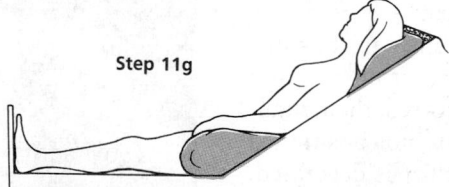

12. Positioning hemiplegic client in supported Fowler's position. a. Elevate head of bed 45°-60°.	Increases comfort, improves ventilation, increases client's opportunity to relax.
b. Sit client up as straight as possible.	Counteracts tendency to slump toward affected side. Improves ventilation, cardiac output; decreases intracranial pressure. Improves client's ability to swallow and helps prevent aspiration of food, liquids, or gastric secretions.
c. Position head with chin slightly forward.	Support reduces risk of joint dislocation. While muscle tone is decreased and muscles do not actively respond, limbs are open to injury.

STEPS	RATIONALE
d. Provide support for both involved arm and hand on an overbed table in front of client; place arm away from client's side and support elbow with pillow.	Paralyzed muscles do not automatically resist pull of gravity as they do normally. As a result, shoulder subluxation, pain, or edema may occur.
e. Position *flaccid* hand in normal resting position with wrist slightly extended, arches of hand maintained, and fingers partially flexed; you may use one section of a rubber ball cut in half; clasp client's hands together.	Maintains hand in functional position. Prevents contractures.
f. Position *spastic* hand with wrist in neutral position or slightly extended; fingers should be extended with the palm down, or may be left in relaxed position with palm up.	Maintains hand in functional position. Inhibits flexor spasticity.
g. Flex knees and hips by using pillow or folded blanket under knees.	Ensures proper alignment. Flexion prevents prolonged hyperextension, which could impair joint mobility.
h. Support feet in dorsiflexion with soft pillow or footboard.	Prevents foot-drop. Stimulation of ball of foot by hard surface has tendency to increase muscle tone in client with extensor spasticity of lower extremity.
13. Positioning client in supine position	
a. Place client on back with head of bed flat.	Necessary for positioning in supine position.
b. Place small rolled towel under lumbar area of back.	Provides support for lumbar spine.
c. Place pillow under upper shoulders, neck, and head.	Maintains correct alignment and prevents flexion contractures of cervical vertebrae.
d. Place trochanter rolls or sandbags parallel to lateral surface of client's thighs.	Reduces external rotation of hip.
e. Place small pillow or roll under ankle to elevate heels.	Reduces pressure on heels, helping to prevent pressure sores.
f. Place footboard or soft pillows against bottom of client's feet.	Maintains feet in dorsiflexion. Prevents foot-drop.
g. Place pillows under pronated forearms, maintaining upper arms parallel to client's body (see illustration).	Reduces internal rotation of shoulder and prevents extension of elbows. Maintains correct body alignment.
h. Place hand rolls in client's hands.	Reduces extension of fingers and abduction of thumb. Maintains thumb slightly adducted and in opposition to fingers.
14. Positioning hemiplegic client in supine position	
a. Place head of bed flat.	Necessary for positioning in supine position.
b. Place folded towel or pillow under shoulder or affected side.	Decreases possibility of pain, joint contracture, or subluxation. Maintains mobility in muscles around shoulder to permit normal movement patterns.

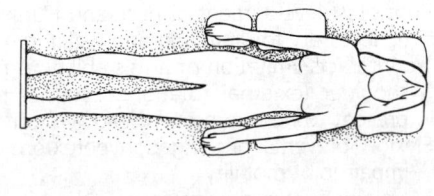

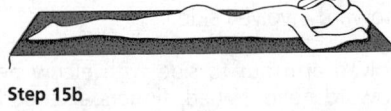

Step 15b

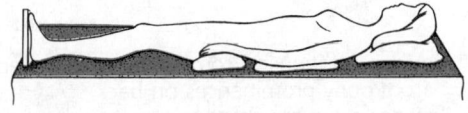

Step 13g

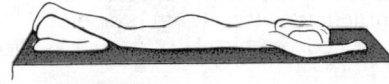

Step 15e

Continued.

PROCEDURE 41-2, cont'd

Positioning Clients in Bed

STEPS	RATIONALE
c. Keep affected arm away from body with elbow extended and palm up. (An alternative is to place arm out to side with elbow bent and hand toward head of bed.)	Maintains mobility in arm, joints, and muscles around shoulder to permit normal movement patterns. (The alternative position counteracts limitation of ability of arm to rotate outward at shoulder [external rotation]. External rotation must be present to raise arm overhead without pain.)
d. Positioning affected hand in one of recommended positions for either flaccid or spastic hand.	Maintains hand in functional position.
e. Place folded towel under hip of involved side.	Diminishes effect of spasticity in entire leg by controlling hip position.
f. Flex affected knee 30° by supporting it on pillow or folded blanket.	Slight flexion breaks up abnormal extension pattern of leg. Extensor spasticity is most severe when client is supine.
g. Support feet with soft pillows at right angle to leg.	Maintains foot in dorsiflexion and prevents footdrop. Soft pillows prevent stimulation to ball of foot by hard surface, which has tendency to increase muscle tone in client with extensor spasticity of lower extremity.
15. Positioning client in prone position a. Roll client over arm positioned close to body with elbow straight and hand under hip. Position on abdomen in center of bed with bed flat.	Positions client correctly so that alignment can be maintained.
b. Turn client's head to one side and support with small pillow (see illustration).	Reduces flexion or hyperextension of cervical vertebrae.
c. Place small pillow under client's abdomen below level of diaphragm.	Reduces pressure on breasts of some female clients, decreases hyperextension of lumbar vertebrae and strain on lower back. Improves breathing by reducing mattress pressure on diaphragm.
d. Support arms in flexed position level at shoulders.	Maintains proper body alignment. Support reduces risk of joint dislocation.
e. Support lower legs with pillow to elevate toes (see illustration).	Prevents foot-drop. Reduces external rotation of legs. Reduces mattress pressure on toes.
16. Positioning hemiplegic client in prone position a. With head of bed flat, move client toward his unaffected side.	Moving client to one side of bed will ensure proper client alignment in center of bed when rolled onto abdomen.
b. Roll client onto his side.	
c. Place pillow on client's abdomen.	Prevents sagging of abdomen when client is rolled over. Decreases hyperextension of lumbar vertebrae and strain on lower back.
d. Roll client onto his abdomen by positioning involved arm close to client's body with elbow straight and hand under hip. Roll client carefully over his arm.	Prevents injury to affected side.
e. Turn head toward involved side.	Promotes development of neck and trunk extension, which is necessary for standing and walking.
f. Position involved arm out to side with elbow bent and hand toward head of bed, fingers extended if possible.	Counteracts limitation of arm's ability to rotate outward at shoulder (external rotation). External rotation must be present to raise arm over head without pain.
g. Flex both knees slightly by placing pillow under both legs from knees to ankles.	Flexion prevents prolonged hyperextension, which could impair joint mobility.
h. Keep feet at right angles to legs by using pillow high enough to keep toes off mattress.	Maintains feet in dorsiflexion.
17. Positioning client in lateral (side-lying) position a. Lower head of bed completely or as low as client can tolerate.	Provides position of comfort for client, removes pressure from bony prominences on back.
b. Position client to side of bed.	Provides room for client to turn to side.

STEPS	RATIONALE
c. Turn client onto side.	
(1) To turn helpless client onto side, flex client's knee that will not be next to mattress. Place one hand on client's hip and one hand on his shoulder.	Prevents injury to client's joints as he is rolled to his side. Client positioned so that leverage on hip makes turning easy.
(2) Roll client onto side.	Rolling client toward you causes less trauma to client's tissues.
d. Place pillow under client's head and neck.	Maintains alignment. Reduces lateral neck flexion. Decreases strain on sternocleidomastoid muscle.
e. Bring shoulder blade forward.	Prevents client's weight from resting directly on shoulder joint.
f. Position both arms in slightly flexed position. Uppermost arm is supported by pillow level with shoulder; other arm by mattress.	Decreases internal rotation and adduction of shoulder. Supporting both arms in slightly flexed position protects joint. Ventilation is improved because chest is able to expand more easily.
g. Place tuck-back pillow behind client's back. (Make tuck-back pillow by folding pillow lengthwise. Smooth area is slightly tucked under client's back.)	Provides support to maintain client on side.
h. Place pillow under semiflexed upper leg level at hip from groin to foot (see illustration).	Flexion prevents hyperextension of leg. Maintains leg in proper alignment. Prevents pressure on bony prominence.
i. Place sandbag parallel to plantar surface of dependent foot.	Maintains dorsiflexion of the foot. Prevents foot-drop.
18. Positioning client in Sims' (semiprone) position	
a. Place head of bed flat.	Provides for proper body alignment while client is lying down.
b. Place client in supine position.	Prepares client for Sims' position.
c. Position client in lateral position lying partially on abdomen.	Client is rolled only partially on abdomen.
d. Place small pillow underneath client's head.	Maintains proper alignment and prevents lateral neck flexion.
e. Place pillow under flexed upper arm, supporting arm level with shoulder.	Prevents internal rotation of shoulder. Maintains proper alignment.
f. Place pillow under flexed upper legs, supporting leg level with hip.	Prevents internal rotation of hip and adduction of leg. Flexion prevents hyperextension of leg. Reduces mattress pressure on knees and ankles.
g. Place sandbags parallel to plantar surface of foot (see illustration).	Maintains foot in dorsiflexion. Prevents foot-drop.
19. Wash hands.	Reduces transmission of infection.
20. Lower bed.	Provides for client safety.
21. Observe client's body alignment position, level of comfort, and potential pressure points.	Determines effectiveness of positioning, maintenance of body alignment, and protection from pressure. Reduces risk of musculoskeletal injury related to improper positioning.
22. Record procedure in nurses' notes, including position assumed, frequency of turning, condition of skin, joint movement, use of supports or splints, client's ability to assist with repositioning, number of staff needed to complete procedure, and client comfort.	Documents effectiveness of nursing care. Provides for consistency among nursing staff.

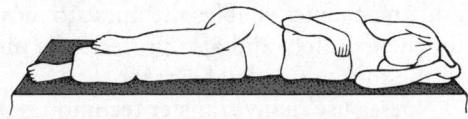

Step 17h

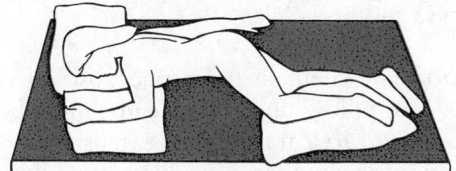

Step 18g

Proper alignment of the body in this position requires support that maintains comfort and reduces the risk of damage to body systems. The angle of head and knee elevation and the length of time that client should remain in the Fowler's position are influenced by the illness and the client's overall condition. Supports must permit flexion of the hips and knees and proper alignment of the normal curves in the cervical, thoracic, and lumbar vertebrae. The following are common trouble areas for the client in the Fowler's position:

1. Increased cervical flexion because the pillow at the head is too thick and the head thrusts forward
2. Extension of knees, allowing the client to slide to the foot of the bed
3. Pressure on the posterior aspect of the knee, decreasing circulation to the feet
4. External rotation of hips
5. Arms hanging unsupported at the client's sides
6. Feet unsupported
7. Unprotected pressure points at the sacrum and heels

Supine Position. The supine position, in which the client rests on the back, is also called the dorsal recumbent position. In the supine position the relationship of body parts is essentially the same as in good standing alignment except that the body is in the horizontal plane. Pillows, trochanter rolls, and hand rolls or arm splints are used to increase comfort and reduce injury to the skin or musculoskeletal system.

The mattress should be firm enough to support the cervical, thoracic, and lumbar vertebrae. Shoulders are supported and the elbows are slightly flexed to control shoulder rotation. A foot support is used to prevent footdrop, maintain proper alignment, and provide freedom of movement for the feet.

There are some common trouble areas for the supine position:

1. Pillow at the head too thick, increasing cervical flexion
2. Head flat on the mattress
3. Shoulders unsupported and internally rotated
4. Elbows extended
5. Thumb not in opposition to the fingers
6. Hips externally rotated
7. Unsupported feet
8. Unprotected pressure points at the lumbar vertebrae, elbows, and heels

Prone Position. The client in the prone position is lying face down. The pillow under the head should be thin enough to prevent cervical flexion or extension and maintain alignment of the lumbar spine. Placing a pillow under the lower leg permits dorsiflexion of the ankles and some knee flexion, which promotes relaxation. If a

pillow is unavailable, the ankles should be in dorsiflexion over the end of the mattress. Body alignment is poor when the ankles are continuously in plantar flexion and the lumbar spine remains in hyperextension.

The nurse should assess for and correct any of these potential trouble points:

1. Neck hyperextension
2. Hyperextension of lumbar spine
3. Plantar flexion
4. Unprotected pressure points at the chin, elbows, hips, knees

Side-Lying Position. In the side-lying (or lateral) position the client is resting on the side, with the major portion of body weight on the dependent hip and shoulder. Trunk alignment should be the same as in good standing position. For example, the structural curves of the spine should be maintained, the head should be supported in line with the midline of the trunk, and rotation of the spine should be avoided, especially in the helpless client (Bilger and Greene, 1973).

The following trouble points are common in the side-lying position:

1. Lateral flexion of the neck
2. Spinal curves out of normal alignment
3. Shoulder and hip joints internally rotated, adducted or unsupported
4. Lack of support for the feet
5. Lack of protection for pressure points at the ear, ilium, knees, and ankles

Sims' Position. The Sims' position differs from the side-lying position in the distribution of the client's weight. In the Sims' position the weight is placed on the anterior ilium and the humerus and clavicle.

Trouble points common in the Sims' position include the following:

1. Lateral flexion of the neck
2. Internal rotation, adduction, or lack of support to the shoulders and hips
3. Lack of support for the feet
4. Lack of protection for pressure points at the ilium, humerus, clavicle, knees, and ankles

TRANSFER TECHNIQUES. Nurses often encounter semihelpless, helpless, or immobilized clients whose position must be changed, who must be moved up in bed, or who must be transferred from bed to chair or bed to stretcher. The nurse learns body mechanics early. Proper body mechanics enables the nurse to move, lift, or transfer clients safely and also protects the nurse from injury to the musculoskeletal system.

Nurses use many transfer techniques. This section details procedures for the most common. However, the nurse follows some general guidelines in any transfer procedure:

1. Raising the side rail on the side of the bed opposite the nurse to prevent the client from falling out of bed.
2. Elevating the level of the bed to a comfortable height
3. Assessing the client's mobility and strength to determine what assistance he or she can offer during transfer
4. Determine need for assistance
5. Explaining the procedure and describing what is expected of the client
6. Assess for correct body alignment and pressure areas following each transfer

Clients who are experiencing pain may require some analgesia before movement to minimize discomfort and to provide relaxation. The nurse who is attempting transfer or moving techniques for the first time should request help to reduce the risk of injury to both client and nurse. The nurse should also recognize personal strength and its limits. Moving a completely immobilized client alone is difficult and dangerous.

Moving a Client in Bed. Clients require various levels of assistance to move up in bed or to the side-lying position or to sit up at the side of the bed. For example, a young, healthy, postpartum woman may need only a little support as she sits at the side of the bed for the first time, while the elderly man 1 day after an appendectomy may need help from one or more nurses to do the same task.

How then does the nurse determine what the client is able to do alone and how many people are needed to help move the client in bed? First the nurse assesses the client to determine if the illness precludes exertion, as with cardiovascular disease. Next, the nurse determines if the client comprehends what is expected. For example, a client recently medicated for postoperative pain may be too lethargic to understand instruction, and to ensure his safety, two nurses are needed to move him in bed. Third, the nurse determines the comfort level of the client. Fourth, the nurse evaluates his or her own strength and knowledge of the procedure. Last is determination of whether the client is too heavy or immobile for the nurse to complete the procedure alone. In doubtful cases the nurse should always request assistance from another person. Procedures 41-3 and 41-4 describe the steps commonly used in moving clients in bed and transferring them to a sitting position at the side of the bed.

Transferring a Client from Bed to Chair. Transfer of a client from bed to chair by one nurse requires assistance from the client and should not be attempted with those who cannot (Procedure 41-4). As with other procedures the nurse explains it to the client before the transfer. The environment is also prepared, with obsta-

cles moved out of the way. The chair is placed next to the bed with the chair back in the same plane as the head of the bed. Placement of the chair allows the nurse to pivot with the client and to transfer the client's weight quickly.

A safe transfer is the first priority. The nurse who is doubtful about his or her strength or the client's ability to help should request assistance. The client should stand at the side of the bed for a minute so he or she can quickly be lowered back into it in case of dizziness or fainting.

Transferring a Client From Bed to Stretcher. An immobilized client who must be transferred from bed to stretcher or bed to bed requires a three-person carry (Procedure 41-4). This technique is best implemented when personnel who are doing the lifting are similar in height. If their centers of gravity are within the same plane, they can lift as a team.

Caution is used when the client has spinal cord trauma. If the client must be moved, the three-person carry is used and spinal alignment is maintained during the transfer.

The client should be prepared for the transfer and asked to help when possible by, for example, folding the arms over the chest. The environment should be free from obstacles, and unnecessary equipment should be removed from the bed. The stretcher should be placed at a right angle to the bed so the lifters can pivot toward the stretcher and transfer the client quickly.

As with all procedures, safety is the priority. Safety is increased in the three-person carry if the lifters work together. Therefore one person should assume the leadership role.

JOINT MOBILITY

To ensure adequate joint mobility the nurse can teach the client about range of joint motion exercises. When the client does not have voluntary motor control, the nurse institutes passive range of motion exercises. Joint mobility is also increased by walking. Occasionally clients need to use mechanical devices such as crutches to help them walk.

RANGE OF JOINT MOTION EXERCISES. Clients with restricted mobility are unable to perform some or all range of joint motion exercises independently. This limitation can be identified in clients in whom one extremity has limited movement or in completely immobilized clients. When caring for clients with actual or potential impaired mobility, the nurse designs interventions directed toward maintaining maximal joint mobility. One such nursing intervention is range of joint motion exercises.

To ensure that clients routinely receive these exercises,

PROCEDURE 41-3

Moving a Client Up in Bed

STEPS	RATIONALE
1. Assess client's comfort level, activity tolerance, muscle strength, and mobility.	Provides baseline data to determine the ability of the client to assist in moving.
2. Raise level of bed to comfortable working height.	Raises level of work toward nurse's center of gravity.
3. Remove all pillows and devices used in previous position.	Reduces interference from bedding during positioning procedure.
4. Get extra help as needed.	Provides for client and nurse safety.
5. Explain procedure to client.	Providing explanation helps decrease client's anxiety and increase cooperation.
6. Wash hands.	Reduces transmission of infection.
7. Provide for client privacy	Ensuring client's mental comfort is as important as ensuring physical comfort.
8. Put bed in flat position.	Provides easy access to client and allows nursing personnel to reposition client without having to work against gravity.
9. Moving helpless client up in bed (one nurse)	
a. Place client on back with head of bed flat. Stand on one side of bed.	Enables nurse to assess body alignment. Reduces gravitational pull on client's upper body.
b. Place pillow at head of bed.	Prevents striking client's head against bed.
c. Begin at client's feet. Face foot of bed at 45° angle. Place feet apart with foot nearest head of bed behind other foot (forward-backward stance). Flex knees and hips as needed to bring your arms level with client's legs. Shift your weight from front to back leg and slide client's legs diagonally toward head of bed.	Positioning is begun at client's legs because they are lighter and easier to move. Facing direction of movement ensures proper balance. Shifting nurse's weight reduces force needed to move load. Diagonal motion permits pull in direction of force. Flexing knees lowers nurse's center of gravity and uses thigh muscles rather than back muscles.
d. Move parallel to client's hips. Flex knees and hips as needed to bring your arms level with client's hips.	Maintains nurse's proper body alignment. Brings nurse closest to object to be moved and lowers the center of gravity. Uses thigh muscles rather than back muscles.
e. Slide client's hips diagonally toward head of bed.	Aligns client's hips and feet.
f. Move parallel to client's head and shoulders. Flex knees and hips as needed to bring arms level with client's body.	Maintains nurse's proper body alignment. Brings nurse closer to object to be moved. Lowers nurse's center of gravity. Uses thigh muscles rather than back muscles.
g. Slide your arm closest to head of bed under client's neck, with your hand reaching under and supporting client's shoulder.	Supports client's head and neck, maintaining proper alignment and preventing injury during movement.
h. Place your other arm under client's chest.	Supports client's body weight and reduces friction during movement.
i. Slide client's trunk, shoulders, head, and neck diagonally toward head of bed.	Realigns client's body on one side of bed.
j. Elevate side rail. Move to other side of bed and lower side rail.	Protects client from falling out of bed.
k. Repeat procedure, switching sides until client reaches desired height in bed.	
l. Center client in middle of bed, moving his body in same three sections.	Maintains proper body alignment. Provides ample room for turning, positioning, or other nursing activities.
m. Lower side rails.	Provides for client safety.
10. Assisting a client to move up in bed (one or two nurses)	
a. Place client on back with head of bed flat.	Enables nurse to assess body alignment. Reduces gravitational pull on client's upper body.
b. Place pillow at head of bed.	Prevents striking client's head against bed.
c. Face head of bed.	
(1) If two nurses assist client, each nurse should have one arm under client's shoulders and one arm under client's thighs.	Facing direction of movement prevents twisting nurse's body while moving client.

STEPS	RATIONALE
(2) Alternate position. Position one nurse at client's upper body. Nurse's arm nearest head of bed should be under client's head and opposite shoulder. Other arm should be under client's closest arm and shoulder. Position other nurse at client's lower torso. This nurse's arms should be under client's lower back and torso.	Prevents trauma to client's musculoskeletal system by supporting shoulder and hip joints and evenly distributing client's weight.
d. Place feet apart with foot nearest head of bed behind other foot (forward-backward stance).	Wide base of support increases nurse's balance. Forward-backward stance enables nurse to shift body weight as client is moved up in bed, thereby reducing force needed to move load.
e. Ask client to flex knees with feet flat on bed	Enables client to use femoral muscles during movement.
f. Instruct client to flex neck, tilting chin toward chest.	Prevents hyperextension of neck when moving client up in bed.
g. Instruct client to assist moving by pushing with the feet on bed surface.	Reduces friction. Increases client's mobility. Decreases nurse's workload.
h. Flex your knees and hips, bringing your forearms closer to level of bed.	Increases balance and strength by bringing nurse's center of gravity closer to client—the "object" to be moved. Uses thigh muscles instead of back muscles.
i. Instruct client to push with the heels and elevate the trunk while breathing out, thus moving toward head of bed on count of 3.	Prepares client for actual move. Reinforces client's assistance in moving up in bed. Increases client cooperation. Breathing out avoids Valsalva maneuver.
j. On count of 3, rock and shift your weight from the front to back leg. At the same time, client pushes with heels and elevates trunk.	Rocking enables nurse to improve balance and overcome inertia. Shifting nurse's weight counteracts client's weight and reduces force needed to move load. Client's assistance reduces friction and nurse's workload.
11. Realign client in supported Fowler's, supine, prone, lateral, or Sims' position.	These positions maintain client's proper body alignment, preventing injury to skin and musculoskeletal system.
12. Wash hands.	Reduces transmission of infection.
13. Lower bed.	Provides for client safety.
14. Observe client's body alignment, position, level of comfort, and potential pressure points.	Maintains support to musculoskeletal system and reduces risk of injury related to improper movement or positioning.
15. Record procedure in nurses' notes, including position assumed, frequency of turning, condition of skin, joint movement, use of supports or splints, client's ability to assist with moving and positioning.	Documents effectiveness of nursing care. Provides for consistency among nursing staff.

the nurse should schedule them at specific times, perhaps along with another nursing activity, such as during the client's bath. This enables the nurse to systematically assess and improve the client's range of joint motion. In addition, bathing or receiving a bed bath usually requires that extremities and joints are put through complete range of motion.

Range of joint motion exercises may be active (the client is able to move all joints through their range of motion unassisted), or passive (the client is unable to move independently and the nurse moves each joint through its range of motion), or somewhere in between. With a weak client, for example, the nurse may merely provide support while the client performs most of the movement, or the client may be able to move some joints actively while the nurse passively moves others. The nurse first assesses the client's ability to engage in active range of motion exercises and the need for support from the nurse. In general, exercises should be as active as health and mobility allow.

Contractures may develop in joints not moved periodically through their range of motion. Contracture is permanent shortening of a muscle and eventual shortening of associated ligaments and tendons. If a contracture occurs because the joint is immobilized for a long time, the joint cannot be used normally and it may become fixed.

Transfer Techniques

STEPS	RATIONALE

1. Assess the following:
  a. Muscle strength
  b. Joint mobility
  c. Presence of paralysis/paresis
  d. Orthostatic hypotension
  e. Activity tolerance
  f. Level of consciousness
  g. Level of comfort
  h. Ability to follow instructions
	Determines client's physiological and cognitive level for participating in transfer technique.

2. Prepare needed equipment and supplies: a. Transfer belt (if needed)	Reduces risk of injury. Transfer belts should be used with all clients who require moderate to maximum assistance or have high risk of falling or injury.
b. If transferring to wheelchair, position chair at 45° angle to bed; lock brakes; remove footrests; lock bed brakes	Position of wheelchair or stretcher facilitates quick transfer from bed to wheelchair or bed to stretcher.
c. If using stretcher position at right angle (90°) to bed; lock brakes on stretcher; lock brakes on bed.	
d. If using Hoyer Lift, use Hoyer frame, canvas strips or chains, and hammock or canvas strips.	Hoyer Lifts safely transfer large immobile clients who are unable to maintain weight bearing.
3. Explain procedure to client. Close door or curtain.	Promotes client cooperation and understanding of procedure and benefits of mobilization. Ensures privacy.
4. Wash hands.	Reduces transfer of infection.
5. Assisting client to sitting position in bed a. Place client in supine position.	Enables nurse to continually assess client's body alignment and to administer additional care, such as suctioning or hygiene needs.
b. Remove pillows from bed.	Decreases interference while sitting client up in bed.
c. Face head of bed.	Reduces twisting of nurse's body when moving client.
d. Place feet apart with foot nearer bed behind other foot.	Improves nurse's balance and allows for transfer of body weight as client is moved to sitting position.
e. Place hand that is farther from client under his shoulders, supporting his head and cervical vertebrae.	Maintains alignment of head and cervical vertebrae and allows for even lifting of client's upper trunk.
f. Place other hand on bed surface.	Provides support and balance.
g. Raise client to sitting position by shifting your weight from front leg to back leg.	Improves nurse's balance, overcomes inertia, and transfers weight in direction in which client is moved.
h. Push against bed using arm that was placed on bed surface.	Divides activity of raising client to sitting position between nurse's arms and legs and protects back from strain. By bracing one hand against mattress and pushing against it as client is lifted, part of weight that would be lifted by nurse's back muscles is transferred through the arms onto mattress (Bilger and Greene, 1973).
6. Assisting client to sitting position on side of bed a. Place client in side-lying position, facing you on side of bed that he will be sitting on.	Prepares client to move to side of bed and protects him from falling.
b. Raise head of bed to highest level client is able to tolerate.	Decreases amount of work needed by client and nurse to raise client to sitting position.
c. Stand opposite client's hips.	Places nurse's center of gravity nearer client.
d. Turn on diagonal so that you are facing client and far corner of foot of bed.	Reduces twisting of nurse's body because nurse is facing direction of movement.
e. Place feet apart with foot closer to head of bed in front of other foot.	Increases balance and allows nurse to transfer weight as client is brought to sitting position at side of bed.
f. Place arm nearer head of bed under client's shoulders, supporting his head and neck.	Maintains alignment of head and neck as nurse brings client to sitting position.

STEPS	RATIONALE
g. Place other arm over client's thighs (see illustration).	Supports hip and prevents client from falling backward during procedure.
h. Move client's lower legs and feet over side of bed.	Decreases friction and resistance.
i. Pivot toward your rear leg, allowing client's upper legs to swing downward.	Allows gravity to lower client's legs.
j. At same time, shift your weight to your rear leg and elevate client (see illustration).	Allows nurse to transfer weight in direction of motion.
k. Remain in front of client until he regains balance.	Reduces risk of falling.
l. Lower level of bed until client's feet touch floor.	Supports client's feet in dorsal flexion and allows client to easily stand at side of bed.
7. Transferring client from bed to chair	
a. Assist client to sitting position on side of bed. Have chair in position at 45° angle to bed.	Positions chair within easy access for transfer.
b. Apply transfer belt if necessary.	Allows nurse to maintain stability of client during transfer, reduces risk of falling.
c. Ensure client has stable nonskid shoes.	Decreases risk of slipping during transfer.
d. Spread your feet apart.	Ensures balance with wide base of support.
e. Flex your hips and knees, aligning your knees with client's.	Lowers nurse's center of gravity to object to be raised and allows for stabilization of knees when client stands.
f. Grasp transfer belt from underneath or reach through client's axilla and place hands on client's scapulae.	Reduces pressure on axilla and maintains client stability.
g. Rock client up to standing on count of 3 while straightening your hips and legs, keeping knees slightly flexed.	Rocking motion gives client's body momentum and requires less muscular effort to lift client. Uses correct body mechanics to raise client to standing position.
h. Maintain stability of weak or paralyzed leg with knee.	Ability to stand can often be maintained in a paralyzed or weak limb with support of knee to stabilize.
i. Pivot on foot that is farther from chair.	Maintains support of client while allowing adequate space for client to move.
j. Instruct client to use arm rests on chair for support.	Increases client's stability.
k. Flex your hips and knees while lowering client into chair.	Prevents injury to nurse resulting from poor body mechanics.
l. Assess client for proper alignment for sitting position.	Prevents injury to client from poor body alignment.
8. Performing three-person carry	
a. Three nurses stand side by side facing side of client's bed. The three people performing the procedure should be of nearly equal height.	Prevents twisting of nurses' bodies. Client's alignment is maintained.
b. Each person assumes responsibility for one of three areas: head and shoulders, hips, thighs and ankles.	Distributes client's body weight.
c. Each assumes wide base of support with foot that is closer to stretcher in front, knees slightly flexed.	Increases balance and lowers lifters' center of gravity.

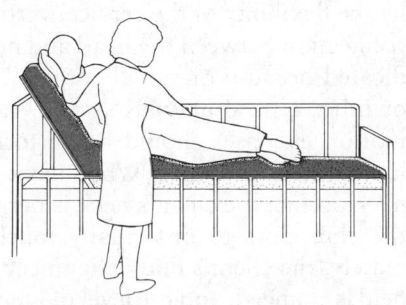

Step 6g

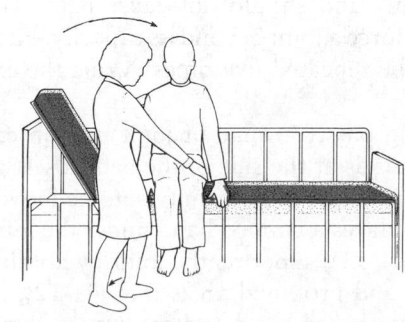

Step 6j

Continued.

PROCEDURE 41-4, cont'd

Transfer Techniques

STEPS	RATIONALE
d. Lifters' arms are placed under client's head and shoulders, hips, and thighs and lower legs, with their fingers securely around other side of client's body (see illustration).	Distributes client's weight over lifters' forearms.

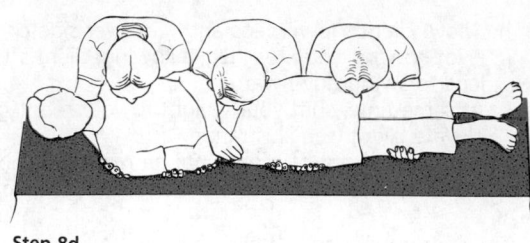

Step 8d

STEPS	RATIONALE
e. Lifters roll client toward their chests.	Moves workload over lifters' base of support.
f. On count of 3, client is lifted and held against nurses' chests.	Enables lifters to work together and safely lift client.
g. On second count of 3, nurses step back and pivot toward stretcher, moving forward if needed.	Transfers weight toward stretcher.
h. Nurses gently lower client onto center of stretcher by flexing their knees and hips until their elbows are level with edge of stretcher.	Maintains nurses' alignment during transfer.
i. Nurses assess client's body alignment, place safety straps across him, and raise side rails.	Reduces risk of injury from poor alignment or falling.
9. Position client in selected position.	Reduces risk of injury to musculoskeletal system from improper positioning.
10. Wash hands.	Reduces transmission of infection.
11. Observe client to determine his response to transfer. Observe for correct body alignment and presence of pressure points.	Reduces risk of injury from subsequent transfers and positioning.
12. Record procedure in nurses' notes.	Documents effectiveness of nursing care. Provides for consistency among nursing staff.

Unless contraindicated, the nursing plan should include moving extremities through as nearly full range of joint motion as possible. Passive range of joint motion exercises should begin as soon as the ability to move the extremity or joint is lost. Movements are carried out slowly and smoothly and should not cause pain. The nurse should never force a joint beyond its capacity. Each movement should be repeated five times during the exercise.

When performing passive range of joint motion exercises, the nurse stands at the side of the bed closest to the joint being exercised. If an extremity is to be moved or lifted, the nurse places a cupped hand under the joint to support it (Fig. 41-11), supports the joint by holding the adjacent distal and proximal areas (Fig. 41-12), or supports the joint with one hand and cradles the distal portion of the extremity with the remaining arm (Fig. 41-13).

The following sections describe specific movements for major joints in the body. Table 41-3 (p. 1216) details range of joint motion for each area and illustrates motion of each joint.

Neck. Range of joint motion for the neck is permitted by the flexibility of the cervical vertebrae and the pivotal connection between the head and neck. Unless contraindicated because of spinal surgery, spinal cord trauma, or other central nervous system trauma, range of joint motion exercises should be performed by clients with limited neck mobility. When flexion contracture of the neck occurs, the client's neck is permanently flexed with the chin close to or actually touching the chest. Ultimately, the client's body alignment is altered, the visual field is changed, and the level of independent functioning is decreased.

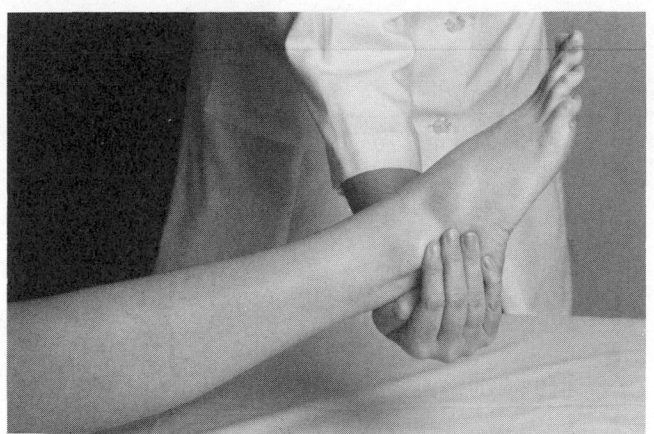

Fig. 41-11   Using a cupped hand to support a joint.

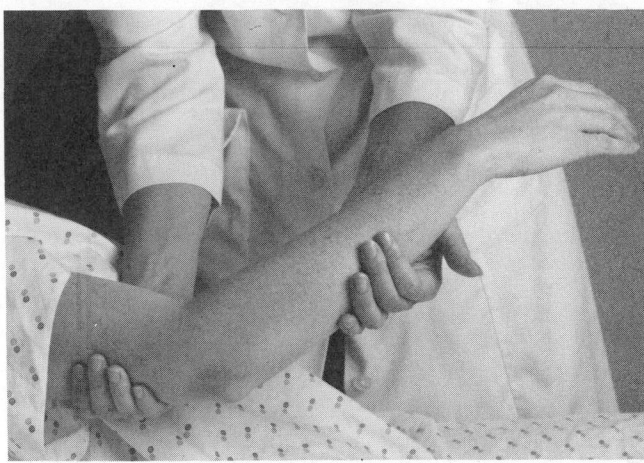

Fig. 41-12   Supporting the joint by holding the distal and proximal areas adjacent to the joint.

Shoulder. One feature of the shoulder that sets it apart from other joints in the body is that the strongest muscle controlling it, the deltoid, is in complete elongation in the normal position. No other muscle exerts its full strength if it begins a movement when in complete elongation. Thus, exercising the shoulder effectively increases the power of the deltoid and range of joint motion; to accomplish this, the shoulder must first be abducted (Bilger and Greene, 1973).

The goal of action in the shoulder is full range of motion. Shoulder movements include flexion, extension, hyperextension, abduction, adduction, internal and external rotation, and circumduction. It is important that the full range of motion in the shoulder be maintained or regained to avoid pain.

When caring for a client with limited voluntary control of the shoulder, the nurse should design interventions to place and support the shoulder in the adducted position. This can be achieved with slings when the client is standing or sitting, or pillows when the client is in bed. Supporting and positioning the shoulder prevent pain, joint dislocation, and further changes in body alignment.

Elbow. The elbow functions optimally at an angle of about 90 degrees. An elbow fixed in full extension is disabling and limits the client's independence. If the elbow becomes contracted in any position, active or passive range of joint motion exercises usually result in increased stiffness.

Forearm. Most functions of the hand are best carried out with the forearm in moderate pronation. When the forearm is fixed in a position of full supination, the client is quite disabled. For optimal functioning the forearm must be able to rotate from supination to pronation.

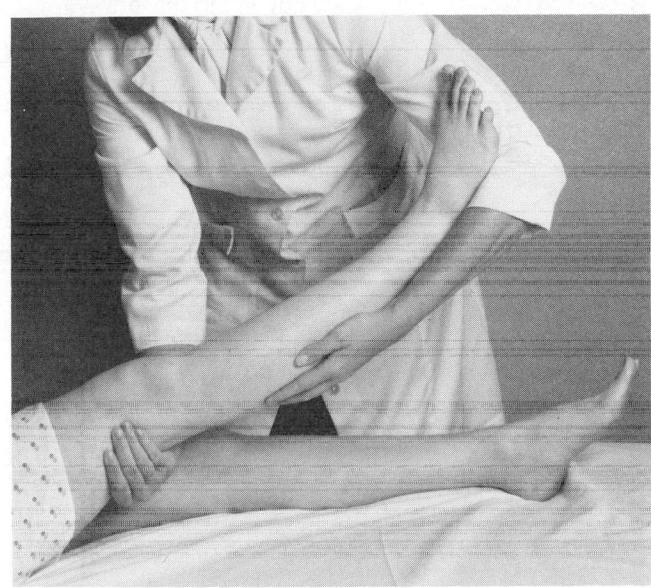

Fig. 41-13   Cradling the distal portion of an extremity.

Wrist. The primary function of the wrist is to place the hand in slight dorsal flexion, the position of functioning. Therefore full range of joint motion is not as great a priority as maintaining the wrist in a functional position. When the wrist is fixed in even a slightly flexed position, grasp is weakened. In the immobilized client the functional position of the wrist can be achieved by using hand and splint rolls.

Fingers and Thumb. The range of motion in fingers and the thumb enables performance of activities of daily living as well as activities requiring fine motor skills such as carpentry, needlework, drawing, or painting.

TABLE 41-3 Range of Joint Motion Exercises

Body Part	Type of Joint	Type of Movement	Range (degrees)	Primary Muscles	
Neck, cervical spine	Pivotal	Flexion: bring chin to rest on the chest Extension: return head to erect position	45 45	Sternocleidomastoid Trapezius	
		Hyperextension: bend head back as far as possible	10	Trapezius	
		Lateral flexion: tilt head as far as possible toward each shoulder	40-45	Sternocleidomastoid	
		Rotation: turn head as far as possible to the right and to the left	180	Sternocleidomastoid, trapezius	
Shoulder	Ball and socket	Flexion: raise arm from side position forward to a position above the head	180	Coracobrachialis, biceps brachii, deltoid, pectoralis major	
		Extension: return arm to position at side of the body	180	Latissimus dorsi, teres major, triceps brachii	
		Hyperextension: move arm behind the body, keeping elbow straight	45-60	Latissimus dorsi, teres major, deltoid	
		Abduction: raise arm to the side to a position above the head with palm away from the head	180	Deltoid, supraspinatus	
		Adduction: lower arm sideways and across the body as far as possible	320	Pectoralis major	

TABLE 41-3—cont'd

Body Part	Type of Joint	Type of Movement	Range (degrees)	Primary Muscles	
		Internal rotation: with elbow flexed, rotate shoulder by moving arm until thumb is turned inward and toward the back	90	Pectoralis major, latissimus dorsi, teres major, subscapularis	
		External rotation: with elbow flexed, move arm until thumb is upward and lateral to the head	90	Infraspinatus, teres major, deltoid	
		Circumduction: move arm in a full circle. Circumduction is a combination of all movements of the ball-and-socket joint	360	Deltoid, coracobrachialis, latissimus dorsi, teres major	
Elbow	Hinge joint	Flexion: bend elbow so that lower arm moves toward its shoulder joint and hand is level with shoulder	150	Biceps brachii, brachialis, brachioradialis	
		Extension: straighten elbow by lowering hand	150	Triceps brachii	
Forearm	Pivotal	Supination: turn lower arm and hand so that palm is up	70-90	Supinator, biceps brachii	
		Pronation: turn lower arm so that palm is down	70-90	Pronator teres, pronator quadratus	
Wrist	Condyloid	Flexion: move palm toward inner aspect of the forearm	80-90	Flexor carpi ulnaris, flexor carpi radialis	
		Extension: move fingers so that fingers, hands, and forearm are in the same plane	80-90	Extensor carpi ulnaris, extensor carpi radialis brevis, extensor carpi radialis longus	
		Hyperextension: bring dorsal surface of hand back as far as possible	89-90	Extensor carpi radialis brevis, extensor carpi radialis longus, extensor carpi ulnaris	

Continued.

TABLE 41-3 Range of Joint Motion Exercises—cont'd

Body Part	Type of Joint	Type of Movement	Range (degrees)	Primary Muscles	
		Abduction (radial flexion): bend wrist medially toward the thumb	Up to 30	Flexor carpi radialis, extensor carpi radialis brevis, extensor carpi radialis longus	
		Adduction (ulnar flexion): bend wrist laterally toward fifth finger	30-50	Flexor carpi ulnaris, extensor carpi ulnaris	
Fingers	Condyloid hinge	Flexion: make a fist	90	Lumbricales, interosseus volaris, interosseus dorsalis	
		Extension: straighten fingers	90	Extensor digiti quinti proprius, extensor digitorum communis, extensor indicis proprius	
		Hyperextension: bend fingers back as far as possible	30-60		
		Abduction: spread fingers apart	30	Interosseus dorsalis	
		Adduction: bring fingers together	30	Interosseus volaris	
Thumb	Saddle	Flexion: move thumb across palmar surface of hand	90	Flexor pollicis brevis	
		Extension: move thumb straight away from hand	90	Extensor pollicis longus, extensor pollicis brevis	
		Abduction: extend thumb laterally (usually done when placing fingers in abduction and adduction)	30	Abductor pollicis brevis	
		Adduction: move thumb back toward hand	30	Adductor pollicis obliquus, adductor pollicis transversus	
		Opposition: touch thumb to each finger of the same hand		Opponeus pollicis, opponeus digiti minimi	

TABLE 41-3—cont'd

Body Part	Type of Joint	Type of Movement	Range (degrees)	Primary Muscles	
Hip	Ball and socket	Flexion: move leg forward and up	90-120	Psoas major, iliacus, iliopsoas, sartorius	
		Extension: move leg back beside the other leg	90-120	Gluteus maximus, semitendinosus, semimembranosus	
		Hyperextension: move leg behind body	30-50	Gluteus maximus, semitendinosus, semimembranosus	
		Abduction: move leg laterally away from body	30-50	Gluteus medius, gluteus minimus	
		Adduction: move leg back toward medial position and beyond if possible	30-50	Adductor longus, adductor brevis, adductor magnus	
		Internal rotation: turn foot and leg toward other leg	90	Gluteus medius, gluteus minimus, tensor fasciae latae	
		External rotation: turn foot and leg away from other leg	90	Obturatorius internus, obturatorius externus	
		Circumduction: move leg in a circle		Psoas major, gluteus maximus, gluteus medius, adductor magnus	

Continued.

TABLE 41-3 Range of Joint Motion Exercises—cont'd

Body Part	Type of Joint	Type of Movement	Range (degrees)	Primary Muscles	
Knee	Hinge joint	Flexion: bring heel back toward back of thigh	120-130	Biceps femoris, semitendinosus, semimembranosus, sartorius	
		Extension: return leg to the floor	120-130	Rectus femoris, vastus lateralis, vastus medialis, vastus intermedius	
Ankle	Hinge joint	Dorsal flexion: move foot so that toes are pointed upward	20-30	Tibialis anterior	
		Plantar flexion: move foot so that toes are pointed downward	45-50	Gastrocnemius, soleus	
Foot	Gliding	Inversion: turn sole of foot medially	10 or less	Tibialis anterior, tibialis posterior	
		Eversion: turn sole of foot laterally	10 or less	Peroneus longus, peroneus brevis	
Toes	Condyloid	Flexion: curl toes downward	30-60	Flexor digitorum, lumbricalis pedis, flexor hallucis brevis	
		Extension: straighten toes	30-60	Extensor digitorum longus, extensor digitorum brevis, extensor hallucis longus	
		Abduction: spread toes apart	15 or less	Abductor hallucis, interosseus dorsalis	
		Adduction: bring toes together	15 or less	Adductor hallucis, interosseus plantaris	

The functional position of the fingers and thumb is slight flexion of the thumb in opposition to the fingers. In clients with restricted mobility, hand rolls help maintain this position.

Hip. Since the lower extremities are concerned chiefly with locomotion and weight bearing, stability of the hip joint may be more important than its mobility. For example, if one hip has no mobility but is fixed in a neutral position and fully extended, it is possible to walk without a significant limp.

Contractures fix the hip in positions of deformity. Excessive abduction makes the affected leg appear too long, whereas excessive adduction makes the affected leg appear too short; in either case the client has limited locomotion and walks with an obvious limp. Flexion contractures result in lordosis when the person is standing. Internal and external rotation contractures cause an unacceptable, unbalanced gait.

Knee. A primary function of the knee is stability, which is achieved by range of joint motion, ligaments, and muscles. However, knees cannot remain stable under weight-bearing conditions unless there is adequate quadriceps power, which maintains the knee in full extension. Range of joint motion exercises should include pulling the knee into full extension.

A stiff knee can result in serious disability, the degree of which depends on the position in which the knee is stiffened. If the knee is fixed in full extension, the person must sit with leg thrust out in front. When the knee is flexed, the person limps while walking. The greater the flexion, the greater the limp. Complete flexion contractures prevent the person from walking without a walker or crutches.

If it is impossible to prevent knee stiffness, the nurse should try to ensure that the knee becomes fixed in a position of slight flexion, 10 to 20 degrees. This permits walking without an excessive limp or sitting without excessive forward thrust of the leg.

Ankle and Foot. During walking, movement of the ankle joint is minimal; however, the joint must be stabilized and able to bear weight or the person will fall. If joint mobility is diminished, the nurse should maintain the joint in a position in which walking can be carried out with a forward rolling motion from the heel onto the forefoot.

When the person relaxes as in sleep or coma, the foot relaxes and assumes a position of plantar flexion. This results from relaxation of the gastrocnemius and soleus muscles, which maintain dorsiflexion. If the foot remains in plantar flexion without support, these two muscles shorten and the dorsiflexion muscles try to compensate by overstretching. As a result the foot becomes fixed in plantar flexion (footdrop), which impairs the ability to walk.

Inversion and eversion must also be avoided in order to allow the foot to rest flat on the floor (Table 41-3). The foot must be flat to allow weight bearing and proper walking.

Toes. Exessive flexion of the toes results in a clawing. When this is a permanent deformity, the foot is unable to rest flat on the floor. Flexion contractures are the most common foot deformity associated with reduced joint mobility.

Adequate range of joint motion gives the necessary mobility to carry out activities of daily living, exercise, and engage in relaxing activities. In addition, adequate range of motion in the lower extremities allows walking.

WALKING

In the normal walking posture the head is erect, the cervical, thoracic, and lumbar vertebrae are aligned, the hips and knees have appropriate flexion, and the arms swing freely in alternation with the legs. Illness or trauma can reduce a client's activity tolerance so that assistance in walking is required. In addition, temporary or permanent damage to the musculoskeletal and nervous systems may necessitate use of a mechanical device for walking.

ASSISTING A CLIENT TO WALK. Like other procedures, assisting the client to walk requires preparation.

First, the nurse assesses the client's activity tolerance, strength, presence of pain, coordination, and balance to determine assistance needed.

Second, the nurse explains how far the client should try to walk, who is going to help, when the walk will take place, and why walking is important. In addition, the nurse and client determine how much independence the client can assume.

Third, the nurse checks the environment to be sure there are no obstacles in the client's path—that chairs, over-the-bed table, and wheelchair are out of the way so the client does not need to expend energy walking an obstacle course.

Fourth, before starting, rest points should be established in case the activity tolerance is less than estimated or the client becomes dizzy.

Fifth, the client should be assisted to a position of sitting at the side of the bed and should rest for 1 to 2 minutes before standing up. Likewise, after standing, the client should remain stationary for a minute or two before moving. It is important to allow the client to stabilize before walking. If the client becomes dizzy, the bed is still nearby and the nurse can quickly ease him back to bed. The longer the period of immobility, the greater the physiological changes, especially changes in circulation. When the person stands, blood pressure may drop (see Chapter 42).

The nurse should provide support at the waist so the client's center of gravity remains midline. This can be achieved when the nurse places both hands at the client's waist or uses a walking belt. This is a leather belt that encircles the waist and has handles attached for the nurse to hold. Clients should not lean to one side because this alters their center of gravity, distorting their balance, and increasing their risk of falling.

The client who at any point appears unsteady or complains of dizziness should be returned to bed or a chair, whichever is closer. If the client faints or begins to fall, the nurse should assume a wise base of support with one foot in front of the other, thus supporting the body weight. Then the nurse gently lowers the client to the floor, protecting the head. Although lowering a client to the floor is not difficult, the student should practice this technique with a friend or classmate before attempting it in a clinical setting.

Occasionally clients with hemiplegia (one-sided paralysis) or hemiparesis (one-sided weakness) need assistance to walk. The nurse always stands on the client's affected side and supports the client by holding one arm around the client's waist and the other arm around the inferior aspect of the client's upper arm so that the nurse's hand is supporting the client's axilla. Providing support by holding the client's arm is incorrect because, if the client should faint or fall, the nurse cannot easily support the weight and lower the client to the floor. In addition, if the client falls with the nurse holding his or her arm, the shoulder joint may be dislocated.

A nurse who does not have the strength and who is unable to ambulate a client alone should request help. The two-nurse method helps to distribute the client's weight evenly. The two nurses stand on either side of the client. Each nurse's near arm is around the client's waist, and the other arm is around the inferior aspect of the client's arm so that both nurses' hands are supporting the client's axillae.

A second method requires that the nurses and client be of similar height. The nurses stand on either side of the client with their near arms slipped under the client's arms toward the back. The nurses then grasp each other's arms. The client's arms are placed over the nurses' shoulders, and the nurses stabilize the client's hands with their free hands. This technique is effective with weakened or heavy clients.

ASSISTIVE DEVICES USED FOR WALKING. Walkers are extremely light, movable devices, about waist high, made of metal tubing. They have four widely placed, sturdy legs. The client holds the handgrips on the upper bars, takes a step, moves the walker forward, and takes another step (Fig. 41-14).

Canes are light, easily movable devices about waist high, made of wood or metal. Two common types of canes are the single straight-legged cane and the quad cane (Fig. 41-15). The first is more common and is used to support and balance a client with decreased leg strength. This cane should be kept on the stronger side of the body. First, for maximum support when walking, the client places the cane forward 15 to 25 cm (6 to 10 inches), keeping body weight on both legs. Second, the weaker leg is moved forward to the cane so the body weight is divided between the cane and the stronger leg. Third, the stronger leg is advanced past the cane so the weaker leg and the body weight are supported by the cane and weaker leg. To walk, the client continually repeats these steps. The client must be taught that two points of support, such as both feet or one foot and cane, are present at all times.

The quad cane provides the most support and is used when there is partial or complete leg paralysis or some hemiplegia. The same three steps used with the straight-legged cane are taught to the client.

Crutches are often needed to increase mobility. Their use may be temporary, such as following ligament damage to the knee. Crutches may be needed permanently, for example, by the client with paralysis of the lower extremities. A crutch is a wooden or metal staff. There are two types of crutches, the double adjustable Lofstrand or forearm crutch (Fig. 41-16), and the axillary wooden crutch (used in Figs. 41-17 through 41-26). The forearm crutch has a handgrip and a metal band that fits around the forearm. Both the metal band and the

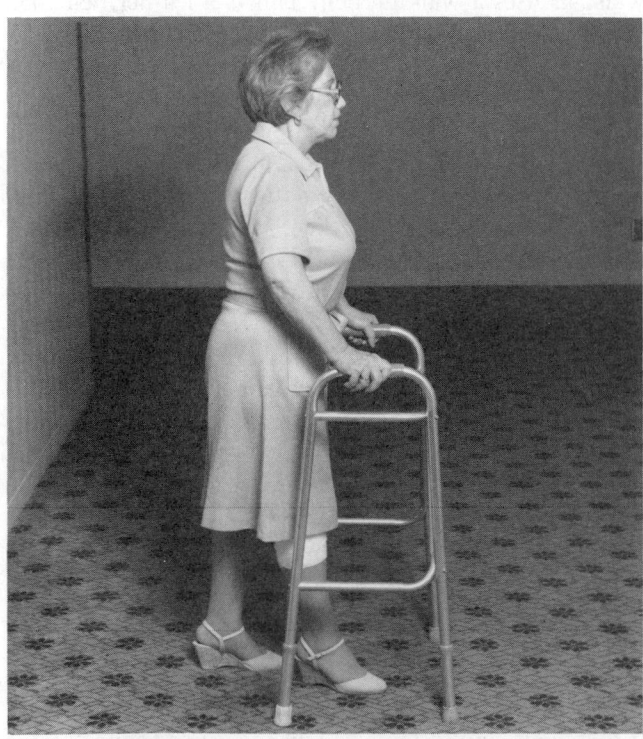

Fig. 41-14   Client using a walker.

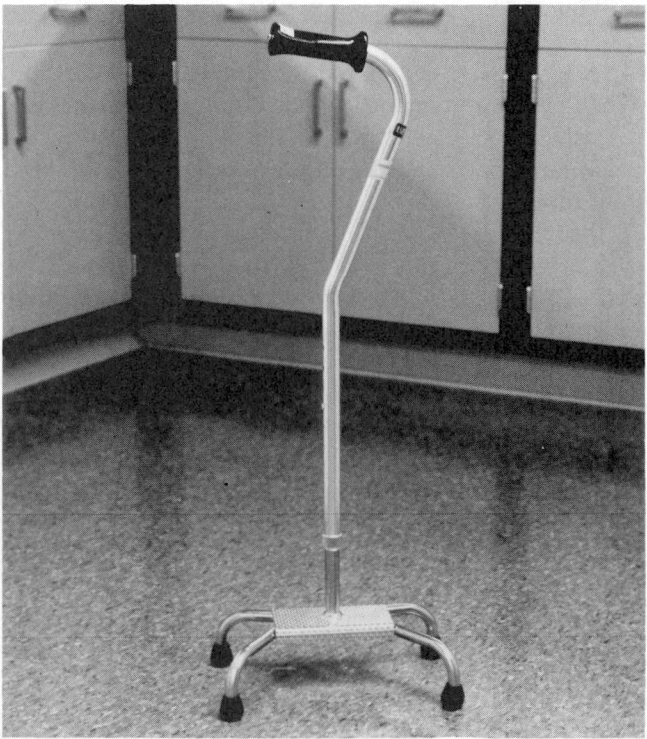

Fig. 41-15   Quad cane.

handgrip are adjusted to fit the client's height. The axillary crutch has a padded curved surface at the top, which fits under the axilla. A handgrip in the form of a crossbar is held at the level of the palms to support the body. It is important that crutches be measured for the appropriate length and that clients be taught how to use their crutches safely, achieve a stable gait, ascend and descend stairs, and rise from a sitting position.

MEASURING FOR CRUTCHES. The axillary crutch is the more common crutch used. Measurements include three areas: the client's height, the angle of elbow flexion, and distance between the crutch pad and axilla. When crutches are fitted, their length should be from three to four finger widths from the axilla to a point 15 cm (6 inches) lateral to the client's heel (Sine et al., 1981) (Fig. 41-17).

It is important that the handgrips be positioned so the body weight is not supported by the axillae. Pressure on the axillae increases risk to underlying nerves, which may cause partial paralysis of the arm. Correct position of the handgrips is determined with the client upright, supporting his weight by the handgrips with elbows slightly flexed (20 to 25 degrees). Elbow flexion is verified with a goniometer (Fig. 41-18). When the height and placement of the handgrips have been determined, the nurse verifies that the distance between the crutch pad and axilla is three to four finger widths (Fig. 41-19).

Crutch Safety. Before walking independently with crutches, the client should be taught these safety guidelines:

1. Clients with axillary crutches must know of the dangers of pressure on the axilla. They must not use crutches that fit improperly or lean on crutches to support their body weight.
2. Crutch tips should be inspected routinely. Rubber tips should be securely attached to the crutches. When tips are worn, they should be replaced. Rubber crutch tips increase surface friction and prevent slipping.

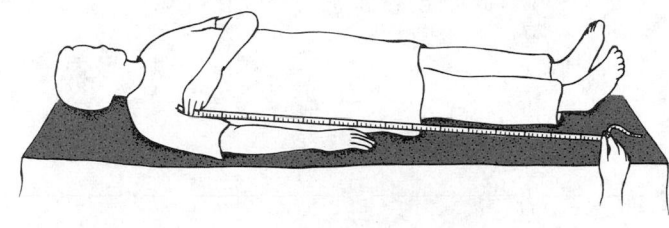

Fig. 41-17   Measuring crutch length.

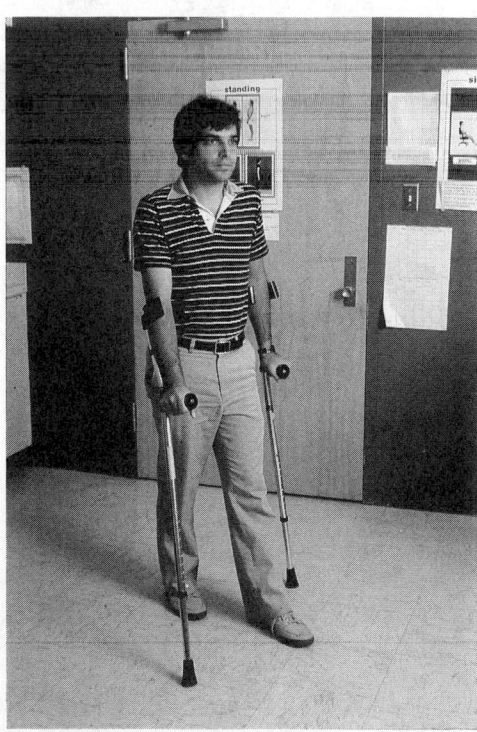

Fig. 41-16   Double adjustable Lofstrand or forearm crutches.

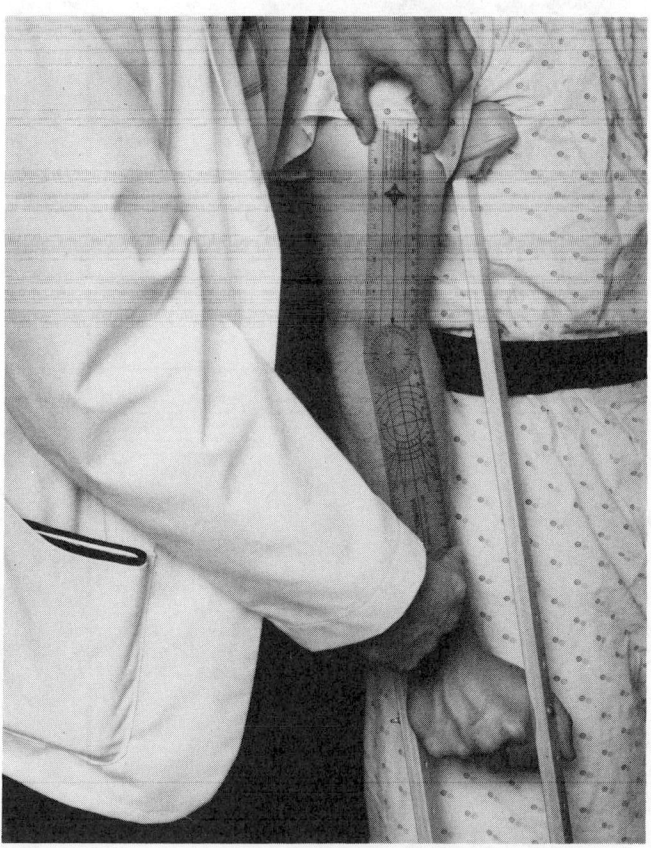

Fig. 41-18   Verifying correct elbow flexion with crutches. Measurement is obtained with a goniometer.

3. Crutch tips should remain dry. If the tips become wet, the client should dry them off. Water decreases surface friction and increases the risk of slipping.
4. The structure of the crutches should also be rou-

tinely inspected. Cracks in a wooden crutch decreases its ability to support weight. Bends in aluminum crutches can alter the body alignment, increasing the risk of further damage to the musculoskeletal system.
5. Clients should be given a list of medical suppliers in their community. This allows them to obtain repairs, new rubber tips, handgrips, and crutch pads.
6. Spare crutches and tips should always be on hand.

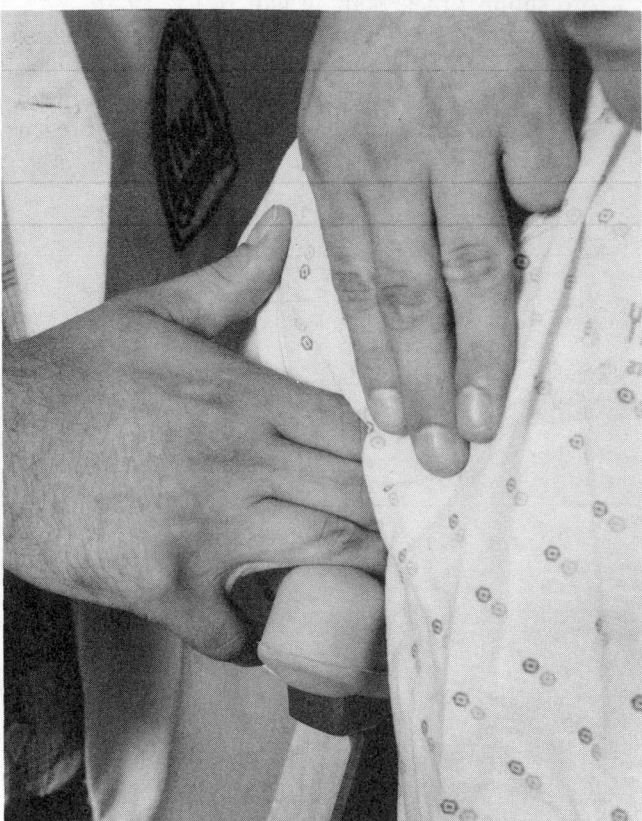

Fig. 41-19 Verifying correct distance between crutch pads and axilla.

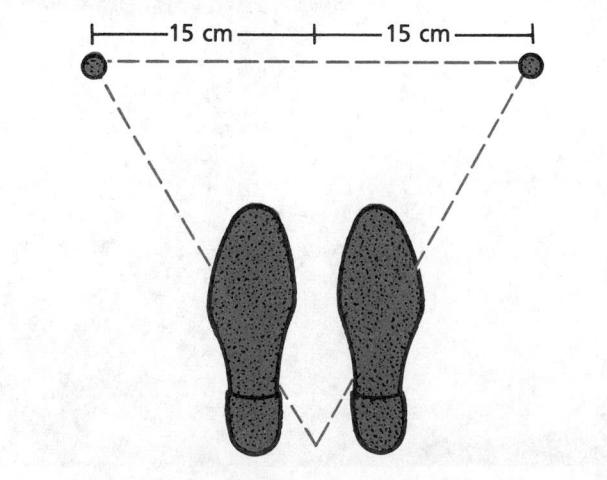

Fig. 41-20 Tripod position, the basic crutch stance.

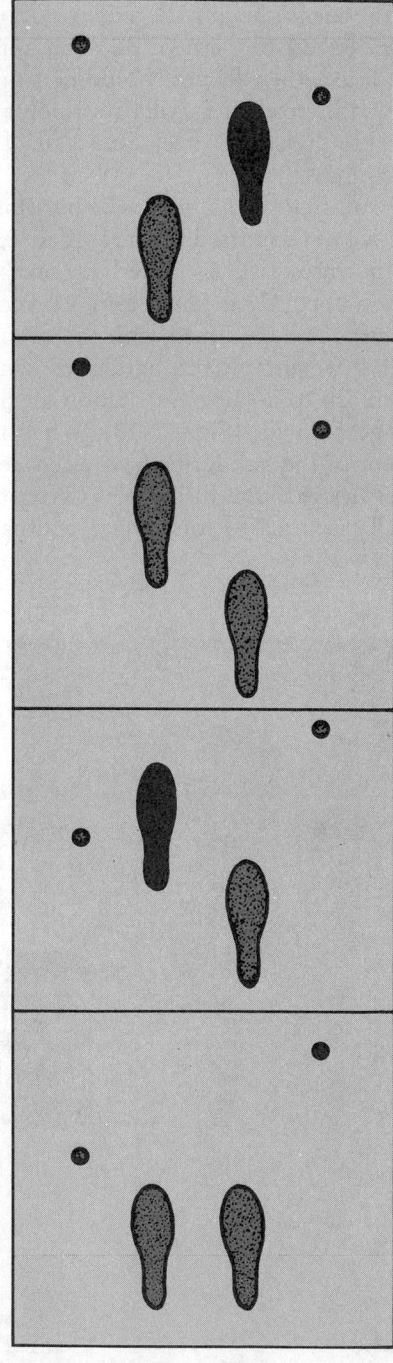

Fig. 41-21 Four-point alternating gait.

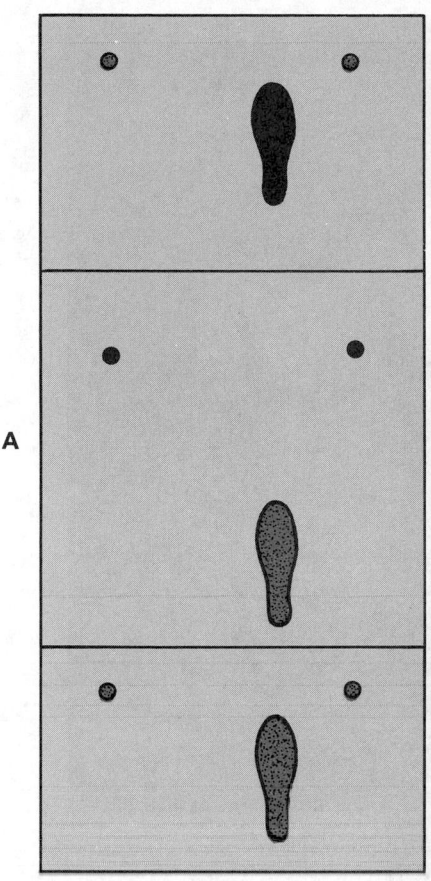
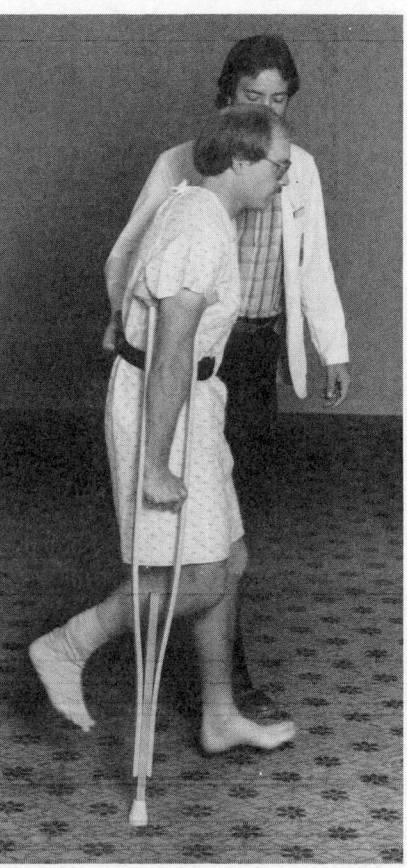
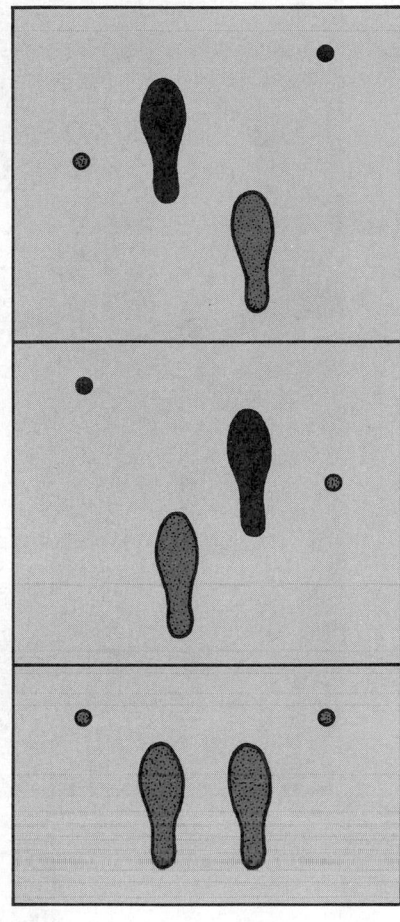

Fig. 41-22 **A,** Three-point alternating gait, with weight borne on the unin-volved leg. Black foot and crutch tips show weight bearing in each phase of the gait. **B,** Weight borne on both crutches.

Fig. 41-23 Two-point alternating gait, with weight borne partially on each foot and crutch advancing with the opposing leg. Black areas indi-cate leg and crutch tips bearing weight.

Crutch Gait. A crutch gait is assumed by alternately bearing weight on one or both legs and on the crutches. The gait selected by the nurse is determined by the assessment of the client's physical and functional abilities and the disease or injury.

The basic crutch stance is the *tripod position,* formed when the crutches are placed 15 cm (6 inches) in front of and 15 cm to the side of each foot (Fig. 41-20). This position improves balance by providing a wider base of support. Body alignment in the tripod position includes erect head and neck, straight vertebrae, and extended hips and knees. No weight should be borne by the axillae. The tripod position is used before crutch walking.

Four-point alternating or *four-point gait* gives stability but requires weight bearing on both legs. Each leg is moved alternately with each crutch so that three points of support are on the floor at all times (Fig. 41-21).

Three-point alternating or *three-point gait* requires the client to bear all of the weight on one foot. In a three-point gait, weight is borne on the uninvolved leg (Fig. 41-22, *A*), then on both crutches (Fig. 41-22, *B*), and the sequence is repeated. The affected leg does not touch the ground during the early phase of the three-point gait.

Gradually the client progresses to touchdown and full weight bearing on the affected leg.

The *two-point gait* requires at least partial weight bearing on each foot (Fig. 41-23). Each crutch is moved at the same time as the opposing leg, so crutch movements are similar to arm motion during normal walking.

The *swing-through* or *swing-to gait* is frequently used by paraplegics who wear weight-supporting braces. With weight placed on the supported legs, the client places the crutches one stride in front and then swings to or through the crutches while they support the body's weight.

Crutch Walking on Stairs. When ascending stairs on crutches, the client usually uses a modified three-point gait (Fig. 41-24). First the client stands at the bottom of the stairs and transfers the body weight to the crutches. Second, the unaffected leg is advanced between the crutches to the stairs. Then weight is shifted from the crutches to the unaffected leg. Last, the client aligns both

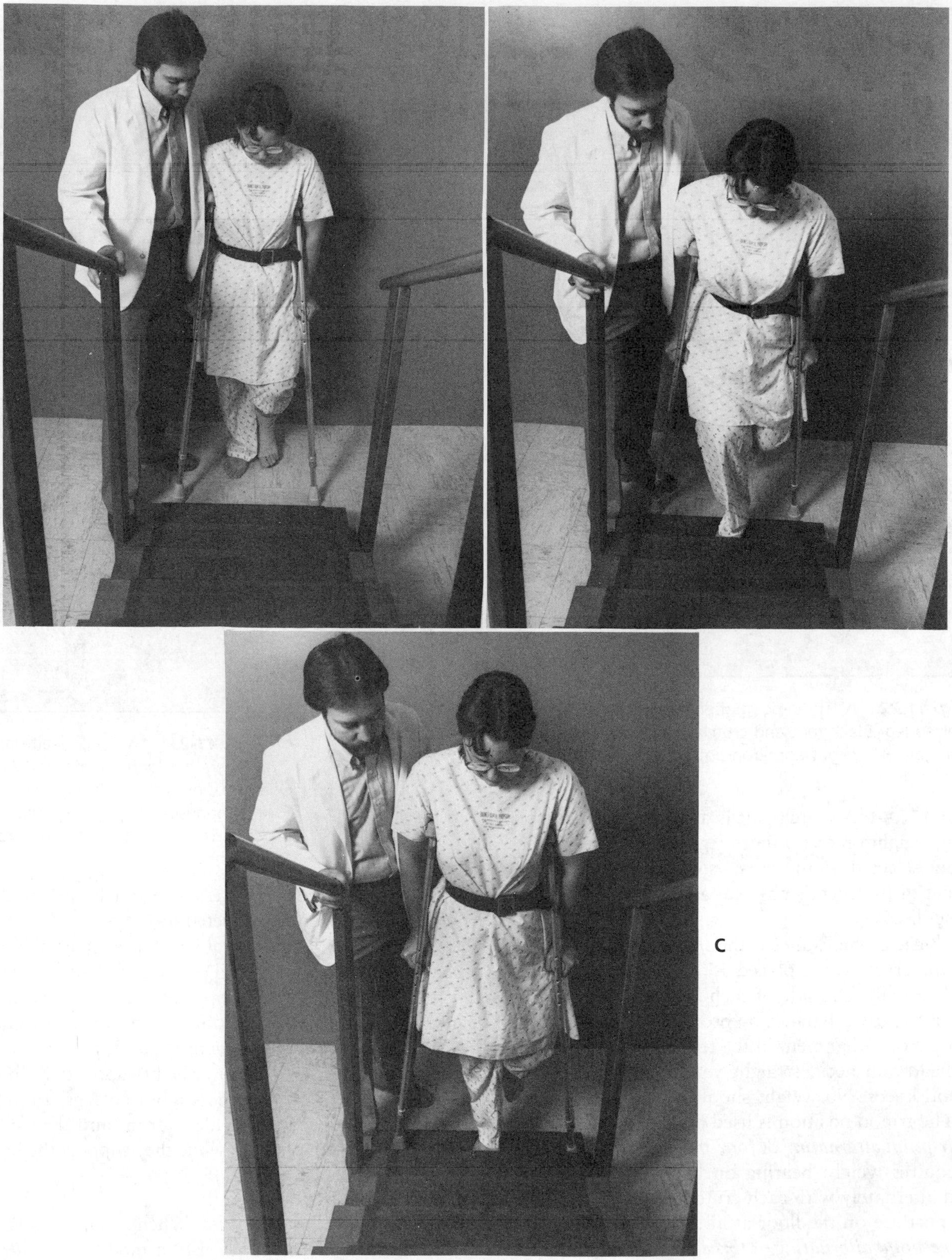

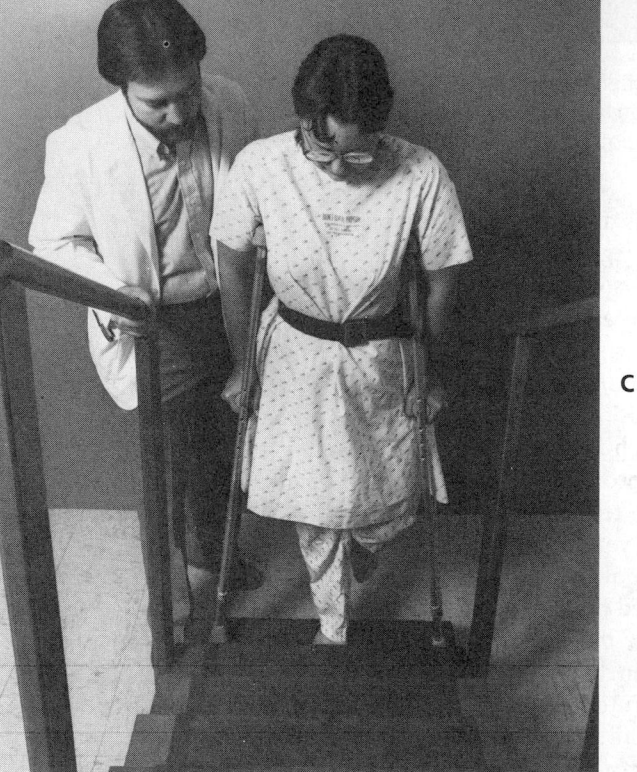

Fig. 41-24 Ascending stairs. **A,** Weight is placed on crutches. **B,** Weight is transferred from crutches to unaffected leg on the stairs. **C,** Crutches are aligned with unaffected leg on the stairs.

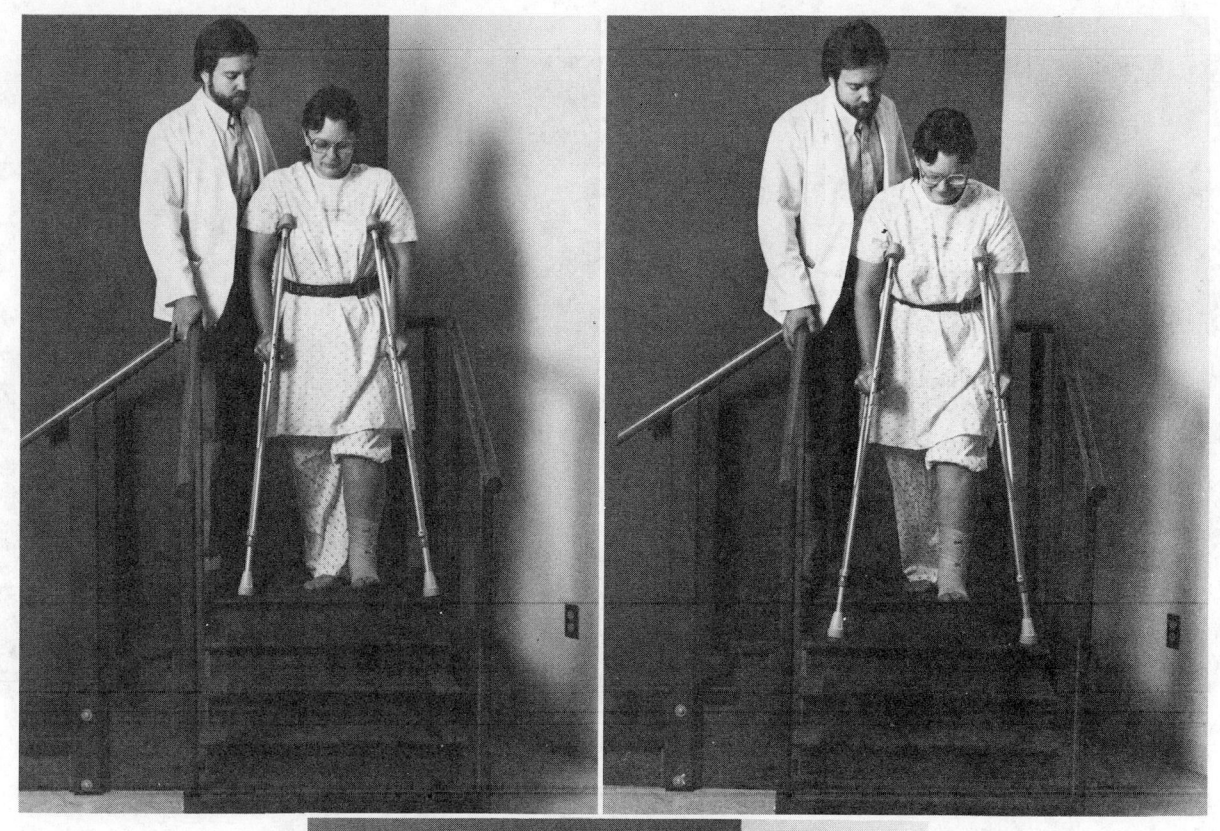

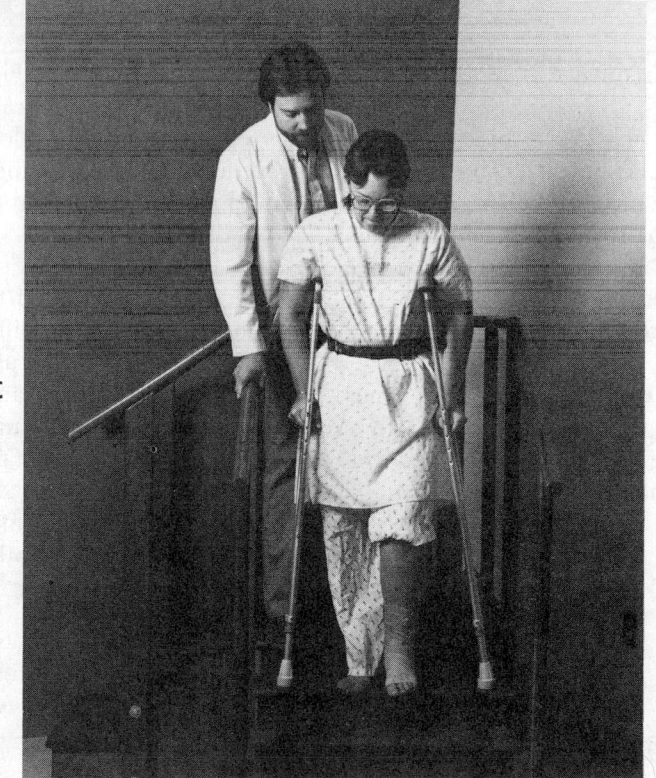

Fig. 41-25 Descending stairs. **A,** Body weight on unaffected leg. **B,** Body weight transferred to crutches. **C,** Unaffected leg aligned on stairs with crutches.

A   B   C

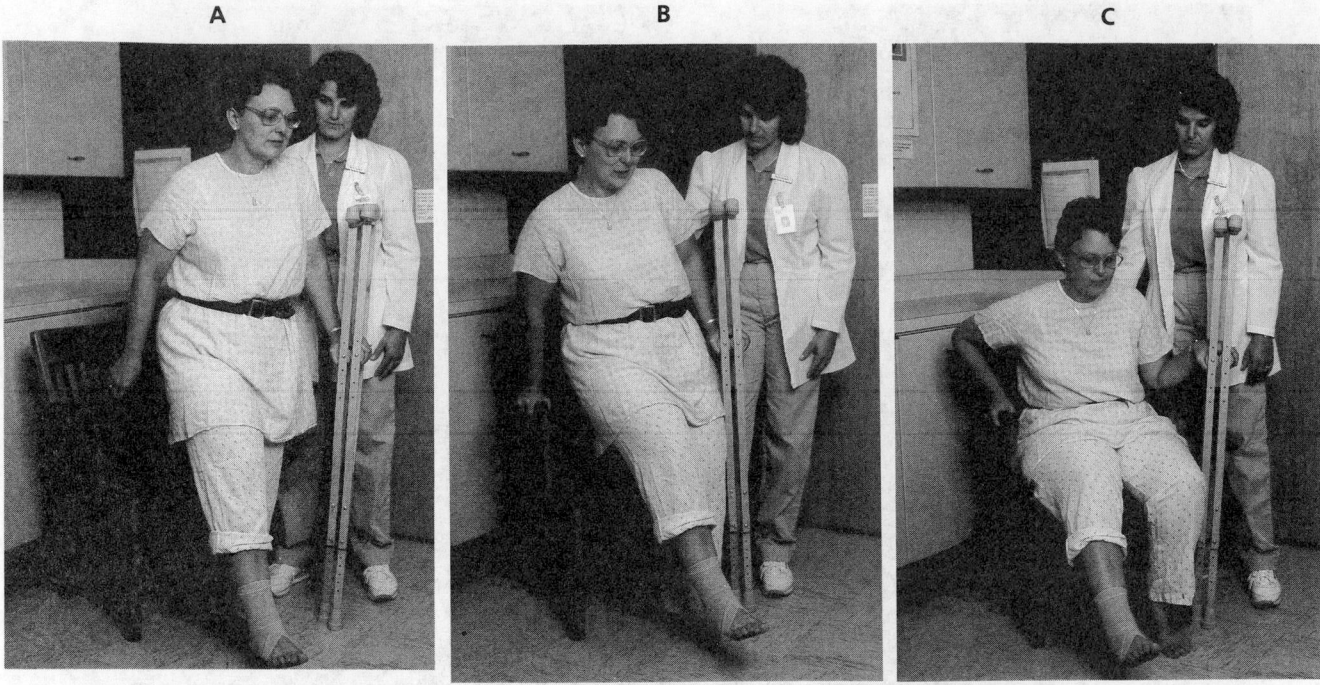

Fig. 41-26 Sitting in a chair. **A,** Both crutches are held by one hand. Client transfers weight to the crutches and the unaffected leg. **B,** Client grasps arm of the chair with the free hand and begins to lower herself into the chair. **C,** Client completely lowers herself into the chair.

crutches on the stairs. This sequence is repeated until the person reaches the top.

To descend the stairs (Fig. 41-25), a three-phase sequence is also used. First, the client transfers body weight to the unaffected leg. Second, the crutches are placed on the stair and the client begins to transfer body weight to the crutches, moving the affected leg forward. Last, the unaffected leg is moved to the stairs with the crutches. Again, the client repeats the sequence until reaching the bottom.

Clients will usually need to use crutches for some time, so they should be taught to use them on stairs before discharge. Instruction applies to all crutch-dependent clients, not only those who have stairs in their homes.

Sitting in a Chair With Crutches. As with crutch walking and crutch walking up and down stairs, the procedure for sitting in a chair involves phases and requires the client to transfer weight. First, the client gets positioned at the center front of the chair with the posterior aspect of the legs touching the chair. Second, the client holds both crutches in the hand opposite the affected leg. If both legs are affected, as with a paraplegic who wears weight-supporting braces, the crutches are held on the client's stronger side. With both crutches in one hand the client supports body weight on the unaf-

fected leg and crutches (Fig. 41-26). While still holding the crutches, the client grasps the arm of the chair with the remaining hand and lowers the body. To stand, the procedure is reversed, and the client when fully erect should assume the tripod position before walking.

■ ■ ■

Interventions designed to maintain the client's body alignment and joint mobility use principles of body mechanics. The nurse also uses body mechanics to avoid self-injury when lifting and transferring clients. When positioning a client, the nurse employs principles of body mechanics to reduce or prevent injury to the client's musculoskeletal system, since the nurse is responsible for protecting clients from damage caused by limitation of movement. This and other hazards of immobility are discussed in Chapter 42.

EVALUATION

Evaluation of nursing care for clients with altered body alignment of joint mobility is based on objective criteria for each of the nursing goals (see evaluation box).

Sample Evaluation of Interventions for Improper Body Mechanics and Impaired Joint Mobility

Goals	Evaluative Measures	Expected Outcomes
Client maintains proper body alignment.	Observe for proper body position.	Client's position reflects proper alignment for standing, sitting, or lying down positions.
	Observe client's position for fatigue or discomfort.	No fatigue or discomfort is expressed or observed.
Proper or optimal body alignment regained.	Observe for improved body alignment.	Body alignment is improved.
	Inspect skin for presence of pressure points.	Skin remains intact and without signs of pressure damage.
	Inspect musculoskeletal system.	Joint contracture or muscle injury is absent.
Injury to skin and underlying musculoskeletal systems is reduced.	Inspect skin and muscles.	Pressure points are absent.
	Palpate soft tissues.	Skin remains intact.
		No joint tenderness observed.
		Muscle tone is present.
Optimal range of joint motion is achieved.	Observe joint through range of joint motion.	Client has improved or full range of joint motion.
	Palpate joint during range of joint motion.	
Joint contractures are prevented.	Measure joint motion.	Joint contractures are absent.

Maintaining good body alignment and joint mobility increases independence and overall mobility. A client with inadequate joint mobility must receive assistance to carry out activities of daily living. The best approach to problems with body alignment and joint mobility is prevention, which begins early in the nursing care plan.

SUMMARY

The nurse incorporates knowledge of the physiology of movement and principles of body mechanics to transfer and position clients safely, as well as assist clients to use walkers and crutches safely. Through the nursing process, the nurse develops a care plan for clients with potential or actual alterations in body alignment. The alteration may be temporary or permanent.

Correct body mechanics protects the nurse and client from injuries to the musculoskeletal system. For example, the nurse can transfer a client from bed to chair without self-injury or injury to the client.

Occasionally, clients with impaired body alignment have restricted mobility or are totally immobilized. Immobilization affects all aspects of the client's life.

KEY CONCEPTS

✓ "Body mechanics" describes coordinated efforts of the musculoskeletal and nervous systems as the person moves, lifts, bends, stands, sits, lies down, and completes activities of daily living.

✓ Coordinated body movement requires integrated functioning of the skeletal system, skeletal muscles, and nervous system.

✓ The skeleton provides bony support structure for movement, for attachment of ligaments and muscles, for protection of vital organs, for some of the regulation of calcium, and for red blood cell production.

✓ The nervous system provides initiation and voluntary control of movement.

✓ A joint is a connection between bones and can be one of four types: synostotic, cartilaginous, fibrous, or synovial.

✓ Ligaments bind joints together and connect bones and cartilages.

✓ Tendons connect muscle to bone.

✓ Cartilage is nonvascular, supportive connective tissue located chiefly in joints and in the thorax, trachea, larynx, nose, and ear.

✓ Muscle contraction is the result of an electrochemical impulse transmitted from nerve to muscle; two types of contraction are possible, isotonic and isometric.

✓ Muscles primarily associated with movement are located near the skeletal region where movement results from leverage, which is characteristic of movements of the upper extremities.

✓ Muscles primarily associated with posture are located in the lower extremities, trunk, neck, and back.

✓ Coordination and regulation of muscle groups depend on muscle tone and activity of antagonistic, synergistic, and antigravity muscles.

✓ The motor strip in the cerebral cortex controls voluntary movement.

✓ Transfer of an impulse from a nerve fiber to a muscle requires a neurotransmitter.

✓ Proprioceptors are nerve endings in muscles, tendons, and joints that respond to stimuli originating from within the body regarding spatial position or movement.

✓ Balance is assisted through nervous system control by the cerebellum and inner ear.

✓ Body alignment is the condition of joints, tendons, ligaments, and muscles in various body positions.

✓ Body balance is achieved when there is a wide base of support, the center of gravity falls within the base of support, and a vertical line falls from the center of gravity through the base of support.

✓ Coordinated body movement can be influenced by physical forces of weight, friction, and leverage.

✓ Developmental stages influence body alignment and mobility; the greatest impact of physiological changes on the musculoskeletal system is observed in children and older adults.

✓ Pathological conditions that affect body alignment and mobility include postural abnormalities, altered bone formation, altered joint mobility, impaired muscle development, damage to the central nervous system, and direct trauma to the musculoskeletal system.

✓ Assessment of a client's body alignment determines normal physiological changes and deviations in alignment; allows the client to observe posture; identifies learning needs as well as the presence of trauma, damage, or dysfunction; and provides other information concerning body alignment.

✓ Assessment of a client's mobility enables the nurse to determine coordination, balance, and ability to complete activities of daily living and makes it possible to evaluate or plan an exercise program.

✓ Range of joint motion is the maximal movement possible at a joint in one of the three planes of the body: sagittal, frontal, and transverse.

✓ Assessing gait allows the nurse to draw conclusions about the client's balance, posture, and ability to walk without assistance.

✓ The nurse's assessment of the client's energy level includes the physiological effects of exercise and activity tolerance.

✓ Activity tolerance is affected by developmental and pathological changes.

✓ When lifting or transferring a client, the nurse considers the basic four principles of lifting: position of weight, height of object, body position, and maximal weight.

✓ Clients with impaired body alignment require nursing interventions to maintain them in the supported Fowler's, supine, prone, side-lying, and Sims' positions.

✓ Transfer techniques require the nurse to use correct body mechanics to move the client in bed, from bed to chair, and from bed to stretcher.

✓ Range of joint motion exercises include one or all of the body joints.

✓ The nurse can cup the joint to be moved, hold the distal and proximal areas adjacent to the joint, or cradle the distal portion of the extremity.

✓ Interventions for impaired joint mobility also entail helping the client walk with one or two nurses.

✓ Mechanical devices to promote walking include canes and walkers, which require specific nursing interventions.

REFERENCES

Bilger, AJ, and Greene, EH: Winger's protective body mechanics: a manual for nurses, New York, 1973, Springer Publishing Co.

Daniels, L, and Worthington, C: Therapeutic exercise for body alignment and function, ed. 2, Philadelphia, 1977, W.B. Saunders Co.

Gordon, M: Assessing activity tolerance, Am J Nurs 76:72, 1976.

Groër, MW, and Shekleton, ME: Basic pathophysiology: a conceptual approach, ed. 2, St. Louis, 1983, The C.V. Mosby Co.

Hudson, MF: Safeguard your elderly patient's health through accurate physical assessment, Nurs 83 (Can. ed.) 13(11):58, 1983.

Owens, BD: How to avoid that aching back, Am J Nurs 80:984, 1980.

Sine, RD, et al.: Basic rehabilitation techniques: a self-instructional guide, ed. 2, Rockville, Md., 1981, Aspen Systems Corp.

Strand, FL: Physiology: a regulatory systems approach, New York, 1978, Macmillan, Inc.

ADDITIONAL READINGS

Bergstrom, N, et al.: The Braden scale for predicting pressure sore risk, Nurs Res 36:205, 1987.

Goldberg, WG, and Fitzpatrick, JJ: Movement with the aged, Nurs Res 29:339, 1980.

Viellion, G: Assessment: examining joints of the upper and lower extremities, Am J Nurs 81:763, 1981.

Winslow, EH, and Weber, TM: Progressive exercises to combat hazards of bedrest, Am J Nurs 80:440, 1980.

Winters, M: Protective body mechanics in daily life and nursing, Philadelphia, 1952, W.B. Saunders Co.

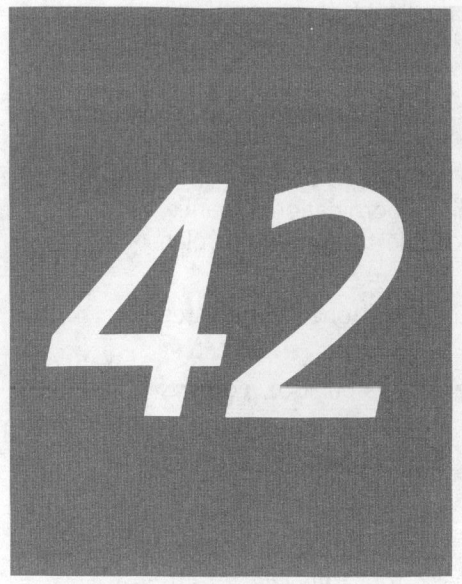

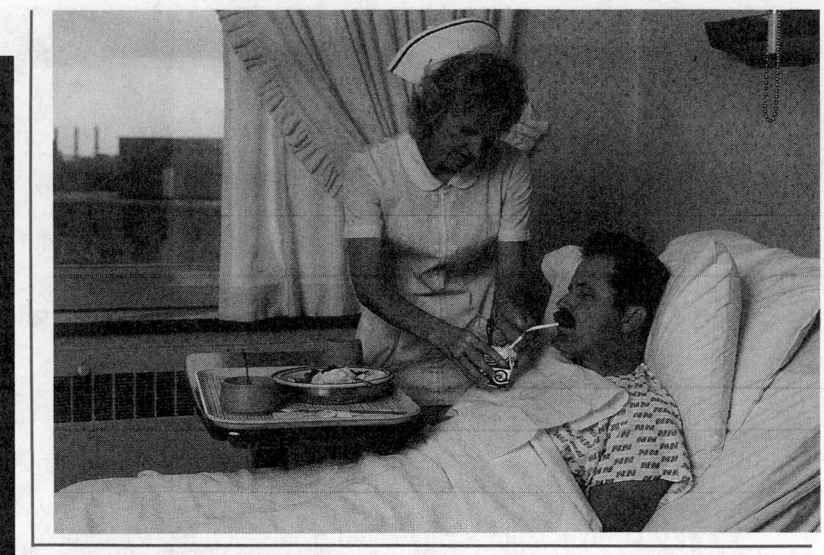

OBJECTIVES

Mastery of content in this chapter will enable the student to:

- Define the key terms listed.
- Discuss benefits and hazards of bed rest.
- Identify changes in metabolism associated with immobility.
- Describe fluid changes associated with immobility.
- Describe alterations in exchange of nutrients and gastrointestinal functioning associated with immobility.
- Describe alterations in respiratory function associated with immobility.
- Discuss the cardiovascular changes caused by immobilization.
- Describe musculoskeletal changes associated with immobility.
- Discuss factors that contribute to decubitus ulcer formation.
- Discuss effects of immobilization on urinary and bowel elimination.
- Describe psychosocial and developmental effects of immobilization.
- Complete an assessment of an immobilized client.
- List nursing diagnoses associated with immobility.
- Develop a nursing care plan for an immobilized client.
- List appropriate nursing interventions for an immobilized client.
- State evaluation criteria for the immobilized client.

KEY TERMS

Anemia
Bed Rest
Bone Resorption
Decubitus Ulcer
Depression
Immobility
Ischemia
Negative Nitrogen Balance
Renal Calculus
Thrombus

Hazards of Immobility

Physical mobility is important in our society. Work, social interaction, development, and relaxation depend on the ability to move body parts freely. In addition, movement of body parts or the entire body is essential for maintenance of total well-being, including physiological, psychosocial, and developmental dimensions.

Movement serves many purposes, such as expression of an emotion with a nonverbal gesture, self-defense, satisfaction of basic needs, the activities of daily living, and recreational activities. To maintain normal physical mobility, the nervous, muscular, and skeletal systems of the body must be intact and functioning.

When a body part or the entire body is immobilized, secondary disabilities may develop in body systems. The greater the degree of immobility and the longer the immobilization, the greater the risk for development of disabilities.

The body's regulation of movement is discussed in Chapter 41. Immobility is described separately here because the many hazards to the immobilized or partially immobilized client require a different and potentially more extensive nursing care plan.

Changes in the client's mobility may result from many health problems. Clients with certain illnesses or injuries become immobilized but return to mobility with rehabilitation. Other clients, such as those with spinal cord injuries and degenerative conditions such as multiple sclerosis, may experience long-term or permanent immobility. A third group of clients is not actually immobilized by an illness or injury but is placed on bed rest or restricted ambulation for therapy such as the client with cardiac or pulmonary conditions.

Both immobility and the return of mobility influence physiological, psychosocial, and developmental dimensions. The nursing process is used to meet the client's needs in all dimensions.

MOBILITY AND IMMOBILITY

Mobility is a person's ability to move about freely. Mobility is often essential to perception of health. Mobility and immobility are best understood as the endpoints of a continuum, with many degrees of mobility between.

Complete, unrestricted mobility requires voluntary motor and complete sensory control of all body regions. Complete mobility has many benefits for the client's physiological and psychosocial well-being. It allows achievement of needs and goals independently and maintenance of social interaction and usual roles.

Immobility is not restricted to clients in bed. The wheelchair-dependent client has a degree of immobility. Rehabilitation teaches this client maximal level of independence for the injury or illness that resulted in the need for a wheelchair.

Clients who are partially mobile usually have a motor or sensory alteration in a region of the body or a therapeutic restriction (for example, a casted extremity). A partial loss of mobility may be temporary (for example, a fractured bone) or permanent (for example, paralysis from a stroke). In some instances, restriction of mobility is beneficial for recovery. This is particularly true with musculoskeletal trauma. Immobilization of the affected area allows healing in proper alignment.

Other clients are capable of mobility but have been placed on bedrest because of illness. While these clients may frequently change position in bed, they can develop health problems as a result of bed rest.

Hazards associated with partial mobility depend on the degree and duration of immobilization. For example, a client whose fractured arm is in a cast for 6 weeks may experience muscle weakness and a reduced ability to carry out daily activities. However, these hazards disappear shortly after the client is able to move the arm again. In contrast, a client with a fractured femur who is placed in traction for a month is more susceptible to the hazards of immobility. The client with permanent partial loss is continually at risk for hazards of immobility and needs to be taught early in rehabilitation how to reduce these hazards.

Five conditions may result in immobility. First, physical inactivity, such as bed rest, is manifested by an overall reduction in body movement. Second, physical restriction or limitation of movement, as by a cast, is manifested by an imposed reduction of movement of a specific body part. Third, restriction in changes in body position and posture results in a loss of the body's ability to adapt to such changes. Fourth, sensory deprivation causes a reduction in the stimulus to move and is manifested by even greater physical inactivity. Last, immobility is the result of regional paralysis. The degree of a client's immobility depends on how many of these five conditions are present (Groër and Shekleton, 1983).

Another factor influencing degree of immobility is its duration. Regardless of the cause, immobility has many negative effects on all body systems.

Bed Rest

Bed rest is an intervention in which the client is restricted to bed for therapy for a prescribed time. Bed rest has different meanings to nurses, physicians, and other health care professionals.

OBJECTIVES OF BED REST

Bed rest can have several therapeutic advantages and clients with many conditions are placed on bed rest (see box). First, it reduces physical activity and oxygen needs

---

Conditions Requiring Bed Rest

CARDIOVASCULAR CONDITIONS

- Acute myocardial infarction
- Congestive heart failure

NEUROLOGICAL CONDITIONS

- Head injuries
- Spinal cord trauma
- Degenerative neurological conditions such as myasthenia gravis

MUSCULOSKELETAL CONDITIONS

- Muscle strains and sprains in lower extremities
- Torn ligaments in lower extremities
- Fractures in lower extremities

INFECTIOUS PROCESSES

- Hepatitis
- Glomerulonephritis

CANCER

- Terminal phase

OPERATIVE CONDITIONS

- First 24 hours following major surgery
- Periodic shorter periods of bed rest after many kinds of surgery

of body tissues. This is beneficial for clients with, for example, recent myocardial infarction so that the myocardium and body tissues do not compete for oxygen. Bed rest also reduces pain and in some cases reduces the need for analgesics.

Bed rest allows ill or debilitated clients to rest and in some instances regain strength. Although febrile clients may be too weak to sit in a chair, when the febrile state is over they can gradually tolerate more activity and require fewer periods of bed rest.

Finally, bed rest can benefit clients psychologically. Overworked and exhausted clients frequently require periods of uninterrupted rest, relaxation, and sleep. Bed rest has physiological and emotional benefits only if the client finds it restful. Clients who resist bed rest may actually expend more energy in fighting it than if allowed to move from bed to chair. Therefore the nurse must continually assess and evaluate the client's physical and emotional responses to bed rest.

HAZARDS OF BED REST

Hazards of bed rest affect the client in all dimensions. A client's response to prolonged bed rest is influenced by psychosocial and developmental factors, prior physical and emotional health, the reason for bed rest, and the duration of bed rest.

Many clients on bed rest have intact motor and sensory tracts that perceive pressure to skin and muscles. As a result, they can change position independently, and their skin may be less susceptible to hazards of immobility than those clients whose immobility results from other conditions. Nonetheless, clients on bed rest, like other immobile clients, must be continually assessed.

EFFECTS OF IMMOBILITY

The effects of immobility are systemic and functional and result from lack of activity. No body system is immune. Experiments have shown that healthy people who are immobilized for a prolonged time suffer the same effects as those whose immobility results from illness. Frequently the effects of immobility occur gradually. The greater the extent and the longer the duration of immobility, the more pronounced are the consequences.

The box lists the effects of immobility in the physiological, psychosocial, and developmental dimensions. This list provides common examples, however, and does not apply to all clients in all situations.

Physiological Responses

Each body system is at risk for impairments resulting from immobility. Severity of the impairment depends on the client's age, overall health, and degree of immobility.

Effects of Immobility

PHYSIOLOGICAL DIMENSION

- Metabolic
  - Fluid and electrolyte changes
  - Bone demineralization
  - Altered exchange of nutrients and gases
  - Altered gastrointestinal functioning
- Respiratory
  - Decreased lung expansion
  - Pooling of secretions
- Cardiovascular
  - Orthostatic hypotension
  - Increased cardiac workload
  - Thrombus formation
- Musculoskeletal
  - Decreased endurance
  - Decreased muscle mass
  - Atrophy
  - Decreased stability
  - Contracture formation
  - Osteoporosis
- Skin
  - Decubitus ulcer formation
- Elimination
  - Renal calculi
  - Stasis of urine
  - Kidney infection
  - Fecal constipation
  - Fecal impaction

PSYCHOSOCIAL DIMENSION

- Depression
- Behavioral changes
- Change in sleep-wake cycles
- Decreased coping abilities
- Decreased problem-solving abilities
- Decreased interest in surroundings
- Increased isolation
- Sensory deprivation

DEVELOPMENTAL DIMENSION

- Young
  - Retardation of developmental states
- Elderly
  - Increased rate of dependence
  - Increased rate of loss of system functions

Elderly clients with chronic illness develop pronounced effects more quickly than younger clients. The following sections detail effects of immobility on each body system.

METABOLIC CHANGES

Immobility disrupts normal metabolic equilibrium in the following ways: reduced metabolic rate, tissue atrophy and protein catabolism, fluid and electrolyte imbalances, bone demineralization, alterations in exchange of nutrients, and gastrointestinal disturbances.

Bed rest or reduced activity results in a decrease from the client's basal metabolic rate (BMR). The client's BMR falls in response to the decreased energy requirement of the body cells, which is directly related to cellular oxygen demands. However, immobilized clients with an infection may have an elevated metabolic rate because infection usually causes fever, which increases tissue oxygen requirements. In addition, immobilized clients with wounds often have an increased metabolic rate necessary for healing.

During immobilization, anabolic processes are decreased and catabolic processes are increased. This alteration is further enhanced by fever or conditions that increase the body's metabolic demands. *Anabolic processes* are constructive metabolic activities that convert simple substances into more complex compounds, as in the conversion of amino acids into muscle mass. *Catabolic processes* are metabolic activities that break down body structures to produce energy, as in the breakdown of protein stores to provide glucose for the body's energy requirements. If the rate of catabolism exceeds anabolism for a prolonged time, the body excretes more nitro-

gen than it takes in and a state of *negative nitrogen balance* occurs (Fig. 42-1). During periods of immobility, urinary excretion of nitrogen increases with the negative nitrogen balance. This occurs on the fifth or sixth day of immobilization in healthy subjects. Nitrogen loss reflects depletion of muscle mass. Certain pathological states and factors accelerate the rate of protein depletion and thus the development of negative nitrogen balance (see box). The major consequence is an inadequate supply of nitrogen for protein synthesis, which promotes rebuilding of muscle mass and wound healing.

When the body's protein stores become depleted, serum protein concentrations decrease. The resultant reduction in osmotic pressure causes fluid shifts from intravascular to interstitial compartments in dependent areas of the body, resulting in edema (see Chapter 37).

During reduced mobility the client's nutritional status is at risk of declining. The decline may be due to an inability to obtain, prepare, or eat food. In addition the client may be febrile or have cancer or another process that increases nutritional demand. Thus, nutritional expenditure exceeds intake.

Because of decreased protein and caloric intake and altered cardiovascular and respiratory functioning, the exchange of nutrients between cells is decreased. The cells do not receive adequate glucose, amino acids, and fats, or necessary oxygen to carry out metabolic activities. In addition, pressure exerted on body tissues because of immobilization decreases local circulation to tissues.

The inactivity of immobility decreases the rate at which food is digested (see Chapter 33). Abdominal dis-

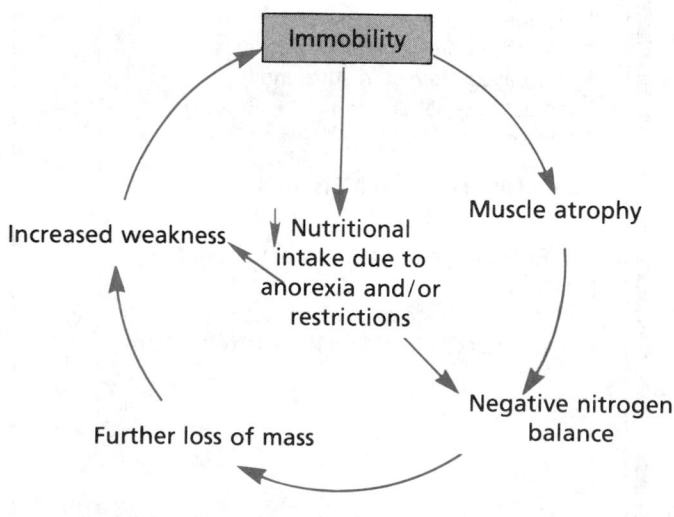

Fig. 42-1 Factors contributing to negative nitrogen balance associated with immobility.

From Groër, MW, and Shekleton, ME: Basic pathophysiology: a conceptual approach, ed. 2, St. Louis, 1983, The C.V. Mosby Co.

Conditions Associated with Negative Nitrogen Balance in Immobilization

- Poor nutrition before immobilization
- Alcohol or drug abuse
- Preexisting gastrointestinal disorder
- Preexisting kidney disorder
- Trauma
- Burns
- Fever
- Cancer
- Infection in one or more body systems
- Coma
- Surgery
- Anorexia
- Restrictions affecting self-feeding, such as traction

tention, nausea, epigastric burning, and food regurgitation may result. Food intake is a second factor that alters gastrointestinal function. An immobilized client may experience a pronounced decrease in food intake if unable to eat independently. Appetite may also be affected by immobilization. Changes in gastrointestinal functioning ultimately affect bowel elimination, often resulting in constipation or fecal impaction (see Chapter 39).

RESPIRATORY CHANGES

Respiratory problems occurring with prolonged immobility are caused by four major factors: decreased hemoglobin, decreased lung expansion, generalized muscle weakness, and stasis of pulmonary secretions.

Altered metabolism decreases the number of red blood cells, which contain hemoglobin. Hemoglobin transports oxygen from alveoli in the lungs to tissues. Decreased hemoglobin results in anemia. When anemia is present, the oxygen-carrying capacity of blood is reduced, so oxygen available to tissues is decreased. Initially the body tries to adapt by increasing the heart rate, but this is a short-term response and ultimately increases cardiac workload.

Immobilization also decreases lung expansion because the bed mattress limits space for expansion. Decreased lung expansion decreases exchange of respiratory gases

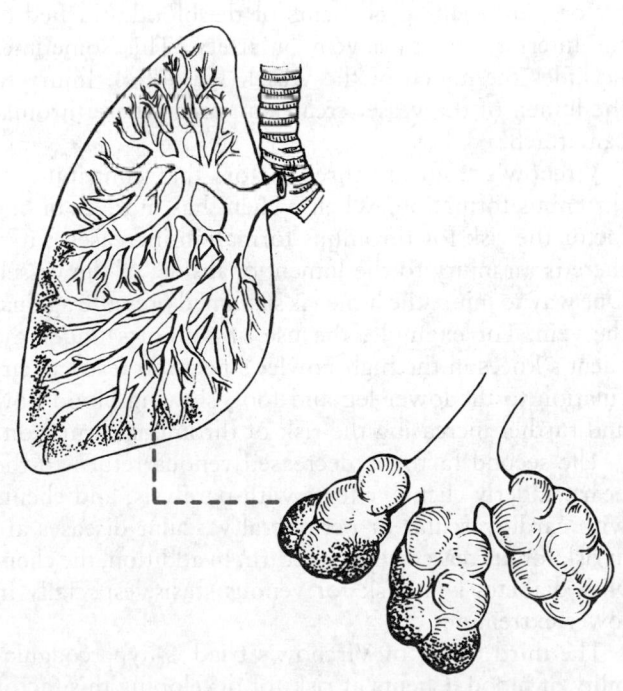

Fig. 42-2 Pooling of secretions in dependent regions of the lungs in the supine position.

between the lungs and circulating blood volume, and increases pooling of respiratory secretions.

Normally, blood is oxygenated in pulmonary circulation when it contacts oxygen-filled alveoli. The carbon dioxide waste product is carried by the blood to the lungs and exhaled. When lung expansion is decreased, the surface area of lung tissue through which the respiratory gases are exchanged is also decreased. Therefore less oxygen is available for the blood, carbon dioxide is retained, and respiratory acidosis develops (see Chapter 36).

With decreased lung expansion and immobilization, secretions stagnate or pool in the dependent region of the lungs (Fig. 42-2). Persons who smoke or who have a chronic lung condition or a productive cough are at risk for increased amounts of secretions. The secretions encourage bacterial growth, which may lead to bronchopneumonia.

The immobilized client with an underlying disease may also experience general muscle weakness, which affects muscles of respiration and muscles needed to cough. Lung expansion declines further and coughing becomes weaker. These two factors increase distribution of mucus in the bronchi, particularly when the client is in a supine, prone, or lateral position. Fig. 42-3 demonstrates gravity's effect on mucus distribution within a bronchus. When the client is in a horizontal position, mucus accumulates in the dependent regions of the bronchial tube. Because mucus is an excellent medium for bacterial growth, hypostatic bronchopneumonia may result.

CARDIOVASCULAR CHANGES

The cardiovascular system is also affected by immobility. The three major changes are orthostatic hypotension, increased cardiac workload, and thrombus formation (Olson, 1967).

Orthostatic or postural hypotension is a drop of 15 mm Hg or more in blood pressure when the client moves from a horizontal to a vertical position. Immobilized clients and those on prolonged bed rest are at risk for orthostatic hypotension because the ability of the autonomic nervous system to equalize blood supply is diminished in a client who has been recumbent for a prolonged period. In an immobilized client, the absence or reduction of peripheral vasoconstriction allows a pooling of venous blood in lower extremities. This in turn decreases venous return to the heart, leading to a decreased cardiac output and lower blood pressure. As a result the client becomes dizzy on rising and may even faint.

Prolonged immobility also decreases muscle tone, contributing to orthostatic hypotension. Because there is a correlation between contractility of muscle with inactivity, vasodilation is increased, and decreased muscle

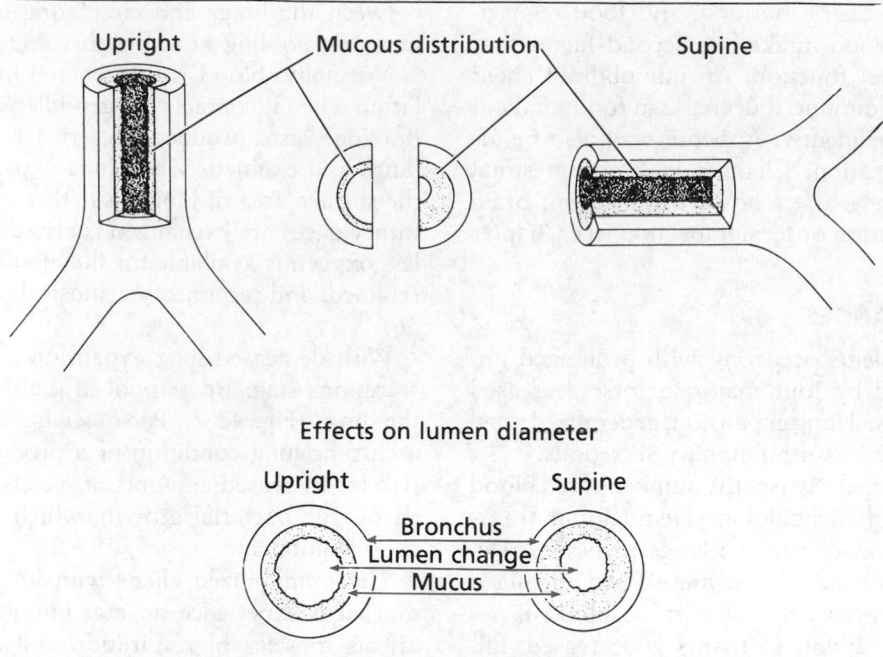

Effects on lumen diameter

Fig. 42-3 Effect of recumbency and gravity on distribution of respiratory tract and diameter of bronchiolar lumen.

From Groër, MW and Shekleton, ME: *Basic pathophysiology: a conceptual approach*, ed. 2, St. Louis, 1983, The C.V. Mosby Co.

tone in the legs reduces the muscular pump's action on the great veins in the lower extremities. Venous return to the heart is decreased, resulting in hypotension.

An immobilized, horizontal client has an increased cardiac workload. In this position, blood that normally pools in lower extremities is mobilized and increases venous return to the heart. As a result, the heart must increase its stroke volume. The overall workload of the heart is increased, and resting pulse rate rises, which further contributes to workload. In immobile clients the workload of the heart is further increased by the Valsalva maneuver. The *Valsalva maneuver* is any forced expiratory effort against a closed airway, as when a person holds the breath and tightens muscles in a strenous effort to move a heavy object or to change position in bed. Clients on bed rest tend to use the Valsalva maneuver when using their arms and upper trunk muscles to move in bed. When the breath is held, intrathoracic pressure increases dramatically, causing blood to pool in the vessels. This markedly diminishes venous return to the heart and the heart rate increases. When a held breath is released, intrathoracic pressure falls dramatically and the venous return to the heart increases significantly, which in turn decreases heart rate. Clients with cardiac illness should be discouraged from doing the Valsalva maneuver because it can cause cardiac dysrhythmias or arrest.

Thrombus formation is another major hazard to the cardiovascular system resulting from immobility. A *thrombus* is an accumulation of platelets, fibrin, clotting factors, and cellular elements of the blood attached to the interior wall of a vein or artery. This sometimes occludes the lumen of the vessel (Fig. 42-4). Injury to the lumen of the vessel creates an area where thrombi can attach.

Virchow's triad are three factors that contribute to thrombus formation. When a client has more than one factor the risk for thrombus formation increases. First, there is an injury to the lumen, or inside, of the vessel. One way to injure the lumen is sustained pressure against the vein. For example, the use of supports under the client's knees in the high Fowler's position restricts circulation to the lower leg and foot, slowing blood flow and further increasing the risk of thrombus formation.

The second factor is decreased venous return to the heart. Elderly clients, clients with paralysis, and clients with cardiovascular or peripheral vascular diseases are at risk for decreased venous return. In addition, the client with diabetes is at risk for venous stasis, especially in lower extremities.

The third factor of Virchow's triad is hypercoagulability of blood. Clients at risk for developing this factor have impaired clotting mechanisms or excessive red blood cells.

The danger of thrombus formation is that the throm-

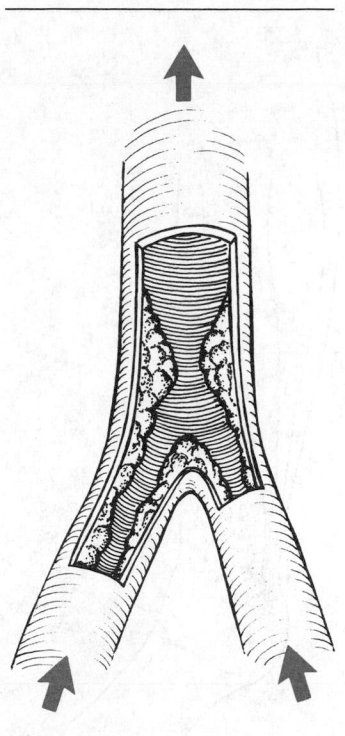

Fig. 42-4 Thrombus formation in a vessel.

bus may break away from the vein to become an emboli or clot that travels to the lungs, heart, or brain, resulting in a pulmonary emboli, heart attack, or stroke.

MUSCULOSKELETAL CHANGES

The effects of immobility on the musculoskeletal system can include permanent impairment of mobility. Immobility can cause gradual changes in the muscles and skeleton.

Restricted mobility affects muscles in four ways: loss of endurance, decreased muscle mass, atrophy, and decreased stability. *Loss of endurance* results primarily from decreased functional capacity of muscles associated with disuse. This is characterized by decreased muscle mass, atrophy, and decreased stability.

Decreased muscle mass and subsequent decreases in strength are directly related to disuse and nutritional alterations associated with immobility. Increased catabolism and reduced anabolism result in a reduction in both cell size and available cellular energy. Decreased muscle mass is often called muscular atrophy.

Muscular atrophy resulting from immobilization is observable and measurable. The size of muscles decreases. Antigravity muscles in the legs appear to be most affected by immobilization, supporting the theory that stresses of gravity are important in maintaining function, development, and therefore mobility (Groër and Shekleton, 1983).

Reduced muscle endurance for physical activity results from changes in the muscles and altered cardiovascular functioning. Immobility increases cardiac workload, and heart rate and cardiac output may actually fall, because of declining myocardial reserve. This further decreases muscular endurance. Manifestations of these muscular effects include weakness, fatigue, and tachycardia. If the immobilized client does not exercise, loss of endurance will lead to greater reduction in physical activity, thus increasing the loss of endurance in a vicious circle. In addition, the immobilized client experiences decreased physical stability. Immobility disrupts muscular stability and reduces ability to move steadily. Such clients are at risk for losing their balance when changing position.

Immobilization causes two major alterations in the skeletal system: joint contractures and osteoporosis. Joint contractures involve the muscles and skeletal system. A *joint contracture* is an abnormal and usually permanent condition of a joint. It is characterized by flexion and fixation and caused by disuse, atrophy, and shortening of muscle fibers. When a contracture occurs, the muscle cannot maintain full range of joint motion. Unfortunately, contractures usually leave the joint in a nonfunctional position. One such condition is permanent flexion of the elbow joint (Fig. 42-5).

A second common contracture is foot-drop (Fig. 42-6). Foot-drop results in the foot being permanently fixed in plantar flexion. Ambulation is difficult with the foot in this position. If foot-drop occurs in both feet, the client is unable to walk without adaptive devices. Nursing care for partially or completely immobilized clients is directed toward preventing contractures through active or passive range of joint motion exercises, proper body alignment, positioning aids, weight bearing activities, such as walking and standing and encouraging independence in activities of daily living (see Chapter 41).

Marked reductions in skeletal mass, or *disuse osteoporosis*, routinely accompany prolonged immobilization or paralysis. The processes of bone formation and resorption (destruction of bone cells) are normally maintained in balance. Immobility, however, causes bone resorption to be relatively greater. Because *bone resorption* causes release of calcium into the blood, immobilized clients become hypercalcemic. Calcium is excreted in large quantities in the urine, which predisposes the immobilized client to renal calculi. The link between disuse osteoporosis and immobility is twofold. Both immobilization and non-weight-bearing activities increase the rate of bone resorption.

The nurse can help maintain joint mobility by performing passive exercises for the immobilized client. Passive range of joint motion alone does not have positive effects on the muscle or bone itself. Active exercise such as walking, aerobics, and jogging are beneficial to muscle and bone.

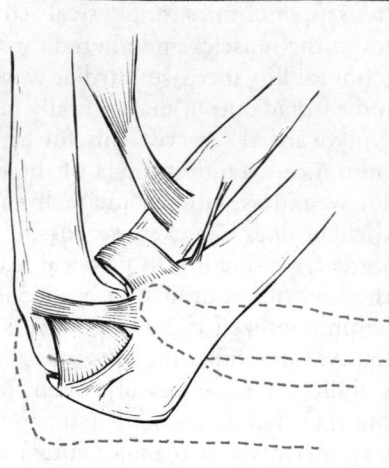

Fig. 42-5 Contracture of the elbow resulting in permanent flexion of the joint. Normally the elbow is able to extend to a 90° angle *(dotted line)* and to a 180° angle (not illustrated).

SKIN CHANGES

The devastating effect of immobility on the skin is compounded by impaired body metabolism and negative nitrogen balance. Any break in the skin is difficult to heal, which may lead to further immobilization. A break in the skin is referred to as a bedsore, pressure sore, or decubitus ulcer.

A *decubitus ulcer* is an inflammation, sore, or ulcer in the skin over a bony prominence. Decubitus ulcers have long been recognized as a hazard for debilitated and immobilized clients. Because the skin—the body's first line of defense against entry of infectious microorganisms—becomes broken, the client is at risk for systemic infection.

In addition, a decubitus ulcer increases loss of body fluids. As the decubitus ulcer invades subcutaneous body tissues, protein- and electrolyte-rich body fluids begin to exit at the site. If fluid loss is significant, the client can develop electrolyte imbalances such as hypokalemia and hypoalbuminemia.

DECUBITUS ULCER FORMATION. Decubitus ulcers form as a result of pressure or from a "shearing force" when moving the client up in bed. The effect of pressure can be increased by an unequal distribution of body weight. Because of gravity, a person is subjected to constant pressures of the body against any surface on which it rests (Berecek, 1975). If the pressure is unevenly distributed on the body, a pressure gradient is increased on those tissues receiving pressure. The cellular metabolism of the skin is altered at the point of pressure.

Normally tissue metabolism depends on receiving oxygen and nutrients from the blood supply and elimi-

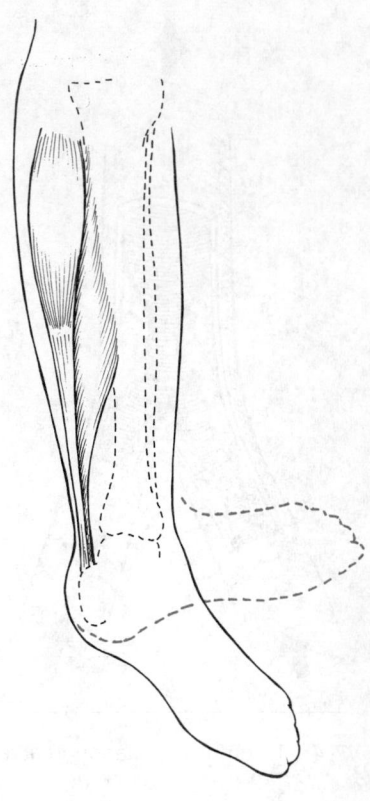

Fig. 42-6 Foot-drop. Ankle is fixed in plantar flexion. Normally the ankle is able to flex *(dotted line)*, which eases walking.

nating metabolites and carbon dioxide. Any factor that interferes with this process clearly affects cellular metabolism and, as a result, the function or life of the cell.

Pressure affects cellular metabolism by decreasing or obliterating tissue circulation. Subsequently, tissue metabolism is changed.

When a client is lying in bed or sitting in a chair, body weight is heavily placed on certain bony prominences. Body surfaces subjected to the greatest weight or pressure are those at greatest risk for decubitus ulcer formation. Researchers have shown that, in people with normal body weight, the following body regions receive the greatest pressures (Linden et al., 1965):

POSITION	POINTS OF PRESSURE
Sitting	Ischial tuberosities, sacrum
Supine	Back of skull, elbows, sacrum, ischial tuberosities, heels
Prone	Elbows, knees, toes
Side-lying	Knees, greater trochanters

The longer pressure is applied, the greater is the risk of skin breakdown. Leaving an immobilized client in a position for longer than 2 hours (and sometimes less) increases risk of skin breakdown.

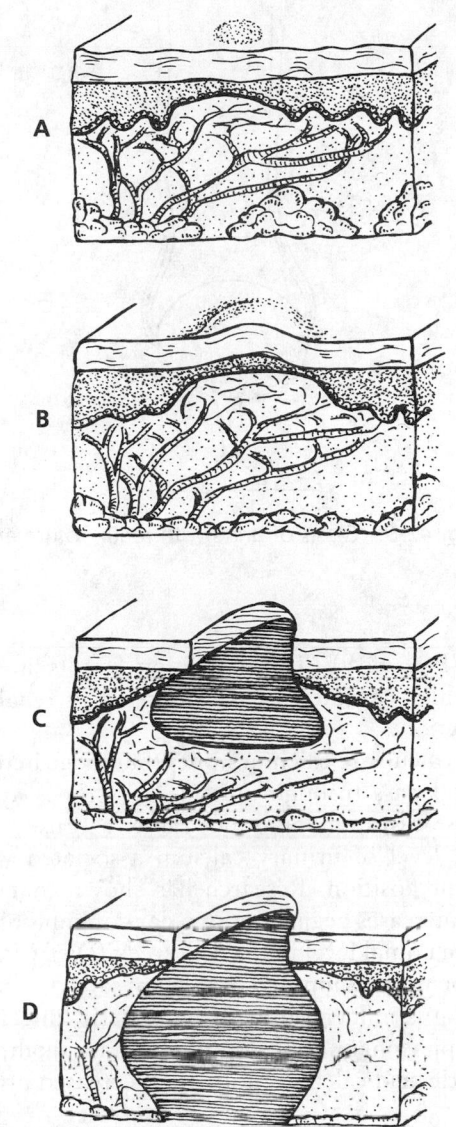

Fig. 42-7   A, Stage I decubitus ulcer. B, Stage II decubitus ulcer. C, Stage III decubitus ulcer. D, Stage IV decubitus ulcer

When blood supply to tissues is diminished, they become ischemic. Ischemia is a decreased blood supply to a body part—in this case the skin. A compensatory response of the tissues to ischemia is reactive hyperemia, an increased blood flow. This permits ischemic tissue to be flooded with blood when pressure is removed. Increased blood flow increases delivery of oxygen and nutrients to tissue. The metabolic debt resulting from pressure can then be met, healthy equilibrium restored, and necrosis of the compressed tissue avoided (Berecek, 1975). Reactive hyperemia is a compensatory response and is effective only if pressure is removed before damage begins in the critical period between 1 and 2 hours.

STAGES OF DECUBITUS ULCERS. Decubitus ulcer formation may occur initially in superficial layers of the skin. The ulcer that is first seen as an area of erythema can progress rapidly to penetrate underlying tissues and can even extend so deep that bony surfaces are exposed. Deep sores do not originate in the skin but are considered to result from a process that begins in deep tissues and spreads to the surface (Berecek, 1975).

Guttmann (1955) defined the following stages in development of a decubitus ulcer (Fig. 42-7):

1. Reddening of skin, which disappears when pressure is relieved
2. Superficial circulatory and tissue damage; reddening and edema that do not disappear; induration of superficial tissue
3. Destruction of subcutaneous layers; necrotic cells; destruction of the underlying capillary bed
4. Advanced destruction of subcutaneous capillaries and muscle mass; if deep enough, exposure of bone

CONTRIBUTING FACTORS TO DECUBITUS ULCER FORMATION. Although many decubitus ulcers are caused by pressure, other factors may contribute to their formation. These include shearing force, moisture, poor nutrition, anemia, infection, and fever.

Shearing force is pressure exerted when a client is moved or repositioned in bed by being pulled or when allowed to slide down in bed (Fig. 42-8). Shearing force

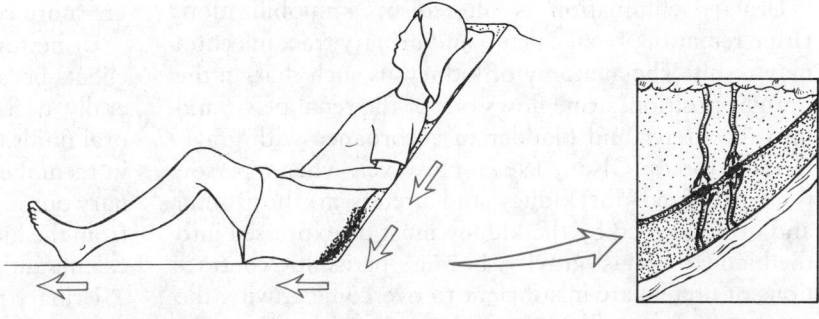

Fig. 42-8   Diagrammatic sketch of shearing force exerted against sacral area.

is the second major cause of decubitus ulcers. With a shearing force the skin and subcutaneous layers adhere to the surface of the bed while the layers of muscle and even the bones slide in the direction of body movement. Underlying capillaries are severed by layers of tissue moving or shearing against each other and create minute layers of bleeding and tissue necrosis deep in tissue layers. Eventually a sinus tract opens to the skin to allow drainage from the necrosis.

The presence of *moisture* on the skin increases the risk of ulcer formation. Moisture reduces the skin's resistance to other physical factors, such as pressure or shearing force. The susceptibility to decubitus ulcers increases proportionally with the duration of skin moisture from perspiration, urine or wound drainage. The immobilized client, unable to meet hygiene needs, depends on the nurse to maintain skin integrity. The nurse must therefore incorporate hygiene into the plan of care.

Clients with *poor nutrition* often experience serious weight loss, muscle atrophy, and decreases in subcutaneous tissue and muscle mass (see Chapter 33). Because of these changes, less tissue is present to serve as padding between the skin and underlying bone. Therefore the effects of pressure are increased on remaining tissue.

Poor nutrition can also alter the client's fluid and electrolyte balance. In clients with severe protein loss, hypoalbuminemia leads to a shift of fluid from the extracellular fluid volume to the tissues, resulting in edema. In addition, clients with poor nutrition generally have impaired wound healing.

Clients with *anemia* are at risk for decubitus ulcer formation because decreased hemoglobin reduces the oxygen-carrying capacity of the blood and the amount of oxygen available to tissues. Anemia also alters cellular metabolism and impairs wound healing.

Infection results from bacteria within the body. When an infection is present, metabolic demands, and therefore oxygen and nutritional demands, of the body increase. In addition, fever that usually accompanies infection results in diaphoresis and increases skin moisture, which further predisposes a client to skin breakdown.

URINARY ELIMINATION CHANGES

Urinary elimination is altered by immobilization. Urine retention, renal calculi, and urinary tract infection may result. The anatomy of kidneys is such that, in the upright position, urine flows out of the renal pelvis and into the ureter and bladder in accordance with gravitational forces (Olson, 1967). However, when a person is immobilized, the kidney and ureters are horizontal and urine formed by the kidney must be expressed into the bladder against gravity. Because peristaltic contractions of ureters are insufficient to overcome gravity, the renal pelvis may fill before urine is expressed into the

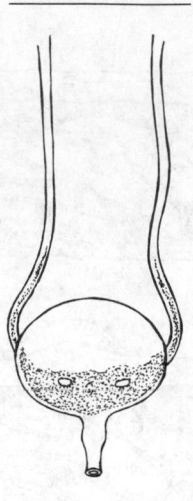

Fig. 42-9 Stasis of urine with reflux to ureters.

ureters (Fig. 42-9). This condition results in urinary stasis, which can increase development of renal calculi and infection.

Renal calculi are calcium stones that lodge in the renal pelvis and pass through ureters. The stones are not a direct result of immobility but rather a consequence of the high level of urinary calcium associated with the recumbent position. Research has shown that urinary calcium increases begin after two days of immobility and reach a maximal level in the fifth week (Dietrick, 1948). Most stones are composed of calcium salts. Calcium salt deposition is influenced by urinary stasis, infection, increased phosphate concentration, urine alkalinity, altered citric acid/calcium ratio, and decreased urine production.

The potential for a urinary tract infection is increased by immobility, which predisposes the kidneys to urinary stasis. This in turn allows bacteria to grow in the stagnant urine. Stagnant urine permits accumulation of deposits within the renal pelvis, resulting in the formation of renal calculi (Fig. 42-10).

Urinary stasis can also occur in the bladder and cause infection. Bladder infections resulting from immobility are more common than renal (kidney) infections.

Urine formation is usually decreased in immobilized clients because of two factors. First, fluid intake is generally decreased because of dependence on others for oral fluids. Second, because cardiac output is decreased in recumbency, renal blood flow is diminished and urinary output declines. When this natural flushing of urine from the kidney and bladder is reduced, the risks of both calculi and infections are increased.

Urinary tract infections result from bacteria in one or more structures of the urinary tract. Most of these in-

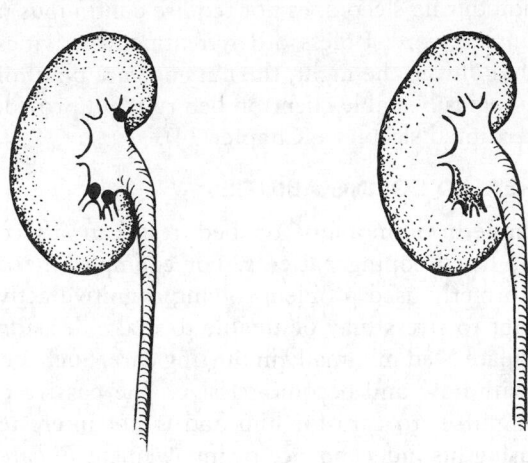

Fig. 42-10 Types of renal calculi in the renal pelvis.

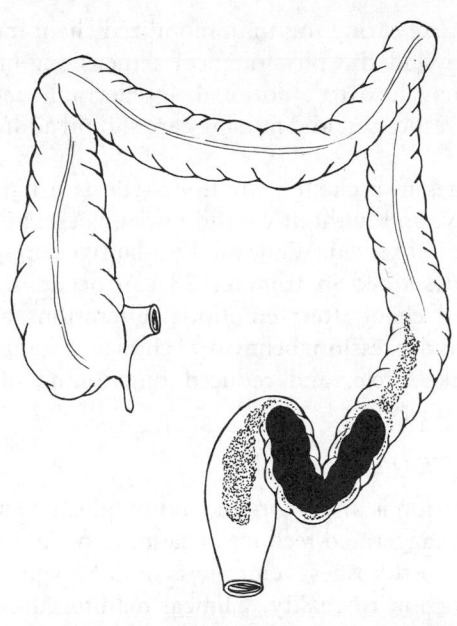

Fig. 42-11 Fecal impaction with liquid stool passing around the impaction.

fections are caused by gram-negative bacteria, especially *Escherichia coli (E. coli)* or species of *Klebsiella, Proteus, Pseudomonas,* or *Enterobacter.* Common urinary tract infections are cystitis, pyelonephritis, and urethritis (see Chapter 38). During immobilization, urinary tract infections can result from three causes: incorrect perineal care, indwelling catheter placement, and urinary reflux into the ureters.

Inadequate perineal care is a major cause of infection, particularly among women who have fecal incontinence. Because of the proximity of the female urethra to the anal region, *E. coli* bacteria may enter the urinary tract, resulting in an infection. Correct perineal care can reduce the risk of infection (see Chapter 32).

Another cause of urinary tract infections in immobilized clients is an indwelling urinary catheter, which provides a pathway for bacteria to ascend into the bladder and occasionally the kidney, causing pyelonephritis.

Urinary tract infections can be the result of retained urine. If the bladder is allowed to overfill, it becomes distended. The bladder of an immobilized client should be palpated to detect distention. Distension may be relieved with the insertion of a sterile catheter or emptied by the Credé method (see Chapter 38).

BOWEL ELIMINATION CHANGES

Bowel elimination is also affected by immobilization. The most common alteration is constipation. Constipation does not result directly from immobility but rather from weakened abdominal and perineal muscles and decreased gastric motility, which are effects of immobilization. Immobility may also cause a decrease in the client's expulsive power and defecation reflex.

Reduction of the defecation reflex as a consequence

of immobility is related to several factors. Primarily the immobilized client may be forced to suppress the need to defecate because no one is available to offer assistance with bedpan placement. Postponing defecation when the stimulus is present may produce an inhibition of colonic motility and a weakening of the gastrocolic, duodenocolic, "mass movements," and defecation reflex.

The nursing care plan should be designed to prevent constipation. Uncorrected constipation can lead to fecal impaction, an accumulation of hardened fecal material in the rectum or sigmoid colon. When fecal material remains in the bowel, water is continually reabsorbed from it through the intestinal wall, and the fecal contents become increasingly drier and harder. Constipation also increases client's use of the Valsalva maneuver, with all the inherent problems previously described.

An early sign of an impaction is frequent passage of liquid stool. This is not diarrhea. The liquid stool is merely passing around the area of impaction. It is usually a small amount of fecal smear or a thin ribbon of diarrheal-like stool (Fig. 42-11). An untreated impaction can lead to a mechanical bowel obstruction that completely or partially occludes the intestinal lumen, blocking normal propulsions of liquid and gas. The resulting fluid stasis within the intestine produces distention and increases intraluminal pressure. Finally, intestinal function becomes depressed, dehydration occurs, and absorption ceases, resulting in fluid and electrolyte imbalance (see Chapter 37).

Psychosocial Responses

The nurse caring for an immobilized client must meet needs beyond the physiological dimension. Immobilization may lead to emotional, intellectual, and socio-cultural responses, and nursing care should address these needs.

Changes in a client's emotional status usually occur gradually, and without careful nursing assessment they may go unobserved. While all the adaptive coping mechanisms described in Chapter 28 can occur in the immobilized client, four emotional alterations are most common: depression, behavioral changes, changes in the sleep-wake cycle, and reduced functioning of coping mechanisms.

DEPRESSION

Depression is an abnormal emotional state characterized by exaggerated feelings of sadness, melancholy, dejection, worthlessness, emptiness, and hopelessness out of proportion to reality. Clinical manifestations range from a slight lack of motivation and inability to concentrate to physiological alterations and severe emotional dysfunction.

The immobilized client is at risk for becoming depressed because of changes in role, self-concept, and other factors. Depression can result from worrying about health, finances, and family needs. Because immobilization removes the client from daily routine, there is more time to worry about disability and level of health. This can quickly increase the client's depression, causing more withdrawal.

BEHAVIORAL CHANGES

Behavioral changes resulting from immobilization vary widely depending on the individual. Moreover, changes in behavior may differ from day to day.

Common behavioral changes include hostility, belligerence, giddiness, withdrawal, confusion, and anxiety. Early in the nursing process family and friends should be interviewed concerning the client's normal behavioral patterns in order to gain baseline data. If nurses later observe unexpected behavior, they can intervene to reduce the effects of immobilization on behavioral patterns.

CHANGES IN SLEEP-WAKE CYCLE

The immobilized client requires round-the-clock nursing care. Because of the physiological hazards, the client cannot be allowed to sleep for 8 hours without having body position changed or other nursing care performed. Disruption of the client's normal sleeping pattern can further potentiate the client's behavioral changes. Nursing interventions should be used to ensure sufficient sleep.

The client who is on bed rest and is able to change position during sleep does not require continuous physical nursing care. Unless other treatment activities are required during the night, the nursing care plan for the physiologically stable client on bed rest can provide for uninterrupted sleep (see Chapter 34).

DECREASED COPING ABILITIES

Long-term immobility or bed rest can affect the client's usual coping patterns. For example, the client who formerly used problem-solving cognitive activities to adapt to stress may be unable to make decisions or participate even minimally in nursing care. Such a client may withdraw and become passive. The passive client allows nurses to care for him and is not interested in increasing his independence or involvement in care.

Early in the care of an immobilized client nurses should determine how the client normally handles stress. Then they design a nursing care plan to allow continued use of these coping abilities or help develop new ones.

Developmental Responses

Developmental changes associated with immobility tend to be greater with clients at each end of the life span: the young and elderly.

The infant, toddler, or preschooler is usually immobilized because of trauma or a congenital skeletal or neuromuscular abnormality. Immobilization can retard the child's motor skill and intellectual development.

Nurses caring for immobilized children should plan activities that provide physical and psychosocial stimuli. Other activities focus on specific effects of immobilization. For example, parents of a 1-year-old with immobilized lower extremities from congenital hip dysplasia need to be reassured that delay in their child's walking is temporary and that, following muscle strengthening exercises, motor development will progress.

Immobilization of elderly clients increases their physical dependence and accelerates functional losses in physiological systems. Usually immobilization of an elderly client results from a fractured hip, osteoarthritis, neurological trauma such as a stroke, or a chronic illness such as cardiopulmonary disease. For some clients immobilization occurs gradually and progressively. For others, especially those who have had a stroke, immobilization is sudden.

When providing care for an elderly client, the nurse should develop a care plan that encourages as many self-care activities as possible, thereby maintaining the client's highest level of mobility.

■ ■ ■

Bed rest and immobilization have beneficial effects and when used appropriately can help restore many clients' level of wellness. However, restriction in mobility is accompanied by many potential hazards that affect the client in all dimensions. If the nurse does not intervene appropriately, the effects of immobility can rapidly worsen, increasing the client's disability and the duration and cost of health care. The nurse continually assesses immobilized clients to minimize these hazards.

ASSESSMENT

Nursing assessment includes the client's level of mobility and potential effects of immobility.

Assessment of Mobility

Assessment of client mobility focuses on range of joint motion, muscle strength, activity tolerance, gait, posture, physical fitness level, muscle endurance, cardiovascular endurance, and ability for activities of daily living. Chapter 41 describes the normal range of movement for joints in the body. Observation of the client during daily activities enables the nurse to estimate fatigability and muscle strength. These assessment data assist in developing a nursing care plan that encourages the client to maintain mobility by increasing the energy level or overall muscle strength.

Finally, observing posture and gait helps the nurse determine what assistance the client may require to change positions or transfer from bed to chair. This information helps the nurse assess overall mobility and coordination.

Assessment of Hazards of Immobility

The nurse assesses the immobilized client for hazards of immobility by performing a head-to-toe physical assessment (see Chapter 13). In addition, the nursing assessment should focus on certain physiological areas, as well as the client's psychosocial and developmental dimensions.

PHYSIOLOGICAL ASSESSMENT

The physiological hazards of immobility that may be identified during a nursing assessment are summarized in Table 42-1.

METABOLIC SYSTEM. When assessing metabolic functioning, the nurse: (1) uses anthropometric measurements to evaluate muscle atrophy, (2) uses intake and output records and laboratory data to evaluate fluid and electrolyte status and serum protein levels (3) assesses wound healing to evaluate alterations in the exchange of nutrients, and (4) assesses the client's food intake and elimination patterns to determine altered gastrointestinal functioning.

Anthropometric measurements include height, weight, mid-upper arm circumference, and triceps skinfold measurements. Ideally, this assessment should be done early in the period of immobilization and should be repeated at 3-week intervals. A decrease in mid-upper arm circumference, measured in centimeters, or triceps skinfold, measured in millimeters, indicates a decline in muscle mass (Blackburn, 1977). This decline, along with decreased serum protein and decreased white cell count, can indicate that more protein is breaking down than building up. As a result the client may be at risk for

TABLE 42-1   Physiological Hazards of Immobility

System	Assessment Techniques	Abnormal Findings
Metabolic	Inspection	Slowed wound healing
	Inspection	Muscle atrophy
	Anthropometric measurements (mid–upper arm circumference, triceps skinfold measurement)	Decreased amount of subcutaneous fat
	Palpation	Generalized edema owing to hypoalbuminemia
Respiratory	Inspection	Asymmetrical chest wall movement
	Auscultation	Presence of crackles, wheezes, increased respiratory rate
Cardiovascular	Auscultation	Orthostatic hypotension
	Auscultation and palpation	Increased heart rate; presence of third heart sound; weak peripheral pulses
Musculoskeletal	Inspection and palpation	Increased diameter in calf or thigh
	Palpation	Decreased joint motion
Skin	Inspection	Break in skin integrity
Elimination	Inspection	Decreased urine output, cloudy or concentrated urine, decreased frequency of bowel movements

severe negative nitrogen imbalance. Measurements of the mid-upper arm circumference and triceps skinfold provide baseline information about subcutaneous fat, which may be lost during immobilization (see Chapter 33).

Intake and output measurements assist the nurse in determining if a fluid imbalance exists. Dehydration and edema can increase the speed of skin breakdown in an immobilized client. Laboratory measurement of serum electrolytes can also indicate an electrolyte imbalance.

If an immobilized client has a wound, the speed of healing indicates how well nutrients are being delivered to tissues. Normal progression of healing indicates that metabolic needs of injured tissues are being met.

Anorexia occurs commonly in immobilized clients. The client's food intake should be assessed before the tray is removed to determine how much is eaten. Nutritional imbalances can be avoided if the nurse learns the client's dietary patterns and food preferences early in his immobilization.

RESPIRATORY SYSTEM. A respiratory assessment should be performed at least every 2 hours for clients with restricted activity. The nurse inspects chest wall movements during the full inspiratory-expiratory cycle. If a client has an atelectatic area, chest movement may be asymmetrical. In addition, the nurse auscultates the entire lung region to identify diminished breath sounds, crackles, or wheezes. Auscultation should focus on the dependent lung fields, since pulmonary secretions tend to collect in these lower regions. A complete respiratory assessment identifies the presence of secretions and can be used to determine the nursing interventions necessary for optimal respiratory function.

CARDIOVASCULAR SYSTEM. Cardiovascular nursing assessment of the immobilized client includes blood pressure monitoring, evaluation of apical and peripheral pulses, and observation for signs of venous stasis (for example, edema, poor wound healing). Because of the risk for orthostatic hypotension, the client's blood pressure should be measured, particularly when changing from a lying (recumbent) to a sitting or standing position. In this way ability to tolerate postural changes can be assessed before the client leaves the safety of the bed.

The nurse also assesses apical and peripheral pulses. Recumbency increases cardiac workload and results in an increased pulse rate. In some clients, particularly the elderly, the heart may not tolerate the increased workload, and a form of cardiac failure may develop. The presence of a third heart sound, heard at the apex, can be an early indication of congestive heart failure. Monitoring peripheral pulses allows the nurse to evaluate the heart's ability to pump blood. The absence of a peripheral pulse in the lower extremities, particularly one that

was previously present, should be documented and reported to the client's physician.

Edema may indicate the heart's inability to handle the increased workload. Because edema moves to dependent body regions, assessment of the immobilized client should include the sacrum, legs, and feet. If the heart is unable to tolerate the increased workload, peripheral body regions, such as the hands, feet, nose, and earlobes, will be colder than central body regions.

Finally, the nurse assesses the venous system because deep vein thrombosis is a hazard of restricted mobility. A dislodged thrombus, called an embolus, may travel through the circulatory system to the lungs or brain and impair circulation. Emboli to the lungs or brain pose a threat to life.

To assess for a deep vein thrombosis, remove the client's elastic stockings every 8 hours and observe the calves for redness, warmth, and tenderness. In addition, calf circumference should be measured daily. To do this the nurse marks a point on each calf 10 cm from the midpatella. The circumference is measured each day using the mark for placement of the tape measure. One-sided increases in calf diameter can be an early indication of thrombosis. Since deep vein thrombosis can also occur in the thigh, thigh measurements should be taken daily if the client is prone to thrombosis. In many clients, deep vein thrombosis can be prevented by active exercise and elastic stockings. Both procedures are detailed in the intervention section later in the chapter.

MUSCULOSKELETAL SYSTEM. Major musculoskeletal abnormalities that may be identified during nursing assessment include decreased muscle tone, loss of muscle mass, contractures, and osteoporosis. The anthropometric measurements described earlier may indicate losses in muscle tone and muscle mass.

Assessment of range of motion is important as a baseline against which later measurements can be compared to evaluate whether a loss in joint mobility has occurred. Range of joint motion is measured with a goniometer (see Chapters 13 and 41).

Disuse osteoporosis cannot be identified by physical assessment. However, postmenopausal women and persons with increased serum and urine calcium levels probably have a greater risk for bone demineralization. The risk of disuse osteoporosis should be considered when planning nursing interventions. For example, rib percussion and vibration should be done cautiously with a client with probable disuse osteoporosis, because of the risk of rib fracture.

SKIN. The nurse must continually assess the client's skin for signs of breakdown. It should be observed each time the client is turned or hygiene measures performed. At the minimum assessment should occur every 2 hours.

In addition, the nurse should be alert for risk factors that increase potential for skin breakdown. First, the nurse assesses the client's position and how position is changed to determine if a shearing force exists. If it does, the position should be changed immediately. Second, the nurse assesses the skin for moisture such as urine or perspiration, which increases the chance of skin breakdown. Third, the nurse assesses possible pressure points to determine if they are protected. Chapter 41 describes body alignments for the Fowler's, supine, prone, side-lying, and Sims' positions. Last, the nurse assesses nutritional and hydration status and looks for evidence of infection, since these are risk factors for skin breakdown.

ELIMINATION SYSTEM. The client's elimination status should be evaluated on each shift, and total intake and output should be evaluated every 24 hours. The nurse should determine that the client is receiving the correct amount and type of fluids orally or parenterally (see Chapter 37).

Inadequate fluid and electrolyte balances or intake and output can increase the risk for renal impairment, ranging from recurrent infections to kidney failure. Dehydration can also increase risk for skin breakdown, thrombi formation, respiratory infections, and constipation. These conditions decrease overall level of mobility and increase duration and cost of care.

Assessment of elimination status should also include the frequency and consistency of bowel movements. Accurate assessment enables the nurse to intervene before constipation and fecal impaction occurs.

PSYCHOSOCIAL ASSESSMENT

Changes in the client's psychosocial status usually occur slowly and are often overlooked by health care personnel. The nurse should observe for inappropriate changes in emotional status. If the client seems depressed, the nurse should observe for several days before concluding that the depression is abnormal. Everyone becomes depressed at some time, especially hospitalized and immobilized clients, but not all depression requires nursing intervention. If the depression is caused by boredom or isolation, it can be alleviated by increasing bedside activities and occupational therapy.

The nurse also observes for behavioral changes, such as the cooperative client who becomes argumentative or the modest client who begins to expose himself repeatedly. The nurse should try to determine the reasons for such alterations to identify specific nursing therapies.

Unexplained changes in the client's sleep-wake cycle must be identified and corrected. Most can be prevented or minimized, such as those occurring because of nursing activities, a noisy environment, or discomfort. They may also occur because of medications such as analgesics, sleeping pills, or cardiovascular drugs.

Finally, the nurse should observe for changes in the client's use of normal coping mechanisms to adapt to immobilization (see Chapter 28). Decreasing coping ability may cause the client to become disoriented, confused, or depressed or to experience other behavioral changes.

Because these psychosocial changes usually occur gradually, the nurse should observe the client's behavior on a daily basis. If behavioral changes do occur, the nurse should determine the causes and evaluate the changes as short or long term. Identifying the cause helps the nurse design appropriate nursing interventions.

DEVELOPMENTAL ASSESSMENT

Assessment of the immobilized client should include developmental considerations to ensure that the client's needs are identified. With a young child the nurse determines whether the child is able to meet developmental tasks and is progressing normally. The child's development may regress or be slowed because of immobilization. By identifying a child's overall developmental needs, the nurse can design nursing therapies to maintain normal development. When developmental delays are temporary, the nurse may also need to assure the parents.

Developmental assessment is as important with the geriatric client as with the young child. The nursing assessment enables the nurse to determine the elderly client's ability to meet needs independently and to adapt to developmental changes, such as declining physical functioning and altered family and peer relationships. A decline in developmental functioning needs prompt investigation to determine why the change occurred and what can be done to return to an optimal level of function as soon as possible.

NURSING DIAGNOSIS

Assessment reveals clusters of data that indicate whether a problem or a potential problem with immobility exists, and a nursing diagnosis is developed (see nursing diagnoses box). In addition, assessment data should contain appropriate defining characteristics to support the diagnostic label. Last, the nursing diagnoses should include a probable cause of the problem (see sample nursing diagnoses box).

A client may have one or more of many problems related to immobility. Many alterations in physiological functioning are related to immobility, and impaired functioning in one system may affect another. For example, urinary stasis in the kidney can quickly lead to a kidney infection, which produces fever and sweating. The resulting increased skin moisture may then increase

---

Examples of Nursing Diagnoses Related to Immobility

NANDA-APPROVED NURSING DIAGNOSES

Impaired physical mobility related to:
- Bed rest
- Decreased strength
- Musculoskeletal impairment

Ineffective airway clearance related to:
- Stasis of pulmonary secretions
- Improper body positioning
- Restricted mobility

Ineffective breathing pattern related to:
- Decreased lung expansion
- Accumulation of pulmonary secretions
- Improper body positioning
- Restricted mobility

Impaired gas exchange related to:
- Asymmetrical breathing patterns
- Decreased lung expansion
- Restricted mobility
- Accumulation of pulmonary secretions

Actual or *potential impaired skin integrity* related to:
- Restricted mobility
- Pressure on skin's surface
- Shearing force

Altered patterns of urinary elimination related to:
- Restricted mobility
- Potential for infection
- Urinary retention

Potential for infection related to:
- Stasis of pulmonary secretions
- Impaired skin integrity
- Stasis of urine

Total incontinence related to:
- Altered elimination patterns
- Restricted mobility
- Infrequent offering of bed pan or urinal by nursing personnel

Potential fluid volume deficit related to:
- Decreased fluid intake

Ineffective individual coping related to:
- Reduced activity
- Social isolation

Sleep pattern disturbance related to:
- Restricted mobility
- Discomfort

Sample Nursing Diagnoses for Immobility

Defining Characteristics	Nursing Diagnoses	Related Factors
Inability to purposefully move Limited range of joint motion Decreased muscle strength Decreased sensation	Impaired physical mobility	• Bed rest • Decreased strength • Musculoskeletal impairment.
Impaired nutrition Altered circulation Decreased skin turgor Edema Body fluids (urine, wound secretions, vomitus) on skin Bony prominence	Actual or potential impaired skin integrity	• Restricted mobility • Pressures on skin's surface
Fever Adventitious lung sounds Wound Urinary catheter in place	Potential for infection	• Stasis of pulmonary secretions • Impaired skin integrity • Stasis of urine

Sample Nursing Care Plan for Immobility			
Nursing Diagnosis	**Goal**	**Expected Outcomes**	**Nursing Interventions**
Potential impaired skin integrity related to bilateral leg casts	Injury to the skin and underlying soft tissue resulting from immobility is prevented.	Skin remains intact.	Reposition client every 2 hours (after casts dry).
		Irritation to ischial tuberosities, sacrum, and heels is absent.	Instruct client to raise buttocks every hour while sitting in wheelchair.
		Circulation to toe remains.	For the first 24 hours after cast application, perform check of capillary refill in the toes every 1 to 2 hours.
		Client will deny skin irritation secondary to casts.	Apply tape and padding to proximal and distal ends of cast.

the potential for skin breakdown. Therefore the nursing diagnosis of "altered patterns of urinary elimination related to infection" should lead the nurse to consider the additional nursing diagnosis of "potential impaired skin integrity related to increased moisture."

Too often the physiological dimension is the sole focus of nursing care for immobilized clients and psychosocial and developmental dimensions are neglected. Yet these can be equally important to health. For example, during immobilization social interaction and stimuli are decreased. Ultimately the client may become isolated, withdrawn, and bored. Such clients may frequently use the nurse's call bell to request minor physical attention, when their real need is greater socialization.

Immobilization changes the family's structure and functioning. For example, if the father is immobilized in traction because of an injury, his role in the family is changed. He is unable to participate in decision making or social activities, and his contributions to the family's income may be decreased. The family's response may lead to problems. The children may resent that their father is unable to attend sports and school activities. Their mother may be frustrated because she must make many of the family's decisions. Any change in family structure of functioning usually results in stress and anxiety for all family members.

PLANNING

Clients at risk for hazards of immobility require a nursing care plan directed toward meeting the actual or potential positioning and mobility needs of the client

(see care plan box). The plan is based on one or more of the following client goals:

1. Regaining proper or optimal body alignment
2. Reducing and preventing injuries to the skin and musculoskeletal system
3. Maintaining a patent airway
4. Achieving optimal lung expansion and gas exchange
5. Mobilizing airway secretions
6. Maintaining cardiovascular function
7. Increasing activity tolerance
8. Achieving normal elimination patterns
9. Maintaining normal sleep-wake patterns
10. Achieving socialization
11. Achieving independent completion of self-care activities
12. Achieving physical and mental stimulation

IMPLEMENTATION

Nursing interventions for an immobilized client focus on preventing or minimizing hazards of immobility. Interventions should therefore be directed toward needs in all dimensions.

Metabolic System

The immobilized client requires a high-protein, high-calorie diet with vitamin B and C supplements. Protein is needed to repair injured tissue and rebuild depleted protein stores. A high calorie intake provides fuel to meet metabolic needs and to replace subcutaneous tissue that may have been destroyed. Supplementation with vitamin C is necessary to replace protein stores. Vitamin B complex is needed for skin integrity and wound healing.

If the client is unable to eat, nutrition must be provided parenterally or enterally. Enteral feedings include delivery through a nasogastric, gastrostomy, or jejunostomy tube of high-protein, high-calorie solutions with complete requirements of vitamins, minerals, and electrolytes (see Chapter 33). Total parenteral nutrition is delivery of nutritional supplements through a central intravenous catheter.

Respiratory System

Nursing interventions for the respiratory system are aimed at promoting expansion of chest and lungs, preventing stasis of pulmonary secretions, maintaining a patent airway, and promoting adequate exchange of respiratory gases.

PROMOTING EXPANSION OF CHEST AND LUNGS

The nurse can counteract reduced chest expansion with several interventions. First, changing the position of the client at least every 2 hours allows the dependent lung to reexpand. This maintains elastic recoil property of lungs and clears the dependent lung of pulmonary secretions.

The nurse should encourage the client to deep breathe and cough every 1 to 2 hours. Alert clients can be taught to deep breathe or yawn every hour. This action expands all lobes of the lungs and prevents atelectasis. Coughing reduces the stasis of pulmonary secretions. For unconscious clients with an artificial airway, the nurse can expand the chest and lungs by using an Ambu bag (see Chapter 36).

The nurse uses discretion when administering postoperative pain medication. These medications can depress the respiratory center so the rate of respiration or expansion of the lungs is decreased. The nurse should ask a postoperative client who has received pain medication to deep breathe and cough at the peak effect of the analgesic, which is 20 to 30 minutes after administration. This reduces the respiratory depressant action of the drug.

If abdominal binders and rib supports are required, they should be removed every 2 hours to allow the client to breathe deeply. Removal may be contraindicated, however, for the newly postoperative or post-trauma client.

PREVENTING STASIS OF PULMONARY SECRETIONS

Stagnant secretions accumulating in the bronchi and lungs may lead to growth of bacteria and subsequent development of pneumonia. Despite interventions to prevent pulmonary secretions, they still develop.

Stagnation of secretions can be reduced by changing the client's position every 2 hours. This change repositions the dependent lung, mobilizing secretions.

Perhaps best for preventing pulmonary secretions is *chest physiotherapy*. This uses positioning techniques to drain secretions from specific segments of the bronchi and lungs into the trachea, from which the client expels them by coughing. Respiratory assessment findings identify areas of the lungs that require chest physiotherapy. Clients are then placed in appropriate positions to promote drainage of pulmonary secretions from affected areas. The nurse uses pillows and slant boards to position clients properly and cupping, clapping, and vibrating techniques to dislodge and mobilize secretions. Chest physiotherapy is a precise procedure requiring specific nursing skills. The complete procedure is presented in Chapter 36.

MAINTAINING A PATENT AIRWAY

Immobilized clients and those on bed rest are generally weakened. If weakness progresses, the cough reflex gradually becomes inefficient. If the client is too weak or unable to cough up secretions, the nurse must maintain a patent airway using suctioning techniques. The stasis of secretions in the lungs may be life threatening for an immobilized client because hypostatic bronchopneumonia can easily develop. Assessment findings that indicate this condition include productive cough with greenish yellow sputum, fever, pain on breathing, and crackles, wheezes, and dyspnea. Dislodging and mobilizing the stagnant secretions reduce the risk of pneumonia.

In the immobilized client an obstructed airway is usually the result of a mucus plug. The nurse can implement several therapies to reduce the risk of mucus plugs and to maintain the patent airway.

First, the nurse can ask the client to deep breathe and cough every 1 to 2 hours. The nurse instructs the client to take in three deep breaths and cough with the third exhalation. This produces a more forceful, productive cough without excessive fatigue.

Second, the nurse may use nasotracheal or orotracheal suction to remove secretions in the upper airways of a client unable to cough productively. This procedure must be performed aseptically. The nurse places a suction catheter in the client's nose or through the mouth and applies suction.

Third, the nurse can maintain a patent airway by suctioning secretions from an artificial airway such as an endotracheal or tracheal tube. The nurse inserts a catheter into the artificial airway in a sterile procedure. This removes pulmonary secretions from the upper and lower airways (see Chapter 36).

Cardiovascular System

The effects of bed rest or immobilization on the cardiovascular system include orthostatic hypotension, increased cardiac workload, and thrombus formation. Nursing therapies are designed to minimize or prevent these alterations.

REDUCING ORTHOSTATIC HYPOTENSION

The causative factors and effects of orthostatic hypotension are described in an earlier section. Nursing interventions can assist in reducing orthostatic hypotension.

First, interventions are directed toward maintaining smooth muscle tone, as by leg exercises. When muscle tone is maintained, venous return to the heart is increased and stasis of blood in lower extremities is prevented.

The client should be encouraged to get out of bed as soon as possible, even if only to a nearby chair. This activity assists in maintaining muscle tone and promotes venous return to the heart. The client should be moved out of bed gradually. To document orthostatic changes, the nurse measures baseline blood pressure in the supine position. The nurse then raises the client to a high Fowler's position and measures blood pressure again to detect lowering of pressure. The client is left in the high Fowler's position for a few moments to allow the body to adapt to any drop in blood pressure. The client's pulse is also assessed. An increase of 20 beats per minute can indicate diminished cardiac reserve, and syncope may occur. The nurse continually assesses the client for signs of dizziness or lightheadedness.

Next the nurse should have the client sit at the side of the bed with feet on the floor. The client should lie down if a dizzy or faint sensation develops. The client sits for a few minutes, and if no dizziness or weakness occurs, stands up at the bedside for a minute before beginning to walk. If the client becomes dizzy or weak, he can be lowered quickly and safely to the bed. If there is no dizziness, the nurse assists the client to a chair. Gradually increasing the frequency and duration of ambulation helps overcome orthostatic hypotension and muscle fatigue resulting from bed rest or immobilization.

REDUCING CARDIAC WORKLOAD

The nurse designs interventions to reduce cardiac workload. The primary intervention is discouraging use of the Valsalva maneuver.

The nurse can provide the alert, partially immobilized client with an overhead trapeze bar that allows a position change without using the Valsalva maneuver, thus increasing intrathoracic pressure. The nurse teaches the client not to hold the breath but to use pursed lip breathing when changing position (see Chapter 36).

The nurse also intervenes to prevent constipation in the inactive client (see Chapter 39). This reduces use of the Valsalva maneuver, which may be used when straining to evacuate a stool.

Inactivity increases venous stasis, hypercoagulability, and external pressure against the veins, which increases the risk of deep vein thrombosis. Three nursing measures can minimize this.

First, the nurse positions the client properly to prevent pressure on the posterior region of the knee and deep veins of the legs. Chapter 41 includes detailed procedures for placing clients in the high Fowler's, supine, prone, Sims', and side-lying positions.

Second, the nurse incorporates routine active, range-of-motion exercises into the care plan. If the client does not have voluntary control of extremities, the nurse performs passive range of joint motion exercises. The nurse can perform such exercises while bathing the client and assess the venous system at the same time.

Third, the use of elastic stockings reduces the risk of thrombus formation. Elastic stockings are available in toe-to-knee and toe-to-midthigh sizes. They promote venous return by maintaining pressure on the muscles. Elastic stockings should be removed and reapplied at least twice a day, and the nurse should make sure they are clean and dry. In addition, "pulsating" (pneumatic) stockings are used in clients at higher risk for deep vein thrombosis. These are composed of cells which alternately deflate and inflate, thereby maintaining venous flow from the lower extremities. (Procedure 42-1).

If the nurse suspects deep vein thrombosis, it should be reported immediately. The leg should be elevated with no pressure on the area of thrombosis. The region should *not* be massaged.

Musculoskeletal System

The immobilized client must receive some exercise to prevent excessive muscle wasting and atrophy and joint contractures.

If the client is unable to move part or all of his body, the nurse must perform passive range of joint motion exercises for all immobilized joints while bathing the client and at least two or three more times a day. If one extremity is paralyzed, the client can be taught to put each joint independently through its range of motion.

Some orthopedic conditions require more frequent passive range of motion exercises to restore the injured joint's function post-operatively. Clients with such conditions may use automatic equipment for passive range of joint motion exercises (Fig. 42-12). The equipment extends an extremity to a prescribed angle for a prescribed period. This is beneficial when the client must gradually increase the degree and duration of extension.

Applying Elastic Stockings

STEPS	RATIONALE

1. Identify need for elastic stockings.
  a. Immobility
  b. Lower extremity edema
  c. Varicose veins
	These conditions increase the risk of thrombus formation.

2. Prepare needed equipment.
  a. Tape measure
  b. Stockings in proper size
  c. Talcum powder
	Stockings must be measured according to directions of specific manufacturer. Measure client's calf circumference length from foot to knee. For thigh-high elastic stockings measure calf circumference, thigh circumference, and length from foot to thigh.

3. Explain procedure to client.	Relieves anxiety and increases cooperation.
4. Wash hands.	Reduces transmission of microorganisms.
5. Elevate bed to comfortable position.	Promotes good body mechanics for nurse.
6. Assist client to supine position.	Eases application.
7. After the legs have been cleansed, apply a small amount of talcum powder to each leg and foot.	Talcum powder reduces friction and allows for easier application of the stocking.
8. Turn elastic stocking inside out by placing one hand into the sock, holding the toe of the sock with other hand, and pulling (see illustration).	Prepares stocking for application.
9. Place the client's toe into the foot of the elastic stocking, making sure that the sock is smooth (see illustration).	Wrinkles in the sock can impede circulation to the lower region of the extremity.
10. Slide the remaining portion of the sock over the client's foot, being sure that the toes are covered. The sock will now be right side out (see illustration).	If the toes remain uncovered, they will become constricted by the elastic and their circulation can be reduced.
11. Slide the sock up over the client's calf until the sock is completely extended. Be sure the sock is smooth and no ridges are present (see illustration).	Ridges impede venous return and can counteract the overall purpose of the elastic stocking.

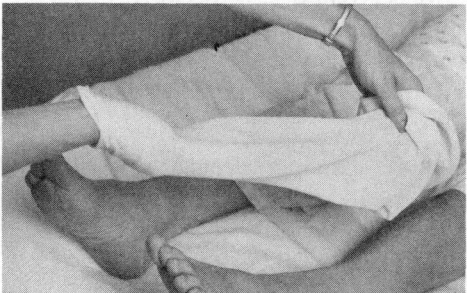

Step 8

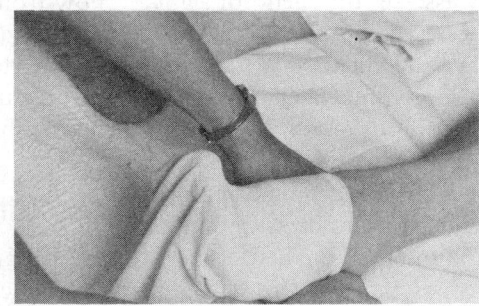

Step 9

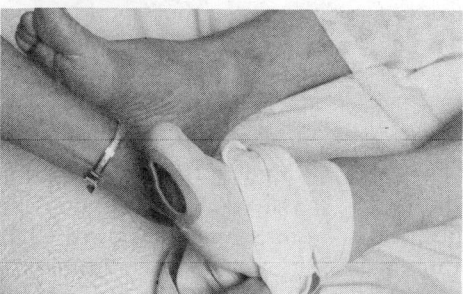

Step 10

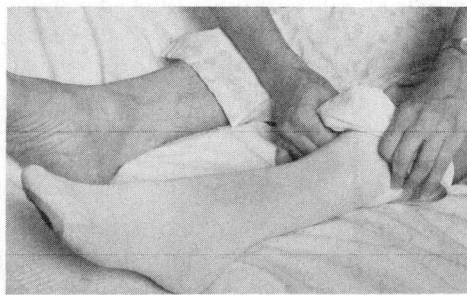

Step 11

STEPS	RATIONALE
12. Instruct the client not to roll socks partially down.	Rolling the sock partially down will have a constricting effect and impede venous return.
13. Reposition client for comfort.	Maintains body alignment and promotes comfort.
14. Wash hands.	Reduces transmission of microorganisms.
15. After 1 hour:	
a. Observe stockings for wrinkles in binding.	Wrinkles increase pressure to skin and impair circulation.
b. Assess capillary refill in toes and palpate pulses in feet.	Ensures circulatory status in lower extremities has not been compromised.
16. Remove stockings at least once a shift.	Provides for assessment of skin and circulatory status.
17. Record in nurses' notes:	
a. Date and time of stocking application and condition of skin before application	Documents condition of lower extremities and performance of procedure.
b. Circulatory status of lower extremities	
c. Stocking length and size	

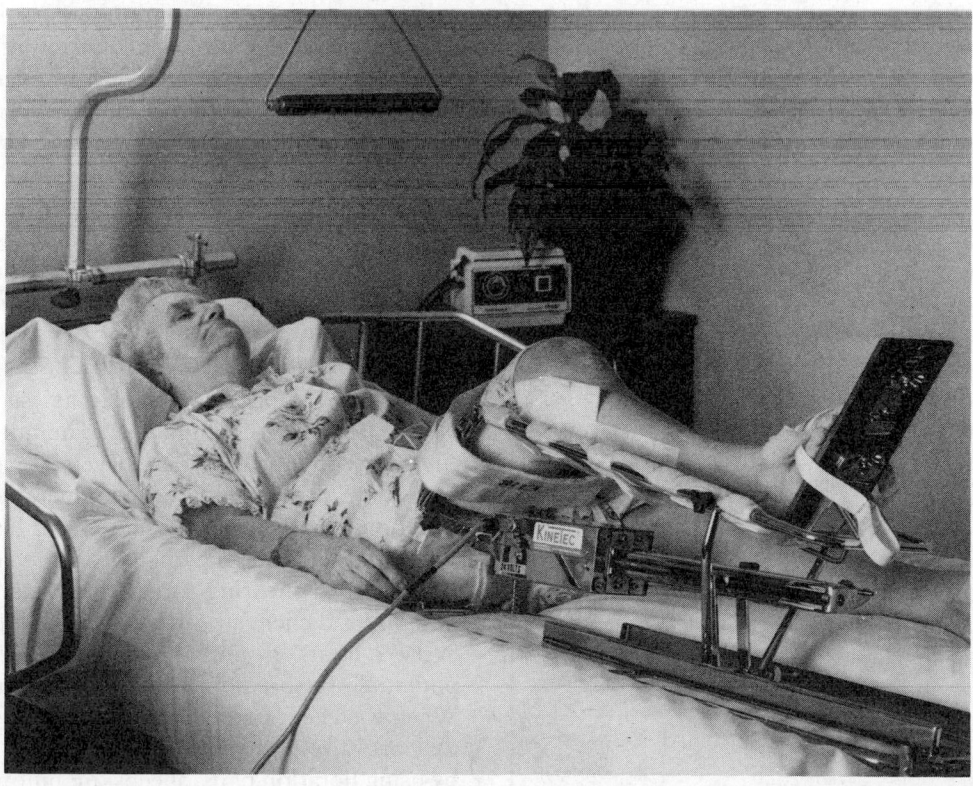

Fig. 42-12 Continuous passive range of motion machine.

Incorporating Active Range of Joint Motion Exercises into Activities of Daily Living

- Nodding head "yes" exercises *neck* (flexion and extension)
- Shaking head "no" exercises *neck* (rotation)
- Moving right ear to right shoulder exercises *neck* (lateral flexion)
- Moving left ear to left shoulder exercises *neck* (lateral flexion)
- Reaching to turn on overhead light exercises *shoulder* (flexion)
- Reaching to bedside stand for book exercises *shoulder* (abduction)
- Scratching back exercises *shoulder* (hyperextension and inward rotation)
- Rotating shoulders toward chest exercises *shoulder*
- Rotating shoulders toward back exercises *shoulder*
- Eating, bathing, shaving, and grooming exercise *elbow* (flexion, extension)

- All activities requiring fine motor coordination, such as writing and eating, exercise *fingers* and *thumb* (flexion, extension, abduction, adduction, opposition)
- Walking exercises *hip* (flexion, extension, hyperextension)
- Rolling toes inward exercises *hip* (internal rotation)
- Rolling toes outward exercises *hip* (external rotation)
- Walking exercises *knee* (flexion, extension)
- Walking exercises *ankle* (dorsiflexion, plantar flexion)
- Pointing toe toward head of bed exercises *ankle* (dorsiflexion)
- Pointing toe toward foot of bed exercises *ankle* (plantar flexion)
- Walking exercises *toes* (extension, hyperextension)
- Wiggling toes exercises *toes* (abduction, adduction)

Clients on bed rest should have active range of joint motion exercises incorporated into the daily schedule (see Chapter 41). The client can perform these exercises during activities of daily living. The box describes joint movements that occur with daily activities.

Active range of joint motion exercises maintain functioning of the musculoskeletal system. The nurse should also plan interventions for the gradual return of mobility in clients who will be able to resume normal activity.

The best nursing intervention is a progressive exercise program individualized to the client's health, age, weight, illness, and motivation. A progressive exercise program gradually increases activity to reverse the deconditioning associated with bed rest (Winslow and Weber, 1980).

Progressive exercise programs are used for clients with musculoskeletal, neurological, cardiopulmonary, renal, and other chronic diseases. Before beginning the program, warm up exercises should be performed, unless they are contraindicated.

SKIN

As discussed previously, the major risk to skin from restricted mobility is decubitus ulcers. Nursing interventions therefore focus on their prevention or treatment.

PREVENTING DECUBITUS ULCERS. The first step in preventing decubitus ulcers is to assess the client's risk factors (see research highlight). The nurse then reduces environmental factors that accelerate decubitus ulcer formation, such as high room temperature (causing perspiration), moisture, or wrinkled bed linen.

The nursing care plan includes interventions to reduce pressure and shearing force to the skin (see box). The immobilized client's position should be changed at least every 2 hours around the clock. Fig. 42-13 illustrates potential pressure points for clients in various positions. When the client is repositioned, the nurse checks to see that pressure points are protected. The nurse does this by using flotation pads, sheepskin, pillows, and bridging techniques.

✄ *Research Highlight* ✄

Bergstrom et al. developed a scale for predicting pressure sore risk to foster early identification of clients at risk for forming pressure sores. The Braden Scale is composed of six subscales: sensory perception, activity, mobility, moisture, friction, and nutrition. Research was conducted to determine the instrument's reliability and validity. The tool is highly reliable when used by nurses. Clinical implications project that it has predictive ability to identify clients at greater risk for pressure sore development. Subsequently, appropriate interventions can be used to reduce or eliminate the risks.

Bergstrom, N, et al.: The Braden Scale for predicting pressure sore risk, Nurs Res 36:205, 1987.

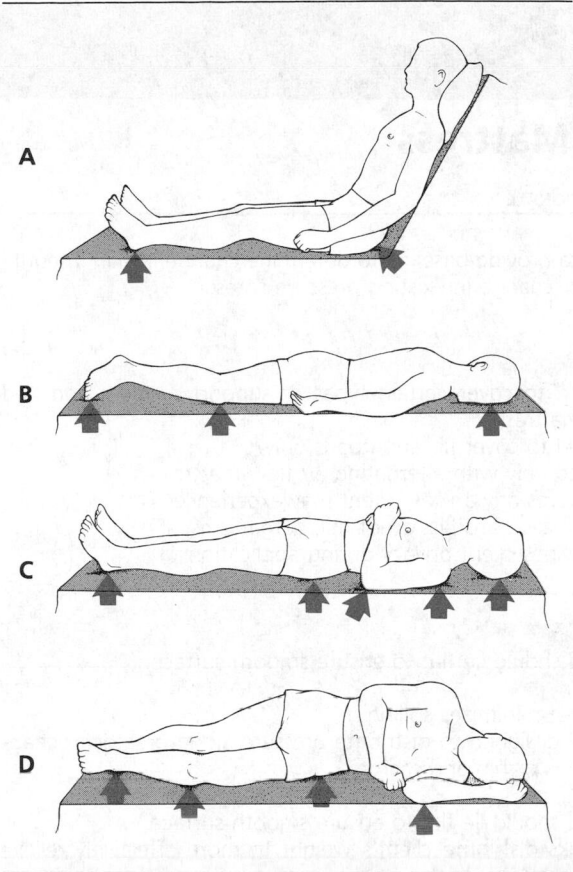

Fig. 42-13 Pressure points *(arrows)* for clients in **A**, high Fowler's, **B**, prone, **C**, supine, and **D**, side-lying positions.

The nurse may use three types of mechanical devices to prevent or treat decubitus ulcers: devices that support specific pressure areas of the body, such as the heels, sacrum, buttocks, and elbows; devices that aid in turning or moving the client; and devices that support the entire body to minimize or equalize pressure (see box and Procedures 42-2 and 42-3).

TREATING DECUBITUS ULCERS. Of primary importance in the treatment of decubitus ulcers is cleanliness

---

Nursing Interventions to Prevent Decubitus Ulcers

- Change client's position at least every 2 hours.
- Maintain smooth bed linens.
- Keep client's skin dry.
- Reposition the client properly.
- Use mechanical devices properly to reduce pressure.

---

of the ulcer area and all skin surfaces. Maintaining cleanliness may be extremely difficult with incontinent, feverish, or confused clients.

Moisture in and around an area of skin breakdown can cause futher ulceration and infection. Many products are available for the care of decubitus ulcers (see box, p. 1266). The nurse should clean the affected area with an antiseptic solution at least every 4 hours or as necessary. Caution is needed because antiseptics can damage tissue unprotected by the dermis and may in-

---

Mechanical Devices Used to Prevent or Treat Decubitus Ulcers

TO SUPPORT PRESSURE AREAS OF THE BODY

- Flotation pads are pliable pads with a consistency like body fat, which disperses pressure over a larger area (Procedure 42-2).
- Natural sheepskin is a resilient substance that disperses pressure over a larger body surface, reduces friction, and absorbs moisture (Procedure 42-2). Synthetic sheepskin does not have the absorptive properties, and should be used cautiously.
- Pillows and bridging techniques lift the pressure site off of the mattress and separate two points of pressure.

TO AID IN TURNING A CLIENT

- A CircOlectric bed is electronically controlled and can be rotated vertically 210 degrees to rotate client from prone to supine position.
- A Guttman bed rotates the client from prone to supine positions and from side to side.
- A Rotokinetic treatment table rotates the client 270 degrees every 3 minutes.
- A Stryker wedge turning frame rotates the client horizontally from the prone to the supine position.

TO MINIMIZE OR EQUALIZE PRESSURE

- Alternating air mattresses made of polyvinyl air cells are attached to a pump that inflates and deflates them every 3 to 7 seconds, alternating pressure points (Procedure 42-2).
- Water mattresses disperse and evenly distribute the client's body weight.
- A Clinitron bed decreases pressure and reduces shearing, friction, and maceration by distributing the client's weight through a gentle flow of temperature-controlled air forced upward through a mass of fine ceramic microsphers (Procedure 42-3).
- An egg crate mattress is a foam rubber pad that rests on the bed mattress and disperses the client's body weight evenly over the mattress (Procedure 42-2).

PROCEDURE 42-2

Placing Client on Support Surface Mattress

STEPS	RATIONALE
1. Assess condition of skin, especially over dependent sites and bony prominences.	Data provide baseline to determine change in skin integrity or change in existing pressure sores.
2. Prepare necessary equipment and supplies:	
a. Flotation pad, foam mattress, air mattress, or sheepskin	
b. Two bed sheets	Used to cover certain types of support surfaces and bed mattress.
c. Pillowcases (optional)	Used to cover flotation pads only.
d. Air flow pumping unit	Used only with alternating air-flow mattresses.
3. Explain purpose and application of mattress or pad.	Relieves any anxiety client may experience.
4. Wash hands.	Reduces transmission of microorganisms.
5. Close room door or bedside curtain.	Provides client privacy during application.
6. Apply support surface to bed (bed may be occupied or unoccupied).	
a. *Flotation pad*	
(1) Apply foam pad over bed mattress by unrolling it fully.	Pad should lie flat to ensure smooth surface.
(2) Apply sheet over foam pad.	Sheet minimizes soiling.
(3) Place flotation pad in center cut-out portion of foam pad.	Pad designed to distribute pressure along greater trochanters of hip and sacrum.
b. *Foam mattress*	
(1) Apply foam mattress over bed.	Pad should lie flat to ensure smooth surface.
(2) With egg crate variety, foam peaks should point up.	Peaks distribute client's weight to more effectively relieve pressure.
(3) Apply bed sheet over mattress, being careful to avoid wrinkles.	Prevents soiling.
c. *Air mattress*	
(1) Apply deflated mattress flat over surface of bed mattress.	Provides smooth, even surface.
(2) Bring any plastic strips or flaps around corners of bed mattress.	Secures air mattress in place.
(3) Attach connector on air mattress to inflation device.	Mattresses vary as to requiring one-time or continuous inflation cycle.
(4) Inflate mattress to proper air pressure determined by air pump or blower.	Manufacturer's directions indicate air pressure to distribute client's body weight evenly.
(5) Place sheet over air mattress, being sure to eliminate all wrinkles.	Prevents soiling of mattress and reduces direct contact of skin against plastic surface.
(6) Check air pumps to be sure pressure cycle alternates.	Alternating air flow mattress produces intermittent cycling, inflating only parts of mattress at any one time. Intermittent cycle continually alternates pressure against skin and soft tissue.
d. *Sheepskin*	
(1) Apply sheepskin flat over desired area of bed mattress.	Provides smooth, even surface.
7. Position client comfortably as desired over support surface. Reposition routinely.	Location of existing decubiti might influence type of positioning. Regular turning is still required.
8. Wash hands.	Reduces transmission of microorganisms.
9. Inspect client's skin and bony prominences routinely.	Determines if pressure sores develop or if condition of existing sores changes.
10. Record transfer of client to support surface and related information in nurses' notes.	Documents safe completion of the procedure and records initial baseline data.

PROCEDURE 42-3

Placing a Client on a Clinitron Bed

STEPS	RATIONALE
1. Assess condition of client's skin; pay particular attention to potential pressure sites and any existing skin lesions.	Data provide baseline to determine any change in client's condition while on bed.
2. Prepare the necessary equipment and supplies: a. Clinitron bed b. Filter sheet	Permeable to rising airflow from mattress and downward flow of fluids (for example, sweat, urine, or wound drainage).
3. Explain procedure and purpose of bed to client and family.	Reduces anxiety and promotes client's cooperation.
4. Obtain any additional personnel needed to transfer client to bed.	Ensures client's safety by having sufficient personnel to assist in transferring.
5. Wash hands.	Reduces transmission of microorganisms.
6. Close client's room door or bedside curtain.	Maintains client's privacy during transfer.
7. For clients with severe to moderate pain, premedicate approximately 30 min. before transfer.	Promotes client's comfort and ability to cooperate during transfer to bed.
8. Transfer client to bed using appropriate transfer techniques (see Chapter 41).	Appropriate transfer techniques maintain alignment and reduce risk of injury during procedure.
9. Turn fluidization cycle on by depressing continuous or intermittent mode switch, regulate temperature in continuous mode.	Fluidization minimizes pressure against skin's surface and reduces friction and shear force when client moves.
10. Position client and perform range of motion (ROM) exercises as appropriate.	Promotes comfort and reduces contracture formation. The bed reduces pressure on skin but clients must still be turned and exercised to avoid joint deformity or contractures.
11. To turn clients, position bed pans, or perform other therapies, set intermittent fluidization mode. Once procedure is completed, set mode to continuous fluidization.	Intermittent fluidization provides firm, molded support that facilitates turning and handling client. Continuous fluidization provides permanent fluid support.
12. In emergencies when resuscitation is required, touch button to defluidize bed immediately.	Creates firm surface against which cardiopulmonary resuscitation can be performed.
13. Wash hands.	Reduces transmission of microorganisms.
14. Inspect condition of client's skin periodically.	Evaluates healing progress of any existing lesions. Determines if any new pressure areas are forming.
15. Assess client for nausea.	Flotation effects of bed can cause sensation of nausea.
16. Measure client's level of consciousness.	Determines onset of perceptual changes.
17. Record transfer of client to bed, tolerance to procedure, and condition of skin in nurses' notes.	Documents safe completion of the procedure and records initial baseline data.

activate certain drugs. The ulcer should be rinsed with normal saline after cleaning to minimize the effect of antiseptic on the tissue (Fowler, 1982).

An ulcer that has necrotic tissue or eschar, or shows signs of sloughing must be debrided. Eschar is the scab or dry crust that results from excoriation of the skin. Sloughing is the shedding of dead tissue as the result of skin ulceration. Debridement is the removal of necrotic tissue so healthy tissue can regenerate.

For reddened areas or skin breaks, skin care products that lubricate and protect, stimulate circulation, and promote wound healing are recommended. When the ulcer bed is pink with granulation tissue throughout, a dressing is indicated to promote healing. A clean, moist environment promotes migration of epithelial cells across the ulcer surface (Fowler, 1982).

Protein and hemoglobin levels are important in treatment of decubitus ulcers. A client can lose as much as 50 g of protein a day from an open, weeping decubitus ulcer. This is a sizable amount of the daily requirement of 60 g for women and 70 g for men (Kavchak-Keyes, 1977).

Increased protein intake, two to four times normal, helps rebuild epidermal tissue. Increased caloric intake,

---

Decubitus Skin Care Products

CLEANSING AGENTS

- Antiseptic agents (povidone-iodine, hypochlorite solution) are used to prevent or reduce microorganisms when necrotic debris is present.
- Oxydizing agents (hydrogen peroxide) debride necrotic tissue from wounds.
- Physiologic saline or water is used to cleanse when there is an ulcer with pink granulation bed and no necrotic debris.
- Enzymes (Travase, Elase, and Collagenase) are used for proteolysis to debride dead tissue or eschar.
- Granulex is used as a mild debriding action to stimulate granulation tissue when there is no necrotic debris. Use is discontinued when ulcer bed is pink with granulation tissue.
- Dextranomer beads (Debrisan) are used for absorption of tissue fluid when there are secretions and no necrotic debris. Use is discontinued when ulcer bed is pink with granulation tissue.
- Bard absorption dressing is used for absorption of tissue fluid and provides a moist environment when there is no necrotic debris. Use is discontinued when ulcer bed is pink with granulation tissue.

WOUND COVERINGS

- Gauze is used for packing when debridement of loose debris is present.
- Absorbent sponges are used to wick drainage when there is absorption and packing.
- Nontransparent occlusive dressing is used to maintain a moist environment when there is no necrotic debris.
- Semipermeable transparent adhesive film is used to maintain a moist environment when there is no necrotic debris.

Modified from Fowler, E: J Gerontol Nurs 8:680, 1982.

---

at least one and one half times normal, helps replace subcutaneous tissue. Increased intake of vitamin C promotes protein synthesis (Kavchak-Keyes, 1977).

A low hemoglobin level decreases delivery of oxygen to the tissues and causes further debilitation. When possible, hemoglobin should be maintained at 12 g/100 ml.

Elimination System

Nursing interventions for maintaining optimal urinary functioning are directed toward keeping the client well hydrated without causing bladder distention and preventing urinary stasis, calculi, and infections.

Adequate hydration (for example, 2000 to 3000 ml of fluids) helps prevent renal calculi and urinary tract infections. The client should void large amounts of dilute urine. If the client is also incontinent, the nurse should modify the care plan so the increased urinary output does not cause skin breakdown.

The nurse must also record the frequency and consistency of bowel movements. A diet rich in fruits, vegetables, and bulk can facilitate normal peristalsis. If a client is unable to maintain normal bowel patterns, the physician may order stool softeners, cathartics, or enemas (see Chapter 39).

Psychosocial Changes

The nursing assessment can identify effects of prolonged immobilization on the client's psychosocial dimension. People who have a tendency toward depression or mood swings are at greater risk for developing these during bed rest or immobilization. There are many nursing interventions to meet the client's psychosocial needs.

First, the nurse should anticipate changes in the client's psychosocial status. The nurse can provide routine and informal socialization. Nursing activities can be planned so the client can talk and interact with staff. If possible the client should be placed in a room with others who are mobile and interactive. If a private room is required, staff members should be asked to visit at least once a shift.

Second, the nurse provides stimuli to maintain orientation and entertain the client. A daily newspaper helps the client keep track of events and time. Bedside chats at appropriate moments orient the client to nursing activities, meals, and visiting hours. Books help occupy the client when alone. If the condition permits, he can participate in craft activities. Radio and television provide stimulation and help pass the time.

Third, clients should be encouraged to wear their glasses or artificial teeth and to shave or apply makeup. These are activities through which people maintain body image. Maintenance of body image can help alleviate depression resulting from immobilization.

Fourth, the client should be involved in care whenever possible. For example, the nurse should encourage the client to determine when the bed should be made. Some clients rest better during the night when fresh sheets are put on in the evening rather than in the morning. The client should provide as much self-care as possible. Hygiene and grooming articles should be kept within easy reach.

Fifth, nursing care between 10 PM and 7 AM should be scheduled to minimize interruptions of sleep. This may involve administering medications and assessing vital signs at times when the client must be turned or receive special skin care.

Last, the nurse should observe for failure to cope with restricted mobility. If the nursing care plan is not improving the client's coping patterns, a clinical nurse specialist, counselor, social worker, clergyman, or other consultant may be needed. Their recommendations should be incorporated into the plan of care.

Developmental Changes

Ideally, immobilized clients continue normal development. However, this is unrealistic for the very young or very old. Nursing interventions can help.

First, particularly with a young child, nursing care should provide mental as well as physical stimulation. Play activities can be incorporated into the nursing care plan. Puzzles, for example, develop fine motor skills, and reading helps the child develop cognitively. An immobilized child should be placed with children of the same

age who are not immobilized unless a contagious disease is present. Nursing activities, such as dressing changes, cast care, and care of traction, can be designed to require participation of the child. The nurse must recognize extreme changes from normal behavioral patterns. If these continue, the nurse should consult with a clinical nurse, counselor, or other health care professional whose specialty is children.

Restricted mobility of the elderly presents unique nursing problems. Elderly clients usually have several chronic illnesses. Because of age and chronic illness, the elderly are at high risk for the hazards of immobility. Once a chronically ill elderly client has been immobilized, it is unlikely that functional abilities will be regained.

Inactive elderly clients are at greater risk for confusion, depression, and disorientation, which result from immobilization, chronic illness, medications, and the ag-

---

Sample Evaluation of Interventions for Immobility

Goals	Evaluative Measures	Expected Outcomes
Injuries to the skin and musculoskeletal system are reduced.	Inspect the skin for presence of pressure points. Inspect the skin's integrity. Inspect the musculoskeletal system for absence of joint contractures. Palpate the integument for absence of tenderness. Palpate muscles for adequate muscle tone.	Skin remains dry and intact. Prolonged erythema is absent. Client has no joint contractures. Severe muscular atrophy and decreased muscular tone are absent.
Activity tolerance is increased.	Observe the client for decreased fatigability. Observe for increased requests by client for self-care and recreational activities. Palpate the pulse for return to resting pulse rate by 10 minutes. Auscultate BP for return to resting BP by 10 minutes.	Client reports decreased fatigability. Tachycardia is absent. Vital signs return to resting values 10 minutes after activity. Client participates in self-care activities.
Socialization is achieved.	Observe the nursing care plan for adequate, uninterrupted time for visitors. Observe the staff for increased social visits to client. Observe the client for assertiveness in interaction with staff, friends, and family.	Client has visits from family, friends, and staff. Prolonged emotional mood swings are absent. Client interacts with health care team.
Physical and mental stimulation are achieved.	Observe the client for absence of prolonged daytime sleeping. Observe the client for increased levels of orientation. Observe the client for increased interaction with environment.	Client returns to near normal sleep-wake cycle. Orientation is improved. Interaction with environment is increased.

ing process. Therefore the elderly may require nursing interventions to orient them to time. A calendar and a clock with a large dial should be in the client's room. The calendar should be marked so the client can immediately identify the day and date. Chapter 25 describes other measures to assist elderly clients in meeting developmental needs.

Nursing care should encourage the elderly immobilized client to perform as many activities of daily living as possible. If the client performs personal grooming before mobility was restricted, this should continue unless contraindicated.

The nurse should remember that the elderly client is extremely susceptible to the hazards of immobility. A nursing care plan should be designed to prevent or minimize these hazards, rather than allowing problems to develop and then treating them. The frail elderly client may need a position change every hour instead of every 2 hours, and need more frequent range of joint motion exercises. Not only are the elderly more susceptible to the hazards of immobility, but the consequences and severity of immobility are more rapid.

EVALUATION

Each client has different risks for the hazards of immobility and subsequent nursing interventions are individualized. Clients with minimal mobility impairments or those whose health status is relatively stable may need only a few measures. Nursing interventions for reducing the risks of immobility are evaluated by determining the client's response to nursing therapies and by determining if each goal was achieved (see evaluation box).

SUMMARY

Immobilization can adversely affect the client in all dimensions. Although in some cases immobilization is necessary to promote wound healing, proper skeletal alignment, or rest after an illness, it involves risks. Nursing care seeks to prevent adverse effects and to minimize them when they do occur. Using the nursing process, the nurse assesses physiological, psychosocial, and developmental health needs, diagnoses actual or potential problems related to immobilization, and plans and delivers nursing care to meet the client's needs. Because effects of immobility can be extensive, nursing care for immobilized clients remains challenging.

KEY CONCEPTS

- ✓ Normal physical mobility depends on intact and functioning nervous and musculoskeletal systems.
- ✓ The risk of disabilities related to immobilization depends on the extent and duration of immobilization.
- ✓ Immobility may result from illness or trauma or may be prescribed for therapeutic reasons, but in any case presents hazards in the physiological, psychological, and developmental dimensions.
- ✓ Decubitus ulcers are one of the most common physiological hazards of immobility, but the nurse can take actions to prevent or treat them.
- ✓ Psychosocial effects of immobility include depression, behavioral changes, changes in the sleep-wake cycle, decreased coping abilities, and developmental effects.
- ✓ The nurse uses the nursing process to provide care for clients experiencing or at risk for the adverse effects of immobility.
- ✓ Assessment focuses on range of joint motion, musculoskeletal status, and complete physical examination for potential adverse effects in all body systems, as well as psychosocial and developmental effects.
- ✓ After identifying nursing diagnoses, the nurse plans and implements interventions to prevent or minimize the hazards and complications of immobilization.

✓ Interventions address the client's psychosocial and developmental needs that result from immobilization.

✓ The primary evaluation criterion for nursing care in the developmental dimension for immobilized clients is prevention of measurable decline in the client's functioning or delay in development.

REFERENCES

Berecek, KH: Etiology of decubitus ulcers, Nurs Clin North Am 10:157, 1975.

Blackburn, GL, et al.: Nutritional and metabolic assessment of the hospitalized patient, J Parental Nutr 1:11, 1977.

Dietrick, J, et al.: Effects of immobilization upon various metabolic and physiologic functions of normal men, Am J Med 4:3, 1948.

Fowler, E: Pressure sores: a deadly nuisance, J Gerontol Nurs 12:680, 1982.

Groër, MW, and Shekleton, ME: Basic pathophysiology: a conceptual approach, ed. 2, St. Louis, 1983, The C.V. Mosby Co.

Guttman, L: The problem of treatment of pressure sores in patients with spinal paraplegia, Br J Plast Surg 8:196, 1955.

Kavchak-Keyes, MA: Treating decubitus ulcers using four proven steps, Nurs 77 7:44, 1977.

Linden, O, et al.: Pressure distribution on the surface of the human body, Arch Phys Med Rehab 46:378, 1965.

Olson, EV: The hazards of immobility, Am J Nurs 67:779, 1967.

Winslow, EH, and Weber, TM: Progressive exercises to combat hazards of bedrest, Am J Nurs 80:440, 1980.

Research Article

Bergstrom, N, et al.: The Braden Scale for predicting pressure sore risk, Nur Res 36:205, 1987.

ADDITIONAL READINGS

Ahmed MC: Opsite for decubitus care, Am J Nurs 82:61, 1982.

Arnell, I: Treating decubitus ulcers: two methods that work, Nurs 83, 13:50, 1983.

Berecek, KH: Treatment of decubitus ulcers, Nurs Clin North Am 10:171, 1975.

Bilger, AJ, and Greene, EH: Winger's protective body mechanics: a manual for nurses, New York, 1973, Springer Publishing Co., Inc.

Byrne, N, and Feld, M: Overcoming the red menace: preventing and treating decubitus ulcers, Nursing 84 14:55, 1984.

Cassell, BL: Treating pressure sores stage by stage, RN 36:41, 1986.

David, JA: Pressure sore treatment: a literature review, Int J Nurs Stud 19:183, 1982.

DiMascio, S: Debrisan for decubitus ulcers, Am J Nurs 79:684, 1979.

Ek, A, and Boman, G: A descriptive study of pressure sores: the prevalence of pressure sore and the characteristics of patient, J Adv Nurs 7:51, 1982.

Fernsebner, B: Sleep deprivation in patients, AORN 37:35, 1983.

Feustel, DE: Pressure sore prevention: age, there is the rub, Nurs 82 12:78, 1982.

Goldberg, WG, and Fitzpatrick, JJ: Movement with the aged, Nurs Res 29:339, 1980.

Hulley, SB, et al.: The effect of supplemental oral phosphate on the bone mineral changes during prolonged bed rest, J Clin Invest 50:2506, 1971.

Jones, PL, and Millman, A: A three-part system to combat pressure sores, Geriatric Nurs 7(2):78, 1986.

Kavchak-Keyes, MA: Four proven steps for preventing decubitus ulcers, Nurs 77 7:58, 1977.

Kosiak, M: Etiology of decubitus ulcers, Arch Phys Med Rehab 42:19, 1961.

Rubin, M: How bedrest changes perception, Am J Nurs 88:55, 1988.

Rubin, M: The physiology of bedrest, Am J Nurs 88:50, 1988.

Steffel, PE, et al.: Reducing devices for pressure sores with respect to nursing care procedures, Nurs Res 29:228, 1980.

Shannon, ML: Five famous fallacies about pressure sores, Nurs 84 13:34, 1984.

Spencer, W, Valbona, C, and Carter, R: Physiologic concepts of immobilization, J Phys Med Rehab 46:89, 1965.

Stewart, AF, et al.: Calcium homeostasis in immobilization: an example of resorptive hypercalciuria, N Engl J Med 306:1136, 1982.

Stoneberg, C, Petcock, N, and Myton, C: Wound care forms pressure sores in the homebound: one solution, Am J Nurs 86:426, 1986.

Tooman, T, and Patterson, J: Decubitus ulcer warfare: product versus process, Geriatric Nurs 5:166, 1984.

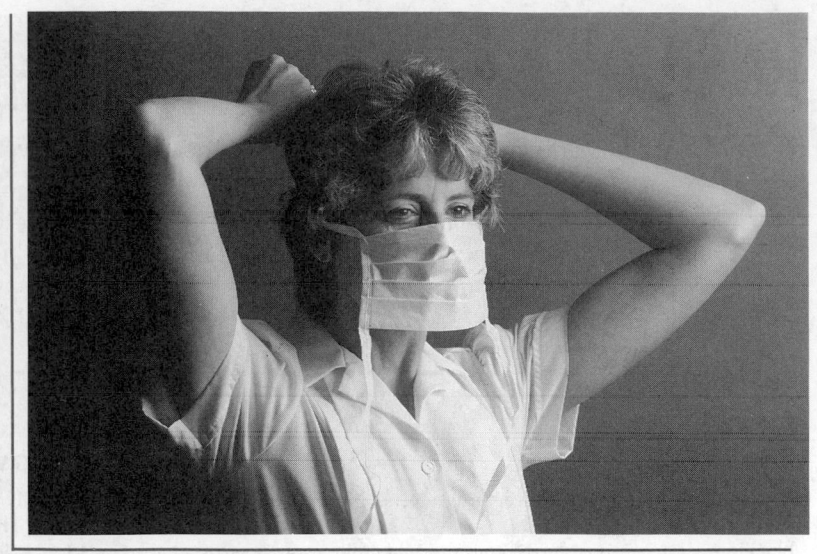

OBJECTIVES

Mastery of content in this chapter will enable the student to:

- Define the key terms listed.
- Identify the body's normal defenses against infection.
- Discuss the events in the inflammatory response
- Explain the difference between cell mediated and humoral immunity
- Describe the nature of signs of a localized and systemic infection.
- Describe characteristics of each link of the infection chain.
- Identify clients most at risk for acquiring an infection.
- Explain conditions that precipitate the onset of nosocomial infections.
- Identify factors to assess a person's risk for infection
- Explain universal blood and body fluid precautions
- Identify principles of surgical asepsis
- Describe nursing interventions designed to break each link in the infection chain.
- Correctly perform protective isolation techniques.
- Perform proper procedures for handwashing.
- Describe the zone of sterility for a sterile gown and sterile field.
- Properly apply a sterile gown, sterile gloves, and surgical mask.

KEY TERMS

Antibody	Immunocompromised
Antigen	Immunoglobulin
Antiseptic	Inflammation
Asepsis	Invasive
Cannulation	Leukocytosis
Carrier	Lymphocyte
Catalytic	Maceration
CDC	Macrophage
Colonized	Microorganism
Communicable Disease	Nosocomial Infection
Contagious	Parasite
Cytotoxic	Pathogen
Endogenous	Phagocytosis
Epidemiology	Prophylactic
Exogenous	Purulent
Expectorate	Rickettsia
Exudate	Sterile
Fomites	Sterile Field
Forceps	Suppurative
Fungus	Virulent
Iatrogenic Disease	Virus

Infection Control

The promotion of health depends in part on the provision of a safe environment. Infection control practices, which control or eliminate sources of infection, help protect clients from disease. A client entering a health care setting is at risk for acquiring infections because of lowered resistance to infectious microorganisms, increased exposure to numbers and types of disease-causing organisms, and invasive procedures performed. The nurse comes in contact with a variety of microorganisms and thus must practice infection control techniques to avoid spreading them to clients.

In the home a client must recognize sources of infection and be able to institute protective measures. The nurse is responsible for teaching clients about infection, methods of transmission, reasons for susceptibility, and methods of control.

The nurse's knowledge of the infectious process, application of infection control principles, and use of common sense help protect clients from infection. Control of infection is an important part of every action the nurse performs.

NATURE OF INFECTION

An infection is an invasion of the body by pathogens or microorganisms capable of producing disease. If the microorganisms fail to cause serious injury to cells or tissues, infection is asymptomatic. Disease results if the pathogens multiply and cause an alteration in normal tissue function. If the infectious disease can be trans-

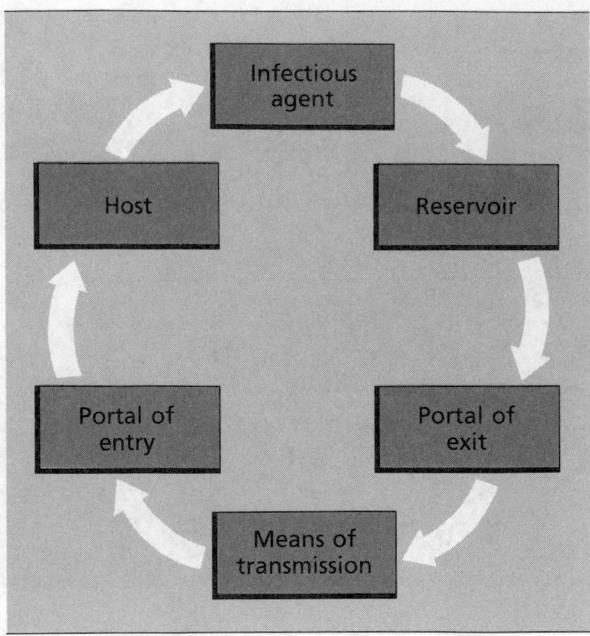

Fig. 43-1 Chain of infection.

mitted directly from one person to another it is a communicable or contagious disease.

Chain of Infection

The mere presence of a pathogen does not mean that an infection will begin. Development of an infection occurs in a cyclical process that depends on six elements: (1) infectious agent or pathogen, (2) reservoir or source for pathogen growth, (3) portal of exit from the reservoir, (4) mode of transmission, (5) portal of entry to host, and (6) susceptible host. An infection will develop if this chain remains intact (Fig. 43-1).

INFECTIOUS AGENT

Pathogenic organisms include bacteria, viruses, fungi, protozoa, and rickettsiae (Table 43-1). All organisms require food and the proper environment for growth. A dark, warm, moist habitat, as in the oral cavity, under a wound dressing, or within a drainage tube, is ideal.

Pathogens on the skin are categorized as resident or transient. Resident pathogens survive and multiply on the skin. Most are found in superficial skin layers but about 10% to 20% inhabit deep epidermal layers (Garner and Favero, 1985). Resident pathogens are not easily removed by handwashing with plain soaps and detergents unless considerable friction is used. Resident microorganisms in deep skin layers are usually killed only by handwashing with products containing antimicrobial ingredients.

Transient pathogens are usually picked up by the hands in normal activities of living. For example, when a nurse touches a bedpan or a contaminated dressing, transient bacteria adhere to the skin. The organisms attach loosely to the skin in dirt and grease or under fingernails. Frequent, thorough handwashing removes transient pathogens easily.

The potential for microorganisms or parasites to cause disease depends on several factors:

1. Number of organisms
2. Virulence or ability to produce disease
3. Ability to enter and survive in the host
4. Susceptibility of host

Many resident skin microorganisms are not highly virulent and cause only minor skin infections. However, they can cause serious infection when surgery or other invasive procedures allow them to enter deep tissues or when a client is severely immunocompromised.

RESERVOIR

Microorganisms have many sources or reservoirs for growth. One of the most common is the body itself. A variety of organisms reside on the surface of the skin and within body cavities, fluids, and discharges. The presence of microorganisms does not always cause a person to be ill. *Carriers* are persons or animals who show no symptoms of illness but who have pathogens on or in their bodies that can be transferred to others. For example, a person can be a carrier of tuberculosis without having manifestations of the disease.

Some areas of the body contain larger populations of resident flora than others. These include the skin, respiratory tract, mouth, vagina, colon, and lower urethra. Areas of the body normally considered sterile, without organism growth, are the bloodstream, spinal fluid, peritoneal cavity, urinary tract, muscles, bones, and chambers of the eye. The entrance of a foreign object into a sterile site leads to a high risk for infection.

Animals, plants, insects, and inanimate objects can also be reservoirs for infectious organisms. Shellfish can become contaminated with *Vibrio cholerae,* the bacterium that causes cholera. The tick is a carrier for the microbe that causes Rocky Mountain spotted fever.

Food, water, and milk are additional reservoirs for pathogens. *Clostridium botulinus* toxin survives in improperly stored food such as nonrefrigerated milk products to cause botulism. The bacterium *Legionella pneumophila,* which causes Legionnaires' disease, lives in contaminated pooled water.

In order to thrive, organisms must survive in the reservoir. Characteristics of an environment that supports organism growth include:

FOOD. Microorganisms require nourishment. Some, such as *Clostridium perfringens,* the microbe that causes gas gangrene, thrive on organic matter. Others, such as

TABLE 43-1   Common Pathogens and Some Infections or Diseases They Produce

Organism	Reservoir	Infection or Disease
BACTERIA		
Staphylococcus aureus	Skin, hair, anterior nares	Wound infection, pneumonia, food poisoning, cellulitis
Streptococcus (beta-hemolytic group A)	Oropharynx, skin, perianal area	"Strep throat," rheumatic fever, scarlet fever, impetigo
Streptococcus (beta-hemolytic group B)	Adult genitalia	Urinary tract infection, wound infection, endometritis
Escherichia coli	Colon	Enteritis
Neisseria gonorrhoeae	Genitourinary tract, rectum, mouth, eye	Gonorrhea, pelvic inflammatory disease, infectious arthritis, conjunctivitis
VIRUSES		
Herpes simplex 1	Lesions of mouth, skin, blood, excretions	Cold sores, aseptic meningitis, sexually transmitted disease
Hepatitis A	Feces, blood, urine	Infectious hepatitis
Hepatitis B	Feces, blood, all body fluids and excretions	Serum hepatitis
HIV	Blood, semen, and vaginal secretions (also isolated in saliva, tears, urine, and breast milk but not proven to be sources of transmission)	Acquired immunodeficiency syndrome.
FUNGI		
Candida albicans	Mouth, skin, colon, genital tract	Thrush, dermatitis
Aspergillus	Soil, dust	Aspergillosis
PROTOZOA		
Plasmodium falciparum	Mosquito	Malaria
RICKETTSIA		
Rickettsia rickettsii	Wood tick	Rocky Mountain spotted fever

Escherichia coli, consume undigested foodstuffs in the bowel. Carbon dioxide and inorganic material such as soil provide nourishment for other organisms.

OXYGEN. Aerobic bacteria require free oxygen for survival and for multiplication sufficient to cause disease. Aerobic organisms tend to cause more infections in humans. Examples of aerobic organisms are *Staphylococcus aureus* and strains of *Streptococcus.*

Anaerobes thrive in environments where little or no free oxygen is available. Infections deep within the pleural cavity, in a joint, or in a deep sinus tract are typically caused by anaerobes. Bacteria that cause tetanus, gas gangrene, and botulism are anaerobes.

WATER. Most organisms require water for survival. The spirochete that causes syphilis, *Treponema pallidum,* lives only in a moist environment. Some bacteria assume a form resistant to drying. These sporeforming bacteria, such as those that cause anthrax, botulism, and tetanus, can live without water.

TEMPERATURE. Microorganisms can live only in certain temperature ranges. However, some can survive temperature extremes that would be fatal to humans. Some viruses are resistant to boiling water. Cold temperatures tend to prevent growth and reproduction of bacteria (bacteriostasis). A temperature that destroys bacteria is bacteriocidal.

pH. Acidity of an environment determines the viability of microorganisms. Most microorganisms prefer an alkaline environment within a pH range of 5 to 8. Bacteria in particular thrive in urine with a high pH. Organisms cannot survive the acid environment of the stomach.

Light. Microorganisms thrive in dark environments such as those under dressings and within body cavities. Ultraviolet light is effective in killing certain forms of bacteria.

PORTAL OF EXIT

Once microorganisms find a site to grow and multiply, they must find a portal of exit if they are to enter another host and cause disease. When the human is the reservoir, microorganisms can exit through a variety of sites.

SKIN AND MUCOUS MEMBRANES. Normally the skin is considered a portal of entry since any break in the integrity of skin and mucous membranes can lead to an infection. However, as pathogenic organisms grow and multiply within a wound, they create purulent drainage. For example, *Staphylococcus aureus* creates a characteristic yellow drainage, whereas *Pseudomonas aeruginosa* causes a greenish cast to drainage. The drainage is a potential portal of exit.

RESPIRATORY TRACT. Pathogens residing in the respiratory tract can be released from the body when a person sneezes, coughs, talks, or even breathes. Microorganisms exit via the mouth and nose in normal clients. In clients with artificial airways such as tracheostomy or endotracheal tubes (see Chapter 36), organisms easily exit through these devices.

URINARY TRACT. Normally urine is sterile. However, in an infected client, microorganisms exit during urination or through urinary diversions such as ileostomies and suprapubic drains (see Chapter 38).

GASTROINTESTINAL TRACT. The mouth is one of the more bacterially contaminated sites of the body even though most of the organisms are normal flora. However, organisms that are normal flora in one person can be pathogens in another. Organisms exist when a person expectorates saliva. Kissing can also provide a means of exit.

Bowel elimination, drainage of bile via surgical wounds or drainage tubes, and escape of gastric contents during vomiting are additional means of exit.

REPRODUCTIVE TRACT. Organisms such as *Neisseria gonorrhoeae* and HIV may exit via the male's urethral meatus or the female's vaginal canal. In the male, urine or semen may be the vehicle of pathogens. Dis-

---

TABLE 43-2 Modes of Transmission

Route and Means	Examples of Organisms (Diseases)
CONTACT	
Direct (direct physical transfer between an infected or colonized person and a susceptible host)—turning clients, giving baths, having sexual contact with an infected person	*Staphylococcus, Treponema* (syphilis), herpes simplex virus
Indirect (personal contact of susceptible host with contaminated inanimate object)—needles, bedpans, intravenous tubing, instruments and dressings, linen, dishes, and silverware	Measles virus, hepatitis B virus, *Enterococcus, Pseudomonas*
Droplet contact (infectious agent coming in contact with conjunctivae, nose, or mouth of susceptible host; droplets travel only up to 3 feet and therefore contact is not airborne)—coughing, sneezing	Influenza virus, *Mycobacterium tuberculosis* (tuberculosis)
AIR	
Droplet nuclei (residue of evaporated droplets remain suspended in air)—coughing, sneezing, talking	Influenza virus, pneumococcus (pneumonia, meningitis, and other infections
Dust (contains infectious agent)	*Aspergillus* (aspergillosis)
VEHICLE	
Contaminated items	
Liquids	
Water	*Vibrio cholerae* (cholera)
Drugs, solutions	*Pseudomonas*
Blood	Hepatitis B virus
Food (improperly handled or stored, fresh fruits and vegetables)	*Salmonella, Staphylococcus, Enterobacter,* and *Klebsiella*
VECTORS	
Insects	
Mosquitoes	*Plasmodium* (malaria)
Fleas, ticks, lice	*Rickettsia typhi* and *R. prowazekii* (typhus)
Animals (cows, pigs)	*Brucella* (brucellosis)

charge from the female's vaginal canal may carry pathogens.

BLOOD. The blood is normally sterile, but in the case of hepatitis or septicemia (presence of bacteria in the circulating blood) it becomes a reservoir for infectious organisms. A break in the skin by needle puncture or a traumatic wound allows pathogens to exit the body in blood.

MODES OF TRANSMISSION

There are many vehicles for transmission of microorganisms from the reservoir to the host. Table 43-2 summarizes common modes of transmission. Certain infectious diseases tend to be transmitted more commonly by specific modes. However, the same microorganisms may be transmitted by more than one route. For example, herpes zoster may be spread by the airborne route in droplet nuclei or by direct contact.

Almost any object within the environment (for example, a stethoscope or thermometer) can become a means of transmitting infection. All hospital personnel providing direct care, such as nurses, physical therapists, and physicians, and those performing diagnostic and support services, such as laboratory technicians, respiratory therapists, and dietary workers, must be free of infection. Each group of health care workers follows procedures for handling equipment and supplies used by clients. For example, respiratory therapists wash their hands before working with each client and dispose of soiled oxygen equipment in a prescribed manner. Certain medical devices and diagnostic procedures provide new avenues for growth and spread of pathogens. Invasive procedures such as cardiac catheterization and cystoscopy (visualization of the bladder) facilitate diagnosis of clients' problems but also increase the risk of transmitting infection. Because so many factors can promote the spread of infection to clients, all health care workers must be conscientious in using infection control practices.

PORTAL OF ENTRY

Organisms can enter a person's body through the same routes they use for exit. Factors that reduce the body's defenses enhance the chances of pathogens entering. For example, when a contaminated needle pierces a client's skin, organisms enter the body. Any obstruction to the flow of urine from a urinary catheter allows organisms to travel up the urethra. Mishandling of sterile bandages over an open wound permits pathogens to enter exposed tissues.

SUSCEPTIBLE HOST

Whether a person acquires an infection depends on susceptibility to an infectious agent. Susceptibility is the degree of resistance an individual has to pathogens. Al-

though everyone is constantly in contact with large numbers of microorganisms, an infection will not develop until an individual becomes susceptible to the strength and numbers of those microorganisms. The more virulent an organism, the greater the likelihood of a person's susceptibility. A person's natural defenses against infection as well as a number of other factors influence susceptibility (see section on risk factors).

Course of Infection

By understanding the infection chain, the nurse can intervene to prevent infections from developing. When the client acquires an infection, the nurse is able to observe early signs and symptoms of infection and to take appropriate actions to prevent its spread. Infections follow a progressive course (Table 43-3). The severity of the client's illness will depend on the extent of the infection, the pathogenicity of the microorganisms, and susceptibility of the host.

If infection is localized or limited to a discrete area such as a wound infection, proper care will control the infection's spread and minimize the client's illness. An infection that affects the entire body instead of just a single organ or part is systemic. A systemic infection can progress to become fatal.

TABLE 43-3 Course of Infection

Stage	Description
Incubation period	Interval between entrance of pathogen into the body and appearance of first symptoms (for example, chickenpox 2-3 weeks, common cold 1-2 days, influenza 1-3 days, mumps 18 days)
Prodromal stage of illness	Interval from the onset of nonspecific signs and symptoms, (malaise, low grade fever, and fatigue) to more specific symptoms; during this time microorganisms grow and multiply and a client is more capable of spreading disease to others
Full stage of illness	Client manifests signs and symptoms specific to type of infection; for example, common cold manifested by sore throat, sinus congestion, rhinitis; mumps manifested by earache, high fever, parotid and salivary gland swelling
Convalescence	Acute symptoms of infection disappear; length of recovery depends on severity of infection and client's general state of health; recovery may take several days to months.

The course of an infection influences the level of nursing care provided. The nurse is responsible for the proper administration of antibiotics and monitoring the client's response to drug therapy (see Chapter 15). Supportive therapy includes providing adequate nutrition and rest to bolster defenses against the infectious process. The complexity of care further depends on body systems affected by the infection.

Regardless of whether infection is localized or systemic, the nurse plays a dominant role in minimizing its spread. A simple wound infection can involve the urinary tract if the nurse uses poor technique during perineal hygiene. Nurses can also acquire infections from clients if their techniques for controlling infection transmission are inadequate.

Defenses Against Infection

The body has normal defenses against infection. Normal body flora that reside in and outside the body protect a person from several pathogens. The body's organ systems each have defense mechanisms that minimize exposure to infectious microorganisms. The inflammatory response is a protective vascular and cellular reaction that neutralizes pathogens and repairs body cells. Normal flora, body system defenses, and inflammation are all nonspecific defenses that protect against microorganisms regardless of prior exposure. The immune system is composed of separate cells and molecules resistant to disease. Certain responses of the immune system are nonspecific, while others are specific defenses against specific pathogens. If any of the body's defenses fail, an infection can quickly progress to a serious health problem.

NORMAL FLORA

The body normally contains microbial flora that reside on the skin, in the mouth, and in the gastrointestinal tract. A person normally excretes trillions of microbes daily through the intestines. The skin also has a large population of resident flora in concentrations greater than 10,000 microbes per square centimenter. Flora reside on the skin's surface as well as deep within epithelial skin structures. Another rich source of flora is saliva and oral mucosa. Normal flora do not cause disease but instead participate in maintaining a person's health.

Flora of the large intestine exist in large numbers without causing injury. These bacterial flora compete with disease-producing microorganisms for food. Flora also secrete antibacterial substances within the intestine's walls. The skin's flora exert a decontaminative action by inhibiting multiplication of organisms landing on the skin. The mouth and pharynx are also protected by flora that impair growth of invading microbes. The mass of normal flora maintains a sensitive balance with other microorganisms to prevent the onslaught of infection. Any factor that disrupts this balance places a person at serious risk for acquiring an infectious disease.

BODY SYSTEM DEFENSES

A number of the body's organ systems have unique defenses against infection (Table 43-4). The skin, respiratory tract, and gastrointestinal tract are easily accessible to microorganisms. Pathogenic organisms can easily adhere to the skin's surface, be inhaled into the lungs, or be ingested with food. Each organ system has defense mechanisms physiologically suited to its structure and function. For example, the lungs cannot completely control the entrance of microorganisms. However, the airways are lined with hairlike projections or cilia, which rhythmically beat to move a blanket of mucus and adherent organisms up to the pharynx to be swallowed. Conditions that impair an organ's specialized defenses increase a person's susceptibility to infection.

INFLAMMATION

The body's cellular response to injury or infection is inflammation (see Chapter 28). Inflammation is a protective vascular reaction that delivers fluid, blood products, and nutrients to interstitial tissues in an area of injury. The process neutralizes and eliminates pathogens or necrotic tissues and establishes a means of repairing body cells and tissues. Signs of inflammation include swelling, redness, heat, pain or tenderness, and loss of function in the affected body part.

The inflammatory response may be triggered by three types of injury: physical agents, chemical agents, and microorganisms. Mechanical trauma, exposure to temperature extremes, and radiation are physical agents. Chemical agents include external and internal irritants such as harsh poisons or gastric acid. Types of microorganisms have been previously discussed in this chapter.

Once injury to the body's tissues occurs, a series of well-coordinated events comes into play. The inflammatory response includes:

1. Vascular and cellular responses
2. Formation of inflammatory exudate
3. Tissue repair

VASCULAR AND CELLULAR RESPONSES. Acute inflammation is an immediate response to cellular injury. Arterioles supplying the infected or injured area dilate, allowing more blood into local circulation. The increase in local blood flow causes the characteristic redness of inflammation. The symptom of localized warmth results from a greater volume of blood at the inflammatory site. If the inflamed area is deep within the body, local

TABLE 43-4 Normal Body System Defense Mechanisms against Infection

System/Organ	Defense Mechanisms	Action	Factors That May Alter Defense
Skin	Intact multilayered surface is the body's first line of defense against infection	Provides mechanical barrier to microorganisms	Cuts, abrasions, puncture wounds, areas of maceration
	Shedding of outer layer of skin cells	Removes organisms that adhere to skin's outer layers	Failure to bathe regularly
	Sebum	Contains fatty acid that kills some bacteria	Excessive bathing
Mouth	Intact multilayered mucosa	Provides mechanical barrier to microorganisms	Lacerations, trauma, extracted teeth
	Saliva	Washes away particles containing microorganisms	Poor oral hygiene, dehydration
		Saliva contains microbial inhibitors (for example, lysozyme)	
Respiratory tract	Cilia lining upper airways, coated by a sticky mucus blanket	Trap inhaled microbes and sweep them outward in mucus to be expectorated or swallowed	Smoking, high concentration of oxygen and carbon dioxide, decreased humidity, cold air
	Macrophages	Engulf and destroy microorganisms that reach the lung's alveoli	Smoking
Urinary tract	Flushing action of urine flow	Washes away microorganisms on lining of bladder and urethra	Obstruction to normal flow by urinary catheter placement, obstruction from growth or tumor, or delayed micturition
	Intact multilayered epithelium	Provides barrier to microorganisms	Introduction of urinary catheter, continual movement of catheter in urethra
Gastrointestinal tract	Acidity of gastric secretions	Chemically destroys microorganisms incapable of surviving low pH	Administration of antacids
	Rapid peristalsis in small intestine	Prevents retention of bacterial contents	Delayed motility owing to impaction of fecal contents in large bowel or mechanical obstruction by masses
Vagina	At puberty, normal flora cause vaginal secretions to achieve a low pH	Acidic secretions inhibit growth of many microorganisms	Antibiotics and birth control pills disrupt normal flora

warmth does not occur, since the maximum body temperature is at the body's core. Local vasodilation delivers blood, as well as leukocytes, to injured tissues.

With tissue necrosis, the body releases histamine, bradykinin, prostaglandin, and serotonin. These chemical mediators increase permeability of small blood vessels. Fluid, protein, and cells enter interstitial spaces. Accumulated fluid appears as localized swelling or edema.

Another sign of inflammation is pain. The swelling of inflamed tissues increases pressure on nerve endings, causing pain. Chemical substances such as histamine stimulate nerve endings. As a result of physiological changes occurring with inflammation, the involved body part undergoes a loss of function, which may be temporary. For example, a localized infection of the hand causes the fingers to become swollen, painful, and dis-

colored. Joints may become stiff as a result of swelling, but function of the fingers returns when inflammation subsides.

The cellular response of inflammation involves leukocytes arriving at the site. White blood cells (WBCs) pass through blood vessels and into the tissues. Through the process of phagocytosis, the neutrophils and monocytes ingest and destroy microorganisms or other small particles. As inflammation becomes systemic, other signs and symptoms develop. Leukocytosis, or an increase in the number of circulating WBCs, is the body's response to leukocytes leaving blood vessels. A serum white blood cell count is normally 5000 to 10,000 cu/mm but may rise to 15,000 to 20,000 cu/mm during inflammation. Fever is caused by phagocytic release of pyrogens from bacterial cells that cause a rise in the hypothalamic set point (see Chapter 12). Other systemic signs and symptoms include malaise, anorexia, and lymph node enlargement.

INFLAMMATORY EXUDATE. Accumulation of fluid and dead tissue cells and WBCs forms an exudate at the inflammation. Exudate may be serous (clear like plasma), or sanguineous (containing red blood cells). Eventually the exudate is cleared away through lymphatic drainage. Platelets and plasma proteins such as fibrinogen form a meshlike matrix at the inflammation to prevent its spread.

TISSUE REPAIR. When there is injury to tissue cells the healing process involves three stages: defensive, reconstructive, and maturative (see Chapter 47). Damaged cells are eventually replaced with healthy new cells. The new cells undergo a gradual maturation until they take on the same structural characteristics and appearance as the previously injured cells. If inflammation is chronic, tissue defects may fill with fragile granulation tissue. Granulation tissue is not as strong as tissue collagen and assumes the form of scar tissue.

IMMUNE RESPONSE

When a foreign material enters the body's tissues, a response similar to inflammation occurs. Certain foreign materials cause a change in the body's biological makeup so that reactions to future exposures are different from the initial reaction. These altered responses are known as immune responses, and the foreign material is called an antigen. In a normal immune response, the antigen is neutralized, destroyed, or eliminated.

Antigens are foreign materials usually composed of proteins that are not normally found in a person's body. Often antigens exist in complex form as part of the structure of a bacterium or virus. Once an antigen enters the body, it travels in the blood or lymph and initiates these two responses:

CELL-MEDIATED IMMUNITY. There are two classes of lymphocytes, T-lymphocytes or T-cells and B-lymphocytes or B-cells. T-cells play a major role in cell-mediated immunity. T-cells have antigen receptors on their surface membrane. When an antigen meets a T-cell whose surface receptors fit the antigen, a binding occurs. This activates the T-cell to divide rapidly to form sensitized T-cells. Sensitized T-cells travel to the area of inflammation or injury, bind with antigens, and release chemical compounds called lymphokines. The lymphokines (for example, chemotactic factor and macrophage activating factor) attract macrophages and stimulate them to attack antigens. Eventually the antigens are killed.

HUMORAL IMMUNITY. Stimulation of B-lymphocytes triggers the humoral immune response, which results in synthesis of immunoglobulins or antibodies that destroy antigens. Once a B-cell binds with an antigen it causes formation of plasma cells, as well as memory B-cells. Plasma cells synthesize and secrete large amounts of antibodies, proteins normally found in the body that provide general immunity. Memory B-cells prepare the body against future antigen invasion. Thus, when an antigen enters the body again, antibodies form more rapidly than during the first exposure and immunoglobulin levels remain high to attack the antigen.

Antibodies are large protein molecules. There are five classes of immunoglobulins identified by letter names as immunoglobulins M, G, A, E, and D. Immunoglobulin M (IgM) is the antibody formed from immature B-cells and the predominant antibody formed after initial contact with an antigen. This initial contact is called the primary immune response. The most abundant circulating antibody is IgG formed after subsequent contacts with antigens or during the secondary immune response. The IgG antibody is important in providing resistance to infection and can cross the placenta from mother to child, giving the infant passive immunity. Formation of antibodies is the basis of immunization against disease. Natural immunity is an inherited resistance to infection. For example, humans are resistant to the distemper virus that attacks dogs and cats. Acquired immunity, which occurs after exposure to a foreign antigen, is the result of antibody production.

COMPLEMENT. Complement is a protein compound found in blood serum. It is inactive enzymes that become activated when an antigen and antibody bind together. Once complement is activated, a rapid sequence of catalytic activity changes the shape of antigenic cells. The foreign bacteria, for example, assumes the shape of a doughnut. The complement actually makes a hole through the antigen's cell membrane. Ions and water enter the cell, causing it to burst. This process is called cytolysis.

INTERFERON. When certain cells are invaded by viruses they synthesize the protein interferon. Interferon interferes with the ability of viruses to cause disease. It is believed that interferon may act to prevent viruses from multiplying in cells.

ASEPSIS AND NOSOCOMIAL INFECTIONS

Clients in health care settings are usually vulnerable to infection because they are in high-risk groups. Nosocomial infections result from delivery of health services in a health care facility. Clients may acquire nosocomial infections during their stay in a facility. Health care workers may also acquire them as a result of contacting infectious organisms in the workplace. The acquisition of hepatitis from contact with a contaminated needle is an example of nosocomial infection. A hospital is one of the most likely places for acquiring an infection, since it harbors a high population of virulent strains of microorganisms that are usually resistant to antibiotics. Iatrogenic infections are a type of nosocomial infection resulting from a diagnostic or therapeutic procedure. Acquisition of a urinary infection after catheter insertion is an example of an iatrogenic nosocomial infection.

Nosocomial infections may be exogenous or endogenous. An exogenous infection arises from microorganisms external to the individual, which do not exist as normal flora, such as *Salmonella*, *Clostridium tetani*, and *Aspergillus*. Endogenous infections can occur when part of the client's flora becomes altered and an overgrowth results. Examples are infections caused by enterococci, yeasts, and streptococci. When sufficient numbers of microorganisms normally found in one body cavity or lining are transferred to another body site, an endogenous infection develops. For example, transmission of enterococci, normally found in fecal material, from the hands to the skin is a common cause of wound infections. The number of microorganisms needed to cause a nosocomial infection depends on the virulence of the organism, the host's susceptibility, and the body site affected.

The number of health care employees having direct contact with clients, type and number of invasive procedures, therapy received, and length of hospitalization all influence the risk of infection. Major sites for nosocomial infection include the urinary tract, surgical or traumatic wounds, respiratory tract, and bloodstream (see box).

Nosocomial infections significantly increase costs of health care. Extended lengths of stay in health care institutions, increased disability, and prolonged recovery times add to expenses of the client, as well as the health care institution and funding bodies (for example, Medicare). Prevention of nosocomial infection has a beneficial financial impact.

The nurse's efforts to minimize the onset and spread of infection are based on the principles of aseptic technique. The term asepsis means the absence of germs or pathogens. The two types of aseptic technique the nurse practices are medical and surgical asepsis.

Medical asepsis or clean technique includes the procedures used to reduce the number of microorganisms and prevent their spread. Changing a client's linen daily, handwashing, and using clean medication cups are examples of medical asepsis. Principles of medical asepsis

---

Sites and Causes for Nosocomial Infections

- **Urinary Tract.** Insertion of urinary catheter; closed drainage system becoming open; catheter and tube becoming disconnected; drainage bag port touching dirty surface; poor specimen collection technique; obstruction or interference with urinary drainage; urine in catheter or drainage tube being allowed to reenter bladder (reflux); poor handwashing technique; repeated catheter irrigations with solutions
- **Surgical or Traumatic Wounds.** Improper skin preparation (shaving and bathing) before surgery; poor handwashing before dressing changes; failure to cleanse skin surface properly; failure to use aseptic technique during dressing changes; use of contaminated antiseptic solutions
- **Respiratory Tract.** Contaminated respiratory therapy equipment; failure to use aseptic technique while suctioning airway; improper disposal of mucous secretions
- **Bloodstream.** Contamination of intravenous (IV) fluids by tubing or needle changes; insertion of drug additives to IV fluid; addition of connecting tube or stopcocks to IV system; improper care of IV needle insertion site; contaminated needles or catheters; failure to change IV site when inflammation first appears

---

are commonly followed in the home as in the case of washing hands before preparing food.

Surgical asepsis or sterile technique includes procedures used to eliminate microorganisms from an area. Sterilization destroys all microorganisms and their spores. Sterile technique is practiced by nurses in the operating room, where only sterile instruments are used.

Once an object becomes unsterile or unclean, it is contaminated. In medical asepsis an area or object is considered contaminated if it contains or is suspected of containing pathogens. For example, a used bedpan, the floor, and a wet piece of gauze are contaminated. In surgical asepsis an area or object is considered contaminated if touched by any object that is not sterile. For example, a tear in a surgical glove exposes the outside of the glove to the skin surface, thus contaminating it.

The nurse is responsible for providing the client with a safe environment. Effectiveness of aseptic practices depends on the nurse's conscientiousness and consistency in using effective aseptic techniques. It is easy to forget key procedural steps or, when hurried, to take shortcuts that break aseptic procedures. However, the nurse's failure to be meticulous will place the client at risk for an infection that can seriously impair recovery.

NURSING PROCESS

ASSESSMENT

The nurse assesses a client's defenses against infection and susceptibility to infection. A review of the client's clinical condition may detect signs and symptoms of infection. An analysis of laboratory findings provides added information about a client's defense against infection. By knowing the factors that increase a client's susceptibility or risk for infection, the nurse is better able to plan preventive therapy that includes aseptic techniques. By recognizing early signs and symptoms of infection, the nurse can alert the physician to the potential need for therapy and initiate supportive nursing measures.

STATUS OF DEFENSE MECHANISMS

A combination of physical assessment findings and review of a client's medical condition will reveal the status of normal defense mechanisms against infection. For example, any break in the skin or mucosa can become a site for infection to develop. Similarly, a chronic smoker is at greater risk for acquiring infection after general surgery (see Chapter 46) since the cilia of the lung are less likely to be active and able to propel retained mucous from the lung's airways. Any reduction in the body's primary or secondary defenses against infection places a client at risk (see box).

Risk Factors for Infection

INADEQUATE PRIMARY DEFENSES

- Broken skin or mucosa
- Traumatized tissue
- Decreased ciliary action
- Obstructed urine outflow
- Altered peristalsis
- Change in pH secretions

INADEQUATE SECONDARY DEFENSES

- Reduced hemoglobin
- Suppression of lymphocytes (drug or disease related)
- Suppressed inflammatory response (drug or disease related)
- Low WBC count (leukopenia)

CLIENT SUSCEPTIBILITY

Many factors influence susceptibility to infection. The nurse gathers information about each factor through a nursing history.

AGE. Throughout the life span susceptibility to infection changes. An infant has reduced defenses against infection. Born with only the antibodies provided by the mother, the infant's immature immune system is incapable of producing necessary immunoglobulins and WBCs. As the child grows, the immune system matures, but the child is still susceptible to organisms that cause the common cold, intestinal infections, and infectious diseases such as mumps, chickenpox, and measles.

The young or middle-aged adult has refined defenses against infection. Normal flora, body system defenses, inflammation, and the immune response provide protection against invading microorganisms. Viruses are the most common cause of infectious illness in adults.

Defenses against infection again change with aging. The immune response, particularly cell-mediated immunity, declines. Alterations in the immune system may even be instrumental in triggering the aging process. Cells of the immune system such as lymphocytes become more diversified with age, and the body undergoes a progressive loss of cellular regulation. When viruses or other antigens and corresponding antibodies lodge in sites such as the kidney and arteries, factors injurious to the tissues are released and deterioration begins. With aging and in autoimmune diseases (alterations of the immune system), cellular changes such as depletion of lymphoid tissues occur. Cancer and adult-onset diabetes mellitus are believed to be diseases of aging that arise from immunodeficiencies. The basic mechanism for the aging process is not understood. However, it is known that with advancing age immunity to infection decreases.

The elderly also undergo alterations in the structure and function of the skin, urinary tract, and lungs. For example, the skin loses its turgor and the epithelium thins. As a result, the skin is more easily abraded or torn. This increases exposure to pathogens.

NUTRITIONAL STATUS. When a person's protein intake is inadequate as a result of poor diet or debilitating disease, the rate of protein breakdown exceeds that of tissue synthesis (see Chapter 33). This deteriorative process results in a negative nitrogen balance; that is, the output of nitrogen sources such as protein exceeds nitrogen intake. A reduction in the intake of protein and other nutrients such as carbohydrates and fats reduces the body's defenses against infection and impairs wound healing (see Chapter 47).

Clients with illness or disease that increases protein requirements are at further risk. These conditions include traumatic injury, postoperative states, extensive burns, and conditions causing fever.

The nurse assesses the client's dietary habits. The ability to tolerate solid foods also influences nutritional status. Clients who have difficulty swallowing, experience alterations in digestion, or are too confused or weak to feed themselves are at risk for inadequate dietary intake.

STRESS. The body responds to emotional or physical stress by what is known as the general adaptation syndrome (see Chapter 28). During the alarm stage the basal metabolic rate increases as the body uses energy stores. Adrenocorticotropic hormone (ACTH) acts to increase serum glucose levels and decrease unnecessary anti-inflammatory responses through release of cortisone. If stress continues or becomes intense, elevated cortisone levels result in decreased resistance to infection. Continued stress leads to exhaustion, wherein energy stores are depleted and the body has no resistance to invading organisms. The same conditions that increase client's nutritional requirements also increase physical stress. After surgery or a traumatic injury the client has a high susceptibility to infection, not only because of trauma to the body but also because of the level of stress endured.

HEREDITY. Certain hereditary conditions impair an individual's response to infection. The client's history of preexisting medical problems should reveal known hereditary disorders. For example, agammaglobulinemia is an inherited or acquired disorder characterized by the absence of serum antibodies. The client's ability to initiate defenses against infection, as by the release of lymphocytes and formation of antibodies, is virtually absent.

DISEASE PROCESS. Clients with diseases of the immune system are at particular risk for infection. Leukemia, AIDS, lymphoma, and aplastic anemia are examples of conditions that compromise a host by weakening defenses against infectious organisms. For example, clients with leukemia are unable to produce sufficient WBCs to ward off infection.

Victims of chronic disease such as diabetes mellitus and multiple sclerosis are also more susceptible to infection because of general debilitation and nutritional impairment. Diseases that impair body system defenses, such as pulmonary emphysema and bronchitis (which impair ciliary action and thicken mucus), cancer (which causes ulceration of previously intact skin and mucous membranes), and peripheral vascular disease (which reduces blood flow to injured tissues), increase susceptibility to infection. Burn clients have a very high susceptibility to infection because of the damage of skin surfaces. The greater the depth and extent of the burns, the higher the risk for infection.

MEDICAL THERAPY. Some drug and medical therapies compromise a person's immunity to infection. The nurse assesses the client's history to determine if the client takes medications at home that increase infection susceptibility. A review of therapies received within the health care setting further reveals risks. Adrenal corticosteroids, prescribed for several conditions, are anti-inflammatory drugs that cause protein breakdown and impair the inflammatory response against bacteria and other pathogens. Cytotoxic or antineoplastic drugs attack cancer cells but cause side effects of bone marrow depression and normal cell toxicity. With bone marrow depression the body is unable to produce lymphocytes and sufficient WBCs. When normal cells become altered by antineoplastic agents, cellular defenses against infection fail.

Cancer clients receiving radiotherapy are also at risk for infection. The massive doses of radiation, which destroy cancerous cells, can also depress the bone marrow and destroy normal cells.

CLINICAL APPEARANCE

A client's signs and symptoms of infection will be either local or systemic. Localized infections are most common in areas of skin or mucous membrane breakdown such as surgical and traumatic wounds, skin ulcers, decubitus ulcers, and mouth lesions. Infections also develop locally in cavities beneath the skin as in an abscess.

To assess an area for localized infection, the nurse first inspects the area for redness and swelling caused by inflammation. There may be drainage from open lesions or wounds. Infected drainage may be yellow, green, or brown, depending on the site of infection. The nurse asks the client if there is pain or tenderness around the site. The client may complain of tightness caused by edema. If the infected area is large enough, movement of a body part may be restricted. Gentle palpation of an infected area usually results in some degree of tenderness.

Systemic infections cause more generalized symptoms than local infection. They usually result in fever, fatigue, and malaise. Lymph nodes that drain the area of infection often become enlarged, swollen, and tender on palpation. For example, an abscess in the peritoneal cavity may cause enlargement of lymph nodes in the groin. An infection of the upper respiratory tract may cause cervical lymph node enlargement. If an infection is serious and widespread, all major lymph nodes may enlarge. Systemic infections commonly cause a loss of appetite, nausea, and vomiting.

Systemic infections often develop after treatment has failed to control a localized infection. The nurse should be alert for changes in the client's level of activity and responsiveness. As systemic infections develop, the client may become lethargic and complain of a loss of energy. During febrile episodes the temperature may become high, leading to episodes of increased heart and respi-

TABLE 43-5 Laboratory Tests to Screen for Infection

Laboratory Value	Normal (Adult Values)	Indication of Infection
WBC count	5,000-10,000 cu/mm	Increased in acute infection. Decreased in certain viral or overwhelming infections.
Erythrocyte sedimentation rate	Up to 15 mm/hour for males and up to 20 mm/hour for females.	Elevated in presence of inflammatory process.
Iron level	60-90 g/dl	Decreased in chronic infection.
Cultures of wound, urine, sputum, throat, and blood	Urine and blood are normally sterile, without microorganism growth. Wound, sputum, and throat cultures may contain normal flora.	Presence of infectious microorganism growth.
Differential count (percentage of each type of WBC)		
Neutrophils	55%-70%	Increased in acute suppurative infection. Decreased in overwhelming bacterial infection (elderly).
Lymphocytes	20%-40%	Increased in chronic bacterial and viral infection. Decreased in sepsis.
Monocytes	2%-8%	Increased in protozoal and rickettsiae infection, also tuberculosis.
Eosinophils	1%-4%	Increased in parasitic infection.
Basophils	0.5%-1%	Remains normal during infection.

ratory rates. Involvement of major body systems produces specific signs. For example, a pulmonary infection results in a productive cough with purulent sputum. A urinary tract infection may result in cloudy, foul-smelling urine.

The nurse uses knowledge of the client's medical condition to anticipate infection and the extent to which body systems might become involved.

LABORATORY DATA

A review of specific laboratory test results may reveal infection (Table 43-5). Laboratory values by themselves are not enough to detect infection. Other clinical signs must be assessed. Factors other than infection may alter test values. For example, trauma and physical stress can cause an elevation in neutrophils.

CLIENTS WITH INFECTION

A client with infection may present a variety of health problems. It is important for the nurse to assess how the infection influences the client's needs, which may be physical, psychological, social, or economic. For example, a client with sexually transmitted disease such as AIDS may experience serious psychological problems as a result of self-imposed isolation or rejection by friends. A client with a chronic infection in need of continuous wound care at home may not be able to afford the cost of medical supplies. The nurse determines the client's ability to adjust to the disease and resources available for managing health problems.

NURSING DIAGNOSIS

The nurse's assessments reveals the client's susceptibility to infection or the presence of infection. These defining characteristics are used to develop nursing diagnoses (see sample nursing diagnoses box). The nurse may also make diagnoses resulting from review of risk factors for infection. For clients with active infection the nurse may identify diagnoses that reflect the overall influence of the infection on life-style. Examples of nursing diagnoses are shown in the nursing diagnoses box.

PLANNING

Before the nurse performs any care, consideration must be given to the risks of exposing the client to infection. Whether a procedure is as simple as giving a bath or administering medications, poor technique can result in injurious effects. The nurse must plan care activities carefully, ensuring that appropriate aseptic techniques are always followed.

For clients with infection, the nurse plans care to maintain the client's dignity and identity. Involvement of the client in decisions regarding care is important. Measures used in infection control such as isolation precautions or cleansing of an infected wound can threaten a client's sense of well-being and control.

Sample Nursing Diagnoses for Clients Susceptible to or Overcome by Infection

Defining Characteristics	Nursing Diagnoses	Related Factors
Broken skin Traumatized tissues Abnormal laboratory values Suppressed inflammatory response	Potential for infection	• Trauma to skin • Malnutrition • Chronic disease • Use of pharmaceutical agents
Abnormal laboratory values Broken skin Tissue hypoxia	Potential for injury	• Altered immunity • Malnutrition • Physical injury
Broken skin or mucosa Reduced capillary refill and edema Inflammation	Impaired tissue integrity	• Altered circulation • Mechanical injury

Examples of Nursing Diagnoses Related to Clients Susceptible to or Overcome by Infection

NANDA-APPROVED NURSING DIAGNOSES

Potential for infection related to:
• Altered immunity
• Tissue destruction
• Invasive procedures
• Malnutrition

Potential for injury related to:
• Altered immunity

Impaired tissue integrity related to:
• Altered circulation
• Mechanical injury
• Exposure to irritants

Altered oral mucous membrane related to:
• Trauma
• Dehydration
• Local pathologies
• Infection

Altered nutrition less than body requirements related to:
• Poor diet habits
• Altered gastrointestinal function

Actual or *potential impaired skin integrity* related to:
• Trauma
• Physical immobilization
• Exposure to irritants

Social isolation related to:
• Misconceptions about sexually transmitted disease

Body image disturbance related to:
• Open wound infection
• Self-perceptions regarding sexually transmitted disease

The care plan box lists a sample care plan for a client at risk for or overcome by infection. With actual or potential infection, goals of care include the following:

1. Preventing exposure to infectious organisms
2. Controlling or reducing the extent of infection
3. Understanding of infection control techniques
4. Maintaining a sense of comfort and self-esteem

IMPLEMENTATION

NURSE'S ROLE IN INFECTION CONTROL

The nurse has two primary responsibilities in controlling infection: (1) preventing the onset and spread of infection, and (2) promoting measures for treatment of infection. To prevent an infection from developing or spreading, the nurse minimizes the numbers and kinds of organisms transmitted to potential infection sites. Eliminating reservoirs of infection, controlling portals of exit and entry, and avoiding actions that transmit microorganisms will prevent bacteria from finding a site to grow. Disinfection and sterilization of supplies and good handwashing are examples of medically aseptic methods the nurse uses to control the spread of microorganisms. A final preventive measure is to strengthen a potential host's defenses against infection. Nutritional support, rest, maintenance of physiological protective mechanisms, and immunization protect a client from invasion by pathogens.

When a client develops an infection, the nurse continues preventive care so health care personnel and other clients do not acquire the infection. Clients with highly communicable diseases require protective aseptic techniques that control the environment by forming barriers against bacterial spread.

Sample Nursing Care Plan for Clients Susceptible to or Overcome by Infection

Nursing Diagnosis	Goals	Expected Outcomes	Nursing Interventions
Potential for infection related to tissue destruction.	Wound remains free of infection.	Surgical incision will stay approximated.	Use strict handwashing technique before surgical dressing changes.
		Wound drainage will be infection free.	Follow surgical aseptic technique during dressing changes.
		Inflammation absent along wound edges.	Administer prophylactic antibiotics on time.
	Normal healing process is promoted.	Incision closes within expected time frame.	Provide well-balanced, high protein meals
	Client understands infection control technique at discharge.	Client correctly demonstrates technique for incision care at home.	Demonstrate and have client practice handwashing. Demonstrate and have client cleanse incision line.

Treatment of an infectious process includes eliminating the infectious organisms and supporting the client's defenses. The nurse must collect specimens of body fluids or drainage from infected body sites for cultures. When the disease process or causative organism has been identified, the physician prescribes the anti-infective or antibiotic drug most effective for the situation. The nurse administers antibiotics judiciously, watching for allergic reactions, assessing the progress of the infection, and administering drugs by proper methods.

Systemic infections require measures to prevent complications of fever (see Chapter 12). Maintaining intake of fluids prevents dehydration resulting from diaphoresis. The client's increased metabolic rate necessitates an adequate nutritional intake. Rest preserves energy for the healing process.

Localized infections often require measures to facilitate removal of infectious organisms. Wet-to-dry dressings (see Chapter 47) are used to remove infected drainage from wound sites. Heat compresses promote blood flow to an infected site and thus the delivery of blood components needed to fight an infection. Drainage tubes are inserted to remove infected drainage from body cavities. The nurse uses medical and surgical aseptic techniques to manage wounds and ensures correct handling of infected drainage or body fluids.

During the course of infection the nurse supports the client's body defense mechanisms. For example, if a client has infectious diarrhea, the nurse must maintain skin integrity to prevent breakdown and entrance of microorganisms. Humidified air maintains function of the lung's protective cilia. Therefore when administering oxygen to a client, the nurse makes sure only humidified gas is used. Routine hygiene measures such as cleansing the oral cavity and bathing protect the skin and mucous membranes from organism spread.

Needs of a client with an infection can be many. By monitoring the infection's course carefully, the nurse can choose the most appropriate measures to maintain or restore health.

MEDICAL ASEPSIS

The nurse follows certain principles and procedures in preventing infection and controlling its spread. The nurse uses basic medical aseptic techniques to break the infection chain. Infections that are readily transmissible between individuals require protective aseptic techniques. Clients with high susceptibility to infection require special precautions to prevent exposure to pathogens.

CONTROL OR ELIMINATION OF INFECTIOUS AGENTS. Proper cleansing, disinfecting, and sterilization of contaminated objects significantly reduce and often eliminate microorganisms. In large health care centers a central supply department does most of the disinfecting and sterilizing of reusable supplies. However, the nurse encounters situations during a client's care that require use of these techniques. Many principles of cleansing and disinfecting also apply to the home setting.

Cleansing. Cleanliness inhibits the growth of microorganisms. When an object used in the care of a client comes in contact with infectious or potentially infectious material the object is contaminated. If the object is disposable, it will be discarded. Reusable objects must be cleansed thoroughly before disinfection and sterilization.

When cleaning equipment is soiled by organic material such as blood, fecal matter, mucus, or pus, it is important to use waterproof gloves, a stiff-bristled brush, and detergent or soap.

These basic steps will ensure that an object is clean:

1. Rinse a contaminated object or article with cold running water to remove organic material. Hot water causes the protein in organic material to coagulate and stick to objects, making removal difficult.
2. After rinsing, wash the object with soap and warm water. Soap or detergent reduces the surface tension of water and emulsifies dirt or remaining material. Few household detergents, however, have disinfectant properties. Rinse the object thoroughly to remove the emulsified dirt.
3. Use a brush to remove dirt or material in grooves or seams. Friction dislodges contaminated material for easy removal.
4. Rinse the object in warm water.
5. Dry the object and prepare it for disinfection or sterilization.
6. The brush, gloves, and sink in which the equipment is cleaned should be considered contaminated and should be cleansed.

Disinfection and Sterilization. Disinfection kills pathogenic organisms that are not spore forming. Noninfectious microorganisms may or may not be killed. Sterilization is the process of destroying all microorganisms, including spores and viruses.

The two primary methods for disinfection and sterilization are physical processes, involving use of heat or radiation, and chemical processes, in which various solutions or gases are used. Both disrupt internal functioning of microorganisms by destroying cell proteins. Sterilization and disinfection occur when heat reaches a level sufficient to destroy organisms or when a concentration of chemicals has adequate exposure to microorganisms.

A disinfectant is a chemical solution that is used when cleaning inanimate objects. Examples of disinfectants are phenols. The solutions can be caustic and toxic to tissues. An antiseptic, for example, silver sulfadiazine (Silvadene) or isopropyl alcohol, is a chemical preparation applied on skin and tissues.

Selection of a method for disinfecting or sterilizing is done after considering the following factors:

1. *Concentration of solution and duration of contact.* A weakened concentration or shortened exposure time may lessen effectiveness.
2. *Type and number of pathogens.* Certain organisms are killed more easily than others by disruption. The greater the number of pathogens on an object the longer the required disinfecting time.
3. *Surface areas to treat.* All dirty surfaces and areas must be fully exposed to disinfecting and sterilizing agents.
4. *Temperature of environment.*Disinfectants tend to work best at room temperature.
5. *Presence of soap.* Soap may cause certain disinfectants to be ineffective. Thorough rinsing of an object is necessary before disinfecting.
6. *Presence of organic materials.* Disinfectants can become inactivated unless blood, saliva, pus, or body excretions are washed off.

Table 43-6 lists methods of disinfection and sterilization and their characteristics.

CONTROL OR ELIMINATION OF RESERVOIRS. To control or eliminate reservoir sites for infection, the nurse eliminates sources of body fluids, drainage, or solutions that might harbor microorganisms. The nurse also carefully discards articles that become contaminated with infectious material (see box).

Infection Control to Reduce Reservoirs of Infection

- **Bathing.** Use soap and water to remove drainage, dried secretions, excess perspiration, or sediment from disinfectants.
- **Dressing changes.** Change dressings that become wet and soiled (see Chapter 47).
- **Contaminated articles.** Place tissues, soiled dressings, or soiled linen in moisture resistant bags for proper disposal.
- **Contaminated needles.** Place syringes and hypodermic needles and intravenous needles in moisture-resistant, puncture-proof containers. (Do not recap needles or attempt to break them.)
- **Bedside unit.** Keep table surfaces clean and dry.
- **Bottled solutions.** Do not leave open for prolonged periods. Keep solutions tightly capped.
- **Surgical wounds.** Keep drainage tubes and collection bags patent to prevent accumulation of serous fluid under the skin surface.
- **Drainage bottles and bags.** Empty and rinse suction bottles according to agency policy. Empty all drainage systems on each shift unless otherwise ordered by a physician. Never raise a drainage system (for example, urinary drainage bag) above the level of the site being drained unless it is clamped off.

TABLE 43-6 Processes for Disinfection and Sterilization

Characteristics	Examples of Use
DRY HEAT	
Not used in health care settings. May be used in home for articles that can't be placed in water. Disinfects only.	Placing articles in oven at 350°F for at least 45 minutes.
BOILING WATER	
Least expensive for use in home. Bacterial spores and some viruses resist boiling.	Boil items for at least 15 minutes (for example, glass baby bottles).
MOIST HEAT	
Includes steam (moist heat under pressure) or free steam. When water vapor is exposed to a high pressure it can attain a temperature above boiling point to kill all pathogens and spores. Free steam used to sterilize objects that would otherwise be destroyed at higher temperature of autoclave.	Autoclave used to sterilize surgical instruments, parenteral solutions, and surgical dressings. Bedpan sterilizers use free steam. Free steam processes for sterilization takes 30 minutes on 3 consecutive days.
RADIATION	
Ionizing radiation penetrates deeply into objects for effective sterilization and disinfection.	Used in sterilizing drugs, foods, and other heat-sensitive items.
CHEMICALS	
An effective chemical disinfectant: attacks all types of microorganisms, acts rapidly, works with water, retains no odor, is stable in light and heat, is inexpensive, is not harmful to body tissues, will not destroy article being disinfected, and is not inactivated by organic material.	Used for disinfection of instruments and equipment such as glass thermometers. Chlorine is useful for disinfecting water and housekeeping purposes.
ETHYLENE OXIDE GAS	
Destroys spores and microorganisms by altering cells metabolic processes. Fumes released within an autoclave-like chamber. Toxic to humans.	Sterilizes rubber, paper, and plastic items.

CONTROL OF PORTALS OF EXIT. To control organisms exiting via the respiratory tract, the nurse should avoid talking directly into a client's face or talking, sneezing, or coughing directly over a surgical wound or sterile dressing field. The nurse should cover mouth or nose when sneezing or coughing. The nurse is also responsible for teaching clients how to protect others when they sneeze or cough and for providing clients with disposable wipes or tissues to control spread of microorganisms.

A nurse who has a mild cold and continues to work with clients should wear a mask, especially when changing a dressing or performing a sterile procedure. The nurse should refrain from working with clients who are highly susceptible to infection.

Another way of controlling the exit of microorganisms is the careful handling of exudate such as urine, feces, and emesis. The nurse should wear disposable gloves if there is a chance of contact with any exudate. Soiled items are appropriately bagged and disposed of.

CONTROL OF TRANSMISSION. Effective control of infection requires a nurse to remain aware of the modes of transmission and how to control them. In the hospital, home, or extended care facility a client should have a personal set of care items. Sharing thermometers, bedpans, urinals, bath basins, and eating utensils can easily lead to transmission of infection. Glass thermometers, even when individually used, warrant special care. Since the client's own mucus can become a source for microorganism growth, after each use the thermometer is washed in soap and water and dried.

Because certain microorganisms travel easily through the air, linens or bedclothes should not be shaken. Dusting with a treated or dampened cloth prevents dust particles from entering the air.

To prevent transmission of microorganisms through indirect contact, soiled items and equipment must be kept from touching the nurse's clothing. A common error is to carry dirty linen in the arms against the uniform. Special linen bags should be used, or soiled linen carried with hand held out from the body. Laundry hampers should not be allowed to overflow.

It is important to remember that anything that touches the floor is contaminated. If the nurse accidentally drops a piece of equipment, it should be discarded. When the nurse stoops or bends, the uniform should not touch the floor, and clean or soiled linen should never be put on the floor.

Handwashing. The most important and most basic technique in preventing and controlling transmission of pathogens is handwashing. Handwashing is a vigorous, brief rubbing together of all surfaces of lathered hands, followed by rinsing under a stream of water (Garner and Favero, 1985).

Contaminated hands are a prime cause of cross-infections. For example, consider a nurse caring for a client who has excessive pulmonary excretions. The nurse assists the client in expectorating mucus and disposes of tissues in a bedside container. The client's roommate asks the nurse to open containers of food on the meal tray. The nurse then leaves the client's room to pour a dose of medication due in 5 minutes. If the nurse fails to wash the hands before each of these actions, organisms from the first client's mucus could easily be transmitted to the roommate's food and to the medication container.

The need for handwashing depends on the type, intensity, duration, and sequence of activity. For example, if a nurse simply touches an object that is not visibly soiled, handwashing is not required. In contrast, prolonged and intense contact with any client, especially one with wound drainage, requires thorough handwashing.

Garner and Favero (1985) recommend that nurses wash their hands in the following situations:

1. Before contact with clients who are susceptible to infection, for example, newborn infants or immunosuppressed clients (with leukemia or organ transplant recipients)
2. After caring for an infected client
3. After touching organic material
4. Before performing invasive procedures, such as administering injections, catheterization, and suctioning
5. Before and after handling dressings or touching open wounds
6. After handling contaminated equipment
7. Between contact with different clients in high-risk units (for example, nursery and critical care units)

The ideal duration of handwashing is not known. The Centers for Disease Control (CDC) and Public Health Service note that washing times of at least 10 to 15 seconds (Garner and Favero, 1985) will remove most transient microorganisms from the skin. If hands are visibly soiled more time may be needed. Agency policies often recommend staff to wash hands for 1 to 2 minutes after working in high-risk areas. Routine handwashing may be performed with bar, liquid, or granule soap, or soap-impregnated tissue.

Use of antimicrobial-containing soaps is encouraged when nurses work in special care units, perform invasive procedures, or care for clients in isolation (see protective asepsis) or clients with known multiple resistant bacteria. Larson (1987) suggests that 1 ml of nonantiseptic liquid soap and 3 to 5 ml of antiseptic soap be used for the respective handwashing procedures. Procedure 43-1 lists the steps for handwashing.

Health care workers' compliance with handwashing is important. Failure to follow good handwashing techniques may be due to concern over the effects repeated handwashing has on the condition of skin. Larson (1986) studied the effects of five different soaps (plain and antimicrobial) on skin damage. The study revealed that although all soaps caused some trauma to the skin, addition of antiseptics to soap caused no greater skin damage. There was no correlation between greater antimicrobial activity and degree of skin damage.

The nurse instructs clients and visitors on the proper technique and times for handwashing. Teaching handwashing is particularly important if the client's health care is to continue at home. Clients should wash their hands before eating or handling food, after handling contaminated equipment, linen, or organic material, and before and after elimination. Visitors are encouraged to wash their hands before eating or handling food, after coming in contact with infected clients, and after handling contaminated equipment or organic material.

CONTROL OF PORTALS OF ENTRY. Many measures that control the exit of microorganisms likewise control the entrance of pathogens. Maintaining the integrity of skin and mucous membranes reduces the chances of microorganisms reaching a host. The client's skin should be kept well lubricated by using hand lotion as appropriate (see Chapter 32). Immobilized and debilitated clients are particularly susceptible to skin breakdown. Clients should not be positioned on tubes or objects that might cause breaks in the skin. Dry, wrinkle-free linen also reduces the chances of skin breakdown. Frequent oral hygiene prevents drying of mucous membranes. A water-soluble ointment will keep the client's lips well lubricated.

After elimination, a woman should clean the rectum and perineum by wiping from the urinary meatus toward

PROCEDURE 43-1

Handwashing

STEPS	RATIONALE
1. Use a sink with warm running water and equipped with soap or disinfectant and paper towels.	Running water facilitates removal of organisms. Paper towels are easy to discard.
2. Push wristwatch and long uniform sleeves up above wrists. Remove jewelry, except a plain band, from fingers and arms.	This provides complete access to fingers, hands, and wrists. Jewelry may harbor microorganisms.
3. Keep fingernails short and filed.	Dirt and secretions that lodge under the fingernails contain microorganisms. Long fingernails can scratch a client's skin.
4. Inspect the surface of the hands and fingers for breaks or cuts in the skin and cuticles. Report such lesions when caring for highly susceptible clients.	Open cuts or wounds can harbor high concentrations of microorganisms. Such lesions may serve as portals of exit, increasing a client's exposure to infection, or as portals of entry, increasing the nurse's risk of acquiring an infection.
5. Stand in front of the sink, keeping hands and uniform away from the sink surface. (If hands touch the sink during handwashing, repeat the process.) Use a sink where it is comfortable to reach the faucet.	The inside of the sink is a contaminated area. Reaching over a sink increases the risk of touching the edge, which is contaminated.
6. Turn on the water. Press foot pedals with the foot to regulate flow and temperature (see illustration). Push knee pedals laterally to control flow and temperature. Turn on hand-operated faucets by covering the faucet with a paper towel.	When the hands come in contact with a faucet, they are considered contaminated. Organisms spread easily from the hands to the faucet.
7. Avoid splashing water against your uniform.	Microorganisms travel and grow in moisture.
8. Regulate flow of water so the temperature is warm.	Warm water is more comfortable. Hot water opens pores of the skin, causing irritation.
9. Wet hands and lower arms thoroughly under running water. Keep the hands and forearms lower than the elbows during washing.	The hands are the most contaminated parts to be washed. Water flows from the least to the most contaminated area, rinsing microorganisms into the sink.
10. Apply 1 ml of regular or 3 ml of antiseptic liquid soap to the hands, lathering thoroughly. If bar soap is used, hold it throughout the lathering period. Soap granules and leaflet preparations may be used.	Bar soap should be rinsed before returning it to soap dish. A soap dish that allows water to drain keeps the soap firm. Jellylike soap permits growth of microorganisms.
11. Wash the hands using plenty of lather and friction for at least 10 to 15 seconds. Interlace the fingers and rub the palms and back of hands with a circular motion at least 5 times each (see illustration).	Soap cleanses by emulsifying fat and oil and lowering surface tension. Friction and rubbing mechanically loosen and remove dirt and transient bacteria. Interlacing fingers and thumbs ensures that all surfaces are cleansed.

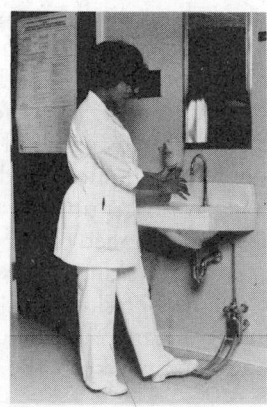

Step 6

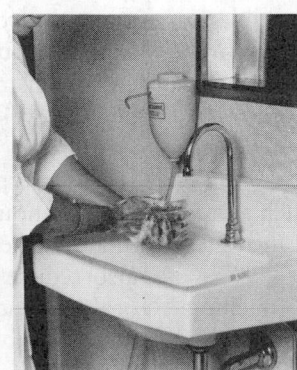

Step 11

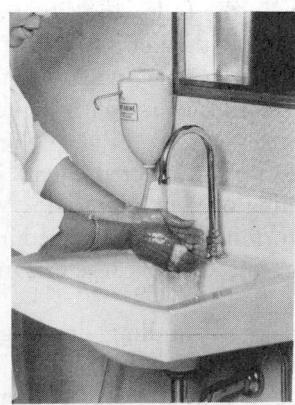

Step 13

STEPS	RATIONALE
12. If areas underlying fingernails are soiled, clean them with fingernails of the other hand and additional soap or a clean orangewood stick. Do not tear or cut the skin under or around the nail.	Mechanical removal of dirt and sediment under nails reduces microorganisms on hands.
13. Rinse hands and wrists thoroughly, keeping hands down and elbows up (see illustration).	Rinsing mechanically washes away dirt and microorganisms.
14. Repeat steps 10 through 12 but extend the actual period of washing for 1-, 2-, and 3-minute handwashings.	The greater the likelihood of the hands being contaminated, the greater the need for thorough handwashing.
15. Dry the hands thoroughly from the fingers up to the wrists and forearms.	Dry from the cleanest area (fingertips) to the least clean (forearms) to avoid contamination. Drying hands prevents chapping and roughened skin.
16. Discard paper towel in proper receptacle.	Proper disposal of contaminated objects prevents transfer of microorganisms.
17. Turn off water with foot and knee pedals. To turn off a hand faucet, use a clean, dry paper towel.	A wet towel and wet hands allow the transfer of pathogens by capillary action.

the rectum. Cleansing in a direction from the least to the most contaminated area helps reduce genitourinary infections.

Clients, health care personnel, and even housekeepers are at risk for acquiring infections from accidental needle sticks. After administering an injection or inserting an intravenous catheter, the nurse should carefully dispose of contaminated needles (see Chapter 15). A stray needle lying in bed linen or carelessly thrown into a wastebasket is a prime source for pathogens. Hepatitis B or serum hepatitis is the infection most commonly transmitted by contaminated needles. A needle stick should be reported immediately. In most health care agencies the victim of a needle stick completes an injury report and sees a physician for treatment. It may be necessary for the person to receive a series of gamma globulin injections.

Another cause for entrance of microorganisms into a host is improper handling and management of catheters and drainage sets. The point of connection between a catheter or drain and tubing should remain closed and intact. As long as such systems are closed, their contents are considered sterile (except for drainage of infectious wounds). When turning, lifting, or moving clients, the nurse should make certain that connecting tubes have enough slack to avoid being pulled apart. At times the nurse obtains specimens from drainage tubes or inserts needles into intravenous tubing ports. The nurse disinfects tubes and ports by wiping them liberally with alcohol or a similar solution before opening the system. Placing squares of sterile gauze around the ends of an opened drainage tube adds further protection against entrance of bacteria.

A final method for reducing the entrance of microorganisms is the technique for cleansing wounds (see Chapter 47). The wound itself is considered to be sterile. To prevent entrance of microorganisms, the nurse should clean outward from a wound site. When applying a disinfectant or cleaning with soap and water, it is important to wipe around the wound edge first and then clean outward. A clean gauze should be used for each revolution around the wound's circumference.

PROTECTION OF THE SUSCEPTIBLE HOST. A client's resistance to infection improves as the nurse protects normal body defenses against infection. The nurse also intervenes to maintain the body's normal reparative processes (see box on p. 1284).

Protective Asepsis. Often clients acquire infectious diseases that can easily be transmitted to other clients, family members, or health care personnel. Communicable diseases, such as measles and tuberculosis, and infections by highly virulent organisms would spread rapidly throughout a health care institution if special precautions were not used for prevention. Clients with low immunity also require special precautions to prevent exposure to organisms that are normally found in a health care environment.

Protective aseptic techniques or isolation precautions are used to control transmission of pathogens. Environ-

TABLE 43-7   Isolation Categories

Type of Isolation (Specific Category)	Purpose	Example of Disease or Condition	Room
Strict	Prevents transmission of highly contagious or virulent infections spread by air and contact	Chickenpox; diphtheria	Private room with door closed
Contact	Prevents transmission of highly transmissible infections spread by close or direct contact, which do not warrant strict precautions	Acute respiratory infections in infants and young children; impetigo; herpes simplex; infections by multiple resistant bacteria	Private room; clients infected with same organism may share a room
Respiratory	Prevents transmission of infectious diseases over short distances via air droplets	Measles; meningitis; mumps; pneumonia; *Haemophilus* influenza (in children)	Private room; clients infected with same organism may share a room
Enteric precautions	Prevents infections transmitted by direct or indirect contact with feces	Cholera; diarrhea of an infectious cause; hepatitis A; gastroenteritis caused by highly infectious organism	Private room if client's hygiene is poor (does not wash hands, shares contaminated items); clients with same organism may share a room
Tuberculosis isolation	Special category for clients with pulmonary tuberculosis who have positive results on sputum or chest x-ray examination indicating active disease	Laryngeal tuberculosis	Private room with special ventilation preferred; door closed
Drainage/secretion precautions	Prevents infections transmitted by direct or indirect contact with purulent material or drainage from an infected body site	Abscess; burn infection; infected wound; minor infections not included in contact isolation	Private room not indicated
Universal blood and body fluid precautions*	Transmitted by direct or indirect contact with infective blood or body fluids	Acquired immune deficiency syndrome (AIDS); hepatitis B; syphillis	Private room indicated if client's hygiene is poor
Care of severely compromised clients†	Protects an uninfected client with lowered immunity and resistance from acquiring infectious organisms	Leukemia; lymphoma; aplastic anemia	Private room with door closed

*Formerly blood and body fluid precautions.
†Formerly protective or reverse isolation.

Gown	Gloves	Mask	Precautions
Required of all persons entering room	Required of all persons entering room	Required of all persons entering room	Discard or bag and label articles contaminated with infective materials. Send reusable articles for disinfection and sterilization.
Indicated if soiling or contact is likely	Indicated for persons touching infective material	Indicated for persons coming close to client	Discard or bag and label articles contaminated with infective material. Send reusable items for disinfection and sterilization.
Not indicated	Not indicated	Indicated for persons who come close to client	Discard or bag and label articles contaminated with infective material. Send reusable items for disinfection and sterilization. Bathroom should not be shared by clients.
Indicated if soiling is likely	Indicated when touching infective material	Not indicated	Discard or bag and label articles contaminated with infective material. Send reusable items for disinfection and sterilization. Bathroom should not be shared by clients.
Indicated only if needed to prevent gross contamination of clothing	Not indicated	Indicated only if client is coughing and does not reliably cover mouth	Articles are rarely involved in transmission of tuberculosis. Articles should be thoroughly cleansed, disinfected, or discarded.
Indicated if soiling or contact with infective material is likely	Indicated for touching infective material	Not indicated	Discard or bag and label articles contaminated with infective material. Send for disinfection or sterilization.
Indicated during procedures that are likely to generate splashes of blood or body fluids	Indicated for touching blood or body fluids, mucous membranes or nonintact skin of all clients; indicated for touching soiled items	Indicated during procedures likely to generate droplets of blood	Discard or bag and label articles contaminated with blood or body fluids. Disinfect and sterilize articles. Avoid needle stick injuries. Dispose of used needles in properly labeled, puncture-resistant container. Clean blood spills promptly with 5.25% solution of sodium hypochloride diluted 1:10 with water.
Required of all persons entering room	Required of all persons entering room	Indicated for persons coming in contact with client	For open wound or burns, use sterile gloves.

Infection Control: Protecting the Susceptible Host

PROTECTING NORMAL DEFENSE MECHANISMS

- Regular bathing removes transient microorganisms from the skin's surface. Lubrication helps to keep the skin hydrated and intact.
- Regular oral hygiene removes proteins in the saliva that attract microorganisms. Flossing removes tartar and plaque that can cause germ infection.
- Maintenance of an adequate fluid intake promotes normal urine formation and a resultant outflow of urine to flush the bladder and urethral lining of microorganisms.
- For physically dependent or immobilized clients encourage routine coughing and deep breathing to keep lower airways clear of mucus.
- Encourage proper immunization of children or adult clients who become exposed to certain infectious microorganisms (for example, tetanus).

MAINTAINING REPARATIVE PROCESSES

- Promote intake of a well-balanced diet containing essential proteins, vitamins, carbohydrates, and fats. Use measures to increase client's appetite (see Chapter 33).
- Promote a client's comfort and sleep so that energy stores are replaced daily (see Chapters 34 and 35).
- Assist client in learning techniques to reduce stress.

---

mental barriers such as a private room, a closed door, a mask, or a protective gown and gloves keep pathogens in a confined area. The extent of protection a client requires depends on how transmissible a disease is. Any person caring for the client follows practices either to prevent organisms from leaving the room of the infected client or to prohibit them from entering the room of a highly susceptible client.

In 1983 the CDC issued specific guidelines for isolating the client within a controlled environment (Garner and Simmons, 1983.) The guidelines establish a balance between ideal and practical isolation precautions and establish scientifically sound and effective precautions that isolate the disease but not the client. In the disease-specific system, certain practices are followed for each infectious disease. This is the less costly and time-consuming system because certain diseases require only minimal precautions. The more commonly used system in hospitals has been the category-specific isolation. Diseases requiring similar isolation precautions, indicated by the manner in which the organisms are transmitted, are grouped in eight categories (Table 43-7).

Hospitals also implement modified or protective isolation precautions for staff working in intensive care units, nurseries, burn units, and organ transplant units. These precautions protect clients who are severely immunosuppressed. Anyone caring for these clients wears a mask, gloves, and gown.

In 1987 the CDC issued recommendations for prevention of human immunodeficiency virus (HIV) transmission in health care settings (CDC, 1987). The HIV that causes AIDS has become a serious enough health risk to warrant special precautions (Table 43-7). The CDC recommends the need for health care workers to consider all clients as potentially infected with HIV and other blood-borne pathogens and to adhere to infection control practices for minimizing risk of exposure to blood and body fluids. The CDC has recommended universal blood and body fluid precautions. These precautions are to be used for all clients, especially those in emergency care settings in which the risk of blood exposure is increased and the infection status of a client is usually unknown. Implementation of universal precautions eliminates the need for use of the isolation category, blood and body fluid precautions, previously recommended by the CDC.

The guidelines for universal precautions include the following (CDC, 1987):

1. Gloves should be worn for touching blood and body fluids, mucous membranes, or nonintact skin of all clients.
2. Gloves should be worn for handling items or surfaces soiled with blood or body fluids and for performing venipuncture and other vascular access procedures.
3. Gloves should be changed after contact with each client.
4. Masks and protective eyewear or face shields should be worn during procedures (for example, irrigations) that are likely to generate droplets of blood or other body fluids to prevent exposure of mucous membranes of the mouth, nose, and eyes.
5. Gowns should be worn during procedures that are likely to generate splashes of blood or other body fluids.
6. Hands and other skin surfaces should be washed immediately and thoroughly if contaminated with blood or other body fluids.
7. To prevent needlestick injuries, needles should be not be recapped, purposely bent, broken, or removed from disposable syringes. Dispose in puncture-resistant containers near the work area.
8. To reduce the need for mouth-to-mouth resuscitation (see Chapter 36) mouthpieces, resuscitator bags, or other ventilation devices should be used.
9. Health care workers who have exudative lesions should refrain from all direct client care and from handling client care equipment.

Regardless of the type of protective asepsis system, the nurse must follow certain basic principles.

1. Hands should be washed thoroughly before entering and leaving the room of a client receiving protective asepsis.
2. Contaminated supplies and equipment should be disposed of in a manner that prevents spread of microorganisms to other persons.
3. Knowledge of the disease process and the means of infection transmission should be applied when using protective barriers.
4. Measures should be implemented to protect other people who might be exposed during transport of the client to locations outside the isolation room.
5. Equipment required in the care of the client and in establishing protective asepsis precautions should be organized and easily accessible.

Psychological Implications of Isolation. Protective asepsis creates a forced solitude that deprives the client of normal social relationships. This situation can be psychologically harmful, especially for children.

As a result of the infectious process the client's body image is altered. He or she may feel unclean, rejected, lonely, or guilty. Aseptic practices the nurse follows further intensify this belief of difference or undesirability. Isolation in a private room limits sensory contact. Unless the nurse acts to minimize feelings of psychological and physical isolation, the client's emotional state can interfere with recovery.

Before protective aseptic measures are instituted, the client and family must understand the nature of the condition, the purposes of protective asepsis, and how to carry out specific precautions. If they are able to participate in maintaining asepsis, the chances of reducing the spread of infection are great. The client and family should be taught how to wash their hands and don gowns, masks, or gloves. Each procedure should be demonstrated, and the client and family should be given an opportunity for practice. It is also important to explain how infectious organisms can be transmitted so the client understands the difference between contaminated and clean objects. Unless family members know that their clothing becomes contaminated by contact with infected secretions, efforts at controlling infection are wasted.

The nurse also takes measures to improve the client's sensory stimulation during isolation. Reading materials, a radio or television set, a clock, and hobby materials should be available. However, if a book or other inanimate object comes in contact with infected material, it must be disinfected or discarded. An object such as a radio can be wrapped in a protective plastic covering. The room environment should be clean and pleasant looking. Drapes or shades should be opened and excess supplies or equipment removed. The nurse must listen to the client's concerns or interests. If the nurse rushes through care or shows a lack of interest, the client will feel rejected and even more isolated. Mealtime is a particularly good opportunity for conversation. Providing comfort measures such as repositioning, a back massage, or a tepid sponge bath increases physical stimulation. If the condition permits, the nurse should encourage the client to walk and sit up in a chair.

It is important for the nurse to explain to family members the client's risk of depression or loneliness. Visiting family members should be encouraged to avoid expressions or actions that convey revulsion or disgust. The nurse advises family members on ways to provide meaningful stimulation.

Protective Environment. A private room reduces the possibility of transmission of infection by separating susceptible clients from those who might be sources of infection and by serving as a reminder for personnel to wash their hands and use aseptic precautions. Many infections do not require isolation in a private room. However, if the client uses poor hygiene or if it would be difficult to separate the client and his or her personal items from a person sharing the room, a private room is preferable. On the door or wall outside the room, the nurse posts a card listing precautions for the client's isolation category. The card is a handy reference for health care personnel and visitors and alerts anyone who

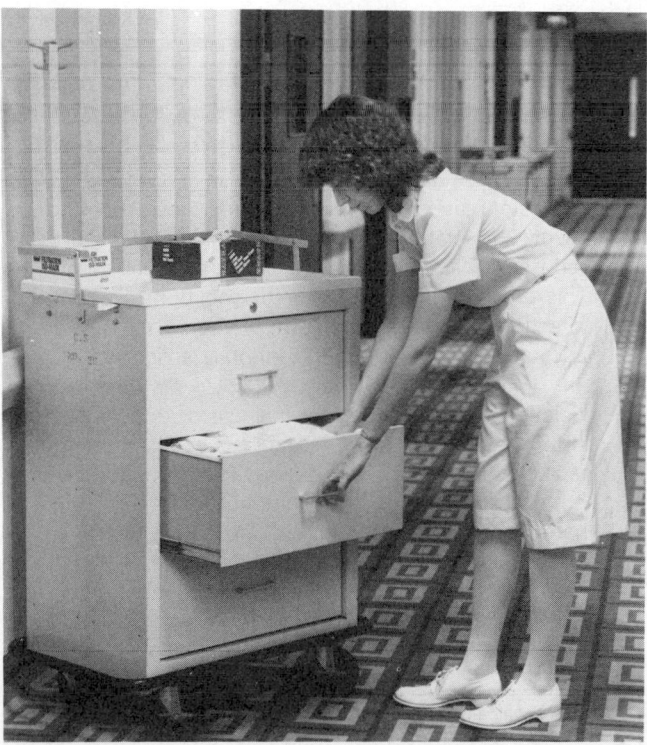

Fig. 43-2 The nurse keeps a supply of gowns, masks, and gloves in a portable isolation unit.

might enter the room accidentally that special precautions must be followed.

The protective environment should contain handwashing, bathing, and toilet facilities. Soap and antiseptic solutions are made available. Personnel and visitors should wash their hands before coming to the client's bedside and again before leaving the room.

When toilet facilities are available, there is no need for portable commodes or special precautions in transporting bedpans, urinals, and emesis basins. Isolation supplies can be stored in an anteroom between the room and hallway or in an isolation cart in the hallway. The nurse keeps ample supplies of gowns, masks, and gloves in the storage area (Fig. 43-2).

Most institutions still follow the double-bag system for removing linen and contaminated articles from rooms of clients in isolation. Maki et al. (1986) suggests that there is no aseptic advantage to double-bagging (see research highlight). The CDC (1987) suggests that a single bag is adequate if it is sturdy and impervious and if the contaminated article can be placed in it without contaminating the outside of the bag. Nevertheless, many hospitals still equip isolation rooms with special impervious bags, in addition to a trash container with plastic liners. These receptacles are designed to prevent transmission of micoorganisms by preventing seepage to and soiling of the outside surface. If a client requires universal blood and body fluid precautions, a disposable container should be available in the room to discard needles and syringes.

⚰ *Research Highlight* ⚰

Waste materials and used linens from rooms of clients in isolation are routinely doubled-bagged to reduce contamination of the bag's external surface. This procedure is aimed at reducing transmission of infection between health care workers. Maki, Alvarado, and Hassemer (1986) randomly assigned waste and linens from the rooms of 42 clients in contact isolation to be transported in single or double bags. After the bags are filled, researchers cultured the surface of the bags in two locations near the knot. Over 2 months, 209 bags were cultured. Surface contamination was infrequent and similar in both the single- and double-bag groups. The study suggests there is no advantage to double-bagging potentially contaminated items compared with a single bag.

Maki, DG, Alvarado, C, and Hassemer, C: Double-bagging of items from isolation rooms is unnecessary as an infection control measure: a comparative study of surface contamination with single and double-bagging, Infect Control 7(11):535, 1986.

The nurse should avoid taking any article or piece of equipment into a client's room that is to be reused outside the isolation area. If such an article becomes contaminated, it must be discarded or disinfected and sterilized. For this reason many hospitals used disposable dishes for clients receiving protective asepsis. A nurse also keeps the chart outside at the nurses' station or on the isolation cart. Equipment such as a sphygmomanometer, stethoscope, or other examination devices should be left in the client's room until protective aseptic precautions are no longer required.

Gowns. The primary reason for gowning is to prevent soiling clothes during contact with the client. Gowns protect health care personnel and visitors from coming in contact with infected material and also protect clients from organisms on other persons' clothing.

Isolation gowns open at the back and have ties at the neck and waist to keep it closed and secure. A gown should be long enough to cover all outer garments. Long sleeves with tight-fitting cuffs provide added protection. There is no technique required for donning a clean gown as long as it is fastened securely. However, the nurse must carefully remove a gown to minimize contamination of the hands and uniform.

To remove a gown, first the waist ties are untied, and then the hands are washed. The neck ties are untied, allowing the gown to fall gently from the shoulders. Care should be taken to remove the hands from the sleeves without touching the outside of the gown. Sleeves should not be allowed to turn inside out. The gown is held inside at the shoulder seams and folded in half with the outside surfaces touching. This minimizes contact with the soiled gown. The gown is then disposed of in the proper receptacle. Then the nurse washes his or her hands. Fig. 43-3 shows the steps for removing a gown.

Masks. A mask protects a nurse from inhaling microorganisms from a client's respiratory tract, and prevents transmission of pathogens from the nurse's respiratory tract.

The mask protects a wearer from inhaling large-particle aerosols that travel short distances (3 feet) and small-particle droplet nuclei that remain suspended in the air and travel longer distances. At times a client who is susceptible to infection wears a mask to prevent inhalation of pathogens. Clients receiving respiratory precautions who are transported outside their rooms should wear masks during transit to protect other clients and personnel.

According to the CDC, masks may prevent transmission of infections by direct contact with mucous membranes (Williams, 1983). A mask discourages the wearer from touching the eyes, nose, or mouth.

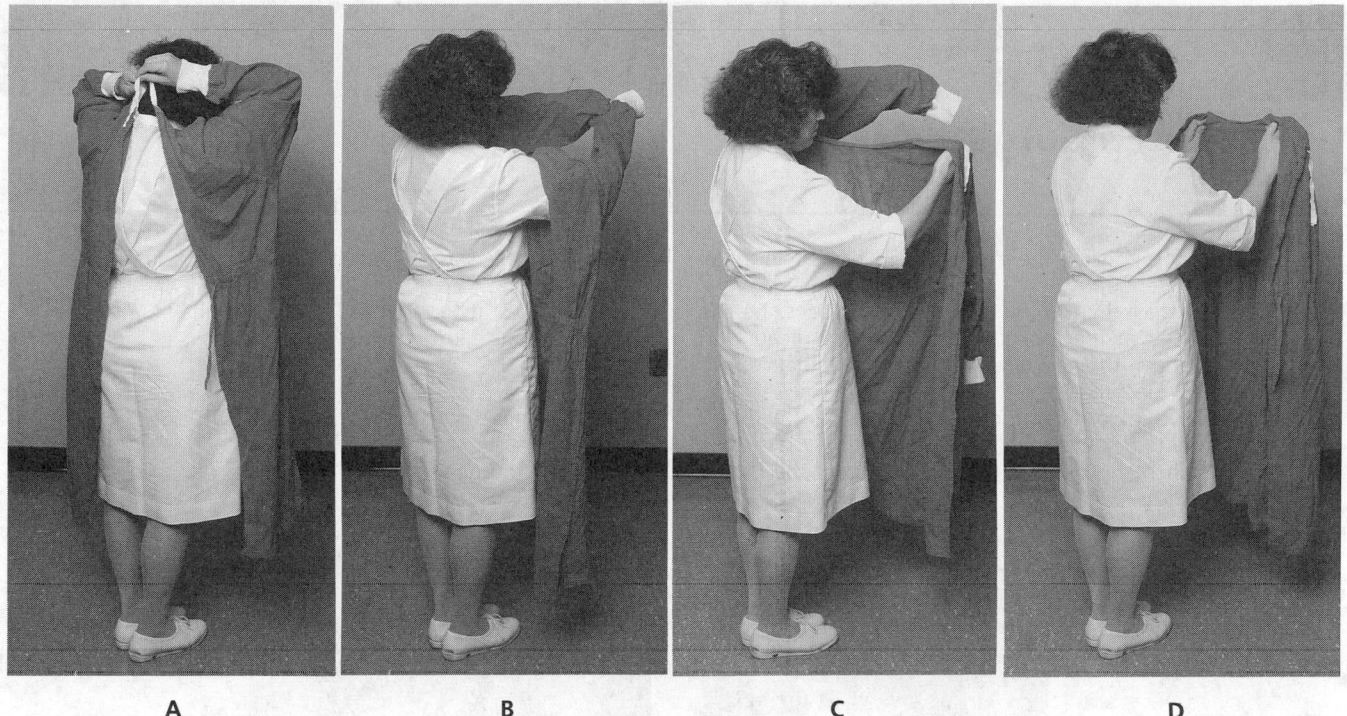

Fig. 43-3   Removing an isolation gown. **A,** Nurse loosens neck ties. **B,** Hands are carefully removed from sleeves. **C,** Sleeves are not allowed to be turned inside out. **D,** Gown is folded with outside surfaces touching.

A properly applied mask fits snugly over the mouth and nose so pathogens and body fluids cannot enter or escape through the sides (Procedure 43-2). If a person wears glasses, the top edge of the mask fits below the glasses so they will not cloud over as the person exhales. Talking should be kept to a minimum while wearing a mask to reduce respiratory air flow. A mask that has become moist is ineffective and should be discarded. A mask should never be reused. A safe rule is to change a mask every hour. Clients and family members should be warned that a mask can cause a sensation of smothering. If family members become uncomfortable, they should leave the room and discard the mask.

Before removing a mask, remove gloves (if worn) or wash hands if in contact with infectious material. Dispose of the mask by folding it in half with the inner surfaces together to control microorganism spread. Place in a waste receptable.

Gloves. Gloves prevent transmission of pathogens by direct and indirect contact. The CDC (Williams, 1983) cites three reasons for wearing gloves:

1. Reduces possibility of personnel coming in contact with infectious organisms that infect clients (for example, handling contaminated dressings, cleaning an incontinent client with hepatitis)
2. Reduces likelihood that personnel will transmit their own endogenous flora to clients
3. Reduces possibility that personnel will become transiently colonized with microorganisms that can be transmitted to other clients (Transient colonization can usually be prevented with handwashing).

Nurses apply gloves when there is risk of handling infected material. In most cases disposable, single-use gloves are worn. Before applying gloves, don a mask (if required), wash and dry hands, and apply a gown. Disposable gloves are easily applied and designed to fit either hand. The glove's thin rubber, however, can be easily torn. The glove cuffs should be pulled up over the wrists or cuffs of a gown.

After coming in contact with any infected material, the nurse should change gloves if care is not completed. If the nurse's actions will not involve more contact with the client, reapplying gloves is unnecessary.

Family members often believe that they can touch any object once they have applied gloves. The nurse should explain that gloves can also become contaminated after

PROCEDURE 43-2

Donning a Surgical Mask

STEPS	RATIONALE
1. Find the top edge of the mask (usually has a thin metal strip along edge).	Pliable metal fits snugly against the bridge of the nose.
2. Hold the mask by the top two strings or loops. Tie the two top ties at the top of the back of your head with the ties above the ears (see illustration) (alternative: slip loops over each ear).	Position of ties at top of head provides tight fit. Ties over ears may cause irritation.
3. Tie the two lower ties snugly around the neck with the mask well under the chin (see illustration).	Prevents escape of microorganisms through sides of mask as nurse talks or breathes.
4. Gently pinch the upper metal band around the bridge of the nose.	Prevents microorganisms from escaping around nose.

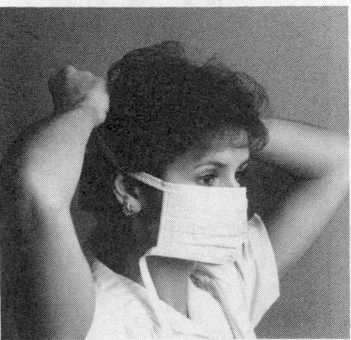

Step 2

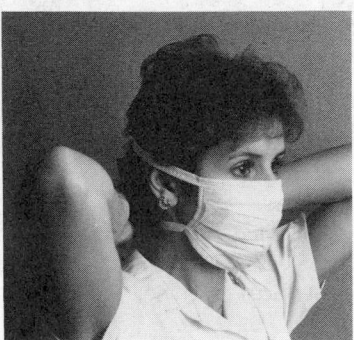

Step 3

touching infected material or another contaminated object.

Delivering Care in an Isolation Room. It is important for the nurse to remain aware of medical aseptic technique while working with a client in a protected environment. If the nurse brings any article into the room or exposes an article to infected material and then touches or removes the article, the risk of transmitting infection to other clients or personnel is increased.

During administration of medications, the medication cart or tray remains outside the client's room. The nurse takes the medication into the room in a cup or its individual wrapper. The nurse need not wear a gown if the isolation precautions do not call for it or if direct client contact is avoided. After the client takes the medication, the cup or wrapper should be discarded in the plastic-lined receptable.

Before administering injections the nurse prepares the syringe in the medication room. Since direct contact with the client is needed, except with respiratory infection, the nurse wears a gown into the room. In most agencies, disposable needles and syringes are used. Otherwise, reusable syringes, such as a Carpuject (see Chapter 15), are

disposed of like any other contaminated reusable object. After administering the injection the nurse discards the contaminated needle and syringe into the appropriate container in the client's room. The nurse never discards needles or syringes into the wastebasket. If containers are not available in the client's room, it is proper for the nurse to carry the syringe and needle in a clean paper towel to the medication room for disposal, although this increases the risk of cross-infection. After administering medication the nurse washes the hands before leaving the client's room and then records the medication.

When hygiene is administered to a client, the gown should not become wet. Carrying a washbasin against the gown or leaning against a wet bedside table soils the gown and provides a direct path for microorganisms to spread to the nurse's uniform. After the gown is removed, anything that comes in contact with the wet uniform, such as fingers or supplies, will be contaminated as well.

The nurse keeps all equipment for assessing vital signs, such as the stethoscope, thermometer, and sphygmomanometer, in the client's room for the duration of protective sepsis. If this is not possible, the nurse uses precautions to prevent cross-contamination. The nurse

TABLE 43-8 Specimen Collection Techniques

Specimen Source	Amount Needed*	Collection Device*	Specimen Collection and Transfer
Wound	As much as possible (after cleaning skin to remove flora)	Cotton-tipped swab or syringe	Have clean test tube or culturette tube on clean paper towel. After swabbing center of wound site, grasp collection tube by holding it with paper towel. Carefully insert swab without touching outside of tube. After washing hands and securing tube's top, transfer tube into bag held by nurse outside room.
Blood	10 ml per culture bottle, from two different venipuncture sites	Syringe and culture media bottles	Perform venipuncture at two different sites to decrease likelihood of both specimens being contaminated by skin flora. Have second nurse at client's door holding culture bottles and swabbing off bottletops with alcohol. Change needles after venipuncture. Inject 10 ml of blood into each bottle. Nurse at doorway secures tops of bottles, labels specimens, and sends to laboratory.
Stool	Small amount, approximate size of a walnut	Clean cup with seal top (not necessary to be sterile) and tongue blade	Place cup on clean paper towel in client's bathroom. Using tongue blade, collect needed amount of feces from client's bedpan. Transfer feces to cup without touching cup's outside surface. Wash hands and place seal on cup. Transfer specimen into clean bag held by nurse outside room.
Urine	1-5 ml	Syringe and sterile cup	Place cup or tube on clean towel in client's bathroom. Use syringe to collect specimen if client has a Foley catheter. Have client follow procedure to obtain a clean voided specimen (see Chapter 38) if not catheterized. Transfer urine into sterile container either by injecting urine from syringe or pouring it from used container. Wash hands and secure top of container. Transfer specimen into clean bag held by nurse outside room.

*Agency policies may differ on type of containers and amount of specimen material required.

carries a clean blood pressure cuff into the room and places it on a clean surface such as a paper towel. The client dons a clean short-sleeved gown that covers the arm above the antecubital fossa. The nurse applies the cuff over the thin gown to prevent contact with the client's skin. After measuring the blood pressure, the nurse removes the cuff and returns it to the clean surface before touching the client or any contaminated article. Then the nurse can safely take the cuff out of the room after handwashing.

A stethoscope can also be worn in and out of an isolation room as long as the nurse does not remove the stethoscope and place it on a contaminated surface. After assessing vital signs, the nurse washes the diaphragm or bell with a disinfectant solution.

If a gown and gloves must be worn while in the client's room, the nurse cannot wear a wristwatch to measure vital signs. The gown's cuffs are to be worn down to the wrist. If the watch fits over the cuff, it will become contaminated. Likewise, if the nurse pushes the cuff up to view the watch, palpates the client's pulse, and then lowers the cuff over the watch, the hand can contaminate the watch. To avoid cross-infection the nurse carries the watch to the client's bedside and places it on a clean paper towel within view. After assessing pulse and respirations the nurse removes the gown and gloves, washes the hands, and picks up the watch by grasping the clean surface of the towel. Once the towel is dicarded, the nurse can put on the watch while leaving the client's room.

Specimen Collection. A client with an infectious disease may require many laboratory studies. Body fluids and secretions suspected of containing infectious organisms are collected for culture and sensitivity tests. The specimen is placed in a medium that promotes growth of organisms. A laboratory technologist then identifies the microorganisms growing in the culture. Additional test results indicate antibiotics to which the organisms are resistant or sensitive. The sensivity reports determine which antibiotics will be used in treatment.

The nurse obtains all culture specimens using disposable gloves and sterile equipment. Collecting fresh material from the site of infection, as in the case of wound drainage, ensures that the specimen will not be contaminated by neighboring microbes. All specimen containers should be sealed tightly to prevent spillage and contamination of the outside of the container. Table 43-8 describes techniques for collecting specimens from the client receiving protective asepsis. In each case a clean container remains outside the room or on a clean paper towel in the client's bathroom. After the specimens are transferred to containers, the nurse labels each with the client's name, type of specimen, and type of protective asepsis. In some institutions nurses place the specimen containers in impervious bags before transporting them to the laboratory.

Bagging Articles. Nurses use special bagging procedures for removing contaminated items from the client's environment. Bagging articles prevents acciden-

tal exposure of personnel to contaminated articles and prevents contamination of the surrounding environment.

Glass bottles or jars are placed in separate plastic or paper containers. Leftover food may be placed in a wet garbage container or flushed down the toilet. Dressings should be placed in either wet or dry waste containers, depending on how much they are soiled. Most institutions require plastic and rubber items to be placed in separate bags from glass and metal equipment since methods of sterilization are different.

Some institutions require double-bagging of linen or trash. To double bag an article such as linen, the nurse puts on a gown to enter the client's room. The nurse places soiled linen within a single linen bag and then ties the top securely (Fig. 43-4, *A*). A second nurse stands outside the room with a clean bag to receive the linen (Fig. 43-4, *B*). The clean bag may bear a special marking for isolation or be color coded to alert laundry workers to its contents. The nurse outside the room holds the clean bag by folding the top edges back to form a cuff over the hands. As the opening of the bag is separated to receive the contaminated bag, the nurse in the room places a hand inside the clean bag to hold the clean bag open fully so the contaminated bag can easily be dropped in (Fig. 43-4, *C*). The goal is to avoid allowing the contaminated bag to touch the clean bag's outer edge. The nurse outside the room secures the outer bag and sends the contents to the laundry, making certain the bag is properly labeled. The outside nurse also hands the nurse inside the room a new bag to collect soiled linen.

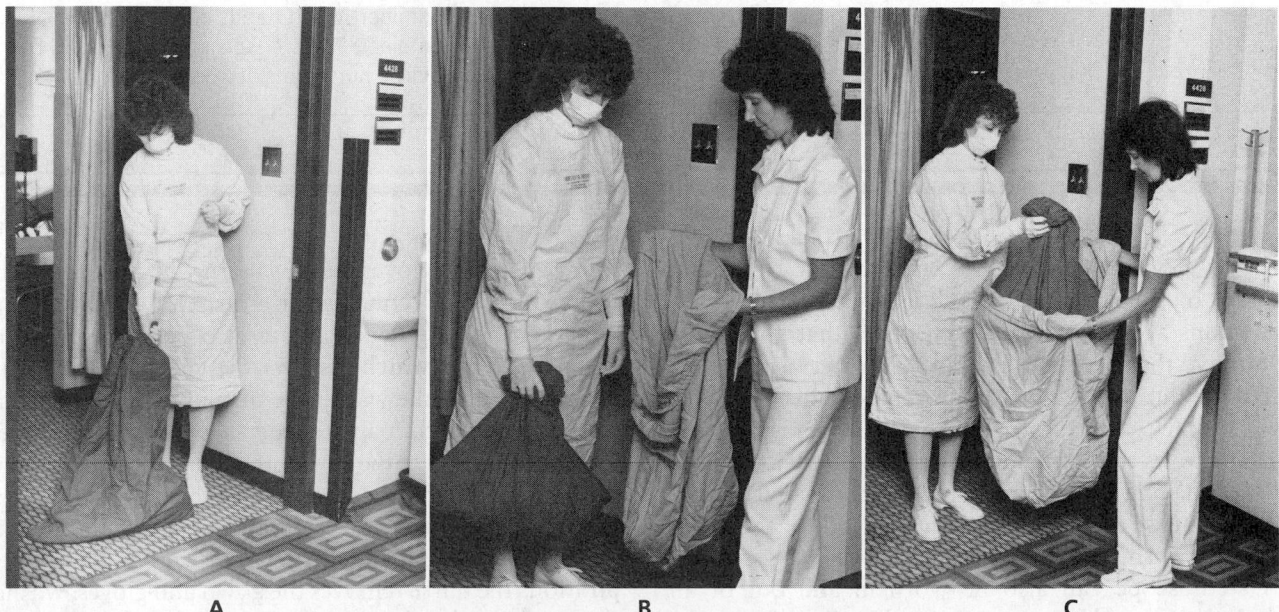

| A | B | C |

Fig. 43-4 Double-bagging. **A**, The nurse secures a linen bag. **B**, A nurse standing outside the client's room receives the soiled linen bag. **C**, The nurse drops the contaminated bag into the clean bag.

Double bagging can be used for any article. The agency's policy should be consulted for the proper procedure.

Removing Protective Clothing. The nurse removes used gloves, mask, and gown before leaving the isolation room. The gloves should be removed first because they are more likely to be contaminated. If the nurse unties a gown with gloves still on, there is a good chance of contaminating hair or a portion of the uniform. When gloves are pulled off, the cuff should be grasped with the other gloved hand and pulled off, turning the glove inside out. With the ungloved hand the nurse tucks the fingers inside the cuff of the remaining glove and pulls it off, turning the glove inside out. Gloves are discarded in a plastic-lined receptacle. Masks are usually disposable and made of a prepared paper or cotton fiber. The wearer removes the mask and discards it in a plastic-lined receptacle.

Linen gowns should be disposed of in the special linen hampers in the client's room. Paper gowns may be discarded in special trash containers. The nurse should never leave a client's room while wearing an isolation gown. When the gown is taken off, it should be turned inside out so hands and clothing do not come in contact with the outside contaminated surface. After the gown is discarded, hands should be washed thoroughly.

Transporting Clients. Clients infected with virulent organisms should leave their rooms only for essential purposes such as diagnostic procedures or surgery. Before transferring the client to a wheelchair or stretcher, the nurse gives the client a clean gown and an isolation gown to serve as a robe. A client who is infected by an organism transmitted via the respiratory tract must also wear a mask. Personnel transporting the client should also wear masks and gowns as needed.

Unless the client is unable to walk, a wheelchair or stretcher should not be brought into the room. If this is impossible, the nurse must be sure to have the equipment disinfected once the client returns to the room. An extra layer of sheets may be used to cover the stretcher or seat of the wheelchair.

Personnel in diagnostic areas or the operating room should be notified that the client is receiving protective asepsis before arrival. The nurse explains ways the client can help prevent transmission of infection during transport. A client on respiratory isolation is given tissues and a bag to allow proper disposal of any secretions. The nurse records the type of isolation on the client's chart.

ROLE OF THE INFECTION CONTROL NURSE. Many hospitals employ nurses who are specially trained in infection control. These nurses are responsible for advising hospital personnel on safe aseptic practices and for monitoring infection outbreaks within the hospital. Duties of an infection control nurse include:

1. Providing staff education on infection control
2. Reviewing infection control policies and procedures
3. Screening clients' laboratory reports for culture results
4. Screening client records for incidence of community-acquired infections
5. Gathering statistics regarding epidemiology of nosocomial infections
6. Notifying public health department of incidence of infections
7. Conferring with support services such as housekeeping and the dietary department
8. Educating clients and their families

An infection control nurse can be a valuable resource for controlling nosocomial infections (Nodolny, 1980).

INFECTION CONTROL IN HOSPITAL PERSONNEL. Hospital workers are continually exposed to infectious microorganisms. An employee who becomes ill can expose clients to infectious diseases. For these reasons the CDC has identified these elements of a personnel health service that assist in infection control:

1. *Placement evaluation*—A health assessment evaluates an employee's risk for acquiring or transmitting an infectious disease in the place of employment. An immunization history, history of previous infectious disease, and a physical examination determine whether an employee is a carrier of a disease (for example, tuberculosis) or has any condition (for example, immunodeficiency) that increases susceptibility to infection.

2. *Personnel health and safety equipment*—A hospital's health service should plan frequent in-service programs to acquaint personnel with the policies and procedures for infection control. An infection control nurse can coordinate such an effort. Written policies and guidelines should be provided for all personnel. Recently the CDC (1987) recommended initial orientation and continuing education of all health care workers on the epidemiology, modes of transmission, and prevention of HIV.

3. *Immunization programs*—Hospital personnel are exposed to vaccine-preventable diseases such as rubella and hepatitis B because of contact with clients or the infected material from clients. An immunization program safeguards personnel and protects clients from becoming infected by personnel. It is especially important to immunize employees who work in high-risk areas. For example, nurses working in intensive care units are more susceptible to hepatitis B because they frequently administer blood. Nurses working in

obstetric clinics should be immunized against rubella to protect pregnant clients.

4. *Work restrictions and control of job-related illnesses*—When an employee is exposed to an infectious disease, the health service determines whether the employee can continue working. The hospital has the responsibility of preventing the spread of infection to clients and employees. It may become necessary to exclude an employee from direct client contact.

5. *Health counseling*—Hospital personnel should know about infection risks. Personnel with certain clinical conditions require health counseling. Female employees who are pregnant or who might become pregnant should know about risks to the fetus from work assignments and measures to reduce these risks.

CLIENT EDUCATION. Often clients must learn to use infection control practices at home. Aseptic technique becomes almost second nature to the nurse practicing it daily. However, the client is less aware of factors that promote spread of infection or of ways to prevent its transmission. The home environment does not always lend itself to the practice of aseptic technique. A nurse must often help a client improvise with the resources available to maintain hygienic techniques. For example, a client may use a laundered washcloth instead of expensive sterile gauze to wash around an open wound.

Once clients are at home, they determine their compliance with infection control practices. It is the nurse's responsibility to educate clients about infection and techniques to prevent or control its spread. Topics the nurse can discuss in a teaching session include:

1. The client's susceptibility to infection
2. The chain of infection with specific reference to means of transmission
3. Basic handwashing practices (when and how)
4. Hygienic practices that minimize organism growth and spread
5. Preventive health care, for example, diet, immunizations, exercise
6. Proper methods for food handling and storage
7. Family members who are at risk for acquiring infections

Except for the need to administer self-injections, it is more practical for clients to learn clean, medical aseptic techniques than strict sterile techniques. Physicians try not to allow clients to return home with open wounds or conditions that require sterile procedures unless home care is available. Family members who must care for such a client, however, must be involved in the nurse's teaching plan. The nurse teaches clients and family members a commonsense approach to controlling and preventing infection.

SURGICAL ASEPSIS

Surgical asepsis or sterile technique requires a nurse to use greater precautions than with medical asepsis. Surgical asepsis requires the absence of all microorganisms, including pathogens and spores, from an object. The nurse working with a sterile field or with sterile equipment must understand that the slightest break in technique results in contamination. The nurse also practices surgical asepsis in an effort to keep microorganisms away from an area, for example, when filling a syringe or changing a dressing on a wound.

Although surgical asepsis is commonly practiced in the operating room, labor and delivery area, and major diagnostic areas, the nurse may also use surgical aseptic techniques at the client's bedside. This would include, for example, inserting intravenous or urinary catheters, suctioning the tracheobronchial airway, and reapplying sterile dressings. A nurse in an operating room will follow a series of steps to maintain sterile techniques, including donning a mask and cap, performing a surgical handwash, and donning a sterile gown and gloves. In contrast, a nurse performing a dressing change may only wash hands and don sterile gloves. A mask would be optional unless there is a risk for body fluids to splash into the nurse's eyes. The box lists guidelines for using sterile technique.

ASSESSMENT. Because surgical asepsis requires exact techniques, the nurse must be able to ensure the client's cooperation. Therefore it is important for the nurse to assess the client's understanding of sterile procedure and to identify whether special precautions are necessary to prevent contamination.

Client Knowledge. Often clients are reluctant to move or touch objects during a sterile procedure because of fear of interfering or of experiencing pain. Clients rarely understand that sterile equipment cannot be touched by unsterile objects or even what an unsterile object is.

The nurse determines if a client has undergone a sterile

Indications for Using Sterile Technique

- During procedures that require intentional perforation of a client's skin (for example, insertion of intravenous catheters, administration of injections)
- When the skin's integrity is broken due to trauma, surgical incision, or burns
- During procedures that involve insertion of catheters or surgical instruments into sterile body cavities

procedure in the past. If not, the nurse explains how it is to be performed and what the client can do to avoid contaminating sterile objects:

1. Avoiding sudden movements of body parts covered by sterile drapes
2. Refraining from touching sterile supplies, drapes, or the nurse's gloves and gown
3. Avoiding coughing, sneezing, or talking over a sterile area

Precautions. Certain sterile procedures may last a long time. The nurse must assess the client's needs and anticipate factors that may disrupt a procedure. If a client is in pain, the nurse tries to administer analgesics no more than half an hour before a sterile procedure begins. Measures are taken to care for elimination needs. Often clients must assume relatively uncomfortable positions during sterile procedures. The nurse helps the client assume the most comfortable position possible. Finally, the client's condition may result in actions or events that contaminate a sterile field, such as the client with a respiratory infection who transmits organisms by coughing or breathing. The nurse anticipates such a problem and offers the client a mask.

PRINCIPLES OF SURGICAL ASEPSIS. When beginning a surgically aseptic procedure, the nurse follows certain principles to ensure maintenance of asepsis. Failure to follow each principle conscientiously endangers the client, placing him or her at risk for an infection. The following principles are important:

1. *A sterile object remains sterile only when touched by another sterile object.* This principle guides the nurse in placement of sterile objects and how to handle them. *Sterile touching sterile remains sterile;* for example, sterile gloves are worn or sterile forceps are used to handle objects on a sterile field. *Sterile touching clean becomes contaminated;* for example, if the tip of a syringe or other sterile object touches the surface of a clean disposable glove, the object is contaminated. *Sterile touching contaminated becomes contaminated;* for example, when the nurse touches a sterile object with an ungloved hand, the object is contaminated. *Sterile touching questionable is considered contaminated;* for example, when a tear or break in the covering of a sterile object is found, it is discarded regardless of whether the object itself appears untouched.
2. *Only sterile objects may be placed on a sterile field.* All items are properly sterilized before use. Sterile objects are kept in clean and dry storage areas for only a prescribed time; thereafter they are considered unsterile. All sterile packages are checked for sterilization dates or time periods on labels before use. The package or container holding a sterile

object must be intact and dry. A package that is torn, punctured, wet, or open is considered unsterile.

3. *A sterile object or field out of the range of vision or an object held below a person's waist is contaminated.* Nurses never turn their backs on a sterile tray or leave it unattended. Contamination can occur accidentally by a dangling piece of clothing, falling hair, or an unknowing client touching a sterile object. If it is necessary to leave a room, the nurse covers a sterile tray with a sterile towel or drape. Any object held below waist level is considered contaminated because it cannot be viewed at all times. Sterile objects should be kept in front with hands as close together as possible.
4. *A sterile object or field becomes contaminated by prolonged exposure to the air.* The nurse avoids activities that may create air currents, such as excessive movements or rearranging linen once a sterile object or field becomes exposed. When sterile packages are being opened, it is important to minimize the number of people walking into the area. Microorganisms also travel by droplet through the air. No one should talk, laugh, sneeze, or cough over a sterile field or when gathering and using sterile equipment. When opening a tray and adding sterile equipment, the nurse should wear a mask. A nurse with a cold or other respiratory ailment should never perform sterile procedures unless a double mask is worn. Microorganisms traveling through the air can fall on sterile items or fields if the nurse reaches over the work area. When opening sterile packages, the nurse holds the item or piece of equipment as close as possible to the sterile field without touching the sterile surface. Minimal movement or rearranging of sterile items also reduces contamination by air transmission.
5. *A sterile object or field becomes contaminated by capillary action when a sterile surface comes in contact with a wet contaminated surface.* If moisture seeps through a sterile package's protective covering, microorganisms travel to the sterile object. Whenever stored sterile packages become wet, the nurse discards the objects immediately or sends the equipment for resterilization. When working with a sterile field or tray, the nurse may have to pour sterile solutions. Any spill can be a source of contamination unless the object or field rests on a sterile surface that cannot be penetrated by moisture. Urinary catheterization trays contain sterile supplies that rest in a sterile plastic container. In this example sterile solutions spilled within the container will not contaminate the catheter or other objects. In contrast, if a nurse places a piece of sterile gauze in its wrapper on a client's bedside table and the table surface is wet, the gauze is considered contaminated.

6. *Fluid flows in the direction of gravity.* A sterile object becomes contaminated if gravity causes a contaminated liquid to flow over the object's surface. In some institutions the nurse uses forceps to transfer sterile objects to a sterile tray or field. Often the forceps are stored in a container of disinfectant solution. The nurse always holds the tips of wet forceps down. If the nurse raised the tips up, fluid would flow toward the hands and become contaminated. Then, as the nurse lowered the forceps, the contaminated fluid would travel down to contaminate the tips. The forceps could no longer be used for transferring sterile objects. For this reason many institutions use dry disposable forceps. The same principle applies to the surgical hand scrub. In contrast to basic handwashing, the surgical nurse holds the hands above the elbows during the surgical hand scrub. This allows water to flow downward without contaminating the nurse's hands and fingers. The principle of water flow by gravity is also the reason for drying from fingers to elbows with hands held up, after the scrub.

7. *The edges of a sterile field or container are considered to be contaminated.* Frequently a nurse places sterile objects on a sterile towel or drape. Since the edge of the drape touches an unsterile surface, such as a table or bed linen, a 2.5 cm (1-inch) border around the drape is considered contaminated. The edges of sterile containers become exposed to air once they are open and are thus contaminated. After a sterile needle is removed from its protective cap, or after forceps are removed from a container, the objects must not touch the container's edge. The lip of an opened bottle of solution also becomes contaminated once it is exposed to the air. When pouring a sterile liquid, the nurse first pours a small amount of solution and discards it. The solution washes away microorganisms on the bottle lip. Then the nurse pours a second time to fill a container with the desired amount of solution.

PERFORMING STERILE PROCEDURES. All equipment that will be needed should be assembled before a procedure. It is important to anticipate what will be required so leaving equipment unattended will not be necessary. A few extra supplies should be available in case objects accidentally become contaminated. Before the sterile procedure, each step should be explained so the client can cooperate fully. Another nurse should be in attendance in case assistance acquiring supplies is needed.

If an object becomes contaminated during the procedure, the nurse should not hesitate to discard it immediately.

Donning and Removing Caps and Masks. For sterile procedures on a general nursing division, the nurse may wear a surgical mask without a cap. For sterile surgical procedures in the operating room the nurse first applies a clean paper or cloth cap that covers all of the hair and then the surgical mask. A mask must fit snugly around the face and nose to prevent contamination by droplet nuclei. After a mask is worn for several hours, the area over the mouth and nose often becomes moist. Moisture promotes the spread of microorganisms. The nurse in the operating room must apply a second mask over the first, since removing a mask in a surgical area results in immediate contamination of surrounding objects. Procedure 43-2 describes the steps for applying a mask. Before removing a mask and cap the nurse removes sterile gloves and washes the hands to prevent contamination of the hair, neck, and facial area.

Opening Sterile Packages. Sterile items such as syringes, gauze dressings, catheters, and sterile liquids are packaged in either paper, plastic, or glass containers. Some institutions wrap reusable supplies in two to four layers of linen or muslin. The wrappers are impervious to microorganisms as long as they are dry and intact. Plastics are pliable and resistant to tearing. Most liquids are usually prepared in amounts needed for one use only, and then leftover liquid is discarded. Paper packages are permeable to steam and thus allow for steam autoclaving. A disadvantage of paper wrappers is that they tear or puncture relatively easily.

Rooms equipped with clean enclosed storage cabinets are the best place to store sterile items. Sterile supplies are never kept in the same room as dirty equipment.

Sterile supplies have dated labels or chemical tapes that indicate the date when the sterilization period expires. The tapes change color during the sterilization process. Failure of the tapes to change color means the item is not sterile. A sterile supply or piece of equipment should never be used after the expiration date. The item is either discarded or returned to the institution's supply area for resterilization.

Before opening a sterile item the nurse washes the hands thoroughly. The nurse assembles the supplies in the work area such as the bedside or treatment room before opening packages. A bedside table or countertop provides a large, clean working area for opening items. The work area should be above waist level. Sterile supplies should not be opened in a confined space where a dirty object might fall on or strike them.

Opening a sterile item on a flat surface. Sterile packaged items are wrapped to allow opening without contaminating the contents. Items are placed flat in the center of the work surface. The nurse tears the top wrapper away from the body and avoids reaching over the sterile

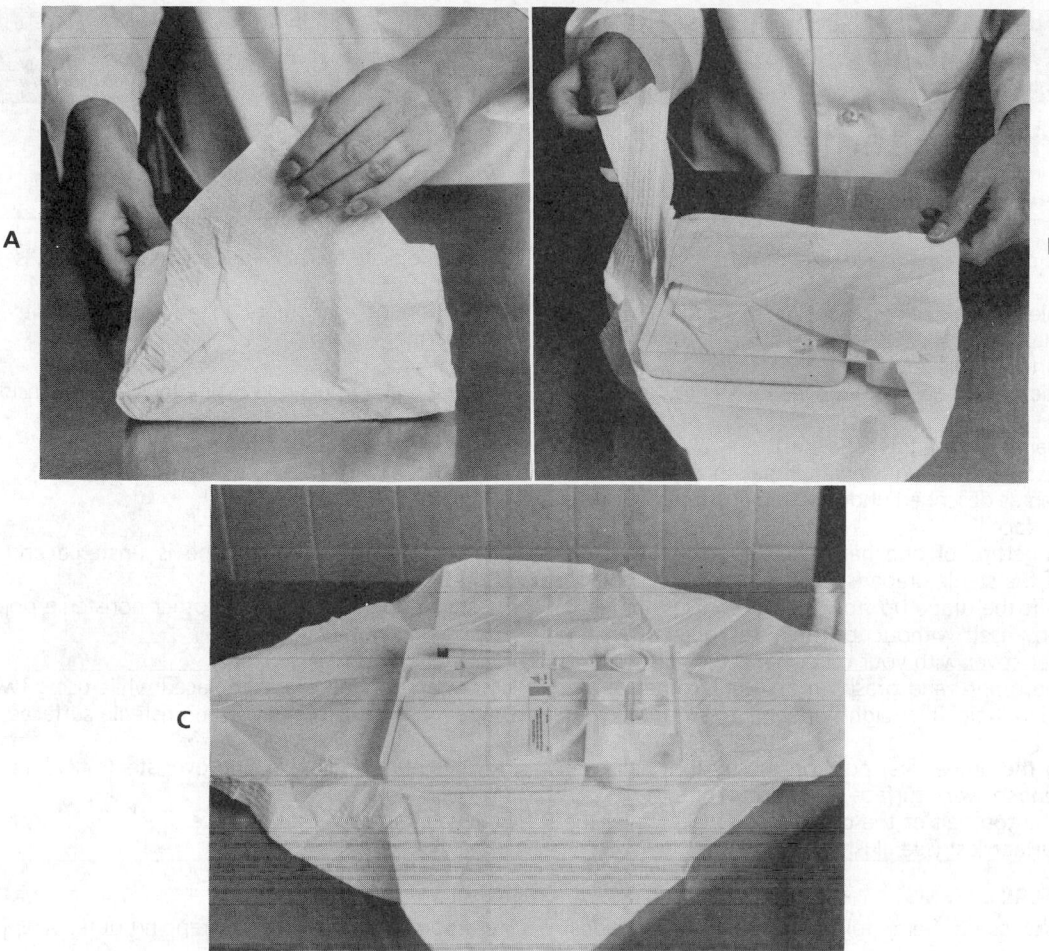

Fig. 43-5   Opening sterile packaged items on a flat surface. **A,** Nurse opens the top flap away from the body. **B,** The nurse's arm is kept out, away from the sterile field while opening side flaps. **C,** The back flap is opened.

contents. One hand can grasp the outside of the wrapper without danger of contamination. While removing wrappers the nurse avoids touching the inside of the wrapper. Once the inside of the wrapper is contaminated it can contaminate the sterile item if the wrapper accidentally slips backward over the item. When opening items on a flat surface the nurse follows these steps:

1. Remove tape or seal indicating sterilization date.
2. Grasp the outer surface of the tip of the outermost flap.
3. Open the flap away from the body, keeping the arm outstretched and away from the sterile field (Fig. 43-5, *A*).
4. Grasp the outside surface of the first side flap.
5. The side flap is then opened, allowing it to lie flat on the table surface. The arm is kept to the side and not over the sterile surface (Fig. 43-5, *B*).
6. Steps 4 and 5 are repeated for the second side of the flap.

7. Grasp the outside surface of the last and innermost flap.
8. Stand away from the sterile package and pull the flap back, allowing it to fall flat on the table (Fig. 43-5, *C*).
9. The inner surface of the linen package (except for the 1-inch border around the edges) is sterile. The sterile field can be used to add additional sterile items. The 1-inch border can be grasped to maneuver the field on the table surface.

If the sterile supplies are not to be used immediately, the nurse can close the sterile package. In this case the nurse should touch only the wrapper's outside surface. To close a package the order of unwrapping is reversed and the nurse does not touch the inside contents or reach over the field.

Opening a sterile item while holding it. To open small sterile items, the package is held in the nondominant hand, while the top flap is opened and pulled away from

PROCEDURE 43-3

Preparing a Sterile Field

STEPS	RATIONALE
1. Select a clean work surface above waist level.	A sterile object held below a person's waist is contaminated.

2. Assemble necessary equipment:
  a. Sterile drape
  b. Assorted sterile supplies
	Preparation of equipment in advance prevents break in technique.

3. Check dates or labels on supplies for sterility of equipment.	Equipment stored beyond expiration date is considered unsterile.
4. Wash hands thoroughly.	Prevents transmission of infection.
5. Place pack containing sterile drape on work surface and open as described under ''opening sterile items on a flat surface.''	Assures sterility of packaged drape.
6. With fingertips of one hand pick up the folded top edge of the sterile drape (see illustration).	One-inch border around drape is unsterile and may be touched.
7. Gently lift the drape up from its outer cover and let it unfold by itself without touching any object. Discard the outer cover with your other hand.	If a sterile object touches any other nonsterile object it becomes contaminated.
8. With the other hand grasp an adjacent corner of the drape and hold it straight up and away from your body.	Drape can now be properly placed while using two hands. Drape must be held away from unsterile surfaces.
9. Holding the drape, first position the bottom half over the intended work surface (see illustration).	Prevents nurse from reaching over sterile field.
10. Allow the top half of the drape to be placed over the work surface last (see illustration).	Creates flat sterile work surface.

ADDING STERILE ITEMS

11. Open the sterile item (following package directions) while holding the outside wrapper in the nondominant hand.	Frees dominant hand for unwrapping outer wrapper.
12. Carefully peel the wrapper onto the nondominant hand.	Item remains sterile. Inner surface of wrapper covers hand, making it sterile.

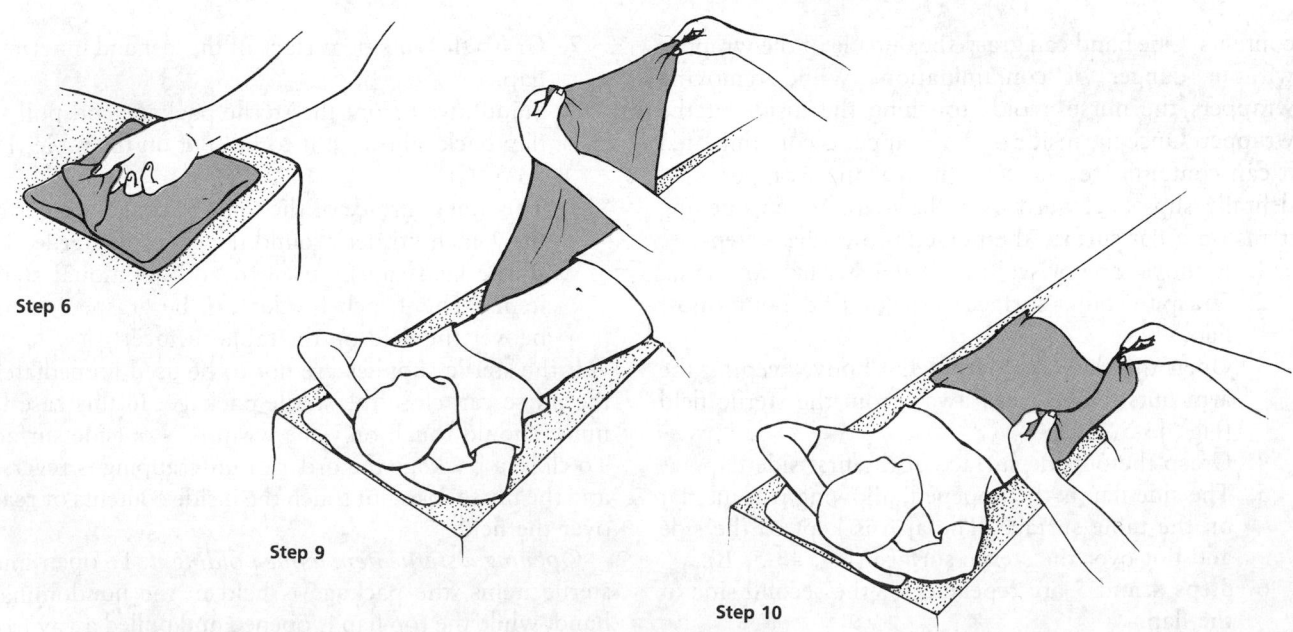

Step 6

Step 9

Step 10

STEPS	RATIONALE
13. Being sure the wrapper does not fall down on the sterile field, place the item onto the field at an angle. Do not hold the arm over the sterile field.	Prevents reaching over field and contaminating its surface.
14. Dispose of the outer wrapper.	Prevents accidental contamination of sterile field.

TRANSFERRING ITEMS WITH A FORCEP

STEPS	RATIONALE
15. Open package containing sterile forceps, allowing forceps to lie on surface of inner sterile cover.	Inner cover of package creates temporary sterile field.
16. Open the sterile item (following package directions) that is to be placed on sterile field.	Keeps contents sterile.
17. Carefully grasp handle of forceps and raise them above the waist and away from your body. (Only handles of forceps are considered contaminated).	Keeping ends of forceps in sight and above waist level prevents their contamination.
18. With the ends of the forceps, grasp the sterile item to be placed on the sterile field. (Do not let forceps touch edge of wrapper.)	If sterile portion of forceps touches any object that is unsterile, the forceps becomes contaminated.
19. Raise the sterile item straight up and lift it over and onto the sterile field. Keep the handles of the forceps outside the sterile area (see illustration).	Reaching over a sterile field with an unsterile object contaminates the field.

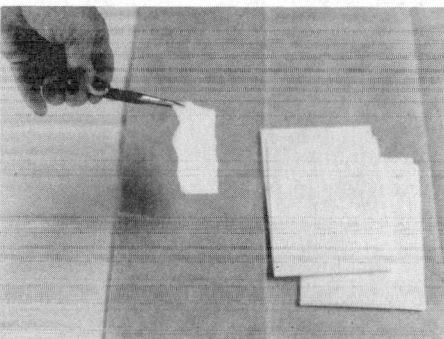

Step 19

the nurse. With the dominant hand the sides and top flaps are carefully opened away from the enclosed sterile item in the same order previously mentioned. The nurse opens items in a hand so that the item can be handed to a person wearing sterile gloves or transferred to a sterile field.

Opening a sterile, commercially packaged item. All commercially packaged, sterile items list directions for correct opening. One technique for opening requires the item to be held in one hand while the wrapper is pulled away with the other (Fig. 43-6). Items that have two flaps sealed together such as gauze dressings are opened by grasping both flaps, one with each hand, and gently pulling them apart.

Preparing a Sterile Field. When performing sterile procedures the nurse needs a work area that provides

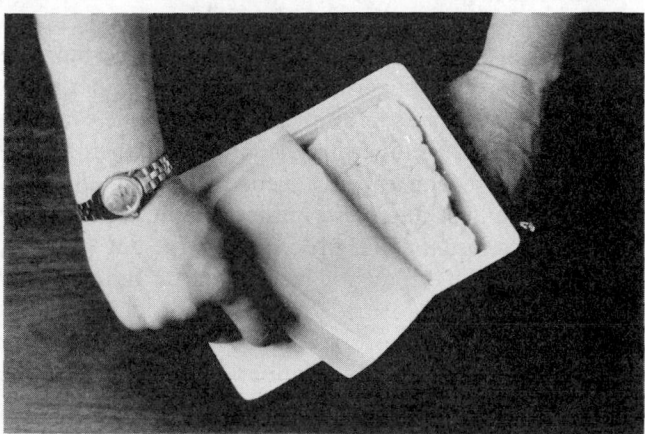

Fig. 43-6 When opening a commercially packaged sterile item, the nurse tears the wrapper away from the body.

room for handling and placement of sterile items. A sterile field is an area free of microorganisms and prepared to receive sterile items. The field may be prepared by using the inner side of a sterile wrapper or by using a sterile drape. Procedure 43-3 (p. 1296) describes preparation of a sterile field. Once a field is created the nurse adds sterile items by placing them directly on the field or by transferring them with a sterile forceps. When transferring sterile items the nurse must carefully place objects onto the sterile field. An object that comes in contact with the edge of the sterile field must be discarded.

Pouring Sterile Solutions. Often the nurse must pour sterile solutions into sterile containers. A bottle containing a sterile solution is sterile on the inside and contaminated on the outside, including the bottle's neck. The inside of the bottle cap is also sterile. After a cap or lid is opened, it is held in the hand or placed sterile side (inside) up on a clean surface. This means that the inside of the lid can be seen as it rests on the table surface. A bottle cap or lid should never rest sterile side down on a sterile surface because the outer edge of the cap is unsterile and would contaminate the surface. Likewise, placing a sterile cap down on an unsterile surface increases the chances of the inside of the cap becoming contaminated.

The bottle should be held with its label in the palm of the hand. This prevents the possibility of the solution wetting and fading the label. Before pouring the solution into the container the nurse pours a small amount (1 to 2 ml) into a disposable cap or plastic-lined waste receptacle. The discarded solution cleans the lip of the bottle. The edge of the bottle is kept away from the edge or inside of the receiving container. The nurse pours the solution slowly to avoid splashing, which would contaminate the underlying drape or field. The bottle should never be held so high above the container that even slow pouring will cause splashing. The bottle should be held outside the edge of the sterile field.

Surgical Handwashing. In surgical handwashing the nurse scrubs from fingertips to elbows with an antimicrobial surgical hand scrub preparation before each operation. Regular handwashing is satisfactory before routine sterile procedures on a general nursing division. Surgical handwashing or scrubbing should take at least 5 minutes before the first procedure of the day (Garner, 1985). The CDC does not recommend a duration for surgical scrubs performed between procedures. However, 2 to 5 minutes is probably acceptable (check agency policies). For maximum elimination of bacteria, the nurse removes all jewelry and keeps fingernails short, clean, and free of polish. Brushes are used during scrubbing. Some experts caution that too much brushing removes outer layers of the epidermis, thereby exposing

bacterial flora in the deeper skin layers. Procedure 43-4 describes the steps of the surgical handwashing procedure.

Applying Sterile Gloves. After thorough handwashing, sterile gloves are an additional barrier to bacterial transfer. There are two gloving methods: open and closed. Nurses who work on general nursing divisions use open gloving before procedures such as dressing changes (see Chapter 47) or urinary catheter insertions (see Chapter 38). The closed gloved method, which requires a nurse to wear a sterile gown, is practiced in operating rooms and special treatment areas. If an operating room nurse contaminates a sterile glove, a new glove is applied using the open technique. Procedures 43-5 and 43-6 review the steps of each gloving technique.

The proper glove size should be selected; the glove should not stretch so tightly that it can easily tear, yet it should be tight enough that objects can be picked up easily.

After a sterile procedure the nurse disposes of gloves in the following manner to minimize hand contamination.

1. The outside of one cuff is grasped with the other gloved hand (taking care not to touch the wrist).
2. The glove is peeled off, turned inside out, and discarded in the proper receptacle.
3. The fingers of the bare hand tuck inside the remaining glove's cuff. (The outside of the glove is not touched.)
4. The glove is peeled off, turned inside out, and disposed of in the proper receptacle.

Donning a Sterile Gown. The nurse must wear a sterile gown in the operating room and delivery room so sterile objects can be comfortably handled with less risk of contamination. The sterile gown acts as a barrier to decrease shedding of microorganisms from skin surfaces into the air and thus prevents wound contamination. Nurses caring for clients with large open wounds or assisting physicians during major invasive procedures (for example, arterial cannulization) may also wear sterile gowns.

The nurse does not don a sterile gown until after surgical handwashing and after applying a mask and surgical cap. The nurse either picks up the gown from a sterile pack or has a gowned assistant hand him or her the gown. Only a certain portion of the gown—the area from the anterior waist to but not including the collar and the anterior surface of the sleeves—is considered sterile. The back of the gown, under the arms, the collar, the area below the waist, and the underside of the sleeves are not sterile, since the nurse cannot keep these areas in constant view and ensure their sterility. Procedure 43-6 reviews the steps for applying a gown.

PROCEDURE 43-4

Surgical Handwashing

STEPS	RATIONALE
1. Use a deep sink with foot pedals or knee controls for the dispensing of soap and control of water temperature and flow.	Minimizes risk of hands and lower arms touching dirty surface.
2. Use an appropriate antiseptic detergent such as chlorhexidine or triclosan.	Antiseptics maximally reduce the number of microorganisms on the hands.
3. Have two hand brushes and an orange stick or disposable nail file available.	Brushes are used to enhance the mechanical friction during handwashing. An orange stick facilitates cleansing under fingernails.
4. Remove all jewelry.	Jewelry harbors microorganisms.
5. Apply a face mask, making certain to cover the nose and mouth snugly.	The mask prevents escape of microorganisms into the air, which can contaminate the hands.
6. Adjust the water flow to a lukewarm temperature.	Hot water removes protective oils from the skin and increases the skin's sensitivity to soap.
7. Wet the hands and forearms liberally, keeping the hands above the level of the elbows during the entire procedure. NOTE: Nurse's scrub dress or uniform must be kept dry.	Water runs by gravity from fingertips to elbows. The hands become the cleanest part of the upper extremity. Keeping the hands elevated allows water to flow from least to most contaminated area.
8. Dispense a liberal amount of soap (2 to 5 ml) into the hands and lather hands and arms to 5 cm (2 inches) above the elbows.	Washing a wide area reduces risk of contaminating the overlying gown that the nurse later applies.
9. Clean nails with orange stick or file under running water.	Removes dirt and organic material that harbor large numbers of microorganisms.
10. Rinse hands and arms thoroughly.	Rinsing removes transient bacteria from fingers, hands, and forearms.
11. Lather hands and arms and scrub each hand with a brush for 45 seconds. Then using the same brush, scrub each arm to 5 cm (2 inches) above the elbow dividing the arm into thirds: scrub each lower forearm 15 seconds, each upper forearm 15 seconds, and 5 cm above each elbow 15 seconds.	Scrubbing loosens resident bacteria that adhere to skin's surface.
12. Discard brush and rinse hands and arms thoroughly.	After touching skin, brush is considered contaminated. Rinsing removes resident bacteria.
13. Using a second brush, scrub each hand for 30 seconds. Then use the same brush to scrub each arm up to the elbow by dividing the arm in half: scrub each lower forearm 15 seconds and each upper forearm 15 seconds.	A second scrubbing ensures thorough cleansing of hands and forearms. The number of resident microorganisms remaining on skin will be minimal.
14. Discard brush and rinse hands and arms thoroughly. Turn off water with foot pedal.	After touching skin, brush is considered to be contaminated. Rinsing removes resident bacteria.
15. Use a sterile towel to dry one hand thoroughly moving from fingers to elbow. Dry in a rotating motion. NOTE: Nurses wishing to apply sterile gloves for use in a regular clinical area need not use brushes or dry hands with sterile towels. Thorough lathering and friction performed twice according to procedure will ensure clean hands. In this situation the nurse may use clean paper towels for drying.	Dry from cleanest to least clean area. Drying prevents chapping and facilitates donning of gloves.
16. Repeat drying method for other hand, using a different area of the towel or a new sterile towel.	
17. Keep hands higher than elbows and away from the body.	Prevents accidental contamination.
18. Proceed into operating room, labor and delivery area, or treatment room.	

PROCEDURE 43-5

Open Gloving

STEPS	RATIONALE
1. Perform thorough handwashing.	Removes bacteria from skin surfaces and reduces transmission of infection.
2. Remove the outer glove package wrapper by carefully peeling apart the sides.	Prevents inner glove package from accidentally opening and touching contaminated objects.
3. Grasp the inner package and lay it on a clean flat surface just above the waist level. Open the package, keeping the gloves on the wrapper's inside surface.	A sterile object held below a person's waist is considered contaminated. The inner surface of the glove package is considered sterile.
4. If gloves are not prepowdered, take the packet of powder and apply lightly to the hands over a sink or wastebasket.	Powder allows gloves to slip on easily. (Some physicians do not use powder for fear of promoting growth of microorganisms.)
5. Identify the right and left glove. Each glove has a cuff approximately 5 cm (2 inches) wide. Glove the dominant hand first.	Proper identification of gloves prevents contamination by improper fit. Gloving of the dominant hand first improves the nurse's dexterity.
6. With the thumb and first two fingers of the nondominant hand, grasp the edge of the cuff of the glove for the dominant hand. Touch only the glove's inside surface (see illustration).	The inner edge of the cuff will lie against the skin and thus is not considered sterile.
7. Carefully pull the glove over the dominant hand, leaving a cuff and being sure the cuff does not roll up the wrist. Be sure the thumb and fingers are in the proper spaces (see illustration).	If the glove's outer surface touches the hand or wrist, it is contaminated.
8. With the gloved dominant hand, slip fingers underneath second glove's cuff (see illustration).	The cuff protects the gloved fingers. Sterile touching sterile prevents glove contamination.
9. Carefully pull the second glove over the nondominant hand. Do not allow the fingers and thumb of the gloved dominant hand to touch any part of the exposed nondominant hand. Keep the thumb of the dominant hand abducted back (see illustration).	Contact of gloved hand with exposed hand results in contamination.
10. Once the second glove is on, interlock the hands together. The cuffs usually fall down after application. Be sure to touch only the sterile sides (see illustration).	Ensures smooth fit over fingers

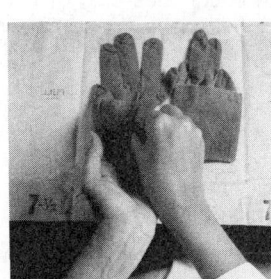
Step 6

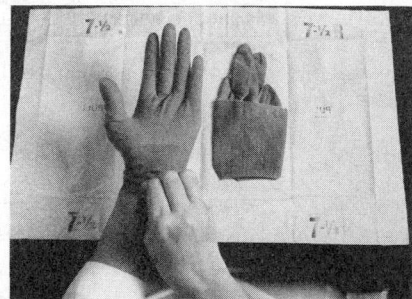
Step 7

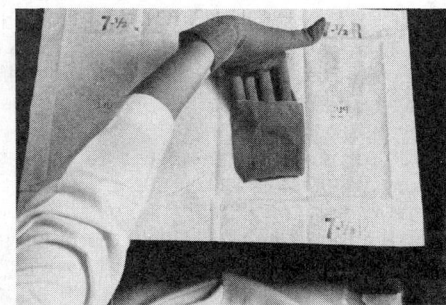
Step 8

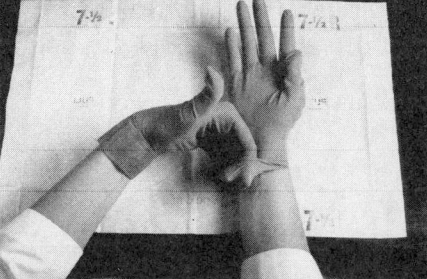
Step 9

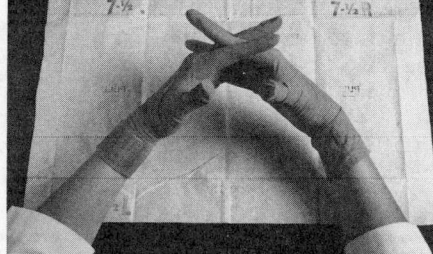
Step 10

Donning a Sterile Gown and Gloves

STEPS	RATIONALE
1. Before entering the operating room (OR) or treatment area, apply a cap and face mask. Foot covers are also required in the OR.	Prevents hair and air droplet nuclei from contaminating sterile work areas. Foot covers are paper or cloth and fit over work shoes.
2. Perform a thorough surgical handwash.	Removes transient and resident bacteria from fingers, hands, and forearms.
3. Dry hands according to Step 15 in Procedure 43-4, p. 1299.	Prevents chapping, facilitates application of gloves, and prevents transmission of microorganisms through moisture.
4. A circulating nurse in the OR assists by opening the sterile pack containing the sterile gown.	Assistance keeps gowns sterile and allows the nurse who has scrubbed to apply a gown without contaminating hands.
5. The circulating nurse prepares the glove package by peeling the outer wrapper open while keeping the inner contents sterile. The inner glove package is then placed on the sterile field created by the sterile outer wrapper.	Keeps gloves sterile and allows nurse who has scrubbed to handle sterile items.
6. Pick up the gown, grasping the inside surface of the gown at the collar.	The hands are not completely sterile. The inside surface of the gown will contact the skin's surface and is thus considered contaminated.
7. Stand away from the sterile pack and table. Hold the gown at arm's length away from your body and allow the gown to unfold by itself. Be careful not to allow the gown to touch the floor (see illustration).	Contact of the outer surface of the gown with a dirty or clean surface would result in gown contamination. Shaking of the gown can cause air currents that increase the risk of contamination.
8. Hold the gown by the inside, open shoulder seams, and insert each hand through the armholes.	The inside of the gown is considered contaminated.
9. Keeping your upper arms in front of you at shoulder height, extend the arms toward the gown cuff. (Do not push the hands through the cuffs if using the closed glove method) (see illustration).	Extension of the arms straight ahead keeps the sterile surface of the gown in view and reduces the risk of touching the floor or a portion of the body.
10. Have a circulating nurse (considered unsterile) tie the collar securely from behind and pull the sleeves onto your arms for proper fit and comfort (see illustration).	Working from behind the gowned person prevents contamination by the circulating nurse.
11. If the waist ties or snaps fall in front of the gown, enclose them within a sterile towel and hand the sterile towel to the circulating nurse standing behind you. (Disposable paper gowns have a special tag the circulating nurse may grasp.)	The towel provides a surface the circulating nurse can grasp without contaminating the gown.
12. Make a three-quarter turn away from the circulating nurse, then grasp the sterile tie and secure it in front of the gown (see illustration),	Back side of gown is considered unsterile. Prevents gown from loosening and touching unsterile objects.

OR

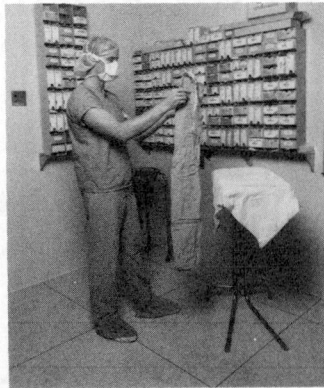 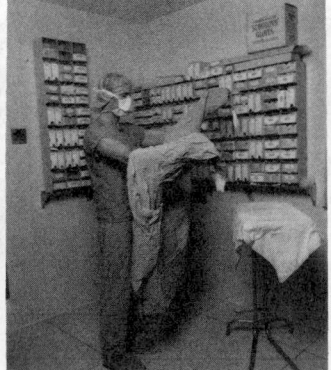 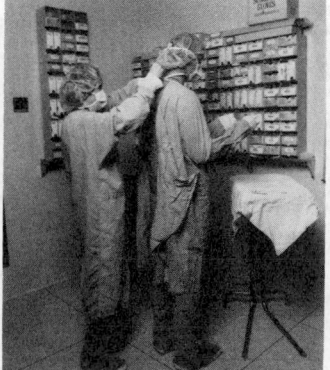 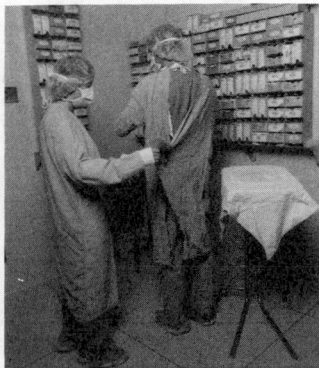

Step 7   Step 9   Step 10   Step 12

Continued.

Donning a Sterile Gown and Gloves

STEPS	RATIONALE
have the circulating nurse, who is wearing sterile gloves, tie or wrap waistband from behind, making certain gown is completely closed.	Reduces air currents and risk of contamination.

CLOSED GLOVING

13. With the hands covered by the gown sleeves, open the inner sterile glove package (see illustration).
14. Grasp the inside of the cuff sleeve covering the nondominant hand. With the same hand pick up the glove for the dominant hand. Place the glove palm side down on the palm of the covered dominant hand, with the glove fingers pointing toward the elbow of the dominant arm (see illustration).
15. The fingers of the covered dominant hand pinch the underside of the glove's cuff. With the covered nondominant hand, grasp the topside of the glove's cuff for the dominant hand. Pull the glove over the gown cuff and fingers of the dominant hand simultaneously (see illustration).
16. Carefully push the fingers into the glove and be sure the glove's cuff covers the gown's cuff.
17. With the gloved dominant hand, place the opposite glove palm side down over the palm of the covered nondominant hand with the glove fingers pointing toward the elbow (see illustration).
18. Repeat steps 15 and 16 for the nondominant hand (see illustration).
19. Interlock the gloved hands.

RATIONALE (column):

Keeps hands clean. Sterile gown touches sterile glove package.
The gown protects the nurse's fingers. Sterile touching sterile is sterile. Positioning of the glove will allow the nurse to slip it over the gown cuff.

Since the fingers do not exit through the gown's cuff, gown and glove contamination is prevented.

This ensures proper fit. The glove fits over the gown cuff to provide extra protection against contamination.
Sterile touching sterile is sterile.

This ensures smooth fit over the fingers.

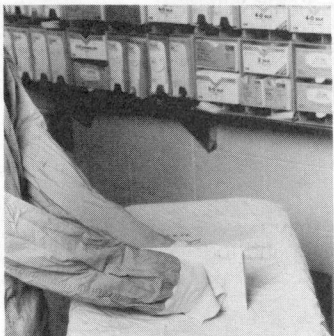

Step 13

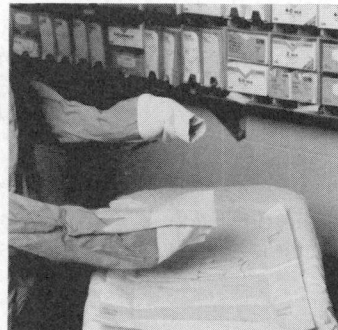

Step 14

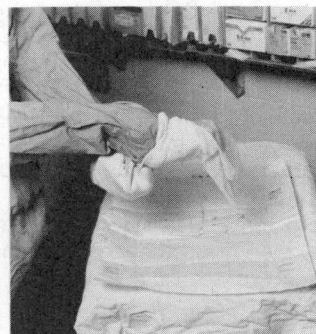

Step 15

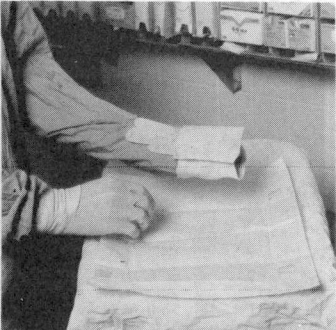

Step 17

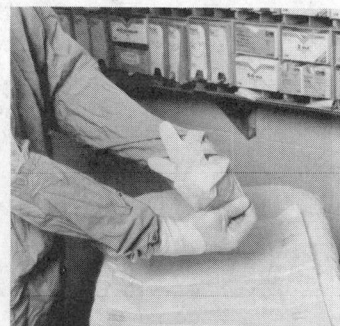

Step 18

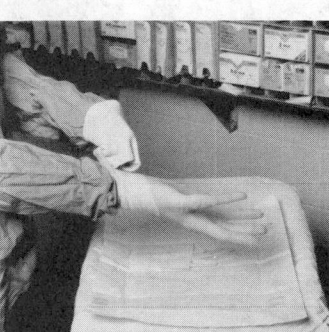

Step 18

Sample Evaluation of Interventions for Clients Susceptible to or Overcome by Infection

Goals	Evaluative Measures	Expected Outcomes
Exposure to infectious organisms is prevented.	Inspect condition of client's wound.	Wound margins are closed, not tender, and without drainage or inflammation.
	Measure client's body temperature.	Client will remain afebrile.
	Assess for systemic symptoms of infection.	Client denies malaise, anorexia, or nausea. Lymph nodes not tender and remain nonpalpable.
Extent of infection is controlled or reduced.	Observe existing wounds for amount of drainage and degree of inflammation.	Amount of drainage declines. Wound edges become less edematous and inflamed.
	Review laboratory values.	White blood cell and other significant laboratory values return to normal.
	Measure client's body temperature.	Client experiences reduction in fever.
Client understands infection control techniques.	Ask client to describe basic infection control measures used in the home.	Client will give examples of infection control (for example, handwashing before meal preparation) and basic hygiene measures.
	Observe client perform medical asepsis procedures.	Client performs procedures such as dressing change, wound cleansing, and correct self-administration of an injection.
Client achieves sense of comfort and self-esteem.	Ask if client experiences pain or discomfort at site of infection.	Client will describe a reduction in pain.
	Ask client in protective isolation if he feels as though staff or family avoids him or treats him differently.	Client will describe family as supportive.

EVALUATION

The nurse monitors clients closely for signs and symptoms of infections, especially clients at risk for nosocomial infection. The evaluation box describes criteria used in determining the effects of infection control techniques. Likewise, if a client has an infection, the nurse will evaluate for return to a normal health state.

SUMMARY

In every aspect of practice the nurse encounters situations that present a risk of an infection developing or being transmitted. Knowledge of the body's normal defenses against infection helps the nurse recognize clients most at risk for acquiring infections. The nature of the infection chain is a useful concept in identifying nursing interventions for infection control.

Nurses use two types of infection control practices, medical and surgical asepsis, to prevent infection transmission. Each set of practices calls for a conscientious and knowledgeable application of infection control principles. The nurse's failure to follow these principles seriously hampers a client's recovery or maintenance of good health.

KEY CONCEPTS

✓ Normal body flora resist infection by releasing antibacterial substances and inhibiting multiplication of pathogenic microorganisms.

✓ The signs of local inflammation and infection are identical.

✓ When pathogens multiply and alter normal tissue function, disease results.

✓ Immunity to infection is measured by the capacity to produce antibodies in response to exposure to an antigen.

✓ An infection can develop as long as the six elements comprising the infection chain are uninterrupted.

✓ A microorganism's virulence depends on its ability to resist attack by the body's normal defense.

✓ Microorganisms are transmitted by direct and indirect contact, by airborne spread, and by vectors and contaminated vehicles.

✓ Increasing age, poor nutrition, stress, inherited conditions, chronic disease, and treatments or conditions that compromise the immune response increase susceptibility to infection.

✓ The major sites for nosocomial infections include the urinary and respiratory tracts, bloodstream, and surgical or traumatic wounds.

✓ Invasive procedures, medical therapies, long hospitalization, and contact with health care personnel increase a hospitalized client's risk for acquiring a nosocomial infection.

✓ Surgical asepsis requires more stringent techniques than medical asepsis and is directed toward eliminating microorganisms.

✓ The CDC recommends health care workers consider all clients as potentially infected with HIV and other blood-borne pathogens and to reduce risk of exposure to blood and body fluids.

✓ Following aseptic principles is the key to a nurse's success in preventing clients from acquiring infections.

✓ Protective aseptic practices prevent personnel and clients from acquiring infections, as well as prevent transmission of microorganisms to other persons.

✓ Proper cleansing requires mechanical removal of all organic material from an object or area.

✓ The nurse does not take an article into an isolation room if the article is to be used by another client.

✓ A client receiving protective asepsis is subject to sensory deprivation because of the restricted environment.

✓ Lack of handwashing is the main cause of nosocomial infections.

✓ An infection control nurse monitors the incidence of infections within an institution and provides educational and consultative services to maintain aseptic practices.

✓ If the skin is broken or if the nurse performs an invasive procedure into a body cavity normally free of microorganisms, surgical aseptic practices are enforced.

✓ A sterile object becomes contaminated by direct contact with a clean or contaminated object, by exposure to airborne microorganisms, and by contact with a wet medium containing microorganisms.

REFERENCES

Centers for Disease Control: Recommendations for prevention of HIV transmission in health care settings, MMWR 36:55, 1987.

Garner, JS: Guidelines for prevention of surgical wound infections, 1985, Hospital Infections Program, CDC, PHS, and U.S. Department of Health and Human Services.

Garner, JS, and Favero, MS: Guidelines for handwashing and hospital environmental control, 1985, Hospital Infections Program, CDC, PH, and U.S. Department of Health and Human Services.

Garner, JS, and Simmons, BP: CDC guidelines for isolation precautions in hospitals, Infect Control 4(4):249, 1983.

Larson, EL, et al.: Physiological and microbiologic changes in skin related to frequent handwashing, Infect Control 7:59, 1986.

Larson, EL, et al.: Quantity of soap as a variable in handwashing, Infect Control 8:371, 1987.

Nodolny, MD: What does the infection control nurse do? Am J Nurs 80:430, 1980.

Williams, WW: CDC guidelines for infection control in hospital personnel, Infect Control 4(4):325, 1983.

Research Article

Maki, DG, Alvarado, C, and Hassemer, C: Double-bagging of items from isolation rooms is unnecessary as an infection control measure: a comparative study of surface contamination with single and double-bagging, Infect Control 7(11):535, 1986.

ADDITIONAL READINGS

Axnick, KJ: Infection control considerations in the care of the immunosuppressed patient, CCQ 3:79, 1980.

Bennett, JV: Incidence and nature of endemic and epidemic nosocomial infections. In Bennett, JV, and Brachman, PS, editors: Hospital infection, Boston, 1979, Little, Brown, & Co., Inc.

Department of Labor: Joint advisory notice: Department of Labor/ Department of Health and Human Services, HBV/HIV 52: October 30, 1987.

Ebersole, P, and Hess, P: Toward healthy aging, ed. 3, St. Louis, 1989, The C.V. Mosby Co.

Garner, JS, and Simmons, BP: CDC Guidelines for the prevention and control of nosocomial infections: guidelines for isolation precautions in hospitals, Am J of Infect Control 12:103, April, 1984.

Gross, PA, et al: Nosocomial infection: decade-specific risk, Infect Control 4(3):145, 1983.

Hargiss, CO: The patient's environment: haven or hazard, Nurs Clin North Am 15(4):671, 1980.

Hargiss, CO, and Larson, E: Infection control guidelines for prevention of hospital acquired infections, Am J Nurs 81:2175, 1981.

Jackson, M, et al.: The body substance isolation system, infection prevention and control manual, San Diego, 1987, University of California, San Diego Medical Center.

Jacobson, G, et al.: Handwashing: ring-wearing and number of microorganisms, Nurs Res 34:186, 1985.

Jaffe, HW: The acquired immunodeficiency syndrome epidemic: issues for health care professionals, Am J Infect Control 14:272, 1986.

Labet, CG, and Roderick, MA: Infection control in the use of intravascular devices, CCQ 3(4):67, 1981.

Larson, EL: Effects of handwashing agent, handwashing frequency, and clinical area on hand flora, Am J Infect Control 12:76, 1984.

Mallison, GF: Decontamination, disinfection, and sterilization, Nurs Clin North Am 15(4):757, 1980.

McCrary, E, and Martone, WJ: Preventing HIV exposure among patients and staff, AIDS Patient Care 1:32, 1987.

Pagana, KD, and Pagana, TJ: Diagnostic testing and nursing implications, ed. 2, St. Louis, 1986, The C.V. Mosby Co.

Simmons, BP: Guidelines for prevention of surgical wound infections, Am J Infect Control 11(4):133, 1983.

Thibodeau, GA: Anatomy and physiology, ed. 12, St. Louis, 1987, The C.V. Mosby Co.

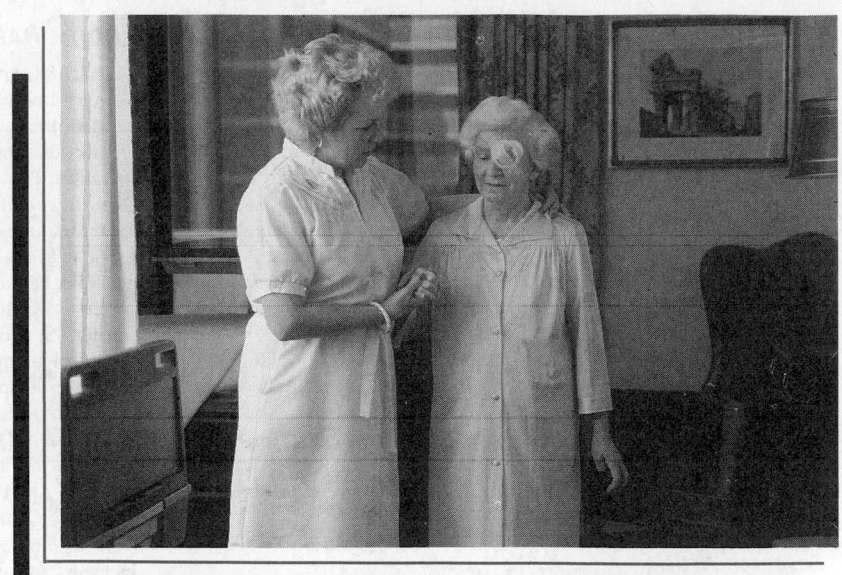

OBJECTIVES

Mastery of content in this chapter will enable the student to:

- Define the key terms listed.
- Differentiate between the processes of reception, perception, and reaction to sensory stimuli.
- Discuss common causes and effects of sensory alterations.
- Discuss common sensory changes that normally occur with aging.
- Identify factors to assess in determining sensory status.
- Describe behaviors indicating sensory alterations.
- Develop a plan of care for clients with visual, auditory, tactile, speech, and olfactory deficits.
- List interventions for preventing sensory deprivation and controlling sensory overload.
- Describe conditions in the health care agency or client's home that can be adjusted to promote meaningful sensory stimulation.
- Discuss ways to maintain a safe environment for clients with sensory deficits.

KEY TERMS

Aphasia

Auditory

Binocular Vision

Cataract

Expressive Aphasia

Gustatory

Kinesthesia

Olfactory

Ototoxic

Presbyopia

Refractive Error

Sensory Deficit

Sensory Deprivation

Sensory Overload

Stereognosis

Sensory Alterations

Part of the uniqueness of human beings is the ability to sense a variety of stimuli within the environment, perceive and organize those stimuli, and respond appropriately. Stimulation comes from many sources in and outside the body, particularly through the senses of sight, hearing, touch (tactile), smell (olfactory), and taste (gustatory). The body also has a kinesthetic sense that enables a person to be aware of the position and movement of body parts without seeing them. Stereognosis is a sense that allows a person to recognize an object's size, shape, and texture. The ability to speak is not considered a sense, but it is similar to the senses in that the client may lack meaningful stimulation from other human beings. Meaningful stimuli allow a person to learn about the environment and are necessary for healthy functioning and for normal development of the sensory organs. When sensory function is altered, the client's ability to relate to and function within the environment changes drastically.

Many clients enter the health care system with preexisting sensory alterations. However, many blind, deaf, or paralyzed clients who have partial or complete loss of a major sensory modality have found alternative ways to function safely within the environment. A client may also enter the health care setting with normal sensory function. However, a health care setting is often a place of unfamiliar sights, sounds, and smells and minimal contact with family or friends. If a client feels depersonalized and is unable to receive meaningful stimuli, serious sensory alterations can develop.

The nurse must understand and help to meet the needs of clients with sensory alterations, as well as to recognize

1307

clients most at risk for developing sensory problems. The nurse helps clients who have sensory alterations learn to react safely and effectively in the environment.

NORMAL SENSATION

Normally, the nervous system continually receives thousands of bits of information from sensory nerve organs, relays the information through appropriate channels, and integrates the information into a meaningful response. Sensory stimuli reach the sensory organs and can elicit an immediate reaction or present information to the brain to be stored for future use. The nervous system must be intact for sensory stimuli to reach appropriate brain centers and for the individual to perceive the sensation. After interpreting the significance of a given sensation, the person can then react to the stimulus.

Reception, perception, and reaction are the three components of any sensory experience (see Chapter 35). Reception begins with stimulation of a nerve cell called a *receptor,* which is usually designed for only one type of stimulus. For example, the retina of the eye receives light, and the surface of the skin receives stimuli from the pressure of tactile contact. Only pain receptors receive several forms of stimuli, such as pressure, chemicals, or heat. With stimulation of receptors, nerve impulses travel along pathways to the spinal cord or directly to the brain. For example, light waves stimulate receptors within the retina of the eye, which cause impulses to travel along the optic nerve directly to the occipital lobe of the brain. The movement of a body part stimulates proprioceptors to send impulses along peripheral spinal nerves to the spinal cord. From the spinal cord a second set of nerve fibers, conducting the sensation of position, travel up the cord, cross over at the medulla, and travel to the thalamus. At the thalamus impulses synapse with a third pathway to eventually be sent to the cerebral cortex. Sensory nerve pathways usually cross over to send stimuli to opposite sides of the brain. For example, if a person touches an object with the right hand, the left side of the brain receives the stimulus.

The actual perception or awareness of unique sensations depends on the receiving region of the cerebral cortex, where specialized brain cells interpret the quality and nature of the sensory stimuli. A person's level of consciousness influences how well stimuli are perceived and interpreted. Any factors lowering consciousness impair sensory perception. Perception includes an integration and interpretation of the stimuli based on the person's experiences. If sensation is incomplete or if past experience is inadequate for understanding the stimuli, the person may react inappropriately.

It is impossible to react to each of the multiple stimuli constantly entering the nervous system. The brain is normally capable of discarding or storing sensory information to prevent sensory bombardment. A person will usually react to stimuli that are most meaningful or significant at the time. After continued reception of the same stimulus, however, a person stops responding and the sensory experience goes unnoticed. For example, a person reading a good book is not aware of the pressure of resting his body against the back of a chair. This adaptability phenomenon occurs with most sensory stimuli except for those of pain.

The balance between sensory stimuli entering the brain and those actually reaching the conscious awareness maintains a person's well-being. If an individual attempts to react to every stimulus within the environment or if a variety and quality of stimuli are lacking, sensory alterations will occur.

TYPES OF SENSORY ALTERATIONS

Many factors alter the capacity to receive or perceive sensations (see box). The types of sensory alterations commonly seen by the nurse are sensory deficits, sensory deprivation, and sensory overload. When a client suffers from more than one sensory alteration, the ability to function and relate effectively within the environment is seriously impaired.

Sensory Deficits

A defect in the normal function of sensory reception and perception is a sensory deficit. A client may no longer be able to receive certain stimuli (for example, the client may be blind or deaf), or stimuli become distorted (for example, the client may have cataracts or be confused). When a deficit develops gradually or when considerable time has passed since the onset of an acute sensory loss, the person learns to rely on unaffected senses. Some senses may even become more acute to compensate for an alteration. For example, a blind client often develops an acute sense of hearing.

Clients with sensory deficits may change behaviors in adaptive or maladaptive ways. For example, one client with a hearing impairment may turn the unaffected ear toward a speaker to hear better, whereas another client may shun other people to avoid the embarrassment of not being able to understand their speech.

Sensory Deprivation

Sensory stimulation must be of sufficient quality and quantity to maintain a person's awareness. When an

Factors that Influence Sensory Function

AGE

- Infants are unable to discriminate sensory stimuli. Nerve pathways are immature.
- Visual changes during adulthood include presbyopia (inability to focus on near objects) and the need for glasses for reading (ages 40 to 50).
- The elderly have reduced visual fields, increased glare sensitivity, and impaired night vision, accommodation, and depth perception.
- Hearing changes include decreased hearing acuity, speech intelligibility, pitch discrimination, and hearing threshold (beginning at age 30). The elderly hear low-pitched sounds the best but have difficulty hearing conversation over background noise.
- The elderly have difficulty discriminating consonants *(f, s, th, ch)*. Speech sounds are garbled, and there is a delayed reception and reaction to speech.
- Gustatory and olfactory changes include atrophy of the taste buds in later years and reduction of olfactory nerve fibers (age 50). Reduced taste discrimination and sensitivity to odors are common.
- Proprioceptive changes include an increased difficulty with balance, spatial orientation, and coordination (age 60).
- Tactile changes include declining sensitivity to pain, pressure, and temperature.

MEDICATIONS

- Some antibiotics (for example, streptomycin and gentamicin) can permanently damage the auditory nerve; chloramphenicol can irritate the optic nerve. Narcotic analgesics, sedatives, and anti depressant medications can alter the perception of stimuli.

ENVIRONMENT

- Excessive environmental stimuli (for example, in an ICU) can result in sensory overload, marked by confusion, disorientation, and inability to make decisions. Restricted environmental stimulation (for example, with protective isolation) can lead to sensory deprivation. Poor quality of environment (for example, lighting, size of walkways, background noise) can worsen sensory impairment.

COMFORT LEVEL

- Pain and fatigue alter how a person perceives and reacts to stimuli.

PREEXISTING ILLNESSES

- Peripheral vascular disease can cause reduced sensation in the extremities and impaired cognition. Chronic diabetes can lead to reduced vision or blindness or peripheral neuropathy. Strokes often produce loss of speech. Some neurological disorders impair motor function and sensory reception.

SMOKING

- Chronic tobacco use can atrophy the taste buds so perception of flavors is lessened.

NOISE LEVELS

- Constant exposure to high noise levels (for example, on the job site) can cause hearing loss.

ENDOTRACHEAL INTUBATION

- Temporary loss of speech results from insertion of an endotracheal tube through the mouth or nose into the trachea.

---

inadequate quality or quantity of stimulation impairs perception, sensory deprivation occurs. Three types of sensory deprivation (Ebersole and Hess, 1989) are reduced sensory input (sensory deficit), elimination of order or meaning from input (for example, clients exposed to strange environment), and restriction of the environment (for example, bedrest) that produces monotony and boredom.

There are many effects of sensory deprivation (Table 44-1). The symptoms can easily cause nurses or physicians to believe a client is psychologically ill, senile, suffering from severe electrolyte imbalance, or under the influence of psychotropic drugs. Therefore the nurse must always be aware of the client's existing sensory function and the quality of stimuli within the environment.

TABLE 44-1   Effects of Sensory Deprivation

Type of Alteration	Associated Symptoms
Cognitive	Reduced capacity to learn, inability to solve problems, poor task performance
Affective	Boredom, restlessness, increased anxiety, emotional lability, increased need for physical stimulation and socialization
Perceptual	Reduced attention span, disorganized visual and motor coordination, temporary loss of color perception, disorientation, confusion of sleeping and waking states

Sensory Overload

When a person receives multiple sensory stimuli and cannot perceptually disregard or selectively ignore some stimuli, sensory overload occurs. Excessive sensory stimulation prevents the brain from appropriately responding to or ignoring certain stimuli. Because of the multitude of stimuli leading to overload, the person no longer perceives the environment in a way that makes sense. Overload thus results in a state similar to that produced by sensory deprivation.

The acutely ill client is a good example of a person who may fall victim to sensory overload. The constant pain from the disease process, the nurse's frequent monitoring of vital signs, and the irritation from drainage tubes protruding from the body combine to cause overload. Even if the nurse offers a comforting word or provides a gentle backrub, the client may not benefit because his or her attention and energy are focused on more stressful stimuli.

Sensory overload differs from deprivation in that the level of stimuli that can cause the condition depends more on individual factors. The point at which stimuli needed for health function become enough to tax endurance changes according to a person's level of fatigue, attitude, or emotional and physical well-being. Continued overload causes a person to eventually develop many of the same symptoms as is found with sensory deprivation.

ASSESSMENT

When assessing clients with or at risk for sensory alterations, the nurse considers all the factors influencing sensory function (see box on p. 1309), particularly age. The nurse collects a history that also assesses the degree to which a sensory deficit affects the client's life-style and ability to relate to the environment. The assessment must also focus on the quality and quantity of environmental stimuli.

Persons at Risk

A nurse can focus on an assessment of sensory function quickly for clients most at risk. The elderly is a high risk group because of normal physiological changes involving sensory organs. Clients immobilized due to bedrest or physical encumbrances (for example, casts or traction) are unable to experience all the normal sensory sensations of free movement. Another group at risk includes clients isolated in a health care setting or at home. For example, the client in protective isolation (see Chapter 43) is often restricted to a hospital room and is unable to enjoy normal interactions with visitors.

A client with a known sensory deficit is at risk for sensory alterations. However, a person's quality of life may differ, depending on the age of onset of the sensory deficit. Magilvy (1985) found that women with a later onset of hearing loss considered themselves to have a lowered quality of life compared with women who experience hearing loss at a younger age.

A hospital environment is full of sensory stimuli, including conversation between staff members, the sounds of electrical monitors and equipment, bright lighting, and the odors of body fluids. A person accustomed to living alone and in a quiet environment may have difficulty coping with hospitalization.

Physical Assessment

To identify sensory deficits the nurse should assess vision, hearing, olfaction, taste, and the ability to discriminate light touch, temperature, pain, and position (see Chapter 13). Table 44-2 summarizes assessment techniques for identifying sensory deficits. As the nurse performs care measures, the client may exhibit behaviors indicating specific sensory alterations.

A neurological assessment of the level of consciousness, orientation, and cognitive thought processes helps to reveal symptoms of sensory deprivation or overload. An assessment of neurological functioning can also reveal level of perception. Of course, factors other than sensory deprivation or overload may cause impaired perception (for example, medications, pain, or reduced oxygenation).

Ability to Perform Self-Care

A client with sensory or perceptual alterations is often unable to perform activities of daily living. The nurse assesses clients' functional abilities in their home environment and the health care setting, including feeding, dressing, grooming, and performing toileting activities. For example, can a client with altered vision find items on a meal tray? Does the loss of balance prevent the client from safely rising from a toilet seat? The nurse also determines a visually impaired client's ability to perform daily routines such as reading bills or writing checks, differentiating money denominations, and driving a vehicle at night. Any alteration in the ability to perform self-care has implications for the nurse in planning the client's discharge from an acute care setting and in providing resources within the home.

Environment

Environment can either minimize or worsen sensory alterations. In some cases the environment is the cause of the problem. The nurse assesses the health care environment and the home environment.

TABLE 44-2   Assessment of Sensory Function

Assessment	Behavior Indicating Deficit (Children)	Behavior Indicating Deficit (Adult)
VISION		
Ask the client to read a newspaper, a magazine, or lettering on a menu. Measure visual acuity with a Snellen chart. Assess visual fields.	Self-stimulation: eye rubbing, body rocking, sniffing or smelling, arm twirling; hitches (uses legs to propel while in sitting position) instead of crawls	Poor coordination; squinting; underreaching or overreaching for objects; uncontrolled eye movements; persistent repositioning of objects, impaired night vision
HEARING		
Perform conventional assessment, including ticking watch, whisper, tuning fork (see Chapter 13). Observe client conversing with others. Assess client's own perception of hearing ability.	Frightened when unfamiliar people approach; no reflex or purposeful response to sounds; failure to be awakened by loud noise; slow or absent development of speech; greater response to movement than to sound; avoidance of social interaction with other children	Blank looks; decreased attention span; lack of reaction to loud noises; increased volume of speech; positioning of head toward sound; smiling and nodding head in approval when someone speaks; using other means of communication such as lip reading or writing
TOUCH		
Assess for sensitivity to light touch and temperature (see Chapter 13). Check the client's ability to discriminate between sharp and dull stimuli. Assess if client can distinguish objects (dime or quarter) in the hand with eyes closed. Ask if client feels any unusual sensations.	Unable to perform developmental tasks related to grasping objects or drawing; repeated injury from the child handling harmful objects (for example, hot stove, sharp knife)	Clumsiness; overreaction or underreaction to painful stimulus; failure to respond when touched; avoidance of touch; feeling sensation of pins and needles
SMELL		
Have client close eyes and identify several nonirritating odors (for example, coffee or mustard).	Difficult to assess until child is 6 or 7 years old; difficulty discriminating noxious odors	Failure to react to noxious or strong odor; increase in body odor
TASTE		
Ask client to sample and distinguish different tastes (lemon, sugar, etc.). (Have client drink a sip of water and wait 1 minute between each taste.) Ask client to detect foods with the same texture (carrots, apples, etc.).	Unable to tell if food is salty or sweet; may eat strange-tasting things	Change in appetite; excessive use of seasoning and sugar; complaints about taste of food; weight loss
POSITION SENSE		
Perform conventional tests for balance and position sense (see Chapter 13).	Children with hyperactivity or learning difficulty may be clumsy, exhibit extraneous movement, or swing their arms excessively	Poor balance and spatial orientation; shuffling gait; reduced response to brace self when falling; becomes more precise and deliberate with movements

HAZARDS

A client with sensory alterations may be at risk for injury if the environment is unsafe. Cluttered furniture, dimly lit corridors or stair steps, and torn carpets pose dangers for clients with visual impairments. If a client has a hearing impairment, the nurse checks to see if the sounds of a doorbell, telephone, smoke alarm, or alarm clock are easy to discriminate. Confusion in sounds may pose a danger.

MEANINGFUL STIMULI

Meaningful stimuli reduce the incidence of sensory deprivation. The nurse observes whether the environment contains stimuli such as pets, a record player or television, pictures of family members, or a calendar and clock. In a hospital the nurse notes whether clients have roommates or visitors. However, a roommate who constantly watches television or persistently tries to talk and prevents the client from resting can be a problem. A client can become disoriented from a barren environment that gives few signals for normal sensory perception. The presence or absence of meaningful stimuli influences alertness and the ability to participate in care. In a hospital setting the nurse checks the environment for bright colors, comfortable furnishings, and good ventilation and clean surroundings.

With infants or young children, the nurse assesses the toys available. Does the play area or crib have toys of different sizes, shapes, and colors? Is the play area clean, pleasantly lit, and decorated attractively?

AMOUNT OF STIMULI

Excessive stimuli in an environment can cause sensory overload. In an acute care setting the nurse assesses the level of care required. The frequency of observations and procedures performed may be stressful. If the client is in pain, has many tubes and dressings, or is restricted by casts or traction, overstimulation can be a problem. If the client's room is near the nurses' station, an elevator, or door leading to stairs, the noise may be excessive.

Family and Significant Others

The amount of contact clients have with supportive family members or significant others can influence the degree of isolation felt. The nurse assesses whether a client lives alone and whether family, friends, or neighbors frequently visit. The absence of visitors while hospitalized can also have a significant impact on sensory status. The ability to discuss fears or concerns with loved ones is an important coping mechanism for most people. The absence of meaningful conversation can cause a person to become sensorially deprived.

A client's inability to socialize with others can be a problem. Older women with hearing losses suffer emotionally when they cannot communicate with companions (Magiluy, 1985). Persons with hearing loss can feel isolated and as though they have a limited choice of social activities.

Communication Methods

Clients with existing sensory deficits often develop alternative ways of communicating. A deaf or hearing-impaired client may read lips, use sign language, or even

---

Aphasia Deficit Checklist

_____ Mild comprehension (understanding) problem

_____ Moderate comprehension (understanding) problem

_____ Severe comprehension (understanding) problem

_____ Nods "yes" and "no" but doesn't really understand what you are saying

_____ Mild speaking (expressing self) problem

_____ Moderate speaking (expressing self) problem

_____ Denies problems in speaking or understanding

_____ Talks in circles because of a problem coming up with names

_____ Difficulty naming objects presented

_____ Difficulty repeating things after others

_____ Difficulty reading single words

_____ Difficulty reading sentences

_____ Difficulty reading paragraphs

_____ Difficulty seeing the right side of the page

_____ Difficulty writing on the right side of the page

_____ Difficulty writing name

_____ Difficulty writing single words

_____ Difficulty writing sentences

_____ Difficulty writing paragraphs

_____ Echoes what others say ("parrots others")

_____ Uses nonsense words (words which do not exist in the English language)

_____ Speaks in jargon or gibberish

_____ Speaks in stuttering manner

_____ Prone to emotional outbursts

_____ Easily frustrated

_____ Difficulty sequencing the sounds or syllables of a word in the right order

_____ Difficulty producing oral (mouth) or facial movements on command

_____ Difficulty imitating oral (mouth) or facial movements

From Pimental, PA: Alterations in communication, Nurs Clin North Am 21(2):329, 1986.

communicate with written notes. The visually impaired often learn to read Braille. Clients who have undergone laryngectomies often write notes, use communication boards, speak with mechanical vibrators, or use esophageal speech. The nurse must understand the client's method of communication to interact with the client and promote interaction with others.

The client with aphasia may be unable to produce or understand language. Expressive aphasia, a motor type of aphasia, is the inability to name common objects or to express simple ideas in words or writing. Sensory or receptive aphasia is an inability to understand written or spoken language, and global aphasia is the inability to understand language or to communicate orally.

To understand the nature of a communication problem, the nurse must know whether a client has trouble speaking, understanding, naming, reading, or writing (see box). Depending on the nature of the communication problem, the nurse selects the best way to interact with the client.

Clients with endotracheal or tracheostomy tubes have a temporary loss of speech. The nurse should observe behavior to determine if the client has developed a sign language or system of symbols to communicate needs.

Self-Perception of Sensory Loss

The nurse should know how sensory losses are perceived by clients. Many clients believe that the quality of their life has been lowered because of sensory alterations. The nurse asks clients questions such as "How have you adjusted to your (hearing, visual, speech) loss?" or "What has changed in your life because of your (hearing, visual, speech) loss?" The nurse then begins to identify individualized measures that will help clients adjust. It also helps to know family members' perceptions of the client's sensory loss.

NURSING DIAGNOSIS

After gathering data about the client's sensory status, the nurse develops specific nursing diagnoses (see nursing diagnoses box). The diagnoses pertain to specific types of sensory alterations or to health care problems created by sensory alterations. The nurse can select nursing diagnoses by predicting how sensory alterations will affect a client's ability to function.

Appropriate defining characteristics are identified to ensure accurate, individualized nursing diagnoses. The sample nursing diagnoses box on p. 1314 lists examples of nursing diagnoses for clients with sensory alterations.

Examples of Nursing Diagnoses Related to Sensory Alterations

NANDA-APPROVED NURSING DIAGNOSES

Sensory/perceptual alterations: visual related to:
- Aging
- Surgical eye patch

Sensory/perceptual alterations: auditory related to:
- Drug side effects
- Neurological disease

Sensory/perceptual alterations: kinesthetic related to:
- Bedrest

Sensory/perceptual alterations: gustatory related to:
- Aging

Bathing/hygiene, dressing/grooming, toileting self-care deficit related to:
- Visual loss
- Reduced tactile sensation

Potential for injury related to:
- Decreased depth perception
- Reduced sense of smell

Impaired verbal communication related to:
- Endotracheal tube
- Motor aphasia

Impaired adjustment related to:
- Sensory overload
- Sensory deficit

Social isolation related to:
- Expressive aphasia

PLANNING

The plan of care (see care plan box on p. 1314) depends on the nurse's understanding of the client's perception and acceptance of the sensory alteration. It also depends on the extent to which the client has adjusted to sensory loss. Every effort should be made to provide care that will enable the client to adapt to the health care setting and to the home. Some sensory alterations are short term (for example, a client suffering sensory-perceptual alterations as a result of sensory overload in an intensive care unit). Sensory alterations such as permanent visual loss require long-term goals of care.

Involvement of family members or friends is important. The family can provide meaningful stimulation and learn to accept the client.

The goals of care for a client with a sensory alteration may include any of the following:
1. Maintaining function of existing senses
2. Maintaining meaningful sensory stimulation
3. Functioning in a safe environment
4. Preventing additional sensory loss

Sample Nursing Diagnoses for Sensory Alterations

Defining Characteristics	Nursing Diagnoses	Related Factors
Reduced visual acuity Reduced depth perception Irritability Lowered perception of body image	Sensory/perceptual alterations: visual	• Aging • Surgical eye patch
Inability to identify common aroma (for example, vanilla) Single living No smoke alarm in home	Potential for injury	• Reduced sense of smell
Inability to unbutton clothing Inability to put on clothing	Dressing/grooming self-care deficit	• Reduced tactile sensation

Sample Nursing Care Plan for Sensory Alterations

Nursing Dianosis	Goals	Expected Outcomes	Nursing Interventions
Sensory/perceptual altera-tions: visual related to aging	Client will maintain optimal visual function.	Client will be able to read the Bible and letters from daughter and identify objects used in self-care.	Provide a pocket magnifier for reading. Offer books printed in large lettering. Discuss purchase of large-print wristwatch and phone-dialer guide.
	Client will function safely in home environment.	Client will be able to discriminate between near and far objects without falls or accidents.	Have client use colors to highlight important visual targets: handrails and light switches yellow, edges of steps orange or yellow. Provide adequate lighting in stairwells or other dark-ened areas. Use rugs color-contrasted with woodwork. Use dishes and cups with colored rims.

5. Communicating effectively with existing sensory alterations
6. Understanding the nature and implications of sensory loss
7. Achieving self-care

IMPLEMENTATION

Nursing interventions involve the client and family so a safe, pleasant, and stimulating sensory environment can be maintained. Effective interventions enable the client with sensory alterations to function effectively with existing deficits.

Promoting Function of Existing Senses

The nurse offers a variety of measures to enhance a client's remaining sensory function to maximize other senses. Sensory testing also detects sensory problems early so corrective devices can be made available.

Promoting Visual Function

Strengthing Visual Stimuli

- Use assistive devices (for example, pocket magnifiers, near vision microscopic glasses, and large-print wristwatch, phone dialers, and books).
- Install two side mirrors on cars for enhancing visual field.

Using Other Senses

- Provide books on taped cassettes.
- Install textual cues on walkways or ramps to alert person to intersections.
- Pour salt and pepper into hand before adding to food.
- Fold money according to value and place in different wallet compartments.

Using Sharp Visual Contrasts

- Use warm colors to highlight visual targets. Orange, red, or yellow can be used on handrails or light switches.
- Color-code the control dials of irons, stoves, dryers, washers, and thermostats. Mark a reference point on dials and on their desired settings.
- Use colored rims around dishes and cups to reduce spills.

Minimizing Glare

- Decrease light contrasts by using diffuse, soft lighting.
- Avoid waxed floors and exposure to bright sunlight.
- Install tinted glass windows with adjustable shades or sheer curtains in large windows.
- Shield eyes with sunglasses, visors, or hats with brims.
- Avoid driving at dusk or night.

VISION

CHILDREN. The most common visual problem during childhood is a refractive error such as nearsightedness. Vision screening of school-age children and adolescents can detect visual impairment early. Parents may need encouragement to pursue eye testing by an ophthalmologist.

ADULTS. Because an adult develops visual changes with aging, the nurse should encourage regular use of corrective contact lenses or eyeglasses. There are many ways the nurse can help the client to maintain existing visual function (see box). The client can be taught to strengthen visual stimuli, use other senses, use sharp visual contrasts, and minimize the effects from glare.

HEARING

CHILDREN. Children with chronic middle ear infections—a common cause of impaired hearing—should undergo auditory testing. Parents must be warned of the risks and should seek medical care when the child has symptoms of earache or respiratory infection. Children should also be immunized against childhood diseases (for example, measles, rubella, and mumps) that can cause hearing loss and should not be treated with ototoxic medications.

ADULTS. To maximize residual hearing function, the nurse suggests ways to modify the environment. Telephone rings can be amplified. Special handsets are available if incoming voices cannot be heard. Important environmental sounds (for example, smoke alarms, doorbells, or alarm clocks) may best be heard if amplified or changed to a more low-pitched, buzzerlike-sound. The elderly may not be able to hear with background noise. The nurse can suggest that clients turn off radios, televisions, or appliances during conversations. If a hearing aid is worn, the client should make sure that it is properly cleaned and adjusted and that it contains functioning batteries, and the client should wear it. The nurse should make sure the client also knows how and when to change the batteries.

TASTE

The nurse can easily promote the sense of taste by using measures to enhance remaining taste perception. Good oral hygiene keeps the taste buds well hydrated. Taste perception will be heightened if foods are well seasoned, differently textured, and eaten separately. If taste perception is improved, food intake and appetite will also improve.

Stimulation of the sense of smell with aromas such as brewed coffee or baked bread can heighten taste sensation. The client should avoid blending or mixing foods because these actions make it difficult to identify tastes. Older persons should chew food thoroughly to allow more food to contact remaining taste buds.

TOUCH

Clients with reduced tactile sensation usually have the impairment over a limited portion of their bodies. The nurse can stimulate existing function by providing touch therapy. If the client is willing to be touched, hairbrushing and combing, backrubbing, and touching on the arms or shoulders are ways of increasing tactile contact. When sensation is reduced, a firm pressure may be necessary for the client to feel the nurse's hand. Turning and repositioning can also improve the quality of tactile sensation.

If a client is overly sensitive to tactile stimuli (hyperesthesia), the nurse must then minimize irritating stimuli. Keeping bed linens loose, minimizing direct contact, and protecting the skin from exposure to irritants also help.

SMELL

Smell can be improved by strengthening olfactory stimulation. A client's environment can be made more pleasant with smells such as cologne, fragrant flowers, or sachets. The nurse encourages clients to sniff food before eating. When the nurse assists clients with eating or sets up a meal tray, naming the foods may help clients imagine the aromas.

Suggestions for Introducing Environmental Stimuli

VISUAL

- Open the drapes to the client's room so outside sights can be seen.
- Raise the head of the bed and draw back any dividing curtains or partitions so the client can see a roommate or movement in the hallway.
- Provide attractive decorations on tables or cabinets, such as fresh flowers, plants, a picture, or greeting cards.
- Encourage family to enrich the client's home environment with clean curtains, familiar objects or keepsakes, and perhaps a fresh coat of paint on bedroom walls.

AUDITORY

- Sit down and speak with the client. Listen to the client's thoughts and experiences. Make the conversation meaningful.
- Turn on a radio with the type of music the *client* (not the nurse) enjoys. A favorite radio or television program can also be stimulating.
- Encourage visitors.

TASTE AND SMELL

- Provide attractive, taste-appealing meals. Be sure tableware and glasses are clean. Foods meant to be served warm should be warm and cold foods cold.
- Provide a variety of textures, aromas, and flavors to enhance appetite.

TOUCH

- The same measures (therapeutic touch) that promote existing sensory function also prove useful in creating meaningful stimuli.

Maintaining Meaningful Stimulation

When a client's environment presents risks of understimulation or overstimulation of the senses, the nurse should provide meaningful stimuli or eliminate confusing or irritating stimuli. When the problem is sensory deprivation, the nurse should introduce meaningful stimuli for all senses based on client preferences (see box). The nurse does not force stimulation if the client is more concerned with basic functions such as comfort or nutrition.

When the problem is sensory overload, the nurse must control excessive stimuli. The client needs time for rest and freedom from stresses caused by frequent monitoring or repeated tests. The nurse may sit quietly with the client or involve him in an undemanding repetitive activity such as combing hair or brushing teeth. A client experiencing stress in the home can find relief in simple activities such as meal planning or household chores. Reorientation to the environment may be provided by wearing name tags on uniforms, addressing the client by name, or using conversational cues as to time or location. The tendency for clients to become confused can be reduced by offering short and simple repeated explanations and reassurance. Helping clients to become as mobile and independent as possible within prescribed limits also provides meaningful stimulation. The nurse can encourage the family not to argue with or contradict the confused client but to calmly explain their location and identity and the time of day.

The nurse can reduce sensory overload by organizing the care plan. Performing a number of activities such as dressing changes, bathing, or vital signs' measurement in one visit prevents the client from becoming overly fatigued. Coordination with laboratory and radiology departments reduces the amount of time needed for tests and examinations. Anticipating client needs such as voiding helps reduce uncomfortable stimuli.

The nurse can also try to control extraneous noise in and around the client's room. It may be necessary to ask a roommate to lower the volume on a television or to move the client to a quieter room. Equipment noise should be kept to a minimum. Bedside equipment not in use, such as suction and oxygen equipment, should be turned off. The nurse also avoids abrupt loud noises such as clattering or rinsing bedpans. Nursing staff should also try to control laughter or conversation at the nurses' station.

Providing a Safe Environment

Clients with existing sensory loss must be protected from injury, whereas clients at risk for sensory loss must learn to avoid injury. The nature of the actual or potential sensory loss determines the safety precautions taken.

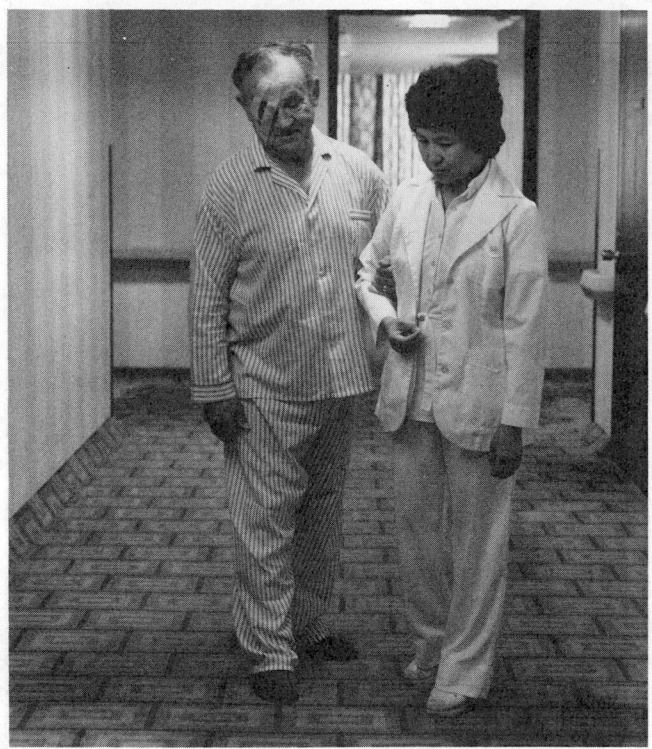

Fig. 44-1   A nurse assists in the ambulation of a client wearing an eye patch.

VISUAL LOSS

The client with recent visual impairment often requires assistance with ambulation. The nurse should stand at the client's nondominant side approximately one step in front of the client (Fig. 44-1). The client can use the nondominant hand to grasp the nurse's arm and reach forward with the dominant hand to feel for any barriers or landmarks. The nurse should describe the course of movement and ensure that obstacles have been removed. A client with visual impairment should never be left standing alone in an unfamiliar area.

A visually impaired client who spends considerable time in bed should have a call light close by. Necessary objects should be placed in front of the client to prevent accidental falls caused by reaching over the bedside. Side rails are also important in this regard.

The nurse removes potential hazards such as furniture that clutters the environment. Adequate lighting should be provided in work areas, corridors, and near steps. More illumination is needed in potentially hazardous areas such as stairs or exits. When possible, steps inside or outside the house should be replaced with ramps.

If a client is partially or totally blind, fire hazards should be removed from the home. For example, flammable items such as paper or cloth should be kept away from the stove. A client who smokes must learn to discard ashes frequently into an ashtray. Water placed in the bottom of an ashtray helps to ensure that cigarette butts are extinguished.

If the client has reduced peripheral vision and difficulty driving in darkness, the nurse should emphasize precautions such as looking to both sides before passing cars or while turning a corner and driving only during the day. When a client's depth perception is poor the edges of steps or driveway curbs should be painted a bright color (for example, orange) to prevent falls. Rugs should be a bright color to contrast with woodwork and walls.

HEARING LOSS

Nurses may rely on clients to report unusual sounds, such as a suction apparatus running improperly or an IV pump alarm sounding. However, the client with a hearing loss may not hear such sounds and thus requires more frequent visits by the nurse. The client can also benefit from learning to use vision to discover sources of danger.

In the home, wake-up and burglar alarms, doorbells, smoke detectors, and telephones can be adapted to set off red or green flashing lights. A computerized mechanism with a printer is available to transfer written words over the telephone to the hearing impaired. Family members or anyone who calls the client regularly should learn to let the phone ring for a longer period.

REDUCED OLFACTION

A reduced sensitivity to odors means the client may be unable to smell leaking gas, a smoldering cigarette or fire, or tainted food. The client should use smoke detectors and other alternative precautions such as checking ashtrays or placing cigarette butts in water. A client can learn to check dates on food packages and the color and texture of food. Pilot gas flames should be checked visually.

REDUCED TACTILE SENSATION

Clients with reduced tactile sensation risk injury when their condition confines them to bed because they are unable to sense pressure on bony prominences or the need to change position. These clients rely on nurses for timely repositioning and turning.

When the ability to sense temperature variations is reduced, the nurse should use extra caution in applying heat and cold therapies (see Chapter 47) and preparing bath water. The nurse must frequently check the condition of the client's skin.

SPEECH ALTERATIONS

A client lacking the ability to speak cannot call out for assistance. Clients with aphasia or a laryngectomy or endotracheal intubation need alternative means of communication such as message boards or note pads.

In the health care agency a call light should always be near. For the client at home a small bell or alarm at the bedside is helpful.

Preventing Sensory Loss

Occupation or life-style may place a person at risk for sensory loss. Persons working around loud noises need to learn potential dangers to hearing function. Protective ear covers are essential if exposure to loud sound is continuous. Ringing of the ears is an early sign of hearing impairment.

Clients exposed to dangerous chemicals or small flying objects should wear eye goggles for protection. A chemical burn to the cornea or a penetrating eye injury can cause permanent blindness. Children should be discouraged from playing with any kind of sharp object because it is common for a child to be blinded accidentally by a playmate.

Promoting Communication

A sensory deficit can cause a person to feel isolated because of an inability to communicate with others. The nature of the sensory loss influences the methods and styles of communication nurses can use. The methods described in the box can also be taught to family members and significant others.

The client with a hearing impairment may be able to speak normally. However, the deaf client's inability to hear his or her own words may cause serious speech alterations. A child born deaf is not able to speak at all. Clients may use sign language or lip reading, write with a pad and pencil, or learn to use a computer for communication. Special communication boards contain common terms used in nursing care and help clients express their needs.

Depending on the type of aphasia, the inability to communicate can be frustrating and frightening. The nurse should initially establish very basic communication and recognize that aphasia does not indicate intellectual impairment or degeneration of personality.

Understanding Sensory Loss

Clients must understand all implications of sensory loss. For example, the client with a hearing impairment must learn that excessive background noise interferes with the ability to hear conversation. Similarly, an older client with visual loss must know to install proper lighting in hazardous areas to reduce risk of injury. Clients can learn to adapt to sensory alterations so their living environment can be safe and appropriately stimulating. All family members should understand the way a client's sensory loss affects normal day-to-day activities. Family

Communication Methods

CLIENTS WITH APHASIA

- Listen to the client and wait for him to communicate.
- Do not shout or speak loudly (hearing loss is not the problem).
- If the client has problems understanding, use simple, short questions and facial gestures to give additional clues.
- If the client has problems speaking, ask questions that require simple yes or no answers or blinking of the eyes. Offer pictures or a communication board so the client can point to them.
- Give the client time to understand.
- Do not pressure or tire the client.

CLIENTS WITH A LARYNGECTOMY

- Use pictures, objects, or word cards so the client can point to them.
- Offer a pad and pencil or magic slate for the client to write messages.
- Do not shout or speak loudly.
- Provide an artificial voice box (vibrator) for the client to use to speak words and phrases.

CLIENTS WITH HEARING IMPAIRMENT

- Get the client's attention. Do not startle him or her when entering a room. Be sure the client knows you wish to speak.
- Face the client. Be sure your face and lips are illuminated to promote lip reading.
- If the client wears glasses, be sure they are clean so your gestures and face can be seen.
- Speak slowly and articulate clearly. Use normal tones of voice and inflections of speech.
- Restate with different words when you are not understood.
- Do not shout. Loud sounds are usually higher pitched. If it is necessary to raise your voice, speak in lower tones.
- Talk toward the client's best or normal ear.
- Use gestures to enhance the spoken word.

and friends can be more supportive when they understand sensory deficits and the types of elements that worsen or lessen sensory problems. If clients feel socially unaccepted, their sensory loss seriously impairs their perceived quality of life.

Promoting Self-Care

The ability to perform self-care is essential for self-esteem. Frequently, family members or nurses believe sensorially impaired persons require assistance, when in fact they can help themselves. Useful guidelines assist clients with visual or tactile impairment when help is required with activities of daily living.

A meal tray can be set up as though food on the tray and condiments or drinks around the tray were numbers on the face of a clock. The visually impaired client can easily become oriented to the items after the nurse explains each item's location.

If tactile sense is diminished, the client will dress more easily with zippers or velcro strips, pullover sweaters or blouses, and elasticized waists. If a client has partial paralysis and reduced sensation, it is always better to dress the affected side first.

Family members responsible for selecting clothing for visually impaired clients should be encouraged to follow the client's preferences. Any sensory impairment has a significant influence on body image, and it is important

Sample Evaluation of Interventions for Sensory Alterations

Goals	Evaluative Measures	Expected Outcomes
Function of existing senses is maintained.	Measure client's ability to read and distinguish objects.	Client will be able to identify objects in environment and read while using visual aids.
	Measure client's ability to hear conversation and identify sounds of alarm clock, doorbell, or smoke alarm.	Client will be able to follow a conversation, respond appropriately to questions, and correctly identify source of sounds in environment.
	Evaluate client's ability to hear with use of hearing aids.	Same as above.
	Observe client's dietary intake.	Food intake and appetite remain or return to normal.
		Weight remains stable.
Meaningful stimulation is maintained.	Observe client for signs and symptoms of sensory deprivation or overload.	Client remains alert and appropriately responsive to stimuli in the environment.
	Measure client's orientation and level of consciousness.	Client remains oriented to person, place, time, and situation.
Client's environment is safe.	Evaluate client's ability to ambulate or climb stairs.	Client is able to walk or climb stairs without fall or other injury.
	Ask client to describe ways to visually identify sources of danger when hearing or olfaction is impaired.	Client identifies appropriate safety measures.
	Evaluate condition of client's skin with reduced tactile sensation.	Skin remains intact without signs of pressure.
Client avoids additional sensory loss	Ask client to identify potential risks to visual or auditory function.	Client is able to describe risks to sensory function in home setting or workplace.
Client communicates effectively.	Evaluate ability of client with aphasia to understand speech or express self.	Client will successfully communicate with nurse.
	Observe use of alternative communication techniques in client with laryngectomy.	Client will successfully write, communicate messages nonverbally, or use an artificial voice box.
	Evaluate the ability of a client with hearing impairment to hear the spoken word and understand lip reading.	Client will respond appropriately to questions and interact spontaneously with nurse.
Client understands sensory loss.	Ask client to discuss implications to health and safety resulting from sensory loss.	Client will describe potential problems posed by sensory loss and ways to minimize their effects.
Client achieves self-care.	Observe the client during feeding, dressing, and toileting.	Client will be able to feed and dress self and perform toileting activities.

for the client to feel well groomed and attractive. The nurse should offer assistance if needed in brushing, combing, and shampooing hair.

The client with visual problems needs assistance in reaching toilet facilities safely. Safety bars should be installed near the toilet. Toilet paper and the call light cord should be within easy reach. Clients with proprioceptive problems may lose their balance when attempting to use the toilet. The nurse must supervise ambulation and sitting, make frequent checks to prevent falls, and caution the client against leaning forward.

EVALUATION

The nature of a client's sensory alteration influences the manner in which the nurse evaluates care. If care is directed at improving sensory acuity the nurse evaluates the integrity of the sensory organs and the client's ability to perceive stimuli. Any interventions designed to relieve problems associated with sensory alterations are evaluated on the basis of the client's ability to function normally without injury. When the nurse attempts to directly or indirectly (through education) alter the client's environment, evaluation is directed at observing environmental changes. The nurse uses evaluative criteria in determining the outcome of therapies (see evaluation box).

SUMMARY

The client with sensory alterations often faces a lonely and frightening world. The inability to interact effectively with the environment leads to a loss of security and self-esteem. A healthy balance between incoming sensory stimuli and those to which the person is able to respond is necessary for the person's well-being.

Nurses work with a variety of clients who have actual or potential sensory alterations. Specific physiological changes can create sensory deficits. Exposure to excessive environmental stimulation causes sensory overload. Isolation within an environment devoid of meaningful stimulation causes sensory deprivation. Clients most at risk for sensory problems include elderly, immobilized, and socially isolated persons.

The nature of any sensory alteration influences the choice of nursing interventions. The nurse promotes the sensorially deprived client's ability to maintain normal function with existing sensory deficits. Likewise, the nurse attempts to make changes within the environment to provide safe and meaningful stimulation for clients. Sensory changes can affect various aspects of a client's life-style. The nurse uses creative intervention to help clients interact effectively with their world.

KEY CONCEPTS

✓ Sensory reception involves the stimulation of sensory nerve fibers and the transmission of impulses to higher centers within the brain.

✓ Sensory perception involves the organization and integration of sensory information into meaningful and conscious awareness.

✓ Because a person learns to rely on unaffected senses after experiencing a sensory loss, the nurse designs interventions to preserve function of these senses.

✓ Sensory deprivation results from an inadequate quality or quantity of sensory stimuli.

✓ Sensory overload differs from sensory deprivation in that the level of stimuli needed to cause overload depends more on individual preferences.

✓ Aging results in a gradual decline of acuity in all senses.

✓ An intensive care unit places a client at risk for sensory overload.

✓ Clients who are elderly, immobilized, or confined in isolated environments are at risk for sensory alterations.

✓ The extent of support from family members or significant others can influence the quality of sensory experiences.

✓ Assessment of sensory function includes a physical examination and measurement of functional abilities.

✓ An assessment of environment includes identifying hazards, sources of meaningful stimuli, and the amount of stimuli.

✓ Nursing care for clients with sensory alterations includes using stronger sensory stimuli, compensating with other senses, and modifying the environment to maximize remaining sensory function.

✓ Clients with existing sensory deficits can learn alternative ways to communicate.

✓ Care of clients at risk for sensory deprivation includes introducing meaningful and pleasant stimuli for all senses.

✓ To prevent sensory overload, the nurse controls stimuli, orients the client to the environment, and promotes rest by minimizing interruptions.

✓ To improve communication with the hearing impaired, the nurse speaks clearly, avoids shouting, and makes sure the client can see facial and lip movements.

✓ Clients with laryngectomy or endotracheal intubation can communicate effectively with communication boards, written messages, and artificial voice devices.

REFERENCE

Ebersole, P, and Hess, P: Toward healthy aging, ed. 3, St. Louis, 1989, The C.V. Mosby Co.

Research Article

Magilvy, JK: Quality of life of hearing-impaired older women, Nurs Res 34:140, 1985.

ADDITIONAL READINGS

Aranosian, RD: Dealing with the deaf, Emergency Med 15:29, 1983.

Blanco, KM: The aphasic patient, J Neurosurg Nurs 14:34, 1982.

Carter, J: The effects of aging upon selected visual functions: color, vision, glare sensitivity, field of vision, and accomodation. In Sekuler, R, Kline, D, and Dismukes, K, editors: Aging and human visual function, vol. 2, New York, 1982, Alan R. Liss, Inc.

Downs, FS: Bedrest and sensory disturbances, Am J Nurs 74:435, 1974.

Foreman, MJ: Acute confessional states in hospitalized elderly: a research dilemma, Nurs Res 35:3, 1986.

Hayter, J: Modifying the environment to help older persons, Nurs Health Care, 4:265, 1983.

Kopac, CA: Sensory loss in the aged: the role of the nurse and the family, Nurs Clin North Am 18:373, 1983.

Kruczek, TM: How hospitals hurt old people, RN 49(2):17, 1986.

Langan, ML, and Yearick, ES: The effects of improved oral hygiene on taste perception and nutrition of the elderly, J Gerontol 31:413, 1976.

Primental, PA: Alteration in communication. In Dudas, S, and Bukowski, L, editors: Nursing care of the stroke patient, Nurs Clin North Am 21:321, 1986.

Schiffman, S: Food recognition by the elderly, J Gerontol 32:586, 1977.

Walsh, C: Common sense nursing care for the patient with poor vision, RN 49(10):24, 1986.

Whaley, LF, and Wong, DL: Nursing care of infants and children, ed. 3, St. Louis, 1987, The C.V. Mosby Co.

Zegeer, LJ: The effects of sensory changes in older persons, J Neurosci Nurs 18:325, 1986.

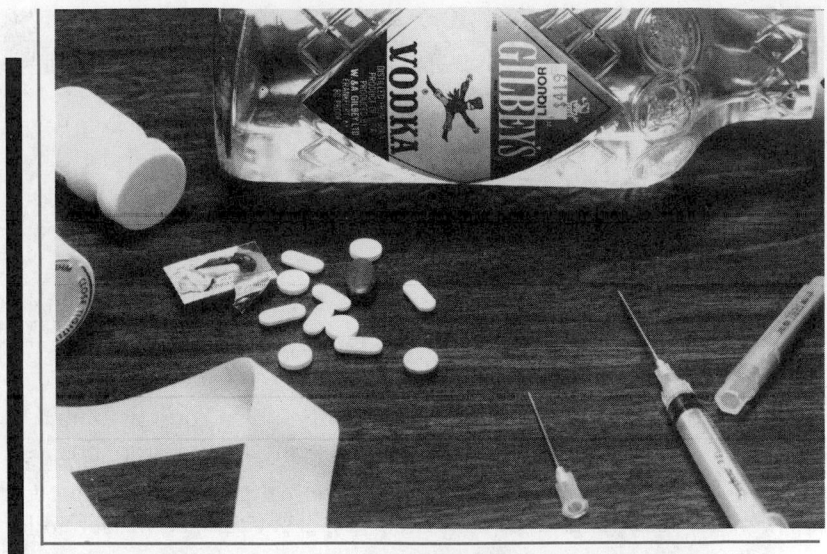

OBJECTIVES

Mastery of content in this chapter will allow the student to:

- Discuss the general health risks related to the abuse of any substance.
- Compare and contrast physiological and psychological dependence.
- List nine major groups of drugs and substances and discuss their major effects.
- Describe several psychosocial causative variables in substance abuse.
- Describe the disease of chemical dependency and its progression.
- Discuss signs and symptoms of chemical dependency and physical, psychological, and social outcomes to the disease.
- Describe the typical course of substance abuse.
- State at least three special groups particularly at risk for substance abuse.
- Describe the nurse's responsibility if a colleague may be abusing a substance.
- Describe special assessment approaches for clients with substance abuse problems.
- List examples of nursing diagnoses related to substance abuse.
- List and discuss seven general types of interventions appropriate for substance abusers.
- Describe major characteristics of the evaluation process for nursing care of substance abusers.

KEY TERMS

Abuse

Addiction

Central Nervous System Sympathomimetic

Chemical Dependency

Chemicals

Escape Mechanism

Fetal Alcohol Syndrome

Hallucinogens

Illegal Chemicals

Impairment

Inhalants

Legal Chemicals

Misuse

Physiological Dependence

Psychological Dependence

Psychotomimetic

Substance

Substance Abuse

Tolerance

Withdrawal Syndrome

Substance Abuse

Substance abuse or chemical dependency is a major problem faced by every society in the world. If it were possible to add up all the direct and indirect results of substance abuse, including automobile accidents, violent crime and behavior, and the full range of health problems associated with the abuse of alcohol and other drugs, substance abuse might be the major health problem in most industrialized countries today. If the economic and social effects of substance abuse are totaled, including the economic costs of health care, job absenteeism, and reduced functioning and effects on the family and other social units, substance abuse can be considered one of the most serious social problems.

A substance is any drug, chemical, or biological entity that can be self-administered. Substance abuse occurs because of the substance's real or perceived effects or benefits. Even substances the general public may consider harmless, such as vitamins, aspirin, and laxatives, can cause health problems if used improperly. The nurse needs to be aware of problems involved in substance abuse because the effects on physiological and psychosocial health have a wide range and can be serious or even life threatening.

Chemical dependency is an "equal opportunity" disease, that is, anyone can get it. Social class, income, education, race, ethnic origin, sex, or occupation does not protect one from the disease. There is one requirement, however, for developing it—a person must use mood-altering chemicals in sufficient quantity for a sufficient length of time for dependency to occur. The person could consume alcohol or drugs in differing patterns, however, and still become chemically dependent. For example, a person could be a "daily drinker," never becoming drunk but consuming regular and increasing amounts, and eventually could not do without the chemical. One could also be a "binge" drinker, consuming large quantities on occasion to the point of drunkenness and then not drink *at all* for a long period of time. The distinguishing characteristic is that once a binge drinker begins drinking, the drinker is unable to control the amount of consumption.

Another characteristic associated with the occurrence of chemical dependency is family history. Offspring of alcoholics often become alcoholic themselves even when they have been raised apart from their natural parents (Goodwin et al., 1973). In addition, males have almost double the chance of acquiring the disease than females, especially when their fathers were alcoholic or drug dependent (Goodwin et al., 1974). Recent research also supports the hereditary nature of chemical dependency (Begleiter et al., 1984).

SUBSTANCE MISUSE, ABUSE, AND DEPENDENCE

Drugs and other substances can be used, misused, or abused, and the nurse must be able to distinguish among these different behaviors when providing care to clients with actual or potential drug or substance problems. These terms are defined in varying ways in different contexts, but the following meanings are generally accepted by health care professionals. A drug or substance is being *used* if it is appropriately taken only as prescribed or generally recommended for its intended physiological or psychological effects. A drug or substance is being *misused* if it is taken indiscriminately, whether as prescribed or self-administered as an over-the-counter medication, or taken improperly by a client who does not clearly understand the correct uses and dosage. A drug or substance is being *abused* if it is regularly taken indiscriminately in excessive quantities to the extent that the person's physiological, psychological, or social functioning is impaired.

The meanings given these terms are related to societal attitudes and values. The ingestion of alcohol to the point of intoxication may be accepted in some groups as a social use but be viewed as misuse or, if chronic, abuse by other groups. In addition, these behaviors exist on a continuum from cautious and appropriate use at one extreme to self-destructive, violent, chronic abuse at the other. We can generally categorize the more extreme cases as clear use or abuse, but it is often more difficult to discriminate between use and misuse or misuse and abuse. For example, it is impossible to draw a line between how many alcoholic drinks a month are acceptable and how many constitute abuse.

Many variables are involved in whether the use of any drug or substance becomes misuse, including personality factors, cultural background, social context, and the person's motivations, values, attitudes, and related behavioral patterns. Although misuse of a drug or substance may not immediately compromise the individual's functioning, misuse has the potential for becoming abuse and therefore can be viewed as a major risk factor. The concept of the health-illness continuum (see Chapter 2) is useful in assessing the client's health status and risk factors related to abuse patterns if physiological changes have not yet begun to occur.

The nurse may encounter substance abuse in two ways. A person may enter the health care system with a complaint directly or indirectly related to substance abuse such as a teenager seen in the emergency room with PCP-induced seizures, or an alcoholic client being treated for liver disease. The nurse may also discover a client's substance abuse while providing care for other conditions, such as learning in a routine nursing history that the client has been using laxatives daily for several months or in a family counseling situation that a father suspects his son frequently smokes marijuana. Because any type of drug or substance abuse threatens the person's health, the nurse who discovers abuse in either way can provide care directed toward resolving the abuse problem.

Two additional concepts are necessary for understanding substance abuse: physiological and psychological dependence. *Physiological dependence* is a condition in which the body has become so accustomed to the drug or substance that functioning is significantly impaired without it. Physiological dependence is present if a withdrawal syndrome occurs when administration of the drug is abruptly stopped. Use of alcohol, opiates, barbiturates, antianxiety drugs, and other agents can lead to physiological dependence.

Psychological dependence is an emotional or psychological reliance on a drug or substance, usually because of its psychological effects. The person prefers the drugged state to a nondrugged state and experiences a desire, craving, or compulsion for the drug or substance. Most physiologically dependent persons are also psychologically dependent on the drug, but psychological dependence can occur alone, as with cocaine, amphetamines, marijuana, and even caffeine.

Any person who is dependent on a drug or substance can be considered to be abusing it because of the actual or potential impairments to functioning related to the chronic use of any drug or substance. Although a person may believe that drugs that do not lead to physiological dependence are safer, as with the teenager who is aware that marijuana is not "addictive" and who believes that he can stop using it whenever he wants, psychological dependence is often at least as powerful a habit. Chronic abuse of these "nonaddictive" drugs can also lead to impaired functioning and physiological damage.

Many clients in a nurse's care who are chemically dependent may be receiving nursing care as a result of their physical problems related to alcohol or drug abuse. For example, the nurse working in obstetrics may care for a mother who is a chronic alcoholic and whose infant is born with fetal alcohol syndrome (FAS). FAS is a permanent disorder characterized by retardation and physical abnormalities. A nurse working in a neighborhood clinic may be a primary care provider for an intravenous substance abuser.

Nurses themselves are at risk for substance abuse. In fact, nurses' problems with chemical dependency have recently been brought to the attention of the profession (Bissell and Haberman, 1984; Sullivan, 1987) with efforts underway to assist nurses with recovery (American Nurses' Association, 1984; Sullivan, Bissell, and Williams, 1988). Because nurses care for clients with substance abuse, because they may be considered as speakers for schools and community programs, and because

they are at risk themselves for substance abuse, they must sort fact from myth (see box).

DRUGS AND SUBSTANCES

The general public often considers only medically prescribed substances and highly publicized illegal substances to be drugs, but chemically active substances such as caffeine, nicotine, and alcohol and nonprescription substances such as aspirin, laxatives, and antacids are also drugs and are commonly abused. The following sections describe the major classes of drugs and chemical substances, their prevalence in society today, and their major physiological and psychological effects.

Alcohol

Estimates of the prevalence of alcoholism have been made by the National Institute on Alcohol Abuse and Alcoholism (NIAAA). In 1979, a national survey was conducted to determine the prevalence of alcoholics and alcohol abusers in the adult population of the United States. The survey revealed that approximately 10% of the population met the criteria for alcoholism, with a higher incidence of males (14%) and fewer females (6%) reporting alcoholism symptoms (Clark and Midanik, 1982).

Based on this research, the trends projected for the future suggest that this percentage will increase by 7% between 1985 and 1995. These increases are based on demographic changes in the population, including the decreasing numbers of young adults, an increase in the large population of "baby boomers," and an increase in the number of elderly.

Although commonly considered a stimulant, alcohol is actually a central nervous system depressant that causes pseudostimulant effects as parts of the brain are released from inhibitory control by the cortex. In the gastrointestinal system, alcohol is an irritant that may cause inflammation, bleeding, and malabsorption at any site. Chronic use of alcohol may lead to gastritis, enteritis, liver disease, and alcoholic pancreatitis. In the neurological system, chronic use may result in brain damage, memory loss and blackouts, sleep disturbances, sensorymotor disturbances, and (with large doses) anesthesia. Cardiovascular effects include diminished cardiac output, arrhythmias, and heat loss as a result of vasodilation of peripheral vessels. In the genitourinary system alcohol has a diuretic effect with rising blood levels and an antidiuretic effect as blood levels fall. Chronic use affects hormone levels and thus primary and secondary sex characteristics. Respiratory effects of chronic use include bronchitis, emphysema, and asthma. In the musculo-

---

Myths and Facts Related to Substance Abuse

Myth: Alcoholics are skid-row bums.
Fact: Only 5% of all alcoholics fit this stereotype. The majority (95%) represent a cross-section of people from all walks of life, all professions and occupations, and all socioeconomic levels.

Myth: Providing information on the dangers of alcohol and drugs will prevent addiction.
Fact: Although information is essential, by itself it will not prevent addiction from occurring. Nurses, physicians, and pharmacists, who are all informed about drugs, become addicted at least as often (if not more so) than others.

Myth: People just *think* they're "addicted" to alcohol or other drugs. They could quit if they had more "willpower."
Fact: Although initial use is under voluntary control, once a person is addicted, either physically or psychologically, it becomes nearly impossible to control one's use.

Myth: Alcoholics (or addicts) must *want* to quit before anything can be done to help them.
Fact: Early treatment is just as beneficial as treating any other disease. By intervening early in a person's addiction, an alcoholic can avoid the long-term complications and consequences that come with extensive use.

skeletal system, chronic alcohol myopathy may produce muscle weakness and wasting.

At intoxicating levels the user's desired effect is often a sense of euphoria produced by depression of the central nervous system. The psychological effects of chronic alcohol use include heightened defense mechanisms, such as denial of reality and rationalization, a tendency to manipulate others, depression, suicidal tendencies, loneliness caused by decreased social skills, dependent behaviors, impulsiveness, and a low frustration tolerance.

Narcotics and Related Drugs

In addition to alcoholism, drug abuse accounts for serious health and economic problems in this country. Determining the incidence of drug abuse is even more difficult than identifying alcoholics but an attempt was also made to estimate these numbers. A community study, conducted in the United States from 1981 to 1983 (American Psychiatric Association, 1987), documented percentages of people who met the criteria for drug abuse (Table 45-1).

Opiates and opiate derivatives, including heroin, morphine, and codeine, are the most commonly abused narcotic drugs. Opiate derivatives are generally administered by sniffing (absorption through the mucous membranes) or subcutaneous or intravenous injection. In addition to physical dependence, opiate abuse leads to severely deteriorated functioning and altered behavioral patterns, often including criminal activities to gain the money for drug purchases.

The opiate derivatives are central nervous system depressants that can lead to tolerance and physical and psychological dependence. The therapeutic effect is the reduction of pain. Depressed respiration is a major side effect, and respiratory arrest can occur with overdose. Nausea and vomiting are common. In the digestive system, motility is delayed, secretions are reduced, and intestinal water absorption is increased. Acute overdosage may result in coma and pulmonary edema.

Opiate derivatives are often abused for their expected effects: mood elevation, relief of tension and anxiety, and a feeling of euphoria and tranquility. The user is generally drowsy and content, with a feeling that all biological needs are met. Usually functioning in all areas is severely impaired, leading to physical problems such as dehydration and malnutrition. As with chronic users of alcohol, social functioning is altered, leading to a range of psychosocial problems.

Sedative-Hypnotics

Sedative-hypnotic drugs include barbiturates, such as pentobarbital, phenobarbital, and primidone, and non-barbiturates, such as ethchlorvynol, glutethimide, and methaqualone. It is not uncommon for individuals who take these prescribed drugs for medical reasons to advance gradually to abuse.

Barbiturates produce central nervous system depression ranging from mild sedation to deep anesthesia. Large doses cause respiratory depression, aspiration pneumonia, hypotension, and reduced gastrointestinal motility. Less common side effects are nausea and skin rashes. Overdose can cause coma, hypoxia, hypothermia, cardiovascular depression or cardiac arrest, and respiratory failure.

Nonbarbiturate sedatives and hypnotics also depress the central nervous system. There is a wide range of additional effects, including headache, ataxia, dizziness, nausea, and vomiting.

Psychological effects include relaxation or sedation, sleepiness, a sense of euphoria that is often followed by depression, and impaired judgment. Chronic users of barbiturates can become both physically and psychologically dependent on these drugs.

Tranquilizers

Tranquilizers include antianxiety and antipsychotic agents such as phenothiazine, benzodiazepine, diazepam, and chlordiazepoxide. Diazepam follows alcohol as the next most commonly abused drug because it is sometimes viewed as harmless and is often freely prescribed. In 1975 diazepam was the most commonly prescribed drug. The risks have since been recognized, and use of the drug has declined considerably. Both physical and psychological dependence can result from chronic use.

The physical effects of tranquilizers in large doses include hypotension, respiratory depression or coma, ataxia, hypothermia or hyperthermia, tachycardia, and reduced coordination such as slurred speech.

TABLE 45-1 **Percentage of People Addicted to Narcotics or Related Drugs**

Drug	Abusers (%)
Cannabis (marijuana)	4.0
Cocaine	.2
Hallucinogens (LSD)	.3
Amphetamines	2.0
Opioids (heroin, morphine, meperidine, analgesics, anesthetics)	.7
Sedatives (tranquilizers, hypnotics, barbiturates)	1.1

Modified from American Psychiatric Association: Diagnostic and statistical manual of mental disorders (DSM III-R), Washington, D.C., 1987, The Association.

Psychological effects include reduced activity, decreased attentiveness or confusion, emotional bluntness, lethargy, somnolence, and a feeling of tranquility and increased self-confidence.

Central Nervous System Sympathomimetics

Central nervous system sympathomimetics include cocaine and amphetamines, which are pharmacologically related to epinephrine and norepinephrine. Both drugs stimulate the central nervous system. Amphetamines are ingested or injected, and cocaine is sniffed, injected intravenously, or smoked in converted base form. Amphetamines produce physical tolerance. Neither drug leads to physical dependence, but both can result in strong psychological dependence.

The physiological effects of amphetamines can include tachycardia, dyspnea, chest pain, and restlessness. Although users report a greater physical and mental energy, this occurs because of more rapid expenditure of energy resources, not with the creation of any new energy. Because the appetite is reduced, malnutrition is common among chronic abusers.

The effects of cocaine are similar to those of amphetamines. Large doses of cocaine can cause nausea, vomiting, muscle spasms, respiratory failure, convulsions, coma, and circulatory collapse.

The psychological effects of amphetamines and cocaine are similar: mood elevation or euphoria, a reduction in fatigue, a sense of greater alertness and increased energy, potential aggressiveness, and hyperactivity. Behaviors may be repetitious and inefficient. Severe depression, often of suicidal proportions, may follow an amphetamine high.

Marijuana

Marijuana and hashish (a powdered form of the plant's resin) are the most common forms of the cannabis drugs and are derived from a species of hemp. The plant is usually dried and smoked but is sometimes ingested. The pharmacological classification of marijuana is not definite, but the drug seems to act as a central nervous system depressant.

The physiological effects of marijuana are less dramatic than with most other drugs affecting the central nervous system. Effects include immediate tachycardia, delayed bradycardia, delayed hypotension, and enhanced appetite. The psychological effects have been the subject of many studies and are still being debated. The drug produces a state of relaxation, distorted perceptions of time and space, moments of excitement or hilarity, impaired decision making, and sometimes fear, panic, or paranoia. Hallucinations occur only with very high doses. Long-term use may be associated with apathy, memory problems, and some loss of mental acuity.

Hallucinogens

Hallucinogens include lysergic acid diethylamide (LSD), mescaline, psilocybin, and phencyclidine (PCP). These drugs generally do not lead to physical or psychological dependence but are of concern because unpredictable, often violent behavior is associated with their use. PCP use has become more widespread in recent years, and it is sometimes smoked in a mixture with marijuana. PCP is particularly dangerous because of its unpredictable behavioral effects.

LSD produces relatively mild autonomic nervous system changes such as tachycardia, hypertension, nausea, and vertigo. The physiological effects of PCP include flushing, sweating, diplopia, nystagmus, analgesia, sedation, ataxia, seizures, hypertension, numbness of extremities, impaired motor skills, respiratory depression, and coma.

LSD causes perceptual changes or hallucinations, impaired judgment, and toxic psychosis characterized by panic, paranoia, and unpredictable behavior. The psychological effects of PCP include perceptual distortions, apathy, disorganized thought processes, impaired attention span, hallucinations that can recur unpredictably for days or weeks after use, paranoid behavior, and self-destructive acts.

Inhalants

Inhalants are substances such as volatile hydrocarbons and aerosols that are abused for their central nervous system depressant effect. Inhalants include toluene, xylene, benzene, gasoline, paint thinner, lighter fluid, and airplane glue.

The physiological effects of inhalants include bronchial and laryngeal irritation, headache, vertigo, and ataxia. Coma may occur with large doses.

The psychological effects of inhalants include inebriation, exhilaration, dizziness, euphoria, abandonment, and aggressiveness. Depression may follow the initial mood elevation.

Nonprescription Substances

Any drug or substance that alters consciousness or physiological functioning in any way has the capacity to be misused or abused. For example, nicotine in cigarettes causes central nervous system changes and can be abused for these effects. Similarly, coffee and soft drinks containing caffeine can be misused. Society is generally becoming more aware of the effects and risks of these substances. Many over-the-counter products,

Classes of Nonprescription Medications Attractive as Drugs of Misuse

- Antacids
- Sedatives and sleep aids
- Cold remedies and antitussives
- Mouthwashes
- Antirheumatics
- Vitamins and minerals
- Laxatives
- Sunburn treatments and preventives
- Stimulants
- Antidiarrheals
- Bronchodilators and antiasthmatics
- Ophthalmics
- Miscellaneous internal products

- Antimicrobials
- Analgesics
- Antihistamines and allergy drugs
- Topical analgesics
- Hematinics
- Antiperspirants
- Dentifrices and dental products
- Contraceptive and vaginal products
- Hemorrhoidals
- Dandruff and athlete's foot preparations
- Antiemetics
- Emetics
- Miscellaneous external products

From Ray, O: Drugs, society, and human behavior, ed. 4, St. Louis, 1987, The C.V. Mosby Co.

however, hold the same potential for misuse and abuse when individuals diagnose their own needs and turn habitually to a commercial product they can easily buy and self-administer. The box lists 26 classes of nonprescription medications having active ingredients that make them attractive as drugs of misuse.

The physiological effects of all nonprescription medications are too numerous and varied to be described here. Unlike other drugs and substances discussed so far, most of these medications are overused or misused not for their psychological effects but because the user becomes psychologically dependent if he feels the medication is necessary for continued good health, even when continued use actually has adverse effects.

SUBSTANCE ABUSE AND PSYCHOSOCIAL HEALTH

Because of their mind- and behavior-altering effects, most abused substances can also have serious effects on a person's psychosocial well-being and family functioning. To understand the relationship between abuse and the client's psychosocial dimension, and thus provide nursing care for a client with a substance abuse problem, the nurse needs to understand the etiological variables that play a causative role in substance abuse, the typical pattern of use, the addiction process, and the psychosocial effects on the abuser's family and other social interactions.

Etiology

Physiological and psychological dependence has a major role in the abuser's pattern of continued use, but the reasons for the person's initial misuse of the substance are more varied. Generally two kinds of conscious or unconscious motivations may explain why a person first misuses a substance (Hahn, Barkin, and Oestreich, 1986). The person using mind-altering drugs may be seeking pleasure, euphoria, a new or unusual experience, or self-discovery; he may be motivated by factors such as curiosity, boredom, peer pressure, or media attention. The person may be consciously or unconsciously seeking to solve or avoid a problem or to cope with stress or other problems. This motivation may apply both to a chronic abuser of self-prescribed laxatives and to a businessman who habitually has three martinis at lunch to relieve tension at the office. Many psychologists have examined substance abuse as an escape mechanism by which the person attempts to reduce inner tensions, depression, self-concept problems, or problems in social interaction with a spouse, family, or peers. Certain theories have been proposed to explain the etiology of substance abuse.

THEORIES OF SUBSTANCE ABUSE

PRIMARY DISEASE. The success of Alcoholics Anonymous (AA) has forced a recognition of the simple fact that when alcoholics stop drinking and adopt abstinence as a goal, many recover from their dependency and their other problems diminish or disappear. This realization has resulted in alcoholism being considered a *primary* disease, for example, one in which the alcohol problem is seen as primary with other problems (psychological or physical) as secondary to the alcoholism. Others have believed that the reverse is true: alcoholism is secondary to other psychiatric or psychological problems.

GENETIC THEORIES. Research evidence is accumulating that indicates the genetic component involved in chemical dependency but environmental influences also seem to be involved. When so many offspring of alcoholics were found to develop the disease, it was assumed that either genetics or the environment were at work (or a combination of both). However, the contributions of each of these (genetics and environment) needed to be examined separately.

In a study in Sweden, it was found that identical twins

had a higher incidence of alcoholism (54%) when one of them was alcoholic than were nonidentical twins who only had a 28% incidence (Kaij, 1960). In addition, a higher incidence was noted when the first twin's alcoholism was more severe. This did not conclude that alcoholism was totally inherited and was not based on environmental factors.

A subsequent study in Denmark attempted to deal with heredity separate from environment (Goodwin et al., 1973). In this study, adoptees (boys) of biological alcoholic parents, who had no knowledge of their alcoholic parents' histories were compared with adoptees without alcoholic parents. Both groups were adopted into nonalcoholic homes. The men were between 25 and 29 at the time of the study. Twenty percent of those with biological alcoholic parents were themselves alcoholic, whereas only 5% of the men without alcoholic parents had developed alcoholism.

In a more recent study, sons of alcoholics were given EEGs at a young age (Begleiter et al., 1984). Their EEGs showed the same abnormal brain wave tracings as EEGs of long-term alcoholics. From these and many other studies, it is apparent that heredity plays a large part in predisposing people to chemical dependency.

PSYCHOLOGICAL THEORIES. Various theories have been studied comparing psychologic factors and alcoholism. One theory suggests that the ability to handle stress contributes to the onset of drinking and to its continuation onto addiction. Since most of these studies were completed after alcoholism developed, it was difficult to know what other factors contributed to the disease. In fact, stressful events in one's life have not been found to be related to alcoholism in one study (Morrissey and Schuckit, 1978).

Other psychological theories are based on reinforcement principles. That is, people begin substance use and continue it because they receive some reward or reinforcement such as feeling good, having fun, or being accepted. Although there is probably some element of truth to this theory, it is not totally supported by research.

SOCIOCULTURAL THEORIES. Sociocultural theories of alcoholism differ from other theories in that instead of examining individuals, they focus on group differences. These theories are based on observation and study of different cultures or groups of people and their drinking practices and the occurrence of alcoholism. Although some differences have been found, there is no way to know why this happens so that such information could be utilized with other groups for preventive action. Theories about how people are socialized in regard to drinking also are included in this area of study. Socialization theories state that values, perceptions, norms, and beliefs are passed on from one generation to another and that the way alcohol is used is part of one's socialization.

Obviously, no one cause of chemical dependency has been clearly identified but rather many possible causes exist. That one can be born with a *predisposition* to develop the disease later in life is apparent, but what is not known is what are the "triggers" that help a social drinker become an alcoholic. Even without knowing the precise mechanism of the cause of chemical dependency, we do know that the disease is progressive and without intervention in this progression, the person is likely to die young or be institutionalized.

Patterns of Use

There are essentially two patterns of alcohol addiction. One is regular daily use and the other is "binge drinking." Binge drinking means that a person will go for long periods of time not drinking at all and then go on a binge of continuous drinking for hours (or even days), not stopping until forced to by unconsciousness, illness, or an accident. Both patterns are common in alcoholics.

Other drugs are used in differing patterns. Amphetamines are often initially used for weight control and later may be used both daily and episodically. Cannabis (marijuana) and cocaine are primarily used recreationally. Episodic use may occur, but as dependence progresses, daily use is common. There are two patterns of use with opioids (heroin and narcotic analgesics). One involves a person who received a prescription for pain relief with a physical problem (trauma or surgery) and continues to use the narcotic, justifying the use on the basis of symptoms long after recovery from the physical problem. Nurses, physicians, pharmacists, and dentists often become addicted in this manner. The second pattern of opioid addiction involves young people who experiment with heroin, cocaine, or crack obtained illegally. Use usually continues in combination with alcohol and other drugs as they are available.

Addiction Process

Alcohol and other drugs of addiction are mood altering, that is, they change the way we feel, usually for the better. Mood-altering chemicals affect the central nervous system (CNS) and alter its functioning. They help people relax, feel "mellow," and enjoy activities. In addition, drugs mediate pain perception, induce sleep, and reduce physical and emotional reactions to stress. Approximately 10% of the population perceive the use of chemicals as necessary for normal daily functioning. These people have become addicted to mood-altering chemicals. They are called alcoholics, drug addicts, or chemical dependents.

Rarely does a person set out to become an alcoholic or addicted to other drugs. Practically all users think they are in control and can stop using the mood-altering drug whenever they wish. What they do not realize is that as addiction progresses, physical and/or psychological dependence on the drug(s) make stopping impossible.

PHYSICAL ADDICTION

Although all drugs cause bodily damage, alcohol is more destructive to tissues than others. Liver damage is the most common, since the liver detoxifies alcohol. Fatty liver, hepatitis, and cirrhosis of the liver are frequent complications of long-term alcohol use. Other body systems are also damaged by long-term use, including the cardiovascular system, musculoskeletal system, and the gastrointestinal system. In fact, every body system is affected when alcohol is ingested in large amounts over a long period of time.

PSYCHOLOGICAL ADDICTION

As the disease of chemical dependency progresses, the afflicted person uses a variety of defense mechanisms to cope with the many problems that the using behaviors cause. Defense mechanisms are unconscious ways people deal with painful events.

The primary defense mechanism used by chemical dependents is denial. The person does not really believe what appears obvious to others. Even in the face of overwhelming evidence that chemical use is impairing a person's life (for example, DWIs, losing jobs and family, or criminal convictions), an addicted person will continue to deny that the chemical use is anything but normal and claim, "I can quit anytime I want."

To try to understand how this works for the alcoholic, see if you can remember a time in your life when you had a shock of some kind, such as a death of someone close to you or the loss of a pet. You probably thought "this can't be true" and even kept "forgetting" it had happened, for instance, when you first woke up in the morning, you may have initially thought the person (or pet) was still alive and any minute you would see him or her coming through the door. This is denial. We actually think what *appears* to be true is not. *We are not lying.* We really believe what we think at the time. Denial helps us deal with difficult and painful events until such time as we are able to assimilate the event into our lives. This is how it works for the alcoholic or drug addict. It is very difficult for anyone to admit to being an alcoholic or drug dependent.

In addition to denial, rationalization is used to explain why they continue to use chemicals. Many recovering alcoholics say good news, bad news, or no news was reason enough to drink. Projection of one's thoughts or feelings on others is also common as a chemically de-

pendent person focuses on faults of others to avoid his own.

Attitudes Toward Substance Abuse

When providing care for a client with a substance abuse problem, to be objective in understanding the problem and to facilitate a therapeutic nurse-client relationship, the nurse should be aware of personal attitudes and values related to use of the substance. The values clarification process is useful in this respect (see Chapter 13). The nurse who adopts a moralistic, judgmental attitude toward drinking might have difficulty understanding how individual factors have contributed to the client's behavior.

The nurse should also assess the client's and family's attitudes toward the abuse problem. A client who views his drinking as a sin, for example, may experience such guilt after drinking that in a vicious circle he continues to drink to escape the guilt, thus causing more guilt and leading to still more drinking. On the other extreme, a client who is convinced his drinking is outside his control may not be motivated to attempt to comply with a treatment program unless counseling or teaching methods first lead to an acceptance of his role in attempting to resolve the problem. As current media announcements for treatment programs emphasize, to admit one has a problem is to take the first step toward solving it.

Impact on Socialization

Because chemical use becomes the major purpose in life and activities are organized around obtaining the drug and using it, the rest of the person's life is affected. Often jobs are lost (or not done well), families leave, and children are neglected or abused. The dependent person is at risk for victimization from robbery, rape, assault, as well as being in trouble for committing such crimes. Prison and heavy fines often result. Even without these serious consequences, the dependent's person's everyday life and functioning become impaired.

SUBSTANCE ABUSE IN SPECIAL GROUPS

Developmental Stages

Because substance abuse involves many physiological and psychosocial effects and causative variables, people in different developmental stages have different susceptibilities and are affected in different ways. For example, a 40-year-old businessman may increase alcohol consumption in response to an awareness that his physical energy is diminishing, or an adolescent may experiment with drugs because of pressures from his peer group. Each developmental stage presents certain kinds of stresses and the potential for maturational crises, and these may influence the individual's behavior related to abuse patterns. In addition, the physiological and psychological effects of substance abuse vary according to the person's developmental stage. Unit 5 discusses the developmental stages in detail and the developmental changes that influence the individual's susceptibilities.

Special attention should be given to the effects of substance abuse in the fetal stage of development. Chapter 22 describes different kinds of teratogens, drugs that cross the placenta into the embryo's or fetus' circulation with a potential effect on normal growth. Many drugs, including prescription and over-the-counter medications and illegal substances, have detrimental effects on fetal development, including low birth weight, high fetal and infant mortality, and congenital abnormalities.

FAS has been recognized only in the last decade, although its effects are wide ranging and can be tragic. Evidence shows that about one third of children of alcoholic mothers will be born with the fetal alcohol syndrome, characterized by growth deficiencies, motor dysfunctions, cranial and cardiac deficiencies, and mental developmental delays or deficiencies. Why some children are affected and others are not is unclear. The teratogenic effects are related to the amount of alcohol consumed and the frequency of consumption, and nurses and pregnant women should understand that alcohol consumption even by nonalcoholics can have adverse effects. Smith (1982) estimates that an average of two drinks a day can affect birth weight and that four to six drinks a day can lead to physical defects and dysfunctions, with the full FAS likely at higher levels of consumption.

The fetal effects of cigarette smoking, caused by the increased level of carbon monoxide in the pregnant woman's blood, have also been recognized increasingly in recent years. Cigarette smoking has been shown to be associated with low-birth-weight infants and higher incidences of stillborn infants and neonatal deaths. Researchers continue to investigate a possible relationship between maternal smoking and a higher incidence of infant bronchitis and pneumonia in the first year. In addition, cigarette smoking has been shown to have an additive effect with the effects of alcohol.

Other drugs associated with congenital malformations include antidepressants, narcotics, and tranquilizers. These effects are generally greater when the drug is taken in the first trimester but are not limited to this period. Drug combinations may intensify the effects. For example, smoking more than triples the risk that tranquilizers will cause malformations.

Much more research is needed to investigate all the potential effects and risks of substances likely to be abused. In addition, more information is needed on the long-term neurological and behavioral effects in the child whose mother engaged in substance abuse during pregnancy. If the nursing history for a pregnant woman or a woman likely to become pregnant indicates the use of any drug or substance with potential fetal effects, the nurse should use teaching and counseling techniques to decrease the health risks, research the current literature on teratogenic effects or obtain a consultation, or make an appropriate referral.

Effects on the Family

The magnitude of the effect on the addict's family is severe. The spouse's response is often one of anger and resentment. As the consequences of substance abuse increase, the spouse may try to cover up to save face or to save the addict's job. The effects of substance abuse on the person's spouse involve all aspects of their relationship and life together. During a nursing history the spouse may mention such matters as sexual maladjustment, thoughts of separation or divorce, quarreling, economic difficulties, feelings of loneliness, confusion, or resentment about increased responsibilities in child rearing and other family roles. All these may be direct or indirect effects of the person's substance abuse, as usual roles and coping mechanisms break down with increasing psychological dependence.

Children who have grown up in alcoholic homes often have severe problems with trust, lack of self-esteem, and dependency. So many people have been affected that self-help groups have formed to assist members in dealing with these issues. These groups are generally associated with Al-Anon and are specified as meetings for adult children of alcoholics.

The effects of substance abuse by either or both parents on their children is often of particular importance to the nurse. The stresses of having an alcoholic parent in the home can have wide-range effects and lead to physical and emotional problems in the early developmental stages. Emotional neglect is the most common problem, and physical neglect may also occur. The child's self-concept may be seriously damaged because most children and adolescents do not understand the complex abuse problem but tend to blame themselves for the parent's emotional neglect. Family conflicts are more likely, and violence often erupts in the presence of children. Children in such families are also at a high risk for child abuse. Sexual child abuse, for example, is often related to alcoholism. Other effects include necessary role changes by the children, a lack of a good role model in the dependent parent, and alterations in the child's relationships with peers. In addition, children of substance abusers, particularly alcoholics, are at greater risk for later becoming substance abusers themselves.

NURSING PROCESS FOR THE CHEMICALLY DEPENDENT CLIENT

ASSESSMENT

Nurses care for clients who have both episodic and chronic use of alcohol or other addictive substances. Episodic care is likely to be acute, short-term intervention to manage a medical emergency, such as a car accident or drug overdose, whereas chronic abuse problems can result in any number of physical and psychological consequences.

The nurse assists clients and their families in primary, secondary, and tertiary care. Primary prevention includes providing accurate information to the health care system and communities regarding chemical dependency. Secondary care is provided when nurses serve as case finders in assisting parents, educators, and other health care professionals in identifying persons with ac-

tual or potential chemical abuse problems. Finally, nurses provide tertiary care to clients in chemical dependency treatment centers, as well as the care of clients in acute care hospitals, home care settings, clinics, and long-term care facilities who have other health care problems.

SCREENING FOR CHEMICAL DEPENDENCY

Identifying the chemically dependent client is the first and most important step in the nursing process. There are a number of assessment tools used to evaluate a client's problems with alcohol or drugs. Several have passed the test of rigorous research and have been found to be reliable and valid predictors of chemical abuse problems. Examples of these include the Michigan Alcoholism Screening Test (MAST) (Table 45-2) and, the Drug Abuse Screening Test (DAST) (see box).

The short MAST is an abbreviated version of the longer one and found to be as reliable. The DAST is similar to the MAST but asks questions about use of drugs other than alcohol. Although not all of these

---

Drug Abuse Screening Test (DAST)

1. Have you used drugs other than those required for medical reasons?
2. Have you abused prescription drugs?
3. Do you abuse more than one drug at a time?
4.* Can you get through the week without using drugs (other than those required for medical reasons)?
5.* Are you always able to stop using drugs when you want to?
6. Do you abuse drugs on a continuous basis?
7.* Do you try to limit your drug use to certain situations?
8. Have you had "blackouts" or "flashbacks" as a result of drug use?
9. Do you ever feel bad about your drug use?
10. Does your spouse (or parents) ever complain about your involvement with drugs?
11. Do your friends or relatives know or suspect you abuse drugs?
12. Has drug abuse ever created problems between you and your spouse?
13. Has any family member ever sought help for problems related to your drug use?
14. Have your ever lost friends because of your use of drugs?
15. Have you ever neglected your family or missed work because of your use of drugs?
16. Have you even been in trouble at work because of drug use?
17. Have you ever lost a job because of drug abuse?
18. Have you gotten into fights when under the influence of drugs?
19. Have you ever been arrested because of unusual behavior while under the influence of drugs?
20. Have you ever been arrested while driving while under the influence of drugs?
21. Have you engaged in illegal activities in order to obtain drugs?
22. Have you ever been arrested for possession of illegal drugs?
23. Have you ever experienced withdrawal symptoms as a result of heavy drug intake?
24. Have you had medical problems as a result of your drug use (e.g., memory loss, hepatitis, convulsions, bleeding, etc.)?
25. Have your ever gone to anyone for help for a drug problem?
26. Have you ever been in a hospital for medical problems related to your drug use?
27. Have you ever been involved in a treatment program specifically related to drug use?
28. Have you been treated as an out-patient for problems related to drug abuse?

Reprinted with permission from Addictive Behaviors 7(4):363, Skinner, HA, The drug abuse screening test, Copyright 1982, Pergamon Press.
*Items 4, 5, and 7 are scored in the "no" or false direction.

TABLE 45-2 Michigan Alcoholism Screening Test (MAST)

Points	Questions	Yes	No
	0. Do you enjoy a drink now and then?	__	__
2	*1. Do you feel you are a normal drinker? (By normal, we mean you drink less or as much as most other people.)	__	__
2	2. Have you ever awakened the morning after some drinking the night before and found that you could not remember a part of the evening?	__	__
1	3. Does your wife, husband, a parent, or other near relative ever worry or complain about your drinking?	__	__
2	*4. Can you stop drinking without a struggle after one or two drinks?	__	__
1	5. Do you ever feel guilty about your drinking?	__	__
2	*6. Do friend or relatives think you are a normal drinker?	__	__
2	*7. Are you able to stop drinking when you want to?	__	__
5	8. Have you ever attended a meeting of Alcoholics Anonymous (AA)?	__	__
1	9. Have you gotten into physical fights when drinking?	__	__
2	10. Has your drinking ever created problems between you and your wife, husband, a parent, or other relative?	__	__
2	11. Has your wife, husband, or other family members ever gone to anyone for help about your drinking?	__	__
2	12. Have you ever lost friends because of your drinking?	__	__
2	13. Have you ever gotten into trouble at work or school because of drinking?	__	__
2	14. Have you ever lost a job because of drinking?	__	__
2	15. Have you ever neglected your obligations, your family, or your work for two or more days in a row because you were drinking?	__	__
1	16. Do you drink before noon fairly often?	__	__
2	17. Have you ever been told you have liver trouble? Cirrhosis?	__	__
2	†18. After heavy drinking have you ever had delirium tremens (DTs) or severe shaking or heard voices or seen things that really weren't there?	__	__
5	19. Have you ever gone to anyone for help about your drinking?	__	__
5	20. Have you ever been in a hospital because of drinking?	__	__
2	21. Have you ever been a patient in a psychiatric hospital or on a psychiatric ward of a general hospital where drinking was part of the problem that resulted in hospitalization?	__	__
2	22. Have you ever been seen at a psychiatric or mental health clinic or gone to any doctor, social worker, or clergyman for help with any emotional problem, where drinking was part of the problem?	__	__
2	†23. Have you ever been arrested for drunk driving, driving while intoxicated, or drinking under the influence of alcoholic beverages? (IF YES, How many times? __)	__	__
2	‡24. Have you ever been arrested, or taken into custody, even for a few hours, because of other drunk behavior? (IF YES, How many times? __)	__	__

SCORING SYSTEM: In general, five points or more would place the subject in an "alcoholic" category. Four points would be suggestive of alcoholism, three points or less would indicate the subject was not alcoholic.

Programs using the above scoring system find it very sensitive at the five-point level, and it tends to find more people alcoholic than anticipated. However, it is a screening test and should be sensitive at its lower levels.

From The American Journal of Psychiatry, *3*:176. Copyright 1971, The American Psychiatric Association. Reprinted with permission.
*Alcoholic response is negative.
†5 points for Delirium Tremens.
‡2 point for *each* arrest.

TABLE 45-3 Summary of Behaviors Associated with Substance Abuse

Substance	Route*	Dependence Physical	Dependence Psychological	Expected Behaviors
Alcohol	Ingestion	Yes	Yes	Euphoria, followed by depression and sometimes hostility; decreased inhibitions; impaired judgment; incoordination; slurred speech
Opiates				
Heroin	Injection, ingestion, inhalation	Yes	Yes	Euphoria, relaxation, relief from pain, lack of concern, detachment from reality, drowsiness, constricted pupils, nausea, constipation, slurred speech, impaired judgment
Morphine	Injection	Yes	Yes	
Meperidine	Ingestion			
Codeine	Ingestion, injection	Yes	Yes	
Opium	Smoking, ingestion	Yes	Yes	
Methadone	Ingestion	Yes	Yes	Relieves craving for drugs without causing impaired functioning
Barbiturates	Ingestion, injection	Yes	Yes	Euphoria, followed by depression and sometimes hostility; decreased inhibitions; impaired judgment; slurred speech; incoordination; drowsiness
Amphetamines	Ingestion, injection	No	Yes	Euphoria, hyperactivity, irritability, hyperalertness, insomnia, anorexia, weight loss, tachycardia, hypertension
Cocaine	Inhalation, smoking, injection	No	Yes	Euphoria, elation, agitation, hyperactivity, irritability, grandiosity, pressured speech, tachycardia, hypertension, diaphoresis, anorexia, weight loss, insomnia
Hallucinogens (psychedelics)	Ingestion, smoking	No	No	Distorted perception, heightened sense of awareness, grandiosity, hallucinations, illusions, distortions of time and space, depersonalization, mystical experiences, dilated pupils, increased blood pressure, increased salivation
Phencyclidine (PCP)	Smoking, ingestion	No	No	Euphoria, perceptual distortion, agitation, violence, delusions, antisocial behavior, elevated blood pressure, increased salivation, diaphoresis, ataxia, nystagmus, decreased pain response
Marijuana	Smoking, ingestion	No	Yes	Relaxation, mild euphoria, loss of inhibition, decreased motivation, red eyes, dry mouth
Antianxiety drugs (benzodiazepines)	Ingestion, injection	Yes	Yes	Relaxation, increased self-confidence, relief of anxiety, drowsiness, ataxia, slurred speech, hypotension

From Stuart, GW, and Sundeen, SJ: Principles and practice of psychiatric nursing, ed 2, St. Louis, 1983, The C.V. Mosby Co.
*Most common listed first.

Behaviors Related to Overdose	Withdrawal Syndrome	Special Considerations
Unconsciousness, coma, respiratory depression, death	Tremors, hallucinosis, seizure disorder, delirium tremens (alcohol withdrawal delirium)	Chronic use leads to serious disruptions in most organ systems; malnutrition and dehydration are common; vitamin deficiency may lead to Wernicke's encephalopathy and alcoholic amnesic syndrome; alcohol dependent people are susceptible to other dependencies as well
Unconsciousness, coma, respiratory depression, circulatory depression, respiratory arrest, cardiac arrest, death	Watery eyes, dilated pupils, anxiety, abdominal cramps, piloerection, yawning, diaphoresis, rhinorrhea, achiness, anorexia, insomnia, fever, nausea, vomiting, diarrhea	Chronic use leads to lack of concern about physical well-being, resulting in malnutrition and dehydration; criminal behavior may take place to acquire money for drugs; injection sites may become infected; multiple drug use is common
Same	Same	
Respiratory depression, coma, death	Postural hypotension, tachycardia, fever, insomnia, tremors, agitation, anxiety; rapid withdrawal causes apprehension, weakness, tremors, postural hypotension, anorexia, grand mal seizures	Frequently used alternately with stimulants; combination with alcohol enhances effects and may lead to overdosage; paradoxical responses of hyperactivity may occur in children and the elderly
Restlessness, tremor, rapid respiration, confusion, assaultiveness, hallucinations, panic	Depression, fatigue	Prolonged use can result in psychotic behavior; a paradoxical depressant reaction occurs in children; frequently used alternately with depressant substances
Restlessness, tremor, rapid respiration, confusion, assaultiveness, hallucinations, panic	Depression, fatigue, anxiety	Psychotic behavior may occur following large doses; prolonged use by inhalation may result in destruction of the mucous membranes in the nose and deterioration of the nasal septum; use in combination with other substances is dangerous
Panic, psychosis	None	A "bad trip" may result in panic, unpredictable behavior, and psychotic behaviors; "flashbacks" may occur for several months after use; self-destructive behavior may occur while under the effect of the drug
Drowsiness, stupor, coma, grand mal seizures, death	None	Use may lead to psychotic behavior, irrationality, panic
Psychosis	None	Physiological consequences of use are under investigation
Drowsiness, confusion, hypotension, coma, death	Tremors, agitation, anxiety, grand mal seizures, abdominal cramps, vomiting, diaphoresis	Dependence may occur insidiously; users may underreport the actual amount taken because of guilt about multiple prescriptions and abuse

screening questionnaires need to be used at the same time, at least one alcoholism screening tool, and preferably the drug abuse screening tool, should be included as part of routine physical examinations in all health care settings.

INTERVIEWING THE CHEMICALLY DEPENDENT CLIENT

Because of the shame and embarrassment regarding chemical use, clients are often reluctant to reveal either the extent of their use or the consequences of it. The man who lost his job because of substance use at work may tell the nurse that he got laid off because of lack of business. It takes a great deal of skill for the nurse to be able to empathize enough with the client so that accurate information can be obtained without encouraging self-pity. It should be noted that it is very difficult to get completely accurate information from the client at this time because often the information is distorted. This is due to the course of the disease. Even skillful nurses sometimes have difficulty getting accurate data. Communication skills are included in nursing education programs at both the beginning and advanced levels. Work with chemically dependent clients requires advanced communications skills. The experienced nurse uses communication skills to interview the client and family to obtain substance abuse history data, thereby assisting in determining patterns of use.

Estes, Smith-DiJulio, and Heinemann (1980) have described four interviewing styles that can direct the interview process productively. With the *empathetic* style, the nurse demonstrates an acceptance and understanding of the client's problem, and the client may respond by speaking more freely about the problem. A *clarifying* style seeks to sort through the client's perception of problems with specific questions. It is particularly useful if the client is having difficulty focusing thoughts or if he or she is denying the extent of the problem. A style based on *giving advice*, although this may seem to move too rapidly to the intervention stage, is occasionally an effective interview approach because many substance abusers tend to look to outside sources for answers. If the client asks frequent questions during the interview process about how he or she might manage the problem, the nurse can incorporate general teaching principles to satisfy this need while continuing to gather assessment data. A fourth style is *confrontation*, in which the nurse confronts elements in the interview that are impeding effective interaction. The nurse may, for example, directly raise the question of the client's lack of motivation or involvement in the interview. This technique runs the risk of seeming to reject the client but is occasionally effective in breaking through relationship barriers.

During the interview and nursing history the nurse should also listen for any misconceptions the client may have about the substance itself or the nature of substance abuse. Later interventions may need to include teaching to provide accurate information so the client can participate more effectively in care. In addition, the nurse should pay attention to the client's nonverbal behaviors during the interview, which may reveal if the client feels threatened, defensive, or angry.

PHYSICAL AND BEHAVIORAL ASSESSMENT

Because of the variety of physiological and psychological effects of chronic substance abuse and the often subtle factors that create the potential for an abuse problem to develop, the nursing assessment should be thorough and explore the client's health status in all dimensions. The goals of the assessment are to determine if a substance abuse problem exists, to explore causative factors and effects in all areas of the client's life, to assess the psychological, behavioral, and physiological impact of the abused substance, and to assess the extent of

---

Examples of Nursing Diagnoses for Substance Abuse

NANDA-APPROVED NURSING DIAGNOSES

Altered thought processes: disorientation related to:
- Drug use
- Alcohol ingestion

Altered nutrition: less than body requirements related to:
- Drinking patterns
- Use of financial resources to purchase alcohol or drugs
- Effects of drugs

Bathing/hygiene self-care deficit related to:
- Intoxication
- Decreased level of consciousness
- Decreased level of awareness
- Decreased self-image

Sleep pattern disturbance related to:
- Substance withdrawal
- Alcohol use
- Nightmares

Ineffective individual coping related to:
- Denial of substance of use or abuse
- Lack of support system
- Fear, anxiety

Ineffective family coping: compromised or *disabled* related to:
- Withdrawal
- Inadequate finances
- Hostility, anger
- Lack of trust

Spiritual distress related to:
- Value conflict
- Perception of punishment by Supreme Being

physiological or psychological dependence. Assessment includes the observation of the client's behaviors that may indicate substance abuse, the interview and nursing history, and the physical examination.

A person under the influence of a drug generally manifests a set of behaviors as a result of the drug's psychological and physiological effects. Table 45-3 (p. 1334) summarizes the behaviors associated with substance abuse and typical behaviors during withdrawal. Observing such behaviors in a client, even when the nurse does not otherwise suspect an abuse problem, should prompt further assessment using interview techniques.

NURSING DIAGNOSIS

The assessment of the chemically dependent client will reveal clusters of data that indicate a variety of problems affecting all areas of the client's life. Many of the nursing diagnoses for chemically dependent clients are closely related to medical diagnoses. The medical diagnoses of chemical dependency are listed and explained in the *Diagnostic and Statistical Manual of Mental Disorders* (DSM III-R).

Because chemically dependent people have so many associated physical, psychological, and social problems,

multiple nursing diagnostic categories are appropriate (see nursing diagnoses box). When developing the nursing diagnostic label, the nurse must be sure that the necessary defining characteristics are present in the client's assessment data base. This ensures an accurate, individualized diagnosis, which is suited to the client's needs. The sample nursing diagnoses box lists examples of nursing diagnoses for clients with substance abuse.

PLANNING

After identifying each nursing diagnosis the nurse develops a plan of care for the chemically dependent client (see care plan box). Nursing is one discipline in the multidisciplinary team used to treat a client with a chemical dependency. Nursing care primarily involves caring for the client's physical health problems, supporting the client and family, and education of the client and family. The goals of care are multiple and include all the client's dimensions. The following are some examples of the goals developed in the planning stage:

1. Cessation of substance use
2. Use of stress management techniques
3. Regaining or returning to ideal body weight
4. Balanced nutritional status
5. Beginning return to normal family dynamics

Sample Nursing Diagnoses for Substance Abuse

Defining Characteristics	Nursing Diagnoses	Related Factors
Disoriented to name, place, time, and self Unable to find way around in familiar environment Sentences incomplete; rambling vocalizations	Altered thought processes: disorientation	▪ Oversedation ▪ Drug use ▪ Drug abuse ▪ Alcoholism
Sleep at inappropriate times Easy arousal Frequent awakening Irritability Difficulty falling asleep Verbalized fatique regardless of sleep patterns	Sleep pattern disturbance: deprivation	▪ Anxiety ▪ Chemical substance use ▪ Withdrawal from chemical substances
Absence of family support Lack of communication Verbalization of dysfunctional family system	Ineffective family coping	▪ Scapegoating ▪ Other family members' drug abuse ▪ Lack of trust ▪ Mood swings ▪ Denial ▪ Impaired communication ▪ Hostility

Sample Nursing Care Plan for Substance Abuse			
Nursing Diagnosis	**Goals**	**Expected Outcomes**	**Nursing Interventions**
Altered nutrition: less than body requirements related to drug abuse	Client regains or returns to ideal body weight.	Client has weekly weight gain of 1 to 2 pounds.	Offer six small meals daily inclusive of client food preferences.
	Client achieves balanced nutritional status.	24-hour diet history shows improving intake and improving nutritional status.	Provide opportunity to prepare food.
			Teach client how to select proper and economical foods.
			Have client plan a menu.

Priorities are set for the goals according to individualized client needs. The withdrawal syndrome of some drugs may be physiologically life threatening, or depression or anxiety may potentially lead to life-threatening behaviors. In some cases emotional support to meet the client's safety and security needs may be as critical as interventions directed toward physiological needs. Modification of goals is an ongoing process when providing care.

IMPLEMENTATION

Treatment for chemical dependency usually takes place in a unit or free-standing treatment center designated for treatment of the disease. Based on the principles of Alcoholics Anonymous (AA), treatment helps the client recognize the disease and how it has affected their lives, teaches them about chemical dependency, and gives them tools for changing their behavior. Treatment is only the beginning of a continuous, lifelong recovery.

An initial intensive phase (inpatient or outpatient) is usually followed by a long-term outpatient follow-up (from 1 to 2 years). Attendance at self-help groups such as AA or Narcotics Anonymous (NA) is usually expected. This approach is supported by those who believe that chemical dependency is a primary disease, that genetics and environment play a role in causing it, and that persons can recover by changing their behavior, including abstaining from use of all mood-altering chemicals.

Those who belive that alcohol or drug use is secondary to other psychological problems or that chemical abuse problems are learned behaviors advocate different treatment. This treatment is based on teaching the person different learned behaviors. This group believes that controlled drinking can be learned if the alcoholic has not developed serious physical problems as a result of drinking.

DETOXIFICATION

Alcohol or other drug withdrawal is a serious and potentially fatal complication of acute intoxication. Detoxification means the removal of mood-altering chemicals from the person's body. Too rapid removal results in seizures, delirium tremens (DTs), and sometimes death. Thus most clients are gradually withdrawn from chemicals, particularly alcohol. The client is kept quiet, stimuli are reduced, and sedative and anticonvulsant medications are given as needed. Good nutrition and fluid balance help the process go smoother.

Detoxification is the first step in treating the chemically dependent client. The client must be free of the immediate effects of chemicals to begin the treatment process. Following initial detoxification, which usually lasts a few days unless serious withdrawal symptoms are expected, other health care professionals become involved in the assessment of the client and the family and begin to plan and implement care. The nurse continues to manage the client's physical health and to participate in other therapeutic activities, depending on the specific agency's policies.

ACUTE CARE INTERVENTIONS

Acute care interventions, which depend on the client's current health status and on the body systems affected by the substance, often involve medical interventions, physiological supportive measures, and a variety of nursing interventions. Emergency therapies may be required in cases of alcoholic coma caused by acute intoxication, hepatic coma related to liver malfunctioning, or trauma caused by falls or accidents while under a drug's effects. Emergency treatments may include the administration of narcotic antagonists for opiate overdose, safety measures in cases of acute toxic psychosis, treatment for respiratory or cardiac depression, or treatment for withdrawal syndromes. In most cases the specific substance that resulted in the acute condition must first be identified, followed by a physical assessment and appropriate diagnostic tests.

In acute situations, nursing and medical care generally focuses on physiological problems. As the initial crisis passes, interventions continue to address physiological problems but increasingly include interventions for the client's psychosocial needs, as described in the following sections.

INTERVENTIONS FOR ABUSIVE BEHAVIORS

When a client enters a health care facility in an intoxicated or drugged state, the nurse often falls victim to the client's verbal abuse and attempts at manipulation. The client should not be held responsible for his behavior, since the substance's effects often cause paranoia, fear, and anger. The verbal attacks on a nurse may simply be a client's expression of self-hatred related to the substance abuse. The challenge nurses face in such circumstances is to keep themselves and their clients in an emotional balance. Too often nurses react to the client's abuses and become angry and resentful. Eventually the nurse's interventions become ineffective because of an inability to provide care with understanding and compassion.

When a client makes critical remarks about the nurse's personality or appearance, such as height, weight, or other distinguishing characteristic, the nurse should not become upset. The client may needle or insult the nurse in an attempt to arouse the nurse's anger, pity, or fear. If the nurse reacts emotionally, the client's verbal attacks are likely to continue. A neutral response by the nurse discourages the client from continuing such manipulative efforts. If the client makes a sexual advance toward the nurse, it is better for the nurse to ignore it and instead direct the client's attention to the present situation, including the reason why he is in the nursing unit or the type of care he will receive. The nurse must have a high level of self-esteem in such cases to be able to ignore the client's physical, mental, or emotional harassment.

It is important also for the nurse to take time out occasionally from caring for abusive clients. A coffee or lunch break helps relieve developing emotional tension. The nurse must remember that the client's abusiveness is the result of intoxication and illness, not the client's personality.

SUPPORT SYSTEMS

Support from family members, friends, and others is often valuable in assisting a person with a substance abuse problem. Such support can be important at any stage, from accepting the problem to learning to live with new coping mechanisms after successful rehabilitation. Helping the client to build a social support system may include family counseling, referral to a self-help group, and other interventions such as those for altered self-concept (see Chapter 29) that can assist the client in adapting positively to interactions with others.

FAMILY INTERVENTIONS

Earlier sections have discussed the potential effects of substance abuse on other family members. Nursing interventions may be required for individual members or for the family as a whole. Family functioning is also affected by the adjustment process of a parent's or spouse's withdrawal or rehabilitation. Because any kind of family health problem may be precipitated or heightened by substance abuse, the nurse assesses and may intervene in substance abuse–related family problems much as with the similar problems in families without substance abuse problems. Interventions for family members include teaching and counseling, values clarification about substance abuse, stress management techniques, interventions adapted to the developmental needs of children, development of support systems, and referral to agencies or self-help groups specializing in family programs.

TEACHING AND COUNSELING

Often a primary nursing role is to provide information about the potential physiological and psychological effects of substance abuse and the effects of withdrawal for the substance-dependent client. Such information should stress positive aspects rather than attempt to frighten the client into changing abuse habits. Portraying in grisly terms the physiological condition of lung cancer, for example, will likely cause stress for the chronic cigarette smoker that may increase rather than decrease the person's desire to smoke. Instead, the nurse can provide information about the success rate of an available treatment program. Other teaching activities include stress management techniques and self-care activities for hygiene, nutrition, and other areas affected by the substance abuse.

Counseling clients with a substance abuse problem often requires specialized experience and skills related to the particular substance. A referral to a qualified health professional is generally appropriate, although the nurse may continue to provide other kinds of care for the client and may engage in counseling activities concurrently. Counseling often follows a pattern based on the extent of the client's problem. The goals of counseling, for example, may be first to assist the client in recognizing and accepting the problem, then in adapting to stresses and other problems associated with the abuse or withdrawal (the client's family may be counseled in this regard), and finally in adapting to a nondependent life-style following successful withdrawal.

COMMUNITY PROGRAMS

In many communities, there are a range of substance withdrawal and other therapy programs to which the nurse can refer the client. AA is a self-help group that assists alcoholics through mutual support to acknowledge the problem and work toward solving it. Similar support groups are Al-Anon, an organization for spouses and relatives of alcoholics, and Alateen, for children and adolescents who have an alcoholic parent. In addition, many inpatient or outpatient alcoholism clinics offer treatment programs independently or in association with hospitals or community mental health centers. As with alcoholism, specialized drug treatment programs offer counseling, health education, and medical services such as methadone maintenance or withdrawal programs for narcotic abusers. Other types of community resources include employee programs within businesses and industries and programs provided by student health clinics in colleges and other schools.

Substance abuse prevention programs are becoming more prominent in community health settings such as schools and mental health clinics. The primary focus of preventive programs is to provide drug education, strengthen family functioning, improve social conditions, and assist individuals in the areas of interpersonal skills and self-esteem. Such a focus helps minimize or eliminate factors that may lead to the abuse of substances as a coping or escape mechanism. On the individual level the nurse can also initiate preventive interventions, such as educating the client about drugs, promoting effective coping mechanisms, and providing support.

EVALUATION

Evaluation of nursing care for clients with substance abuse problems is based on goals of care and expected outcomes (see evaluation box). The evaluation process, like the setting of goals, must be realistic and avoid unreasonable hopes, such as expecting a psychologically dependent client to achieve abstinence overnight. Often a more important criterion is that the client make significant progress toward long-term goals. Other evaluation criteria typically include gaining increased self-esteem, learning to use more effective coping mechanisms and internal resources when confronted by stress, and forming behavioral patterns and activities that replace substance-related behaviors.

The client must be involved in evaluation. Even if the nurse evaluates the client's progress as satisfactory, the client may return to former habits if he has unrealistically high personal goals and thus views his progress with frustration. By involving the client and family in evaluation, the nurse can provide further support, reinforcement, and reassurance. Evaluation may also reveal the need for changes in the nursing care plan.

Sample Evaluation of Interventions for Substance Abuse

Goals	Evaluative Measures	Expected Outcomes
Client ceases substance use.	Observe client for signs of substance use. Obtain urine specimens.	Symptoms of substance use absent. Urine tests are negative for chemicals.
Client uses stress management techniques.	Observe client for signs of stress. Ask client about techniques used for stress mediation.	Signs of stress are absent. Client reports using stress mediation techniques.
Ideal body weight is achieved.	Weigh client weekly.	Client has steady weight gain, and no weight loss
Client achieves a balanced nutritional status.	Observe client's food intake patterns. Ask client about nutritional value of selected foods.	Client improves type and quality of food selected. Client correctly states nutritional value of selected food.
Client begins to return to normal family dynamics.	Observe family interaction. Ask family members about family activities.	There is observable improvement in family interaction. Client reports improvement in family's interactions.

SUMMARY

Substance abuse takes a variety of forms and may be encountered by the nurse in any setting. Because substance abuse affects the client in all dimensions, the nurse should be alert to both actual and potential health problems associated with abuse patterns. Although any person at any age and in any life situation may become physiologically or psychologically dependent on a drug or substance, including nurses and other health professionals, certain groups may be more susceptible to the problem of abuse at certain developmental stages. The client's family may also be affected in a variety of ways, and the nurse should include the family in the total plan of care.

The nurse's choice of the appropriate interventions for the client with a substance abuse problem depends on both the causative variables and the client's individual health status. Because society is increasingly aware of substance abuse as a health problem, it carries less stigma than in the past, and individuals with abuse problems are now more likely to seek help before physiological problems bring them to the attention of health care professionals. With increasing societal recognition of the problem has come a wider variety of support and treatment services, including prevention programs. Substance abuse remains a sensitive area for many clients, however, and the nurse needs to be particularly aware of communication skills and other aspects of the nurse-client relationship when providing care to clients experiencing the wide range of psychosocial stresses commonly associated with substance abuse.

KEY CONCEPTS

✓ Chemical dependency is a major health care problem in the world today.

✓ There are many myths surrounding chemical dependency.

✓ Any substance that produces physiological or psychological effects can potentially be misused or abused.

✓ Substance abuse is the indiscriminate, usually chronic abuse of a substance to the extent that the person's physiological and psychosocial functioning is impaired.

✓ The major groups of abused drugs include alcohol, narcotics, sedative-hypnotics, tranquilizers, central nervous system sympathomimetics, hallucinogens, inhalants, and nonprescription substances, each of which produces distinct psychological and physiological effects.

✓ The cause of chemical dependency is not known but heredity has been found to be a predisposing factor.

✓ Substance abusers are more likely to experience health problems as a result of drug interactions.

✓ Many psychosocial variables have a causative role in substance abuse, including pleasure-seeking and problem-solving or avoidance behaviors, personality factors, sociocultural factors, and stressors.

✓ No one cause or set of causes affects all or most persons who abuse a substance.

✓ To facilitate the therapeutic relationship and work toward solving the problems of substance abuse, both the client and the nurse should be aware of their attitudes toward the abused substance and the causes of the abuse.

✓ The course of substance abuse varies but typically progresses from social misuse or experimentation through a gradually increasing pattern of abuse to a state of dependence in which all aspects of the person's life are affected.

✓ Substance abuse affects family functioning, roles, and responsibilities, often with seriously detrimental psychosocial effects on spouse and children.

✓ Causative variables in substance abuse vary among developmental stages, as do the effects of the abuse, and therefore a developmental perspective should be included when the client's abuse problem is assessed.

✓ The fetus is susceptible to the effects of substance abuse by the mother.

✓ Certain patterns of substance abuse are more common in particular groups sharing common stresses.

✓ Nurses and other health professionals are highly susceptible to abuse problems and need to be aware of how such problems can develop and what interventions may be necessary.

✓ The assessment of a client with a substance abuse problem may include a tactfully obtained history, observation of behaviors linked to substance abuse, and a complete psychosocial and physical assessment.

✓ Nursing diagnoses for clients with abuse problems identify needs for physiological support as well as problems involving stress, interpersonal conflicts, altered work or family roles, and self-concept deficits.

✓ Intervention and treatment provide an opportunity for the chemically dependent person to alter behavior regarding use of chemicals, as well as begin life-style changes.

✓ Interventions may address the client's needs in all dimensions and may include acute care, teaching and counseling, support systems, family interventions, and the use of community resources.

✓ Evaluation of the care of substance abusers should be based on realistic goals and often focuses on day-to-day progress toward long-term goals rather than on the expectation that the client will immediately overcome the problems associated with abuse.

REFERENCES

American Nurses' Association: Addictions and psychological dysfunctions in nursing: the profession's response to the problem, Kansas City, Mo., 1984, The Association.

American Psychiatric Association: Diagnostic and statistical manual of mental disorders (DSM III-R), Washington, D.C., 1987, The Association.

Begleiter, H, et al.: Event-related brain potentials in boys at risk for alcoholism, Science 225:1493, 1984.

Bissell, L, and Haberman, PW: Alcoholism in the professions, New York, 1984, Oxford University Press.

Estes, NJ, Smith-DiJulio, K, and Heinemann, ME, editors: Nursing diagnosis of the alcoholic person, St. Louis, 1980, The C.V. Mosby Co.

Goodwin, DW, et al.: Alcohol problems in adoptees raised apart from alcoholic biological parents, Arch Gen Psy 31:238, 1973.

Goodwin, DW, et al.: Drinking problems in adopted and nonadopted sons of alcoholics, Arch Gen Psy 31:164, 1974.

Hahn, AB, Barkin, RL, and Oestreich, SJK: Pharmacology in nursing, ed. 16, St. Louis, 1986, The C.V. Mosby Co.

Kaij, L: Alcoholism in twins, Stockholm, 1960, Almqvist & Wiksell, Publishers.

Morrissey, ER, and Schuckit, MA: Stressful life events and alcohol problems among women seen at a detoxification center, J Stud Alcohol 39(6):1559, 1978.

Smith, JW: Fetal alcohol syndrome: a tragic and preventable disorder. In Estes, NJ, and Heinemann, ME, editors: Alcoholism: development consequences, and interventions, ed. 2, St. Louis, 1982, The C.V. Mosby Co.

Sullivan, EJ: Cost savings of retaining chemically dependent nurses, Nurs Econ 4(4):179, 1987.

Sullivan, EJ, Bissell, L, and Williams, E: Chemical dependency in nursing: the deadly diversion, Menlo Park, Calif., 1988, Addison-Wesley Publishing Co., Inc.

ADDITIONAL READINGS

Cody, B: Alcohol and other drug abuse among adolescents, Stat Bull Metropol Life Insur Co 65(1):4, 1984.

Dusek, D, and Girdano, DA: Drugs: a factual account, Reading, Mass., 1980, Addison-Wesley Publishing Co., Inc.

Estes, NJ, and Heinemann, ME: Alcoholism: development, consequences, and interventions, ed. 3, St. Louis, 1986, The C.V. Mosby Co.

Freedman, AM: Opiate dependence. In Kaplan, HI, Freedman, AM, and Sadock, BJ: Comprehensive textbook of psychiatry, ed. 3, Baltimore, 1980, The Williams & Wilkins Co.

Greene, MH, et al.: Evolving patterns of drug abuse, Ann Intern Med 83:402, 1975.

Hughes, R, and Brewin, R: The tranquilizing of America: pill popping and the American way of life, New York, 1979, Harcourt Brace Jovanovich, Inc.

Isler, C: The alcoholic nurse: what we try to deny, RN 41:48, 1978.

Lawrence, F, et al.: Admitting an intoxicated patient, Am J Nurs 84(5):617, 1984.

Ray, O: Drugs, society, and human behavior, ed. 4, St. Louis, 1987, The C.V. Mosby Co.

Sullivan, EJ: A descriptive study of 139 recovering chemically dependent nurses, Arch Psy Nurs 1(3):1984, 1987.

Sullivan, EJ: Comparison of chemically dependent and nondependent nurses on familial, personal, and professional characteristics, J Stud Alcohol 48(6):563, 1987.

Yowell, S, and Brose, C: Working with drug abuse patients in the ER, Am J Nurs 77:82, 1977.

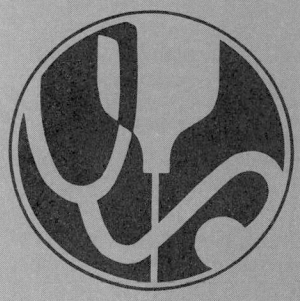

UNIT 9

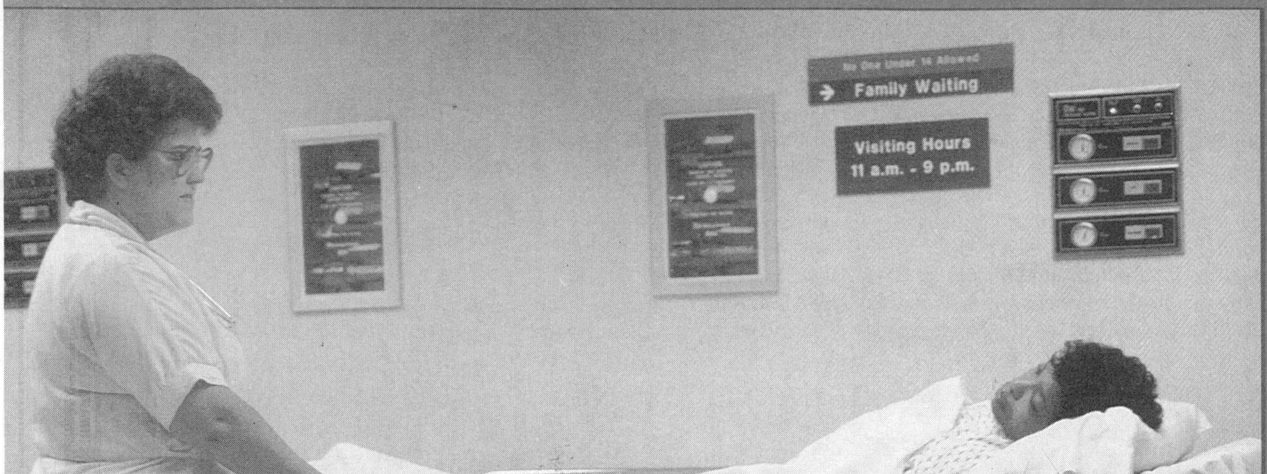

Caring for the Perioperative Client

In hospitals, clinics, and other health care settings, nurses provide care for clients before and after surgical procedures. Special skills are required for the care of these clients, as well as preparatory teaching activities. Because the anticipation of surgery creates emotional stresses for many clients and families, the nurse also provides care to promote successful coping with these stresses and to help clients and families adapt to changes after surgery during the recovery and rehabilitation stages. Specific nursing skills are also required to care for the surgical wound, thus this unit includes a chapter on wound healing in which nursing care for other types of wounds is also discussed.

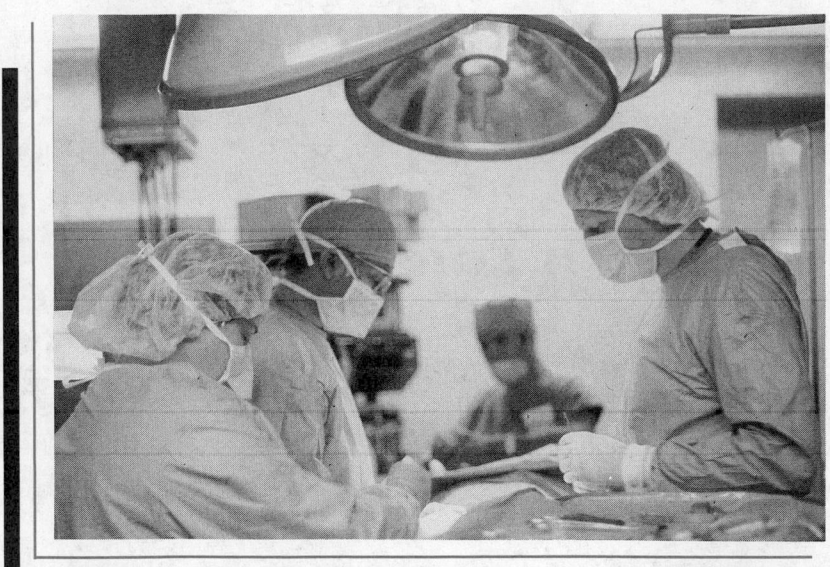

OBJECTIVES

Mastery of content in this chapter will enable the student to:

- Define the key terms listed.
- Explain the concept of perioperative nursing care.
- Differentiate between classifications of surgery.
- List factors to include in the preoperative assessment of a surgical client.
- Properly witness a client's informed consent for surgery.
- Demonstrate postoperative exercises: diaphragmatic breathing, coughing , turning, leg exercises.
- Design a preoperative teaching program.
- Prepare a client for surgery on the morning of a scheduled operation.
- Compare and contrast the actions and side effects of general, regional, and local anesthesia.
- Explain the nurse's role in the operating room.
- Describe the nurse's role in phase I and II recovery.
- Identify factors to include in the postoperative assessment of a client in recovery.
- Describe the rationale for nursing interventions designed to prevent postoperative complications.
- Explain the difference and similarities in caring for outpatient versus inpatient surgical clients.

KEY TERMS

Ambulatory Surgery

Anesthesia

Autopsy

Cholecystectomy

Convalescence

Dehiscence

Depilatory

Embolus

Evisceration

Excise

Gangrene

Induction of Anesthesia

Intraoperative

Intubation

Local Anesthesia

Necrotic

Petechiae

Postoperative

Recovery Room

Regional Anesthesia

Serosanguineous

Suture

Vascularization

Venous Stasis

The Surgical Client

A client faces a variety of stressors when confronting surgery. Anticipating surgery leads to fear and anxiety since it is often associated with pain, possible disfigurement, dependence, and perhaps even loss of life. Family members often fear a disruption in life-style and experience a sense of powerlessness as the client's surgery approaches. The trauma a client sustains during an operation creates physical needs requiring close supervision and skilled intervention by the nurse and physician. The client is better able to cooperate and participate in the care plan if the nurse has provided information about events occurring before and after surgery.

Many surgical procedures are performed in hospitals. However, ambulatory out-patient surgical units are increasingly common. A client enters the unit, undergoes surgery, and returns home the same day. Nurses working in many settings must understand the principles of caring for surgical clients.

HISTORY OF SURGICAL NURSING

In the mid-nineteenth century, surgery became a medical specialty. Surgery gave physicians the means to treat conditions that were difficult or impossible to manage only by pure medicine. However, early surgeons had little knowledge of the principles of asepsis, and anesthesia techniques were primitive and unsafe. Nurses working in the first operating rooms cleaned the rooms and equipment, performed such technical tasks as obtaining supplies, and occasionally accompanied the client to the surgical ward to deliver nursing care.

With the advent of antiseptic and later aseptic practices, surgery became a treatment of choice for many conditions. The development of safer anesthetic gases allowed surgeons to conduct longer operative procedures. All surgery was conducted in hospital settings. Operating room nurses required special training for new responsibilities (for example, assisting the surgeon during surgery, preparing sterile equipment, and caring for the surgical client). Massachusetts General Hospital provided the first operating room education for nurses in 1876 (Metzger, 1976). This trend continued into the 1900s as nursing schools included operating room experience in each nurse's clinical instruction.

In 1956 the Association of Operating Room Nurses (AORN) was formed to gain knowledge and explore methods to improve nursing care of surgical clients. The association met many challenges, including overcoming the idea that operating room nurses were only technically skilled practitioners. The organization developed standards of nursing practice in the operating room to establish the need for registered nurses in the operating room.

During the 1970s a change occurred in nursing education. A focus on the importance of nurses' acquiring a broad knowledge resulted in less emphasis on operating room techniques. Many schools eliminated operating room experience from curriculums. As a result, nurses missed practicing strict aseptic techniques and observing the delicate anatomy of the human body.

Today many nursing schools have reinstituted clinical operating room experience. There has also been a new development in the setting for operative procedures. Ambulatory surgery, sometimes referred to as outpatient surgery or one-day surgery, is a health care service that is growing rapidly in numbers and types of procedures performed. Ambulatory surgery can be defined as scheduled surgical procedures provided for clients who do not remain overnight in a hospital. Small biopsies, cosmetic surgery, tubal ligations, and cataract extractions are just a few examples.

Discovery of anesthetic drugs that metabolize rapidly with few after effects allowed shorter operative times. Surgeons recognized the benefit of early postoperative ambulation and encouraged clients to assume a more active role in recovery. Ambulatory surgery also offers cost savings by eliminating the need for hospital stays. Many ambulatory surgical settings have emerged over the past 10 years, but there are the following four basic types:
1. *Hospital based*—outpatient procedures are done in main operating room suites, along with inpatient procedures.
2. *Hospital affiliated*—a separate, self-contained area that is in or next to an inpatient facility.
3. *Hospital satellite*—a unit that is owned by a hospital, but is physically separated from it.

4. *Private or free-standing*—owned and operated by surgeons or private investors.

In addition to traditional inpatient surgical stays that may last several days, and outpatient ambulatory surgery, most hospitals have same day surgical programs. In a same day surgical program a client is admitted early on the morning of surgery and stays one or more nights during recovery.

Ambulatory and same-day surgical programs provide challenges for surgical nurses. Before surgery, nurses must find creative ways to educate clients and family members. The preparation time before surgery is shortened, so nurses must perform complete assessments efficiently. The surgical procedures that clients in ambulatory surgery undergo also require special considerations by the nurse. Changing trends in care of surgical clients has changed the nurse's role.

PERIOPERATIVE NURSING CARE

Perioperative nursing refers to the role of the operating room nurse during the preoperative, intraoperative, and postoperative phases of surgery. Perioperative nursing stresses the importance of providing continuity of care. In many hospitals, operating room nurses assess a client's health status preoperatively, identify specific needs, teach and counsel, attend to the client's needs in the operating room, and then follow recovery. However, in other institutions different nurses care for the surgical client during each phase of the surgical experience. Involving the operating room nurse in each phase of the client's care provides a smooth course for therapy. The nurse's major responsibility in whatever role, is to provide safe, consistent, and effective nursing care during each phase of surgery.

CLASSIFICATION OF SURGERY

Classification for types of surgical procedures relates to the seriousness, urgency, or purpose of surgery (Table 46-1). A procedure may fall into more than one classification. For example, surgical removal of a disfiguring scar is minor in seriousness, elective in urgency, and reconstructive in purpose. Frequently, the classes overlap. A procedure that is urgent is also considered major in seriousness. The same operation may be performed for different reasons on different clients. For example, a gastrectomy may be performed as an emergency procedure to resect a bleeding ulcer or as an urgent procedure to remove a cancerous growth. The classification indicates to the nurse the level of care a client might require.

TABLE 46-1 Classification for Surgical Procedures

Classification	Type	Description	Example
Seriousness	Major	Involves extensive reconstruction or alteration in body parts; poses great risks to a client's well-being	Coronary artery bypass, colon resection, laryngectomy, mastectomy
	Minor	Involves minimal alteration in body parts; often designed to correct deformities; physical risks minimal compared with major procedures	Cataract extraction, facial plastic surgery, skin graft, tooth extraction, arthrotomy
Urgency	Elective	Performed on the basis of a client's choice; is not essential and may not be necessary for physical health	Bunionectomy, facial plastic surgery, hernia repair, breast reconstruction
	Urgent	Necessary for the client's health; may prevent additional problems from developing, (for example, tissue destruction or impaired organ function); not necessarily an emergency	Excision of cancerous tumor, removal of gallbladder for stones, vascular repair for obstructed artery (for example, coronary artery bypass)
	Emergency	Must be done immediately to save life or preserve function of a body part	Repair of perforated appendix, repair of traumatic amputation, control of internal hemorrhaging
Purpose	Diagnostic	Surgical exploration that allows a physician to confirm a diagnosis; may involve removal of tissue for further diagnostic testing	Exploratory laparotomy (incision into peritoneal cavity to inspect abdominal organs), breast mass biopsy
	Ablative	Excision or removal of a diseased body part	Amputation, appendectomy, cholecystectomy
	Palliative	Designed to relieve or reduce intensity of disease symptoms; will not produce a cure	Colostomy, debridement of necrotic tissue, resection of nerve roots
	Reconstructive	Restores function or appearance to traumatized or malfunctioning tissues	Internal fixation of fractures, scar revision
	Transplant	Performed to replace malfunctioning organs or structures	Kidney, cornea, or liver transplant, total hip replacement
	Constructive	Restores function lost or reduced as a result of congenital anomalies	Repair of cleft palate, closure of atrial septal defect in the heart

PREOPERATIVE SURGICAL PHASE

Surgical clients enter the health care setting in different stages of health. A client may enter the hospital or ambulatory satellite unit on a predetermined day feeling relatively healthy and prepared to face elective surgery. In contrast, a victim of a vehicle accident may face emergency surgery with no time to prepare.

The surgical client undergoes tests and procedures to confirm or rule out alterations requiring surgery. Many can be performed in the physician's office or an outpatient laboratory, preventing the need for hospitalization before surgery. Usually clients scheduled for ambulatory surgery have tests done several days in advance of surgery. However, the tests can also be done the morning of surgery.

Once it is clear that surgery is necessary, the client meets many health care personnel, including surgeons, nurse anesthetists or anesthesiologists, therapists, and nurses. All play a role in the client's care and recovery. Family members attempt to provide support through their presence, yet face many of the same stressors as the client.

The nurse's role in the preoperative surgical phase is to assess the client's physical and emotional well-being, recognize the degree of surgical risk, coordinate diagnostic tests, identify nursing diagnoses reflecting the client's and family members' needs, prepare the client physically and mentally for surgery, and communicate pertinent information to the surgical team.

ASSESSMENT

The nurse's assessment of the surgical client involves collecting a nursing history, performing a physical ex-

TABLE 46-2 Medical Conditions That Increase the Risks of Surgery

Type of Condition	Reason for Risk
Bleeding disorders (thrombocytopenia, leukemia, hemophilia, bone marrow depression following use of chemotherapeutic drugs)	Increases risk of hemorrhaging during and after surgery
Diabetes mellitus	Impairs wound healing and increases risk of infection from altered glucose metabolism and associated circulatory impairment; blood sugar levels may cause CNS malfunction during anesthesia
Heart disease (recent myocardial infarction, dysrhythmias, congestive heart failure)	Stress of surgery causing increased demands on myocardium to maintain cardiac output; general anesthetic agents that depress cardiac function
Upper respiratory infection	Increases risk of respiratory complications during anesthesia (for example, pneumonia and spasm of the laryngeal muscles)
Liver disease	Alters metabolism and elimination of drugs administered during surgery; impairs wound healing because of alterations in protein metabolism
Fever	Predisposes client to fluid and electrolyte imbalances; may indicate underlying infection
Chronic respiratory disease (emphysema, bronchitis, asthma)	Reduces client's means to compensate for acid-base alterations (see Chapter 37); anesthetic agents reduce respiratory function, increasing risk for severe hypoventilation.

amination, reviewing the client's and family members' emotional health, and analyzing risk factors and diagnostic data. The length of the preoperative period will determine how thorough the nurse's assessment will be.

For example, if a client is a same-day admission, it may be difficult to do a comprehensive physical examination. In this case, the nurse focuses on key measurements for all body systems, to ensure that no obvious problems are overlooked. Even though the physician will have screened the client before scheduling surgery, preoperative assessment occasionally reveals an abnormality that delays or cancels surgery. Usually, however, the assessment establishes what is normal for the client and alerts the nurse to possible postoperative complication.

NURSING HISTORY

The nurse conducts an initial interview to collect a history similar to that described in Chapter 6. In the ambulatory surgical setting the history may be shorter than what is collected when the client is hospitalized the evening before surgery. If a client is unable to relate all necessary information, the nurse may interview family members.

MEDICAL HISTORY. A review of the client's medical history should include past illnesses and the primary reason for seeking medical care. One valuable source of data is medical records from past hospitalizations. When the nurse first assesses the client, the reasons for surgery

may be unclear or it may not yet be known if surgery will be required. Preexisting illnesses can influence the client's ability to tolerate surgery and reach full recovery (Table 46-2). Candidates for ambulatory surgery must be carefully screened to minimize the risk for complications during or after surgery. They should be healthy with no anesthesia or major medical risks.

PREVIOUS SURGERIES. A client's past experience with surgery can significantly influence both physical and psychological responses to a procedure. The type of previous surgery, level of discomfort, extent of disability, and overall level of care provided are some factors the client may recall. The nurse determines the client's unpleasant experiences and if complications developed. This helps the nurse anticipate the client's needs preoperatively and postoperatively.

Previous surgery may also influence the level of physical care required after a surgical procedure. For example, a client who has had a thoracotomy for resection of a lung lobe is at a greater risk for postoperative pulmonary complications than one with normal lungs.

CLIENTS' AND FAMILY MEMBERS' PERCEPTIONS AND UNDERSTANDING OF SURGERY. The nurse must prepare clients and their families for the surgical experience. Identification of the client's knowledge, expectations, and perceptions allows the nurse to plan teaching and emotional preparation measures. If a client

TABLE 46-3 Drugs with Special Implications for the Surgical Client

Drug Class	Effects during Surgery
Antibiotics	Potentiate action of anesthetic agents; if taken within 2 weeks preoperatively, aminoglycosides (gentamicin, tobramycin, neomycin) may cause mild respiratory depression from depressed neuromuscular transmission
Antidysrhythmics	Have potential for reducing cardiac contractility and impairing conduction during anesthesia
Anticoagulants	Alter normal clotting factors and thus increase risk of hemorrhaging; should be discontinued at least 48 hours preoperatively. Aspirin is a commonly used medication that can alter clotting mechanisms.
Anticonvulsants	Long-term use of certain anticonvulsants—for example phenytoin (Dilantin) and phenobarbital—alters metabolism of anesthetic agents
Antihypertensives	Interact with anesthetic agents to cause bradycardia, hypotension, and impaired circulation; inhibit synthesis and storage of norepinephrine in sympathetic nerve endings
Corticosteroids	With prolonged use cause adrenal atrophy, which reduces body's ability to withstand stress; before and during surgery dosages may be temporarily increased
Insulin	Diabetic client's need for insulin preoperatively is reduced since client fasts; postoperatively, stress response and IV administration of glucose solutions can increase dosage requirements
Diuretics	Potentiate electrolyte imbalances postoperatively (particularly potassium)

is scheduled for ambulatory surgery the nurse's assessment may be performed in a physician's office or the client's home.

Each client brings fears to the surgical setting. Some are due to past hospital experiences, warnings from friends and family, or simply lack of knowledge. If a client has had previous surgery, the nurse assesses what the experience was like. The course of recovery, occurrence of complications, or the perception of the quality of care given by nurses can influence how a client feels about upcoming surgery. The nurse faces an ethical dilemma when a client is misinformed of the reason for surgery. The nurse asks for a description of the client's understanding of what surgery is planned and its implications. The nurse might ask questions such as, "Tell me about what you think will happen before and after surgery" or, "Explain to me what you know about surgery." The nurse should confer with the physician before revealing information related to the medical diagnosis. The nurse should also determine if the physician explained procedures that are routinely performed before and after surgery. When a client is well prepared and knows what to expect, the nurse reinforces the knowledge and maintains accuracy and consistency.

MEDICATION HISTORY. If a client regularly uses prescription or over-the-counter drugs, the physician may temporarily discontinue them before surgery or adjust the dosages (Table 46-3). Prescription drugs taken preoperatively are automatically discontinued postoperatively unless a physician reorders them.

ALLERGIES. The nurse is particulary alert for allergies to drugs that may be given during surgery. If one or

more exists the client receives an allergy identification band to be worn on the wrist before going to surgery. The nurse also makes sure that the front of the client's chart contains a list of allergies.

SMOKING HABITS. The client who smokes is at a greater risk for postoperative pulmonary complications than a nonsmoker. The chronic smoker already has an increased amount and thickness of mucous secretions in the lungs. General anesthetics stimulate pulmonary secretions, which are retained as a result of reduction in ciliary activity during anesthesia. After surgery the client who smokes has greater difficulty clearing the airways of mucous secretions. Smoke also causes local irritation to the tracheobronchial mucosa. Exposure to general anesthetic agents worsens the irritated airways of a smoker.

ALCOHOL INGESTION. Habitual use of alcohol predisposes the client to adverse reactions to anesthetic drugs. The client also experiences a cross-tolerance to anesthetic drugs, necessitating higher than normal doses. In addition, the physician may need to increase postoperative dosages of analgesics.

FAMILY SUPPORT. It is important for the nurse to determine the extent of the client's support from family or friends. Surgery often results in temporary or permanent disability that requires added assistance during recovery. The client cannot always immediately assume the same level of physical activity enjoyed before an illness. Often a client returns home with dressings to change or medications to administer. With ambulatory surgery it is especially important for clients and their families to assume responsibility for postoperative care.

OCCUPATION. Surgery may result in physical alterations that hinder or prevent a person from returning to work. The nurse assesses the client's occupational history to anticipate the effects surgery might have on convalescence and eventual work performance. This prepares the nurse to explain any restrictions the client will have before returning to work. When a client is unable to return to a job, the nurse may confer with a social worker for referral to job-training programs or to help seek economic assistance.

REVIEW OF EMOTIONAL HEALTH

Surgery is psychologically stressful. The client is anxious in anticipation of what will happen during surgery and whether it will improve health. Clients often feel they have little control over their situation. Family members perceive the surgery as a disruption in life-style. Hospitalization, as well as the recovery period at home, may be lengthy. The family is usually concerned about the client returning to a normal productive life. When the client has chronic illness, the family becomes fearful that surgery may result in further disability. To understand the impact surgery has on a client and family's emotional health, the nurse assesses the client's feelings about surgery as well as self-concept, coping resources, and body image.

FEELINGS. The nurse may be able to detect the client's feelings about surgery from mannerisms or behaviors. A fearful client often asks many questions, seems uneasy when strangers enter the room, or actively seeks the company of friends and relatives. It is often difficult to assess feelings thoroughly when ambulatory surgery is scheduled. The nurse usually has limited time for establishing a relationship with the client. In some outpatient surgical programs the nurse may visit with a client in the home or on the phone before surgery. In a hospital room the nurse should choose a time for discussion after admitting or diagnostic tests are completed. It should be explained that it is normal to have fears and concerns. The client's ability to share feelings depends on the nurse's willingness to listen, be supportive, and clarify misconceptions.

If the client feels powerless, the nurse determines the reason. Perhaps the client's medical diagnosis generates apprehension of increased dependence and loss of physical or mental function. The thought of being "put to sleep" under anesthesia creates concern about loss of control. It is also important for many clients to retain the power to make decisions about treatment. The nurse must assure clients of their right to ask questions and seek information.

A client may be angry about the need for surgery. A young person may feel it is unfair to have a disorder that typically affects older people. Surgery may occur at a time when it is inconvenient or potentially disruptive. The client may occasionally express anger by verbally attacking the nurse or physician. Being argumentative or overly demanding, refusing to cooperate, and criticizing the nurse's efforts to provide care are manifestations of anger and anxiety.

SELF-CONCEPT. A client with a positive self-concept is more likely to approach the surgical experience appropriately. The nurse can assess self-concept by asking the client to identify personal strengths and weaknesses. The client who is quick to criticize or scorn personal characteristics is likely either to have little self-regard or to be testing the nurse's opinion of his or her character. A poor self-concept hinders the ability to adapt to the stress of surgery and aggravates feelings of guilt or inadequacy.

COPING RESOURCES. Assessment of a client's feelings and self-concept will help reveal whether the client has the ability to cope with the stress of surgery. It is also valuable to ask the client about past anxiety management. If the client has had previous surgery, the nurse determines what behaviors helped resolve tension or nervousness. The nurse may instruct the client on relaxation exercises (see Chapter 35), which can help control anxiety.

The nurse should inquire if family members or friends can provide support. The client may want someone else present when the nurse provides instructions or explanations. Often a family member can become the client's coach, offering valuable support during the postoperative period when the client's participation in care is vital.

BODY IMAGE. Surgical removal of a diseased body part often leaves permanent disfigurement or alteration in body function. Concern over mutilation or loss of a body part compounds a client's fears.

The nurse determines what body image alterations the client perceives will result from surgery. Individuals will react differently, depending on occupation, self-image, and degree of self-esteem.

Often surgery changes the physical or psychological aspects of a client's sexuality. Excision of breast tissue, a colostomy or a ureterostomy (see Chapter 38), or removal of the prostate gland may permanently affect sexuality. Surgery such as a hernia repair or cataract extraction forces clients to refrain from sexual intercourse until they return to normal physical activity.

The nurse should encourage clients to express concerns about sexuality. The client facing even temporary sexual dysfunction requires understanding and support. Discussions about the client's sexuality should be held with the client's sexual partner so they can gain a shared understanding of how to cope with limitations in sexual function.

PHYSICAL EXAMINATION

The nurse conducts a partial or complete physical examination depending on available time and the client's preoperative condition. Chapter 13 describes techniques used in physical assessment. The assessment focuses on findings related to the client's medical history and on body systems to be affected by the surgery.

GENERAL SURVEY. The nurse observes the client's general appearance. Gestures and body movements may reflect energy or weakness caused by illness. The client may appear malnourished. Height and body weight are important indicators of nutritional status.

The nurse carefully measures vital signs, including blood pressure while sitting and standing. Preoperative assessment of vital signs provides an important baseline with which to compare alterations that occur during and after surgery. Anxiety and fear commonly cause elevations in heart rate and blood pressure. Anesthetic agents typically depress all vital functions; however, adverse drug reactions may include elevations in heart rate and blood pressure. As the effects of the anesthesia diminish after surgery, the nurse closely monitors vital signs and compares findings with preoperative baselines.

Preoperative assessment of vital signs is also important to rule out fluid and electrolyte abnormalities (see Chapter 37). An elevated heart rate may result from a plasma fluid volume deficit, potassium deficit, or sodium excess. If the pulse is full and bounding, a fluid volume excess may be the cause. Cardiac dysrhythmias are commonly caused by electrolyte imbalances.

An elevated temperature preoperatively is a cause for concern. If the client has an underlying infection, the surgeon may choose to postpone surgery until the infection has been treated. An increased body temperature increases the risk of fluid and electrolyte imbalance postoperatively.

HEAD AND NECK. The condition of oral mucous membranes reveals the level of hydration. A dehydrated client is at risk for developing serious fluid and electrolyte imbalances during surgery.

Inspection of the soft palate and nasal sinuses can reveal sinus drainage indicative of respiratory or sinus infection. To rule out the possiblity of local or systemic infection the nurse palpates for cervical lymph node enlargement.

The nurse inspects the jugular veins for distention. An excess of fluid within the circulatory system or failure of the heart to contract efficiently may lead to jugular vein distention. A client with known heart disease poses risks by having surgery.

INTEGUMENT. The nurse carefully inspects the skin overlying all body parts. Particular attention is paid to bony prominences such as elbows, the sacrum, or scapula. During surgery a client must lie in a fixed position, often for several hours. Thus a client is susceptible to pressure sores (see Chapter 42) if the skin is thin and dry and has poor turgor. The overall condition of the skin also reveals the client's level of hydration.

THORAX AND LUNGS. Assessment of the breathing pattern and chest excursion will aid the nurse in determining the client's ventilatory capacity. Clients are encouraged to breathe deeply and cough postoperatively (see section on preoperative teaching). A decline in ventilatory function preoperatively or postoperatively places the client at risk for respiratory complications. For example, a client who has high abdominal surgery will have difficulty breathing deeply because of a painful abdominal incision. Auscultation of breath sounds will detect pulmonary congestion or narrowing of airways. Serious pulmonary congestion may cause postponement of surgery. Certain anesthetics can cause laryngeal muscle spasm. If the nurse auscultates wheezing in the airways preoperatively, the client is at risk for further airway narrowing during surgery.

HEART AND VASCULAR SYSTEM. If the client has known cardiac disease, the nurse must assess the character of the apical pulse. Postoperatively the nurse compares the rate and rhythm of the pulse with preoperative baselines. Anesthetic agents, alterations in fluid balance, and stimulation from the surgical stress response can cause cardiac dysrhythmias.

The nurse assesses peripheral pulses and the color and temperature of extremities to determine a client's circulatory status.

This is particularly important for the client having vascular surgery or one who may have casts or constricting bandages applied to the extremities postoperatively. Postoperative development of a weak or absent pulse in contrast to adequate circulation before surgery indicates impaired circulation.

ABDOMEN. The nurse assesses the abdomen for size, shape, symmetry, and distention. If the client has abdominal surgery, the nurse makes frequent postoperative assessments of the abdominal incision and compares findings with preoperative data. Alteration in gastrointestinal function postoperatively may be manifest by distention. The nurse should know whether the client is simply obese or the abdomen has become distended after surgery.

Assessment of preoperative bowel sounds is useful as a baseline. The nurse also determines whether the client has regular bowel movements. If the surgery requires manipulation of portions of the gastrointestinal tract or if general anesthetic is used, normal peristalsis will not return and bowel sounds will be absent or diminished for several days postoperatively.

NEUROLOGICAL STATUS. During the health history and physical assessment the nurse observes the client's level of orientation, alertness, and mood, noting whether the client answers questions appropriately and is able to recall recent and past events. Clients who are to have surgery for neurological disease (for example, brain tumor or aneurysm) are likely to demonstrate an impaired level of consciousness or altered behavior. A client's level of consciousness will change as a result of general anesthesia. However, once the effects of anesthesia disappear, the client should either return to the preoperative level of responsiveness or show improvement.

If the client is to have spinal anesthesia, preoperative assessment of gross motor function and strength is important. Spinal anesthesia causes temporary paralysis of the lower extremities. If the client enters surgery with weakness or impaired mobility of the lower extremities, the nurse should be aware of this to avoid becoming alarmed when full motor function does not return immediately postoperatively.

RISK FACTORS

Various conditions and factors increase a person's risk in surgery. Knowledge of risk factors enables the nurse to take necessary precautions in planning a client's care.

AGE. Very young and elderly clients are surgical risks as a result of an immature or a declining physiological status. During surgery nurses and physicians are especially concerned with maintaining an infant's normal body temperature. The infant's shivering reflex is underdeveloped, and often wide temperature variations occur. Anesthesia adds to the risk, because anesthetics can cause vasodilation and heat loss.

During surgery an infant has difficulty maintaining a normal circulatory blood volume. The total blood volume of infants is considerably less than that of older children and adults. Even a small amount of blood loss can be serious. A reduced circulatory volume makes it difficult for the infant to respond to the need for increased oxygen during surgery. Thus the infant is highly susceptible to dehydration. However, if blood or fluids are replaced too quickly, overhydration may occur.

With advancing age a client's physical capacity to adapt to the stress of surgery is hampered because of deterioration in certain body functions. Despite the risk, the majority of clients undergoing surgery are elderly. Table 46-4 summarizes physiological factors that place elderly clients at risk for surgery.

NUTRITION. Normal tissue repair and resistance to infection depend on adequate nutrients. Surgery intensifies this need. Postoperatively a client requires at least 1500 kcal per day just to maintain energy reserves (Keithley, 1982). A malnourished client is prone to improper wound healing, reduced energy stores, and infection following surgery. If a client has elective surgery, nutrient imbalances can be corrected beforehand (see Chapter 33). However, if a malnourished client must have emergency surgery, efforts to restore nutrients occur postoperatively.

Obesity increases a client's surgical risk. The obese client usually has reduced ventilatory and cardiac function and has difficulty resuming normal physical activity after surgery. The obese client is susceptible to poor wound healing and wound infection because of the structure of fatty tissue, which contains a poor blood supply. This slows delivery of essential nutrients, antibodies, and enzymes needed for wound healing (see Chapter 47). It is often difficult to close the surgical wound of an obese client because of the thick adipose layer.

RADIOTHERAPY. For the client with cancer, radiotherapy is often given preoperatively to reduce the size of the cancerous tumor so it can be removed surgically. Radiation has some unavoidable effects on normal tissue, such as excess thinning of skin layers, destruction of collagen, and impaired vascularization of tissue. Ideally the surgeon waits to perform surgery 4 to 6 weeks after completion of radiation treatments, otherwise the client may have wound healing problems postoperatively.

FLUID AND ELECTROLYTE BALANCE. The body responds to surgery as a form of trauma. As a result of the adrenocortical stress response, hormonal reactions cause sodium and water retention and potassium loss within the first 2 to 5 days after surgery. Severe protein breakdown causes a negative nitrogen balance. The severity of the stress response influences the degree of fluid and electrolyte imbalance. The more extensive the surgery, the more severe the stress. A client who is hypovolemic or who has serious electrolyte alterations preoperatively is at significant risk during and after surgery. For example, an excess or depletion of potassium preoperatively increases the chance of dysrhythmias developing during or after surgery. If the client has preexisting renal, gastrointestinal, or cardiovascular abnormalities, the risk of fluid and electrolyte alterations is even greater.

DIAGNOSTIC SCREENING

Before a client undergoes surgery, the surgeon will order diagnostic tests to screen for preexisting abnormalities. Many clients are able to be tested on an outpatient basis before surgery. However, a client may also enter the hospital several days in advance to complete

TABLE 46-4   Physiological Factors that Place an Elderly Client at Risk for Surgery

System	Alterations	Risks	Preoperative Nursing Implications
Cardiovascular	Degenerative change in myocardium and valves	Reduced cardiac reserve	Assessing baseline vital signs
	Rigidity of arterial walls and reduction in sympathetic and parasympathetic innervation to heart	Predisposes client to postoperative hemorrhage and rise in systolic and diastolic blood pressure	
	Increase in calcium and cholesterol deposits within small arteries; arterial walls thickened	Predisposes client to clot formation in lower extremities	Instructing client on techniques for performing leg exercises and proper turning
Pulmonary	Rib cage stiffened and reduced in size	Reduced vital capacity	Instructing client on proper technique for coughing and deep breathing exercises
	Reduced range of movement in diaphragm	Greater residual capacity or volume of air left in lung after normal breath increases, reducing amount of new air brought into lungs with each inspiration	
	Lung tissue stiffened and airspaces enlarged	Reduced blood oxygenation	
Renal	Reduced blood flow to kidneys	Increases danger of shock when blood loss occurs	Determining baseline urinary output for 24-hour period
	Reduced glomerular filtration rate and excretory times	Limits ability to remove drugs or toxic substances	
	Reduced bladder capacity	Voiding frequency increases, and larger amount of urine stays in the bladder after voiding	Instructing client to notify nurse immediately when sensation of bladder fullness develops
		Sensation of need to void may not occur until bladder is filled	Keeping call light and/or bedpan within easy reach
Neurological	Sensory losses: reduced tactile sense, increased pain tolerance	Client less able to respond to early warning signs of surgical complications	Orienting client to surrounding environment
	Decreased reaction time	Becomes easily confused following anesthesia	
Metabolic	Lower basal metabolic rate	Reduced total oxygen consumption	
	Reduced number of red blood cells and hemoglobin levels	Reduced ability to carry adequate oxygen to tissues	Administering necessary blood products preoperatively
	Change in total amounts of body potassium and water volume	Greater risk for fluid or electrolyte imbalance	Monitoring electrolyte levels preoperatively

testing procedures. If diagnostic tests reveal severe problems, the surgeon may cancel surgery until the condition stabilizes.

The nurse is responsible for coordinating completion of tests and for being sure clients are prepared for the diagnostic studies. The nurse also reviews diagnostic results as they become available to alert physicians to findings and plan appropriate therapy.

Routine screening tests include a complete blood count (CBC), serum electrolytes, coagulation studies, serum creatinine, urinalysis, and a chest x-ray study.

COMPLETE BLOOD COUNT. A CBC is an analysis of a peripheral venous blood specimen that includes measurement of red blood cell count, hemoglobin concentration, and hematocrit (packed red cell volume). The laboratory of each health institution has a standard for normal values. An abnormal CBC may be indicative of a number of alterations (for example, dietary deficiency and chronic blood loss), placing the client at risk for cardiovascular and pulmonary complications. In such a case the surgeon may administer blood products before surgery.

TABLE 46-5 Common Laboratory Test Values

Test	Values
Sodium (Na^+)	135-145 mEq/L
Potassium (K^+)	3.5-5.0 mEq/L
Chloride (Cl^+)	100-106 mEq/L
Bicarbonate	24-32 mEq/L
Creatinine	0.6-1.5 mg/100 ml
Prothrombin time	Less than 2-second deviation from control
Partial thromboplastin time	25-27 seconds
Platelet count	150,000-350,000/mm^3

SERUM ELECTROLYTES. Analysis of serum electrolytes also requires a peripheral venous blood sample. Batteries of tests are available to reveal a client's electrolyte balance (Table 46-5). Because of the potential for fluid and electrolyte imbalances following surgery, the surgeon determines if electrolyte replacement is needed before surgery.

COAGULATION STUDIES. The ability of blood to clot or coagulate is essential for minimizing a surgical client's risk of hemorrhaging. The prothrombin time (PT), partial thromboplastin time (PTT), and platelet counts are routine tests for the clotting ability of blood (Table 46-5). Coagulation studies allow the nurse and physician to identify clients at risk for bleeding tendencies and thrombus formation.

SERUM CREATININE. To assess the client's renal function the physician orders a serum creatinine test. Creatinine is the by-product of muscle metabolism. The body excretes a constant amount through the kidneys, which serves as an excellent measure of the glomerular filtration rate. The creatinine level can be a sensitive indicator of renal failure when the value rises. (Table 46-5)

URINALYSIS. Analysis of a urine specimen consists of screening for urinary infection, renal disease, and diabetes mellitus. The nurse collects a clean voided specimen. Included in a urinalysis is measurement of urine color, pH, and specific gravity. Also determined is the presence of protein, glucose, ketones, and blood. Chapter 38 discusses normal values in a urinalysis.

CHEST X-RAY STUDY. A chest film allows the physician to examine the condition of the heart and lungs before surgery. Although the x-ray study does not always detect subtle pathological changes, it can reveal the overall size and shape of the heart, presence of lung lesions and chest wall abnormalities, and position of the diaphragm and aorta. If the physician detects lung abnormalities, a different type and dosage of sedatives or anesthetic agents may be used. Before sending the female client for an x-ray examination, the nurse should be sure she is not pregnant. Exposure of the fetus to radiation may cause injury.

ADDITIONAL SCREENING TESTS. If a client is over the age of 40 or has heart disease, the physician orders an electrocardiogram (ECG). The test involves painless application of electrodes to the chest and extremities. An ECG measures the heart's electrical activity to determine if the heart rate, rhythm, and other factors are normal. The procedure takes less than 5 minutes and requires the client simply to lie flat and relax.

Depending on the type of surgery the client will undergo, there are several diagnostic tests for specific anatomical structures and physiological functions.

If the client is likely to lose a significant amount of blood during surgery, the physician orders a blood spec-

---

Examples of Nursing Diagnoses for Preoperative Client

NANDA-APPROVED NURSING DIAGNOSES

Ineffective airway clearance related to:
- Diminished cough
- Increased pulmonary congestion

Anxiety related to:
- Impending surgery
- Threat of loss of body part

Ineffective family coping: compromised related to:
- Temporary role change of client
- Impending severity of surgery

Fear related to:
- Impending surgery
- Anticipation of postoperative pain

Knowledge deficit regarding implications of surgery related to:
- First experience with surgery
- Inadequate preparation by physician

Altered nutrition: less than body requirements related to:
- Preoperative malnourishment

Altered nutrition: more than body requirements related to:
- Obesity

Powerlessness related to:
- Emergency nature of surgery

Potential impaired skin integrity related to:
- Preoperative radiation
- Immobilization during surgery

Sleep pattern disturbance related to:
- Fear of surgery
- Preoperative hospital routines

imen for type and cross-matching. This enables the laboratory to determine the proper blood type and Rh factor. The surgeon usually designates the number of blood units to have available during surgery.

NURSING DIAGNOSIS

The nurse clusters defining characteristics gathered during the assessment to identify nursing diagnoses for the surgical client (see sample nursing diagnoses box). The diagnoses establish direction for care that will be provided during one or all surgical phases. Preoperative nursing diagnoses allow the nurse to take precautions and actions, so care provided during the intraoperative and postoperative phases is consistent with the client's needs.

Nursing diagnoses made preoperatively may also focus solely on the potential risks a client may face postoperatively. Preventive care is essential to manage the surgical client effectively. The nature and type of surgery, as well as the client's health status, will pose characteristics for a number of nursing diagnoses. The nursing diagnoses box lists typical nursing diagnoses that have implications for clients during the surgical experience.

PLANNING

It is essential to include any client in health care planning, especially the surgical client. Involving the client early in developing the surgical plan of care will minimize surgical risks and postoperative complications. For example, nursing research has shown that structured preoperative teaching can reduce the client's hospital stay (Lindemann and VanAernam, 1971). A client informed about the surgical experience is less likely to be fearful and is able to prepare for expected outcomes. The care plan box provides a sample care plan for a preoperative surgical client.

For the ambulatory surgical client, the preoperative planning phase occurs either in the home or in the outpatient surgery unit on the morning of surgery. Ideally, it is done in the home. This gives the client time to think about the surgical experience, make necessary physical preparations (for example, altering diet or discontinuing medication use), and ask questions about postoperative procedures. The ambulatory surgical client returns home on the day of surgery. Thus well-planned, preoperative care ensures that the client is well informed and able to be an active participant during recovery. The family or significant others can also play an active supportive role for the client.

Sample Nursing Diagnoses for Preoperative Client

Defining Characteristics	Nursing Diagnoses	Related Factors
No previous surgical experience Very alert and apprehensive when staff enter room Asks same questions several times Wife reports client fearful of being in pain	Fear	▪ Impending surgery
No previous surgical experience either personally or involving family Asks questions about what to expect Has received minimal preparation by physician Alert and responsive to discussion	Knowledge deficit regarding implications of surgery	▪ First experience with surgery
Abnormal breath sounds History of smoking Scheduled for anesthesia Scheduled for abdominal surgery	Potentially, ineffective airway clearance	▪ Diminished cough ▪ Increased pulmonary congestion

Sample Nursing Care Plan for Preoperative Client

Nursing Diagnoses	Goals	Expected Outcomes	Nursing Interventions
Knowledge deficit related to first surgical experience	Client understands intraoperative and postoperative events.	Client and family will describe routine procedures that nurses perform postoperatively. Client will describe ways to participate in care postoperatively. Client and family will describe events that commonly occur in the holding area and operating room.	Offer teaching booklet "Your surgical experience." Provide planned teaching session to explain common events that occur postoperatively (monitoring, IV care, exercise). Explain events that will occur in holding area (IV insertion, vital sign check) and in operating room (positioning, anesthesia).
Potentially ineffective airway clearance	Client will achieve and maintain normal ventilatory function.	Client will ventilate to maximum ability. Client will be able to cough forcefully and effectively.	Demonstrate proper deep breathing exercises. Explain how history of smoking and an abdominal incision are factors that can impair airway clearance postoperatively. Demonstrate proper technique for controlled coughing. Explain implications postoperatively if ventilatory function is not maintained.

The preoperative plan of care is based on nursing diagnoses and is thus individualized for each client. However, there are basic preparations each must undergo. Goals of care for the preoperative client include the following:

1. Understanding physiological and psychological responses to surgery
2. Understanding intraoperative and postoperative events
3. Acquiring emotional comfort
4. Gaining a return of normal physiological function postoperatively
5. Maintaining a normal fluid and electrolyte balance intraoperatively and postoperatively
6. Achieving comfort and rest
7. Remaining free of postoperative surgical wound infection
8. Remaining safe from physical harm intraoperatively

IMPLEMENTATION

Preoperative nursing interventions give the client an understanding of the surgical experience and prepare the client physically for surgical intervention.

INFORMED CONSENT

A surgeon cannot legally perform surgery until a client understands the need for a procedure, what is involved, risks, expected results, and alternative treatments. Primary responsibility for informing the client rests with the surgeon. Consent is not informed if the client is confused, unconscious, mentally incompetent, or under the influence of sedatives. All consent forms (Fig. 46-1) must be signed before the nurse administers preoperative medications. Ideally a surgeon will obtain consent before a client is admitted to the hospital or satellite surgical setting.

The surgeon's explanation should be witnessed by a

**CONSENT FOR SURGERY OR DIAGNOSTIC PROCEDURE
BY PHYSICIANS ON THE STAFF OF
BARNES HOSPITAL OR
ST. LOUIS CHILDREN'S HOSPITAL**

STAMP ADDRESSOGRAPH PLATE HERE

PATIENT_____ DATE_____

(1) I authorize performance on _____ of the following operation or proce-
(Myself or name of patient)

dure*_____ by _____ and such persons
from the staffs of either hospital who may be present.

(2) I also consent to the performance of such other unforseen operations or procedures as are indicated.

(3) The nature and purpose of the operation or diagnostic procedure, possible alternative methods of treatment, the risks involved, and the possibility of complications despite precautions have been explained to me. I understand that all procedures are associated with certain risks and acknowledge that no guarantee or assurance has been made as to the results that may be obtained.

(4) I consent to the administration of such anesthetic procedures as may be considered reasonable and understand that certain risks attend all anesthetics. I also consent to the administration of blood, drugs, medications, and other substances reasonably considered advisable and the use of x-ray and other procedures and devices that my physician considers to be reasonably useful.

(5) For the purpose of advancing medical education, I also consent to the admittance of observers to the operating and procedure rooms and to the taking of any photographs in the course of the operation or procedure.

(6) My physician or the hospital staff may examine, use (including use in other patients), or dispose of any bones, organs, tissues, fluids, or parts removed from my body.

We/I certify that we/I have read and understand the above consent to operation or diagnostic procedure, that the explanations therein referred to were made and to my satisfaction, and that all blanks or statements requiring insertion or completion were filled in and inapplicable paragraphs, if any, were stricken before we/I signed.

Witness to signature:

Signature of patient _____

Signature of patient's parent
or guardian: _____

_____
(Physician or nurse)

SUMMARY OF SIGNATURE REQUIREMENTS

(1) If the patient is an unemancipated minor, the parents or only available parent should sign. If the minor has a court appointed guardian, he/she must sign, and his/her signature alone will suffice.

(2) If non compos adult, legal guardian (if any); if none, spouse (if any); if none, adult children should sign.

(3) If emergency operation is immediately necessary and signature is unavailable, get consultation and proceed.

(4) In the event that the patient or the person who must sign for the patient refuses to consent to a procedure, refusal should be noted in the record, and beneath the refusal, the patient or person who must sign for the patient should sign the note relating to the refusal.

(5) On minors, when parents or legal guardians refuse to sign a permit and the procedure is urgently needed by the patient, the refusal is to be referred to the administrator on duty by the surgeon. The administrator on duty will refer the matter to the Juvenile Court.

I consent to have additional people present in the room during my procedure to observe the procedure or to provide technical consultation to the physician. My physician has explained to me why the additional individual(s) will be present.

Witness to signature:

Signature of patient: _____

Signature of patient's parent
or guardian: _____

_____
(Physician or nurse)

*State nature and extent of operation or procedure using laymen's language (for example, "exploratory operation in...")

Fig. 46-1 Surgical consent form.
Courtesy Barnes Hospital, St. Louis.

qualified member of the health care team. The form's structure allows the physician to write in information related to the surgery. A client's signature on a consent form implies that the client has been thoroughly informed about the procedure. The nurse frequently witnesses signing of the form and examines the document for the correct date, time, and signature, which must be in ink. A client who is illiterate can sign by making a mark as long as it is properly witnessed. As a witness the nurse is able to attest that the client's signature is on the form but not that the client was properly informed. In many institutions a time limit is placed on consent forms, for example, 30 days.

Individuals must personally sign the consent form if they are (1) of legal age (varies among states and Canadian provinces), (2) under legal age but have a valid marriage certificate, (3) designated as an emancipated minor (certain states), and (4) not at present under legal guardianship. In some Canadian provinces a teenager may sign a consent form under certain conditions. If the client is a minor or legally considered to be incompetent and is not included in these categories, a parent or legal guardian signs the consent form. A spouse or next of kin signs for an adult who is unconscious or mentally incompetent.

In emergency situations the client may be unable to sign and family members may be unavailable. The surgeon is legally permitted to perform surgery without consent in such a case; however, every effort must be made to obtain permission from a responsible family member by telephone, telegram or in some states by court order. A telephone consent must be witnessed by two persons who hear the family member's oral consent. The two witnesses sign the consent with the name of the family member, noting that an oral consent was obtained. Informed consent is critical to protect not only the client but also health personnel so the surgical team can practice without fear of legal reprisal.

Once the client's consent form has been completed, the nurse makes sure the form is placed in the client's record. The record goes to the operating room with the client. Chapter 18 discusses in detail the nurse's responsibilities for informed consent.

PREOPERATIVE TEACHING

Structured preoperative teaching has proven benefits. Preoperative teaching concerning a client's expected postoperative behaviors has a positive influence on the client's recovery. It should be provided in a systematic and structured format with teaching and learning principles. Structured preoperative teaching can influence such postoperative factors as the following:

1. *Ventilatory function.* Teaching improves the client's ability to cough and deep breathe effectively.
2. *Physical functional capacity.* Teaching improves the client's ability to ambulate and resume activities of daily living early.
3. *Sense of well-being.* Clients who are prepared for surgery experience less anxiety and report a greater sense of psychological well-being.
4. *Length of hospital stay.* Structured preoperative teaching can reduce the length of stay.

The most effective teaching program for surgical clients is planned so all clients receive the same information. However, if a client has previously undergone surgery, the nurse makes sure the client understands the information required. Detailed discussion and demonstration of postoperative exercises are vital. If the client understands why these exercises are important to postoperative recovery and knows how to perform them correctly, the recovery period will be less complicated. Today, since many clients come to the hospital on the day of surgery, preoperative teaching may occur in the home setting. Printed literature, instructions, and videotapes are made available to clients (Fig. 46-2). Preadmission nurses may call clients the evening before surgery to clarify questions and reinforce explanations. Including family members in the client's preoperative preparation is advised. Often a family member is the coach for postoperative exercises when the client returns from surgery. If anxious relatives do not understand routine postoperative events, it is likely their anxiety will heighten the client's fears or concerns. Preoperative preparation of family members minimizes anxiety and misunderstanding.

The nurse should provide the client with information about sensations typically experienced after surgery. Preparatory information helps clients anticipate what will happen during a procedure and thus helps them form a realistic image of the surgical experience. When events occur as predicted, the client is better able to cope and attend to the experiences. For example, in the operating room the anesthesiologist may apply petrolatum ointment to the client's eyes to prevent corneal damage. Warning the client about the sensation of blurred vision will reduce the client's anxiety on awakening from surgery. Sensations the nurse may describe include the expected pain at the surgical site, the tightness of dressings, dryness of the mouth, or the sensation of a sore throat resulting from an endotracheal tube.

It is best to begin preoperative teaching well in advance of a client's scheduled surgery. If the nurse is able to teach a client 1 or 2 days before surgery, the client will be better able to learn. Anxiety and fear are barriers to learning, and both emotions are heightened as surgery approaches. The nurse assesses the surgical client's readiness and ability to learn. If the client is capable and receptive to learning, the nurse presents information in a logical sequence beginning with preoperative events

INSTRUCTIONS FOR OUTPATIENT SURGERY

Your surgery will take place at:

DATE: _____ SURGERY TIME: _____ ARRIVE: _____

Anesthesia: Local _____ General _____ Block _____

1. Please be at the facility one to one and a half hours prior to scheduled time of operation.
2. You should have nothing to eat or drink for eight to twelve hours before surgery.
3. Register at the Reception Desk when you arrive.
4. It is best to leave valuables at home. However, any valuables you do have will be checked with the receptionist for safe keeping. You will then change into a hospital gown. Your clothing will be placed in a locker until after surgery.
5. After the operation, you will recover in the Recovery Room, if necessary, and then be discharged to your home.
6. Someone must accompany you. They should wait for you in the Outpatient Waiting Room until you come out of the OR.
7. When riding home in your car or a taxi, use shoulder belts, seat straps, or ride in the rear seat.
8. Routine laboratory tests, cardiogram and/or x-rays will be ordered as needed. The patient will be asked for a urine specimen the morning of surgery.
9. We request that you take *no aspirin* for two weeks before surgery. You may take aspirin substitute (non-aspirin compound).
10. If facial surgery is indicated, *DO NOT WEAR cosmetics to surgery*. Wash your face the night before and the morning of surgery. Cosmetics in the area of surgery could cause infection.
11. If surgery of the hand is indicated, the hand should be clean and the nails trimmed. *DO NOT wear nail polish.*
12. Hand surgery patients should wear clothing with large sleeves that will fit over a bulky dressing.
13. It is imperative that your insurance forms be in order for surgery. If forms are requested, be sure to have them with you the day of surgery.
14. You will be called the night before surgery. The main purpose of this call is to confirm your time on the schedule. If you cannot be reached, your surgery may be cancelled. If you have any questions, please call our office.
15. You will also be called the evening after your surgery. If you are not going to be home, leave the number where you can be reached with the nurse.

Fig. 46-2 Instructions for outpatient surgery.
From Kasdan, AS, et al.: Taking the extra step: the nursing role in same day surgery, Today's OR Nurse, December 1984, vol. 6, No. 12, p. 19.

and advancing to intraoperative and postoperative routines. Preoperative teaching checklists give nurses useful guidelines for presenting comprehensive instructions.

The Association of Operating Room Nurses (AORN) (1982) has established criteria by which the client demonstrates understanding of the surgical experience. Extensive preoperative teaching will not only improve the client's understanding but will also promote return of the client's normal physiological function. The criteria and a discussion of each follow.

1. *The client cites reasons for each of the preoperative instructions provided and exercises explained or practiced.* Given a rationale for preoperative and postoperative procedures, the client is better prepared to participate in care. Every preoperative teaching program includes explanation and demonstration of the four postoperative exercises: diaphragmatic breathing, coughing, turning, and leg exercises. These exercises are designed to prevent postoperative complications (Procedure 46-1).

Demonstrating Postoperative Exercises

STEPS	RATIONALE
1. Assess client's risk for postoperative respiratory complications. Review client's medical history to identify: presence of chronic pulmonary condition (for example, emphysema or asthma); any condition that affects chest wall movement; history of smoking; and presence of reduced hemoglobin.	General anesthesia predisposes client to respiratory problems because lungs are not fully inflated during surgery; cough reflex is suppressed and mucous collects within airway passages. Postoperatively, client may have reduced lung volume and require greater efforts to cough and deep breathe; inadequate lung expansion can lead to atelectasis and pneumonia; client is at greater risk to develop respiratory complications if other chronic lung conditions are present; smoking damages ciliary clearance and increases mucous secretion.
2. Assess client's ability to cough and deep breathe by having him or her take a deep breath and observing movement of shoulders and chest wall. Measure chest excursion during deep breath. Ask client to cough after taking a deep breath.	Reveals maximum potential for chest expansion and ability to cough forcefully; serves as baseline to measure client's ability to perform exercises postoperatively.
3. Assess client's risk for postoperative thrombus formation (elderly, immobilized clients are most at risk).	Following general anesthesia circulation is slowed and when rate of blood flow is slowed, there is greater tendency for clot formation. Immobilization results in decreased muscular contraction in lower extremities, which promotes venous stasis.
4. Prepare necessary supplies: a. Pillow (optional)	Client may prefer to use a pillow to splint incision when coughing to reduce discomfort.
5. Explain postoperative exercises to the client, including their importance to recovery, and physiological benefits.	Information allows client to attend and can motivate client to learn. Persons tend to learn new skills when benefits can be gained.

Diaphragmatic Breathing

6. Assist client to comfortable sitting or standing position. If client chooses to sit, assist to side of bed or to upright position in chair.	Upright position facilitates diaphragmatic excursion.

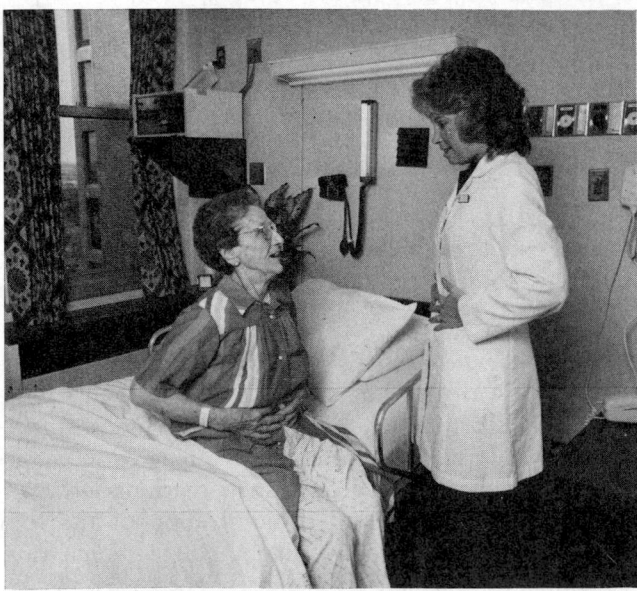

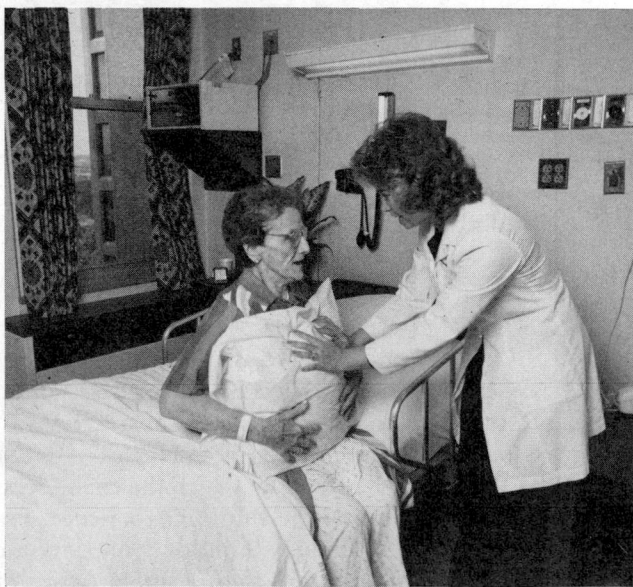

Step 8

Step 20

STEPS	RATIONALE
7. Stand or sit facing client.	Client will be able to observe breathing exercise performed by nurse.
8. Instruct client to place palms of the hands across from each other, down, and along lower borders of anterior rib cage; place tips of third fingers lightly together (see illustration). Demonstrate for client.	Position of hands allows client to feel movement of chest and abdomen as diaphragm descends and lungs inside chest wall expand.
9. Have client take slow, deep breaths, inhaling through nose. Tell client to feel the middle fingers separate as he or she inhales. Demonstrate for client.	Slow deep breath prevents panting or hyperventilation. Inhaling through nose warms, humidifies, and filters air.
10. Explain that client will feel normal downward movement of diaphragm during inspiration. Explain that abdominal organs descend and chest wall expands.	Explanation and demonstration focus on normal ventilatory movement of chest wall. Client develops understanding of how diaphragmatic breathing feels.
11. Avoid using chest and shoulders while inhaling and instruct client in same manner.	Using auxiliary chest and shoulder muscles during breathing increases useless energy expenditures.
12. Have client hold slow, deep breath for count of 3 and then slowly exhale through mouth. Tell client he or she will feel middle finger tips touch as chest wall contracts.	Allows for gradual expulsion of all air.
13. Repeat breathing exercise three to five times.	Allows client to observe slow, rhythmical breathing pattern.
14. Have client practice exercise. Client is instructed to take 10 slow, deep breaths every 2 hr while awake during postoperative period until he or she is mobile.	Repetition of exercise reinforces learning. Regular deep breathing will prevent postoperative complications.

Controlled Coughing

STEPS	RATIONALE
15. Explain importance of maintaining an upright position.	Position facilitates diaphragm excursion and enhances thorax expansion.
16. Demonstrate coughing. Take two slow, deep breaths, inhaling through nose and exhaling through mouth.	Deep breaths expand lungs fully so that air moves behind mucus and facilitates effects of coughing.
17. Inhale deeply a third time and hold breath to count of 3. Cough fully for two to three consecutive coughs without inhaling between coughs. (Tell client to push all air out of lungs.)	Consecutive coughs help remove mucus more effectively and completely than one forceful cough.
18. Caution client against just clearing throat instead of coughing.	Clearing throat does not remove mucus from deep in airways.
19. If surgical incision is to be either abdominal or thoracic, teach client to place one hand over incisional area and other hand on top of first. During breathing and coughing exercises, client presses gently against incisional area to splint or support it. (Pillow over incision is optional.)	Surgical incision cuts through muscles, tissues, and nerve endings. Deep breathing and coughing exercises place additional stress on suture line and cause discomfort. Splinting incision with hands provides firm support and reduces incisional pulling. Some clients prefer to have pillow to place over incision.
20. Client continues to practice coughing exercises, splinting imaginary incision. The client is instructed to cough two to three times every 2 hr while awake (see illustration).	Value of deep coughing with splinting is stressed to effectively expectorate mucus with minimal discomfort.

Turning

STEPS	RATIONALE
21. Instruct client to assume supine position to right side of bed. Side rails on both sides of bed should be in up position.	Positioning begins on right side of bed so that turning to left side will not cause client to roll toward bed's edge.
22. Instruct client to place the left hand over incisional area to splint it.	Splinting incision supports and minimizes pulling on suture line during turning.
23. Instruct client to keep left leg straight and flex right knee up and over left leg.	Straight leg stabilizes the client's position. Flexed right leg shifts weight for easier turning.
24. Have client grab left side rail with right hand, pull toward left, and roll onto left side.	Pulling toward side rail reduces effort needed for turning.
25. Instruct client to turn every 2 hr while awake.	Reduces risk of vascular and pulmonary complications.

Continued.

PROCEDURE 46-1, cont'd

Demonstrating Postoperative Exercises

STEPS	RATIONALE

Leg Exercises

26. Have client assume supine position in bed. Demonstrate leg exercises by performing passive range of motion exercises and simultaneously explaining exercise.

Provides normal anatomical position of lower extremities.

27. Rotate each ankle in complete circle. Instruct client to draw imaginary circles with big toe. Repeat five times.

Leg exercises maintain joint mobility and promote venous return.

28. Alternate dorsiflexion and plantar flexion of both feet. Direct client to feel calf muscles contract and relax alternately (see illustration).

Stretches and contracts gastrocnemius muscles.

29. Client continues leg exercises by alternately flexing and extending knees. Repeat five times (see illustration).

Contracts muscles of upper legs and maintains knee mobility.

30. Client alternately raises each leg straight up from bed surface, keeping legs straight.

Promotes contraction and relaxation of quadriceps muscles.

31. Have client continue to practice exercises at least every 2 hr while awake. Client is instructed to coordinate turning and leg exercises with diaphragmatic breathing and coughing exercises.

Repetition of sequence of performing exercises reinforces learning. Establishes routine for exercises that develops habit for performance. Sequence of exercises should be leg exercises, turning, breathing, and coughing.

32. Observe client's ability to perform all four exercises independently.

Ensures client has learned correct technique.

33. Record the exercises that have been demonstrated to client and whether client can perform them independently.

Documents client's education and provides data for instructional follow-up.

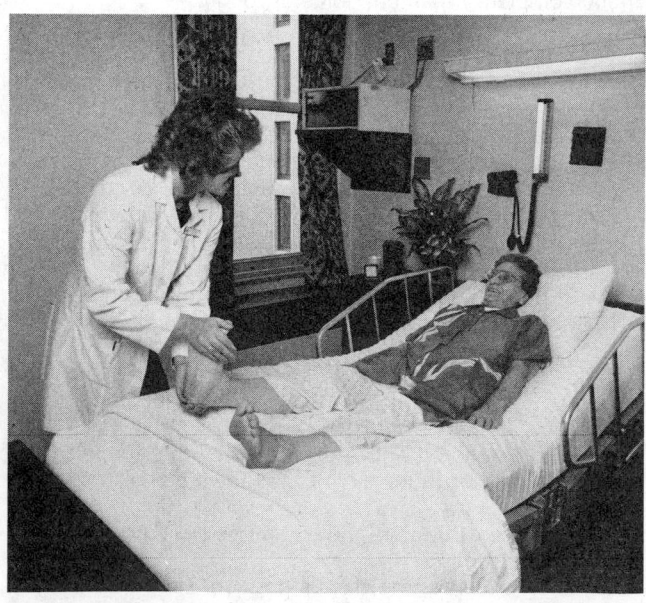

Step 28

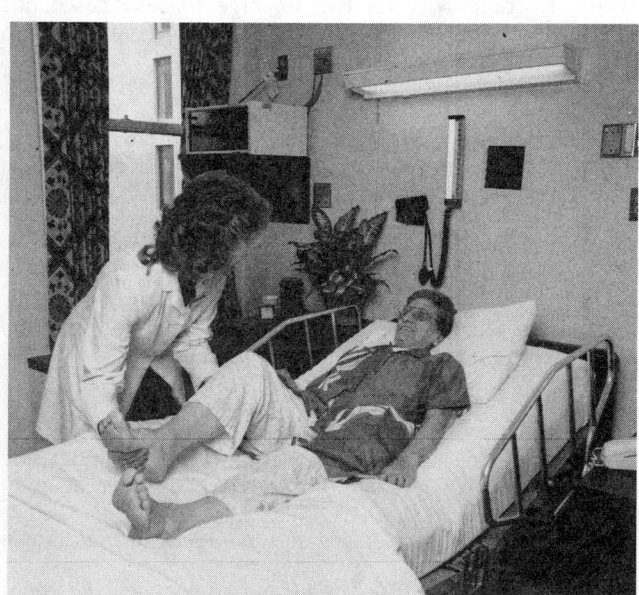

Step 29

While a client is under general anesthesia, the lungs do not ventilate fully. Postoperatively the client has a reduced lung volume and needs greater effort to breathe. During surgery venous blood flow to the legs slows. Stasis of circulation may lead to thrombi or clots. A clot can break off and travel to the brain, heart, or lungs to cause potentially fatal complications.

Diaphragmatic breathing improves lung expansion and oxygen delivery without using excess energy. The client learns how to use the diaphragm during deep breathing to take slow, deep, and relaxed breaths. Eventually the client's lung volume improves postoperatively. Deep breathing also helps to clear out anesthetic gases remaining in the airways. To facilitate deep breathing the physician may order an incentive spirometer for the client, which encourages effective deep breathing through sustained maximal inspiration (see Chapter 36).

Coughing assists in removing retained mucus in the airways. A deep productive cough is more beneficial than merely clearing the throat. Postoperative incisional pain makes coughing difficult. The client must anticipate the pain and understand the importance of coughing. The nurse also teaches the client how to splint an incision to minimize pain during coughing. Nurses direct clients to cough and deep breathe at least every 2 hours while awake.

Leg exercises and turning improve blood flow to the extremities and thus reduce stasis. Contraction of lower leg muscles promotes venous return, making it difficult for clots to form. When a client has learned how to turn and perform leg exercises, the nurse encourages the client to perform each at least every 2 hours while awake.

After explaining each exercise, the nurse demonstrates it. The nurse acts as a coach, guiding the client through each exercise. For example, the nurse says whether the client is sitting properly and helps the client place the hands in the proper position during breathing. The nurse then allows the client time (at least 15 minutes) for independent practice. The nurse can attend to other duties before returning to watch each exercise independently. The nurse gives feedback, telling the client what aspect of each exercise is done correctly and what needs improvement.

2. *The client states the time surgery is scheduled.* The client and family should be told the approximate time when surgery will begin. If the hospital has a busy operating room schedule, it is best to let them know how many procedures are scheduled before the client's. It is unwise to tell the client and family the anticipated length of surgery. Unanticipated delays may occur for many unharmful reasons. If the client fails to return at the time expected, the family will be highly anxious. Family members should be told that nurses in the postoperative sur-

gical division will inform them of the client's arrival in the recovery room.

3. *The client states the unit to which he or she will return after surgery and the location of family during the intraoperative and immediate recovery periods.* The unit to which the client is admitted before surgery may be different from the postoperative unit. The family needs to know where the client will be taken after surgery. The nurse also explains where the family can wait and where the surgeon will attempt to find family members after surgery. If the client is to be taken to a special unit, it helps to orient the client and family members to it through a tour before surgery.

4. *The client discusses anticipated monitoring and therapeutic devices or materials likely to be used postoperatively.* The client and family want to know what to expect. If they understand about routine postoperative vital sign monitoring before surgery, they will not be apprehensive when nurses make these checks. The nurse can also explain whether the client is likely to have intravenous lines, dressings, or drainage tubes. The nurse should neither overprepare nor underprepare the client and family. The nurse cannot predict all that the client will require, because each surgeon tends to follow different practices for each type of surgery. Although the nurse becomes familiar with each surgeon's preferences, it is easy to misinform a client about a therapy that may not be initiated. Contradictions between what the nurse explains and what actually occurs postoperatively can cause great anxiety.

5. *The client describes in general terms the surgical procedures and subsequent treatment plan.* After the surgeon has explained the basic purpose of a surgical procedure and what it involves, the client may ask the nurse additional questions to clarify misunderstandings. The nurse is careful to avoid saying anything that contradicts the surgeon. One way to avoid problems is to first ask what the client has been told. When the client has little or no understanding about the surgery, the nurse first checks with the physician to determine what explanation can be given. Postoperatively certain predictable aspects of the client's treatment plan (dressing changes, respiratory therapy) and level of supportive nursing care are explained. The nurse can also describe plans for postoperative rehabilitation and drug therapy.

6. *The client describes anticipated steps in postoperative activity resumption.* The type of surgery a client undergoes will affect the speed with which normal physical activity and regular eating habits can be resumed. The nurse explains that it is normal to progress gradually in activity and eating. If the client tolerates activity and diet well, they will progress more quickly.

7. *The client verbalizes expectations about pain relief*

and the measures likely to be taken to alleviate pain. One of the surgical client's greatest fears is pain. The family also has a primary concern for the client's comfort. Pain after surgery is normal. The nurse informs the client and family of therapies available for pain relief, for example, analgesics, positioning, splinting, and relaxation exercises. The client needs to know how often pain-killing drugs will be available, how they are administered, and the drugs' effects.

The client should be encouraged to inform the nurses as soon as pain becomes a constant discomfort. If a client waits until postoperative pain becomes excruciating, an analgesic will not provide relief. The client should also know that it takes time for a drug to act and rarely will all discomfort be eliminated.

Often surgical clients avoid taking pain drugs for fear of becoming dependent. But most drug dosages and the required intervals between "as needed" are not sufficient to cause dependence. The nurse should encourage the client to use analgesics as needed. Unless the pain is controlled, it will be difficult for the client to participate in postoperative therapy. Hospitalized clients initially receive parenteral injections. As they become able to tolerate food, the physician replaces parenteral analgesics with oral forms.

8. *The client expresses feelings regarding surgical intervention and its expected outcomes.* The client may feel like part of an assembly line during the preoperative surgical phase. Frequent visits by staff, diagnostic testing, and physical preparation for surgery consume a lot of time, and the client has few opportunities to reflect on what is happening. The nurse makes sure the client feels like an individual. The client and family need time to express feelings about surgery. The client's level of anxiety will influence how often the nurse should provide time for discussion. While delivering routine care the nurse can encourage expression of concerns. The family may wish to discuss concerns without the client so that their fears will not frighten the client.

PHYSICAL PREPARATION

The degree of preoperative physical preparation depends on the client's health status, the surgery to be performed, and the surgeon's preferences. A seriously ill client will recieve more supportive care in the form of medications, intravenous fluid therapy, and monitoring than the client facing a minor elective procedure. The nurse's responsibilities include:

1. *Maintenance of normal fluid and electrolyte balance.* The surgical client is vulnerable to fluid and electrolyte imbalances as a result of inadequate preoperative intake or excessive fluid losses intraoperatively. A client takes nothing by mouth (NPO) after midnight before

the morning of surgery. After 6 to 8 hours of fasting the client's gastrointestinal tract will be relatively empty, so the risks of vomiting or aspirating emesis during surgery are minimal. General anesthetics typically cause slowing of gastrointestinal peristalsis. The nurse removes fluids and solid foods from the client's bedside and posts a sign over the bed to alert hospital personnel and family members about fasting restrictions.

A client who is at home the evening before surgery must understand the importance of not taking food or fluids and be willing to follow restrictions.

The nurse can allow the client to rinse the mouth with water or mouthwash and brush the teeth as long as the client does not swallow water. In the hospital the nurse notifies the surgeon if the client eats or drinks during the fasting period.

During surgery, normal mechanisms for controlling fluid and electrolyte balance, including respiration, digestion, circulation, and elimination, are disturbed. The surgical procedure itself may cause extensive losses of blood and other body fluids. The surgical stress response aggravates any fluid and electrolyte imbalance. The nurse determines if the client eats and drinks sufficient amounts preoperatively before fasting to ensure adequate fluid and nutrition intake.

This prevents fluid and electrolyte imbalances and reduces the risk of infection postoperatively. The client's diet should include foods high in protein, with sufficient carbohydrates, fat, and vitamins. If a client cannot eat because of gastrointestinal alterations or impairments in consciousness, an intravenous route for fluid replacement is started. The physician relies on serum electrolyte levels to determine the type of intravenous fluids and elctrolyte additives to administer. Clients with severe nutritional imbalances may require intravenous supplements that contain concentrated protein and glucose (see Chapter 33).

2. *Minimize risk of surgical wound infection.* The risk of developing a surgical wound infection is determined by three factors: (1) amount and type of microorganisms contaminating a wound, (2) susceptibility of the host, and (3) condition of the wound at the end of the operation (largely determined by the surgeon's operative technique). All three factors may interact to cause infection.

The skin is a favorite site for microorganisms to grow and multiply. Without proper skin preparation (Procedure 46-2), the risk of postoperative wound infection is high. Bathing the evening before surgery with an antimicrobial soap (for example hexachlorophene or chlorhexidine) is believed to be effective in reducing the incidence of postoperative wound infections (Ayliffe et al., 1983). Many surgeons have clients bathe or shower the evening prior to surgery. Some may order clients to bathe

PROCEDURE 46-2

Skin Preparation For Surgery

STEPS	RATIONALE
1. Inspect general condition of skin.	If lesions, irritations, or signs of skin infection are present, shaving should not be done. These conditions increase chances for postoperative wound infections.
2. Review physician's order for area to be clipped (Review institution's operating room manual as needed.)	Extent of area for hair removal depends upon site of incision, nature of surgery, and physician's preference. Area is always larger than actual incision to ensure wide perimeter with minimal bacteria.
3. Prepare necessary equipment and supplies:	Ensures smooth procedure.
a. Portable lamp	Needed if room light is not sufficient. Good lighting important to inspect skin condition.
b. Bath blanket	Used for draping client to provide privacy.
c. Towel or waterproof pad	
Clipping:	
a. Electric clippers	Used ro remove short hair.
b. Scissors	Used to cut long body hair.
c. Towel	
d. Cotton balls, applicators, and antiseptic solution (optional)	
Wet shave:	
a. Razor with extra blade	Sharp blade minimizes skin abrasion.
b. Clean basin with warm water	
c. Gauze sponges	
d. Basin with liquid antiseptic soap mixed with water. (Avoid using iodophor for clients with allergies.)	
e. Waterproof underpad or towels	
f. Washcloth, bath blanket	
g. Cotton balls, cotton applicators, and antiseptic solution (optional)	Used to cleanse skin in body crevices (optional).
h. Disposable gloves (optional)	
4. Explain procedure and rationale for removal of hair over large surface area.	Promotes cooperation and minimizes anxiety because client may think incision will be as large as clipped site.
5. Wash hands.	Reduces transmission of infection.
6. Close room doors or bedside curtains.	Provides client privacy.
7. Raise bed to high position.	Avoids need to bend over for long periods of time.
8. Position client comfortably with surgical site accessible.	Hair removal and skin preparation can take several minutes. Nurse should have easy access to hard-to-reach areas.
9. Hair clipping:	
a. Lightly dry area to be clipped with towel.	Removes moisture, which interferes with clean cut of clippers.
b. Hold clippers in dominant hand, about 1 cm above skin, and cut hair in direction it grows. Clip small area at time.	Prevents pulling on hair and abrasion of skin.
c. Arrange drapes as necessary.	Prevents unnecessary exposure of body parts.
d. Lightly brush off cut hair with towel.	Removes contaminated hair and promotes client's comfort. Improves visibility of area being clipped.
e. When clipped area is over body crevices, (for example, umbilicus or groin), clean crevices with cotton-tipped applicators or cotton ball dipped in antiseptic solution, then dry.	Removes secretions, dirt, and any remaining hair clippings, which harbor microorganisms.
10. Wet shave	
a. Place towel or waterproof pads under body part to be shaved.	Prevents soiling of bed linen.

Continued.

Skin Preparation For Surgery

STEPS	RATIONALE
b. Drape client with bath blanket, leaving only area to be shaved at one time (10-20 cm [4-8 in]) exposed.	Prevents unnecessary exposure of body parts and reduces client's anxiety.
c. Adjust lamp.	Provides maximum skin illumination.
d. Apply gloves if desired.	Prevents exposure to blood resulting from accidental cuts.
e. Lather skin with gauze sponges dipped in antiseptic soap.	Softens hair and reduces friction from razor.
f. Shave small area at a time. With nondominant hand hold gauze sponge to stabilize skin. Hold razor at 45-degree angle in dominant hand and shave hair in direction it grows. Use short, gentle strokes.	Shaving small areas minimizes cutting skin; shaving in direction hair grows prevents pulling.
g. Rinse razor in basin of water as soap and hair accumulate on the blade. Change and discard blades as they become dull.	Maintains clean, sharp razor edge to promote client's comfort.
h. Rearrange bath blanket as each portion of shave is completed.	Maintains client's comfort and privacy.
i. Use washcloth and warm water to rinse away remaining hair and soap solution. Change water as needed.	Reduces skin irritation and improves visibility of skin.
j. If shaved area is over body crevices (for example, umbilicus or groin), cleanse with cotton tipped applicators or cotton balls dipped in antiseptic solution.	Removes secretions, dirt, and other remaining hair clippings, which harbor microorganisms.
k. Dry crevices with cotton balls or applicators.	Reduces maceration of skin from retained moisture.
l. Discard waterproof towel or pad.	Reduces spread of microorganisms.
m. Observe skin closely for nicks or cuts.	Any break in skin integrity increases risk of wound infection.
11. Tell client that procedure is completed.	Relieves client's anxiety.
12. Clean and dispose of equipment according to policy and dispose of gloves.	Proper disposal of soiled equipment prevents spread of infection and reduces risk of injury from razor blades.
14. Inspect condition of skin after completion of hair removal.	Determines if there is remaining hair or if skin was cut.
15. Record procedure, area clipped or shaved, and condition of skin before and after in nurse's notes.	Documents procedure performed and condition of skin before surgery.

or shower more than once while others may have clients give special attention to cleansing the proposed operative site. Depending on the surgical procedure, a client may repeat a shower the morning of surgery.

If the surgical procedure involves the head, neck, or upper chest area, the client may also be required to shampoo the hair. Cleansing and trimming of fingernails and toenails are necessary when the surgeon desires strict asepsis, as in the case of certain transplant procedures.

In the past a surgical client's skin was thoroughly shaved to remove hair around the incision site. The rationale for the procedure was to remove microorganisms residing in body hair. However, studies have shown that shaving the surgical site increases the incidence of

postoperative wound infection (Cruse and Foord, 1980). Shaving with a razor can cause superficial cuts and nicks in the skin that allow microorganisms to grow. The CDC recommends avoiding hair removal or, if necessary, shaving only immediately before to the operation. (Garner, 1985). Clippers are preferred over shaving. However, there are hospitals and surgical clinics that still perform shaving. The nurse should consult an institution's policy and procedure manual.

Another way to reduce the risk of a postoperative wound infection is to keep a client's preoperative hospital stay short. A number of researchers have shown that this is associated with low wound infection rates (Cruse, and Foord, 1980; Halsey, 1981). Clients are less likely to acquire pathogens from the hospital environment.

3. *Prevent bowel and bladder incontinence.* At one time clients routinely received enemas before surgery because general anesthesia slows gastrointestinal motility. Emptying the client's intestinal tract reduces the chance that constipation will develop postoperatively.

Today a client may not receive a bowel preparation unless surgery involves the gastrointestinal system. Manipulation of portions of the gastrointestinal tract during surgery results in absence of peristalsis for 24 hours and sometimes longer. Enemas and cathartics cleanse the gastrointestinal tract to prevent postoperative constipation, as well as incontinence during surgery. An empty bowel reduces risk of injury to the intestines and prevents contamination of the operative wound should a portion of the bowel be incised or opened. The surgeon's order may read "give enemas until clear." This means the nurse is to administer enemas until the enema return contains no fecal material (see Chapter 39). Too many enemas given over a short period of time, however, can cause serious fluid and electrolyte imbalances. Most agencies recommend a limit to the number of enemas a nurse may administer successively.

4. *Promoting rest and comfort.* Rest is essential for normal healing. Anxiety about surgery can easily interfere with the client's ability to relax or sleep. The underlying condition necessitating surgery may be painful, further impairing rest.

The nurse should attempt to make the client's environment quiet and comfortable. Frequently, the physician orders a sedative-hypnotic or antianxiety agent for the night before surgery. Sedative-hypnotics (for example, flurazepam [Dalmane]) effect and promote sleep. Antianxiety agents (for example, alprazolam [Xanax] and diazepam [Valium]) act on the cerebral cortex and limbic system to relieve anxiety.

An advantage to ambulatory surgery or same-day surgical admissions is that the client is able to sleep at home the night before surgery. The client is likely to get more rest in a familiar environment.

DAY OF SURGERY

On the morning before surgery the nurse completes a number of routine procedures before releasing the client for surgery.

1. *The nurse checks medical record contents and completes recording.* Before the client goes to the operating room, the nurse checks the contents of the medical record to be sure pertinent laboratory and test results are present. The nurse checks consent forms for accuracy of information. A preoperative checklist (Fig. 46-3) provides the nurse with guidelines for ensuring completion of nursing interventions. The nurse also checks the

BEND PEEL TAB - FORM #52-1 REVISED 1/77			
BARNES HOSPITAL SURGICAL CHECK LIST			
NAME:		DATE:	
ITEM	YES	NO	NURSE SIGNATURE
I.D. band on			
Face sheet in chart			
Name plate in chart			
Operative Permit signed			
History & Physical in chart			
Patient on proper service			
Operative area prepped and checked			
Blood work in chart and within normal limits			
Urinalysis in chart			
Allergies noted as to whether or not present			
Chest X-ray done if ordered EKG			
V.S. taken & charted			
Jewelry removed or secured to patient			
Dentures, eyeglasses, contact lenses, nail polish, hairpins, or prothesis removed			
Patient in hospital pajamas			
Voided or catheterized			
Has patient been NPO			
Pre-op med given			
TIME_____			

Fig. 46-3 Preoperative checklist.
Courtesy Barnes Hospital, St. Louis.

nurse's notes to be sure documentation of nursing care is current. This is especially important if the hospitalized client experienced unpredicted problems the night before surgery.

2. *The nurse checks vital signs.* The nurse makes a final preoperative assessment of vital signs. The anesthesiologist will use these values as a baseline for comparing intraoperative vital signs. If preoperative vital signs prove to be abnormal, there may be a need to postpone surgery. For example, an elevated temperature increases the client's surgical risk. The nurse notifies the physician of vital sign abnormalities before sending the client to the operating room.

3. *The nurse provides hygiene.* Basic hygiene measures provide an additional level of comfort before surgery. If the hospitalized client is unwilling to take a complete bath, a partial bath is refreshing and removes irritating secretions or drainage from the skin. Since the client

cannot wear personal nightwear to the operating room, the nurse provides a clean hospital gown. After being allowed nothing by the mouth throughout the night, the client usually has a very dry mouth. The nurse may offer mouthwash and toothpaste, again cautioning the client not to swallow water.

4. *The nurse checks hair and cosmetics.* During surgery under general anesthesia the anesthesiologist positions the client's head in order to introduce an endotracheal tube into the airway (see Chapter 36). This procedure may involve manipulation of the client's hair and scalp. To avoid injury the nurse asks the client to remove hairpins or clips before leaving for surgery. Hairpieces or wigs should also be removed. Long hair can be braided to keep it in place. The client will wear a paper hair net before entering the operating room.

During and after surgery the anesthesiologist and nurses assess skin and mucous membranes to determine oxygenation and circulation. The client must remove all makeup (lipstick, powder, blush, nail polish) to expose normal skin and nail coloring.

5. *The nurse checks removal of prosthetics.* It is easy for any type of prosthetic device to become lost or damaged during surgery. The client must remove all prosthetics including partial or complete dentures, artificial limbs, artificial eyes, and contact lenses. Hearing aids, false eyelashes, and eyeglasses must also be removed. If a client has a brace or splint, the nurse checks with the physician to determine if it should remain with the client.

For many clients it is embarrassing to remove dentures or other devices that enhance appearance. Thus privacy should be offered as the dentures are removed. Dentures must be placed in special containers for safekeeping to prevent breakage, and the client assessed for any loose teeth. A broken tooth can become dislodged during insertion of an endotracheal tube and obstruct the airway.

In many agencies nurses must inventory all prosthetic devices and have them locked away for safekeeping. It is also common practice for nurses to give prosthetics to family members or to keep the devices at the client's bedside.

6. *The nurse prepares the bowel and bladder.* The client may require an enema or cathartic the morning of surgery. If so, it should be given at least an hour before the client is scheduled to leave, allowing time for the client to defecate and void without rushing. If the client is unable to void, it should be noted on the preoperative checklist.

7. *The nurse checks antiembolic stockings.* Many physicians prefer clients to wear antiembolic stockings during surgery. The stockings provide support to the lower extremities and maintain compression of small veins and capillaries. The constant compression forces blood into larger vessels, thus promoting venous return and preventing circulatory stasis. When correctly sized and applied properly, antiembolism stockings can prevent formation of thrombi. Chapter 42 reviews the procedure for sizing and application.

8. *The nurse promotes the client's dignity.* During preoperative preparations a client's care can become depersonalized unless the nurse maintains the client's privacy and reduces sources of anxiety. Ambulatory and same-day surgical admission clients often must sit in a waiting room before surgery. To protect client's modesty the nurse allows them to wear underclothes whenever possible and provide cover robes. Hospitalized clients should be ensured privacy by closing room curtains or doors during preoperative preparation. Family may be allowed to stay until it is time for transport to the operating room.

9. *The nurse performs special procedures.* A client's condition may warrant special interventions before leaving for the operating room. The surgeon's orders inform nurses of the need to start intravenous infusions, insert Foley catheters, or administer medications preoperatively.

One special procedure involves insertion of a nasogastric tube, a pliable plastic tube, through the client's nasopharynx into the stomach (Procedure 46-3). The tube has a hollow lumen that allows removal of gastric secretions, as well as introduction of solutions into the stomach. There are several purposes and types of tubes for nasogastric intubation (Table 46-6). For a surgical

TABLE 46-6   Purposes of Nasogastric Intubation

Purpose	Description	Type of Tube
Decompression	Removal of secretions and gaseous substances from the gastrointestinal tract; prevention or relief of abdominal distention	Salem sump, Levin, Miller-Abbott
Feeding (gavage)	Instillation of liquid nutritional supplements or feedings into the stomach for clients unable to swallow fluid	Duo, Dobhoff, Levin
Compression	Internal application of pressure by means of an inflated balloon to prevent internal gastrointestinal hemorrhage	Sengstaken-Blakemore
Lavage	Irrigation of stomach in cases of active bleeding, poisoning, or gastric dilation	Levin, Ewald, Salem sump

PROCEDURE 46-3

Inserting and Maintaining a Nasogastric (NG) Tube

STEPS	RATIONALE
1. Inspect condition of client's oral cavity. (Use of gloves is recommended.)	Determines baseline condition of oral cavity so as to determine need for special nursing measures for oral hygiene following tube placement.
2. Palpate client's abdomen.	Baseline determination of level of abdominal distention will later serve as comparison once tube is inserted.
3. Check medical record for surgeon's order, type of NG tube to be placed, and whether tube is to be attached to suction or drainage bag.	Procedure requires physician's order. Adequate decompression depends on suction.
4. Prepare necessary equipment and supplies:	
a. #14 or #16 Fr NG tube (smaller lumen for child)	For decompression, smaller lumen catheters are not used because they must be able to remove thick secretions.
b. Water-soluble lubricating jelly	Lubricates tube for insertion.
c. Stethoscope	Determines tube placement.
d. Tongue blade	
e. Flashlight	
f. Asepto blub or cone tip syringe	Irrigate or instill fluid into tube.
g. 1 in (2.5 cm) wide hypoallergenic tape	Hypoallergenic tape prevents loss of skin on nose.
h. Safety pin and rubber band	
i. Clamp, drainage bag, or suction machine	NG tube may be open or closed to drainage.
j. Bath towel	
k. Emesis basin with ice (optional)	
l. Glass of water with straw	
m. Facial tissues	
n. Normal saline	For irrigation of tube.
o. Tincture of Benzoin (optional)	Increases adhesion of tape to nose.
5. Identify client and explain procedure	Identification prevents error and gains client's cooperation to facilitate passage of tube and lessen possibility that client will remove tube.
6. Position client in high Fowler's position with pillows behind head and shoulders. Raise bed to its highest horizontal level.	Promotes client's ability to swallow during procedure. Good body mechanics prevents injury to nurse or client.
7. Wash hands.	Reduces transmission of infection.
8. Assemble equipment at bedside and place on side of bed nearest nurse.	Procedure should be organized to limit client's discomfort.
9. Pull curtain around bed or close room door.	Provides privacy.
10. Stand on client's right side if right-handed; left side if left-handed.	Allows easiest manipulation of tubing.
11. If NG tube is too pliable, place in emesis basin and cover with ice (optional).	Stiffens tube for easier insertion.
12. Place bath towel over client's chest; give facial tissues to client.	Prevents soiling of client's gown. Tube insertion through nasal passages may cause tearing.
13. Instruct client to relax and breathe normally while occluding one naris. Then repeat this action for other naris. Select nostril with greater air flow.	Tube passes more easily through naris that is more patent.
14. Measure distance to insert tube by placing tip of tube at client's nose and extending tube first to tip of earlobe and then from earlobe down to xiphoid process of sternum (see illustration).	Tube should extend from nares to stomach; distance varies with each client.
15. Mark length of tube to be inserted with piece of tape or note distance of point from next tube marking.	Marks amount of tube to be inserted from nares to stomach.
16. Curve 4-6 in (10-15 cm) of end of tube tightly around index finger; then release.	Curving tube tip aids insertion.
17. Lubricate 3-4 in (7.5-10 cm) of end of tube with water-soluble lubricating jelly.	Minimizes friction against nasal mucosa.

Continued.

Inserting and Maintaining a Nasogastric (NG) Tube

STEPS	RATIONALE
18. Initially instruct client to extend the neck back against pillow; insert tube slowly through naris with curved end pointing downward.	Facilitates initial passage of tube through naris and maintains clear airway for open naris.
19. Continue to pass tube along floor of nasal passage aiming down toward ear. When resistance is felt, apply gentle downward pressure to advance tube (do not force past resistance).	Minimizes discomfort of tube rubbing against upper nasal turbinates. Resistance is caused by posterior nasopharynx. Downward pressure helps tube curl around corner of nasopharynx.
20. If resistance is met, withdraw tube, allow client to rest, relubricate tube and insert into other naris.	Forcing against resistance can cause trauma to mucosa. Helps relieve client's anxiety.
21. Continue insertion of tube until just past nasopharynx by gently rotating tube toward opposite nares.	
a. Stop tube advancement, allow client to relax, and provide tissues.	Relieves client's anxiety; tearing is natural response to mucosal irritation.
b. Explain to client that next step requires him or her to swallow.	Tube about to enter esophagus.
22. With tube just above oropharynx, instruct client to flex head forward and dry swallow or suck in air through straw. Advance tube 2.5-5 cm (1-2 in) with each swallow. If client has trouble swallowing and is allowed fluids, offer glass of water. Advance tube with each swallow of water.	Flexed position closes off upper airway to trachea and opens esophagus. Swallowing closes epiglottis over trachea and helps move the tube into the esophagus. Swallowing water reduces gagging or choking.
23. If client begins to cough, gag, or choke, stop tube advancement. Instruct client to breathe easily and take sips of water.	Tubing may accidentally enter larynx and initiate cough reflex. Gagging is eased by swallowing water.
24. If client continues to cough, pull tube back slightly.	Tube may enter larynx and obstruct airway.
25. If client continues to gag, check back of pharynx using flashlight and tongue blade.	Tube may coil around itself in back of throat.
26. After client relaxes, continue to advance tube desired distance.	Tip of tube should be within stomach to decompress properly.
Checking Tube Placement	
27. Ask client to talk.	Client would be unable to talk if NG tube has passed through vocal cords.
28. Check posterior pharynx for presence of coiled tube.	Tube is pliable and can coil up back of pharynx instead of advancing into esophagus.
29. Attach cone-tipped syringe to end of NG tube. Place diaphragm of stethoscope over upper left quadrant of abdomen just below costal margin. Inject 10-20 cc of air while auscultating abdomen (see illustration).	Air entering stomach creates "whooshing" sound and confirms tube placement in stomach. Absence of sound indicates tip of tube is still in esophagus.

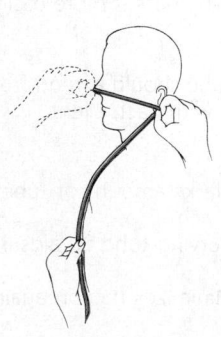

Step 14

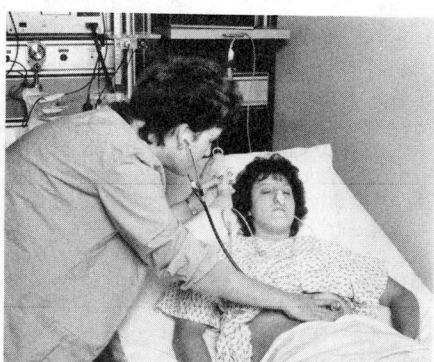

Step 29

STEPS	RATIONALE
30. Aspirate gently back on syringe to obtain gastric contents. (optional—check pH of gastric contents).	Placement of tube in stomach should result in return of gastric contents. Gentle suction prevents collapse and closure of tube tip. (Gastric contents are acidic and intestinal contents are basic)
31. If tube is not in stomach, advance another 1-2 in (2.5-5 cm) and repeat Steps 29 and 30 to check tube position.	NG tube must be in stomach to provide decompression.

Anchoring Tube

32. After tube is properly inserted, either clamp end or connect it to drainage bag or suction machine.	Drainage bag is used for gravity drainage. Intermittent suction is most effective for decompression. Client going to operating room often will have tube clamped.
33. Tape NG tube to client's nose; avoid putting pressure on nares. Cut 10 cm (4 in) long piece of tape. Split the bottom 2 in of tape in half lengthwise. Apply small amount of tincture of benzoin to lower end of nose and allow to dry (optional). Place top end of tape over nose and carefully wrap the two split ends around the tube (see illustration).	Prevents tissue necrosis. Tape anchors tube securely. Benzoin prevents loosening of tape if client perspires.
34. Fasten end of NG tube to client's gown by looping rubber band around tube in slip knot. Pin rubber band to gown (provides slack for movement).	Reduces pressure on the nares if tube moves.
35. Unless physician orders otherwise, head of bed should be elevated 30 degrees.	Helps prevent esophageal reflux and minimizes irritation of tube against posterior pharynx.
36. Explain to client that sensation of tube will decrease somewhat.	Adaptation to continued sensory stimulus.
37. Wash hands.	Reduces transmission of microorganisms.
38. Record time and type of NG tube inserted, client's tolerance to procedure, confirmation of placement, character of gastric contents and whether tube is changed or connected to drainage device in nurse's notes.	Documents procedure performed correctly. Description of gastric contents provides baseline to determine change.

Tube Irrigation

39. Check tube placement.	Prevents accidental entrance of irrigating solution into lungs.
40. Draw up 30 ml of normal saline into Asepto or cone-tipped syringe.	Use of saline minimizes loss of electrolytes from stomach fluids.
41. Clamp connection tubing proximal to connection site for drainage or suction apparatus. Disconnect tubing and lay end on towel.	Reduces backflow of secretions and soiling of client's gown and bed linen.

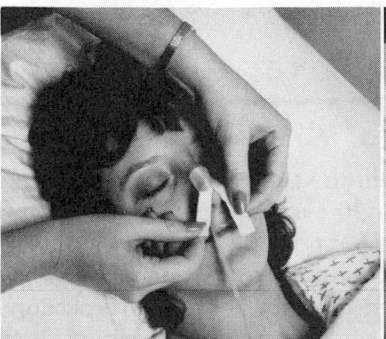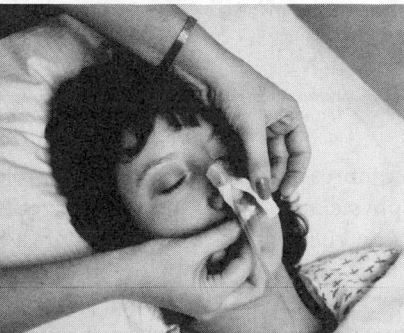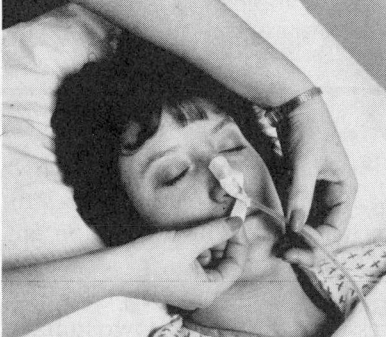

Step 33

Continued

Inserting and Maintaining a Nasogastric (NG) Tube

STEPS	RATIONALE
42. Insert tip of irrigating syringe into end of NG tube. Hold syringe with tip pointed at floor and inject saline slowly and evenly. (Do not force solution).	Position of syringe prevents introduction of air into vent tubing, which could cause gastric distention. Solution introduced under pressure can cause gastric trauma.
43. If resistance occurs, check for kinks in tubing. Turn client onto left side. Repeated resistance should be reported to surgeon.	Tip of tube may lie against stomach lining. Buildup of secretions will cause distention.
44. After instilling saline, immediately aspirate or pull back slowly on syringe to withdraw fluid. Measure volume returned as output.	Irrigation clears tubing so stomach should remain empty. Fluid remaining in stomach is measured as intake.
45. Reconnect NG tube to drainage or suction. (If solution does not return, repeat irrigation.)	Reestablishes drainage collection; may repeat irrigation or repositioning of tube until NG tube drains properly.
46. Wash hands.	Reduces transmission of microorganisms.
47. Record each irrigation; type and amount of solution used, character, and volume of aspirate.	Documents procedure and results.

Discontinuation of NG Tube

STEPS	RATIONALE
48. Turn off suction and disconnect NG tube from drainage bag or suction. Remove tape from bridge of nose and unpin tube from gown.	Have tube free of connections before removal.
49. Explain procedure to client and reassure that removal is less distressing than insertion.	Minimizes anxiety and increases cooperation. Tube passes out smoothly.
50. Hand the client facial tissue; place clean towel across his chest. Instruct him to take and hold deep breath.	Airway will be temporarily obstructed during tube's removal. Client may wish to blow nose after tube is removed.
51. Clamp or kink tubing securely and then pull tube out steadily and smoothly while client holds breath.	Reduces trauma to mucosa and minimizes client's discomfort. Clamping prevents tube contents from draining into oropharynx.
52. Measure unit of drainage and note character of content. Dispose of tube and drainage equipment. Measure unit of drainage.	Reduces transfer of microorganisms. Provides accurate measure of fluid output.
53. Clean nares and provide mouth care.	Promotes comfort.
54. Position client comfortably and explain procedure for drinking fluids.	Depends on physician's order; usually begins with small amount of ice chips each hour and increases as client is able to tolerate more.
55. Clean equipment and return to proper place. Place soiled linen in "dirty" utility room or proper receptacle.	Proper disposal of equipment prevents spread of microorganisms and ensures proper exchange procedures.
56. Wash hands.	Reduces spread of infection.
57. Palpate client's abdomen periodically, noting any distention.	Determines success of abdominal decompression.
58. Inspect condition of nares and nose.	Evaluates status of skin and tissue integrity.
59. Record removal of nasogastric tube, client's tolerance of the procedure, presence of bowel sounds, and abdominal assessment.	Documents procedure and provides baseline information regarding abdominal assessment and presence of bowel sounds.

client the main purpose is stomach decompression to prevent abdominal distention. Often the physician waits to order nasogastric tube insertion until the client is in the operating room.

The Salem sump tube is preferable for stomach decompression. The tube has two lumina: one for removal of gastric contents and one to provide an air vent. A blue "pigtail" is the air vent that connects with the second lumen. When the sump tube's main lumen is connected to suction, the air vent permits free, continuous drainage of secretions. The air vent should never be clamped off or connected to suction.

The procedure for tube insertion (Procedure 46-3) does not require sterile technique. The nurse simply uses good clean technique. The procedure is uncomfortable. The client experiences a burning sensation as the tube passes through the sensitive nasal mucosa. When the tube reaches the back of the pharynx, the client may begin to gag. The nurse must help the client try to relax to make tube insertion easier.

One of the greatest problems in caring for a client with a nasogastric tube is maintaining comfort. The tube is a constant irritation to nasal mucosa. The nurse must assess the condition of the nares and mucosa daily for inflammation and excoriation. As the tape used to anchor the tube becomes soiled, the nurse changes it to lessen irritation. Frequently lubrication of the nares also minimizes excoriation. With one naris occluded, the client may breathe through the mouth. Frequent mouth care (at least every 2 hours) helps minimize dehydration. Keeping a glass of cool water for rinsing the mouth close to the client's reach is useful, but the client who is to receive nothing by mouth should not swallow the water. The client will frequently complain of a sore throat. An ice bag applied externally to the throat sometimes helps.

Once the client is intubated, the nurse must maintain the tube's patency. If the tip of the tubing rests against the stomach wall or if the tube becomes blocked with thick secretions, it is necessary for the nurse to irrigate the tube regularly. Flushing the tube with normal saline by way of a cone-tipped syringe clears blockage within the tube (Procedure 46-3). If a nasogastric tube continues to drain improperly after irrigation, the nurse must reposition it by advancing or withdrawing it slightly. Any change in position requires reassessment of tube placement.

The nasogastric tube can actually cause distention unless the nurse manages the client correctly. Presence of the tube in the nose causes many clients to swallow large volumes of air. Channels of gastric secretions also form along the walls of the stomach and bypass the suction holes. Turning the client regularly helps to collapse the channels and promote emptying of stomach contents.

10. *The nurse safeguards valuables.* If a client has any valuables, the nurse should either turn them over to family members or secure them for safekeeping. Many hospitals require clients to sign a release to free the institution of responsibility for lost valuables. Valuables can usually be stored and locked in a designated location. Often clients are reluctant to remove wedding rings or religious medals. A wedding band can be taped in place; however, if there is a risk that the client will experience swelling of the hand or fingers, the band should be removed. Many hospitals allow clients to pin religious medals to their gowns, although the risk of loss increases.

11. *The nurse administers preoperative medications.* The anesthesiologist or surgeon will order preanesthetic drugs that reduce the client's anxiety, the amount of general anesthesia required, and respiratory tract secretions. Tranquilizers such as chlorpromazine (Thorazine)

or diazepam (Valium) reduce anxiety and relax skeletal muscles. Narcotic analgesics such as meperidine (Demerol) or morphine provide sedation, reduce pain and anxiety, and reduce the amount of anesthetic required during surgery. Drugs such as glycopyrrolate (Robinul) or atropine create anticholinergic effects to inhibit mucous secretions in the oral and respiratory passages and prevent spasm of laryngeal muscles.

Typically the physician orders preoperative medications to be administered when the client leaves for the operating room or at an earlier prescribed time. The nurse provides all nursing care measures before giving the client preoperative medications. Since the drugs cause sedation, the client should not be allowed to leave the bed or stretcher until surgical orderlies and nurses arrive to transport the client to the operating room. The client should be warned to anticipate drowsiness and dry mouth, although the medications usually do not induce sleep. The side rails should be raised and the bed or stretcher kept in the low position for client safety.

EVALUATION

Often there is limited time to evaluate the outcomes of the nurse's preoperative plan of care. The client's surgery may be an emergency, or performance of various procedures may make it difficult for the nurse to find time for evaluation. The nurse's interventions may continue intraoperatively and postoperatively so that evaluation does not occur until after surgery. For example, the nurse will not be able to evaluate the success of reducing postoperative wound infection or promoting return of normal physiological function until a few days after surgery.

The nurse can evaluate success at preoperative teaching, as well as promoting the client's physiological function and achievement of rest and physical comfort (see evaluation box). However, evaluation of these interventions must also continue postoperatively.

Transport to the Operating Room

Personnel in the operating room notify the nursing division or ambulatory surgical waiting area when it is time for surgery. In many hospitals a nursing orderly or transporter brings a stretcher for transporting the client. The transporter checks the client's identification bracelet against the client's chart to be sure the right person is going to surgery. Because the client has already received preoperative drugs, the nurses and transporter will assist the client in transferring from bed to stretcher to prevent falls.

Sample Evaluation of Interventions for Preoperative Client

Goals	Evaluative Measures	Expected Outcomes
Client understands physiological and psychological responses to surgery.	Ask client and family to identify basic purpose of surgery and changes to expect postoperatively.	Client describes purpose for having surgery and physical or psychological changes to expect.
Client understands intraoperative and postoperative events.	Ask client and family to identify: appropriate times of surgery; routine types of postoperative monitoring and treatment.	Client and family will describe events that will occur postoperatively.
Cient achieves return of normal physiological function postoperatively.	Have client demonstrate deep breathing, coughing, splinting, foot and leg exercises, and turning.	Client is able to ventilate to maximum ability, cough forcibly, perform exercises and turn correctly postoperatively.
Client achieves rest and comfort.	Observe time client falls asleep after bedtime. Ask if client feels rested upon awakening in morning.	Client falls asleep within 30 minutes after bedtime. Client reports feeling rested and at ease.

The family gets one last opportunity to visit before the client is transported to the operating room. Nurses then direct the family to a waiting area.

Once the client leaves the nursing division, the nurse prepares the bed and room for the client's return, if returning to the same nursing division. A postoperative bedside unit should include:

1. Sphygmomanometer, stethoscope, and thermometer
2. Emesis basin
3. Clean gown
4. Washcloth, towel, and facial tissues
5. Intravenous pole
6. Suction equipment
7. Oxygen equipment
8. Extra pillows for positioning the client comfortably
9. Bed pads to protect bed linen from drainage

The nurse will be better prepared to care for the client postoperatively if the room is readied well in advance of the client's return.

INTRAOPERATIVE SURGICAL PHASE

Care of the client during surgery requires careful preparation and knowledge of the events that occur during the surgical procedure.

Holding Area

In most hospitals the client enters a holding area outside the operating room. Here the nurse explains the steps to be taken in preparing the client for surgery. Nurses in the holding area are usually part of the operating room staff and wear surgical scrub suits, hats, and footwear in accordance with infection control policies. In some ambulatory surgical settings a perioperative primary nurse admits the client, circulates for the operative procedure, recovers, and discharges the client.

In the holding area the nurse or anesthesiologist will insert an intravenous catheter into the arm to establish a route for fluid replacement and intravenous drugs. A large-bore intravenous catheter is used for easy infusion of fluids. The nurse will also apply a blood pressure cuff. It will remain in place throughout surgery for the anesthesiologist to assess blood pressure readings.

By this time the client begins to feel drowsy. Because the temperature in the holding area and adjacent operating room suites is usually cool, the client should be offered an extra blanket. The stay in the holding area should be brief.

Admission to the Operating Room

Nurses transfer the client to the operating room via stretcher. The client is usually still awake and will notice nurses and physicians wearing complete surgical masks and gowns. The staff carefully transfers the client to the operating table, being sure both the stretcher and table are locked in place. Once the client is on the table, the nurse fastens a safety strap around the client.

The operating room nurse goes through a checklist, checking the client's identification and chart, reviewing consent forms, medical history, physical assessment findings, and test results, making sure prosthetic devices and valuables have been removed, and reviewing the nursing care plan to establish an intraoperative care plan.

The nurse may apply monitoring devices to the client before surgery begins. Clients receiving general and regional anesthesia undergo continuous electrocardiographic monitoring during surgery. Small plastic electrodes are placed on the chest and extremities to record electrical activity of the heart. A monitor in the operating room displays the heart's electrical activity.

Many ambulatory surgical clients remain awake during the procedure since only local anesthetic is used. The nurse supports the client by explaining procedures and encouraging the client to ask questions. Sights and sounds in the surgical suite can frighten clients.

Introduction of Anesthesia

Clients undergoing surgical procedures will receive anesthesia in one of three ways: general, regional, or local.

GENERAL ANESTHESIA

Under general anesthesia a client loses all sensation and consciousness. Muscles relax to ease manipulation of body parts. The client also experiences amnesia of all surgical events. Surgery using general anesthesia involves major procedures requiring extensive tissue manipulation.

An anesthesiologist gives general anesthetics by intravenous and inhalation routes through the four stages of anesthesia:

Stage 1   Begins with client awake; client gradually becomes drowsy and loses consciousness; state of analgesia begins

Stage 2   Stage of excitement; client's muscles are often tense and almost spasmodic; swallowing and vomiting reflexes remain intact; client may have an irregular breathing pattern

Stage 3   Begins with onset of regular rhythmical breathing; vital functions depressed; reflexes are depressed or temporarily lost; surgeon begins operation during this phase

Stage 4   Stage of complete respiratory depression; can be fatal

To move the client quickly to stage 3 of general anesthesia the anesthesiologist usually gives an intravenous dose of a barbiturate. To prevent possible aspiration and other respiratory complications the anesthesiologist puts an endotracheal tube into the client's airway. Succinylcholine causes temporary paralysis of vocal cords and respiratory muscles while the client is intubated. The anesthesiologist then provides artificial ventilation until succinylcholine's effects wear off and the client again breathes spontaneously. From that point anesthetic gases

or vapors are usually delivered by inhalation through the endotracheal tube. The client also receives a continuous supply of oxygen.

The duration of anesthesia depends on the length of surgery. Surgical risks influence how long a surgeon is willing to prolong surgery. The greatest risks from general anesthesia are the side effects of anesthetic agents, including cardiovascular depression or irritability, respiratory depression, and liver and kidney damage.

REGIONAL ANESTHESIA

Induction of regional anesthesia results in loss of sensation in an area of the body. The method of induction influences which portion of sensory pathways is anesthetized. The anesthesiologist gives regional anesthetics by infiltration and local application (see Chapter 35). In major surgery, such as a hernia repair, vaginal hysterectomy, or vascular repair of leg blood vessels, only infiltrative induction is used.

Infiltration of anesthetic agents may involve one of three induction methods:

1. *Nerve block.* Local anesthetic is injected into a nerve (for example, brachial plexus to the arm) blocking the nerve supply to the operative site.
2. *Spinal anesthesia.* The anesthesiologist performs a lumbar puncture and introduces local anesthetic into the cerebrospinal fluid in the spinal subarachnoid space. Anesthesia can extend from the tip of the xiphoid process down to the feet. Positioning of the client influences movement of the anesthetic agent up or down the spinal cord.
3. *Epidural anesthesia.* This is a safer procedure than spinal anesthesia, because the anesthetic agent is injected into the epidural space outside the dura mater, and the level of anesthesia is not as great as spinal anesthesia. Because epidural anesthesia provides an effective loss of sensation in the vaginal and perineal areas, it is the best anesthetic for obstetrical procedures.
4. *Caudal anesthesia.* A form of epidural anesthesia achieved by giving the local anesthetic at the base of the spine. The extent of anesthesia only affects the pelvic region and legs.

There are risks involved with infiltrative anesthetics, particularly in the case of spinal anesthesia, because the level of anesthesia may rise. The client may have a sudden fall in blood pressure, which results from extensive vasodilation caused by the anesthetic block to sympathetic vasomotor nerves, pain, and motor fibers. If the level of anesthesia rises, respiratory paralysis may develop, necessitating resuscitation by the anesthesiologist. The client requires careful monitoring during and immediately after surgery.

The client under regional anesthesia is awake throughout the surgery unless the physician orders a tranquilizer that allows sleep. Because the client is responsive and capable of breathing voluntarily, it is not necessary for the anesthesiologist to use an endotracheal tube. Operating room personnel often gain a false sense of security because of the client's relative alertness. Nurses must remember that burns and other trauma can occur on the anesthetized part of the body without the client being aware of the injury. It is therefore necessary to frequently observe the position of extremities, as well as condition of the skin.

LOCAL ANESTHESIA

Local anesthesia involves loss of sensation at the desired site (for example, a growth on the skin or the cornea of the eye). The anesthetic agent (for example, lidocaine) inhibits nerve conduction until the drug diffuses into the circulation. The client experiences a loss in pain sensation as well as touch, motor, and autonomic activities (for example, bladder emptying). Local anesthesia is commonly used for minor procedures performed in ambulatory surgery.

Positioning the Client for Surgery

During general anesthesia the nursing personnel and surgeon often do not position the client until the stage of complete relaxation. The position is usually determined by the surgical approach. Ideally the client's position provides good access to the operative site and sustains adequate circulatory and respiratory function; it should not impair neuromuscular structures. The client's comfort and safety must be considered.

It is sometimes difficult for nurses in postoperative divisions to appreciate the discomfort a client may feel after surgery (for example, discomfort of the right arm or side of a client whose left kidney was removed) (Fig. 46-4). Normal range of motion is maintained in an alert person by pain and pressure receptors. If a joint is extended too far, pain stimuli provide a warning that muscle and joint strain are too great. In a client who is anesthetized, normal defense mechanisms cannot guard against joint damage, muscle stretch, and strain. The mucles are so relaxed that it is relatively easy to place the client in a position the individual normally could not assume while awake. The client often remains in a given position for several hours. Although it may be necessary to place a client in an unusual position, the nurse should attempt to maintain correct physiological alignment and protect the client from pressure, abrasion, and other injuries. Attachments to the operating table allow for protection and padding of extremities and bony prominences. Positioning should not impede normal movement of the diaphragm or interfere with circulation to body parts. If restraints are necessary, the nurse uses blankets to prevent trauma to the skin.

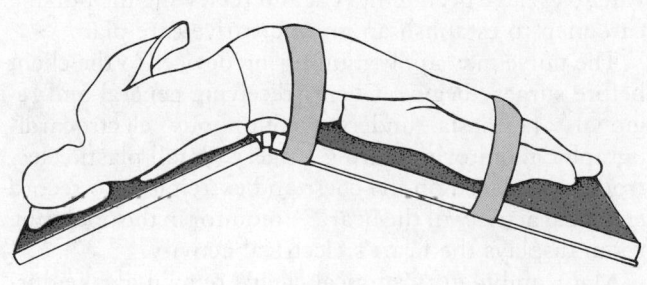

Fig 46-4 Client's position on operating room table for a nephrectomy.

Nurse's Role during Surgery

The nurse assumes one of two roles during the surgical procedure: scrub nurse or circulating nurse. The scrub nurse provides the surgeon with instruments and supplies, which requires strict surgical asepsis (see Chapter 43), as well as familiarity with surgical instruments. Each instrument is designed for a specific purpose during a phase or step in surgery. It takes knowledge and skill to anticipate which instrument the surgeon requires and to pass it quickly and smoothly. The scrub nurse also disposes of soiled gauze sponges and accounts for sponges, needles, and instruments on the surgical field and in body cavities. Since few schools of nursing provide clinical scrub nurse training, most learn on the job.

The circulating nurse is an assistant to the scrub nurse and surgeon. When the client first enters the operating room, the circulator helps position the client and apply necessary equipment and surgical drapes. During surgery the circulator provides the scrub nurse with supplies, disposes of soiled equipment and sponges, and keeps a count of instruments, needles, and sponges used. If there is a need to help reposition the client or move the operating room lights, the circulating nurse is available to assist. Like all members of the surgical team the circulator follows surgical aseptic technique. If a break in asepsis occurs, the circulator assists team members with regowning and regloving.

At the end of each surgical procedure the scrub nurse and circulator count the number of used instruments, needles, and gauze sponges. This procedure prevents the accidental loss of such items within the client's surgical wound. It is not difficult for a sponge saturated with blood to be overlooked within a wound. Careful monitoring of items is essential for the client's safety. The nurse who fails to make accurate counts can be held legally accountable. If a client is injured by a misplaced needle or instrument the nurse may be judged negligent (see Chapter 18).

Barnes Hospital
Nursing Service
Operative Nursing Note

C-22

130658 Rev. 7/86

	Serv.	OpRm #	Anest. Code	Operation			
				Time In		Time Out	
				hr.	min.	hr.	min.
	Flat Rate	Factor					

Date: ___ / ___ / ___

☐ Scheduled ☐ Emergency ☐ Clean ☐ Clean/Contaminated ☐ Contaminated ☐ Dirty

Pre-Op Diagnosis: _____

Procedure: _____
_____
_____

Post-Op Diagnosis: _____

Surgeon: _____
Phys. #: _____
First Asst. _____
Second Asst. _____
Third Asst. _____

Anesthesiologist: _____

Anesthetist: _____
Anesthetic Route: ☐ General ☐ Spinal/Epi.
☐ Local,
☐ Regional

Observers: _____
Scrub Nurse: _____
Circulating Nurse: _____

Initial Counts: _____ Sponge _____ Sharps

C.N. _____
S.N. _____

1st Count: Sponge ☐ Correct Sharp ☐ Correct ☐ Incorrect, Explain _____
C.N. _____ S.N.

2nd Count: Sponge ☐ Correct Sharp ☐ Correct ☐ Incorrect, Explain _____
C.N. _____ S.N.

1. Implants/Prosthesis: _____
   Mftr: _____
   Lot/SN: _____
   Size: _____
   Location: _____
Other:

2. Implants/Prosthesis: _____
   Mftr: _____
   Lot/SN: _____
   Size: _____
   Location: _____

3. Implants/Prosthesis: _____
   Mftr: _____
   Lot/SN: _____
   Size: _____
   Location: _____

Specimens: _____

PREOPERATIVE ASSESSMENT

☐ Operative Permit Verified ☐ Pt. I.D. Verified ☐ Chart Reviewed Allergies: ☐ None Known ☐ Yes, _____
R.N.

Level of Consciousness: ☐ Alert/Oriented ☐ Drowsy ☐ Confused ☐ Unconscious ☐ Sedated
Physical Abnormalities/Limitations: _____
Skin Condition: ☐ Intact ☐ Other, _____
☐ IV _____ ☐ O2 _____ ☐ Foley Catheter _____ ☐ NG _____ ☐ Other, _____ ☐ N/A
Remarks: _____

INTRAOPERATIVE ASSESSMENT

Position: ☐ Supine ☐ Prone ☐ Lithotomy ☐ L. Lateral ☐ R. Lateral ☐ Jacknife ☐ Other, _____
Positioning Aids/Devices: _____
Positioned By: _____ ☐ Safety Strap Applied ☐ Electrosurgical Grounding Plate, Location: _____
Applied By: _____ Cautery Unit Serial Number: _____
Surgical Shave Prep: ☐ Pre-Op ☐ Holding Area ☐ O.R. ☐ N/A
Surgical Skin Prep: _____ Prepped By: _____
Foley Catheter: ☐ N/A ☐ Yes, Size: _____ Description: _____ Inserted By: _____
Irrigation Solutions: ☐ N/A _____

Tourniquet Times: ☐ N/A _____
Medications: ☐ N/A _____

Remarks: _____

POSTOPERATIVE ASSESSMENT

Wound Appearance: ☐ Dry/ Approximated ☐ Other, _____
Dressing: _____ Packing: _____
Drains: ☐ N/A ☐ Yes, Size/Location: _____

Tubes/Drains: ☐ IV _____ ☐ O2 via _____ ☐ Foley Catheter _____
☐ NG _____ ☐ Other _____
Disposition: ☐ PAR ☐ ICU, _____ ☐ O.P. ☐ Pt. Room ☐ Home ☐ Other, _____
Via: ☐ Stretcher ☐ Bed ☐ W.C. ☐ Amb. Accompanied By: _____
Remarks: _____
R.N.

Fig. 46-5 Operative nursing note.
Courtesy Barnes Hospital, St. Louis.

Documentation of Intraoperative Care

During the intraoperative phase the nursing staff continue the plan of care established preoperatively. For example, strict asepsis must be followed to minimize the risk of surgical wound infection (see Chapter 43). Intravenous fluid infusion and monitoring urinary and nasogastric output are actions the nurse takes to maintain fluid balance. Throughout the surgical procedure the nurse keeps an accurate record of client care activities and procedures performed by operating room personnel (Fig. 46-5). Documentation of intraoperative care provides useful data for the nurse who cares for the client postoperatively.

POSTOPERATIVE SURGICAL PHASE

Postoperatively a client's care can become complex as a result of physiological changes that may occur. Clients who have undergone general anesthesia are more likely to face complications than those who have only had local anesthesia. The client who requires general anesthesia usually has undergone extensive surgery as well. In contrast an ambulatory surgical client who had local anesthesia with no sedation and has stable vital signs may be discharged immediately.

To assess a client's postoperative condition the nurse relies on information from the preoperative nursing assessment and on knowledge regarding the surgical procedure performed and events occurring intraoperatively. The nurse must be able to detect change. A slight variation in respiratory rhythm, an increase in wound drainage, or increased restlessness may indicate onset of surgically-related complications.

A client's postoperative course involves two phases: the immediate recovery period and postoperative convalescence. For an ambulatory surgical client recovery normally lasts only one to two hours and convalescence will take place at home. For a hospitalized client recovery may last a few hours with convalescence taking one or more days, depending on the extent of surgery and the client's response.

Immediate Postoperative Recovery

Before the arrival of the client in the recovery room (RR), or postanesthesia room (PAR), the recovery room nurse determines from the surgical team in the operating room the client's general status and need for special equipment and nursing care. Careful planning allows the nursing staff to consider placement of clients in the recovery room. For example, clients who undergo spinal anesthesia are aware of their surroundings and may benefit from being in a quieter part of the recovery room, away from clients needing frequent monitoring. The client with a serious infection should be isolated from other clients.

When the client enters the recovery room, the nurse and members of the surgical team confer about the client's status. The surgical team's report includes a review of anesthetic agents administered so the recovery room nurse can anticipate the ease with which a client should regain consciousness. A report on intravenous fluids or blood products administered during surgery alerts the nurse to the fluid and electrolyte balance. The surgeon often reports special concerns, for example, if the client is at risk for hemorrhaging or infection. The operating room nurse discusses whether there were complications during surgery such as excessive blood loss or cardiac irregularities.

After reviewing events in the operating room, the recovery room nurse makes a complete assessment of the client's status. Until stabilized, the client remains in the recovery room.

The recovery room personnel notify the nursing division of the client's arrival. This allows the nursing staff to inform family members of the client's operative course. The nurse usually advises family members to remain in the designated waiting area so they can be found when the surgeon arrives to explain the client's condition.

Anxiety can arise if the surgeon informs the family preoperatively of the anticipated length of surgery and the client remains in the operating room past this time. Nurses can help relieve family members' concerns by explaining normal delays that occur, such as room preparation or delay in the previous surgery. If the client's stay in recovery is extended, the nurses can explain to the family that the client is being held longer for observation. Should the client have complications, it is the surgeon's responsibility to explain to family members what occurred during surgery.

If the client's surgery was unsuccessful or the surgeon discovered an inoperable condition (for example, a malignant tumor), it is the nurse's responsibility to provide support to the family. Directing the family to the location of public telephones, providing a cup of coffee, or encouraging expression of fears in a private location are a few ways to help the family cope with the waiting period. The family's initial shock requires the nurse to be available and serve as a resource for the family.

After the initial assessment on the client's arrival to recovery, the nurse repeats evaluation of vital signs and other key observations at least every 15 minutes.

RESPIRATION

Certain anesthetic agents may continue to cause respiratory depression. For this reason the nurse is especially alert for shallow, slow breathing and a weak cough. The nurse assesses respiratory rate, rhythm, depth of ventilation, symmetry of chest wall movement, breath sounds, and color of mucous membranes. If the client's breathing is unusually shallow, placement of the hand over the client's face or mouth allows the nurse to feel exhaled air.

The client often has an oral or nasal airway (see Chapter 36) inserted to maintain a patent airway until comfortable breathing at a normal rate resumes. As respiratory function returns, the nurse will ask the client to spit out the airway. The ability to do so signifies the return of a normal gag reflex.

One of the nurse's greatest concerns is airway obstruction resulting from (1) aspirations of emesis, (2) accumulation of mucous secretions in the pharynx, or (3) swelling or spasm of the larynx. The following measures maintain airway patency:

1. The nurse positions the client on one side with the face down and the neck slightly extended. A small folded towel supports the head. The neck extension prevents occlusion of the airway at the pharynx. When the face is kept turned downward, the tongue moves forward and mucous secretions flow out of the mouth instead of accumulating in the pharynx. If the nature of the surgery prevents turning the client on one side, the head of the bed is slightly elevated and the client's neck slightly extended, with the head turned to the side. The client should never be positioned with arms over or across the chest because this reduces maximal chest expansion.

2. The nurse begins coughing and deep breathing exercises as soon as the client is responsive.

3. The nurse suctions artificial airways and the oral cavity for mucous secretions. Care must be taken to avoid continually eliciting the gag reflex, which might cause vomiting. Before the nurse or client removes an airway, the back of the airway should be suctioned so mucous plugs and secretions are not retained.

4. The nurse administers oxygen as ordered.

CIRCULATION

The client is at risk for cardiovascular complications resulting from actual or potential blood loss from the surgical site, side effects of anesthesia, electrolyte imbalances, and depression of normal circulatory regulating mechanisms. Careful assessment of heart rate and rhythm along with blood pressure reveals the client's cardiovascular status. The values are monitored at least every 15 minutes throughout the recovery phase. The nurse compares preoperative vital signs with postoperative values. The surgeon's postoperative orders may specify when vital sign changes should be reported. For example, a heart rate above 110 per minute or below 60 usually should be reported immediately. However, the nurse must use judgement in reporting vital sign changes. If the client's blood pressure drops progressively after each check or if the heart rate becomes more irregular, the physician should be notified.

The nurse assesses circulatory perfusion by noting the color of nail beds and skin. If the client has had vascular surgery or has casts or constricting devices that may impair circulation, the nurse assesses peripheral pulses distal to the site of surgery. For example, after surgery to the femoral artery, the nurse assesses popliteal and dorsalis pedis pulses. The nurse also compares pulses in the affected extremity with those in the nonaffected extremity.

A common circulatory problem to observe for is hemorrhage. A client's blood loss may occur externally through a drain or incision or internally within the surgical wound. Either type of hemorrhage may manifest itself by the classic signs of fall in blood pressure, elevated heart and respiratory rate, thready pulse, cool, clammy, pale skin, and restlessness. If hemorrhage is external, the nurse will note increased bloody drainage on dressings or through drains. If a dressing becomes saturated, the blood will ooze down the client's sides and collect in a pool under bedclothes. An alert nurse always checks under the client for drainage. When hemorrhage is internal, the operative site becomes swollen and tight. For example, if a client bleeds within the abdomen, the abdomen becomes tight and distended. The first signs of suspected hemorrhaging should be reported to the physician immediately. The nurse will maintain intravenous fluid infusion and monitor vital signs every 15 minutes or more frequently until the client's condition stabilizes.

TEMPERATURE CONTROL

The operating room and recovery room environments are extremely cool. The client's depressed level of body function results in a lowering of metabolism and fall in body temperature. When clients begin to awaken, they complain of feeling cold and uncomfortable.

The nurse measures the client's body temperature and provides warmed blankets. Increasing body warmth causes the client's metabolism to rise and circulatory and respiratory functions to improve.

Often clients exhibit postoperative shivering. This may not be a sign of hypothermia but rather a side effect of certain anesthetic agents. Deep breathing and coughing will help expel retained anesthetic gases. In rare instances the complication malignant hyperpyrexia develops. A life-threatening complication of anesthesia, the condition causes a high fever, tachycardia, metabolic changes, and even convulsions. Without proper treatment it can be fatal.

NEUROLOGICAL FUNCTIONS

The client on arrival in the recovery room is usually asleep or reacting to verbal commands. However, medications, electrolyte and metabolic changes, pain, and emotional factors can influence the client's level of consciousness. The nurse rouses the client by calling his or her name in a moderate tone of voice. The nurse notes if the client responds appropriately or seems confused and disoriented. If the client remains asleep or unresponsive, the nurse attempts arousal through touch or by gently moving a body part. If a painful stimulus is needed to arouse the client, the nurse should notify the anesthesiologist.

As the effects of the anesthetic wear off, the client's reflexes return, muscle strength is regained, and a normal level of orientation returns. The nurse can easily check for pupillary and gag reflexes (see Chapter 13). If a client has had surgery involving a portion of the neurological system, the nurse conducts a more thorough neurological assessment. For example, if the client had low back surgery, the nurse assesses leg movement, sensation, and strength. Clients with regional anesthesia begin to experience a return in motor function before tactile sensation returns.

Orientation to the recovery room environment is important in maintaining the client's alertness. The nurse explains that surgery is completed and describes procedures and nursing measures within the recovery area. The client who was properly prepared preoperatively is less likely to be as anxious when recovery nurses begin their care.

SKIN INTEGRITY AND CONDITION OF WOUND

In the recovery room, the nurse assesses the condition of the client's skin, noting rashes, petechiae, abrasions, or burns. A rash may indicate a drug sensitivity or allergy. Abrasions or petechiae may result from inappropriate positioning or restraining that injures skin layers. Burns may indicate that an electrical cautery grounding pad was incorrectly placed on the client's skin. Burns or serious injury to the skin should be communicated by an incident report (see Chapter 14).

Following surgery most surgical wounds are covered with a dressing that protects the wound site and collects drainage. The nurse observes the amount, color, odor, and consistency of drainage on dressings. The nurse estimates the amount of drainage by noting the number of saturated gauze sponges. If drainage appears on the outer surface of a dressing, another way of assessing drainage is by drawing a circle around the outer perimeter of the drainage. If the perimeter expands, drainage is increasing (see Chapter 47). However, this is not the most accurate measure of volume of fluid lost.

Many physicians prefer to change a client's dressing the first time so they can inspect the incisional area.

Therefore the recovery room nurse may simply add an extra layer of gauze on top of the original dressing.

GENITOURINARY FUNCTION

A client may not regain voluntary control over urinary function for 6 to 8 hours after anesthesia. An epidural or spinal anesthetic may prevent the client from feeling bladder fullness or distention. The nurse palpates the lower abdomen just above the symphysis pubis for bladder distention. Because a full bladder can be painful and is often the cause of a client's restlessness in recovery, it may become necessary to catheterize a client. If the client has a Foley catheter, there should be a continuous flow of urine of at least 2 cc/kg/hr in adults. The nurse observes the color and odor of urine. Surgery involving portions of the urinary tract normally causes bloody urine for at least 12 to 24 hours, depending on the type of surgery.

GASTROINTESTINAL FUNCTION

Anesthetics slow gastrointestinal motility and cause nausea. Normally during the immediate recovery phase a nurse will hear faint or absent bowel sounds in all four quadrants. Inspection of the abdomen rules out distention that may be caused by accumulation of gas. In a client who has had abdominal surgery, distention will develop if internal bleeding occurs.

To minimize nausea the nurse avoids sudden movement of the client. If the client has a nasogastric tube, it is important to keep the tube patent by regular irrigations. Occlusion of nasogastric tubes results in accumulation of gastric contents within the stomach. Since stomach emptying slows under anesthesia, the accumulated contents cannot escape and nausea and vomiting develop. Normally a client does not receive fluids to drink in the recovery room because of the risk of vomiting.

FLUID AND ELECTROLYTE BALANCE

Becuse of the surgical client's risk for fluid and electrolyte abnormalities, the nurse assesses the hydration status and monitors cardiac and neurological function for signs of electrolyte alterations (see Chapter 37). The nurse also has an important responsibility for maintaining patency of intravenous infusions. The client's only source of fluid intake immediately after surgery is through intravenous catheters. The nurse inspects a catheter insertion site to be sure it is properly positioned within a vein so fluid flows freely. The physician orders a prescribed rate for each infusion. To ensure adequate fluid intake the nurse should not allow infusion of fluids to fall behind. The client may also receive blood products postoperatively depending on the blood loss during surgery.

Accurate recording of intake and output helps assess

renal and circulatory function. The nurse measures all sources of output including urine, gastric drainage, drainage from wounds, and any insensible loss from diaphoresis. Mucus suctioned from airways is not included in output measurements.

COMFORT

As a client awakens from general anesthesia, the sensation of pain becomes prominent. Pain can be perceived before full consciousness is regained. Acute incisional pain causes the client to become restless and may be responsible for changes in vital signs. It is difficult for clients to begin coughing and deep breathing exercises when they experience pain. The client who had regional or local anesthesia usually does not experience pain initially, since the incisional area is still anesthetized.

It is common to administer intravenous narcotic analgesics immediately after surgery to expedite pain relief and minimize respiratory depression. Once a hospitalized client is transferred to a hospital room, patient controlled analgesia (PCA) given intravenously may be continued (see Chapter 35). Intramuscular injections may initially be given in divided doses but this is not the preferred route of administration immediately postoperatively.

Recovery in Ambulatory Surgery

The thoroughness and extent of a nurse's postoperative assessment will depend on the ambulatory client's condition, type of surgery, and anesthesia. In many cases the assessment will be identical to that conducted for hospitalized clients. However, if the client has undergone minor surgery, (for example, cosmetic removal of a mole) the postoperative recovery phase requires minimal assessment.

If an ambulatory client has received general or regional anesthesia or intensive intravenous sedation, the client will be transferred to the recovery room. In phase I recovery, clients in need of close monitoring are frequently assessed for vital sign changes and respiratory and circulatory status, level of consciousness, condition of the surgical wound, or pain level.

The time a client spends in phase I recovery depends on several factors. Outpatient anesthesia is gauged to provide a quick recovery time, few after effects, and a speedy return to daily routines. The average time spent in phase I is 1 hour, without complications. Clients are encouraged to gradually sit up on the stretcher or bed and begin to take ice chips or sips of water while regaining full alertness. Once clients become stable and no longer require close monitoring the nurse transfers them to phase II recovery. Clients who have undergone minor surgery may be transferred directly to phase II recovery.

Postoperative Instructions for Ambulatory Surgical Clients

- Physician's office phone number
- Surgery center's phone number
- Follow-up appointment, date and time
- Review prescribed medications
- Guidelines related to specific surgery, for example:
  Dressing and wound care
  Activity restrictions
- Warning signs of complications

Phase II recovery consists of a room equipped with medical recliner chairs, side tables, and foot rests. Kitchen facilities for preparing light snacks and beverages are usually located in the area, along with bathrooms. The phase II environment is designed to promote the client's and families' comfort and well-being until discharge. The nurse monitors clients but not at the same intensity as phase I. In phase II recovery, nurses initiate postoperative teaching with clients and family members (see box).

Postoperative Convalescence

Once the hospitalized client's condition stabilizes, it is time to return to the postoperative nursing division. Ambulatory surgical clients will, in contrast, be discharged. Nursing care focuses on returning the client to a relatively functional level of wellness as soon as possible. The speed of convalescence will depend on the type or extent of surgery, risk factors, postoperative complications, and the nurse's care plan.

DISCHARGE FROM THE RECOVERY ROOM

The nurse evaluates readiness for discharge from recovery on the basis of vital signs stability, body temperature control, good ventilatory function, orientation to surroundings, absence of complications, minimal pain and nausea, controlled wound drainage, adequate urine output, and fluid-electrolyte balance. If the client's condition is still poor after 2 to 3 hours, the stay will lengthen or the surgeon may transfer the client to an intensive care unit (ICU).

When the client is discharged from recovery, the nurse calls the nursing division to report vital signs, the type of surgery and anesthesia performed, blood loss, level of consciousness, general physical condition, and whether there are intravenous lines or drainage tubes. The nurse's report helps the nurse on the division anticipate special client needs and obtain necessary equipment.

A nurse and transporter bring the client on a stretcher. Staff members assist in safely transferring the client to a bed (see Chapter 41). The recovery room nurse shows the division nurse the recovery room record and reviews the client's course. The recovery room nurse also points out physician orders that require attention. Before the recovery nurse leaves, the division nurse takes a complete set of vital signs to compare with recovery room findings. Minor vital sign variations normally occur after transporting the client.

POSTOPERATIVE ASSESSMENT

The nurse's assessment includes an initial check of the client's general condition, including vital signs, level of consciousness, condition of dressings and drains, intravenous fluid status, comfort level, and skin integrity.

The same physical measurements and observations performed in the recovery room are also carried out on the postoperative division. The nurse routinely assesses the client at least every 15 minutes the first hour, every 30 minutes for 1 to 2 hours, every hour for 4 hours, and then every 4 hours. Frequency of assessment depends on the client's condition. A nurse should not assume that further monitoring is unnecessary if the client appears normal during the initial assessment. A client's condition can change rapidly. A nurse is guilty of neglect when failing to follow the assessment schedule.

The nurse thoroughly documents the initial assessment and makes entries in the nurse's notes. Vital signs, intravenous fluid intake, and urinary output can be entered on flowsheets. The nurse's initial findings are a baseline for comparing postoperative changes.

After the nurse completes the first assessment and has attended to immediate needs, the family is allowed to visit. Now the nurse can explain the purpose of procedures or equipment. The family will want to know how the client is doing. The nurse explains if vital signs are stable and if the client seems to be awakening without difficulty. The family should know that the client will fall in and out of sleep for most of the rest of the day from the effects of general anesthesia. The family should also be reminded that frequent assessments of the client's condition are to be expected and that, if the client had spinal anesthesia, loss of sensation and movement in the extremities remains for several hours.

NURSING DIAGNOSIS

The nurse determines the status of problems identified from preoperative nursing diagnoses and clusters new relevant data to identify new diagnoses postoperatively

---

Examples of Nursing Diagnoses for Postoperative Client

NANDA-APPROVED NURSING DIAGNOSES

Ineffective airway clearance related to:
* Diminished cough
* Retained secretions
* Prolonged sedation

Ineffective breathing pattern related to:
* Incisional pain
* Analgesia effects on ventilation

Pain related to:
* Surgical incision
* Nasogastric tube placement

Ineffective individual coping related to:
* Constraints imposed by surgery
* Numerous postoperative therapies

Potential fluid volume deficit related to:
* Wound drainage
* Inadequate fluid intake

Potential or actual impaired skin integrity related to:
* Wound drainage
* Impaired mobility

Anticipatory grieving related to:
* Client's critical condition

Impaired physical mobility related to:
* Pain
* Postoperative activity restrictions
* Casts or dressings

Altered oral mucous membrane related to:
* Presence of nasogastric or endotracheal tube
* NPO status

Feeding, bathing/hygiene, dressing/grooming, toileting self-care deficit related to:
* Postoperative activity restrictions

Potential altered body temperature related to:
* Lowered metabolism

Potential for infection related to:
* Surgical wound incision

Impaired verbal communication related to:
* Endotracheal or airway tube placement

Sample Nursing Diagnoses for Postoperative Client

Defining Characteristics	Nursing Diagnoses	Related Factors
Abnormal breath sounds Ineffective cough Dyspnea Elevated respiratory rate Shallow respirations	Ineffective airway clearance	• Incisional pain • Decreased energy
Grimaces when coughs or breathes deeply Abdominal incision of 6 in Attempts to splint abdomen during moving Verbalizes sharp pain present in abdomen	Pain	• Surgical incision
Wound draining copious secretions Client allergic to adhesive tape Client diaphoretic Nutritional intake reduced two days postoperatively	Potential impaired skin integrity	• Exposure of skin to secretions

(see nursing diagnoses box). Previously defined diagnoses such as impaired skin integrity may continue as a postoperative problem. The nurse may also identify risk factors leading to identification of potential nursing diagnoses (see sample nursing diagnoses box). For example, an elderly client, who has undergone major abdominal surgery and who has a preexisting problem of reduced hip mobility due to arthritis will be at risk for the diagnosis of potential impaired physical mobility. The nurse also considers needs of a client's family when making diagnoses. For example, the inability of the family to cope with the client's condition requires the nurse's intervention.

PLANNING

At the convalescent phase the nurse has much information to plan the client's care. Current physical assessment data coupled with analysis of the preoperative nursing history allows the nurse to plan specific nursing interventions. The surgeon's postoperative orders also offer guidelines. Typical postoperative orders include:

1. Frequency of vital signs and special assessments
2. Types of intravenous fluids and rate of infusion
3. Postoperative drugs
4. Fluids and food allowed by mouth
5. Level of activity the client is allowed to resume
6. Position the client is to maintain while in bed
7. Intake and output
8. Laboratory tests and x-ray studies
9. Special directions

The nurse considers effects of the stress of surgery and limitations it produces when establishing goals of care for the client. Likewise, the nurse considers goals of care established during the preoperative surgical phase. Typical goals of care postoperatively include:

1. Gaining a return of normal physiologic function
2. Remaining free of postoperative surgical wound infection
3. Achieving rest and comfort
4. Maintaining self-concept
5. Returning to a functional state of health within limitations posed by surgery

The care plan box outlines a typical sample care plan for a postoperative surgical client.

IMPLEMENTATION

REGAINING NORMAL PHYSIOLOGICAL FUNCTION. A surgical wound, the effects of prolonged immobilization during surgery and convalescence, and the influence of anesthesia and analgesics are the principal causes for postoperative complications. Nursing interventions are directed at preventing complications so that the client returns to the highest level of functioning possible. Failure of the client to become actively involved

Sample Nursing Care Plan for Postoperative Client

Nursing Diagnoses	Goals	Expected Outcomes	Nursing Interventions
Ineffective airway clearance related to incisional pain	Client achieves normal ventilatory function with patent airway.	Client is able to breathe deeply.	Have client perform diaphragmatic breathing using incentive spirometer every 2 hours while awake.
		Cough is clear and nonproductive.	Have client splint abdominal incision while performing coughing exercises.
			Offer preferred fluids (iced tea and cranberry juice), 1500 ml per day minimum.
		Lung sounds are clear.	Turn client side to side every 1 to 2 hours while awake.
Pain	Client achieves comfort.	Client denies discomfort.	Keep surgical dressings dry.
		Client performs ambulation and self-care activities without pain.	Avoid positioning client on drainage tubes.
		Client shows no nonverbal signs of discomfort.	Administer PRN analgesic ½ hour before ambulation or self-care activity.
			Have client splint incisional area during movement.

in recovery adds to the risk of complications (Table 46-7). Virtually any body system can be affected. The nurse must consider the interrelationship of all systems, as well as therapies provided.

Maintaining Respiratory Function. To prevent respiratory complications the nurse begins aggressive pulmonary hygiene measures early. The benefits of thorough preoperative teaching are realized when the client is able to participate actively. The following measures promote expansion of the lungs:
1. The nurse encourages diaphragmatic breathing exercises at least every 2 hours while the client is awake. Maximal inspirations lasting 3 to 5 seconds open up alveoli.
2. The nurse instructs the client to use an incentive spirometer for maximum inspiration (see Chapter 36).
3. The nurse encourages early ambulation. Walking causes the client to assume a position that does not restrict chest wall expansion and stimulates an increased respiratory rate.
4. The nurse assists clients who are restricted to bed to turn on their sides every 1 to 2 hours while awake and to sit when possible. Turning permits expansion

of the lungs. Sitting causes lowering of abdominal organs, thus facilitating diaphragmatic movement and lung expansion.

The following measures promote removal of pulmonary secretions:
1. The nurse encourages coughing exercises every 2 hours while the client is awake and maintains pain control to promote a full productive cough.
2. The nurse provides oral hygiene to expectorate mucus. Oral mucosa becomes dry when the client is allowed nothing by mouth or placed on limited fluid intake.
3. The nurse initiates orotracheal or nasotracheal suction for clients who are too weak or unable to cough (see Chapter 36).

Preventing Circulatory Stasis. Early measures directed at preventing circulatory complications prevent circulatory stasis. Some clients are at greater risk of venous stasis because of the nature of their surgery. The following measures promote normal venous return and circulatory blood flow.
1. The nurse encourages clients to perform leg exercises at least every hour while awake. Exercise may be

contraindicated in an affected extremity involving vascular repair or realignment of fractured bones and torn cartilage.

2. The nurse applies elastic antiembolism stockings as ordered by the physician. The stockings should be removed every 8 hours and left off for 1 hour (see Chapter 42)

3. The nurse applies pneumatic antiembolism stockings. Each stocking wraps around a client's leg and is kept

in place with a velcro attachment. Compressed air inflates the padded plastic stocking systematically from ankle to calf to thigh and then deflates. The stocking reduces venous stasis.

4. The nurse encourages early ambulation. Most clients are ordered to ambulate the evening of surgery depending on the severity of surgery and the client's condition. The degree of activity allowed progresses as the condition improves. Before ambulation the

TABLE 46-7   Postoperative Complications

Complication	Cause
RESPIRATORY SYSTEM	
Atelectasis is a collapse of alveoli with retained mucous secretions; signs and symptoms include elevated respiratory rate, dyspnea, fever, crackles auscultated over involved lobes of lungs, productive cough	Inadequate lung expansion; anesthesia, analgesics, and immobilized position prevent full lung expansion; greater risk in clients with upper abdominal surgery who have pain during inspiration and repress deep breathing
Pneumonia is an inflammation of alveoli caused by infectious process; it may involve one or several lobes of lung; development of pneumonia in lower dependent lobes of lung is common in immobilized surgical client; signs and symptoms include fever, chills, productive cough, chest pain, purulent mucus, dyspnea	Poor lung expansion with retained secretion; common resident bacteria in respiratory tract is *Diplococcus pneumoniae*, which causes most cases of pneumonia
Hypoxia is the inadequate concentration of oxygen in arterial blood; signs and symptoms include restlessness, dyspnea, high blood pressure, tachycardia, diaphoresis, cyanosis	Respirations depressed by anesthetics or analgesics; increased retention of mucus with impaired ventilation because of pain or poor positioning
Pulmonary embolism is an embolus blocking pulmonary artery and disrupting blood flow to one or more lobes of lung; signs and symptoms include dyspnea, sudden chest pain, cyanosis, tachycardia, drop in blood pressure	Same factors that lead to formation of thrombus or embolus; immobilized surgical client with preexisting circulatory or coagulation disorders is at high risk
CIRCULATORY SYSTEM	
Hemorrhage is a loss of a large amount of blood either externally or internally in short period of time; signs and symptoms same as hypovolemic shock	Slipping of suture or dislodged clot at incisional site, clients with coagulation disorders at greater risk
Hypovolemic shock is the inadequate perfusion of tissues and cells from loss of circulatory fluid volume; signs and symptoms include hypotension, weak and rapid pulse, cool clammy skin, rapid breathing, restlessness, reduced urine output	In surgical client usually caused by hemorrhage
Thrombophlebitis is an inflammation of vein often accompanied by clot formation; veins in legs most commonly affected; signs and symptoms include swelling and inflammation of involved site, aching or cramping pain; vein feels hard, cordlike, and sensitive to touch; pain in calf when client walks or dorsiflexes foot (Homans' sign)	Venous stasis aggravated by prolonged sitting or immobilization; trauma to vessel wall and hypercoagulability of blood increase risk of vessel inflammation
Thrombus is a formation of clot attached to interior wall of a vein or artery, which can occlude the vessel lumen	Venous stasis (see thrombophlebitis) and vessel trauma; venous injury common following surgery of legs, abdomen, pelvis, and major vessels; thrombi also form from increased coagulability of blood (for example, polycythemia and use of birth control pills containing estrogen)
Embolus is a piece of thrombus that has dislodged and circulates in bloodstream until it lodges in another vessel, commonly the lungs, hearts, or brain	

Continued.

TABLE 46-7 Postoperative Complications—cont'd

Complication	Cause
GASTROINTESTINAL SYSTEM	
Abdominal distention is retention of air within intestines; signs and symptoms include increased abdominal growth and tympanic percussion note over abdominal quadrants; client complains of fullness and "gas pains"	Slowed peristalsis from anesthesia, bowel manipulation, or immobilization
Constipation is the infrequent passage of stools; should not be a concern immediately postoperatively, especially if client has a preoperative bowel preparation; after client resumes a solid diet, failure to pass a stool within 48 hours is cause for concern	Slowed peristalsis (see causes of distention) and delay in resuming normal diet
Nausea and vomiting are symptoms of improper gastric emptying or chemical stimulation of vomiting center; client complains of gagging, feeling full or sick to the stomach	Severe pain, abdominal distention, fear, medications, eating, or drinking before peristalsis returns, initiating gag reflex
GENITOURINARY SYSTEM	
Urinary retention is the involuntary accumulation of urine in the bladder as result of loss of muscle tone; signs and symptoms include inability to void, restlessness, bladder distention; common 6-8 hours after surgery	Effects of anesthesia and narcotic analgesics; local manipulation of tissues surrounding bladder and edema interfere with bladder tone; poor positioning of client impairs voiding reflexes
INTEGUMENTARY SYSTEM	
Wound infection is an invasion of deep or superficial wound tissues by pathogenic microorganisms; signs and symptoms include skin around incision warm to touch, red, and tender; client may have fever and chills; purulent material may exit from drains or from separated wound edges; appears 3-6 days postoperatively	Poor aseptic technique; contaminated wound before surgical exploration
Wound dehiscence is a separation of wound edges at the suture line; signs and symptoms include increased drainage and appearance of underlying tissues, usually occurs 6-8 days after surgery	Malnutrition; obesity; preoperative radiation to surgical site; old age; poor circulation to tissues; unusual strain on suture line from coughing
Wound evisceration is a protrusion of internal organs and tissues through incision; usually occurs 6-8 days after surgery	See dehiscence; client with dehiscence is at risk for developing evisceration

nurse assesses vital signs. Abnormalities may contraindicate ambulation. If vital signs are normal, the nurse first assists the client to sit on the side of the bed. If the client complains of dizziness, this is a sign of postural hypotension. A recheck of blood pressure will determine if ambulation is safe. The nurse assists with ambulation by standing at the client's side, making sure the client is able to walk steadily. The first few times out of bed the client may be able to walk only a few feet. This will improve each time. The nurse evaluates the client's tolerance to activity by periodically assessing the pulse rate.

5. The nurse avoids positioning the client in a manner that interrupts blood flow to extremities. While in bed the client should not have pillows or rolled blankets placed under the knees. Compression of the popliteal vessels can cause a thrombus. When sitting in a chair, the client's legs should be elevated on a footstool. The client should never be allowed to sit with one leg crossed over the other.

6. The nurse gives anticoagulant drugs as ordered. Physicians often order small doses of anticoagulants such as heparin for clients at greatest risk for thrombus formation. Orthopedic clients often receive aspirin for anticoagulation.

7. The nurse promotes adequate fluid intake orally or intravenously. Adequate hydration prevents concentrated buildup of formed blood elements such as platelets and red blood cells. When a client's plasma volume is low, these may gather to form small clots within blood vessels.

Promoting Normal Elimination and Adequate Nutrition. The nurse's interventions for preventing gastrointestinal complications promote return of normal elimination and faster resumption of normal nutritional intake. It takes several days for a client who has had surgery on gastrointestinal structures (for example, a colon resection) to resume a normal dietary intake. Normal peristalsis may not return for 2 to 3 days. In contrast, the client whose gastrointestinal tract is unaffected directly by surgery must simply endure the effects of anesthesia before resuming dietary intake.

The following measures promote return of normal elimination:

1. The nurse assesses for return of peristalsis. The nurse routinely auscultates the abdomen to detect return of normal bowel sounds: 5 to 30 loud gurgles per minute over each quadrant indicates that peristalsis has returned. High-pitched tinkling sounds accompanied by abdominal distention suggests the bowel is not functioning properly. The nurse asks if the client is passing flatus. This is an important sign indicating normal bowel function.

2. The nurse maintains a gradual progression in dietary intake. For the first few hours postoperatively a client receives only intravenous fluids. If the physician orders a normal diet the first evening postoperatively, the nurse first provides clear liquids such as water, apple juice, or tea after nausea subsides. Overloading with large amounts of fluids may lead to distention and vomiting. If the client tolerates liquids without nausea, the diet is advanced as ordered. Clients who have had abdominal surgery are usually allowed nothing by mouth the first 24 to 48 hours. As peristalsis returns, the nurse provides clear liquids, followed by full liquids, a light diet of solid foods, and finally a regular diet.

3. The nurse promotes ambulation and exercise. Physical activity stimulates a return of peristalsis. The client who suffers abdominal distention and "gas pain" will often obtain relief while walking.

4. The nurse maintains an adequate fluid intake. Fluids keep fecal material soft for easy passage. Fruit juices and warm liquids are especially effective.

5. The nurse administers enemas, rectal suppositories, and rectal tubes as ordered. If constipation or distention develops, the physician will attempt to stimulate peristalsis with cathartics or enemas. A rectal tube or return flow enema promotes passage of flatus (see Chapter 39).

The following measures maintain an adequate dietary intake:

1. The nurse removes sources of noxious odors.

2. The nurse assists the client to a comfortable position during mealtime. The client should sit if possible to minimize pressure on the abdomen.

3. The nurse provides small servings of food. A client will be more willing to face the first meal when servings are not large.

4. The nurse provides frequent oral hygiene. Adequate hydration and cleansing of the oral cavity eliminate dryness and bad tastes.

5. The nurse provides meals when the client is rested and free from pain. Often a client will lose interest in eating if mealtime has been preceded by exhausting activities such as ambulation, coughing and deep breathing exercises, or extensive dressing changes. When a client has pain, the associated nausea often causes a loss of appetite.

Promoting Urinary Elimination. The depressant effects of anesthetics and analgesics impair the sensation of bladder fullness. If bladder tone is reduced, the client has difficulty starting urination. Clients who undergo surgery of the urinary system frequently have Foley catheters inserted to maintain free urinary flow until voluntary control of urination returns.

The following measures promote normal urinary elimination (see Chapter 38):

1. The nurse assists clients to assume normal positions during voiding. The male client may need assistance to stand to void. Bedpans make voiding difficult. A female client will have better results if she is able to use a toilet.

2. The nurse checks the client frequently for the need to void. A surgical client restricted to bed will need assistance in handling and using bedpans or urinals. Often the client acquires a sudden feeling of bladder fullness and urgency to void, and the nurse must respond quickly when the client calls for help.

3. The nurse assesses for bladder distention. If a client does not void within 8 hours of surgery, it may be necessary to insert a urinary catheter. A physician's order is needed.

4. The nurse monitors intake and output. An accepted level of urine output is at least 2 ml/kg/hr for adults. If the client's urine is dark, concentrated, and low in volume, a physician should be notified. A client can easily become dehydrated as a result of fluid loss from the surgical wound. The nurse will measure intake and output for several days postoperatively until normal fluid intake and urinary output are achieved.

PREVENTING INFECTION. A surgical wound undergoes considerable stress during convalescence. The stress of inadequate nutrition, impaired circulation, and metabolic alterations increases the risk for delayed healing. A wound may also undergo considerable physical stress. Strain on sutures from coughing, vomiting, distention, and movement of body parts can disrupt the wound layers. The nurse is responsible for protecting the wound and promoting the healing process. A critical time for wound healing is 24 to 72 hours following surgery. If a wound becomes infected, it usually occurs 3 to 6 days after surgery. A clean surgical wound usually does not regain strength against normal stress for 15 to 20 days postoperatively. The nurse uses aseptic technique during dressing changes and wound care (see Chapter 43). Surgical drains must remain patent so accumulated secretions may escape from the wound bed (see Chapter 47). Ongoing observation of the wound will identify early signs and symptoms of infection.

ACHIEVING REST AND COMFORT. A surgical client's pain increases as the effects of anesthesia wear off. The client becomes more aware of the surroundings and more perceptive of discomfort. The incisional area may be only one source of pain. Irritation from drainage tubes, tight dressings, or casts and the muscular strains caused from positioning on the operating room table are facts that can make the client feel miserable.

Pain can significantly slow recovery. The client becomes reluctant to cough, breathe deeply, turn, ambulate, or perform necessary exercises. It is important for the nurse to assess the client's pain thoroughly (see Chapter 35). It should not be assumed that the pain is incisional. When the client calls for a pain drug, the nature and character of the pain should be determined. The nurse should provide p.r.n. analgesics as often as allowed the first 24 to 48 hours after surgery to improve pain control. The "patient-controlled analgesia" system allows clients to administer their own intravenous analgesics from a specially prepared intravenous pump (Bast and Hayes, 1986). If clients gain a sense of control over their pain, they usually have fewer postoperative problems.

MAINTAINING SELF-CONCEPT. The appearance of wounds, bulky dressings, and extruding drains and tubes are just some factors that threaten a client's self-concept. The nature of the surgery may create permanent change, such as disfiguring scars in the client's body image. If surgery leads to impairment in body function, the client's role within the family can change significantly.

It is important for the nurse to observe the client for alterations in self-concept. Clients may show a revulsion toward their apperance by refusing to look at an incision, carefully covering dressings with bedclothes, or refusing to get out of bed because of tubes and devices. The fear of not being able to return to a functional role in the family may even cause the client to avoid participating in the nurse's plan of care.

The family becomes an important part of the nurse's efforts to improve the client's self-concept. The nurse explains to the family when the client's appearance is like and how to avoid nonverbal expressions of revulsion or surprise. The family needs to be accepting of the client's needs and still encourage the client's independence. If the condition is terminal, the family learns how to assist the client through the grieving process so the client and family can reach a stage of acceptance.

The following measures maintain the client's self-concept:

1. The nurse provides privacy during dressing changes or inspection of the wound. Room curtains are kept closed around the bed and the client is draped so only the dressing or incisional area is exposed.
2. The nurse maintains the client's hygiene. Wound drainage and antiseptic solutions from the surgical skin preparation dry on the skin's surface and act as sources of irritation. A complete bath the first day after surgery can make the client feel renewed. Whenever the gown becomes soiled by wound drainage, the nurse offers a clean gown and washcloth. The nurse keeps the client's hair neatly combed and offers frequent oral hygiene, especially for the client who is allowed nothing by mouth.
3. The nurse prevents drainage sets from overflowing. Typically the physician orders contents of drainage sets to be measured every 8 hours for output recording. The client sometimes becomes preoccupied with observing the gradual collection of drainage, and some drainage sets can leak contents if they become too full. The nurse should empty the sets periodically to prevent accidental spills and hampering the client's movement.
4. The nurse maintains a pleasant environment. A client's self-concept is heightened by being in pleasant, comfortable surroundings. Frequently the room of a surgical client becomes cluttered with extra dressings, rolls of tape, and bottles of antiseptic solution. If the client requires frequent dressing changes, the room may take on the appearance of a supply room. The nurse should store or remove unused supplies and keep the client's bedside orderly and clean.
5. The nurse offers opportunities for clients to discuss feelings about their appearance. If the nurse notices that the client avoids looking at an incision, the client may need to discuss any fears or concerns. A client having surgery for the first time is often more anxious than one who has had multiple surgeries. Both male and female clients may worry about permanent scarring. A client is more apt to look at an incision several days after surgery when healing is occurring and the client begins to gain more energy and a feeling of well-being. If the client chooses to look at an incision for the first time, the area should be clean. Eventually the client should be able to care for the incision site by applying simple dressings or bathing the affected area.
6. The nurse provides the family with opportunities to discuss ways to promote the client's self-concept.

Promoting Return to a Functional State of Health. Throughout the postoperative convalescent period the nurse promotes the client's independence and active participation in care. When a client is in pain or suffers from postoperative complications, there is little motive for self-care. The nurse must maintain a balance of providing for clients' needs when they are physically dependent and promoting more involvement when their conditions allow it.

The goals a nurse sets for a client's involvement in care must be realistic. Surgery may limit the ability to participate effectively. It is unrealistic for the nurse to involve the client if movement is highly restricted or if participation increases discomfort.

The nurse should keep the client and family informed of recovery progress. Many clients become depressed if they think recovery is slow. The nurse explains that it normally takes many days to reach a level of maximal recovery. Surgery may also cause permanent physical limitations that will require time for acceptance.

The nurse plans care daily, keeping in mind the ultimate goals for a client's recovery. From the moment the client enters the hospital, through surgery, and during the postoperative phase, the nurse anticipates the client's return home.

Involvement of family members in the client's care plan can facilitate recovery. If the client requires additional care at home such as dressing changes, assistance with ambulation, or drug administration, the nurse instructs family members on proper care techniques. If family members are unable to assist the client, the nurse works with the physician in making plans for home care. The client will be more able to assume a functional state of health when family members understand the limitations a client faces.

EVALUATION

The nurse evaluates effectiveness of care provided to the surgical client on the basis of expected outcomes of nursing interventions. In all surgical settings the nurse consults with the client and family to gather data. One way the nurse evaluates the ambulatory surgical client's outcomes is by making a postoperative telephone call to the client's home. The call is usually placed 24 hours after surgery and reassures the client that the nurse is concerned and allows the nurse to evaluate the progress of recovery. The evaluation box outlines criteria used for postoperative clients.

Sample Evaluation of Interventions for Postoperative Client

Goals	Evaluative Measures	Expected Outcomes
Normal physiological function returns.	Measure client's ventilatory capacity.	Client is able to breathe deeply. Cough is non-productive.
	Assess lung sounds.	Lung sounds are clear.
	Assess vital signs.	Vital signs stabilize to preoperative norms.
	Assess color, temperature, and pulses of extremities.	Extremities are warm; pulses are strong bilaterally.
	Measure urinary output.	Output averages 2 ml/kg/hr.
	Assess client's dietary intake and measure body weight.	Body weight stabilizes or improves from preoperative level.
Client remains free of surgical wound infection.	Inspect condition of wound edges and character of any drainage.	Wound edges are approximated, slightly reddened, with drainage minimal and clear.
	Assess client's body temperature.	Client remains afebrile.
Client achieves rest and comfort.	Evaluate client for verbal and nonverbal behaviors indicative of pain.	Client denies discomfort. Client able to perform activities of living without signs of discomfort.
Client maintains self-concept.	Observe client inspecting and caring for wound or dressing.	Client will observe and care for wound openly and freely.
	Observe client discussing changes experienced as a result of surgery.	Client will talk about physical changes with others.
	Note client's personal appearance.	Client maintains personal grooming.
Client returns to functional state of health.	Observe client participate in self-care activities.	Client will initiate self-care independently.
	Observe client's level of ambulation.	Client exercises progressively.

SUMMARY

Care for the client during all phases of the surgical experience needs to be continuous and integrated. Preoperatively, the nurse prepares the client and family for the surgery and performs diagnostic tests and assessments in preparation for the operation. Intraoperatively, the nurse assists surgeons and operating room nurses to ensure that the client receives optimal care. Postoperatively, the nurse assists the client to physical stability and wakefulness and institutes measures to help the client achieve maximal recovery. Through all phases of care, the nurse involves the client and family as much as possible in the care plan and helps maintain the client's dignity.

KEY CONCEPTS

✓ With the evolution of surgical asepsis and development of modern anesthetic practices, the nurse's role in the operating room expanded.

✓ Perioperative nursing is professional nursing care afforded the surgical client before, during, and after surgery.

✓ Surgery is classified by level of severity, urgency, and purpose.

✓ In addition to the nature of nursing care provided, previous illnesses and past surgeries influence the client's ability to tolerate surgery.

✓ The duration of the preoperative period may be several days or only a few hours.

✓ All medications taken preoperatively are automatically discontinued postoperatively unless a physician reorders the drugs.

✓ Family members are important in assisting clients with any physical limitations and in providing emotional support during postoperative recovery.

✓ Preoperative assessment of vital signs and physical findings provides an important baseline with which to compare postoperative assessment data.

✓ A client's feelings about surgery can have significant impact on relationships with nursing staff and the client's ability to participate in care.

✓ Surgical removal of a body part may permanently alter a person's body image as well as the individual's sexuality.

✓ Routine diagnostic tests used to screen for preexisting abnormalities preoperatively include a complete blood count (CBC), serum electrolytes, coagulation studies, urinalysis, ECG, and chest x-ray study.

✓ Nursing diagnoses of the surgical client may pose implications for nursing care during one or all phases of surgery.

✓ Primary responsibility for informed consent rests with the client's surgeon.

✓ Informed consent should not be obtained if a client is confused, unconscious, mentally incompetent, or under the influence of sedatives.

✓ Structured preoperative teaching has a positive influence on a client's postoperative recovery.

✓ Basic to preoperative teaching is explanation of all preoperative and postoperative routines, as well as demonstration of postoperative exercises.

✓ Shaving of a surgical site should be done as close as possible to the time of surgery to minimize infection.

✓ In ambulatory surgery, nurses must use the limited time available to educate clients, assess their health status, and prepare them for surgery.

✓ A routine preoperative checklist provides a guide for final preparation of the client before surgery.

✓ Many responsibilities of nurses within the operating room focus on protecting the client from potential harm.

✓ The nurse's assessment of the postoperative client centers on the body systems most likely to be affected by anesthesia, immobilization, and surgical trauma.

✓ Because a surgical client's condition may change rapidly in recovery, the nurse monitors the client's status every 15 minutes.

✓ The recovery room nurse reports to the nurse on the postoperative division information pertaining to the client's current physical status and risk for postoperative complications.

✓ From the time of admission to the hospital the nurse plans for the surgical client's discharge.

REFERENCES

Bast, C, and Hayes, P: Patient-controlled analgesia, Nurs 86 16:25, 1986.

Cruse, PJE, and Foord, R: The epidemiology of wound infection: a ten-year prospective study of 62,939 wounds, Surg Clin North Am 60:1, 1980.

Garner, JS: Guidelines for prevention of surgical wound infections, 1985, Hospital Infections Program, CDC, PHS, and U.S. Department of Health and Human Services.

Halsey, RW, et al.: Nosocomial infections in U.S. hospitals, 1975-1976: estimated frequency by selected characteristics of patients, Am J Med 70:947, 1981.

Keithley, JK: Wound healing in malnourished patients, J Am Assoc OR Nurs 35:1094, 1982.

Lindeman, C, and VanAernam, B: Nursing intervention with the pre-surgical patient—the effects of structured and unstructured preoperative teaching, Nurs Res 20:319, 1971.

Metzger, RS: The beginning of OR nursing education, J Am Assoc OR Nurs 24:73, 1976.

Research Article

Ayliffe, GAJ, et al.: A comparison of preoperative bathing with chlorhexidine detergent and non-medicated soap in the prevention of wound infection, J Hosp Infect 237, 1983.

ADDITIONAL READINGS

American Nurses' Association and Association of Operating Room Nurses: Standards of perioperative nursing care, Kansas City, Mo., 1972, The Associations.

Andrews, DR, and Taylor, C: Documenting post-anesthesia recovery, Am J Nurs 85:290, 1985.

Blackwood, S: Back to basics, the preop exam, Am J Nurs 86:39, 1986.

Breslin, EF: Prevention and treatment of pulmonary complications in patients after surgery of the upper abdomen, Heart Lung 10:511, 1981.

Burtman, F, and Salminer, CA: Back to basics: controlling postoperative infection, Nurs 84 14:43, 1984.

Croushore, TM: Postoperative assessment: the key to avoiding the most common nursing mistakes, Nurs 79 9:47, 1979

Cummings C: Taking the fear out of surgery, Nurs 87 17:64b, 1987.

Faherty, BS, and Grien, MR: Analgesic medication for elderly people post-surgery, Nurs Res 33:369, 1984.

Fortin, F, and Kirovac, S: A randomized controlled trial of preoperative patient education, Int J Nurs Stud 13:11, 1976.

Frogge, MH: Promoting wound healing in the irradiated patient, J Am Assoc OR Nurs 35:1088, 1982.

Gruendemann, BJ, and Meeker, MH: Alexander's care of the patient in surgery, ed. 8, St. Louis, 1987, The C.V. Mosby Co.

Hathaway, A: Effect of preoperative instruction on postoperative outcomes: a meta-analysis, Nurs Res 35:269, 1986.

Hogan, P, and Bell, S: How to handle postanesthetic hypertension, Nurs 86 16:58, 1986.

Horsley, J, and Crane, J: Structured preoperative teaching, New York, 1981, Grune & Stratton, Inc.

Kneedler, J, and Dodge, G: Perioperative patient care, Boston, 1987, Blackwell Scientific Publications, Inc.

Lynch, S: Ambulatory surgery: families can watch surgery while they wait, AORN J 46:522, 1987.

McHugh, NG, et al.: Preparatory information: what helps and why, Am J Nurs 82:780, 1982.

Metheny, N: Preoperative fluid balance assessment, J Am Assoc OR Nurs 33:51, 1981.

Pagana, KD, and Pagana, TJ: Diagnostic testing and nursing implications, ed. 2, St. Louis, 1986, The CV Mosby Co.

Podjasek, JH: Which postop patient faces the greatest respiratory risk? RN 48:44, 1985.

Ross, R: Overcoming fear: a review on research on patient, family instruction, AORN J 43:1107, 1986.

Seneca, CM: How we streamlined preop paperwork, RN 49:42, 1986.

Volden, C, and Grinde J: Taking the trauma out of nasogastric intubation, Nurs 80 10:64, 1980.

Wells, N: The effect of relaxation on postoperative muscle tension and pain, Nurs Res 31:236, 1982.

Ziemer, MM: Effects of information on postsurgical coping, Nurs Res 32:232, 1983.

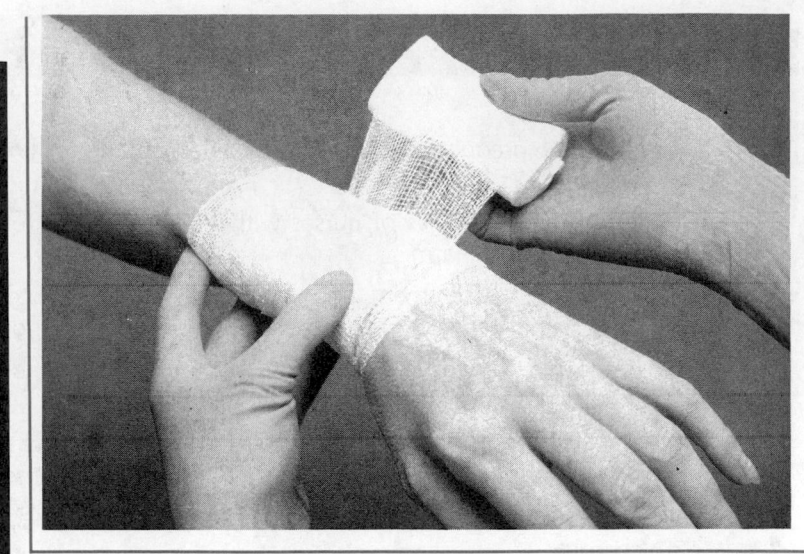

OBJECTIVES

Mastery of content in this chapter will enable the student to:

- Define the key terms listed.
- Discuss normal stages of wound healing by primary intention.
- Describe complications of wound healing and their usual time of occurrence.
- Explain the factors that impair or promote wound healing.
- Describe differences in assessing a wound in a stable versus emergency setting.
- Conduct an assessment of a closed and open wound.
- Identify nursing diagnoses related to clients with wounds.
- Discuss principles of first aid in wound care.
- Explain nursing care implications in the use of dressings.
- Apply a sterile dry and wet-to-dry dressing.
- Discuss the purpose of bandages and binders.
- Describe the effects of hot and cold on wound healing.
- Apply warm and cold applications safely to an injured body part.

KEY TERMS

Approximate

Binder

Compress

Debridement

Desquamation

Drainage Tube

Ecchymosis

Fibrin

Fistula

Granulation Tissue

Hematoma

Hemostasis

Hypercoagulability

Laceration

Primary Intention

Purulent

Secondary Intention

Sitz Bath

Steri-Strip

Superinfection

Nursing Care of Clients with Wounds

The body's integument is a protective barrier against disease-causing organisms and a sensory organ for pain, temperature, and touch. Injury to the integument poses risks to safety and triggers a complex healing response. Knowing the normal healing pattern helps the nurse recognize alterations that require intervention. The nurse's main responsibilities are to prevent invasion of microorganisms into wounds and to support the body's defenses in achieving wound repair. In choosing interventions, the nurse considers the type of wound, pain associated with it, conditions that affect healing, and the client's psychological well-being.

NORMAL INTEGUMENT

In relation to wound healing the integument has two principal layers: the epidermis and the dermis (Fig. 47-1). The epidermis or outer skin layer has two layers. The stratum corneum is the thin, outermost layer of the epidermis. It consists of flattened, dead cells. The cells originate from the second epidermal layer, the stratum malpighii. Cells in the stratum malpighii divide, proliferate, and migrate toward the epidermal surface. Once cells reach the stratum corneum they flatten and die. This constant movement of epidermal cells ensures replacement of surface cells sloughed off during normal desquamation. The thin stratum corneum protects underlying cells and tissues from dehydration and prevents entrance of certain chemical agents. However, the stratum corneum does allow evaporation of water from the skin and permits absorption of certain topically applied medications.

The dermal skin layer differs from the epidermis in that the dermis contains no skin cells. Collagen (a tough fibrous protein), blood vessels, and nerves comprise the dermis. Fibroblasts, which are responsible for collagen formation, are the only distinctive cell type within the dermis.

Understanding the integument's layers helps the nurse promote wound healing. The epidermis functions to resurface wounds and restore the barrier to invading organisms. The dermis responds during wound healing to restore the structural integrity and physical properties of the skin. Even though a wound may close in the upper epidermal layer, the client is at risk for infection, circulatory impairment, and tissue breakdown if the underlying dermis fails to heal.

WOUND CLASSIFICATIONS

There are many ways to classify wounds. Wound classification systems describe the status of skin integrity, cause of the wound, severity of tissue injury, cleanliness of the wound, or descriptive qualities of the wound. These classifications overlap. For example, a penetrating knife wound is also an open wound, and a contused wound is a closed wound. Table 47-1 outlines wound classifications. Wound classifications enable the nurse to understand the potential risks associated with a wound and implications for wound care. An open wound, for example, presents a greater risk of infection than a closed wound, while an abrasion will require less extensive dressings than a deep penetrating wound.

WOUND HEALING PROCESS

Wound healing involves a series of integrated physiological processes. The nature of healing is the same for all wounds with variations depending on the location, severity, and extent of injury. The ability of cells and tissues to regenerate or return to normal structure by cell growth also affects healing. Cells of the liver, renal tubules, and neurons of the central nervous system typically regenerate slowly or not at all.

There are two types of wounds with respect to tissue loss: those with loss and those without. A clean surgical incision is an example of a wound with little tissue loss. The surgical wound heals by *primary intention*. The skin edges approximate, or close together, and the risk of infection developing is lower. In contrast, a wound involving loss of tissue, such as a burn, pressure ulcer, or severe laceration, heals by *secondary intention*. The wound edges do not approximate. The wound is left open until it becomes filled by scar tissue. It takes longer

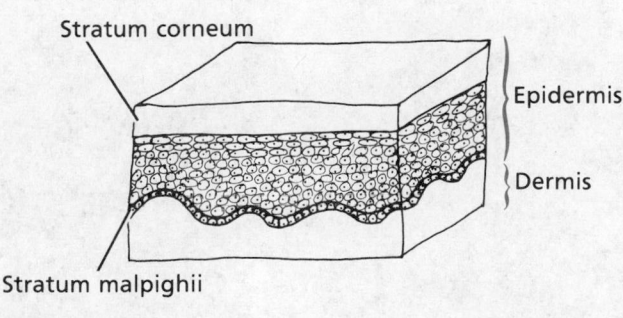

Fig. 47-1 Layers of the integument.

for a wound to heal by secondary intention, and thus the chance of infection is greater. If scarring from secondary intention is severe, there may be permanent loss of tissue function.

Healing by Primary Intention

An example of the normal healing process is repair of a clean surgical wound. The healing process occurs in four stages as described by Westaby (1986): inflammatory, destructive, proliferative, and maturation.

INFLAMMATORY PHASE

The stage of inflammation begins within minutes of injury and lasts about 3 days. Reparative processes control bleeding (hemostasis), deliver blood and cells to the injured area (inflammation), and form epithelial cells at the injury site (epithelial cell migration). During hemostasis, injured blood vessels constrict and platelets gather to stop bleeding. Clots form a fibrin matrix that later provides a framework for cellular repair. Damaged tissue and mast cells secrete histamine, resulting in vasodilation of surrounding capillaries and exudation of serum and white blood cells into damaged tissues. This results in localized redness, edema, warmth, and throbbing. The inflammatory response is a beneficial one and there is no value in attempting to cool the area or reduce the swelling unless the swelling occurs within a closed compartment (fascial compartment or neck).

Leukocytes reach the wound within a few hours. The primary acting white blood cell is the neutrophil, which begins to ingest bacteria and small debris. The neutrophils die in a few days and leave behind an enzyme exudate that either attacks bacteria or interferes with tissue repair. In chronic inflammation the dying neutrophils create wound pus. The second important leukocyte is the monocyte, which transforms into macrophages. The macrophages are "garbage cells" that clean a wound of bacteria, dead cells, and debris by phagocytosis. The macrophages also digest and recycle substances such as amino acids and sugars that aid in wound repair.

TABLE 47-1 Wound Classifications

Description	Causes	Implications for Healing
STATUS OF SKIN INTEGRITY		
Open. Wound involving a break in skin or mucous membranes	Trauma by sharp object or blow (surgical incision, venipuncture, gunshot wound)	Break in skin exposes body to invasion by microorganisms; loss of blood and body fluids through wound; reduced function of body part
Closed. Wound involving no break in skin integrity	Part of body being struck by a blunt object; twisting, straining, or deceleration force against the body (bone fracture, tear of visceral organ)	May predispose person to internal hemorrhage; reduced function of affected body part
CAUSE		
Intentional. Wound resulting from therapy	Surgical incision; introduction of needle into body part	Usually performed under aseptic technique to minimize chance of infection; wound edges usually smooth, clean
Unintentional. Wound that occurs unexpectedly	Traumatic injury (knife wound, burn)	Occurs under unsterile conditions; wound edges often jagged
SEVERITY OF INJURY		
Superficial. Wound that involves only epidermal layer of skin	Result of friction applied to skin surface (abrasion, first-degree burn, shearing)	Break creates risk of infection; does not involve underlying injury to tissues or organs; blood supply to area intact
Penetrating. Wound involving break in epidermal skin layer as well as dermis and deeper tissues or organs	Foreign object or instrument entering deep into body tissues; usually unintentional (gunshot wound, stab wound)	High risk of infection, since foreign object is contaminated; may cause internal and external hemorrhage; damage to organs causes temporary or permanent loss of function
Perforating. Penetrating wound in which foreign object enters and exits an internal organ	(see above entry)	High risk of infection; nature of injury depends on organ perforated: lung, compromised oxygenation; major vessel, hemorrhage; intestine, contamination of abdominal cavity by feces
CLEANLINESS		
Clean. Wound containing no pathogenic organisms	Closed surgical wound not entering gastrointestinal, respiratory, genital, or uninfected urinary tracts or oropharyngeal cavity	Low risk of infection
Clean-contaminated. Wound made under aseptic conditions but involving body cavity that normally harbors microorganisms	Surgical wound entering gastrointestinal, respiratory, genital, or urinary tracts or oropharyngeal cavity under controlled conditions	Greater risk of infection than with clean wound
Contaminated. Wound existing under conditions in which presence of microorganisms is likely	Open, traumatic, accidental wounds; surgical wound in which a break in asepsis occurred	Tissues often not healthy and show inflammation; high risk of infection
Infected. Bacterial organisms present in wound site usually above 10^5 organisms per gram of tissue	Any wound that does not properly heal and grows organisms; old traumatic wound; surgical incision into area infected (for example, ruptured bowel)	Wound presents signs of infection (inflammation, purulent drainage, skin separation)
Colonized. Wound containing microorganisms (usually multiple)	Chronic wound (vascular stasis ulcer, pressure ulcer)	Wound healing is slow and high risk of infection exists
DESCRIPTIVE QUALITIES		
Laceration. Tearing of tissues with irregular wound edges	Severe traumatic injury (knife wound, industrial accident involving machinery, tissues cut by broken glass)	Wound usually created by a contaminated object; depth of wound determines other complications
Abrasion. Superficial wound involving scraping or rubbing of skin's surface by friction	Often results from a fall (skinned knee or elbow); also result of a dermatological procedure for removing scar tissue	Painful owing to exposure of superficial nerves; deeper tissues uninvolved; risk of infection from exposure to contaminated surface
Contusion. Closed wound caused by a blow to the body by a blunt object; contusion or bruise characterized by swelling, discoloration, and pain	Bleeding in underlying tissues caused by blunt force against body part	More severe if internal organ contused; may cause temporary loss of function of body part; localized bleeding into the tissues may form a hematoma, or collection of blood

After the macrophages clean the wound and make it ready for tissue repair, epithelial cells move from the wound margins under the base of the clot or scab. Epithelial cells continue to gather under the wound space for about 48 hours. Eventually a thin layer of epithelial tissue forms over the wound as a barrier against infectious organisms and toxic materials.

The inflammatory phase will be prolonged and repair processes slowed if too little inflammation occurs as in debilitating disease or after administration of steroids. Too much inflammation also prolongs healing as arriving cells compete for available nutrients.

DESTRUCTIVE PHASE

The destructive phase (2 to 5 days) begins before inflammation ends. The macrophage continues the process of clearing the wound of unwanted debris, attracting further macrophages, and stimulating formation of fibroblasts—the cells that synthesize collagen. Collagen can be found as early as the second day and is the main component of scar tissue. Fibroblasts require vitamins B and C, oxygen, and amino acids to function properly. Collagen provides strength and structural integrity to a wound.

PROLIFERATIVE PHASE

With the appearance of new blood vessels as reconstruction progresses, the proliferative phase lasting from 3 to 24 days begins. During this period, the wound begins to close with new tissue. As reconstruction progresses, the tensile strength of the wound increases and the risk of wound separation or rupture is less likely. The degree of stress on a wound influences the amount of scar tissue formed. For example, more scar tissue forms in an extremity wound than in a less mobile area such as the scalp or chest. Impairment of healing during this stage usually results from systemic factors such as age, anemia, hypoproteinemia, and zinc deficiency.

MATURATION

Maturation, the final stage of healing, may take more than a year, depending on the depth and extent of the wound. The collagen scar continues to gain strength for several months. However, a healed wound usually does not have the strength of the tissue it replaces. Collagen fibers undergo remodeling or organization before assuming their normal appearance. Usually scar tissue contains fewer pigmented cells (melanocytes) and has a lighter color than normal skin.

Healing by Secondary Intention

When tissue loss in a wound is extensive, wound healing takes longer. A large open wound typically drains more fluid than a closed wound. Inflammation is often chronic, and tissue defects become filled with fragile granulation tissue rather than collagen. Granulation tissue is a form of connective tissue that has a more abundant blood supply than collagen. Since the wound is larger, the amount of connective tissue scarring is larger.

When epithelial and connective tissue cells are unable to close a wound defect, contraction may occur. Wound contraction involves movement of the dermis and epidermis on each side of the wound. The mechanism of contracture is not completely understood. However, it is known that collagen is not essential and any event that interferes with cell viability at the wound margin will inhibit contraction. Wound contraction begins on about the 4th day and occurs simultaneously with epithelialization. The cell that provides the motive force is the myofibroblast. Wound contraction results in thinning of surrounding tissues and the size and shape of the final scar corresponds to tension lines in the damaged area. For example, a square wound in the abdomen assumes the shape of two Y's, end to end. There are areas of the body where contraction gives poor results such as wounds on the face, sternum, and anterior lower leg. Wound contraction is not the same as a contracture or deformity resulting from muscle shortening and joint fixation.

Nutrition in Wound Healing

Wound healing does not occur normally unless a client is properly nourished. Physiological processes of wound healing depend on the ready availability of protein, vitamins (especially A and C), and the trace minerals, zinc and copper. Collagen is a protein formed from amino acids acquired by fibroblasts from protein ingested in food. Vitamin C is needed for synthesis of collagen. Vitamin A reduces the negative effects steroids can have on wound healing (Table 47-2). Trace elements are needed for epithelialization (zinc), collagen synthesis (zinc), and collagen fiber linking (copper).

For clients weakened or debilitated by illness, nutritional therapy is especially important. A client who has undergone surgery (see Chapter 46) and is well-nourished still requires at least 1500 kcal per day for nutritional maintenance. Alternatives such as enteral feedings (see Chapter 33) and parenteral nutrition (see Chapter 37) are made available for clients unable to maintain normal food intake.

COMPLICATIONS OF WOUND HEALING

When a wound fails to heal properly, a number of complications may develop.

TABLE 47-2   Factors that Impair Wound Healing

Factor	Physiological Effects	Nursing Implications
Age	Aging alters all phases of the wound healing process. Vascular changes impair circulation to wound site. Reduced liver function alters synthesis of clotting factors. Inflammatory response is slowed. Reduced formation of antibodies and lymphocytes. Collagen tissue is less pliable. Scar tissue is less elastic.	Instruct client on safety precautions to avoid injuries. Wound care may be needed for longer time period. Support persons in home setting must learn wound care techniques.
Malnutrition	All phases of wound healing are impaired. Stress from burns or severe trauma increases nutritional requirements.	Provide balanced diet rich in protein, carbohydrates, lipids, vitamins A and C, and minerals (for example, zinc and copper).
Obesity	Fatty tissue lacks adequate blood supply to resist bacterial infection or deliver nutrients and cellular elements for healing.	Nurse observes obese client for signs of wound infection and evisceration.
Impaired oxygenation	Low arterial oxygen tension alters synthesis of collagen and formation of epithelial cells. If local circulating blood flow is poor, tissues fail to receive needed oxygen. Decreased hemoglobin in the blood (anemia) reduces arterial oxygen levels in capillaries and interferes with tissue repair.	Provide diet adequate in iron. Monitor hematocrit and hemoglobin levels of clients with wounds.
Smoking	Reduces amount of functional hemoglobin in blood, thus decreasing tissue oxygenation. May increase platelet aggregation and cause hypercoagulability. Interferes with normal cellular mechanisms that promote release of oxygen to tissues.	Discourage client from smoking by explaining its effects on wound healing.
Drugs	Steroids reduce the inflammatory response and slow collagen synthesis. Antiinflammatory drugs suppress protein synthesis, wound contraction, epithelialization and inflammation. Prolonged antibiotic use may increase risk of superinfection. Chemotherapeutic drugs can depress bone marrow function, lower the number of leukocytes, and impair inflammatory response.	Clients receiving these drugs must be observed carefully since signs of inflammation may not be obvious.
Diabetes	Chronic disease causes small blood vessel disease that impairs tissue perfusion. Causes hemoglobin to have a greater affinity for oxygen so it fails to release oxygen to tissues. Hyperglycemia alters ability of leukocytes to perform phagocytosis and also supports overgrowth of fungal and yeast infection.	Instruct diabetic clients to take preventive measures to avoid cuts or breaks in skin. Preventive foot care is essential. Control of blood sugar will reduce the physiological changes associated with diabetes.
Radiation	Fibrosis and vascular scarring eventually develop in the irradiated skin layers. Tissues become fragile and poorly oxygenated.	Clients who have surgery following radiation should be observed closely for wound complications.
Wound stress	Vomiting, abdominal distention, and respiratory effort may stress suture line and disrupt wound layer. Sudden unexpected tension on an incision inhibits formation of endothelial cell and collagen networks.	Control nausea with ordered antiemetics. Keep nasogastric tubes patent and draining to avoid accumulation of secretions. Instruct and assist client to splint abdominal wound during coughing.

Hemorrhage

Bleeding from a wound site is normal during and immediately after the initial trauma. Hemostasis occurs within several minutes unless large blood vessels are involved or the client has poor clotting function. Hemorrhage occurring after the period of hemostasis indicates a slipped surgical suture, a dislodged clot, infection, or erosion of a blood vessel by a foreign object (for example, a drain). Hemorrhage may occur externally or internally. For example, if a surgical suture slips off a blood vessel, bleeding will occur within the tissues and there will be no visible signs of blood unless a surgical drain is present. (The surgeon often inserts a drain into tissues beneath a wound to remove fluid that collects in underlying tissues.) The nurse can detect internal bleeding by looking for distention or swelling of the affected body part, a change in the type and amount of drainage from a surgical drain, or signs of hypovolemic shock (fall in blood pressure, increased thready pulse, increased respirations, restlessness, and diaphoresis). A hematoma is a localized collection of blood underneath the tissues. It will appear as a swelling or mass that often takes on a bluish discoloration. A hematoma near a major artery or vein is dangerous because pressure from the expanding hematoma may obstruct blood flow.

External hemorrhaging is more obvious. The nurse observes dressings covering the wound for bloody drainage. If bleeding is extensive, the dressing soon becomes saturated and frequently blood escapes along the sides of the dressing and pools beneath the client. The nurse observes all wounds closely, particularly surgical wounds in which the risk of hemorrhage is great during the first 24 to 48 hours after surgery.

Infection

Wound infection is the second most common nosocomial (hospital-related) infection. According to the Centers for Disease Control (Garner, 1985), a wound is infected if purulent material drains from it, even if a culture is not taken or has negative results. A sample of drainage from an infected wound may not reveal bacteria in a culture because of poor culture technique or because the client has already received antibiotics. Positive culture findings do not always indicate an infection, since many wounds contain colonies of noninfective resident bacteria. The chances of wound infection are greater when the wound contains dead or necrotic tissue, when there are foreign bodies in or near the wound, and when blood supply and local tissue defenses are reduced. Bacterial wound infection inhibits wound healing.

A contaminated or traumatic wound may show signs of infection early, within 2 to 3 days. A surgical wound infection usually does not develop until the fourth or fifth day. The client will have a fever, tenderness and pain at the wound site, and an elevated white blood cell count. The edges of the wound may appear inflamed. If drainage is present, it is purulent, odorous, and has a yellow, green, or brown color, depending on the causative organism.

Dehiscence

When a wound fails to heal properly, the layers of skin and tissue may separate. This most commonly occurs before collagen formation (3 to 11 days after injury). Dehiscence is the partial or total separation of wound layers. Any client with poor wound healing is at risk for dehiscence. However, obese clients have a high risk because of the constant strain placed on their wounds and the poor healing qualities of fatty tissue. Dehiscence most often involves abdominal surgical wounds and occurs after a sudden strain such as coughing, vomiting, or sitting up in bed. Clients often report feeling as though something had given way. When there is an increase in serosanguineous drainage from a wound, the nurse should be alert for dehiscence.

Evisceration

With total separation of wound layers, evisceration (protrusion of visceral organs through a wound opening) may occur.

The condition is a medical emergency that requires surgical repair. When evisceration occurs, the nurse places sterile towels soaked in sterile saline over the extruding tissues to reduce chances of bacterial invasion and drying. If the organs protrude through the wound, blood supply to the tissues is compromised.

Fistulas

A fistula is an abnormal passage between two organs or between an organ and the outside of the body. A surgeon may create a fistula for therapeutic purposes,

---

Risks for Skin Breakdown from Body Fluids

LOW RISK
- Saliva
- Serosanguineous

HIGH RISK
- Gastric
- Pancreatic

MODERATE RISK
- Bile
- Stool
- Urine
- Ascitic Fluid
- Purulent exudate

for example, making an opening between the stomach and the outer abdominal wall to insert a gastrostomy tube for feeding purposes. Most fistulas, however, form as a result of poor wound healing. Trauma, infection, radiation exposure, and diseases such as cancer prevent tissue layers from closing properly and allow the fistula tract to form. Fistulas increase the risk of infection, as well as fluid-electrolyte imbalances from fluid loss. Chronic drainage of fluids through a fistula can also predispose a person to skin breakdown (see box).

FACTORS INFLUENCING WOUND HEALING

A number of factors influence the rate of wound healing. A client with any factors listed in Table 47-2 is at risk for wound complications. The nurse's knowledge of factors influencing healing will help in providing preventive care and selecting appropriate wound care therapies.

ASSESSMENT

The nurse often assesses wounds under two conditions: (1) at the time of injury before the initiation of treatment and (2) after therapy when the wound is relatively stable. Each condition requires the nurse to make different observations and to take different actions.

Emergency Setting

The nurse may see wounds in any setting: clinic, emergency room, a rural Girl Scout camp, or the nurse's own backyard. The type of wound determines the criteria for inspection. For example, the nurse need not inspect for signs of internal bleeding after an abrasion but should do so in the event of a puncture wound.

When a client's condition is judged to be stable because of the presence of spontaneous breathing, a clear airway, and a strong carotid pulse (see Chapter 36), the nurse inspects the wound for bleeding. An *abrasion* is usually superficial with little bleeding. The wound may appear "weepy" because of leakage of plasma from damaged capillaries. A *laceration* may bleed more profusely depending on the wound's depth and location. For example, minor scalp lacerations tend to bleed profusely because of the rich blood supply to the scalp. Lacerations greater than 5 cm (2 inches) long or 2.5 cm (1 inch) deep can cause serious bleeding. *Puncture* wounds bleed in relation to the depth and size of the wound; obviously

a nail puncture does not cause as much bleeding as a knife wound. The primary dangers of puncture wounds are internal bleeding and infection.

The nurse next inspects the wound for foreign bodies or contaminant material. Most traumatic wounds are dirty. Soil, broken glass, shreds of cloth, and foreign substances clinging to penetrating objects can become embedded in the wound.

The size of the wound is the next criterion for inspection. A deep laceration will require suturing by a physician. A large open wound may expose bone or tissue that should be protected.

When the injury is the result of trauma from a dirty penetrating object, the nurse inquires when the client last received a tetanus toxoid injection. Tetanus bacteria reside in soil and in the gut of man and animals. A tetanus antitoxin injection is necessary if the client has not had one within 5 years.

Stable Setting

When the client's condition is stabilized (for example, after surgery or treatment) the nurse assesses the wound to determine its progress toward healing. If the wound is covered by a dressing and the physician has not ordered it changed, the nurse should not directly inspect the wound unless serious complications are suspected. In such a situation the nurse should inspect only the dressing and any external drains. If the physician prefers to change the dressing, the physician will assess the wound at least daily. When the nurse removes dressings, care is taken to avoid accidentally removing or displacing underlying drains. Since removal of dressings can be painful, it may be helpful to give an analgesic at least 30 minutes before exposing a wound.

WOUND APPEARANCE

The nurse notes if wound edges are closed. A surgical incision should have clean, well-approximated edges. Crusts often form along the wound edges from exudate. A puncture wound is usually a small circular wound with the edges coming together toward the center. If a wound is open, the wound edges will be separated and the nurse inspects the condition of underlying tissue such as adipose and connective tissue. This is also the time to look for complications such as dehiscence and evisceration. The outer edges of a wound normally appear inflamed for the first 2 to 3 days, but this slowly disappears. Within 7 to 10 days a normally-healing wound fills with epithelial cells and edges close. If infection develops, the wound edges become brightly inflamed and swollen.

Skin discoloration usually results from bruising of interstitial tissues or possibly hematoma formation. Blood collecting beneath the skin first takes on a bluish or purple appearance. Gradually, as the clotted blood is broken down, shades of brown and yellow appear.

CHARACTER OF WOUND DRAINAGE

The nurse notes the amount, color, odor, and consistency of drainage. The amount of drainage depends on the location and extent of the wound. For example, drainage is minimal after a simple appendectomy. In contrast, wound drainage is moderate for 1 to 2 days after resection of a portion of the small bowel. If the nurse needs an accurate measurement of the amount of drainage within a dressing, the dressing can be weighed and compared with the weight of the same dressing when clean and dry. A rule of thumb is 1 gm of drainage equals 1 cc.

The color and consistency of drainage vary depending on the components. Types of drainage include:

1. Serous—Clear, watery plasma
2. Sanguineous—Fresh bleeding
3. Serosanguineous—Pale, more watery than sanguineous
4. Purulent—Thick, yellow, green, or brown

If the drainage has a pungent or strong odor, an infection should be suspected.

The nurse objectively records the integrity of a wound and character of drainage. Phrases such as "appears to be healing well" or "minimal drainage" do not give a clear picture of the wound's condition. The nurse should describe the wound's appearance according to characteristics observed. An example of accurate recording includes:

Abdominal incision is approximately 5 cm long across RLQ [right lower quadrant]; edges well approximated without inflammation or exudate. 1.2 cm diameter circle of serous drainage present on one 4 × 4 gauze.

DRAINS

The physician inserts a drain into or close to a surgical wound if a large amount of drainage is expected and if keeping wound layers closed is especially important. If fluid is allowed to accumulate under tissues, the inner wound edges may never close.

A drain such as a penrose may lie under a dressing, extend through a dressing, or be connected to a drainage bag or a suction apparatus. The physician often places a pin or clip through the drain to prevent it from slipping farther into a wound (Fig. 47-2). It is usually the physician's responsibility to pull or advance the drain as drainage decreases to permit healing deep within the drain site.

The nurse assesses drain placement, character of drainage, and condition of collecting apparatus. First, the nurse observes the security of the drain and its location with respect to the wound. Next the nurse notes the character of drainage. If there is a collecting device,

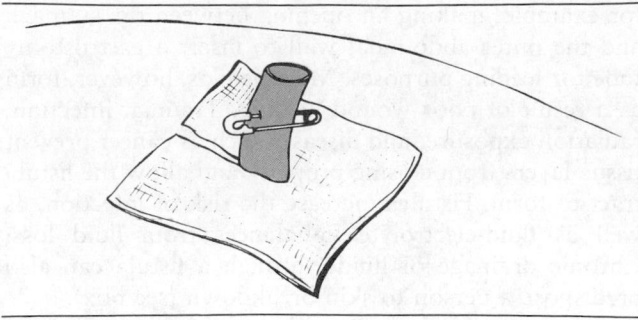

Fig. 47-2 Penrose drain.

the nurse measures the volume of drainage. Since a drainage system must be patent, the nurse looks for flow of drainage through the tubing. A sudden decrease may indicate a blocked drain, and the physician should be notified. When a drain is connected to suction, the nurse assesses the system to be sure the pressure ordered is being exerted. Evacuator units such as a Hemovac or

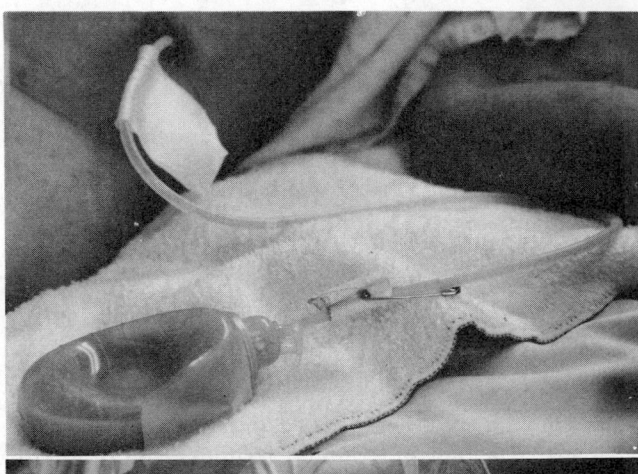

A

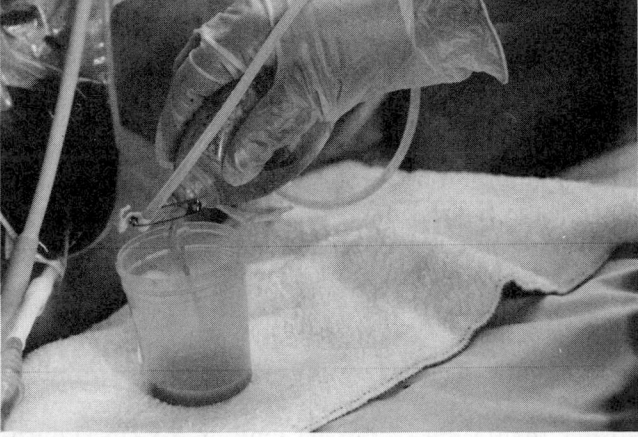

B

Fig. 47-3 Jackson-Pratt drainage device. **A,** Drainage tubes and reservoir. **B,** Emptying drainage reservoir.

Jackson-Pratt (Fig. 47-3) exert a constant low pressure as long as the suction bladder or bag is fully compressed.

WOUND CLOSURES

Surgical wounds are closed with *staples, sutures,* or *wound closures.* A popular skin closure is the stainless steel staple. The staple provides more strength than nylon or silk sutures and tends to cause less irritation to the skin. The nurse looks for irritation around staple or suture sites and notes if closures are intact. The nurse may choose to count sutures when the physician has removed a portion of them. Normally for the first 2 to 3 days postoperatively the skin around sutures or staples is swollen. Continued swelling may indicate that the closures are too tight. The skin can be cut by overly tight suture material, leading to wound separation. Sutures that are too tight are a common cause of wound dehiscence. Early suture removal reduces formation of defects along the suture line and minimizes chances of unattractive scar formation.

PALPATION OF WOUND

When inspecting a wound the nurse may observe swelling or separation of wound edges. With light *palpation* to wound edges the nurse can detect localized areas of tenderness or drainage collection. The nurse should don sterile gloves before palpating any wound. The nurse gently applies the fingertips along the wound edges. If pressure causes fluid to be expressed, the nurse notes the character of the drainage. It may be necessary to collect the drainage for culturing. The client is normally sensitive to palpation of wound edges. Extreme tenderness may indicate infection.

PAIN

Pain assessment is an important part of wound assessment, in terms of detecting complications as well as planning for future wound care. If the client experiences serious discomfort while the nurse inspects or palpates the wound, the nurse should look for underlying problems. If the wound is extensive and discomfort seems to be related to dressing removal or application, the nurse plans to administer analgesics before future dressing changes. If discomfort is related to tape removal, use of an adhesive removal may make it painless.

Wound Cultures

If the nurse detects purulent or suspicious-looking drainage, collecting a specimen for culture may be necessary (see Chapter 43). The nurse never collects a wound culture sample from old drainage. Resident colonies of bacteria from the skin grow within exudate and may not be the true causative organisms of a wound infection. The nurse cleans a wound first to remove skin

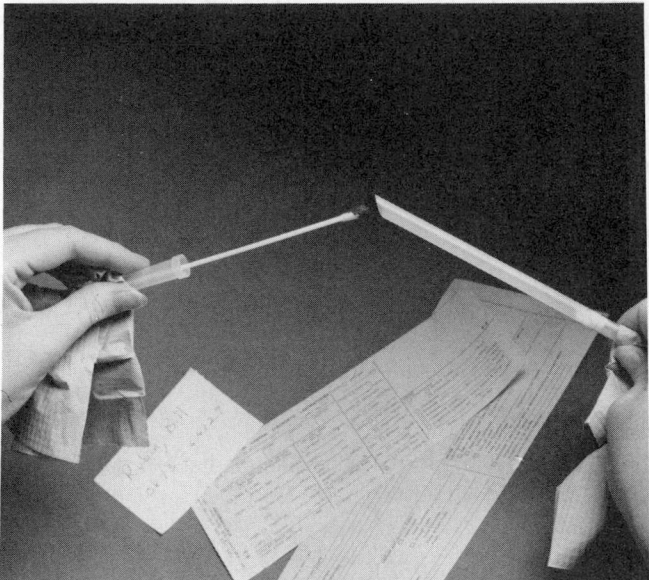

Fig. 47-4 Wound culturette tube.

flora. Aerobic organisms grow in superficial wounds exposed to the air, and anaerobic organisms tend to grow within body cavities. The nurse uses a different method of specimen collection for each type of organism.

To collect an aerobic specimen the nurse uses a sterile swab from a culturette tube (Fig. 47-4). If wound edges are separated, the nurse slowly and gently inserts the tip of the swab into the wound to collect deeper secretions. After collecting the specimen the nurse returns the swab to the culturette tube, caps the tube, and crushes the inner ampule containing the medium for organism growth. The medium must moisten and coat the swab tip. The nurse immediately sends the labeled specimen to the lab.

If drainage from a deep body cavity has a foul odor, there is a chance of anaerobic organism growth. The nurse uses a sterile syringe tip to aspirate drainage from the *inner* wound. After collecting the specimen the nurse applies a sterile needle to the syringe, expels air from the syringe and needle, and places a cork over the needle to prevent entrance of air. In some institutions the nurse may inject the specimen into a special vacuum container with a culture medium.

NURSING DIAGNOSIS

After completing an assessment of the client's wound, the nurse identifies nursing diagnoses that will direct both supportive and preventive care (see nursing diag-

Examples of Nursing Diagnoses Related to Wound Healing

NANDA-APPROVED NURSING DIAGNOSES

Impaired skin integrity related to:
- Surgical incision
- Pressure
- Chemical injury
- Secretions/excretions

Potential impaired skin integrity related to:
- Physical immobilization
- Exposure to secretions

Potential for infection related to:
- Malnutrition
- Tissue loss and increased environmental exposure

Acute pain related to:
- Abdominal incision
- Fear

Impaired physical mobility related to:
- Pain of surgical wound

Altered nutrition: less than body requirements related to:
- Inability to ingest food

Ineffective breathing pattern related to:
- Pain of abdominal incision

Altered peripheral tissue perfusion related to:
- Interruption of arterial flow
- Interruption of venous flow

noses box). Existence of a wound clearly indicates a diagnosis for actual impaired skin integrity. This diagnosis directs the nurse to initiate interventions that promote the healing process, since these clients are at risk for wound infection.

The client may be at risk for poor wound healing because of previously defined factors that impair healing. Thus, even though the client's wound may appear normal, the nurse identifies diagnoses such as "altered nutrition" or "altered peripheral tissue perfusion," which direct nursing care toward support of wound repair.

The nature of a wound can cause problems unrelated to wound healing. Alteration in comfort and impaired mobility are problems that have implications for the client's eventual recovery. For example, a large abdominal incision can cause enough pain to interfere with the client's ability to turn in bed effectively. The sample nursing diagnoses box lists nursing diagnoses related to problems of wound healing.

PLANNING

The nurse's priorities in wound care depend on whether the client's condition is stable or emergent. The care plan box shows a sample nursing care plan. The type of wound care administered will depend on the type of wound, its size and location, and complications. Nursing interventions will be both dependent and independent. Dependent interventions are those resulting from the physician's wound care orders. Goals of care for clients with wounds include the following:

1. Promoting wound hemostasis
2. Preventing infection
3. Preventing further tissue injury
4. Promoting wound healing
5. Maintaining skin integrity
6. Regaining normal function
7. Gaining comfort

Sample Nursing Diagnoses for Wound Healing

Defining Characteristics	Nursing Diagnoses	Related Factors
Disruption of skin surface Destruction of skin layers	Impaired skin integrity	- Physical immobility - Altered nutritional state - Altered circulation - Presence of secretions
Guarding behavior Altered muscle tone Verbal description of pain Changes in vital signs	Acute pain	- Inadequate pain relief from analgesics - Fear of drug dependence
Broken skin Malnutrition Wound drainage	Potential for infection	- Abdominal incision - Suppressed immune system

Sample Nursing Care Plan for Wound Healing

Nursing Diagnoses	Goals	Expected Outcomes	Nursing Interventions
Impaired skin integrity related to abdominal incision, wound drainage, and inadequate nutrition	Client's incision heals without complication.	Client will maintain adequate dietary intake for healing.	Instruct client in the importance of adequate dietary intake.
		Wound drainage will be contained in the dressing.	Monitor dressing weight. Monitor dressings for integrity and change or reinforce as needed.
		Client will deny irritation around incisional site.	Cleanse skin around abdominal incision to remove drainage or wound cleansing solution.
		Client is free of infection.	Wash hands thoroughly before and after dressing changes.
Acute pain related to abdominal incision, anxiety, and fear	Client achieves a sense of well-being and comfort.	Client will remain mobile and verbalize less discomfort with breathing exercises.	Instruct client to splint incisional area with flat of hands or a small pillow while changing position.
		Client will state minimal discomfort during dressing change.	Administer prescribed pain medication 30 minutes before dressing change.
		Client will deny irritation from dressing.	Monitor skin around wound for signs of irritation from drainage, solutions used, or tape.

IMPLEMENTATION

In an emergency setting the nurse uses first aid measures for wound care. Under more stable conditions the nurse is able to use a variety of interventions to ensure wound healing.

First Aid for Wounds

When a client suffers a traumatic wound, first aid interventions include stabilizing cardiopulmonary function (see Chapter 36), promoting hemostasis, cleansing the wound, and protecting the wound from further injury.

HEMOSTASIS

After assessing the type and extent of the wound the nurse controls bleeding of a laceration by applying direct pressure on the wound with a sterile or clean dressing, such as a washcloth. Once bleeding subsides, an adhesive bandage strip or gauze dressing taped over the laceration allows skin edges to close and a blood clot to form. If a dressing becomes saturated with blood, the nurse adds another layer of dressing, continues to apply pressure, and elevates the affected part. Further disruption of skin layers should be avoided. More serious lacerations should be sutured by a physician. Pressure dressings used the first 24 to 48 hours after trauma help maintain hemostasis.

A puncture wound is allowed to bleed to remove dirt and other contaminants such as saliva from a dog bite. If a penetrating object such as a knife blade is in a client's body, removal could cause massive, uncontrolled bleeding. Therefore the penetrating object should not be removed. The nurse may apply pressure around the object but not on it and the client should be transported to an emergency clinic or hospital.

CLEANSING

Gentle cleansing of a wound removes contaminants that might serve as sources of infection. However, vigorous cleaning can cause bleeding or further injury. For abrasions, minor lacerations, and small puncture wounds the nurse first rinses the wound in running water, cleans it with mild soap and water, and may apply an over-the-counter antiseptic. Topical antibiotics applied to wound edges may slow microorganism growth. However, prolonged application of topical antibiotics can foster growth of nonsusceptible organisms. When a laceration is bleeding profusely, the nurse should only brush away surface contaminants and concentrate on hemostasis until the client can be cared for in a clinic or hospital.

PROTECTION

Regardless of whether bleeding has stopped, the nurse protects the wound from further injury by applying sterile or clean dressings and immobilizing the body part. A light dressing applied over minor wounds prevents entrance of microorganisms. In the case of small abrasions it is acceptable to leave the wound open to air so a scab can form.

The more extensive the wound, the larger the bandage required. In the home setting a clean towel or diaper may be the best dressing. A bulky dressing applied with pressure minimizes movement of underlying tissues and helps immobilize the entire body part. A bandage or cloth wrapped around a penetrating object should immobilize it adequately.

Dressings

The use of dressings requires an understanding of wound healing. A variety of dressing materials are commercially available. Unless a dressing is suited to the characteristics of a wound, the dressing can hinder wound repair.

The choice of dressings and the method of dressing a wound influence the progress of wound healing. The proper dressing should not allow a draining wound to become overly dry with extensive scab formation. When this occurs, the dermis dehydrates and crusts. As a result, a barrier forms against normal epidermal cell growth, leaving a depression or defect in the new epidermal surface. Furthermore, dryness of the wound may increase the client's discomfort. Ideally a dressing leaves a wound slightly moist to promote normal epithelial cell migration. The dressing should also absorb drainage to prevent pooling of exudate that may promote bacterial growth.

For surgical wounds that heal by primary intention, it is common to remove dressings as soon as drainage stops. In contrast, when the nurse dresses an open wound

healing by secondary intention, the dressing material becomes a means for mechanically removing exudate and necrotic tissue.

PURPOSES OF DRESSINGS

A dressing may serve several purposes:
1. Protecting a wound from microorganism contamination
2. Aiding hemostasis
3. Promoting healing by absorbing drainage and debriding a wound
4. Supporting or splinting the wound site
5. Protecting the client from seeing the wound (if perceived as unpleasant)
6. Promoting thermal insulation to the wound surface
7. Providing maintenance of high humidity between the wound and dressing

When the skin becomes broken, a dressing helps reduce exposure to microorganisms. However, when wound drainage is minimal, the healing process forms a natural fibrin seal that can eliminate the need for a dressing. A dressing is always needed for extensive wounds.

Pressure dressings promote hemostasis. Applied with elastic bandages, a pressure dressing exerts localized downward pressure over an actual or potential bleeding site.

A pressure dressing eliminates dead space in underlying tissues so wound healing progresses normally. The nurse checks pressure dressings to be sure they do not interfere with circulation of a body part. The nurse assesses skin color, pulses in distal extremities, the client's comfort, and changes in sensation. Pressure dressings are not routinely removed.

A primary function of a dressing is to absorb drainage. Most surgical dressings have three layers: (1) a contact or primary dressing, (2) an absorbent dressing, and (3) an outer protective layer. The contact dressing covers the incision and part of the adjacent skin. Fibrin, blood products, and debris adhere to the contact dressing's surface. A problem occurs if the wound drainage dries, causing the dressing to stick to the suture line. Early or improper removal of the dressing can cause tearing of the healing epidermal surface. The nurse must either remove the dressing gently and moisten the attached area with sterile normal saline before removal or leave the dressing unchanged for several days. When wounds require debriding, such as infected or necrotic wounds, the contact dressing serves to debride necrotic tissue and debris. In this case, the contact dressing sticks to underlying tissue and debridement occurs during removal. Dressings applied to a draining wound require frequent changing to prevent microorganism growth and skin breakdown. Bacteria grow readily in the dark, warm, moist environment underneath a dressing. Skin surfaces become macerated and irritated. Skin breakdown can be minimized by keeping the skin clean and dry and reducing the use of tape.

The absorbent dressing layer serves as a reservoir for additional secretions. The wicking action of gauze dressings pulls excess drainage into the dressing and away from the wound.

The final outer layer of a dressing helps to prevent bacteria and other external contaminants from reaching the wound surface. Usually the outer dressing is made of a thicker dressing material.

A firmly taped or wrapped dressing supports or immobilizes a body part, minimizing movement of the underlying incision and injured tissues. Finally, a dressing insulates and keeps a wound's surface well hydrated. The humidity between a dressing and the skin's surface promotes normal epithelial cell growth.

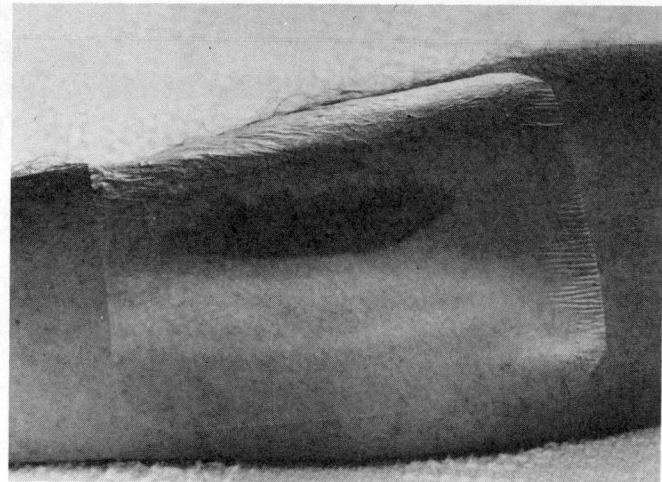

Fig. 47-5 Transparent film dressing.

TYPES OF DRESSINGS

Dressings vary by type of material and mode of application (wet or dry). They should be easy to apply, comfortable, and made of materials that promote wound healing.

Gauze dressings are the most common. They do not interact with wound tissues and thus cause little wound irritation. Gauze is available in different textures and in squares of 10×10 cm (4×4 inches) or 5×5 cm (2×2 inches), rectangles of 10×20 cm (4×8 inches), and rolls of various lengths.

Wet dressings are preferred in treating wounds that require debridement (see research highlight). The nurse moistens the contact dressing layer, increasing the gauze's ability to collect exudate and wound debris, and then applies a dry second layer of absorbent dressing. This wet-to-dry dressing effectively cleanses infected and necrotic wounds.

Nonadherent gauze dressings such a Telfa are used over clean wounds. Telfa gauze has a shiny, nonadherent surface that does not stick to incisions or wound openings but allows drainage to pass through to the softened gauze above.

Another type of dressing is a self-adhesive, transparent film that acts as a temporary second skin (Fig. 47-5). It has several advantages: (1) it adheres to undamaged skin, (2) it serves as a barrier to external fluids and bacteria but still allows the wound surface to "breathe," (3) it promotes a moist environment that speed epithelial cell growth, (4) it can be removed without damaging underlying tissues, and (5) it permits viewing the wound. The transparent dressing is ideal for small, superficial wounds or those that do not require debridement.

Hydrocolloid (HCD) and hydrogel dressings (Comfeel Ulcus, Duoderm, Vigilon) are occlusive dressings. This type of dressing has several functions: (1) it absorbs drainage through the use of exudate absorbers (Duod-

erm granules, Bard Absorption dressing, Comfeel Ulcus powder) beneath the dressing, (2) it maintains wound humidity, (3) it slowly liquefies necrotic debris, and (4) it provides protective cushioning. This type of dressing is most useful on shallow to moderately deep dermal ulcers.

CHANGING DRESSINGS

To prepare for changing a dressing, the nurse must know what type of dressing it is, whether there are underlying drains or tubing, and the type of supplies needed for wound care. Poor preparation may cause a break in

---

⚘ *Research Highlight* ⚘

Oleske et al. evaluated two dressing methods (wet-to-dry normal saline and polyurethane dressings) used in treating low-grade (stage one and two) pressure ulcers. Low-grade ulcers were chosen, since they are the most common and this type of ulcer is most often deferred to nursing for treatment recommendations. A total of 16 clients were placed in two study groups. Although the number of clients treated was small, the authors noted a significant reduction in wound size in the group using the self-adhesive polyurethane dressing. The authors suggest the need for further studies looking at reducing the healing time of grade I and II ulcers and addressing supportive nutritional protocols.

Oleske, DM, et al.: A randomized clinical trial of two dressing methods for the treatment of low-grade pressure ulcers, J Entero Therapy 13(3):90, 1986.

PROCEDURE 47-1

Applying Dry and Wet-to-Dry Dressings

STEPS	RATIONALE
1. Assess size and location of wound to be dressed.	Assists nurse to plan for proper type and amount of supplies needed. Alerts nurse when assistance is needed to hold dressings in place.
2. Assess client's level of comfort.	Removal of dry dressing can be painful; client may require pain medication.
3. Review medical orders for dressing change procedure.	Indicates type of dressing or applications to use.
4. Prepare necessary equipment and supplies:	
a. Sterile gloves	
b. Dressing set (sterile); scissors; forceps	Used to apply dressing and cut gauze to size.
c. Sterile drape (optional)	
d. Gauze dressings and pads	
e. Fine-mesh gauze (wet-to-dry only)	
f. Sterile basin	For antiseptic or cleansing solution.
g. Antiseptic ointment (optional for dry dressing)	
h. Cleansing solution	
i. Sterile solution to moisten dressing (wet-to-dry only)	
j. Clean disposable gloves	
k. Tape, ties, or bandage as needed	
l. Waterproof bag	For disposal of old dressing and supplies
m. Extra gauze dressings, surgi-pads, or ABD pads	
n. Bath blanket	
o. Adhesive remover (optional)	
p. Disposable mask (optional)	
5. Explain procedure to client and instruct client not to touch wound area or sterile supplies.	Decreases client's anxiety. Sudden unexpected movement on client's part could result in contamination of wound and supplies.
6. Close room or cubicle curtains; close open windows.	Provides privacy and reduces airborne microorganisms.
7. Position client comfortably and drape with bath blanket to expose only wound site.	Draping provides access to the wound yet minimizes unnecessary exposure.
8. Place disposable bag within reach of work area. Fold top of bag to make cuff.	Ensures easy disposal of soiled dressings. Prevents soiling of bag's outer surface.
9. Apply face mask, if required, and wash hands thoroughly	Reduces transmission of pathogens to exposed tissues.
10. Put on clean disposable gloves and remove tape, bandage, or ties.	Prevents transmission of infectious organisms from soiled dressings to nurse's hands.
11. Remove tape: pull parallel to skin; pull toward dressing; remove remaining adhesive from skin.	Pulling tape toward dressing reduces stress on suture line or wound edges.
12. With gloved hand carefully remove gauze dressings, taking care not to dislodge drains or tubes. Keep soiled undersurface away from client's sight. (If dressing sticks on a wet-to-dry dressing, do not moisten it; instead gently free dressing and warn client of discomfort.)	Appearance of drainage may be upsetting to client. (Wet-to-dry dressing should debride wound.)
13. Observe character and amount of drainage on dressing and appearance of wound.	Provides estimate of drainage amount and assessment of wound's condition.
14. Dispose of soiled dressings in disposable bag.	Reduces transmission of microorganisms.
15. Remove gloves by pulling them inside out. Dispose in bag.	Prevents contact of nurse's hands with material on gloves.
16. Open sterile dressing tray or individually wrapped sterile supplies. Place on bedside table (see illustration).	Sterile dressings remain sterile while on or within sterile surface. Preparation of supplies prevents break in technique during dressing change.
17. **Dry Dressing**	
a. Open bottle of antiseptic solution and pour into sterile basin.	Keeps supplies sterile.
b. Put on sterile gloves.	Sterile gloves allow handling of sterile supplies without contamination.

STEPS	RATIONALE
c. Inspect wound for appearance, drains, drainage, and integrity (see illustration). Avoid contact with contaminated material.	Indicates status of healing.
d. Cleanse wound with antiseptic solution:	
(1) Use separate swab for each cleansing stroke.	Prevents contaminating previously cleaned area.
(2) Clean from least contaminated area to most contaminated (Fig. 47-8).	Cleansing in proper direction prevents introduction of organisms into wound.
e. Use dry gauze to swab in same manner as Step d to dry wound.	Drying reduces excess moisture, which could eventually harbor microorganisms.
f. Apply antiseptic ointment if ordered, using same technique as for cleansing.	Helps reduce growth of microorganisms. Ointment may be applied to dressing if direct application causes discomfort.
g. Apply dry sterile dressings to incision or wound site	
(1) Apply loose woven gauze as contact layer.	Promotes proper absorption of drainage.
(2) Cut 4 x 4 gauze flat to fit around drain, if present. Precut gauze also is available.	Secures drain and promotes drainage absorption at site.
(3) Apply second layer of gauze.	Layering ensures proper coverage and optimal absorption.
(4) Apply thicker woven pad (surgi-pad).	Protects wound from external environment.
18. Wet-to-dry dressing	
a. Pour prescribed solution into sterile basin and add fine-mesh gauze.	Contact layer must be totally moistened to increase dressing's absorptive abilities.
b. Put on sterile gloves.	Allows handling of sterile supplies without contamination.
c. Inspect wound for color, character of drainage, presence and type of sutures, presence of any drains.	Provides assessment of wound healing.
d. Cleanse wound with prescribed antiseptic solution or normal saline. Clean from least to most contaminated area.	Assists in debridement and cleanses wound of debris.

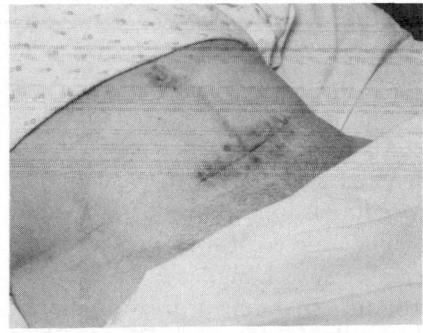

Step 17c

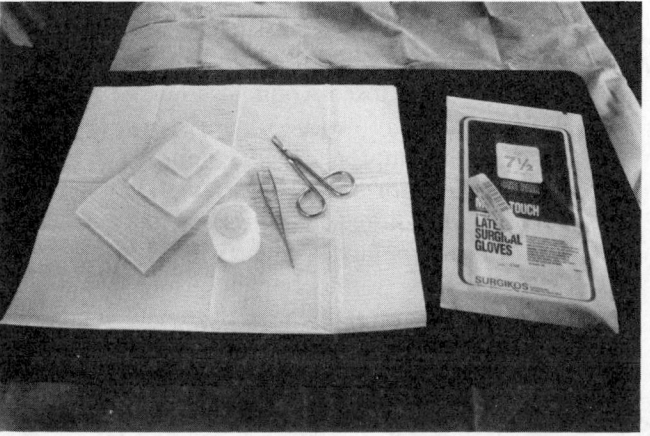

Step 16

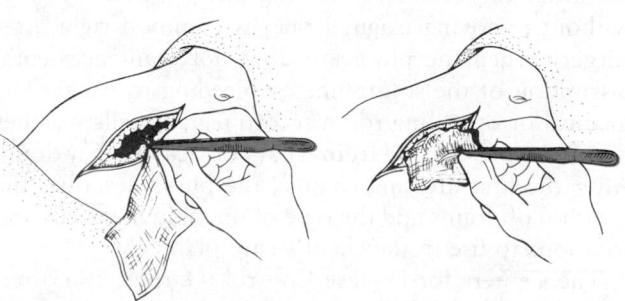

Step 18e

Continued.

PROCEDURE 47-1, cont'd

Applying Dry and Wet-to-Dry Dressings

STEPS	RATIONALE
e. Apply moist fine-mesh gauze directly onto wound surface. If wound is deep, gently pack gauze into wound with forceps until all wound surfaces are in contact with moist gauze (see illustration).	Moist gauze absorbs drainage and adheres to debris. Wound should be loosely packed to facilitate wicking of drainage into absorbent outer layer of dressing.
f. Apply dry sterile 4 x 4's over wet gauze.	Dry layer pulls moisture from wound.
g. Cover with ABD pad, surgi-pad, or gauze.	Protects wound from the entrance of microorganisms.
19. Apply tape over dressing, Kling roll (for circumferential dressings), or Montgomery ties. For application of Montgomery ties:	Secures dressing in place.
a. Expose adhesive surface of tape on end of each tie.	Montgomery tie allows for frequent dressing changes without removal of adhesive tape.
b. Place ties on opposite sides of dressing.	
c. Adhesive may be placed directly on client's skin or skin barrier may be used.	
d. Secure dressing by lacing ties across it.	Ensures dressing remains intact and covers wound.
20. Remove gloves and dispose in bag.	Reduces transmission of infection.
21. Assist client to comfortable position.	Promotes client's sense of well-being.
22. Dispose of all supplies.	Clean environment enhances client's comfort.
23. Wash hands.	Reduces transmission of infection.
24. Reassess client to determine response to dressing change.	Determines client's comfort level.
25. Monitor status of dressing at least every shift.	Evaluates extent of drainage and integrity of dressing.
26. Record appearance of wound and drainage, client's tolerance, and type of dressing applied in nurses' notes.	Documents progress of wound healing and promotes continuity in dressing change techniques.
27. Record frequency of dressing change and supplies needed on Kardex.	Alerts staff members to dressing change times and supplies needed.

aseptic technique (see Chapter 43) or an accidental dislodging of a drain. The nurse's judgment in modifying a dressing change procedure is important during wound care, particularly if the character of a wound changes. Notifying the physician of any change is essential.

The physician's order for changing a dressing should indicate the dressing type, the frequency of changing and any solutions or ointments to be applied to the wound. An order to "reinforce dressing p.r.n." (add dressings without removing original one) is common right after surgery when the physician does not want accidental disruption of the suture line or bleeding to occur. The medical or operating room record usually tells whether drains are present and from what body cavity they drain. After the first dressing change, the nurse describes the location of drains and the type of dressing materials and solutions to use in the client's care plan.

The Centers for Disease Control (Garner, 1985) recommends the following guidelines during dressing change procedure:

1. The nurse should perform thorough handwashing before and after wound care.
2. Personnel should not touch an open or fresh wound directly without wearing sterile gloves (see Chapter 43).
3. If a wound is sealed, dressings may be changed without gloves.
4. Dressings over closed wounds should be removed or changed when they become wet or if the client has signs or symptoms of infection.

To prepare a client for a dressing change the nurse:

1. Administers required analgesics so that peak effects occur during the dressing change
2. Describes steps of the procedure to lessen anxiety
3. Describes normal signs of healing
4. Answers questions about the procedure or the wound

Often the physician orders clients to learn how to change dressings so they will be prepared for home care. In this situation the nurse must demonstrate dressing change to the client and family and then provide an opportunity for the client or family member to practice. Usually in this situation wound healing has progressed to the point that risks of complications such as dehiscence or evisceration are minimal. The client should be able to change a dressing independently or with assistance from a family member before discharge. Procedure 47-1 outlines the steps for changing dry and wet-to-dry dressings.

SECURING DRESSINGS

The nurse may use tape, ties, or bandages and cloth binders to secure a dressing over a wound site. The choice of anchoring depends on the wound size, location, presence of drainage, frequency of dressing changes, and client's level of activity.

The nurse most often uses strips of tape to secure dressings if the client is not allergic to tape. Nonallergenic paper and plastic tapes minimize skin reactions. Common adhesive tape adheres well to the skin's surface, while elastic adhesive tape compresses closely around pressure bandages and permits more movement of a body part. Skin sensitive to adhesive tape can become severely inflamed and excoriated and may even slough when the tape is removed.

Tape is available in various widths such as 1.2 cm, 2.5 cm, 5 cm, and 7.5 cm (½ inch, 1 inch, 2 inch, and 3 inch). The nurse chooses the size that sufficiently secures the dressing. For example, a large abdominal wound dressing must remain secure over a large area despite frequent stress from movement, respiratory effort, and possibly abdominal distention. Strips of 7.5 cm (3-inch) adhesive will better stabilize such a large dressing so it will not continually slip off. Whenever a nurse applies tape, it is important that the tape adhere to several inches of skin on both sides of the dressing, in addition to being placed across the middle of the dressing. When securing the dressing the nurse presses the tape gently, exerting pressure away from the wound. This way tension occurs in both directions away from the wound, minimizing skin distortion and irritation. Tape is never applied over irritated or broken skin.

To remove tape safely the nurse loosens the tape ends and gently pulls the outer end parallel with the skin surface toward the wound. The nurse applies light traction to the skin away from the wound as the tape is loosened and removed. The traction minimizes pulling of the skin. If tape covers area of hair growth, the client will experience less discomfort if the nurse pulls the tape in the direction of hair growth.

To avoid repeated removal of tape from sensitive skin, the nurse can secure dressings with pairs of reuseable Montgomery ties (Fig. 47-6). Each tie consists of a long strip; half contains an adhesive backing to apply to the

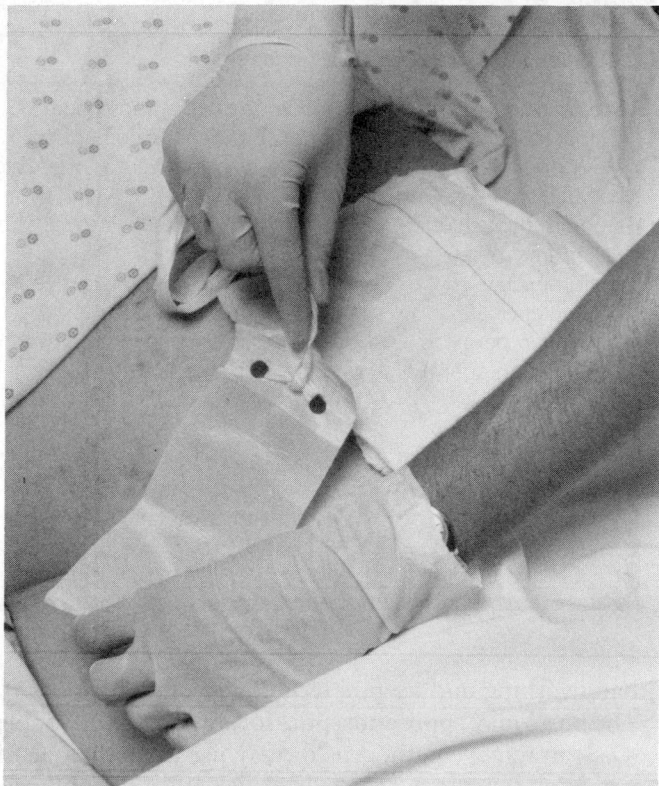

Fig. 47-6 Montgomery ties.

skin and the other half folds back and contains a cloth tie to be tied across a dressing and untied at dressing changes. A large, bulky dressing may require two or more sets of Montgomery ties.

To provide even support to a wound and immobilize a body part the nurse may apply elastic gauze or cloth bandages and binders over a dressing.

COMFORT MEASURES

Any wound can be painful, depending on the extent of tissue injury. The nurse uses several techniques to minimize discomfort during wound care. Careful removal of tape, gentle cleansing of wound edges, and careful manipulation of dressings and drains minimize stress on sensitive tissues. Careful turning and positioning also reduce strain on a wound. Administration of analgesic medications 30 to 60 minutes before dressing changes (depending on a drug's time of peak action) also reduces discomfort.

Cleansing Skin and Drain Sites

Although a moderate amount of wound exudate promotes epithelial cell growth, the physician may order cleansing of a wound or drain site if a dressing does not properly absorb drainage or if an open drain deposits drainage onto the skin. Wound cleansing requires good

TABLE 47-3 Cleansing Agents

Solution	Indications	Effects
Acetic acid (bactericidal)	*Pseudomonas aeruginosa,* some Gram-positive and Gram-negative organisms	May change the color of the wound exudate, does not significantly aid healing
Povidone-iodine (antibacterial)	Reported to be active against bacteria, spores, fungi, and viruses	Liberates 10% free iodine
Sodium hypochloride (antimicrobial)	Effective against staphylococci, streptococci, and pyocyareu	Releases elemental chlorine, which is a tissue irritant
Chlorhexidine (bactericidal)	Effective against Gram-negative and Gram-positive organisms and some fungi	
Hydrogen peroxide (oxidizing agent)	Useful for softening and removal of crusted exudate and debris	Should not be used in the presence of granulation tissue
Normal saline (irrigant)	Irrigation of clean or noninfected wounds	May be used under gentle pressure (35 cc syringe with 19-gauge needle) to assist in wound debridement
Cara-Klenz (cleanser)		Does not delay wound healing
PharmaClens (cleanser)	Cleans dead tissue and secretions	Does not delay wound healing

handwashing and aseptic techniques (see Chapter 43). The nurse may apply antiseptics locally to the skin (Table 47-3) to remove pathogens or may use the technique of irrigation to remove debris. The most effective antiseptic solutions for skin cleansing are tincture of chlorhexidine (Hibiclens) and the iodophors (such as Betadine), which persist in acting against bacteria as they remain on the skin. Alcohol 70% acts rapidly on bacteria but has no persistent effect since it evaporates. Hydrogen peroxide is useful when cleaning open wounds containing necrotic debris. The oxidizing property of peroxide exerts a mechanical cleansing effect, although its antiseptic action is slight. Its use should be avoided in the presence of granulation tissue.

BASIC SKIN CLEANSING

The nurse cleanses surgical or traumatic wounds by applying antiseptic solutions with sterile gauze or by irrigation. The following three principles are important when cleaning an incision or the area surrounding a drain:

1. Cleanse in a direction from the least contaminated area such as from the wound or incision to the surrounding skin (Fig. 47-7) or from an isolated drain site to the surrounding skin (Fig. 47-8).
2. Use gentle friction when applying antiseptics locally to the skin.
3. When irrigating, allow the solution to flow from the least to most contaminated area.

A wound is thought to be less contaminated than the surrounding skin. After applying an antiseptic solution to sterile gauze the nurse cleans away from the wound. The nurse never uses the same piece of gauze to cleanse across an incision or wound twice.

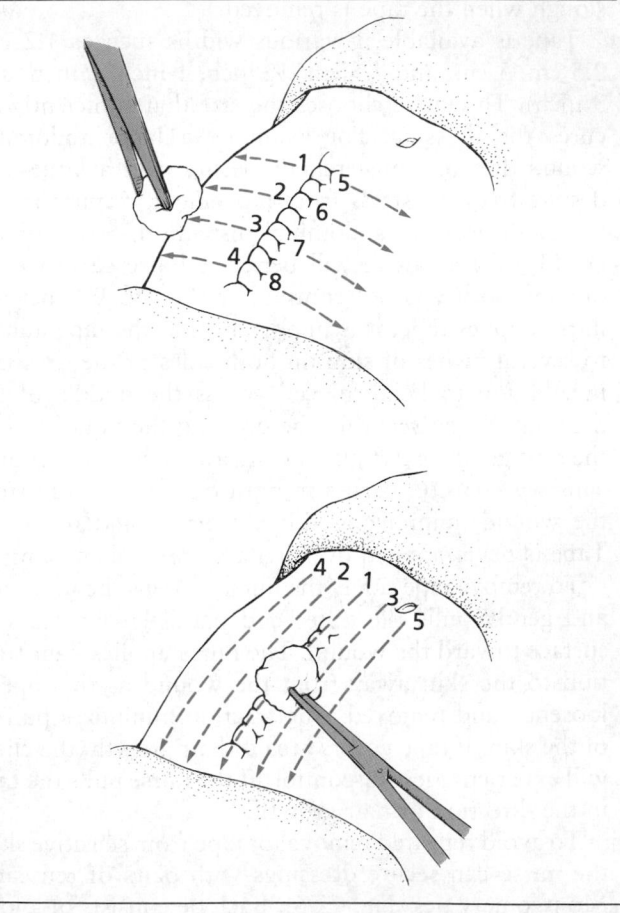

Fig. 47-7 Methods for cleansing a wound site.

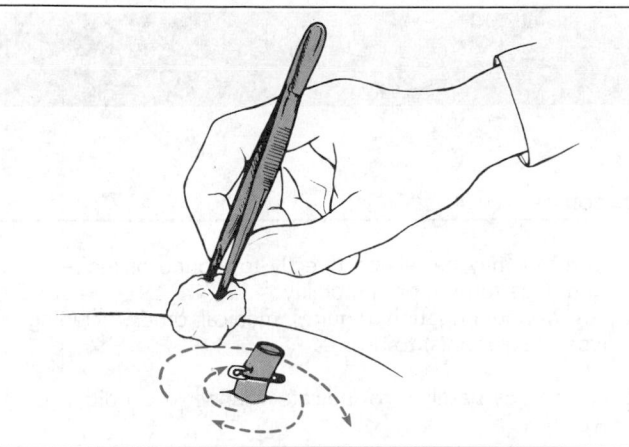

Fig. 47-8 Cleansing a drain site.

A drain site is highly contaminated, since the moist drainage harbors microorganisms. If a wound has a dry incisional area and a moist drain site, cleansing moves from the incisional area toward the drain. The nurse uses two separate swabs; one to clean from the top of the incision toward the drain and one to clean from the bottom of the incision toward the drain. To cleanse the area of an isolated drain site the nurse swabs around the drain, moving in circular rotations outward from a point closest to the drain. In this situation the skin near the site is more contaminated than the site itself. To cleanse circular wounds the nurse uses the same technique as cleansing around a drain.

IRRIGATIONS

Irrigations are a special way of cleansing wounds. The nurse uses an irrigating syringe to flush the area with a constant flow of solution. The gentle washing action of the irrigation cleans a wound of exudate and debris. Irrigations are particularly useful for open deep wounds, involving an inaccessible body part such as the ear canal or when cleansing sensitive body parts such as the conjunctival lining of the eye.

In addition to wound cleansing, irrigations serve to (1) apply heat to an affected area and (2) apply locally acting medications in the form of sterile solutions. The prescribed solution is usually sterile water, saline, or an antiseptic solution. Administration of irrigating solutions at body temperature enhances the client's comfort and provides the added benefit of local heat application.

WOUND IRRIGATIONS. Irrigation of an open wound requires sterile technique. The nurse uses a large Asepto or cone-tipped syringe to deliver the solution, since large volumes of solution are often necessary. It is important never to occlude a wound opening with a syringe, since

this would result in the introduction of irrigating fluid into a closed space. The pressure of the fluid could cause tissue damage and discomfort to the client. A wound should always be irrigated with the syringe tip over but not in the drainage site. Fluid should flow directly into the wound and not over a contaminated area before entering the wound. Procedure 47-2 lists steps for wound irrigation.

Suture Care

A surgeon closes a wound by bringing the wound edges as close together as possible to reduce scar formation. Proper wound closure involves minimal trauma and tension to tissues with control of bleeding.

Sutures are threads of wire used to sew body tissues together. The client's history of wound healing, site of surgery, tissues involved, and purpose of the sutures determine the suture material to be used. For example, if the client has had repeated surgery for an abdominal hernia, the physician might choose wire sutures to provide greater strength for wound closure. In contrast, a small laceration of the face calls for the use of very fine Dacron (polyester) sutures to minimize scar formation.

Sutures are available in a variety of materials, including silk, steel, cotton, linen, wire, nylon, and Dacron. Sutures come with or without sharp surgical needles attached. Growing in popularity are steel staples, a type of outer skin closure that causes less trauma to tissues than sutures, yet provides extra strength. It is also common to see wounds closed with steri-strips (Fig. 47-9). A steri-strip is a sterile butterfly tape, applied along both sides of a wound to keep the edges closed.

Sutures are placed within tissue layers in deep wounds

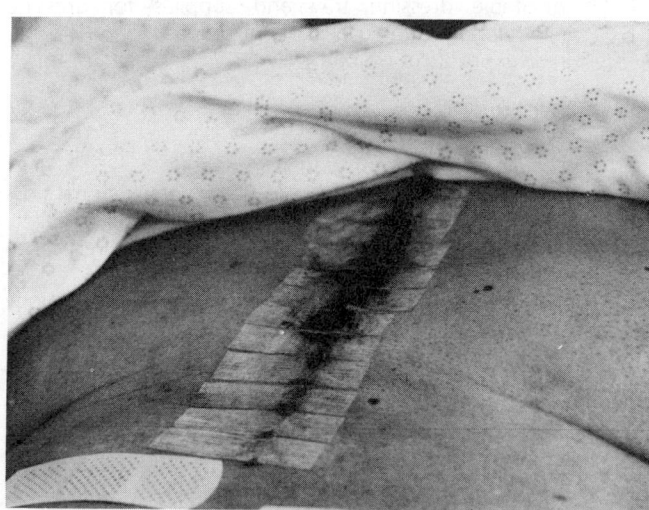

Fig. 47-9 Steri-Strips placed over an incision for closure.

Performing Wound Irrigation

STEPS	RATIONALE
1. Assess client's level of pain.	Discomfort may be related directly to wound or indirectly to muscle tension or immobility.
2. Review client's medical record for physician's prescription for irrigation of open wound and type of solution to be used.	Open wound irrigation requires medical order including type of solution(s) to use.
3. Identify recent recording of signs and symptoms related to client's open wound:	Data used as baseline to indicate change in condition of wound.
a. Extent of impairment of skin integrity	
b. Elevation of body temperature	May indicate response to infection.
c. Drainage from wound (amount, color)	Expect amount to decrease as healing takes place; serous drainage is clear; bright red drainage indicates fresh bleeding; purulent drainage is thick and yellow, pale green or white.
d. Odor	Strong odor indicates infectious process.
e. Consistency of drainage	Leukocytes produce thick drainage.
f. Size of wound	Measure depth, length, and width to assess client's stage of healing.
4. Administer prescribed analgesic 30-45 min before starting wound irrigation procedure.	Increased comfort level will permit client to move more easily and be positioned to facilitate infection control during wound irrigation.
5. Gather equipment at bedside:	Increases efficiency.
a. Sterile basin	To hold sterile irrigation solution in preparation for irrigation.
b. 150-500 ml prescribed sterile irrigating solution warmed to body temperature	Warming adds to client's comfort level.
c. Sterile irrigation syringe, sterile soft catheter, if needed	To prevent introduction of additional pathogens during procedure; soft catheter is used to irrigate deep wounds with small openings.
d. Clean basin	Basin collects contaminated irrigating solution.
e. Clean gloves (check policy of institution)	Gloves will protect nurse from infection while removing wound dressing.
f. Sterile gloves	To maintain asepsis during irrigation and redressing procedures.
g. Waterproof underpad	Prevents soiling of bed linen; is both cost and time effective.
h. Sterile dressing tray and supplies for dressing change including packing, if ordered	Prevents infection and promotes wound healing.
i. Leakproof refuse bag	Used to gather soiled and contaminated dressings and prevent cross-infection.
j. Gown	Gown may or may not be indicated to protect nurse's uniform from contamination.
6. Explain procedure of wound irrigation.	Providing necessary information will reduce client anxiety.
7. Position client comfortably to permit gravitational flow of irrigating solution through wound and into collection basin. Position client so that wound is vertical to collection basin.	Directing solution from top to bottom of wound and from clean area to contaminated area will prevent further infection. Positioning client during planning stage provides bed surfaces for later preparation.
8. Warm sterile irrigating solution to approximate body temperature.	Warmed solution increases comfort and reduces vascular constriction response in tissues.
9. Form cuff on leakproof refuse bag and place it near bed.	Helps maintain large opening, thereby permitting placement of contaminated dressing without soiling bag's outer surface.
10. Close room door or bed curtains.	Maintains privacy.

STEPS	RATIONALE
11. Place waterproof underpad on bed surface in front of wound.	Protection of bedding eliminates need to change linens.
12. Place clean basin directly under wound.	Collects contaminated irrigating solution.
13. Wash hands.	Reduces transmission of infection.
14. If gown is needed, put it on now.	Protects nurse's clothing and prevents cross-infection.
15. Prepare sterile field using sterile dressing set and supplies.	Reduces risk of introducing microorganisms into wound.
16. Add sterile basin and pour in estimated volume of warm sterile irrigating solution and set irrigating syringe in basin with solution.	Prepares solution for wound irrigation.
17. Place several strips of adhesive tape within reach and *not* on sterile field.	Provides easy access to tape for securing dressing.
18. Put on clean gloves and remove soiled dressing and discard in leakproof refuse bag.	Reduces transmission of microorganisms.
19. Remove and discard gloves.	
20. Inspect wound and make mental note of healing process, inflammation, presence of drainage or purulent matter.	Facilitates accurate description later.
21. Put on sterile gloves.	Reduces transmission of microorganisms.
22. To irrigate wound with wide opening:	Flushing wound will aid in removal of debris and facilitate healing by secondary intention.
a. Fill syringe with irrigating solution.	
b. Hold syringe tip 2.5 cm (1 in) above upper end of wound.	Prevents trauma to granulation tissue from syringe.
c. Using slow, continuous pressure, flush wound.	Ensures removal of all debris.
d. Repeat Steps 22 a, b, and c until solution draining into basin is clear.	
23. To irrigate deep wound with very small opening:	
a. Attach soft catheter to filled irrigating syringe.	Catheter permits direct flow of irrigant into wound.
b. Lubricate tip of catheter with irrigating solution; then gently insert tip of catheter until resistance is felt, then pull out about 1.2 cm (½ in) to remove tip from fragile inner wall of wound.	
c. Using slow, continuous pressure, flush wound.	Ensures removal of debris without traumatizing new granulation tissue.
d. Pinch off catheter just below syringe.	Avoids contamination of sterile solution or basin.
e. Remove syringe, fill and reattach to catheter; repeat process until return is clear.	
24. Dry wound edges with sterile gauze.	Prevents maceration of surrounding tissue from excess moisture.
25. Apply sterile dressing.	Maintains sterile protective barrier over wound.
26. Remove and dispose of gloves.	Facilitates placement of adhesive tape.
27. Secure dressing with adhesive tape.	
28. Assist client to comfortable position.	Relieves tension on wound site.
29. Dispose of equipment and refuse; retain remaining bottle of sterile solution.	Sterile solution can be used for subsequent irrigations.
30. Wash hands.	Reduces transmission of infection.
31. Inspect dressing periodically.	Determines client's response to wound irrigation and need to modify plan of care.
32. Evaluate skin integrity.	Determines if extension of wound has occurred.
33. Record wound appearance, irrigation, and client response on nurses' notes.	Recording fulfills legal responsibility of nurse and provides information needed to ensure continuity of care.

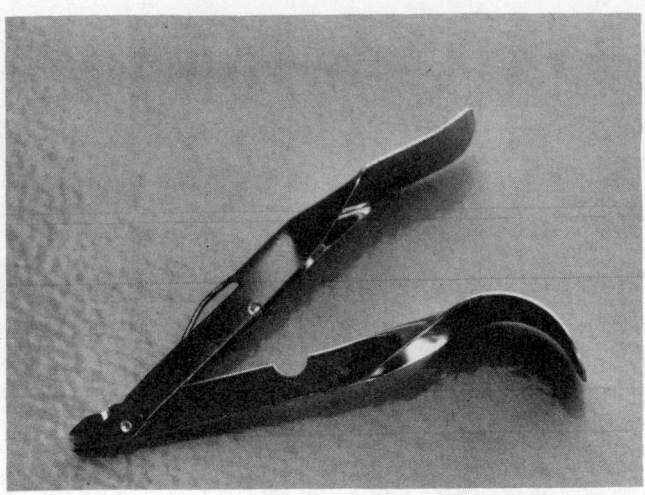

Fig. 47-10 Staple remover.

and superficially as the final means for wound closure. The deeper sutures are usually an absorbable material that disappears in several days. Sutures are foreign bodies and thus are capable of causing local inflammation. The surgeon can minimize tissue injury by using the finest suture possible and the smallest number necessary.

Policies vary within institutions as to who may remove sutures. If the nurse is allowed to remove them, a physician's order is required. An order for suture removal will not be written until the physician believes the wound has closed (usually 7 to 10 days). Special scissors with curved cutting tips or special staple removers slide under the skin closures for their removal (Fig. 47-10). The physician usually signifies the number of sutures or staples to remove. If the suture line appears to be healing

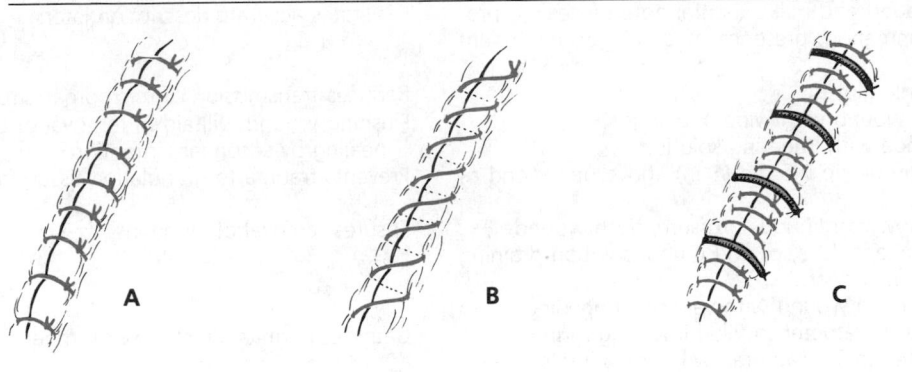

Fig. 47-11 Examples of suturing methods. **A,** Intermittent. **B,** Continuous. **C,** Retention.

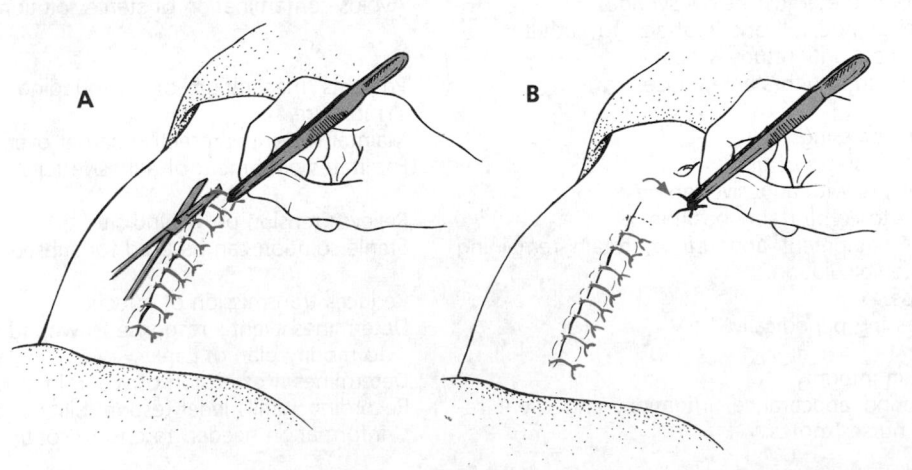

Fig. 47-12 Removal of intermittent suture. **A,** The nurse cuts the suture as close to the skin as possible, away from the knot. **B,** The nurse removes the suture and never pulls the contaminated stitch through tissues.

in certain locations better than in others, the physician may choose to have only some sutures removed (for example, every other one).

To remove staples, the nurse simply inserts the tips of the staple remover under each wire staple. While slowly closing the ends of the staple remover together the tips squeeze the center of the staple, freeing it from the skin.

To remove sutures the nurse first checks the type of suturing used (Fig. 47-11). With interrupted suturing the surgeon ties each individual suture made in the skin. Continuous suturing, as the name implies, is a series of sutures with only two knots, one at the beginning and one at the end of the suture line. Retention sutures are placed more deeply than skin sutures and may or may not be removed by the nurse depending on agency policy. The manner in which the suture crosses and penetrates the skin determines the method for removal. The most important principle in suture removal is *never pull the visible portion of a suture through underlying tissue.* Sutures on the skin's surface harbor microorganisms and debris. The portion of the suture beneath the skin is sterile. Pulling the contaminated portion of the suture through tissues may lead to infection. The nurse clips suture materials as close to the skin edge on one side as possible and then pulls the suture through from the other side (Fig. 47-12).

Drainage Evacuation

When drainage interferes with healing, drainage evacuation can be achieved by using either a drain alone or a drainage tube with continuous suction. The nurse may apply special skin barriers, similar to those used with ostomies (see Chapter 39), around drain sites. The barriers are a soft, waferlike, plastic material that apply to the skin with adhesive. Drainage flows on the barrier but not directly on the skin. Drainage evacuators (Fig. 47-13) are convenient portable units that connect to tubular drains lying within a wound bed and exert a safe, constant, low-pressure vaccuum to remove and collect drainage. The nurse ensures that suction is exerted and that connection points between the evacuator and tubing are intact. The evacuator collects drainage that the nurse assesses for volume and character every shift and as needed. When the evacuator fills, the nurse measures output by emptying the contents into a graduated cylinder and immediately resets the evacuator to apply suction.

Bandages and Binders

A simple gauze dressing is often not enough to immobilize or provide support to a wound. Binders and bandages applied over or around dressings can provide extra protection and therapeutic benefits by: (1) creating pressure over a body part, for example, an elastic pressure bandage applied over an arterial puncture site; (2) immobilizing a body part, for example, an elastic bandage applied around a sprained ankle; (3) supporting a wound, for example, an abdominal binder applied over a large abdominal incision and dressing; (4) reducing or preventing edema, for example, a breast binder used to minimize swelling between skin and tissue layers following a mastectomy; (5) securing a splint, for example, a bandage applied around hand splints for correction of deformities, or (6) securing dressings, for example, elas-

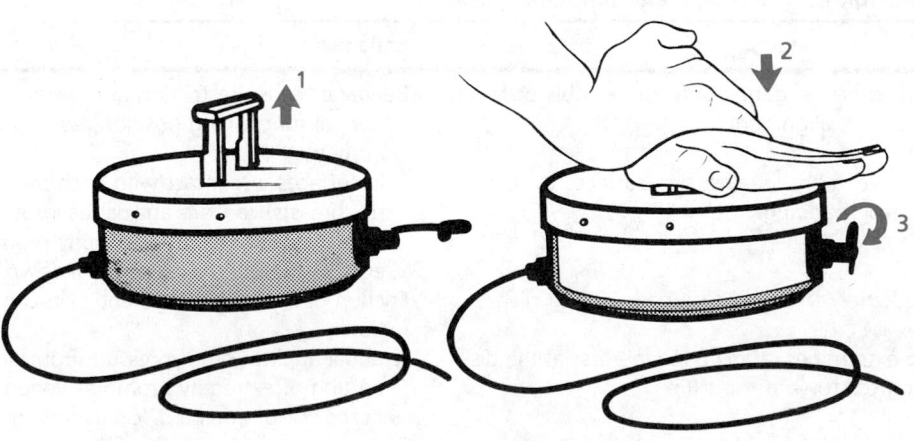

Fig. 47-13 Setting the suction on a drainage evacuator. **1,** With drainage port open, the lever to the vacuum diaphragm is raised. **2,** The nurse pushes straight down on the lever to lower the diaphragm. **3,** Closure of the port prevents escape of air and creates vacuum pressure.

tic webbing applied around leg dressings following a vein stripping.

Bandages are available in rolls of various widths and materials, including gauze, elasticized knit, elastic webbing, flannel, and muslin. Gauze bandages are lightweight and inexpensive, mold easily around contours of the body, and permit air circulation to prevent skin maceration. Elastic bandages conform well to body parts but can also be used to exert pressure over a body part. Flannel and muslin bandages are thicker than gauze and thus stronger for supporting or applying pressure. A flannel bandage also insulates to provide warmth.

Binders are bandages made of large pieces of material to fit a specific body part. Most binders are made of cotton, muslin, or flannel. An abdominal binder and a breast binder are examples.

PRINCIPLES FOR APPLYING BANDAGES AND BINDERS

Correctly applied bandages and binders do not cause injury to underlying and nearby body parts or create discomfort for the client. For example, a chest binder must not be so tight as to restrict chest wall expansion. Before a bandage or binder is applied, the nurse's responsibilities include the following:

1. Inspecting the skin for abrasions, edema, discoloration, or exposed wound edges
2. Covering exposed wounds or open abrasions with a sterile dressing
3. Assessing the condition of underlying dressings and changing them if soiled.
4. Assessing the skin of underlying body parts and parts that will be distal to the bandage for signs of circulatory impairment (coolness, pallor or cy-

anosis, diminished or absent pulses, swelling, numbness, and tingling) to provide a means for comparing changes in circulation after bandage application.

Table 47-4 outlines the principles of bandage and binder application. Once a bandage is applied, the nurse assesses, documents, and immediately reports changes in circulation, skin integrity, comfort level, and body function such as ventilation or movement. The nurse who applies a bandage can loosen or readjust it as necessary. The nurse should have a physician's order before loosening or removing a bandage applied by a physician. The nurse explains to the client that any bandage or binder will feel relatively firm or tight. A bandage should be carefully assessed to be sure it is properly applied and is providing therapeutic benefit, and soiled bandages should be replaced. Like a damp dressing, a bandage or binder can harbor microorganisms.

BINDER APPLICATION

Binders are especially designed for the body part to be supported. The most common types of binders are the breast binder, abdominal binders (Scultetus and straight) and T binder (Procedure 47-3).

BREAST BINDER. A breast binder looks like a tight-fitting sleeveless vest. It conforms to the shape of the chest wall and is available in different sizes. Breast binders can provide support after breast surgery or exert pressure to reduce lactation in a woman after childbirth. It is essential that excess pressure be avoided when clients or family members are learning how to apply a binder. Chest expansion should remain unimpaired.

TABLE 47-4 Principles for Bandage and Binder Application

Principle	Rationale
Position body part to be bandaged in a comfortable position of normal anatomical alignment	Bandages cause restriction in movement. Immobilization in a normal functioning position reduces the risks of deformity or injury.
Prevent friction between and against skin surfaces by applying gauze or cotton padding.	Skin surfaces in contact with each other (between toes, under breasts) can rub against each other to cause abrasion or chafing. Bandages over bony prominences may rub against the skin to cause breakdown.
Apply bandages securely to prevent slippage during client's movement.	Friction between bandage and skin can cause skin breakdown.
When bandaging extremities, apply bandage first at the distal end and progress toward the trunk.	Gradual application of pressure from distal toward proximal portion of extremity promotes venous return and minimizes risk of edema or circulatory impairment.
Apply bandages firmly with equal tension exerted over each turn or layer. Avoid excess overlapping of bandage layers.	Prevents unequal pressure distribution over bandaged body part. Localized pressure causes circulatory impairment.
Position pins, knots, or ties away from the wound or sensitive skin areas.	Can exert localized pressure and irritation.

PROCEDURE 47-3

Applying an Abdominal Binder, T Binder, or Breast Binder

STEPS	RATIONALE
1. Observe client with need for support of thorax or abdomen. Observe ability to breathe deeply and cough effectively.	Baseline assessment determines client's ability to breathe and cough. Impaired ventilation of lung can lead to alveolar atelectasis and inadequate arterial oxygenation.
2. Inspect skin for actual or potential alterations in integrity. Observe for irritation, abrasions; skin surfaces that rub against each other; allergic response to adhesive tape used to secure dressing.	Actual impairments in skin integrity can be worsened with application of a binder. Binder can cause pressure and excoriation.
3. Review medical record if medical prescription for particular binder is required and reasons for application.	Application of supportive binders may be based on nursing judgment. In some situations physician input is required.
4. Gather necessary data regarding size of client and appropriate binder.	Ensures proper fit of binder.
5. Prepare the necessary equipment and supplies:	
a. Abdominal binder:	
(1) Correct size cloth/elastic straight binder or scultetus binder	Binder must be large enough to surround client's abdomen and overlap to secure closure.
(2) Safety pins (unless Velcro closure is attached)	
b. T and double-T binder:	
(1) Correct size	
(2) Safety pins: 2 pins for T binders; 3 pins for double-T binder	One pin secures horizontal waistband. One pin secures each tail, placing pin through all thicknesses at horizontal level.
c. Breast binders:	
(1) Correct size binder	Binder must be large enough to overlap to secure Velcro closure.
6. Explain procedure to client.	Promotes client's understanding.
7. Wash hands.	Maintains medical asepsis and infection control.
8. Close curtains or room door.	Provides privacy.
9. **Abdominal binder (straight and Scultetus)** Apply abdominal binder as follows:	
a. Position client in supine position with head slightly elevated and knees slightly flexed.	Minimizes muscular tension on abdominal organs.
b. Fanfold far side of binder toward midline of binder.	Reduces time client remains in uncomfortable position.
c. Instruct and assist client to roll away from nurse toward raised side rail while firmly supporting abdominal incision and dressing with hands.	Reduces pain and discomfort.
d. Place fanfolded ends of binder under client.	Permits placement and centering of binder with minimal discomfort.
e. Instruct/assist client to roll over folded ends.	
f. Unfold and stretch ends out smoothly on far side of bed. (Binder should extend from just above symphysis pubis to just below costal margin.)	Maintains skin integrity and comfort.
g. Instruct client to roll back into supine position.	Facilitates chest expansion and adequate wound support when the binder is closed.
h. Adjust binder so that supine client is centered over binder using symphysis pubis and costal margins as low and upper landmarks.	Centers support from binder over abdominal structures.
i. Close binder.	
(1) Straight binder: Pull distal end of binder over center of client's abdomen. While maintaining tension on that end of binder, pull opposite end of binder over center and secure with Velcro closure tabs or safety pins.	Provides continuous wound support and comfort.
(2) Scultetus binder: With left hand bring bottom tail at client's left side over center of abdomen. Maintain tension on the tail and overlap it with bottom right tail. Repeat with each pair of tails, moving toward top of binder. Secure each end of top set of tails with safety pins.	Provides continuous wound support and comfort. For postsurgical application, binders are applied upward from bottom to minimize pull on suture line.

Continued.

PROCEDURE 47-3, cont'd

Applying an Abdominal Binder, T Binder, or Breast Binder

STEPS	RATIONALE
j. Assess client's ability to breathe deeply and cough effectively.	Determines ventilation and clears the airways of pulmonary secretions.
k. Ask client about comfort level.	Excess discomfort may inhibit expirations.
l. Adjust binder as necessary.	

10. **T and double-T binders**
    Apply T or double-T binder as follows:
    a. Assist client to dorsal recumbent position.
    b. Have client raise hips and place horizontal band around client's waist (or above iliac crests) with vertical tails extending past buttocks. Overlap wasteband in front and secure with safety pins.

    Minimizes muscular tension on perineal organs. Secures binder around client.

    c. Complete binder application:

    Single-T and double-T binders provide support to perineal muscles and organs.

    (1) T *binder:* Bring remaining vertical strip over perineal dressing and continue up and under center front of horizontal band. Bring ends over waistband and secure all thicknesses with safety pin.
    (2) *Double*-T *binder:* Bring remaining vertical strips over perineal or suprapubic dressing with each tail supporting one side of scrotum and proceeding upward on either side of penis. Continue drawing ends behind and then downward in front of horizontal band. Secure all thicknesses with one safety pin.
    d. Assess client's comfort level with client in lying, sitting, and standing positions. Readjust front pins as necessary. Increase padding if any area rubs against surrounding tissues.

    Determines efficacy of binder to maintain dressings and support perineal structures.

    e. Instruct client regarding removal of binder before defecating or urinating and need to replace binder after these bodily functions.

    Cleanliness of binder reduces infection risk.

11. **Breast binder**
    Apply breast binder as follows:
    a. Assist client in placing arms through binder's armholes.

    Eases binder placement process.

    b. Assist client to supine position in bed.

    Supine positioning facilitates normal anatomical situation of breasts. Maintains normal anatomical alignment of breasts, facilitates healing and comfort.

    c. Pad area under breasts if necessary.

    Prevents skin contact with undersurface.

    d. Using Velcro closure tabs secure binder at nipple level first. Continue closure process above and then below nipple line until entire binder is closed.

    Reduces risk of uneven pressure or localized irritation.

    e. Make appropriate adjustments including individualizing fit of shoulder straps.

    Maintains support to client's breasts.

    f. Instruct and observe skill development in self-care related to reapplying breast binder.

    Self-care is an integral aspect of discharge planning. Skin integrity and comfort level goals are assured.

    g. Wash hands.

    Prevents cross-infections.

12. Observe site for skin integrity, circulation, characteristics of the wound.

    Determines that binder has not resulted in irritation to skin or underlying organs.

13. Note comfort level of client.

    Binders should not impede breathing or increase discomfort.

14. Record application of binder, condition of skin and circulation, integrity of dressings, and client's comfort level.

    Documents procedure. Baseline data ensures continuity of care.

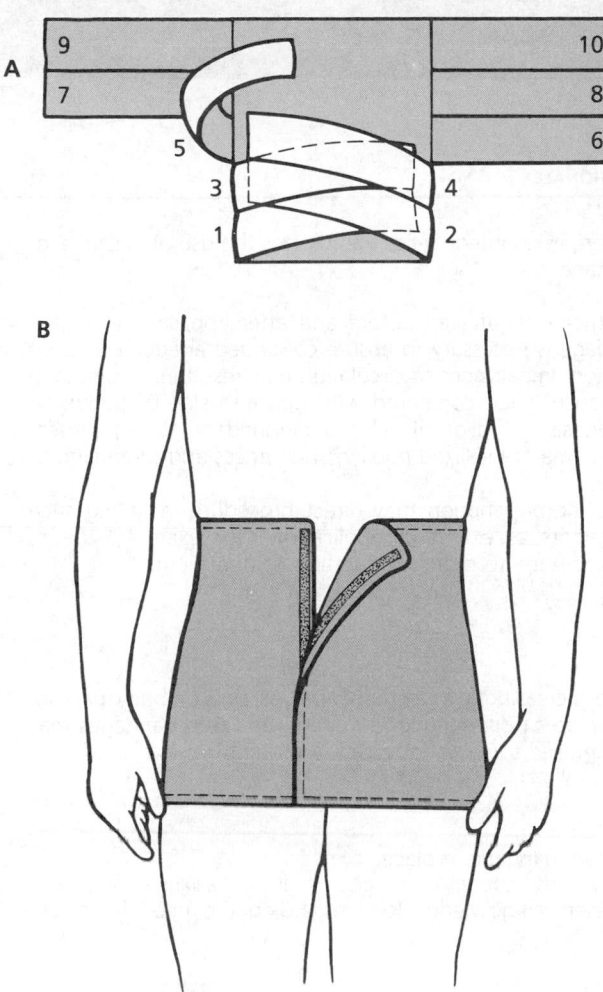

Fig. 47-14 A, Scultetus binder. Each successive tail overlaps and secures the previous tail. B, An abdominal binder secures with velcro.

ABDOMINAL BINDERS. An abdominal binder supports large abdominal incisions that are vulnerable to tension or stress as the client moves or coughs. It is a rectangular piece of cotton or elasticized material that has many tails attached to the two longer sides or has long extensions on each side to surround the abdomen (Fig 47-14). The nurse secures an abdominal binder with safety pins, Velcro strips, or metal stays. Procedure 47-3 describes steps for an abdominal binder application.

T BINDERS. As the name implies, the T binder looks like the letter T (Fig. 47-15) and is used to secure rectal or perineal dressings. The single T is for female clients and the double T fits male clients.

The belt of the binder fits securely around the client's waist with the tail passing between the client's legs from back to front and attaching to the belt's front. It is important for the nurse to be sure the tail fits smoothly

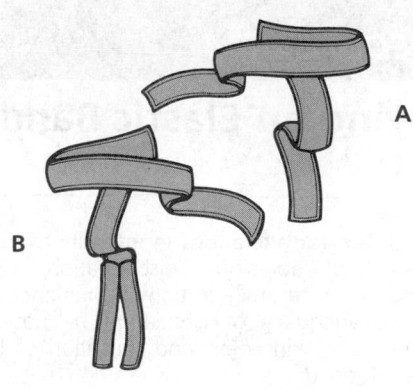

Fig. 47-15 T binders. **A**, Female. **B**, Male.

and against the dressing. T binders become soiled easily and often require frequent changing. Irritation to the urethra or scrotum must be avoided.

SLINGS

Slings support arms with muscular sprains or fractures. A commercially made sling consists of a long sleeve that extends above the elbow, with a strap that fits around the neck. In the home setting a large triangular piece of cloth can be used. The client may sit or lie supine during sling application (Fig. 47-16). The nurse instructs the client to bend the affected arm, bringing the forearm straight across the chest. The open sling fits under the

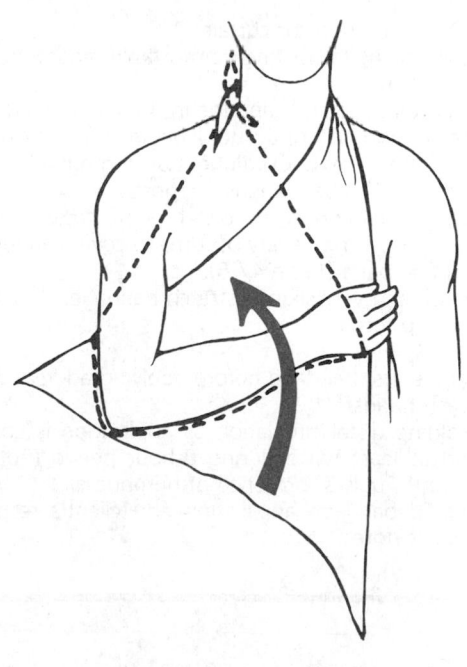

Fig. 47-16 Application of a sling.

PROCEDURE 47-4

Applying an Elastic Bandage

STEPS	RATIONALE
1. Inspect skin for alterations in integrity as indicated by presence of abrasions, discoloration, chafing, or edema. (Look carefully at bony prominences.)	Altered skin integrity contraindicates the use of elastic bandage.
2. Observe adequacy of circulation by noting surface temperature, skin color, and sensation of body parts to be wrapped.	Comparison of area before and after application of bandage is necessary to ensure continued adequate circulation. Impairment of circulation may result in: coolness to touch when compared with opposite side of body; cyanosis or pallor of skin; diminished or absent pulses; edema or localized pooling; numbness and/or tingling of part.
3. Review client's medical record for specific orders related to application of elastic bandage. Note area to be covered, type of bandage required, frequency of change, previous response to treatment.	Specific prescription may direct procedure including such factors as extent of application, (for example, toe to knee, toe to groin) or duration of treatment.
4. Obtain necessary equipment and supplies (determine if present bandage is to be reused or a replacement is to be obtained):	
a. Correct widths and number of bandages; elastic bandages are available in 2 in (5 cm), 2½ in (6.25 cm), 3 in (7.5 cm), 4 in (10.0 cm), 6 in (15.0 cm), and 8 in (20.0 cm) and in 3 yd (270 cm) and 1½ yd (135 cm) lengths; 3- and 4-width bandages are most often appropriate.	Use increasingly wider bandages as size of body part increases (for example, 3-in, 4-in, and 6-in bandages may be used to cover foot, calf, and thigh).
b. Safety pins, tape.	Secure bandage in place.
5. Explain procedure to client. Reinforce teaching that smooth, even, light pressure will be applied to improve venous circulation; prevent clot formation; reduce or prevent swelling, immobilize arms; secure surgical dressings; provide pressure.	Promotes cooperation and reduces anxiety. Improves client's knowledge level regarding the need for elastic bandages.
6. Wash hands.	Reduces transmission of infection.
7. Close room door or curtains.	Maintains client's comfort and dignity.
8. Assist client to assume comfortable, anatomically correct position.	Maintains alignment. Prevents musculoskeletal deformity.
9. Hold roll of elastic bandage in dominant hand and use other hand to lightly hold beginning of bandage at distal body part. Continue transferring roll to dominant hand as bandage is wrapped.	Maintains appropriate and consistent bandage tension.
10. Apply bandage from distal point toward proximal boundary using variety of turns to cover various shapes of body parts (Table 47-5).	Bandage applied in manner that conforms evenly to body part and promotes venous return.
11. Unroll and very slightly stretch bandage.	Maintains uniform bandage tension.
12. Overlap turns.	Prevents uneven bandage tension and circulatory impairment.
13. Secure first bandage before applying additional rolls.	To prevent wrinkling or loose ends.
14. Wash hands.	Reduces transmission of microorganisms.
15. Evaluate distal circulation as application is completed and at least twice during 8-hour period (note color, warmth, pulses, presence of numbness).	Early detection of circulatory difficulties ensures healthy neuromuscular status.
16. Record bandage application and client's response in nurse's notes.	Documents procedures and ensures continuity of care.

TABLE 47-5 Types of Bandage Turns

Type	Description	Purpose or Use
Circular	Bandage turn overlapping previous turn completely	Anchors a bandage at the first and final turn; covers a small part (finger or toe)
Spiral	Bandage ascending body part with each turn overlapping previous one by one-half or two-thirds width of bandage	Covers cylindrical body parts such as wrist or upper arm
Spiral—reverse	Turn requires a twist (reversal) of bandage halfway through each turn	Covers cone-shaped body parts such as the forearm, thigh, or calf; useful with nonstretching bandages such as gauze or flannel.
Figure-eight	Oblique overlapping turns alternately ascending and descending over bandaged part; each turn crossing previous one to form a figure-eight	Covers joints; snug fit provides excellent immobilization
Recurrent	Bandage first secured with two circular turns around proximal end of body part; half turn made perpendicular up from bandage edge; body of bandage brought over distal end of body part to be covered with each turn folded back over on itself	Covers uneven body parts such as head or stump.

client's arm and over the chest, with the base of the triangle under the wrist and the triangle's point at the client's elbow. One end of the sling fits around the back of the client's neck. The nurse brings the other end up and over the affected arm while supporting the extremity. The nurse ties the two ends at the side of the neck so the knot does not press against the cervical spine. The loose material at the elbow can be folded evenly around the elbow and pinned. The lower arm and hand should always be supported at a level above the elbow to prevent formation of dependent edema.

BANDAGE APPLICATION

Rolls of bandage can secure or support dressings over irregularly shaped body parts. Each roll has a free outer end and a terminal end at the center of the roll. The rolled portion of the bandage is its body, and its outer surface is placed against the client's skin or dressing. Procedure 47-4 describes the steps for applying an elastic bandage. The nurse may use a variety of bandage turns depending on the body part to be bandaged (Table 47-5). Care must be taken to prevent the applied bandage from exerting a tourniquet effect.

Heat and Cold Therapy

Local application of heat and cold to an injured body part can be therapeutic. Before using these therapies, however, the nurse must understand normal body responses to local temperature variations, assess the integrity of the body part, determine the client's ability to sense temperature variations, and ensure proper operation of equipment. The nurse is legally responsible for safe administration of heat and cold applications.

BODILY RESPONSES TO HEAT AND COLD

Exposure to heat and cold can cause both systemic and local responses. Systemic responses occur through heat loss mechanisms (sweating, vasodilation) or mechanisms promoting heat conservation (vasoconstriction, piloerection) and heat production (shivering) (see Chapter 12). Local responses to heat and cold occur through stimulation of temperature-sensitive nerve endings within the skin. This stimulation sends impulses from the periphery to the hypothalamus, which becomes aware of local temperature sensations and triggers adaptive responses for maintenance of normal body temperature. If alterations occur along temperature sensation

pathways, the reception and eventual perception of stimuli will be altered.

The body also possesses a protective reflex response so that when a person touches an extremely hot or cold stimulus, impulses travel to the spinal cord, synapse within the cord, and return by way of a motor nerve to cause withdrawal from the stimulus. The person simultaneously becomes aware of the discomfort.

The body can tolerate wide variations in temperature. The normal temperature of the skin's surface is 34° C (93.2° F), but temperature receptors usually adapt quickly to local temperatures between 45° C (113° F) and 15° C (59° F). Pain develops when local temperatures exceed this range. Excessive heat causes a burning sensation. Cold produces a numbing sensation prior to the pain.

The body's adaptive ability creates the major problem in protecting clients from injury resulting from temperature extremes. A person initially feels an extreme change in temperature but within a short time hardly notices it. This can be dangerous, since a person insensitive to heat and cold extremes can suffer serious tissue injury. The nurse must recognize clients most at risk for injuries from heat and cold applications (Table 47-6).

LOCAL EFFECTS OF HEAT AND COLD

Heat and cold stimuli create different physiological responses. The choice of heat or cold therapy depends on local responses desired for wound healing.

EFFECTS OF HEAT APPLICATION. Table 47-7 summarizes the benefits of heat application. Heat generally is quite therapeutic, improving blood flow to an injured part. If heat is applied for 1 hour or more, however, blood flow is reduced by a reflex vasoconstriction as the body attempts to control heat loss from the area. Peri-

TABLE 47-6 Conditions That Increase Risk of Injury from Heat and Cold Application

Condition	Risk Factors
Very young; elderly	Thinner skin layers in children increase risk of burns; the elderly have reduced sensitivity to pain.
Open wounds, broken skin, stomas	Subcutaneous and visceral tissues are more sensitive to temperature variations; also contain no temperature and fewer pain receptors.
Areas of edema or scar formation	Reduced sensation to temperature stimuli because of thickening of skin layers from fluid buildup or scar formation.
Peripheral vascular disease (for example, diabetes or arteriosclerosis)	Body's extremities are less sensitive to temperature and pain stimuli because of circulatory impairment and local tissue injury; cold application would further compromise blood flow.
Confusion or unconsciousness	Reduced perception of sensory or painful stimuli.
Spinal cord injury	Alterations in nerve pathways preventing reception of sensory or painful stimuli.
Abscessed tooth or appendix	Infection highly localized; application of heat may cause rupture with spread of microorganisms systemically.

TABLE 47-7   Therapeutic Effects of Heat and Cold Applications

Therapy	Physiological Response	Therapeutic Benefit	Examples of Conditions Treated
Heat	Vasodilation	Improves blood flow to injured body part; promotes delivery of nutrients and removal of wastes; lessens venous congestion in injured tissues	Inflamed or edematous body part; new surgical wound; infected wound; arthritis, degenerative joint disease; localized joint pain, muscle strains; low back pain; menstrual cramping; hemorrhoidal, perianal, and vaginal inflammation; local abscesses
	Reduced blood viscosity	Improved delivery of leukocytes and antibiotics to wound site	
	Reduced muscle tension	Promotes muscle relaxation and reduces pain from spasm or stiffness	
	Increased tissue metabolism	Increases blood flow; provides local warmth	
	Increased capillary permeability	Promotes movement of waste products and nutrients	
Cold	Vasoconstriction	Reduces blood flow to injured body part, preventing edema formation; reduces inflammation	Immediately after direct trauma (sprains, strains, fractures, muscle spasms); superficial laceration or puncture wound; minor burn; when malignancy is suspected in area of injury or pain; after injections; arthritis, joint trauma
	Local anesthesia	Reduces localized pain	
	Reduced cell metabolism	Reduces oxygen needs of tissues	
	Increased blood viscosity	Promotes blood coagulation at injury site	
	Decreased muscle tension	Relieves pain	

odic removal and reapplication of local heat will restore vasodilation. Continuous exposure to heat damages epithelial cells, causing redness, localized tenderness, and even blistering of the skin.

EFFECTS OF COLD APPLICATION. Table 47-7 also summarizes the benefits of cold application. Prolonged exposure of the skin to cold results in a reflex vasodilation. The cell's inability to receive adequate blood flow and nutrients results in tissue ischemia. The skin initially takes on a reddened appearance, followed by a bluish purple mottling with numbness and a burning type of pain. The skin's tissues can freeze from exposure to extreme cold.

FACTORS INFLUENCING HEAT AND COLD TOLERANCE

The body's response to heat and cold therapies depends on a number of factors.
1. *Duration of application*—A person is better able to tolerate short exposure to temperature extremes.
2. *Body part*—Certain areas of the skin are more sensitive to temperature variations. These include the neck, inner aspect of the wrist and forearm, and perineal region. The foot and palm of the hand are less sensitive.
3. *Damage to body surface*—Exposed skin layers are more sensitive to temperature variations.

4. *Prior skin temperature*—The body responds best to minor temperature adjustments. If a body part is cool and a hot stimulus touches the skin, the response is greater than if the stimulus were only warm.
5. *Body surface area*—A person has less tolerance to temperature changes when a large area of the body is exposed to heat or cold.
6. *Age and physical condition*—Tolerance to temperature variations changes with age. The very young and elderly are most sensitive to heat and cold. If a client's physical condition reduces the reception or perception of sensory stimuli, tolerance to temperature extremes is high but the risk of injury is also high.

ASSESSMENT FOR TEMPERATURE TOLERANCE

Before applying heat or cold therapies the nurse assesses the client's physical condition for signs of potential intolerance to heat and cold. The nurse first observes the area to be treated. Alterations in skin integrity, such as abrasions, open wounds, edema, bruising, bleeding, or localized areas of inflammation, increase the client's risk of injury. Since the physician commonly orders heat and cold applications to be placed on traumatized areas, the nurse's baseline assessment provides a guide for evaluating skin changes that might occur during therapy.

The nurse's assessment includes identification of conditions that contraindicate heat or cold therapy. An active area of bleeding should not be covered by a warm application, since bleeding will continue. Warm applications are contraindicated when the client has an acute localized inflammation such as appendicitis, since the heat could cause the appendix to rupture. If a client has cardiovascular problems, it is unwise to apply heat to large portions of the body as the resulting massive vasodilation may disrupt blood supply to vital organs.

Cold is contraindicated if the site of injury is already edematous. Cold will further retard circulation to the area and prevent absorption of the interstitial fluid. If the client has impairment in circulation, for example, arteriosclerosis, cold will further reduce blood supply to the affected area. One other contraindication for cold therapy is the presence of shivering. Cold applications may intensify shivering and dangerously increase the client's body temperature. The nurse also assesses the client's response to stimuli. Sensation to light touch, pinprick, and mild temperature variations (see Chapter 13) will reveal the ability of the client to recognize when heat or cold becomes excessive. If a client has peripheral vascular disease, the nurse pays particular attention to the integrity of extremities. For example, if the physician's order is to apply a cold compress to a lower extremity, the nurse should assess circulation to the leg by observing skin color and palpating skin temperatures, distal pulses, and any edematous areas. If signs of circulatory inadequacy are present, the nurse should question the order.

Safety Suggestions for Applying Heat or Cold Therapy

- *Do* explain to the client sensations to be felt during the procedure.
- *Do* instruct the client to report changes in sensation or discomfort immediately.
- *Do* provide a timer, clock, or watch so the client can help the nurse time the application.
- *Do* keep the call light within the client's reach.
- *Do* refer to the institution's policy and procedure manual for safe temperatures.
- *Do not* allow the client to adjust temperature settings.
- *Do not* allow the client to move an application or place hands on the wound site.
- *Do not* place the client in a position that prevents movement away from the temperature source.
- *Do not* leave unattended a client who is unable to sense temperature changes or move from the temperature source.

A client's level of consciousness will influence the ability to perceive heat, cold, or pain. If a client is confused or unresponsive, the nurse must make frequent observations of skin integrity once therapy begins.

The nurse must also assess the condition of equipment being used. Electrical equipment should be checked for cracked cords, frayed wires, damaged insulation, or exposed heating components. Equipment containing circulating fluids should not have leaks. The nurse also checks equipment for evenness of temperature distribution. Uneven temperature distribution suggests that the equipment is functioning improperly.

CLIENT EDUCATION AND SAFETY

A prerequisite to using any heat or cold application is a physician's order which should include the body site to be treated and the type, frequency, and duration of application. The nurse should consult the agency's procedure manual for correct temperatures to use.

APPLYING HEAT AND COLD

Before application of heat or cold therapy the client should understand its purpose, the symptoms of temperature exposure, and precautions taken to prevent injury. The box provides hints for safely applying heat and cold therapy.

CHOICE OF MOIST OR DRY. Both heat and cold applications can be administered in dry or moist forms. The type of wound or injury, the location of the body part, and the presence of drainage or inflammation are factors considered in selecting dry or moist applications. Table 47-8 (p. 1429) summarizes advantages and disadvantages of both.

HOT MOIST COMPRESSES. For open wounds, sterile hot moist compresses improve circulation, relieve edema, and promote consolidation of pus and drainage. A compress is a piece of gauze dressing moistened in a prescribed warmed solution. A pack is a larger cloth or dressing applied to a larger body area.

Heat from hot compresses dissipates quickly. To maintain a constant temperature the nurse must either change the compress often or apply a warm aquathermic pad or waterproof heating pad over the compress. Since moisture *conducts heat,* any device's temperature setting should be lower for a moist compress than for a dry application. A layer of plastic wrap or a dry towel can also be used to insulate the compress and retain heat. Moist heat promotes vasodilation and evaporation of heat from the skin's surface. For this reason a client may feel chilly. The nurse controls drafts within the room and keeps the client covered with a blanket or robe. Procedure 47-5 describes the steps for applying a hot, moist compress.

PROCEDURE 47-5

Applying a Hot, Moist Compress to an Open Wound

STEPS	RATIONALE
1. Inspect condition of exposed skin and wound on which compress is to be applied.	Provides baseline to determine changes in skin during heat application. Very thin or damaged skin is more susceptible to injury from heat.
2. Assess client's extremities for sensitivity to temperature and pain by measuring light touch, pin prick, and temperature sensation tests.	Determines if client is insensitive to heat and cold extremes.
3. Refer to physician's order for type of compress, location and duration of application, desired temperature.	Ensures likelihood of safe application.
4. Prepare the necessary equipment and supplies:	
a. Prescribed solution warmed to proper temperature, approximately 43-46° C (110-115° F)	Correct temperature prevents accidental burns.
b. Sterile gauze dressings	
c. Sterile container for solution	
d. Commercially prepared compresses (optional)	Premoistened compress reduces preparation.
e. Sterile gloves	
f. Petrolatum jelly, if desired	Protects untreated skin surface.
g. Sterile cotton swabs	
h. Waterproof pad	Prevents soiling of bed linen.
i. Tape or ties	
j. Dry bath towel	
k. Aquathermic or heating pad (optional)	Provides continuous source of heat.
l. Disposable gloves	
m. Bath thermometer	Measures solution temperature.
n. Bath blanket	
5. Explain steps of procedure and purpose to client. Describe sensation to be felt (for example, feeling of warmth and wetness). Explain precautions to prevent burning.	Minimizes client's anxiety and promotes cooperation during procedure.
6. Assist client in assuming comfortable position in proper body alignment.	Compress remains in place for several minutes. Limited mobility in uncomfortable position causes muscular stress.
7. Place waterproof pad under area to be treated.	Prevents soiling of bed linen.
8. Expose body part to be covered with compress and drape client with bath blanket. Close bedside curtains.	Prevents unnecessary cooling and exposure of body part. Provides privacy.
9. Wash hands.	Reduces transmission of infection.
10. Assemble equipment. Pour warmed solution into sterile container. (If using portable heating source, keep solution warm. Commercially prepared compresses may remain under infrared lamp until just before use). Open sterile packages and drop gauze into container to become immersed in solution. Turn aquathermia pad (if desired) to correct temperature.	Compresses must retain warmth for therapeutic benefit.
11. Apply disposable gloves. Remove any existing dressing covering wound. Dispose of gloves and dressings in proper receptacle.	Reduces transmission of microorganisms.
12. If wound was covered, assess condition of it and surrounding skin.	Provides baseline to determine skin changes following compress application.
13. Apply sterile gloves.	Allows nurse to manipulate sterile dressing and touch open wound.
14. Apply sterile petrolatum jelly, if desired, with cotton swab to skin surrounding wound. Do not apply jelly on broken areas of skin.	Jelly protects skin from possible burns and maceration.
15. Pick up one layer of immersed gauze and wring out excess water.	Excess moisture macerates skin and increases risk of burns and infection.

Continued.

Applying a Hot, Moist Compress to an Open Wound

STEPS	RATIONALE
16. Apply gauze lightly to open wound. Watch client's response and ask if client feels discomfort. In a few seconds lift edge of gauze to assess for redness.	Skin is sensitive to sudden change in temperature. Redness indicates burn.
17. If client tolerates compress, pack gauze snugly against wound. Be sure all wound surfaces are covered by hot compress.	Packing of compress prevents rapid cooling from underlying air currents.
18. Wrap or cover moist compress with dry bath towel. If necessary, pin or tie in place.	Towel insulates compress to prevent heat loss.
19. Change hot compress every 5 min or as ordered.	Prevents cooling and maintains therapeutic benefit of compress.
20. Apply aquathermic or waterproof heating pad over towel (optional). Keep it in place for desired duration of application (about 20-30 min).	Provides constant temperature to compress. Local application of heat for greater than 60 min often results in reflex vasoconstriction. Removing hot compress after 30 min and then reapplying in 15 min, if desired, maintains vasodilation and positive therapeutic effects.
21. Ask client periodically if there is discomfort or burning sensation. Observe area of skin not covered by compress.	Continued exposure to heat can cause burning of skin.
22. Remove pad, towel, and compress in 30 min. Again assess wound and condition of skin.	Continued exposure to moisture will macerate skin.
23. Replace dry sterile dressing as ordered.	Prevents entrance of microorganisms into wound site.
24. Assist client to preferred comfortable position.	Maintains client's comfort.
25. Dispose of equipment and soiled compress. Wash hands.	Reduces transmission of infection.
26. Inspect affected area covered by compress and heating pad.	Assists in determining effects of application.
27. Ask client if any unusual burning sensation is noticed that was not felt before.	It may be difficult to assess burn merely by color changes if wound is inflamed or drainage is present.
28. Record type, location, and duration of application. Note temperature used in nurses' notes.	Documents therapy administered.
29. Describe condition of wound, skin, and client's response.	Documents client's response to therapy.

WARM SOAKS. Immersion of a body part in a warmed solution promotes circulation, lessens edema, increases muscle relaxation, and can provide a means to debride wounds and apply medicated solution. A soak can also be accompanied by wrapping the body part in dressings and saturating them with the warmed solution.

The nurse positions the client comfortably, places waterproof pads under the area to be treated, and heats the solution to about 40.5° to 43° C (105° to 110° F). After immersing the body part the nurse covers the container and extremity with a towel to reduce heat loss. It is usually necessary to remove the cooled solution and the body part and add heated solution after about 10 minutes. The problem is to keep the solution at a constant temperature. Never add a hotter solution while the body part remains immersed. After any soak the nurse dries the body part thoroughly to prevent maceration.

SITZ BATHS. The client who has had rectal surgery, an episiotomy during childbirth, painful hemorrhoids, or vaginal inflammation may benefit from a sitz bath, a bath in which only the pelvic area is immersed in warm fluid. The client sits in a special tub or chair or in a basin that fits on the toilet seat so that the legs and feet remain out of the water. Immersing the entire body causes widespread vasodilation and nullifies the effect of local heat application to the pelvic area.

The desired temperature for a sitz bath depends on whether the purpose is to promote relaxation or to clean a wound. It may be necessary to carefully add warm

TABLE 47-8   Choice of Dry or Moist Applications

Advantages	Disadvantages
MOIST APPLICATIONS	
Moist application reduces drying of skin and softens wound exudate.	Prolonged exposure can cause maceration of the skin.
Moist compresses conform well to body area being treated.	Moist heat will cool rapidly because of moisture evaporation.
Moist heat penetrates deeply into tissue layers.	Moist heat creates a greater risk for burns to the skin since moisture conducts heat.
Warm moist heat does not promote sweating and insensible fluid loss.	
DRY APPLICATIONS	
Dry heat has less risk of burns to skin than moist applications.	Dry heat increases body fluid loss through sweating.
Dry application does not cause skin maceration.	Dry applications do not penetrate deep into tissues.
Dry heat retains temperature longer, since it is not influenced by evaporation.	Dry heat causes increased drying of skin.

water during the procedure, which normally lasts 20 minutes, to maintain a constant temperature. Agency procedure manuals recommend safe water temperatures. A disposable sitz basin contains an attachment resembling an enema bag that allows gradual introduction of warmer water (Fig. 47-17).

The nurse prevents overexposure of the client by draping bath blankets around the client's shoulders and thighs and controlling drafts. The client should be able to sit in the basin or tub with feet flat on the floor and without pressure on the sacrum or thighs. Since exposure of a large portion of the body to heat can cause extensive vasodilation, the nurse should assess the pulse and facial color and ask if the client feels light-headed or nauseated.

PARAFFIN BATHS. A paraffin bath consists of a mixture of heated paraffin wax and mineral oil (1 part oil to 5 parts paraffin). Clients with painful arthritis or other joint discomforts of the hands and feet benefit most from the baths. In many institutions only physical therapists administer the applications. Clients often heat paraffin baths at home in double boilers (53.3° to 54.4° C [128° to 130° F]).

AQUATHERMIA (WATER FLOW) PADS. A popular device in health care institutions is the aquathermia (water flow) pad (Fig. 47-18), used for treating muscle sprains and areas of mild inflammation or edema. The aquathermia unit consists of a waterproof plastic or rubber pad connected by two hoses to an electrical control unit that has a heating element and motor. Distilled water circulates through hollowed channels within the pad to the control unit where water is heated or cooled (depending on temperature setting). Some pads have an

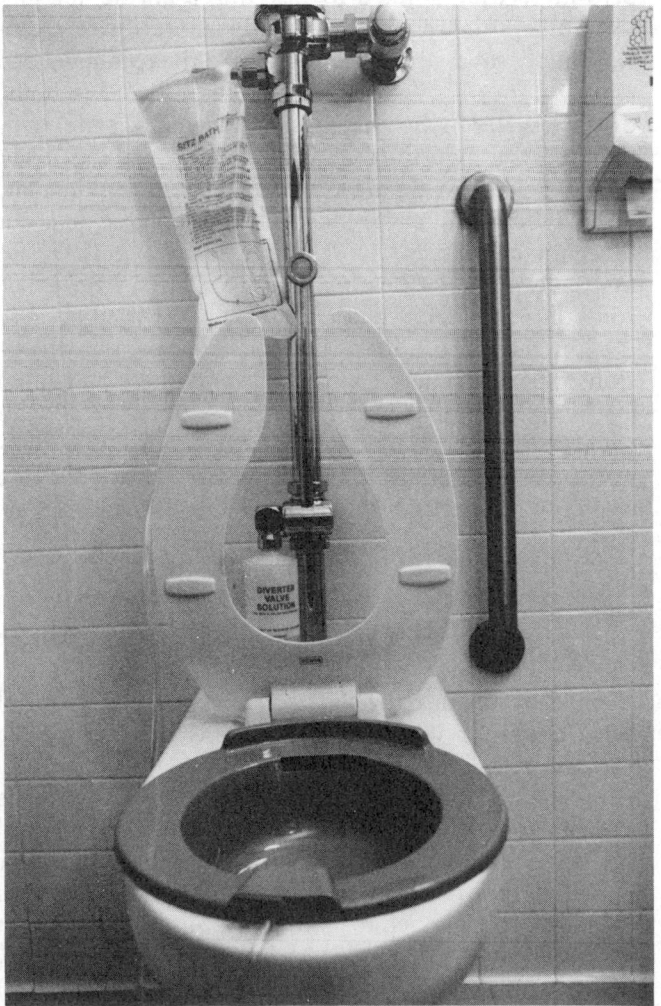

Fig. 47-17   Disposable sitz bath.

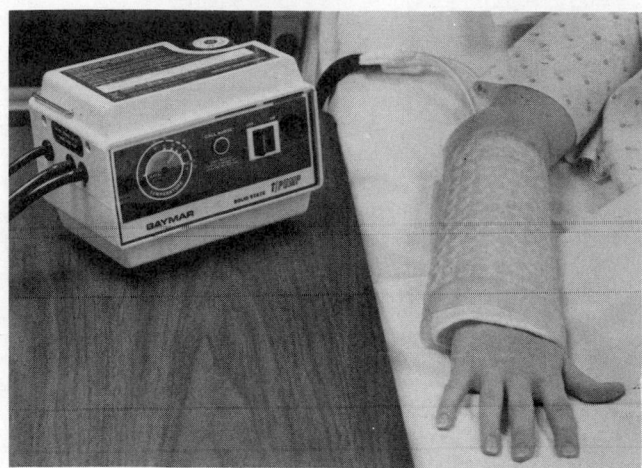

Fig. 47-18 Aquathermia pad.

absorbent surface to apply moist heat. The units are safer than conventional heating pads. However, the nurse should still check for equipment malfunctions. The temperature setting is fixed by inserting a plastic key into the temperature regulator. In many institutions the central supply room sets the regulators to the recommended temperature (40.5° to 43° C [110° to 115° F]). If the distilled water in the unit runs low, the nurse simply fills the reservoir two-thirds full. Plain tap water is never added, since it might leave mineral deposits in the unit.

To avoid burning the client's skin the nurse does not place the pad directly on it. A thin towel or pillow case fits easily over the heating pad. Tape, ties, or a gauze roll holds the pad in place. Pins are never used because they might cause a leak. The nurse checks the client's skin often for signs of burning. An application should last only 20 to 30 minutes. The nurse does not allow a client to lie on a pad. Pressure against a mattress prevents normal heat dissipation. If the pad is to be applied to a region of the back, the client should lie prone or on one side.

HEAT LAMPS. Heat lamps use infrared or regular (40 to 75 watt) light bulbs to expose superficial layers of the skin to heat. Since nothing touches the skin surface, this therapy is valuable for clients with sensitive or painful skin lesions or wounds. The lamp is used mainly to increase circulation to a wound.

After explaining the procedure, the nurse provides the client privacy, covers any scars or stomas, cleans and dries the area to be heated, positions the lamp a safe distance from the exposed body surface, and instructs the client not to touch the lamp's hot surface. A 60-watt bulb should be placed at least 50 cm (24 inches) away. A larger watt bulb should be about 75 cm (30 inches) away. Treatments last about 20 minutes with the nurse

checking the condition of the client's skin at least every 5 minutes.

HEAT CRADLES. A heat cradle is a long, metal, half-circle frame that fits over a large body part such as a leg or the lower trunk. A series of small (25-watt) light bulbs emits heat over a broad area to promote circulation.

The nurse takes precautions to protect the client's skin, but these low-watt bulbs can be positioned closer to the skin and left on longer than can heat lamps. The bulb should be at least 40 to 45 cm (16 to 18 inches) away from the client's skin. The nurse checks the client for discomfort or redness of the skin every 5 to 10 minutes.

COMMERICAL HOT PACKS. Commercially prepared, disposable hot packs apply warm dry heat to an injured area. By striking, kneading, or squeezing the pack, chemicals are mixed that releases heat. Package directions recommend the time for heat application.

HOT WATER BOTTLES. Hot water bottles are rarely used in hospital or other health care settings because of the risk of causing serious burns. In the home the hot water bottle is still economical to use. Nurses must give clients and family members the following instructions on the safe use of water bottles:

1. First ensure there are no leaks. Fill the bottle with tap water, secure the cap, and turn the bottle upside down.
2. Use tap water at a temperature of 40.5° to 46° C (105° to 115° F).
3. Fill the bag only two-thirds full, expel any air at the top, and secure the cap. The bag is then easier to mold over a body part.
4. Wipe off any moisture on the outside of the bag.
5. Never apply a water bottle directly to the skin surface. Cover it with a towel or pillow case.
6. Keep the bottle in place for 20 to 30 minutes.
7. Never apply a water bottle if the client has sensorineural deficits.

ELECTRIC HEATING PADS. Another conventional form of heat therapy is the heating pad, an electric coil enclosed within a water-proof pad covered with cotton or flannel cloth. The pad is connected to an electric cord that has a temperature-regulating unit for a high, medium, or low setting. Nurses should advise clients to avoid using the high setting and to never lie on the pad. Another precaution to note is that a safety pin inserted through a pad can result in an electrical shock.

COLD MOIST AND DRY COMPRESSES. The procedure for applying cold moist compresses is the same as that for warm compresses. Cold compresses should be applied for 20 minutes at a temperature of 15° C (59° F) to relieve inflammation and swelling. They may be clean or sterile.

There are commercially prepared cold packs similar to the disposable hot packs for dry applications. They come in various shapes and sizes to fit different body parts. When using cold compresses, the nurse observes for adverse reactions such as burning or numbness, mottling of the skin, redness, extreme paleness, or a bluish skin discoloration.

COLD SOAKS. The procedure for preparing cold soaks and immersing a body part is the same as for warm soaks. The desired temperature for a 20-minute cold soak is 15° C (59° F). The nurse controls drafts and uses outer coverings to protect the client from chilling. It may be necessary to add cold water during the procedure to maintain a constant temperature.

ICE BAGS OR COLLARS. For a client who has a muscle sprain, localized hemorrhage or hematoma, or has undergone dental surgery, an ice bag is ideal to prevent edema formation, control bleeding, and anesthetize the body part. Proper use of the bag requires these steps:

1. Fill the bag with water, secure the cap, invert to check for leaks, and pour out the water.
2. Fill the bag two-thirds full with crushed ice, so the bag can mold easily over a body part.
3. Release any air from the bag by squeezing its sides before securing the cap (since excess air interferes with conduction of cold).
4. Wipe off excess moisture.
5. Cover the bag with a flannel cover, towel, or pillow case.
6. Apply the bag to the injury site for 30 minutes; the bag can be reapplied in an hour.

EVALUATION

The nurse evaluates wound healing on an on going basis (see evaluation box). This occurs during dressing changes, when therapies are administered, or as a client attempts to perform self-care in the presence of a wound. The nurse instructs clients and family members on how to evaluate wound healing following discharge from a health care setting. For example, clients should be warned to notify a physician if signs of infection develop.

Sample Evaluation of Interventions for Wound Healing

Goals	Evaluative Measures	Expected Outcomes
Hemostasis is promoted. Wound healing is promoted. Infection is prevented.	Observe condition of wound and character of any drainage.	Client will exhibit incision line that is clean, approximated, without drainage and nontender. Client is afebrile. Inflammation will diminish progressively.
Normal function is regained.	Observe client perform self-care activities and/or ambulate.	Client will perform self-care activities independently (unless there is presence of complicating disease). Range of motion and movement will return to normal.
Client is comfortable.	Observe nonverbal responses as client moves or places stress on wound. Ask client if discomfort is experienced at wound site.	Client will deny discomfort around wound site.
Skin integrity is maintained.	Inspect skin surfaces next to wound and around drain sites.	Skin surrounding wound is clean and intact without maceration or inflammation.

SUMMARY

The nurse delivers various forms of therapy to clients with surgical or traumatic wounds. The type of wound determines the types of dressing used, their method of application, the manner of caring for drains and sutures, and observations to make for monitoring wound repair. Clients most at risk for impaired wound healing require close observation and may benefit from the use of bandages and binders to support and protect wounds, or the use of heat and cold therapies.

Principles the nurse follows to promote wound healing include use of aseptic technique, protection of the wound from further injury, and promotion of the stages of healing. These principles are also used in the application of hot and cold therapies. In addition, the nurse uses knowledge of the effects of heat and cold to recognize wounds that will benefit from heat or cold applications.

KEY CONCEPTS

✓ In normal wound healing the epidermal skin layer resurfaces wounds while the dermis restores the structural integrity and physical properties of the skin.

✓ A clean surgical incision with little tissue loss heals by primary intention.

✓ Healing by primary intention proceeds through four stages: inflammation, destruction, proliferation, and maturation.

✓ When there is extensive tissue loss, a wound heals by secondary intention.

✓ Hemorrhaging most often occurs during the destructive stage of wound healing.

✓ The chances of wound infection are greater when the wound contains dead or necrotic tissue, when foreign bodies lie on or near the wound, and when blood supply and tissue defenses are reduced.

✓ Any factor that lowers a client's immune response impairs wound healing.

✓ Physical stress from vomiting, coughing, or sudden muscular contraction can cause separation of wound edges.

✓ Wound assessment requires a description of the appearance of the wound, palpation of the area, character of drainage, presence of drains and wound closures, and presence of pain.

✓ Wound drains remove secretions within tissue layers to promote wound closure.

✓ The nurse never collects a wound culture from old drainage.

✓ Principles of wound first aid include control of bleeding, wound cleansing, and wound protection.

✓ The type of dressing chosen for a wound depends on the character of the wound and the goal of wound care.

✓ The layers of a dry dressing protect the wound edges, absorb drainage, and prevent entrance of bacteria.

✓ The wet-to-dry dressing mechanically removes dead tissue and wound exudate to debride the wound.

✓ When cleaning wounds or drain sites, an important principle is to clean from the least to most contaminated area, away from wound edges.

✓ The type of suture securing a wound influences the method of suture removal.

✓ A bandage or binder should be applied in a manner that does not impair circulation or irritate the skin.

✓ The safe use of heat and cold therapy requires an assessment of the client's sensory function, identification of risk factors, and understanding of the physiological effects of heat and cold.

✔ An acute sprain, fracture, or bruise responds best to cold applications.

✔ Warm applications are effective for improving circulation to wound sites and promoting muscle relaxation.

✔ The choice of moist or dry applications depends on the type of wound, location of body part, and presence of drainage or inflammation.

REFERENCES

Garner, JS: Guidelines for prevention of surgical wound infections, Atlanta, 1985, Centers for Disease Control.

Westaby, S, editor: Wound care, St. Louis, 1986, The C.V. Mosby Co.

ADDITIONAL READINGS

Alterescu, V: Toward a physiologic approach to the topical treatment of opened wounds, J Enterostomal Ther 10:101, 1983.

Bonier, P: Wound care forum, an unusual alternative, Am J Nurs 85:418, 1985.

Boykin, A, and Winland-Brown, J: Pressure sores: nursing management, J Gerontol Nurs 12(12):17, 1986.

Brubacher, LL: To heal a draining wound, RN 45:30, 1982.

Bruno, P, and Craven, RF: Age challenges to wound healing, J Gerontol Nurs 8:686, 1982.

Cooper, DM, et al.: Guide to wound care, Libertyville, Ill., 1983, Hollister, Inc.

Cuzzell, JZ: Artful solutions to chronic problems, Am J Nurs 85:163, 1985.

Cuzzell, JZ: Wound care forum, a dialogue on wound care, Am J Nurs 85:715, 1985.

Flynn, ME, and Rovee, DT: Wound healing mechanisms, Am J Nurs 82:1544, 1982.

Fowler, EM: Equipment and products used in management and treatment of pressure ulcers, Nurs Clin North Am 22(2):449, 1987.

Greenburg, AG, et al.: Wound dehiscence, pathophysiology and prevention, Arch Surg 114:143, 1979.

Greenhalgh, DG, and Garnelli, RA: Is impaired wound healing caused by infection or nutritional depletion? Surgery 102(2):306, 1987.

Hotter, AN: Physiologic aspects and clinical implications of wound healing, Heart Lung 11:522, 1982.

Lanyon, S, Van Nieuwenhuyzen, J, and Wearing, J: Leg ulcers: frustration or challenge? Can Nurse 80(48):33, 1987.

Johnson, A: Toward rapid tissue healing, Nurs Times, p. 39, 1984.

Oleske, DM, et al.: A randomized clinical trial of two dressing methods for the treatment of low-grade pressure ulcers, J Entero Therapy 13(3):90, 1986.

Pollack, S: Wound healing: a review. I. The biology of wound healing, J Entero Therapy 8:16, 1981.

Pollack, S: Wound healing: a review. II. Environmental factors affecting wound healing, J Entero Therapy 9:14, 1982.

Pollack, S: Wound healing: a review. III. Nutritional factors affecting wound healing, J Entero Therapy 9:28, 1982.

Preston, KM: Dermal ulcers: simplifying a complex problem, Rehabil Nurs 12(10):17, 1987.

Randolph, MS, and Still, JM: Contemporary wound management with natural and synthetic dressings, Ostomy/Wound Management 15:14, 1987.

Schumann, D: Preoperative measures to promote wound healing, Nurs Clin North Am 14:683, 1979.

Shira, L: Seeking an optimum dressing: a nursing intervention implemented and evaluated, Ostomy/Wound Management 15:72, 1987.

Sieggren, MY: Healing of physical wounds, Nurs Clin North Am 22(2):439, 1987.

Strauss, MB: Wound hypoxia, Curr Conc Wound Care 9(4):16, 1986.

Sutherland, D: Wound healing, Can Nurse 83(6):36, 1987.

Timberlake, GA: Wound healing: the physiology of scar formation, Curr Conc Wound Care 9(2):4, 14, 1986.

Wroblewski, JR: Ointments, creams, gels: working with topical skin care preparations, Ostomy/Wound Management 15:46, 1987.

Yve, DK, et al.: Effects of experimental diabetes, uremia, and malnutrition on wound healing, Diabetes 36:295, 1987.

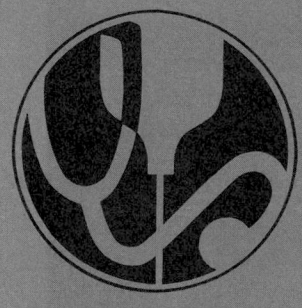

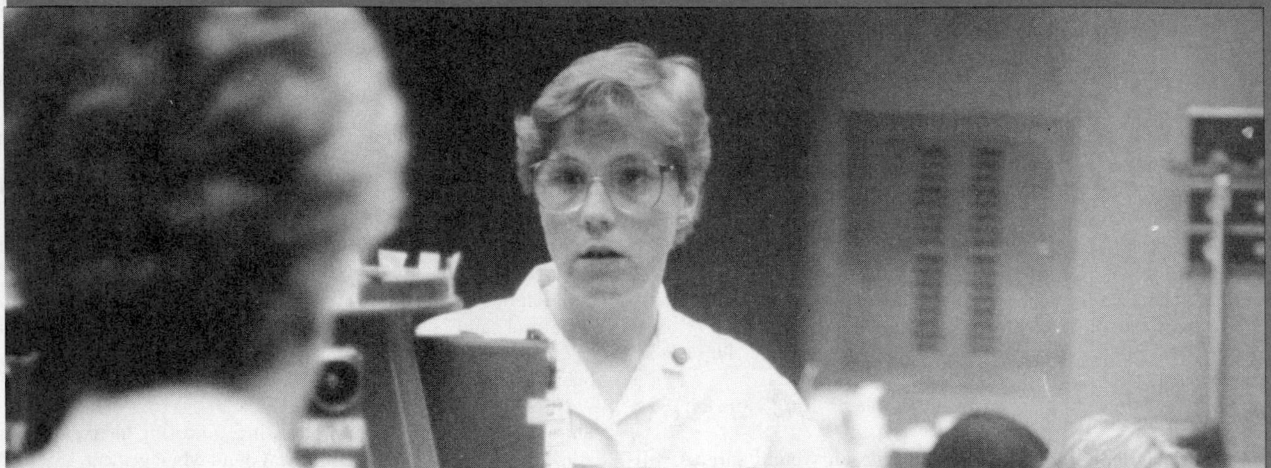

Contemporary Issues

Contemporary nursing, as a profession, involves more than the day-to-day care of individuals. Because nurses work with other nurses and health care professionals, leadership skills are often needed to ensure successful cooperation and direction of groups to provide high quality health care. Similarly, nurses may often be agents of change, both in direct client care and in the health care delivery system, and thus can gain from an understanding of the change process. The chapters in this unit address these dimensions of the profession and their dynamic relationship with the world around us.

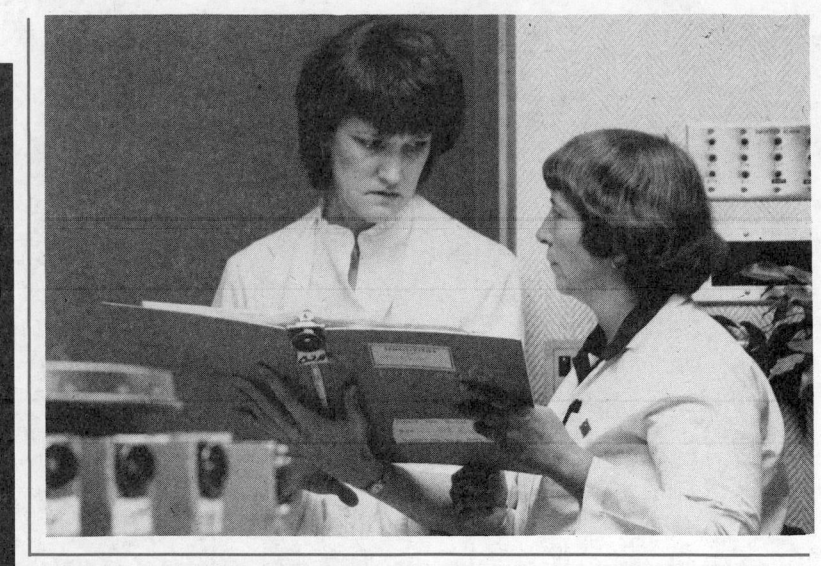

OBJECTIVES

Mastery of content in this chapter will enable the student to:

- Define the key terms listed.
- Differentiate between leadership and management.
- Compare and contrast the scientific management theory and the human relations movement in their perspectives for improving productivity.
- Identify the primary principles of situational leadership theories.
- Describe and give examples of the four classic leadership styles: authoritarian, democratic, laissez-faire, and situational.
- Explain why leadership is important for nursing.
- List and give examples of the four primary types of leadership skills student nurses can begin to develop.

KEY TERMS

Authoritarian Style
Democratic Style
Human Relations Movement
Laissez-Faire Style
Leader
Leadership Style
Manager
Scientific Management Theory
Situational Theory
Trait Development Theory

Nursing Leadership and Management

Successful organizations have effective and dynamic leadership. In hospitals and other health care facilities, certain nursing units have a reputation for delivering superior nursing care. These units generally have head nurses who are recognized leaders within their institutions and who motivate the nursing staff to maintain higher standards of nursing care. Effective nursing leaders such as these head nurses are generally successful because of their early commitment to developing leadership skills.

Drucker (1954), a well-known authority on management, identifies a need for effective leaders in many areas of modern society. Effective leaders are the most basic and scarcest resource in any business, as well as in government and religious, educational, and health care institutions. According to other authorities in this area, there is not only a shortage of leaders who can get the job done effectively but also a scarcity of people willing to assume significant leadership roles in our society (Hersey and Blanchard, 1977). Leadership is needed in nursing as in other areas.

Leadership skills are usually developed by individuals early in their careers. To meet the need for more effective leaders in nursing, it is important for nursing students to understand leadership concepts, to begin to develop leadership skills early in their careers, and to commit themselves to exercising leadership skills in their everyday nursing activities.

DEFINITIONS OF LEADERSHIP AND MANAGEMENT

Leadership is the ability to influence others toward the accomplishment of a goal. Currently, most authorities agree that leadership is a community of feelings between the leader and the group that promotes the group's desire to follow the leader's directions. Leadership is required when a group of people need to work toward a common goal. Leadership occurs in all areas of life, including the family, the classroom, the dormitory, the hospital, and the nursing division.

Effective leaders have different capabilities and styles. However, effective leaders demonstrate the ability to guide others on an ongoing, daily basis in a wide variety of situations and circumstances.

A manager directs, coordinates, and supervises a group's activities. Managers accomplish their work through others. Experience and research have shown that the effective manager can also be an effective leader. The manager has been selected by the organization to direct and supervise a group. This direction and supervision should inspire willingness and cooperation.

This chapter focuses on the study and development of leadership styles. A nurse manager will select the leadership style that is likely to be the most effective. A beginning student will observe a variety of situations in which managers apply leadership skills.

LEADERSHIP AND MANAGEMENT THEORIES

Leadership has been studied since the turn of the century, when psychological testing became popular and provided tools for objective research. A number of theories about the qualities of leadership have been developed. The review of these theories in the following sections can help the student nurse better understand what is involved in leadership.

Early leadership studies concentrated on the traits and qualities of leaders. Trait development theorists generally believed that the leader was born with certain qualities that determined leadership ability and success. These qualities include intelligence, aggressiveness, high energy level, and friendliness. The trait theorists believed that these leadership traits could be applied to all situations. Effective leaders were studied to identify the traits they had in common. Many attempts were made to put this theory into practice. From a group of job applicants, for example, only those possessing the identified traits were considered potential leaders and were selected for positions requiring leadership. Leadership training was provided only for those who possessed the desired leadership traits. This method of selecting and developing leaders, however, was not particularly effective.

As more research has been conducted in the area of leadership, the theory that a leader possesses certain traits has been shown to be incorrect. Research into necessary leadership traits revealed few consistent findings. The list of traits grew to over 100 traits that were considered essential to successful leadership. Gradually it became clear that very few successful leaders could possess all these traits identified as essential for the successful leader. In a review of this research, Jennings (1961) concluded, "Fifty years of study have failed to produce one personality trait or set of qualities that can be used to discriminate leaders and non-leaders."

Scientific Management Theory

Another approach to the study of leadership was developed by Taylor in the early 1900s. Taylor's scientific management theory emphasized technology as the basis for increasing the productivity of employees. Taylor used the principles of observation, measurement, and scientific comparison to develop work standards. He introduced time-and-motion studies to analyze tasks, based on the belief that improving the performance of tasks would improve the efficiency of the organization. Taylor recommended careful selection and training of workers that could meet the established work standards. Before Taylor's studies, workers selected their own jobs and trained themselves. Attempts were made to satisfy the needs of employees through various incentives, including increasing wages. If this approach were applied to nursing, a staff could secure cash bonuses for providing efficient client care.

Some critics of this theory believe that the incentives approach is ineffective and simplistic because it emphasizes the performance of the workers and ignores complex human needs. It also encourages shortcuts and short-term goals at the expense of long-term goals.

In the scientific management theory, the leader creates and enforces performance criteria through close supervision. The leader provides direction in an authoritarian manner, focusing on the needs of the organization rather than the needs of the employees.

Human Relations Movement

Mayo and his associates in the 1920s and 1930s argued that managers attempting to improve productivity must be concerned with human affairs and technological methods. The human relations theorists believed that the real power centers within an organization were the interpersonal relationships established within the work environment. They suggested that organizations be developed around human relationships, including those between leaders and employees. The human relations movement focused on human feelings and attitudes of the employees.

The leader ensured that employees cooperated to attain their goals and also encouraged the employees' personal growth and development. The leader focused more on the workers' needs than the needs of the organization. In this respect the human relations movement directly opposed the scientific management movement.

Michigan Leadership Studies

University of Michigan researchers studied leadership to identify clusters of characteristics related to the leader's effectiveness. According to their studies the two primary kinds of leaders are those who are employee oriented and those who are production oriented. Production-oriented leaders are more concerned about the technical aspects of the job, whereas employee-oriented leaders stress the importance of the employees' needs.

Theory X and Theory Y

McGregor described two kinds of management theories, which he called theory X and theory Y. Managers who believe in theory X assume that people inherently dislike work and will avoid it whenever possible. The manager therefore must force employees to work, control and direct them continually, and threaten them with punishment if they are to work toward the accomplishment of organizational goals. Theory X assumes that human beings prefer to be directed, have little ambition, reject responsibility, and are most concerned about job security. McGregor believed that managers who used the theory X approach would never be able to reach high levels of production because only employees' low-level needs were satisfied.

Theory Y, in contrast, assumes that employees can enjoy physical and mental work just as they enjoy play and rest. Employees are capable of self-motivation and job satisfaction if they are happy in the organization and committed to its goals. Most human beings want responsibility, and if employees have responsibility rather than being controlled authoritatively, many organizational problems can be solved through group interaction. Theory Y managers believe that the organization is more successful when employees are self-directed and exercise self-control in their work. For this to occur, the employee must share the organization's goals and feel a commitment to the organization. McGregor suggests that theory Y organizations will satisfy higher human needs, resulting in greater employee responsibility and, in turn, higher productivity.

Ohio State Leadership Studies

The Bureau of Business Research at Ohio State University conducted studies in the 1940s to identify various dimensions of leadership behaviors. Leadership behaviors were described in terms of two dimensions: structure and consideration. Consideration behaviors reflect friendship, mutual trust, respect, and warmth between the leader and employee. Structure behaviors are those that clearly define the structured organizational relationship between the leader and employees.

Researchers collected data on the behaviors of leaders through a specially designed questionnaire. The results of the research indicated that structure and consideration behaviors are separate and distinct dimensions, each on a continuum that ranges from low to high. Any leader may have any combination of characteristics in these two dimensions. A high level in one dimension does not necessarily mean a low level in the other. Thus there are four general types of leaders, with many variations in specific characteristics:

1. High consideration, high structure
2. High consideration, low structure
3. Low consideration, high structure
4. Low consideration, low structure

Fig. 48-1 describes the characteristics of these four types of leaders. This study is particularly important because it represents the first multidimensional approach to leadership behavior.

These types of leadership behaviors involve different approaches to the manager-employee relationship. For example, a head nurse who believes the staff's scheduling requests are more important than the needs of the nursing unit would rate high in consideration and low in structure. A head nurse who considers only the needs of the nursing unit and not the needs of the staff would rate low in consideration and high in structure. The first head nurse may achieve a more harmonious working relationship with staff nurses, but the second head nurse may be more effective in ensuring that short-staffing does not occur. Neither is necessarily a better leader because effective leadership also depends on many other factors and skills.

Managerial Grid

The managerial grid theory of Blake and Mouton focuses on management purposes and organizational improvement. Organizations are seen to have three universal characteristics: organizational purposes, employees, and a power structure or hierarchy. The power structure involves the supervision of employees by leaders. Management styles in this approach involve two concerns: task accomplishment and the development of human relationships. As in the Ohio State Study, these two concerns exist on continuums, here represented with

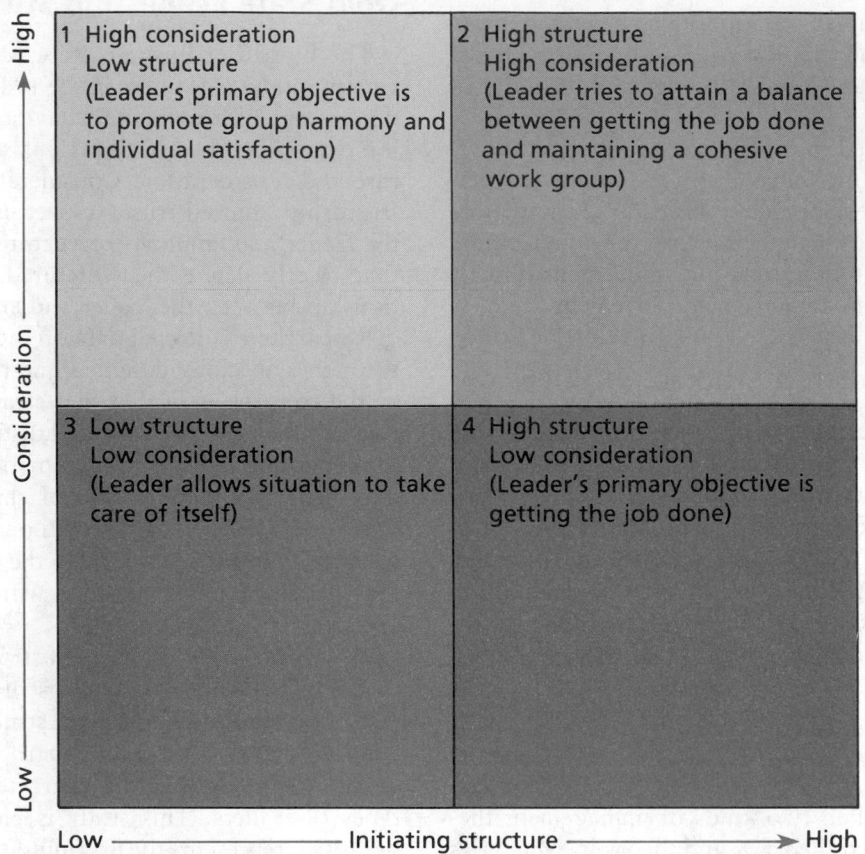

Fig. 48-1 Ohio State leadership quadrants.

a grid (Fig. 48-2). The position of a manager on this grid is determined by the extent of concern for employees and for organizational goals. There are four extreme types of leadership styles:

1. Impoverished
2. Country club
3. Task
4. Team management

The ultimate management style in this theory is the team management style. The team manager is both committed to the organization and concerned for the employees. The team manager makes decisions through employee involvement, participation, and exchange of ideas. Team managers are even tempered, maintain a sense of humor, are dependable in difficult situations, and are willing to change their ideas.

Situational Theories

In recent years human relations theorists have influenced how managers deal with the needs, feelings, and general working conditions of employees. Because of this humanistic approach to management the modern manager must maintain a balance between managing in a "democratic" manner and exercising the necessary control and authority to complete the specified tasks or goals.

Management style can be described on a continuum that ranges from highly autocratic leadership to a democratic process in which the group makes decisions within prescribed limits (Tannenbaum and Schmidt, 1958). The leader chooses a style on this continuum that reflects what is practical and desirable for the situation. According to situational theory, the manager's traits, employee factors, and situational factors must be considered in this choice. Managerial factors include confidence in employees, leadership philosophy, values, and feelings of security in any given situation. Employee factors include the need for independence, readiness to accept responsibility, understanding of the organizational goals, and previous knowledge and experience to manage the problem. Situational factors are important in the manager's choice of leadership style. One key factor is the extent of employee's understanding of organizational values within the situation. Other situational factors include the effectiveness of the working group, the problems under consideration, time limitations, and available resources.

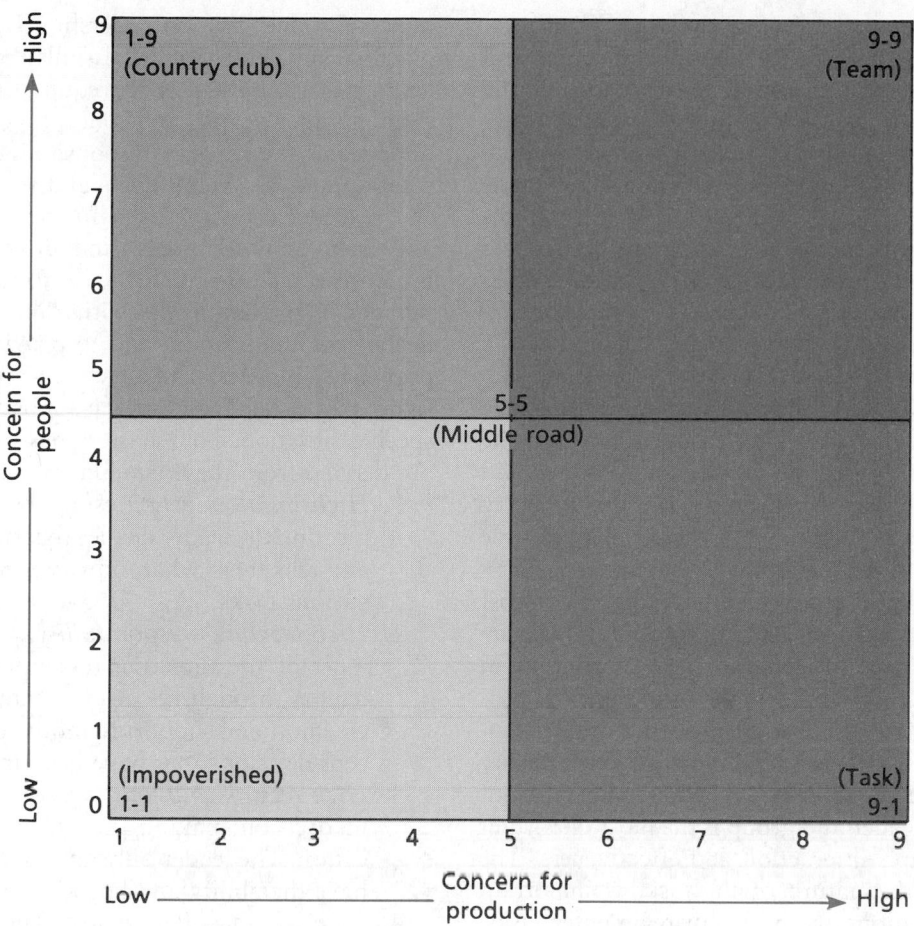

Fig. 48-2 Managerial grid leadership styles.

Managers are concerned about their responsibilities and the effectiveness and productivity of the employees they supervise. They are also concerned about the motivation and needs of employees. Several theorists have analyzed this double concern in leadership with a situational approach.

Redden (1970) developed an approach to managerial effectiveness based on the Ohio State studies. In this approach no one style of leadership is seen as always effective. Effectiveness depends, instead, on the leader's qualities and skills. Three managerial skills are necessary for effective leadership: situational sensitivity, style flexibility, and situational management. Situational sensitivity is the manager's ability to read and diagnose a working situation. Style flexibility is the leader's ability to choose from a variety of management styles the most appropriate style for a given situation; this does not involve avoiding pressure or simply keeping employees happy but rather maintaining efficiency, even in a stressful situation, by balancing the needs of employees and the organization. Situational mangement is the process of working to change from an unfavorable situation to a more favorable one.

Another situational management theorist, Likert (1961, 1967), addresses human factors while recognizing the impact of situational variables. This approach suggests that managers who are helpful and oriented to employees achieve higher productivity and greater effectiveness within the organization. Management style is based on supportive relationships, group decision making, group methods of supervision, and high performance goals. Each employee views the institution as supportive and interested in developing the employee's personal worth and importance. The organization is arranged in working groups rather than the usual structure in which one manager supervises many employees working individually.

Working groups overlap within the organizational structure to promote communication. Important decisions are made by the group. The group's goals include high productivity, high quality, and low costs. The manager is accountable for the group's decisions, productivity, and results.

Likert's System 4 Management theory is effective only if each person within the organization belongs to one or more effectively functioning work groups characterized by strong group loyalty, effective skills, and high performance goals. Situational factors are important and can affect the group decision-making process. If the group is unable to reach a united decision, the leader must make the decision. If the leader disagrees with the group's decision, an attempt may be made to persuade the group to act in another direction. If the group's decision is followed, the leader is responsible for the outcome. The leader must also make decisions when time or other factors restrict the use of the group decision-making process.

The situational approach of Fiedler (1967) emphasizes fitting the job to the style of the leader rather than the leader changing styles according to the situation. The two major styles of leadership are the task-oriented and employee-oriented styles. According to this theory, every leader has a certain predominant style, and effective management should not attempt to change a leader's style but should choose a leader with the style most appropriate to the situation. Three major situational variables affect what type of leader is most appropriate in a particular situation: the acceptance and personal feelings of the group for the leader, the structured or unstructured nature of the task, and the need for authority to accomplish the group's task. The personal relationship between the leader and group is the most important factor in the group's interaction and effectiveness. The second variable, the nature of the task, is important because some situations involve highly regimented tasks, whereas others require more creativity and personal or group initiative. Finally, in some situations groups require directive leadership to accomplish the job, while in others the group requires more permissive leadership.

Fiedler describes eight possible combinations of these situational variables. In a difficult situation in which the tasks must be accomplished by group effort, for example, the autocratic, task-oriented manager produces the most favorable results. In less difficult or less structured situations, the nondirective, permissive leader is more successful. Based on studies showing that leaders are generally unaware of their own leadership styles, Fiedler concludes that the most effective approach teaches leaders how to identify their styles and to diagnose the working situation to match the leader to the situation. This has been applied successfully in various organizations.

Hersey and Blanchard's situational leadership theory (1977), originally called the life cycle theory of leadership, is concerned with the extent of structure and socioemotional support from the leader necessary according to the maturity of employees. As the leader and group develop a working relationship based on mutual trust and respect, the process encourages mature and effective followers. The effective leader must be flexible in using more than one style of leadership. Leadership depends on three key skills: technical skills required to perform definite tasks, human skills required to work with and through other people, and conceptual skills necessary to understand the leader's responsibility within the organization and its overall goals and structures.

The leader uses task behaviors to organize the group and task, establish goals, and direct employees. The leader uses relationship behavior to establish and maintain personal relationships with followers, to open channels of communication, and to provide emotional support for employees. The effective leader combines these two types of behaviors in ways most appropriate for a specific situation. Four basic types of leadership styles are derived from these combinations:

1. *High task/low relationship.* By one-way communication the leader defines the roles of the followers and tells them what, how, when, and where to do various tasks.
2. *High task/high responsibility.* The leader provides most of the direction to employees but also attempts through two-way communication and socioemotional support to motivate employees to accept decisions that have been made.
3. *High relationship/low task.* Employees participate in decision making through two-way communication. The leader only guides the employees, who have the ability and knowledge to do the task.
4. *Low relationship/low task.* The leader allows employees to make their own decisions with only general supervision. In this case the employees are mature in terms of both the task and the ability to accept responsibility.

Leadership style therefore depends on the maturity of the employee group in relation to specific work situations. An employee may be mature and capable of accepting responsibility in one situation but immature and requiring directive management in another. The concept of maturity applies to both individuals and groups. In addition, maturity depends on both job maturity (technical skill and ability to do the task) and psychological maturity (feeling of self-confidence needed to complete the task). The leader's responsibility is to diagnose the situation, determine the maturity of employees, and select the appropriate leadership style. As the maturity of the followers increases, the leader should gradually move from a task style into a relationship style. The reverse is true in situations where the individual or group demonstrates immaturity. As followers develop higher maturity levels, the leader should be able to reduce both task and relationship behaviors. Employees who achieve a high level of maturity in their performance can provide their own direction and achieve on their own the necessary psychological satisfaction.

LEADERSHIP AND MANAGEMENT STYLE

A leader is not necessarily a manager, nor is a manager necessarily a leader. A manager is a person whose official position within an organization is to guide and direct the work of others. The manager has been given authority and responsibility by the organization to enforce decisions and policies. A manager may or may not have leadership abilities. Examples of management positions in nursing are head nurses and charge nurses for specific shifts. In contrast, a leader must possess the ability to direct the actions of others. The leader may or may not hold an official management position within the organization. There are two types of leaders. The formal leader is appointed by the organization and therefore is a manager. The informal leader does not have an official appointment within the organization but nonetheless influences the behaviors of others. If that influence is lost, the person is no longer a leader. In the following discussion on leadership styles, the term "leader" refers to a formal leader who is a manager, but many of the general qualities of leadership styles are true of informal leaders as well.

Leadership style is an important factor influencing the extent to which a leader is effective. Style in general involves the ways in which something is said or done, including particular behaviors associated with an individual. Leadership style specifically refers to how the leader influences the group to accomplish goals. Leadership styles, like other behaviors, can be learned, regulated, and developed. Research indicates that no one leadership style is effective in all situations but that each has unique strengths for different situations. The three classical styles of leadership are the authoritarian, democratic, and laissez-faire.

Authoritarian Style

The authoritarian leader retains all authority and responsibility and is concerned primarily with tasks and goal accomplishment. This type of leader assigns people to clearly defined tasks and establishes one-way communication patterns with the group. The authoritarian leader is firm, insistent, self-assured, and dominating. Such a leader stresses prompt, orderly, and predictable performance from employees or followers. The leader displays little trust or confidence in employees, and generally employees are fearful of this type of manager. The authoritarian leader tends to stifle individual initiative and creativity.

The authoritarian leader may also be benevolent and value employees both as people and for their capabilities. This kind of authoritarian leader issues orders but allows employees to comment on them. Employees are permitted some flexibility to carry out their tasks within specific limits and procedures. A benevolent authoritarian leader may give orders, praise employees, demand their loyalty, and make followers feel they are participating in the decision process even though they continue to do as the leader directs. The benevolent authoritarian leader generally has a condescending attitude toward employees, who therefore tend to be cautious when dealing with the leader.

Authoritarian leaders have always been present in nursing. The authoritarian nurse leader manages by giving orders and expecting staff members to accept them. The authoritarian manager stresses adherence to hospital policies and procedures. Staff members are expected to conform in nursing practice to the example and direction of the manager (Douglass, 1980).

The authoritarian style of leadership is appropriate in some situations. Some nursing staff members function more productively under the direction of authoritarian leaders because this leadership style meets their needs for security and job satisfaction. In situations when immediate action is required and there is no time for a group decision-making process, the authoritarian leader is able to take action quickly. Authoritarian leaders excel in times of crisis and in situations of disorder; they often can remain calm while others falter. Authoritarian leaders have the reputation for being able to get difficult assignments completed.

Democratic Style

The democratic leadership style is a people-centered approach. The democratic leader allows greater individual participation in the decision-making process. The leader delegates authority but retains ultimate responsibility. The democratic leader maintains active communication that is open, friendly, and trusting with employees.

This style of management enhances employees' personal commitment to the organization through group participation. The manager encourages goal setting by the group and has a sense of responsibility for the good of the group and for individual achievements. The democratic manager uses performance standards to assist the group in knowing job responsibilities rather than to control employees.

In nursing practice, democratic nurse managers have introduced a variety of mechanisms to promote staff involvement in the management of the nursing unit. Some examples are staff involvement in the development of the time schedule, group problem solving through quality control circles, and mutual goal setting during performance appraisals.

Laissez-Faire Style

The last classical leadership style is called laissez-faire. Laissez-faire leadership is also referred to as the free-run style or as permissive leadership. This type of leader denies responsibility and abdicates authority to the group. The laissez-faire manager may simply tell group members to work things out themselves and do the best they can. Communication between the manager and employees is open and lacks control and direction.

The laissez-faire manager wants everyone to feel good, including himself. This management style allows the group to drift aimlessly because the leader provides no direction. The principal management functions, such as decision making, planning, structuring, and controlling organization goals, are carried out by the group.

This style is not generally useful in the health care system because organization and control are necessary for day-to-day operation. Laissez-faire leadership may be beneficial for employees involved in research projects, however, because self-direction assists in the creative process (Douglass, 1980). This style is probably most beneficial to a staff of highly motivated professionals who have shown the capacity for independent work.

■ ■ ■

There is no one best leadership style. The effectiveness of each of the three classical leadership styles depends on the situation. As the situation changes, the effective manager adapts by changing leadership behaviors. Hersey (1967) concludes about differences in leadership styles, "The more managers adapt their style of leader behaviors to meet the particular situations and the needs of their followers, the more effective they will tend to be in reaching personal and organizational goals."

Situational Leadership

Situational leadership combines the style of the leader, skills needed in the situation, and the maturity of the employees. Situational leadership uses the following four different leadership styles:

Style 1: Directing. The leader provides specific instructions and supervises task accomplishment.

Style 2: Coaching. The leader directs and closely supervises task accomplishment. The leader also explains decisions, seeks suggestions, and supports progress.

Style 3: Supporting. The leader facilitates and supports the efforts of the subordinates toward task accomplishment. The leader shares responsibility for decision-making with employees.

Style 4: Delegating. The leader gives the responsibility for decision making and problem solving to subordinates (Blanchard, Zigarmi, and Zigarmi, 1975).

Employees who have limited technical skills or who are unwilling or unable to take responsibility require an authoritarian or directive leadership style. Employees with appropriate skills and who are willing to take responsibility are effectively managed with a democratic or participatory style. This style encourages participation in decision making. In the delegating leadership style, the leader allows employees to make decisions and manage the daily operations. The leader diagnoses the particular situation to determine the correct leadership style.

The following example applies situational leadership to a specific situation: A nursing service institutes a new client-classification system. The head nurse uses the directing style (1) to introduce the staff to the form. As the nursing staff becomes familiar with the new task, the head nurse solicits staff participation in working through the details of implementation. Using the coaching (2) and supporting (3) styles, the head nurse en-

---

Primary Leadership Skills for Nurses

SKILLS OF PERSONAL BEHAVIOR

The effective leader:
- Is sensitive to feelings of the group
- Identifies self with the needs of the group
- Listens attentively
- Does not ridicule or criticize another's suggestions
- Helps others feel important and needed
- Does not argue

SKILLS OF COMMUNICATION

The effective leader:
- Makes sure everyone understands what is needed and the reason why
- Establishes positive communication with the group as a routine part of the job
- Recognizes that everyone's contributions are important

SKILLS OF ORGANIZATION

The effective leader helps the group to:
- Develop long-range and short-range objectives
- Break big problems into small ones
- Share responsibilities and opportunities
- Plan, act, follow-up, and evaluate
- Be attentive to details

SKILLS OF SELF-EXAMINATION

The effective leader:
- Is aware of personal motivations
- Is aware of group members' level of hostility so that appropriate countermeasures are taken
- Helps the group be aware of their attitudes and values

courages the group decision-making process to resolve problems. Finally, when all staff members have demonstrated they have the knowledge and ability to continue using the system without direction, the head nurse uses the delegating style (4), which allows staff nurses to continue using the new system on their own. If problems occur, the head nurse returns to a directing or coaching style as needed to resolve the problem. While the nurse uses a delegating style with this situation, another situation may require a directive style to accomplish the task.

LEADERSHIP SKILLS FOR STUDENT NURSES

Nursing continues to need new effective leaders in all practice areas. Leadership is most important when changes are occurring in health care, such as the current changes being implemented in financing of the health care system. Changes are coming about in both Medicare and private health care insurance programs (see Chapter 3). For this and other reasons, it is imperative that student nurses begin early to prepare for future leadership and management roles. The box lists skills in four areas that are important for effective leadership and that the student nurse can begin to develop. These skills can be applied by leaders using any leadership style in any situation.

SUMMARY

As the nursing profession and health care agencies become increasingly specialized and complex, the need for effective leadership in nursing is even more important than in the past. Many nursing roles and responsibilities involve group activities, and for a group to function optimally, the leader must be able to motivate and influence the behavior of others. Successful leadership, whether in nursing, business, or other areas of group effort, depends on an effective leadership style. For this reason many theorists have analyzed the components of leadership that result in success. Although these theories do not agree entirely about the components of successful leadership, it is clear that the leader must remain flexible and adapt the leadership style to the particular group situation and goals.

In any situation the nurse in a leadership role needs certain skills, including skills related to personal behavior, communication skills, organization skills, and the skills of self-examination. These are all skills the nursing student can begin to develop while learning other nursing skills. By developing these skills early in their careers, individual nurses will be better prepared to meet the needs for leadership in professional groups, health care agencies, and practice settings.

KEY CONCEPTS

✓ Leadership is the ability to influence the behaviors of others toward the accomplishment of a goal.

✓ Studies of leadership have demonstrated that the effective leader is concerned with both the needs of employees and the needs of the organization.

✓ No single set of personality traits is true of all effective leaders.

✓ Situational leadership theory proposes that the leader should adapt the style of leadership to the needs of the situation.

✓ A leader may or may not have an official appointment within the organization.

✓ A manager has authority and responsibility to enforce decisions and policies of the organization but is not necessarily an effective leader.

✓ The three classical leadership styles are the authoritarian, the democratic, and the laissez-faire.

✓ There is no one best leadership style because effective leaders alter their behaviors to fit the situation.

✓ Leadership style is important in all nursing practice areas just as in other types of organizations.

✓ Leadership skills the nurse can begin to develop while still a student include those of personal behaviors, communication, organization, and self-examination.

REFERENCES

Blanchard, K, Zigarmi, P, and Zigarmi, D: Leadership and the one minute manager, New York, 1985, William Morrow & Co., Inc.

Douglass, LM: The effective nurse: leader and manager, ed. 3, St. Louis, 1988, The C.V. Mosby Co.

Drucker, PF: The practice of management, New York, 1954, Harper & Row, Publishers, Inc.

Fiedler, F: A theory of leadership effectiveness, New York, 1967, McGraw-Hill Book Co.

Hersey, P: Management concepts and behavior: programmed instruction for managers, Little Rock, Ark., 1967, Mancin Publishing Co.

Hersey, P, and Blanchard, KH: Management of organizational behavior: utilizing human resources, ed. 3, Englewood Cliffs, N.J., 1977, Prentice-Hall, Inc.

Jennings, EE: The anatomy of leadership, Management Personnel Quarterly 1(1):1, 1961.

Likert, R: New patterns of management, New York, 1961, McGraw-Hill Book Co.

Likert, R: The human organization, New York, 1967, McGraw-Hill Book Co.

Redden, W: Managerial effectiveness, New York, 1970, McGraw-Hill Book Co.

Tannenbaum, R, and Schmidt, W: How to choose a leadership pattern, Harvard Business Review 36:95, 1958.

ADDITIONAL READINGS

Blake, RR, and Mouton, JS: The new managerial grid, Houston, 1964, Gulf Publishing Co.

Fiedler, F: Engineer the job to fit the manager, Harvard Business Review 43:115, 1965.

Fiedler, F: Responses to Sergiovanni, Educational Leadership 36:394, 1979.

Grammatteo, M, and Grammatteo, D: Forces on leadership, Reston, Va., 1981, The National Association of Secondary School Principals.

McMurry, R: The case for the benevolent autocrat, Harvard Business Review 36:82, 1958.

Stagdill, RM, and Coons, AE, editors: Leader behaviors: its description and measurement, Research Monogr 88, Columbus, 1957, Bureau of Business Research, The Ohio State University.

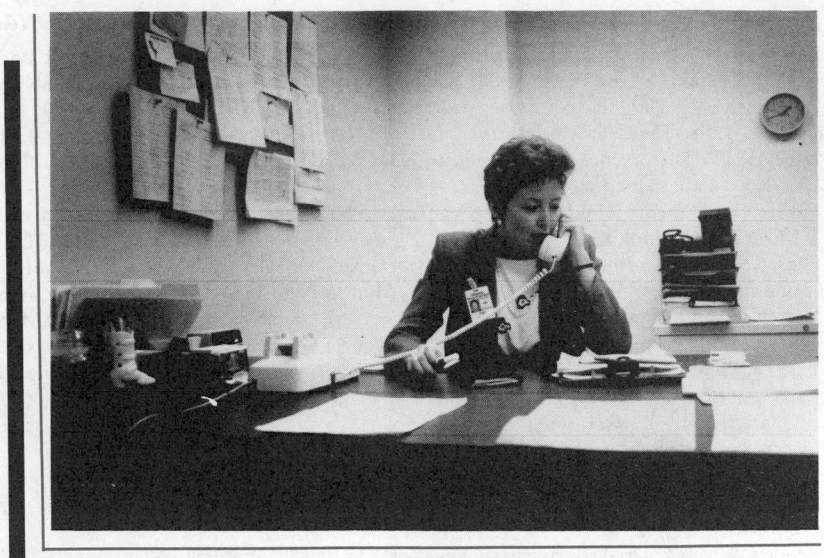

OBJECTIVES

Mastery of content in this chapter will enable the student to:

- Define the key terms listed.
- Compare and contrast theories of change formulated by Lewin, Lippitt, and Rogers and describe examples of application.
- Compare and contrast the systems, developmental, change and confrontation models of change and describe examples of application.
- Describe the major concept(s) and examples of application for other models of change: traditional, elite corps, psychoanalytical, and scholarly consultation.
- Analyze response to change, including interference and resistance, and factors that contribute to various reactions.
- Compare steps of the nursing process to steps of the change process.
- Describe characteristics, skills, and behaviors of the effective nurse change agent.
- Relate the concept of power to skills and behavior of the nurse change agent.
- Relate the role of change agent to other nursing roles.

KEY TERMS

Change
Change Agent
Coercive Change
Developmental Change
Driving Forces
Interference
Moving
Planned Change
Power
Refreezing
Resistance
Restraining Forces
Situational Change
Unfreezing

Change Process and the Nurse

Change is a natural and inevitable characteristic of all modern societies. Many people view change as a sign of progress, but others perceive it as a threat to their equilibrium. Therefore, nurses must recognize and evaluate the need for change as well as plan and implement change effectively. Successful change will depend on the change agent's ability to use the steps of the change process. Thus nurses should be familiar with change theory to facilitate a helping relationship with a client system.

DEFINITION OF CHANGE

Change is a process by which alterations occur within the behavior and function of an individual, family, group, or community (Mauksch and Miller, 1981). Change ultimately will have an impact on all behavioral patterns within a system. It can be viewed as natural, constantly occurring, and dynamic in nature.

Types of Change

Several types of change are evident: developmental, coercive, situational (unplanned), and planned. Developmental change refers to the normal biopsychosocial changes that occur within the life cycle experiences. Examples may be an adolescent during puberty, the young adult entering marriage, or retirement for the older adult (Murray and Huelskoetter, 1987). The nurse and client also experience developmental changes.

Coercive changes occur when an individual or group must carry out another's will without choice (for example, the long-term employee must relocate to another city or risk losing employment or the staff nurse is changed from full-time to part-time status because of a lower client census in the hospital).

Situational (unplanned) changes occur accidentally without any control by the individual, group, or community (Murray and Huelskoetter, 1987). Consider the changes that occur in the family uprooted after a tornado because of extensive property damage to their home. Conversely, not all unplanned changes need be viewed negatively. The young executive or the nurse who receives a job promotion unexpectedly is often pleased and considers the opportunity favorably, although the new employment status means change and may be a potential stressor.

Ideally, change occurs after a well-planned course of action has been developed. Planned change is a deliberate and collaborative attempt to alter the environment with specific consideration given to the mutual goals of those involved. The difference between unplanned and planned change is that unplanned change occurs spontaneously without intent for change. See the box for further characteristics of planned change (Murray and Huelskoetter, 1987).

The nurse uses the planned change process when asking the client about current dietary habits before exploring with the client how diet can be modified to maintain diabetic control. The target of planned change may be an individual who consults the nurse for information on how to quit smoking. However, change can occur within families, communities, small organizations, and large companies, and the nurse may be a key member in the planned change process. Change will have an impact not only on the individual or group directly involved in the change but will invariably affect all who are peripherally involved as well.

Theories of Change

Many people believe that most changes do not happen without effort. Some changes within a client, group, or organization may occur because of the aging process, longevity, or by coincidence (drift theory), although most change involving the nurse can be understood through the use of various theories.

Several theories of change are useful to the nurse change agent. Kurt Lewin (1951) developed the classical change theory on which all other theories have evolved. Lewin's theory of change identified three stages of change: unfreezing, moving, and refreezing. During the unfreezing stage, one becomes aware of the need for change and identifies the problem. Need for change comes about because previous expectations have not been met; because of guilt, anxiety, or discomfort with the status quo; or because a previous obstacle has been removed, making it psychologically safe to change. After seeking information from a variety of sources, change is planned in detail. It is during the moving stage that change is then initiated. The refreezing stage is when the new changes become operational within the value system, and new behaviors, policies, or procedures become standard. Some time is necessary before equilibrium stabilizes (Lewis, 1951, 1958; Olson, 1979),

Lewin also identified forces that either facilitate or impede change, referred to as driving and restraining forces. He recommended that these factors be identified during the planning phase to benefit from the driving or positive forces, as well as prevent interference from restraining or resisting forces (Lewin, 1951, 1958; Olson, 1979). Driving forces may simply be the approval of the nursing director for a proposed change within a health care organization, and staff nurses that resist the change could be the restraining forces because they feel their ideas were not solicited before the change that affects them.

Lippitt's theory of planned change is an expansion of Lewin's three phases. Lippitt outlined several stages: diagnosis, investigation of potential solutions, implementation, and evaluation. An accurate diagnosis of the problem should be stated, including the involvement of all who will be affected by the change. All possible solutions should be investigated with particular consideration given to driving and limiting factors plus financial concerns. Specifics on how, when, and where the change will occur should be planned. A possible trial period may be considered before a full-scale implementation occurs. The role of the change agent should be delineated within the plan. It is important that an open line of communication be established to allow for frequent feedback after the change has been evaluated (Lippitt, Watson, and Westley, 1958; Olson, 1979). Lippitt's theory of planned change is advantageous, since it defines the role of the change agent and emphasizes the termination of the change agent and client system at a mutually agreeable time. Lippitt believed that the ability of the change agent is crucial, whether it is someone in or out of the organization (Olson, 1979).

Characteristics of Planned Change

- Conscious
- Deliberate
- Collaborative
- Goal-oriented
- Improvement
- Problem solving
- Uses scientific knowledge
- Purposeful

Rogers' theory of change states that the individual should be motivated and committed to the proposed changes. Rogers identified five stages of planned change: awareness, interest, evaluation, trial, and adoption. First the need for change must be realized and become the key impetus. Second, the individual's or group's interest in change must be determined and, the impact of the proposal and the alternatives for change must be evaluated. Rogers believed that after a trial period, adoption of the change can be either presently accepted, rejected, or used at a later date (Rogers, 1962). The characteristics of a successfully planned change are relative advantage, compatibility, complexity, divisibility, and communicability. In other words, if the alternative is considered an advantageous improvement, acceptable in the value system, simple to implement, tried on a sample basis, and easily communicated, the chance for success is great (Olson, 1979).

MODELS OF CHANGE

Along with the existence of several change theories are several models of change. Three models of change elaborate on the theories described by Lewis, Lippitt, and Rogers. These are systems, developmental, and confrontation theories.

Systems Theory Model

According to systems theory, any entity (person, family, agency, or health care unit) is a functioning dynamic whole and is considered an open system, attempting to maintain a state of equilibrium as it maintains life or function (Murray and Huelskoetter, 1987). The system is considered to be in a steady state when the dynamics operating within and on the system are in a balanced relationship to one another.

Chin (1961) and Murray and Huelskoetter (1987) concluded that the systems theory emphasizes the following concepts in the change process:

1. Organization—the entity, organism, structure, or agency follows a pattern of organization. A change in one aspect of the organization affects the entire organization.
2. Interdependency—any system is made up of parts that are interdependent in their function. A change in one part affects the function of every other part.
3. Integration of parts—all parts or components of a system are interrelated and integrated in the function of the whole. Communications and feedback between parts of the system maintain integration.
4. Change in any system depends on how well the parts fit or are interrelated or integrated in function.

The source or the motivating force and need for change generally grow out of structural stress or dysfunction in some part of the system and may come from within or outside the client or agency system. When dysfunction occurs, efforts at solution are directed to tension reduction as certain goals are imposed externally or internally on the system. When using systems theory the nurse as change agent defines or diagnoses the dysfunction, problem, or tension state in a part or between parts of the system (client). The nurse occupies a position outside the client system and thereby perceives self in the role of change agent, as in the role of motivating or assisting the individual or family client to make changes that will result in a more balanced health state. However, the nurse is also part of the agency system, and thus is within that system. Being a part of the system may enable the nurse to move accurately or quickly to identify problem areas or dysfunction in nursing care delivery and to propose solutions. Or, it may hinder the nurse in either identifying dysfunction or in proposing or implementing action to correct problems. The systems theory resolves problems of leadership, power, communication, organizational conflict, and intergroup relations (Murray and Heulskoetter, 1987).

The following situation is an example of change using systems theory:

An open psychiatric unit was changed to a stress center, day hospital, and a geropsychiatric treatment area in response to new and increasing client needs. The change was planned by the hospital administrator and the directors of Nursing Service, Marketing, and Psychiatry. Several staff nurses served as nursing representatives on the committee. The actual change process was initiated and presented to the nursing staff by the Director of Nursing. Implementation of the plan required maximum efforts in cooperation and communication between everyone involved. The motivating factors to create change in this situation were a decreased census of clients who had primary diagnoses of psychiatric disorders and an increase in clients who were frail and elderly with many physical illnesses and secondary diagnoses that were psychiatric-related. Physicians, as well as nurses, were the major sources of information that convinced the administration of the need for change. The system had become dysfunctional and no longer met its stated goals or provided effective psychiatric care for its clients. The total change process took 2 years from problem identification to the actual beginning implementation.

Developmental Model

Constant change and development are important elements underlying the developmental theory of change. Many difficulties arise when there is a discrepancy between potential growth and actual growth, development, or change (Murray and Huelskoetter, 1987). The conflict that surfaces usually has developed over an extended period of time and its source is generally natural, end-related, and purposeful. The process is also natural, and difficulties are automatic and characterized by major blocks leading to conflict between actual and potential change. The nurse change agent defines and diagnoses conflict areas, proposing actions to remove obstacles and engaging in actions to promote growth and development. The nurse is external and thereby may be objective in the role of promoting change or development with the client. As a part of the health care system, the nurse may experience conflict between desired, expected, and

actual development of self or may fail to perceive developmental needs or conflicts within self or with others.

The following example describes an individual developmental change:

A 16-year-old male client in a long-term adolescent facility told the nurse assigned to him that he no longer wanted to be called "Benjy," a nickname, because it showed that the staff had not acknowledged his growth and maturity. The client stood well over 6-feet tall and the nickname did not reflect any forward development. The staff nurse served as the change

TABLE 49-1 Summary of Other Models of Change

Model	Concept	Applications	Problems in Application
Traditional approach	Change occurs by exposition, teaching, or promotion of ideas and accumulated knowledge.	Client teaching, workshops, or in-service education for staff nurses in an agency, or advertising of a product or idea is used to change behavior.	The process of change is a multifaceted phenomenon that affects and is affected by all parts of the client system (individual, agency, family). These facets must be considered in this approach.
Elite corps approach	Change occurs when the people in charge, the power person, or leader uses knowledge or power maneuvers.	The nurse takes on an elitist or power position with the client, impressing the client with knowledge in an effort to get the client to change. The head nurse, executive, or administrator mandates change in an agency, stating rationale. The expectation is that others will automatically change behavior.	Change does not come about only with positions of knowledge and power as a basis. Improved media enlighten the masses of people, and they are no longer highly impressed by superior knowledge.
Psychoanalytical approach	Change occurs through the use of power and knowledge, but the leader or powerful person uses insights about self, others, and the change process to institute change.	The nurse is sensitive to client needs and uses insight about the client when proposing a change in behavior. The head nurse or administrator uses understanding of the people involved in the change and is sensitive or responsive to psychological factors when proposing change.	One person cannot impose change by the use of power and knowledge. Attitudes about authority have changed negatively.
Scholarly consultation approach	Change occurs when an expert or consultant uses scientific findings or sociological information as a basis for proposing a solution. The client, group, or agency can better select proposed solutions that best fit the need or situation as the result of the consultation.	The nurse acts as a consultant to the client, using knowledge of physiology, psychodynamics, or family process when discussing with the client why behavior should be changed. Generally, the administrator of an agency hires a consultant to propose solutions based on research findings and expert knowledge.	The nurse change agent who assumes the role of consultant must know personal limitations and boundaries and be aware of the policy covering such action. An outsider needs to gather complete data so that proposals have a chance to work in an individual agency.

agent by passing on to the hospital community Benjy's concern about how he was perceived. The change and development had been constant, gradual, natural, and not readily observed as something outside of the ordinary. Therefore the conflict that surfaced had developed over an extended period of time. When the care givers were made aware of Benjy's feelings, the change process was met with no resistance, and every effort was made to call him Benjamin as he had requested.

Confrontation Model

Smoyak's confrontation theory (1979) proposes that change occurs by direct confrontation, challenge, or criticism. The confronter or change agent position is determined by the status and power positions of the change agent. This theory is useful when there is a clearly identified issue or situation that must be changed. The decision for change must be supported by group consensus. This theory has three phases: planning, confrontation or implementation, and rebuilding. In the planning phase, the nurse as change agent must clearly identify the issue or concern, gather facts and ideas, and plan strategies for confrontation or challenge in a specific time dimension. Group members who oppose the plan of strategy for change should be confronted individually. However, all information or plans should be conveyed to the group as a whole. Repetition in describing ideas, facts, and plans is essential. The confrontation or implementation phase occurs when the change process is initiated. During this phase, progress reports or reviews are described to the group, whether or not the plan is currently progressing. The nurse change agent must remain calm and objective. The rebuilding phase involves strengthening relationships among the people involved in the confrontation. New images, new insights into roles and relationships, results of successful confrontation with others, and success in the change process are shared by the change agent with the group.

The following is an example of the use of confrontation theory:

Clients on a rehabilitation unit confronted staff nurses and complained about the room where group therapy sessions were held. Clients vowed to discontinue participating in the sessions until another room with windows was used. The nurses had reported to the head nurse, at varying times, about the clients' desires for a room with windows and a view. The administration had urged the head nurse and supervisor to encourage staff and clients to continue using the present room because a room change would be costly. The nurses on the unit elected a spokesperson from among them. The nurse change agent confronted the head nurse, supervisor, and administration about the need to change the room where the group sessions were held. Each member was presented supporting documentation from the client and nurses groups. The 50% decline in client participation in group therapy and a list of comments expressing a desire for a room change by clients were tactfully presented. The nurse change agent applied the principles of

good interpersonal relationship skills and convinced the opposition to agree to the change. In addition, the change agent helped to rebuild and strengthen relationships among the people involved in the confrontation. The change brought about a new awareness for all involved. Administration began to include more client input when planning for the clients' therapeutic milieu.

The various approaches used when applying change theory are presented in Table 49-1. The base concept, an example of application of the model, and problems in application are described for the traditional, elite corps, psychoanalytical, and scholarly consultation approaches or models (Reinkemeyer, 1970).

RESPONSE TO CHANGE

Change is usually accompanied by feelings of uneasiness, fear, and anxiety, even when change is desired. Some theorists believe that resistance is the most universal response of an individual or group to the change process. Resistance can be defined as any behavior that will inhibit or impede the movement toward change. This can be either through active or passive behavior. Active resistance occurs when one responds to change by openly refusing to comply with the proposed changes. Passive resistance occurs when one avoids or delays participation in the change process through deliberate strategies. Resistance can occur for several reasons (see box). It may also be an indication that the goals and reasons for change have not been clearly stated or that communication is distorted. On the positive side, change may be perceived as a hope for improvement, thus invoking good feelings. How one elects to deal with any anticipated resistance will strongly affect the overall success of the change (Murray and Huelskoetter, 1987; Olson, 1979).

Reasons for Resistance to Planned Change

- Effort, time, or money investment
- Threat to present values or norms
- Skewed power relationships, loss of status or power
- Fear of failure in the new situation
- Anxiety or stress from loss of routine or security
- Risk of losing the group's wholeness
- Loss of the familiar pattern of behavior
- Loss of familiar roles or status
- Insufficient consideration to consequent problems

THE CHANGE PROCESS

The change process has been compared to the steps of the nursing process. The components of the nursing process—assessment, nursing diagnosis, planning, implementation, and evaluation—can be used to facilitate change within the client system. A description of how the nursing process and the change process are parallel is shown in Table 49-2.

Assessment

Assessment is the first step in the process. The nurse change agent must be an effective and active listener, as well as an accurate recorder, while collecting information about the client or organizational system. The nurse must take note of how people relate to one another. Murray and Huelskoetter (1987) concluded that it is important to be able to identify signs of stress that may be harmful to the client system. Emphasis must be placed on listening and observing for indications of trust, respect, confidence, openness, commitment, and cohesiveness, or the opposite of these feelings. In addition, feelings and suggestions expressed by others should be listened to closely to determine centers of resistance. The relationship between the change agent and client or organizational system must be defined. Assessment of the group's motivating capacity for change should be determined. All possible alternatives and solutions should be examined to accomplish mutually acceptable goals within the group. All people affected by the change should be observed, interviewed, and encouraged to participate in assessment of the situation designated for change, as well as alternative solutions.

TABLE 49-2 Comparison of the Change Process and the Nursing Process

Change Process	Nursing Process
Collection of information about the client system	Assessment
Problem identification	Nursing diagnosis
Goal formulation and planning	Identification of nursing care goals and formulation of plan of care
Implementation	Intervention or implementation
Evaluation of the affected change	Evaluation of the effectiveness of the outcomes of intervention as compared to short-term and long-term goals

Nursing Diagnosis

Diagnosis of the problem should be specifically stated with consideration given to any possible ramifications of change for all key individuals. To formulate a clear definition of a problem, the nurse change agent must work back and forth between initial assessment information, tentatively stated problems, and newly gathered information. During the change process, interpersonal issues should be clearly stated, since these may influence diagnosis of the problem.

Planning

Goals should be stated as desired outcomes. Input from all people involved in the change should be gathered to formulate short-term objectives to in turn attain the stated long-term or overall goals and plans of action. How the course of action would be implemented is an important aspect of the planning phase. All people affected by the change should be involved. Consideration of each suggested solution's advantages and drawbacks is helpful in selecting the most efficient plan. The key to a successful transition is a comprehensive plan that has looked at benefits, costs, and risks for each proposed change. Some results are not anticipated, but it is important to try to consider every possible outcome from the proposed solutions before implementation of a plan.

Resistance to change can be reduced if restraining forces are identified during the assessment and planning steps before the implementation. Restraining forces may simply be rules and regulations within an organization, financial limitations, or a group of disgruntled employees. Therefore it is important to identify the anticipated resistances and devise a method to deal with them. On the other hand, enlisting individuals who view the change favorably may positively influence the outcome. In an attempt to "sell" the proposed change, the change agent must be genuinely sincere, highly motivated, and demonstrate professional expertise. Involve those who are resistant by gradually involving them in the goal setting if at all possible to gain their commitment to the change.

Plan specific interventions through collaboration with others. Acknowledging the feelings and suggestions of all involved will help prevent the client, family, group, or agency from thinking that the change agent is not providing all of the possible solutions to the problem.

Implementation

When a specific course of action has been chosen, an outline detailing steps in the change process and a time frame should be developed. Some experts recommend that the change be piloted by a small group in an effort to identify any unexpected problems. Thus the environment and key personnel would be adequately prepared before a full-scale implementation. As the change is initiated, open lines of communication and a support system are essential. A therapeutic climate should be created that is conducive to bringing about a successful improvement or change for the client or any component of the client system. The nurse must use effective interpersonal and communication skills to collaborate with the client, family, or agency during the change process (see research highlight). The change must be accepted as permanent and standard for the system to return to a stable state with the change accomplished.

Evaluation

When the change has been activated, the outcomes should be examined to see if the goals have been accomplished. It is possible that further modifications may need to be developed. Analysis of the negative and the positive elements produced by the change must be made and reported to the client or organizational system. For example, analysis may reveal that a client changed his attitude and stopped resisting attempts by the nurse change agent who had explained the benefits of and encouraged his active participation in group therapy. The need and the desire to change behavior are now perceived by the client as a benefit rather than as a move to satisfy staff. The nursing administration may issue a memorandum describing the effectiveness and success of a specific change that alleviated a problem. It is important to remember that change takes time. In some cases, it may take years to plan, implement, and evaluate the change process.

⚜ *Research Highlight* ⚜

Feldman and Ventura designed a study to assess the influence of an intervention program on health and health promoting behaviors of patients with peripheral vascular disease. The purpose of this VA-funded Health Services research and development study was to help clients reduce smoking, increase exercise, and improve foot-care habits. The hypothesis that clients who worked with professionals on this intervention program would show more improvement than the control group who received the usual care was significant at $p < .005$. The experimental group improved more in each area than the control group, per chi-square analysis.

Feldman, M, and Ventura, M: Evaluating changes in using non-interval data, Nurs Res 33(3):182, 1984.

In addition, every system must also maintain a balanced relationship with surrounding systems. A health care agency both influences and is influenced by the total community (federal, state, and local communities). Nursing administration must appreciate how this extension can affect operations because change can originate in these other systems in the forms of new legislation, new ideas about client rights, or a new kind of care equipment (Spradley, 1980).

When using a person-centered approach to effect positive change, the change agent must be aware of personal reactions to change and be able to change behavior accordingly (Murray and Huelskoetter, 1987). A collaborative relationship between the nurse change agent and the client system can then be developed. The nursing process provides a foundation for a humanistic, knowledgeable, organized, and holistic client care system and a framework for the change process. The change process can be used with any theoretical framework, any type of client system, and in any situation or environment.

CHARACTERISTICS OF THE NURSE CHANGE AGENT

Change agent refers to the person or group that is responsible for instituting change or alterations. The nurse change agent must possess a combination of expertise and skills to be effective. The key component in being an effective change agent is competence in use of communication principles and interpersonal relationships. Being aware as one's own, as well as others', attitudes, beliefs, and values regarding the change is essential to the outcome. Remember that being an initiator and a catalyst for motivation carries a great responsibility to the client system and all of its components. The nurse change agent must try to understand personal motivation for participating in the change process by asking the following questions:

1. Is there a genuine desire to improve something?
2. Does the motivation arise from a personal desire for power or recognition? Or is the change simply being done for the sake of change?
3. Will there be an improvement as a result of the change?

Other questions that may need to be asked by the nurse change agent and the client system (individuals, family, or agency) include the following:

1. How much experience has the change agent had with the particular problem?
2. Does the nurse change agent have the credentials of an expert in the situation as defined by the key people involved in the problem?
3. Will the personality of the change agent be con-

ducive to promoting effective change? Can this person be the facilitator for change in this situation?

4. Is the nurse change agent sensitive to what can or cannot be changed?
5. What is the approach or orientation of the change agent? What model of change is used by the change agent?

Regardless of the size or kind of group, similarities exist in the relationships between the members (parts or subsystems) that are conducive to health, growth, and collaboration or that promote dysfunction and conflict when change is planned and instituted (Bennis, Benne, and Chin, 1969).

Constructive criticism can help promote the change process. Be prepared to rebuild and leave the individual's ego intact whenever you give instruction or suggestions. The purpose of criticism is to facilitate, clarify, keep focused on the situation undergoing change, and continue having support for the change from members of the client system. Therefore it is important to identify unfavorable forces and to postpone or to modify a planned presentation or activity related to the change process. The degree to which a client can change is limited. To appropriately give and receive constructive criticism, the change agent must know about the goals and norms of the client's orientation and philosophy and key people to work within the system.

The greatest risk involved in change is that the client system may lose its identity and may become so disorganized with change that the system is unable to function effectively or meet goals because of the way the change was effected. The competent interpersonal or relationship skills of the nurse change agent are crucial during this phase. Relationships may need rebuilding because of disagreements or conflicts that may have arisen during the change process. An evaluation and comparison of the situation before and after the change and observing a clear difference in the situation may help those who participated in the change to continue practicing the new concepts or procedures. Giving praise to others while personally sharing the success of the change often helps in rebuilding and raising the self-esteem of those involved in the change.

USE OF POWER

The nurse change agent throughout the process must be cautious and sensitive to the effective and constructive utilization of power. Power is the ability to influence, produce, or control to exert authority. Within the change process, power refers to the person or persons directing or controlling the change. Power may be categorized as expert power, managerial or line power, elected power, and appointed power (Ivancevich and Donnelly, 1970).

Expert Power

Expert power is technical advanced knowledge about the area requiring the change. Experts are called on for information or clarification on limitations and boundaries found within the area to be changed or for their performance skills (Calkin, 1980).

Line Power

Line power refers to influence that the change agent can exert because of position in the organizational chart. Certain positions in nursing carry multidirectional movement. The nurse change agent in some positions can communicate directly to staff, administration, interdisciplinary team members, as well as auxiliary personnel. The staff nurse is in a position to exert influence with other staff nurses, auxiliary personnel, and interdisciplinary team members. The unique position of the staff nurse affords the opportunity to be a participant observer and gather pertinent information from all levels of staff. The nurse reports those data into a meaningful analysis necessary to successfully affect the proposed changes (Calkin, 1980).

Managerial Power

Managerial power is similar to line power. The ability to get others to perform is the key component of nurses in managerial levels such as head nurse or supervisor because of this position in the organization. Power from these sources is authorized by administration and requires an upward direction of accountability and responsibility for the changes that are proposed and implemented (Calkin, 1980). The staff nurse is responsible for managing those changes involving the individual client, family, or significant others. Managerial power exerted by the staff nurse may involve teaching the client discharge planning. It is the responsibility of the nurse change agent to implement management directives related to discharge planning. Implementation could involve teaching the client the importance of the proposed changes on life-style, the specific components of these changes, and effect—when, where, how, and for how long—these changes will have (Calkin, 1980). Staff positions often advise the nurse manager on testing and final selection of new equipment for client care, arrangement of a nursing unit, or the best approach for policy implementation.

Elected Power

Elected power generally exists as a result of group members empowering an individual to serve as spokesperson and to make decisions without the group being present. At the time of the election, the individual is given the key components of what is desired within the change process, as well as the feelings and expectations of others involved in the change. Goals are usually specifically stated. However, the change agent is usually free to suggest possible objectives for goal attainment (Calkin, 1980; Spradley, 1980).

Appointed Power

Appointed power infers that some level of administration has selected an individual to act as a change agent. This appointment may be the result of some observed evidence of competency or successful interaction with members involved in the change. This individual may at some earlier time have served as spokesperson for the group. An example of appointed power is a staff nurse who may act as a unit-wide consultant for institution of a specific procedure and yet not have responsibility for other managerial aspects of the unit (Calkin, 1980).

AUTHORITY AND POWER ASPECTS OF THE NURSE CHANGE AGENT

Both the authority and power aspects of the nurse change agent should be considered. Authority is the influence that is generated from possessing a position in the organizational hierarchy (Ivancevich and Donnelly, 1970). Head nurse and supervisor positions carry such authority. Power is the source that alters the behavior and decisions of others. The individual who is an expert in the area of the change certainly exerts such power, since knowledge of the area is necessary to effectively effect the change.

The nurse change agent should know who occupies power positions. The change agent may need to reorganize the distribution of power, either by encouraging new sources of influence or by making old power centers more responsive and representative of the client system. Changing intergroup competition to intergroup collaboration can be effective and productive for a client system and is derived from a combination of two sources, expert and line power.

Resistance to Change

When there is resistance to change, the following precautions may be applied by the change agent to all elements of a client system (individuals, families, significant others, and organizations/agencies). The theoretical framework identified and selected for use by the nurse change agent should fit the specific situation. Often a combination of approaches is required to effect a change.

Knowing values and opinions of the opponents, as well as allies, to the change in progress is vitally important. The nurse change agent needs to analyze the adversarial position from the opposition's point of view. For example, in the case of the individual client, the nurse must know if discharge plans for the client are being resisted by the family members and which family member may be the lead of opposition. The advantages are that the change agent is provided a better perspective and greater insight into ways of coping with and resolving resistance to the change process. When a change affects the nursing staff, resistance can be manifested by absenteeism, resignations, requests for transfers, reduction in performance, drifting back into old patterns of behavior, postponing deadlines for action, communication breakdown, or uncooperative, aggressive, and defensive behavior (Murray and Huelskoetter, 1987). These signs of resistance must be acknowledged by the change agent and efforts made to overcome the resistance through use of communication and relationship skills referred to earlier in the chapter.

To keep the change process moving in a positive direction, the nurse change agent must be able to differentiate between interference and resistance. Olson (1979) defines interference as behavior intended to protect the individual or group from the effects of real or imagined change. Interference interrupts the change process because the change is not a priority item. Resistance is more forceful, and individuals or groups take on defensive postures of hostility and aggression. Interfering members may react overtly in a favorable way to the change, although they do not actively participate in implementaton of the change. Resistance forces are generally decreased when (1) the project has support from the administrative level, (2) participants are actively involved in the process, (3) group decisions are reached by consensus, (4) provisions are made for immediate feedback, and (5) there are open and objective feelings and attitudes about testing revisions and reconsiderations (Olson, 1979).

Nursing Roles as a Change Agent

The staff nurse change agent is reflected in the efforts to return the individual client to a favorable health state. Involving the client's family and significant others in teaching during hospitalization and discharge planning, more often than not, requires the nurse change agent to use knowledge and interpersonal relationship skills at the highest possible level.

Often, positive change comes about for the client because the nurse has become an advocate for the client. The nurse change agent as a client advocate requires a reassessment of personal values and beliefs and an assurance that advocacy is appropriate for the client. For the most part, an investigation must be made to be sure that the issue is not detrimental to the health of the client and that it does not interfere with prescribed therapy. The client must be made aware of known and potential consequences of the advocacy. The role of client advocate, assisting the client in obtaining the best possible care in the situation with informed consent and knowledge of alternatives, may cut across all positions and levels.

At any point in time, the staff nurse may respond to a request for change. The administration may insist that some nursing routine be discontinued because they may have received overwhelming complaints from the hospital population. For example, efforts to reduce or eliminate the noise that results from activities of early morning procedures and diagnostic testing at 5 or 6 AM is an example of client advocacy that could be initiated by a staff nurse, nurse manager, or vice-president of nursing.

SUMMARY

The nurse in any position or any care setting is a change agent when working with a client, family, or group to change behavior or institute a new self-care procedure. The nurse is a change agent when working with colleagues to implement a change in policy or procedure within a nursing unit or agency. The steps of the nursing process are similar to the steps of the change process. To institute any change, the nurse must do the following:

1. Understand theories of and approaches to change.
2. Use the theory or approach that is most applicable to the situation.
3. Recognize and work with the normal reactions to changes.
4. Acknowledge and work with interference and resistance that is normally found during any change.
5. Use carefully and appropriately the level of power or influence that is personally and professionally available during the change process.
6. Use the principles of communication and interpersonal relationships with patience and skill.

KEY CONCEPTS

✓ Change is a dynamic process that results in an alteration in ideas, behavior, or functions of an individual, family, or group or in functions, policies, or procedures of an organization.

✓ Change may be developmental, coercive, situational (unplanned), or planned.

✓ Lewin's theory of change defines the change process in three steps: unfreezing, moving, and refreezing. Change involves either driving or restraining forces.

✓ The steps of the change process involve (1) *unfreezing* (recognizing a need for change, diagnosing the problem, investigating alternatives, planning), (2) *moving* (implementing the planned strategies or modifications, working with driving forces, and overcoming restraining forces, interference, or resistance), and (3) *refreezing*, incorporating the alterations or modifications as normal behavior, regular function, or standard policy or procedure.

✓ Lippett's theory of change defines the change process as involving diagnosis, investigation of potential solutions, and evaluation.

✓ Roger's theory of change defines five stages in the change process: awareness, interest, evaluation, trial, and adoption.

✓ Systems theory of change describes the change process or alteration in behavior as involving the entire unit or organization, as well as its component parts in an interdependent, integrated manner.

✓ Developmental theory of change refers to purposeful alterations that occur overtime as a part of the natural expansion, growth, or development of an individual, family, group, organization, or community, based on aspirations or potential for movement.

✓ The change process often combines aspects of the systems and developmental theories.

✓ Confrontation theory of change refers to an individual with power and status who can direct modifications in behavior or function through a process of planned challenge, criticism, review, and direction of others.

✓ Power, the ability to influence, direct, produce, or control, may be categorized as (1) expert (based on knowledge or skill), (2) managerial (based on position in the organization, (3) elected (being voted by the group as the person to represent them and to be in charge), and (4) appointed (being selected as the spokesman).

✓ Change occurs regularly in the health care setting and is a consistent aspect of the nursing process.

✓ The steps of the change process are comparable to the steps of the nursing process.

✓ The role of change agent is incorporated into any level or position of nursing.

✓ The effective change agent uses knowledge of the model that is appropriate to the situation.

✓ The effective change agent uses interpersonal skills, as well as expertise in knowledge and skill to work with others, either as a consultant or as the person(s) primarily responsible, to modify or alter.

✓ The effective change agent understands and appropriately uses the power base in the change process.

REFERENCES

Bennis W, Benne, K, and Chin, R: The planning of change, ed. 2, New York, 1969, Holt, Rinehart & Winston.

Calkin, J: Using management literature to enhance new leadership roles, J Nurs Admin 10:24, 1980.

Chin, R: The utility of system models and developmental models for practitioners in the planning of change. In Bennis, W, Benne, K, and Chin R, editors: Applied behavior science, New York, 1961, Holt, Rinehart & Winston.

Ivancevich, J, and Donnelly, J: Leader influence and performance, Pers Psychiatr 23:538, 1970.

Lewin, K: Field theory in social science, New York, 1951, Harper & Row Publishers.

Lewin, K: Group decision and social change. In Maccoby, E, editor: Readings in social psychology, ed. 3, New York, 1958, Holt, Rinehart & Winston.

Lippitt, R, Watson, J, and Westley, B; The dynamics of planned change, New York, 1958, Harcourt, Brace, Jovanovich, Inc.

Mauksch, I, and Miller, M: Implementing change in nursing, St. Louis, 1981, The C.V. Mosby Co.

Murray, R, and Huelskoetter, M: Psychiatric/mental health nursing: Giving emotional care, ed. 2, Englewood Cliffs, N.J., 1987, Prentice-Hall, Inc.

Olson, E: Strategies and techniques for the nurse change agent, Nurs Clin North Am 14(2):323, 1979.

Reinkemeyer, A: Commitment to an idealogy of change, Nurs Forum 9(4):341, 1970.

Rogers, E: Diffusion of innovations, New York, 1962, The Free Press.

Smoyak, S: Confrontation model. In Olson, EW, editor: Strategies and techniques for the nurse change agent, Nurs Clin North Am 14(2):330, 1979.

Spradley, B: Managing change creatively, J Nurs Admin 10:32, 1980.

Welch, L: Planned change in nursing: the theory, Nurs Clin North Am 14(2):307, 1979.

Research Article

Feldman, M, and Ventura, M: Evaluating changes in using non-interval data, Nurs Res 33(3):182, 1984.

ADDITIONAL READINGS

Green, C: Teaching strategies for the process of planned change, Contin Educ Nurs 14:16, 1983.

Levenstein, A: Effective change requires change agent, Hospitals: J Am Hosp Assoc 50(24): 71, 1976.

McGovern, W, and Rogers, J: Change theory, Am J Nurs 86(5):556, 1986.

National League for Nursing: Developing strategies to effect change, Publ. No. 52-1537, New York, 1974, National League for Nursing.

Oromaner, D: Overcoming employee resistance to technological change, St. Louis Manager, November 1985.

Rodgers, J: Theoretical considerations involved in the process of change, Nurs Forum 12(2):161, 1973.

Ward, M, and Moran, S: Resistance to change: recognize, respond, overcome, Nurs Manag 15(1):30, 1984.

Appendix A
Professional Nursing Organizations in the United States

NATIONAL ORGANIZATIONS

Alpha Tau Delta National Fraternity
for Professional Nurses
489 Serento Circle
Thousand Oaks, California 91360

American Association of
Colleges of Nursing
1 Dupont Circle, Suite 530
Washington, DC 20036

American Hospital Association
Division of Nursing
840 N. Lake Shore Drive
Chicago, IL 60611

American Indian/Alaska Native Nurses
Association, Inc.
P.O. Box 1588
Norman, OK 73070

American Nurses' Association
2420 Pershing Road
Kansas City, MO 64108

Committee on Nursing of the
Catholic Hospital Association
1438 S. Grand Boulevard
St. Louis, MO 63104

Gay Nurses' Alliance
P.O. Box 115
Brownsville, TX 78520

Lutheran Hospital
Association of America
Room 607 W
840 N. Lake Shore Drive
Chicago, IL 60611

National Black Nurses
Association, Inc.
P.O. Box 18358
Boston, MA 02118

National Center for
Nursing Ethics
P.O. Box 2237
Cincinnati, OH 45201

National League for Nursing
10 Columbus Circle
New York, NY 10019

National Male Nurses'
Association
2308 State Street
Saginaw, MI 48602

National Nurses for Life
1998 Menold
Allison Park, PA 15101

National Student Nurses'
Association, Inc.
555 West 57th Street
Suite 1325
New York, NY 10019

Nurses Christian Fellowship
233 Langdon Street
Madison, WI 53703

Nurses Educational Funds
10 Columbus Circle
New York, NY 10019

Sigma Theta Tau
National Honor Society of Nursing
1200 Waterway Blvd.
Indianapolis, IN 46202

SPECIALTY ASSOCIATIONS

American Association for
Respiratory Therapy
1720 Regal Row
Dallas, TX 75235

American Association of
Critical Care Nurses
One Civic Plaza
Newport Beach, CA 92660

American Nephrology
Nurses' Association
North Woodbury Road
Box 56
Pitman, NJ 08071

American Association of
Neuroscience Nurses
218 N. Jefferson
Suite 204
Chicago, IL 60606

American Association of
Neurosurgical Nurses
Suite 1519
625 North Michigan Avenue
Chicago, IL 60611

American Association of Nurse
Anesthetists
216 Higgins Road
Park Ridge, IL 60068

American Association of
Occupational Health Nurses
50 Lenox Pointe
Atlanta, GA 30324

American Urological Association
Allied
6845 Lake Shore Drive
Raytown, MO 64133

American Burn Association
Burn Treatment Center
Crozier-Chester Medical Center
15th and Upland Avenue
Chester, PA 19013

American College of Nurse-Midwives
1522 K Street
Suite 1120
Washington, DC 20005

American Geriatric Society
Room 1470
10 Columbus Circle
New York, NY 10019

Association for Practitioners in
Infection Control
505 E. Hawley Street
Mundelein, IL 60060

Association of Operating
Room Nurses, Inc.
10170 East Mississippi Avenue
Denver, CO 80231

Association of Pediatric
Oncology Nurses
Pacific Medical Center
P.O. Box 7999
San Francisco, CA 94120

Association of Rehabilitation Nurses
2506 Gross Point Road
Evanston, IL 60201

Emergency Nurses Association
230 East Ohio
6th Floor
Chicago, IL 60611

International Association for
Enterostomal Therapy
5000 Birch
P.O. Box 2690-175
Newport Beach, CA 92660

National Association of Orthopaedic
Nurses
North Woodbury Road
Box 56
Pitman, NJ 08071

National Association of Pediatric
Nurse Associates and Practitioners
1000 Maplewood Drive
Suite 104
Maple Shade, NJ 08052

National Flight Nurses' Association
P.O. Box 68395
Virginia Beach, VA 23455

National Intravenous Therapy
Association
87 Blanchard Road
Cambridge, MA 02138

Nurses Association of the American
College of Obstetricians and
Gynecologists
409 12th Street, S.W.
Washington, DC 20024-2191

Oncology Nursing Society
North Woodbury Road, Box 56
Pitman, NJ 08071

American Organization of
Nurse Executives
840 N. Lake Shore Drive
Chicago, IL 60611

Nurse Consultants Association
P.O. Box 2587
Colorado Springs, CO 80936

American Society of Ophthalmic
Registered Nurses, Inc.
P.O. Box 3030
San Francisco, CA 94119

American Society of Post Anesthesia
Nurses (ASPAN)
P.O. Box 11083
Richmond, VA 23230

Public Health Nursing Association
1015 15th Street, N.W.
Washington, DC 20005

American Society of Plastic and
Reconstructive Surgical Nurses, Inc.
North Woodbury Road, Box 56
Pitman, NJ 08071

National Association of
School Nurses, Inc.
Lamplighter Lane
P.O. Box 1300
Scarborough, ME 04074

Dermatology Nurses' Association
North Woodbury Road, Box 56
Pitman, NJ 08071

American Holistic Nurses Association
205 St. Louis Street
Suite 506
Springfield, MO 65806

National Association of Hispanic
Nurses
2014 Johnson Street
Los Angeles, CA 90031

National Association for Health Care
Recruitment
P.O. Box 93851
Cleveland, OH 44101-5851

Nurses' Environmental
Health Watch, Inc.
33 Columbus Avenue
Somerville, MA 02143

Nurses House, Inc.
10 Columbus Circle
New York, NY 10019

Professional Nursing Organizations in Canada

NATIONAL ORGANIZATIONS

Canadian Association of Practical and Nursing Assistants

R.R. No. 4
St. Stephen, New Brunswick
E3L 2Y2

Canadian Association of University Schools of Nursing

1200-151 Slater
Ottawa, Ontario
K1P 5N1

Canadian Nurses Association

50 The Driveway
Ottawa, Ontario
K2P 1E2

Canadian Nurses Foundation

50 The Driveway
Ottawa, Ontario
K2P 1E2

Nursing Sisters Association of Canada

8500 Francis Road
Richmond, British Columbia
V6Y 1A6

Canadian University Nursing Students Association

School of Nursing
Université de Montréal
C.P. 6128
Montréal, Québec
H3T 1J4

Registered Nurses of Canadian Indian Ancestry

500-222 Queen St.
Ottawa, Ontario
K1P 5V9

SPECIALTY ASSOCIATIONS

Canadian Association of Enterostomal Therapy

4389 Prospect Rd.
North Vancouver, B.C.
V7N 3L8

Canadian Association of Quality Care Coordinators

Nursing Practice
Surrey Memorial Hospital
King George Highway
Surrey, British Columbia
V3V 1Z2

Canadian Association of Neurological and Neurosurgical Nurses

296 Palace Road
Kingston, Ontario
K7L 4T3

Canadian Nurses Respiratory Society Nurses Section Canadian Lung Association

908-75 Albert Street
Ottawa, Ontario
K1P 5E7

Canadian Orthopedic Nurses Association

43 Wellesley Street E.
Toronto, Ontario
M4Y 1H1

Canadian Council of Cardiovascular Nurses

1200-1 Nicholas Street
Ottawa, Ontario
K1N 7B7

Psychiatric Nurses Association of Canada

1854 Portage Avenue
Winnipeg, Manitoba
R3J 0G9

Canadian Association of Critical Care Nurses

P.O. Box 61
Welland, Ontario
L3B 5N9

Professional Health Workers Section Canadian Diabetes Association

601-123 Edward St.
Toronto, Ontario
M5G 1E2

Canadian Hospital Infection Control Association

Mount Sinai Hospital
600 University Ave.
Toronto, Ont.
M5G 1X5

Canadian Intravenous Nurses Association

200-4433 Sheppard Ave. E.
Agincourt, Ontario
M1S 1V3

Canadian Society of Dialysis Perfusionists

Dialysis Unit
Health Sciences Centre
700 William Ave.
Winnipeg, Manitoba
R3E 0Z3

Dynamics of Critical Care Association of Canada

CNSC
200-4433 Sheppard Ave. E.
Agincourt, Ontario
M1S 1V3

Operating Room Nurses Association of Canada

213-52377 Range Rd.
Sherwood Park, Alberta
T8G 1B9

TPN Nurses Association of Canada

P.O. Box 62
Station K
Toronto, Ont.
M4P 2G1

INTERNATIONAL ASSOCIATIONS

Association for The Care of Children's Health Canadian Institute of Child Health

202-17 York St.
Ottawa, Ontario
K1M 5S7

Appendix B

Normal Reference Laboratory Values

Blood, Plasma, or Serum Values

Determination	Reference Range Conventional	SI
Acetoacetate plus acetone	0.3-2.0 mg/100 ml	3-20 mg/l
Aldolase	1.3-8.2 mU/ml	12-75 nmol · s^{-1}/l
Alpha amino nitrogen	3.0-5.5 mg/100 ml	2.1-3.9 mmol/l
Ammonia	80-110 μg/100 ml	47-65 μmol/l
Ascorbic acid	0.4-1.5 mg/100 ml	23-85 μmol/l
Barbiturate	0	0 μmol/l
	Coma level: phenobarbital, approximately 10 mg/100 ml; most other drugs, 1-3 mg/100 ml	
Bilirubin (van den Bergh test)	One minute: 0.4 mg/100 ml	Up to 7 μmol/l
	Direct: 0.4 mg/100 ml	Up to 17 μmol/l
	Total: 1.0 mg/100 ml Indirect is total minus direct	
Blood volume	8.5-9.0% of body weight in kg	80-85 ml/kg
Bromide	0	0 mmol/l
	Toxic level: 17 mEq/l	
Bromsulfalein (BSP)	Less than 5% retention 45 min after 5 mg/kg IV	<0.05l
Calcium	8.5-10.5 mg/100 ml (slightly higher in children)	2.1-2.6 mmol/l
Carbon dioxide content	24-30 mEq/l	24-30 mmol/l
	20-26 mEq/l in infants (as HCO$_3^-$)	
Carbon monoxide	Symptoms with over 20% saturation	0(1)
Carotenoids	0.8-4.0 μg/ml	1.5-7.4 μmol/l
Ceruloplasmin	27-37 mg/100 ml	1.8-2.5 μmol/l
Chloride	100-106 mEq/l	100-106 mmol/l
Cholinesterase (pseudocholinesterase)	0.5 pH U or more/h	0.5 or more arb. unit
	0.7 pH U or more/h for packed cells	

Modified from Kaye, DA, and Rose, LF: Fundamentals of internal medicine, St. Louis, 1983, The C.V. Mosby Co. Adapted by permission from the New England Journal of Medicine, Vol. 302, pages 37-48, 1980.
Abbreviations used: SI, Système international d'Unités (The SI for the Health Professions. World Health Organization, Office of Publications, Geneva, Switzerland, 1977); d, 24 hours; P, plasma; S, serum; B, blood; U, urine; l, liter; h, hour; and s, second.

Blood, Plasma, or Serum Values, cont'd

Determination	Reference Range Conventional	SI
Copper	Total: 100-200 µg/100 ml	16-31 µmol/l
Creatine phosphokinase (CPK)	Female 5-35 mU/ml	0.08-0.58 µmol · s⁻¹/l
	Male 5-55 mU/ml	
Creatinine	0.6-1.5 mg/100 ml	60-130 µmol/l
Ethanol	0.3-0.4%, marked intoxication; 0.4-0.5%, alcoholic stupor; 0.5% or over, alcoholic coma	65-87 mmol/l 87-109 mmol/l >109 mmol/l
Glucose	Fasting: 70-110 mg/100 ml	3.9-5.6 mmol/l
Iron	50-150 µg/100 ml (higher in males)	9.0-26.9 µmol/l
Iron-binding capacity	250-410 µg/100 ml	44.8-73.4 µmol/l
Lactic acid	0.6-1.8 mEq/l	0.6-1.8 mmol/l
Lactic dehydrogenase	60-120 U/ml	1.00-2.00 µmol · s⁻¹/l
Lead	50 µg/100 ml or less	Up to 2.4 µmol/l
Lipase	2 U/ml or less	Up to 2 arb. unit
Lipids		
Cholesterol	120-220 mg/100 ml	3.10-5.69 mmol/l
Cholesterol esters	60-75% of cholesterol	
Phospholipids	9-16 mg/100 ml as lipid phosphorus	2.9-5.2 mmol/l
Total fatty acids	190-420 mg/100 ml	1.9-4.2 g/l
Total lipids	450-1000 mg/100 ml	4.5-10.0 g/l
Triglycerides	40-150 mg/100 ml	0.4-1.5 g/l
Lithium	Toxic level 2 mEq/l	2 mmol/l
Magnesium	1.5-2.0 mEq/l	0.8-1.3 mmol/l
5'Nucleotidase	0.3-3.2 Bodansky U	30-290 nmol · s⁻¹/l
Osmolality	285-295 mOsm/kg water	285-295 mmol/kg
Oxygen saturation (arterial)	96-100%	0.96-1.00 l
Pco₂	35-43 mm Hg	4.7-6.0 kPa
pH	7.35-7.45	Same
Po₂	75-100 mm Hg (dependent on age) while breathing room air	
	Above 500 mm Hg while on 100% O₂	10.0-13.3 kPa
Phenylalanine	0-2 mg/100 ml	0-120 µmol/l
Phenytoin (Dilantin)	Therapeutic level, 5-20 µg/ml	19.8-79.5 µmol/l
Phosphorus (inorganic)	3.0-4.5 mg/100 ml (infants in 1st yr up to 6.0 mg/100 ml)	1.0-1.5 mmol/l
Potassium	3.5-5.0 mEq/l	3.5-5.0 mmol/l
Primidone (Mysoline)	Therapeutic level 4-12 µg/ml	18-55 µmol/l
Protein: Total	6.0-8.4 g/100 ml	60-84 g/l
Albumin	3.5-5.0 g/100 ml	35-50 g/l
Globulin	2.3-3.5 g/100 ml	23-35 g/l
Electrophoresis	% of total protein	Of total protein
Albumin	52-68	0.52-0.68
Globulin:		
Alpha₁	4.2-7.2	0.042-0.072
Alpha₂	6.8-12	0.068-0.12
Beta	9.3-15	0.093-0.15
Gamma	13-23	0.13-0.23
Pyruvic acid	0-0.11 mEq/l	0-0.11 mmol/l
Quinidine	Therapeutic: 1.5-3 µg/ml	4.6-9.2 µmol/l
	Toxic: 5-6 µg/ml	15.4-18.5 µmol/l
Salicylate:	0	
Therapeutic	20-25 mg/100 ml; 25-30 mg/100 ml to age 10 yr 3 h post dose	1.4-1.8 mmol/l 1.8-2.2 mmol/l

Blood, Plasma, or Serum Values, cont'd

Determination	Reference Range Conventional	SI
Toxic	Over 30 mg/100 ml	Over 2.2 mmol/l
	Over 20 mg/100 ml after age 60	Over 1.4 mmol/l
Sodium	135-145 mEq/l	135-145 mmol/l
Sulfate	0.5-1.5 mg/100 ml	0.05-1.2 mmol/l
Sulfonamide	0 mg/100 ml	0 mmol/l
	Therapeutic: 5-15 mg/100 ml	
Transaminase (SGOT) (aspartate amino-transferase)	10-40 U/ml	0.08-0.32 μmol $\cdot$ s^{-1}/l
Urea nitrogen (BUN)	8-25 mg/100 ml	2.9-8.9 mmol/l
Uric acid	3.0-7.0 mg/100 ml	0.18-0.42 mmol/l
Vitamin A	0.15-0.6 μg/ml	0.5-2.1 μmol/l
Vitamin A tolerance test	Rise to twice fasting level in 3 to 5 h	

Urine Values

Determination	Reference Range Conventional	SI
Acetone plus acetoacetate (quantitative)	0	0 mg/l
Alpha amino nitrogen	64-199 mg/d; not over 1.5% of total nitrogen	4.6-14.2 mmol/d
Amylase	24-76 U/ml	24-76 arb. unit
Calcium	150 mg/d or less	3.8 or less mmol/d
Catecholamines	Epinephrine: under 20 μg/d	<55 nmol/d
	Norepinephrine: under 100 μg/d	<590 nmol/d
Copper	0-100 μg/d	0-1.6 μmol/d
Coproporphyrin	50-250 μg/d	80-380 nmol/d
	Children under 80 lb 0-75 μg/d	0-115 nmol/d
Creatine	Under 100 mg/d or less than 6% of creatinine. In pregnancy: up to 12%. In children under 1 yr: may equal creatinine. In older children: up to 30% of creatinine	<0.75 mmol/d
Cystine or cysteine	0	0
Follicle-stimulating hormone:		
Follicular phase	5-20 IU/d	Same
Midcycle	15-60 IU/d	
Luteal phase	5-15 IU/d	
Menopausal	50-100 IU/d	
Men	5-25 IU/d	
Hemoglobin and myoglobin	0	
5-Hydroxyindole acetic acid	2-9 mg/d (women lower than men)	10-45 μmol/d
Lead	0.08 μg/ml or 120 μg or less/d	0.39 μmol/l or less
Phenolsulfonphthalein (PSP)	At least 25% excreted by 15 min; 40% by 30 min; 60% by 120 min	0.25 l
Phosphorus (inorganic)	Varies with intake; average 1 g/d	32 mmol/d

Urine Values, cont'd

Determination	Reference Range		
	Conventional		SI
Porphobilinogen	0		0
Protein:			
Quantitative	<150 mg/d		<0.15 g/d
Steroids			
17-Ketosteroids (per day)	*Age* *Male* *Female*		*Male* *Female*
	(yr) (mg) (mg)		(μmol/d) (μmol/d)
	10 1-4 1-4		3-14 3-14
	20 6-21 4-16		21-73 14-56
	30 8-26 4-14		28-90 14-49
	50 5-18 3-9		17-62 10-31
	70 2-10 1-7		7-35 3-24
17-Hydroxysteroids	3-8 mg/d (women lower than men)		8-22 μmol/d as hydrocortisone
Sugar:			
Quantitative glucose	0		0 mmol/l
Identification of reducing substances			
Fructose	0		0 mmol/l
Pentose	0		0 mmol/l
Titratable acidity	24-40 mEq/d		20-40 mmol/d
Urobilinogen	Up to 1.0 Ehrlich U		To 1.0 arb. unit
Uroporphyrin	0		0 nmol/d
Vanillylmandelic acid (VMA)	Up to 9 mg/d		Up to 45 μmol/d

Special Endocrine Tests

Determination	Reference Range	
	Conventional	SI
STEROID HORMONES		
Aldosterone	Excretion: 5-19 μg/d	14-53 nmol/d
Fasting, at rest, 210 mEq sodium diet	Supine: 48 ± 29 pg/ml	180 ± 64 pmol/l
	Upright: (2 h) 65 ± 23 pg/ml	
Fasting, at rest, 110 mEq sodium diet	Supine: 107 ± 45 pg/ml	279 ± 125 pmol/l
	Upright: (2 h) 239 ± 123 pg/ml	663 ± 341 pmol/l
Fasting, at rest, 10 mEq sodium diet	Supine: 175 ± 75 pg/ml	485 ± 208 pmol/l
	Upright: (2 h) 532 ± 228 pg/ml	1476 ± 632 pmol/l
Cortisol		
Fasting	8 AM: 5-25 μg/100 ml	0.14-0.69 μmol/l
At rest	8 PM: Below 10 μg/100 ml	0-0.28 μmol/l
20 U ACTH	4 h ACTH test: 30-45 μg/100 ml	0.83-1.24 μmol/l
Dexamethasone at midnight	Overnight suppression test: Below 5 μg/100 ml	<0.14 nmol/l
	Excretion: 20-70 μg/d	
		55-193 nmol/d
11-Deoxycortisol	Responsive; over 7.5 μg/100 ml (after metyrapone)	>0.22 μmol/l
Testosterone	Adult male: 300-1100 ng/100 ml	10.4-38.1 nmol/l
	Adolescent male: over 100 ng/100 ml	>3.5 nmol/l
	Female: 25-90 ng/100 ml	0.87-3.12 nmol/l
Unbound testosterone	Adult male: 3.06-24.0 ng/100 ml	106-832 pmol/l
	Adult female: 0.09-1.28 ng/100 ml	3.1-44.4 pmol/l

Special Endocrine Tests, cont'd

Determination	Reference Range Conventional	SI
POLYPEPTIDE HORMONES		
Adrenocorticotropin (ACTH)	15-70 pg/ml	3.3-15.4 pmol/l
Calcitonin	Undetectable in normals	0
	>100 pg/ml in medullary carcinoma	>29.3 pmol/l
Growth hormone		
Fasting, at rest	Below 5 ng/ml	<233 pmol/l
After exercise	Child: Over 10 ng/ml	>465 pmol/l
	Male: Below 5 ng/ml	<233 pmol/l
	Female: Up to 30 ng/ml	0-1395 pmol/l
After glucose	Male: Below 5 ng/ml	<233 pmol/l
	Female: Below 10 ng/ml	0-465 pmol/l
Insulin		
Fasting	6-26 μU/ml	43-187 pmol/l
During hypoglycemia	Below 20 μU/ml	<144 pmol/l
After glucose	Up to 150 μU/ml	0-1078 pmol/l
Leuteinizing hormone	Male: 6-18 mU/ml	6-18 u/l
Pre- or postovulatory	Female: 5-22 mU/ml	5-22 u/l
Midcycle peak	30-250 mU/ml	30-250 u/l
Parathyroid hormone	<10 μl equiv/ml	<10 ml equiv/l
Prolactin	2-15 ng/ml	0.08-6.0 nmol/l
Renin activity		
Normal diet	Supine: 1.1 ± 0.8 ng/ml/h	0.9 ± 0.6 (nmol/l)h
	Upright: 1.9 ± 1.7 ng/ml/h	1.5 ± 1.3 (nmol/l)h
Low-sodium diet	Supine: 2.7 ± 1.8 ng/ml/h	2.1 ± 1.4 (nmol/l)h
	Upright: 6.6 ± 2.5 ng/ml/h	5.1 ± 1.9 (nmol/l)h
Low-sodium diet	Diuretics: 10.0 ± 3.7 ng/ml/h	7.7 ± 2.9 (nmol/l)h
THYROID HORMONES		
Thyroid-stimulating hormone (TSH)	0.5-3.5 μU/ml	0.5-3.5 mU/l
Thyroxine-binding globulin capacity	15-25 μg T_4/100 ml	193-322 nmol/l
Total triiodothyronine by radioimmunoassay (T_3)	70-190 ng/100 ml	1.08-2.92 nmol/l
Total thyroxine by RIA (T_4)	4-12 μg/100 ml	52-154 nmol/l
T_3 resin uptake	25-35%	0.25-0.35
Free thyroxine index (FT_4I)	1-4 ng/100 ml	12.8-51.2 pmol/l

Cerebrospinal Fluid Values

Determination	Reference Range Conventional	SI	Determination	Reference Range Conventional	SI
Bilirubin	0	0 μmol/l	Glucose	50-75 mg/100 ml	2.8-4.2 mmol/l
Chloride	120-130 mEq/l (20 mEq/l higher than serum)			(30-50% less than blood)	
			Pressure (initial)	70-180 mm of water	70-80 arb. units
Albumin	Mean: 29.5 mg/100 ml ±2 SD: 11-48 mg/100 ml	0.295 g/l ±2 SD: 0.11-0.48	Protein:		
			Lumbar	15-45 mg/100 ml	0.15-0.45 g/l
IgG	Mean: 4.3 mg/100 ml ±2 SD: 0-8.6 mg/100 ml	0.043 g/l ±2 SD: 0-0.086	Cisternal	15-25 mg/100 ml	0.15-0.25 g/l
			Ventricular	5-15 mg/100 ml	0.05-0.15 g/l

Hematologic Values

Determination	Reference Range	
	Conventional	SI
Coagulation factors:		
Factor I (fibrinogen)	0.15-0.35 g/100 ml	4.0-10.0 μmol/l
Factor II (prothrombin)	60-140%	0.60-1.40
Factor V (accelerator globulin)	60-140%	0.60-1.40
Factor VII-X (proconvertin-Stuart)	70-130%	0.70-1.30
Factor X (Stuart factor)	70-130%	0.70-1.30
Factor VIII (antihemophilic globulin)	50-200%	0.50-2.0
Factor IX (plasma thromboplastic cofactor)	60-140%	0.60-1.40
Factor XI (plasma thromboplastic antecedent)	60-140%	0.60-1.40
Factor XII (Hageman factor)	60-140%	0.60-1.40
Coagulation screening tests:		
Bleeding time (Simplate)	3-9 min	180-540 s
Prothrombin time	Less than 2-s deviation from control	Less than 2-s deviation from control
Partial thromboplastin time (activated)	25-37 s	25-37 s
Whole-blood clot lysis	No clot lysis in 24 h	0/d
Fibrinolytic studies:		
Euglobin lysis	No lysis in 2 h	0 (in 2 h)
Fibrinogen split products	Negative reaction at greater than 1:4 dilution	0 (at >1:4 dilution)
Thrombin time	Control ± 5 s	Control ± 5 s
"Complete" blood count:		
Hematocrit	Male: 45-52%	Male: 0.42-0.52
	Female: 37-48%	Female: 0.37-0.48
Hemoglobin	Male: 13-18 g/100 ml	Male 8.1-11.2 mmol/l
	Female: 12-16 g/100 ml	Female: 7.4-9.9 mmol/l
Leukocyte count	4300-10,800/mm^3	4.3-10.8 × 10^9/l
Erythrocyte count	4.2-5.9 million/mm^3	4.2-5.9 × 10^{12}/l
Mean corpuscular volume (MCV)	80-94 μm^3	80-94 fl
Mean corpuscular hemoglobin (MCH)	27-32 pg	1.7-2.0 fmol
Mean corpuscular hemoglobin concentration (MCHC)	32-36%	19-22.8 mmol/l
Erythrocyte sedimentation rate (Westergren method)	Male: 1-13 mm/h	Male: 1-13 mm/h
	Female: 1-20 mm/h	Female: 1-20 mm/h
Erythrocyte enzymes:		
Glucose-6-phosphate dehydrogenase	5-15 U/gHb	5-15 U/g
Pyruvate kinase	13-17 U/gHb	13-17 U/g
Ferritin (serum)		
Iron deficiency	0-20 ng/ml	0-20 μg/l
Iron excess	Greater than 400 ng/l	>400 μg/l
Folic acid		
Normal	Greater than 1.9 ng/ml	>4.3 mmol/l
Borderline	1.0-1.9 ng/ml	2.3-4.3 mmol/l
Haptoglobin	100-300 mg/100 ml	1.0-3.0 g/l
Hemoglobin studies:		
Electrophoresis for A$_2$ hemoglobin	1.5-3.5%	0.015-0.035
Hemoglobin F (fetal hemoglobin)	Less than 2%	<0.02
Hemoglobin, met- and sulf-	0	0
Serum hemoglobin	2-3 mg/100 ml	1.2-1.9 μmol/l
Thermolabile hemoglobin	0	0

Hematologic Values, cont'd

Determination	Reference Range	
	Conventional	SI
L.E. (lupus erythematosus) preparation:		
Heparin as anticoagulant	0	0
Defibrinated blood	0	0
Leukocyte alkaline phosphatase:		
Quantitative method	15-40 mg of phosphorus liberated/h/ 10^{10} cells	15-40 mg/h
Qualitative method	Males: 33-188 U	33-188 U
	Females (off contraceptive pill): 30-160 U	30-160 U
Muramidase	Serum, 3-7 μg/ml	3-7 mg/l
	Urine, 0-2 μg/ml	0-2 mg/l
Osmotic fragility of erythrocytes	Increased if hemolysis occurs in over 0.5% NaCl; decreased if hemolysis is incomplete in 0.3% of NaCl	
Peroxide hemolysis	Less than 10%	<0.10
Platelet count	150,000-350,000/mm³	150-350 × 10^9/l
Platelet function tests:		
Clot retraction	50-100%/2 h	0.50-1.00/2 h
Platelet aggregation	Full response to ADP, epinephrine, and collagen	1.0
Platelet factor 3	33-57 s	33-57 s
Reticulocyte count	0.5-1.5% red cells	0.005-0.015
Vitamin B$_{12}$	90-280 pg/ml (borderline: 70-90)	66-207 pmol/l (borderline: 52-66)

Miscellaneous Values

Determination	Reference Range	
	Conventional	SI
Autoantibodies in serum		
Thyroid colloid and microsomal antigens	Absent	
Stomach parietal cells	Absent	
Smooth muscle	Absent	
Kidney mitochondria	Absent	
Rabbit renal collecting ducts	Absent	
Cytoplasm of ova, theca cells, testicular interstitial cells	Absent	
Skeletal muscle	Absent	
Adrenal gland	Absent	
Carcinoembryonic antigen (CEA) in blood	0-2.5 ng/ml, 97% healthy nonsmokers	0-2.5 μg/l, 97% healthy nonsmokers
Cryoprecipitable proteins in blood	0	0 arb. unit
Digitoxin in serum	17 ± 6 ng/ml	22 ± 7.8 nmol/l
Digoxin in serum		
0.25 mg/d	1.2 ± 0.4 ng/ml	1.54 ± 0.5 nmol/l
0.5 mg/d	1.5 ± 0.4 ng/ml	1.92 ± 0.5 nmol/l
Duodenal drainage:		
pH	5.5-7.5	5.5-7.5
Amylase	Over 1200 U/total sample	>1.2 arb. unit
Trypsin	Values from 35 to 160% "normal"	0.35-1.60
Viscosity	3 min or less	180 s or less

Miscellaneous Values, cont'd

Determination	Reference Range Conventional	SI
Gastric analysis	Basal:	
	Females 2.0 ± 1.8 mEq/h	0.6 ± 0.5
	Males 3.0 ± 2.0 mEq/h	0.8 ± 0.6 μmol/s
	Maximal: (after histalog or gastrin)	
	Females 16 ± 5 mEq/h	4.4 ± 1.4 μmol/s
	Males 23 ± 5 mEq/h	6.4 ± 1.4 μmol/s
Gastrin-I in blood	0-200 pg/ml	0-95 pmol/l
Immunologic tests		
Alpha-feto-globulin	Abnormal if present	
Alpha 1-antitrypsin	200-400 mg/100 ml	2.0-4.0 g/l
Antinuclear antibodies	Positive if detected with serum diluted 1:10	
Anti-DNA antibodies	Less than 15 units/ml	
Complement, total hemolytic	150-250 U/ml	
C3	Range 55-120 mg/100 ml	0.55-1.2 g/l
C4	Range 20-50 mg/100 ml	0.2-0.5 g/l
Immunoglobulins in blood:		
IgG	1140 mg/100 ml	11.4 g/l
	Range 540-1663	5.5-16.6 g/l
IgA	214 mg/100 ml	2.14 g/l
	Range 66-344	0.66-3.44 g/l
IgM	168 mg/100 ml	1.68 g/l
	Range 39-290	0.39-2.9 g/l
Viscosity	1.4-1.8 expressed as relative viscosity of serum compared to water	
Iontophoresis	Children: 0-40 mEq sodium/l	0-40 mmol/l
	Adults: 0-60 mEq sodium/l	0-60 mmol/l
Propranolol (includes bioactive 4-OH metabolite) in serum 4h after last dose	100-300 ng/ml	386-1158 nmol/l
Stool fat	Less than 5 g in 24 h or less than 4% of measured fat intake in 3-d period	<5 g/d
Stool nitrogen	Less than 2 g/d or 10% of urinary nitrogen	<2 g/d
Synovial fluid:		
Glucose	Not less than 20 mg/100 ml lower than simultaneously drawn blood sugar	See blood glucose mmol/l
Mucin	Type 1 or 2	1-2 arb. unit
	Grades as:	
	Type 1-tight clump	
	Type 2-soft clump	
	Type 3-soft clump that breaks up	
	Type 4-cloudy, no clump	
D-Xylose absorption	5-8 g/5 h in urine	33-53 mmol
	40 mg/100 ml in blood 2 h after ingestion of 25 g of D-xylose	2.7 mmol/l

Glossary

abdominal-diaphragmatic breathing Respiration in which the abdomen moves out while the diaphragm descends on inspiration.

abortion Spontaneous or induced termination of pregnancy before the fetus has developed enough to be expected to live if born.

abstract thought Final stage in the development of the cognitive thought processes that occurs between the ages of 12 and 15 years; it is characterized by adaptability, flexibility, the use of abstractions and generalizations, and logical problem-solving based on observations.

abuse Indiscriminate chronic or acute use of a drug or other substance such that physiological or psychosocial functioning is impaired.

accommodation Process of responding to the environment through new activity and thinking.

accommodation reflex Adjustment of the eyes for near vision, comprised of pupillary constriction, convergence of the visual axes, and increased convexity of the lens.

accountability State of being answerable for one's actions—the professional nurse answers to herself, the client, the profession, the employing institution, and society for the effectiveness of nursing care performed.

Achilles tendon Thickest and strongest tendon in the body.

acidemia Increased concentration of hydrogen ions in the blood, causing a reduced pH.

acne Inflammatory, papulopustular skin eruption, usually occurring on the face, neck, shoulders, and upper back.

acromegaly Chronic metabolic condition caused by overproduction of growth hormone and characterized by gradual, marked enlargement and elongation of bones of the face, jaw, and extremities.

active strategies of health promotion Activities that depend on the client being motivated to adopt a specific health program.

active transport Movement of materials across the cell membrane by means of chemical activity that allows the cell to admit larger molecules than would otherwise be possible.

activities of daily living Activities usually performed in the course of a normal day in the client's life, such as eating, dressing, bathing, brushing the teeth, or grooming.

activity tolerance Kind and amount of exercise or work that a person is able to perform.

actual health care problem Health problem currently being perceived or experienced by the client.

acuity Intensity of nursing care required to meet the needs of a client; higher acuity usually requires longer and more frequent visits and more supplies and equipment.

acute illness Illness characterized by symptoms that are of relatively short duration, are usually severe, and affect the functioning of the client in all dimensions.

adaptation Process by which changes occur in any of a person's dimensions in response to stress.

addiction Compulsive, uncontrollable, physical and psychological dependence on a substance or habit, for example, a narcotic, to the point that withdrawal causes severe emotional, mental, and physiological reactions.

ADH Hormone affecting fluid and electrolyte balance; decreases the production of urine by increasing reabsorption of water by the kidney tubules.

adherence Process in which a client follows the prescriptions and recommendations of a regimen of care.

adverse reaction Harmful or unintended effect of a medication, diagnostic test, or therapeutic intervention.

advocacy Process whereby a nurse objectively provides a client with the information he needs to make decisions and supports the client in whatever decisions he makes.

aerobic metabolism Production of energy and body fuels by the tissues in the presence of oxygen.

affective learning Acquisition of behaviors involved in expressing feelings in attitudes, appreciations, and values.

afferent Proceeding a center, as with nerves, arteries, and veins.

ageism Attitude that disadvantages, separates, and stigmatizes older adults on the basis of age-related characteristics.

agent Element of the agent-host-environment model of health and illness; any biological, chemical, physical or mechanical, or psychosocial factor whose presence or absence can lead to disease or illness.

air pollution Contamination of the environmental atmosphere with substances known as pollutants that are not normally found in the air.

Alcoholics Anonymous International, nonprofit organization of recovering alcoholics whose purpose is to help alcoholics stop drinking and maintain sobriety through group support, shared experiences, and a faith in a power greater than themselves.

aldosterone Mineral corticoid, produced by the adrenal cortex, that regulates sodium and potassium balance.

algor mortis Reduction in body temperature after death accompanied by loss of skin elasticity.

alkalemia Decreased concentration of hydrogen ions in the blood, causing an elevated pH.

alopecia Partial or complete loss of hair; baldness.

alveolar hyperventilation Respiratory rate in excess of that required to maintain normal carbon dioxide levels in the body tissues.

alveolar hypoventilation Respiratory rate insufficent to prevent carbon dioxide retention.

Alzheimer's disease A brain disorder that causes gradual and progressive decline in cognitive functioning. The most frequent cause of irreversible dementia; also known as senile dementia of the Alzheimer type, or SDAT.

ambiguous genitalia Newborn genitalia that are not clearly identifiable as female or male; external genitalia may appear male in an infant with female internal sex organs or vice versa.

ambulatory surgery Scheduled outpatient procedures provided for clients who do not remain overnight in a hospital.

American Nurses' Association (ANA) Organization of professional nurses in the United States that focuses on standards of health care, nurses' professional development, and economic and general welfare of nurses.

ampule Small sterile glass or plastic ontainer that usually contains a single dose of solution to be administered parenterally.

amylase Enzyme secreted in saliva and pancreatic juice to digest starch.

anabolism Constructive metabolism characterized by conversion of simple substances into more complex compounds of living matter.

anaerobic metabolism Production of energy and body fuels by the tissues without oxygen.

analgesic Relieving pain; a drug that relieves pain.

analogy Resemblance made between things otherwise unlike.

anemia Disorder characterized by a decrease in hemoglobin in the blood.

anesthesia Absence of normal sensation, especially sensitivity to pain.

aneurysm Localized dilatation of the wall of a blood vessel, usually caused by atherosclerosis, hypertension, or a congenital weakness in the vessel wall.

angina Episodic chest pain caused most often by myocardial anoxia, resulting from atherosclerosis of the coronary arteries. Pain radiates down inner aspect of left arm and is often accompanied by feeling of suffocation and impending death.

anions Negatively charged electrolytes.

anlingus Sexual stimulation by licking the anus. Anal-oral sexual activity.

anonymity Nondisclosure of a client's or other person's name or identification, such as is used in research to ensure the privacy of research subjects.

anorexia Lack or loss of appetite resulting in the inability to eat.

anoxia Condition characterized by a relative or total lack of oxygen; may be local or systemic.

antagonistic muscles Group of muscles that work together to bring about movement at the joint.

antibody Immunoglobulin, essential to the immune system, which is produced by lymphoid tissue in response to bacteria, viruses, or other antigens.

anticipatory grief Grief response in which the person begins the grieving process before an actual loss.

anticipatory guidance Pscyhological and physical preparation of a client to help relieve fear and anxiety of an event or outcome that is expected to be stressful.

antidiuretic hormone (ADH) Hormone that decreases the production of urine by increasing reabsorption of water by the kidney tubules.

antiemetic Medication that prevents or alleviates nausea and vomiting.

antigen Substance, usually a protein, that causes the formation of an antibody and reacts specifically with that antibody.

antigravity muscles Muscles involved with stabilization of joints by opposing the effect of gravity on the body.

antipyretic Of or pertaining to a substance or procedure that reduces fever.

antiseptic Tending to inhibit the growth and reproduction of microorganisms.

anuria Cessation of urine production.

anxiety Feeling of apprehension, uneasiness, agitation, uncertainty, and fear resulting from the anticipation of something perceived as negative.

Apgar scale Assessment tool that rates the newborn's physiological status 1 to 5 minutes after birth.

aphasia Neurological disorder concerning the production and understanding of language.

apnea Cessation of air flow through the nose and mouth.

apocrine gland One of the large, deep exocrine glands located in the axillary, anal, genital, and mammary areas of the body; secretes sweat having a strong odor.

approximate To come close together, as in the edges of a wound.

ariboflavinosis Condition caused by dietary deficiency of vitamin B_2.

arterial blood gases Oxygen and carbon dioxide concentrations, pH, and oxygen saturation of the hemoglobin in arterial blood; also refers to the laboratory tests that measure these levels.

ascites Abnormal accumulation of fluid in the intraperitoneal space.

asepsis Absence of germs of microorganisms.

assault Unlawful threatening or inflicting of harm on another.

assimilation To become absorbed into another culture and to adopt its characteristics.

atelectasis Collapse of alveoli, preventing the normal respiratory exchange of oxygen and carbon dioxide.

atherosclerosis Common arterial disorder characterized by yellowish plaques of cholesterol, lipids, and cellular debris in the inner layers of the walls of the large and medium-sized arteries.

atrophy Wasting or diminution of size or physiological activity of a part of the body caused by disease or other influences.

attachment Initial psychosocial relationship that develops between parents and the neonate.

attitudinal isolation Social isolation that occurs because of the older adult's personal or cultural values.

audit Methodical examination or review of written records with the intent to verify or deny the accuracy of information based on established standards.

auditory Related to, or experienced through, hearing.

auscultation Act of listening for sounds within the body to evaluate the condition of body organs; usually performed with a stethoscope.

authoritarian style Leadership style in which the leader retains all authority and responsibility and is concerned primarily with tasks and goal achievement.

autonomy Ability or tendency to function independently.

autopsy Examination performed after a person's death to confirm or determine the cause of death.

autotransfusion The collection, anticoagulation, filtration, and reinfusion of blood from an active bleeding site.

bacteriuria Presence of bacteria in the urine.

basal metabolism rate (BMR) Amount of energy used in a unit of time by a fasting, resting subject to maintain vital functions.

basic human needs Needs for things, such as food, water, safety, and love, that people require to survive and be healthy.

battery Legal term for touching of another's body without consent.

bed rest Placement of the client in bed for therapeutic reasons for a prescribed period.

behavioral isolation Social isolation that occurs because of the older adult's socially unacceptable behaviors.

bereavement Response to loss through death; a subjective experience that a person suffers after losing a person with whom there has been a significant relationship.

beriberi Disease of the peripheral nerves caused by a deficiency of or an inability to assimilate thiamin.

bias Prejudice or mental inclination to collect or interpret data according to a person's opinions or beliefs.

bilirubin Orange-yellow pigment of bile formed principally by the breakdown of hemoglobin in red blood cells.

binder Bandage made of a large piece of material to fit a specific body part.

binocular vision Vision involving the use of both eyes.

bioethics Study of the ethical problems in health care delivery and the obligations of health professionals.

biological clock Cyclical nature of body functions; functions controlled from within the body are synchronized with environmental factors; same meaning as biorhythm.

biological identity (sex) Chromosomal masculinity or feminity (xy or xx)

biopsy Removal of a small piece of living tissue from an organ or other part of the body for microscopic examination.

bisexual Sexual orientation involving erotic preferences for members of either sex.

blastocyst Embryonic form that arises as a cavity within the morula, where cellular differentiation begins.

blended family Family formed when parents bring together unrelated children from previous marriages.

body image Mental picture of one's body internally and externally.

body mechanics Coordinated efforts of the musculoskeletal and nervous systems to maintain proper balance, posture, and body alignment.

bolus Round mass of chewed food ready to be swallowed.

bone resorption Destruction of bone cells and release of calcium into the blood.

borborygmus Audible abdominal sound produced by hyperactive intestinal peristalsis.

bradycardia Slower than normal heart rate; heart contracts fewer than 60 times per minute.

brain death Irreversible, complete loss of brain function while the heart continues to beat.

bronchoscopy Visual examination of the tracheal and bronchial tree using the standard rigid, tubular metal bronchoscope or the narrower, flexible fiberoptic bronchoscope.

bruit Abnormal sound or murmur heard while auscultating an organ, gland, or artery.

buccal Of or pertaining to the inside of the cheek or the gum next to the cheek.

buffer Substance of group of substances that can absorb or release hydrogen ions to correct an acid-base imbalance.

cachexia General ill health and malnutrition marked by weakness and emaciation.

calorie Amount of heat required to raise 1 gram of water 1° centigrade at atmospheric pressure; a kilocalorie or large calorie, used to represent energy values of food, is 1000 times as large as the small calorie, the unit used in physics to describe energy exchange in the body.

Canadian Nurses Association (CNA) Organization of professional nurses in Canada that focuses on standards of health care, nurses' professonal development, and economic and general welfare of nurses.

cannulation Insertion of a flexible tube (cannula) into a body duct or cavity, such as the bladder or a blood vessel.

carbon dioxide Respiratory gas formed in the body as an end product of tissue metabolism.

carbon monoxide Colorless, odorless, poisonous gas produced by the combustion of carbon or organic fuels.

carbon monoxide poisoning Toxic condition in which carbon monoxide gas has been inhaled and absorbed in the lungs, displacing oxygen from hemoglobin and decreasing the capacity of the blood to carry oxygen.

carcinoma Malignant epithelial neoplasm that tends to invade surrounding tissue and spread to distant regions of the body.

cardiac arrest Sudden cessation of cardiac output and effective circulation.

cardiac telemetry Transmission of a client's ECG signals by way of a small battery powered unit connected to the client. Signals travel to a receiving location near a nurses' station where the ECG is displayed on a monitor.

cardiopulmonary rehabilitation Process of actively assisting the cardiopulmonary client to achieve and maintain an optimal level of health through controlled physical exercise, nutritional counseling, relaxation and stress management techniques, prescribed medication and oxygen therapy, and adherence to the prescribed rehabilitation program.

cardiopulmonary resuscitation Basic emergency procedures for life support consisting of artifical respiration and manual external cardiac massage.

carrier Animal or person who harbors and spreads a disease-causing organism but who does not become ill.

cartilage Nonvascular, supporting connective tissue located mainly in the joints and in the thorax, trachea, larynx, nose, and ear.

cartilaginous joint Slightly movable, highly elastic cartilage that unites bony surfaces.

case management Organized system for delivering health care to an individual client or group of clients; includes assessment and development of a plan of care, coordination of all services, referral, and follow-up; and usually assigned to one professional.

catabolism Complex metabolic process in which energy is liberated for use in work, energy, storage, or heat production by oxidation of carbohydrates, lipids, and proteins; carbon dioxide and water, as well as energy, are produced.

catalyst Substance that influences the rate of a chemical reaction without being permanently altered by the process.

catalytic Pertaining to a chemical reaction caused by an agent unchanged by the reaction.

cataplexy Condition characterized by sudden muscular weakness and loss of muscle tone.

cataract Abnormal opacity of the lens of the eye causing interference with light reaching the retina.

cathartic Drug that acts to promote bowel evacuation.

cations Positively charged electrolytes.

Centers for Disease Control (CDC) Agency of the U.S. government that provides facilities and services for the investigation, identification, prevention, and control of disease.

centigrade Denotes a temperature scale in which 0° is the freezing point of water and 100° is the boiling point of water at sea level; also called Celsius.

central sleep apnea Sleep disorder characterized by the absence of attempts to breathe; person is momentarily unable to move respiratory muscles or maintain airflow through the nose and mouth.

cerebellum Portion of the brain located in the posterior cranial fossa behind the brainstem.

certified nurse-midwife Nurse who is educated in midwifery and possesses certification in accordance with criteria of the American College of Midwives.

cerumen Waxy substance secreted in the ear.

change Dynamic process by which alterations occur within the behavior and function of a person, family, group, or community.

change agent A person or group who identifies need, initiates strategies, and implements alterations.

chart *n.*, Informal term for the client's record; *v.*, to enter data into a client's record.

chemicals Substances that alter senses, emotions, physical condition, or mood when ingested by mouth, injected, or inhaled; includes both legal and illegal drugs: alcohol, narcotics, tranquilizers, barbiturates, amphetamines, cocaine, marijuana, and others.

chemical dependencey Continued use of mood-altering chemicals despite the emotional, physical, social, and legal problems created.

chemotherapy Medication used for the treatment of cancer. The actions and side effects of these drugs can lead to serious physical problems. The knowledge required to safely administer these medications is quite specialized. Nurses may be required to have special training and certification before giving these drugs.

chest percussion Striking the chest wall with a cupped hand to promote mobilization and drainage of pulmonary secretions.

chest physiotherapy Group of therapies used to mobilize pulmonary secretions.

cholecystectomy Surgical removal of the gallbladder.

chordotomy Surgical resection of the anterolateral nerve tracts in the spinal cord for pain relief.

chromosomes Strands of DNA from the ovum and sperm that carry genes and thus determine genetic inheritance.

chronic illness Illness that persists over a long period of time and affects physical, emotional, intellectual, social, and spiritual functioning.

chyme Viscous, semifluid contents of the stomach present during digestion of a meal, which eventually pass into the intestines.

circadian rhythm Repetition of certain physiological phenomena within a 24-hour cycle.

cirrhosis Chronic degenerative disease of the liver.

citation Reference notation to the source of an idea or quotation.

client-centered goal Specific measurable objective designed to reflect the client's highest level of wellness and independence in function.

climacteric Physiological, developmental change that occurs in the male reproductive system between the ages of 45 and 60.

clinical nurse specialist Nurse with a master's degree in nursing and expertise in a specific area of practice.

clinical reasoning Cognitive skills by which the nurse gathers relevant data about the client, analyzes the client's response to the health care problem, organizes the data, and formulates the nursing diagnosis.

CNS sympathomimetic Drug, such as cocaine and amphetamines, whose effects mimic the effects of sympathetic nervous system stimulation.

coccidioidomycosis Infectious fungal disease caused by the inhalation of windborne spores of the bacterium *Coccidioides immits,* also called valley fever.

code of ethics Formal statement that delineates a profession's guidelines for ethical behavior; a code of ethics sets standards or expectations for the professional to achieve.

coercive change Alterations in behavior or life-style that is forced on the person, family, or group.

cognitive learning Acquisition of intellectual skills that encompass behaviors such as thinking, understanding, and evaluating.

coitus interruptus Withdrawal of the penis from the vagina during intercourse before ejaculation. While ineffective, it is often practiced by adolescents as a method of contraception.

colic Sharp visceral pain resulting from obstruction or smooth muscle spasm of a hollow organ, such as the ureter or the intestines.

colitis Inflammatory condition of the large intestine.

collagen Substance that combines to form the white, glistening, inelastic fibers of tendons, ligaments, and fasciae.

colon Portion of the large intestine from the cecum to the rectum.

colonized Referring to the establishment of a mass of microorganisms, often nonpathogenic, in or on the body.

communal family Form of family comprised of unrelated adults rearing their children together in a communal living arrangement.

communicable disease Any disease that can be transmitted from one person or animal to another by direct or indirect contact, or by vectors.

communication Ongoing, dynamic series of events that involves the transmission of information or feelings from sender to receiver.

comparison group Group of subjects in a study who are equivalent to the subjects in the experimental group but do not receive the treatment or intervention the study is examining; also known as a control group.

compensation Action by the body's chemical, biological, or physiological buffering systems to correct an acid-base imbalance. Also an adaptive ego-defense mechanism in which a person avoids feelings of inferiority or inadequacy in one area through achievement in another area.

compliance Person's fulfillment of prescribed course of treatment.

compress Soft pad of gauze or cloth used to apply heat, cold, or medications to the surface of a body part.

computer-assisted instruction (CAI) Self-instructed teaching method utilizing computers.

concept Abstract idea summarized in a word or phrase.

concomitant symptoms Symptoms that accompany a primary symptom.

concrete thought Stage in the development of cognitive thought processes that occurs in ages 7 to 11 years; it is characterized by increasingly logical and coherent thought, the ability to classify, sort, order, and organize facts, and an inability to generalize or think in abstractions.

concurrent nursing audit Evaluation of nursing care while the client is receiving the care.

confabulation Defense mechanism in which the person fabricates experiences or situations and often recounts them in a detailed and plausible way in order to fill in and cover up gaps in memory.

confidentiality Privacy; a nurse must maintain the confidentiality of information related to a client's health care.

Congress for Nursing Practice Unit of the ANA whose activities concern the scope of nursing practice, legal aspects of nursing

practice, public recognition of the significance of nursing in health care, and implications of health care trends for nursing practice.

consensual light reflex Constriction of the pupil of one eye when the other eye is illuminated.

constipation Condition characterized by difficulty in passing stool or an infrequent passage of hard stool.

consultation Process in which the help of a specialist is sought to identify ways to handle problems in client management or in the planning and implementation of programs.

contagious Communicable, as a disease.

continuing education Formal educational programs designed to further the knowledge, skills, and professional attitudes of practicing nurses.

contraception Prevention of pregnancy by means of a medication, device, or method that blocks or alters one or more of the processes of reproduction in such a way that sexual union can occur without impregnation.

contrast medium Radiopaque substance injected into the body to improve visualization of internal structures that are otherwise difficult to see on x-ray examination.

control To regulate or limit error or distortion of information.

convalescence Period of recovery after an illness, injury, or surgery.

coping mechanism Any effort directed toward stress management, including task-oriented and ego-defense mechanisms.

corpus luteum Ovarian site of ruptured Graffian follicle after ovulation. The corpus luteum is maintained through the secretory phase of the menstrual cycle and produces progesterone.

costal Of or referring to the ribs.

cough Sudden, audible expulsion of air from the lungs.

counseling Implementation method that helps the client use a problem-solving process to recognize and manage stress and that facilitates interpersonal relationships between the client and the family, significant others, or the health care team.

crackle Fine bubbling sound heard on auscultation of the lung; produced by air entering distal airways and alveoli containing serous secretions.

cretinism Condition characterized by severe congenital hypothyroidism.

crime Act that violates a law and that may include criminal intent.

crisis Stressful encounter with a change or obstacle to life goals that is perceived as insurmountable.

crisis intervention Use of therapeutic techniques directed toward helping a client resolve a particular and immediate problem.

crisis intervention centers Agencies providing emergency psychiatric and counseling assistance to clients experiencing extreme stress or conflict, often involving attempted suicide, drug or alcohol abuse, or other crisis behaviors.

critical period of development Time span during which the environment has its greatest impact on an individual's environment.

Crohn's disease Disease involving inflammation of the small intestine.

crutch gait Gait assumed by a person on crutches by alternately bearing weight on one or both legs and on the crutches.

culture Nonphysical traits such as values, beliefs, attitudes, customs shared by a group and passed from one generation to the next.

culture shock Disorder that occurs in response to transition from one setting to another; former behavior patterns are ineffective in such an unfamiliar situation and basic cues for social behavior are absent.

cunnilingus Oral stimulation of the female external genitalia; oral-genital sex.

curing Traditionally, a two-dimensional phenomena that results in ridding disease from the body or mind.

cutaneous stimulation Stimulation of a person's skin to prevent or reduce pain perception. A massage, warm bath, application of liniment, hot and cold therapies, and transcutaneous electric nerve stimulation are some ways to reduce pain perception.

cyanosis Bluish discoloration of the skin and mucus membranes caused by an excess of deoxygenated hemoglobin in the blood or a structural defect in hemoglobin.

cystitis Inflammation of the urinary bladder, characterized by pain, urgency, and frequency of urination.

cytotoxic Pharmacological compound that inhibits the proliferation of cells within the body.

data clustering Grouping of related information from the nursing health history, physical examination, and laboratory results as part of the process of determining the nursing diagnosis.

data source Origin of information relevant to the client's level of wellness and health patterns.

data validation Process of determining if information gathered during assessment is complete and accurate.

day-care centers Agencies that provide health care during the day to children or adults with special needs.

debridement Removal of dead tissue from a wound.

decibel Unit of measure of the intensity of sound.

decubitus ulcer Inflammation, sore, or ulcer in the skin over a bony prominence.

defecation Passage of feces from the digestive tract through the rectum.

defining characteristic Cluster of signs and symptoms that are observed in the client having a specific nursing diagnosis.

dehiscence Separation of a wound's edges, revealing underlying tissues.

dehydration Excessive loss of water from the body tissues, accompanied by a disturbance of body electrolytes.

delirium Syndrome involving impairment of memory and other cognitive abilities, and characterized by clouding of consciousness.

delusion Persistent belief or perception held by a person even though it is illogical and probably wrong.

dementia Irreversible mental state characterized by decreased impairment of memory, intellectual function, and other cognitive abilities that can have a variety of causes.

democratic style People-centered leadership style in which the group participates openly in decision making for group goals.

denial Defense mechanism by which a person avoids emotional conflicts and anxiety by refusing to acknowledge thoughts, feelings, desires, impulses, and other factors that would cause intolerable pain.

dependent intervention Action completed with a physician's order but requiring nursing judgment or decision-making.

depersonalization Extreme form of identity confusion in which a person is unable to distinguish between inner and outer realities or between himself and others.

depilatory Substance that removes hair.

depression Abnormal emotional state characterized by exaggerated or inappropriate feelings of sadness, melancholy, dejection, worthlessness, emptiness, and hopelessness.

dermatitis Inflammation of skin characterized by itching, redness, and skin lesions.

dermis Layer of skin just below the epidermis, containing blood and lymphatic vessels, nerves and nerve endings, glands and hair follicles.

desquamation Normal process in which the dead cells of the epidermal skin layer slough off.

development Qualitative or observable aspects of the progressive changes an individual makes in adapting to the environment.

developmental change Biopsychosocial alterations that occur normally within the life cycle of the person or family.

diagnosis Identification of a health problem by analyzing the assessment data about a client's health status.

diagnostic process Process of determining a client's health status and evaluating the factors influencing that status.

diagnostic related groups (DRGs) Group of patients classified for measuring a hospital's delivery of care; classification is based on the following variables: primary and secondary diagnosis, primary and secondary procedures, age, and length of stay.

diaphoresis Secretion of sweat, especially profuse secretion associated with an elevated body temperature, physical exertion, or emotional stress.

diarrhea Increase in the number of stools and the passage of liquid, unformed feces.

diffusion Movement of molecules from an area of high concentration to an area of lower concentration.

direct-question interview Type of inquiry that requires one- or two-word answers.

discharge planning Set of decisions and activities involved in providing continuity and coordination of nursing care when a client is discharged from a health care agency.

diuresis Increased formation and excretion of urine.

diurnal Daily.

diverticula Pouchlike herniations through the muscular wall of tubular organ; may be present in the stomach, small intestine, or, most commonly, the colon.

documentation Act of authenticating events or activities by keeping written records.

domains of learning Areas in which learning occurs cognitive, affective, and psychomotor.

dorsal Pertaining to the back or posterior.

drainage tube Catheter used for evacuation of air or fluid from a cavity or wound in the body.

driving forces for change Motivating or facilitating factors in the change process.

drug allergy Hypersensitivity to a pharmacologic agent, manifested by reactions ranging from a mild rash to anaphylactic shock.

drug dependence Psychological or physiological reliance on a chemical agent.

drug rehabilitation centers Agencies providing long-term care for a gradual return to the community of a person with chemical or drug dependency.

dysarthria Difficulty in articulating speech.

dyspareunia Painful intercourse in a woman.

dysphagia Difficulty in swallowing.

dysrhythmia Deviation from the normal pattern of the heart beat.

dysuria Painful urination resulting from bacterial infection of the bladder and obstructive conditions of the urethra.

ear oximeter Continuous measurement of capillary oxygen saturation through the use of a cutaneous monitoring system attached to a client's ear lobe.

ecchymosis Discoloration of skin or bruise caused by leakage of blood into subcutaneous tissues as a result of trauma to underlying vessels.

edema Abnormal accumulation of fluid in interstitial spaces of tissues.

efferent Directed away from a center, as with nerves, arteries, and veins.

ego-defense mechanism Unconscious behavior that protects a person from an emotional stress.

electrolyte Element or compound that, when melted or dissolved in water or other solvent, dissociates into ions and can carry an electric current.

emaciation Excessive leanness caused by disease or malnutrition.

embolus Small amount of air, fat, or other substance that circulates in the blood until becoming lodged in a blood vessel.

embyro Stage of human development from implantation of the fertilized ovum to the eighth week of intrauterine life.

emphysematous Of or pertaining to emphysema, an abnormal condition of the lungs, characterized by overinflation and destructive changes of alveolar walls.

empirical data Information that has been collected through the human senses and can be verified through research.

endocrine Pertaining to one of the ductless glands in the endocrine system.

endogenous Produced within a cell or organism.

endorphin Naturally occurring neuropeptide with morphine-like properties secreted within the CNS to inhibit pain impulse transmission.

endoscopy Visualization of the interior of body organs and cavities with an endoscope.

enema Procedure involving introduction of a solution into the rectum for cleansing or therapeutic purposes.

enterostomal therapist Specially trained nurse for care of patients with ostomies.

enucleation Removal of the eyeball; a procedure used in corneal tissue recovery.

enuresis Involuntary passage of urine; incontinence.

enzyme Protein produced by living cells that catalyzes chemical reactions in organic matter.

epidemiology Study of the occurrence, distribution, and causes of disease.

epidermis Superficial, avascular layers of the skin, made up of an outer, dead, cornified portion of cells and a deeper, living cellular portion.

epidural Type of nerve block local anesthesia, in which an anesthetic is injected in the lumbosacral region of the spinal cord to prevent or eliminate pain in the lower trunk and extremities.

erectile dysfunction Inability of a male to attain or maintain an erection sufficient to achieve penetration during sexual contact; the dysfunction may be primary or secondary.

error of commission Mistake resulting from over-diagnosis or diagnosing a nonexistent health problem.

error of omission Mistake resulting from failure of the nurse to diagnose a health problem.

erythema Redness or inflammation of the skin or mucous membranes that is a result of dilation and congestion of superficial capillaries; sunburn is an example.

erythrocyte Red blood cell.

escape mechanism Behavioral response by which a person consciously or unconsciously attempts to avoid a problem or stressor.

estrogen Hormonal steroid compound that promotes the development of female secondary sex characteristics.

ethics Principles or standards that govern proper conduct as they apply to professional issues or problems.

ethnicity Cultural group's sense of identification associated with the group's common social and cultural heritage.

ethnocentrism Tendency of members of one cultural group to view the members of other cultural groups in terms of the standards of behavior, attitudes, and values of their own group.

etiological factor Probable cause contributing to or maintaining the nursing diagnosis.

eupnea Normal respiration that is quiet, effortless, and rhythmical.

evaluation Category of nursing behavior in which a determination is made and recorded regarding the extent to which the client's goals have been met.

evisceration Protrusion of visceral organs through a surgical wound.

exacerbation Increase in the seriousness of a disease or disorder as marked by greater intensity in signs or symptoms.

excise To remove completely, as in the surgical excision of the appendix.

excoriation Injury to the skin's surface caused by abrasion.

exercise Performance of any physical activity for the purpose of conditioning the body, improving health, maintaining fitness, or as a therapeutic measure.

exogenous Originating outside an organ or part.

exophthalmos Abnormal protrusion of one or both eyeballs.

expected outcome Expected condition of a client at the end of therapy or of a disease process, including the degree of wellness and the need for continuing care, medications, support, counseling or education.

expectorate Eject mucus, sputum, or fluids from the trachea and lungs by coughing or spitting.

experiment Research study designed to examine a cause-and-effect relationship.

expressive aphasia Inability to name common objects or to express simple ideas in words or writing.

extended care facility Institution providing medical, nursing, or custodial care for clients over a prolonged period.

extended family Form of family comprised of the nuclear family and all other relatives in both of the couple's families.

external environment Set of factors outside and distinct from a person that may influence his health, including the physical environment, social relationships, economic variables, and so on.

external stressor Stressor originating outside a person.

extracellular fluid Portion of the body fluid comprised of the interstitial fluid and blood plasma.

exudate Fluid, cells, or other substances that have been slowly discharged from cells or blood vessels through small pores or breaks in cell membranes.

family Group of interacting individuals composing a basic unit of society. Although concepts of what constitutes a family vary, the family usually has some degree of permanence, commitment, and attachment.

family as client Nursing perspective in which the family is viewed as a unit of interacting members having attributes, function, and goals separate from those of the individual family members; the nurse provides care to the family as a whole.

family as environment Nursing perspective in which the family is viewed as the significant provider of physical, psychosocial, and emotional support to individual family members; the nurse provides care primarily to one of the family members.

family functions Processes by which the family operates as a whole, including communication and manipulation of the environment for problem solving.

family health Phenomenon that is more than the sum of the health of individual family members, including the achievement of satisfying family functioning and the attainment of family goals.

family of origin Family into which a person is born, as distinct from the person's family of procreation.

family of procreation Family a person forms through marriage and/or having children, as distinct from the person's family of origin.

family stress Stress related to the individual's roles, relationships, or functions within the family.

family structure Composition of the family organization of relationships among family members.

fatigue State of exhaustion or loss of strength or endurance.

febrile Pertaining to or characterized by an elevated body temperature

feces Waste or excrement from the gastrointestinal tract.

fellatio Sexual stimulation by licking, sucking, or placing the penis in the mouth; oral-genital sex.

female genitalia Female's external sex organs (vulva, mons veneris, labia majora, labia minora, clitoris, and vaginal opening or introitus) and internal sex organs (vagina, uterus, fallopian tubes, and ovaries).

fetal alcohol syndrome Fetal abnormalities associated with heavy alcohol consumption by the pregnant woman.

fetus Stage of human development from the end of the embryonic period until birth.

fever Elevation in the hypothalamic set-point, so that body temperature is regulated at a higher level.

fibrin Protein product formed from the action of thrombin on fibrinogen in the clotting process.

fibrous joint Tough layer of fibrous connective tissue that binds bones firmly together.

fistula Abnormal passage from an internal organ to the body surface or between two internal organs.

flail chest Condition caused by multiple rib fractures, resulting in instability in part of the chest wall and paradoxical breathing. The chest wall underlying the injured area contracts on inspiration and expands on expiration.

flat bones Bones providing for structural contours of the skeleton.

flatulence Condition characterized by the accumulation of gas within the lumen of the intestines.

"flight-or-fight" syndrome Set of sympathetic physiological responses to a stressor that prepares a person to attempt to overcome or avoid stress.

follicular phase First part of the menstrual cycle, in which ovarian follicles grow to prepare for ovulation and the menstrual flow signifies that the uterus has shed its lining from the preceding cycle.

fomites Inanimate substances or objects, such as clothing and paper, that absorb and transmit infectious material.

Food and Drug Administration (FDA) Federal agency responsible for the enforcement of federal regulations regarding the manufacture and distribution of food, drugs, and cosmetics to ensure protection against the sale of impure or dangerous substances.

food poisoning Toxic processes resulting from the ingestion of a food contaminated by toxic substances or by bacteria containing toxins.

footboard Board placed perpendicular to the mattress, parallel to and touching the plantar surface of the client's foot, and used to maintain dorsiflexion of the feet.

forceps Pair of any of a large variety and number of surgical instruments, with two handles or sides each attached to a blade.

formulary Listing of drugs and information about them used by health practitioners to prescribe appropriate therapy.

fracture Breakage of bone caused by violence to the body; disruption of bone tissue continuity.

friction Effect of rubbing or the resistance that a moving body meets from the surface on which it moves; a force that occurs in a direction to oppose movement.

friction rub Dry, grating sound heard during auscultation, caused by rubbing of tissue surfaces.

frostbite Traumatic effect of extreme cold on the skin and subcutaneous tissues, first manifested by distinct pallor.

fungus Simple parasitic plant dependent on other life forms for food.

gait Manner or style of walking, including rhythm, cadence, and speed.

gangrene Necrosis or death of tissue, usually the result of loss of blood supply.

gender identity Awareness of being male or female that develops from infancy.

gender role (sex role) Expression of one's maleness or femaleness to both oneself and others.

general adaptation syndrome (GAS) Generalized defense response of the body to stress, consisting of three stages: alarm, resistance, and exhaustion.

generalization Application of findings from a research study in a broader situation.

geographic isolation Social isolation of the older adult resulting from urban crime, institutional barriers, and distance from family.

geriatrics Branch of health care dealing with the physiology and psychology of aging and with the diagnosis and treatment of illnesses affecting the aged.

gerontology Study of all aspects of the aging processes and their consequences.

gingiva Gum of the mouth; a mucous membrane with supporting fibrous tissue that overlies the crowns of unerupted teeth and encircles the necks of those that have erupted.

glaucoma Abnormal condition of elevated pressure within the anterior chamber of the eye caused by obstructed outflow of aqueous humor.

glomerulus Cluster or collection of capillary vessels within the kidney involved in the initial formation of urine.

gluconeogenesis Formation of glucose or glycogen from substances that are not carbohydrate, such as protein or lipid.

glycerol Alcohol that is a component of lipids and that is soluble in ethyl alcohol and water.

glycogen Polysaccharide that is the major carbohydrate stored in animal cells.

glycolysis Series of enzymatically catalyzed reactions within cells by which glucose and other sugars are broken down to yield lactic acid or pyruvic acid, releasing energy in the form of adenosine triphosphate.

glycosuria Abnormal presence of glucose in the urine.

gonadotropic hormones Substances that are produced and secreted by the anterior pituitary gland and stimulate the function of the testes and ovaries.

governmental agencies Clinics, hospitals, and health services that are supported by local, state or provincial, or national taxes.

Graafian follicle Ovarian follicle that continues to mature through a given menstrual cycle and ruptures to release an ova at the time of ovulation.

granulation tissue Soft, pink, fleshy projections of tissue that form during the healing process in a wound not healing by primary intention.

gravity Heaviness of an object resulting from the universal effect of the attraction of a planetary body.

grief Form of sorrow involving the person's thoughts, feelings, and behaviors, occurring as a response to an actual or perceived loss.

grieving process Sequence of affective, cognitive, and physiological states through which the person responds to and finally accepts an irretrievable loss.

growth Quantitative or measureable aspect of an individual's increase in physical measurements.

guaiac test Test of feces for the presence of occult (hidden) blood.

gurgle Abnormal coarse sound heard during auscultation of the lung; produced by air entering large mucus-containing airways.

gustatory Pertaining to the sense of taste.

half-life Time required for elimination processes to reduce the blood concentration of a drug by half.

halitosis Offensive breath resulting from poor oral hygiene, dental or oral infection, ingestion of certain foods, or systemic disease.

hallucinogens Drugs such as LSD and PCP that cause excitation of the central nervous system, including hallucinations, sensory distortions, and other effects.

hand rolls A roll of cloth that keeps the thumb slightly adducted and in oppostion to the fingers.

hand-wrist splints Splints individually molded for the client to maintain proper alignment of the thumb, slight adduction of the wrist, and slight dorsiflexion.

haustral contraction Type of peristaltic contraction that occurs in the large intestine; produces a large sac in the colon's wall to increase surface area for nutrient absorption.

healing Traditionally, a holistic or three-dimensional phenomena that results in the restoration of balance or harmony to the body, mind, and spirit.

health Dynamic state in which an individual adapts to his internal and external environments so that there is a state of physical, emotional, intellectual, social, and spiritual well-being.

health behavior Activities through which a person maintains, attains, or regains good health and prevents illness.

health belief model Conceptual framework that predicts a person's health behavior as an expression of his health beliefs.

health care delivery system Total complex of preventive, remedial, and therapeutic services provided by hospitals and other institutions, governmental and voluntary agencies, health care professionals, pharmaceutical and medical equipment manufacturers, and governmental and private insurance agencies.

health care need Condition or problem that results when clients are unable to meet their physiological, psychological, sociocultural, developmental, and spiritual needs within the context of daily living.

health-illness continuum Scale by means of which a person's level of health can be described, ranging from high-level wellness to severe illness. The scale takes into account the presence of risk factors.

health maintenance organization (HMO) Group health care agency that provides basic and supplemental health maintenance and treatment services to voluntary enrollees who prepay a fixed periodic fee that is set without regard to the amount or kind of services received.

health promotion Activities directed toward maintaining or enhancing the health and well-being of clients.

hematemesis Vomiting or blood indicating upper gastrointestinal bleeding.

hematocrit Measure of the packed cell volume of red cells, expressed as a percentage of the total blood volume.

hematoma Collection of blood trapped in the tissues of the skin or an organ.

hematuria Abnormal presence of blood in the urine.

hemodynamics Study of the circulation of the blood.

hemolysis Breakdown of red blood cells and release of hemoglobin as may result by administration of hypotonic intravenous solutions that cause progressive swelling and rupture of the erythrocytes.

hemoptysis Coughing up of blood from the respiratory tract.

hemorrhage External or internal loss of a large amount of blood in a short period of time.

hemorrhoids Permanent dilation and engorgement of veins within the lining of the rectum.

hemosiderin Iron-rich pigment that is the product of red blood cell hemolysis.

hemosiderosis Abnormal deposition of iron in a variety of tissues.

hemostasis Termination of bleeding by mechanical or chemical means or by the coagulation process of the body.

hemothorax Accumulation of blood and fluid in the pleural cavity between the parietal and visceral pleurae.

heredity Primary natural force influencing an individual's genetic development.

heterosexual Sexual orientation involving erotic preference for members of the opposite sex.

hierarchy of basic human needs Categorization of human needs from the most basic to those at a higher level.

hirsutism Excessive body hair in a masculine distribution caused by heredity, hormonal dysfunction, or medication.

Holter monitor Portable ECG device, similar to the size of a miniature tape recorder; records a continuous ECG over 24 hours or longer.

home health agency Public or private organization that complies with all conditions or participation of government insurance programs. Services provided may include nursing, rehabilitation, social work, home health aides, or homemakers.

home health care Professional and paraprofessional services and equipment provided to clients and families in their place of residence for purposes of health promotion and maintenance, patient and family education, illness prevention, diagnosis and treatment of disease, and palliation and rehabilitation.

homosexual Sexual orientation involving erotic preference for members of one's own sex.

hope Confident, yet uncertain, expectation of achieving a future goal.

hospice Philosophy of patient care that advocates physical and psychosocial support for palliative care of persons in the last months of an incurable illness so that life can be lived as fully and comfortably as possible.

host Element of the agent-host-environment model of health and illness. A host is a person or group who, because of risk factors, may be susceptible to disease or illness.

human relations movement Leadership theory that emphasizes the role of interpersonal relationships and human needs for improving productivity in the workplace.

hydrostatic pressure Pressure exerted by a liquid.

hygiene Science of health.

hypercarbia Greater than normal amounts of carbon dioxide in the blood; also called hypercapnia.

hypercoagulability Increased tendency for blood to clot.

hypermetabolism Increased metabolism, producing above normal body heat.

hyperpigmentation Unusual darkening of the skin.

hypertension Disorder characterized by an elevated blood pressure persistently exceeding 140/90 mm Hg.

hyperthermia Situation in which body temperature exceeds the set-point.

hypervolemia Increase in the amount of fluid in the circulating blood volume.

hypnotic Class of drug that causes insensibility to pain and induces sleep.

hypotension Abnormal lowering of blood pressure, which is inadequate for normal perfusion and oxygenation of tissues.

hypothermia Abnormal lowering of body temperature below 93° F or 35° C, usually caused by prolonged exposure to cold.

hypoventilation Reduction in the volume of air that enters the lung for gas exchange; oxygen exchange is insufficient to meet metabolic demands of the body.

hypovolemia Decreased circulatory blood volume resulting from extracellular fluid losses.

hypoxia Inadequate cellular oxygenation that may result from a deficiency in the delivery or use of oxygen at the cellular level.

iatrogenic disease Disease caused by a treatment or diagnostic procedure.

identification Internalizing beliefs, values, and behavior of another through imitation and introjection with a unique individual expression.

identity Component of self-concept; sense of continuity and sameness; one's persisting consciousness of being oneself, separate, unique, and distinct from others.

identity confusion Form of self-concept disturbance in which a person does not maintain a clear consciousness of a consistent and continuous self; sense of fragmentation or distortion.

illegal chemicals Mood-altering substances not available on open market, including cocaine, marijuana, heroin, and prescription drugs sold without a prescription.

illiterate Having little education, especially in relation to the ability to read or write.

illness Abnormal process in which any aspect of a person's functioning is diminished or impaired as compared with his previous condition.

illness behavior Ways in which people monitor their bodies, define and interpret their symptoms, take remedial actions, and use the health care system.

illness prevention Health education programs or activities directed toward protecting clients from threats or potential threats to health and toward minimizing risk factors.

immobility Inability to move about freely, caused by any condition in which movement is impaired or therapeutically restricted.

immunocompromised Abnormal condition of the immune system in which cellular or humoral immunity is inadequate.

immunoglobulin Humoral antibody produced by the body and present in serum and external secretions; formed in response to specific antigens.

impairment A reduction in a person's physical and/or mental functioning as a result of chemical dependency.

implementation Category of nursing behavior in which the action necessary for achieving the projected outcomes of the health care plan are initiated and completed.

incentive spirometry Method of encouraging voluntary deep breathing by providing visual feedback to clients of the inspiratory volume they have achieved.

incident report Confidental document that describes any client accident while the person is on the premises of a health care agency.

independent intervention Nursing action that can solve the client's problems without consultation or collaboration with physicians or other nonnursing health professionals.

individual practice association Prospective payment plans requiring the client to pay a fixed annual payment; the plan pays the provider when the services are used.

induction of anesthesia All portions of the anesthetic process that occur before attaining the desired stage of anesthesia, including premedication, intubation, and administration of oxygen.

induration Hardening of a tissue, particularly the skin, because of edema or inflammation.

industry Diligence in the pursuit of a goal.

infancy Stage of life from 1 month to 1 year of age.

infertility Man's, woman's, or couple's involuntary inability to conceive.

infestation Presence of animal parasites on the skin or in the hair of a host (person or animal).

inflammation Protective response of body tissues to irritation or injury.

informed consent Process of obtaining permission from a client to perform a specific test or procedure, after describing all risks, side effects, and benefits.

infradian rhythm Repetition of certain physiological phenomena within a cycle exceeding 24 hours.

infusion Introduction of a substance, such as a fluid, drug, electrolyte, or nutrient, directly into a vein by means of gravity flow.

inhalants Medications administered via the nasal passage.

inhibition Process of socialization in which one learns to refrain from a behavior even when motivated to engage in that behavior.

initiative Energy displayed in starting an action.

injection Act of introducing a liquid into the body by means of a syringe.

inpatient Client admitted for treatment within a hospital over the course of more than 1 day.

insensible water loss Loss of fluid from the body by evaporation, as normally occurs during respiration.

in-service education Instruction or training provided by an agency or institution to nurses practicing within the agency or institution.

insomnia Condition characterized by chronic inability to sleep or remain asleep through the night.

inspection Assessment process during which the nurse observes the client.

instillation Procedure in which a fluid is slowly introduced into a cavity or passage of the body (for example, rectum) and allowed to remain for a specific length of time before being withdrawn or drained.

integument Skin and its appendages: hair, nails, and sweat and sebaceous glands.

interdependent intervention Action with or without a physician's order or written at a nurse's suggestion that can provide the solution to the client's problem in a collaborative manner with judgment and recommendations of the interdisciplinary health team.

interference Behavior(s) that deliberately delays or impedes the change process.

internal environment Set of factors inside a person that may influence his health, including genetic factors, physiological processes, psychological variables, and intellectual and spiritual dimensions.

internal stressor Stress-causing stimulus that arises within a person.

International Council of Nurses (ICN) International organization for professional nurses; the ANA and CNA are members.

interpersonal communication Exchange of information between two persons or among persons in a small group.

interstitial fluid Fluid that fills the spaces between most of the cells of the body and provides a substantial portion of the liquid environment of the body.

interview Type of communication with a client initiated for a specific purpose and focused on a specific content area.

intonation Rise and fall in pitch of the voice in speech.

intra-arterial Within an artery.

intra-articular Within a joint.

intracardiac Within the myocardium.

intracellular fluid Liquid within the cell membrane.

intractable pain Pain not easily relieved, as may occur with some types of cancer.

intradermal injection Form of injection in which the solution is introduced into the dermis of the skin.

intramuscular (IM) injection Form of injection in which the solution is introduced into the body of a muscle.

intraoperative Pertaining to the period of time during a surgical procedure.

intrapersonal communication Communication that occurs within an individual, for example, a person "talks with himself" silently or forms an idea in his own mind.

intrathecal Within the sheath surrounding the spinal cord.

intravenous (IV) injection Form of injection in which the solution is introduced into a vein.

intravenous therapy Delivery of fluids, medications, and nutrients through a small catheter placed in a vein. Home IV therapy usually involves electronic control devices (infusion pumps) to regulate the rate of infusion of the fluids and medications.

intrinsic factor Substance that is secreted by the gastric mucosa and is essential for the intestinal absorption of vitamin B$_{12}$.

Intubation Passage of a tube into a body opening, for example, insertion of a breathing tube through the mouth or nose into the trachea.

invasive Referring to procedures that involve puncture, incision, or insertion of a foreign object, such as a needle or catheter, into the body.

irregular bones Bones of the vertebral column and some bones of the skull.

irrigation Process of washing out a body cavity or wounded area with a stream of fluid.

ischemia Decreased blood supply to a body part such as skin tissue, or to an organ such as the heart.

isometric contraction Increased muscle tension without muscle shortening.

isotonic contraction Increased muscle tension resulting in muscle contraction and muscle shortening.

jaundice Yellow discoloration of the skin, mucous membranes, and sclera, caused by greater than normal amounts of bilirubin in the blood.

job stress Condition in which some factor or combination of factors at work disrupts the worker's psychological or physiological balance.

joints Connections between bones; classified according to structure and degree of mobility.

Kardex Trade name for card-filing system that allows quick reference to the particular need of the client for certain aspects of nursing care.

keratosis Any skin condition in which there are overgrowth and thickening of the cornified epithelium; types are actinic and seborrheic.

ketoacidosis Acidosis accompanied by an accumulation of ketones in the body, resulting from faulty carbohydrate metabolism.

ketonuria Presence in the urine of excessive amounts of ketone bodies (products of fat metabolism) such as occurs in diabetes mellitus.

kinesthesia Perception of position of body parts, weight, and movement.

Korsakoff's syndrome Psychosis characterized by disorientation of time, place, and person, by amnesia for recent events, and by confabulation.

laceration Torn, jagged wound.

lactation Process and period in which the mother produces milk for the infant.

laissez-faire Philosophy characterized by an individual freedom of choice and action.

laissez-faire style Leadership style in which the leader denies responsibility, abdicates authority, and allows the group to direct themselves.

lanugo Fine hair that normally covers the fetus after the fifth month of intrauterine life and is mostly shed by birth.

laxative Drug that acts to promote bowel evacuation.

leader Person with the ability to influence the behavior of others toward the accomplishment of common goals; not necessarily a manager.

leadership style Specific means by which a leader influences a group to accomplish goals.

learning Acquisition of new knowledge and skills as a result of reinforcement, practice, and experience.

learning objectives Written statement that describes the behavior a teacher expects from an individual following a learning activity.

legal chemicals Mood-altering substances that may be purchased legally, including alcohol, prescription drugs, and over-the-counter medications.

legal right Claim that is due according to legal guarantees.

legume Fruit or pod of beans, peas, and lentils.

lesbian Female with homosexual partner preference.

leukocytosis Abnormal increase in the number of circulating white blood cells.

libel Written false statement about a person that may injure his reputation.

libido Psychological term for sexual desire.

licensed practical or vocational nurse Person trained in basic nursing techniques and direct client care who practices under the supervision of a registered nurse.

lifesaving measure Independent, dependent, or interdependent nursing intervention that is implemented when a client's physiological or psychological status is threatened.

ligaments White, shiny, flexible bands of fibrous tissues binding joints together and connecting various bones and cartilage.

litigation Practice of taking legal action.

living will Instrument by which a dying person makes his wishes known to those who are caring for him: a living will has no legal validity in most states.

livor mortis Purple discoloration of the skin in dependent body parts after death; results from red blood cell destruction.

local adaptation syndrome (LAS) Localized response of tissue, an organ, or a system that occurs as a direct reaction to stress.

local anesthesia Loss of sensation at the desired site of action.

localized pain Pain caused by injury in a specific location and perceived in that location, in contrast to diffuse, radiating, or referred pain.

long bones Bones that contribute to height of the person or to the length of an extremity such as the arm, or to the length of a portion of an extremity such as the hand.

luteal phase Third and final phase of the menstrual cycle, in which the corpus luteum develops, preparing for implantation of the egg, and deteriorates if an egg is not implanted.

lymphocyte One type of leukocyte developing in the bone marrow; responsible for synthesizing antibodies and T cells that attack antigens.

maceration Softening something solid, such as the skin, by soaking.

macrophage Large phagocytic cell of the reticuloendothelial system.

malabsorption syndrome Set of symptoms resulting from disorders in the intestinal absorption of nutrients, characterized by anorexia, weight loss, bloating of the abdomen, and muscle cramps.

male genitalia Male external sex organs (penis and scrotum) and internal sex organs (testicles, epididymis, vas deferens, prostate gland, seminal vesicles, and Cowper's gland).

malignant tumor Neoplasm that is anaplastic and invasive and that spreads to other body tissues.

malnutrition Any nutritional disorder such as unbalanced, insufficient, or excessive diet or impaired absorption, assimilation, or utilization of food.

malpractice Injurious or unprofessional actions that harm another.

manager Person with an official organizational position to guide and direct the work of subordinate employees.

mastication Chewing, tearing, or grinding food with the teeth while it becomes mixed with saliva.

masturbation Erotic self-stimulation by touching the genitals.

maturation Process of becoming fully developed and grown, involving the individual's biological ability and environmental opportunities to alter functions and learning.

maturational loss Loss, usually of an aspect of self, resulting from the normal changes of growth and development.

maturity State of adulthood in which the person has attained independence with a balanced development in physiological, psychosocial, and cognitive dimensions.

meatus Opening through any part of the body, for example, the urethral meatus.

Medicaid State medical assistance based on Title XIX of the Social Security Act. States receive 50% in matching federal funds to provide medical care and services to people meeting categorical and income requirements. Covers home health services based on Medicare guidelines. Many innovative home health programs can be covered by Medicaid as long as they meet the recipient's needs and cost less than institutionalization.

medical diagnosis Identification of a specific disease or pathological process.

Medicare Federal government insurance coverage for persons over 65 years of age (or disabled and under 65) who have paid into the Social Security or Railroad Retirement system. Covers inpatient hospital charges and some home health services.

medulla oblongata Portion of the brain that controls vital functions necessary for homeostasis and survival.

megadose Dose greatly in excess of that usually prescribed.

melanin Black or dark brown pigment that occurs naturally in the skin, hair, and iris.

melena Abnormal black, tarry stool containing digested blood; indicative of gastrointestinal bleeding.

menarche Onset of a girl's first menstruation, usually occurring between 9 and 16 years of age.

meniscus Interface between a liquid, for example, mercury and air that causes a convex shape to the liquid.

menopause Natural cessation of menses by the ovaries, normally occurs in women between ages 45 and 60.

menses Normal flow of blood, secretions, and tissue debris that occurs during menstruation, beginning on the first day of the menstrual cycle.

menstrual cycle Recurring cycle of changes in the ovaries, uterus, and hormone levels, involving the development of an egg, ovulation, and implantation of the egg or sloughing of the corpus luteum and lining. The cycle can be divided into proliferative and secretory phases by uterine changes or follicular, ovulation, and luteal phases based on ovarian activity.

menstruation Time of menstrual flow during the menstrual cycle.

message Information sent or expressed by sender in the communication process.

metabolism Aggregate of all chemical processes that take place in living organisms, resulting in growth, generation of energy, elimination of wastes, and other functions concerned with the distribution of nutrients in the blood after digestion.

metacognition Act of reflecting on one's own thought processes.

microorganism Any microscopic entity capable of carrying on living processes, such as bacteria, viruses, and fungi.

micturition Urination; act of passing or expelling urine voluntarily through the urethra.

mild stress situation Type of stress situation that is encountered by most people on a daily or weekly basis.

milliequivalent Number of grams of a specific electrolyte dissolved in 1 liter of plasma.

misuse Indiscriminate use of a drug or substance but a lesser extent than with chronic abuse and dependence.

modeling Technique in which a person learns a desired response by observing it performed.

moderate stress situation Stress situation that lasts from several hours to a number of days.

modern Present day beliefs and practices of the providers within the American, or western, health-care delivery system.

molding Overlapping and shaping of the soft skull bones during birth, usually resolved during the first few days of life.

morality Behavior involving judgment, attitudes, and actions based on nationally conceived norms.

moralize Explain or interpret behavior on the basis of rigid principles of right or wrong.

morning sickness Pregnant woman's symptoms of nausea and vomiting related to changes in serum hormone levels.

mortician Person trained in the care of the dead.

morula Early stage of human development in which a solid mass of cells forms from the zygote approximately 3 days after fertilization.

motivation Internal impulse that causes a person to take action.

moving stage of change Initiation of new behaviors or functions as a result of information gathered and deliberate planning.

muscle tone Normal state of balanced muscle tension.

myalgia Diffuse muscle pain.

myoneural junction Point at which impulses traveling along motor nerves are transferred to muscle fibers.

narcolepsy Syndrome involving sudden sleep attacks that a person cannot inhibit; uncontrollable desire to sleep may occur several times during a day.

narcotic Drug substance, derived from opium or produced synthetically, that alters perception of pain and that with repeated use may result in physical and psychological dependence.

nasal Of or pertaining to the nose and the nasal cavity.

National League for Nursing (NLN) Organization of nurses and lay people concerned with improving nursing education, nursing service, and the delivery of health care in the United States. The NLN is the official accrediting agency for nursing schools.

nebulization Process of adding moisture to inspired air by the addition of water droplets.

necrotic Of or pertaining to the death of tissue in response to disease or injury.

negative nitrogen balance Condition occurring when the body excretes more nitrogen than it takes in.

negligence Careless act of omission or commission that results in injury to another.

neonate Stage of life from birth to 1 month of age.

nephron Structural and functional unit of the kidney containing a renal glomerulus and tubule.

neurogenic bladder Dysfunctional urinary bladder resulting from impaired neurological innervation.

neuropathy Abnormal condition characterized by inflammation and degeneration of peripheral nerves that alter sensory or motor function.

neurotransmitter Chemical that transfers the electrical impulse from the nerve fiber to the muscle fiber.

nocturia Urination at night; can be a symptom of renal disease or may occur in persons who drink excessive amounts of fluids before bedtime.

nocturnal enuresis Incontinence of urine during the night.

noise pollution Noise level in an environment when it becomes uncomfortable to its inhabitants.

nonREM or NREM sleep Abbreviation for nonrapid eye movement, which occurs during the first four stages of normal sleep.

norm Measure of a phenomenon generally accepted as the ideal standard performance against which other measures of the phenomenon may be measured.

nosocomial infection Infection acquired during hospitalization or stay in a health care facility.

noxious   Painful or harmful to health.

nuclear family   Form of family consisting of husband and wife and their children.

nurse administrator   Nurse in management position with an agency who focuses on the delivery of nursing services.

nurse anesthetist   Nurse with advanced training and accreditation in the speciality of nurse anesthesia; manages the anesthetic care of clients in certain surgical situations.

nurse-client relationship   Association between the nurse and the client that has as a mutual concern the well-being of the client.

nurse educator   Nurse with a background in clinical nursing who works in a school of nursing as a faculty member, in a staff development department of a health care agency, or in an inpatient education department.

nurse practice acts   Statutes enacted by the legislature of any state delineating the legal scope of the practice of nursing within the geographical boundaries of the jurisdiction.

nurse practitioner   Nurse with advanced training or education who provides primary care for nonemergency clients, usually in an outpatient or community setting.

nurse researcher   Nurse with graduate nursing education who investigates problems related to nursing practice.

nursing   Profession concerned with the diagnosis and treatment of human responses to actual and potential health problems.

nursing audit   Thorough investigation designed to identify, examine, or verify the performance of certain specified aspects of nursing care using established professional standards.

nursing care plan   Written guidelines of nursing care, documenting specific nursing diagnoses for the client and goals, interventions, and projected outcomes.

nursing care strategy   Detailed nursing care plans that include direct and indirect care for the client.

nursing diagnosis   Statement of the client's potential or actual health problem that the nurse is licensed and competent to treat.

nursing health history   Data collected about a client's present level of wellness, changes in the life patterns, sociocultural role, and mental and emotional reactions to illness.

nursing intervention   Any action by a nurse that implements the nursing care plan or any specific objective of the plan.

nursing research   A detailed process in which a systematic study of a problem in the field of nursing is performed.

nursing theory   Organized framework of concepts and purposes designed to guide the practice of nursing.

objective data   Data relating to a client's health problem that is obtained through observation or diagnostic measurements.

observation   Report of what is seen or noticed about the client.

obstructive sleep apnea   Temporary cessation of airflow (apnea) but with continuation of chest and abdominal movements; occurs while a person is sleeping.

occupational therapist   Health care professional certified to develop and use adaptive devices that help the chronically ill or handicapped carry out activities of daily living.

olfactory   Pertaining to the sense of smell.

oliguria   Diminished capacity to form and pass urine.

open-ended question interview   Inquiry aimed at obtaining a full client response and discussion between the client and the nurse.

ophthalmic   Of or pertaining to the eye.

oral hygiene   Condition or practice of maintaining the tissues and structures of the mouth.

oral report   Verbal exchange of information.

organic foods   Foods grown in soils that have been treated only with organic matter (manure or compost).

orgasm   Climax phase of sexual response, in which reflex muscular contractions, genital vasocongestion, and increased heart and respiratory rates occur.

orgasmic maturity   Physiological maturity of the reproductive system enabling completion of the adult sexual response cycle.

orthopnea   Abnormal condition in which a person must sit or stand to breathe deeply or comfortably.

orthostatic hypotension   Abnormally low blood pressure occurring when a person stands up/sits down.

osmosis   Movement of a pure solvent through a semipermeable membrane from a solution with a lower solute concentration to one with a higher solute concentration.

osmotic pressure   Drawing power for water, which depends on the number of molecules in the solution.

ostomate   Person with an ostomy.

ostomy   Surgical procedure in which an opening is made into the abdominal wall to allow the passage of intestinal contents from the bowel (colostomy) or urine from the bladder (urostomy).

ototoxic   Having a harmful effect on the eighth cranial (auditory) nerves or the organs of hearing and balance.

outcome   Condition of a client at the end of therapy, including the degree of wellness and the need for continuing care, medication, support, counseling, or education.

outpatient   Client who has not been admitted to a hospital but receives treatment in a clinic or facility associated with the hospital.

outpatient setting   Physician's office, clinic, or other ambulatory care facility for the provision of health care services.

overhydration   Excess of water in the extracellular fluid.

over-the-counter drug   Drug available to a consumer without a prescription.

ovulation   Second phase of the menstrual cycle, in which a mature egg is released from the ovary and moves down the fallopian tubes.

oxidation   Any process in which the oxygen content of a compound is increased.

oxygen therapy   Administration of oxygen to a client by any route to prevent or relieve hypoxia.

pain   Subjective, unpleasant sensation caused by noxious stimulation of sensory nerve endings.

pain perception   Threshold or point at which a person experiences pain.

palliative therapy   Treatment designed to relieve or reduce intensity of uncomfortable symptoms but not to produce a cure.

pallor   Unnatural paleness or absence of color in the skin.

palpation   Use of the hands and the sense of touch to gather data.

palpebra   Portion of the conjunctiva that lines the inner surface of the eyelids; it is thick, opaque, and highly vascular.

paralytic ileus   Usually temporary paralysis of intestinal wall causing cessation of peristalsis. Leads to abdominal distention and symptoms of obstruction.

paranoia   Disorder characterized by a system of thinking with delusions of persecution and grandeur, usually centered on one major theme.

paraphrasing   Restating a passage or phrase to give the same meaning in another form.

parasite   Organism living in or on another organism and obtaining nourishment from it.

parenteral   Not in or through the digestive system; typically refers to administering medications by injection.

paronychia   Infection of the fold of skin at the margin of a nail.

partial bed bath   Bath in which body parts that might cause the client discomfort if left unbathed, that is, face, hands, axillary areas, back, and perineum, are washed in bed.

passive smoking   Smoke and toxic fumes inhaled by a nonsmoker from a smoker's cigarette, cigar, or pipe.

passive strategies of health promotion   Activities that involve the client as the recipient of actions by health care professonals.

pathogen   Any microorganism capable of producing disease.

pathological fractures   Fractures resulting from weakened bone tissue; frequently caused by osteoporosis or neoplasms.

peer review   Appraisal, by professional co-workers of equal status, of the way a nurse conducts practice, education, or research.

pellagra   Disorder resulting from a deficiency of niacin or tryptophan.

perception   Person's mental image or concept of elements in his environment, including information gained through the senses.

percussion   Tapping of various body organs and structures to produce vibration and sound.

perineal care   Cleansing procedure prescribed for cleaning the genital and anal areas as part of the daily bath or after various obstetrical and gynecological procedures.

periodontal disease (pyorrhea)   Disease of the tissues around the tooth, such as an inflammation of the periodontal membrane or ligament.

peristalsis   Coordinated, rhythmical, serial contractions of smooth muscle that force food through the digestive tract.

PERRLA   Acronym for "pupils equal, round, reactive to light, accommodative"; the acronym is recorded in the physical examination if eye and pupil assessment is normal.

petechiae Tiny purple or red spots that appear on skin as minute hemorrhages within dermal layers.

phagocytosis Process by which certain cells, such as macrophages, engulf and dispose of microorganisms.

pharmacist Licensed professional who formulates and dispenses medications.

phenomena Data than can be observed in reality.

phlebitis Inflammation of a vein.

physical examination Scrutinization of all body parts through the use of inspection, palpation, percussion, and auscultation.

physical therapist Health care professional licensed to assist in the management of physically disabled or handicapped clients through techniques such as special exercise, application of heat and cold, and sonar wave methods.

physician Health care professional who has the degree of Doctor of Medicine (MD) or Doctor of Osteopath (DO) and is licensed to provide medical, surgical, and other treatment.

physician assistant Health care professional trained in aspects of the practice of medicine to provide support to physicians.

physiological dependence Condition in which the body is so accustomed to a drug or substance that functioning is impaired without it.

physiological needs Needs necessary for human survival, including those for oxygen, fluid, nutrition, temperature, elimination, and shelter.

PIE (Problem-Intervention-Evaluation) A format for documenting client care that unifies the care plan and progress notes into a complete record.

pigmentation Organic coloring material, such as melanin, that gives color to the skin.

pituitary gland Small gland attached to the hypothalamus that supplies numerous hormones for the control of vital functions and the maintenance of homeostasis.

placebo Dosage form that contains no pharmacologically active ingredients but may relieve pain through psychological effects.

placenta Organ surrounding the embryo and fetus through which nutrients and other substances from the mother and waste products from the fetus pass.

planned change Goal-directed, collaborated efforts to alter a situation or environment.

plantar wart Painful lesion on the sole of the foot, primarily at pressure points, caused by the common wart virus.

plasma Watery, colorless, fluid portion of the lymph and blood.

plasma proteins Albumin, fibrinogen, prothrombin, and the gamma globulins, which constitute about 6% to 7% of the blood plasma in the body.

pleura Delicate serous membrane enclosing the lung.

pleural cavity Cavity within the thorax that contains the lungs.

pneumothorax Collection of air or gas in the pleural space.

podiatrist Practitioner trained to diagnose and treat diseases and other disorders of the feet.

point of maximal impulse (PMI) Anatomic point along the fourth to fifth intercostal space at the midclavicular line where the heartbeat can most easily be palpated through the chest wall.

poison Any substance that impairs health or destroys life when ingested, inhaled, or absorbed by the body in relatively small amounts.

poison control center One of a network of facilities that provides information regarding all aspects of poisoning or intoxication, maintains records of their occurrence, and refers clients to treatment centers.

pollutant A harmful chemical or waste material discharged into the water or atmosphere.

polycythemia Abnormal increase in the number of erythrocytes in the blood.

polysomnogram Monitoring device that involves placement of electrodes on the scalp, face, chin, and legs to measure brain waves, eye movements, and muscle activity; used to diagnose sleep disorders.

polyuria Excretion of an abnormally large volume of urine.

postoperative Pertaining to the period of time after surgery.

postural drainage Use of positioning along with percussion and vibration to drain secretions from specific segments of the lungs and bronchi into the trachea.

posture Position of the body in relation to the surrounding space.

potential health care problem Health problem for which the client is at risk.

potentiation Synergistic action in which the effect of two drugs given simultaneously is greater than the effect of the drugs given separately.

power Ability to influence, direct, produce, or control; to exert authority force, or strength.

precipitating factor Element that causes or contributes to the occurrence of a symptom.

preferred provider organization (PPO) Group of physicians or hospital that provides company employees and their dependents with comprehensive health services at a discount.

premenstrual syndrome Complex of physical and psychological symptoms experienced by some women just before menstruation.

prenatal Stage of life from conception to birth.

preoperative Pertaining to the period of time before surgery.

presbycusis Condition that affects the client's ability to hear high-pitched sounds and sibilant consonants such as "s," "sh," and "ch" because of the aging process.

presbyopia Farsightedness with inability to focus on near objects, resulting from loss of elasticity of the lens; occurs with age.

preschooler Stage of life from 3 to 5 years of age.

prescription Authorized order for medication, therapy, or a therapeutic device.

presentational isolation Social isolation that occurs because of the older adult's socially unacceptable appearance or presentation of self to others.

preventive nursing action Interventions directed toward preventing illness and promoting health to avoid the need for secondary or tertiary health care.

primary intention Primary union of the edges of a wound, progressing to complete scar formation without granulation.

primary nursing System of nursing care in which the care of a client is managed for the entire day by one nurse, who directs and coordinates other nurses and other personnel and schedules all tests, procedures, and daily activities for the client. When on duty, the primary nurse cares for the client personally.

primary prevention Activities directed toward decreasing the probability of specific illnesses or dysfunctions.

primary source Research report written by an investigator in an original study.

private duty agencies Organizations that provide professional and paraprofessional home health care services on a continuous basis.

private insurance Health insurance other than government coverage. Insurance provided for profit by citizen-owned companies.

proactive decision Decision made by an individual directed at attaining a goal.

problem-oriented record (POR) Method of recording data about the health status of a client that fosters a collaborative problem-solving approach by all members of the health care team.

problem-seeking interview Type of inquiry that focuses on gathering data to identify problems the client needs to resolve.

problem-solving interview Type of inquiry that focuses on specific problems that have been identified by the client or nurse.

profession Vocation requiring specialized knowledge and intensive academic preparation.

professional organization Association of professionals created to deal with issues of concern to the profession as a whole.

prophylactic Preventing the spread of infection.

proposition Statement that defines or explains a relationship between two or more concepts.

proprioception Sensation achieved through stimuli from within the body regarding spatial position and muscular activity.

proprioceptors Nerve endings located in muscles, tendons, and joints that respond to stimuli originating from within the body regarding spatial position or movement.

prospective payment Procedure by which the federal government sets rates for hospitals in advance for treatment of specific illnesses;

this replaces the previous policy of reimbursing each hospital based on actual cost.

prospective reimbursement Predetermined amount of payment before delivery of services.

protocol Written and approved plan specifying the procedures to be followed during an assessment or in providing treatment.

pruritus Symptom of itching, an uncomfortable sensation leading to the urge to scratch, which may result in secondary infections.

psychiatric hospital Institution providing inpatient and outpatient counseling services to clients with behavioral or emotional illnesses.

psychological dependence Chronic emotional or psychological reliance on a drug or substance such that the person feels unable to handle stress without it.

psychomotor learning Acquisition of ability to perform motor skills.

psychosurgery Surgical interruption of certain nerve pathways in the brain; performed in selected cases of agitation, unremitting anxiety, and other forms of abnormal behavior.

psychotherapy Treatment of mental and emotional disorders by any of a large number of psychological techniques rather than by physical means.

psychotomimetic Drug or substance whose effects mimic the symptoms of psychosis, such as hallucinations.

ptosis Abnormal condition of one or both upper eyelids in which the eyelid droops, caused by weakness of the levator muscle or paralysis of the third cranial nerve.

puberty Developmental period of emotional and physical changes, including the development of secondary sex characteristics and the onset of menstruation and ejaculation.

public communication Interaction between one person and a large group of people.

puerperium Period of approximately 6 weeks after childbirth during which the woman's reproductive system is in transition to the nonpregnant state.

pulmonary function tests Procedures for determining the capacity of the lungs to exchange oxygen and carbon dioxide efficiently.

pursed-lip breathing Deep inspiration through the nose and mouth, not using pursed lips, followed by prolonged expiration through pursed lips.

purulent Producing or containing pus.

pyrogen Any substance that causes a rise in body temperature, as in the case of bacterial toxins.

quality assurance Evaluation of the quality and appropriateness of nursing care provided and the results achieved as compared with accepted standards.

radiating pain A sensation of pain extending from the initial site of injury to another body part.

random selection Method of choosing subjects for a research study in which all members of a particular group are equally likely to be included.

reaction Component of the pain experience that may include both physiological responses such as in the general adaptation syndrome and behavioral responses.

reactive decision Decision made by an individual in response to the influence of others.

reality orientation Therapeutic modality for restoring an individual's sense of the present.

receiver Person to whom message is sent during the communication process.

reception Neurophysiological components of the pain experience, in which nervous system receptors receive painful stimuli and transmit them through peripheral nerves to the spinal cord and brain.

recommended daily allowances (RDAs) Suggested or recommended amounts of various nutrients used in planning diets.

record Written form of communication that permanently documents information relevant to health care management.

recovery room Area adjoining the operating room to which surgical clients are taken while still under anesthesia.

recumbent Lying down or leaning backward.

referent Factor that motivates a person to communicate with another individual.

referred pain Pain perceived in an area separate from and unaffected by the source of pain, as sensory neurons from the affected organ meet neurons in the spinal cord from organs where the pain is perceived.

reflux Abnormal backward flow of fluid, as in the case of gastric contents reentering the esophagus.

refractive error Defect in the ability of the lens of the eye to focus light, such as occurs in nearsightedness and farsightedness

refractory period Postejaculation recovery time during which further ejaculation is physiologically impossible.

refreezing stage of change Incorporation of modifications as standard procedure or function.

regional anesthesia Loss of sensation in an area of the body supplied by sensory nerve pathways.

registered nurse Health care professional who has completed a course of study at an accredited school of professional nursing and has passed an examination administered by a state board of nursing or the Canadian Nurses Association Testing Service.

regurgitation Return of swallowed food into the mouth.

rehabilitation Restoration of an individual to normal or near-normal function following a physical or mental illness, injury, or chemical addiction.

rehabilitation center Facility that provides therapy and training to restore a client to his optimal level of functioning and independence.

reinforcement Provision of a contingent response to a learner's behavior that increases the probability of the behavior recurring.

reinforcement-extinction Process of socialization in which one learns to engage in certain behaviors (reinforcement) or to avoid certain behaviors (extinction).

relative humidity Amount of moisture in the air as compared with the maximum amount that the air could contain at the same temperature.

relieving factor Element that alleviates a symptom.

religion Belief in a divine or superhuman power or powers to be obeyed and worshipped as the creator(s) and ruler(s) of the universe.

remission Partial or complete disappearance of the clinical and subjective characteristics of a chronic or malignant disease; remission may be spontaneous or the result of therapy.

REM sleep Abbreviation for rapid eye movement, occurring during stage of sleep in which dreaming and rapid eye movements are prominent; important for mental restoration.

reminiscence Recalling the past for the purpose of assigning new meaning to past experiences.

remission Partial or complete disappearance of the clinical and subjective characteristics of a chronic or malignant disease; remission may be spontaneous or the result of therapy.

renal Of or pertaining to the kidney.

renal calculus Calcium stone in the renal pelvis.

research process Systematic collection and analysis of data to obtain new knowledge, add to existing knowledge, or find solutions to problems.

research utilization Systematic process for determining the scientific worth of a group of conceptually related nursing research studies and whether or not the findings can be used to solve a nursing care problem with a particular group of clients in a setting other than the one in which the studies were conducted.

residual urine Volume of urine remaining in the bladder after a normal voiding; the bladder normally is almost completely empty after micturition.

resistance An overtly active or covertly passive set of behaviors whether conscious or unconscious in motivation, to avoid or to prevent the change process.

resocialization Technique that assists the older adult to expand his social network within his community.

respiratory therapist Health care professional licensed to deliver treatment to improve ventilatory function or oxygenation.

respite Temporary relief services for the primary caregiver of a dependent older adult in the home or institutional setting.

responsibility Carrying out duties associated with a particular role.

restraining forces against change Factors that resist, slow, or interfere with the occurrence of the change process.

restraint Device to aid in the immobilization of a client or client's extremity.

resuscitation Process of sustaining the vital functions of a person in respiratory or cardiac arrest while reviving him.

reticular activating system Group of specialized nerve cells located in the brainstem, upper spinal cord, and cerebral cortex.

reticular formation Small cluster of neurons in the brainstem and spinal cord that continuously monitor and control vital functions to maintain homeostasis

retroperitoneal Of or pertaining to organs closely attached to the posterior abdominal wall and partly covered by peritoneum.

Rickettsia Group of microorganisms that occupy an intermediate position between viruses and bacteria.

rigidity Condition of stiffness or inflexibility, as in muscle rigidity.

rigor mortis Stiffening of the body shortly after death because of the contraction of skeletal and smooth muscle.

Rinne's test Method of assessing auditory acuity useful in distinguishing conductive from sensorineural hearing loss.

role A person's pattern of behavior in a particular social group or situation.

role ambiguity State in which a person has unclear role expectations and feels unable to predict the outcomes of his behavior.

role conflict State in which a person experiences incongruent or incompatible expectations within one role or between two or more simultaneously held roles.

role overload State in which a person experiences conflicting role priorities and must decide with which pressures to comply.

role strain Generalized state of frustration or anxiety produced by the stress of role conflict and ambiguity.

safety and security needs Needs for freedom from threats to one's physical and psychological well-being.

sample Portion of a larger group of subjects.

satiety Satisfied feeling of being full.

scientific management theory Leadership theory that emphasizes technology and task analysis, rather than human factors, as a means of improving productivity.

scientific rationale Reason, based on supporting literature, why a specific nursing action was chosen.

sebaceous gland One of the small organs in the dermis that secretes an oily substance (sebum) on the skin's surface and in the hair.

sebum Normal secretion of the sebaceous glands of the skin; when combined with sweat, forms a moist, oily, acidic film that protects the skin from drying.

secondary intention Wound closure in which the edges are separated, granulation tissue develops to fill the gap, and finally, epithelium grows in over the granulation, producing a larger scar than results with healing by primary intention.

secondary prevention Activities directed toward early diagnosis and prompt intervention, thereby shortening severity and enabling the client to return to his highest level of health at the earliest possible point.

secondary sex characteristics Physical characteristics other than genitals that distinguish females from males, for example, the breasts.

secondary source Report that interprets research data written by someone not involved in the original research.

sedative Medication that produces a calming effect by decreasing functional activity, diminishing irritability, and allaying excitement.

sedative-hypnotics Drugs, such as barbiturates, that depress the central nervous system and produce a sense of euphoria or relaxation.

self-actualization State of being in which one is fully achieving one's potential and is able to cope realistically with problems.

self-concept Complex, dynamic integration of conscious and unconscious feelings, attitudes, and perceptions about one's identity, physical being, worth, and roles; how a person perceives and defines himself.

self-esteem Feeling of self-worth characterized by feelings of achievement, adequacy, self-confidence, and usefulness.

self-ideal Aspirations, goals, values, and standards of behavior that a person considers ideal and strives to attain.

sender Person who initiates interpersonal communication by conveying a message.

sensate exercises Series of pleasurable touching exercises that focus on sensual (not sexual) activities.

sensory deficit Defect in the function of one or more of the senses, resulting in visual, auditory, or olfactory impairments.

sensory deprivation State in which stimulation to one or more of the senses is lacking, resulting in impaired sensory perception.

sensory overload State in which stimulation to one or more of the senses is so excessive that the brain disregards or does not meaningfully respond to stimuli.

separation anxiety Behavioral manifestation created by fear of being apart from primary caretaker.

serosanguineous Thin red drainage composed of serum and blood.

serous fluid Clear fluid that reduces friction between structures covered by serous membranes, such as the lung.

severe stress situation Chronic stress situation that may last from several weeks to years.

sex Classification of male or female based on many criteria, among them anatomical and chromosomal characteristics; refers also to biological aspects of sexuality and genital sexual activity.

sex skin Term used for the labia minora because of the distinctive color changes that occur during sexual arousal.

sexual dysfunction Inability or diffculty in sexual functioning caused by physiological or psychological factors or both.

sexual orientation Clear, persistent desire of a person for one sex rather than the other.

sexual response cycle Four phases of biological sexual response: excitement, plateau, orgasm, and resolution as defined by Masters and Johnson.

sexuality Dynamic and diverse facet of the personality involving the biological, psychological, sociological, spiritual, and cultural dimensions, depending in part on the person's sense of sexual identity and affecting the person's values, attitudes, behaviors, and relationships with others.

sexually transmitted diseases (STDs) Infectious diseases transmitted to any part of the body through contact with body fluids during sexual activities.

sign Objective finding perceived by an examiner, such as a fever, rash, abnormal reflex, or abnormal breath sound.

single-parent family A form of family composed of a single, divorced or widowed parent and his or her children.

situational change Unplanned events that alter behavior of a person, family, group, or community.

situational crisis Crisis occurring suddenly in response to a specific external event or conflict.

situational loss Loss of a person, thing, or quality resulting from a change in a life situation, including changes related to illness, body image, environment, and death.

situational theory Leadership theory in which the manager chooses a leadership style to match the particular situation.

sitz bath Bath in which only the hips or buttocks are immersed in fluid.

slander Utterance of a false statement about another that harms his reputation.

sleep deprivation Condition resulting from a decrease in the amount, quality, and consistency of sleep.

SOAP Acronym for *subjective, objective, assessment,* and *plan,* the four parts of the written account of a client's health problem in a problem-oriented record.

socialization Process that begins in infancy by which a person acquires values, behavior, skills, and roles from social norms and significant others.

social worker Professional trained to counsel clients and families to help them seek community and financial resources and to assist them in selecting long-term and extended care facilities.

sodium pump Physiological mechanism that transports sodium ions across cellular membranes against an opposing concentration gradient.

somnolence Condition characterized by constant sleepiness or drowsiness.

spasm Involuntary muscle contraction of sudden onset.

specific gravity Measurement of the degree of concentration of a liquid.

spiritual distress State of being out of harmony with a system of beliefs, a Supreme being, or God.

spiritual health Awareness and openness to a system of beliefs, a Supreme Being, or God; a presence with or in each person and in the world.

spirituality Spiritual dimension of a person, including the relationship with humanity, nature, and a system of beliefs, a supreme being, or God.

spirometer Instrument that measures and records the volume of inhaled and exhaled air; used to assess pulmonary function.

standard Measure or guide that serves as a basis for comparison when evaluating similar phenomena or substances.

standardized care plan (SCP) Written care plan to be used for groups of patients that have similar health care problems.

standing order Written and approved document containing rules, policies, procedures, regulations, and orders for the conduct of client care in various stipulated clinical settings.

statistics Mathematical science concerned with measuring, classifying, and analyzing objective information.

stereognosis Ability to recognize objects by the sense of touch.

sterile Aseptic.

sterile field Specified area, such as within a tray or on a sterile towel, that is considered free of microorganisms.

sterilization Rendering a person unable to produce children; accomplished by surgical, chemical, or other means.

Steri-strip Trade name for butterfly tape used as a wound closure.

stoma Artificially created opening between a body cavity and the body's surface—for example, a colostomy, formed from a portion of the colon pulled through the abdominal wall.

stomatitis Any inflammatory condition of the mouth.

stress Physiological or psychological tension that threatens homeostasis or a person's psychological equilibrium.

stress behaviors Changes from a person's normal behaviors in response to a stressor.

stressor Any event, situation, or other stimulus encountered in a person's external or internal environment that necessitates change or adaptation by the person.

stridor An abnormal, high-pitched, musical respiratory sound, caused by an obstruction in the trachea or larynx.

subcutaneous injection Form of injection in which the solution is introduced into subcutaneous tissues.

subjective data Data relating to a client's health problem described in the client's own words.

subjects People or events selected for a study in order to examine a particular variable or condition.

substance Any drug, chemical, or biological entity; specifically, any material capable of being self-administered or abused because of its physiological or psychological effects.

substance abuse Commonly used as synonymous for chemical dependency; a less precise term that only indicates abuse of a substance, not dependence on it.

Sundown syndrome Nocturnal confusion in clients who are usually not confused at other times during the day. Institutional tempo changes, sensory deficit, and environmental change are major contributors to this confusion.

superinfection Infection occurring during antimicrobial treatment for another infection; usually caused by a change in normal tissue flora.

suppurative Producing or associated with formation of pus.

sustained maximal inspiration Alveolar inflation to total lung capacity produced by high negative transpulmonary pressures.

suture Surgical stitch taken to repair an incision or wound.

symptom Subjective indication of a disease or a change in condition as perceived by a client; some symptoms, such as numbness of a body part, may be objectively confirmed.

synapse Region surrounding the point of contact between two neurons or between a neuron and an effector organ.

synergistic agent Substance that augments or adds to the activity of another substance or agent.

syntax Arrangement of words as elements in a phrase, clause, or sentence.

system Unit made up of separate parts or elements; the parts rely on each other, are interrelated, have a common purpose, and together form a collective whole.

systemic Of or pertaining to the whole body rather than to a localized area.

tachycardia Rapid regular heart rate ranging between 100 and 150 beats per minute.

tactile Relating to the sense of touch.

tarry Sticky quality of feces containing blood.

teaching Interaction between a teacher and a student that promotes learning.

teaching-learning process Interaction between the teacher and learner in which specific learning objectives are presented.

technique Method followed in performing a specific procedure such as administering medications, changing a client's dressing, or inserting a Foley catheter.

teratogenic Any chemical or physiological agent that may produce adverse effects in the embryo or fetus.

terminal illness Condition of a client for whom medical technology cannot offer curative treatment.

territoriality Persistent attachment of a person to a specific area or space.

tertiary prevention Activities directed toward rehabilitation, rather than diagnosis and treatment.

testosterone Naturally occurring male sex hormone.

theory General statement about relationships among concepts or facts, based on existing information.

therapeutic Of or pertaining to a treatment or beneficial act.

thermoregulation Internal control of body temperature.

thoracentesis Surgical perforation of the chest wall and pleural space with a needle for the aspiration of fluid or to obtain a specimen for diagnostic or therapeutic purposes.

threshold Point at which a person first perceives a painful stimulus as being painful.

thrombus Accumulation of platelets, fibrin, clotting factors, and the cellular elements of the blood attached to the interior wall of a vein or artery, sometimes occluding the lumen of the vessel.

tidal volume Amount of air inhaled and exhaled during normal ventilation.

toddlerhood Stage of life from 1 to 3 years of age.

tolerance (pain) Point at which a person is not willing to accept pain of greater severity or duration.

tolerance (chemical substance) Need for increasingly larger amounts of a drug (alcohol or other) to achieve the same physical and/or psychological effect.

topical Pertaining to a drug or treatment applied to the surface of a part of the body.

tort Act that causes injury for which the injured party can bring civil action.

tracheostomy Opening through the neck into the trachea with an indwelling tube inserted, which is created surgically to produce an airway.

traditional Ancient ethnocultural-religious beliefs and practices handed down through the generations.

trait development theory Leadership theory that analyzes successful leadership in terms of the leader's personal qualities, including intelligence, energy level, aggressiveness, and friendliness.

tranquilizer Medication that calms agitated or anxious persons without causing loss of consciousness.

transcutaneous electrical nerve stimulation (TENS) Technique in which a battery-powered device blocks pain impulses from reaching the spinal cord by delivering weak electrical pulses directly to the skin's surface.

transplantation Transfer of an organ or tissue from one person to another or from one part of the body to another in order to replace a diseased structure or to restore function.

transsexual Person whose gender identity is opposite his or her biological sex identity.

transvestism Tendency to achieve psychic and sexual relief by dressing in clothing of the opposite sex.

Trendelenburg position Position in which the body and legs are on an inclined plane with the head lowermost.

tryptophan Essential amino acid, precursor of serotonin and niacin.

tumescence To become swollen, as with genital vasocongestion during sexual arousal.

turgor Normal resiliency of the skin caused by the outward pressure of the cells and interstitial fluid.

ultradian rhythm Repetition of certain physiological phenomena within a cycle lasting less than 24 hours.

unfreezing stage of change Identifying the problem and need for alterations.

unresolved grief Severe chronic grief reaction in which the person does not complete the resolution stage of the grieving process within a reasonable time.

uremia Presence of excessive amounts of urea and other nitrogenous wastes in the blood; occurs in renal failure.

ureterostomy Diversion of urine away from a diseased or defective bladder through an artificial opening in the skin.

urgency Sensation of the need to void soon.

urinary frequency Symptom involving increased voiding.

urinary incontinence Inability to control urination.

urinometer Device for determining the specific gravity of urine.

value Personal belief about the worth of a given idea or behavior.

values clarification Technique for clarifying values, developed by Louis Raths; process designed to give an individual the opportunity to find meaning and significance in personal values.

values clarification strategy Exercise used to clarify one's values.

varicosity Abnormal condition of a vein, characterized by swelling and irregular shape or course.

vascular access devices Catheters, cannulas, or infusion ports designed for long-term, repeated access to the vascular system.

vascularization Process by which body tissue becomes vascular and develops proliferating capillaries.

venipuncture Technique in which a vein is punctured transcutaneously by a sharp, rigid stylet or by a needle attached to a syringe.

venous stasis Disorder in which the normal flow of blood through a vein is slowed or halted.

ventilation Respiratory process by which gases are moved into and out of the lungs.

ventilators Mechanical devices used to artifically support breathing in patients with ventilatory failure. Small electronic ventilators with battery back-up have been specifically designed for home use.

ventral Of or pertaining to an anterior position, toward the abdomen.

vernix caseosa A grayish-white cheeselike substance consisting of sebaceous gland secretions, lanugo, and epithelial cells that coats the skin of the fetus and newborn.

vial Glass container with a metal-enclosed rubber seal.

vibration Fine, shaking pressure applied by hands to the chest wall only during exhalation.

virulent Of or pertaining to a very pathogenic or rapidly progressive condition.

virus Minute microorganism (smaller than a bacterium) having no independent metabolic activity, which may only replicate within a cell of a living animal or plant host.

viscera Internal organs of the abdominal cavity.

visual Of or pertaining to the sense of sight.

vital signs Temperature, pulse, respirations, and blood pressure.

vitiligo Benign acquired skin disease consisting of irregular patches of various sizes totally lacking in pigment; exposed areas of skin are most affected.

volunteer agencies Not-for-profit health care agencies established within a community to meet specific needs.

water pollution Contamination of lakes, rivers, and streams by industrial pollutants.

Wernicke's syndrome Illness occurring with advanced stages of vitamin B_1 depletion and accompanied by nystagmus, papillary abnormalities, ataxia, tremor, and stupor.

withdrawal syndrome Physiological and psychological responses that occur when a person physiologically dependent on a substance abruptly withdraws from its use.

witness Person who is present and can testify that he has observed something (such as the signing of a will or consent form).

xenophobia Morbid fear of strangers.

zygote Fertilized ovum created by the joining of the mother's ovum and father's sperm.

Index